BONE MARROW ASPIRATE REFERENCE INTERVALS (ADULT)

WBC Differential	Reference Intervals (%)	Erythrocyte Series	Reference Intervals (%)
Blasts	0–3		
Promyelocytes	1–5	Pronormoblasts	0–1
N. myelocytes	6–17	Basophilic NB	1–4
N. metamyelocytes	3–20	Polychromatophilic NB	10–20
N. bands	9–32	Orthochromic NB	6–10
N. segmented (polymorphonuclear)	7–30		
Eosinophils	0–3	**Other**	
Basophils	0–1	M:E ratio	1.5–3.3:1
Lymphocytes	5–18	Megakaryocytes	2–10/lpf
Plasma cells	0–1		
Monocytes	0–1		
Histiocytes (macrophages)	0–1		

COMPLETE BLOOD COUNT REFERENCE INTERVALS (PEDIATRIC)

Assay	Units	0–1 d	2–4 d	5–7 d	8–14 d	15–30 d	1–2 mo	3–5 mo	6–11 mo	1–3 y	4–7 y	8–13 y
RBC	× 10⁶/µL	4.10–6.10	4.36–5.96	4.20–5.80	4.00–5.60	3.20–5.00	3.40–5.00	3.65–5.05	3.60–5.20	3.40–5.20	4.00–5.20	4.00–5.40
	(× 10¹²/L)											
HGB	g/dL (g/L)	16.5–21.5	16.4–20.8	15.2–20.4	15.0–19.6	12.2–18.0	10.6–16.4	10.4–16.0	10.4–15.6	9.6–15.6	10.2–15.2	12.0–15.0
		(165–215)	(164–208)	(152–204)	(150–196)	(122–180)	(106–164)	(104–160)	(104–156)	(96–156)	(102–152)	(120–150)
HCT	%	48–68	48–68	50–64	46–62	38–53	32–50	35–51	35–51	34–48	36–46	35–49
MCV	fL	95–125	98–118	100–120	95–115	93–113	83–107	83–107	78–102	76–92	78–94	80–94
MCH	pg	30–42	30–42	30–42	30–42	28–40	27–37	25–35	23–31	23–31	23–31	26–32
MCHC	g/dL	30–34	30–34	30–34	30–34	30–34	31–37	32–36	32–36	32–36	32–36	32–36
RDW	%	*	*	*	*	*	*	*	11.5–14.5	11.5–14.5	11.5–14.5	11.5–14.5
RETIC	%	1.8–5.8	1.3–4.7	0.2–1.4	0–1.0	0.2–1.0	0.8–2.8	0.5–1.5	0.5–1.5	0.5–1.5	0.5–1.5	0.5–1.5
RETIC	× 10³/µL	73.8–353.8	56.7–280.1	8.4–81.2	0.0–56.0	6.4–50.0	27.2–140.0	18.3–75.8	18.0–78.0	17.0–78.8	20–78.0	20–124.2
	(× 10⁹/L)											
NRBC	/100 WBC	2–24	5–9	0–1	0	0	0	0	0	0	0	0
WBC	× 10³/µL	9.0–37.0	8.0–24.0	5.0–21.0	5.0–21.0	5.0–21.0	6.0–18.0	6.0–18.0	6.0–18.0	5.5–17.5	5.0–17.0	4.5–13.5
	(× 10⁹/L)											
NEUT (ANC)	× 10³/µL (× 10⁹/L)	3.7–30.0	2.6–17.0	1.5–12.6	1.2–11.6	1.0–9.5	1.2–8.1	1.1–7.7	1.2–8.1	1.2–8.9	1.5–11.0	1.6–9.5
LYMPH	× 10³/µL (× 10⁹/L)	1.6–14.1	1.3–11.0	1.2–11.3	1.5–13.0	2.1–12.8	2.5–13.0	2.7–13.5	2.9–14.0	2.0–12.8	1.5–11.1	1.0–7.2
MONO	× 10³/µL (× 10⁹/L)	0.1–4.4	0.2–3.4	0.2–3.6	0.2–3.6	0.1–3.2	0.2–2.5	0.1–2.0	0.1–2.0	0.1–1.9	0.1–1.9	0.1–1.5
EO	× 10³/µL (× 10⁹/L)	0.0–1.5	0.0–1.2	0.0–1.3	0.0–1.1	0.0–1.1	0.0–0.7	0.0–0.7	0.0–0.7	0.0–0.7	0.0–0.7	0.0–0.5
BASO	× 10³/µL (× 10⁹/L)	0.0–0.7	0.0–0.5	0.0–0.4	0.0–0.4	0.0–0.4	0.0–0.4	0.0–0.4	0.0–0.4	0.0–0.4	0.0–0.3	0.0–0.3
PLT	× 10³/µL (× 10⁹/L)	150–450	150–450	150–450	150–450	150–450	150–450	150–450	150–450	150–450	150–450	150–450

*The RDW is markedly elevated in newborns, with a range of 14.2% to 19.9% in the first few days of life, gradually decreasing until it reaches adult levels by 6 months of age. Pediatric reference intervals are from Riley Hospital for Children, Indiana University Health, Indianapolis, IN.

Some reference intervals are listed in common units and in international system of units (SI units) in parenthesis.
ANC, absolute neutrophil count (includes segmented neutrophils and bands); BAND, neutrophil bands; BASO, basophils; d, days; EO Hb, hemoglobin fraction; HCT, hematocrit; HGB, hemoglobin; lpf, low power field; LYMPH, lymphocytes; MCH, mean cell hemoglobin; , mean cell volume; M:E, myeloid:erythroid; mo, month; MONO, monocytes; MPV, mean platelet volume; N, neutrophilic; NB, normobla cells; PLT, platelets; RBC, red blood cells; RDW, red blood cell distribution width; RETIC, reticulocytes; WBC, white blood cells; y, year.

Please see inside back cover for additional reference interval tables.

BMA

RODAK'S
Hematology
CLINICAL PRINCIPLES AND APPLICATIONS

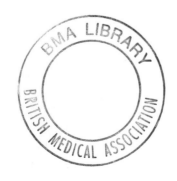

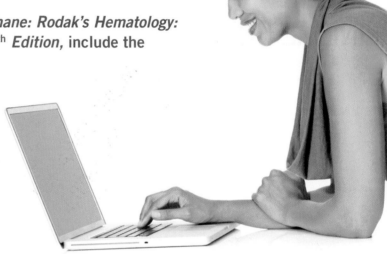

Fifth Edition

RODAK'S
Hematology
CLINICAL PRINCIPLES AND APPLICATIONS

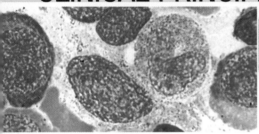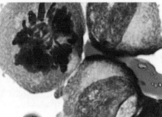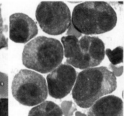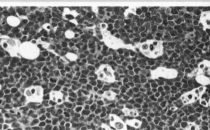

Elaine M. **Keohane**, PhD, MLS
Chair and Professor, Department
  of Clinical Laboratory Sciences
School of Health Related Professions
Rutgers, The State University of New Jersey
Newark, New Jersey

Larry J. **Smith**, PhD, SH(ASCP),
HCLD/CC(ABB)
Assistant Attending Scientist and Director,
  Coagulation Laboratory
Department of Laboratory Medicine
Memorial Sloan-Kettering Cancer Center
New York, New York
Adjunct Professor, Department of Health Professions
York College, The City University of New York
Jamaica, New York
Adjunct Associate Professor, Department of Clinical
  Laboratory Sciences
School of Health Related Professions
Rutgers, The State University of New Jersey
Newark, New Jersey

Jeanine M. **Walenga**, PhD,
MT(ASCP)
Professor, Thoracic-Cardiovascular Surgery, Pathology,
  and Physiology
Co-Director, Hemostasis and Thrombosis Research Unit
Stritch School of Medicine
Loyola University Chicago
Maywood, Illinois
Director, Clinical Coagulation Core Laboratory and
  Special Coagulation Laboratory
Director, Urinalysis and Medical Microscopy
Associate Director, Point of Care Testing
Loyola University Hospital
Maywood, Illinois

ELSEVIER

ELSEVIER
SAUNDERS

3251 Riverport Lane
St. Louis, Missouri 63043

Executive Content Strategist: Kellie White
Content Development Manager: Laurie Gower
Content Development Specialist: Rebecca Corradetti
Publishing Services Manager: Julie Eddy
Project Manager: Sara Alsup
Design Direction: Teresa McBryan
Text Designer: Ashley Miner

Printed in Canada

Last digit is the print number: 9   8   7   6   5   4   3   2   1

Working together
to grow libraries in
developing countries

www.elsevier.com • www.bookaid.org

To my students for being great teachers, and to Camryn, Riley, Harper, Stella, Jackie, Alana, Ken, and Jake for reminding me about the important things in life.

EMK

To my wonderful mentors and students who have taught me so much about laboratory medicine.

LJS

To my teachers, both formal and informal, for all this fascinating knowledge in clinical laboratory sciences which made possible my interesting career.

JMW

Special Dedication

To **Bernadette "Bunny" F. Rodak**, *with great admiration and gratitude for your vision, perseverance, and courage to first publish* Hematology: Clinical Principles and Applications *in 1995; for your over 20-year commitment to publish the highest quality text through five editions; for your mentorship and guidance of five co-editors and over 50 authors; and for sharing your great enthusiasm for hematology and hemostasis and lifelong learning that has inspired a generation of students and faculty in this country and around the world.*

Special Acknowledgment

To **George A. Fritsma**, *with our sincere gratitude for your dedication and reasoned approach that has kept* Hematology: Clinical Principles and Applications *at the leading edge as a comprehensive, state-of-the-art, yet practical textbook, guided by you as co-editor for two editions and through the multiple number of chapters that you have authored. We are indebted to you for sharing your vast knowledge in hematology and hemostasis and for your unwavering commitment to the profession of clinical laboratory science.*

Reviewers

Keith Bellinger, PBT(ASCP)
Medical Technologist
The United States Department of Veterans Affairs New Jersey
    Health Care System
East Orange, New Jersey;
Adjunct Assistant Professor, Clinical Laboratory Sciences
Rutgers, The State University of New Jersey
Newark, New Jersey

Susan Conforti, EdD, MLS(ASCP)SBB
Associate Professor, Medical Laboratory Technology
Farmingdale State College
Farmingdale, New York

Shamina Davis, MS, MT(ASCP)
Faculty, College of Biomedical Sciences and Health
    Professions
University of Texas at Brownsville
Brownsville, Texas

Kathleen Doyle, PhD, M(ASCP), MLS(ASCP)CM
Medical Laboratory Scientist, Consultant
Professor Emeritus, Clinical Laboratory and Nutritional
    Sciences
University of Massachusetts Lowell
Lowell, Massachusetts

Michele Harms, MS, MLS(ASCP)
Program Director, School of Medical Technology
WCA Hospital
Jamestown, New York

Jeanne Isabel, MS, MT(ASCP), CLSpH(NCA)
Associate Professor and Program Director,
    Allied Health and Communicative Disorders
Northern Illinois University
DeKalb, Illinois

Steve Johnson, MS, MT(ASCP)
Program Director, School of Medical Technology
Saint Vincent Health Center
Erie, Pennsylvania

Haywood B. Joiner, Jr., EdD, MT(ASCP)
Chair, Department of Allied Health
Louisiana State University at Alexandria
Alexandria, Louisiana

Amy R. Kapanka, MS, MT(ASCP)SC
MLT Program Director
Hawkeye Community College
Waterloo, Iowa

Linda Kappel, MLT(FCP, CAET)
Instructor, Medical Diagnostics
Saskatchewan Polytechnic, Saskatoon Campus
Saskatoon, Saskatchewan, Canada

Linda J. McCown, PhD, MLS(ASCP)CM
Chair and Program Director, Clinical Laboratory Science
University of Illinois Springfield
Springfield, Illinois

Christine Nebocat, MS, MT(ASCP)CM
Assistant Professor
Farmingdale State College
Farmingdale, New York

Tania Puro, CLS, MS, MT(ASCP)
Instructor, Clinical Lab Science Program
San Francisco State University
San Francisco, California

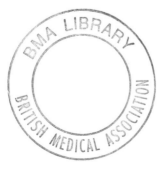

Contributors

Sameer Al Diffalha, MD
Pathology Resident PGY3
Loyola University Medical Center
Maywood, Illinois

Larry D. Brace, PhD, MT(ASCP)SH
Clinical Pathology/Laboratory Consultant
Emeritus Professor of Pathology
University of Illinois at Chicago
Chicago, Illinois;
Scientific Director of Laboratories
Laboratory and Pathology Diagnostics at Edward Hospital
Naperville, Illinois

Karen S. Clark, BS, MT(ASCP)SH
Point of Care Manager
Baptist Memorial Hospital
Memphis, Tennessee

Magdalena Czader, MD, PhD
Director, Division of Hematopathology
Director, Clinical Flow Cytometry Laboratory
Department of Pathology and Laboratory Medicine
Indiana University School of Medicine
Indianapolis, Indiana

Kathryn Doig, PhD, MLS(ASCP)CMSH(ASCP)CM
Professor, Biomedical Laboratory Diagnostics
College of Natural Science
Michigan State University
East Lansing, Michigan

Sheila A. Finch, CHSP, CHMM, MS, BS, MT(ASCP)
Executive Director, Environment of Care/Emergency
    Management
Detroit Medical Center
Detroit, Michigan

George A. Fritsma, MS, MLS
Manager
The Fritsma Factor, Your Interactive Hemostasis Resource
Birmingham, Alabama

Margaret G. Fritsma, MA, MT(ASCP)SBB
Associate Professor, Retired
School of Health Professions
Division of Laboratory Medicine,
    Department of Pathology
University of Alabama at Birmingham
Birmingham, Alabama

Pranav Gandhi, MD, MS
Hematopathology Fellow
Scripps Clinic
La Jolla, California

Bertil Glader, MD, PhD
Professor, Pediatric Hematology/Oncology
Stanford University
Palo Alto, California

Linda H. Goossen, PhD, MT(ASCP)
Professor, Medical Laboratory Science
Associate Dean, College of Health Professions
Grand Valley State University
Grand Valley, Michigan

Teresa G. Hippel, BS, MT(ASCP)SH
Laboratory Manager
Baptist Memorial Hospital
Memphis, Tennessee

**Debra A. Hoppensteadt, BS, MT(ASCP),
    MS, PhD, DIC**
Professor of Pathology and Pharmacology
Loyola University Chicago
Maywood, Illinois

Cynthia L. Jackson, PhD
Director of Clinical Molecular Biology
Lifespan Academic Medical Center
Associate Professor of Pathology
Warren Alpert Medical School at Brown University
Providence, Rhode Island

Ameet R. Kini, MD, PhD
Director, Division of Hematopathology
Medical Director, Hematology & Flow Cytometry
Associate Director, Molecular Diagnostics
Associate Professor of Pathology,
    Stritch School of Medicine
Loyola University Medical Center
Maywood, Illinois

Clara Lo, MD
Instructor, Pediatric Hematology/Oncology
Stanford University
Palo Alto, California

Sharral Longanbach, MT, SH(ASCP)
Senior Technical Application Specialist
Siemens Healthcare Diagnostics
Deerfield, Illinois

Lynn B. Maedel, MS, MLS(ASCP)^CMSH^CM
Executive Director
Colorado Association for Continuing Medical
    Laboratory Education, Inc. (CACMLE)
Denver, Colorado

Naveen Manchanda, MBBS
Associate Professor of Clinical Medicine, Division of
    Hematology-Oncology
Indiana University School of Medicine
Indianapolis, Indiana

Steven Marionneaux, MS, MT(ASCP)
Manager, Clinical Hematology Laboratories
Memorial Sloan Kettering Cancer Center
New York, New York
Adjunct Assistant Professor, Clinical Laboratory Sciences
Rutgers, The State University of New Jersey
Newark, New Jersey

Richard C. Meagher, PhD
Section Chief, Cell Therapy Laboratory
Department of Laboratory Medicine
Memorial Sloan Kettering Cancer Center
New York, New York

Shashi Mehta, PhD
Associate Professor, Clinical Laboratory Sciences
School of Health Related Professions
Rutgers University, The State University of New Jersey
Newark, New Jersey

Martha K. Miers, MS, MBA
Assistant Professor, Division of Medical Education
    and Administration
Vice Chair, Finance and Administration
Department of Pathology, Microbiology, and Immunology
Vanderbilt University School of Medicine
Nashville, Tennessee

JoAnn Molnar, MT(ASCP)
Core Laboratory Technical Specialist
Loyola University Medical Center
Maywood, Illinois

Kim A. Przekop, MBA, MLS(ASCP)^CM
Assistant Professor, Clinical Laboratory Sciences
School of Health Related Professions
Rutgers, The State University of New Jersey
Newark, New Jersey

Tim R. Randolph, PhD, MT(ASCP)
Chair and Associate Professor, Department of Biomedical
    Laboratory Science
Doisy College of Health Sciences
Saint Louis University
St. Louis, Missouri

Bernadette F. Rodak, MS, CLSpH(NCA),
    MT(ASCP)SH
Professor, Clinical Laboratory Science Program
Department of Pathology and Laboratory Medicine
Indiana University School of Medicine
Indianapolis, Indiana

Woodlyne Roquiz, DO
Hematopathology Fellow
Loyola University Medical Center
Maywood, Illinois

Kathleen M. Sakamoto, MD, PhD
Professor and Chief, Division of Hematology/Oncology
Department of Pediatrics
Stanford University School of Medicine
Lucile Packard Children's Hospital at Stanford
Stanford, California

Gail H. Vance, MD
Sutphin Professor of Cancer Genetics
Department of Medical and Molecular Genetics
Indiana University School of Medicine
Indianapolis, Indiana
Staff Physician
Indiana University Health Hospitals
Carmel, Indiana

Instructor and Student Ancillaries

Case Studies, Instructor's Guide, Test Bank
Susan Conforti, EdD, MLS(ASCP)SBB
Associate Professor, Medical Laboratory Technology
Farmingdale State College
Farmingdale, New York

PowerPoint Slides
Kathleen Doyle, PhD, M(ASCP), MLS(ASCP)^CM
Medical Laboratory Scientist, Consultant
Professor Emeritus, Clinical Laboratory and
    Nutritional Sciences
University of Massachusetts Lowell
Lowell, Massachusetts

PowerPoint Slides
Carolina Vilchez, MS, MLS(ASCP)H
Assistant Professor, Clinical Laboratory Sciences
School of Health Related Professions
Rutgers, The State University of New Jersey
Newark, New Jersey

The science of *clinical laboratory hematology* provides for the analysis of normal and pathologic peripheral blood cells, hematopoietic (blood-producing) tissue, and the cells in non-vascular body cavities such as cerebrospinal and serous fluids. Laboratory hematology also includes the analysis of the cells and coagulation proteins essential to clinical hemostasis. Hematology laboratory assay results are critical for the diagnosis, prognosis, and monitoring treatment for primary and secondary hematologic disorders. Similarly, hematology results are used to establish safety in the perioperative period, monitor treatments during surgical procedures, and monitor transfusion needs in trauma patients.

Clinical laboratory hematology has been enhanced by profound changes as reflected in the numerous updates in the fifth edition of *Rodak's Hematology: Clinical Principles and Applications*. Automation and digital data management have revolutionized the way blood specimens are transported and stored, how assays are ordered, and how results are validated, reported, and interpreted.

Molecular diagnosis has augmented and in many instances replaced long-indispensable laboratory assays. Hematologic disorders have been reclassified on the basis of phenotypic, cytogenetic, and molecular genetic analyses. Diagnoses that once depended on the analysis of cell morphology and cytochemical stains now rely on flow cytometry, cytogenetic testing, fluorescence in situ hybridization (FISH), end-point and real-time polymerase chain reaction assays, gene sequencing, and microarrays. Traditional chemotherapeutic monitoring of leukemias and lymphomas at the cellular level has shifted to the management of biologic response modifiers and detection of minimal residual disease at the molecular level. Hemostasis has grown to encompass expanded thrombophilia testing, methods that more reliably monitor newly available antiplatelet and anticoagulant drugs, molecular analysis, and a shift from clot-based to functional and chromogenic assays.

Rodak's Hematology: Clinical Principles and Applications systematically presents basic to advanced concepts to provide a solid foundation of normal and pathologic states upon which readers can build their skills in interpreting and correlating laboratory findings in anemias, leukocyte disorders, and hemorrhagic and thrombotic conditions. It provides key features for accurate identification of normal and pathologic cells in blood, bone marrow, and body fluids. The focus, level, and detail of hematology and hemostasis testing, along with the related clinical applications, interpretation, and testing algorithms, make this text a valuable resource for all healthcare professionals managing these disorders.

ORGANIZATION

Rodak's Hematology: Clinical Principles and Applications fifth edition is reorganized into 7 parts and 45 chapters for enhanced pedagogy. Chapter highlights and new content are described as follows:

Part I: Introduction to Hematology

Chapters 1 to 5 preview the science of clinical laboratory hematology and include laboratory safety, blood specimen collection, microscopy, and quality assurance. The quality assurance chapter was significantly updated to include enhanced sections on statistical significance; assay validation with applications of the Student's t test, ANOVA, linear regression, and Bland-Altman difference plots; and assessment of diagnostic efficacy.

Part II: Blood Cell Production, Structure, and Function

Chapters 6 and 7 use photomicrographs and figures to describe general cellular structure and function and the morphologic and molecular details of hematopoiesis. Chapters 8, 12, and 13 discuss erythropoiesis, leukopoiesis, and megakaryopoiesis using numerous photomicrographs demonstrating ultrastructure and microscopic morphology. Chapters 9 and 10 examine mature red blood cell metabolism, hemoglobin structure and function, and red blood cell senescence and destruction. Iron kinetics and laboratory assessment in Chapter 11 was substantially updated with new figures and updated coverage of systemic and cellular regulation of iron. Chapter 13 includes detailed descriptions of platelet adhesion, aggregation, and activation with updated figures.

Part III: Laboratory Evaluation of Blood Cells

Chapter 14 describes manual procedures such as microscopy-based cell counts, hemoglobin and hematocrit determinations, and point-of-care technology. Chapter 15 has been substantially updated to include descriptions and figures of the latest automated hematology analyzers. Chapter 16 describes peripheral blood film examination and the differential count correlation to the complete blood count. New figures correlate red blood cell and platelet histograms to their morphology. Chapter 17 follows up with bone marrow aspirate and biopsy collection, preparation, examination, and reporting. Chapter 18 describes methods for analyzing normal and pathologic cells of cerebrospinal fluid, joint fluid, transudates, and exudates, illustrated with many excellent photomicrographs.

Part IV: Erythrocyte Disorders

Chapter 19 provides an overview of anemia and describes cost-effective approaches that integrate patient history, physical examination, and symptoms with the hemoglobin, red blood cell indices, reticulocyte count, and abnormal red blood cell morphology. Chapters 20 to 22 describe disorders of iron and DNA metabolism and bone marrow failure. New algorithms help the reader to distinguish types of microcytic and macrocytic anemias. Chapters 23 to 26 discuss hemolytic anemias due to intrinsic or extrinsic defects. Chapter 23 is fully updated with new figures that detail extravascular and intravascular hemolysis and hemoglobin catabolism. Chapters 27 and 28 provide updates in pathophysiology, diagnosis, and treatment of hemoglobinopathies (such as sickle cell disease) and the thalassemias.

Part V: Leukocyte Disorders

Chapter 29 is significantly updated with many excellent photomicrographs and summary boxes of nonmalignant systemic disorders manifested by the abnormal distribution or morphology of leukocytes. These include bacterial and viral infections, various systemic disorders, and benign lymphoproliferative disorders. Chapter 30 provides details on traditional cytogenetic procedures for detection of quantitative and qualitative chromosome abnormalities and more sensitive methods such as FISH and genomic hybridization arrays. Chapter 31 covers molecular diagnostics and was fully updated with new and enhanced figures on basic molecular biology, end-point and real-time polymerase chain reaction, microarrays, and DNA sequencing, including next generation sequencing. Chapter 32 describes flow cytometry and its diagnostic applications. It includes numerous scatterplots of normal and leukemic conditions. Chapters 33 to 36, with significant updating, provide the latest classifications and pathophysiologic models for myeloproliferative neoplasms, myelodysplastic syndromes, acute lymphoblastic and myeloid leukemias, chronic lymphocytic leukemia, and solid tumor lymphoid neoplasms, such as lymphoma and myeloma, with numerous full-color photomicrographs and illustrations.

Part VI: Hemostasis and Thrombosis

Chapter 37 provides the plasma-based and cell-based coagulation models and the interactions between primary and secondary hemostasis and fibrinolysis with updated illustrations. Chapter 38 details hemorrhagic disorders, including the management of the acute coagulopathy of trauma and shock. Chapter 39 updates the currently recognized risk factors of thrombosis and describes laboratory tests that identify venous and arterial thrombotic diseases, particularly for lupus anticoagulant and heparin-induced thrombocytopenia (HIT) testing. Chapters 40 and 41 detail the quantitative and qualitative platelet disorders using additional tables and figures, and Chapter 42 details laboratory assays of platelets and the coagulation mechanisms with helpful new figures and diagrams. Chapter 43 covers the mechanisms and monitoring methods of the traditional warfarin and heparin-derived antithrombotic drugs, as well as all thrombin and factor Xa inhibitor drugs. It also includes methods for monitoring the different classes of antiplatelet drugs, including aspirin. Chapter 44 reviews the latest coagulation analyzers and point of care instrumentation.

Part VII: Hematology and Hemostasis in Selected Populations

Chapter 45 provides valuable information on the hematology and hemostasis laboratory findings in the pediatric and geriatric populations correlated with information from previous chapters.

READERS

Rodak's Hematology: Clinical Principles and Applications is designed for medical laboratory scientists, medical laboratory technicians, and the faculty of undergraduate and graduate educational programs in the clinical laboratory sciences. This text is also a helpful study guide for pathology and hematology-oncology residents and fellows and a valuable shelf reference for hematologists, pathologists, and hematology and hemostasis laboratory managers.

TEXTBOOK FEATURES

Elaine M. Keohane, PhD, MLS, Professor, Rutgers University, School of Health Related Professions, Department of Clinical Laboratory Sciences, co-editor in the fourth edition, and lead editor in the fifth edition, is joined by **Larry J. Smith**, PhD, Coagulation and Satellite Laboratory Director, Memorial Sloan Kettering Cancer Center, Adjunct Professor at Rutgers University, School of Health Related Professions and York College, CUNY, Department of Health Professions, and **Jeanine M. Walenga**, PhD, MT(ASCP), Professor, Loyola University Chicago, Stritch School of Medicine, Clinical Coagulation Laboratories Director, Loyola University Health System.

The outstanding value and quality of *Rodak's Hematology: Clinical Principles and Applications* reflect the educational and clinical expertise of its current and previous authors and editors. The text is enhanced by nearly 700 full-color digital photomicrographs, figures, and line art. Detailed text boxes and tables clearly summarize important information. Reference intervals are provided on the inside front and back covers for quick lookup.

Each chapter contains the following pedagogical features:
- **Learning objectives** at all taxonomy levels in the cognitive domain.
- One or two **case studies** with open-ended discussion questions at the beginning of the chapter that stimulate interest and provide opportunities for application of chapter content in real-life scenarios.
- A bulleted **summary** at the end of each chapter that provides a comprehensive review of essential material.
- **Review questions** at the end of each chapter that correlate to chapter objectives and are in the multiple-choice format used by certification examinations.
- **Answers** to case studies and review questions that are provided in the Appendix.

The Evolve website has multiple features **for the instructor:**
- An **ExamView test bank** contains multiple-choice questions with rationales and cognitive levels.
- **Instructor's manuals** for every chapter contain key terms, objectives, outlines, and study questions.
- **Learning Objectives with taxonomy levels** are provided to supplement lesson plans.
- **Case studies** have been updated and feature discussion questions and photomicrographs when applicable.
- **PowerPoint presentations** for every chapter can be used "as is" or as a template to prepare lectures.
- The **Image Collection** provides electronic files of all the chapter figures that can be downloaded into PowerPoint presentations.

For the student, a Glossary is available as a quick reference to look up unfamiliar terms electronically.

Acknowledgments

The editors express their immense gratitude to Bernadette F. (Bunny) Rodak, who laid the foundation for this textbook with her expert writing, editing, detailed figures, and especially her contribution of over 200 outstanding digital photomicrographs over the past 2 decades. Now in its fifth edition, she has authored three chapters, provided invaluable contributions and assistance with additional photomicrographs and figures, and provided the opportunity for us to continue her work on this outstanding textbook. We sincerely thank George A. Fritsma for his significant contribution to this text as a previous coeditor and author, for sharing his immense expertise in hemostasis, for updating and authoring ten chapters in the fifth edition, and for his constant support and encouragement. We thank Kathryn Doig for her contributions as coeditor for the third edition; author in previous editions; and for her tenaciousness, creativity, and care in updating the five chapters authored in the fifth edition. The editors also thank the many authors who have made and continue to make significant contributions to this work. All of these outstanding professionals have generously shared their time and expertise to make *Rodak's Hematology: Clinical Principles and Applications* into a worldwide educational resource and premier reference textbook for medical laboratory scientists and technicians, as well as pathology and hematology practitioners, residents, and fellows.

We also express our appreciation to Elsevier, especially Ellen Wurm-Cutter, Laurie Gower, Kellie White, Sara Alsup, Megan Knight, and Rebecca Corradetti, whose professional support and reminders kept the project on track, and to Debbie Prato for her editorial assistance.

Finally, and with the utmost gratitude, we acknowledge our families, friends, and professional colleagues who have supported and encouraged us through this project.

Elaine M. Keohane, PhD, MLS
Larry J. Smith, PhD, SH(ASCP), HCLD/CC(ABB)
Jeanine M. Walenga, PhD, MT(ASCP)

Contents

PART V   Leukocyte Disorders

PART VI   Hemostasis and Thrombosis

PART VII   Hematology and Hemostasis in Selected Populations

APPENDIX

An Overview of Clinical Laboratory Hematology

1

George A. Fritsma

The average human possesses 5 liters of blood. Blood transports oxygen from lungs to tissues; clears tissues of carbon dioxide; transports glucose, proteins, and fats; and moves wastes to the liver and kidneys. The liquid portion is plasma, which, among many components, provides coagulation enzymes that protect vessels from trauma and maintain the circulation.

Plasma transports and nourishes blood cells. There are three categories of blood cells: red blood cells (RBCs), or *erythrocytes*; white blood cells (WBCs), or *leukocytes*; and platelets (PLTs), or *thrombocytes*.[1] Hematology is the study of these blood cells. By expertly staining, counting, analyzing, and recording the appearance, phenotype, and genotype of all three types of cells, the medical laboratory professional (technician or scientist) is able to predict, detect, and diagnose blood diseases and many systemic diseases that affect blood cells. Physicians rely on hematology laboratory test results to select and monitor therapy for these disorders; consequently, a complete blood count (CBC) is ordered on nearly everyone who visits a physician or is admitted to a hospital.

HISTORY

The first scientists such as Athanasius Kircher in 1657 described "worms" in the blood, and Anton van Leeuwenhoek in 1674 gave an account of RBCs,[2] but it was not until the late 1800s that Giulio Bizzozero described platelets as "petites plaques."[3] The development of Wright stain by James Homer Wright in 1902 opened a new world of visual blood film examination through the microscope. Although automated instruments now differentiate and enumerate blood cells, Wright's Romanowsky-type stain (polychromatic, a mixture of acidic and basic dyes), and refinements thereof, remains the foundation of blood cell identification.[4]

In the present-day hematology laboratory, RBC, WBC, and platelet appearance is analyzed through automation or visually using 500× to 1000× light microscopy examination of cells fixed to a glass microscope slide and stained with *Wright* or *Wright-Giemsa stain* (Chapters 15 and 16). The scientific term for cell appearance is *morphology*, which encompasses cell color, size, shape, cytoplasmic inclusions, and nuclear condensation.

RED BLOOD CELLS

RBCs are anucleate, biconcave, discoid cells filled with a reddish protein, hemoglobin (HGB), which transports oxygen and carbon dioxide (Chapter 10). RBCs appear pink to red and measure 6 to 8 μm in diameter with a zone of pallor that occupies one third of their center (Figure 1-1, *A*), reflecting their biconcavity (Chapters 8 and 9).

Since before 1900, physicians and medical laboratory professionals counted RBCs in measured volumes to detect anemia or polycythemia. *Anemia* means loss of oxygen-carrying capacity and is often reflected in a reduced RBC count or decreased RBC hemoglobin concentration (Chapter 19). *Polycythemia* means an increased RBC count reflecting increased circulating RBC mass, a condition that leads to hyperviscosity (Chapter 33). Historically, microscopists counted RBCs by carefully pipetting a tiny aliquot of whole blood and mixing it with 0.85% (normal) saline. Normal saline matches the osmolality of blood; consequently, the suspended RBCs retained their intrinsic morphology, neither swelling nor shrinking. A 1:200 dilution was typical for RBC counts, and a glass

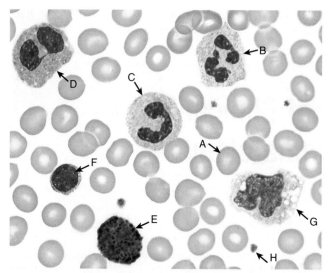

Figure 1-1 Normal cells in peripheral blood: A, Erythrocyte (red blood cell, RBC); **B,** Neutrophil (segmented neutrophil, NEUT, SEG, polymorphonuclear neutrophil, PMN); **C,** Band (band neutrophil, BAND); **D,** Eosinophil (EO); **E,** Basophil (BASO); **F,** Lymphocyte (LYMPH); **G,** Monocyte (MONO); **H,** Platelet (PLT).

pipette designed to provide this dilution, the Thoma pipette, was used routinely until the advent of automation.

The diluted blood was transferred to a glass counting chamber called a hemacytometer (Figure 14-1). The microscopist observed and counted RBCs in selected areas of the hemacytometer, applied a mathematical formula based on the dilution and on the area of the hemacytometer counted (Chapter 14), and reported the RBC count in cells per microliter (μL, mcL, also called *cubic millimeter*, mm³), milliliter (mL, also called *cubic centimeter*, or cc), or liter (L).

Visual RBC counting was developed before 1900 and, although inaccurate, was the only way to count RBCs until 1958, when automated particle counters became available in the clinical laboratory. The first electronic counter, patented in 1953 by Joseph and Wallace Coulter of Chicago, Illinois, was used so widely that today automated cell counters are often called *Coulter counters*, although many high-quality competitors exist (Chapter 15).[5] The Coulter principle of direct current electrical impedance is still used to count RBCs in many automated hematology profiling instruments. Fortunately, the widespread availability of automated cell counters has replaced visual RBC counting, although visual counting skills remain useful where automated counters are unavailable.

Hemoglobin, Hematocrit, and Red Blood Cell Indices

RBCs also are assayed for hemoglobin concentration (HGB) and hematocrit (HCT) (Chapter 14). Hemoglobin measurement relies on a weak solution of potassium cyanide and potassium ferricyanide, called *Drabkin reagent*. An aliquot of whole blood is mixed with a measured volume of Drabkin reagent, hemoglobin is converted to stable *cyanmethemoglobin* (hemiglobincyanide), and the absorbance or color intensity of the solution is measured in a spectrophotometer at 540 nm wavelength.[6] The color intensity is compared

with that of a known standard and is mathematically converted to hemoglobin concentration. Modifications of the cyanmethemoglobin method are used in most automated applications, although some automated hematology profiling instruments replace it with a formulation of the ionic surfactant (detergent) *sodium lauryl sulfate* to reduce environmental cyanide.

Hematocrit is the ratio of the volume of packed RBCs to the volume of whole blood and is manually determined by transferring blood to a graduated plastic tube with a uniform bore, centrifuging, measuring the column of RBCs, and dividing by the total length of the column of RBCs plus plasma.[7] The normal ratio approaches 50% (refer to inside front cover for reference intervals). Hematocrit is also called *packed cell volume* (PCV), the packed cells referring to RBCs. Often one can see a light-colored layer between the RBCs and plasma. This is the *buffy coat* and contains WBCs and platelets, and it is excluded from the hematocrit determination. The medical laboratory professional may use the three numerical results—RBC count, HGB, and HCT—to compute the RBC indices *mean cell volume* (MCV), *mean cell hemoglobin* (MCH), and *mean cell hemoglobin concentration* (MCHC) (Chapter 14). The MCV, although a volume measurement recorded in femtoliters (fL), reflects RBC diameter on a Wright-stained blood film. The MCHC, expressed in g/dL, reflects RBC staining intensity and amount of central pallor. The MCH in picograms (pg) expresses the mass of hemoglobin and parallels the MCHC. A fourth RBC index, *RBC distribution width* (RDW), expresses the degree of *variation* in RBC volume. Extreme RBC volume variability is visible on the Wright-stained blood film as variation in diameter and is called *anisocytosis*. The RDW is based on the standard deviation of RBC volume and is routinely reported by automated cell counters. In addition to aiding in diagnosis of anemia, the RBC indices provide stable measurements for internal quality control of counting instruments (Chapter 5).

Medical laboratory professionals routinely use light microscopy at 500× or 1000× magnification (Chapters 4 and 16) to visually review RBC morphology, commenting on RBC diameter, color or hemoglobinization, shape, and the presence of cytoplasmic inclusions (Chapters 16 and 19). All these parameters—RBC count, HGB, HCT, indices, and RBC morphology—are employed to detect, diagnose, assess the severity of, and monitor the treatment of anemia, polycythemia, and the numerous systemic conditions that affect RBCs. Automated hematology profiling instruments are used in nearly all laboratories to generate these data, although visual examination of the Wright-stained blood film is still essential to verify abnormal results.[8]

Reticulocytes

In the Wright-stained blood film, 0.5% to 2% of RBCs exceed the 6- to 8-μm average diameter and stain slightly blue-gray. These are *polychromatic (polychromatophilic)* erythrocytes, newly released from the RBC production site: the bone marrow (Chapters 8 and 17). Polychromatic erythrocytes are closely observed because they indicate the ability of the bone marrow to increase RBC production in anemia due to blood loss or excessive RBC destruction (Chapters 23 to 26).

Methylene blue dyes, called *nucleic acid stains* or *vital stains,* are used to differentiate and count these young RBCs. Vital (or "supravital") stains are dyes absorbed by live cells.[9] Young RBCs contain ribonucleic acid (RNA) and are called *reticulocytes* when the RNA is visualized using vital stains. Counting reticulocytes visually by microscopy was (and remains) a tedious and imprecise procedure until the development of automated reticulocyte counting by the TOA Corporation (presently Sysmex Corporation, Kobe, Japan) in 1990. Now all fully automated profiling instruments provide an *absolute reticulocyte count* and, in addition, an especially sensitive measure of RBC production, the *immature reticulocyte count* or *immature reticulocyte fraction* (Chapter 15). However, it is still necessary to confirm instrument counts visually from time to time, so medical laboratory professionals must retain this skill.

WHITE BLOOD CELLS

WBCs, or leukocytes, are a loosely related category of cell types dedicated to protecting their host from infection and injury (Chapter 12). WBCs are transported in the blood from their source, usually bone marrow or lymphoid tissue, to their tissue or body cavity destination. WBCs are so named because they are nearly colorless in an unstained cell suspension.

WBCs may be counted visually using a microscope and hemacytometer. The technique is the same as RBC counting, but the typical dilution is 1:20, and the diluent is a dilute acid solution. The acid causes RBCs to *lyse* or rupture; without it, RBCs, which are 500 to 1000 times more numerous than WBCs, would obscure the WBCs. The WBC count ranges from 4500 to 11,500/μL. Visual WBC counting has been largely replaced by automated hematology profiling instruments, but it is accurate and useful in situations in which no automation is available. Medical laboratory professionals who analyze body fluids such as cerebrospinal fluid or pleural fluid may employ visual WBC counting.

A decreased WBC count (fewer than 4500/μL) is called *leukopenia,* and an increased WBC count (more than 11,500/μL) is called *leukocytosis,* but the WBC count alone has modest clinical value. The microscopist must differentiate the categories of WBCs in the blood by using a Wright-stained blood film and light microscopy (Chapter 16). The types of WBCs are as follows:

- Neutrophils (NEUTs, segmented neutrophils, SEGs, polymorphonuclear neutrophils, PMNs; Figure 1-1, *B*). Neutrophils are phagocytic cells whose major purpose is to engulf and destroy microorganisms and foreign material, either directly or after they have been labeled for destruction by the immune system. The term *segmented* refers to their multilobed nuclei. An increase in neutrophils is called *neutrophilia* and often signals bacterial infection. A decrease is called *neutropenia* and has many causes, but it is often caused by certain medications or viral infections.
- Bands (band neutrophils, BANDs; Figure 1-1, *C*). Bands are less differentiated or less mature neutrophils. An increase in bands also signals bacterial infection and is customarily called a *left shift.* The cytoplasm of neutrophils and bands

contains submicroscopic, pink- or lavender-staining granules filled with bactericidal secretions.
- Eosinophils (EOs; Figure 1-1, *D*). Eosinophils are cells with bright orange-red, regular cytoplasmic granules filled with proteins involved in immune system regulation. An elevated eosinophil count is called *eosinophilia* and often signals a response to allergy or parasitic infection.
- Basophils (BASOs; Figure 1-1, *E*). Basophils are cells with dark purple, irregular cytoplasmic granules that obscure the nucleus. The basophil granules contain histamines and various other proteins. An elevated basophil count is called *basophilia.* Basophilia is rare and often signals a hematologic disease.
- The distribution of basophils and eosinophils in blood is so small compared with that of neutrophils that the terms *eosinopenia* and *basopenia* are theoretical and not used. Neutrophils, bands, eosinophils, and basophils are collectively called *granulocytes* because of their prominent cytoplasmic granules, although their functions differ.
- Leukemia is an uncontrolled proliferation of WBCs. Leukemia may be chronic—for example, *chronic myelogenous* (granulocytic) *leukemia*—or acute—for example, *acute myeloid leukemia.* There are several forms of granulocytic leukemias that involve any one of or all three cell lines, categorized by their respective genetic aberrations (Chapters 30, 33 to 35). Medical laboratory scientists are responsible for their identification using Wright-stained bone marrow smears, cytogenetics, flow cytometric immunophenotyping, molecular diagnostic technology, and occasionally, cytochemical staining (Chapter 17 and Chapters 30 to 32).
- Lymphocytes (LYMPHs; Figure 1-1, *F*). Lymphocytes comprise a complex system of cells that provide for host immunity. Lymphocytes recognize foreign antigens and mount *humoral* (antibodies) and *cell-mediated* antagonistic responses. On a Wright-stained blood film, most lymphocytes are nearly round, are slightly larger than RBCs, and have round featureless nuclei and a thin rim of nongranular cytoplasm. An increase in the lymphocyte count is called *lymphocytosis* and often is associated with viral infections. Accompanying lymphocytosis are often variant or reactive lymphocytes with characteristic morphology (Chapter 29). An abnormally low lymphocyte count is called *lymphopenia* or *lymphocytopenia* and is often associated with drug therapy or immunodeficiency. Lymphocytes are also implicated in leukemia; *chronic lymphocytic leukemia* is more prevalent in people older than 65 years, whereas *acute lymphoblastic leukemia* is the most common form of childhood leukemia (Chapters 35 and 36). Medical laboratory scientists and hematopathologists classify lymphocytic leukemias largely based on Wright-stained blood films, flow cytometric immunophenotyping, and molecular diagnostic techniques (Chapters 31 to 32).
- Monocytes (MONOs; Figure 1-1, *G*). The monocyte is an immature *macrophage* passing through the blood from its point of origin, usually the bone marrow, to a targeted tissue location. Macrophages are the most abundant cell type in the body, more abundant than RBCs or skin cells, although monocytes comprise a minor component of peripheral

blood WBCs. Macrophages occupy every body cavity; some are motile and some are immobilized. Their tasks are to identify and *phagocytose* (engulf and consume) foreign particles and assist the lymphocytes in mounting an immune response through the assembly and presentation of immunogenic *epitopes*. On a Wright-stained blood film, monocytes have a slightly larger diameter than other WBCs, blue-gray cytoplasm with fine azure granules, and a nucleus that is usually indented or folded. An increase in the number of monocytes is called *monocytosis*. Monocytosis may be found in certain infections, collagen-vascular diseases, or in acute and chronic leukemias (Chapters 29, 33, and 35). Medical laboratory professionals seldom document a decreased monocyte count, so the theoretical term *monocytopenia* is seldom used.

PLATELETS

Platelets, or thrombocytes, are true blood cells that maintain blood vessel integrity by initiating vessel wall repairs (Chapter 13). Platelets rapidly adhere to the surfaces of damaged blood vessels, form aggregates with neighboring platelets to plug the vessels, and secrete proteins and small molecules that trigger *thrombosis*, or clot formation. Platelets are the major cells that control *hemostasis*, a series of cellular and plasma-based mechanisms that seal wounds, repair vessel walls, and maintain vascular patency (unimpeded blood flow). Platelets are only 2 to 4 μm in diameter, round or oval, anucleate (for this reason some hematologists prefer to call platelets "cell fragments"), and slightly granular (Figure 1-1, *H*). Their small size makes them appear insignificant, but they are essential to life and are extensively studied for their complex physiology. Uncontrolled platelet and hemostatic activation is responsible for deep vein thrombosis, pulmonary emboli, acute myocardial infarctions (heart attacks), cerebrovascular accidents (strokes), peripheral artery disease, and repeated spontaneous abortions (miscarriages).

The microscopist counts platelets using the same technique used in counting WBCs on a hemacytometer, although a different counting area and dilution is usually used (Chapter 14). Owing to their small volume, platelets are hard to distinguish visually in a hemacytometer, and phase microscopy provides for easier identification (Chapter 4). Automated profiling instruments have largely replaced visual platelet counting and provide greater accuracy (see Chapter 15).

One advantage of automated profiling instruments is their ability to generate a mean platelet volume (MPV), which is unavailable through visual methods. The presence of predominantly larger platelets generates an elevated MPV value, which sometimes signals a regenerative bone marrow response to platelet consumption (Chapters 13 and 40).

Elevated platelet counts, called *thrombocytosis*, signal inflammation or trauma but convey modest intrinsic significance. *Essential thrombocythemia* is a rare malignant condition characterized by extremely high platelet counts and uncontrolled platelet production. Essential thrombocythemia is a life-threatening hematologic disorder (Chapter 33).

A low platelet count, called *thrombocytopenia*, is a common consequence of drug treatment and may be life-threatening. Because the platelet is responsible for normal blood vessel maintenance and repair, thrombocytopenia is usually accompanied by easy bruising and uncontrolled hemorrhage (Chapter 40). Thrombocytopenia accounts for many hemorrhage-related emergency department visits. Accurate platelet counting contributes to patient safety because it provides for the diagnosis of thrombocytopenia in many disorders or therapeutic regimens.

COMPLETE BLOOD COUNT

A complete blood count (CBC) is performed on automated hematology profiling instruments and includes the RBC, WBC, and platelet measurements indicated in Box 1-1. The medical laboratory professional may collect a blood specimen for the CBC, but often a phlebotomist, nurse, physician assistant, physician, or patient care technician may also collect the specimen (Chapters 3 and 42). No matter who collects, the medical laboratory professional is responsible for the integrity of the specimen and ensures that it is submitted in the appropriate anticoagulant and tube and is free of clots and hemolysis (red-tinted plasma indicating RBC damage). The specimen must be of sufficient volume, as "short draws" result in incorrect anticoagulant-to-specimen ratios. The specimen must be tested or prepared for storage within the appropriate time frame to ensure accurate analysis (Chapter 5) and must be accurately registered in the work list, a process known as specimen *accession*. Accession may be automated, relying on bar code or radio-frequency identification technology, thus reducing instances of identification error.

Although all laboratory scientists and technicians are equipped to perform visual RBC, WBC, and platelet counts

---

BOX 1-1 Complete Blood Count Measurements Generated by Automated Hematology Profiling Instruments

RBC Parameters	WBC Parameters
RBC count	WBC count
HGB	NEUT count: % and absolute
HCT	LYMPH count: % and absolute
MCV	MONO count: % and absolute
MCH	EO and BASO counts: % and
MCHC	absolute
RDW	
RETIC	

Platelet Parameters
PLT count
MPV

BASO, Basophil; *EO*, eosinophil; *HGB*, hemoglobin; *HCT*, hematocrit; *LYMPH*, lymphocyte; *MCH*, mean cell hemoglobin; *MCHC*, mean cell hemoglobin concentration; *MCV*, mean cell volume; *MONO*, monocyte; *MPV*, mean platelet volume; *NEUT*, segmented neutrophil; *PLT*, platelet; *RBC*, red blood cell; *RDW*, RBC distribution width; *RETIC*, reticulocyte; *WBC*, white blood cell.

using dilution pipettes, hemacytometers, and microscopes, most laboratories employ automated profiling instruments to generate the CBC. Many profiling instruments also provide comments on RBC, WBC, and platelet morphology (Chapter 15). When one of the results from the profiling instrument is abnormal, the instrument provides an indication of this, sometimes called a *flag*. In this case, a "reflex" *blood film examination* is performed (Chapter 16).

The blood film examination (described next) is a specialized, demanding, and fundamental CBC activity. Nevertheless, if all profiling instrument results are normal, the blood film examination is usually omitted from the CBC. However, physicians may request a blood film examination on the basis of clinical suspicion even when the profiling instrument results fall within their respective reference intervals.

BLOOD FILM EXAMINATION

To accomplish a blood film examination, the microscopist prepares a "wedge-prep" blood film on a glass microscope slide, allows it to dry, and fixes and stains it using Wright or Wright-Giemsa stain (Chapter 16). The microscopist examines the RBCs and platelets by light microscopy for abnormalities of shape, diameter, color, or inclusions using the 50× or 100× oil immersion lens to generate 500× or 1000× magnification (Chapter 4). The microscopist then visually estimates the WBC count and platelet count for comparison with their respective instrument counts and investigates discrepancies. Next, the microscopist systematically reviews, identifies, and tabulates 100 (or more) WBCs to determine their percent distribution. This process is referred to as determining the *WBC differential* ("diff"). The WBC differential relies on the microscopist's skill, visual acuity, and integrity, and it provides extensive diagnostic information. Medical laboratory professionals pride themselves on their technical and analytical skills in performing the blood film examination and differential count. Visual recognition systems such as the Cellavision® DM96 or the Bloodhound automate the RBC and platelet morphology and WBC differential processes, but the medical laboratory professional or the hematopathologist is the final arbiter for all cell identification. The results of the CBC, including all profiling and blood film examination parameters and interpretive comments, are provided in paper or digital formats for physician review with abnormal results highlighted.

ENDOTHELIAL CELLS

Because they are structural and do not flow in the bloodstream, endothelial cells—the endodermal cells that form the inner surface of the blood vessel—are seldom studied in the hematology laboratory. Nevertheless, endothelial cells are important in maintaining normal blood flow, in tethering (decelerating) platelets during times of injury, and in enabling WBCs to escape from the vessel to the surrounding tissue when needed. Increasingly refined laboratory methods are becoming available to assay and characterize the secretions (cytokines) of these important cells.

COAGULATION

Most hematology laboratories include a blood coagulation–testing department (Chapters 42 and 44). Platelets are a key component of hemostasis, as previously described; plasma coagulation is the second component. The coagulation system employs a complex sequence of plasma proteins, some enzymes, and some enzyme cofactors to produce clot formation after blood vessel injury. Another 6 to 8 enzymes exert control over the coagulation mechanism, and a third system of enzymes and cofactors digests clots to restore vessel patency, a process called *fibrinolysis*. Bleeding and clotting disorders are numerous and complex, and the coagulation section of the hematology laboratory provides a series of plasma-based laboratory assays that assess the interactions of hematologic cells with plasma proteins (Chapters 42 and 44).

The medical laboratory professional focuses especially on blood specimen integrity for the coagulation laboratory, because minor blood specimen defects, including clots, hemolysis, lipemia, plasma bilirubin, and short draws, render the specimen useless (Chapters 3 and 42). High-volume coagulation tests suited to the acute care facility include the platelet count and MPV as described earlier, *prothrombin time* and *partial thromboplastin time* (or activated partial thromboplastin time), *thrombin time* (or thrombin clotting time), *fibrinogen assay*, and *D-dimer* assay (Chapter 42). The prothrombin time and partial thromboplastin time are particularly high-volume assays used in screening profiles. These tests assess each portion of the coagulation pathway for deficiencies and are used to monitor anticoagulant therapy. Another 30 to 40 moderate-volume assays, mostly clot-based, are available in specialized or tertiary care facilities. The specialized or tertiary care coagulation laboratory with its interpretive complexities attracts advanced medical laboratory scientists with specialized knowledge and communication skills.

ADVANCED HEMATOLOGY PROCEDURES

Besides performing the CBC, the hematology laboratory provides *bone marrow examinations, flow cytometry immunophenotyping, cytogenetic analysis,* and *molecular diagnosis assays*. Performing these tests may require advanced preparation or particular dedication by medical laboratory scientists with a desire to specialize.

Medical laboratory scientists assist physicians with bedside *bone marrow* collection, then prepare, stain, and microscopically review bone marrow smears (Chapter 17). Bone marrow *aspirates* and *biopsy specimens* are collected and stained to analyze nucleated cells that are the immature precursors to blood cells. Cells of the *erythroid* series are precursors to RBCs (Chapter 8); *myeloid* series cells mature to form bands and neutrophils, eosinophils, and basophils (Chapter 12); and *megakaryocytes* produce platelets (Chapter 13). Medical laboratory scientists, clinical pathologists, and hematologists review Wright-stained aspirate smears for morphologic abnormalities, high or low bone marrow cell concentration, and inappropriate cell line distributions. For instance, an increase in the erythroid cell line may indicate bone marrow compensation for excessive RBC destruction or blood loss (Chapter 19 and Chapters 23 to 26). The biopsy specimen, enhanced by *hematoxylin and eosin* (H&E) staining, may reveal abnormalities in bone marrow architecture indicating leukemia, bone marrow failure, or one of a host of additional hematologic disorders. Results of examination of bone marrow aspirates and biopsy specimens are compared with CBC results generated from the peripheral blood to correlate findings and develop pattern-based diagnoses.

In the bone marrow laboratory, cytochemical stains may occasionally be employed to differentiate abnormal myeloid, erythroid, and lymphoid cells. These stains include *myeloperoxidase, Sudan black B, nonspecific and specific esterase, periodic acid–Schiff, tartrate-resistant acid phosphatase,* and *alkaline phosphatase.* The cytochemical stains are time-honored stains that in most laboratories have been replaced by flow cytometry immunophenotyping, cytogenetics, and molecular diagnostic techniques (Chapters 30 to 32). Since 1980, however, *immunostaining* methods have enabled identification of cell lines by detecting lineage-specific antigens on the surface or in the cytoplasm of leukemia and lymphoma cells. An example of immunostaining is a visible dye that is bound to antibodies to CD42b, a membrane protein that is present in the megakaryocytic lineage and may be diagnostic for megakaryoblastic leukemia (Chapter 35).

Flow cytometers may be *quantitative,* such as clinical flow cytometers that have grown from the original Coulter principle, or *qualitative,* including laser-based instruments that have migrated from research applications to the clinical laboratory (Chapters 15 and 32). The former devices are automated clinical profiling instruments that generate the quantitative parameters of the CBC through application of electrical impedance and laser or light beam interruption. Qualitative laser-based flow cytometers are mechanically simpler but technically more demanding. Both qualitative and quantitative flow cytometers are employed to analyze cell populations by measuring the effects of individual cells on laser light, such as *forward-angle fluorescent light scatter* and *right-angle fluorescent light scatter,* and by *immunophenotyping* for cell membrane epitopes using monoclonal antibodies labeled with fluorescent dyes. The qualitative flow cytometry laboratory is indispensable to leukemia and lymphoma diagnosis.

Cytogenetics, a time-honored form of molecular technology, is employed in bone marrow aspirate examination to find gross genetic errors such as the Philadelphia chromosome, a reciprocal translocation between chromosomes 9 and 22 that is associated with chronic myelogenous leukemia, and t(15;17), a translocation between chromosomes 15 and 17 associated with acute promyelocytic leukemia (Chapter 30). Cytogenetic analysis remains essential to the diagnosis and treatment of leukemia.

Molecular diagnostic techniques, the fastest-growing area of laboratory medicine, enhance and even replace some of the advanced hematologic methods. Real-time polymerase chain reaction, microarray analysis, fluorescence in situ hybridization, and DNA sequencing systems are sensitive and specific methods that enable medical laboratory scientists to detect various chromosome translocations and gene mutations that confirm specific types of leukemia, establish their therapeutic profile and prognosis, and monitor the effectiveness of treatment (Chapter 31).

ADDITIONAL HEMATOLOGY PROCEDURES

Medical laboratory professionals provide several time-honored manual whole-blood methods to support hematologic diagnosis. The *osmotic fragility* test uses graduated concentrations of saline solutions to detect spherocytes (RBCs with proportionally reduced surface membrane area) in *hereditary spherocytosis* or *warm autoimmune hemolytic* anemia (Chapters 24 and 26). Likewise, the *glucose-6-phosphate dehydrogenase assay* phenotypically detects an inherited RBC enzyme deficiency causing severe episodic hemolytic anemia (Chapter 24). The sickle cell solubility screening assay and its follow-up tests, hemoglobin electrophoresis and high performance liquid chromatography, are used to detect and diagnose sickle cell anemia and other inherited qualitative hemoglobin abnormalities and thalassemias (Chapters 27 and 28). One of the oldest hematology tests, the *erythrocyte sedimentation rate,* detects inflammation and roughly estimates its intensity (Chapter 14).

Finally, the medical laboratory professional reviews the cellular counts, distribution, and morphology in body fluids other than blood (Chapter 18). These include cerebrospinal fluid, synovial (joint) fluid, pericardial fluid, pleural fluid, and peritoneal fluid, in which RBCs and WBCs may be present in disease and in which additional malignant cells may be present that require specialized detection skills. Analysis of nonblood body fluids is always performed with a rapid turnaround, because cells in these hostile environments rapidly lose their integrity. The conditions leading to a need for body fluid analysis are invariably acute.

HEMATOLOGY QUALITY ASSURANCE AND QUALITY CONTROL

Medical laboratory professionals employ particularly complex quality control systems in the hematology laboratory (Chapter 5). Owing to the unavailability of weighed standards, the measurement of cells and biological systems defies chemical standardization and requires elaborate calibration, validation, matrix effect examination, linearity, and reference interval determinations. An internal standard methodology known as the *moving average* also supports hematology laboratory applications.[10] Medical laboratory professionals in all disciplines compare methods through clinical efficacy calculations that produce clinical sensitivity, specificity, and positive and negative predictive values for each assay. They must monitor specimen integrity and test ordering patterns and ensure the integrity and delivery of reports, including numerical and narrative statements and reference interval comparisons. As in most branches of laboratory science, the hematology laboratory places an enormous responsibility for accuracy, integrity, judgment, and timeliness on the medical laboratory professional.

REFERENCES

1. Perkins, S. L. (2009). Examination of the blood and bone marrow. In Greer, J. P., Foerster, J, Rodgers, G. M., et al, (Eds.), *Wintrobe's Clinical Hematology.* (12th ed.). Philadelphia: Lippincott Williams and Wilkins.

2. Wintrobe, M. M. (1985). *Hematology, the Blossoming of a Science: A Story of Inspiration and Effort.* Philadelphia: Lea & Febiger.

3. Bizzozero, J. (1882). Über einem neuen formbestandtheil des blutes und dessen rolle bei der Thrombose und der Blutgerinnung. *Virchows Arch Pathol Anat Physiol Klin Med, 90,* 261–332.

4. Woronzoff-Dashkoff, K. K. (2002). The Wright-Giemsa stain. Secrets revealed. *Clin Lab Med, 22,* 15–23.

5. Blades, A. N., Flavell, H. C. (1963). Observations on the use of the Coulter model D electronic cell counter in clinical haematology. *J Clin Pathol, 16,* 158–163.

6. Klungsöyr, L., Stöa, K. F. (1954). Spectrophotometric determination of hemoglobin oxygen saturation: the method of Drabkin & Schmidt as modified for its use in clinical routine analysis. *Scand J Clin Lab Invest, 6,* 270–276.

7. Mann, L. S. (1948). A rapid method of filling and cleaning Wintrobe hematocrit tubes. *Am J Clin Pathol, 18,* 916.

8. Barth, D. (2012). Approach to peripheral blood film assessment for pathologists. *Semin Diagn Pathol, 29,* 31–48.

9. Biggs, R. (1948). Error in counting reticulocytes. *Nature, 162,* 457.

10. Gulati, G. L., Hyun, B. H. (1986). Quality control in hematology. *Clin Lab Med, 6,* 675–688.

2 Safety in the Hematology Laboratory

Sheila A. Finch

OBJECTIVES

After completion of this chapter, the reader will be able to:

1. Define standard precautions and list infectious materials included in standard precautions.
2. Describe the safe practices required in the Occupational Exposure to Bloodborne Pathogens Standard.
3. Identify occupational hazards that exist in the hematology laboratory.
4. Describe appropriate methods to decontaminate work surfaces after contamination with blood or other potentially infectious material.
5. Identify the regulatory requirements of the Occupational Exposure to Hazardous Chemicals in Laboratories standard.
6. Describe the principles of a fire prevention program, including details such as the frequency of testing equipment.
7. Name the most important practice to prevent the spread of infection.
8. Given a written laboratory scenario, assess for safety hazards and recommend corrective action for any deficiencies or unsafe practices identified.
9. Select the proper class of fire extinguisher for a given type of fire.
10. Explain the purpose of *Safety Data Sheets* (SDSs), list information contained on SDSs, and determine when SDSs would be used in a laboratory activity.
11. Name the specific practice during which most needle stick injuries occur.
12. Describe elements of a safety management program.

CASE STUDY

After studying the material in this chapter, the reader should be able to respond to the following case study:

Hematology Services, Inc., had a proactive safety program. Quarterly safety audits were conducted by members of the safety committee. The following statements were recorded in the safety audit report. Which statements describe good work practices, and which statements represent deficiencies? List the corrective actions required for identified unsafe practices.

1. A hematology laboratory scientist was observed removing gloves and immediately left the laboratory for a meeting. She did not remove her laboratory coat.
2. Food was found in the specimen refrigerator.
3. Hematology laboratory employees were seen in the lunchroom, wearing laboratory coats.
4. Fire extinguishers were found every 75 feet of the laboratory.
5. Fire extinguishers were inspected quarterly and maintained annually.
6. Unlabeled bottles were found at a workstation.
7. A 1:10 solution of bleach was found near an automated hematology analyzer. Further investigation revealed that the bleach solution was made 6 months ago.
8. Gloves were worn by the staff receiving specimens.
9. Safety data sheets were obtained by fax.
10. Chemicals were stored alphabetically.

Many conditions in the laboratory have the potential for causing injury to staff and damage to the building or to the community. Patients' specimens, needles, chemicals, electrical equipment, reagents, and glassware all are potential causes of accidents or injury. Managers and employees must be knowledgeable about safe work practices and incorporate these practices into the operation of the hematology laboratory. The key to prevention of accidents and laboratory-acquired infections is a well-defined safety program.

Safety is a broad subject and cannot be covered in one chapter. This chapter simply highlights some of the key safe practices that should be followed in the hematology laboratory. Omission of a safe practice from this chapter does not imply that it is not important or that it should not be considered in the development of a safety curriculum or a safety program.

STANDARD PRECAUTIONS

One of the greatest risks associated with the hematology laboratory is the exposure to blood and body fluids. In December 1991, the Occupational Safety and Health Administration (OSHA) issued the final rule for the Occupational Exposure to Bloodborne Pathogens Standard. The rule that specifies standard precautions to protect laboratory workers and other health care professionals became effective on March 6, 1992. *Universal precautions* was the original term; OSHA's current terminology is *standard precautions*. Throughout this text, the term *standard precautions* is used to remind the reader that all blood, body fluids, and unfixed tissues are to be handled as though they were potentially infectious.

Standard precautions must be adopted by the laboratory. Standard precautions apply to blood, semen, vaginal secretions, cerebrospinal fluid, synovial fluid, pleural fluid, any body fluid with visible blood, any unidentified body fluid, unfixed slides, microhematocrit clay, and saliva from dental procedures. Adopting standard precautions lessens the risk of health care worker exposures to blood and body fluids, decreasing the risk of injury and illness.

Bloodborne pathogens are pathogenic microorganisms that, when present in human blood, can cause disease. They include, but are not limited to, hepatitis B virus (HBV), hepatitis C virus (HCV), and human immunodeficiency virus (HIV). This chapter does not cover the complete details of the standard; it discusses only the sections that apply directly to the hematology laboratory. Additional information can be found in the references at the end of this chapter.

Applicable Safety Practices Required by the OSHA Standard

The following standards are applicable in a hematology laboratory and must be enforced:

1. *Hand washing* is one of the most important safety practices. Hands must be washed with soap and water. If water is not readily available, alcohol hand gels (minimum 62% alcohol) may be used. Hands must be thoroughly dried. The proper technique for hand washing is as follows:
   a. Wet hands *and wrists* thoroughly under running water.
   b. Apply germicidal soap and rub hands vigorously for at least 15 seconds, including between the fingers and around and over the fingernails (Figure 2-1, *A*).
   c. Rinse hands thoroughly under running water in a downward flow from wrist to fingertips (Figure 2-1, *B*).
   d. Dry hands with a paper towel (Figure 2-1, *C*). Use the paper towel to turn off the faucet handles (Figure 2-1, *D*).
   Hands must be washed:
   a. Whenever there is visible contamination with blood or body fluids
   b. After completion of work
   c. After gloves are removed and between glove changes
   d. Before leaving the laboratory
   e. Before and after eating and drinking, smoking, applying cosmetics or lip balm, changing a contact lens, and using the lavatory
   f. Before and after all other activities that entail hand contact with mucous membranes, eyes, or breaks in skin
2. Eating, drinking, smoking, and applying cosmetics or lip balm must be prohibited in the laboratory work area.
3. Hands, pens, and other fomites must be kept away from the mouth and all mucous membranes.
4. Food and drink, including oral medications and tolerance-testing beverages, must not be kept in the same refrigerator as laboratory specimens or reagents or where potentially infectious materials are stored or tested.
5. Mouth pipetting must be prohibited.
6. Needles and other sharp objects contaminated with blood and other potentially infectious materials should not be manipulated in any way. Such manipulation includes resheathing, bending, clipping, or removing the sharp object. Resheathing or recapping is permitted only when there are no other alternatives or when the recapping is required by specific medical procedures. Recapping is permitted by use of a method other than the traditional two-handed procedure. The one-handed method or a resheathing device is often used. Documentation in the exposure control plan should identify the specific procedure in which resheathing is permitted.
7. *Contaminated sharps* (including, but not limited to, needles, blades, pipettes, syringes with needles, and glass slides) must be placed in a puncture-resistant container that is appropriately labeled with the universal biohazard symbol (Figure 2-2) or a red container that adheres to the standard. The container must be leakproof (Figure 2-3).
8. Procedures such as removing caps when checking for clots, filling hemacytometer chambers, making slides, discarding specimens, making dilutions, and pouring specimens or fluids must be performed so that splashing, spraying, or production of droplets of the specimen being manipulated is prevented. These procedures may be performed behind a barrier, such as a plastic shield, or protective eyewear should be worn (Figure 2-4).

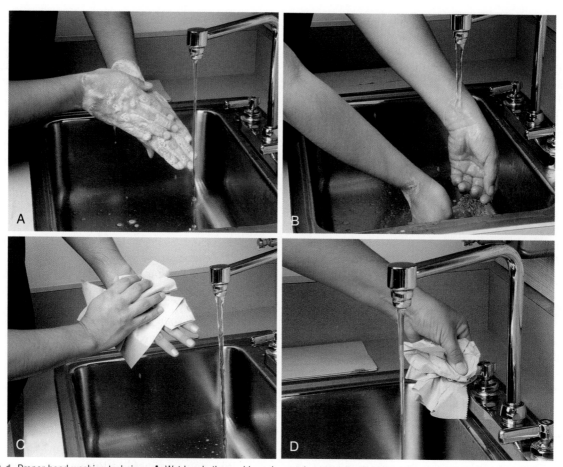

Figure 2-1 Proper hand washing technique. **A,** Wet hands thoroughly under running water, apply soap, and rub hands vigorously for at least 15 seconds. **B,** Rinse hands thoroughly under running water in a downward flow from wrist to fingertips. **C,** Dry hands with a paper towel. **D,** Turn off faucet with paper towel. (From Young AP, Proctor DB: Kinn's the medical assistant, ed 11, St Louis, 2011, Saunders.)

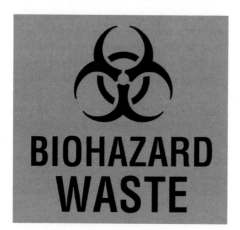

Figure 2-2 Biohazard symbol.

9. *Personal protective clothing* and equipment must be provided to the laboratory staff. The most common forms of personal protective equipment are described in the following section:

   a. *Outer coverings,* including gowns, laboratory coats, and sleeve protectors, should be worn when there is a chance of splashing or spilling on work clothing. The outer covering must be made of fluid-resistant material, must be long-sleeved, and must remain buttoned at all times. If contamination occurs, the personal protective equipment should be removed immediately and treated as infectious material.

Cloth laboratory coats may be worn if they are fluid resistant. If cloth coats are worn, the coats must be laundered inside the laboratory or hospital or by a contracted laundry service. Laboratory coats used in the laboratory while performing laboratory analysis are considered personal protective equipment and are not to be taken home.

All protective clothing should be removed before leaving the laboratory; it should not be worn into public areas. Public areas include, but are not limited to, break rooms, storage areas, bathrooms, cafeterias, offices, and meeting places outside the laboratory.

A second laboratory coat can be made available for use in public areas. A common practice is to have a different-colored laboratory coat that can be worn in public areas. This second laboratory coat could be laundered by the employee.

   b. *Gloves* must be worn when the potential for contact with blood or body fluids exists (including when removing and handling bagged biohazardous material and when decontaminating bench tops) and when venipuncture or skin puncture is performed. One of the limitations of gloves is that they *do not* prevent needle sticks or other puncture wounds. Provision of gloves to laboratory staff must accommodate latex allergies. Alternative gloves must be readily accessible to any laboratory employee with a latex

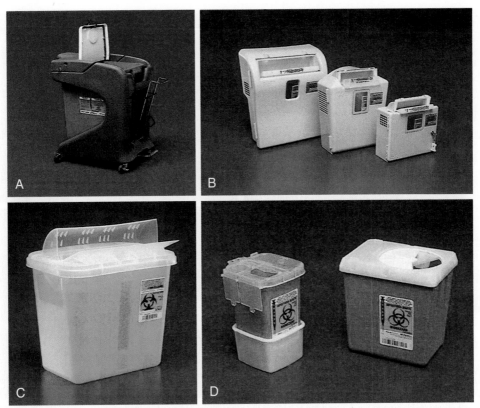

Figure 2-3 Examples of sharps disposal systems. **A,** Molded foot pedal cart with hinged or slide top lid. **B,** In-room system wall enclosures. **C,** Multipurpose container with horizontal drop lid. **D,** Phlebotomy containers. (Courtesy Covidien, Mansfield, MA.)

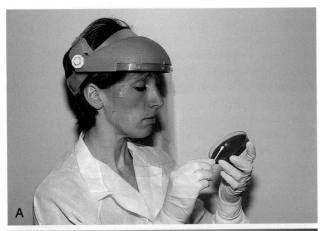

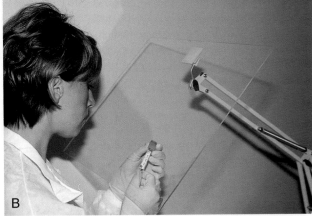

Figure 2-4 Examples of safety shields. **A,** Face shield. **B,** Adjustable swing arm shield. (Courtesy Steve Kasper.)

allergy. Gloves must be changed after each contact with a patient, when there is visible contamination, and when physical damage occurs. Gloves should not be worn when "clean" devices, such as a copy machine or a "clean" telephone, are used. Gloves must not be worn again or washed. After one glove is removed, the second glove can be removed by sliding the index finger of the ungloved hand between the glove and the hand and slipping the second glove off. This technique prevents contamination of the "clean" hand by the "dirty" second glove (Figure 2-5).[1] Contaminated gloves should be disposed of according to applicable federal or state regulations.

   c. *Eyewear*, including face shields, goggles, and masks, should be used when there is potential for aerosol mists, splashes, or sprays to mucous membranes (mouth, eyes, or nose). Removing caps from specimen tubes, working at an automated hematology analyzer, and centrifuging specimens are examples of tasks that could produce an aerosol mist.

10. *Phlebotomy trays* should be appropriately labeled to indicate potentially infectious materials. Specimens should be placed into a secondary container, such as a resealable biohazard-labeled bag.

11. If a *pneumatic tube system* is used to transport specimens, the specimens should be transported in the appropriate tube (primary containment), and placed into a special self-sealing leakproof bag appropriately labeled with the biohazard symbol (secondary containment). Requisition forms should be placed outside of the secondary container to prevent contamination if the specimen leaks. Foam

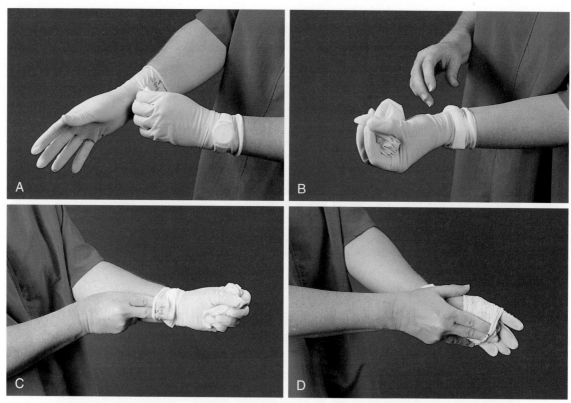

Figure 2-5 Removal of gloves. **A,** Using one hand, grasp the outside of the other glove and slowly pull it off the hand, turning it inside out as you remove it. **B,** Scrunch the removed glove into a ball. **C,** Place the index and middle finger of the ungloved hand on the inside of the other glove. **D,** Pull the second glove off of the hand, turning it inside out as it is removed and enclosing the balled-up glove. (From Bonewit-West K: Clinical procedures for medical assistants, ed 9, St Louis, 2015, Saunders.)

inserts for the pneumatic tube system carrier prevent shifting of the sample during transport and also act as a shock absorber, thus decreasing the risk of breakage.

When specimens are received in the laboratory, they should be handled by an employee wearing gloves, a laboratory coat, and other protective clothing, in accordance with the type and condition of specimen. Contaminated containers or requisitions must be decontaminated or replaced before being sent to the work area.

12. When *equipment* used to process specimens becomes visibly contaminated or requires maintenance or service, it must be decontaminated, whether service is performed within the laboratory or by a manufacturer repair service. Decontamination of equipment consists of a minimum of flushing the lines and wiping the exterior and interior of the equipment. If it is difficult to decontaminate the equipment, it must be labeled with the biohazard symbol to indicate potentially infectious material. *Routine cleaning* should be performed on equipment that has the potential for receiving splashes or sprays, such as inside the lid of the microhematocrit centrifuge.

Housekeeping

Blood and other potentially infectious materials can contaminate work surfaces easily. Contamination can be caused by splashes, poor work practices, and droplets of blood on the work surface. To prevent contamination, all work surfaces should be cleaned when procedures are completed and whenever the bench area or floor becomes visibly contaminated. An appropriate disinfectant solution is household bleach, used in a 1:10 volume/volume dilution (10%), which can be made by adding 10 mL of bleach to 90 mL of water or 1½ cups of bleach to 1 gallon of water to achieve the recommended concentration of chlorine (5500 ppm). Because this solution is not stable, it must be made fresh *daily.* The container of 1:10 solution of bleach should be labeled properly with the name of the solution, the date and time prepared, the date and time of expiration (24 hours), and the initials of the preparer. Bleach is not recommended for aluminum surfaces. Other solutions used to decontaminate include, but are not limited to, a phenol-based disinfectant such as Amphyl®, tuberculocidal disinfectants, and 70% ethanol. All paper towels used in the decontamination process should be disposed of as biohazardous waste. Documentation of the disinfection of work areas and equipment after each shift is required.

Laundry

If nondisposable laboratory coats are used, they must be placed in appropriate containers for transport to the laundry at the facility or to a contract service and not taken to the employee's home.

Hepatitis B Virus Vaccination

Laboratory employees should receive the HBV vaccination series at no cost before or within 10 days after beginning work in the laboratory. An employee must sign a release form if he or she refuses the series. The employee can request and receive the hepatitis vaccination series at any time, however. If an exposure incident (needle puncture or exposure to skin, eye, face, or mucous membrane) occurs, postexposure evaluation and follow-up, including prophylaxis and medical consultation, should be made available at no cost to the employee. Employees should be encouraged to report all exposure incidents, and such reporting should be enforced as standard policy.

Training and Documentation

Hematology staff should be properly educated in epidemiology and symptoms of bloodborne diseases, modes of transmission of bloodborne diseases, use of protective equipment, work practices, ways to recognize tasks and other activities that may result in an exposure, and the location of the written exposure plan for the laboratory. Education should be documented and should occur when new methods, equipment, or procedures are introduced; at the time of initial assignment to the laboratory; and at least annually thereafter.

Regulated Medical Waste Management

Specimens from the hematology laboratory are identified as regulated waste. There are different categories of regulated medical waste, and state and local regulations for disposal of medical waste must be followed. OSHA regulates some aspects of regulated medical waste such as needle handling, occupational exposure, labeling of containers, employee training, and storing of the waste. The Occupational Exposure to Bloodborne Pathogens Standard provides information on the handling of regulated medical waste. Detailed disposal guidelines are specific to the state disposal standards. When two regulations conflict, the more stringent standard is followed.

OCCUPATIONAL HAZARDS

Four important occupational hazards in the laboratory are discussed in this chapter: fire hazard, chemical hazards, electrical hazard, and needle puncture. There are other hazards to be considered when a safety management program is developed, and the reader is referred to the Department of Labor section of the Code of Federal Regulations for detailed regulations.[2]

Fire Hazard

Because of the numerous flammable and combustible chemicals used in the laboratory, fire is a potential hazard. Complying with standards established by the National Fire Protection Association, OSHA, the Joint Commission, the College of American Pathologists, and other organizations can minimize the dangers. A good fire safety/prevention plan is necessary and should consist of the following:

1. Enforcement of a no-smoking policy.
2. Installation of appropriate fire extinguishers. Several types of extinguishers, most of which are multipurpose, are available for use for specific types of fires.
3. Placement of fire extinguishers every 75 feet. A distinct system for marking the locations of fire extinguishers enables quick access when they are needed. Fire extinguishers should be checked monthly and maintained annually. Not all fire extinguishers are alike. Each fire extinguisher is rated for the type of fire that it can suppress. It is important to use the correct fire extinguisher for the given class of fire. Hematology laboratory staff should be trained to recognize the class of extinguisher and use a fire extinguisher properly. Table 2-1 summarizes the fire extinguisher classifications. The fire extinguishers used in the laboratory are portable extinguishers and are not designed to fight large fires. In the event of a fire in the laboratory, the local fire department must be contacted immediately.
4. Placement of adequate fire detection and suppression systems (alarms, smoke detectors, sprinklers), which should be tested every 3 months.
5. Placement of manual fire alarm boxes near the exit doors. Travel distance should not exceed 200 feet.
6. Written fire prevention and response procedures, commonly referred to as the *fire response plan*. All staff in the laboratory should be knowledgeable about the procedures. Employees should be given assignments for specific responsibilities in case of fire, including responsibilities for patient care, if applicable. Total count of employees in the laboratory should be known for any given day, and a buddy system should be developed in case evacuation is necessary. Equipment shutdown procedures should be addressed in the plan, as should responsibility for implementation of those procedures.
7. Fire drills, which should be conducted so that response to a fire situation is routine and not a panic response. Frequency of fire drills varies by type of occupancy of the building and by accrediting agency. Overall governance can be by the local or state fire marshal. All laboratory employees should participate in the fire drills. Proper documentation should be maintained to verify that all phases of the fire response plan were activated. If patients are in areas adjacent to the hematology laboratory, evacuation can be simulated, rather than evacuating actual patients. The entire evacuation route should be walked to verify the exit routes and clearance of the corridors. A summary of the laboratory's fire response plan can be copied onto a quick reference card and attached to workers' identification badges to be readily available in a fire situation.

TABLE 2-1   Fire Extinguisher Classifications and Use

Class/Type of Extinguisher	Type of Fire
A	Ordinary combustibles such as wood, cloth, or paper.
B	Flammable liquids, gases, or grease.
C	Energized (plugged-in) electrical fires. Examples are fires involving equipment, computers, fuse boxes, or circuit breakers.
ABC	Multipurpose for type A, B, and C fires.

8. Written storage requirements for any flammable or combustible chemicals stored in the laboratory. Chemicals should be arranged according to hazard class and not alphabetically. A master chemical inventory should be maintained and revised when new chemicals are added or deleted from the laboratory procedures.

9. A well-organized fire safety training program. This program should be completed by all employees. Activities that require walking evacuation routes and locating fire exit boxes in the laboratory area should be scheduled. Types of fires likely to occur and use of the fire extinguisher should be discussed. Local fire departments may request a tour of the laboratory or facility to become familiar with the potential fire hazards prior to an actual fire occurring in the laboratory.

Chemical Hazards

Some of the chemicals used in the hematology laboratory are considered hazardous and are governed by the Occupational Exposure to Hazardous Chemicals in Laboratories Standard. This regulation requires laboratories to develop a chemical hygiene plan that outlines safe work practices to minimize exposures to hazardous chemicals. The full text of this regulation can be found in 29 CFR (Code of Federal Regulations) 1910.1450.[2]

General principles that should be followed in working with chemicals are as follows:

1. Label all chemicals properly, including chemicals in secondary containers, with the name and concentration of the chemical, preparation or fill date, expiration date (time, if applicable), initials of preparer (if done in-house), and chemical hazards (e.g., poisonous, corrosive, flammable). Do not use a chemical that is not properly labeled as to the identity or content.

2. Follow all handling and storage requirements for the chemical.

3. Store alcohol and other flammable chemicals in approved safety cans or storage cabinets at least 5 feet away from a heat source (e.g., Bunsen burners, paraffin baths). Limit the quantity of flammable chemicals stored on the workbench to 2 working days' supply. Do not store chemicals in a hood or in any area where they could react with other chemicals.

4. Use adequate ventilation, such as fume hoods, when working with hazardous chemicals.

5. Use personal protective equipment, such as gloves (e.g., nitrile, polyvinyl chloride, rubber—as appropriate for the chemical in use), rubber aprons, and face shields. Safety showers and eye wash stations should be available every 100 feet or within 10 seconds of travel distance from every work area where the hazardous chemicals are used.

6. Use bottle carriers for glass bottles containing more than 500 mL of hazardous chemical.

7. Use alcohol-based solvents, rather than xylene or other particularly hazardous substances, to clean microscope objectives.

8. The wearing of contact lenses should not be permitted when an employee is working with xylene, acetone, alcohols, formaldehyde, and other solvents. Many lenses are permeable to chemical fumes. Contact lenses can make it difficult to wash the eyes adequately in the event of a splash.

9. Spill response procedures should be included in the chemical safety procedures, and all employees must receive training in these procedures. Absorbent material should be available for spill response. Multiple spill response kits and absorbent material should be stored in various areas and rooms rather than only in the area where they are likely to be needed. This prevents the need to walk through the spilled chemical to obtain the kit.

10. Safety Data Sheets (SDS), formerly known as Material Safety Data Sheets (MSDS), are written by the manufacturers of chemicals to provide information on the chemicals that cannot be put on a label. In 2012, the Hazard Communication Standard (29 CFR 1910.1200(g)) was revised to align with the United Nations Globally Harmonized System (GHS) of Classification and Labeling of Chemicals. The significant revisions required the use of new labeling elements and a standardized format for Safety Data Sheets (SDS). The standardized information on the SDS uses a 16-section format, and the implementation date is June 1, 2015. The OSHA website on Hazard Communication Safety Data Sheets specifies the content for the 16 sections of the SDS as follows:[3]

- Section 1. *Identification* includes product identifier, manufacturer or distributor (name, address, emergency phone number), recommended use, and restrictions on use.

- Section 2. *Hazard(s) identification* includes all hazards of the chemical and required label information.

- Section 3. *Composition/information on ingredients* includes information on chemical ingredients and trade secret claims.

- Section 4. *First-aid measures* includes symptoms, acute and delayed effects, and required treatment.

- Section 5. *Firefighting measures* provides extinguishing techniques and equipment and chemical hazards from fire.

- Section 6. *Accidental release measures* lists emergency procedures, protective equipment, and methods of containment and cleanup.

- Section 7. *Handling and storage* lists precautions for safe handling and storage and incompatibilities with other chemicals.

- Section 8. *Exposure controls and personal protection* lists OSHA's permissible exposure limits, threshold limit values, engineering controls, and personal protective equipment.

- Section 9. *Physical and chemical properties* includes properties such as boiling point, vapor pressure, evaporation rate, appearance, and odor.

- Section 10. *Stability and reactivity* lists chemical stability and the possibility of hazardous reactions.

- Section 11. *Toxicological information* lists the routes of exposure, related symptoms, acute and chronic effects, and measures of toxicity.

- Section 12. *Ecological information* (nonmandatory) provides information to evaluate the environmental impact if chemical was released.
- Section 13. *Disposal consideration* (nonmandatory) provides guidance on proper disposal practices and recycling or reclamation of the chemical.
- Section 14. *Transport information* (nonmandatory) provides classification information for shipping and transporting the chemical.
- Section 15. *Regulatory information* (nonmandatory) lists safety, health, and environmental regulations for the chemical that are not listed in the other sections.
- Section 16. *Other information* includes the date of SDS preparation or last revision.

A SDS management system should be considered to track the incoming SDSs received in the laboratory. A notice should be posted to alert the hematology staff when new or revised SDSs have been received. SDSs may be obtained electronically by means of computer, fax, or Internet. If an electronic device is used in the laboratory to receive and store SDSs, each employee must be trained on the use of the device. The training must include emergency procedures in case of power outages or malfunctions of the device. The device must be reliable and readily accessible during the hours of operation. In the event of emergency, hard copies of the SDSs must be accessible to medical staff. SDSs are required to be kept for 30 years after employment of the last employee who used the chemicals in the work area, and they should be documented with the date when the chemical was no longer used in the laboratory.

Electrical Hazard

Electrical equipment and outlets are other sources of hazard. Faulty wiring may cause fires or serious injury. Guidelines include the following:

1. Equipment must be grounded or double insulated. (Grounded equipment has a three-pronged plug.)
2. Use of "cheater" adapters (adapters that allow three-pronged plugs to fit into a two-pronged outlet) should be prohibited.
3. Use of gang plugs (plugs that allow several cords to be plugged into one outlet) should be prohibited.
4. Use of extension cords should be avoided.
5. Equipment with loose plugs or frayed cords should not be used.
6. Stepping on cords, rolling heavy equipment over cords, and other abuse of cords should be prohibited.
7. When cords are unplugged, the plug, not the cord, should be pulled.
8. Equipment that causes shock or a tingling sensation should be turned off, the instrument unplugged and identified as defective, and the problem reported.
9. Before repair or adjustment of electrical equipment is attempted, the following should be done:
   a. Unplug the equipment.
   b. Make sure the hands are dry.
   c. Remove jewelry.

Needle Puncture

Needle puncture is a serious occupational hazard for laboratory personnel. Needle-handling procedures should be written and followed, with special attention to phlebotomy procedures and disposal of contaminated needles (Chapter 3). Other items that can cause a puncture similar to a needle puncture include sedimentation rate tubes, applicator sticks, capillary tubes, glass slides, and transfer pipettes.

Disposal procedures should be followed and enforced. The most frequent cause of a needle puncture or a puncture from other sharp objects is improper disposal. Failure to check sharps containers on a regular basis and to replace them when they are no more than three-quarters full encourages overstuffing, which sometimes leads to injury. Portable bedside containers are available for personnel when performing venipunctures or skin punctures. Wall-mounted needle disposal containers also are available and make disposal convenient. All needle punctures should be reported to the health services or proper authorities within the institution.

DEVELOPING A SAFETY MANAGEMENT PROGRAM

Every accredited laboratory is required to have a safety management program. A safety management program is one that identifies the guidelines necessary to provide a safe working environment free from recognizable hazards that can cause harm or injury. Many medical laboratory scientists assume positions as supervisors or laboratory safety officers. Responsibilities in these positions require knowledge of the safety principles and the development, implementation, and maintenance of a laboratory safety program. This section provides an overview of the elements that should be considered in developing a safety program.

Planning Stage: Hazard Assessment and Regulatory Review

Assessment of the hazards found in the laboratory and awareness of the standards and regulations that govern laboratories is a required step in the development of a safety program. Taking the time to become knowledgeable about the regulations and standards that relate to the procedures performed in the hematology laboratory is an essential first step. Examples of the regulatory agencies that have standards, requirements, and guidelines that are applicable to hematology laboratories are given in Box 2-1. Sorting through the regulatory maze can be challenging, but the government agencies and voluntary standards organizations are willing to assist employers in complying with their standards.

Safety Program Elements

A proactive program should include the following elements:

- *Written safety plan.* Written policies and procedures should be developed that explain the steps to be taken for all of the occupational and environmental hazards that exist in the hematology laboratory.

BOX 2-1 Government Regulatory Agencies Providing Laboratory Safety Standards

Department of Labor: 29 Code of Federal Regulations Part 1910

Hazard Communication Standard (right to know): 29 CFR 1910.1200

Occupational Exposure to Bloodborne Pathogens Standard: 29 CFR 1910.1030

Occupational Exposure to Hazardous Chemicals in Laboratories Standard: 29 CFR 1910.1450

Formaldehyde Standard: 29 CFR 1910.1048

Air Contaminants: Permissible Exposure Limits: 29 CFR 1910.1000

Occupational Noise Level Standard: 29 CFR 1910.95

Hazardous Waste Operations and Emergency Response Standard: 29 CFR 1910.120

Personal Protective Equipment: 29 CFR 1910.132

Eye and Face Protection: 29 CFR 1910.133

Respiratory Protection: 29 CFR 1910.134

Medical Waste Standards Regulated by the State

State medical waste standards

Department of the Interior, Environmental Protection Agency: 40 Code of Federal Regulations Parts 200-399

Resource Conservation and Recovery Act (RCRA)

Clean Air Act

Clean Water Act

Toxic Substances Control Act (TSCA)

Comprehensive Environmental Response, Compensation, and Liability Act (CERCLA)

Superfund Amendments and Reauthorization Act (SARA)

SARA Title III: Community Right to Know Act

Voluntary Agencies/Accrediting Agencies/Other Government Agencies

The Joint Commission

College of American Pathologists (CAP)

State public health departments

Centers for Disease Control and Prevention (CDC)

Clinical and Laboratory Standards Institute

National Fire Protection Association (NFPA)

Department of Transportation (DOT): Regulated Medical Waste Shipment Regulations: 49 CFR 100-185

CFR, Code of Federal Regulations.

- *Training programs.* Conducted annually for all employees. New employees should receive safety information on the first day that they are assigned to the hematology laboratory.
- *Job safety analysis.* Identifies all of the tasks performed in the hematology laboratory, the steps involved in performing the procedures, and the risk associated with the procedures.

- *Safety awareness program.* Promotes a team approach and encourages employees to take an active part in the safety program.
- *Risk assessment.* Proactive risk assessment (identification) of all the potential safety, occupational, or environmental hazards that exist in the laboratory should be conducted at least annually and when a new risk is added to the laboratory. After the risk assessment is conducted, goals, policies, and procedures should be developed to prevent the hazard from injuring a laboratory employee. Some common risks are exposure to bloodborne pathogens; exposure to chemicals; needle punctures; slips, trips, and falls; and ergonomics issues.
- *Safety audits and follow-up.* A safety checklist should be developed for the hematology laboratory for use during scheduled and unscheduled safety audits. Any unsafe practices should be corrected. Actions taken to correct the unsafe practice should be documented and monitored to verify the actions are effective in correcting the practice.
- *Reporting and investigating of all accidents, "near misses," or unsafe conditions.* The causes of all incidents should be reviewed and corrective action taken, if necessary.
- *Emergency drill and evaluation.* Periodic drills for all potential internal and external disasters should be conducted. Drills should address the potential accident or disaster event before it occurs and test the preparedness of the hematology personnel for an emergency situation. Planning for disaster events and practicing the response to a disaster event reduce the panic that results when the correct response procedure is not followed.
- *Emergency management plan.* Emergencies, sometimes called disasters (anything that prevents normal operation of the laboratory) do not occur only in the hospital-based laboratories. Freestanding laboratories, physician office laboratories, and university laboratories can be affected by emergencies that occur in the building or in the community. Emergency planning is crucial to being able to experience an emergency situation and recover enough to continue the daily operation of the laboratory. In addition to the safety risk assessment, a hazard vulnerability analysis should be conducted. Hazard vulnerability analysis helps to identify all of the potential emergencies that may have an impact on the laboratory. Emergencies such as a utility failure—loss of power, water, or telephones—can have a great impact on the laboratory's ability to perform procedures. Emergencies in the community, such as a terrorist attack, plane crash, severe weather, flood, or civil disturbances, can affect the laboratory employee's ability to get to work and can affect transportation of crucial supplies or equipment. When the potential emergencies are identified, policies and procedures should be developed and practiced so that the laboratory employee knows the backup procedures and can implement them quickly during an emergency or disaster situation. The emergency management plan should cover the four phases of response to an emergency, as follows:
  1. *Mitigation* includes measures to prevent or reduce the adverse effects of the emergency.

BOX 2-2 Emergency Management Activities: Planning for Response to a Fire

Mitigation Tools
Fire alarm pull box
Emergency code to notify workers
Smoke detectors
Fire/smoke doors
Audible and visual alarms
Fire exit lights
Sprinkler system

Preparedness Activities
Training of workers
Fire drills
Fire response procedure development
Annual and monthly fire extinguisher checks

Response Activities
Fire response plan implementation
Assignment of specific tasks during the actual event

Recovery Activities
Communication of "all clear"
Documentation of response to the fire
Damage assessment
Financial accounting of response activities
Replenishment of supplies
Stress debriefing for employees

---

2. *Preparedness* includes the design of procedures, identification of resources that may be used, and training in the procedures.
3. *Response* includes the actions that will be taken when responding to the emergency.
4. *Recovery* includes the procedures to assess damage, evaluate response, and replenish supplies so that the laboratory can return to normal operation.

An example of an emergency management plan is shown in Box 2-2.

The key to prevention of accidents and laboratory-acquired infections is a well-defined safety program that also includes:

- *Safety committee/department safety meetings* to communicate safety policies to the employees.
- *Review of equipment and supplies purchased for the laboratory* for code compliance and safety features.
- *Annual evaluation of the safety program* for review of goals and performance as well as a review of the regulations to assess compliance in the laboratory.

SUMMARY

- The responsibility of a medical laboratory professional is to perform analytical procedures accurately, precisely, and safely.
- Safe practices must be incorporated into all laboratory procedures and should be followed by every employee.
- The laboratory must adopt standard precautions that require that all human blood, body fluids, and unfixed tissues be treated as if they were infectious.
- One of the most important safety practices is hand washing.
- Occupational hazards in the laboratory include fire, chemical and electrical hazards, and needle puncture.
- Some commonsense rules of safety are as follows:
- Be knowledgeable about the procedures being performed. If in doubt, ask for further instructions.

- Wear protective clothing and use protective equipment when required.
- Clean up spills immediately, if the substance is low hazard and the spill is small; otherwise, contact hazardous materials team (internal or vendor) for spill reporting and appropriate spill management.
- Keep workstations clean and corridors free from obstruction.
- Report injuries and unsafe conditions. Review accidents and incidents to determine their fundamental cause. Take corrective action to prevent further injuries.
- Maintain a proactive safety management program.

Now that you have completed this chapter, go back and read again the case study at the beginning and respond to the questions presented.

REVIEW QUESTIONS

Answers can be found in the Appendix.

1. Standard precautions apply to all of the following *except*:
   a. Blood
   b. Cerebrospinal fluid
   c. Semen
   d. Concentrated acids

2. The *most important* practice in preventing the spread of disease is:
   a. Wearing masks during patient contact
   b. Proper hand washing
   c. Wearing disposable laboratory coats
   d. Identifying specimens from known or suspected HIV- and HBV-infected patients with a red label

3. The appropriate dilution of bleach to be used in laboratory disinfection is:
   a. 1:2
   b. 1:5
   c. 1:10
   d. 1:100

4. How frequently should fire alarms and sprinkler systems be tested?
   a. Weekly
   b. Monthly
   c. Quarterly
   d. Annually

5. Where should alcohol and other flammable chemicals be stored?
   a. In an approved safety can or storage cabinet away from heat sources
   b. Under a hood and arranged alphabetically for ease of identification in an emergency
   c. In a refrigerator at 2° C to 8° C to reduce volatilization
   d. On a low shelf in an area protected from light

6. The most frequent cause of needle punctures is:
   a. Patient movement during venipuncture
   b. Improper disposal of phlebotomy equipment
   c. Inattention during removal of needle after venipuncture
   d. Failure to attach needle firmly to syringe or tube holder

7. Under which of the following circumstances would a SDS be helpful?
   a. A phlebotomist has experienced a needle puncture with a clean needle.
   b. A fire extinguisher failed during routine testing.
   c. A pregnant laboratory employee has asked whether she needs to be concerned about working with a given reagent.
   d. During a safety inspection, an aged microscope power supply is found to have a frayed power cord.

8. It is a busy evening in the City Hospital hematology department. One staff member called in sick, and there was a major auto accident that has one staff member tied up in the blood bank all evening. Mary, the medical laboratory scientist covering hematology, is in a hurry to get a stat sample on the analyzer but needs to pour off an aliquot for another department. She is wearing gloves and a lab coat. She carefully covers the stopper of the well-mixed ethylenediaminetetraacetic acid (EDTA) tube with a gauze square and tilts the stopper toward her so it opens away from her. She pours off about 1 mL into a prelabeled tube, replaces the stopper of the EDTA tube, and puts it in the sample rack and sets it on the conveyor. She then brings the poured sample off to the other department. How would you assess Mary's safety practice?
   a. Mary was careful and followed all appropriate procedures.
   b. Mary should have used a shield when opening the tube.
   c. Mary should have poured the sample into a sterile tube.
   d. Mary should have wiped the tube with alcohol after replacing the stopper.

9. What class fire extinguisher would be appropriate to use on a fire in a chemical cabinet?
   a. Class A
   b. Class B
   c. Class C
   d. Class D

10. According to OSHA standards, laboratory coats must be all of the following *except*:
    a. Water resistant
    b. Made of cloth fabric that can be readily laundered
    c. Long-sleeved
    d. Worn fully buttoned

11. Which one of the following would NOT be part of a safety management plan?
    a. Job safety analysis
    b. Risk assessment of potential safety hazards
    c. Mechanism for reporting accidents
    d. Budget for engineering controls and personal protective equipment

REFERENCES

1. Garza, D., Becan-McBride, K. (2010). *Phlebotomy handbook,* (8th ed.). Upper Saddle River, NJ: Pearson Education, Inc.
2. United States Department of Labor. *29 Code of Federal Regulations Part 1910.* Available at: http://www.osha.gov/law-regs.html. Accessed 22.11.13.
3. United States Department of Labor. *Occupational Safety and Health Administration, Hazard Communication Safety Data Sheets.* https://www.osha.gov/Publications/HazComm_QuickCard_SafetyData.html. Accessed 20.10.13.

Blood Specimen Collection

3

*Elaine M. Keohane**

OBJECTIVES

After completion of this chapter, the reader will be able to:

1. Describe the application of standard precautions to the collection of blood specimens.
2. List collection equipment used for venipuncture and skin puncture.
3. Correlate tube stopper color with additive, if any, and explain the purpose of the additive and use of that tube type for laboratory tests.
4. Explain reasons for selection of certain veins for venipuncture and name the veins of choice in the antecubital fossa in order of preference.
5. Describe the steps recommended by the Clinical and Laboratory Standards Institute for venipuncture, including the recommended order of draw for tubes with additives.
6. Describe complications encountered in blood collection and the proper response of the phlebotomist.
7. Describe the steps recommended by the Clinical and Laboratory Standards Institute for skin puncture, including collection sites for infants, children, and adults, and the order of draw for tubes with additives.
8. Describe components of quality assurance in specimen collection.
9. List reasons for specimen rejection.
10. Given a description of a specimen and its collection, determine specimen acceptability.
11. Recognize deviations from the recommended venipuncture practice in a written scenario and describe corrective procedures.
12. State the most important step in the phlebotomy procedure.
13. List reasons for inability to obtain a blood specimen.
14. Summarize legal issues that need to be considered in blood specimen collection and handling.

CASE STUDIES

After studying the material in this chapter, the reader should be able to respond to the following case studies:

Case 1
A phlebotomist asks an outpatient, "Are you Susan Jones?" After the patient answers yes, the phlebotomist proceeds by labeling the tubes and drawing the blood. What is wrong with this scenario?

Case 2
A patient must have blood drawn for a complete blood count (CBC), potassium level, prothrombin time (PT), and type and screen. The phlebotomist draws blood into the following tubes in this order:
1. Serum separation tube
2. Light blue stopper tube for PT
3. Lavender stopper tube for CBC
4. Green stopper tube for the potassium
   Which of the results will be affected by the incorrect order of draw? Explain.

*The author extends appreciation to Carole A. Mullins, whose work in prior editions provided the foundation for this chapter.

SAFETY

Standard precautions must be followed in the collection of blood, and all specimens must be treated as potentially infectious for bloodborne pathogens. Regulations of the Occupational Safety and Health Administration (OSHA) that took effect on March 6, 1992, outlined in detail what must be done to protect health care workers from exposure to bloodborne pathogens, such as the pathogens that cause hepatitis C, hepatitis B, hepatitis D, syphilis, malaria, and human immunodeficiency virus (HIV) infection.[1]

Bloodborne pathogens may enter the body through an accidental injury by a sharp object, such as a contaminated needle, a scalpel, broken glass, or any other object that can pierce the skin. Cuts, skin areas with dermatitis or abrasions, and mucous membranes of the mouth, eyes, and nose may also provide a portal of entry. Indirect transmission can occur when a person touches a contaminated surface or object and then touches the mouth, eyes, nose, or nonintact skin without washing the hands. Hepatitis B virus can survive on inanimate or dried surfaces for at least 1 week.[2]

Hand washing is the most important practice to prevent the spread of infectious diseases. The phlebotomist should wash his or her hands with soap and running water between patients and every time gloves are removed. An alcohol-based hand rub may be used if hands are not visibly contaminated.[3] Antimicrobial wipes or towelettes are less effective for hand sanitation.[3] *Gloves* are essential personal protective equipment and must be worn during blood collection procedures. When gloves are removed, no blood from the soiled gloves should come in contact with the hands. Glove removal is covered in detail in Chapter 2.

Contaminated sharps and infectious wastes should be placed in designated puncture-resistant containers. The red or red-orange biohazard sign (Figure 2-2) indicates that a container holds potentially infectious materials. Biohazard containers should be easily accessible and should not be overfilled.

RESPONSIBILITY OF THE PHLEBOTOMIST IN INFECTION CONTROL

Because phlebotomists interact with patients and staff throughout the day, they potentially can infect numerous people. Phlebotomists should become familiar with and observe infection control and isolation policies. Violations of policies should be reported. A phlebotomist must maintain good personal health and hygiene, making sure to have clean clothes, clean hair, and clean, short fingernails. Standard precautions must be followed at all times, with special attention to the use of gloves and hand washing.

PHYSIOLOGIC FACTORS AFFECTING TEST RESULTS

Certain physiologic variables under the control of the patient or the phlebotomist may introduce preanalytical variation in laboratory test results. Examples of these factors include posture (supine or erect), diurnal rhythms, exercise, stress, diet (fasting or not), and smoking (Box 3-1).[4-8] The phlebotomist must adhere to the specific schedule for timed specimen collections and accurately record the time of collection.

BOX 3-1 Some Physiologic Factors That Can Contribute to Preanalytical Variation in Test Results

Posture

Changing from a supine (lying) to a sitting or standing position results in a shift of body water from inside the blood vessels to the interstitial spaces. Larger molecules, such as protein, cholesterol, and iron cannot filter into the tissues, and their concentration increases in the blood.[4,5]

Diurnal Rhythm

Diurnal rhythm refers to daily body fluid fluctuations that occur with some constituents of the blood. For example, levels of cortisol, thyroid-stimulating hormone, and iron are higher in the morning and decrease in the afternoon.[4,5] Other test values, such as the eosinophil count, are lower in the morning and increase in the afternoon.[4,5]

Exercise

Exercise can increase various constituents in the blood such as creatinine, total protein, creatine kinase, myoglobin, aspartate aminotransferase, white blood cell count, and HDL-cholesterol.[6] The extent and duration of the increase depend on the intensity, duration, and frequency of the exercise and the time the blood specimen was collected postexercise.

Stress

Anxiety and excessive crying in children can cause a temporary increase in the white blood cell count.[4]

Diet

Fasting means no food or beverages except water for 8 to 12 hours before a blood draw. If a patient has eaten recently (less than 2 hours earlier), there will be a temporary increase in glucose and lipid content in the blood. In addition, the increased lipids may cause turbidity (lipemia) in the serum or plasma, affecting some tests that require photometric measurement, such as the hemoglobin concentration and coagulation tests performed on optical detection instruments.

Smoking

Patients who smoke before blood collection may have increased white blood cell counts and cortisol levels.[7,8] Long-term smoking can lead to decreased pulmonary function and result in increased hemoglobin levels.

VENIPUNCTURE

This chapter only covers an overview of blood specimen collection; sources that provide detailed information are listed in the reference section.

Equipment for Venipuncture

Tourniquet

A tourniquet is used to provide a barrier against venous blood flow to help locate a vein. A tourniquet can be a disposable elastic strap, a heavier Velcro strap, or a blood pressure cuff. The tourniquet should be applied 3 to 4 inches above the venipuncture site and left on for no longer than 1 minute before the venipuncture is performed.[9] Latex-free tourniquets are available for individuals with a latex allergy.

Collection Tubes

The most common means of collecting blood specimens is through the use of an evacuated tube system. The system includes an evacuated tube, which can be either plastic or glass; a needle; and an adapter that is used to secure the needle and the tube. When the needle is inserted into a vein and a tube is inserted into the holder, the back of the needle pierces the stopper, allowing the vacuum pressure in the tube to automatically draw blood into the tube. For safety, OSHA recommends the use of plastic tubes whenever possible. Most glass tubes are coated with silicone to help decrease the possibility of hemolysis and to prevent blood from adhering to the sides of the tube. Evacuated tubes are available in various sizes and may contain a variety of premeasured additives.

Manufacturers of evacuated tubes in the United States follow a universal color code in which the stopper color indicates the type of additive contained in the tube. Figure 3-1 provides a summary of various types of evacuated collection tubes.

Additives in Collection Tubes

Clot activators. Blood specimens for serum testing must first be allowed to clot for 30 to 60 minutes prior to centrifugation and removal of the serum.[10] A clot activator accelerates the clotting process and decreases the specimen preparation time. Examples of clot activators include glass or silica particles (activates factor XII in the coagulation pathway) and thrombin (an activated coagulation factor that converts fibrinogen to fibrin) (Chapter 37).

Anticoagulants. An anticoagulant prevents blood from clotting. Ethylenediaminetetraacetic acid (EDTA), citrate, and oxalate remove calcium needed for clotting by forming insoluble calcium salts. Heparin prevents clotting by binding to antithrombin in the plasma and inhibiting thrombin and activated coagulation factor X (Chapter 37). Tubes with anticoagulant must be gently inverted *immediately* after collection according to the manufacturer's directions to ensure proper mixing. Tubes with anticoagulant are either tested as whole blood or are centrifuged to yield plasma.

Antiglycolytic Agent. An antiglycolytic agent inhibits the metabolism of glucose by blood cells. Such inhibition may be necessary if testing for the glucose level is delayed. The most commonly used antiglycolytic agent is sodium fluoride.[4,5] Tubes containing sodium fluoride alone yield serum. Tubes containing sodium fluoride and an anticoagulant (such as EDTA or oxalate) yield plasma. Anticoagulated blood can be centrifuged immediately to obtain plasma for testing, thus decreasing the specimen preparation time.

Separator Gel. Separator gel is an inert material that undergoes a temporary change in viscosity during the centrifugation process; this enables it to serve as a separation barrier between the liquid (serum or plasma) and cells. Because this gel may interfere with some testing, serum or plasma from these tubes cannot be used with certain instruments or for blood bank procedures.

Needles

Venipuncture needles are sterile and are available in a variety of lengths and gauges (bore or opening size). Needles used with evacuated tube systems screw into a plastic needle holder and are double pointed. The end of the needle that is inserted into the vein is longer and has a point with a slanted side or *bevel*. A plastic cap covers this end of the needle and is removed prior to insertion. The end of the needle that pierces the stopper of the evacuated tube is shorter and is covered by a rubber sleeve in multiple-sample needles. The rubber sleeve prevents blood from dripping into the holder when changing tubes (Figure 3-2). Needles used with syringes are discussed below.

The gauge number of a needle is inversely related to the bore size: the smaller the gauge number, the larger the bore. Needles for drawing blood range from 19 to 23 gauge.[9] The most common needle size for adult venipuncture is 21 gauge with a length of 1 inch. The advantage of using a 1-inch needle is that it provides better control during venipuncture.

Needle Holders

Needles and holders are designed to comply with OSHA's revised Occupational Exposure to Bloodborne Pathogens Standard (effective April 18, 2001) and its requirement for implementation of safer medical devices.[11] Needles and holders have safety features to prevent accidental needle sticks. Needle holders are made to fit a specific manufacturer's needles and tubes and should not be interchanged. The holders are disposable and must be discarded after a single use with the needle still attached as required by OSHA.[12]

The following are some examples of safety needles and holders:

1. The Vacutainer® Eclipse™ Blood Collection System (BD Medical, Franklin Lakes, NJ) allows single-handed activation after the venipuncture is performed by pushing the safety shield forward with the thumb until it is over the needle and an audible click is heard. The BD Eclipse needle is used with a single-use needle holder. After the safety shield is activated, the entire assembly is discarded intact into a sharps container.

2. The Jelco multisample blood collection needle used with the Venipuncture Needle-Pro® Device (Smiths Medical ASD,

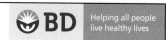

BD Vacutainer® Venous Blood Collection

Tube Guide

For the full array of BD Vacutainer® Blood Collection Tubes, visit www.bd.com/vacutainer.
Many are available in a variety of sizes and draw volumes (for pediatric applications). Refer to our website for full descriptions.

BD Vacutainer® Tubes with BD Hemogard™ Closure	BD Vacutainer® Tubes with Conventional Stopper	Additive	Inversions at Blood Collection*	Laboratory Use	Your Lab's Draw Volume/Remarks
Gold	Red/Gray	• Clot activator and gel for serum separation	5	For serum determinations in chemistry. May be used for routine blood donor screening and diagnostic testing of serum for infectious disease.** Tube inversions ensure mixing of clot activator with blood. Blood clotting time: 30 minutes.	
Light Green	Green/Gray	• Lithium heparin and gel for plasma separation	8	For plasma determinations in chemistry. Tube inversions ensure mixing of anticoagulant (heparin) with blood to prevent clotting.	
Red	Red	• Silicone coated (glass) • Clot activator, Silicone coated (plastic)	0 5	For serum determinations in chemistry. May be used for routine blood donor screening and diagnostic testing of serum for infectious disease.** Tube inversions ensure mixing of clot activator with blood. Blood clotting time: 60 minutes.	
Orange		• Thrombin-based clot activator with gel for serum separation	5 to 6	For stat serum determinations in chemistry. Tube inversions ensure mixing of clot activator with blood. Blood clotting time: 5 minutes.	
Orange		• Thrombin-based clot activator	8	For stat serum determinations in chemistry. Tube inversions ensure mixing of clot activator with blood. Blood clotting time: 5 minutes.	
Royal Blue		• Clot activator (plastic serum) • K_2EDTA (plastic)	8 8	For trace-element, toxicology, and nutritional-chemistry determinations. Special stopper formulation provides low levels of trace elements (see package insert). Tube inversions ensure mixing of either clot activator or anticoagulant (EDTA) with blood.	
Green	Green	• Sodium heparin • Lithium heparin	8 8	For plasma determinations in chemistry. Tube inversions ensure mixing of anticoagulant (heparin) with blood to prevent clotting.	
Gray	Gray	• Potassium oxalate/sodium fluoride • Sodium fluoride/Na_2 EDTA • Sodium fluoride (serum tube)	8 8 8	For glucose determinations. Oxalate and EDTA anticoagulants will give plasma samples. Sodium fluoride is the antiglycolytic agent. Tube inversions ensure proper mixing of additive with blood.	
Tan		• K_2EDTA (plastic)	8	For lead determinations. This tube is certified to contain less than .01 μg/mL(ppm) lead. Tube inversions prevent clotting.	
	Yellow	• Sodium polyanethol sulfonate (SPS) • Acid citrate dextrose additives (ACD): **Solution A -** 22.0 g/L trisodium citrate, 8.0 g/L citric acid, 24.5 g/L dextrose **Solution B -** 13.2 g/L trisodium citrate, 4.8 g/L citric acid, 14.7 g/L dextrose	8 8 8	SPS for blood culture specimen collections in microbiology. ACD for use in blood bank studies, HLA phenotyping, and DNA and paternity testing. Tube inversions ensure mixing of anticoagulant with blood to prevent clotting.	
Lavender	Lavender	• Liquid K_3EDTA (glass) • Spray-coated K_2EDTA (plastic)	8 8	K_2EDTA and K_3EDTA for whole blood hematology determinations. K_2EDTA may be used for routine immunohematology testing, and blood donor screening.*** Tube inversions ensure mixing of anticoagulant (EDTA) with blood to prevent clotting.	
White		• K_2EDTA and gel for plasma separation	8	For use in molecular diagnostic test methods (such as, but not limited to, polymerase chain reaction [PCR] and/or branched DNA [bDNA] amplification techniques.) Tube inversions ensure mixing of anticoagulant (EDTA) with blood to prevent clotting.	
Pink	Pink	• Spray-coated K_2EDTA (plastic)	8	For whole blood hematology determinations. May be used for routine immunohematology testing and blood donor screening.*** Designed with special cross-match label for patient information required by the AABB. Tube inversions prevent clotting.	
Light Blue / Clear	Light Blue	• Buffered sodium citrate 0.105 M (≈3.2%) glass 0.109 M (3.2%) plastic • Citrate, theophylline, adenosine, dipyridamole (CTAD)	3-4 3-4	For coagulation determinations. CTAD for selected platelet function assays and routine coagulation determination. Tube inversions ensure mixing of anticoagulant (citrate) to prevent clotting.	
Clear	New Red/Light Gray	• None (plastic)	0	For use as a discard tube or secondary specimen tube.	

Note: BD Vacutainer® Tubes for pediatric and partial draw applications can be found on our website.

BD Diagnostics
Preanalytical Systems
1 Becton Drive
Franklin Lakes, NJ 07417 USA

BD Global Technical Services: 1.800.631.0174
BD Customer Service: 1.888.237.2762
www.bd.com/vacutainer

* Invert gently, do not shake
** The performance characteristics of these tubes have not been established for infectious disease testing in general; therefore, users must validate the use of these tubes for their specific assay-instrument/reagent system combinations and specimen storage conditions.
*** The performance characteristics of these tubes have not been established for immunohematology testing in general; therefore, users must validate the use of these tubes for their specific assay-instrument/reagent system combinations and specimen storage conditions.

BD, BD Logo and all other trademarks are property of Becton, Dickinson and Company. © 2010 BD

Printed in USA   07/10   VS5229-13

Figure 3-1 Vacutainer® tube guide. (Courtesy and © Becton, Dickinson and Company.)

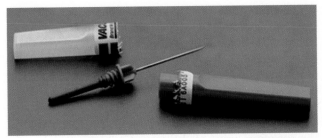

Figure 3-2 Multisample needle. The rubber sleeve prevents blood from dripping into the holder when tubes are changed. (Courtesy and © Becton, Dickinson and Company.)

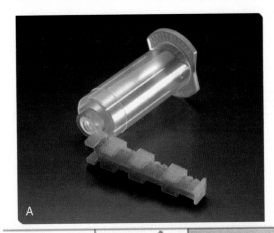

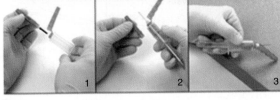

B

Figure 3-3 A, Jelco Needle-Pro®. **B,** Use of Jelco Needle-Pro®. (1) Attach needle. (2) Remove cap and draw blood from patient. (3) After collection press sheath on flat surface. (Courtesy Smiths Medical ASD, Norwell MA.)

Norwell, MA) allows the Needle-Pro® sheath to be snapped over the needle by pushing it against a flat, firm surface after the venipuncture is completed. The entire device is discarded into the sharps container (Figure 3-3).

3. The Greiner Bio-One (Monroe, NC) VACUETTE® QUICK-SHIELD has a sheath that locks into place over the needle after use. The QUICKSHIELD Complete PLUS is a system that incorporates a holder with an attached VACUETTE® Visio PLUS multisample needle. The flash window in the needle hub indicates when a successful venipuncture has been achieved (Figure 3-4).

Winged Blood Collection Set (Butterfly)

A winged blood collection set or butterfly consists of a short needle with plastic wings connected to thin tubing (Figure 3-5). The other end of the tubing can be connected to a needle holder for an evacuated tube, a syringe, or a blood culture bottle with the use of special adapters. Winged blood collection sets are useful in collecting specimens from children or other patients from whom it is difficult to draw blood. They also have sheathing

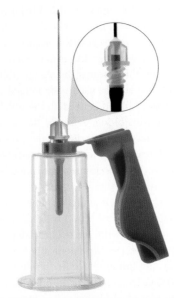

Figure 3-4 QUICKSHIELD Complete PLUS with flash window. Blood in the flash window indicates successful venipuncture. (Courtesy Greiner Bio-One, Monroe, NC.)

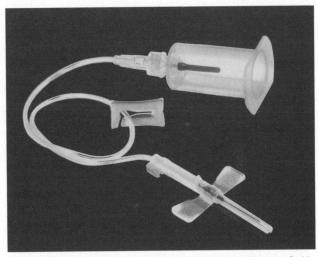

Figure 3-5 Jelco Saf-T Wing® Blood Collection set. (Courtesy Smiths Medical ASD, Norwell, MA.)

devices to minimize the risk of needle stick injury. Examples include MONOJECT™ ANGEL WING™ Blood Collection Set (Covidien, Mansfield, MA), Vacutainer® Safety-Lok™ and Vacutainer® Push Button Blood Collection Set (BD Medical, Franklin Lakes, NJ), VACUETTE® Safety Blood Collection Set (Greiner Bio-One, Monroe, NC), and Jelco Saf-T Wing® Blood Collection set (Smiths Medical ASD, Norwell, MA).

Syringes

A syringe consists of a barrel, graduated in milliliters, and a plunger. Syringe needles have a point at one end and an open hub at the other end that attaches to the barrel of the syringe. Syringes are available with different types of needle attachments and in different sizes. It is important to attach the needle securely to the syringe to prevent air from entering the system.

Syringes may be useful in drawing blood from pediatric, geriatric, or other patients with tiny, fragile, or "rolling" veins that would not be able to withstand the vacuum pressure from evacuated tubes. With a syringe, the amount of pressure exerted is controlled by the phlebotomist by slowly pulling back the plunger. Syringes may also be used with winged infusion sets.

If only one tube of blood is needed, the phlebotomist fills the syringe barrel with blood, removes the needle from the arm, activates the needle safety device, removes and discards the needle in a sharps container, and attaches the hub of the syringe to a transfer device to transfer the blood into an evacuated tube. An example is the BD Vacutainer® Blood Transfer Device with Luer adapter. If multiple tubes are needed, the phlebotomist can use a closed blood collection system such as the Jelco Saf-T Holder® with male Luer adapter with Saf-T Wing® butterfly needle (Smiths Medical ASD) (Figure 3-6). With this system, the butterfly needle tubing branches into a Y shape and attaches to the syringe on one side and an evacuated tube in a holder on the other side. Clamps in the tubing control the flow of blood from the arm to the syringe and then from the syringe to the evacuated tube. To prevent hemolysis when using transfer devices, only the tube's vacuum (and not the plunger) should be used to transfer the blood from the syringe into the evacuated tube.

Solutions for Skin Antisepsis

The most common skin antiseptic is 70% isopropyl alcohol in a commercially prepared pad. The phlebotomist cleans the phlebotomy site in a circular motion, beginning in the center and working outward. The area is allowed to air-dry before the venipuncture is performed so that the patient does not experience a burning sensation after needle insertion and to prevent contamination of the specimen with alcohol. The phlebotomist must use a non-alcohol-based antiseptic to collect blood for a legal blood alcohol level.[9] When a sterile site is prepared for collection of specimens for blood culture, a two-step procedure with a 30- to 60-second scrub is used in which cleansing with 70% isopropyl alcohol is followed by cleansing with 1% to 10% povidone-iodine pads, tincture of iodine, chlorhexidine

compounds, or another isopropyl alcohol prep.[9] Some health care facilities use a one-step application of chlorhexidine gluconate/isopropyl alcohol or povidone-70% ethyl alcohol.[9] Whatever method is used, the antiseptic agent should be in contact with the skin for at least 30 seconds to minimize the risk of accidental contamination of the blood culture.

Selection of a Vein for Routine Venipuncture

The superficial veins of the antecubital fossa (bend in the elbow) are the most common sites for venipuncture. There are two anatomical patterns of veins in the antecubital fossa[4,9] (Figure 3-7). In the "H" pattern, the three veins that are used, in the order of preference, are (1) the median cubital vein,

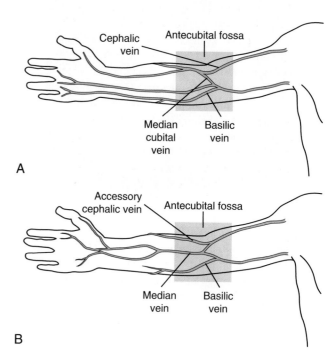

Figure 3-7 Superficial veins of the anterior right arm in the antecubital fossa (two views). **A,** "H" pattern of veins. **B,** "M" pattern of veins. The preferred vein for venipuncture is the median cubital vein in the H pattern and the median vein in the M pattern. (Adapted from McCall RE, Tankersley CM. Phlebotomy Essentials, ed. 5, Philadelphia, 2012, Lippincott, Williams & Wilkins.)

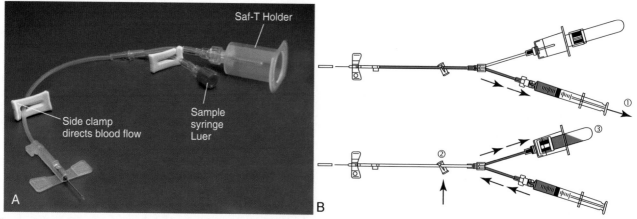

Figure 3-6 A, Jelco closed blood collection system. (Courtesy Smiths Medical ASD, Norwell, MA.) **B,** Device for transferring blood from syringe to vacuum tube. (1) Draw blood with syringe. (2) Close clamp. (3) Insert tube to transfer blood from syringe to tube. To fill additional tubes, open clamp, draw blood with syringe again, close clamp, and transfer. (Courtesy Smiths Medical ASD, Norwell, MA.)

which connects the basilic and cephalic veins in the antecubital fossa; (2) the cephalic vein, located on the outside (lateral) aspect of the antecubital fossa on the thumb side of the hand; and (3) the basilic vein, located on the inside (medial) aspect of the antecubital fossa. In the "M" pattern, the order of preference is the (1) median vein, (2) accessory cephalic vein, and (3) the basilic vein. The cephalic and basilic veins should only be used if the median cubital or median veins are not prominent after checking both arms. The basilic vein is the last choice due to the increased risk of injury to the median nerve and/or accidental puncture of the brachial artery, both located in close proximity to the basilic vein.[9]

If necessary, the phlebotomist should have the patient make a fist after application of the tourniquet; the veins should become prominent. The patient should not pump the fist because it may affect some of the test values. The phlebotomist should palpate (examine by touching) the vein with his or her index finger to determine vein depth, direction, and diameter. If a vein cannot be located in either arm, it may be necessary to examine the veins on the dorsal surface of the hand.

The veins in the feet should not be used without physician permission. The policy in some institutions is to request that a second phlebotomist attempt to locate a vein in the arm or the hand before a vein in the foot is used. The veins in the inner wrist should never be used due to the high risk of injury to tendons and nerves in that area.[9]

Venipuncture Procedure

The phlebotomist uses standard precautions, which include washing hands and applying gloves at the beginning of the procedure and removing gloves and washing hands at the end of the procedure. The Clinical and Laboratory Standards Institute (CLSI) recommends the following steps:[9]

1. Prepare the accession (test request) order.
2. Greet the patient and identify the patient by having the patient verbally state his or her full name and confirm with the patient's unique identification number, address, and/or birth date. Ensure the same information is on the request form.
3. Sanitize hands.
4. Verify that any dietary restrictions have been met (e.g., fasting, if appropriate) and check for latex sensitivity.
5. Assemble supplies and appropriate tubes for the requested tests. Verify paperwork and tube selection.
6. Reassure and position the patient.
7. If necessary to help locate a vein, request that the patient clench his or her fist.
8. Apply the tourniquet and select an appropriate venipuncture site, giving priority to the median cubital or median vein. Ensure the tourniquet is on for no longer that 1 minute.
9. Put on gloves.
10. Cleanse the venipuncture site with 70% isopropyl alcohol using concentric circles from the inside to outside. *Allow skin to air-dry.*
11. Inspect the equipment and needle tip for burrs and bends.
12. Perform the venipuncture by anchoring the vein with the thumb 1 to 2 inches *below* the site and inserting the needle, bevel up, with an angle less than 30 degrees between the needle and the skin. Collect tubes using the correct order of draw, and invert each tube containing any additive *immediately* after collection. CLSI recommends a particular order of draw when collecting blood in multiple tubes from a single venipuncture.[9] Its purpose is to avoid possible test result error because of cross-contamination from tube additives. The recommended order of draw is as follows: (Box-3-2)
    a. Blood culture tube (yellow stopper)
    b. Coagulation tube (light blue stopper)
    c. Serum tube with or without clot activator or gel (red, gold, red-gray marbled, orange, or yellow-gray stopper)
    d. Heparin tube (green or light green stopper)
    e. EDTA tube (lavender or pink stopper)
    f. Sodium fluoride tube with or without EDTA or oxalate (gray stopper)
13. Release and remove the tourniquet as soon as blood flow is established or after no longer than 1 minute.
14. Ensure that the patient's hand is open.
15. Place gauze lightly over the puncture site without pressing down.
16. After the last tube has been released from the back of the multisample needle, remove the needle and activate the safety device according to the manufacturer's directions.
17. Apply direct pressure to the puncture site using a clean gauze pad.
18. Bandage the venipuncture site *after* checking to ensure that bleeding has stopped.
19. If a syringe has been used, fill the evacuated tubes using a syringe transfer device.
20. Dispose of the puncture equipment and other biohazardous waste.
21. Label the tubes with the correct information. The minimal amount of information that must be on each tube is as follows:
    a. Patient's full name
    b. Patient's unique identification number
    c. Date of collection
    d. Time of collection (military time)
    e. Collector's initials or code number

NOTE: Compare the labeled tube with the patient's identification bracelet or have the patient verify that the information on the labeled tube is correct whenever possible.

BOX 3-2   Order of Draw for Venipuncture[9]

1. Blood culture tube (*yellow stopper*)
2. Coagulation tube (*light blue stopper*)
3. Serum tube with or without activator (*red, gold, red-gray marbled, orange, or yellow-gray stopper*)
4. Heparin tube (*green or light green stopper*)
5. EDTA tube (*lavender or pink stopper*)
6. Sodium fluoride with or without EDTA or oxalate (*gray stopper*)

EDTA, ethylenediaminetetraacetic acid

22. Carry out any special handling requirements (e.g., chilling or protecting from light).
23. Cancel any phlebotomy-related dietary restrictions and thank the patient.
24. Send the properly labeled specimens to the laboratory.

The most crucial step in the process is patient identification. The patient must verbally state his or her full name, or someone must identify the patient for the phlebotomist. In addition, at least one additional identifier needs to be checked such as the address, birth date, or the unique number on the patient's identification bracelet (for hospitalized patients). The phlebotomist must match the patient's full name and unique identifier with the information on the test requisition. Any discrepancies must be resolved before the venipuncture can continue. Failure to confirm proper identification can result in a life-threatening situation for the patient and possible legal ramifications for the facility. The phlebotomist must also label all tubes immediately after the blood specimen has been drawn, with the label attached to the tube, before leaving the patient's side.

Coagulation Testing

If only a light blue stopper coagulation tube is to be drawn for determination of the prothrombin time or activated partial thromboplastin time, the *first* tube drawn may be used for testing. It is no longer necessary to draw a 3-mL discard nonadditive tube before collecting for routine coagulation testing. The phlebotomist must fill tubes for coagulation testing to full volume (or to the minimum volume specified by the manufacturer) to maintain a 9:1 ratio of blood to anticoagulant. Underfilling coagulation tubes results in prolonged test values. When a winged blood collection set is used to draw a single light blue stopper tube, the phlebotomist must first partially fill a nonadditive tube or another light blue stopper tube to clear the dead air space in the tubing before collecting the tube to be used for coagulation testing. For special coagulation testing, however, a second-drawn light blue stopper tube may be required.[9] Chapter 42 covers specimen collection for hemostasis testing in more detail.

Venipuncture in Children

Pediatric phlebotomy requires experience, special skills, and a tender touch. Excellent interpersonal skills are needed to deal with distraught parents and with crying, screaming, or frightened children. Ideally, only experienced phlebotomists should draw blood from children; however, the only way to gain experience is through practice. Through experience, one learns what works in different situations. Smaller gauge (22- to 23-gauge) needles are employed.[9] Use of a syringe or winged blood collection set may be advantageous for accessing small veins in young children. The child's arm should be immobilized as much as possible so that the needle can be inserted successfully into the vein and can be kept there if the child tries to move. Use of special stickers or character bandages as rewards may serve as an incentive for cooperation; however, the protocol of the institution with regard to their distribution must be followed.

Complications Encountered in Venipuncture
Ecchymosis (Bruise)

Bruising is the most common complication encountered in obtaining a blood specimen. It is caused by leakage of a small amount of blood in the tissue around the puncture site. The phlebotomist can prevent bruising by applying direct pressure to the venipuncture site with a gauze pad. Bending the patient's arm at the elbow to hold the gauze pad in place is not effective in stopping the bleeding and may lead to bruising.

Hematoma

A hematoma results when leakage of a large amount of blood around the puncture site causes the area to rapidly swell. If swelling begins, the phlebotomist should remove the needle immediately and apply pressure to the site with a gauze pad for at least 2 minutes. Hematomas may result in bruising of the patient's skin around the puncture site. Hematomas can also cause pain and possible nerve compression and permanent damage to the patient's arm. Hematomas most commonly occur when the needle goes through the vein or when the bevel of the needle is only partially in the vein (Figure 3-8, *B* and *C*) and when the phlebotomist fails to remove the tourniquet before removing the needle or does not apply enough pressure to the site after venipuncture. Hematomas can also form after inadvertent puncture of an artery.

Fainting (Syncope)

Fainting is also a common complication encountered. Before drawing blood, the phlebotomist should always ask the patient whether he or she has had any prior episodes of fainting during or after blood collection. The CLSI does not recommend the use of ammonia inhalants to revive the patients because they may trigger an adverse response that could lead to patient injury.[9] The phlebotomist should follow the protocol at his or her facility.

If the patient begins to faint, the phlebotomist should remove and discard the needle immediately, apply pressure to the site with a gauze pad, lower the patient's head, and loosen any constrictive clothing. The phlebotomist should also notify the designated first-aid providers at the facility. The incident should be documented.

Hemoconcentration

Hemoconcentration is an increased concentration of cells, larger molecules, and analytes in the blood as a result of a shift in water balance. Hemoconcentration can be caused by leaving the tourniquet on the patient's arm for too long. The tourniquet should not remain on the arm for longer than 1 minute. If it is left on for a longer time because of difficulty in finding a vein, it should be removed for 2 minutes and reapplied before the venipuncture is performed.[9]

Hemolysis

The rupture of red blood cells with the consequent escape of hemoglobin—a process termed *hemolysis*—can cause the plasma or serum to appear pink or red. Hemolysis can occur if

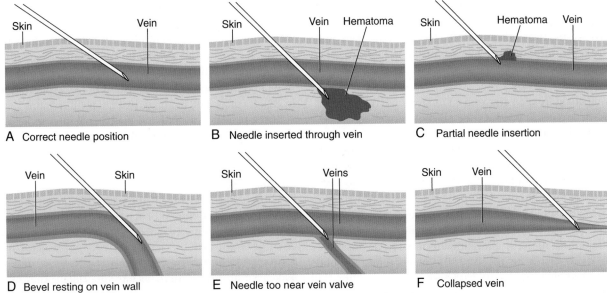

Figure 3-8 Proper and improper needle insertion for venipuncture.

the phlebotomist used too small a needle during a difficult draw; drew the blood through an existing hematoma; pulled back too quickly on the plunger of a syringe; forced blood into a tube from a syringe by pushing the plunger; mixed a tube too vigorously; or contaminated the specimen with alcohol or water at the venipuncture site or in the tubes. Hemolysis also can occur physiologically as a result of hemolytic anemias. Hemolyzed specimens can alter test results, such as levels of potassium, lactate dehydrogenase, and aspartate aminotransferase, which can result in patient treatment errors.[10]

Petechiae

Petechiae are small red spots indicating that small amounts of blood have escaped into the skin. Petechiae indicate a possible hemostasis abnormality and should alert the phlebotomist to be aware of possible prolonged bleeding.

Allergies

Some patients may be allergic to skin antiseptic substances and adhesive bandages and tape. The phlebotomist should use hypoallergenic tape or apply pressure manually until the bleeding has stopped completely. The phlebotomist should also determine if the patient has a latex sensitivity before the phlebotomy procedure.

Nerve Damage

The phlebotomist must select the appropriate veins for venipuncture and should not blindly probe the arm with the needle or try to laterally relocate the needle. If a nerve has been affected, the patient may complain about shooting or sharp pain, tingling, or numbness in the arm. The phlebotomist should immediately remove and discard the needle, apply pressure with a gauze pad, and collect the blood from the other arm.

Seizures

Patients occasionally experience seizures because of a preexisting condition or as a response to the needle stick. If a seizure occurs, the phlebotomist should immediately remove and discard the needle, apply pressure with a gauze pad, and notify the nurse or designated first-aid providers at the facility. The phlebotomist should also ensure the patient's safety by preventing injury from nearby objects.

Vomiting

If the patient begins vomiting, the phlebotomist should provide the patient an appropriate container and tissues, notify the nurse or designated first-aid providers at the facility, and ensure the patient's head is positioned so that he or she does not aspirate vomit.

Venipuncture in Special Situations
Edema

Swelling caused by an abnormal accumulation of fluid in the intercellular spaces of the tissues is termed *edema*. The most common cause is infiltration of the tissues by the solution running through an incorrectly positioned intravenous catheter. Edematous sites should be avoided for venipuncture because the veins are hard to find and the specimens may become contaminated with tissue fluid.

Obesity

In obese patients, veins may be neither readily visible nor easy to palpate. Sometimes the use of a blood pressure cuff can aid in locating a vein. The cuff should not be inflated any higher than 40 mm Hg and should not be left on the arm for longer than 1 minute.[9] The phlebotomist should not probe blindly in the patient's arm because nerve damage may result.

Burned, Damaged, Scarred, and Occluded Veins

Burned, damaged, scarred, and occluded veins should be avoided because they do not allow the blood to flow freely and may make it difficult to obtain an acceptable specimen.

Intravenous Therapy

Drawing blood from an arm with an intravenous (IV) infusion should be avoided if possible; the phlebotomist should draw the blood from the opposite arm without the IV. If there is no alternative, blood should be drawn *below* the IV with the tourniquet also placed *below* the IV site. Prior to venipuncture, the phlebotomist should ask an authorized caregiver to stop the infusion for 2 minutes before the specimen is drawn. The phlebotomist should note on the requisition and the tube that the specimen was obtained from an arm into which an IV solution was running, indicating the arm and the location of the draw relative to the IV.[4,9] The phlebotomist should always follow the protocol established at his or her facility.

Mastectomy Patients

The CLSI requires physician consultation before blood is drawn from the same side as a prior mastectomy (removal of the breast), even in the case of bilateral mastectomies.[9] The pressure on the arm that is on the same side as the mastectomy from a tourniquet or blood pressure cuff can lead to pain or lymphostasis from accumulating lymph fluid. The other arm on the side without a mastectomy should be used.

Inability to Obtain a Blood Specimen
Failure to Draw Blood

One reason for failure to draw blood is that the vein is missed, often because of improper needle positioning. The needle should be inserted completely into the vein with the bevel up and at an angle of less than 30 degrees.[9] Figure 3-8 shows reasons for unsatisfactory flow of blood. It is sometimes possible to reposition the needle in the vein by *slightly* withdrawing or advancing the needle, but only an experienced phlebotomist should attempt this. The phlebotomist should never attempt to relocate the needle in a lateral direction because such manipulation can cause pain and risk a disabling nerve injury to the patient.

Occasionally an evacuated tube has insufficient vacuum, and insertion of another tube yields blood. Keeping extra tubes within reach during blood collection can avoid a recollection when the problem is a technical issue associated with the tube.

Each institution should have a policy covering the proper procedure when a blood specimen cannot be collected. If two unsuccessful attempts at collection have been made, the CLSI recommends that the phlebotomist seek the assistance of another practitioner with blood collection expertise.[9] Another individual can make two attempts to obtain a specimen. If a second person is unsuccessful, the physician should be notified.

Patient Refusal

The patient has the right to refuse to give a blood specimen. If gentle urging does not persuade the patient to allow blood to be drawn, the phlebotomist should alert the nurse, who will either talk to the patient or notify the physician. The phlebotomist must not force an uncooperative patient to have blood drawn; it can be unsafe for the phlebotomist and for the patient. In addition, forcing a patient of legal age and sound mind to have blood drawn against his or her wishes can result in charges of assault and battery or unlawful restraint.

If the patient is a child and the parents offer to help hold the child, it is usually acceptable to proceed. Any refusals or problems should be documented for legal reasons.

Missing Patient

For hospitalized patients, if the patient is not in his or her room, the absence should be reported to the nursing unit so that the nurses are aware that the specimen was not obtained.

SKIN PUNCTURE

Skin puncture is the technique of choice to obtain a blood specimen from newborns and pediatric patients. In adults skin puncture may be used in patients who are severely burned and whose veins are being reserved for therapeutic purposes; in patients who are extremely obese; and in elderly patients with fragile veins.

Blood obtained from skin puncture is a mixture of blood from venules, arterioles, capillaries, and interstitial and intracellular fluids.[9] After the puncture site is warmed, the specimen more closely resembles arterial blood. The phlebotomist should note that the specimen was obtained by skin puncture because those specimens may generate slightly different test results.[13] For example, higher glucose values are found in specimens obtained by skin puncture compared with those obtained by venipuncture, and this difference can be clinically significant.[13] It is especially important to note the specimen type when a glucose tolerance test is performed or when glucometer results are compared with findings from venous specimens.

Collection Sites

The site of choice for skin puncture in infants under 1 year of age is the lateral (outside) or medial (inside) plantar (bottom) surface of the heel (Figure 3-9, *A*). In children older than 1 year of age and in adults, the palmar surface of the distal portion of the third (middle) or fourth (ring) finger on the nondominant hand may be used.[13] The puncture on the finger should be made perpendicular to the fingerprint lines (Figure 3-9, *B*). Fingers of infants should not be punctured because of the risk of serious bone injury.

Warming the site can increase the blood flow sevenfold.[13] The phlebotomist should warm the site with a commercial heel warmer or a warm washcloth to a temperature no greater than 42° C and for no longer than 3 to 5 minutes.[13] The phlebotomist should clean the skin puncture site with 70% isopropyl alcohol and allow it to air-dry. Povidone-iodine should not be used because of possible specimen contamination, which could falsely elevate levels of potassium, phosphorus, or uric acid.[13]

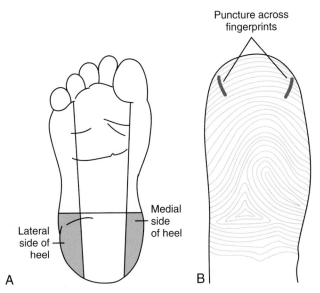

Puncture across fingerprints

Lateral side of heel

Medial side of heel

A

B

Figure 3-9 Areas for skin puncture: **A,** Heel of infant less than 1 year old. Puncture is made on the lateral or medial plantar surface of the heel, in the shaded area demarcated by lines from the middle of the big toe to the heel, and from between the fourth and fifth toe to the heel.[12,13] **B,** Finger. Puncture is made on the palmar surface of the distal portion of the third or fourth finger, perpendicular to the fingerprint lines.

Precautions with Skin Puncture

The finger or heel must be securely immobilized. Heel punctures in infants should not be made more than 2 mm deep because of the risk of bone injury and possible infection (osteomyelitis).[13] In premature infants, a puncture device that makes an incision with even less depth is preferred.

The phlebotomist should not puncture an area that is swollen, bruised, infected, or already has been punctured. In addition phlebotomists should not perform skin puncture in patients with edema, dehydration, or poor peripheral circulation because specimen integrity and test accuracy may be compromised. The first drop of blood should be wiped away with a clean gauze pad to prevent contamination of the specimen with tissue fluid and to facilitate the free flow of blood.[13]

Equipment for Skin Puncture

Devices for skin puncture contain sterile lancets that puncture or sterile blades that make a small incision in the skin. The lancet or blade is spring-loaded in the device, and when activated by the phlebotomist, pierces the skin. Devices are single-use, disposable, and have retractable blades in compliance with OHSA safety standards.[11] Devices are available for newborns, children, and adults that produce punctures or incisions of varying depths in the skin.

Containers for collecting blood from skin puncture include capillary tubes and microcollection tubes.[13] *Capillary tubes* of various sizes are available with or without heparin. OSHA recommends the use of plastic tubes or Mylar-coated glass tubes to avoid injury by broken glass and exposure to bloodborne pathogens. *Microcollection tubes* are preferred and are available with or without additives. The cap colors on microcollection tubes correspond with the color coding system for evacuated tubes. The order of draw, however, is different for microcollection tubes (Box 3-3). The EDTA microcollection tube should be filled first to ensure adequate volume and accurate hematology results, especially for platelets, which tend to aggregate at the site of puncture.[13] Skin puncture specimens should be labeled with the same information as required for evacuated tubes. Examples of skin puncture equipment are shown in Figure 3-10.

Skin Puncture Procedure

The phlebotomist uses standard precautions that include washing hands and applying gloves at the beginning of the procedure and removing gloves and washing hands at the end of the procedure. CLSI recommends the following steps:[13]

1. Prepare the accession (test request) order.
2. Greet the patient (and parents); identify the patient by having the patient (or parent in the case of a child) verbally

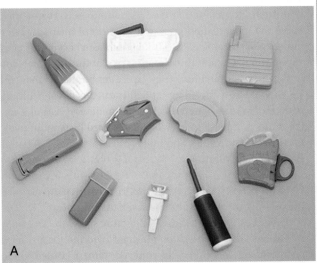

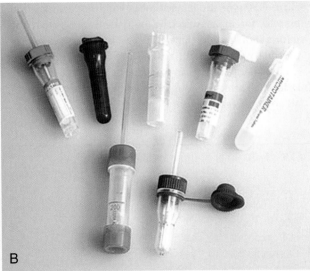

Figure 3-10 Examples of equipment used for skin puncture. **A,** Various puncture devices. **B,** Various microcollection tubes. (A, B Courtesy Dennis J. Ernst, MT[ASCP], Director, Center for Phlebotomy Education, Inc.)

state his or her full name and confirm with patient's identification number, address, and/or birth date. Ensure that the same information is on the requisition form.

3. Position the patient and the parents (or individual designated to hold an infant or small child) as necessary.
4. Verify that any dietary restrictions have been met (e.g., fasting), and check for latex sensitivity.
5. Wash hands and put on gloves.
6. Assemble supplies and appropriate tubes for the requested tests. Check paperwork and tube selection.
7. Select the puncture site.
8. Warm the puncture site.
9. Cleanse the puncture site with 70% isopropyl alcohol using concentric circles, working from the inside to outside. *Allow skin to air-dry.*
10. Open and inspect the sterile disposable puncture device, and perform the puncture while firmly holding the heel or finger. Discard the device in the appropriate sharps container.
11. *Wipe away the first drop of blood* with a clean, dry gauze pad. This removes any residual alcohol and any tissue fluid contamination.
12. Make blood films if requested.
13. Collect blood in the appropriate collection tubes and mix as needed. If an insufficient specimen has been obtained because the blood flow has stopped, repeat the puncture at a different site with all new equipment. CLSI recommends the following order of draw:[13] (Box 3-3)
    a. Tube for blood gas analysis
    b. Slides, unless made from a specimen in the EDTA microcollection tube
    c. EDTA microcollection tube
    d. Other microcollection tubes with anticoagulants
    e. Serum microcollection tubes
14. Apply pressure and elevate the puncture site until bleeding has stopped.
15. Label each specimen with the required information and indicate skin puncture collection.
    NOTE: Compare the labeled tubes with the identification bracelet for inpatients; have outpatients verify that the information on the labeled tubes is correct, whenever possible.
16. Handle the specimens appropriately.
17. Discard all puncture equipment and biohazardous materials appropriately.

BOX 3-3 Order of Draw for Skin Puncture[13]

1. Tube for blood gas analysis
2. Slides, unless made from specimen in the EDTA microcollection tube
3. EDTA microcollection tube
4. Other microcollection tubes with anticoagulants
5. Serum microcollection tubes

EDTA, ethylenediaminetetraacetic acid

18. Remove gloves and wash hands.
19. Deliver the properly labeled specimens to the laboratory.

Preparation of Peripheral Blood Films

Peripheral blood films can be made directly from skin puncture blood or from a tube of EDTA-anticoagulated venous blood. With a skin puncture, the phlebotomist must remember to wipe away the first drop of blood and use the second drop to make the blood film. Chapter 16 covers preparation of blood films in detail.

QUALITY ASSURANCE IN SPECIMEN COLLECTION

To ensure accurate patient test results, it is essential that the blood collection process, which includes specimen handling, be monitored. Patient diagnosis and medical care are based on the outcomes of these tests. The following areas should be monitored.

Technical Competence

The individual performing phlebotomy should be trained properly in all phases of blood collection. Certification by an appropriate agency is recommended. Continuing education is required to keep current on all the changes in the field. Competency should be assessed and documented on an annual basis for each employee performing phlebotomy.

Collection Procedures

Periodic review of collection procedures is essential to maintaining the quality of specimens. This includes a review of policies on the allowable number of blood collection attempts for unsuccessful blood draws, procedures for what to do when the patient is unavailable for a blood draw, or when the patient refuses a draw. Proper patient preparation and correct patient identification are crucial. The correct tube or specimen container must be used.

Anticoagulants and Other Additives

The phlebotomist must follow the manufacturer's instructions with regard to mixing *all* tubes with additives to ensure proper specimen integrity and prevent formation of microclots in the anticoagulated tubes. All tubes should be checked for cracks, expiration dates, and discoloration or cloudiness, which could indicate contamination. New lot numbers of tubes must be checked to verify draw and fill accuracy. When blood is collected in the light blue stopper tube for coagulation, a 9:1 ratio of blood to anticoagulant must be maintained to ensure accurate results. Specimens must be stored and handled properly before testing.

Requirements for a Quality Specimen

Requirements for a quality specimen are as follows:
1. Patient properly identified
2. Patient properly prepared for draw
3. Specimens collected in the correct order and labeled correctly
4. Correct anticoagulants and other additives used
5. Specimens properly mixed by inversion, if required

6. Specimens not hemolyzed
7. Specimens requiring patient fasting collected in a timely manner
8. Timed specimens drawn at the correct time

Collection of Blood for Blood Culture

Each facility should monitor its blood culture contamination rate and keep that rate lower than 3% as recommended by the CLSI and the American Society for Microbiology.[14,15] Higher blood culture contamination rates should prompt an investigation of the causes and implementation of the appropriate corrective action. False-positive blood culture results lead to unnecessary testing and treatment for patients and increased costs for the institution.[14,15] A 2012 CDC-funded Laboratory Medicine Best Practices systematic review and meta-analysis concluded that the use of well-trained phlebotomy teams and proper venipuncture technique was an effective way to reduce blood culture contamination rates.[15]

Quality Control and Preventive Maintenance for Specimen Processing and Storage Equipment

Thermometers used in refrigerators and freezers in which specimens are stored should be calibrated annually, or only thermometers certified by the National Bureau of Standards should be used. Centrifuges should be maintained according to the manufacturer's instructions for cleaning and timing verification.

Reasons for Specimen Rejection

A laboratory result is only as good as the integrity of the specimen provided. Specimens are rejected for conditions that may result in identification errors or inaccurate results. Box 3-4 lists some reasons for specimen rejection.

SPECIMEN HANDLING

Proper handling of specimens begins with the initiation of the test request and ends when the specimen is tested. Accurate test results depend on what happens to the specimen during that time. This pretesting period is called the *preanalytical phase* of the total testing process (Chapter 5).

Blood collected into additive tubes must be inverted to mix the additive and blood according to manufacturer's instructions. Shaking can result in hemolysis of the specimen and lead to specimen rejection or inaccurate test results. Specimens should be transported in an upright position to ensure complete clot formation and reduce agitation, which can also result in hemolysis.

Exposure of the blood specimen to light can cause falsely decreased values for bilirubin, beta-carotene, vitamin A, and porphyrins.[9] For certain tests, the specimens need to be chilled, not frozen, and should be placed in an ice-water bath to slow down cellular metabolism. Examples of these tests include ammonia, lactic acid, parathyroid hormone, and gastrin.[9] Other tests, such as the cold agglutinin titer, require that specimens be kept warm to ensure accurate results. If the specimen is refrigerated before the serum is removed, the antibody in the serum will bind to the red blood cells, thus falsely decreasing the serum cold agglutinin titer. To ensure accurate results, cells and serum must be separated within 2 hours of collection for tests such as those measuring glucose, potassium, and lactate dehydrogenase.[10] The CLSI provides recommendations to laboratories for the maximum time uncentrifuged specimens are stable at room temperature for various tests based on studies in the literature.[10]

LEGAL ISSUES IN PHLEBOTOMY

There are many daily practices in health care that, if performed without reasonable care and skill, can result in a lawsuit. Facilities have been and will continue to be held legally accountable for the actions of those who collect blood for diagnostic testing. Two areas of particular concern to phlebotomists are breach of patient confidentiality and patient misidentification. Unless there is a clinical need to know or a patient has given written permission, no one has a right to patient information. A patient will not be misidentified if correct procedures for specimen collection are followed. Phlebotomists often are called to testify in court in cases involving blood alcohol levels. The phlebotomist is asked about patient identification procedures and skin antisepsis. Only alcohol-free antiseptics should be used for skin antisepsis in such cases. Soap and water may be used if no other cleaners are available.

To minimize the risk of legal action, the phlebotomist should do the following:

1. Follow up on all incident reports.
2. Participate in continuing education.
3. Become certified in the profession.
4. Acknowledge the extent of liability coverage.
5. Follow established procedures.
6. Always exhibit professional, courteous behavior.
7. Always obtain proper consent.
8. Respect and honor the Patients' Bill of Rights.
9. Maintain proper documentation.

BOX 3-4 Reasons for Specimen Rejection

- Test order requisition and the tube identification do not match.
- Tube is unlabeled, or the labeling, including patient identification number, is incorrect.
- Specimen is hemolyzed.
- Specimen was collected at the wrong time.
- Specimen was collected in the wrong tube.
- Specimen was clotted, and the test requires whole blood or plasma.
- Specimen was contaminated with intravenous fluid.
- Specimen is lipemic.*

*Lipemic specimens cannot be used for certain tests; however, the phlebotomist has no control over this aspect. Collection of a specimen after patient fasting may be requested to try to reduce the potential for lipemia.

SUMMARY

- Laboratory test results are only as good as the integrity of the specimen tested.
- Standard precautions must be followed in the collection of blood to prevent exposure to bloodborne pathogens.
- Some physiologic factors affecting test results include posture, diurnal rhythm, exercise, stress, diet, and smoking.
- U.S. manufacturers of evacuated tubes follow a universal color coding system in which the stopper color indicates the type of additive contained in the tube.
- The gauge numbers of needles relate inversely to bore size: the smaller the gauge number, the larger the bore. Needle safety devices are required for venipuncture equipment.
- For venipuncture in the antecubital fossa, the median cubital vein (H-shaped vein pattern) or median vein (M-shaped vein pattern) is preferred to avoid accidental arterial puncture and nerve damage. If those veins are not available after checking both arms, the cephalic, then the basilic veins are the second and third choices.
- CLSI guidelines should be followed for venipuncture and skin puncture.
- Sites for skin puncture include the lateral or medial plantar surface of the heel (infants), or the palmar surface of the distal portion of the third or fourth finger on the nondominant hand (children and adults). Heel punctures are used for infants less than 1 year old; the puncture must be less than 2 mm deep to avoid injury to the bone.
- Common complications of blood collection include bruising, hematoma, and fainting.
- Each institution should establish a policy covering proper procedure when a blood specimen cannot be obtained.
- Following established procedures and documenting all incidents minimize the risk of liability when performing phlebotomy.

Now that you have completed this chapter, go back and read again the case studies at the beginning and respond to the questions presented.

REVIEW QUESTIONS

Answers can be found in the Appendix.

1. Which step in the CLSI procedure for venipuncture is part of standard precautions?
   a. Wearing gloves
   b. Positively identifying the patient
   c. Cleansing the site for the venipuncture
   d. Bandaging the venipuncture site

2. Select the needle most commonly used in standard venipuncture in an adult:
   a. One inch, 18 gauge
   b. One inch, 21 gauge
   c. One-half inch, 23 gauge
   d. One-half inch, 25 gauge

3. For a complete blood count (hematology) and measurement of prothrombin time (coagulation), the phlebotomist collected blood into lavender stopper and green stopper tubes. Are these specimens acceptable?
   a. Yes, EDTA is used for hematologic testing and heparin is used for coagulation testing.
   b. No, although EDTA is used for hematologic testing, citrate, not heparin, is used for coagulation testing.
   c. No, although heparin is used for hematologic testing, citrate, not EDTA, is used for coagulation testing.
   d. No, hematologic testing requires citrate and coagulation testing requires a clot, so neither tube is acceptable.

4. The vein of choice for performing a venipuncture is the:
   a. Basilic, because it is the most prominent vein in the antecubital fossa
   b. Cephalic or accessory cephalic, because it is the least painful site
   c. Median or median cubital, because it has the lowest risk of damaging nerves in the arm
   d. One of the hand veins, because they are most superficial and easily accessed

5. The most important step in phlebotomy is:
   a. Cleansing the site
   b. Identifying the patient
   c. Selecting the proper needle length
   d. Using the correct evacuated tube

6. The venipuncture needle should be inserted into the arm with the bevel facing:
   a. Down and an angle of insertion between 15 and 30 degrees
   b. Up and an angle of insertion less than 30 degrees
   c. Down and an angle of insertion greater than 45 degrees
   d. Up and an angle of insertion between 30 and 45 degrees

7. Failure to obtain blood by venipuncture may occur because of all of the following *except:*
   a. Incorrect needle positioning
   b. Tying the tourniquet too tightly
   c. Inadequate vacuum in the tube
   d. Collapsed vein

8. What is the recommended order of draw when the evacuated tube system is used?
   a. Gel separator, nonadditive, coagulation, and blood culture
   b. Additive, nonadditive, gel separator, and blood culture
   c. Nonadditive, blood culture, coagulation, and other additives
   d. Blood culture, coagulation, nonadditive, and gel separator or other additives

9. Which one of the following is an acceptable site for skin puncture on infants:
   a. Back curvature of the heel
   b. Lateral or medial plantar surface of the heel
   c. Plantar surface of the heel close to the arch of the foot
   d. Middle of the plantar surface of the heel

10. An anticoagulant is an additive placed in evacuated tubes to:
    a. Make the blood clot faster
    b. Dilute the blood before testing
    c. Prevent the blood from clotting
    d. Ensure the sterility of the tube

11. Which one of the following is a reason for specimen rejection:
    a. Clot in a red stopper tube
    b. Specimen collected for blood cortisol in the morning
    c. Specimen in lavender stopper tube grossly hemolyzed
    d. Room number is missing from the specimen tube label

12. One legal area of concern for the phlebotomist is:
    a. Breach of patient confidentiality
    b. Failure to obtain written consent for phlebotomy
    c. Entering a patient's room when the family is present
    d. Asking an outpatient for his or her full name in the process of identification

REFERENCES

1. Department of Labor OSHA. (1991). Occupational exposure to bloodborne pathogens; final rule. *Fed Reg, 56*, 64175–64182.
2. Centers for Disease Control and Prevention. (2014, March 21). *Hepatitis B FAQs for Health Professionals.* http://www.cdc.gov/hepatitis/hbv/hbvfaq.htm. Accessed 10.10.14.
3. Centers for Disease Control. (2002, October 25). *Guideline for hand hygiene in Health-Care Settings. MMWR, 51*, 1–44.
4. McCall, R. E., Tankersley, C. M. (2012). *Phlebotomy Essentials.* (5th ed.). Philadelphia: Lippincott Williams & Wilkins.
5. Garza, D., Becan-McBride, K. (2010). *Phlebotomy Handbook.* (8th ed.). Upper Saddle River, NJ: Pearson Prentice Hall.
6. Foran, S. E., Lewandrowski, K. B., Kratz, A. (2003). Effects of exercise on laboratory test results. *Lab Med, 34*, 736–742.
7. Badrick, E., Kirschbaum, C., Kumari, M. (2007). The relationship between smoking status and cortisol secretion. *J Clin Endocrinol Metab, 92*, 819–824.
8. Johnson, A. A., Piper, M. E., Fiore, M. C., et al. (2010). Effects of smoking intensity and cessation on inflammatory markers in large cohort of active smokers. *Am Heart J, 160*, 458–463.
9. Clinical and Laboratory Standards Institute. (2007). *Procedures for the Collection of Diagnostic Blood Specimens by Venipuncture; Approved Standard.* (6th ed.). CLSI document H3–A6, Wayne, PA: Clinical and Laboratory Standards Institute.
10. Clinical and Laboratory Standards Institute. (2010). *Procedures for Handling and Processing of Blood Specimens for Common Laboratory Tests, Approved Standard.* (4th ed.). CLSI document H18–A4, Wayne, PA: Clinical and Laboratory Standards Institute.
11. Department of Labor OSHA. (2001). Occupational exposure to bloodborne pathogens; needle sticks and other sharps injuries: final rule. *Fed Reg, 66*, 5317–5325.
12. Occupational Safety and Health Administration (OSHA), US Department of Labor. (2003, October 15). *Disposal of Contaminated Needles and Blood Tube Holders Used for Phlebotomy.* OSHA Safety and Health Information Bulletin https://www.osha.gov/dts/shib/shib101503.pdf. Accessed 10.10.14.
13. Clinical and Laboratory Standards Institute. (2008). *Procedures and Devices for the Collection of Diagnostic Capillary Blood Specimens; Approved Standard.* (6th ed.). CLSI document H04–A6, Wayne, PA: Clinical and Laboratory Standards Institute.
14. Clinical and Laboratory Standards Institute. (2007). *Principles and Procedures for Blood Cultures; Approved Guideline.* CLSI document M47–A, Wayne, PA: Clinical and Laboratory Standards Institute.
15. Snyder, S. R., Favoretto, A. M., Baetz, R. A., et al. (2012). Effectiveness of practices to reduce blood culture contamination: a laboratory medicine best practices systematic review and meta-analysis. *Clin Biochem, 45*, 999–1011.

4

Care and Use of the Microscope

Bernadette F. Rodak

OBJECTIVES

After completion of this chapter, the reader will be able to:

1. Given a diagram of a brightfield light microscope, identify the component parts.
2. Explain the function of each component of a brightfield light microscope.
3. Define *achromatic, plan achromatic, parfocal,* and *parcentric* as applied to lenses and microscopes; explain the advantages and disadvantages of each; and recognize examples of each from written descriptions of microscope use and effects.
4. Explain the purpose of and proper order of steps for adjusting microscope light using Koehler illumination.
5. Describe the proper steps for viewing a stained blood film with a brightfield light microscope, including use of oil immersion lenses, and recognize deviations from these procedures.
6. Describe the proper care and cleaning of microscopes and recognize deviations from these procedures.
7. Given the magnification of lenses in a compound microscope, calculate the total magnification.
8. Given a problem with focusing a blood film using a brightfield light microscope, suggest possible causes and their correction.
9. For each of the following, describe which components of the microscope differ from those of a standard light microscope, what the differences accomplish, and what are the uses and benefits of each type in the clinical laboratory:
   - Phase-contrast microscope
   - Polarized light microscope
   - Darkfield microscope

CASE STUDY

After studying the material in this chapter, the reader should be able to respond to the following case study:

A Wright-stained peripheral blood film focuses under 10× and 40× but does not come into focus under the 100× oil objective. What steps should be taken to identify and correct this problem?

---

icroscopes available today reflect improvement in every aspect from the first microscope of Anton van Leeuwenhoek (1632-1723).[1] Advanced technology as applied to microscopy has resulted in computer-designed lens systems, sturdier stands, perfected condensers, and built-in illumination systems. Microscopes can be fitted with multiple viewing heads for teaching or conferences, or they can be attached to a computer to allow an object to be projected onto a monitor or a large screen. Regular care and proper cleaning ensure continued service from this powerful diagnostic instrument. The references listed at the end of this chapter address the physical laws of light and illumination as applied to microscopy.

PRINCIPLES OF MICROSCOPY

In the compound microscope, a magnified intermediate image of the illuminated specimen is formed in the optical tube by each objective lens. This image is then magnified again and viewed through the eyepiece as an enlarged virtual image that appears to be located about 10 inches from the eye (Figure 4-1). Microscopists must focus their eyes in that more distant plane, rather than trying to focus at the distance of the microscope stage.

An example of a *simple microscope* is a magnifying lens that enlarges objects that are difficult to view with the unaided eye. Movie theater projection units incorporate this system efficiently.

The *compound microscope* employs two separate lens systems, objective and eyepiece, the product of which produces the final magnification. Standard microscopes use brightfield illumination in which light passes through the thin specimen.

COMPONENT PARTS AND THEIR FUNCTIONS

Component parts and the function of each part of the microscope are summarized as follows (Figure 4-2):

1. The *eyepieces*, or *oculars*, usually are equipped with 10× lenses (degree of magnification is 10×). The lenses magnify the intermediate image formed by the objective lenses in the optical tube; they also limit the area of visibility. Microscopes may have either one or two adjustable eyepieces. All eyepieces should be used correctly for optimal focus (see section on operating procedure). Eyepieces should not be interchanged with the eyepieces of the same model or other models of microscopes, because the eyepieces in a pair are optically matched.

2. The *interpupillary control* is used to adjust the lateral separation of the eyepieces for each individual. When it is properly adjusted, the user should be able to focus both eyes comfortably on the specimen and visualize *one* clear image.

3. The *optical tube* connects the eyepieces with the objective lens. The intermediate image is formed in this component. The standard length is 160 mm, which, functionally, is the distance from the real image plane (eyepieces) to the objective lenses.

4. The *neck*, or *arm*, provides a structural site of attachment for the revolving nosepiece.

5. The *stand* is the main vertical support of the microscope. The stage assembly, together with the condenser and base, is supported by the stand.

6. The *revolving nosepiece* holds the objectives and allows for easy rotation from one objective lens to another. The working distance (WD) between the objectives and the slide varies with the make and model of the microscope.

7. There are usually three or four *objective lenses* (Figure 4-3), each with a specific power of magnification. Engraved on the barrel of each objective lens is the power of magnification and the numerical aperture (NA). The NA is related to the angle of light collected by the objective; in essence, it indicates the light-gathering ability of the objective lens. Functionally, the larger the NA, the greater the *resolution* or the ability to distinguish between fine details of two closely situated objects.

Four standard powers of magnification and NA used in the hematology laboratory are 10×/0.25 (low power), 40×/0.65 or 45×/0.66 (high power, dry), 50×/0.90 (oil immersion), and 100×/1.25 (oil immersion). The smaller the magnification, the larger the viewing field; the larger the magnification, the smaller the viewing field. Total magnification is calculated by multiplying the magnification of the eyepiece by the magnification of the objective lens; for example, 10× (eyepiece) multiplied by 100× (oil immersion) is 1000× total magnification.

Microscopes employed in the clinical laboratory are used with achromatic or plan achromatic objective lenses, whose

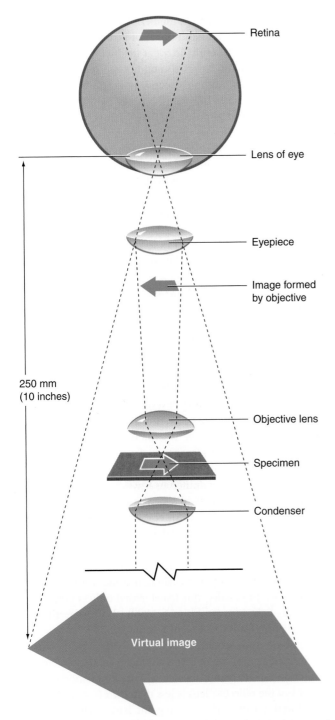

Figure 4-1 Compound microscope. Two separate lens systems are used (objective and eyepiece). Each objective lens forms a magnified image of the illuminated specimen in the optical tube. The eyepiece lenses further magnify this image so that the microscopist sees an enlarged virtual image that appears to be approximately 10 inches from the eye. (From Abramowitz M: The microscope and beyond, vol 1, Lake Success, NY, 1985, Olympus Corp, p. 2. Reprinted courtesy Eastman Kodak Company, Rochester, NY.)

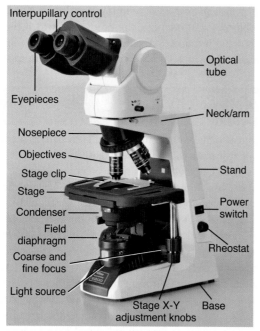

Figure 4-2 Components of a compound microscope. (Courtesy Nikon Instruments, Inc., Melville, NY.)

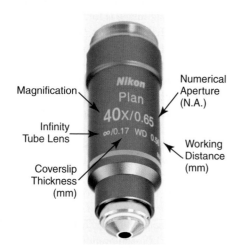

Figure 4-3 Microscope objective lens. The numerical aperture (NA) indicates the light-gathering ability of the objective lens and reflects its ability to distinguish between fine details of two closely situated objects. The working distance (WD) is the distance in millimeters between the lens of the objective and the cover glass when the specimen is in focus. (Courtesy Nikon Instruments, Inc., Melville, NY.)

function is to correct for chromatic and spheric aberrations. *Chromatic aberrations* are caused by the spheric surface of the lens, which acts as a prism. As the various wavelengths pass through the lens, each focuses at a different point, which gives rise to concentric rings of color near the periphery of the lens. *Spheric aberrations* result as light waves travel through the varying thicknesses of the lens, blurring the image. The *achromatic objective lens* brings light of two colors into focus, partially correcting for the aberrations. When achromatic objective lenses are used, the center of the

field is in focus, whereas the periphery is not. A *plan achromatic lens* provides additional corrections for curvature of the field, which results in a flat field with uniform focus.[2] Plan achromatic lenses sometimes are referred to as *flat field* lenses. Critical microscopy applications may require a *plan apochromatic lens,* which brings light of three colors into focus and almost completely corrects for chromatic aberration. This type of objective lens is more expensive and is rarely needed for routine laboratory use.

A set of lenses with corresponding focal points all in the same plane is said to be *parfocal.* As the nosepiece is rotated from one magnification to another, the specimen remains in focus, and only minimal fine adjustment is necessary.

8. The *stage* supports the prepared microscope slide to be reviewed. A spring assembly secures the slide to the stage.
9. The *focus controls* (or adjustments) can be incorporated into one knob or can be two separate controls. When a single knob is used, moving it in one direction engages the coarse control, whereas moving it in the opposite direction engages the fine control. One gradation interval of turning is equivalent to 2 μm. Many microscopes are equipped with two separate adjustments: one coarse and one fine. The order of usage is the same: engage the coarse adjustment first and then fine-tune with the fine adjustment.
10. The *condenser,* consisting of several lenses in a unit, may be permanently mounted or vertically adjustable with a rack-and-pinion mechanism. It gathers, organizes, and directs the light through the specimen. Attached to and at the bottom of the condenser is the *aperture diaphragm,* an adjustable iris containing numerous leaves that control the angle and amount of the light sent through the specimen. The angle, also expressed as an NA, regulates the balance between *contrast* (ability to enhance parts within a cell) and *resolution* (ability to differentiate fine details of two closely situated objects). The best resolution is achieved when the iris is used fully open, but there is some sacrifice of image contrast. In practice, this iris is closed only enough to create a slight increase in image contrast. Closing it beyond this point leads to a loss of resolution.

Some microscopes are equipped with a swing-out lens immediately above or below the main condenser lens. This lens is used to permit a wider field of illumination when the NA of the objective lens is less than 0.25 (e.g., the 4×/0.12 objective lens).[3] If the swing-out lens is *above* the main condenser, it should be *out* for use with the 4× objective lens and *in* for lenses with magnification of 10× and higher. If it is *below* the condenser, it should be *in* for use with the 4× objective lens and *out* for lenses of magnification of 10× and higher. The 4× objective is not used routinely for examination of peripheral blood films.

The stage and condenser (Figure 4-4) consist of a swing-out lens, an aperture diaphragm, a control for vertical adjustment of the condenser, and two centering screws for adjustment of the condenser.

11. The condenser top lens can swing out of position.
12. The *stage controls* located under the stage move it along an x- or a y-axis.

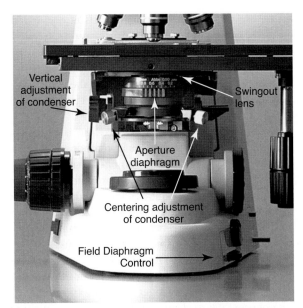

Figure 4-4 Condenser. (Courtesy Nikon Instruments, Inc., Melville, NY.)

Labels in figure:
- Vertical adjustment of condenser
- Swingout lens
- Aperture diaphragm
- Centering adjustment of condenser
- Field Diaphragm Control

13. The *field diaphragm* is located below the condenser within the base. When it is open, it allows a maximally sized circle of light to illuminate the slide. Almost closing the diaphragm, when low power is used, assists in centering the condenser apparatus by the use of two centering screws. Some microscopes have permanently centered condensers, whereas in others the screws are used for this function. The glass on top of the field diaphragm protects the diaphragm from dust and mechanical damage.

14. Microscopes depend on electricity as the primary source for illumination power. There are two types of *brightfield illumination:* (1) critical illumination, in which the light source is focused at the specimen, which results in increased but uneven brightness; and (2) the Koehler (or Köhler) system, in which the light source and the condenser are properly aligned. The end result of Koehler illumination is a field of evenly distributed brightness across the specimen. This is especially important when using the oil objectives or when taking photomicrographs. Tungsten-halogen light bulbs are used most frequently as the illumination source. They consist of a tungsten filament enclosed in a small quartz bulb that is filled with a halogen gas. Tungsten possesses a high melting point and gives off bright yellowish light. A blue (daylight) filter should be used to eliminate the yellow color produced by tungsten.[4,5] The *rheostat* or light control knob or lever turns on the light and should be used to regulate the brightness of the light needed to visualize the specimen. The aperture diaphragm control lever should never be used for this purpose, because closing it reduces resolving ability.[3]

OPERATING PROCEDURE WITH KOEHLER ILLUMINATION

The procedure outlined here applies to microscopes with a nonfixed condenser. The following steps should be performed at the start of each laboratory session in which the oil objectives will be used:

1. Connect the microscope to the power supply.
2. Turn on the light source with the power switch.
3. Open the condenser aperture and field diaphragms.
4. Revolve the nosepiece until the 10× objective lens is directly above the stage.
5. Place a stained blood film on the stage and focus on it, using the fixed eyepiece, while covering the other eye. (Do not simply close the other eye, because this would necessitate adjustment of the pupil when you focus with the other eyepiece.)
6. Adjust the interpupillary control so that looking through both eyepieces yields one clear image.
7. Using the adjustable eyepiece and covering the opposite eye, focus on the specimen. Start with the eyepiece all the way out, and adjust inward. If using two adjustable eyepieces, focus each individually.
8. Raise the condenser to its upper limit.
9. Focus the field so that the cells become sharp and clear. Concentrate on one cell and place it in the center of the field.
10. Close the field (lower) diaphragm. Look through the eyepieces. A small circle of light should be seen. If the light is not in the center of the field, center it by using the two centering screws located on the condenser. This step is essential, because an off-center condenser will result in uneven distribution of light. Adjust the vertical height of the substage condenser so that you see a sharp image of the field diaphragm, ringed by a magenta halo. If the condenser is raised too much, the halo is orange; if it is lowered too far, the halo is blue.
11. Reopen the field diaphragm until it is nearly at the edge of the field, and fine-tune the centering process.
12. Open the field diaphragm slightly until it just disappears from view.
13. Remove one eyepiece and, while looking through the microscope (without the eyepiece), close the condenser aperture diaphragm completely. Reopen the condenser aperture diaphragm until the leaves just disappear from view. Replace the eyepiece.
14. Rotate the nosepiece until the 40× objective lens is above the slide. Adjust the focus (the correction should be minimal) and find the cell that you had centered. If it is slightly off center, center it again with the stage x-y control. Note the greater amount of detail that you can see.
15. Move the 40× objective out of place. Place a drop of immersion oil on top of the slide. Rotate the nosepiece until the 100× objective lens is directly above the slide. Avoid moving a non–oil immersion objective through the drop of oil. Adjust the focus (the correction should be minimal) and observe the detail of the cell: the nucleus and its chromatin pattern; the cytoplasm and its color and texture. The objective lens should dip into the oil slightly.

Considerations

1. When revolving the nosepiece from one power to another, rotate it in such a direction that the 10× and 40× objective lenses never come into contact with the oil on a slide. If oil

inadvertently gets onto the high dry objective, clean the objective immediately.

2. *Parcentric* refers to the ability to center a cell in question in the microscopic field and rotate from one magnification power to another while retaining the cell close to the center of the viewing field. Recentering of the cell at each step is minimal. Most laboratory microscopes have this feature.

3. In general, when the 10× and 40× objective lenses are used, the light intensity should be low. When the 50× and 100× objective lenses are used, increase the intensity of the light by adjusting *only* the rheostat (light control knob or lever) or by varying neutral density filters. Neutral density filters are used to reduce the amplitude of light and are available in a variety of densities.[3]

4. Do not change the position of the condenser or the aperture diaphragm control lever to regulate light intensity when viewing specimens with the oil immersion objectives. The condenser should always be in its upward position as set during the Koehler illumination adjustment. The aperture diaphragm may be adjusted to achieve proper contrast of the features of the specimen being viewed.

5. After setting the Koehler illumination, when a new slide is to be examined, always bring the specimen into focus with the 10× objective first, and then move to the higher magnifications.

IMMERSION OIL AND TYPES

Immersion oil is required to increase the *refractive index* when either the 50× or the 100× oil immersion objective lens is used. The refractive index is the speed at which light travels in air divided by the speed at which light travels through a substance. This oil, which has the same properties as glass, allows the objective lens to collect light from a wide NA, which provides high resolution of detail.

Three types of immersion oil, differing in viscosity, are employed in the clinical laboratory:

1. *Type A* has very low viscosity and is used in fluorescence and darkfield studies.

2. *Type B* has high viscosity and is used in brightfield and standard clinical microscopy. In hematology, this oil is routinely used.

3. *Type C* has very high viscosity and is used with inclined microscopes with long-focus objective lenses and wide condenser gaps.

Bubbles in the oil tend to act as prisms and consequently reduce resolution. Bubbles may be created when oil is applied to the slide. They are caused by lowering the objective immediately into the oil. Sweeping the objective from right to left in the oil eliminates bubbles.[5]

CARE OF THE MICROSCOPE

Care of the microscope involves the following details:

1. When not in use for an extended period of time, always cover the microscope to protect it from dust.

2. Before use, inspect the component parts. If dust is found, use an air syringe, a camel hair brush, or a soft lint-free cloth to remove it. Using lens paper directly on a dirty lens without first removing the dust may scratch the lens. Do not use laboratory wipes or facial tissue to clean the lenses.[6]

3. Avoid placing fingers on the lens surface. Fingerprints affect the contrast and resolution of the image.

4. Use solvent sparingly. The use of xylene is discouraged, because it contains a carcinogenic component (benzene). Xylene is also a poor cleaning agent, leaving an oily film on the lens. Lens cleaner or 70% isopropyl alcohol employed sparingly on a cotton applicator stick can be used to clean the objective lenses. Alcohol should be kept away from the periphery of the lenses, because alcohol can dissolve the cement and seep into the back side of the lens.

5. When fresh oil is added to residual oil on the 100× objective lens, there may be loss of contrast. Clean off all residual oil first.

6. Do not use water to clean lenses. If no lens cleaner is available, use a clean microfiber cloth.

7. When transporting the microscope, place one hand under the base as support and one hand firmly around the arm.

In addition to daily care of the microscope, semiannual or annual maintenance with thorough cleaning should be done by a professional. Microscope professionals may recognize and correct problems with mechanics or optics before they are detected by the microscope user. They can correct problems such as sticking of stage controls or incorrect optical alignment that can lead to physical problems like carpal tunnel syndrome and headaches.

BASIC TROUBLESHOOTING

Most common problems are related to inability to focus. Once the operator has ensured that he or she is not trying to obtain a "flat field" using an objective lens that is not plan achromatic, the following checklist can aid in identifying the problem:

- Eyepieces
  Clean?
  Securely assembled?
- Objective lens
  Screwed in tightly?
  Dry objective free of oil?
- Condenser
  Adjusted to proper height?
  Free of oil?
- Slide
  Correct side up?
- Coverslip
  Correct side of blood film?
  Only one coverslip on slide?
  Free of mounting media?
- Light source
  Fingerprints on bulb?
  Bulb in need of changing?
  Light source aligned correctly?

OTHER MICROSCOPES USED IN THE CLINICAL LABORATORY

Phase-Contrast Microscope

The ability to view a stained specimen by the use of brightfield microscopy is affected by two features: (1) the ability of the specimen to absorb the light hitting it, and (2) the degree to which light waves traveling through the specimen remain in phase (∿∿∿).

Specimens that are transparent or colorless, such as unstained cells, are not clearly visualized with brightfield microscopy. Phase-contrast microscopy, through the installation of an *annular diaphragm* in the condenser, together with a *phase-shifting element*, creates excellent contrast of a cell against its surrounding background.

The principle of phase contrast is related to the index of refraction and the thickness of a specimen, which produce differences in the optical path. Light passing through a transparent specimen travels slightly slower than light that is unobstructed. The difference is so small that it is not noticeable to the viewer. When a transparent phase plate is placed into the microscope, however, the change in phase can be increased to half a wavelength, which makes the otherwise transparent objective visible (∿∿∿).

This phase difference produces variation in light intensity from bright to dark, creating contrast in the image. Often the objects appear to have "haloes" surrounding them.

In hematology, phase-contrast microscopy is employed in counting platelets in a hemacytometer, since they are difficult to visualize and count using brightfield microscopy. It also can be used to view formed elements in unstained urine sediments.

Polarized Light Microscope

Polarized light microscopy is another contrast-enhancing technique used to identify substances such as crystals in urine and other body fluids (Chapter 18). With brightfield microscopy, light vibrates in all directions. If a polarizer (filter) is placed in the light path, the light vibrates in only one direction or plane, which creates polarized light. To convert a brightfield microscope to a polarizing one, two filters are needed. One filter (the polarizer) is placed below the condenser and allows only light vibrating in the east-west direction perpendicular to the light path to pass through the specimen. The second filter (the analyzer) is placed between the objective and the eyepiece and allows only light vibrating in a north-south direction to pass to the eyepiece. When the transmission axes of these two filters are oriented at right angles, no light can pass through the pair to the eyepieces. When polarized light (vibrating in an east-west direction) passes through an optically active substance such as a monosodium urate crystal, however, the light is refracted into two beams, one vibrating in the original direction (east-west) and one vibrating in a plane 90 degrees to it (i.e., north-south). The refracted light vibrating in the north-south direction can pass through the second filter (the analyzer) and is visible at the eyepiece. The magnified crystal appears white against a black background. If a first-order red compensator filter also is placed in the light path below the stage, the background becomes pink-red, and the crystal appears yellow or blue, depending on its physical orientation relative to the incident light path (east-west). Some crystals can be specifically identified based on their unique birefringent (doubly refractive) characteristics when polarizing microscopy is used (Figures 18-22 and 18-23).

Darkfield Microscope

Darkfield microscopy is a contrast-enhancing technique that employs a special condenser. The condenser sends light upward the specimen in a hollow cone. Because of the high angle of this cone, none of the illuminating rays enters the objective lens. Without the specimen in place, the field would appear black because of the absence of light. When the specimen is in place, and if fine detail exists in the specimen, light is diffracted in all directions. This diffracted light is picked up by the objective lens and appears as bright detail on a black background. Darkfield microscopy is helpful in microbiology in the identification of spirochetes.

SUMMARY

- The compound microscope, through the use of an objective lens in the optical tube, forms an intermediate image of the illuminated specimen. The image is then magnified and viewed through the eyepiece lenses.
- The numerical aperture or NA, which is engraved on the barrel of objective lenses, designates the light-gathering ability of the lens. The larger the NA, the greater the resolution.
- Achromatic lenses maintain the center of the field in focus, whereas plan achromatic lenses correct for the curvature of a field, providing a flat field uniform focus.
- The condenser gathers the light and directs it through a thin specimen.
- Koehler illumination establishes a field of evenly distributed brightness across the specimen; the microscope should be adjusted for proper Koehler illumination with each use.
- Only the rheostat (light control knob or lever) should be used to regulate the light intensity needed to visualize a specimen. Light intensity should not be regulated by adjusting the position of the aperture diaphragm or the height of the condenser when using the oil immersion lenses.

- The aperture diaphragm control lever may be adjusted to achieve proper contrast of the features of the specimen being viewed.
- The use of oil immersion for the 50× and 100× oil immersion objectives improves the resolution of the image; type B oil is typically used with brightfield microscopy in hematology.
- Microscopes should be carefully handled and maintained. Solvents should not be used to clean lenses; lens cleaner or 70% isopropyl alcohol is recommended.
- Phase-contrast microscopy relies on the effect of index of refraction and the thickness of the specimen; these two features affect light by retarding a fraction of the light waves, resulting in a difference in phase. This allows transparent or colorless objects to become visible.

- Polarizing microscopes use two polarizing filters to cancel the light passing through the specimen. If the object is able to polarize light, as are some crystals, the light passing through is rotated and the object becomes visible.
- Darkfield microscopes use condensers that send light to the specimen at a high angle, directing the light away from the objective lens. If the specimen has fine detail, it causes the light to bend back toward the objective, which allows it to be viewed against an otherwise dark background.

Now that you have completed this chapter, go back and read again the case study at the beginning and respond to the question presented.

REVIEW QUESTIONS

Answers can be found in the Appendix.

1. Use of which one of the following type of objective lens causes the center of the microscope field to be in focus, whereas the periphery is blurred?
   a. Plan achromatic
   b. Achromatic
   c. Plan apochromatic
   d. Flat field

2. Which of the following gathers, organizes, and directs light through the specimen?
   a. Eyepiece
   b. Objective lens
   c. Condenser
   d. Optical tube

3. After focusing a specimen by using the 40× objective, the laboratory professional switches to a 10× objective. The specimen remains in focus at 10×. Microscopes with this characteristic are described as:
   a. Parfocal
   b. Parcentric
   c. Compensated
   d. Parachromatic

4. Which objective has the greatest degree of color correction?
   a. Achromatic
   b. Plan apochromatic
   c. Bichromatic
   d. Plan achromatic

5. In adjusting the microscope light using Koehler illumination, which one of the following is *true*?
   a. Condenser is first adjusted to its lowest position
   b. Height of the condenser is adjusted by removing the eyepiece
   c. Image of the field diaphragm iris is used to center the condenser
   d. Closing the aperture diaphragm increases the resolution of the image

6. The total magnification obtained when a 10× eyepiece and a 10× objective lens are used is:
   a. 1×
   b. 10×
   c. 100×
   d. 1000×

7. After a microscope has been adjusted for Koehler illumination, and the specimen is being viewed with an oil immersion objective lens, light intensity should *never* be regulated by adjusting the:
   a. Rheostat
   b. Neutral density filter
   c. Light control knob
   d. Condenser

8. The recommended cleaner for removing oil from objectives is:
   a. 70% alcohol or lens cleaner
   b. Xylene
   c. Water
   d. Benzene

9. Which of the following types of microscopy is valuable in the identification of crystals that are double refractive?
   a. Compound brightfield
   b. Darkfield
   c. Polarizing
   d. Phase-contrast

10. A laboratory science student has been reviewing a hematology slide using the 10× objective to find a suitable portion of the slide for examination. He moves the 10× objective out of place, places a drop of oil on the slide, rotates the nosepiece so that the 40× objective passes through the viewing position, and continues to rotate the 100× oil objective into viewing position. This practice should be corrected in which way?
   a. The stage of a parfocal microscope should be lowered before the objectives are rotated.
   b. The 100× oil objective should be in place for viewing before the oil is added.

   c. The drop of oil should be in place and the 100× objective lowered into the oil, rather than swinging the objective into the drop.
   d. The objectives should be rotated in the opposite direction so that the 40× objective does not risk entering the oil.

11. Darkfield microscopes create the dark field by:
   a. Using two filters that cancel each other out, one above and the other below the condenser
   b. Angling the light at the specimen so that it misses the objective unless something in the specimen bends it backward
   c. Closing the condenser diaphragm entirely, limiting light to just a tiny ray in the center of the otherwise dark field
   d. Using a light source above the specimen and collecting light reflected from the specimen, rather than transmitted through the specimen, so that when there is no specimen in place, the field is dark

REFERENCES

1. Asimov, I. (1966). *Understanding Physics: Light, Magnetism, and Electricity.* London: George Allen & Unwin.
2. Microscope terms. Available at: http://www.microscope.com/microscope-terms. The Microscope Store, LLC. Accessed 06.04.14.
3. Olympus Microscopy Resource Center: Anatomy of the Microscope. Available at: http://www.olympusmicro.com/primer/anatomy/anatomy.html. Accessed 06.04.14.
4. Microscope Illumination. Olympus Microscope primer. Available at: http://micro.magnet.fsu.edu/primer/anatomy/illumination.html. Accessed 06.04.14.
5. Centonze Frohlich, V. (2008, July 30). Major components of the light microscope. *J Vis Exp* 17. Available at: http://www.jove.com/index/details.stp?ID=843. Accessed 06.04.14. doi:10.3791/843.
6. Centonze Frohlich, V. (2008, August 11). Proper care and cleaning of the microscope. *J Vis Exp* 18. Available at: http://www.jove.com/index/details.stp?ID=842. Accessed 06.04.14. doi:10.3791/842.

ADDITIONAL RESOURCES

Nikon Microscopy U, http://www.microscopyu.com/
Brunzel N. A. (2013). Microscopy. In *Fundamentals of Urine and Body Fluid Analysis.* (3rd ed.). St Louis. Saunders, Chapter 1.

Gill G. W. (2005). Köhler illumination. *Lab Med 36(9)*, 530.

5

Quality Assurance in Hematology and Hemostasis Testing

George A. Fritsma*

OBJECTIVES

After completion of this chapter, the reader will be able to:

1. Describe the procedures to validate and document a new or modified laboratory assay.
2. Compare a new or modified assay to a reference using statistical tests to establish accuracy.
3. Select appropriate statistical tests for a given application and interpret the results.
4. Define and compute precision using standard deviation and coefficient of variation.
5. Determine assay linearity using graphical representations and transformations.
6. Discuss analytical limits and analytical sensitivity and specificity.
7. Explain Food and Drug Administration clearance levels for laboratory assays.
8. Compute a reference interval and a therapeutic range for a new or modified assay.
9. Interpret internal quality control using controls and moving averages.
10. Explain the benefits of participation in periodic external quality assessment.
11. Measure and describe assay clinical efficacy.
12. Interpret relative and absolute risk ratios.
13. Interpret receiver operating characteristic curves.
14. Describe methods to enhance and assess laboratory staff competence.
15. Describe a quality assurance plan to control for preanalytical and postanalytical variables.
16. List the agencies that regulate hematology and hemostasis quality.

CASE STUDY

After studying the material in this chapter, the reader should be able to respond to the following case study:

On an 8:00 AM assay run, the results for three levels of a preserved hemoglobin control specimen are 2 g/dL higher than the upper limit of the target interval. The medical laboratory scientist reviews δ-check data on the hemoglobin results for the last 10 patients in sequence and notices that the results are consistently 1.8 to 2.2 g/dL higher than results generated the previous day.
1. What do you call the type of error detected in this case?
2. Can you continue to analyze patient specimens as long as you subtract 2 g/dL from the results?
3. What aspect of the assay should you first investigate in troubleshooting this problem?

In medical laboratory science, *quality* implies the ability to provide *accurate, reproducible* assay results that offer clinically useful information.[1] Because physicians base 70% of their clinical decision making on laboratory results, assay results must be *reliable*.[2] Reliability requires vigilance and effort on the part of all laboratory staff members.[3] An experienced medical laboratory scientist who is a quality assurance and quality control specialist often directs this effort.

*The author acknowledges David McGlasson, M.S., MLS (ASCP)^CM, Clinical Research Scientist, Wilford Hall Ambulatory Surgical Center, JBSA, San Antonio, Texas, for his assistance in preparing this chapter.

Of the terms *quality control* and *quality assurance*, quality assurance is the broader concept, encompassing *preanalytical, analytical,* and *postanalytical* variables (Box 5-1). Quality control processes are employed to document assay validity, accuracy, and precision, including external quality assessment, reference interval preparation and publication, and lot-to-lot validation.[4]

Preanalytical variables, listed further in this chapter in Table 5-11, are addressed in Chapter 3, which discusses blood specimen collection, and in Chapter 42, which includes a section on coagulation specimen management. Postanalytical variables are discussed briefly at the end of this chapter and are listed in Table 5-12. Quality assurance further encompasses laboratory assay utilization and physician test ordering patterns, nicknamed "pre-pre" analytical variables, and the appropriate application of laboratory assay results, sometimes called "post-post" analytical variables. There exists a combined 17% medical error rate associated with the pre-pre and post-post analytical phases of laboratory test utilization and application, prompting laboratory directors and scientists to develop *clinical query systems* that guide clinicians in laboratory assay selection.[5] Clinical query systems are enhanced by *reflex assay algorithms* developed in collaboration with the affiliated medical and surgical staff.[5] Equally important, a system of narrative reports that accompany and augment numerical laboratory assay output, authored by medical laboratory scientists and directors, is designed to assist physicians with case management.[6] A discussion of pre-pre and post-post analytical variables extends beyond the scope of this textbook but may be found in the references listed at the end of this chapter.[7,8] Quality control relies on the initial computation of central tendency and dispersion.

STATISTICAL SIGNIFICANCE AND EXPRESSIONS OF CENTRAL TENDENCY AND DISPERSION

Statistical Significance

When applying a statistical test such as the *Student's t-test* of means or the *analysis of variance* (ANOVA), the statistician begins with a *null hypothesis*. The null hypothesis states that there is no difference between or among the means or variances of the populations being compared.[9] The *alternative (research) hypothesis* is the logical opposite of the null hypothesis.[10] For example, the null hypothesis may state there is no difference between *t*-test means, but the alternative hypothesis states that the null hypothesis is rejected and a statistical difference between the means does indeed exist (Table 5-2). In medical research, the null and alternative hypotheses may go unstated but are always implied.[11]

The power of a statistical test is defined as its ability to reject the null hypothesis when the null hypothesis is indeed false. Power is expressed as *p*, which stands for the *probability* that the test is able to detect an effect. The *p* scale ranges from 0 to 1. Power is determined by the sample size (number of data points, *n*), the design of the research study, and the study's ability to control for extraneous variables.

The conventional levels for significance, or for rejecting the null hypothesis, are $p \leq 0.05$ (5%) or $p \leq 0.01$ (1%). In the former instance, there exists a 5% chance that the effect has occurred by chance alone; in the latter instance, there exists a more stringent 1% chance. Often researchers combine the statistical results, and thus the powers of several studies, to compute a common *p*-value, a process called *meta-analysis*.

BOX 5-1 Examples of Components of Quality Assurance

1. *Preanalytical* variables: selection of assay relative to patient need; implementation of assay selection; patient identification and preparation; specimen collection equipment and technique; specimen transport, preparation, and storage; monitoring of specimen condition
2. *Analytical* variables: laboratory staff competence; assay and instrument selection; assay validation, including linearity, accuracy, precision, analytical limits, and specificity; internal quality control; external quality assessment
3. *Postanalytical* variables: accuracy in transcription and filing of results; content and format of laboratory report, narrative report; reference interval and therapeutic range; timeliness in communicating critical values; patient and physician satisfaction; turnaround time; cost analysis; physician application of laboratory results

The term *significant* has a specific meaning based on the *p*-value, and it should not be generalized to imply *practical* or *clinical* significance.[12] A statistical test result may indicate a statistically significant difference that is based on a selected study condition and power, but the difference may not possess practical importance because the clinical difference may be inconsequential. Experience and clinical judgment help when analyzing data, as does asking the question "Will this result generate a change in the prognosis, diagnosis, or treatment plan?"

Computing the Mean

The arithmetic mean ($\bar{x}$), or average, of a data series is the sum (Σ) of the individual data values divided by the number (*n*) of data points. A data series that represents a single population, for instance, a series of prothrombin time results from a population, is called a *sample*. Often clinical laboratory personnel apply the terms *sample* and *specimen* interchangeably. A specimen may be defined as a single data point within a data series (sample). In the clinical laboratory, of course, a specimen often means a tube of blood or a piece of tissue collected from a patient, which provides a single data point. The sum of sample data values above the mean is equal to the sum of the data values below the mean; however, the actual numbers of points above and below the mean are not necessarily equal.[13] The mean is a standard expression of central tendency employed in most scientific applications; however, it is profoundly affected by outliers and is unreliable in a skewed population. This is the formula for computing the arithmetic mean:

$$\text{Mean } (\bar{x}) = \frac{\left(\sum x \right)}{n};$$

where $\bar{x}$ = mean; Σx = sum of data point values; and n = number of data points

The *geometric* mean is the *n* root of the product of *n* individual data points and is used to compute means of unlike data series. The geometric mean of the prothrombin time reference interval is used to compute the prothrombin time international normalized ratio (Chapter 43). This is the formula for computing the geometric mean:

Geometric mean of *n* instances of $a = \sqrt[n]{a_1 a_2 ... a_n}$.

Determining the Median

The median is the data point that separates the upper half from the lower half of a data series (sample). To find the median, arrange the data series in numerical order and select the central data point. If the data series has an even number of data points, the median is the mean of the two central points. The median is a robust expression of central tendency in a skewed distribution because it minimizes the effects of outliers.

Determining the Mode

The mode of a data series (sample) is the data point that appears most often in the sample. The mode is not a true measure of central tendency because there is often more than one mode in a data series. For instance, a typical white blood cell histogram may be trimodal, with three modes, one each for lymphocytes, monocytes, and neutrophils. Conversely, in a Gaussian, "normal" sample, in which the data points are distributed symmetrically, the mean, median, and mode coincide at a single data point.

Computing the Variance

Variance (σ^2) expresses the deviation of each data point from its expected value, usually the mean of the data series (sample) from which the data point is drawn. The difference between each data point from the mean is squared, the squared differences are summed, and the sum of squares is divided by n – 1. Variance is expressed in the units of the variable squared as follows:

$$\sigma^2 = \frac{\sum (x_i - \bar{x})^2}{(n-1)},$$

where σ^2 = sample variance; x_i = value of each data point; $\bar{x}$ = mean; and n = number of data points

Computing the Standard Deviation

Standard deviation (SD), a commonly used measure of dispersion, is the square root of the variance and is the mean distance of all the data points in a sample from the sample mean (Figure 5-1). The larger the SD of a sample, the greater the deviation from the mean. In clinical analyses, the SD of an assay is an expression of its quality based on its inherent dispersion or variability. The formula for SD is:

$$SD = \sqrt{\left[\frac{\sum (X_i - \bar{X})^2}{(n-1)} \right]},$$

where SD = standard deviation; x_i = each data point value; $\bar{x}$ = mean; and n = number of observations

SD states the confidence, or degree of *random error*, for statistical conclusions. Dispersion is typically expressed as $\bar{x} \pm 2$ SD or the 95.5% *confidence interval* (CI). Data points that are over 2 SD from the mean are outside the 95.5% CI and may be considered abnormal. The dispersion of data points within $\bar{x} \pm 2$ SD is considered the expression of random or chance variation. Typically, $\bar{x} \pm 2$ SD is used to establish biological reference intervals (normal ranges), provided the frequency of the data points is "Gaussian," or normally distributed, meaning symmetrically distributed about the mean.

Computing the Coefficient of Variation

The coefficient of variation (CV) is the *normalized expression* of the SD, ordinarily articulated as a percentage (CV%). CV% is the most commonly used measure of dispersion in laboratory medicine. CV% is expressed without units (except percentage), thus making it possible to compare data sets that use different units. The computation formula is:

$$CV\% = 100 \frac{SD}{\bar{x}}$$

where CV% = coefficient of variation expressed as a percentage; SD = standard deviation; and $\bar{x}$ = mean

VALIDATION OF A NEW OR MODIFIED ASSAY

All new laboratory assays and all assay modifications require *validation*.[14] Validation is an activity comprised of procedures to determine accuracy, specificity, precision, limits, and linearity.[15] The results of these procedures are faithfully recorded and made available to on-site assessors upon request.[16]

Accuracy

Accuracy is the measure of agreement between an assay value and the theoretical "true value" of its analyte (Figure 5-1). Some statisticians prefer to define accuracy as the magnitude of error separating the assay result from the true value. By comparison, *precision* is the expression of reproducibility or dispersion about the mean, often expressed as SD or CV%, as discussed in a subsequent section, "Precision." Accuracy is easy to define but difficult to establish and maintain; precision is relatively easy to measure and maintain.

For many analytes, laboratory professionals employ *primary standards* to establish accuracy. A primary standard is a material of known, fixed composition that is prepared in pure form, often by determining its mass on an analytical balance. The practitioner dissolves the weighed standard in an aqueous solution, prepares suitable dilutions, calculates the anticipated concentration for each dilution, and assigns the calculated concentrations to assay outcomes. For example, he or she may obtain pure glucose, weigh 100 mg, dilute it in 100 mL of buffer, and assay an aliquot of the solution using photometry. The resulting absorbance would then be assigned the value of 100 mg/dL. The practitioner may repeat this procedure using a series of four additional glucose solutions at 20, 60, 120, and 160 mg/dL to produce a five-point *standard curve*. The curve may be reassayed several times to generate means for each concentration. Standard curve generation is automated, however laboratory professionals retain the ability to generate curves manually when necessary. The assay is then employed

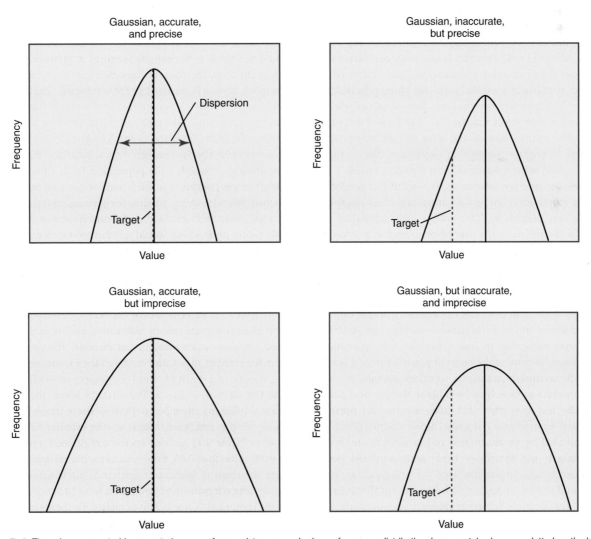

Figure 5-1 The values generated by repeated assays of an analyte are graphed as a frequency distribution. Incremental values are plotted on the horizontal (x) scale and number of times each value was obtained (frequency) on the vertical (y) scale. In this example, the values are normally distributed about their mean (symmetric, Gaussian distribution). Results from an accurate assay generate a mean that closely duplicates the reference target value. Results from a precise assay generate small dispersion about the mean, whereas imprecision is reflected in a broad curve. The ideal assay is both accurate and precise.

on human serum or plasma, with absorbance compared with the standard curve to generate a result. The matrix of a primary standard need not match the matrix of the patient specimen; the standard may be dissolved in an aqueous buffer, whereas the test specimen may be human serum or plasma.

To save time and resources, the laboratory professional may employ a secondary standard, perhaps purchased, that the vendor has previously calibrated to a primary standard. The secondary standard may be a preserved plasma preparation at a certified known concentration. The laboratory professional merely thaws or reconstitutes the secondary standard and incorporates it into the test series during validation or revalidation. Manufacturers often match secondary standards as closely as possible to the test specimen's matrix, for instance, serum to serum, plasma to plasma, and whole blood to whole blood. Primary and secondary standards are seldom assayed during routine patient specimen testing, only during calibration or when the assay tends to be unstable.

Regrettably, in hematology and hemostasis, where the analytes are often cell suspensions or enzymes, there are just a handful of primary standards: cyanmethemoglobin, fibrinogen, factor VIII, protein C, antithrombin, and von Willebrand factor.[17] For scores of analytes, the hematology and hemostasis practitioner relies on *calibrators*. Calibrators for hematology may be preserved human blood cell suspensions, sometimes supplemented with microlatex particles or nucleated avian red blood cells (RBCs) as surrogates for hard-to-preserve human white blood cells (WBCs). In hemostasis, calibrators may be frozen or lyophilized plasma from healthy human donors. For most of these analytes, it is impossible to prepare "weighed-in" standards; instead, calibrators are assayed using *reference methods* ("gold standards") at selected *independent expert laboratories*. For instance, a vendor may prepare a 1000-L lot of preserved human blood cell suspension, assay for the desired analytes within their laboratory ("in-house"), and send aliquots to five laboratories that employ well-controlled reference instrumentation and methods. The vendor obtains blood count results from all five, averages the results, compares them to their in-house values, and publishes the averages as the reference calibrator values. The vendor then distributes sealed aliquots to customer laboratories with the calibrator values published in the accompanying package inserts. Vendors often market calibrators in sets of three or five, spanning the range of assay linearity or the range of potential clinical results.

As with secondary standards, vendors attempt to match their calibrators as closely as possible to the physical properties of the test specimen. For instance, human preserved blood used to calibrate complete blood count (CBC) analytes generated by an automated cell counter is prepared to closely match the matrix of fresh anticoagulated patient blood specimens, despite the need for preservatives, refrigeration, and sealed packaging. Vendors submit themselves to rigorous certification by governmental or voluntary standards agencies in an effort to verify and maintain the validity of their products.

The laboratory practitioner assays the calibration material using the new or modified assay and compares results with the vendor's published results. When new results parallel published results within a selected range, for example ±10%, the results are recorded and the assay is validated for accuracy. If they fail to match, the new assay is modified or a new reference interval and therapeutic range is prepared.

Medical laboratory professionals may employ locally collected fresh blood from a healthy donor as a calibrator; however, the process for validation and certification is laborious, so few attempt it. The selected specimens are assayed using reference instrumentation and methods, calibration values are assigned, and the new or modified assay is calibrated (adjusted) from these values.

New or modified assays may also be compared to reference methods. A reference method may be a previously employed, well-controlled assay or an assay currently being used by a neighboring laboratory. Several statistics are available to compare results of the new or modified assay to a reference method, including the Student's *t*-test, analysis of variance (ANOVA), linear regression, Pearson correlation coefficient, and the Bland-Altman plot.

Statistical Tests
Comparing Means of Two Data Series Using Student's t-Test

The Student's *t*-test compares the sample *mean* of a new or modified assay to the sample mean of a reference assay.[18] In a standard *t*-test the operator assumes that population distributions are normal (Gaussian), the SDs are equal, and the assays are independent. Often laboratory professionals use the more robust *paired* t-*test* in which the new and reference assays are performed using specimens from the same donors (aliquots). Laboratory scientists also choose between the *one-tailed* and *two-tailed* t-*test*, depending on whether the population being sampled has one (high *or* low) versus two (high *and* low) critical values. For instance, when assaying plasma for glucose, clinicians are concerned about both elevated and reduced glucose values, so the laboratory professional would use the two-tailed *t*-test; however, when assaying for bilirubin, clinical concern focuses only on elevated bilirubin concentrations, so the laboratory professional would apply the more robust one-tailed *t*-test in method comparison studies.

The laboratory professional generates *t*-test data by entering the paired data sets side by side into columns of a spreadsheet and applying an automated *t*-test formula. The program generates the number, mean, and variance for each data series (sample; n_1, n_2; $\bar{x}_1$, $\bar{x}_2$; σ^2_1, σ^2_2), and the "degrees of freedom" (df) for the test: df = $n_1 + n_2 - 2$. The operator selects the appropriate critical value (*p*), often $p \leq 0.05$. The computer uses df and *p* to compare the computed *t*-value to the *standard table of critical t-values* (Table 5-1) and reports the corresponding *p*-value. If the *p*-value is less than 0.05, the means of the two samples are unequal and the result is "*statistically significant.*" For instance, if the two assays are each performed on aliquots from 10 donors, the df is 18. If the computed *t*-value is 2.10 or higher, the means are unequal at $p \leq 0.05$. Applying a stricter critical value, the computed *t*-value would have to be 2.88 or higher for the means to be considered unequal at $p \leq 0.01$. Table 5-2 illustrates a typical *t*-test result.

When the *t*-test indicates that two sample means are *not unequal*, the operator may choose to implement the new or modified assay. However, statistically, if two means are adjudged "not

TABLE 5-1 Excerpt from the Standard Table of Critical *t*-Values for a Two-tailed Test

df	$p \leq 0.05$	$p \leq 0.01$	df	$p \leq 0.05$	$p \leq 0.01$	df	$p \leq 0.05$	$p \leq 0.01$
2	$t = 4.30$	$t = 9.93$	12	2.18	3.06	22	2.07	2.82
4	2.78	4.60	14	2.15	2.98	24	2.06	2.80
6	2.45	3.71	16	2.12	2.92	26	2.06	2.78
8	2.31	3.36	18	2.10	2.88	28	2.05	2.76
10	2.23	3.17	20	2.09	2.85	30	2.04	2.75

The operator matches the degrees of freedom (df) with the test and looks up the critical *t*-value at the selected level of significance, often $p \leq 0.05$ or $p \leq 0.01$. If the computed *t*-value exceeds the critical value from the table, the null hypothesis is rejected and the difference between method means is statistically significant.

TABLE 5-2 Typical Student's *t*-Test Results

Example 1	Reference Method	New or Modified Method
n	10	10
$\overline{X}$	0.45	0.46
SD	0.01	0.02
Null hypothesis	$\overline{X}$ of control = $\overline{X}$ of test	
Selected *p*-value	0.01	—
Computed *p*-value	0.085	—
Two-tail *t*	0.99	Null hypothesis is supported, means are not unequal
Critical two-tail *t*	2.88	—

Example 2	Reference Method	New or Modified Method
n	10	10
$\overline{X}$	0.40	0.44
SD	0.07	0.07
Null hypothesis	$\overline{X}$ of control = $\overline{X}$ of test	
Selected *p*-value	0.01	—
Computed *p*-value	0.008	—
Two-tail *t*	3.89	Null hypothesis is rejected, means are unequal
Critical two-tail *t*	2.88	—

In the first example of a two-tail *t*-test, the difference in the means does not rise to statistical significance, the computed *p*-value exceeds the selected *p*-value, and the means are "not unequal." In the second example, the selected *p*-value exceeds the computed *p*-value, and the means are unequal.
$\overline{X}$, mean; SD, standard deviation; n, number of data points.

unequal," that is not the same as "equal." To increase the power of the validation, the scientist often chooses to compute the *Pearson correlation coefficient* and to apply *linear regression* and the *Bland-Altman plot*.

Using Analysis of Variance to Compare Variances of More Than Two Data Series

ANOVA accomplishes the same outcomes as the *t*-test; however, ANOVA may be applied to more than two series of data. A laboratory scientist may often choose to compare two, three, or four new methods with a reference method. The ANOVA computes variance (σ^2) for each group (between-group σ^2), an overall σ^2 (within-group σ^2), and an *F*-statistic (similar to the *t*-statistic) based on the within-group σ^2. The *F*-statistic is compared with a table of critical *F*-statistic values to determine significance analogous to the *t*-statistic as shown in Table 5-1.

Like the Student's *t*-test, ANOVA is available on computer spreadsheets. The operator enters the data in one column per data series (group or sample) and applies the ANOVA formula. The test reports *between-groups* df (the number of groups – 1)

and the *within-group* df (total of observations – 1 per group). The test also computes and reports the sum of squares within and between groups, the total sum of squares, the mean squares within and between groups, and the *F*-statistic. Spreadsheet programs compare the *F*-statistic to the table of critical *F*-values and report the *p*-value, which the operator then compares to the selected *p*-value limit to determine significance. Table 5-3 illustrates typical ANOVA results.

Comparing Data Series Using the Pearson Correlation Coefficient

In addition to comparing means by *t*-test or ANOVA, the laboratory professional compares a series of paired data to learn if the data points agree with adequate precision throughout the measurable range. For instance, to validate a new prothrombin time reagent, the scientist or technician assembles 100 plasma aliquots, assays them in sequence using first the new and then the current reagents, and records the paired data points in two spreadsheet columns, *x* and *y*. He or she then applies the spreadsheet's *Pearson product-moment correlation coefficient*

TABLE 5-3 Typical ANOVA Results

SUMMARY OF DESCRIPTIVE STATISTICS (PROVIDED WITH EVERY ANOVA)				
Group	n	Σ	$\bar{x}$	σ^2
Reference	25	63.74	2.55	1.07
Test 1	25	61.17	2.45	0.60
Test 2	25	65.08	2.60	0.68

ANOVA
In this example, the F-value does not exceed the critical F-value from the table of critical values; there is no significant difference among the groups.

Variation source	df	SS	MS	F	p-value	Critical F
Between groups	2	0.32	0.17	0.20	0.82	3.12
Within groups	72	56.37	0.78			
Total	74	56.69	This test fails significance at $p \le 0.05$; null hypothesis is supported			

ANOVA = analysis of variance; df = degrees of freedom; SS = sum of squares; MS = mean squares.

formula to generate a Pearson *r*, or *correlation coefficient*, which may range from –1.0 to +1.0. The spreadsheet uses this formula:

$$r = \frac{\left(\sum xy/n - \bar{x}\bar{y}\right)}{SD_X \, SD_Y},$$

where *r* = Pearson correlation coefficient; $\sum xy$ = sum of the products of each pair of scores; n = number of values; $\bar{x}$ = mean of the X distribution; $\bar{y}$ = mean of the Y distribution; SD_X = SD of the X distribution; and SD_Y = SD of the Y distribution.

Pearson *r*-values from 0 to +1.0 represent positive correlation; 1.0 equals perfect correlation. Laboratorians employ the Pearson formula to assess the range of values from two like assays or to compare assay results to previously assigned standard or calibrator results. Most operators set an *r*-value of 0.975 (or r^2-value of 0.95) as the lower limit of correlation; any Pearson *r*-value less than 0.975 is considered invalid because it indicates unacceptable variability of the reference method.

When the Pearson *r*-value result indicates the adequacy of the range of values, the linear regression *r*-value equation described in the next section is applied. Linear regression finds the line that best predicts *x* from *y* but its equation does not account for dispersion. The Pearson correlation coefficient formula quantifies how *x* and *y* vary together while documenting dispersion.

Comparing Data Series Using Linear Regression
If a series of five calibrators is used, results may be analyzed by the following regression equation:

$$y = a + bx$$

$$\text{Slope } (b) = \left[n\sum XY - \left(\sum X\right)\left(\sum Y\right)\right] / \left[n\sum X^2 - \left(\sum X\right)^2\right]$$

$$\text{Intercept } (a) = \left[\sum Y - b\left(\sum X\right)\right] / n$$

where *x* and *y* are the variables; *a* = the intercept between the regression line and the *y*-axis; *b* = the slope of the regression line; *n* = number of values or elements; *X* = first calibrator value; *Y* = second calibrator value; $\sum XY$ = sum of the product of first and second calibrator values; $\sum X$ = sum of first calibrator values; $\sum Y$ = sum of second calibrator values; and $\sum X^2$ = sum of squared first calibrator values.

Perfect correlation generates a *slope* of 1 and a *y intercept* of 0. Local policy based on total error calculation establishes limits for slope and y intercept; for example, many laboratory directors reject a slope of less than 0.9 or an intercept of more than 10% above or below zero (Figure 5-2).

Slope measures *proportional systematic error*; the higher the analyte value, the greater the deviation from the line of identity. Proportional errors are caused by malfunctioning instrument components or a failure of some part of the testing process. The magnitude of the error increases with the concentration or activity of the analyte. An assay with proportional error may be invalid.

Intercept measures *constant systematic error* (or *bias*, in laboratory vernacular), a constant difference between the new and reference assay regardless of assay result magnitude. A laboratory director may choose to adopt a new assay with systematic error but must modify the published reference interval.

Regression analysis gains sufficient power when 40 or more patient specimens are tested using both the new and reference assay in place of or in addition to calibrators. Data may be entered into a spreadsheet program that offers an automatic regression equation.

Comparing Data Series Using the Bland-Altman Difference Plot
Linear regression and the Pearson correlation coefficient are essential tests of accuracy and performance; however, both are influenced by dispersion. The Bland-Altman difference plot, also known as the Tukey mean-difference plot, provides a graphical representation of agreement between two assays.[19] Similar to the *t*-test, Pearson correlation, and linear regression,

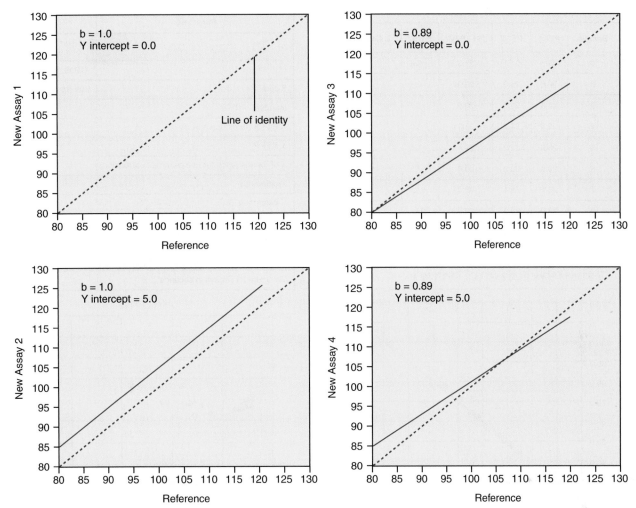

Figure 5-2 Linear regression comparing four new assays with a reference method. Assay 1 is a perfect match. The y intercept of assay 2 is 5.0, which illustrates a constant systematic error, or bias. The slope (*b*) value for assay 3 is 0.89, which illustrates a proportional systematic error. New assay 4 has both bias and proportional error.

paired assay results are tabled in automated spreadsheet columns. This formula is applied:

$$S\ (x,y) = (S_1 + S_2)/2,\ \text{and}\ S_1 - S_2,$$
where S = individual coordinates

The operator computes the mean of the assays and the signed difference between the values. A chart is prepared with the means plotted on the *x*-axis and the numerical or % differences on the *y*-axis. Difference limits are provided, characteristically at $\bar{x} \pm 2$ SD (Figure 5-3). The plot visually illustrates the magnitude of the differences. In a normal distribution, 95.5% of the values are expected to fall within the limits; when more than 5% of data points fall outside the limits, the assay is rejected.

Precision

Unlike the determination of accuracy, assessment of precision (dispersion, reproducibility, variation, random error) is a simple validation effort, because it merely requires performing a series of assays on a single specimen or lot of reference

material (Figure 5-1).[20] Precision studies always assess both *within-day* and *day-to-day* variation about the mean and are usually performed on three to five calibration specimens, although they may also be performed using a series of patient specimens. To calculate within-day precision, the scientist assays a single specimen at least 20 consecutive times using one reagent batch and one instrument run. For day-to-day precision, 20 assays are required on at least 10 runs on 10 consecutive days. The day-to-day precision study employs the same source specimen and instrument but separate aliquots. Day-to-day precision accounts for the effects of different operators, reagents, and environmental conditions such as temperature and barometric pressure.

The collected data from within-day and day-to-day sequences are reduced by formula to the mean and a measure of dispersion such as standard deviation or, most often, coefficient of variation in percent (CV%), as described in "Statistical Significance and Expressions of Central Tendency and Dispersion". The CV% documents the degree of dispersion or random error generated by an assay, a function of assay stability.

Sample	PTT 1	PTT 2	(S1+S2)/2	S1-S2	Difference, %
1	31.5	31.1	31.3	−0.4	−1.3
2	30.0	29.9	30.0	−0.1	−0.3
3	34.3	33.5	33.9	−0.8	−2.4
4	35.6	34.7	35.2	−0.9	−2.6
5	28.6	28.2	28.4	−0.4	−1.4
6	30.8	30.3	30.6	−0.5	−1.6
7	28.1	28.4	28.3	0.3	1.1
8	28.0	28.0	28.0	0.0	0.0
9	28.6	28.1	28.4	−0.5	−1.8
10	29.4	29.2	29.3	−0.2	−0.7

There was a total of 31 data points, 10 of which are shown.

A

Parameter	Value
n	31 (see table A for 10 of the data points)
r^2	0.999 (target = 0.95)
Slope	1.05 (target = 0.9–1.1)
Intercept	1.08
$\bar{X}$ PTT 1 (reference assay)	48.09
$\bar{X}$ PTT 2	47.73
$\bar{X}$ of means (used for Bland-Altman correlation)	47.91
$\bar{X}$ difference	0.36
$\bar{X}$ difference, %	0.98
$\bar{X}$ difference, %/A versus B	0.8 (target = ±8%)
Minimum difference, %	3.92
Maximum difference, %	3.95
Maximum PTT result in seconds	110.02

B

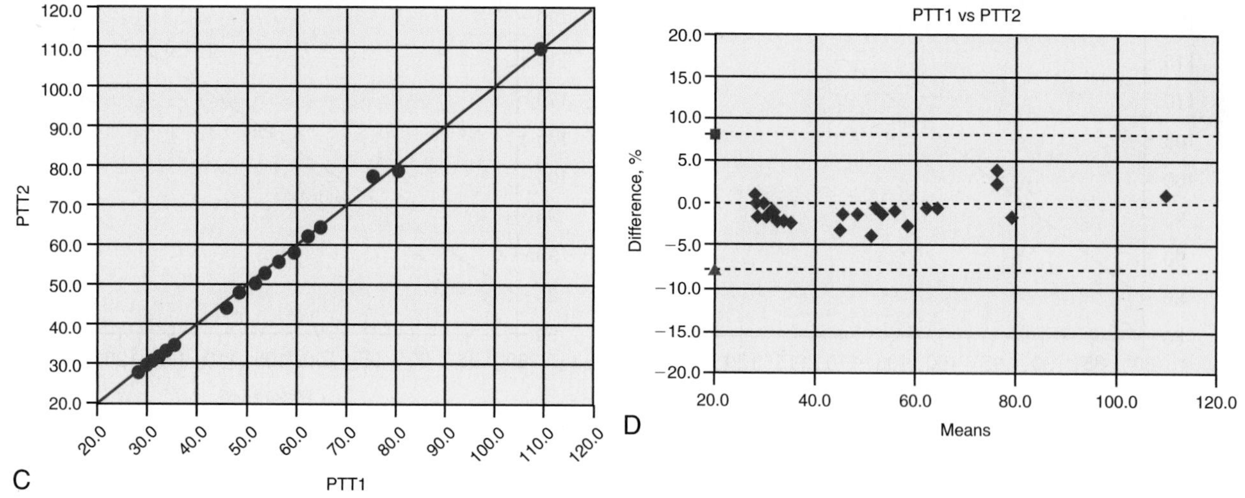

C

D

Figure 5-3 Bland-Altman data and plot. **A,** Excerpt illustrating 10 of the 31 PTT result data points from a current and new reagent; **B,** preliminary correlation data; **C,** identity line; and **D,** Bland-Altman plot based on data given above. The difference between the results from each assay are within the acceptance limits; the new PTT assay is validated. PTT, partial thromboplastin time.

CV% limits are established locally. For analytes based on primary standards, the within-run CV% limit may be 5% or less, and for hematology and hemostasis assays, 10% or less; however, the day-to-day run CV% limits may be as high as 30%, depending on the stability and complexity of the assay. Although accuracy, linearity, and analytical specificity are just as important, medical laboratory professionals often equate the quality of an assay with its CV%. The best assay, of course, is one that combines the smallest CV% with the greatest accuracy.

Precision for visual light microscopy leukocyte differential counts on stained blood films is immeasurably broad, particularly for low-frequency eosinophils and basophils.[21] Most visual differential counts are performed by reviewing 100 to 200 leukocytes. Although impractical, it would take differential counts of 800 or more leukocytes to improve precision to measurable though inadequate levels. Automated differential counts generated by profiling instruments, however, provide CV% levels of 5% or lower because these instruments count thousands of cells.

Linearity

Linearity is the ability to generate results proportional to the calculated concentration or activity of the analyte.[22] The laboratory professional dilutes a high-end calibrator or elevated patient specimen to produce at least five dilutions spanning the full range of the assay. The dilutions are then assayed. Computed and assayed results for each dilution are paired and plotted on a linear graph, x-scale, and y-scale, respectively. The line is inspected visually for nonlinearity at the highest and lowest dilutions (Figure 5-4). The acceptable range of linearity is established just above the low value and below the high value at which linearity loss is evident. Although formulas exist for computing the limits of linearity, visual inspection is an accepted practice. Nonlinear graphs may be transformed using semilog or log-log graphs when necessary.

Patient specimens with results above the linear range must be diluted and reassayed. Results from diluted specimens that fall within the linear range are valid; however, they must be multiplied by the dilution factor (reciprocal of the dilution) to

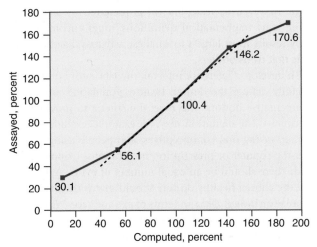

Figure 5-4 Determination of linearity. At least five dilutions of standard or calibrator are prepared. Dilutions must span the expected range of analyte measurements (analytical measurement range, AMR). The concentration of the analyte for each of the five dilutions is calculated. The assayed values are plotted on the y scale and the computed concentrations on the x scale. The linear range is selected by visual inspection, including the dilutions for which assayed values vary in a linear manner. In this example, the limits of linearity are 56.1% to 146.2%. Assay results that fall outside these limits are inaccurate.

produce the final concentration. Laboratory personnel never report results that fall below or above the linear limits, because accuracy is compromised in the nonlinear regions of the assay. Lower limits are especially important when counting platelets or assaying coagulation factors. For example, the difference between 1% and 3% coagulation factor VIII activity affects treatment options and the potential for predicting coagulation factor inhibitor formation. Likewise, the difference between a platelet count of 10,000/μL and 5000/μL affects the decision to treat with platelet concentrate.

Lower Limit of Detection

Linearity studies are coupled with the *lower limit of detection* study.[23] A "zero calibrator," or blank, is assayed 20 times, and the mean and standard deviation are computed from the results. The lower limit of detection is determined from the computed standard deviation. The limit is three standard deviations above the mean of blank assay results. This cutoff prevents false-positive results generated by low-end assay interference, commonly called *noise*. The manufacturer or distributor typically performs limit assays and provides the results on

the package insert; however, local policies often require that results of the manufacturer's limit studies be confirmed.

Analytical Specificity

Analytical specificity is the ability of an assay to distinguish the analyte of interest from anticipated interfering substances within the specimen matrix. The laboratory practitioner "spikes" identical specimens with potential interfering substances and measures the effects of each upon the assay results. Analytical specificity is determined by the manufacturer and need not be confirmed at the local laboratory unless there is suspicion of interference from a particular substance not assayed by the manufacturer. Manufacturer specificity data are transferred from the package insert to the laboratory validation report.

Levels of Laboratory Assay Approval

The U.S. Food and Drug Administration (FDA) categorizes assays as *cleared, analyte-specific reagent* (ASR) assays, *research use only* (RUO), and laboratory-developed (home-brew) assays. FDA-cleared assays are approved for the detection of specific analytes and should not be used for non-cleared (off-label) applications. ASRs that are bundled with other ASRs or other general reagents and labeled with an intentional use are subject to premarket review requirements. RUO kits may be used on a trial basis, but the institution or a clinical trial typically bears their expense, not the third-party payer or the patient. The FDA monitors in-house assays by regulating the main components, which include, but are not limited to, ASRs, locally prepared reagents, and laboratory instrumentation. Details are given in Table 5-4.

Documentation and Reliability

Validation is recorded on standard forms available from commercial sources, for example, Data Innovations LLC EP Evaluator®. Validation records are stored for 7 to 10 years in readily accessible databases and made available to laboratory assessors upon request.[24]

Precision and accuracy records document assay reliability over specified periods. The recalibration interval may be once every 6 months or in accordance with operators' manual recommendations. Recalibration is necessary whenever reagent lots are updated unless the laboratory professional can demonstrate that the reportable range is unchanged using lot-to-lot comparison. When control results demonstrate a shift or consistently fall outside action limits, or when an instrument

TABLE 5-4 Categories of Laboratory Assay Approval by the United States Food and Drug Administration

Assay Category	Comment
FDA-cleared assay	The local institution may use package insert data for linearity and specificity but must establish accuracy and precision.
Analyte-specific reagent	Manufacturer may provide individual reagents but not in kit form, and may not provide package insert validation data. Local institution must perform all validation steps.
Research use only	Local institution must perform all validation steps. Research use only assays are intended for clinical trials, and carriers are not required to pay.
Laboratory-developed assay	Assays devised locally, Food and Drug Administration evaluates using criteria developed for FDA-cleared assay kits.

is repaired, the laboratory professional repeats the validation procedure.[25]

Regularly scheduled validity rechecks, lot-to-lot comparisons, instrument preventive maintenance, staff competence, and scheduled performance of internal quality control and external quality assessment procedures ensure continued reliability and enhance the value of a laboratory assay to the patient and physician.

LOT-TO-LOT COMPARISONS

Laboratory managers reach agreements with vendors to sequester kit and reagent lots, thereby ensuring infrequent lot changes, optimistically no more than once a year.[26] The new reagent lot must arrive approximately a month before the laboratory runs out of the old lot so that *lot-to-lot comparisons* may be completed and differences resolved, if necessary. The scientist uses control or patient specimens and prepares a range of analyte dilutions, typically five, spanning the limits of linearity. If the reagent kits provide controls, these are also included, and all are assayed using the old and new reagent lots. Results are charted as illustrated in Table 5-5.

Action limits vary by laboratory, but many managers reject the new lot when more than one specimen (data point pair) generates a variance greater than 10% or when all variances are positive or negative. In the latter case, the new lot may be rejected or it may be necessary to use the lot but develop a new reference interval and therapeutic range.

For several analytes, lot-to-lot comparisons include revalidation of the analytical measurement range (AMR) or reportable range. AMR is the range of results a method produces without any specimen pre-treatment, such as dilution, and is similar to a linearity study.

DEVELOPMENT OF THE REFERENCE INTERVAL AND THERAPEUTIC RANGE

Once an assay is validated, the laboratory professional develops the *reference interval* (reference range, normal range).[26] Most laboratory professionals use the vernacular phrase *normal*

range; however, *reference interval* is preferred by statisticians. Using strict mathematical definitions, *range* encompasses all assay results from largest to smallest, whereas *interval* is a statistic that trims outliers.

To develop a reference interval, the laboratory professional carefully defines the desired healthy population and recruits representative donors who meet the criteria to provide blood specimens. The definition may, for example, exclude smokers, women taking oral contraceptives, and people using specified over-the-counter or prescription medications. Donors may be paid. There should be an equal number of males and females, and the chosen healthy donors should match the institution's population *demographics* in terms of age and race. When practical, large-volume blood specimens are collected, aliquotted, and placed in long-term storage. For instance, plasma aliquots for coagulation reference interval development are stored indefinitely at –70° C. It may be impractical to develop local reference intervals for infants, children, or geriatric populations. In these cases the laboratory director may choose to use published (textbook) intervals.[27] In general, although published reference intervals are available for educational and general discussion purposes, local laboratories must generate their own reference intervals for adults to most closely match the demographics of the area served by their institution.

The minimum number of subject specimens (data points) required to develop a reference interval may be determined using statistical power computations; however, practical limitations prevail.[28] For a new assay with no currently established reference interval, a minimum of 120 data points is necessary. In most cases, however, the assay manufacturer provides a reference interval on the package insert, and the local laboratory practitioner need only assay 30 specimens, approximately 15 male and 15 female, to validate the manufacturer's reference interval, a process called *transference.* Likewise, the practitioner may refer to published reference intervals and, once they are locally validated, transfer them to the institution's report form.

Scientists assume that the population specimens employed to generate reference intervals will produce frequency distributions (in laboratory vernacular, *histograms*) that are normal bell-shaped (Gaussian) curves (Figure 5-5). In a Gaussian frequency distribution the mean is at the center; the mean, median, and mode coincide; and the dispersion about the mean is identical in both directions. In many instances, however, biologic frequency distributions are "log-normal" with a "tail" on the high end. For example, laboratory professionals assumed for years that the visual reticulocyte percentage reference interval in adults is 0.5% to 1.5%; however, repeated analysis of healthy populations in several locations has established the interval to be 0.5% to 2%, owing to a subset of healthy donors whose reticulocyte counts fall at the high end of the interval.[29] Scientists may choose to live with a log-normal distribution, or they may transform it by replotting the curve using a semilog or log-log graphic display. The decision to transform may arise locally but eventually becomes adopted as a national practice standard.

In a normal distribution, the mean ($\bar{x}$) is computed by dividing the sum of the observed values by the number of data

TABLE 5-5 Example of a Lot-to-Lot Comparison

Specimen	Old Lot Value	New Lot Value	% Difference
Low	7	6	−14.3%
Low middle value	12	12	0
Middle	20.5	19.4	−5%
High middle	31	27	−12.9%
High	48	48	0
Old kit control 1	9	11	22%
Old kit control 2	22	24	9%
New kit control 1	10	10	0
New kit control 2	24	24	0

Negative % difference indicates the new lot value is below the old lot (reference) value. The new lot is rejected because the low and high middle value results differ by more than 10%.

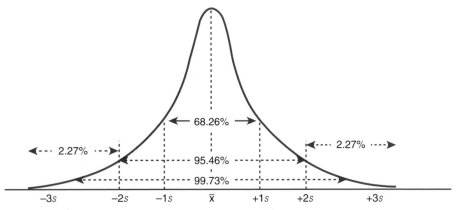

Figure 5-5 Normal (Gaussian) distribution. When the test values obtained for a given subject population are normally distributed, the mean is at the peak and the mean, mode, and median coincide. The segments of the population distribution representing ±1, ±2, and ±3 standard deviations are illustrated. In developing the reference interval, laboratory directors often use ±2 standard deviations to establish the 95.5% confidence interval. This means that 95.46% of the test values from the healthy population are included within ±2 standard deviations. Consequently, 4.54%, or approximately 1 in 20 test results from theoretically healthy donors, fall outside the interval, half (2.27%) above and half below.

points, *n*, as shown in the equation in the section entitled "Statistical Significance and Expressions of Central Tendency and Dispersion." The standard deviation is calculated using the formula provided in the same section. A typical reference interval is computed as ±2 standard deviations and assumes that the distribution is normal (Gaussian). The limits at ±2 standard deviations encompass 95.46% of results from healthy individuals, known as the *95.5% confidence interval*. This implies that 4.54% of results from theoretically healthy individuals fall outside the interval. A standard deviation computed from a non-Gaussian distribution may turn out to be too narrow to reflect the true reference interval and may thus encompass fewer than 95.5% of results from presumed healthy donors and generate a number of false positives. Assays with high CV% values have high levels of random error reflected in a broad curve; low CV% assays with "tight" dispersal have smaller random error and generate a narrow curve, as illustrated in Figure 5-1. The breadth of the curve may also reflect biologic variation in values of the analyte.

A few hematology and hemostasis assays are used to monitor drug therapy. For instance, the international normalized ratio (INR) for prothrombin time is used to monitor the effects of oral Coumadin (warfarin) therapy, and the therapeutic range is universally established at an INR of 2 to 3. On the other hand, the therapeutic range for monitoring treatment with unfractionated heparin using the partial thromboplastin time (PTT) assay must be established locally by graphically comparing regression of the PTT results in seconds against the results of the *chromogenic anti-Xa heparin assay*, whose therapeutic range is established empirically as 0.3 to 0.7 international heparin units. The PTT therapeutic range is called the *Brill-Edwards curve* and is described in Chapter 42.

If assay revalidation or lot-to-lot comparison reveals a systematic change caused by reagent or kit modifications, a new reference interval (and therapeutic range, when applicable) is established. The laboratory director must advise the hospital staff of reference interval and therapeutic range changes because failure to observe new intervals and ranges may result in diagnosis and treatment errors.

INTERNAL QUALITY CONTROL

Controls

Laboratory managers prepare, or more often purchase, assay *controls*. Although it may appear similar, a control is wholly distinct from a calibrator. Indeed, cautious laboratory directors may insist that controls be purchased from distributors different from those who supply their calibrators. As discussed in the section "Validation of a New or Modified Assay," calibrators are used to adjust instrumentation or to develop a standard curve. Calibrators are assayed by a reference method in expert laboratories, and their assigned value is certified. Controls are used independently of the calibration process so that systematic errors caused by deterioration of the calibrator or a change in the analytical process can be detected through internal quality control. This process is continuous and is called *calibration verification*.[29] Compared with calibrators, control materials are inexpensive and are prepared from the same matrix as patient specimens except for preservatives, lyophilization, or freezing necessary to prolong shelf life. Controls provide known values and are sampled alongside patient specimens to accomplish within-run assay validation. In nearly all instances, two controls are required per test run: one within the reference interval and one above or below the reference interval. For some assays there is reason to select controls whose values are just outside the upper or lower limit of the reference interval, "slightly" abnormal. In institutions that perform continuous runs, the controls should be run at least once per shift, for instance, at 7 AM, 3 PM, and 11 PM. In laboratories where assay runs are discrete events, two controls are assayed with each run.

Control results must fall within predetermined dispersal limits, typically ±2 SD. Control manufacturers provide limits; however, local laboratory practitioners must validate and transfer manufacturer limits or establish their own, usually

TABLE 5-6 Steps Used to Correct an Out-of-Control Assay Run

Step	Description
1. Reassay	When a limit of ±2 standard deviations is used, 5% of expected assay results fall above or below the limit.
2. Prepare new control and reassay	Controls may deteriorate over time when exposed to adverse temperatures or subjected to conditions causing evaporation.
3. Prepare fresh reagents and reassay	Reagents may have evaporated or become contaminated.
4. Recalibrate instrument	Instrument may require repair.

by computing standard deviation from the first 20 control assays. Whenever the result for a control is outside the established limits, the run is rejected and the cause is found and corrected. The steps for correction are listed in Table 5-6.

Control results are plotted on a Levey-Jennings chart that displays each data point in comparison to the mean and limits (Figure 5-6).[30] The Levey-Jennings chart assumes that the control results distribute in a Gaussian manner and provide limits at 1, 2, and 3 SD above and below the mean. In addition to being analyzed for single-run errors, the data points are examined for sequential errors over time (Figure 5-7). Both single-run and long-term control variation are a function of assay dispersion or random error and reflect the CV% of an assay.

Dr. James Westgard has established a series of internal quality control rules that are routinely applied to long-term deviations, called the *Westgard rules*.[31] The rules were developed for assays that employ primary standards, but a few Westgard rules

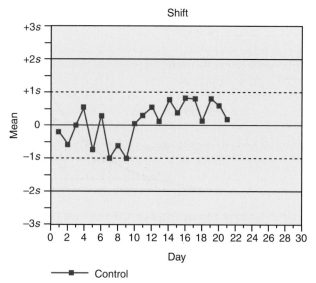

Figure 5-7 Levey-Jennings chart that illustrates a systematic error or *Westgard 10x* condition (shift, Table 5-7). Control results from 21 runs in 22 days all fall within the action limits established as ±2 standard deviations (*s*); however, the final 11 control results are above the mean. When 10 consecutive control results fall on one side of the mean, the assay has been affected by a systematic error (shift). The operator troubleshoots and recalibrates the assay.

TABLE 5-7 Westgard Rules Employed in Hematology and Hemostasis

1_{3s}	A single control value is outside the ±3 SD limit.
2_{2s}	Two control values are outside the ±2 SD limit.
R_{4s}	Two consecutive control values within a run are more than 4 SD apart.
4_{1s}	Four consecutive control values within a run exceed the mean by ±1 SD.
10_X	Also called a "shift." A series of 10 consecutive control values remain within the dispersal limits but are consistently above or below the mean.
7_T	Also called a "trend." A series of at least 7 control values trend in a consistent direction.

10_X or 7_T may indicate an instrument calibration issue that has introduced a constant systematic error (bias). Shifts or trends may be caused by deterioration of reagents, pump fittings, or light sources. Abrupt shifts may reflect a reagent or instrument fitting change.

In all cases, assay results are rejected and the error is identified using the steps in Table 5-6.

that are the most useful in hematology and hemostasis laboratories are provided in Table 5-7, along with the appropriate actions to be taken.[32]

Moving Average ($\bar{X}_B$) of the Red Blood Cell Indices

In 1974, Dr. Brian Bull proposed a method of employing *patient* RBC indices to monitor the stability of hematology analyzers, recognizing that the RBC indices mean cell volume (MCV), mean cell hemoglobin (MCH), and mean cell hemoglobin

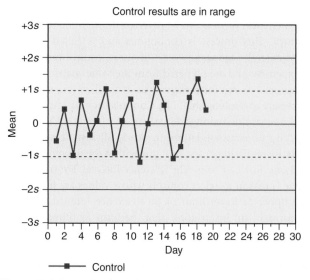

Figure 5-6 Levey-Jennings chart illustrating acceptable control results. Control results from 19 runs in 20 days all fall within the action limits established as ±2 standard deviations (*s*). Results distribute evenly about the mean.

concentration (MCHC) remain constant on average despite individual patient variations.[33] Each consecutive sequence of 20 patient RBC index assay results is collected and treated by the moving average formula (see reference), which accumulates, "smooths," and "trims" data to reduce the effect of outliers. Each trimmed 20-specimen mean, $\overline{X}_{B'}$ is plotted on a Levey-Jennings chart and tracked for trends and shifts using Westgard rules. The formula has been automated and embedded in the circuitry of all hematology analyzers, which provide a Levey-Jennings chart for MCV, MCH, and MCHC. The moving average concept has been generalized to WBC and platelet counts and to some clinical chemistry analytes, albeit with moderate success.

To begin, 500 consecutive specimens are analyzed for the mean MCV, MCH, and MCHC. A Levey-Jennings chart is prepared using ±3% of the mean or one SD as the action limits, and subsequent data accumulation commences in groups of 20.

The moving average method requires a computer to calculate the averages, does not detect within-run errors, and is less sensitive than the use of commercial controls in detecting systematic shifts and trends. It works well in institutions that assay specimens from generalized populations that contain minimal numbers of sickle cell or oncology patients. A population that has a high percentage of abnormal hematologic results, as may be seen in a tertiary care facility, may generate a preponderance of moving average outliers.[34] Moving average systems do not replace the use of control specimens but provide additional means to detect shifts and trends.

Delta Checks

The δ-check system compares a current analyte result with the result from the most recent previous analysis for the same patient.[35] Certain patient values remain relatively consistent over time unless there is an intervention. A result that fails a δ-check, often a 20% deviation, is investigated for intervention such as a transfusion or surgery, or a profound change in the patient's condition subsequent to the previous analysis. If there is no ready explanation, the failed δ-check may indicate an analytical error or mislabeled specimen. Results that fail a δ-check are sequestered until the cause is found. Laboratory directors may require δ-checks on MCV, RDW, HGB, PLT, PT, INR, and PTT. Action limits for δ-checks are based on clinical impression and are assigned by hematology and hemostasis laboratory directors in collaboration with clinicians and laboratory staff. Computerization is essential, and δ-checks are designed only to identify gross errors, not changes in random error, or shifts or trends. There is no regulatory requirement for δ-checks.

EXTERNAL QUALITY ASSESSMENT

External quality assessment further validates the accuracy of hematology and hemostasis assays by comparing results from identical aliquots of specimens distributed at regular intervals among laboratories nationwide or worldwide. The aliquots are often called *survey* or *proficiency testing* specimens and include preserved human donor plasma and whole blood, stained peripheral blood films and bone marrow smears, and photomicrographs of cells or tissues.

In most proficiency testing systems, target (true or reference) values for the test specimens are established in-house by their manufacturer or distributor and are then further validated by preliminary distribution to a handful of "expert" laboratories. Separate target values may be assigned for various assay methods and instruments, as feasible.

Laboratories that participate in external quality assessment are directed to manage the survey specimens using the same principles as those employed for patient specimens—survey specimens should not receive special attention. Turnaround is swift, and results are sent electronically to the provider.

In addition to establishing a target value, agencies that administer surveys reduce the returned data to statistics, including the mean, median, and standard deviation of all participant results. Provided the survey is large enough, the statistics may be computed individually for the various instruments and assay methods. The statistics collected from participants should match the predetermined targets. If they do not, the agency troubleshoots the assay and assigns the most reliable statistics, usually the group mean and standard deviations.

The agency provides a report to each laboratory, illustrating its result in comparison with the target value and appending a comment if the laboratory result exceeds the established limits, usually ±2 standard deviations from the mean. If the specimen is a blood or bone marrow smear, a photomicrograph, or a problem that requires a binary (positive/negative, yes/no) response, the local laboratory comment is compared with expert opinion and consensus.

Although a certain level of error is tolerated, error rates that exceed established limits result in corrective recommendations or, in extreme circumstances, loss of laboratory accreditation or licensure.

There are a number of external quality assessment agencies; however, the College of American Pathologists (CAP, cap.org) and the American Proficiency Institute (API, api-pt.com) provide the largest survey systems. Survey packages are provided for laboratories offering all levels of service. API and CAP are nongovernmental agencies; however, survey participation is necessary to meet the accreditation requirements of the Joint Commission (jointcommission.org) and to qualify for Medicare reimbursement. The North American Specialized Coagulation Laboratory Association (nascola.org) provides survey systems for specialty coagulation laboratories in the United States and Canada and is affiliated with the ECAT (external quality control of diagnostic assays and tests, ecat.nl) Foundation External Quality Assessment Program of the Netherlands, which provides survey materials throughout Europe. Many state health agencies provide proficiency testing surveys, requiring laboratories to participate as a condition of licensure.

ASSESSING DIAGNOSTIC EFFICACY

Since the 1930s, surgeons have used the *bleeding time* test to predict the risk of intraoperative hemorrhage. The laboratory scientist, technician, or phlebotomist activates an automated lancet to make a 5-mm long, 1-mm deep incision in the volar surface of the forearm and uses a clean piece of filter paper to meticulously absorb drops of blood in 30-second intervals. The time interval from initial incision to bleeding cessation is recorded, normally 2 to 9 minutes. The test is simple and logical, and experts have claimed for over 50 years that if the incision bleeds for longer than 9 minutes, there is a risk of surgical bleeding. In the 1990s clinical researchers compared within-range and prolonged bleeding times with instances of intraoperative bleeding and found to their surprise that prolonged bleeding time results predicted fewer than 50% of intraoperative bleeds.[36,37] Many bleeds occurred despite a bleeding time shorter than 9 minutes. Thus, the positive predictive value of the bleeding time for intraoperative bleeding was less than 50%, which is the probability of turning up heads in a coin toss. Today the bleeding time test is widely agreed to have no clinical efficacy and is obsolete, though still available.

Like the bleeding time test, many time-honored hematology and hemostasis assays gain credibility on the basis of logic and expert opinion. Now, however, besides being valid, accurate, linear, and precise, a new or modified assay must be diagnostically effective.[38] To compute diagnostic efficacy, the laboratory professional obtains a series of specimens from healthy subjects, volunteers who do not have the particular disease or condition being measured, called *controls*; and from patients who *conclusively possess a disease or condition*. The patients' diagnosis is based on downstream clinical outcomes, discharge notes, or the results of valid existing laboratory tests, excluding the new assay. The new assay is then applied to specimens from both the healthy control and disease patient groups to assess its efficacy.

In a perfect world, the laboratory scientist sets the *discrimination threshold* at the 95.5% confidence interval limit (± 2 SD) of the mean. When this threshold, also called the limit or "cut point," is used, the test hopefully yields a positive result, meaning a level elevated beyond the upper limit or reduced below the lower limit, in every instance of disease and a negative result, within the reference interval, in all subjects (controls) without the disease. In reality, there is always some overlap: a "gray area" in which some positive test results are generated from non-disease specimens (*false positives*) and some negative results are generated from specimens taken from patients with proven disease (*false negatives*). False positives cause unnecessary anxiety, follow-up expense, and erroneous diagnostic leads—worrisome, expensive, and time consuming, but seldom fatal. False negatives fail to detect the disease and may delay treatment which can be potentially life threatening. The laboratory scientist employs diagnostic efficacy computations to establish the effectiveness of laboratory assays and to minimize both false-positive and false-negative results (Table 5-8). Diagnostic efficacy testing includes determination of diagnostic sensitivity and specificity, positive and negative predictive value, and receiver operating characteristic analysis.

To start a diagnostic efficacy study, the scientist selects control specimens from healthy subjects and specimens from patients proven to have the disease or condition addressed

TABLE 5-8 Diagnostic Efficacy Definitions and Binary Display

True positive	Assay correctly identifies a disease or condition in those who have it.
False positive	Assay incorrectly identifies disease when none is present.
True negative	Assay correctly excludes a disease or condition in those without it.
False negative	Assay incorrectly excludes disease when it is present.

	Individuals Unaffected by the Disease or Condition	Individuals Affected by the Disease or Condition
Assay is negative	True negative	False negative
Assay is positive	False positive	True positive

by the assay. To make this discussion simple, assume that 50 specimens of each are chosen. All are assayed, and the results are shown in Table 5-9.

The scientist next computes diagnostic sensitivity and specificity and positive and negative predictive value as shown in Table 5-10. These values are then used to consider the conditions in which the assay may be effectively used.

The Effects of Population Incidence and Odds Ratios on Diagnostic Efficacy

Epidemiologists describe population events using the terms *prevalence* and *incidence*. Prevalence describes the total number of events or conditions in a broadly defined population, for instance, the total number of patients with chronic heart disease in the United States. Prevalence quantitates the burden of a disease on society but is not qualified by time intervals and does not predict disease risk.

Incidence describes the number of events occurring within a randomly selected number of subjects representing a population, over a defined time, for instance, the number of new cases of heart disease per 100,000 U.S. residents per year. Incidence numbers are non-cumulative. Incidence can be further defined, for instance by the number of heart disease cases per 100,000 nonsmokers, 100,000 women, or 100,000 people ages 40 to 50. Scientists use incidence, not prevalence, to select

TABLE 5-9 Diagnostic Efficacy Study

	Individuals Unaffected by the Disease or Condition	Individuals Affected by the Disease or Condition
Assay is negative	True negative: 40	False negative: 5
Assay is positive	False positive: 10	True positive: 45

Data on specimens from 50 individuals who are unaffected by the disease or condition and 50 individuals who are affected by the disease or condition.

TABLE 5-10 Diagnostic Efficacy Computations

Statistic	Definition	Formula	Example*
Diagnostic sensitivity	Proportion with the disease who have a positive test result	Sensitivity (%) = TP/(TP + FN) × 100	45/(45 + 5) × 100 = 90%
Distinguish diagnostic sensitivity from analytical sensitivity. Analytical sensitivity is a measure of the smallest increment of the analyte that can be distinguished by the assay.			
Diagnostic specificity	Proportion without the disease who have a negative test result	Specificity (%) = TN/(TN + FP) × 100	40/(40 +10) × 100 = 80%
Distinguish diagnostic specificity from analytical specificity. Analytical specificity is the ability of the assay to distinguish the analyte from interfering substances.			
Positive predictive value (PPV)	Proportion with a disease who have a positive test result compared with all individuals who have a positive test result	PPV (%) = TP/(TP + FP) × 100	45/(45 + 10) × 100 = 82%
The positive predictive value predicts the probability that an individual with a positive assay result has the disease or condition.			
Negative predictive value (NPV)	Proportion without a disease who have a negative test result compared with all individuals who have a negative test result	NPV (%) = TN/(TN + FN) × 100	40/(40 + 5) × 100 = 89%
The negative predictive value predicts the probability that an individual with a negative assay result does not have the disease or condition.			

FN, false negative; FP, false positive; TN, true negative; TP, true positive.
*Using data from Table 5-9.

laboratory assays for specific applications such as screening or confirmation.

For all assays, as diagnostic sensitivity rises, specificity declines. A *screening test* is an assay that is applied to a large number of subjects within a convenience sample where the participant's condition is unknown, for example, lipid profiles offered in a shopping mall. Assays that possess high sensitivity and low specificity make effective screening tests, although they produce a number of false positives. For instance, if the condition being studied has an incidence of 0.0001 (1 in 10,000 per year) and the false-positive rate is a modest 1%, the assay will produce 99 false-positive results for every true-positive result. Clearly such a test is useful only when the consequence of a false-positive result is minimal and follow-up confirmation is readily available.

Conversely, as specificity rises, sensitivity declines. Assays with high specificity provide effective confirmation when used in follow-up to positive results on screening assays. High-specificity assays produce a number of false negatives and should not be used as initial screens. A positive result on both a screening assay and a confirmatory assay provides a definitive conclusion. A positive screening result followed by a negative confirmatory test result generates a search for alternative diagnoses.

Laboratory assays are most effective when chosen to assess patients with high clinical pretest probability. In such instances, the incidence of the condition is high enough to mitigate the effects of false positives and false negatives. For instance, when a physician orders hemostasis testing for patients who are experiencing easy bruising, there is a high pretest probability, which raises the assays' diagnostic efficacy. Conversely, ordering hemostasis assays as screens of healthy individuals prior to elective surgery introduces a low pretest probability and reduces the efficacy of the test profile, raising the relative rate of false positives.

Epidemiologists further assist laboratory professionals by designing prospective randomized control trials to predict the relative odds ratio (or relative risk ratio, RRR) and the absolute odds ratio (or absolute risk ratio, ARR) of an intervention that is designed to modify the incidence of an event within a selected population, as illustrated in the following example.[38]

You design a 5-year study in which you select 2000 obese smokers ages 40 to 60 who have no heart disease. You randomly select 1000 for intervention: periodic laboratory assays for inflammatory markers, with follow-up aspirin for those who have positive assay results. The 1000 controls are tested with the same lab assays but are given a placebo that resembles aspirin. The primary endpoint is acute myocardial infarction (AMI). No one dies or drops out, and at the end of five years, 100 of the 1000 controls and 50 of the 1000 members of the intervention arm have suffered AMIs. The control arm ratio is 100/1000 = 0.1; the intervention arm ratio is 50/1000 = 0.05; and the RRR is 0.05/0.1 = 0.5 (50%). You predict from your study that the odds (RRR) of having a heart attack are cut in half by the intervention. You repeat the study using 2000 slim nonsmokers ages 20 to 40. In this sample, 10 of the 1000 controls and 5 in the intervention group suffer AMIs, the computation is 0.01/0.005 = 0.5, same as in the obese smoker group, thus enabling you to generalize your results to slim non-smokers. RRR has been used extensively to support widespread medical interventions, often without regard to control arm incidence or the risks associated with generalizing to non-studied populations.

You go on to compute the ARR, which is the absolute value of the arithmetic *difference* in the event rates of the control and intervention arms.[39] In our example using the obese smokers group, the ARR = 0.1 − 0.05 = 0.05, or 5% (not 50%, as reported in the example using RRR above). The ARR is often expressed as the number necessary to treat (NNT), the inverse of ARR. In our example, for everyone whose AMI is prevented by the laboratory test and subsequent treatment, you would have to treat 20 total donors over a 5-year period. Further, if you reduce the ARR to an annual rate, 0.05/5 years = 0.01, or a 1% annual reduction. You conclude from your study that 100 interventions per year are required to prevent one AMI.

Finally, your RRR and ARR are not discrete integers but means computed from samples of 1000, so they must include an expression of dispersion, usually ±2 SD or a 95.5% confidence interval. Suppose the 95.5% confidence interval for the RRR turns out to be relatively broad: −0.1 to +1.1. A ratio of 1 implies no effect from the intervention, that is, the rate of change in the intervention arm is equal to the rate of change in the control arm. Given that the 95.5% confidence interval embraces the number 1, the intervention has failed to provide any benefit.

In summary, once a laboratory assay is verified to be accurate and precise, it must then be revealed to possess diagnostic efficacy and to provide for effective intervention as determined by favorable RRR and ARR or NNT values. Application of the receiver operating characteristic (ROC) curve may help achieve these goals.

RECEIVER OPERATING CHARACTERISTIC CURVE

A ROC curve is a further refinement of diagnostic efficacy testing that may be employed to determine the decision limit (cutoff, threshold) for an assay when the assay generates a *continuous variable*.[40] In diagnostic efficacy testing as described in the previous section, the ±2 SD limits of the reference interval are used as the thresholds for discriminating a positive from a negative test result. Often the "true" threshold varies from the ±2 SD limit. Using ROC analysis, the limit is adjusted by increments of 1 (or other increments depending upon the analytical range), and the true-positive and false-positive rates are recomputed for each new threshold level using the same formulas provided in the section named "Assessing Diagnostic Efficacy." The limit that is finally selected is the one that provides the largest true-positive and smallest false-positive rate (Figure 5-8). The operator generates a line graph plotting true positives on the *y*-axis and false positives on the *x*-axis. Measuring the *area under the curve* (a computer-based calculus function) assesses the overall efficacy of the assay. If the area under the curve is 0.5, the curve is at the line of identity between false and true positives and provides no discrimination. Most agree that a clinically useful assay should have an area under the curve of 0.85 or higher.[41]

ASSAY FEASIBILITY

Most laboratory managers and directors review assay feasibility before launching complex validation, efficacy, reference interval, and quality control initiatives. Feasibility studies include a review of assay throughput (number of assays per unit time), dwell time (length of assay interval from specimen sampling to report), cost per test, cost/benefit ratio, turnaround time, and the technical skill required to perform the assay. To select a new instrument, the manager reviews issues of operator safety, footprint, overhead, compatibility with laboratory utilities and information system, the need for middleware, frequency and duration of breakdowns, and distributor support and service.

LABORATORY STAFF COMPETENCE

Staff integrity and professional staff competence are the keys to assay reliability. In the United States, California, Florida, Georgia, Hawaii, Louisiana, Montana, Nevada, New York, North Dakota, Rhode Island, Tennessee, West Virginia, and Puerto Rico enforce licensure laws. In these states, only licensed laboratory professionals may be employed in medical center or reference laboratories. Legislatures in Alaska, Illinois, Massachusetts, Minnesota, Missouri, Vermont, and Virginia have considered and rejected licensure bills, the bills having been opposed by competing health care specialty associations and for-profit entities. In non-licensure states, conscientious laboratory directors employ only nationally certified professionals. Certification is available from the American Society for Clinical Pathology Board of Certification in Chicago, Illinois. Studies of laboratory errors and outcomes demonstrate that laboratories that employ only licensed or certified professionals produce the most reliable assay results.[42,43]

Competent laboratory staff members continuously watch for and document errors by inspecting the results of internal validation and quality control programs and external quality assessment. Error is inevitable, and incidents should be documented and highlighted for quality improvement and instruction. When error is associated with reprimand, the opportunity for improvement may be lost to cover-up. Except in cases of negligence, the analysis of error without blame is consistently practiced in an effort to improve the quality of laboratory service.

Proficiency Systems

Laboratory managers and directors assess and document professional staff skills using proficiency systems. The hematology laboratory manager may, for instance, maintain a collection of normal and abnormal blood films, case studies, or laboratory assay reports that technicians and scientists are required to examine at regular intervals. Personnel who fail to reproduce the target values on examination of the blood film are provided remedial instruction. The proficiency set may also be used to assess applicants for laboratory positions. Proficiency testing systems are available from external quality assessment agencies, and proficiency reports are made accessible to laboratory assessors.

Continuing Education

The American Society for Clinical Pathology Board of Certification and state medical laboratory personnel licensure boards require technicians and scientists to participate in and document

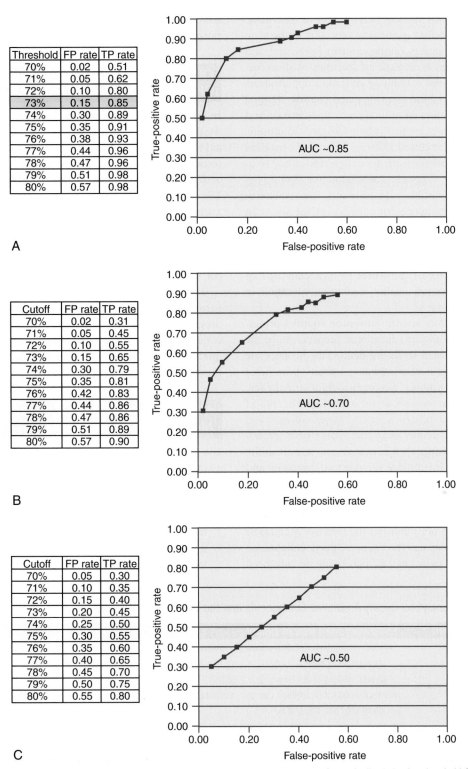

Threshold	FP rate	TP rate
70%	0.02	0.51
71%	0.05	0.62
72%	0.10	0.80
73%	0.15	0.85
74%	0.30	0.89
75%	0.35	0.91
76%	0.38	0.93
77%	0.44	0.96
78%	0.47	0.96
79%	0.51	0.98
80%	0.57	0.98

A

Cutoff	FP rate	TP rate
70%	0.02	0.31
71%	0.05	0.45
72%	0.10	0.55
73%	0.15	0.65
74%	0.30	0.79
75%	0.35	0.81
76%	0.42	0.83
77%	0.44	0.86
78%	0.47	0.86
79%	0.51	0.89
80%	0.57	0.90

B

Cutoff	FP rate	TP rate
70%	0.05	0.30
71%	0.10	0.35
72%	0.15	0.40
73%	0.20	0.45
74%	0.25	0.50
75%	0.30	0.55
76%	0.35	0.60
77%	0.40	0.65
78%	0.45	0.70
79%	0.50	0.75
80%	0.55	0.80

C

Figure 5-8 A, Receiver operating characteristic curve. The false-positive and true-positive rates for each discrimination threshold from 70% to 80% are computed and graphed as paired variables on a linear scale, false-positive rate on the horizontal (x) scale and true-positive rate on the vertical (y) scale. The assay has acceptable discrimination between affected and non-affected individuals; with an area under the curve (AUC) of 0.85, and 73% is the threshold that produces the most desirable false-positive and true-positive rates. **B,** This assay has unacceptable discrimination between affected and unaffected individuals, with an AUC of 0.70. It is difficult to find the threshold that produces the most desirable false-positive and true-positive rates. **C,** This assay, with an AUC of 0.50, has no ability to discriminate. *FP,* false positive; *TP,* true positive.

continuing education for *periodic recertification* or *relicensure.* Educators and experts deliver continuing education in the form of journal articles, case studies, online seminars (webinars), and seminars and workshops at professional meetings. Medical centers offer periodic internal continuing education opportunities (in-service education) in the form of grand rounds, lectures, seminars, and participative educational events. Presentation and discussion of current cases are particularly effective. Continuing education maintains the critical skills of laboratory personnel and provides opportunities to learn about new clinical and technical approaches. The Colorado Association for Continuing Medical Laboratory Education (cacmle.org), the American Society for Clinical Laboratory Science (ascls.org), the American Society for Clinical Pathology (ascp.org), the American Society of Hematology (hematology.org), the National Hemophilia Foundation (hemophilia.org), and the Fritsma Factor (fritsmafactor.com) are examples of the scores of organizations that direct their activities toward quality continuing education in hematology and hemostasis.

The medical laboratory science profession stratifies professional staff responsibilities by educational preparation. In the United States, professional levels are defined as the associate (2-year) degree level, or *medical laboratory technician;* bachelor (4-year) degree level, or *medical laboratory scientist;* and the levels of advanced degrees: master's degree or doctorate in clinical laboratory science and related sciences. Many colleges and universities offer articulation programs that enable professional personnel to advance their education and responsibility levels. Several of these institutions provide undergraduate and graduate distance-learning opportunities. A current list is maintained by the National Accrediting Agency for Clinical Laboratory Sciences (naacls.org), and the American Society for Clinical Laboratory Science publishes the *Directory of Graduate Programs for Clinical Laboratory Practitioners,* 5th ed. Enlightened employers encourage personnel to participate in advanced educational programs, and many provide resources for this purpose. Education contributes to quality laboratory services.

QUALITY ASSURANCE PLAN: PREANALYTICAL AND POSTANALYTICAL

In addition to keeping analytical quality control records, U.S. regulatory agencies such as the Centers for Medicare and Medicaid Services (cms.gov) require laboratory directors to maintain records of preanalytical and postanalytical quality assurance and quality improvement efforts.[44] Although not exhaustive, Table 5-11 lists and characterizes a number of examples of preanalytical quality efforts, and Table 5-12 provides a review of postanalytical components. All quality assurance plans provide objectives, sources of authority, scope of services, an activity calendar, corrective action, periodic evaluation, standard protocol, personnel involvement, and methods of communication.[45]

API Paperless Proficiency Testing™ and CAP Q-PROBES® are subscription services that provide model quality assurance programs. Experts in quality assurance continuously refine the consensus of appropriate indicators of laboratory medicine quality. Quality assurance programs search for events that provide improvement opportunities.

AGENCIES THAT ADDRESS HEMATOLOGY AND HEMOSTASIS QUALITY

The following are agencies that are concerned with quality assurance in hematology and hemostasis laboratory testing:
- Data Innovations North America (datainnovations.com), 120 Kimball Avenue, Suite 100, South Burlington, VT 05403: Quality assurance management software: instrument management middleware, laboratory production management software, EP Evaluator®, reference interval tables, allowable total error tables.

TABLE 5-11 Preanalytical Quality Assurance Components and the Laboratory's Responsibility

Preanalytical Component	Laboratory Staff Responsibility
Test orders	Conduct continuous utilization reviews to ensure that physician laboratory orders are comprehensive and appropriate to patient condition. Inform physician about laboratory test availability and ways to avoid unnecessary orders. Reduce unnecessary repeat testing.
Test request forms	Are requisition forms legible? Can you confirm patient identity? Are physician orders promptly and correctly interpreted and transcribed?
	Is adequate diagnostic, treatment, and patient preparation information provided to assist the laboratory in appropriately testing and interpreting results?
Stat orders and timeliness	Do turnaround time expectations match clinical necessity and ensure that stat orders are reserved for medical emergencies?
Specimen collection	Is the patient correctly identified, prepared, and available for specimen collection? Is fasting and therapy status appropriate for laboratory testing?
	Is the tourniquet correctly applied and released at the right time? Are venipuncture sites appropriately cleansed? Are timed specimens collected at the specified intervals? Are specimen tubes collected in the specified order? Are additive tubes properly mixed? Are specimen tubes labeled correctly?
Specimen transport	Are specimens delivered intact, sealed, and in a timely manner? Are they maintained at the correct temperature?
Specimen management	Are specimens centrifuged correctly? Are tests begun within specified time frames? Are specimens and aliquots stored properly? Are coagulation specimens platelet-poor when specified?

TABLE 5-12 Postanalytical Quality Assurance Components and the Laboratory's Responsibility

Postanalytical Component	Laboratory Staff Responsibility
Publication of reports	Are results accurately transcribed into the information system? Are they reviewed for errors by additional laboratory staff? If autoverification is in effect, are the correct parameters employed?
	Do reports provide reference intervals? Do they flag abnormal results? Are result narratives appended when necessary? Does the laboratory staff conduct in-service education to support test result interpretation?
	Are critical values provided to nursing and physician staff? Are verbal reports confirmed with feedback? Are anomalous findings resolved?
Timeliness	Are turnaround times recorded and analyzed? Are laboratory reports being posted to patient charts in a timely fashion?
Patient satisfaction	Does the institution include laboratory care in patient surveys? Was specimen collection explained to the patient?

- Clinical and Laboratory Standards Institute (CLSI, clsi .org), 940 West Valley Road, Suite 1400, Wayne, PA 19087. International guidelines and standards for laboratory practice. Hematology and hemostasis guidelines and standards include CLSI H02-A4, H07-A3, and H21–H48, method evaluation and assessment of diagnostic accuracy, mostly EP-prefix standards; quality assurance and quality management systems, mostly QMS-prefix standards are available.
- Centers for Medicare and Medicaid Services (CMS, cms.gov), 7500 Security Boulevard, Baltimore, MD 21244. Administers the laws and rules developed from the *Clinical Laboratory Improvement Amendments of 1988*. Establishes Current Procedural Terminology (CPT) codes, reimbursement rules, and classifies assay complexity.

- American Proficiency Institute (API, api-pt.com), 1159 Business Park Drive, Traverse City, MI 49686. Laboratory proficiency testing and quality assurance programs, continuing education programs and summaries, tutorials, special topics library.
- College of American Pathologists (CAP, cap.org), 325 Waukegan Road, Northfield, IL 60093. Laboratory accreditation, proficiency testing, and quality assurance programs; laboratory education, reference resources, and e-lab solutions.
- Joint Commission (jointcommission.org), One Renaissance Boulevard, Oakbrook Terrace, IL 60181. Medical center-wide accreditation and certification programs.
- Laboratory Medicine Quality Improvement (cdc.gov/osels/ lspppo/Laboratory_Medicine_Quality_Improvement/ index.html), an initiative of the U.S. Centers for Disease Control and Prevention.

SUMMARY

- Hematology and hemostasis laboratory quality assurance relies on basic statistics describing measures of central tendency, measures of dispersion, and significance.
- Each new assay or assay modification must be validated for accuracy, precision, linearity, specificity, and lower limit of detection ability. In the hematology and hemostasis laboratory, accuracy validation usually requires a series of calibrators. Accuracy is established using the Student's *t*-test, ANOVA, Pearson product-moment correlation, linear regression, and the Bland-Altman distribution.
- Precision is established by using repeated within-day and day-to-day assays, then computing the mean, standard deviation, and coefficient of variation of the results.
- Vendors usually provide assay linearity, specificity, and lower limit of detection; however, laboratory managers may require that these parameters be revalidated locally.
- Internal quality control is accomplished by assaying controls with each test run. Control results are compared with action limits, usually the mean of the control assay ± 2 SD. When a specified number of control values are outside the limits, the use of the

assay is suspended and the practitioner begins troubleshooting. Control results are plotted on Levey-Jennings charts and examined for shifts and trends. Internal quality control is enhanced through the use of the moving average algorithm and ∂-checks.
- All conscientious laboratory directors subscribe to an external quality assessment system, also known as *proficiency testing* or *proficiency surveys*. External quality assessment enables the director to compare selected assay results with other laboratory results, nationally and internationally, as a further check of accuracy. Maintaining a good external quality assessment record is essential to laboratory accreditation. Most U.S. states require external quality assessment for laboratory licensure.
- All laboratory assays are analyzed for diagnostic efficacy, including diagnostic sensitivity and specificity, their true-positive and true-negative rates, and positive and negative predictive values. Highly sensitive assays may be used for population screening but may poorly discriminate between the healthy and diseased population. Specific assays may be used to confirm a condition, but generate a number of false negatives. Assays are chosen on the basis of the value of their intervention, based on relative or

absolute risk ratios. Diagnostic efficacy computations expand to include receiver operating characteristic curve analysis.

- Conscientious laboratory managers hire only certified or licensed medical laboratory scientists and technicians and provide regular individual proficiency tests that are correlated with in-service education. They encourage staff members to participate in continuing education activities and in-house discussion of cases. Quality laboratories provide resources for staff to pursue higher education.

- The laboratory director maintains a protocol for assessing and improving upon preanalytical and postanalytical variables and finds means to communicate enhancements to other members of the health care team.

Now that you have completed this chapter, go back and read again the case study at the beginning and respond to the questions presented.

REVIEW QUESTIONS

Answers can be found in the Appendix.

1. What procedure is employed to validate a new assay?
   a. Comparison of assay results to a reference method
   b. Test for assay precision
   c. Test for assay linearity
   d. All of the above

2. You validate a new assay using linear regression to compare assay calibrator results with the distributor's published calibrator results. The slope is 0.99 and the y intercept is +10%. What type of error is present?
   a. No error
   b. Random error
   c. Constant systematic error
   d. Proportional systematic error

3. Which is a statistical test comparing means?
   a. Bland-Altman
   b. Student's *t*-test
   c. ANOVA
   d. Pearson

4. The acceptable hemoglobin control value range is 13 ± 0.4 g/dL. The control is assayed five times and produces the following five results:

   12.0 g/dL   12.3 g/dL   12.0 g/dL   12.2 g/dL   12.1 g/dL

   These results are:
   a. Accurate but not precise
   b. Precise but not accurate
   c. Both accurate and precise
   d. Neither accurate nor precise

5. A WBC count control has a mean value of 6000/μL and a standard deviation of 300/μL. What is the 95.5% confidence interval?
   a. 3000 to 9000/μL
   b. 5400 to 6600/μL
   c. 5500 to 6500/μL
   d. 5700 to 6300/μL

6. The ability of an assay to distinguish the targeted analyte from interfering substances within the specimen matrix is called:
   a. Analytical specificity
   b. Analytical sensitivity
   c. Clinical specificity
   d. Clinical sensitivity

7. The laboratory purchases reagents from a manufacturer and develops an assay using standard references. What FDA category is this assay?
   a. Cleared
   b. Home-brew
   c. Research use only
   d. Analyte-specific reagent

8. A laboratory scientist measures prothrombin time for plasma aliquots from 15 healthy males and 15 healthy females. She computes the mean and 95.5% confidence interval and notes that they duplicate the manufacturer's statistics within 5%. This procedure is known as:
   a. Confirming linearity
   b. Setting the reference interval
   c. Determining the therapeutic range
   d. Establishing the reference interval by transference

9. You purchase a preserved whole blood specimen from a distributor who provides the mean values for several complete blood count analytes. What is this specimen called?
   a. Normal specimen
   b. Calibrator
   c. Control
   d. Blank

10. You perform a clinical efficacy test and get the following results:

	Unaffected by Disease or Condition	Affected by Disease or Condition
Assay is negative	40	5
Assay is positive	10	45

What is the number of false-negative results?
a. 40
b. 10
c. 5
d. 45

11. What agency provides external quality assurance (proficiency) surveys and laboratory accreditation?
a. Clinical Laboratory Improvement Advisory Committee (CLIAC)
b. Centers for Medicare and Medicaid Services (CMS)
c. College of American Pathologists (CAP)
d. Joint Commission

12. What agency provides continuing medical laboratory education?
a. Colorado Association for Continuing Medical Laboratory Education (CACMLE)
b. Clinical Laboratory Improvement Advisory Committee (CLIAC)
c. Centers for Medicare and Medicaid Services (CMS)
d. College of American Pathologists (CAP)

13. Regular review of blood specimen collection quality is an example of:
a. Postanalytical quality assurance
b. Preanalytical quality assurance
c. Analytical quality control
d. External quality assurance

14. Review of laboratory report integrity is an example of:
a. Preanalytical quality assurance
b. Analytical quality control
c. Postanalytical quality assurance
d. External quality assurance

15. When performing a receiver operating curve analysis, what parameter assesses the overall efficacy of an assay?
a. Area under the curve
b. Performance limit (threshold)
c. Positive predictive value
d. Negative predictive value

16. You require your laboratory staff to annually perform manual lupus anticoagulant profiles on a set of plasmas with known values. This exercise is known as:
a. Assay validation
b. Proficiency testing
c. External quality assessment
d. Pre-pre analytical variable assay

REFERENCES

1. Westgard, J. O. (2007). *Assuring the Right Quality Right: Good Laboratory Practices for Verifying the Attainment of the Intended Quality of Test Results.* Madison, WI: Westgard QC.
2. Becich, M. J. (2000). Information management: moving from test results to clinical information. *Clin Leadership Manag Rev, 14,* 296–300.
3. Clinical and Laboratory Standards Institute (CLSI) (2011). *Quality Management System: Continual Improvement, Approved Guideline.* (3rd ed.). Wayne, PA: CLSI document QMS06–A3.
4. Clinical and Laboratory Standards Institute (CLSI) (2007). *Procedures for the Collection of Diagnostic Blood Specimens by Venipuncture, Approved Standard.* (6th ed.). Wayne, PA: CLSI document H3–A6.
5. Stroobants, A. K., Goldschmidt, H. M., Piebani, M. (2003). Error budget calculations in laboratory medicine: linking the concepts of biological variation and allowable medical errors. *Clin Chim Acta, 333,* 169–176.
6. Laposata, M. E., Laposata. M., Van Cott, E. M., et al. (2004). Physician survey of a laboratory medicine interpretive service and evaluation of the influence of interpretations on laboratory test ordering. *Arch Pathol Lab Med, 128,* 1424–1427.
7. Hickner, J., Graham, D. G., Elder, N. C., et al. (2008). Testing practices: a study of the American Academy of Family Physicians National Research Network. *Qual Saf Health Care, 17,* 194–200.
8. Laposata, M., Dighe, A. (2007). "Pre-pre" and "post-post" analytical error: high-incidence patient safety hazards involving the clinical laboratory. *Clin Chem Lab Med, 45,* 712–719.
9. Isaac, S., Michael, W. B. (1995). *Handbook in Research and Evaluation: A Collection of Principles, Methods, and Strategies useful in the Planning, Design, and Evaluation of Studies in Education and the Behavioral Sciences.* (3rd ed. p. 262). San Diego: EdITS Publishers.
10. Huck, S. W. (2011). *Reading Statistics and Research.* (6th ed. p 592). New York: Pearson.
11. Fritsma, G. A., McGlasson, D. L. (2012). *Quick Guide to Laboratory Statistics and Quality Control.* Washington, DC: AACC Press.
12. McGlasson, D. L., Plaut, D., Shearer, C. (2006). *Statistics for the Hemostasis Laboratory, CD-ROM.* McLean, VA: ASCLS Press.
13. Westgard, J. O. (2008). *Basic Method Validation.* (3rd ed.). Madison, Wisc: Westgard QC.
14. Clinical and Laboratory Standards Institute (CLSI) (2010). *Method Comparison and Bias Estimation using Patient Samples; Approved Guideline.* (2nd ed.). (interim revision). Wayne, PA: CLSI document EP09–A2.
15. McGlasson, D., Plaut, D., Shearer, C. (2006). *Statistics for the Hemostasis Laboratory.* McLean, VA: ASCLS Press.
16. Clinical Laboratory Improvement Amendments (CLIA). *Calibration and Calibration Verification.* Brochure No. 3. Available at: http://www.cms.gov/Regulations-and-Guidance/Legislation/CLIA/CLIA_Brochures.html. Accessed 24.05.13.
17. Clinical and Laboratory Standards Institute (CLSI): (2009). *Laboratory Instrument Implementation, Verification, and Maintenance; Approved Guideline.* Wayne, PA: CLSI document GP31–A.

18. Bartz, A. E. (1988). *Basic Statistical Concepts.* (3rd ed.). New York: MacMillan Publishing.

19. Bland, J. M., Altman, D. G. (1986). Statistical methods for assessing agreement between two methods of clinical measurement. *Lancet, 327,* 307–310.

20. Westgard, J. O., Quam, E. F., Barry, P. L., et al. (2010). *Basic QC practices.* (3rd ed.). Madison, WI: Westgard QC.

21. Koepke, J. A., Dotson, M. A., Shifman, M. A. (1985). A critical evaluation of the manual/visual differential leukocyte counting method. *Blood Cells, 11,* 173–186.

22. Henderson, M. P. A., Cotten, S. W., Rogers, M. W., et al. (2013) Method evaluation. In Bishop, M. L., Fody, E. P., Schoeff, L. E. (Eds.), *Clinical Chemistry: Principles, Techniques, and Applications* (7th ed.) Philadelphia: Lippincott Williams & Wilkins.

23. Schork, M. A., Remington, R. D. (2000). *Statistics with Applications to the Biological and Health Sciences.* (3rd ed.). Upper Saddle River, NJ: Prentice-Hall.

24. Data Innovations EP Evaluator. Available at http://www.datainnovations.com/products/ep-evaluator. Accessed 25.05.13.

25. Burns, C., More, L. (2010). Quality assessment in the hematology laboratory. In: McKenzie, S. B., Williams, J. L., (Eds.), *Clinical Laboratory Hematology.* Boston: Prentice-Hall.

26. Clinical and Laboratory Standards Institute (CLSI). (2010). *Defining, Establishing and Verifying Reference Intervals in the Clinical Laboratory; Approved Guideline.* (3rd ed.). Wayne, PA: CLSI document C28–A3.

27. Malone, B. (2012). The quest for pediatric reference ranges: why the national children's study promises answers. *Clin Lab News, 38,* 3–4.

28. Krejcie, R. V., Morgan, D. W. (1970). Determining sample size for research activities. *Educ Psychological Measurement, 30,* 607–610.

29. Bachner, P. (1987). Quality assurance in hematology. In Howanitz, J. F., Howanitz, J. H., (Eds.), *Laboratory Quality Assurance.* New York: McGraw-Hill.

30. Levey, S., Jennings, E. R. (1950). The use of control charts in the clinical laboratory. *Am J Clin Pathol, 20,* 1059–1066.

31. Westgard, J. O. (2010). *Basic QC Practices.* (3rd ed.). Madison, WI: Westgard QC.

32. Westgard, J. O., Barry, P. L., Hunt, M. R., et al. (1981). A multirule Shewhart chart for quality control in clinical chemistry. *Clin Chem, 27,* 493–501.

33. Bull, B. S., Elashoff, R. M., Heilbron, D. C., et al. (1974). A study of various estimators for the derivation of quality control procedures from patient erythrocyte indices. *Am J Clin Pathol, 61,* 473–481.

34. Cembrowski, G. S., Smith, B., Tung, D. (2010). Rationale for using insensitive quality control rules for today's hematology analyzers. *Int J Lab Hematol, 32,* 606–615.

35. Ovens, K., Naugler, C. (2012). How useful are delta checks in the 21st century? A stochastic-dynamic model of specimen mix-up and detection. *J Pathol Inform, 3,* 5.

36. Lind, S. E. (1991). The bleeding time does not predict surgical bleeding. *Blood, 77,* 2547–2552.

37. Gewirtz, A. S., Miller, M. L., Keys, T. F. (1996). The clinical usefulness of the preoperative bleeding time. *Arch Pathol Lab Med, 120,* 353–356.

38. Tripepi, G., Jager, K. J., Dekker, F. W., Zoccali, C. (2010). Measures of effect in epidemiological research. *Clin Practice, 115,* 91–93.

39. Replogle, W. H., Johnson, W. D. (2007). Interpretation of absolute measures of disease risk in comparative research. *Fam Med, 39,* 432–435.

40. Fardy, J. M. (2009). Evaluation of diagnostic tests. *Methods Mol Biol, 473,* 127–136.

41. Søreide, K. (2009). Receiver-operating characteristic curve analysis in diagnostic, prognostic and predictive biomarker research. *J Clin Pathol, 62,* 1–5.

42. Novis, D. A. (2004). Detecting and preventing the occurrence of errors in the practices of laboratory medicine and anatomic pathology: 15 years' experience with the College of American Pathologists' Q-PROBES and Q-TRACKS programs. *Clin Lab Med, 24,* 965–978.

43. Winkelman, J. W., Mennemeyer, S. T. (1996). Using patient outcomes to screen for clinical laboratory errors. *Clin Lab Manage Rev, 10,* 134–136, 139–142.

44. Westgard, J. O., Ehrmeyer, S. S., Darcy, T. P. (2004). *CLIA Final Rule for Quality Systems, Quality Assessment Issues and Answers,* Madison, WI: Westgard QC.

45. Howanitz, P. J., Hoffman, G. G., Schifman, R. B., et al. (1992). A nationwide quality assurance program can describe standards for the practice of pathology and laboratory medicine. *Qual Assur Health Care, 3,* 245–256.

Cellular Structure and Function 6

Elaine M. Keohane*

OBJECTIVES

After completion of this chapter, the reader will be able to:

1. Describe the structure, composition, and general function of cellular membranes.
2. Describe the structure, composition, and function of components of the nucleus, including staining qualities visible by light microscopy.
3. Describe the structure, composition, and general function of the cytoplasmic organelles in the cell, including staining qualities visible by light microscopy, if applicable.
4. Describe the general structure and function of the hematopoietic microenvironment.
5. Associate the stages of the cell cycle with activities of the cell.
6. Describe the role of cyclins and cyclin-dependent kinases in cell cycle regulation.
7. Discuss the function of checkpoints in the cell cycle and where in the cycle they occur.
8. Differentiate between apoptosis and necrosis.

Knowledge of the normal structure, composition, and function of cells is fundamental to the understanding of blood cell pathophysiology covered in later chapters. From the invention of the microscope and the discovery of cells in the 1600s to the present-day highly sophisticated analysis of cell ultrastructure with electron microscopy and other technologies, a remarkable body of knowledge is available about the structure of cells and their varied organelles. Complementing these discoveries were other advances in technology that enabled detailed understanding of the biochemistry, metabolism, and genetics of cells at the molecular level. Today, highly sophisticated analysis of cells using flow cytometry, cytogenetics, and molecular genetic testing (Chapters 30, 31, and 32) has become the standard of care in diagnosis and management of many malignant and non-malignant blood cell diseases. This new and ever-expanding knowledge has revolutionized the diagnosis and treatment of hematologic diseases resulting in a dramatic improvement in patient survival for many conditions that previously had a dismal prognosis. With all these advances, however, the visual examination of blood cells on a peripheral blood film by light microscopy still remains the hallmark for the initial evaluation of hematologic abnormalities.

This chapter will provide an overview of the structure, composition, and function of the components of the cell, the hematopoietic microenvironment, the cell cycle and its regulation, and the process of cell death by apoptosis and necrosis.

CELL ORGANIZATION

Cells are the structural units that constitute living organisms (Figures 6-1 and 6-2). Cells have specialized functions and contain the components necessary to perform and perpetuate these

---

*The author extends appreciation to Keila B. Poulsen, whose work in prior editions provided the foundation for this chapter.

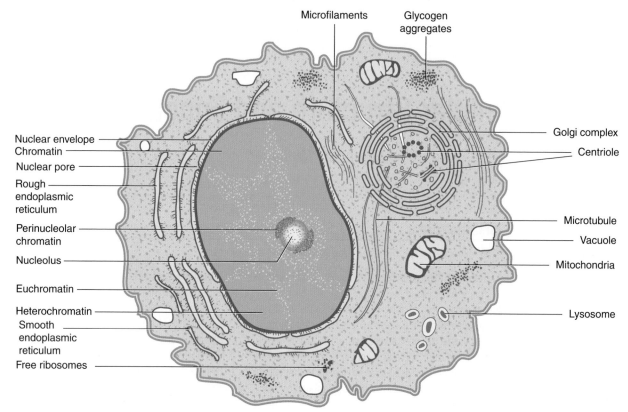

Figure 6-1 Cell organization and components.

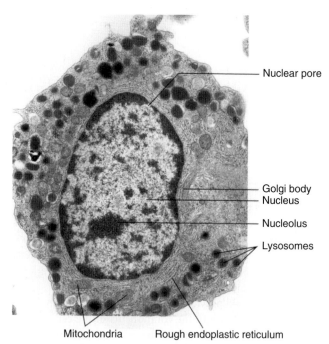

Figure 6-2 Electron micrograph of a cell. (From Carr JH, Rodak BF: Clinical hematology atlas, ed 4, St. Louis, 2013, Saunders.)

functions. Regardless of shape, size, or function, human cells contain:

- *A plasma membrane* that separates the *cytoplasm* and cellular components from the extracellular environment;
- A membrane-bound *nucleus* (with the exception of mature red blood cells and platelets); and

- Other unique subcellular structures and organelles that support the various cellular functions.[1]

Table 6-1 summarizes the cellular components and their functions, which are explained in more detail later.

PLASMA MEMBRANE

The plasma membrane serves as a semipermeable outer boundary separating the cellular components from their surrounding environment. The cell membrane serves four basic functions: (1) it provides a physical but flexible barrier to contain and protect cell components from the extracellular environment; (2) it regulates and facilitates the interchange of substances with the environment by endocytosis, exocytosis, and selective permeability (using various membrane channels and transporters); (3) it establishes electrochemical gradients between the interior and exterior of the cell; and (4) it has receptors that allow the cell to respond to a multitude of signaling molecules through signal transduction pathways.[2]

Relevant to hematology, the membrane is also the location of cell surface glycoprotein and glycolipid molecules (surface markers or antigens) used for blood cell identity. Each type of blood cell expresses a unique repertoire of surface markers at different stages of differentiation.[3] Monoclonal antibodies are used to identify a blood cell's surface antigens using flow cytometry (Chapter 32). An international nomenclature was developed, called the *cluster of differentiation,* or *CD,* system, in which a CD number was assigned to each identified blood cell surface antigen.[4] Over 350 CD antigens have been identified on blood

TABLE 6-1 Summary of Cellular Components and Functions

Organelle	Location	Appearance and Size	Function
Plasma membrane	Outer boundary of cell	Lipid bilayer consisting of phospholipids, cholesterol, proteins; glycolipids and glycoproteins form a glycocalyx	Provides physical barrier for cell; facilitates and restricts cellular exchange of substances; maintains electrochemical gradient and receptors for signal transduction
Nucleus	Within cell	Round or oval; varies in diameter; composed of DNA and proteins	Controls cell division and functions; and contains genetic code
Nucleolus	Within nucleus	Usually round or irregular in shape; 2-4 μm in diameter; composed of ribosomal RNA and the genes coding it, and accessory proteins; there may be one to several within the nucleus	Synthesizes ribosomal RNA and assembles ribosome subunits
Ribosomes	Free in cytoplasm; also on outer surface of rough endoplasmic reticulum	Macromolecular complex composed of protein and ribosomal RNA; composed of large and small subunits	Synthesizes proteins
Rough endoplasmic reticulum	Membranous network throughout cytoplasm	Membrane-lined tubules that branch and connect to nuclear membrane; studded with ribosomes	Synthesizes most membrane-bound proteins
Smooth endoplasmic reticulum	Membranous network throughout cytoplasm	Membrane-lined tubules contiguous with rough endoplasmic reticulum; does not have ribosomes	Synthesizes phospholipids and steroids; detoxifies drugs; stores calcium
Golgi apparatus	Next to nucleus and rough endoplasmic reticulum	System of stacked, membrane-bound, flattened sacs	Modifies and packages macromolecules for other organelles and for secretion
Mitochondria	Randomly distributed in cytoplasm	Round or oval structures; 3-14 nm in length, 2-10 nm in width; membrane has two layers; inner layer has folds called *cristae*	Produces most of the cell's ATP by oxidative phosphorylation
Lysosomes	Randomly distributed in cytoplasm	Membrane-bound sacs; diameter varies	Contains hydrolytic enzymes that degrade unwanted material in the cell
Microfilaments	Near nuclear envelope, plasma membrane, and mitotic processes	Double-stranded, intertwined solid structures of actin; 5-7 nm in diameter	Supports cytoskeleton and motility
Intermediate filaments	Cytoskeleton	Solid structures 8-10 nm in diameter; self-assemble into larger bundles	Provides strong structural support
Microtubules	Cytoskeleton and centrioles, near nuclear envelope and Golgi apparatus	Hollow cylinder of α- and β-tubulin forming 13 protofilaments; 20-25 nm in diameter	Maintains cell shape, motility, and mitotic process
Centrosome	Near nucleus	Composed of two centrioles, each having nine sets of triplet microtubules; 150 nm in diameter, 300-500 nm in length	Contains centrioles that serve as insertion points for mitotic spindle fibers

cells.[3] The CD nomenclature allows scientists, clinicians, and laboratory practitioners to communicate in a universal language for hematology research and diagnostic and therapeutic practice.

In addition to the plasma membrane, many components found within the cell (e.g., the mitochondria, Golgi apparatus, nucleus, and endoplasmic reticulum) have similarly constructed membrane systems. The red blood cell membrane has been the most widely studied and serves as an example of a cell membrane (Figure 9-2).

To accomplish its many requirements, the cell membrane must be resilient and elastic. It achieves these qualities by being a fluid structure of proteins floating in lipids. The lipids are phospholipids and cholesterol arranged in two layers. The phosphate end of the phospholipid and the hydroxyl radical of cholesterol are polar-charged hydrophilic (water-soluble) structures that orient toward the extracellular and cytoplasmic surfaces of the cell membrane. The fatty acid chains of the phospholipids and the steroid nucleus of cholesterol are non-polar-charged hydrophobic (water-insoluble) structures and are directed toward each other in the center of the bilayer (Figure 13-10).[2] The phospholipids are distributed asymmetrically in the membrane with mostly phosphatidylserine and phosphatidylethanolamine in the inner layer and sphingomyelin and phosphatidylcholine in the outer layer (Chapters 9 and 13). In the outer layer, carbohydrates (oligosaccharides) are covalently linked to some membrane proteins and phospholipids (forming glycoproteins and glycolipids, respectively).[2] These also contribute to the membrane structure and function.

Membrane Proteins

Cell membranes contain two types of proteins: transmembrane and cytoskeletal. Transmembrane proteins may traverse the entirety of the lipid bilayers in one or more passes and penetrate the plasma and cytoplasmic layers of the membrane. The transmembrane proteins serve as channels and transporters of water, ions, and other molecules between the cytoplasm and the external environment. They also function as receptors and adhesion molecules. Cytoskeletal proteins are found only on the cytoplasmic side of the membrane and form the lattice of the cytoskeleton. The cytoplasmic ends of transmembrane proteins attach to the cytoskeletal proteins at junctional complexes to provide structural integrity to the cell and vertical support in linking the membrane to the cytoskeleton (Figure 9-4).[5] Inherited mutations in genes coding for transmembrane or cytoskeletal proteins can disrupt membrane integrity, decrease the life span of red blood cells, and lead to a hemolytic anemia. An example is hereditary spherocytosis (Chapter 24).

Membrane Carbohydrates

The carbohydrate chains of the glycoproteins and glycolipids extend beyond the outer cell surface, giving the cell a carbohydrate coat often called the *glycocalyx*. These carbohydrate moieties function in cell-to-cell recognition and provide a negative surface charge, surface receptor sites, and cell adhesion capabilities. The function of the red blood cell membrane is discussed in detail in Chapter 9.

NUCLEUS

The nucleus is composed of three components: the chromatin, the nuclear envelope, and the nucleoli. It is the control center of the cell and the largest organelle within the cell. The nucleus is composed largely of deoxyribonucleic acid (DNA) and is the site of DNA replication and transcription (Chapter 31). It is responsible for the chemical reactions within the cell and the cell's reproductive process. The nucleus has an affinity for basic dyes because of the nucleic acids contained within it; it stains deep purple with Wright stain (Chapters 8 and 12).

Chromatin

The chromatin consists of one long molecule of double-stranded DNA in each chromosome that is tightly folded with histone and nonhistone proteins. The first level of folding is the formation of *nucleosomes* along the length of the DNA molecule (Figure 30-3). Each nucleosome is 11 nm in length and consists of approximately 150 base pairs of DNA wrapped around a histone protein core.[6] The positive charge of the histones facilitates binding with the negatively charged phosphate groups of DNA. The nucleosomes are folded into 30 nm chromatin fibers, and these fibers are further folded into loops, then supercoiled chromatin fibers that greatly condense the DNA (Figure 30-3). This highly structured folding allows the long strands of DNA to be tightly condensed in the nucleus when inactive and enables segments of the DNA to be rapidly unfolded for active transcription when needed. This complex process of gene expression is controlled by transcription factors and other regulatory proteins and processes. Inappropriate silencing of genes needed for blood cell maturation contributes to the molecular pathophysiology of myelodysplastic syndromes and acute leukemias (Chapters 34 and 35).

Morphologically, chromatin is divided into two types: (1) the *heterochromatin*, which is represented by the more darkly stained, condensed clumping pattern and is the transcriptionally inactive area of the nucleus, and (2) the *euchromatin*, which has diffuse, uncondensed, open chromatin and is the genetically active portion of the nucleus where DNA transcription into mRNA occurs. The euchromatin is loosely coiled and turns a pale blue when stained with Wright stain. More mature cells have more heterochromatin because they are less transcriptionally active.

Nuclear Envelope

Surrounding the nucleus is a nuclear envelope consisting of two phospholipid bilayer membranes. The inner membrane surrounds the nucleus, and the outer membrane is continuous with an extension of the endoplasmic reticulum.[1] Between the two membranes is a 30- to 50-nm perinuclear space that is continuous with the lumen of the endoplasmic reticulum.[6] Nuclear pore complexes penetrate the nuclear envelope, which allows passage of molecules between the nucleus and the cytoplasm.

Nucleoli

The nucleus contains one to several nucleoli. The nucleolus is the site of ribosomal RNA (rRNA) production and assembly into ribosome subunits. Because the ribosomes synthesize proteins, the number of nucleoli in the nucleus is proportional to the amount of protein synthesis that occurs in the cell. As blood cells mature, protein synthesis decreases, and the nucleoli eventually disassemble.

Nucleoli contain a large amount of rRNA, the genes that code for rRNA (or rDNA), and ribosomal proteins. In ribosome biogenesis, rDNA is first transcribed to rRNA precursors. The rRNA precursors are processed into smaller RNA molecules and subsequently complexed with proteins forming the small and large ribosome subunits.[6] The ribosomal proteins enter the nucleus through the nuclear pores after being synthesized in the cytoplasm. After the ribosome subunits are synthesized and assembled, they are transported out of the nucleus through the nuclear pores. Once in the cytoplasm, the large and small ribosome subunits self-assemble into a functional ribosome during protein synthesis (Chapter 31).[6]

CYTOPLASM

The cytoplasmic matrix is a homogeneous, continuous, aqueous solution called the *cytosol*. It is the environment in which the organelles exist and function. These organelles are discussed individually.

Ribosomes

Ribosomes are macromolecular complexes composed of a small and large subunit of rRNA and many accessory ribosomal proteins. Ribosomes are found free in the cytoplasm or on the surface of rough endoplasmic reticulum. They may exist singly or form chains (polyribosomes). Ribosomes serve as the site of protein synthesis. This is accomplished with transfer RNA (tRNA) for amino acid transport to the ribosome, and specific messenger RNA (mRNA) molecules. The mRNA provides the genetic code for the sequence of amino acids for the protein being synthesized (Chapter 31). Cells that actively produce proteins have many ribosomes in the cytoplasm which give it a dark blue color (basophilia) when stained with Wright stain. Cytoplasmic basophilia is particularly prominent in RBC precursor cells when hemoglobin and other cell components are actively synthesized (Chapter 8).

Endoplasmic Reticulum

The endoplasmic reticulum (Figure 6-3) is a membranous network found throughout the cytoplasm and appears as flattened sheets, sacs, and tubes of membrane. The outer membrane of the nuclear envelope is continuous with the endoplasmic reticulum membrane and it specializes in making and transporting lipids and membrane proteins.

Rough endoplasmic reticulum (RER) has a studded look on its outer surface caused by the presence of ribosomes engaged in the synthesis of mainly membrane-bound proteins.[2] Smooth endoplasmic reticulum (SER) is contiguous with the RER, but it does not contain ribosomes. It is involved in synthesis of phospholipids and steroids, detoxification or inactivation of harmful compounds or drugs, and calcium storage and release.[2]

Golgi Apparatus

The Golgi apparatus is a system of stacked, membrane-bound, flattened sacs called *cisternae* that are involved in modifying, sorting, and packaging macromolecules for secretion or delivery to other organelles. It contains numerous enzymes for these activities. The Golgi apparatus is normally located in close proximity to the rough endoplasmic reticulum (RER) and the nucleus. In stained bone marrow smears of developing white blood cell precursors, the Golgi area may be observed as an unstained region next to the nucleus.

Vesicles containing membrane-bound and soluble proteins from the RER enter the Golgi network on the "cis face" and are directed through the stacks where the proteins are modified, as needed, by enzymes for glycosylation, sulfation, or phosphorylation.[1,2] Vesicles with processed proteins exit the Golgi on the "trans face" to form lysosomes or secretory vesicles bound for the plasma membrane.[1,2]

Mitochondria

The mitochondrion (Figure 6-4) has a continuous outer membrane. Running parallel to the outer membrane is an inner membrane that invaginates at various intervals, giving the interior a shelflike or ridgelike appearance. These internal ridges, termed *cristae*, are where oxidative enzymes are attached. The convolution of the inner membrane increases the surface area to enhance the respiratory capability of the cell. The interior of the mitochondrion consists of a homogeneous material known as the *mitochondrial matrix*, which contains many enzymes for the extraction of energy from nutrients.

The mitochondria generate most of the adenosine triphosphate (ATP) for the cell. Mitochondrial enzymes oxidize pyruvate and fatty acids to acetyl CoA, and the citric acid cycle oxidizes the acetyl CoA producing electrons for the electron-transport pathway. This pathway generates ATP through oxidative phosphorylation.[2]

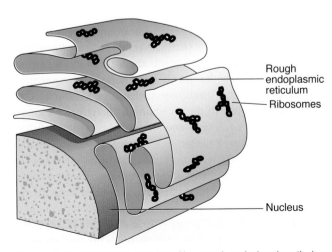

Figure 6-3 Endoplasmic reticulum. Note rough endoplasmic reticulum with attached ribosomes.

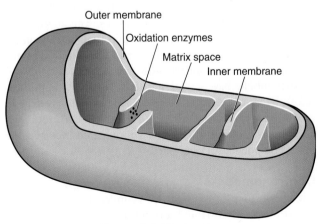

Figure 6-4 Mitochondrion.

The mitochondria are capable of self-replication. This organelle has its own DNA and RNA for the mitochondrial division cycle. There may be fewer than 100 or up to several thousand mitochondria per cell. The number is directly related to the amount of energy required by the cell.

Lysosomes

Lysosomes contain hydrolytic enzymes bound within a membrane and are involved in the cell's intracellular digestive process. The membrane prevents the enzymes from digesting cellular components and macromolecules. Lysosomal enzymes are active at the acidic pH of the lysosome and are inactivated at the higher pH of the cytosol.[2] This also protects the cell in case lysosomal enzymes are released into the cytoplasm. Lysosomes fuse with endosomes and phagosomes (Chapter 12); this allows the lysosome hydrolytic enzymes to safely digest their contents.[1] With Wright stain, lysosomes are visualized as granules in white blood cells and platelets (Chapters 12 and 13). Lysosomal lipid storage diseases result from inherited mutations in genes for enzymes that catabolize lipids. Gaucher disease and Tay-Sachs disease are examples of these disorders (Chapter 29).

Microfilaments and Intermediate Filaments

Actin microfilaments are double-stranded, intertwined solid structures approximately 5 to 7 nm in diameter. They associate with myosin to enable cell motility, contraction, and intracellular transport. They locate near the nuclear envelope or in the proximity of the nucleus and assist in cell division. They also are present near the plasma membrane and provide cytoskeletal support.

Intermediate filaments, with a diameter of approximately 8 to 10 nm, self-assemble into larger bundles.[2] They are the most durable element of the cytoskeleton and provide structural stability for the cells, especially those subjected to more physical stress, such as the epidermal layer of skin.[1] Examples include the keratins and lamins.

Microtubules

Microtubules are hollow cylindrical structures that are approximately 25 nm in diameter and vary in length. These organelles are organized from α- and β-tubulin through self-assembly.[2] The tubulin polypeptides form protofilaments, and the microtubule usually consists of 13 protofilaments.[1] This arrangement gives the microtubules structural strength. Tubulins can rapidly polymerize and form microtubules and then rapidly depolymerize them when no longer needed by the cell.

Microtubules have several functions. They help support the cytoskeleton to maintain the cell's shape and are involved in the movement of some intracellular organelles. Microtubules also form the mitotic spindle fibers during mitosis and are the major components of centrioles.

Centrosomes

The centrosome consists of two cylinder-shaped centrioles that are typically oriented at right angles to each other. A centriole consists of nine bundles of three microtubules each. They serve as insertion points for the mitotic spindle fibers during mitosis.

HEMATOPOIETIC MICROENVIRONMENT

Hematopoiesis occurs predominantly in the bone marrow from the third trimester of fetal life through adulthood (Chapter 7). The bone marrow microenvironment must provide for hematopoietic stem cell self-renewal, proliferation, differentiation, and apoptosis and support the developing progenitor cells. This protective environment is provided by stromal cells, which is a broad term for specialized endothelial cells; reticular adventitial cells (fibroblasts); adipocytes (fat cells); lymphocytes and macrophages; osteoblasts; and osteoclasts.[7] The stromal cells secrete substances that form an extracellular matrix, including collagen, fibronectin, thrombospondin, laminin, and proteoglycans (such as hyaluronate, chondroitin sulfate, and heparan sulfate).[7,8] The extracellular matrix is critical for cell growth and for anchoring developing blood cell progenitors in the bone marrow. Hematopoietic progenitor cells have many receptors for cytokines and adhesion molecules. One purpose of these receptors is to provide a mechanism for attachment to extracellular matrix. This provides an avenue for cell-cell interaction, which is essential for regulated hematopoiesis.

Stromal cells also secrete many different growth factors required for stem, progenitor, and precursor cell survival (Chapter 7). Growth factors participate in complex processes to regulate the proliferation and differentiation of progenitor and precursor cells. Growth factors must bind to specific receptors on their target cells to exert their effect. Most growth factors are produced by cells in the hematopoietic microenvironment and exert their effects in local cell-cell interactions. One growth factor, erythropoietin, has a hormone-type stimulation in that it is produced in another location (kidney) and exerts its effect on erythroid progenitors in the bone marrow (Chapter 8). An important feature of growth factors is their use of synergism to stimulate a cell to proliferate or differentiate. In other words, several different growth factors work together to generate a more effective response.[9] Growth factors are specific for their corresponding receptors on target cells.

Growth factor receptors are transmembrane proteins.[9] When the growth factor (or ligand) binds the extracellular domain of the receptor, a signal is transmitted to the nucleus in the cell through the cytoplasmic domain. For example, when erythropoietin binds with its receptor, it causes a conformational change in the receptor which activates a kinase (Janus kinase 2 or JAK2) associated with its cytoplasmic domain.[9] The activated kinase in turn activates other intracellular signal transduction molecules that ultimately interact with the DNA in the nucleus to promote expression of genes required for cell growth and proliferation (Figure 33-9).

CELL CYCLE

The purpose of the cell cycle is to replicate DNA once and distribute identical chromosome copies equally to two daughter cells during mitosis.[10] The cell cycle is a biochemical and morphologic four-stage process through which a cell passes when it is stimulated to divide (Figure 6-5). These stages are G_1 (gap 1), S (DNA synthesis), G_2 (gap 2), and M (mitosis). G_1 is a period of cell growth and synthesis of components necessary for replication. G_1 lasts about 10 hours.[10] In the S stage, DNA replication takes place, a process requiring about 8 hours (Chapter 31). An exact copy of each chromosome is produced and they pair together as *sister chromatids*. The centrosome is also duplicated during the S stage.[10] In G_2, the tetraploid DNA is checked for proper replication and damage (discussed later). G_2 takes approximately 4 hours. The time spent in each stage can be variable, but mitosis takes approximately 1 hour.[10] During G_0 (quiescence) the cell is not actively in the cell cycle.

The mitosis or M stage involves the division of chromosomes and cytoplasm into two daughter cells. It is divided into six phases (Figure-6-5):[10]

1. *Prophase:* the chromosomes condense, the duplicated centrosomes begin to separate, and mitotic spindle fibers appear.
2. *Prometaphase:* the nuclear envelope disassembles, the centrosomes move to opposite poles of the cell and serve as a point of origin of the mitotic spindle fibers; the sister chromatids (chromosome pairs) attach to the mitotic spindle fibers.
3. *Metaphase:* the sister chromatids align on the mitotic spindle fibers at a location equidistant from the centrosome poles.

4. *Anaphase:* the sister chromatids separate and move on the mitotic spindles toward the centrosomes on opposite poles.
5. *Telophase:* the nuclear membrane reassembles around each set of chromosomes and the mitotic spindle fibers disappear.
6. *Cytokinesis:* the cell divides into two identical daughter cells

Interphase is a term used for the non-mitosis stages of the cell cycle, that is, G_1, S, and G_2.

Regulation of the Cell Cycle

A regulatory mechanism is needed to prevent abnormal or mutated cells from going through the cell cycle and producing an abnormal clone. The cell cycle is a highly complicated process that can malfunction. There are four major checkpoints in the cell cycle (Figure 6-5).[1,10] The first is a *restriction point* late in G_1 that checks for the appropriate amount of nutrients and appropriate cell volume. The second checkpoint at the end of G_1 (called the G1 DNA damage checkpoint) checks the DNA for damage and makes the cell wait for DNA repair or initiates apoptosis. The third checkpoint, G2 DNA damage checkpoint, takes place after DNA synthesis at the end of G_2, and its purpose is to verify that replication took place without error or damage. If abnormal or malformed replication occurred, then mitosis is blocked. The last checkpoint is during mitosis at the time of metaphase (*metaphase checkpoint*). Here the attachment and alignment of chromosomes on the mitotic spindle and the integrity of the spindle apparatus are checked.[1,10] Anaphase will be blocked if any defects are detected.

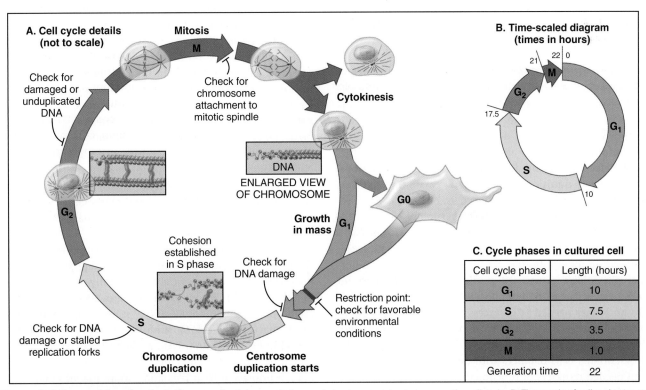

Figure 6-5 Stages of the cell cycle. **A,** Diagrams of cellular morphology and chromosome structure across the cell cycle; **B,** Time scale of cell cycle stages; **C,** Length of cell cycle stages in cultured cells. (From Pollard TD, Earnshaw WC. Chapter 40 Introduction to the cell cycle. In: Cell Biology, e2. Philadelphia, 2008, Saunders, An imprint of Elsevier.)

Cell cycle control is under the direction of cyclin and cyclin-dependent kinases (CDKs). The cyclin/CDK complexes phosphorylate key substrates that assist the cell through the cell cycle. Cyclin is named appropriately because the concentration of the cyclin/CDK complex moves the cell through the different stages of the cell cycle. G_1 begins with a combination of the cyclin D family (D1, D2, D3) with CDK4 and CDK6.[10] To transition the cell from G_1 to S, cyclin E increases and binds to CDK2, producing the cyclin E/CDK2 complex. In the S stage cyclin E decreases and cyclin A increases and complexes with CDK2, forming cyclin A/CDK2. This complex takes the cell through the S and G_2 stage. Cyclin A also partners with CDK1 (cyclin A/CDK1). For mitosis to occur, cyclin B must replace cyclin A and bind to CDK1, forming the cyclin B/CDK1 complex. This complex takes the cell through the intricate process of mitosis.[10,11] Inhibitors of the cyclin/CDK complexes also play a primary role in cell cycle regulation.[11]

Tumor suppressor proteins are needed for the proper function of the checkpoints. One of the first tumor suppressor genes recognized was *TP53*. It codes for the TP53 protein that detects DNA damage during G_1. It can also assist in triggering apoptosis. Many tumor suppressor genes have been described.[11] When these genes are mutated or deleted, abnormal cells are allowed to go through the cell cycle and replicate. Some of these cells simply malfunction, but others form neoplasms, often with aggressive characteristics. For example, patients with chronic lymphocytic leukemia have a more aggressive disease with a shorter survival time when their leukemic cells lose TP53 activity either through gene mutation or deletion (Chapter 36). Patients whose leukemia cells have normal TP53 function have a better prognosis.

CELL DEATH BY NECROSIS AND APOPTOSIS

Cell death occurs as a normal physiologic process in the body or as a response to injury. Events that injure cells include ischemia (oxygen deprivation), mechanical trauma, toxins, drugs, infectious agents, autoimmune reactions, genetic defects including acquired and inherited mutations, and improper nutrition.[12] There are two major mechanisms for cell death: necrosis and apoptosis. *Necrosis* is a pathologic process caused by direct external injury to cells—for example, from burns, radiation, or toxins.[12] *Apoptosis* is a self-inflicted cell death originating from the activation signals within the cell itself.[13] Most apoptosis occurs as a normal physiologic process to eliminate potentially harmful cells (e.g., self-reacting lymphocytes [Chapter 7]), cells that are no longer needed (e.g., excess erythroid progenitors in oxygen-replete states (Chapter 8) or neutrophils after phagocytosis), and aging cells.[12] Apoptosis of older terminally differentiated cells balances with new cell growth to maintain needed numbers of functional cells in organs, hematopoietic tissue, and epithelial cell barriers, particularly in skin and the intestines. On the other hand, apoptosis also initiates in response to internal or external pathologic injury to

a cell. For example, if DNA damage occurred during the replication phase of the cell cycle and the damage is beyond the capability of the DNA repair mechanisms, the cell will activate apoptosis to prevent its further progression through the cell cycle. Apoptosis can also be triggered in virally infected cells by the virus itself or by the body's immune response.[12] This is one of the mechanisms to remove virally infected cells from the body.

The first morphologic manifestation of necrosis is a swelling of the cell. The cell may be able to recover from minor injury at that point. More severe damage, however, disrupts organelles and membranes; enzymes leak out of lysosomes that denature and digest DNA, RNA, and intracellular proteins; and ultimately the cell lyses.[12] An inflammatory response usually accompanies necrosis due to the release of cell contents into the extracellular space.

The morphologic manifestation of apoptosis is shrinkage of the cell. The nucleus condenses and undergoes systematic fragmentation due to cleavage of the DNA between nucleosome subunits (multiples of 180 to 200 base pairs). The plasma membrane remains intact, but the phospholipids lose their asymmetric distribution and "flip" phosphatidylserine (PS) from the inner to the outer leaflet.[14] The cytoplasm and nuclear fragments bud off in membrane-bound vesicles. Macrophages, recognizing the PS and other signals on the membranes, rapidly phagocytize the vesicles. Thus, cellular products are not released into the extracellular space and an inflammatory response is not elicited.[12] Figure 6-6 and Table 6-2 summarize the differences between necrosis and apoptosis.

Activation of apoptosis occurs through extrinsic and intrinsic pathways. Both pathways involve the activation of proteins called *caspases*. The extrinsic pathway, also called the *death receptor pathway*, initiates with the binding of ligand to a death receptor on the cell membrane. Examples of death receptors and their ligands include Fas and Fas ligand, and tumor necrosis factor receptor 1 (TNFR1) and tumor necrosis factor.[15] The binding activates caspase-8. The intrinsic pathway is initiated by intracellular stressors (such as hypoxia, DNA damage, or membrane disruption) that stimulate the release of cytochrome c from mitochondria.[15] Cytochrome c binds to apoptotic protease-activating factor-1 (APAF-1) and caspase-9, forming an *apoptosome*, which activates caspase-9. Both pathways converge when the "initiator" caspases (8 or 9) activate "executioner" caspases 3, 6, and 7, which leads to apoptosis.[13,15]

Various cellular proapoptotic and antiapoptotic proteins tightly regulate apoptosis. Examples of antiapoptotic proteins include some members of the BCL-2 family of proteins (such as Bcl-2, Bcl-XL) as well as various growth factors (such as erythropoietin, granulocyte-colony stimulating factor, granulocyte-macrophage-colony stimulating factor, interleukin-3, and FLT3 ligand).[14] BAX, BAK, and BID are examples of proapoptotic proteins.[14] The ratio of these intracellular proteins plays a primary role in regulating apoptosis. Any dysregulation, mutation, or translocation can cause inhibition or overexpression of apoptotic proteins, which can lead to hematopoietic malignancies or malfunctions.[12,14]

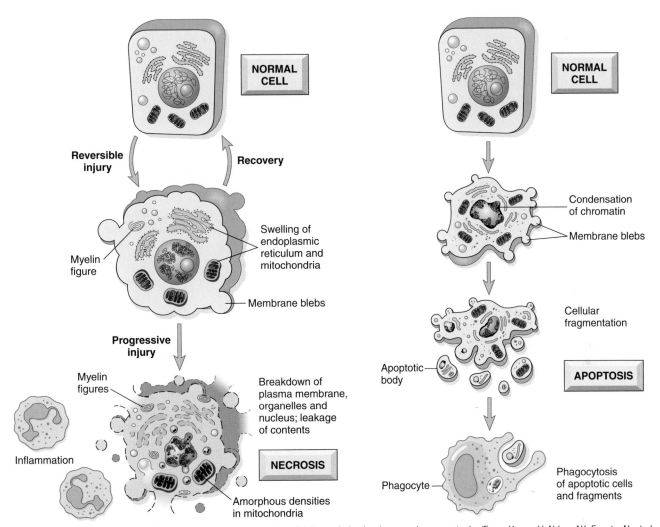

Figure 6-6 Schematic illustration of the morphologic changes in cell injury culminating in necrosis or apoptosis. (From: Kumar V, Abbas AK, Fausto, N, et al. Chapter 1 Cellular Responses to Stress and Toxic Insults: Adaptation, Injury, and Death. In: Robbins and Cotran Pathologic Basis of Disease, e8. Philadelphia, 2009, Saunders, an Imprint of Elsevier.)

TABLE 6-2 Comparison of Necrosis and Apoptosis[12,13]

	Necrosis	Apoptosis
Cell size	Enlarged due to swelling	Reduced due to shrinkage
Nucleus	Random breaks and lysis (karyolysis)	Condensation and fragmentation between nucleosomes
Plasma membrane	Disrupted with loss of integrity	Intact with loss phospholipid asymmetry
Inflammation	Enzyme digestion and leakage of cell contents; inflammatory response occurs	Release of cell contents in membrane-bound apoptotic bodies which are phagocytized by macrophages; no inflammation occurs
Physiologic or pathologic function	Pathologic; results from cell injury	Mostly physiologic to remove unwanted cells; pathologic in response to cell injury

SUMMARY

- The cell contains cytoplasm that is separated from the extracellular environment by a plasma membrane; a membrane-bound nucleus (with the exception of mature red blood cells and platelets); and other unique subcellular structures and organelles.

- The plasma membrane is a bilayer of phospholipids, cholesterol, and transmembrane proteins. Glycolipids and glycoproteins on the outer surface form the glycocalyx.

- The cytoplasm contains ribosomes for protein synthesis, which can be free in the cytoplasm or located on rough endoplasmic reticulum (RER). The RER makes most of the membrane proteins. Smooth endoplasmic reticulum (SER) lacks ribosomes; the SER is involved in synthesis of phospholipids and steroids, detoxification or inactivation of harmful compounds or drugs, and calcium storage and release.
- The Golgi apparatus modifies and packages macromolecules for secretion and for other cell organelles. Mitochondria make ATP to supply energy for the cell. Lysosomes contain hydrolytic enzymes involved in the cell's intracellular digestive process.
- The bone marrow provides a suitable microenvironment for hematopoietic stem cell self-renewal, proliferation, differentiation, and apoptosis. Stromal cells secrete substances that form an extracellular matrix to support cell growth and function and help to anchor developing cells in the bone marrow. Growth factors participate in complex processes to regulate the proliferation and differentiation of hematopoietic stem and progenitor cells.
- The cell cycle involves four active stages: G_1 (gap 1), S (DNA synthesis), G_2 (gap 2), and M (mitosis). The cell cycle is under the direction of cyclins and CDKs. Checkpoints in the cell cycle recognize abnormalities and initiate apoptosis.
- Two major mechanisms for cell death are necrosis and apoptosis. Necrosis is a pathologic process caused by direct external injury to cells, while apoptosis is a self-inflicted cell death originating from the activation signals within the cell itself. Most apoptosis occurs as a normal physiologic process to eliminate unwanted cells, but it can also be initiated in response to internal or external pathologic injury to a cell.

REVIEW QUESTIONS

Answers can be found in the Appendix.

1. The organelle involved in packaging and trafficking of cellular products is the:
   a. Nucleus
   b. Golgi apparatus
   c. Mitochondria
   d. Rough endoplasmic reticulum

2. The glycocalyx is composed of membrane:
   a. Phospholipids and cholesterol
   b. Glycoproteins and glycolipids
   c. Transmembrane and cytoskeletal proteins
   d. Rough and smooth endoplasmic reticulum

3. The "control center" of the cell is the:
   a. Nucleus
   b. Cytoplasm
   c. Membrane
   d. Microtubular system

4. The nucleus is composed largely of:
   a. RNA
   b. DNA
   c. Ribosomes
   d. Glycoproteins

5. Protein synthesis occurs in the:
   a. Nucleus
   b. Mitochondria
   c. Ribosomes
   d. Golgi apparatus

6. The shape of a cell is maintained by which of the following?
   a. Microtubules
   b. Spindle fibers
   c. Ribosomes
   d. Centrioles

7. Functions of the cell membrane include all of the following *except*:
   a. Regulation of molecules entering or leaving the cell
   b. Receptor recognition of extracellular signals
   c. Maintenance of electrochemical gradients
   d. Lipid production and oxidation

8. The energy source for cells is the:
   a. Golgi apparatus
   b. Endoplasmic reticulum
   c. Nucleolus
   d. Mitochondrion

9. Ribosomes are synthesized by the:
   a. Endoplasmic reticulum
   b. Mitochondrion
   c. Nucleolus
   d. Golgi apparatus

10. Euchromatin functions as the:
    a. Site of microtubule production
    b. Transcriptionally active DNA
    c. Support structure for nucleoli
    d. Attachment site for centrioles

11. The cell cycle is regulated by:
    a. Cyclins and CDKs
    b. Protooncogenes
    c. Apoptosis
    d. Growth factors

12. The transition from the G_1 to S stage of the cell cycle is regulated by:
    a. Cyclin B/CDK1 complex
    b. Cyclin A/CDK2 complex
    c. Cyclin D1
    d. Cyclin E/CDK2 complex

13. Apoptosis is morphologically identified by:
    a. Cellular swelling
    b. Nuclear condensation
    c. Rupture of the cytoplasm
    d. Rupture of the nucleus

14. Regulation of the hematopoietic microenvironment is provided by the:
    a. Stromal cells and growth factors
    b. Hematopoietic stem cells
    c. Liver and spleen
    d. Cyclins and caspases

REFERENCES

1. Pollard, T. D., Earnshaw, W. C. (2008). Introduction to cells. In *Cell Biology.* (2nd ed.). Philadelphia: Saunders, An imprint of Elsevier.
2. Mescher, A. L. (2013). The cytoplasm. In Mescher, A. L., (Ed.), *Junqueira's Basic Histology.* (13th ed.). New York: McGraw-Hill. http://www.accessmedicine.com.libproxy2.umdnj.edu/content .aspx?aID=57330175. Accessed January 5.01.14.
3. Kipps, T. J. (2010). The cluster of differentiation antigens. In Prchal, J. T., Kaushansky, K., Lichtman, M. A., Kipps, T. J., Seligsohn, U., (Eds.), *Williams Hematology.* (8th ed.). New York: McGraw-Hill.
4. Zola, H., Swart, B., Nicholson, I., et al. (2005). *CD molecules 2005: human cell differentiation molecules. 106,* 3123–3126.
5. Mohandas, N., Gallagher, P. G. (2008). Red cell membrane: past, present, and future. *Blood, 112,* 3939–3948.
6. Mescher, A. L. (2013). The nucleus. In: Mescher, A. L., (Ed.), *Junqueira's Basic Histology.* (13th ed.). New York: McGraw-Hill.
7. Koury, M. J., Lichtman, M. A. (2010). Structure of the marrow and the hematopoietic microenvironment. In Prchal, J. T., Kaushansky, K., Lichtman, M. A., Kipps, T. J., Seligsohn, U., (Eds.), *Williams Hematology.* (8th ed.). New York: McGraw-Hill.
8. Kaushansky, K. (2010). Hematopoietic stem cells, progenitors, and cytokines. In Prchal, J. T., Kaushansky, K., Lichtman, M. A., Kipps, T. J., Seligsohn, U., (Eds.), *Williams Hematology.* (8th ed.). New York: McGraw-Hill.
9. Kaushansky, K. (2010). Signal transduction pathways. In Prchal, J. T., Kaushansky, K., Lichtman, M. A., Kipps, T. J., Seligsohn, U., (Eds.), *Williams Hematology.* (8th ed.). New York: McGraw-Hill.
10. Pollard, T. D., Earnshaw, W. C. (2008). Introduction to the cell cycle. In *Cell Biology.* (2nd ed., Chapter 40). Philadelphia: Saunders, An imprint of Elsevier.
11. Schmid, M., Carson, D. A. (2010). Cell-cycle regulation and hematologic disorders. In Prchal, J. T., Kaushansky, K., Lichtman, M. A., Kipps, T. J., Seligsohn, U., (Eds.), *Williams Hematology.* (8th ed.). New York: McGraw-Hill.
12. Kumar, V., Abbas, A. K., Fausto, N., et al. (2009). Cellular responses to stress and toxic insults: adaptation, injury, and death. In *Robbins and Cotran Pathologic Basis of Disease.* (8th ed., Chapter 1). Philadelphia: Saunders, an Imprint of Elsevier.
13. Danial, N. K., Hockenbery, D. M. (2013). Cell death. In Hoffman, R., Benz, E. J., Jr., Silberstein, L. E., et al., (Eds.), *Hematology: Basic Principles and Practice.* (6th ed.). Philadelphia: Saunders, an imprint of Elsevier.
14. Gottlieb, R. A. (2010). Apoptosis. In Prchal, J. T., Kaushansky, K., Lichtman, M. A., Kipps, T. J., Seligsohn, U., (Eds.) *Williams Hematology.* (8th ed., Chapter 12). New York: McGraw-Hill.
15. McIlwain, D. R., Berger, T., Mak, T. W. (2013). Caspase functions in cell death and disease. *Cold Spring Harb Perspect Biol, 5,* 1–28.

7

Hematopoiesis

Richard C. Meagher

OBJECTIVES

After completion of this chapter, the reader will be able to:

1. Define hematopoiesis.
2. Describe the evolution and formation of blood cells from embryo to fetus to adult, including anatomic sites and cells produced.
3. Predict the likelihood of encountering active marrow from biopsy sites when given the patient's age.
4. Relate normal and abnormal hematopoiesis to the various organs involved in the hematopoietic process.
5. Explain the stem cell theory of hematopoiesis, including the characteristics of hematopoietic stem cells, the names of various progenitor cells, and their lineage associations.
6. Discuss the roles of various cytokines and hematopoietic growth factors in differentiation and maturation of hematopoietic progenitor cells, including nonspecific and lineage-specific factors.
7. Describe general morphologic changes that occur during blood cell maturation.
8. Define apoptosis and discuss the relationship between apoptosis, growth factors, and hematopoietic stem cell differentiation.
9. Discuss therapeutic applications of cytokines and hematopoietic growth factors.

HEMATOPOIETIC DEVELOPMENT

Hematopoiesis is a continuous, regulated process of blood cell production that includes cell renewal, proliferation, differentiation, and maturation. These processes result in the formation, development, and specialization of all of the functional blood cells that are released from the bone marrow to the circulation. The hematopoietic system serves as a functional model to study stem cell biology, proliferation, maturation and their contribution to disease and tissue repair. Rationale for this assumption is founded on the observations that mature blood cells have a limited lifespan (e.g., 120 days for RBC), a cell population capable of renewal is present to sustain the system, and the demonstration that the cell renewal population is unique in this capacity. A hematopoietic stem cell is capable of self-renewal (i.e., replenishment) and directed differentiation into all required cell lineages.[1]

Hematopoiesis in humans can be characterized as a select distribution of embryonic cells in specific sites that rapidly change during development.[2] In healthy adults hematopoiesis is restricted primarily to the bone marrow. During fetal development, the restricted, sequential distribution of cells initiates in the yolk sac and then progresses in the aorta-gonad mesonephros (AGM) region (*mesoblastic phase*), then to the fetal liver (*hepatic phase*), and finally resides in the bone marrow (*medullary phase*). Due to the different locations and resulting microenvironmental conditions (i.e., niches) encountered, each of these locations has distinct but related populations of cells.

Mesoblastic Phase

Hematopoiesis is considered to begin around the nineteenth day of embryonic development after fertilization.[3] Early in embryonic development, cells from the mesoderm migrate to the yolk sac. Some of these cells form primitive erythroblasts in the central cavity of the yolk sac, while the others (*angioblasts*) surround the cavity of the yolk sac and eventually form blood vessels.[4-7] These primitive but transient yolk sac erythroblasts are important in early embryogenesis to produce hemoglobin (Gower-1, Gower-2, and Portland) needed for delivery of oxygen to rapidly developing embryonic tissues (Chapter 10).[8] Yolk sac hematopoiesis differs from hematopoiesis that occurs later in the fetus and the adult in that it occurs intravascularly, or within developing blood vessels.[8]

Cells of mesodermal origin also migrate to the aorta-gonad-mesonephros (AGM) region and give rise to hematopoietic stem cells (HSCs) for definitive or permanent adult hematopoiesis.[4,7] The AGM region has previously been considered to be the only site of definitive hematopoiesis during embryonic development. However, more recent evidence suggests that HSC development and definitive hematopoiesis occur in the yolk sac. Metcalf and Moore performed culture experiments using 7.5-day mouse embryos lacking the yolk sac and demonstrated that no hematopoietic cells grew in the fetal liver after several days of culture.[9] They concluded that the yolk sac was the major site of adult blood formation in the embryo.[9] This view is supported by Weissman and colleagues in transplant experiments demonstrating that T cells could be recovered following transplantation of yolk sac into fetuses.[10] However, others have postulated de novo production of HSCs could occur at different times or locations.[11] Reports indicate that Flk1[+] HSCs separated from human umbilical cord blood could generate hematopoietic as well as endothelial cells in vitro.[12] Others have shown that purified murine HSCs generate endothelial cells following in vivo transplantation.[13] More recently, others have challenged the AGM origin of HSCs based on transgenic mouse data showing that yolk sac hematopoietic cells in 7.5-day embryos express *Runx*1 regulatory elements

needed for definitive hematopoiesis.[14] This suggests that the yolk sac contains either definitive HSCs or cells that can give rise to HSCs.[14] The precise origin of the adult HSC remains unresolved.

Hepatic Phase

The hepatic phase of hematopoiesis begins at 5 to 7 gestational weeks and is characterized by recognizable clusters of developing erythroblasts, granulocytes, and monocytes colonizing the fetal liver, thymus, spleen, placenta, and ultimately the bone marrow space in the final medullary phase.[8] These varied niches support development of HSCs that migrate to them. However, the contribution of each site to the final composition of the adult HSC pool remains unknown.[15,16] The developing erythroblasts signal the beginning of definitive hematopoiesis with a decline in primitive hematopoiesis of the yolk sac. In addition, lymphoid cells begin to appear.[17,18] Hematopoiesis during this phase occurs extravascularly, with the liver remaining the major site of hematopoiesis during the second trimester of fetal life.[8] Hematopoiesis in the aorta-gonad-mesonephros region and the yolk sac disappear during this stage. Hematopoiesis in the fetal liver reaches its peak by the third month of fetal development, then gradually declines after the sixth month, retaining minimal activity until 1 to 2 weeks after birth[8] (Figure 7-1). The developing spleen, kidney, thymus, and lymph nodes contribute to the hematopoietic process during this phase. The thymus, the first fully developed organ in the fetus, becomes the major site of T cell production, whereas the kidney and spleen produce B cells.

Production of megakaryocytes also begins during the hepatic phase. The spleen gradually decreases granulocytic

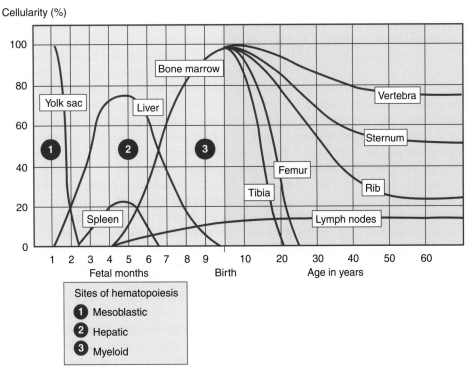

Figure 7-1 Sites of hematopoiesis by age.

production and involves itself solely in lymphopoiesis. During the hepatic phase, fetal hemoglobin (Hb F) is the predominant hemoglobin, but detectable levels of adult hemoglobin (Hb A) may be present (Chapter 10).[8]

Medullary (Myeloid) Phase

Prior to the fifth month of fetal development, hematopoiesis begins in the bone marrow cavity.[3] This transition is called *medullary hematopoiesis* because it occurs in the medulla or inner part of the bone. During the myeloid phase, HSCs and mesenchymal cells migrate into the core of the bone.[8] The mesenchymal cells, which are a type of embryonic tissue, differentiate into structural elements (i.e, stromal cells such as endothelial cells and reticular adventitial cells) that support the developing blood cells.[19,20] Hematopoietic activity, especially myeloid activity, is apparent during this stage of development, and the myeloid-to-erythroid ratio gradually approaches 3:1 (adult levels).[8] By the end of 24 weeks' gestation, the bone marrow becomes the primary site of hematopoiesis.[8] Measurable levels of erythropoietin (EPO), granulocyte colony-stimulating factor (G-CSF), granulocyte-macrophage colony-stimulating factor (GM-CSF), and hemoglobins F and A can be detected.[8] In addition, cells at various stages of maturation can be seen in all blood cell lineages.

ADULT HEMATOPOIETIC TISSUE

In adults, hematopoietic tissue is located in the bone marrow, lymph nodes, spleen, liver, and thymus. The bone marrow contains developing erythroid, myeloid, megakaryocytic, and lymphoid cells. Lymphoid development occurs in primary and secondary lymphoid tissue. Primary lymphoid tissue consists of the bone marrow and thymus and is where T and B lymphocytes are derived. Secondary lymphoid tissue, where lymphoid cells respond to foreign antigens, consists of the spleen, lymph nodes, and mucosa-associated lymphoid tissue.

Bone Marrow

Bone marrow, one of the largest organs in the body, is the tissue located within the cavities of the cortical bones. Resorption of cartilage and endosteal bone creates a central space within the bone. Projections of calcified bone, called *trabeculae,* radiate out from the bone cortex into the central space, forming a three-dimensional matrix resembling a honeycomb. The trabeculae provide structural support for the developing blood cells.

Normal bone marrow contains two major components: *red marrow,* hematopoietically active marrow consisting of the developing blood cells and their progenitors, and *yellow marrow,* hematopoietically inactive marrow composed primarily of adipocytes (fat cells), with undifferentiated mesenchymal cells and macrophages. During infancy and early childhood, all the bones in the body contain primarily red (active) marrow. Between 5 and 7 years of age, adipocytes become more abundant and begin to occupy the spaces in the long bones previously dominated by active marrow. The process of replacing the active marrow by adipocytes (yellow marrow) during

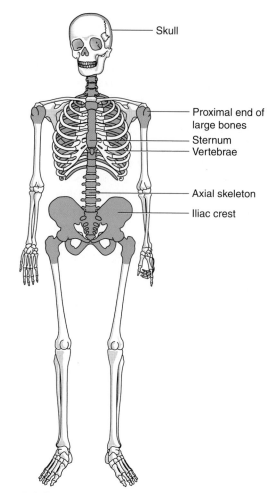

Figure 7-2 The adult skeleton, in which darkened areas depict active red marrow hematopoiesis.

development is called *retrogression* and eventually results in restriction of the active marrow in the adult to the sternum, vertebrae, scapulae, pelvis, ribs, skull, and proximal portion of the long bones (Figure 7-2). Hematopoietically inactive yellow marrow is scattered throughout the red marrow so that in adults, there is approximately equal amounts of red and yellow marrow in these areas (Figure 7-3). Yellow marrow is capable of reverting back to active marrow in cases of increased demand on the bone marrow, such as in excessive blood loss or hemolysis.[3]

The bone marrow contains hematopoietic cells, stromal cells, and blood vessels (arteries, veins, and vascular sinuses). Stromal cells originate from mesenchymal cells that migrate into the central cavity of the bone. *Stromal cells* include endothelial cells, adipocytes (fat cells), macrophages and lymphocytes, osteoblasts, osteoclasts, and reticular adventitial cells (fibroblasts).[3] *Endothelial cells* are broad, flat cells that form a single continuous layer along the inner surface of the arteries, veins, and vascular sinuses.[21] Endothelial cells regulate the flow of particles entering and leaving hematopoietic spaces in the vascular sinuses. *Adipocytes* are large cells with a single fat vacuole; they play a role in regulating the volume of the marrow in which active hematopoiesis occurs. They also secrete cytokines or growth factors that

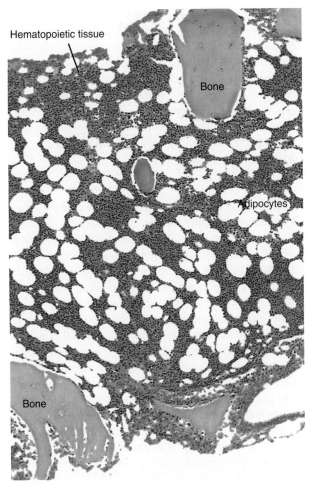

Figure 7-3 Fixed and stained bone marrow biopsy specimen (hematoxylin and eosin stain, ×100). The extravascular tissue consists of blood cell precursors and various tissue cells with scattered fat tissue. A normal adult bone marrow displays 50% hematopoietic cells and 50% fat.

located in spaces between the vascular sinuses and are supported by trabeculae of spongy bone.[3] The cords are separated from the lumen of the vascular sinuses by endothelial and reticular adventitial cells (Figure 7-4). The hematopoietic cells develop in specific *niches* within the cords. *Erythroblasts* develop in small clusters, and the more mature forms are located adjacent to the outer surfaces of the vascular sinuses[3] (Figures 7-4 and 7-5); in addition, erythroblasts are found surrounding iron-laden macrophages (Figure 7-6). *Megakaryocytes* are located adjacent to the walls of the vascular sinuses, which facilitates the release of platelets into the lumen of the sinus.[3] Immature *myeloid (granulocytic) cells* through the metamyelocyte stage are located deep within the cords. As these maturing granulocytes proceed along their differentiation pathway, they move closer to the vascular sinuses.[19]

The mature blood cells of the bone marrow eventually enter the peripheral circulation by a process that is not well understood. Through a highly complex interaction between the maturing blood cells and the vascular sinus wall, blood cells pass between layers of adventitial cells that form a discontinuous layer along the abluminal side of the sinus. Under the layer of

may positively stimulate HSC numbers and bone homeostasis.[22,23] Macrophages function in phagocytosis, and both macrophages and lymphocytes secrete various cytokines that regulate hematopoiesis; they are located throughout the marrow space.[3,24] Other cells involved in cytokine production include endothelial cells and reticular adventitial cells. *Osteoblasts* are bone-forming cells, and *osteoclasts* are bone-resorbing cells. *Reticular adventitial cells* form an incomplete layer of cells on the abluminal surface of the vascular sinuses.[3] They extend long, reticular fibers into the perivascular space that form a supporting lattice for the developing hematopoietic cells.[3] Stromal cells secrete a semifluid extracellular matrix that serves to anchor developing hematopoietic cells in the bone cavity. The extracellular matrix contains substances such as *fibronectin, collagen, laminin, thrombospondin, tenascin,* and *proteoglycans* (such as *hyaluronate, heparan sulfate, chondroitin sulfate,* and *dermatan*).[3,25] Stromal cells play a critical role in the regulation of hematopoietic stem and progenitor cell survival and differentiation.[21]

Red Marrow

The red marrow is composed of the hematopoietic cells and macrophages arranged in *extravascular cords*. The cords are

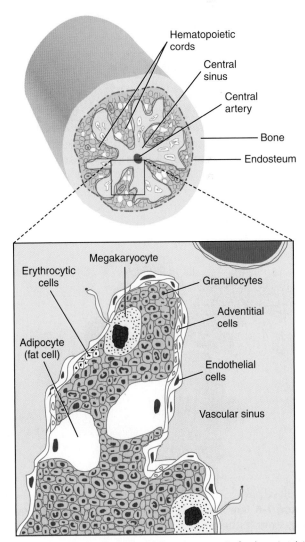

Figure 7-4 Graphic illustration of the arrangement of a hematopoietic cord and vascular sinus in bone marrow.

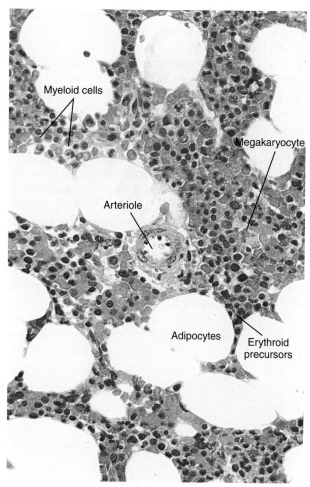

Figure 7-5 Fixed and stained bone marrow biopsy specimen (hematoxylin and eosin stain, ×400). Hematopoietic tissue reveals areas of granulopoiesis (lighter-staining cells), erythropoiesis (with darker-staining nuclei), and adipocytes (unstained areas).

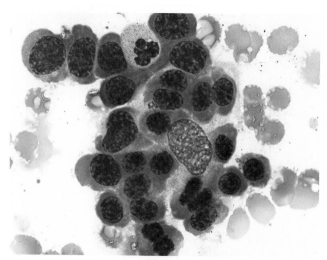

Figure 7-6 Bone marrow aspirate smear (Wright-Giemsa stain). Macrophage surrounded by developing erythroid precursors. (Courtesy of Dr. Peter Maslak, Memorial Sloan Kettering Cancer Center, NY.)

adventitial cells is a *basement membrane* followed by a continuous layer of *endothelial cells* on the luminal side of the vascular sinus. The adventitial cells are capable of contracting, which allows mature blood cells to pass through the basement membrane and interact with the endothelial layer.

As blood cells come in contact with endothelial cells, they bind to the surface through a receptor-mediated process. Cells pass through pores in the endothelial cytoplasm, are released into the vascular sinus, and then move into the peripheral circulation.[3,26]

Marrow Circulation

The nutrient and oxygen requirements of the marrow are supplied by the *nutrient* and *periosteal arteries,* which enter via the bone *foramina.* The nutrient artery supplies blood only to the marrow.[20] It coils around the central longitudinal vein, which passes along the bone canal. In the marrow cavity, the nutrient artery divides into ascending and descending branches that also coil around the central longitudinal vein. The arteriole branches that enter the inner lining of the cortical bone (*endosteum*) form *sinusoids* (endosteal beds), which connect to periosteal capillaries that extend from the periosteal artery.[3] The *periosteal arteries* provide nutrients for the osseous bone and the marrow. Their capillaries connect to the venous sinuses located in the endosteal bed, which empty into a larger collecting sinus that opens into the central longitudinal vein.[3] Blood exits the marrow via the central longitudinal vein, which runs the length of the marrow. The central longitudinal vein exits the marrow through the same foramen where the nutrient artery enters. Hematopoietic cells located in the endosteal bed receive their nutrients from the nutrient artery.[3]

Hematopoietic Microenvironment

The *hematopoietic inductive microenvironment,* or *niche,* plays an important role in nurturing and protecting HSCs and regulating a balance among their quiescence, self-renewal, and differentiation.[21,27] As the site of hematopoiesis transitions from yolk sac to liver, then to bone marrow, so must the microenvironmental niche for HSCs. The adult bone marrow HSC niche has received the most attention, although its complex nature makes studying it difficult. Stromal cells form an extracellular matrix in the niche to promote cell adhesion and regulate HSCs through complex signaling networks involving cytokines, adhesion molecules, and maintenance proteins. Key stromal cells thought to support HSCs in bone marrow niches include osteoblasts, endothelial cells, mesenchymal stem cells, CXCL12-abundant reticular cells, perivascular stromal cells, glial cells, and macrophages.[28,29]

Recent findings suggest that HSCs are predominantly quiescent, maintained in a nondividing state by intimate interactions with thrombopoietin-producing osteoblasts.[30] Opposing studies suggest that vascular cells are critical to HSC maintenance through CXCL12, which regulates migration of HSCs to the vascular niche.[31] These studies suggest a heterogeneous microenvironment that may impact the HSC differently, depending on location and cell type encountered.[32] Given the close proximity of cells within the bone marrow cavity, it is likely that niches may overlap, providing multiple signals simultaneously and thus ensuring tight regulation of HSCs.[32] Although the cell-cell interactions are complex and multifactorial, understanding these relationships is critical to the advancement of cell therapies based on HSCs such as clinical marrow transplantation.

Recent reviews, which are beyond the scope of this chapter, discuss and help to delineate between transcription factors required for HSC proliferation or function and those that regulate HSC differentiation pathways.[33,34] The importance of transcription factors and their regulatory role in HSC maturation and redeployment in hematopoietic cell lineage production are demonstrated by their intimate involvement in disease evolution, such as in leukemia. Ongoing study of hematopoietic disease continues to demonstrate the complex and delicate nature of normal hematopoiesis.

Liver

The liver serves as the major site of blood cell production during the second trimester of fetal development. In adults, the hepatocytes of the liver have many functions, including protein synthesis and degradation, coagulation factor synthesis, carbohydrate and lipid metabolism, drug and toxin clearance, iron recycling and storage, and hemoglobin degradation in which bilirubin is conjugated and transported to the small intestine for eventual excretion.

The liver consists of two lobes situated beneath the diaphragm in the abdominal cavity. The position of the liver with regard to the circulatory system is optimal for gathering, transferring, and eliminating substances through the bile duct.[35,36] Anatomically, the hepatocytes are arranged in radiating plates emanating from a central vein (Figure 7-7). Adjacent to the longitudinal plates of hepatocytes are vascular sinusoids lined with endothelial cells. A small noncellular space separates the endothelial cells of the sinusoids from the plates of hepatocytes. This spatial arrangement allows plasma to have direct access to the hepatocytes for two-directional flow of solutes and fluids.

The lumen of the sinusoids contains *Kupffer cells* that maintain contact with the endothelial cell lining. Kupffer cells are macrophages that remove senescent cells and foreign debris from the blood that circulates through the liver; they also secrete mediators that regulate protein synthesis in the hepatocytes.[37] The particular anatomy, cellular components, and location in the body enables the liver to carry out many varied functions.

Liver Pathophysiology

The liver is often involved in blood-related diseases. In *porphyrias*, hereditary or acquired defects in the enzymes involved in heme biosynthesis result in the accumulation of the various intermediary *porphyrins* that damage hepatocytes, erythrocyte precursors, and other tissues. In severe hemolytic anemias, the liver increases the conjugation of *bilirubin* and the storage of iron. The liver sequesters membrane-damaged RBCs and removes them from the circulation. The liver can maintain hematopoietic stem and progenitor cells to produce various blood cells (called *extramedullary hematopoiesis*) as a response

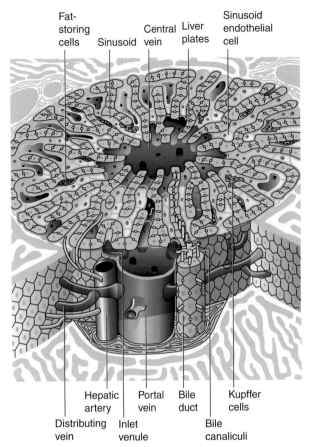

Fat-storing cells Sinusoid Central vein Liver plates Sinusoid endothelial cell

Hepatic artery Portal vein Bile duct Kupffer cells

Distributing vein Inlet venule Bile canaliculi

Figure 7-7 Three-dimensional schematic of the normal liver.

to infectious agents or in pathologic myelofibrosis of the bone marrow.[38] It is directly affected by storage diseases of the monocyte/macrophage (Kupffer) cells as a result of enzyme deficiencies that cause hepatomegaly with ultimate dysfunction of the liver (Gaucher disease, Niemann-Pick disease, Tay-Sachs disease; Chapter 29).

Spleen

The spleen is the largest lymphoid organ in the body. It is located directly beneath the diaphragm behind the fundus of the stomach in the upper left quadrant of the abdomen. It is vital but not essential for life and functions as an indiscriminate filter of the circulating blood. In a healthy individual, the spleen contains about 350 mL of blood.[35]

The exterior surface of the spleen is surrounded by a layer of *peritoneum* covering a connective tissue capsule. The capsule projects inwardly, forming trabeculae that divide the spleen into discrete regions. Located within these regions are three types of splenic tissue: *white pulp*, *red pulp*, and a *marginal zone*. The white pulp consists of scattered follicles with germinal centers containing lymphocytes, macrophages, and dendritic cells. Aggregates of T lymphocytes surround arteries that pass through these germinal centers, forming a region called the *periarteriolar lymphatic sheath*, or *PALS*. Interspersed along the periphery of the PALS are lymphoid nodules containing primarily B lymphocytes. Activated B lymphocytes are found in the germinal centers.[37]

The marginal zone surrounds the white pulp and forms a reticular meshwork containing blood vessels, macrophages, memory B cells, and CD4+ T cells.[39] The red pulp is composed primarily of vascular sinuses separated by cords of reticular cell meshwork (*cords of Billroth*) containing loosely connected specialized macrophages. This creates a sponge-like matrix that functions as a filter for blood passing through the region.[37] As RBCs pass through the cords of Billroth, there is a decrease in the flow of blood, which leads to stagnation and depletion of the RBCs' glucose supply. These cells are subject to increased damage and stress that may lead to their removal from the spleen. The spleen uses two methods for removing senescent or abnormal RBCs from the circulation: *culling*, in which the cells are phagocytized with subsequent degradation of cell organelles, and *pitting*, in which splenic macrophages remove inclusions or damaged surface membrane from the circulating RBCs.[40] The spleen also serves as a storage site for platelets. In a healthy individual, approximately 30% of the total platelet count is sequestered in the spleen.[41]

The spleen has a rich blood supply receiving approximately 350 mL/min. Blood enters the spleen through the *central splenic artery* located at the *hilum* and branches outward through the trabeculae. The branches enter all three regions of the spleen: the white pulp with its dense accumulation of lymphocytes, the marginal zone, and the red pulp. The venous sinuses, which are located in the red pulp, unite and leave the spleen as splenic veins (Figure 7-8).[42]

Spleen Pathophysiology

As blood enters the spleen, it may follow one of two routes. The first is a slow-transit pathway through the red pulp in which the RBCs pass circuitously through the macrophage-lined cords before reaching the sinuses. Plasma freely enters the sinuses, but the RBCs have a more difficult time passing through the tiny openings created by the *interendothelial junctions* of adjacent endothelial cells (Figure 7-9). The combination of the slow passage and the continued RBC metabolism creates an environment that is acidic, hypoglycemic, and hypoxic. The increased environmental stress on the RBCs circulating through the spleen leads to possible hemolysis.

In the rapid-transit pathway, blood cells enter the splenic artery and pass directly to the sinuses in the red pulp and continue to

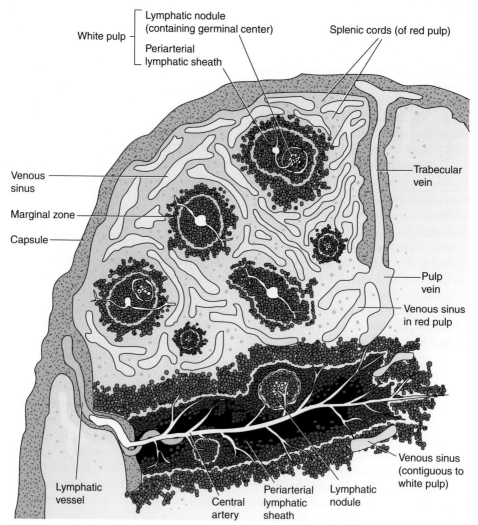

Figure 7-8 Schematic of the normal spleen. (From Weiss L, Tavossoli M: Anatomical hazards to the passage of erythrocytes through the spleen, Semin Hematol 7:372-380, 1970.)

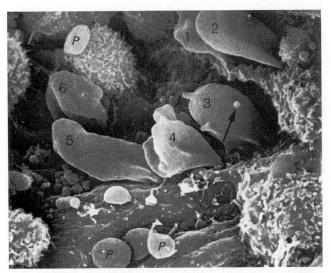

Figure 7-9 Scanning electron micrograph of the spleen shows erythrocytes (numbered 1 to 6) squeezing through the fenestrated wall in transit from the splenic cord to the sinus. The view shows the endothelial lining of the sinus wall, to which platelets (*P*) adhere, along with white blood cells, probably macrophages. The arrow shows a protrusion on a red blood cell (×5000). (From Weiss L: A scanning electron microscopic study of the spleen, Blood 43:665, 1974.)

the venous system to exit the spleen. When *splenomegaly* occurs, the spleen becomes enlarged and is palpable. This occurs as a result of many conditions, such as chronic leukemias, inherited membrane or enzyme defects in RBCs, hemoglobinopathies, Hodgkin disease, thalassemia, malaria, and the myeloproliferative disorders. *Splenectomy* may be beneficial in cases of excessive destruction of RBCs, such as autoimmune hemolytic anemia when treatment with corticosteroids does not effectively suppress hemolysis or in severe hereditary spherocytosis.[40,43] Splenectomy also may be indicated in severe refractory immune thrombocytopenic purpura or in storage disorders with portal hypertension and splenomegaly resulting in peripheral cytopenias.[40] After splenectomy, platelet and leukocyte counts increase transiently.[40] In sickle cell anemia, repeated splenic infarcts caused by sickled RBCs trapped in the small-vessel circulation of the spleen cause tissue damage and necrosis, which often results in *autosplenectomy* (Chapter 27).

Hypersplenism is an enlargement of the spleen resulting in some degree of pancytopenia despite the presence of a hyperactive bone marrow. The most common cause is congestive splenomegaly secondary to cirrhosis of the liver and portal hypertension. Other causes include thrombosis, vascular stenosis, other vascular deformities such as aneurysm of the splenic artery, and cysts.[44]

Lymph Nodes

Lymph nodes are organs of the lymphatic system located along the *lymphatic capillaries* that parallel, but are not part of, the circulatory system. The nodes are bean-shaped structures (1 to 5 mm in diameter) that occur in groups or chains at various intervals along lymphatic vessels. They may be superficial (inguinal, axillary, cervical, supratrochlear) or deep (mesenteric, retroperitoneal). Lymph is the fluid portion of blood that escapes into the connective tissue and is characterized by a low protein concentration and the absence of RBCs. *Afferent* lymphatic vessels carry circulating lymph to the lymph nodes. Lymph is filtered by the lymph nodes and exits via the *efferent* lymphatic vessels located in the hilus of the lymph node.[39]

Lymph nodes can be divided into an outer region called the *cortex* and an inner region called the *medulla*. An outer capsule forms trabeculae that radiate through the cortex and provide support for the macrophages and lymphocytes located in the node. The trabeculae divide the interior of the lymph node into follicles (Figure 7-10). After antigenic stimulation, the cortical region of some follicles develop foci of activated B cell proliferation called *germinal centers*.[19,35] Follicles with germinal centers are called *secondary follicles*, while those without are called *primary follicles*.[39] Located between the cortex and the medulla is a region called the *paracortex*, which contains predominantly T cells and numerous macrophages. The *medullary cords* lie toward the interior of the lymph node. These cords consist primarily of plasma cells and B cells.[43] Lymph nodes have three main functions: they are a site of lymphocyte proliferation from the germinal centers, they are involved in the initiation of the specific immune response to foreign antigens, and they filter particulate matter, debris, and bacteria entering the lymph node via the lymph.

Lymph Node Pathophysiology

Lymph nodes, by their nature, are vulnerable to the same organisms that circulate through the tissue. Sometimes increased numbers of microorganisms enter the nodes, overwhelming the macrophages and causing *adenitis* (infection of the lymph node). More serious is the frequent entry into the lymph nodes of malignant cells that have broken loose from malignant tumors. These malignant cells may grow and metastasize to other lymph nodes in the same group.

Thymus

To understand the role of the thymus in adults, certain formative intrauterine processes that affect function must be considered. First, the thymus tissue originates from endodermal and mesenchymal tissue. Second, the thymus is populated initially by primitive lymphoid cells from the yolk sac and the liver. This increased population of lymphoid cells physically pushes the epithelial cells of the thymus apart; however, their long processes remain attached to one another by desmosomes. In adults, T cell progenitors migrate to the thymus from the bone marrow for further maturation.

At birth, the thymus is an efficient, well-developed organ. It consists of two lobes, each measuring 0.5 to 2 cm in diameter, and is further divided into lobules. The thymus is located in the upper part of the anterior mediastinum at about the level of the great vessels of the heart. It resembles other lymphoid tissue in that the lobules are subdivided into two areas: the cortex (a peripheral zone) and the medulla (a central zone) (Figure 7-11). Both areas are populated with the same cellular components—lymphoid cells, mesenchymal cells, reticular cells, epithelial cells, dendritic cells, and many macrophages—although in different proportions.[45] The cortex

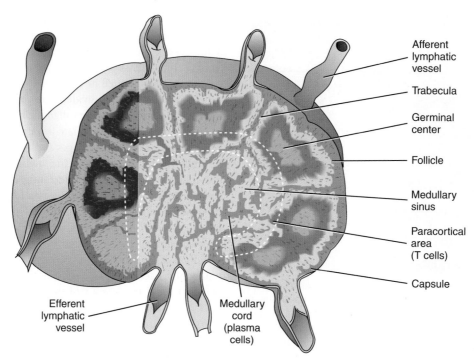

Afferent lymphatic vessel

Trabecula

Germinal center

Follicle

Medullary sinus

Paracortical area (T cells)

Capsule

Efferent lymphatic vessel

Medullary cord (plasma cells)

Figure 7-10 Histologic structure of a normal lymph node. Trabeculae divide the lymph node into follicles with an outer cortex (predominantly B cells) and a deeper paracortical zone (predominantly T cells). A central medulla is rich in plasma cells. After antigenic stimulation, secondary follicles develop germinal centers consisting of activated B cells. Primary follicles (not shown) lack germinal centers.

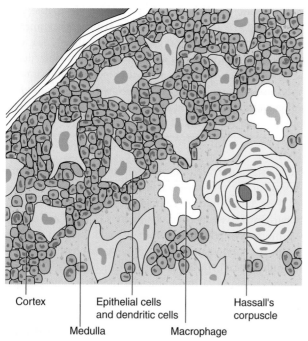

Cortex

Medulla

Epithelial cells and dendritic cells

Macrophage

Hassall's corpuscle

Figure 7-11 Schematic diagram of the edge of a lobule of the thymus, showing cells of the cortex and medulla. (From Abbas AK, Lichtman AH, Pober JS: Cellular and molecular immunology, Philadelphia, 1991, Saunders.)

is characterized by a blood supply system that is unique in that it consists only of capillaries. Its function seems to be that of a "waiting zone" densely populated with progenitor T cells. When these progenitor T cells migrate from the bone marrow and first enter the thymus, they have no identifiable CD4 and CD8 surface markers (*double negative*), and they locate to the corticomedullary junction.[45] Under the influence of chemokines, cytokines, and receptors, these cells move to the cortex and express both CD4 and CD8 (*double positive*).[45] Subsequently they give rise to mature T cells that express either CD4 or CD8 surface antigen as they move toward the medulla.[45] Eventually, the mature T cells leave the thymus to populate specific regions of other lymphoid tissue, such as the T cell-dependent areas of the spleen, lymph nodes, and other lymphoid tissues. The lymphoid cells that do not express the appropriate antigens and receptors, or are self-reactive, die in the cortex or medulla as a result of apoptosis and are phagocytized by macrophages.[45] The medulla contains only 15% mature T cells and seems to be a holding zone for mature T cells until they are needed by the peripheral lymphoid tissues.[45] The thymus also contains other cell types, including B cells, eosinophils, neutrophils, and other myeloid cells.[37]

Gross examination indicates that the size of the thymus is related to age. The thymus weighs 12 to 15 g at birth, increases to 30 to 40 g at puberty, and decreases to 10 to 15 g at later ages. It is hardly recognizable in old age due to atrophy (Figure 7-12). The thymus retains the ability to produce new T cells, however, as has been shown after irradiation treatment that may accompany bone marrow transplantation.

Thymus Pathophysiology

Nondevelopment of the thymus during gestation results in the lack of formation of T lymphocytes. Related manifestations seen in patients with this condition are failure to thrive, uncontrollable infections, and death in infancy. Adults with thymic disturbance are not affected because they have developed and maintained a pool of T lymphocytes for life.

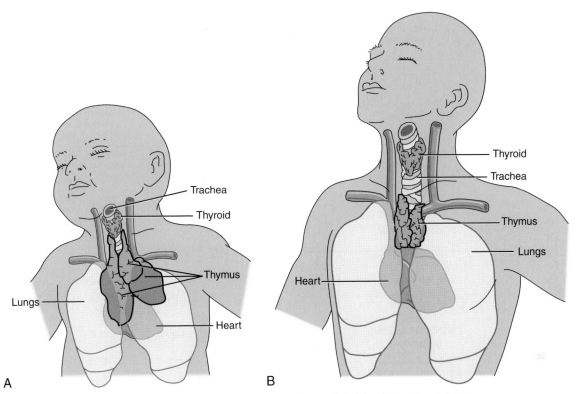

Figure 7-12 Differences in the size of the thymus of the infant **(A)** and the adult **(B)**.

HEMATOPOIETIC STEM CELLS AND CYTOKINES

Stem Cell Theory

In 1961, Till and McCulloch[46] conducted a series of experiments in which they irradiated spleens and bone marrow of mice, creating a state of aplasia. These aplastic mice were given an intravenous injection of marrow cells. Colonies of HSCs were seen 7 to 8 days later in the spleens of the irradiated (recipient) mice. These colonies were called *colony-forming units–spleen* (CFU-S). These investigators later showed that these colonies were capable of self-renewal and the production of differentiated progeny. The CFU-S represents what we now refer to as *committed myeloid progenitors* or *colony-forming unit–granulocyte, erythrocyte, monocyte, and megakaryocyte* (CFU-GEMM).[46,47] These cells are capable of giving rise to multiple lineages of blood cells.

Morphologically unrecognizable hematopoietic progenitor cells can be divided into two major types: noncommitted or undifferentiated hematopoietic stem cells, and committed progenitor cells. These two groups give rise to all of the mature blood cells. Originally there were two theories describing the origin of hematopoietic progenitor cells. The *monophyletic theory* suggests that all blood cells are derived from a single progenitor stem cell called a *pluripotent hematopoietic stem cell*. The *polyphyletic theory* suggests that each of the blood cell lineages is derived from its own unique stem cell. The monophyletic theory is the most widely accepted theory among experimental hematologists today.

Hematopoietic stem cells by definition are capable of self-renewal, are pluripotent and give rise to differentiated progeny, and are able to reconstitute the hematopoietic system of a lethally irradiated host. The undifferentiated HSCs can differentiate into progenitor cells committed to either lymphoid or myeloid lineages. These lineage-specific progenitor cells are the *common lymphoid progenitor*, which proliferates and differentiates into T, B, and natural killer lymphocyte and dendritic lineages; and the *common myeloid progenitor*, which proliferates and differentiates into individual granulocytic, erythrocytic, monocytic, and megakaryocytic lineages. The resulting limited lineage-specific progenitors give rise to morphologically recognizable, lineage-specific precursor cells (Figure 7-13 and Table 7-1). Despite the limited numbers of HSCs in the bone marrow, 6 billion blood cells per kilogram of body weight are produced each day for the entire life span of an individual.[3] Most of the cells in normal bone marrow are precursor cells at various stages of maturation.

HSCs are directed to one of three possible fates: self-renewal, differentiation, or apoptosis.[48] When the HSC divides, it gives rise to two identical daughter cells. Both daughter cells may follow the path of differentiation, leaving the stem cell pool (*symmetric division*), or one daughter cell may return to the stem cell pool and the other daughter cell may follow the path of differentiation (*asymmetric division*) or undergo apoptosis. Many theories have been proposed to describe the mechanisms that determine the fate of the stem cell. Till and McCulloch proposed that hematopoiesis is a random process whereby the HSC randomly commits to self-renewal or differentiation.[46] This model is also called the *stochastic* model of hematopoiesis. Later studies suggested that the microenvironment in the bone marrow determines whether the HSC will self-renew or differentiate (*instructive*

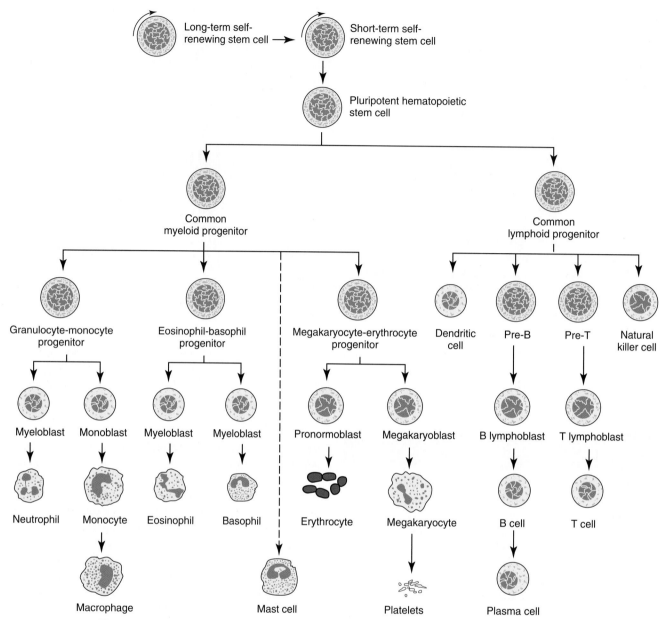

Figure 7-13 Diagram of hematopoiesis shows derivation of cells from the pluripotent hematopoietic stem cell.

TABLE 7-1 Culture-Derived Colony-Forming Units (CFUs)

Abbreviation	Cell Line
CFU-GEMM	Granulocyte, erythrocyte, megakaryocyte, monocyte
CFU-E	Erythrocyte
CFU-Meg	Megakaryocyte
CFU-M	Monocyte
CFU-GM	Granulocyte, monocyte
CFU-BASO	Myeloid to basophil
CFU-EO	Myeloid to eosinophil
CFU-G	Myeloid to neutrophil
CFU-pre-T	T lymphocyte
CFU-pre-B	B lymphocyte

model of hematopoiesis).[48] Current thinking is that the ultimate decision made by the HSC can be described by both the stochastic and instructive models of hematopoiesis. The initial decision to self-renew or differentiate is probably stochastic, whereas lineage differentiation that occurs later is determined by various signals from the hematopoietic inductive microenvironment in response to specific requirements of the body.

The multilineage priming model suggests that HSCs receive low-level signals from the *hematopoietic inductive microenvironment* to amplify or repress genes associated with commitment to multiple lineages. The implication is that the cell's fate is determined by intrinsic and extrinsic factors. Extrinsic regulation involves proliferation and differentiation signals from specialized niches located in the hematopoietic inductive microenvironment via direct cell-to-cell or cellular-extracellular signaling molecules.[48] Some of the cytokines released from the hematopoietic inductive microenvironment include factors that regulate proliferation and differentiation, such as KIT ligand, thrombopoietin (TPO), and FLT3 ligand. Intrinsic regulation involves genes such as *TAL1*, which is expressed in cells in the *hemangioblast*, a bipotential progenitor cell of mesodermal origin that gives rise to hematopoietic and endothelial lineages; and *GATA2*, which is expressed in later-appearing HSCs. Both of these genes are essential for primitive and definitive hematopoiesis.[48] In addition to factors involved in differentiation and regulation, there are regulatory signaling factors, such as Notch-1 and Notch-2, that allow HSCs to respond to hematopoietic inductive microenvironment factors, altering cell fate.[49]

As hematopoietic cells differentiate, they take on various morphologic features associated with maturation. These include an overall decrease in cell volume and a decrease in the ratio of nucleus to cytoplasm. Additional changes that take place during maturation occur in the cytoplasm and nucleus. Changes in the nucleus include loss of nucleoli, decrease in the diameter of the nucleus, condensation of nuclear chromatin, possible change in the shape of the nucleus, and possible loss of the nucleus. Changes occurring in the cytoplasm include decrease in basophilia, increase in the proportion of cytoplasm, and possible appearance of granules in the cytoplasm. Specific changes in each lineage are discussed in subsequent chapters.

Stem Cell Cycle Kinetics

The bone marrow is estimated to be capable of producing approximately 2.5 billion erythrocytes, 2.5 billion platelets, and 1 billion granulocytes per kilogram of body weight daily.[3] The determining factor controlling the rate of production is physiologic need. HSCs exist in the marrow in the ratio of 1 per 1000 nucleated blood cells.[4] They are capable of many mitotic divisions when stimulated by appropriate cytokines. When mitosis has occurred, the cell may reenter the cycle or go into a resting phase, termed G_0. Some cells in the resting phase reenter the active cell cycle and divide, whereas other cells are directed to terminal differentiation (Figure 7-14).

From these data, a mitotic index can be calculated to establish the percentage of cells in mitosis in relation to the total number of cells. Factors affecting the mitotic index include the duration of mitosis and the length of the resting state. Normally, the mitotic index is approximately 1% to 2%. An increased mitotic index implies increased proliferation. An exception to this rule is in the case of megaloblastic anemia, in which mitosis is prolonged.[50] An understanding of the mechanism of the generative cycle aids in understanding the mode of action of specific drugs used in the treatment and management of proliferative disorders.

Stem Cell Phenotypic and Functional Characterization

The identification and origin of HSCs can be determined by immunophenotypic analysis using flow cytometry. The earliest identifiable human HSCs capable of initiating long-term cultures

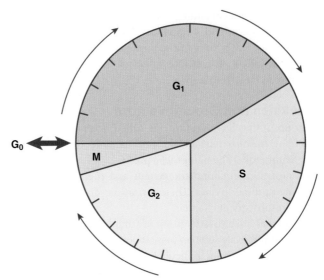

Figure 7-14 Cell cycle schematic. G_0, Resting stage; G_1, cell growth and synthesis of components necessary for cell division; *S*, DNA replication; G_2, premitotic phase; *M*, mitosis.

are CD34[+], CD38[−], HLA-DR[low], Thy$_1$[low], and Lin[−].[49] This population of marrow cells is enriched in primitive progenitors. The expression of CD38 and HLA-DR is associated with a loss of "stemness." The acquisition of CD33 and CD38 is seen on committed myeloid progenitors, and the expression of CD10 and CD38 is seen on committed lymphoid progenitors.[49] The expression of CD7 is seen on T-lymphoid progenitor cells and natural killer cells, and the expression of CD19 is seen on B-lymphoid progenitors (Chapter 32).[45]

Functional characterization of HSCs can be accomplished through in vitro techniques using long-term culture assays. These involve the enumeration of colony-forming units (e.g., CFU-GEMM) on semisolid media, such as methylcellulose. Primitive progenitor cells, such as the *high proliferative potential colony-forming cell* and the *long-term colony initiating cell*, also have been identified. These hematopoietic precursor cells give rise to colonies that can survive for 5 to 8 weeks and be replated.[49] In vivo functional assays also are available and require transplantation of cells into syngeneic, lethally irradiated animals, followed by transference of the engrafted bone marrow cells into a secondary recipient.[49] These systems promote the proliferation and differentiation of HSCs, thus allowing them to be characterized; they may serve as models for developing clinically applicable techniques for gene therapy and hematopoietic stem cell transplantation.

From our rudimentary knowledge of stem cell biology, it has been possible to move from the bench to the bedside with amazing speed and success. Hematopoietic stem cell transplantation (HSCT) is over a half-century old, and we have witnessed tremendous growth in the field due to the reproducibility of clinical procedures to produce similar outcomes. However, caution must be exercised because the cells capable of these remarkable clinical events are still not well defined, the niche that they inhabit is poorly understood, and the signals that they potentially respond to are plentiful and diverse in action. Current treatment of hematologic disorders is based on fundamental understanding of the biologic principles of HSC proliferation and maturation. The control mechanisms that regulate HSCs, and the requisite processes necessary to manipulate them to generate sufficient numbers for clinical use, remain largely unknown.

Cytokines and Growth Factors

A group of specific glycoproteins called *hematopoietic growth factors* or *cytokines* regulate the proliferation, differentiation, and maturation of hematopoietic precursor cells.[51] Figure 7-15 illustrates the hematopoietic system and the sites of action of some of the cytokines. These factors are discussed in more detail in subsequent chapters.

Cytokines are a diverse group of soluble proteins that have direct and indirect effects on hematopoietic cells. Classification of cytokines has been difficult because of their overlapping and redundant properties. The terms *cytokine* and *growth factor*

are often used synonymously; cytokines include *interleukins (ILs), lymphokines, monokines, interferons, chemokines,* and *colony-stimulating factors (CSFs).*[51] Cytokines are responsible for stimulation or inhibition of production, differentiation, and trafficking of mature blood cells and their precursors.[52] Many of these cytokines exert a positive influence on hematopoietic stem cells and progenitor cells with multilineage potential (e.g., KIT ligand, FLT3 ligand, GM-CSF, IL-1, IL-3, IL-6, and IL-11).[52] Cytokines that exert a negative influence on hematopoiesis include transforming growth factor-β, tumor necrosis factor-α, and the interferons.[49]

Hematopoietic progenitor cells require cytokines on a continual basis for their growth and survival. Cytokines prevent hematopoietic precursor cells from dying by inhibiting apoptosis; they stimulate them to divide by decreasing the transit time from G_0 to G_1 of the cell cycle; and they regulate cell differentiation into the various cell lineages.

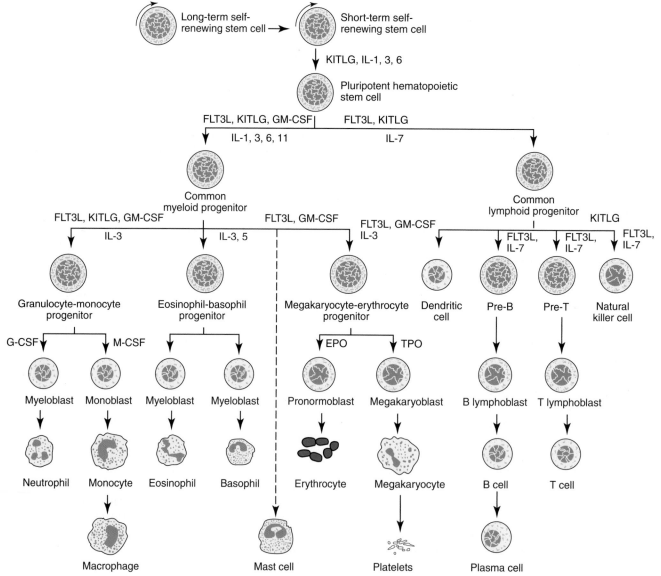

Figure 7-15 Diagram of derivation of hematopoietic cells, illustrating sites of action of cytokines. *EPO,* Erythropoietin; *FLT3L,* FLT3 ligand; *G-CSF,* granulocyte colony-stimulating factor; *GM-CSF,* granulocyte-macrophage colony-stimulating factor; *IL-1,* interleukin-1; *IL-3,* interleukin-3; *IL-5,* interleukin-5; *IL-6,* interleukin-6; *IL-7,* interleukin-7; *IL-11,* interleukin-11; *KITLG,* KIT ligand; *M-CSF,* macrophage colony-stimulating factor; *TPO,* thrombopoietin.

Apoptosis refers to programmed cell death, a normal physiologic process that eliminates unwanted, abnormal, or harmful cells. Apoptosis differs from necrosis, which is accidental death from trauma (Chapter 6). When cells do not receive the appropriate cytokines necessary to prevent cell death, apoptosis is initiated. In some disease states, apoptosis is "turned on," which results in early cell death, whereas in other states apoptosis is inhibited, which allows uncontrolled proliferation of cells.[52,53]

Research techniques have accomplished the purification of many of these cytokines and the cloning of pure recombinant growth factors, some of which are discussed in detail later in this chapter. The number of cytokines identified has expanded greatly in recent years and will further increase as research continues. This chapter focuses primarily on CSFs, KIT ligand, FLT3 ligand, and IL-3. A detailed discussion is beyond the scope of this text, and the reader is encouraged to consult current literature for further details.

Colony-Stimulating Factors

CSFs are produced by many different cells. They have a high specificity for their target cells and are active at low concentrations.[51] The names of the individual factors indicate the predominant cell lines that respond to their presence. The primary target of G-CSF is the granulocytic cell line, and GM-CSF targets the granulocytic-monocytic cell line. The biologic activity of CSFs was first identified by their ability to induce hematopoietic colony formation in semisolid media. In addition, it was shown in cell culture experiments that although a particular CSF may show specificity for one cell lineage, it is often capable of influencing other cell lineages as well. This is particularly true when multiple growth factors are combined.[54] Although GM-CSF stimulates the proliferation of granulocyte and monocyte progenitors, it also works synergistically with IL-3 to enhance megakaryocyte colony formation.[54]

Early-Acting Multilineage Growth Factors

Ogawa[55] described early-acting growth factors (multilineage), intermediate-acting growth factors (multilineage), and late-acting growth factors (lineage restricted). KIT ligand, also known as *stem cell factor* (SCF), is an early-acting growth factor; its receptor is the transmembrane protein, KIT. KIT is a receptor-type tyrosine-protein kinase that is expressed on HSCs and is down-regulated with differentiation. The binding of KIT ligand to the extracellular domain of the KIT receptor triggers its cytoplasmic domain to induce a series of signals that are sent via signal transduction pathways to the nucleus of the HSC, stimulating the cell to proliferate. As HSCs differentiate and mature, the expression of KIT receptor decreases. Activation of the KIT receptor by KIT ligand is essential in the early stages of hematopoiesis.[52,56]

FLT3 is also a receptor-type tyrosine-protein kinase. KIT ligand and FLT3 ligand work synergistically with IL-3, GM-CSF, and other cytokines to promote early HSC proliferation and differentiation. In addition, IL-3 regulates blood cell production by controlling the production, differentiation, and function of

granulocytes and macrophages.[57] GM-CSF induces expression of specific genes that stimulate HSC differentiation to the common myeloid progenitor.[58]

Interleukins

Cytokines originally were named according to their specific function, such as lymphocyte-activating factor (now called IL-1), but continued research showed that a particular cytokine may have multiple actions. A group of scientists began calling some of the cytokines *interleukins*, numbering them in the order in which they were identified (e.g., IL-1, IL-2). Characteristics shared by interleukins include the following:

1. They are proteins that exhibit multiple biologic activities, such as the regulation of autoimmune and inflammatory reactions and hematopoiesis.
2. They have synergistic interactions with other cytokines.
3. They are part of interacting systems with amplification potential.
4. They are effective at very low concentrations.

LINEAGE-SPECIFIC HEMATOPOIESIS

Erythropoiesis

Erythropoiesis occurs in the bone marrow and is a complex, regulated process for maintaining adequate numbers of erythrocytes in the peripheral blood. The CFU-GEMM gives rise to the earliest identifiable colony of RBCs, called the *burst-forming unit–erythroid* (BFU-E). The BFU-E produces a large multiclustered colony that resembles a cluster of grapes containing brightly colored hemoglobin. These colonies range from a single large cluster to 16 or more clusters. BFU-Es contain only a few receptors for EPO, and their cell cycle activity is not influenced significantly by the presence of exogenous EPO. BFU-Es under the influence of IL-3, GM-CSF, TPO, and KIT ligand develop into *colony-forming unit–erythroid* (CFU-E) colonies.[47] The CFU-E has many EPO receptors and has an absolute requirement for EPO. Some CFU-Es are responsive to low levels of EPO and do not have the proliferative capacity of the BFU-E.[25] EPO serves as a differentiation factor that causes the CFU-E to differentiate into pronormoblasts, the earliest visually recognized erythrocyte precursors in the bone marrow.[59]

EPO is a lineage-specific glycoprotein produced in the *renal peritubular interstitial cells*.[25] In addition, a small amount of EPO is produced by the liver.[56] Oxygen availability in the kidney is the stimulus that activates production and secretion of EPO.[60] EPO exerts it effects by binding to transmembrane receptors expressed by erythroid progenitors and precursors.[60] EPO serves to recruit CFU-E from the more primitive BFU-E compartment, prevents apoptosis of erythroid progenitors, and induces hemoglobin synthesis.[59,61] Erythropoiesis and EPO's actions are discussed in detail in Chapter 8.

Leukopoiesis

Leukopoiesis can be divided into two major categories: *myelopoiesis* and *lymphopoiesis*. Factors that promote differentiation of the CFU-GEMM into neutrophils, monocytes, eosinophils, and basophils include GM-CSF, G-CSF, macrophage colony-stimulating factor (M-CSF), IL-3, IL-5, IL-11, and KIT ligand. GM-CSF stimulates the proliferation and differentiation of neutrophil and macrophage colonies from the colony-forming unit–granulocyte-monocyte. G-CSF and M-CSF stimulate neutrophil differentiation and monocyte differentiation from the colony-forming unit–granulocyte and colony-forming unit–monocyte.[25] IL-3 is a multilineage stimulating factor that stimulates the growth of granulocytes, monocytes, megakaryocytes, and erythroid cells. Eosinophils require GM-CSF, IL-5, and IL-3 for differentiation. The requirements for basophil differentiation are less clear, but it seems to depend on the presence of IL-3 and KIT ligand. Growth factors promoting lymphoid differentiation include IL-2, IL-7, IL-12, and IL-15 and to some extent IL-4, IL-10, IL-13, IL-14, and IL-16.[53] Leukopoiesis is discussed further in Chapter 12.

Megakaryopoiesis

Earlier influences on megakaryopoiesis include GM-CSF, IL-3, IL-6, IL-11, KIT ligand, and TPO.[53] The stimulating hormonal factor TPO (also known as MPL ligand), along with IL-11, controls the production and release of platelets. The liver is the main site of production of TPO.[62,63] Megakaryopoiesis is discussed in Chapter 13.

THERAPEUTIC APPLICATIONS

Clinical use of growth factors approved by the U.S. Food and Drug Administration has contributed numerous options in the treatment of hematologic malignancies and solid tumors. In addition, growth factors can be used as priming agents to increase the yield of HSCs during apheresis for transplantation protocols. Advances in molecular biology have resulted in cloning of the genes that are responsible for the synthesis of various growth factors and the recombinant production of large quantities of these proteins. Table 7-2 is an overview of selected cytokines and their major functions and clinical applications. Many more examples can be found in the literature.

In addition to the cytokines previously mentioned, it is important to recognize another family of low-molecular-weight proteins known as chemokines (chemotactic cytokines) that complement cytokine function and help to regulate the adaptive and innate immune system. These interacting biological mediators have amazing capabilities, such as controlling growth and differentiation, hematopoiesis, and a number of lymphocyte functions like recruitment, differentiation, and inflammation.[64-66] The chemokine field has rapidly developed and is beyond the scope of this chapter. Nevertheless, a classification

TABLE 7-2 Selected Cytokines, Characteristics, Current and Potential Therapeutic Applications

Cytokine	Primary Cell Source	Primary Target Cell	Biological Activity	Current/Potential Therapeutic Applications
EPO	Kidney (peritubular interstitial cell)	Bone marrow erythroid progenitors (BFU-E and CFU-E)	Simulates proliferation of erythroid progenitors and prevents apoptosis of CFU-E	Anemia of chronic renal disease (in predialysis, dialysis dependent, and chronic anemia patients) Treatment of anemia in cancer patients on chemotherapy Autologous predonation blood collection Anemia in HIV infection to permit use of zidovudine (AZT) Post autologous hematopoietic stem cell transplant
G-CSF	Endothelial cells Placenta Monocytes Macrophages	Neutrophil precursors Fibroblasts Leukemic myeloblasts	Stimulates granulocyte colonies Differentiation of progenitors toward neutrophil lineage Stimulation of neutrophil maturation	Chemotherapy-induced neutropenia Stem cell mobilization Peripheral blood/bone marrow transplantation Congenital neutropenia Idiopathic neutropenia Cyclic neutropenia
GM-CSF	T cells Macrophages Endothelial cells Fibroblasts Mast cells	Bone marrow progenitor cells Dendritic cells Macrophages NKT cells	Promotes antigen presentation T cell homeostasis Hematopoietic cell growth factor	Chemotherapy-induced neutropenia Stem cell mobilization Peripheral blood/bone marrow transplantation Leukemia treatment
IL-2	CD4$^+$ T cells NK cells B cells	T cells NK cells B cells Monocytes	Cell growth/activation of CD4$^+$ and CD8$^+$ T cells Suppress T$_{reg}$ responses Mediator of immune tolerance	Metastatic melanoma Renal cell carcinoma Non-Hodgkin lymphoma Asthma

TABLE 7-2 Selected Cytokines, Characteristics, Current and Potential Therapeutic Applications—cont'd

Cytokine	Primary Cell Source	Primary Target Cell	Biological Activity	Current/Potential Therapeutic Applications
IL-3	Activated T cells NK cells	Hematopoietic stem cells and progenitors	Proliferation of hematopoietic progenitors	Stem cell mobilization Postchemotherapy/transplantation Bone marrow failure states
IL-6	T cells Macrophages Fibroblasts	T cells B cells Liver	Costimulation with other cytokines Cell growth/activation of T cells and B cells Megakaryocyte maturation Neural differentiation Acute phase reactant	Stimulation of platelet production, but not at tolerable doses Melanoma Renal cell carcinoma IL-6 inhibitors may be promising
IL-10	CD4+, Th2 T cells CD8+ T cells Monocytes Macrophages	T cells Macrophages	Inhibits cytokine production Inhibits macrophages	Target lymphokines in prevention of B cell lymphoma and Epstein-Barr virus lymphomagenesis Human immunodeficiency virus infection
IL-12	Macrophages	T cells	T cell, Th1 differentiation	Allergy treatment Adjuvant for infectious disease therapy Asthma Possible role for use in vaccines
IL-15	Activated CD4+ T cells	CD4+ T cells CD8+ T cells NK cells	CD4+/CD8+ T cell proliferation CD8+/NK cell cytotoxicity	Melanoma Rheumatoid arthritis Adoptive cell therapy Generation of antigen-specific T cells
IFN-α	Dendritic cells NK cells T cells B cells Macrophages Fibroblasts Endothelial cells Osteoblasts	Macrophages NK cells	Antiviral Enhances MHC expression	Adjuvant treatment for stage II/III melanoma Hematologic malignancies: Kaposi sarcoma, hairy cell leukemia, and chronic myelogenous leukemia

BFU-E, Burst-forming unit–erythroid; *CFU-E,* colony-forming unit–erythroid; *EPO,* erythropoietin; *G-CSF,* granulocyte colony-stimulating factor; *GM-CSF,* granulocyte-macrophage colony-stimulating factor; *HIV,* human immunodeficiency virus; *IFN,* interferon; *IL,* interleukin; *MHC,* major histocompatibility complex; *NK,* natural killer; *NKT,* natural killer T cells; *Th1,* T helper, type 1; *Th2,* T helper, type 2; *T reg,* regulatory T cells. (Adapted from Lee S and Margolin K: Cytokines in cancer immunotherapy. cancer 3:3856-3893, 2011; Kurzrock R. Chapter 64 Hematopoietic Growth Factors. In Bast RC, Kufe DW, Pollock RE, et al, editors: Holland-Frei Cancer Medicine, 5e, Hamilton [ON], 2000, BC Decker; and Cutler A, Brombacher F: Cytokine therapy. Ann NY Acad Sci 1056:16-29, 2005; and Cazzola M, Mercuriall F, Bruguara C. Use of recombinant human erythropoietin outside the setting of uremia. Blood, 1997;89:4248-4267.)

system has been developed based on the positions of the first two cysteine residues in the primary structure of these molecules, and the classification system divides the chemokine family into four groups. References provide a starting point for further investigation of chemokines.[64-67]

A recent chemokine-related discovery with clinical implications has led to a successful transplantation-based HSC collection strategy targeting the HSC-microenvironment niche interaction to cause release of HSCs from the bone marrow compartment (referred to a stem cell mobilization) into the peripheral circulation so that they may be harvested by apheresis techniques.[68]

Experimental studies conducted in the 1990s identified a critical role for CXCL12 and its receptor CXCR4 in the migration of HSCs during early development.[69] Further investigation in adult bone marrow demonstrated that CXCL12 is a key factor in the retention of HSCs within the stem cell niche. It was also shown that inhibiting the CXCL12-CXCR4 interaction permitted release of HSCs into the peripheral circulation for harvesting by apheresis.[69] Plexifor (a CXCR4 antagonist) is currently being used as a single agent and in conjunction with G-CSF in novel mobilization strategies to optimize donor stem cell collection.[68,69]

SUMMARY

- Hematopoiesis is a continuous, regulated process of blood cell production that includes cell renewal, proliferation, differentiation, and maturation. These processes result in the formation, development, and specialization of all the functional blood cells.
- During fetal development, hematopoiesis progresses through the mesoblastic, hepatic, and medullary phases.
- Organs that function at some point in hematopoiesis include the liver, spleen, lymph nodes, thymus, and bone marrow.
- The bone marrow is the primary site of hematopoiesis at birth and throughout life. In certain situations, blood cell production may occur outside the bone marrow; such production is termed *extra-medullary*.
- The *hematopoietic inductive microenvironment* in the bone marrow is essential for regulating hematopoietic stem cell maintenance, self-renewal, and differentiation.
- Monophyletic theory suggests that all blood cells arise from a single stem cell called a *pluripotent hematopoietic stem cell*.
- Hematopoietic stem cells (HSCs) are capable of self-renewal. They are pluripotent and can differentiate into all the different types of blood cells. One HSC is able to reconstitute the entire hematopoietic system of a lethally irradiated host.

- As cells mature, certain morphologic characteristics of maturation allow specific lineages to be recognized. General characteristics of maturation include decrease in cell diameter, decrease in nuclear diameter, loss of nucleoli, condensation of nuclear chromatin, and decreased basophilia in cytoplasm. Some morphologic changes are unique to specific lineages (e.g., loss of the nucleus in RBCs).
- Cytokines or growth factors play a major role in the maintenance, proliferation, and differentiation of HSCs and progenitor cells; they are also necessary to prevent premature apoptosis. Cytokines include interleukins, colony stimulating factors, chemokines, interferons, and others.
- Cytokines can exert a positive or negative influence on HSCs and blood cell progenitors; some are lineage specific, and some function only in combination with other cytokines.
- Cytokines have provided new options in the treatment of hematologic malignancies and solid tumors. They are also used as priming agents to increase the yield of HSCs during apheresis for transplantation protocols.

REVIEW QUESTIONS

Answers can be found in the Appendix.

1. The process of formation and development of blood cells is termed:
   a. Hematopoiesis
   b. Hematemesis
   c. Hematocytometry
   d. Hematorrhea

2. During the second trimester of fetal development, the primary site of blood cell production is the:
   a. Bone marrow
   b. Spleen
   c. Lymph nodes
   d. Liver

3. Which one of the following organs is responsible for the maturation of T lymphocytes and regulation of their expression of CD4 and CD8?
   a. Spleen
   b. Liver
   c. Thymus
   d. Bone marrow

4. The best source of active bone marrow from a 20-year-old would be:
   a. Iliac crest
   b. Femur
   c. Distal radius
   d. Tibia

5. Physiologic programmed cell death is termed:
   a. Angiogenesis
   b. Apoptosis
   c. Aneurysm
   d. Apohematics

6. Which organ is the site of sequestration of platelets?
   a. Liver
   b. Thymus
   c. Spleen
   d. Bone marrow

7. Which one of the following morphologic changes occurs during normal blood cell maturation:
   a. Increase in cell diameter
   b. Development of cytoplasm basophilia
   c. Condensation of nuclear chromatin
   d. Appearance of nucleoli

8. Which one of the following cells is a product of the CLP?
   a. Megakaryocyte
   b. T lymphocyte
   c. Erythrocyte
   d. Granulocyte

9. What growth factor is produced in the kidneys and is used to treat anemia associated with kidney disease?
   a. EPO
   b. TPO
   c. G-CSF
   d. KIT ligand

10. Which one of the following cytokines is required very early in the differentiation of a hematopoietic stem cell?
    a. IL-2
    b. IL-8
    c. EPO
    d. FLT3 ligand

11. When a patient has severe anemia and the bone marrow is unable to effectively produce red blood cells to meet the increased demand, one of the body's responses is:
    a. Extramedullary hematopoiesis in the liver and spleen
    b. Decreased production of erythropoietin by the kidney
    c. Increased apoptosis of erythrocyte progenitor cells
    d. Increase the proportion of yellow marrow in the long bones

12. Hematopoietic stem cells produce all lineages of blood cells in sufficient quantities over the lifetime of an individual because they:
    a. Are unipotent
    b. Have the ability of self-renewal by asymmetric division
    c. Are present in large numbers in the bone marrow niches
    d. Have a low mitotic potential in response to growth factors

REFERENCES

1. Orkin, S. (2000). Diversification of haematopoietic stem cells to specific lineages. *Nat Rev Genet, 1,* 57–64.
2. Galloway, J. L., Zon, L. I. (2003). Ontongeny of hematopoiesis: examining the emergence of hematopoietic cells in the vertebrate embryo. *Curr Top Dev Biol, 53,* 139–158.
3. Koury, M. J., Lichtman, M. A. (2010). Structure of the marrow and the hematopoietic microenvironment. In Prchal, J. T., Kaushansky, K., Lichtman, M. A., et al. (Eds.), *Williams Hematology.* (8th ed.). New York: McGraw-Hill.
4. Chute, J. P. (2013). Hematopoietic stem cell biology. In Hoffman, R., Benz, E. J., Silberstein, L. E., et al. (Eds.), *Hematology Basic Principles and Practice.* (8th ed.). Philadelphia: Saunders-Elsevier.
5. Peault, B. (1996). Hematopoietic stem cell emergence in embryonic life: developmental hematology revisited. *J Hematotherapy, 5,* 369–378.
6. Tavian, M., Coulombel, L., Luton, D., et al. (1996). Aorta-associated CD34+ hematopoietic cells in the early human embryo. *Blood, 87,* 67–72.
7. Ivanovs, A., Rybtsov, S., Welch, L., Anderson, R. A., et al. (2011). Highly potent human hematopoietic stem cells first emerge in the intraembryonic aorta-gonad-mesonephros region. *J Exp Med, 208,* 2417–2427.
8. Palis, J., Segal, G. B. (2010). Hematology of the fetus and newborn. In Prchal, J. T., Kaushansky, K., Lichtman, M. A., et al. (Eds.), *Williams Hematology.* (8th ed.). New York: McGraw-Hill.
9. Moore, M. A., Metcalf, D. (1970). Ontogeny of the haematopoietic system: yolk sac origin of in vivo and in vitro colony forming cells in the developing mouse embryo. *Br J Haematol, 18,* 279–296.
10. Weissman, I. L., Papaloannou, V., Gardner, R. L. (1978). Fetal hematopoietic origins of the adult hematolymphoid system. In Clarkson, B., Marks, P. A., Till, J. E., (Eds.), *Differentiation of Normal and Neoplastic Hematopoietic Cells.* Cold Spring Harbor, NY: Cold Spring Harbor Laboratory Press.
11. Bailey, A. S., Fleming, W. H. (2003). Converging roads: evidence for an adult hemangioblast. *Exp Hematol, 31,* 987–993.
12. Pelosi, E., Valtieri, M., Coppola, S., Botta, R., et al. (2002). Identification of the hemangioblast in postnatal life. *Blood, 100,* 3203–3208.
13. Bailey, A. S., Jiang, S., Afentoulis, M., Baumann, C. I., et al. (2004). Transplanted adult hematopoietic stems cells differentiate into functional endothelial cells. *Blood, 103,* 13–19.
14. Samokhvalov, I. M., Samokhvalov, N. I., Nishikawa, S. (2007). Cell tracing shows the contribution of the yolk sac to adult haematopoiesis. *Nature, 446,* 1056–1061.
15. Delassus, S., Cumano, A. (1996). Circulation of hematopoietic progenitors in the mouse embryo. *Immunity, 4,* 97–106.
16. DeWitt, N. (Published online 2007, June 21). Rewriting in blood: blood stem cells may have a surprising origin. *Nat Rep Stem Cells.* 10.1038/stem-cells.2007.42.
17. Dieterlen-Lievre, F., Godin, I., Pardanaud, I. (1997). Where do hematopoietic stem cells come from? *Arch Allergy Immunol, 112,* 3–8.
18. Chang, Y., Paige, C. J., Wu, G. E. (1992). Enumeration and characterization of DJH structures in mouse fetal liver. *EMBO J, 11,* 1891–1899.
19. Mescher, A. L. (2010). *Junqueira's Basic Histology.* (12th ed.). Stamford, Conn: Appleton & Lange.
20. Ross, M. H., Pawlina, W. (2006). *Histology: a Text and Atlas: with Correlated Cell and Molecular Biology.* (5th ed.). Philadelphia: Lippincott Williams & Wilkins.
21. Gupta, P., Blazar, B., Gupta, K., et al. (1998). Human CD34+ bone marrow cells regulate stromal production of interleukin-6 and granulocyte colony-stimulating factor and increase the colony-stimulating activity of stroma. *Blood, 91,* 3724–3733.
22. Rosen, C. J., Ackert-Bicknell, C., Rodriguez, J. P., Pino, A. M. (2009). Marrow fat and bone marrow microenvironment: developmental, functional, and pathological implications. *Crit Rev Eukaryot Gene Expr, 19,* 109–124.
23. Silberstein, L., Scadden, D. (2013). Hematopoietic microenvironment. In Hoffman, R., Benz, E. J., Silberstein, L. E., et al. (Eds.), *Hematology Basic Principles and Practice.* (6th ed.). Philadelphia: Saunders-Elsevier.
24. Sadahira, Y., Mori, M. (1999). Role of the macrophage in erythropoiesis. *Pathol Int, 10,* 841–848.
25. Kaushansky, K. (2009). Hematopoietic stem cells, progenitors, and cytokines. In Prchal, J. T., Kaushansky, K., Lichtman, M. A., et al. (Eds.), *Williams Hematology.* (8th ed.). New York: McGraw-Hill.
26. Warren, J. S., Ward, P. A. (2010). The inflammatory response. In Prchal, J. T., Kaushansky, K., Lichtman, M. A., et al. (Eds.), Williams Hematology. (8th ed.). New York: McGraw-Hill.
27. Klein, G. (1995). The extracellular matrix of the hematopoietic microenvironment. *Experientia, 51,* 914–926.

28. Ehninger, A., Trumpp, A. (2011). The bone marrow stem cell niche grows up: mesenchymal stem cells and macrophages move in. *J Exp Med, 208,* 421–428.

29. Smith, J. N. P., Calvi, L. M. (2013). Current concepts in bone marrow microenvironmental regulation of hematopoietic stem and progenitor cells. *Stem Cells, 31,* 1044–1050.

30. Yoshihara, H., Arai, F., Hosokawa, K., Hagiwara, T., et al. (2007). The niche regulation of quiescent hematopoietic stem cells through thrombopoietin/Mpl signaling. *Cell Stem Cell, 1,* 685–697.

31. Morrison, S. J., Spradling, A. C. (2008). Stem cells and niches: mechanisms that promote stem cell maintenance throughout life. *Cell, 132,* 598–611.

32. Ema, H., Suda, T. (2012). Anatomically distinct niches regulate stem cell activity. *Blood, 120,* 2174–2181.

33. Iwasaki, H., Akashi, K. (2007). Myeloid lineage commitment from the hematopoietic stem cell. *Immunity, 26,* 726–740.

34. Kim, S. I., Bresnick, E. H. (2007). Transcriptional control of erythropoiesis: emerging mechanisms and principles. *Oncogene, 26,* 6777–6794.

35. Thibodeau, G. A., Patton, K. T. (2003). *Anatomy and Physiology.* (5th ed.). St Louis: Mosby.

36. Roy-Chowdhury, N., Roy-Chowdhury, J. (2012). Liver physiology and energy metabolism. In Feldman, M., Friedman, L. S., Brandt, L. J., (Eds.), *Sleisenger and Fordtran's Gastrointestinal and Liver Disease.* (9th ed.). Philadelphia: Saunders-Elsevier.

37. Taylor, G. A., Weinberg, J. B. (2009). Mononuclear phagocytes. In Greer, J. P., Foerster, J., Rodgers, G. M., et al. (Eds.), *Wintrobe's Clinical Hematology.* (12th ed.). Philadelphia: Wolters Kluwer Health/Lippincott Williams & Wilkins.

38. Kim, C. H. (2010). Homeostatic and pathogenic extramedullary hematopoiesis. *J Blood Med, 1,* 13–19.

39. Kipps, T. J. (2010). The organization and structure of lymphoid tissues. In Prchal, J. T., Kaushansky, K., Lichtman, M. A., et al. (Eds.), *Williams Hematology.* (8th ed.). New York: McGraw-Hill.

40. Connell, N. T., Shurin, S. B., Schiffman, F. J. (2013). The spleen and its disorders. In Hoffman, R., Benz, E. J., Silberstein, L. E., et al. (Eds.), *Hematology basic principles and practice.* (6th ed.). Philadelphia: Saunders, Elsevier.

41. Warkentin, T. E. (2013). Thrombocytopenia caused by platelet destruction, hypersplenism, or hemodilution. In Hoffman, R., Benz, E. J., Silberstein, L. E., et al. (Eds.), *Hematology Basic Principles and Practice.* (6th ed.). Philadelphia: Saunders, Elsevier.

42. Seeley, R. R., Stephens, D., Tate, P. (1995). *Anatomy and physiology.* (3th ed.). St Louis: Mosby.

43. Ware, R. E. (2009). The autoimmune hemolytic anemias. In Nathan, D. G., Orkin, S. H., (Eds.), *Nathan and Oski's Hematology of Infancy and Childhood.* (3th ed.). Philadelphia: Saunders.

44. Porembka, M. R., Majella, Doyl, M. B., Chapman, W. C. (2009). Disorders of the spleen. In Greer, J. P., Foerster, J., Rodgers, G. M., et al, (Eds.), *Wintrobe's Clinical Hematology.* (12th ed.). Philadelphia: Wolters Kluwer Health/Lippincott Williams & Wilkins.

45. Paraskevas, F. (2009). T lymphocytes and NK cells. In Greer, J. P., Foerster, J., Rodgers, G. M., et al, (Eds.), *Wintrobe's Clinical Hematology.* (12th ed.). Philadelphia: Wolters Kluwer Health/Lippincott Williams & Wilkins.

46. Till, T. E., McCulloch, E. A. (1961). A direct measurement of the radiation sensitivity of normal mouse marrow cells. *Radiat Res, 14,* 213–222.

47. Dessypris, E. N., Sawyer, S. T. (2009). Erythropoiesis. In Greer, J. P., Foerster, J., Rodgers, G. M., et al, (Eds.), *Wintrobe's Clinical Hematology.* (12th ed.). Philadelphia: Wolters Kluwer Health/Lippincott Williams & Wilkins.

48. Metcalf, D. (2007). On hematopoietic stem cell fate. *Immunity, 26,* 669–673.

49. Verfaillie, C. (2003). Regulation of hematopoiesis. In Wickramasinghe, S. N., McCullough, J., (Eds.), *Blood and Bone Marrow Pathology.* New York: Churchill Livingstone.

50. Antony, A. C. (2013). Megaloblastic anemias. In Hoffman, R., Benz, E. J., Silberstein, L. E., et al, (Eds.), *Hematology Basic Principles and Practice.* (6th ed.). Philadelphia: Saunders, Elsevier.

51. Horst Ibelfault's COPE. (Spring 2013). *Cytokines Online Pathfinder Encyclopedia,* version 31.4. Available at: http://www .copewithcytokines.org/cope.cgi. Accessed 12.10.13.

52. Mathur, S. C., Schexneider, K. I., Hutchison, R. E. (2011). Hematopoiesis. In McPherson, R. A., Pincus, M. R., (Eds.), *Henry's Clinical Diagnosis and Management by Laboratory Methods.* (22nd ed.). Philadelphia: Saunders, Elsevier.

53. Shaheen, M., Broxmeyer, H. E. (2013). Principles of cytokine signaling. In Hoffman R, Benz EJ, Silberstein LE, et al, (Eds.), *Hematology Basic Principles and Practice.* (6th ed.). Philadelphia: Saunders, Elsevier.

54. Sieff, C., Zon, L. I. (2009). The anatomy and physiology of hematopoiesis. In Nathan, D. G., Orkin, S. H., (Eds.), *Nathan and Oski's Hematology of Infancy and Childhood.* (7th ed.). Philadelphia: Saunders, pp 195–273.

55. Ogawa, M. (1993). Differentiation and proliferation of hematopoietic stem cells. *Blood, 81,* 2844–2853.

56. Koury, M. J., Mahmud, N., Rhodes, M. M. (2009). Origin and development of blood cells. In Greer, J. P., Foerster, J., Rodgers, G. M., et al, (Eds.), *Wintrobe's Clinical Hematology.* (12th ed.). Philadelphia: Wolters Kluwer Health/Lippincott Williams & Wilkins.

57. Dorssers, L., Burger, H., Bot, F., et al. (1987). Characterization of a human multilineage-colony-stimulating factor cDNA clone identified by a conserved noncoding sequence in mouse interleukin-3. *Gene, 55,* 115–124.

58. Lin, E. Y., Orlofsky, A., Berger, M. S., et al. (1993). Characterization of A1, a novel hemopoietic-specific early-response gene with sequence similarity to bcl-s. *J Immunol, 151,* 1979–1988.

59. Sawada, K., Krantz, S. B., Dai, C. H. (1990). Purification of human burst-forming units-erythroid and demonstration of the evolution of erythropoietin receptors. *J Cell Physiol, 142,* 219–230.

60. Rizzo, J. D., Seidenfield, J., Piper, M., Aronson, N., Lictin, A., Littlewood, T. J. (2001). Erythropoietin: a paradigm for the development of practice guidelines. *Haematology, 1,* 10–30.

61. Cazzola, M., Mercuriall, F., Bruguara, C. (1997). Use of recombinant human erythropoietin outside the setting of uremia. *Blood, 89,* 4248–4267.

62. Wolber, E. M., Ganschow, R., Burdelski, M., et al. (1999). Hepatic thrombopoietin mRNA levels in acute and chronic liver failure of childhood. *Hepatology, 29,* 1739–1742.

63. Wolber, E. M., Dame, C., Fahnenstich, H., et al. (1999). Expression of the thrombopoietin gene in human fetal and neonatal tissues. *Blood, 94,* 97–105.

64. Scales, W. E. (1992). Structure and function of interleukin-1. In Kunkel, S. L., Remick, D. G., (Eds.), *Cytokines in Health and Disease.* New York: Marcel Dekker.

65. Zlotnik, A., Yoshie, O. (2000). Chemokines: a new classification system and their role in immunity. *Immunity, 12,* 121–127.

66. Baggiolini, M., Dewald, B., Moser, B. (1997). Human c hemokines: an update. *Annu Rev Immunol, 15,* 675–705.

67. Murphy, P. M., Baggiolini, M., Charo, I. F., et al. (2000). International union of pharmacology. XXII. Nomenclature for chemokine receptors. *Pharmacol Rev, 52,* 145–176.

68. Luster, A. D. (1998). Chemokines—Chemotactic cytokines that mediate inflammation. *N Engl J Med, 338,* 436–445.

69. DiPersio, J. F., Uy, G. L., Yasothan, U., Kirkpatrick, P. (2009). Plerixafor. *Nat Rev Drug Discov, 8,* 105–106.

Erythrocyte Production and Destruction 8

Kathryn Doig

OBJECTIVES

After completion of this chapter, the reader will be able to:

1. List and describe the erythroid precursors in order of maturity, including the morphologic characteristics, cellular activities, normal location, and length of time in the stage for each.
2. Correlate the erythroblast, normoblast, and rubriblast nomenclatures for red blood cell (RBC) stages.
3. Name the stage of erythroid development when given a written description of the morphology of a cell in a Wright-stained bone marrow preparation.
4. List and compare the cellular organelles of immature and mature erythrocytes and describe their specific functions.
5. Name the erythrocyte progenitors and distinguish them from precursors.
6. Explain the nucleus-to-cytoplasm (N:C) ratio, describe the appearance of a cell when given the N:C ratio, and estimate the N:C ratio from the appearance of a cell.
7. Explain how reticulocytes can be recognized in a Wright-stained peripheral blood film.
8. Define and differentiate the terms *polychromasia, diffuse basophilia, punctate basophilia,* and *basophilic stippling.*
9. Discuss the differences between the reticulum of reticulocytes and punctate basophilic stippling in composition and conditions for microscopic viewing.

10. Define and differentiate *erythron* and *RBC* mass.
11. Explain how hypoxia stimulates RBC production.
12. Describe the general chemical composition of erythropoietin (EPO) and name the site of production.
13. Discuss the various mechanisms by which EPO contributes to erythropoiesis.
14. Define and explain apoptosis resulting from Fas/FasL interactions and how this regulatory mechanism applies to erythropoiesis.
15. Explain the effect of Bcl-XL (Bcl-2 like protein 1) and the general mechanism by which it is stimulated in red blood cell progenitors.
16. Describe the features of the bone marrow that contribute to establishing the microenvironment necessary for the proliferation of RBCs, including location and arrangement relative to other cells, with particular emphasis on the role of fibronectin.
17. Discuss the role of macrophages in RBC development.
18. Explain how RBCs enter the bloodstream and how premature entry is prevented and, when appropriate, promoted.
19. Describe the characteristics of senescent RBCs and explain why RBCs age.
20. Explain and differentiate the two normal mechanisms of erythrocyte destruction, including location and process.

CASE STUDY

After studying the material in this chapter, the reader should be able to respond to the following case study:

A 42-year-old premenopausal woman has emphysema. This lung disease impairs the ability to oxygenate the blood, so patients experience significant fatigue and shortness of breath. To alleviate these symptoms, oxygen is typically prescribed, and this patient has a portable oxygen tank she carries with her at all times, breathing through nasal cannulae. Before she began using oxygen, her red blood cell (RBC) count was 5.8×10^{12}/L. After

oxygen therapy for several months, her RBC count dropped to 5.0×10^{12}/L.
1. What physiologic response explains the elevation of the first RBC count?
2. What hormone is responsible? How is its production stimulated? What is the major way in which it acts?
3. What explains the decline in RBC count with oxygen therapy for this patient?

The red blood cell (RBC), or erythrocyte, provides a classic example of the biological principle that cells have specialized functions and that their structures are specific for those functions. The erythrocyte has one true function: to carry oxygen from the lung to the tissues, where the oxygen is released. This is accomplished by the attachment of the oxygen to hemoglobin (HGB), the major cytoplasmic component of mature RBCs. The role of the RBC in returning carbon dioxide to the lungs and buffering the pH of the blood is important but is quite secondary to its oxygen-carrying function. To protect this essential life function, the mechanisms controlling development, production, and normal destruction of RBCs are fine-tuned to avoid interruptions in oxygen delivery, even under adverse conditions such as blood loss with hemorrhage. This chapter and subsequent chapters discussing iron, RBC metabolism, membrane structure, and hemoglobin constitute the foundation for understanding the body's response to diminished oxygen-carrying capacity of the blood, called *anemia*.

The mammalian erythrocyte is unique among animal cells in having no nucleus in its mature, functional state. While amphibians and birds possess RBCs, their nonmammalian RBCs retain the nuclei throughout the cells' lives. The implications of this unique mammalian adaptation are significant for cell function and life span.

NORMOBLASTIC MATURATION

Terminology

RBCs are formally called *erythrocytes*. The nucleated precursors in the bone marrow are called *erythroblasts*. They also may be called *normoblasts*, which refers to developing nucleated cells (i.e., blasts) with normal appearance. This is in contrast to the abnormal appearance of the developing nucleated cells in megaloblastic anemia, in which the erythroblasts are called *megaloblasts* because of their large size.

Three nomenclatures are used for naming the erythroid precursors (Table 8-1). The erythroblast terminology is used primarily in Europe. Like the normoblastic terminology used more often in the United States, it has the advantage of being descriptive of the appearance of the cells. Some prefer the *rubriblast* terminology because it parallels the nomenclature used for granulocyte development (Chapter 12). Normoblastic terminology is used in this chapter.

Maturation Process
Erythroid Progenitors

As described in Chapter 7, the morphologically identifiable erythrocyte precursors develop from two functionally identifiable progenitors, burst-forming unit–erythroid (BFU-E) and colony-forming unit–erythroid (CFU-E), both committed to the erythroid cell line. Estimates of time spent at each stage suggest that it takes about one week for the BFU-E to mature to the CFU-E and another week for the CFU-E to become a pronormoblast,[1] which is the first morphologically identifiable RBC precursor. While at the CFU-E stage, the cell completes approximately three to five divisions before maturing further.[1] As seen later, it takes approximately another 6 to 7 days for the precursors to become mature enough to enter the circulation, so approximately 18 to 21 days are required to produce a mature RBC from the BFU-E.

Erythroid Precursors

Normoblastic proliferation, similar to the proliferation of other cell lines, is a process encompassing replication (i.e., division) to increase cell numbers and development from immature to mature cell stages (Figure 8-1). The earliest morphologically recognizable erythrocyte precursor, the pronormoblast, is derived via the BFU-E and CFU-E from the pluripotential stem cells, as discussed in Chapter 7. The pronormoblast is able to divide, with each daughter cell maturing to the next stage of development, the basophilic normoblast. Each of these cells can divide, with each of its daughter cells maturing to the next stage, the polychromatic normoblast. Each of these cells also can divide and mature. In the erythrocyte cell line, there are typically three and occasionally as many as five divisions[2] with subsequent nuclear and cytoplasmic maturation of the daughter cells, so from a single pronormoblast, 8 to 32 mature RBCs usually result. The conditions under which the number of divisions can be increased or reduced are discussed later.

The cellular activities at each stage of development described below occur in an orderly and sequential process. It is often likened to a computer program that once activated runs certain processes in a specified order at specified times. The details of the developmental program are becoming clearer, and selected details are provided in these descriptions.

TABLE 8-1 Three Erythroid Precursor Nomenclature Systems

Normoblastic	Rubriblastic	Erythroblastic
Pronormoblast	Rubriblast	Proerythroblast
Basophilic normoblast	Prorubricyte	Basophilic erythroblast
Polychromatic (polychromatophilic) normoblast	Rubricyte	Polychromatic (polychromatophilic) erythroblast
Orthochromic normoblast	Metarubricyte	Orthochromic erythroblast
Polychromatic (polychromatophilic) erythrocyte*	Polychromatic (polychromatophilic) erythrocyte*	Polychromatic (polychromatophilic) erythrocyte*
Erythrocyte	Erythrocyte	Erythrocyte

*Polychromatic erythrocytes are called reticulocytes when observed with vital stains.

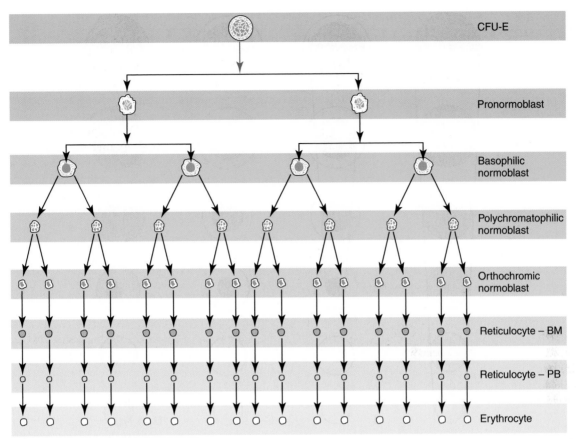

Figure 8-1 Typical production of erythrocytes from two pronormoblasts illustrating three mitotic divisions among precursors. *BM,* Bone marrow; *CFU,* colony forming unit–erythroid; *PB,* peripheral blood.

Criteria Used in Identification of the Erythroid Precursors

Morphologic identification of blood cells depends on a well-stained peripheral blood film or bone marrow smear (Chapters 16 and 17). In hematology, a modified Romanowsky stain, such as Wright or Wright-Giemsa, is commonly used. The descriptions that follow are based on the use of these types of stains.

The stage of maturation of any blood cell is determined by careful examination of the nucleus and the cytoplasm. The qualities of greatest importance in identification of RBCs are the nuclear chromatin pattern (texture, density, homogeneity), nuclear diameter, nucleus:cytoplasm (N:C) ratio (Box 8-1), presence or absence of nucleoli, and cytoplasmic color.

As RBCs mature, several general trends affect their appearance. Figure 8-2 graphically represents these trends.

1. The overall diameter of the cell decreases.
2. The diameter of the nucleus decreases more rapidly than does the size of the cell. As a result, the N:C ratio also decreases.
3. The nuclear chromatin pattern becomes coarser, clumped, and condensed. The nuclear chromatin of RBCs is inherently coarser than that of myeloid precursors. It becomes even coarser and more clumped as the cell matures, developing a raspberry-like appearance, in which the dark staining of the chromatin is distinct from the almost white appearance of the

parachromatin. This chromatin/parachromatin distinction is more dramatic than in other cell lines. Ultimately, the nucleus becomes quite condensed, with no parachromatin evident at all, and the nucleus is said to be *pyknotic.*

4. Nucleoli disappear. Nucleoli represent areas where the ribosomes are formed and are seen early in cell development as cells begin actively synthesizing proteins. As RBCs mature, the nucleoli disappear, which precedes the ultimate cessation of protein synthesis.

BOX 8-1 Nucleus-to-Cytoplasm (N:C) Ratio

The nucleus-to-cytoplasm (N:C) ratio is a morphologic feature used to identify and stage red blood cell and white blood cell precursors. The ratio is a visual estimate of what area of the cell is occupied by the nucleus compared with the cytoplasm. If the areas of each are approximately equal, the N:C ratio is 1:1. Although not mathematically proper, it is common for ratios other than 1:1 to be referred to as if they were fractions. If the nucleus takes up less than 50% of the area of the cell, the proportion of nucleus is lower, and the ratio is lower (e.g., 1:5 or less than 1). If the nucleus takes up more than 50% of the area of the cell, the ratio is higher (e.g., 3:1 or 3). In the red blood cell line, the proportion of nucleus shrinks as the cell matures and the cytoplasm increases proportionately, although the overall cell diameter grows smaller. In short, the N:C ratio decreases.

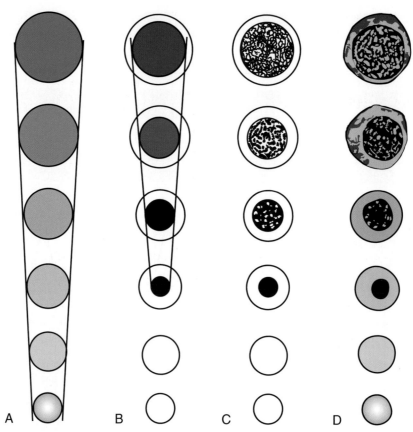

Figure 8-2 General trends affecting the morphology of red blood cells during the developmental process. **A,** Cell diameter decreases and cytoplasm changes from blue to salmon pink. **B,** Nuclear diameter decreases and color changes from purplish-red to a very dark purple-blue. **C,** Nuclear chromatin becomes coarser, clumped, and condensed. **D,** Composite of changes during developmental process. (Modified from Diggs LW, Sturm D, Bell A: The morphology of human blood cells, ed 5, Abbott Park, Ill, 1985, Abbott Laboratories.)

5. The cytoplasm changes from blue to gray-blue to salmon pink. Blueness or basophilia is due to acidic components that attract the basic stain, such as methylene blue. The degree of cytoplasmic basophilia correlates with the amount of ribosomal RNA. These organelles decline over the life of the developing RBC, and the blueness fades. Pinkness called *eosinophilia* or *acidophilia* is due to accumulation of more basic components that attract the acid stain eosin. Eosinophilia of erythrocyte cytoplasm correlates with the accumulation of hemoglobin as the cell matures. Thus the cell starts out being active in protein production on the ribosomes that make the cytoplasm basophilic, transitions through a period in which the red of hemoglobin begins to mix with that blue, and ultimately ends with a thoroughly salmon pink color when the ribosomes are gone and only hemoglobin remains.

Maturation Sequence

Table 8-2 lists the stages of RBC development in order and provides a convenient comparison. The listing makes it appear that these stages are clearly distinct and easily identifiable. The process of cell maturation is a gradual process, with changes occurring in a generally predictable sequence but with some variation for each individual cell. The identification of a given cell's stage depends on the preponderance of characteristics, although the cell may not possess all the features of the archetypal descriptions that follow. Essential

TABLE 8-2 Normoblastic Series: Summary of Stage Morphology

Cell or Stage	Diameter	Nucleus-to-Cytoplasm Ratio	Nucleoli	% in Bone Marrow	Bone Marrow Transit Time
Pronormoblast	12–20 μm	8:1	1–2	1%	24 hr
Basophilic normoblast	10–15 μm	6:1	0–1	1%–4%	24 hr
Polychromatic normoblast	10–12 μm	4:1	0	10%–20%	30 hr
Orthochromic normoblast	8–10 μm	1:2	0	5%–10%	48 hr
Bone marrow polychromatic erythrocyte*	8–10 μm	No nucleus	0	1%	24–48 hr

*Also called reticulocyte.

features of each stage are in italics in the following descriptions. The cellular functions described subsequently also are summarized in Figure 8-3.

Pronormoblast (Rubriblast)

Figure 8-4 shows the pronormoblast.

Nucleus.   The nucleus takes up much of the cell (N:C ratio of 8:1). The nucleus is round to oval, *containing one or two nucleoli. The purple red chromatin is open* and contains few, if any, fine clumps.

Cytoplasm.   *The cytoplasm is dark blue* because of the concentration of ribosomes. The Golgi complex may be visible next to the nucleus as a pale, unstained area. Pronormoblasts may show small tufts of irregular cytoplasm along the periphery of the membrane.

Division.   The pronormoblast undergoes mitosis and gives rise to two daughter pronormoblasts. More than one division is possible before maturation into basophilic normoblasts.

Location.   The pronormoblast is present only in the bone marrow in healthy states.

Cellular Activity.   The pronormoblast begins to accumulate the components necessary for hemoglobin production. The proteins and enzymes necessary for iron uptake and protoporphyrin synthesis are produced. Globin production begins.[3]

Length of Time in This Stage.   This stage lasts slightly more than 24 hours.[3]

Basophilic Normoblast (Prorubricyte)

Figure 8-5 shows the basophilic normoblast.

Nucleus.   *The chromatin begins to condense,* revealing clumps along the periphery of the nuclear membrane and a few in the interior. As the chromatin condenses, the parachromatin areas become larger and sharper, and the N:C ratio decreases to about 6:1. The chromatin stains deep purple-red. Nucleoli may be present early in the stage but disappear later.

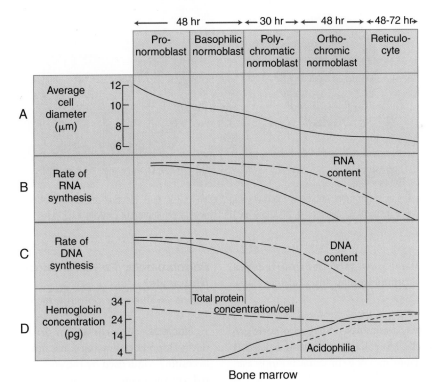

Bone marrow

Figure 8-3 Changes in cellular diameter, RNA synthesis and content, DNA synthesis and content, protein and hemoglobin content during red blood cell development. **A**, Red blood cell diameter (solid line) shrinks from the pronormoblast to the reticulocyte stage. **B**, The rate of RNA synthesis (solid line) for protein production is at its peak at the pronormoblast stage and ends in the orthochromic normoblast stage. The RNA accumulates so that the RNA content (dashed line) remains relatively constant into the orthochromic normoblast stage when it begins to degrade, being eliminated by the end of the reticulocyte stage. **C**, The rate of DNA synthesis (solid line) correlates to those stages of development that are able to divide; the pronormoblast, basophilic normoblast, and early polychromatic normoblast stages. DNA content (dashed line) of a given cell remains relatively constant until the nucleus begins to break up and be extruded during the orthochromic normoblast stage. There is no DNA, i.e., no nucleus, in reticulocytes. **D**, The dashed line represents the total protein concentration which declines slightly during maturation. Proteins other than hemoglobin predominate in early stages. The hemoglobin concentration (solid line) begins to rise in the basophilic normoblast stage, reaching its peak in reticulocytes and representing most of the protein in more mature cells. Hemoglobin synthesis is visible as acidophilia (dotted line) that parallels hemoglobin accumulation but is delayed since the earliest production of hemoglobin in basophilic normoblasts is not visible microscopically. (Modified from Granick S, Levere RD: Heme synthesis in erythroid cells. In Moore CV, Brown EB, editors: Progress in hematology, New York, 1964, Grune & Stratton.)

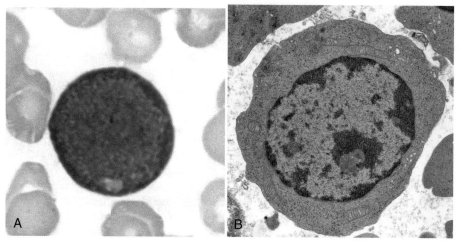

Figure 8-4 **A**, Pronormoblast (rubriblast), bone marrow (Wright stain, ×1000). **B**, Electron micrograph of pronormoblast (×15,575). (**B** from Rodak BF, Carr JH: Clinical hematology atlas, ed 4, St. Louis, 2013, Saunders, an imprint of Elsevier Inc.)

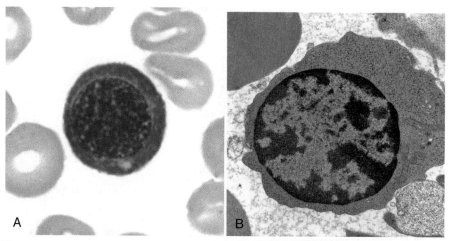

Figure 8-5 **A**, Basophilic normoblast (prorubricyte), bone marrow (Wright stain, ×1000). **B**, Electron micrograph of basophilic normoblast (×15,575). (**B** from Rodak BF, Carr JH: Clinical hematology atlas, ed 4, St. Louis, 2013, Saunders, an imprint of Elsevier Inc.)

Cytoplasm. When stained, *the cytoplasm may be a deeper, richer blue* than in the pronormoblast—hence the name *basophilic* for this stage.

Division. The basophilic normoblast undergoes mitosis, giving rise to two daughter cells. More than one division is possible before the daughter cells mature into polychromatic normoblasts.

Location. The basophilic normoblast is present only in the bone marrow in healthy states.

Cellular Activity. Detectable hemoglobin synthesis occurs,[3] but the many cytoplasmic organelles, including ribosomes and a substantial amount of messenger ribonucleic acid (RNA; chiefly for hemoglobin production), completely mask the minute amount of hemoglobin pigmentation.

Length of Time in This Stage. This stage lasts slightly more than 24 hours.[3]

Polychromatic (Polychromatophilic) Normoblast (Rubricyte)

Figure 8-6 shows the polychromatic normoblast.

Nucleus. The chromatin pattern varies during this stage of development, showing some openness early in the stage but becoming condensed by the end. *The condensation of chromatin reduces the diameter of the nucleus considerably, so the N:C ratio decreases from 4:1 to about 1:1 by the end of the stage.* Notably, *no nucleoli are present.*

Cytoplasm. This is the first stage in which the pink color associated with stained hemoglobin can be seen. The stained color reflects the accumulation of hemoglobin pigmentation over time and concurrent decreasing amounts of RNA. The color produced is a mixture of pink and blue, resulting in a *murky gray-blue.* The stage's name refers to this combination of multiple colors, because *polychromatophilic* means "many color loving."

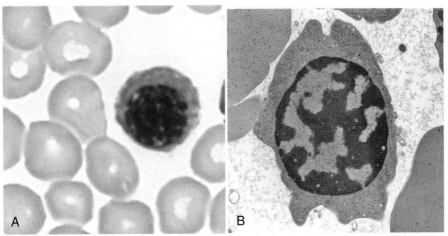

Figure 8-6 A, Polychromatic normoblast (rubricyte), bone marrow (Wright stain, ×1000). **B,** Electron micrograph of polychromatic normoblast (×15,575). (**B** from Rodak BF, Carr JH: Clinical hematology atlas, ed 4, St. Louis, 2013, Saunders, an imprint of Elsevier Inc.)

Division.   This is the last stage in which the cell is capable of undergoing mitosis, although likely only early in the stage. The polychromatic normoblast goes through mitosis, producing daughter cells that mature and develop into orthochromic normoblasts.

Location.   The polychromatic normoblast is present only in the bone marrow in healthy states.

Cellular Activity.   Hemoglobin synthesis increases, and the accumulation begins to be visible in the color of the cytoplasm. Cellular organelles are still present, particularly ribosomes, which contribute a blue aspect to the cytoplasm. The progressive condensation of the nucleus and disappearance of nucleoli are evidence of progressive decline in transcription of deoxyribonucleic acid (DNA).

Length of Time in This Stage.   This stage lasts approximately 30 hours.[3]

Orthochromic Normoblast (Metarubricyte)

Figure 8-7 shows the orthochromic normoblast.

Nucleus.   *The nucleus is completely condensed* (i.e., pyknotic) or nearly so. As a result, the N:C ratio is low or approximately 1:2.

Cytoplasm.   The increase in the *salmon-pink color* of the cytoplasm reflects nearly complete hemoglobin production. The residual ribosomes react with the basic component of the stain and contribute a slightly bluish hue to the cell, but that fades toward the end of the stage as the organelles are degraded.

Division.   The orthochromic normoblast is not capable of division due to the condensation of the chromatin.

Location.   The orthochromic normoblast is present only in the bone marrow in healthy states.

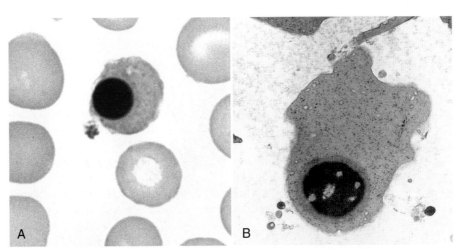

Figure 8-7 A, Orthochromic normoblast (metarubricyte), bone marrow (Wright stain, ×1000). **B,** Electron micrograph of orthochromic normoblast (×20,125). (**B** from Rodak BF, Carr JH: Clinical hematology atlas, ed 4, St. Louis, 2013, Saunders, an imprint of Elsevier Inc.)

Cellular Activity. Hemoglobin production continues on the remaining ribosomes using messenger RNA produced earlier. Late in this stage, the nucleus is ejected from the cell. The nucleus moves to the cell membrane and into a pseudopod-like projection. As part of the maturation program, loss of vimentin, a protein responsible for holding organelles in proper location in the cytoplasm, is probably important in the movement of the nucleus to the cell periphery.[1] Ultimately, the nucleus-containing projection separates from the cell by having the membrane seal and pinch off the projection with the nucleus enveloped by cell membrane.[4] Nonmuscle myosin of the membrane is important in this pinching process.[5] The enveloped extruded nucleus, called a *pyrenocyte*,[1] is then engulfed by bone marrow *macrophages*. The macrophages recognize phosphatidlyserine on the pyrenocyte surface as an "eat me" flag.[6] Other organelles are extruded and ingested in similar fashion. Often, small fragments of nucleus are left behind if the projection is pinched off before the entire nucleus is enveloped. These fragments are called *Howell-Jolly bodies* when seen in peripheral blood cells (Table 19-3 and Figure 19-1) and are typically removed from the cells by the splenic macrophage pitting process once the cell enters the circulation.

Length of Time in This Stage. This stage lasts approximately 48 hours.[3]

Polychromatic (Polychromatophilic) Erythrocyte or Reticulocyte

Figure 8-8 shows the polychromatic erythrocyte.

Nucleus. Beginning at the polychromatic erythrocyte stage, there is *no nucleus*. The polychromatic erythrocyte is a good example of the prior statement that a cell may not have all the classic features described but may be staged by the preponderance of features. In particular, when a cell loses its nucleus, regardless of cytoplasmic appearance, it is a polychromatic erythrocyte.

Cytoplasm. The cytoplasm can be compared with that of the late orthochromic normoblast in that the predominant color is that of hemoglobin. By the end of the polychromatic erythrocyte stage, *the cell is the same color as a mature RBC, salmon pink*. It remains *larger than a mature cell*, however. The shape of the cell is not the mature biconcave disc but is *irregular* in electron micrographs (Figure 8-8, *B*).

Division. Lacking a nucleus, the polychromatic erythrocyte cannot divide.

Location. The polychromatic erythrocyte resides in the bone marrow for 1 day or longer and then moves into the peripheral blood for about 1 day before reaching maturity. During the first several days after exiting the marrow, the polychromatic erythrocyte is retained in the spleen for pitting of inclusions and membrane polishing by splenic macrophages, which results in the biconcave discoid mature RBC.[7]

Cellular Activity. The polychromatic erythrocyte completes production of hemoglobin from residual messenger RNA using the remaining ribosomes. The cytoplasmic protein production machinery is simultaneously being dismantled. Endoribonuclease, in particular, digests the ribosomes. The acidic components that attract the basophilic stain decline during this stage to the point that the polychromatophilia is not readily evident in the polychromatic erythrocytes on a normal peripheral blood film stained with Wright stain. A small amount of residual ribosomal RNA is present, however, and can be visualized with a vital stain such as new methylene blue, so called because the cells are stained while alive in suspension (i.e., vital), before the film is made (Box 8-2). The residual ribosomes appear as a mesh of small blue strands, a reticulum, or, when more fully digested, merely blue dots (Figure 8-9). When so stained, the polychromatic erythrocyte is called a *reticulocyte*. However, the name reticulocyte is often used to refer to the stage immediately preceding the mature

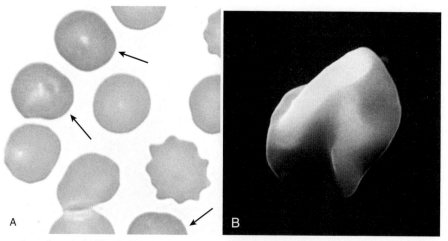

Figure 8-8 A, Polychromatic erythrocyte (shift reticulocyte), peripheral blood (Wright stain, ×1000). **B,** Scanning electron micrograph of polychromatic erythrocyte (×5000). (**B** from Rodak BF, Carr JH: Clinical hematology atlas, ed 4, St. Louis, 2013, Saunders, an imprint of Elsevier Inc.)

BOX 8-2 Cellular Basophilia: Diffuse and Punctate

The *reticulum* of a polychromatic erythrocyte (reticulocyte) is not seen using Wright stain. The residual RNA imparts the bluish tinge to the cytoplasm seen in Figure 8-8, *A*. Based on the Wright-stained appearance, the reticulocyte is called a *polychromatic erythrocyte* because it lacks a nucleus and is no longer an erythroblast but has a bluish tinge. When polychromatic erythrocytes are prominent on a peripheral blood film, the examiner uses the comment *polychromasia* or *polychromatophilia*. Wright-stained polychromatic erythrocytes are also called *diffusely basophilic erythrocytes* for their regular bluish tinge. This term distinguishes polychromatic erythrocytes from red blood cells with *punctate basophilia*, in which the blue appears in distinct dots throughout the cytoplasm. More commonly known as *basophilic stippling* (Table 19-3 and Figure 19-1), punctate basophilia is associated with some anemias. Similar to the basophilia of polychromatic erythrocytes, punctate basophilia is due to residual ribosomal RNA, but the RNA is degenerate and stains deeply with Wright stain.

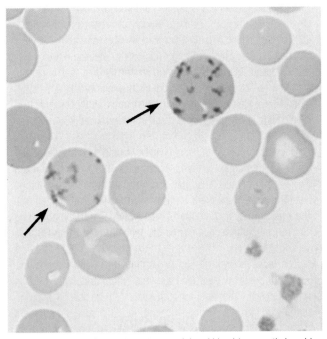

Figure 8-9 Reticulocytes at arrows, peripheral blood (new methylene blue stain, ×1000).

erythrocyte, even when stained with Wright stain and without demonstrating the reticulum.

A second functional change in polychromatic erythrocytes is the reduced production of receptors for the adhesive molecules that hold developing RBCs in the marrow (see details later).[8-10] As these receptors decline, cells are freed to leave the marrow.

Length of Time in This Stage. The cell typically remains a polychromatic erythrocyte for about 3 days,[3] with the first 2 days spent in the marrow and the third spent in the peripheral blood, although possibly sequestered in the spleen.

Erythrocyte

Figure 8-10 shows the erythrocyte.

Nucleus. *No nucleus* is present in mature RBCs.

Cytoplasm. The mature circulating erythrocyte is a biconcave disc measuring 7 to 8 μm in diameter, with a thickness of about 1.5 to 2.5 μm. On a stained blood film, it appears as a *salmon pink-staining cell* with a *central pale area* that corresponds to the concavity. The central pallor is about one third the diameter of the cell.

Division. The erythrocyte cannot divide.

Location and Length of Time in This Stage. Mature RBCs remain active in the circulation for approximately 120 days.[11] Aging leads to their removal by the spleen as described subsequently.

Cellular Activity. The mature erythrocyte delivers oxygen to tissues, releases it, and returns to the lung to be reoxygenated. The dynamics of this process are discussed in detail in Chapter 10. The interior of the erythrocyte contains mostly hemoglobin, the oxygen-carrying component. It has a surface-to-volume ratio and shape that enable optimal gas exchange to occur. If the cell were to be spherical, it would have hemoglobin at the center of the cell that would be relatively distant from the membrane and would not be readily oxygenated and deoxygenated. With the biconcave shape, even hemoglobin molecules that are toward the center of the cell are not distant from the membrane and are able to exchange oxygen.

The cell's main function of oxygen delivery throughout the body requires a membrane that is flexible and deformable—that is, able to flex but return to its original shape. The interaction of various membrane components described in Chapter 9 creates these properties. RBCs must squeeze through small spaces such as the basement membrane of the bone marrow venous sinus. Similarly, when a cell enters the red pulp of the spleen, it must squeeze between epithelial cells to move into the venous outflow. Deformability is crucial for RBCs to enter and subsequently remain in the circulation.

ERYTHROKINETICS

Erythrokinetics is the term describing the dynamics of RBC production and destruction. To understand erythrokinetics, it is helpful to appreciate the concept of the *erythron*. Erythron is the name given to the collection of all stages of erythrocytes throughout the body: the developing precursors in the bone marrow and the circulating erythrocytes in the peripheral blood and the vascular spaces within specific organs such as the spleen. When the term *erythron* is used, it conveys the concept of a unified functional tissue. The erythron is distinguished from the RBC *mass*. The erythron is the entirety of erythroid cells in the body, whereas the RBC mass refers only to the cells in circulation. This discussion of erythrokinetics begins by looking at the erythrocytes in the bone marrow and

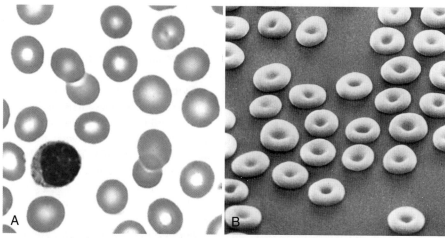

Figure 8-10 A, Mature erythrocytes and one lymphocyte, peripheral blood (Wright stain, ×1000). **B,** Scanning electron micrograph of mature erythrocytes. (A from Rodak BF, Carr JH. Clinical hematology atlas, ed 4, St. Louis, 2013, Saunders, an imprint of Elsevier Inc.)

the factors that affect their numbers, their progressive development, and their ultimate release into the blood.

Hypoxia—the Stimulus to Red Blood Cell Production

As mentioned previously, the role of RBCs is to carry oxygen. To regulate the production of RBCs for that purpose, the body requires a mechanism for sensing whether there is adequate oxygen being carried to the tissues. If not, RBC production and the functional efficiency of existing cells must be enhanced. Thus a second feature of the oxygen-sensing system must be a mechanism for influencing the production of RBCs.

The primary oxygen-sensing system of the body is located in peritubular fibroblasts of the kidney.[12-14] Hypoxia, too little tissue oxygen, is detected by the peritubular cells, which produce *erythropoietin* (EPO), the major stimulatory cytokine for RBCs. Under normal circumstances, the amount of EPO produced fluctuates very little, maintaining a level of RBC production that is sufficient to replace the approximately 1% of RBCs that normally die each day (see section on erythrocyte destruction). When there is hemorrhage, increased RBC destruction, or other factors that diminish the oxygen-carrying capacity of the blood (Box 8-3), the production of EPO is increased.

Hypoxia increases EPO production in peritubular cells mainly by transcriptional regulation. The EPO gene has a hypoxia-sensitive region (enhancer) in its 3′ regulatory component.[15] When oxygen tension in the cell decreases, hypoxia-inducible factor-1, a transcription factor, is assembled in the cytoplasm,[16] migrates to the nucleus, and interacts with the 3′ enhancer of the gene. This results in transcription of more EPO messenger RNA molecules, and production of more EPO.

Erythropoietin

Structure.   EPO is a thermostable, nondialyzable, glycoprotein hormone with a molecular weight of 34 kD.[17] It consists of a *carbohydrate unit* that reacts specifically with RBC receptors and a *terminal sialic acid unit*, which is necessary for biological activity in vivo.[18] On desialation, EPO activity ceases.[19]

BOX 8-3   Hypoxia and Red Blood Cell Production

Teleologically speaking, the location of the body's hypoxia sensor in the kidney is practical,[1] because the kidney receives approximately 20% of the cardiac output[2] with little loss of oxygen from the levels leaving the heart. The location provides early detection when oxygen levels decline. Making the hypoxia sensor the cell that is able to stimulate red blood cell (RBC) production also is practical, because regardless of the cause of hypoxia, having more RBCs should help to overcome it. The hypoxia might result from decreased RBC numbers, as with hemorrhage.

Decreased RBC number, however, is only one cause of hypoxia. Another cause is the failure of each RBC to carry as much oxygen as it should. This can occur because the hemoglobin is defective or because there is not enough hemoglobin in each cell. The hypoxia may be unrelated to the RBCs in any way; poor lung function resulting in diminished oxygenation of existing RBCs is an example.

The kidney's hypoxia sensor cannot know why there is hypoxia, but it does not matter. Even when there are plenty of RBCs compared with the reference interval, if there is still hypoxia, stimulation of RBC production is warranted because the numbers present are not meeting the oxygen need. An elevation of RBC numbers above the reference interval, erythrocytosis, is seen in conditions such as lung disease and cardiac disease in which the blood is not being well oxygenated. Newborns have higher numbers of RBCs because the fetal hemoglobin in their cells does not unload oxygen to the tissues readily, so newborns are slightly hypoxic compared with adults. To compensate, they make more RBCs.

1. Donnelly S: Why is erythropoietin made in the kidney? The kidney functions as a "critmeter" to regulate the hematocrit, Adv Exp Med Biol 543:73-87, 2003.
2. Stewart P: Physiology of the kidney, Update in Anaesthesia 9:24-28, 1998. http://www.wfsahq.org/archive-update-in-anaesthesia/update-in-anaesthesia/update-009/detail. Accessed October 6, 2014.

Action.   EPO is a true hormone, being produced at one location (the kidney) and acting at a distant location (the bone marrow). It is a growth factor (or cytokine) that initiates an intracellular message to the developing RBCs; this process is called *signal transduction*. EPO must bind to its receptor on the surface of cells to initiate the signal or message (Figure 33-9). The receptor is a transmembrane homodimer consisting of two identical polypeptide chains.[20] EPO-responsive cells vary in their sensitivity to EPO.[21] Some are able to respond to low levels of EPO,[22] whereas others require higher levels. In healthy circumstances when RBC production needs to proceed at a modest but regular rate, the cells requiring only low levels of EPO respond. If EPO levels rise secondary to hypoxia, however, a larger population of EPO-sensitive cells is able to respond.

The binding of EPO, the ligand, to its receptor on erythrocyte progenitors initiates a cascade of intracellular events ("the program") that ultimately leads to cell division, maturation, and more red blood cells entering the circulation. EPO's effects are mediated by Janus-activated tyrosine kinase 2 (JAK2) signal transducers that are associated with the cytoplasmic domain of the EPO receptor and ultimately affect gene expression in the RBC nucleus (Figure 33-9).[23] EPO has three major effects: allowing early release of reticulocytes from the bone marrow, preventing apoptotic cell death, and reducing the time needed for cells to mature in the bone marrow. These processes are described in detail in the following sections. The essence is that EPO puts more RBCs into the circulation at a faster rate than occurs without its stimulation.

Early Release of Reticulocytes.   EPO promotes early release of developing erythroid precursors from the marrow by two mechanisms. EPO induces changes in the adventitial cell layer of the marrow/sinus barrier that increase the width of the spaces for RBC egress into the sinus.[24] This mechanism alone, however, is insufficient for cells to leave the marrow. RBCs are held in the marrow because they express surface membrane receptors for adhesive molecules located on the bone marrow stroma. EPO downregulates the expression of these receptors so that cells can exit the marrow earlier than they normally would.[8-10] The result is the presence in the circulation of reticulocytes that are still very basophilic because they have not spent as much time degrading their ribosomes or making hemoglobin as they normally would before entering the bloodstream. These are called *shift reticulocytes* because they have been shifted from the bone marrow early (Figure 8-8, *A*). Their bluish cytoplasm with Wright stain is evident, so the overall blood picture is said to have polychromasia. Even nucleated RBCs (i.e., normoblasts) can be released early in cases of extreme anemia when the demand for RBCs in the peripheral circulation is great. Releasing cells from the marrow early is a quick fix, so to speak; it is limited in effectiveness because the available precursors in the marrow are depleted within several days and still may not be enough to meet the need in the peripheral blood for more cells. A more sustained response is required in times of increased need for RBCs in the circulation.

Inhibition of Apoptosis.   A second, and probably more important, mechanism by which EPO increases the number of circulating RBCs is by increasing the number of cells that will be able to mature into circulating erythrocytes. It does this by decreasing apoptosis, the programmed death of RBC progenitors.[25,26] To understand this process, an overview of apoptosis in general is helpful.

Apoptosis: programmed cell death.   As noted previously, it takes about 18 to 21 days to produce an RBC from stimulation of the earliest erythroid progenitor (BFU-E) to release from the bone marrow. In times of increased need for RBCs, such as when there is loss from the circulation during hemorrhage, this time lag would be a significant problem. One way to prepare for such a need would be to maintain a store of mature RBCs in the body for emergencies. RBCs cannot be stored in the body for this sort of eventuality, however, because they have a limited life span. Therefore, instead of storing mature cells for emergencies, the body produces more CFU-Es than needed at all times. When there is a basal or steady-state demand for RBCs, the extra progenitors are allowed to die. When there is an increased demand for RBCs, however, the RBC progenitors have about an 8- to 10-day head start in the production process. This process of intentional wastage of cells occurs by apoptosis, and it is part of the cell's genetic program.

Process of apoptosis.   Apoptosis is a sequential process characterized by, among other things, the degradation of chromatin into fragments of varying size that are multiples of 180 to 185 base pairs long; protein clustering; and activation of transglutamase. This is in contrast to necrosis, in which cell injury causes swelling and lysing with release of cytoplasmic contents that stimulate an inflammatory response (Chapter 6). Apoptosis is not associated with inflammation.[27]

During the sequential process of apoptosis, the following morphologic changes can be seen: condensation of the nucleus, causing increased basophilic staining of the chromatin; nucleolar disintegration; and shrinkage of cell volume with concomitant increase in cell density and compaction of cytoplasmic organelles, while mitochondria remain normal.[28] This is followed by a partition of cytoplasm and nucleus into membrane-bound apoptotic bodies that contain varying amounts of ribosomes, organelles, and nuclear material. The last stage of degradation produces nuclear DNA fragments consisting of multimers of 180 to 185 base pair segments. Characteristic blebbing of the plasma membrane is observed. The apoptotic cell contents remain membrane-bound and are ingested by macrophages, which prevents an inflammatory reaction. The membrane-bound vesicles display so-called "eat me" signals on the membrane surface (discussed later) that promote macrophage ingestion.[29]

Evasion of apoptosis by erythroid progenitors and precursors.   Thus, under normal circumstances, many red cell progenitors will undergo apoptosis. However, when increased numbers of red cells are needed, apoptosis can be avoided. One effect of EPO is an indirect avoidance of apoptosis by removing an apoptosis induction signal. Apoptosis of RBCs is a cellular process that depends on a signal from either the inside or outside of the cell. Among the crucial molecules in the external messaging system is the death receptor Fas on the membrane of the earliest RBC precursors, while its ligand, FasL, is expressed by more mature RBCs.[28,30] When EPO levels are low, cell production should be at a low rate because hypoxia is not present. The excess early erythroid precursors should undergo apoptosis. This occurs when the older FasL-bearing erythroid precursors, such as polychromatic normoblasts, cross-link with Fas-marked immature erythroid precursors, such as pronormoblasts and basophilic normoblasts, which are then stimulated to undergo apoptosis.[28] As long as the more mature cells with FasL are present in the marrow, erythropoiesis is subdued. If the FasL-bearing cells are depleted, as when EPO stimulates early marrow release, the younger Fas-positive precursors are allowed to develop, which increases the overall output of RBCs from the marrow. Thus early release of older cells in response to EPO indirectly allows more of the younger cells to mature.

A second mechanism for escaping apoptosis exists for RBC progenitors: direct EPO rescue from apoptosis. This is the major way in which EPO is able to increase RBC production. When EPO binds to its receptor on the CFU-E, one of the effects is to reduce production of Fas ligand.[31] Thus the younger cells avoid the apoptotic signal from the older cells. Additionally, EPO is able to stimulate production of various anti-apoptotic molecules, which allows the cell to survive and mature.[31,32] The cell that has the most EPO receptors and is most sensitive to EPO rescue is the CFU-E, although the late BFU-E and early pronormoblast have some receptors.[33] Without EPO, the CFU-E does not survive.[34]

The binding of EPO to its transmembrane receptors on erythroid progenitors and precursors activates JAK2 protein associated with its cytoplasmic domain (Figure 33-9). Activated JAK2 then phosphorylates (activates) the signal transduction and activator of transcription (STAT) pathway, leading to the production of the anti-apoptotic molecule Bcl-XL (now called Bcl-2 like protein 1).[31,32] EPO-stimulated cells develop this molecule on their mitochondrial membranes, preventing release of cytochrome c, an apoptosis initiator.[35] EPO's effect is mediated by the transcription factor GATA-1, which is essential to red cell survival.[36]

Reduced marrow transit time. Apoptosis rescue is the major way in which EPO increases RBC mass—by increasing the number of erythroid cells that survive and mature to enter the circulation. Another effect of EPO is to increase the rate at which the surviving precursors can enter the circulation. This is accomplished by two means: increased rate of cellular processes and decreased cell cycle times.

EPO stimulates the synthesis of RBC RNA and effectively increases the rate of the developmental "program." Among the processes that are accelerated is hemoglobin production.[37] As mentioned earlier, another accelerated process is bone marrow egress with the loss of adhesive receptors and the acquisition of egress-promoting surface molecules.[38] The other process that is accelerated is the cessation of division. Cell division takes time and would delay entry of cells to the circulation, so cells enter cell cycle arrest sooner. As a result, the cells spend less time maturing in the marrow. In the circulation, such cells are larger due to lost mitotic divisions, and they do not have time before entering the circulation to dismantle the protein production machinery that gives the

bluish tinge to the cytoplasm. These cells are true shift reticulocytes similar to those in Figure 8-8, *A*, recognizable in the stained peripheral blood film as especially large, bluish cells typically lacking central pallor. They also are called *stress reticulocytes* because they exit the marrow early during conditions of bone marrow "stress," such as in certain anemias.

EPO also can reduce the time it takes for cells to mature in the marrow by reducing individual cell cycle time, specifically the length of time that cells spend between mitoses.[39] This effect is only about a 20% reduction, however, so that the normal transit time in the marrow of approximately 6 days from pronormoblast to erythrocyte can be shortened by only about 1 day by this effect.

With the decreased cell cycle time and fewer mitotic divisions, the time it takes from pronormoblast to reticulocyte can be shortened by about 2 days total. If the reticulocyte leaves the marrow early, another day can be saved, and the typical 6-day transit time is reduced to fewer than 4 days under the influence of increased EPO.

Measurement of Erythropoietin. Quantitative measurements of EPO are performed on plasma and other body fluids. EPO can be measured by chemiluminescence. Although the reference interval for each laboratory varies, an example reference interval is 4 to 27 mU/L.[40] Increased amounts of EPO in the urine are expected in most patients with anemia, with the exception of patients with anemia caused by renal disease.

Therapeutic Uses of Erythropoietin. Recombinant erythropoietin is used as therapy in certain anemias such as those associated with chronic kidney disease and chemotherapy. It is also used to stimulate RBC production prior to autologous blood donation and after bone marrow transplantation. The indications for EPO therapy are summarized in Table 7-2.

Unfortunately, some athletes illicitly use EPO injections to increase the oxygen-carrying capacity of their blood to enhance endurance and stamina, especially in long-distance running and cycling. The use of EPO is one of the methods of *blood doping*, and aside from being banned in organized sports events, it increases the RBC count and blood viscosity to dangerously high levels and can lead to fatal arterial and venous thrombosis.

Other Stimuli to Erythropoiesis

In addition to tissue hypoxia, other factors influence RBC production to a modest extent. It is well documented that testosterone directly stimulates erythropoiesis, which partially explains the higher hemoglobin concentration in men than in women.[41] Also, pituitary[42] and thyroid[43] hormones have been shown to affect the production of EPO and so have indirect effects on erythropoiesis.

MICROENVIRONMENT OF THE BONE MARROW

The microenvironment of the bone marrow is described in Chapter 7, and the cytokines essential to hematopoiesis are discussed there. Here, the details pertinent to erythropoiesis (i.e., the erythropoietic inductive microenvironment) are emphasized, including the locale and arrangement of erythroid cells and the anchoring molecules involved.

Hematopoiesis occurs in marrow cords, essentially a loose arrangement of cells outside a dilated sinus area between the arterioles that feed the bone and the central vein that returns blood to efferent veins. Erythropoiesis typically occurs in what are called *erythroid islands* (Figure 7-6). These are macrophages surrounded by erythroid precursors in various stages of development. It was previously believed that these macrophages provided iron directly to the normoblasts for the synthesis of hemoglobin. This was termed the *suckling pig* phenomenon. However, since developing RBCs obtain iron via transferrin (Chapter 11), no direct contact with macrophages is needed for this. Macrophages are now known to elaborate cytokines that are vital to the maturation process of the RBCs.[44-46] RBC precursors would not survive without macrophage support via such stimulation.

A second role for macrophages in erythropoiesis also has been identified. Although movement of cells through the marrow cords is sluggish, developing cells would exit the marrow prematurely in the outflow were it not for an anchoring system within the marrow that holds them there until development is complete. There are three components to the anchoring system: a stable matrix of accessory and stromal cells to which normoblasts can attach, bridging (adhesive) molecules for that attachment, and receptors on the erythrocyte membrane.

The major cellular anchor for the RBCs is the macrophage. Several systems of adhesive molecules and RBC receptors tie the developing RBCs to the macrophages.[44] At the same time, RBCs are anchored to the extracellular matrix of the bone marrow, chiefly by *fibronectin*.[9]

When it comes time for the RBCs to leave the marrow, they cease production of the receptors for the adhesive molecules.[9] Without the receptor, the cells are free to move from the marrow into the venous sinus. Entering the venous sinus requires the RBC to traverse the barrier created by the adventitial cells on the cord side, the basement membrane, and the endothelial cells lining the sinus. Egress through this barrier occurs between adventitial cells, through holes (fenestrations) in the basement membrane, and through pores in the endothelial cells[19] (Figure 8-11).[24,47,48]

ERYTHROCYTE DESTRUCTION

All cells experience the deterioration of their enzymes over time due to natural catabolism. Most cells are able to replenish needed enzymes and continue their cellular processes. As a nonnucleated cell, however, the mature erythrocyte is unable to generate new proteins, such as enzymes, so as its cellular functions decline, the cell ultimately approaches death. The average RBC has sufficient enzyme function to live 120 days. Because RBCs lack mitochondria, they rely on glycolysis for production of adenosine triphosphate (ATP). The loss of glycolytic enzymes is central to this process of cellular aging, called

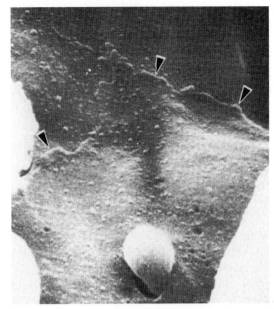

Figure 8-11 Egress of a red blood cell through a pore in an endothelial cell of the bone marrow venous sinus. Arrowheads indicate the endothelial cell junctions. (From DeBruyn PPH: Structural substrates of bone marrow function, Semin Hematol 18:182, 1981.)

senescence, which culminates in phagocytosis by macrophages. This is the major way in which RBCs die normally.

Macrophage-Mediated Hemolysis (Extravascular Hemolysis)

At any given time, a substantial volume of blood is in the spleen, which generates an environment that is inherently stressful on cells. Movement through the red pulp is sluggish. The available glucose in the surrounding plasma is depleted quickly as the cell flow stagnates, so glycolysis slows. The pH is low, which promotes iron oxidation. Maintaining reduced iron is an energy-dependent process, so factors that promote iron oxidation cause the RBC to expend more energy and accelerate the catabolism of enzymes.

In this hostile environment, aged RBCs succumb to the various stresses. Their deteriorating glycolytic processes lead to reduced ATP production, which is complicated further by diminished amounts of available glucose. The membrane systems that rely on ATP begin to fail. Among these are enzymes that maintain the location and reduction of phospholipids of the membrane. Lack of ATP leads to oxidation of membrane lipids and proteins. Other ATP-dependent enzymes are responsible for maintaining the high level of intracellular potassium while pumping sodium out of the cells. As this system fails, intracellular sodium increases and potassium decreases. The effect is that the selective permeability of the membrane is lost and water enters the cell. The discoid shape is lost and the cell becomes a sphere.

RBCs must remain highly flexible to exit the spleen by squeezing through the so-called *splenic sieve* formed by the endothelial cells lining the venous sinuses and the basement membrane. Spherical RBCs are rigid and are not able to squeeze through the narrow spaces; they become trapped

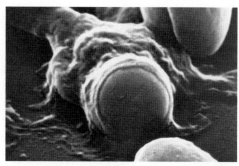

Figure 8-12 Macrophage ingesting a spherocytic erythrocyte. (From Bessis M: Corpuscles, atlas of RBC shapes, New York, 1974, Springer-Verlag.)

against the endothelial cells and basement membrane. In this situation, they are readily ingested by macrophages that patrol along the sinusoidal lining (Figure 8-12).

Some researchers view erythrocyte death as a nonnucleated cell version of apoptosis, termed *eryptosis,*[49] that is precipitated by oxidative stress, energy depletion, and other mechanisms that create membrane signals that stimulate phagocytosis. It is highly likely that there is no single signal but rather that macrophages recognize several. Examples of the signals generating continuing research interest include binding of autologous immunoglobulin G (IgG) to band-3 membrane protein clusters, exposure of phosphatidylserine on the exterior (plasma side) of the membrane, and inability to maintain cation balance.[50] Senescent changes to leukocyte surface antigen CD47 (integrin-associated protein) may also be involved by binding thrombospondin-1, which then provides an "eat me" signal to macrophages.[51] Whatever the signal, macrophages are able to recognize senescent cells and distinguish them from younger cells; thus the older cells are targeted for ingestion and lysis.

When an RBC lyses within a macrophage, the major components are catabolized. The iron is removed from the heme. It can be stored in the macrophage as ferritin until transported out. The globin of hemoglobin is degraded and returned to the metabolic amino acid pool. The protoporphyrin component of heme is degraded through several intermediaries to bilirubin, which is released into the plasma and ultimately excreted by the liver in bile. The details of bilirubin metabolism are discussed in Chapter 23.

Mechanical Hemolysis (Fragmentation or Intravascular Hemolysis)

Although most natural RBC deaths occur in the spleen, a small portion of RBCs rupture *intravascularly* (within the lumen of blood vessels). The vascular system can be traumatic to RBCs, with turbulence occurring in the chambers of the heart or at points of bifurcation of vessels. Small breaks in blood vessels and resulting clots can also trap and rupture cells. The intravascular rupture of RBCs from purely mechanical or traumatic stress results in fragmentation and release of the cell contents into the plasma; this is called *fragmentation* or *intravascular hemolysis.*

When the membrane of the RBC has been breached, regardless of where the cell is located when it happens, the cell contents enter the surrounding plasma. Although mechanical lysis is a relatively small contributor to RBC demise under normal circumstances, the body still has a system of plasma proteins, including haptoglobin and hemopexin, to salvage the released hemoglobin so that its iron is not lost in the urine. Hemolysis and the functions of haptoglobin and hemopexin are discussed in Chapter 23.

SUMMARY

- RBCs develop from committed erythroid progenitor cells in the bone marrow, the BFU-E and CFU-E.
- The morphologically identifiable precursors of mature RBCs, in order from youngest to oldest, are the pronormoblast, basophilic normoblast, polychromatic normoblast, orthochromic normoblast, and polychromatic erythrocyte or reticulocyte.
- As erythroid precursors age, the nucleus becomes condensed and ultimately is ejected from the cell, which produces the polychromatic erythrocyte or reticulocyte stage. The cytoplasm changes color from blue, reflecting numerous ribosomes, to salmon-pink as hemoglobin accumulates and the ribosomes are degraded. Each stage can be identified by the extent of these nuclear and cytoplasmic changes.
- It takes approximately 18 to 21 days for the BFU-E to mature to an RBC, of which about 6 days are spent as identifiable precursors in the bone marrow. The mature erythrocyte has a life span of 120 days in the circulation.
- Hypoxia of peripheral blood is detected by the peritubular fibroblasts of the kidney, which upregulates transcription of the EPO gene to increase the production of EPO.

- EPO, the primary hormone that stimulates the production of erythrocytes, is able to rescue the CFU-E from apoptosis, shorten the time between mitoses of precursors, release reticulocytes from the marrow early, and reduce the number of mitoses of precursors.
- Apoptosis is the mechanism by which an appropriate normal production level of cells is controlled. Fas, the death receptor, is expressed by young normoblasts, and FasL, the ligand, is expressed by older normoblasts. As long as older cells mature slowly in the marrow, they induce the death of unneeded younger cells.
- EPO rescues cells from apoptosis by stimulating the production of anti-apoptotic molecules that counteract the effects of Fas and FasL and simultaneously decreasing Fas production by young normoblasts.
- Survival of RBC precursors in the bone marrow depends on adhesive molecules, such as fibronectin, and cytokines that are elaborated by macrophages and other bone marrow stromal cells. RBCs are found in erythroid islands, where erythroblasts at various stages of maturation surround a macrophage.
- As RBC precursors mature, they lose adhesive molecule receptors and can leave the bone marrow. Egress occurs between

- adventitial cells but through pores in the endothelial cells of the venous sinus.
- Aged RBCs, or senescent cells, cannot regenerate catabolized enzymes because they lack a nucleus. The semipermeable membrane becomes more permeable to water, so the cell swells and becomes spherocytic and rigid. It becomes trapped in the splenic sieve.
- Extravascular or macrophage-mediated hemolysis accounts for most normal RBC death. The signals to macrophages that initiate RBC ingestion may include binding of autologous IgG, expression of phosphatidylserine on the outer membrane, cation balance changes, and CD47-thrombospondin 1 binding.
- Fragmentation or intravascular hemolysis results when mechanical factors rupture the cell membrane while the cell is in the peripheral circulation. This pathway accounts for a minor component of normal destruction of RBCs.

Now that you have completed this chapter, go back and read again the case study at the beginning and respond to the questions presented.

REVIEW QUESTIONS

Answers can be found in the Appendix.

1. Which of the following is an erythrocyte progenitor?
   a. Pronormoblast
   b. Reticulocyte
   c. CFU-E
   d. Orthochromic normoblast

2. Which of the following is the most mature normoblast?
   a. Orthochromic normoblast
   b. Basophilic normoblast
   c. Pronormoblast
   d. Polychromatic normoblast

3. What erythroid precursor can be described as follows: the cell is of medium size compared with other normoblasts, with an N:C ratio of nearly 1:1. The nuclear chromatin is condensed and chunky throughout the nucleus. No nucleoli are seen. The cytoplasm is a muddy, blue-pink color.
   a. Reticulocyte
   b. Pronormoblast
   c. Orthochromic normoblast
   d. Polychromatic normoblast

4. Which of the following is *not* related to the effects of erythropoietin?
   a. The number of divisions of a normoblast
   b. The formation of pores in sinusoidal endothelial cells for marrow egress
   c. The time between mitoses of normoblasts
   d. The production of antiapoptotic molecules by erythroid progenitors

5. Hypoxia stimulates RBC production by:
   a. Inducing more pluripotent stem cells into the erythroid lineage
   b. Stimulating EPO production by the kidney
   c. Increasing the number of RBC mitoses
   d. Stimulating the production of fibronectin by macrophages of the bone marrow

6. In the bone marrow, RBC precursors are located:
   a. In the center of the hematopoietic cords
   b. Adjacent to megakaryocytes along the adventitial cell lining
   c. Surrounding fat cells in apoptotic islands
   d. Surrounding macrophages in erythroid islands

7. Which of the following determines the timing of egress of RBCs from the bone marrow?
   a. Maturing normoblasts slowly lose receptors for adhesive molecules that bind them to stromal cells.
   b. Stromal cells decrease production of adhesive molecules over time as RBCs mature.
   c. Endothelial cells of the venous sinus form pores at specified intervals of time, allowing egress of free cells.
   d. Periodic apoptosis of pronormoblasts in the marrow cords occurs.

8. What single feature of normal RBCs is most responsible for limiting their life span?
   a. Loss of mitochondria
   b. Increased flexibility of the cell membrane
   c. Reduction of hemoglobin iron
   d. Loss of the nucleus

9. Intravascular or fragmentation hemolysis is the result of trauma to RBCs while in the circulation.
   a. True
   b. False

10. Extravascular hemolysis occurs when:
    a. RBCs are mechanically ruptured
    b. RBCs extravasate from the blood vessels into the tissues
    c. Splenic macrophages ingest senescent cells
    d. Erythrocytes are trapped in blood clots outside the blood vessels

11. A pronormoblast in its usual location belongs to the RBC mass of the body, but not to the erythron.
    a. True
    b. False

12. A cell has an N:C ratio of 4:1. Which of the following statements would describe it?
    a. The bulk of the cell is composed of cytoplasm.
    b. The bulk of the cell is composed of nucleus.
    c. The proportions of cytoplasm and nucleus are roughly equal.

REFERENCES

1. Papayannopoulou, T., & Mighaccio, A. R. (2012). Biology of erythropoiesis, erythroid differentiation, and maturation. In Hoffman, R., Benz, E. J., Silberstein, L. E., Heslog, H., Weitz, J., & Anastasi, J. (Eds.), *Hematology: Basic Principles and Practice*. (6th ed., pp. 258–279). Philadelphia: Elsevier/Saunders.
2. Shumacher, H. R., & Erslev, A. J. (1956). Bone marrow kinetics. In Szirmani, E., (Ed.), *Nuclear Hematology*. (pp. 89–132). New York: Academic Press.
3. Granick, S., & Levere, R. D. (1964). Heme synthesis in erythroid cells. In Moore, C. V., & Brown, E.B., (Eds.), *Progress in Hematology*. (vol 4., pp. 1–47). New York: Grune & Stratton.
4. Skutelsky, E., & Danon, D. (1967). An electron microscopic study of nuclear elimination from the late erythroblast. *J Cell Biol, 33*, 625–635.
5. Ubukawa, K., Guo, Y. M., Takahashi, M., et al. (2012). Enucleation of human erythroblasts involves non-muscle myosin IIB. *Blood, 119*, 1036–1044.
6. Yoshida, H., Kawane, K., Koike, M., et al. (2005). Phosphatidylserine-dependent engulfment by macrophages of nuclei from erythroid precursor cells. *Nature, 437*, 754–758.
7. Song, S. H., & Groom, A. C. (1972). Sequestration and possible maturation of reticulocytes in the normal spleen. *Can J Physiol Pharmacol, 50*, 400–406.
8. Patel, V. P., & Lodish, H. F. (1986). The fibronectin receptor on mammalian erythroid precursor cells: characterization and developmental regulation. *J Cell Biol, 102*, 449–456.
9. Vuillet-Gaugler, M. H., Breton-Gorius, J., Vainchenker, W., et al. (1990). Loss of attachment to fibronectin with terminal human erythroid differentiation. *Blood, 75*, 865–873.
10. Goltry, K. L., & Patel, V. P. (1997). Specific domains of fibronectin mediate adhesion and migration of early murine erythroid progenitors. *Blood, 90*, 138–147.
11. Ashby, W. (1919). The determination of the length of life of transfused blood corpuscles in man. *J Exp Med, 29*, 268–282.
12. Jacobson, L. O., Goldwasser, E., Fried, W., et al. (1957). Role of the kidney in erythropoiesis. *Nature, 179*, 633–634.
13. Lacombe, C., DaSilva, J. L., Bruneval, P., et al. (1988). Peritubular cells are the site of erythropoietin synthesis in the murine hypoxic kidney. *J Clin Invest, 81*, 620–623.
14. Maxwell, P. H., Osmond, M. K., Pugh, C. W., et al. (1993). Identification of the renal erythropoietin-producing cells using transgenic mice. *Kidney Int, 44*, 1149–1162.
15. Semenza, G. L., Nejfelt, M. K., Chi, S. M., et al. (1991). Hypoxia-inducible nuclear factors bind to the enhancer element located 3′ to the human erythropoietin gene. *Proc Natl Acad Sci U S A, 88*, 5680–5684.
16. Wang, G. L., & Semenza, G. L. (1993). Characterization of hypoxia inducible factor 1 and regulation of DNA binding by hypoxia. *J Biol Chem, 268*, 21513–21518.
17. Shelton, R. N., Ichiki, A. T., & Lange, R. D. (1975). Physicochemical properties of erythropoietin: isoelectric focusing and molecular weight studies. *Biochem Med, 12*, 45–54.
18. Dordal, M. S., Wang, F. F., & Goldwasser, E. (1985). The role of carbohydrate in erythropoietin action. *Endocrinology, 116*, 2293–2299.
19. Goldwasser, E. (1974). On the mechanism of erythropoietin-induced differentiation: XIII. The role of sialic acid in erythropoietin action. *J Biol Chem, 249*, 4202–4206.
20. Schneider, H., Chaovapong, W., Matthews, D. J., et al. (1997). Homodimerization of erythropoietin receptor by a bivalent monoclonal anibody triggers cell proliferation and differentiation of erythroid precursors. *Blood, 89(2)*, 473–482.
21. Kaushansky, K. (2001). Hematopoietic growth factors and receptors. In Stamatoyannopoulos, G., Majerus, P. W., Perlmutter, R. M., et al. (Eds.), *The Molecular Basis of Blood Diseases*. (3rd ed., pp 25–79). Philadelphia: Saunders.
22. Broudy, V. C., Lin, N., Brice, M., et al. (1991). Erythropoietin receptor characteristics on primary human erythroid cells. *Blood, 77*, 2583–2590.
23. Parganas, E., Wang, D., Stravopodis, D., et al. (1998). Jak2 is essential for signaling through a variety of cytokine receptors. *Cell, 93*, 385–395.
24. Chamberlain, J. K., Leblond, P. F., & Weed, R. I. (1975). Reduction of adventitial cell cover: an early direct effect of erythropoietin on bone marrow ultrastructure. *Blood Cells, 1*, 655–674.
25. Sieff, C. A., Emerson, S.G., Mufson, A., et al. (1986). Dependence of highly enriched human bone marrow progenitors on hemopoietic growth factors and their response to recombinant erythropoietin. *J Clin Invest, 77*, 74–81.
26. Eaves, C. J., & Eaves, A. C. (1978). Erythropoietin (Ep) dose-response curves for three classes of erythroid progenitors in normal human marrow and in patients with polycythemia vera. *Blood, 52*, 1196–1210.
27. Allen, P. D., Bustin, S. A., & Newland, A.C. (1993). The role of apoptosis (programmed cell death) in haemopoiesis and the immune system. *Blood Rev, 7*, 63–73.
28. DeMaria, R., Testa, U., Luchetti, L., et al. (1999). Apoptotic role of Fas/Fas ligand system in the regulation of erythropoiesis. *Blood, 93*, 796–803.
29. Martin, S. J., Reutelingsperger, C. P., McGahon, A. J., et al. (1995). Early redistribution of plasma membrane phosphatidylserine is a general feature of apoptosis regardless of the initiating stimulus: inhibition by overexpression of Bcl-2 and Abl. *J Exp Med, 182*, 1545–1556.
30. Zamai, L., Burattini, S., Luchetti, F., et al. (2004). In vitro apoptotic cell death during erythroid differentiation. *Apoptosis, 9*, 235–246.
31. Elliott, S., Pham, E., & Mcdougall, I. C. (2008). Erythropoietins: a common mechanism of action. *Exp Hematol, 36*, 1573–1584.
32. Dolznig, H., Habermann, B., Stangl, K., et al. (2002). Apoptosis protection by the Epo target Bcl-X(L) allows factor-independent differentiation of primary erythroblasts. *Curr Biol, 12*, 1076–1085.
33. Sawada, K., Krantz, S. B., Dai, C. H., et al. (1990). Purification of human blood burst-forming units–erythroid and demonstration of the evolution of erythropoietin receptors. *J Cell Physiol, 142*, 219–230.

34. Koury, M. J., & Bondurant, M. C. (1988). Maintenance by erythropoietin of viability and maturation of murine erythroid precursor cells. *J Cell Biol, 137,* 65–74.

35. Basanez, G., Soane, L., & Hardwick, J. M. (2012). A new view of the lethal apoptotic pore. *PLoS Biol, 10(9),* e100139.

36. Gregory, T., Yu, C., Ma, A., et al. (1999). GATA-1 and erythropoietin cooperate to promote erythroid cell survival by regulating bcl-xL expression. *Blood, 94,* 87–96.

37. Gross, M., & Goldwasser, E. (1969). On the mechanism of erythropoietin-induced differentiation: V. Characterization of the ribonucleic acid formed as a result of erythropoietin action. *Biochem, 8,* 1795–1805.

38. Sathyanarayana, P., Menon, M. P., Bogacheva, O., et al. (2007). Erythropoietin modulation of podocalyxin and a proposed erythroblast niche. *Blood, 110(2),* 509–518.

39. Hanna, I. R., Tarbutt, R. O., & Lamerton, L. F. (1969). Shortening of the cell-cycle time of erythroid precursors in response to anaemia. *Br J Haematol, 16,* 381–387.

40. ARUP Laboratories. Laboratory Test Directory. *Erythropoietin.* Available at: http://ltd.aruplab.com/Tests/Pub/0050227. Accessed 24.11.13.

41. Jacobson, W., Siegman, R. L., & Diamond, L. K. (1968). Effect of testosterone on the uptake of tritiated thymidine in bone marrow of children. *Ann N Y Acad Sci, 149,* 389–405.

42. Golde, D, W., Bersch, N., & Li, C. H. (1977). Growth hormone: species-specific stimulation of in vitro erythropoiesis. *Science, 196,* 1112–1113.

43. Popovic, W, J., Brown J. E., & Adamson, J. W. (1977). The influence of thyroid hormones on in vitro erythropoiesis: mediation by a receptor with beta adrenergic properties. *J Clin Invest, 60,* 908–913.

44. Chasis, J. A., & Mohandas, N. (2008). Erythroblastic islands: niches for erythropoiesis. *Blood, 112,* 470–478.

45. Sadahira, Y., & Mori, M. (1999). Role of the macrophage in erythropoiesis. *Pathol Int, 49,* 841–848.

46. Obinata, M., & Yanai, N. (1999). Cellular and molecular regulation of an erythropoietic inductive microenvironment (EIM). *Cell Struct Funct, 24,* 171–179.

47. Chamberlain, J. K., & Lichtman, M. A. (1978). Marrow cell egress: specificity of the site of penetration into the sinus. *Blood, 52,* 959–968.

48. DeBruyn, P. P. H. (1981). Structural substrates of bone marrow function. *Semin Hematol, 18,* 179–193.

49. Lang, F., & Qadri, S. M. (2012). Mechanisms and significance of eryptosis, the suicidal death of erythrocytes. *Blood Purif, 33(1-3),* 125–130.

50. Rifkind, J. M., & Nagababu, E. (2013). Hemoglobin redox reactions and red blood cell aging. *Antiox Redox Signal, 18(17),* 2274–2283.

51. Burger, P., Hilarius-Stokman, P., de Korte, D., van den berg, T. K., & van Bruggen, R. (2012). CD47 functions as a molecular switch for erythrocyte phagocytosis. *Blood, 119(23),* 5512–5521.

9

Erythrocyte Metabolism and Membrane Structure and Function

*George A. Fritsma**

OBJECTIVES

After completion of this chapter, the reader will be able to:

1. List the erythrocyte metabolic processes that require energy.
2. Diagram the Embden-Meyerhof anaerobic glycolytic pathway (EMP) in the red blood cell (RBC), highlighting adenosine triphosphate (ATP) consumption and generation.
3. Name the components of the hexose-monophosphate pathway that detoxify peroxide and the process that accomplishes detoxification.
4. Describe the RBC metabolic pathway that generates 2,3-BPG, state the effect of its formation on ATP production, and explain its importance in oxygen transport.
5. Diagram the methemoglobin reductase pathway and explain its importance in maintaining functional hemoglobin.
6. Explain the importance of semipermeability of biological membranes.
7. Describe the arrangement and function of lipids in the RBC membrane.
8. Explain cholesterol exchange between the RBC membrane and plasma, including factors that affect the exchange.
9. Define, locate, and explain the role of RBC transmembrane proteins in maintaining membrane stability and provide examples.
10. Cite the relative concentrations of RBC cytoplasmic potassium, sodium, and calcium, and name the structures that maintain those concentrations.
11. Discuss how ankyrin, protein 4.1, actin, adducin, tropomodulin, dematin, and band 3 interact with α- and β-spectrin and the lipid bilayer.
12. Name conditions caused by abnormalities of vertical linkages and horizontal (lateral) linkages in RBC transmembrane and cytoskeletal proteins.

CASE STUDY

After studying the material in this chapter, the reader should be able to respond to the following case study:

Cyanosis is blue skin coloration, visible in Caucasians, that occurs when the blood does not deliver enough oxygen to the tissues. It is a common sign of heart or lung disease, in which the blood fails to become oxygenated or is distributed improperly throughout the body. In the 1940s, Dr. James Deeny, an Irish physician, was experimenting with the use of vitamin C (ascorbic acid), a potent reducing agent, as a treatment for heart disease.[1] To his disappointment, it was ineffective for nearly all patients. However, he discovered two brothers with the distinction of being truly blue men. When he treated them with vitamin C, each turned a healthy pink. Neither man was determined to have either heart or lung disease.

1. What does it mean to say that vitamin C is a reducing agent?
2. What must be happening if vitamin C was able to cure the cyanosis?
3. What is the significance of finding this condition in brothers?

*The author acknowledges the contribution of Kathryn Doig, who is the previous author of this chapter.

The erythrocyte (red blood cell, RBC) is the primary blood cell, circulating at 5 million RBCs per microliter of blood on average. It is anucleate and biconcave and has an average volume of 90 fL. The cytoplasm provides abundant hemoglobin, a complex of globin, protoporphyrin, and iron that transports elemental oxygen (O_2) from high partial pressure to low partial pressure environments, that is, from lung capillaries to the capillaries of organs and tissues. Hemoglobin, plasma proteins, and additional RBC proteins also transport molecular carbon dioxide (CO_2) and bicarbonate (HCO_3^-) from the tissues to the lungs. Hemoglobin is composed of four globin molecules, each supporting one heme molecule; each heme molecule contains a molecule of iron (Chapters 10 and 11). The biconcave RBC shape supports deformation, enabling the circulating cell to pass smoothly through capillaries, where it readily exchanges O_2 and CO_2 while contacting the vessel wall.[2,3]

RBCs are produced through erythrocytic (normoblastic) maturation in bone marrow tissue (Chapter 8). The nucleus, while present in maturing marrow normoblasts, becomes extruded as the cell passes from the bone marrow to peripheral blood. Cytoplasmic ribosomes and mitochondria disappear 24 to 48 hours after bone marrow release, eliminating the cells' ability to produce proteins or support oxidative metabolism. Adenosine triphosphate (ATP) is produced within the cytoplasm through anaerobic glycolysis (Embden-Meyerhof pathway, EMP) for the lifetime of the cell. ATP drives mechanisms that slow the destruction of protein and iron by environmental peroxides and superoxide anions, maintaining hemoglobin's function and membrane integrity. Oxidation, however, eventually takes a toll, limiting the RBC circulating life span to 120 days, whereupon the cell becomes disassembled into its reusable components globin, iron, and the phospholipids and proteins of the cell membrane, while the protoporphyrin ring is excreted as bilirubin (Chapters 8 and 23).

This chapter is one of a series of four that present the physiology of normal RBC production, structure, function, and senescence. These include Chapter 8, Erythrocyte Production and Destruction; Chapter 10, Hemoglobin Metabolism; and Chapter 11, Iron Kinetics and Laboratory Assessment. This chapter describes RBC energy production, the protective mechanisms that preserve structure and function, and the structure, function, deformability, and maintenance of the cell membrane. Taken as a unit, these four chapters form the basis for understanding RBC disorders (anemias), as described in Chapters 19 through 28.

ENERGY PRODUCTION—ANAEROBIC GLYCOLYSIS

Lacking mitochondria, the RBC relies on anaerobic glycolysis for its energy.[4] The hemoglobin exchange of O_2 and CO_2 is a passive function, however the cells' metabolic processes listed in Box 9-1 require energy. As energy production slows, the RBC grows senescent and is removed from the circulation (Chapter 8). Hematologists have identified hereditary deficiencies of nearly every glycolytic enzyme, and their common result

> **BOX 9-1 Erythrocyte Metabolic Processes Requiring Energy**
>
> Intracellular cationic gradient maintenance
> Maintenance of membrane phospholipid distribution
> Maintenance of skeletal protein deformability
> Maintenance of functional hemoglobin with ferrous iron
> Protecting cell proteins from oxidative denaturation
> Glycolysis initiation and maintenance
> Glutathione synthesis
> Nucleotide salvage reactions

is shortened RBC survival, known collectively as *hereditary non-spherocytic hemolytic anemia* (Chapter 24).

Glucose enters the RBC without energy expenditure via the transmembrane protein *Glut-1*.[5] Anaerobic glycolysis, the EMP (Figure 9-1), requires glucose to generate ATP, a high-energy phosphate source. With no cytoplasmic glycogen organelles, RBCs lack internal energy stores and rely on plasma glucose for glycolysis-generated ATP. Through the EMP, glucose is catabolized to pyruvate (pyruvic acid), consuming two molecules of ATP per molecule of glucose and maximally generating four molecules of ATP per molecule of glucose, for a net gain of two molecules of ATP.

The sequential list of biochemical intermediates involved in glucose catabolism, with corresponding enzymes, is given in Figure 9-1. Tables 9-1 through 9-3 organize glycolysis into three phases.

The first phase of glycolysis employs glucose phosphorylation, isomerization, and diphosphorylation to yield fructose 1,6-bisphosphate (F1,6-BP). *Fructose-bisphosphate aldolase* cleaves F1,6-BP to produce glyceraldehyde-3-phosphate (G3P; Figure 9-1 and Table 9-1). Intermediate stages employ, in order, the enzymes *hexokinase, glucose-6-phosphate isomerase,* and *6-phosphofructokinase.* The initial hexokinase and 6-phosphofructokinase steps consume a total of 2 ATP molecules and limit the rate of glycolysis.

The second phase of glucose catabolism converts G3P to 3-phosphoglycerate (3-PG). The substrates, enzymes, and products for this phase of glycolytic metabolism are summarized in Table 9-2. In the first step, G3P is oxidized to 1,3-bisphosphoglycerate (1,3-BPG) through the action of *glyceraldehyde-3-phosphate dehydrogenase* (G3PD). 1,3-BPG is dephosphorylated by *phosphoglycerate kinase,* which generates 2 ATP molecules and 3-PG.

The third phase of glycolysis converts 3-PG to pyruvate and generates ATP. Substrates, enzymes, and products are listed in Table 9-3. The product 3-PG is isomerized by *phosphoglycerate mutase* to 2-phosphoglycerate (2-PG). *Enolase (phosphopyruvate hydratase)* then converts 2-PG to phosphoenolpyruvate (PEP). *Pyruvate kinase* (PK) splits off the phosphates, forming 2 ATP molecules and pyruvate. PK activity is allosterically modulated by increased concentrations of F1,6-BP, which enhances the affinity of PK for PEP.[5] Thus, when the F1,6-BP is plentiful, increased activity of PK favors pyruvate production. Pyruvate may diffuse from the erythrocyte or may become a substrate for

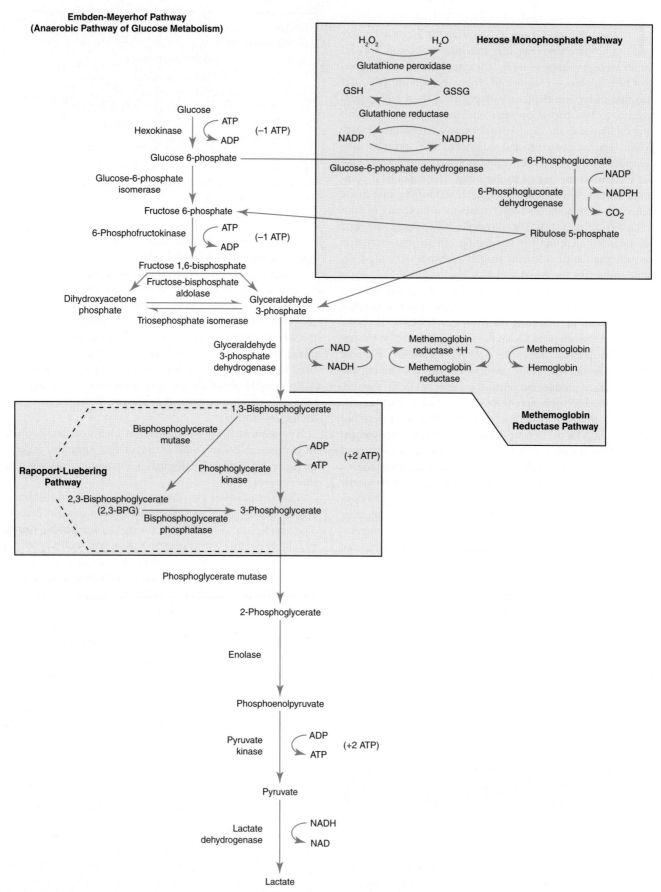

Figure 9-1 Glucose metabolism in the erythrocyte. *ADP,* Adenosine diphosphate; *ATP,* adenosine triphosphate; *G6PD,* glucose-6-phosphate dehydrogenase; *NAD,* nicotinamide adenine dinucleotide (oxidized form); *NADH,* nicotinamide adenine dinucleotide (reduced form); *NADP,* nicotinamide adenine dinucleotide phosphate (oxidized form); *NADPH,* nicotinamide adenine dinucleotide phosphate (reduced form).

TABLE 9-1 Glucose Catabolism: First Phase

Substrates	Enzyme	Products
Glucose, ATP	Hexokinase	G6P, ADP
G6P	Glucose-6-phosphate isomerase	F6P
F6P, ATP	6-Phosphofructokinase	F1,6-BP, ADP
F1,6-BP	Fructose-bisphosphate adolase	DHAP, G3P

ADP, Adenosine diphosphate; *ATP*, adenosine triphosphate; *DHAP*, dihydroxyacetone phosphate; *F1,6-BP*, fructose-1,6-bisphosphate; *F6P*, fructose-6-phosphate; *G3P*, glyceraldehyde-3-phosphate; *G6P*, glucose-6-phosphate.

TABLE 9-2 Glucose Catabolism: Second Phase

Substrates	Enzyme	Product
G3P	Glyceraldehyde-3-phosphate dehydrogenase	1,3-BPG
1,3-BPG, ADP	Phosphoglycerate kinase	3PG, ATP
1,3-BPG	Bisphosphoglycerate mutase	2,3-BPG
2,3-BPG	Bisphosphoglycerate phosphatase	3-PG

1,3-BPG, 1,3-bisphosphoglycerate; *2,3-BPG*, 2,3-bisphosphoglycerate; *3-PG*, 3-phosphoglycerate; *ADP*, adenosine diphosphate; *ATP*, adenosine triphosphate; *G3P*, glyceraldehye-3-phosphate.

TABLE 9-3 Glucose Catabolism: Third Phase

Substrates	Enzyme	Product
3-PG	Phosphoglycerate mutase	2-PG
2-PG	Enolase (phosphopyruvate hydratase)	PEP
PEP, ADP	Pyruvate kinase	Pyruvate, ATP

2-PG, 2-phosphoglycerate; *3-PG*, 3-phosphoglycerate; *ADP*, adenosine diphosphate; *ATP*, adenosine triphosphate; *PEP*, phosphoenolpyruvate.

lactate dehydrogenase with regeneration of the oxidized form of nicotinamide adenine dinucleotide (NAD^+). The ratio of NAD^+ to the reduced form (NADH) modulates the activity of this enzyme.

GLYCOLYSIS DIVERSION PATHWAYS (SHUNTS)

Three alternate pathways, called diversions or shunts, branch from the glycolytic pathway. The three diversions are the *hexose monophosphate pathway* (HMP) or aerobic glycolysis, the *methemoglobin reductase pathway*, and the *Rapoport-Luebering pathway*.

Hexose Monophosphate Pathway

Aerobic or oxidative glycolysis occurs through a diversion of glucose catabolism into the HMP, also known as the *pentose phosphate shunt* (Figure 9-1). The HMP detoxifies peroxide (H_2O_2), which arises from O_2 reduction in the cell's aqueous environment, where it oxidizes and destroys heme iron, proteins, and lipids, especially lipids containing thiol groups.[5] By detoxifying peroxide, the HMP extends the functional life span of the RBC.

The HMP diverts glucose-6-phosphate (G6P) to ribulose 5-phosphate by the action of *glucose-6-phosphate dehydrogenase*

(G6PD). In the process, oxidized nicotinamide adenine dinucleotide phosphate (NADP) is converted to its reduced form (NADPH). NADPH is then available to reduce oxidized glutathione (GSSG) to reduced glutathione (GSH) in the presence of *glutathione reductase*. Glutathione is a cysteine-containing tripeptide, and the designation GSH highlights the sulfur in the cysteine moiety. Reduced glutathione becomes oxidized as it reduces peroxide to water and oxygen via *glutathione peroxidase*.

During steady-state glycolysis, 5% to 10% of G6P is diverted to the HMP. After oxidative challenge, HMP activity may increase up to thirtyfold.[6] The HMP catabolizes G6P to ribulose 5-phosphate and carbon dioxide by oxidizing G6P at carbon 1. The substrates, enzymes, and products of the HMP are listed in Table 9-4.

G6PD provides the only means of generating NADPH for glutathione reduction, and in its absence erythrocytes are particularly vulnerable to oxidative damage (Chapter 24).[7] With normal G6PD activity, the HMP detoxifies oxidative compounds and safeguards hemoglobin, sulfhydryl-containing enzymes, and membrane thiols, allowing RBCs to safely carry O_2. However, in G6PD deficiency, the most common inherited RBC enzyme deficiency worldwide, the ability to detoxify is hampered, resulting in hereditary nonspherocytic anemia.

Methemoglobin Reductase Pathway

Heme iron is constantly exposed to oxygen and peroxide.[8] Peroxide oxidizes heme iron from the ferrous (+2) to the ferric (+3) state. The affected hemoglobin molecule is called *methemoglobin*. Although the HMP prevents hemoglobin oxidation by reducing peroxide, it is not able to reduce methemoglobin once it forms. NADPH is able to do so, but only slowly. The reduction of methemoglobin by NADPH is rendered more efficient in the presence of *methemoglobin reductase*, also called *cytochrome b_5 reductase*. Using H^+ from NADH formed when G3P is converted to 1,3-BPG, cytochrome b_5 reductase acts as an intermediate electron carrier, returning the oxidized ferric iron to its ferrous, oxygen-carrying state. This enzyme accounts for more than 65% of the methemoglobin-reducing capacity within the RBC.[8]

Rapoport-Luebering Pathway

A third metabolic shunt generates 2,3-bisphosphoglycerate (2,3-BPG; also called 2,3-diphosphoglycerate or 2,3-DPG). 1,3-BPG is diverted by *bisphosphoglycerate mutase* to form 2,3-BPG. 2,3-BPG regulates oxygen delivery to tissues by competing with oxygen for the oxygen-binding site of hemoglobin

TABLE 9-4 Glucose Catabolism: Hexose Monophosphate Pathway

Substrates	Enzyme	Product
G6P	Glucose-6-phosphate dehydrogenase and 6-Phosphogluconolactonase	6-PG
6-PG	6-Phosphogluconate dehydrogenase	R5P

6-PG, 6-phosphogluconate; *G6P*, glucose-6-phosphate; *R5P*, ribulose 5-phosphate.

(Chapter 10). When 2,3-BPG binds heme, oxygen is released, which enhances delivery of oxygen to the tissues.

2,3-BPG forms 3-PG by the action of *bisphosphoglycerate phosphatase*. This diversion of 1,3-BPG to form 2,3-BPG sacrifices the production of two ATP molecules. There is further loss of two ATP molecules at the level of PK, because fewer molecules of PEP are formed. Because two ATP molecules were used to generate 1,3-BPG and production of 2,3-BPG eliminates the production of four molecules, the cell is put into ATP deficit by this diversion. There is a delicate balance between ATP generation to support the energy requirements of cell metabolism and the need to maintain the appropriate oxygenation and deoxygenation status of hemoglobin. Acidic pH and low concentrations of 3-PG and 2-PG inhibit the activity of *bisphosphoglycerate mutase*, thus inhibiting the shunt and retaining 1,3-BPG in the EMP. These conditions and decreased ATP activate *bisphosphoglycerate phosphatase*, which returns 2,3-BPG to the glycolysis mainstream. In summary, these conditions favor generation of ATP by causing the conversion of 1,3-BPG directly to 3-PG and returning 2,3-BPG to 3-PG for ATP generation downstream by PK.

RBC MEMBRANE

RBC Membrane Deformability

RBCs are biconcave and average 90 fL in volume.[9] Their average surface area is 140 μm^2, a 40% excess of surface area compared with a 90-fL sphere. This excess surface-to-volume ratio enables RBCs to stretch undamaged up to 2.5 times their resting diameter as they pass through narrow capillaries and through splenic pores 2 μm in diameter; this property is called RBC *deformability*.[10] The RBC plasma membrane, which is 5 μm thick, is 100 times more elastic than a comparable latex membrane, yet it has tensile (lateral) strength greater than that of steel. The deformable RBC membrane provides the broad surface area and close tissue contact necessary to support the delivery of O_2 from lungs to body tissue and CO_2 from body tissue to lungs.

RBC deformability depends not only on RBC *geometry* but also on relative cytoplasmic (hemoglobin) *viscosity*. The normal mean cell hemoglobin concentration (MCHC) ranges from 32% to 36% (Chapter 14 and inside front cover), and as MCHC rises, internal viscosity rises.[11] MCHCs above 36% compromise deformability and shorten the RBC life span because viscous cells become damaged as they stretch to pass through narrow capillaries or splenic pores. As RBCs age, they lose membrane surface area, while retaining hemoglobin. As the MCHC rises, the RBC, unable to pass through the splenic pores, is destroyed by splenic macrophages (Chapter 8).

RBC Membrane Lipids

Besides geometry and viscosity, membrane *elasticity* (pliancy) also contributes to deformability. The RBC membrane consists of approximately 8% carbohydrates, 52% proteins, and 40% lipids.[12] The *lipid* portion, equal parts of cholesterol and phospholipids, forms a bilayer universal to all animal cells (Figure 13-10). Phospholipids form an impenetrable fluid barrier as their *hydrophilic polar head groups* are arrayed upon the membrane's surfaces, oriented toward both the aqueous plasma and the cytoplasm, respectively.[13] Their *hydrophobic nonpolar acyl tails* arrange themselves to form a central layer dynamically sequestered (hidden) from the aqueous plasma and cytoplasm. The membrane maintains extreme differences in osmotic pressure, cation concentrations, and gas concentrations between external plasma and the cytoplasm.[14] Phospholipids reseal rapidly when the membrane is torn.

Cholesterol, esterified and largely hydrophobic, resides parallel to the acyl tails of the phospholipids, equally distributed between the outer and inner layers, and evenly dispersed within each layer, approximately one cholesterol molecule per phospholipid molecule. Cholesterol's β-hydroxyl group, the only hydrophilic portion of the molecule, anchors within the polar head groups, while the rest of the molecule becomes *intercalated* among and parallel to the acyl tails. Cholesterol confers *tensile strength* to the lipid bilayer.[15]

The ratio of cholesterol to phospholipids remains relatively constant and balances the need for deformability and strength. Membrane enzymes maintain the cholesterol concentration by regularly exchanging membrane and plasma cholesterol. Deficiencies in these enzymes are associated with membrane abnormalities such as *acanthocytosis*, as the membrane loses tensile strength (Chapter 24). Conversely, as cholesterol concentration rises, the membrane gains strength but loses elasticity.

The *phospholipids* are asymmetrically distributed. *Phosphatidylcholine* and *sphingomyelin* predominate in the outer layer; *phosphatidylserine (PS)* and *phosphatidylethanolamine* form most of the inner layer. Distribution of these four phospholipids is energy dependent, relying on a number of membrane-associated enzymes, whimsically termed *flippases, floppases,* and *scramblases,* for their positions.[16] When phospholipid distribution is disrupted, as in sickle cell anemia and thalassemia (Chapters 27 and 28) or in RBCs that have reached their 120-day life span, PS, the only negatively charged phospholipid, redistributes (flips) to the outer layer. Splenic macrophages possess receptors that bind PS and destroy *senescent* and damaged RBCs.

Membrane phospholipids and cholesterol may also *redistribute laterally* so that the RBC membrane may respond to stresses and deform within 100 milliseconds of being challenged by the presence of a narrow passage, such as when arriving at a capillary. Redistribution becomes limited as the proportion of cholesterol increases. Plasma bile salt concentration also affects cholesterol exchange.[17] In liver disease with low bile salt concentration, membrane cholesterol concentration becomes reduced. As a result, the more elastic cell membrane shows a "target cell" appearance when the RBCs are layered on a glass slide (Figure 19-1).

Glycolipids (sugar-bearing lipids) make up 5% of the external half of the RBC membrane.[18] They associate in clumps or *rafts* and support *carbohydrate side chains* that extend into the aqueous plasma to anchor the *glycocalyx*. The glycocalyx is a layer of carbohydrates whose net negative charge prevents microbial attack and protects the RBC from mechanical damage caused by adhesion to neighboring RBCs or to the endothelium. Glycolipids may bear copies of carbohydrate-based blood group antigens, for example, antigens of the ABH and the Lewis blood group systems.

RBC Membrane Proteins

Although cholesterol and phospholipids constitute the principal RBC membrane structure, *transmembrane (integral)* and *cytoskeletal (skeletal, peripheral)* proteins make up 52% of the membrane structure by mass.[19] A proteomic study reveals there are at least 300 RBC membrane proteins, including 105 transmembrane proteins. Of the purported 300 membrane proteins, about 50 have been characterized and named, some with a few hundred copies per cell, and others with over a million copies per cell.[20]

Transmembrane Proteins

The *transmembrane* proteins serve a number of RBC functions, as listed in Table 9-5.[21] Through *glycosylation* they support *surface carbohydrates,* which join with glycolipids to make up the protective *glycocalyx.*[22] They serve as *transport* and *adhesion* sites and *signaling receptors.* Any disruption in transport protein function changes the osmotic tension of the cytoplasm, which leads to a rise in viscosity and loss of deformability. Any change affecting adhesion proteins permits RBCs to adhere to one another and to the vessel walls, promoting fragmentation (vesiculation), reducing membrane flexibility, and shortening the RBC life span. Signaling receptors bind plasma ligands and trigger activation of intracellular signaling proteins, which then initiate various energy-dependent cellular activities, a process called *signal transduction.*

The transmembrane proteins assemble into one of two macromolecular complexes named by their respective cytoskeletal anchorages: *ankyrin* or *protein 4.1* (Figure 9-2). These complexes and their anchorages provide RBC membrane structural integrity, because the membrane relies on the cytoskeletal proteins positioned immediately within (underneath) the lipid bilayer for its ability to retain (and return to) its biconcave shape despite deformability. The transmembrane proteins provide vertical membrane structure.

Blood Group Antigens. Transmembrane proteins support carbohydrate-defined *blood group antigens.*[23] For instance, band 3 (anion transport) and Glut-1 (glucose transport) support the majority of *ABH system carbohydrate determinants* by virtue of their high copy numbers.[24] ABH system determinants are also found on several low copy number transmembrane proteins. Certain transmembrane proteins provide *peptide epitopes.* For instance, glycophorin A carries the peptide-defined M and N determinants, and glycophorin B carries the Ss determinants, which together comprise the MNSs system.[25,26]

The Rh system employs two *multipass* transmembrane lipoproteins and a multipass glycoprotein, each of which crosses the membrane 12 times.[27-30] The two lipoproteins present the D and CcEe epitopes, respectively, but expression of the D and

TABLE 9-5 Names and Properties of Selected Transmembrane RBC Proteins

Transmembrane Protein	Band	Molecular Weight (D)	Copies per Cell (×10³)	% of Total Protein	Function
Aquaporin 1					Water transporter
Band 3 (anion exchanger 1)	3	90,000–102,000	1200	27%	Anion transporter, supports ABH antigens
Ca²⁺-ATPase					Ca²⁺ transporter
Duffy		35,000–43,000			G protein-coupled receptor, supports Duffy antigens
Glut-1	4.5	45,000–75,000		5%	Glucose transporter, supports ABH antigens
Glycophorin A	PAS-1	36,000	500–1000	85% of glycophorins	Transports negatively charged sialic acid, supports MN determinants
Glycophorin B	PAS-4	20,000	100–300	10% of glycophorins	Transports negatively charged sialic acid, supports Ss determinants
Glycophorin C	PAS-2	14,000–32,000	50–100	4% of glycophorins	Transports negatively charged sialic acid, supports Gerbich system determinants
ICAM-4					Integrin adhesion
K⁺-Cl⁻ cotransporter					
Kell		93,000			Zn²⁺-binding endopeptidase, Kell antigens
Kidd		46,000–50,000			Urea transporter
Na⁺,K⁺-ATPase					
Na⁺-K⁺-2Cl⁻ cotransporter					
Na⁺-Cl⁻ cotransporter					
Na⁺-K⁺ cotransporter					
Rh		30,000–45,500			D and CcEe antigens
RhAG		50,000			Necessary for expression of D and CcEe antigens; gas transporter, probably of CO_2

ATPase, Adenosine triphosphatase; *Duffy,* Duffy blood group system protein; *ICAM,* intracellular adhesion molecule; *Kell,* Kell blood group system protein; *PAS,* periodic acid–Schiff dye; *RBC,* red blood cell; *Rh,* Rh blood group system protein; *RhAG,* Rh antigen expression protein.

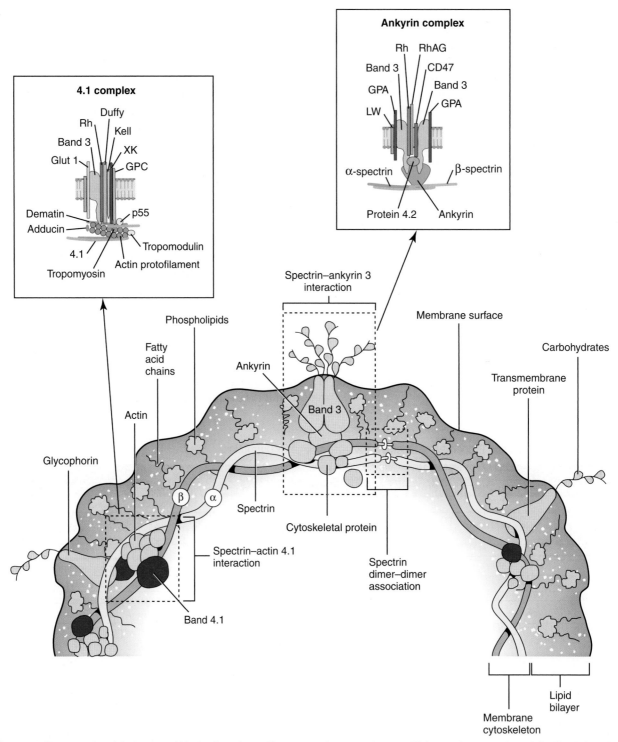

Figure 9-2 Representation of the human red blood cell membrane. The transmembrane proteins assemble in one of two complexes defined by their anchorage to skeletal protein ankyrin and skeletal protein 4.1. Band 3 is the most abundant transmembrane protein. In the ankyrin complex band 3 and protein 4.2 anchor to ankyrin, which is bound to the spectrin backbone. In the 4.1 complex, band 3, Rh, and other transmembrane proteins bind the complex of dematin, adducin, actin, tropomyosin, and tropomodulin through protein 4.1. *CD47,* Signaling receptor; *Duffy,* Duffy blood group system protein; *GPA,* glycophorin A; *GPC,* glycophorin C; *Kell,* Kell blood group system protein; *LW,* Landsteiner-Weiner blood group system protein; *Rh,* Rh blood group system protein; *RhAG,* Rh antigen expression protein; *XK,* X-linked Kell antigen expression protein.

CcEe antigens requires the separately inherited glycoprotein RhAG, which localizes near the Rh lipoproteins in the ankyrin complex. Loss of the RhAG glycoprotein prevents expression of both the D and CcEe antigens (Rh-null) and is associated with RBC morphologic abnormalities (Chapter 24). Additional blood group antigens localize to the 4.1 complex or specialized proteins.[28-30]

The GPI Anchor and Paroxysmal Nocturnal Hemoglobinuria. A few copies of the phospholipid _phosphatidylinositol_ (PI), not mentioned in the RBC Membrane Lipids section, reside in the outer, plasma-side layer of the membrane. PI serves as a base upon which a glycan core of sugar molecules is synthesized, forming the glycosylphosphatidylinositol (GPI) anchor. Over 30 surface proteins bind to the GPI anchor including _decay-accelerating factor_ (DAF, or CD55) and _membrane inhibitor of reactive lysis_ (MIRL, or CD59).[31,32] These proteins appear to float on the surface of the membrane as they link to the GPI anchor. The _phosphatidylinositol glycan anchor biosynthesis, class A_ (_PIGA_) gene codes for a glycosyltransferase required to add _N_-acetylglucosamine to the PI base early in the biosynthesis of the GPI anchor on the membrane. In paroxysmal nocturnal hemoglobinuria (Chapter 24), an acquired mutation in the _PIGA_ gene affects the cells' ability to synthesize the GPI anchor. Without the GPI anchor on the membrane, CD55 and CD59 become deficient, and the cells are susceptible to complement-mediated hemolysis.

Nomenclature. Numerical naming, for instance, band 3, protein 4.1, and protein 4.2, derives from historical (pre-proteomics) protein identification techniques that distinguished 15 membrane proteins using _sodium dodecyl sulfate-polyacrylamide gel electrophoresis_ (SDS-PAGE), as illustrated in Figure 9-3.[33] Bands migrate through the gel, with their velocity a property of their molecular weight and net charge, and are identified using Coomassie blue dye. The glycophorins, with abundant carbohydrate side chains, are stained using periodic acid–Schiff (PAS) dye.

Band 3, protein 4.2, and RhAG, members of the ankyrin complex, link their associated proteins and the bilayer membrane to the cytoskeletal proteins through ankyrin.[34-36] Likewise, glycophorin C, Rh, and blood group Duffy link the 4.1 complex through protein 4.1.[37] The 4.1 anchorage also includes the more recently defined proteins _adducin_ and _dematin_, which link with band 3 and Glut-1, respectively.[38]

Cytoskeletal Proteins

The principal cytoskeletal proteins are the filamentous α-spectrin and β-spectrin (Table 9-6), which assemble to form an _antiparallel_ heterodimer held together with a series of lateral bonds.[39] Antiparallel means that the carboxyl (COOH) end of one strand associates with the amino (NH_3) end of the other, and the two heterodimers associate head-to-head to form a tetramer (Figure 9-2). The spectrins form a hexagonal lattice (Figure 9-4) that is immediately adjacent to the cytoplasmic membrane lipid layer and provides _lateral or horizontal_ membrane stability.[40] Because the skeletal proteins do not penetrate the bilayer, they are also called _peripheral_ proteins.

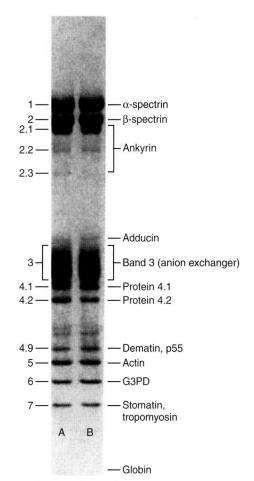

Figure 9-3 Sodium dodecyl sulfate-polyacrylamide gel electrophoresis of RBC membrane proteins stained with Coomassie blue dye. Lane A illustrates numerical band naming based on migration. Lane B names and illustrates the positions of some of the major proteins. (Adapted from Costa FF, Agre P, Watkins PC, et al: Linkage of dominant hereditary spherocytosis to the gene for the erythrocyte membrane-skeleton protein ankyrin, N Engl J Med 323:1046, 1990.)

Spectrin Stabilization. The secondary structure of both α- and β-spectrin features triple-helical repeats of 106 amino acids each; 20 such repeats make up α-spectrin, and 16 make up β-spectrin.[41] Essential to the cytoskeleton are the previously mentioned ankyrin, protein 4.1, adducin and dematin, and, in addition, _actin, tropomyosin_, and _tropomodulin_ (Figure 9-4).[35] A single helix at the amino terminus of α-spectrin consistently binds a pair of helices at the carboxyl terminus of the β-spectrin chain, forming a stable triple helix that holds together the ends of the heterodimers.[42] Joining these ends are actin and protein 4.1. Actin forms short filaments of 14 to 16 monomers whose length is regulated by tropomyosin. Adducin and tropomodulin cap the ends of actin, and dematin appears to stabilize actin in a manner that is the subject of current investigation.[43]

Membrane Deformation. Spectrin dimer bonds that appear along the length of the molecules disassociate and reassociate (open and close) during RBC deformation.[44] Likewise, the 20 α-spectrin and 16 β-spectrin repeated helices unfold and refold.

TABLE 9-6 Names and Properties of Selected Skeletal RBC Proteins

Skeletal Protein	Band	Molecular Weight (D)	Copies per Cell (×10³)	% of Total Protein	Function
α-spectrin	1	240,000–280,000	240	16%	Filamentous antiparallel heterodimer,
β-spectrin	2	220,000–246,000	240	14%	primary cytoskeletal proteins
Adducin	2.9	80,000–103,000	60	4%	Caps actin filament
Ankyrin	2.1	206,000–210,000	120	4.5%	Anchors band 3 and protein 4.2
Dematin	4.9	43,000–52,000	40	1%	Actin bundling protein
F-actin	5	42,000–43,000	400–500	5.5%	Binds β-spectrin
G3PD	6	35,000–37,000	500	3.5%	
Protein 4.1	4.1	66,000–80,000	200	5%	Anchors 4.1 complex
Protein 4.2 (protein kinase)	4.2	72,000–77,000	200	5%	Anchors ankyrin complex
Tropomodulin	5	41,000–43,000	30	—	Caps actin filament
Tropomyosin	7	27,000–38,000	80	1%	Regulates actin polymerization

G3PD, Glucose-3-phosphate dehydrogenase glyceraldehyde; *RBC,* red blood cell.

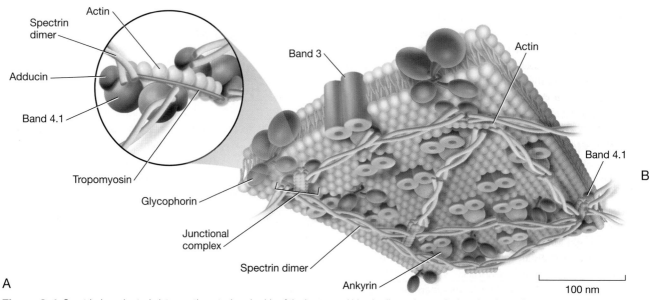

Figure 9-4 Spectrin-based cytoskeleton on the cytoplasmic side of the human red blood cell membrane. **A,** Junctional complex composed of actin filaments containing 14 to 16 actin monomers, band 4.1, adducin, and tropomyosin, which probably determines the length of the actin filaments. **B,** Spectrin dimers form a lattice that binds band 3 and protein 4.2 (not shown) via ankyrin and band 3, Glut-1 and Duffy (not shown), and glycophorin via protein 4.1.

These flexible interactions plus the spectrin-actin-protein 4.1 junctions between the tetramers are key regulators of membrane elasticity and mechanical stability, and abnormalities in any of these proteins result in deformation-induced membrane fragmentation. For instance, *hereditary elliptocytosis* (ovalocytosis) arises from one of several autosomal dominant mutations affecting spectrin dimer-to-dimer lateral bonds or the spectrin–ankyrin–protein 4.1 junction.[45] In hereditary elliptocytosis, the membrane fails to rebound from deformation, and RBCs progressively elongate to form visible elliptocytes, which causes a mild to severe hemolytic anemia.[46] Conversely, autosomal dominant mutations that affect the integrity of band 3, ankyrin, protein 4.2, or α- or β-spectrin are associated with *hereditary*

spherocytosis (Chapter 24).[47,48] In these cases there are too few *vertical anchorages* to maintain membrane stability. The lipid membrane peels off in small fragments called *"blebs,"* or *vesicles,* whereas the cytoplasmic volume remains intact. This generates spherocytes with a reduced membrane-to-cytoplasm ratio.

Osmotic Balance and Permeability

The RBC membrane is impermeable to cations Na^+, K^+, and Ca^{2+}. It is permeable to water and the anions bicarbonate (HCO_3^-) and chloride (Cl^-), which freely exchange between plasma and RBC cytoplasm.[49] *Aquaporin 1* (Table 9-5) is a transmembrane protein that forms pores or channels whose surface charges create inward water flow in response to internal osmotic changes.

The ATP–dependent cation pumps *Na⁺-ATPase* and *K⁺-ATPase* (Table 9-5) regulate the concentrations of Na⁺ and K⁺, maintaining intracellular-to-extracellular ratios of 1:12 and 25:1, respectively.[50,51] *Ca²⁺-ATPase* extrudes calcium, maintaining low intracellular levels of 5 to 10 μmol/L. Calmodulin, a cytoplasmic Ca²⁺-binding protein, controls the function of Ca²⁺-ATPase.[52] These enzymes, in addition to aquaporin, maintain osmotic balance.

The cation pumps consume 15% of RBC ATP production. ATP loss or pump damage permits Ca²⁺ and Na⁺ influx, with water following osmotically. The cell swells, becomes spheroid, and eventually ruptures. This phenomenon is called *colloid osmotic hemolysis*.

Sickle cell disease provides an example of increased cation permeability. When crystallized sickle hemoglobin deforms the cell membranes, internal levels of Na⁺, K⁺, and especially Ca²⁺ rise, which results in hemolysis.[52]

SUMMARY

- Glucose enters the RBC with no energy expenditure via the transmembrane protein Glut-1.
- The anaerobic Embden-Meyerhof pathway (EMP) metabolizes glucose to pyruvate, consuming two ATP molecules. The EMP subsequently generates four ATP molecules per glucose molecule, a net gain of two.
- The hexose-monophosphate pathway (HMP) pathway aerobically converts glucose to pentose and generates NADPH. NADPH reduces glutathione. Reduced glutathione reduces peroxides and protects proteins, lipids, and heme iron from oxidation.
- The methemoglobin reductase pathway converts ferric heme iron (valence 3⁺ iron, methemoglobin) to reduced ferrous (valence 2⁺ form), which binds O₂.
- The Rapoport-Luebering pathway generates 2,3-BPG and enhances O₂ delivery to tissues.
- The RBC membrane is a lipid bilayer whose hydrophobic components are sequestered from aqueous plasma and cytoplasm. The membrane provides a semipermeable barrier separating plasma from cytoplasm and maintaining an osmotic differential.
- RBC membrane phospholipids are asymmetrically distributed. Phosphatidylcholine and sphingomyelin predominate in the outer layer; phosphatidylserine and phosphatidylethanolamine form most of the inner layer.
- Enzymatic plasma to membrane exchange maintains RBC membrane cholesterol.
- Acanthocytosis and target cells are associated with abnormalities in the concentration or distribution of membrane cholesterol and phospholipids.
- RBC transmembrane proteins channel ions, water, and glucose and anchor cell membrane receptors. They also provide the

vertical support connecting the lipid bilayer to the underlying cytoskeleton to maintain membrane integrity.
- RBC cytoplasm K⁺ concentration is higher than plasma K⁺, whereas Na⁺ and Ca²⁺ concentrations are lower. Disequilibria are maintained by membrane enzymes K⁺-ATPase, Na⁺-ATPase, and Ca²⁺-ATPase. Pump failure leads to Na⁺ and water influx, cell swelling, and lysis.
- The shape and flexibility of the RBC, which are essential to its function, depend on the cytoskeleton. The cytoskeleton is derived from a group of peripheral proteins on the interior of the lipid membrane. The major structural proteins are α- and β-spectrin, which are bound together and connected to transmembrane proteins by ankyrin, actin, protein 4.1, adducin, tropomodulin, dematin, and band 3. Cytoskeletal proteins provide the horizontal or lateral support for the membrane.
- Hereditary spherocytosis arises from defects in proteins that provide vertical support for the membrane. Hereditary elliptocytosis is due to defects in cytoskeletal proteins that provide horizontal support for the membrane.
- Membrane proteins are extracted using sodium dodecyl sulfate, separated using polyacrylamide gel electrophoresis, and stained with Coomassie blue. They are numbered from the point of application; lower numbers correlate to high protein molecular weight and lower net charge.

Now that you have completed this chapter, go back and read again the case study at the beginning and respond to the questions presented.

REVIEW QUESTIONS

Answers can be found in the Appendix.

1. Which RBC process does *not* require energy?
   a. Oxygen transport
   b. Cytoskeletal protein deformability
   c. Preventing the peroxidation of proteins and lipids
   d. Maintaining cytoplasm cationic electrochemical gradients

2. What pathway anaerobically generates energy in the form of ATP?
   a. Hexose monophosphate pathway
   b. Rapoport-Luebering pathway
   c. Embden-Meyerhof pathway
   d. 2,3-BPG pathway

3. Which is true concerning 2,3-BPG?
   a. The least abundant of RBC organophosphates
   b. Enhances O_2 release from hemoglobin
   c. Source of RBC glucose
   d. Source of RBC ATP

4. To survive, the RBC must detoxify peroxides. What hexose-monophosphate shunt product(s) accomplishes detoxification?
   a. ATP
   b. 2,3-BPG
   c. Pyruvic and lactic acid
   d. NADPH and reduced glutathione

5. Which of the following helps maintain RBC shape?
   a. Membrane phospholipids
   b. Cytoskeletal proteins
   c. GPI anchor
   d. Glycocalyx

6. The glycolipids of the RBC membrane:
   a. Provide flexibility.
   b. Carry RBC antigens.
   c. Constitute ion channels.
   d. Attach the cytoskeleton to the lipid layer.

7. RBC membranes block passage of most large molecules such as proteins, but allow passage of small molecules such as the cations Na+, K+, and Ca++. What is the term for this membrane property?
   a. Semipermeable
   b. Deformable
   c. Intangible
   d. Flexible

8. RBC membrane phospholipids are arranged:
   a. In a hexagonal lattice.
   b. In chains beneath a protein exoskeleton.
   c. In two layers whose composition is asymmetric.
   d. So that hydrophobic portions are facing the plasma.

9. RBC membrane cholesterol is replenished from the:
   a. Plasma.
   b. Mitochondria.
   c. Cytoplasm.
   d. EMB pathway.

10. The hemoglobin iron ion may become oxidized to the +3 valence state by several pathological mechanisms. What portion of the Embden-Meyerhof pathway reduces iron to the physiologic +2 valence state?
    a. Methemoglobin reductase pathway
    b. Hexose monophosphate pathway
    c. Rapoport-Luebering pathway
    d. The 2,3-BPG shunt

11. Which of the following is an example of a transmembrane or integral membrane protein?
    a. Glycophorin A
    b. Ankyrin
    c. Spectrin
    d. Actin

12. Abnormalities in the horizontal and vertical linkages of the transmembrane and cytoskeletal RBC membrane proteins may be seen as:
    a. Shape changes.
    b. Methemoglobin increase.
    c. Reduced hemoglobin content.
    d. Enzyme pathway deficiencies.

REFERENCES

1. Percy, M. J., & Lappin, T. R. (2008). Recessive congenital methaemoglobinaemia: cytochrome b_5 reductase deficiency. *Brit J Haem, 141,* 298–308.
2. Bull, B., & Hermann, P. C. (2010). Morphology of the erythron. In Kaushansky, K., Lichtman, M., Beutler, E., et al. *Williams Hematology.* (8th ed., pp. 409–429). New York: McGraw Hill.
3. Quigley, J. G., Means, R. T., & Glader, B. (2013). The birth, life, and death of red blood cells, erythropoiesis, the mature red blood cell, and cell destruction. In Greer, J. P., Arber, D. A., Glader, B., et al. (Eds.), *Wintrobe's Clinical Hematology.* (13th ed.). Philadelphia: Wolters Kluwer Health/Lippincott Williams & Wilkins.
4. Von Solinge, W. W., & Van Wijk, R. (2010). Disorders of red cells resulting from enzyme abnormalities. In Kaushansky, K., Lichtman, M., Beutler, E., et al. *Williams Hematology.* (8th ed., pp. 647–674). New York: McGraw Hill.
5. Kondo, T., & Beutler, E. (1980). Developmental changes in glucose transport of guinea pig erythrocytes. *J Clin Invest, 65,* 1–4.
6. Price, E. A., Otis, S., & Schrier, S. L. (2013). Red blood cell enzymopathies. In Hoffman, R., Benz, E. J. Jr., Silberstein, L. E., et al. (Eds.), *Hematology.* (6th ed.). St Louis: Elsevier.
7. Beutler, E. (1990). Disorders of red cells resulting from enzyme abnormalities. *Semin Hematol, 27,* 137–167.
8. Agarwal, N., & Prchal, J. (2010). Methemoglobinemia and other dyshemoglobinemias. In Kaushansky, K., Lichtman, M., Beutler, E., et al. *Williams Hematology* (8th ed., pp. 743–754). New York: McGraw Hill.
9. Mohandas, N., & Gallagher, P. G. (2008). Red cell membrane: past, present, and future. *Blood, 112,* 3939–3948.
10. Schmid-Schönbein, H. (1975). Erythrocyte rheology and the optimization of mass transport in the microcirculation. *Blood Cell, 1,* 285–306.
11. Mohandas, N., & Chasis, J. A. (1993). Red blood cell deformability, membrane material properties, and shape: regulation by transmembrane, skeletal and cytosolic proteins and lipids. *Semin Hematol, 30,* 171–192.
12. Cooper, R. A. (1970). Lipids of human red cell membrane: normal composition and variability in disease. *Semin Hematol, 7,* 296–322.
13. Singer, S. J., & Nicolson, G. L. (1972). The fluid mosaic model of the structure of cell membranes. *Science, 175,* 720–731.
14. Discher, D. E. (2000). New insights into erythrocyte membrane organization and microelasticity. *Curr Opin Hematol, 7,* 117–122.

15. Cooper, R. A. (1978). Influence of the increased membrane cholesterol on membrane fluidity and cell function in human red blood cells. *J Supramol Struct, 8,* 413–430.
16. Zhou, Q., Zhao, J., Stout, J. G., et al. (1997). Molecular cloning of human plasma membrane phospholipid scramblase. A protein mediating transbilayer movement of plasma membrane phospholipids. *J Biol Chem, 272,* 18240–18244.
17. Cooper, R. A., & Jandl, J. H. (1968). Bile salts and cholesterol in the pathogenesis of target cells in obstructive jaundice. *J Clin Invest, 47,* 809–822.
18. Alberts, B., Johnson, A., Lewis, J., et al. (2007). Membrane structure. In Alberts, B., Johnson, A., Lewis, J., et al. (Eds.), *Molecular Biology of the Cell.* (5th ed.). Garland: Science.
19. Steck, T. (1974). The organization of proteins in the human red blood cell membrane. *J Cell Biol 62,* 1–19.
20. Pasini, E. M., Kirkegaard, M., Mortensen, P., et al. (2006). In-depth analysis of the membrane and cytosolic proteome of red blood cells. *Blood, 108,* 791–801.
21. Bennett, V. (1985). The membrane skeleton of human erythrocytes and its implications for more complex cells. *Annu Rev Biochem, 54,* 273–304.
22. Furthmayr, H. & Glycophorins, A., B., and C. (1979). A family of sialoglycoproteins, isolation and preliminary characterization of trypsin derived peptides. In Lux, S. E., Marchesi, V. T., & Fox, C. J., (Eds.), *Normal and Abnormal Red Cell Membranes* (pp. 195–211). New York: Alan R Liss.
23. Reid, M. E., & Mohandas, N. (2004). Red blood cell blood group antigens: structure and function. *Semin Hematol, 41,* 93–117.
24. Daniels, G. (2013). ABO, H, and Lewis systems. In *Human Blood Groups.* (3rd ed., pp. 11–95). Wiley-Blackwell.
25. Daniels, G. (2013). MNS blood group system. In *Human Blood Groups.* (3rd ed., pp. 96–161). Wiley-Blackwell.
26. Daniels, G. (2013). Gerbich blood group system. In *Human Blood Groups.* (3rd ed., pp. 410–425). Wiley-Blackwell.
27. Daniels, G. (2013). Rh and RHAG blood group systems. In *Human Blood Groups.* (3rd ed., pp. 183–258). Wiley-Blackwell.
28. Daniels, G. (2013). Duffy blood group system. In *Human Blood Groups.* (3rd ed., pp. 306–324). Wiley-Blackwell.
29. Daniels, G. (2013). Kell and KX blood group systems. In *Human Blood Groups.* (3rd ed., pp. 278–305). Wiley-Blackwell.
30. Daniels, G. (2013). Kidd blood group system. In *Human Blood Groups.* (3rd ed., pp. 325–335). Wiley-Blackwell.
31. Parker, C. (2010). Chapter 40: Paroxysmal nocturnal hemoglobinuria. In Kaushansky, K., Lichtman, M., Beutler, E., et al. *Williams Hematology.* (8th ed., pp. 521–532). New York: McGraw Hill.
32. Fairbanks, G., Steck, T. L., & Wallach, D. F. (1971). Electrophoretic analysis of the major polypeptides of the human erythrocyte membrane. *Biochemistry, 10,* 2606–2617.
33. Jennings, M. L. (1984). Topical review: oligometric structure and the anion transport function of human erythrocyte band 3 protein. *J Membr Biol, 80,* 105–117.
34. Kay, M. M., Bosman, G. J., Johnson, G. J., et al. (1988). Band 3 polymers and aggregates and hemoglobin precipitates in red cell aging. *Blood Cells, 14,* 275–295.
35. Bennett, V. (1983). Proteins involved in membrane-cytoskeleton association in human erythrocytes: spectrin, ankyrin, and band 3. *Methods Enzymol, 96,* 313–324.
36. Anderson, R. A., & Lovrien, R. E. (1984). Glycophorin is linked by band 4.1 protein to the human erythrocyte membrane skeleton. *Nature, 307,* 655–658.
37. Khan, A. A., Hanada, T., Mohseni, M, et al. (2008). Dematin and adducin provide a novel link between the spectrin cytoskeleton and human erythrocyte membrane by directly interacting with glucose transporter-1. *J Biol Chem, 283,* 14600–14609.
38. Shotton, D. M., Burke, B. E., & Branton, D. (1979). The molecular structure of human erythrocyte spectrin: biophysical and electron microscope studies. *J Mol Biol, 131,* 303–329.
39. Liu, S. C., Drick, L. H., & Palek, J. (1987). Visualization of the hexagonal lattice in the erythrocyte membrane skeleton. *J Cell Biol, 104,* 527–536.
40. Speicher, D. W., & Marchesi, V. T. (1984). Erythrocyte spectrin is composed of many homologous triple helical segments. *Nature, 311,* 177–180.
41. Shen, B. W., Josephs, R., & Steck, T. L. (1984). Ultrastructure of unit fragments of the skeleton of the human erythrocyte membrane. *J Cell Biol, 99,* 810–821.
42. An, X., Guo, X., Zhang, X., et al. (2006). Conformational stabilities of the structural repeats of erythroid spectrin and their functional implications. *J Biol Chem, 281,* 10527–10532.
43. DeSilva, T. M., Peng, K. C., Speicher, K. D., et al. (1992). Analysis of human red cell spectrin tetramer (head-to-head) assembly using complementary univalent peptides. *Biochemistry, 31,* 10872–10878.
44. An, X., Lecomte, M. C., Chasis, J. A., et al. (2002). Shear-response of the spectrin dimer-tetramer equilibrium in the red blood cell membrane. *J Biol Chem, 277,* 31796–31800.
45. Coetzer, T., & Zail, S. (1982). Spectrin tetramer-dimer equilibrium in hereditary elliptocytosis. *Blood, 59,* 900–905.
46. Brugnara, C. (1997). Erythrocyte membrane transport physiology. *Curr Opin Hematol, 4,* 122–127.
47. Costa, F. F., Agre, P., Watkins, P. C., et al. (1990). Linkage of dominant hereditary spherocytosis to the gene for the erythrocyte membrane-skeleton protein ankyrin. *N Engl J Med, 323,* 1046–1050.
48. Gallagher, P. G., & Forget, B. G. (1998). Hematologically important mutations: spectrin and ankyrin variants in hereditary spherocytosis. *Blood Cells Mol Dis, 24,* 539–543.
49. Jorgensen, P. L. (1982). Mechanism of the Na^+, K^+ pump: protein structure and conformation of the pure (Na^+ K^+)-ATPase. *Biochim Biophys Acta, 694,* 27–68.
50. James, P. H., Pruschy, M., Vorherr, T. E., et al. (1989). Primary structure of the cAMP-dependent phosphorylation site of the plasma membrane calcium pump. *Biochemistry, 28,* 4253–4258.
51. Takakuwa, Y., & Mohandas, N. (1988). Modulation of erythrocyte membrane material properties by Ca^{2+} and calmodulin: implications for their role in skeletal protein interaction. *J Clin Invest, 82,* 394–400.
52. Rhoda, M. D., Aprovo, N., Beuzard, Y., et al. (1990). Ca^{2+} permeability in deoxygenated sickle cells. *Blood, 75,* 2453–2458.

10

Hemoglobin Metabolism

*Elaine M. Keohane**

OBJECTIVES

After completion of this chapter, the reader will be able to:

1. Describe the components and structure of hemoglobin.
2. Describe steps in heme synthesis that occur in the mitochondria and the cytoplasm.
3. Name the genes and the chromosome location and arrangement for the various polypeptide chains of hemoglobin.
4. Describe the polypeptide chains produced and the hemoglobins they form in the embryo, fetus, newborn, and adult.
5. List the three types of normal hemoglobin in adults and their reference intervals.
6. Describe mechanisms that regulate hemoglobin synthesis.
7. Describe the mechanism by which hemoglobin transports oxygen to the tissues and transports carbon dioxide to the lungs.
8. Explain the importance of maintaining hemoglobin iron in the ferrous state (Fe^{2+}).
9. Explain the significance of the sigmoid shape of the oxygen dissociation curve.
10. Correlate right and left shifts in the oxygen dissociation curve with conditions that can cause shifts in the curve.
11. Differentiate T and R forms of hemoglobin and the effect of oxygen and 2,3-bisphosphoglycerate on those forms.
12. Explain the difference between adult Hb A and fetal Hb F and how that difference impacts oxygen affinity.
13. Compare and contrast the composition and the effect on oxygen binding of methemoglobin, carboxyhemoglobin, and sulfhemoglobin.

CASE STUDY

After studying the material in this chapter, the reader should be able to respond to the following case study:

Hemoglobin and hemoglobin fractionation and quantification using high performance liquid chromatography (HPLC) were performed on a mother and her newborn infant, both presumed to be healthy. The assays were part of a screening program to establish reference intervals. The mother's hemoglobin concentration was 14 g/dL, and the newborn's was 20 g/dL. The mother's hemoglobin fractions were quantified as 97% Hb A, 2% Hb A_2, and 1% Hb F by HPLC. The newborn's results were 88% Hb F and 12% Hb A.

1. Were these hemoglobin results within expected reference intervals?
2. Why were the mother's and the newborn's hemoglobin concentration so different?
3. What is the difference between the test to determine the hemoglobin concentration and the test to analyze hemoglobin by HPLC?
4. Why were the mother's and newborn's hemoglobin fractions so different?

---

*The author extends appreciation to Mary Coleman, whose work in prior editions provided the foundation for this chapter.

Hemoglobin (Hb) is one of the most studied proteins in the body due to the ability to easily isolate it from red blood cells (RBCs). It comprises approximately 95% of the cytoplasmic content of RBCs.[1] The body very efficiently carries hemoglobin in RBCs, which provides protection from denaturation in the plasma and loss through the kidneys. Free (non-RBC) hemoglobin, generated from RBCs through hemolysis, has a short half-life outside of the RBCs. When released into the plasma, it is rapidly salvaged to preserve its iron and amino acid components; when salvage capacity is exceeded, it is excreted by the kidneys (Chapter 23). The concentration of hemoglobin within RBCs is approximately 34 g/dL, and its molecular weight is approximately 64,000 Daltons.[2] Hemoglobin's main function is to transport oxygen from the lungs to tissues and transport carbon dioxide from the tissues to the lungs for exhalation. Hemoglobin also contributes to acid-base balance by binding and releasing hydrogen ions and transports nitric oxide (NO), a regulator of vascular tone.[1,3]

This chapter covers the structure, biosynthesis, ontogeny, regulation, and function of hemoglobin. The formation, composition, and characteristics of several dyshemoglobins—namely, methemoglobin, carboxyhemoglobin, and sulfhemoglobin—are also discussed at the end of the chapter.

HEMOGLOBIN STRUCTURE

Hemoglobin is the first protein whose structure was described using x-ray crystallography.[4] The hemoglobin molecule is a globular protein consisting of two different pairs of polypeptide chains and four heme groups, with one heme group imbedded in each of the four polypeptide chains (Figure 10-1).

Heme Structure

Heme consists of a ring of carbon, hydrogen, and nitrogen atoms called *protoporphyrin IX*, with a central atom of divalent ferrous iron (Fe^{2+}) (Figure 10-2). Each of the four heme groups is positioned in a pocket of the polypeptide chain near the surface of the hemoglobin molecule. The ferrous iron in each heme molecule reversibly combines with one oxygen molecule. When the ferrous irons are oxidized to the ferric state (Fe^{3+}), they no longer can bind oxygen. Oxidized

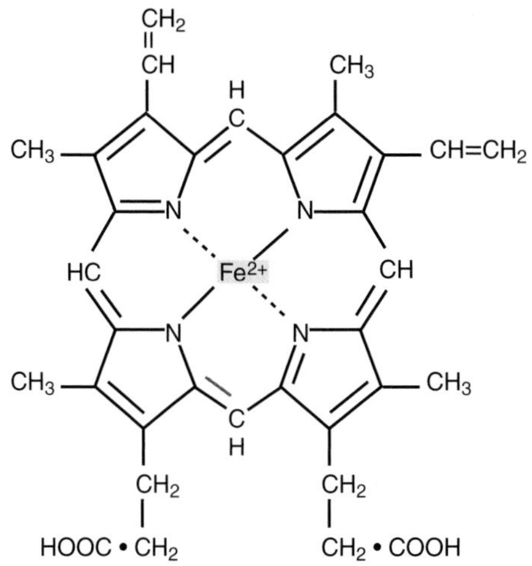

Figure 10-2 Heme is protoporphyrin IX that carries a central ferrous ion (Fe^{2+}).

hemoglobin is also called *methemoglobin* and is discussed later in this chapter.

Globin Structure

The four globin chains comprising each hemoglobin molecule consist of two identical pairs of unlike polypeptide chains, 141 to 146 amino acids each. Variations in amino acid sequences give rise to different types of polypeptide chains. Each chain is designated by a Greek letter (Table 10-1).[1,3]

TABLE 10-1 Globin Chains

Symbol	Name	Number of Amino Acids
α	Alpha	141
β	Beta	146
γ_A	Gamma A	146 (position 136: alanine)
γ_G	Gamma G	146 (position 136: glycine)
δ	Delta	146
ϵ	Epsilon	146
ζ	Zeta	141
ϑ	Theta	Unknown

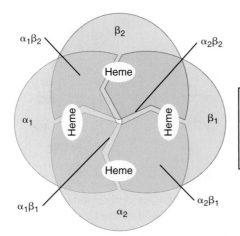

$\alpha_1\beta_2$ bonds and $\alpha_2\beta_1$ bonds are located between the dimers, $\alpha_1\beta_1$ bonds are in the front, $\alpha_2\beta_2$ bonds are behind.

Figure 10-1 Hemoglobin: a tetramer of four globin polypeptide chains, with a heme molecule attached to each chain.

Each globin chain is divided into eight helices separated by seven nonhelical segments (Figure 10-3).[3] The helices, designated A to H, contain subgroup numberings for the sequence of the amino acids in each helix and are relatively rigid and linear. Flexible nonhelical segments connect the helices, as reflected by their designations: NA for the sequence between the N-terminus and the A helix, AB between the A and B helices, and so forth, with BC, CD, DE, EF, FG, GH, and finally HC between the H helix and the C-terminus.[3]

Complete Hemoglobin Molecule

The hemoglobin molecule can be described by its primary, secondary, tertiary, and quaternary protein structures. The *primary structure* refers to the amino acid sequence of the polypeptide chains. The *secondary structure* refers to chain arrangements in helices and nonhelices. The *tertiary structure* refers to the arrangement of the helices into a pretzel-like configuration.

Globin chains loop to form a cleft pocket for heme. Each chain contains a heme group that is suspended between the E

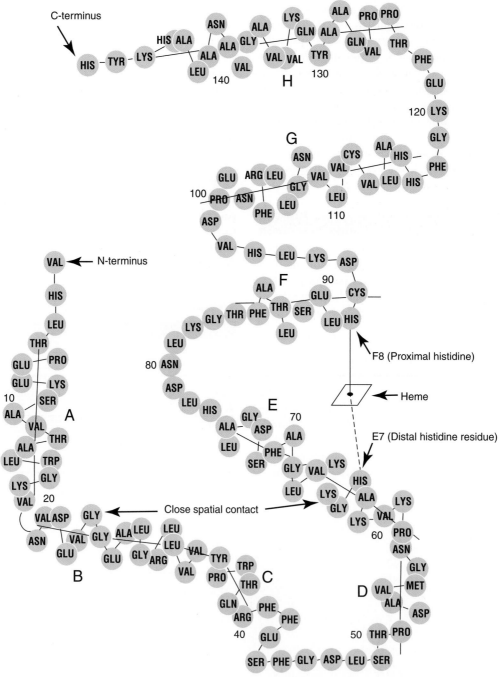

Figure 10-3 A β-globin chain: a polypeptide with helical (labeled A through H) and nonhelical segments. Heme (protoporphyrin IX with a central iron atom) is suspended in a pocket between the E and F helices. The iron atom of heme is linked to the F8 proximal histidine on one side of the heme plane (solid line). Oxygen binds to the iron atom on the other side of the plane and is close (but not linked) to the E7 distal histidine (dotted line). (Modified from Huisman TH, Schroder WA: New aspects of the structure, function, and synthesis of hemoglobins, Boca Raton, Fla, 1971, CRC Press; modified from Stamatoyannopoulos G: The molecular basis of blood diseases, ed 2, Philadelphia, 1994, Saunders.)

and F helices of the polypeptide chain (Figure 10-3).[2,3] The iron atom at the center of the protoporphyrin IX ring of heme is positioned between two histidine radicals, forming a proximal histidine bond within F8 and, through the linked oxygen, a close association with the distal histidine residue in E7.[3] Globin chain amino acids in the cleft are hydrophobic, whereas amino acids on the outside are hydrophilic, which renders the molecule water soluble. This arrangement also helps iron remain in its divalent ferrous form regardless of whether it is oxygenated (carrying an oxygen molecule) or deoxygenated (not carrying an oxygen molecule).

The *quaternary structure* of hemoglobin, also called a *tetramer*, describes the complete hemoglobin molecule. The complete hemoglobin molecule is spherical, has four heme groups attached to four polypeptide chains, and may carry up to four molecules of oxygen (Figure 10-4). The predominant adult hemoglobin, Hb A, is composed of two α-globin chains and two β-globin chains. Strong α_1–β_1 and α_2–β_2 bonds hold the dimers in a stable form. The α_1–β_2 and α_2–β_1 bonds are important for the stability of the quaternary structure in the oxygenated and deoxygenated forms (Figure 10-1).[1,2]

A small percentage of Hb A is *glycated*. Glycation is a posttranslational modification formed by the nonenzymatic binding of various sugars to globin chain amino groups over the life span of the RBC. The most characterized of the glycated hemoglobins is Hb A_{1c}, in which glucose attaches to the N-terminal valine of the β chain.[1] Normally, about 4% to 6% of Hb A circulates in the A_{1c} form. In uncontrolled diabetes mellitus, the amount of A_{1c} is increased proportionally to the mean blood glucose level over the preceding 2 to 3 months.

HEMOGLOBIN BIOSYNTHESIS

Heme Biosynthesis

Heme biosynthesis occurs in the mitochondria and cytoplasm of bone marrow erythrocyte precursors, beginning with the pronormoblast through the circulating polychromatic (also known as polychromatophilic) erythrocyte (Chapter 8). As they lose their ribosomes and mitochondria (location of the citric/tricarboxylic acid cycle), mature erythrocytes can no longer make hemoglobin.[5]

Heme biosynthesis begins in the mitochondria with the condensation of *glycine* and *succinyl coenzyme A* (CoA) catalyzed by *aminolevulinate synthase* to form *aminolevulinic acid* (ALA) (Figure 10-5).[5] In the cytoplasm, *aminolevulinic acid dehydratase* (also known as *porphobilinogen synthase*) converts ALA to *porphobilinogen* (PBG). PBG undergoes several transformations in the cytoplasm from *hydroxylmethylbilane* to *coproporphyrinogen III*. This pathway then continues in the mitochondria until, in the final step of production of heme, Fe^{2+} combines

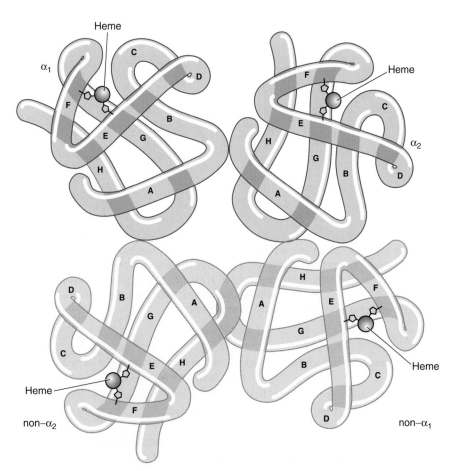

Figure 10-4 Hemoglobin molecule illustrating tertiary folding of the four polypeptide chains. Heme is suspended between the E and F helices of each polypeptide chain. Pink represents α_1 (*left*) and α_2 (*right*); yellow represents non-α_2 (*left*) and non-α_1 (*right*). The polypeptide chains first form α_1 - non-α_1 and α_2-non-α_2 dimers, and then assemble into a tetramer (quaternary structure) with α_1-non-α_2 and α_2-non-α_1 bonds.

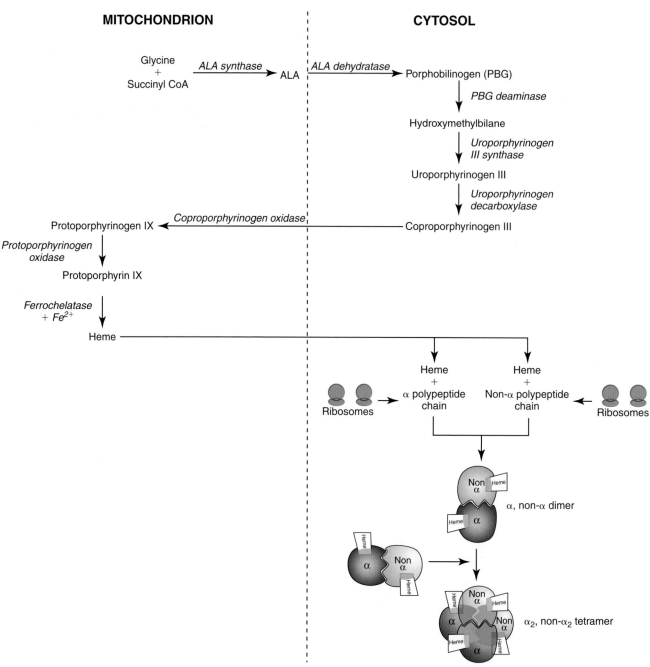

Figure 10-5 Hemoglobin assembly begins with glycine and succinyl coenzyme A (CoA), which assemble in the mitochondria catalyzed by aminolevulinate synthase to form aminolevulinic acid (ALA). In the cytoplasm, ALA undergoes several transformations from porphobilinogen (PBG) to coproporphyrinogen III, which, catalyzed by coproporphyrinogen oxidase, becomes protoporphyrinogen IX. In the mitochondria, protoporphyrinogen IX is converted to protoporphyrin IX by protoporphyrinogen oxidase. Ferrous (Fe^{2+}) ion is added, catalyzed by ferrochelatase to form heme. In the cytoplasm, heme assembles with an α chain and non-α chain, forming a dimer, and ultimately two dimers join to form the hemoglobin tetramer.

with *protoporphyrin IX* in the presence of *ferrochelatase* (*heme synthase*) to make heme.[5]

Transferrin, a plasma protein, carries iron in the ferric (Fe^{3+}) form to developing erythroid cells (Chapter 11). Transferrin binds to transferrin receptors on erythroid precursor cell membranes and the receptors and transferrin (with bound iron) are brought into the cell in an endosome (Figure 11-5). Acidification of the endosome releases the iron from transferrin. Iron is transported out of the endosome and into the

mitochondria where it is reduced to the ferrous state, and is united with protoporphyrin IX to make heme. Heme leaves the mitochondria and is joined to the globin chains in the cytoplasm.

Globin Biosynthesis

Six structural genes code for six globin chains. The α- and ζ-globin genes are on the short arm of chromosome 16; the ε-, γ-, δ-, and β-globin gene cluster is on the short arm of chromosome 11

(Figure 28-1). In the human genome, there is one copy of each globin gene per chromatid, for a total of two genes per diploid cell, with the exception of α and γ. There are two copies of the α- and γ-globin genes per chromatid, for a total of four genes per diploid cell.

The production of globin chains takes place in erythroid precursors from the pronormoblast through the circulating polychromatic erythrocyte, but not in the mature erythrocyte.[5] Transcription of the globin genes to messenger ribonucleic acid (mRNA) occurs in the nucleus, and translation of mRNA to the globin polypeptide chain occurs on ribosomes in the cytoplasm. Although transcription of the α-globin genes produces more mRNA than the β-globin gene, there is less efficient translation of the α-globin mRNA.[2] Therefore, the α and β chains are produced in approximately equal amounts. After translation is complete, the chains are released from the ribosomes in the cytoplasm.

Hemoglobin Assembly

After their release from ribosomes, each globin chain binds to a heme molecule, then forms a heterodimer (Figure 10-5). The non-α chains have a charge difference that determines their affinity to bind to the α chains. The α chain has a positive charge and has the highest affinity for a β chain due to its negative charge.[1,2] The γ-globin chain has the next highest affinity, followed by the δ-globin chain.[2] Two heterodimers then combine to form a tetramer. This completes the hemoglobin molecule.

Two α and two β chains form Hb A, the major hemoglobin present from 6 months of age through adulthood. Hb A_2

contains two α and two δ chains. Owing to a mutation in the promoter region of the δ-globin gene, production of the δ chain polypeptide is very low.[6] Consequently, Hb A_2 comprises less than 3.5% of total hemoglobin in adults. Hb F contains two α and two γ chains. In healthy adults, Hb F comprises 1% to 2% of total hemoglobin, and it is present only in a small proportion of the RBCs (uneven distribution). These RBCs with Hb F are called *F* or *A/F cells*.[1,2]

The various amino acids that comprise the globin chains affect the net charge of the hemoglobin tetramer. Electrophoresis and high performance liquid chromatography (HPLC) are used for fractionation, presumptive identification, and quantification of normal hemoglobins and hemoglobin variants (Chapter 27). Molecular genetic testing of globin gene DNA provides definitive identification of variant hemoglobins.

HEMOGLOBIN ONTOGENY

Hemoglobin composition differs with prenatal gestation time and postnatal age. Hemoglobin changes reflect the sequential activation and inactivation (or switching) of the globin genes, progressing from the ζ- to the α-globin gene on chromosome 16 and from the ε- to the γ-, δ-, and β-globin genes on chromosome 11. The ζ- and ε-globin chains normally appear only during the first 3 months of embryonic development. These two chains, when paired with the α and γ chains, form the embryonic hemoglobins (Figure 10-6). During the second and third trimesters of fetal life and at

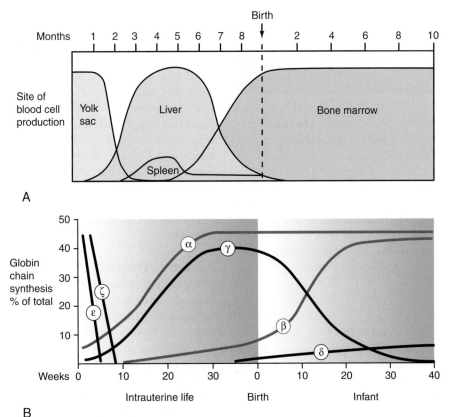

Figure 10-6 Timeline of globin chain production from intrauterine life to adulthood. See also Table 10-2.

TABLE 10-2 Normal Hemoglobins

Stage	Globin Chain	Hemoglobin
Intrauterine		
Early embryogenesis (product of yolk sac erythroblasts)	$\zeta_2 + \epsilon_2$	Gower-1
	$\alpha_2 + \epsilon_2$	Gower-2
	$\zeta_2 + \gamma_2$	Portland
Begins in early embryogenesis; peaks during third trimester and begins to decline just before birth	$\alpha_2 + \gamma_2$	F
Birth		
	$\alpha_2 + \gamma_2$	F, 60% to 90%
	$\alpha_2 + \beta_2$	A, 10% to 40%
Two Years through Adulthood		
	$\alpha_2 + \gamma_2$	F, 1% to 2%
	$\alpha_2 + \delta_2$	A_2, <3.5%
	$\alpha_2 + \beta_2$	A, >95%

birth, Hb F ($\alpha_2\gamma_2$) is the predominant hemoglobin. By 6 months of age and through adulthood, Hb A ($\alpha_2\beta_2$) is the predominant hemoglobin, with small amounts of Hb A_2 ($\alpha_2\delta_2$) and Hb F.[2] Table 10-2 presents the reference intervals for the normal hemoglobin fractions at various ages.

Mechanisms that control the switching from γ chain production to β chain production (γ-β switching) are discussed in the next section.

REGULATION OF HEMOGLOBIN PRODUCTION

Heme Regulation

The key rate-limiting step in heme synthesis is the initial reaction of glycine and succinyl CoA to form ALA, catalyzed by ALA synthase (Figure 10-5). Heme inhibits the transcription of the ALA synthase gene, which leads to a decrease in heme production (a negative feedback mechanism). Heme inhibits other enzymes in the biosynthesis pathway, including ALA dehydrase and PBG deaminase. A negative feedback mechanism by heme or substrate inhibition by protoporphyrin IX is believed to inhibit the ferrochelatase enzyme.[5] Conversely, an increased demand for heme induces an increased synthesis of ALA synthase.[5]

Globin Regulation

Globin synthesis is highly regulated so that there is a balanced production of globin and heme. This is critical because an excess of globin chains, protophophyrin IX, or iron can accumulate and damage the cell, reducing its life span.

Globin production is mainly controlled at the transcription level by a complex interaction of deoxyribonucleic acid (DNA) sequences (cis-acting promoters, enhancers, and silencers) and soluble transcription factors (trans-acting factors) that bind to DNA or to one another to promote or suppress transcription.[2] Initiation of transcription of a particular globin gene requires (1) the promoter DNA sequences immediately before the 5' end or the beginning of the gene; (2) a key transcription factor called *Krüppel-like factor 1* (KLF1); (3) a number of other transcription factors (such as GATA1, Ikaros, TAL1, p45-NF-E2, and LDB1); and (4) an enhancer region of DNAse 1 hypersensitive nucleic acid sequences located more than 20 kilobases upstream (before the 5' start site of the gene) from the globin gene called the *locus control region* or *LCR*.[7] For example, to activate transcription of the β-globin gene in the β-globin gene cluster on chromosome 11, the LCR, the promoter for the β-globin gene, and various transcription factors join together to form a three-dimensional active chromosome hub (ACH), with KLF1 playing a key role in connecting the complex.[7,8] Because the LCR is located a distance upstream from the β-globin gene complex, a loop of DNA is formed when the LCR and β-globin gene promoter join together in the chromosome hub.[8] The other globin genes in the cluster (ϵ-, γ-, and δ-) are maintained in the inactive state in the DNA loop, so only the β-globin gene is transcribed.[7,8]

Krüppel-like factor 1 also plays a key regulatory role in the switch from γ chain to β chain production (γ-β switching) that begins in late fetal life and continues through adulthood. The KLF1 is an exact match for binding to the DNA promoter sequences of the β-globin gene, while the γ-globin gene promoter has a slightly different sequence.[7] This results in a preferential binding to and subsequent activation of transcription of the β-globin gene.[7] KLF1 also regulates the expression of repressors of γ-globin gene transcription, such as BCL11A and MYB.[7,9]

Globin synthesis is also regulated during translation when the mRNA coding for the globin chains associates with ribosomes to produce the polypeptide. Many protein factors are required to control the initiation, elongation, and termination steps of translation. Heme is an important regulator of globin mRNA translation at the initiation step by promoting the activation of a translation initiation factor and inactivating its repressor.[5] Conversely, when the heme level is low, the repressor accumulates and inactivates the initiation factor, thus blocking translation of the globin mRNA.[2,5]

Systemic Regulation of Erythropoiesis

When there is an insufficient quantity of hemoglobin or if the hemoglobin molecule is defective in transporting oxygen, tissue hypoxia occurs. The hypoxia is detected by the peritubular cells of the kidney, which respond by increasing the production of erythropoietin (EPO). EPO increases the number of erythrocytes produced and released into the periphery; it also accelerates the rate of synthesis of erythrocyte components, including hemoglobin (Chapter 8).

Although each laboratory must establish its own reference intervals based on their instrumentation, methodology, and patient population, in general, reference intervals for hemoglobin concentration are as follows:

Men:	14 to 18 g/dL (140 to 180 g/L)
Women:	12 to 15 g/dL (120 to 150 g/L)
Newborns:	16.5 to 21.5 g/dL (165 to 215 g/L)

Reference intervals for infants and children vary according to age group. Individuals living at high altitudes have slightly higher levels of hemoglobin as a compensatory mechanism to provide more oxygen to the tissues in the oxygen-thin air. Tables on the inside front cover of this text provide reference intervals for all age-groups.

HEMOGLOBIN FUNCTION

Oxygen Transport

The function of hemoglobin is to readily bind oxygen molecules in the lung, which requires high oxygen affinity; to transport oxygen; and to efficiently unload oxygen to the tissues, which requires low oxygen affinity. During oxygenation, each of the four heme iron atoms in a hemoglobin molecule can reversibly bind one oxygen molecule. Approximately 1.34 mL of oxygen is bound by each gram of hemoglobin.[1]

The affinity of hemoglobin for oxygen relates to the partial pressure of oxygen (PO_2), often defined in terms of the amount of oxygen needed to saturate 50% of hemoglobin, called the P_{50} *value*. The relationship is described by the oxygen dissociation curve of hemoglobin, which plots the percent oxygen saturation of hemoglobin versus the PO_2 (Figure 10-7). The curve is *sigmoidal*, which indicates low hemoglobin affinity for oxygen at low oxygen tension and high affinity for oxygen at high oxygen tension.

Cooperation among hemoglobin subunits contributes to the shape of the curve. Hemoglobin that is completely deoxygenated has little affinity for oxygen. However, with each oxygen molecule that is bound, there is a change in the conformation of the tetramer that progressively increases the oxygen affinity of the other heme subunits. Once one oxygen molecule binds, the remainder of the hemoglobin molecule quickly becomes fully oxygenated.[2] Therefore, with the high oxygen tension in the lungs, the affinity of hemoglobin for oxygen is high, and hemoglobin becomes rapidly saturated with oxygen. Conversely, with the relatively low oxygen tension in the tissues, the affinity of hemoglobin for oxygen is low, and hemoglobin rapidly releases oxygen.

Normally, a PO_2 of approximately 27 mm Hg results in 50% oxygen saturation of the hemoglobin molecule. If there is a shift of the curve to the left, 50% oxygen saturation of hemoglobin occurs at a PO_2 of less than 27 mm Hg. If there is a shift of the curve to the right, 50% oxygen saturation of hemoglobin occurs at a PO_2 higher than 27 mm Hg.

The reference interval for arterial oxygen saturation is 96% to 100%. If the oxygen dissociation curve shifts to the left, a patient with arterial and venous PO_2 levels in the reference intervals (80 to 100 mm Hg arterial and 30 to 50 mm Hg venous) will have a higher percent oxygen saturation and a

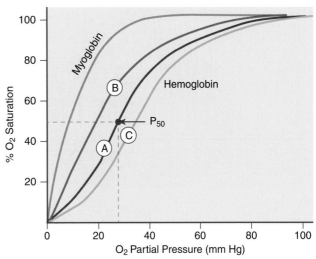

Figure 10-7 Oxygen dissociation curves. **A,** Normal hemoglobin-oxygen dissociation curve. P_{50} is the partial pressure of oxygen (O_2) needed for 50% O_2 saturation of hemoglobin. **B,** Left-shifted curve with reduced P_{50} can be caused by decreases in 2,3-bisphosphoglycerate (2,3-BPG), H^+ ions (raised pH), partial pressure of carbon dioxide (PCO_2), and/or temperature. A left-shifted curve is also seen with hemoglobin F and hemoglobin variants that have increased oxygen affinity. **C,** Right-shifted curve with increased P_{50} can be caused by elevations in 2,3-BPG, H^+ ions (lowered pH), PCO_2, and/or temperature. A right-shifted curve is also seen with hemoglobin variants that have decreased oxygen affinity. Myoglobin, a muscle protein, produces a markedly left-shifted curve indicating a very high oxygen affinity. It is not effective in releasing oxygen at physiologic oxygen tensions.

higher affinity for oxygen than a patient for whom the curve is normal. With a shift in the curve to the right, a lower oxygen affinity is seen.

In addition to the PO_2, shifts of the curve to the left or right occur if there are changes in the pH of the blood. In the tissues, a lower pH shifts the curve to the right and reduces the affinity of hemoglobin for oxygen, and the hemoglobin more readily releases oxygen. A shift in the curve due to a change in pH (or hydrogen ion concentration) is termed the *Bohr effect*. It facilitates the ability of hemoglobin to exchange oxygen and carbon dioxide (CO_2) and is discussed later.

The concentration of 2,3-bisphosphoglycerate (2,3-BPG, formerly 2,3-diphosphoglycerate) also has an effect on oxygen affinity. In the deoxygenated state, the hemoglobin tetramer assumes a *tense* or *T* conformation that is stabilized by the binding of 2,3-BPG between the β-globin chains (Figure 10-8). The formation of salt bridges between the phosphates of 2, 3-BPG and positively charged groups on the globin chains further stabilizes the tetramer in the T conformation.[1] The binding of 2, 3-BPG shifts the oxygen dissociation curve to the right, favoring the release of oxygen.[1] In addition, a lower pH and higher PCO_2 in the tissues further shifts the curve to the right, favoring the release of oxygen.[1]

As hemoglobin binds oxygen molecules, a change in conformation of the hemoglobin tetramer occurs with a change in hydrophobic interactions at the $\alpha_1\beta_2$ contact point, a disruption of the salt bridges, and release of 2, 3-BPG.[1] A 15-degree rotation of the $\alpha_1\beta_1$ dimer, relative to the $\alpha_2\beta_2$ dimer, occurs

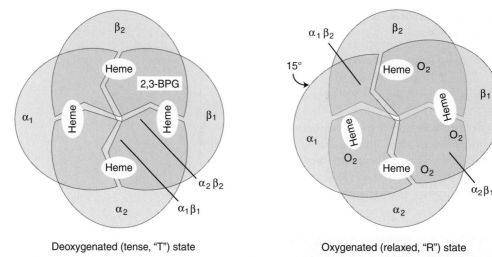

Figure 10-8 Tense (T) and relaxed (R) forms of hemoglobin. The tense form incorporates one 2,3-bisphosphoglycerate (2,3-BPG) molecule, bound between the β-globin chains with salt bridges. It is unable to transport oxygen. As hemoglobin binds oxygen molecules, the $\alpha_1\beta_1$ and $\alpha_2\beta_2$ dimers rotate 15° relative to each other as a result of the change in hydrophobic interactions at the $\alpha_1\beta_2$ contact point, disruption of salt bridges, and release of 2, 3-BPG.

along the $\alpha_1\beta_2$ contact point.[2] When the hemoglobin tetramer is fully oxygenated, it assumes a *relaxed* or R state (Figure 10-8).

Clinical conditions that produce a shift of the oxygen dissociation curve to the left include a lowered body temperature due to external causes; multiple transfusions of stored blood with depleted 2,3-BPG; alkalosis; and the presence of hemoglobin variants with a high affinity for oxygen. Conditions producing a shift of the curve to the right include increased body temperature; acidosis; the presence of hemoglobin variants with a low affinity for oxygen; and an increased 2,3-BPG concentration in response to hypoxic conditions, such as high altitude, pulmonary insufficiency, congestive heart failure, and severe anemia (Chapter 19).

The sigmoidal oxygen dissociation curve generated by normal hemoglobin contrasts with myoglobin's hyperbolic curve (Figure 10-7). Myoglobin, present in cardiac and skeletal muscle, is a 17,000-Dalton, monomeric, oxygen-binding heme protein. It binds oxygen with greater affinity than hemoglobin. Its hyperbolic curve indicates that it releases oxygen only at very low partial pressures, which means it is not as effective as hemoglobin in releasing oxygen to the tissues at physiologic oxygen tensions. Myoglobin is released into the plasma when there is damage to the muscle in myocardial infarction, trauma, or severe muscle injury, called *rhabdomyolysis*. Myoglobin is normally excreted by the kidney, but levels may become elevated in renal failure. Serum myoglobin levels aid in diagnosis of myocardial infarction in patients who have no underlying trauma, rhabdomyolysis, or renal failure. Myoglobin in the urine produces a positive result on the urine dipstick test for blood; this must be differentiated from a positive result caused by hemoglobin.

Hb F (fetal hemoglobin, the primary hemoglobin in newborns) has a P_{50} of 19 to 21 mm Hg, which results in a left shift of the oxygen dissociation curve and increased affinity for oxygen relative to that of Hb A. This increased affinity for oxygen is due to its weakened ability to bind 2,3-BPG.[2] There is only one amino acid difference in a critical 2,3-BPG binding site

between the γ chain and the β chain that accounts for this difference in binding.[2]

In fetal life, the high oxygen affinity of Hb F provides an advantage by allowing more effective oxygen withdrawal from the maternal circulation. At the same time, Hb F has a disadvantage in that it delivers oxygen less readily to tissues. The bone marrow in the fetus and newborn compensates by producing more RBCs to ensure adequate oxygenation of the tissues. This response is mediated by erythropoietin (Chapter 8). Consequently, the RBC count, hemoglobin concentration, and hematocrit of a newborn are higher than adult values (values are on the inside front cover), but they gradually decrease to normal physiologic levels by 6 months of age as the γ-β switching is completed and most of the Hb F is replaced by Hb A.

Carbon Dioxide Transport

A second crucial function of hemoglobin is the transport of carbon dioxide. In venous blood, the carbon dioxide diffuses into the red blood cells and combines with water to form carbonic acid (H_2CO_3). This reaction is facilitated by the RBC enzyme carbonic anhydrase. Carbonic acid then dissociates to release H^+ and bicarbonate (HCO_3^-) (Figure 10-9).

The H^+ from the second reaction binds oxygenated hemoglobin (HbO_2), and the oxygen is released from the hemoglobin due to the Bohr effect. The oxygen then diffuses out of the cell into the tissues. As the concentration of the negatively charged bicarbonate increases, it diffuses across the RBC membrane into the plasma. Chloride (Cl^-), also negatively charged, diffuses from the plasma into the cell to maintain electroneutrality across the membrane; this is called the *chloride shift* (Figure 10-9).

In the lungs, oxygen diffuses into the cell and binds to deoxygenated hemoglobin (HHb) due to the high oxygen tension. H^+ is released from hemoglobin and combines with bicarbonate to form carbonic acid. Carbonic acid is converted to water and CO_2; the latter diffuses out of the cells and is expelled by the lungs. As more bicarbonate diffuses into the cell to produce carbonic acid, chloride diffuses back out into

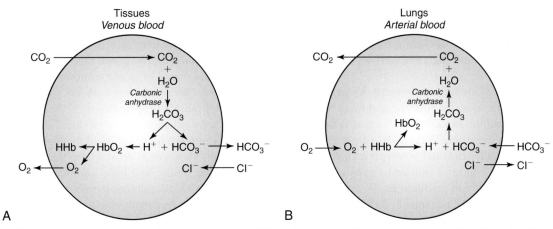

Figure 10-9 Transport and release of oxygen (O_2) and carbon dioxide (CO_2) in the tissues and lungs. **A,** In the tissues, CO_2 diffuses into the red blood cell and combines with water (H_2O) to form carbonic acid (H_2CO_3). This reaction is catalyzed by carbonic anhydrase. H_2CO_3 disassociates to hydrogen (H^+) and bicarbonate (HCO_3^-) ions. H^+ binds to oxyhemoglobin (HbO_2). resulting in the release of O_2 due to the Bohr effect. The O_2 diffuses out of the cell into the tissues. The HCO_3^- diffuses out of the cell as its concentration increases and is replaced by chloride (Cl^-) to maintain electroneutrality (chloride shift). Some CO_2 directly binds to the globin chains of hemoglobin. **B,** In the lungs, O_2 binds to deoxygenated hemoglobin (HHb) due to the high oxygen tension. The H^+ dissociates from HbO_2, combines with HCO_3^- to form H_2CO_3, which then dissociates into CO_2 and H_2O. The CO_2 diffuses out of the red blood cells and is exhaled by the lungs.

the plasma. Approximately 85% of the CO_2 produced in the tissues is transported by hemoglobin as H^+.[1] In this capacity, hemoglobin provides a buffering effect by binding and releasing H^+.[1] A small percentage of CO_2 remains in the cytoplasm and the remainder binds to the globin chains as a carbamino group.

Nitric Oxide Transport

A third function of hemoglobin involves the binding, inactivation, and transport of nitric oxide (NO).[10] Nitric oxide is secreted by vascular endothelial cells and causes relaxation of the vascular wall smooth muscle and vasodilation.[11] When released, free nitric oxide has a very short half-life, but some enters the RBCs and can bind to cysteine in the β chain of hemoglobin, forming S-nitrosohemoglobin.[10,11] Some investigators propose that hemoglobin preserves and transports nitric oxide to hypoxic microvascular areas, which stimulates vasodilation and increases blood flow (hypoxic vasodilation).[10] In this way, hemoglobin may work with other systems in regulating local blood flow to microvascular areas by binding and inactivating nitric oxide (causing vasoconstriction and decreased blood flow) when oxygen tension is high and releasing nitric oxide (causing vasodilation and increased blood flow) when oxygen tension is low.[10] This theory is not universally accepted, and the roles of hemoglobin, endothelial cells, and nitric oxide in regulating blood flow and oxygenation of the microcirculation are still being investigated.[11]

DYSHEMOGLOBINS

Dyshemoglobins (dysfunctional hemoglobins that are unable to transport oxygen) include methemoglobin, sulfhemoglobin, and carboxyhemoglobin. Dyshemoglobins form and may accumulate to toxic levels, after exposure to certain drugs or environmental chemicals or gasses. The offending agent modifies the structure of the hemoglobin molecule, preventing it

from binding oxygen. Most cases of dyshemoglobinemia are acquired; a small fraction of methemoglobinemia cases are hereditary.

Methemoglobin

Methemoglobin (MetHb) is formed by the reversible oxidation of heme iron to the ferric state (Fe^{3+}). Normally, a small amount of methemoglobin is continuously formed by oxidation of iron during the normal oxygenation and deoxygenation of hemoglobin.[11,12] However, methemoglobin reduction systems, predominantly the NADH-cytochrome b_5 reductase 3 (NADH-methemoglobin reductase) pathway, normally limit its accumulation to only 1% of total hemoglobin (Chapter 9 and Figure 9-1).[11-13]

Methemoglobin cannot carry oxygen because the oxidized ferric iron cannot bind it. An increase in the methemoglobin level results in decreased delivery of oxygen to the tissues. Individuals with methemoglobin levels less than 25% are generally asymptomatic.[14] If the methemoglobin level increases to more than 30% of total hemoglobin, cyanosis (bluish discoloration of skin and mucous membranes) and symptoms of hypoxia (dyspnea, headache, vertigo, change in mental status) occur.[12,13] Levels of methemoglobin greater than 50% can lead to coma and death.[12,13]

An increase in methemoglobin, called *methemoglobinemia*, can be acquired or hereditary. The acquired form, also called *toxic methemoglobinemia*, occurs in normal individuals after exposure to an exogenous oxidant, such as nitrites, primaquine, dapsone, or benzocaine.[12,14] As the oxidant overwhelms the hemoglobin reduction systems, the level of methemoglobin increases, and the patient may exhibit cyanosis and symptoms of hypoxia.[11] In many cases, withdrawal of the offending oxidant is sufficient for a recovery, but if the level of methemoglobin increases to 30% or more of total hemoglobin, intravenous methylene blue is administered. The methylene blue reduces the methemoglobin ferric iron to the ferrous state through the NADPH-methemoglobin reduction pathway that involves glutathione reductase and glucose-6-phosphate dehydrogenase (Figure 9-1).[11] In life-threatening cases, exchange transfusion may be required.[12]

Hereditary causes of methemoglobinemia are rare and include mutations in the gene for NADH-cytochrome b$_5$ reductase 3 (*CYB5R3*), resulting in a diminished capacity to reduce methemoglobin, and mutations in the α-, β-, or γ-globin gene, resulting in a structurally abnormal polypeptide chain that favors the oxidized ferric form of iron and prevents its reduction.[11,12] The methemoglobin produced by the latter group is called *M hemoglobin* or *Hb M*. (Chapter 27). Hb M is inherited in an autosomal dominant pattern, with methemoglobin comprising 30% to 50% of total hemoglobin.[12] There is no effective treatment for this form of methemoglobinemia.[11,12] Cytochrome b$_5$ reductase deficiency is an autosomal recessive disorder, and methemoglobin elevations occur in individuals who are homozygous or compound heterozygous for a *CYB5R3* mutation.[11,12] Most individuals with Hb M or homozygous cytochrome b$_5$ reductase deficiency maintain methemoglobin levels below 50%; they have cyanosis but only mild symptoms of hypoxia that do not require treatment.[11-13] Individuals heterozygous for the *CYB5R3* mutation have normal levels of methemoglobin but develop methemoglobinemia, cyanosis, and hypoxia when exposed to an oxidant drug or chemical.[12,14]

Methemoglobin is assayed by spectral absorption analysis instruments such as the CO-oximeter. Methemoglobin shows an absorption peak at 630 nm.[12] With high levels of methemoglobin, the blood takes on a chocolate brown color and does not revert back to the normal red color after oxygen exposure.[12,13] The methemoglobin in Hb M disease has different absorption peaks, depending on the variant.[11] Hemoglobin electrophoresis, high performance liquid chromatography, and DNA mutation testing are used for identification of Hb M variants. Cytochrome b$_5$ reductase 3 deficiency is diagnosed by enzyme assays and DNA mutation testing.[11]

Sulfhemoglobin

Sulfhemoglobin is formed by the irreversible oxidation of hemoglobin by drugs (such as sulfonilamides, phenacetin, nitrites, and phenylhydrazine) or exposure to sulfur chemicals in industrial or environmental settings.[11,12] It is formed by the addition of a sulfur atom to the pyrrole ring of heme and has a greenish pigment.[11] Sulfhemoglobin is ineffective for oxygen transport, and patients with elevated levels present with cyanosis. Sulfhemoglobin cannot be converted to normal Hb A; it persists for the life of the cell. Treatment consists of prevention by avoidance of the offending agent.

Sulfhemoglobin has a similar peak to methemoglobin on a spectral absorption instrument. The sulfhemoglobin spectral curve, however, does not shift when cyanide is added, a feature that is used to distinguish it from methemoglobin.[11]

Carboxyhemoglobin

Carboxyhemoglobin (COHb) results from the combination of carbon monoxide (CO) with heme iron. The affinity of carbon monoxide for hemoglobin is 240 times that of oxygen.[11] Once one molecule of carbon monoxide binds to hemoglobin, it shifts the hemoglobin-oxygen dissociation curve to the left, further increasing its affinity and severely impairing release of oxygen to the tissues.[11,15] Carbon monoxide has been termed the *silent killer* because it is an odorless and colorless gas, and victims may quickly become hypoxic.[15]

Some carboxyhemoglobin is produced endogenously, but it normally comprises less than 2% of total hemoglobin.[11] Exogenous carbon monoxide is derived from the exhaust of automobiles, tobacco smoke, and from industrial pollutants, such as coal, gas, and charcoal burning. In smokers, COHb levels may be as high as 15%.[14] As a result, smokers may have a higher hematocrit and polycythemia to compensate for the hypoxia.[11,14]

Exposure to carbon monoxide may be coincidental, accidental, or intentional (suicidal). Many deaths from house fires are the result of inhaling smoke, fumes, or carbon monoxide.[15] Even when heating systems in the home are properly maintained, accidental poisoning with carbon monoxide may occur. Toxic effects, such as headache, dizziness, and disorientation, begin to appear at blood levels of 20% to 30% COHb.[11,14] Levels of more than 40% of total hemoglobin may cause coma, seizure, hypotension, cardiac arrhythmias, pulmonary edema, and death.[11,15]

Carboxyhemoglobin may be detected by spectral absorption instruments at 540 nm.[12] It gives blood a cherry red color, which is sometimes imparted to the skin of victims.[15] A diagnosis of carbon monoxide poisoning is made if the COHb level is greater than 3% in nonsmokers and greater than 10% in smokers.[15] Treatment involves removal of the patient from the carbon monoxide source and administration of 100% oxygen.[11] The use of hyperbaric oxygen therapy is controversial.[15] It is primarily used to prevent neurologic and cognitive impairment after acute carbon monoxide exposure in patients whose COHb level exceeds 25%.[15]

HEMOGLOBIN MEASUREMENT

The *cyanmethemoglobin* method is the reference method for hemoglobin assay.[16] A lysing agent present in the cyanmethemoglobin reagent frees hemoglobin from RBCs. Free hemoglobin combines with potassium ferricyanide contained in the cyanmethemoglobin reagent, which converts the hemoglobin iron from the ferrous to the ferric state to form methemoglobin. Methemoglobin combines with potassium cyanide to form the stable pigment cyanmethemoglobin. The cyanmethemoglobin color intensity, which is proportional to hemoglobin concentration, is measured at 540 nm spectrophotometrically and compared with a standard (Chapter 14). The cyanmethemoglobin method is performed manually but has been adapted for use in automated instruments.

Many instruments now use sodium lauryl sulfate (SLS) to convert hemoglobin to SLS-methemoglobin. This method does not generate toxic wastes (Chapter 15).

Hemoglobin electrophoresis and HPLC are used to separate the different types of hemoglobins such as Hb A, A$_2$, and F (Chapters 27 and 28).

SUMMARY

- The hemoglobin molecule is a tetramer composed of two pairs of unlike polypeptide chains. A heme group (protoporphyrin IX + Fe^{2+}) is bound to each of the four polypeptide chains.
- Hemoglobin, contained in RBCs, carries oxygen from the lungs to the tissues. Oxygen binds to the ferrous iron in heme. Each hemoglobin tetramer can bind four oxygen molecules.
- Six structural genes code for the six globin chains of hemoglobin. The α- and ζ-globin genes are on chromosome 16; the ϵ-, γ-, δ-, and β-globin gene cluster is on chromosome 11. There is one copy of the δ-globin gene and one β-globin gene per chromosome, for a total of two genes per diploid cell. There are two copies of the α- and γ-globin genes per chromosome, for a total of four genes per diploid cell.
- The three hemoglobins found in normal adults are Hb A, Hb A$_2$, and Hb F. Hb A ($\alpha_2\beta_2$), composed of two $\alpha\beta$ heterodimers, is the predominant hemoglobin of adults. Hb F ($\alpha_2\gamma_2$) is the predominant hemoglobin in the fetus and newborn. Hb A$_2$ ($\alpha_2\delta_2$) is present from birth through adulthood, but at low levels.
- Hemoglobin ontogeny describes which hemoglobins are produced by the erythroid precursor cells from the fetal period through birth to adulthood.
- Complex genetic mechanisms regulate the sequential expression of the polypeptide chains in the embryo, fetus, and adult. Heme provides negative feedback regulation on protoporphyrin and globin chain production.
- The hemoglobin-oxygen dissociation curve is sigmoid owing to cooperativity among the hemoglobin subunits in binding and releasing oxygen.
- 2,3-BPG produced by the glycolytic pathway facilitates the delivery of oxygen from hemoglobin to the tissues. The Bohr effect is the influence of pH on the release of oxygen from hemoglobin.
- In the tissues, carbon dioxide diffuses into the RBCs and combines with water to form carbonic acid (H_2CO_3). The carbonic acid is then converted to bicarbonate and hydrogen ions (HCO_3^- and H^+). Most of the carbon dioxide is carried by hemoglobin as H^+.
- Methemoglobin, sulfhemoglobin, and carboxyhemoglobin cannot transport oxygen. They can accumulate to toxic levels due to exposure to certain drugs, industrial or environmental chemicals, or gases. A small fraction of methemoglobinemia cases are hereditary. Cyanosis occurs in patients with increased levels of methemoglobin or sulfhemoglobin.

Now that you have completed this chapter, go back and read again the case study at the beginning and respond to the questions presented.

REVIEW QUESTIONS

Answers can be found in the Appendix.

1. A hemoglobin molecule is composed of:
   a. One heme molecule and four globin chains
   b. Ferrous iron, protoporphyrin IX, and a globin chain
   c. Protoporphyrin IX and four globin chains
   d. Four heme molecules and four globin chains

2. Normal adult Hb A contains which polypeptide chains?
   a. α and β
   b. α and δ
   c. α and γ
   d. α and ϵ

3. A key rate-limiting step in heme synthesis is suppression of:
   a. Aminolevulinate synthase
   b. Carbonic anhydrase
   c. Protoporphyrin IX reductase
   d. Glucose 6-phosphate dehydrogenase

4. Which of the following forms of hemoglobin molecule has the lowest affinity for oxygen?
   a. Tense
   b. Relaxed

5. Using the normal hemoglobin-oxygen dissociation curve in Figure 10-7 for reference, predict the position of the curve when there is a decrease in pH.
   a. Shifted to the right of normal with decreased oxygen affinity
   b. Shifted to the left of normal with increased oxygen affinity
   c. Shifted to the right of normal with increased oxygen affinity
   d. Shifted to the left of normal with decreased oxygen affinity

6. The predominant hemoglobin found in a healthy newborn is:
   a. Gower-1
   b. Gower-2
   c. A
   d. F

7. What is the normal distribution of hemoglobins in healthy adults?
   a. 80% to 90% Hb A, 5% to 10% Hb A$_2$, 1% to 5% Hb F
   b. 80% to 90% Hb A$_2$, 5% to 10% Hb A, 1% to 5% Hb F
   c. >95% Hb A, <3.5% Hb A$_2$, 1% to 2% Hb F
   d. >90% Hb A, 5% Hb F, <5% Hb A$_2$

8. Which of the following is a description of the structure of oxidized hemoglobin?
   a. Hemoglobin carrying oxygen on heme; synonymous with oxygenated hemoglobin
   b. Hemoglobin with iron in the ferric state (methemoglobin) and not able to carry oxygen
   c. Hemoglobin with iron in the ferric state so that carbon dioxide replaces oxygen in the heme structure
   d. Hemoglobin carrying carbon monoxide; hence "oxidized" refers to the single oxygen

9. In the quaternary structure of hemoglobin, the globin chains associate into:
   a. α tetramers in some cells and β tetramers in others
   b. A mixture of α tetramers and β tetramers
   c. α dimers and β dimers
   d. Two αβ dimers

10. How are the globin chain genes arranged?
    a. With α genes and β genes on the same chromosome, including two α genes and two β genes
    b. With α genes and β genes on separate chromosomes, including two α genes on one chromosome and one β gene on a different chromosome
    c. With α genes and β genes on the same chromosome, including four α genes and four β genes
    d. With α genes and β genes on separate chromosomes, including four α genes on one chromosome and two β genes on a different chromosome

11. The nature of the interaction between 2,3-BPG and hemoglobin is that 2,3-BPG:
    a. Binds to the heme moiety, blocking the binding of oxygen
    b. Binds simultaneously with oxygen to ensure that it stays bound until it reaches the tissues, when both molecules are released from hemoglobin
    c. Binds to amino acids of the globin chain, contributing to a conformational change that inhibits oxygen from binding to heme
    d. Oxidizes hemoglobin iron, diminishing oxygen binding and promoting oxygen delivery to the tissues

REFERENCES

1. Telen, M. J. (2009). The mature erythrocyte. In Greer, J. P., Foerster, J., Rodgers, G. M., et al. (Eds.), *Wintrobe's Clinical Hematology.* (12th ed., pp. 126–155). Philadelphia: Wolters Kluwer Health/Lippincott Williams & Wilkins.
2. Steinberg, M. H., Benz, E. J. Jr, Adewoye, A. H., et al. (2013). Pathobiology of the human erythrocyte and its hemoglobins. In Hoffman, R., Benz, E. J., Silberstein, L. E., et al. (Eds.), *Hematology Basic Principles and Practice.* (6th ed., pp. 406–417). Philadelphia: Saunders, an imprint of Elsevier Inc.
3. Natarajan, K., Townes, T. M., & Kutlar, A. (2010). Chapter 48. Disorders of hemoglobin structure: sickle cell anemia and related abnormalities. In Lichtman, M. A., Kipps, T. J., Seligsohn, U., Kaushansky, K., & Prchal, J. T. (Eds.), *Williams Hematology.* (8th ed.). New York: McGraw-Hill. http://accessmedicine.mhmedical.com.libproxy2.umdnj.edu/content.aspx?bookid=358&Sectionid=39835866. Accessed 11.01.14.
4. Perutz, M. F., Rossmann, M. G., Cullis, A. F., et al. (1960). Structure of hemoglobin: a three dimensional Fourier synthesis at 5.5A resolution obtained by x-ray analysis. *Nature, 185,* 416–422.
5. Dessypris, E. N., & Sawyer, S. T. (2009). Erythropoiesis. In Greer, J. P., Foerster, J., Rodgers, G. M., et al. (Eds.), *Wintrobe's Clinical Hematology.* (12th ed., pp. 106–125). Philadelphia: Wolters Kluwer Health/Lippincott, Williams & Wilkins.
6. Donze, D., Jeancake, P. H., & Townes, T. M. (1996). Activation of delta-globin gene expression by erythroid Krüpple-like factor: a potential approach for gene therapy of sickle cell disease. *Blood, 88,* 4051–4057.
7. Tallack, M. R., & Perkins, A. C. (2013). Three fingers on the switch: Krüppel-like factor 1 regulation of α-globin to β-globin gene switching. *Curr Opin Hematol, 20,* 193–200.
8. Tolhuis, B., Palstra, R-J., Splinter, E., et al. (2002). Looping and interaction between hypersensitive sites in the active β-globin locus. *Molecular Cell, 10,* 1453–1465.
9. Zhou, D., Liu, K., Sun, C. W. et al. (2010). KLF1 regulates BCL11A expression and gamma to beta-globin switching. *Nat Genet, 42,* 742–744.
10. Allen, B. W., Stamler, J. S., & Piantadosi, C. A. (2009). Hemoglobin, nitric oxide and molecular mechanisms of hypoxic vasodilation. *Trends Mol Med, 15,* 452–460.
11. Steinberg, M. H. (2009). Hemoglobins with altered oxygen affinity, unstable hemoglobins, M-hemoglobins, and dyshemoglobinemias. In Greer, J. P., Foerster, J., Rodgers, G. M., et al. (Eds.), *Wintrobe's Clinical Hematology.* (12th ed., pp. 1132–1142). Philadelphia: Wolters Kluwer Health/Lippincott Williams & Wilkins.
12. Benz, E. J., Jr., & Ebert, B. L. (2013). Hemoglobin variants associated with hemolytic anemia altered oxygen affinity, and methemoglobinemias. In Hoffman, R., Benz, E. J., Silberstein, L. E., et al. (Eds.), *Hematology Basic Principles and Practice.* (6th ed., pp. 573–580). Philadelphia: Saunders, an imprint of Elsevier Inc.
13. Skold, A., Cosco, D. I., & Klein, R. (2011). Methemoglobinemia: pathogenesis, diagnosis, and management. *South Med J, 104,* 757–761.
14. Vajpayee, N., Graham, S. S., & Bem, S. (2011). Basic examination of blood and bone marrow. In McPherson, R. A., & Pincus, M. R. (Eds.), *Henry's Clinical Diagnosis and Management by Laboratory Methods.* (22nd ed., pp. 509–512). Philadelphia: Saunders, an imprint of Elsevier Inc.
15. Guzman, J. A. (2012). Carbon monoxide poisoning. *Crit Care Clin, 28,* 537–548.
16. Clinical and Laboratory Standards Institute (CLSI). (2000). Reference and selected procedures for the quantitative determination of hemoglobin in blood; approved guideline. (3rd ed.). Wayne, PA: CLSI document H15–A3.

Iron Kinetics and Laboratory Assessment

11

*Kathryn Doig**

OBJECTIVES

After completion of this chapter, the reader will be able to:

1. Describe the essential metabolic processes in which iron participates.
2. State whether body iron is regulated by excretion or absorption.
3. Describe the compartments in which body iron is distributed, including the relative amounts in each site.
4. Trace a molecule of iron from its absorption through the enterocyte to transport into mitochondria and then recycling via macrophages, including the names of all proteins with which it interacts and that control its kinetics.
5. Name the ionic form and number of molecules of iron that bind to one molecule of apotransferrin.
6. Explain how hepcidin regulates body iron levels.
7. Explain how individual cells absorb iron.
8. Explain how individual cells regulate the amount of iron they absorb.
9. Describe the role of each of the following in the kinetics of iron:
   a. Divalent metal transporter 1 (DMT1)
   b. Ferroportin
   c. Transferrin (Tf)
   d. Transferrin receptor (TfR)
   e. Hepcidin
10. For the proteins listed in objective 9, distinguish those that are involved in the regulation of iron within individual cells versus those involved in systemic body iron regulation.
11. Recognize the names of proteins involved in hepatocyte iron sensing and regulation of hepcidin production.
12. List factors that increase and decrease the bioavailability of iron.
13. Name foods high in iron, both heme-containing and ionic.
14. For each of the following assays, describe the principle of the assay and the iron compartment assessed:
    a. Total serum iron (SI)
    b. Total iron-binding capacity (TIBC)
    c. Percent transferrin saturation
    d. Serum ferritin
    e. Soluble transferrin receptor (sTfR)
    f. Measures of the hemoglobin content of reticulocytes
    g. Prussian blue staining of tissues and cells
    h. Zinc protoporphyrin (ZPP)
15. Plot given patient values on a Thomas plot and interpret the patient's iron status.
16. Calculate the percent transferrin saturation when given total serum iron and TIBC.
17. When given reference intervals, interpret the results of each of the assays in objective 14 plus a Thomas plot and sTfR/log ferritin and recognize results consistent with decreased, normal, and increased iron status.
18. Identify instances in which sTfR, hemoglobin content of reticulocytes, sTfR/log ferritin, and Thomas plots may be needed to improve diagnosis of iron deficiency.

CASE STUDY

After studying the material in this chapter, the reader will be able to respond to the following case study:

In 1995, Garry, Koehler, and Simon assessed changes in stored iron in 16 female and 20 male regular blood donors aged 64 to 71.[1] They measured hemoglobin, hematocrit, serum ferritin concentration, and % transferrin saturation in specimens from the donors, who gave an average of 15 units (approximately 485 mL/unit) of blood over 3.5 years. The investigators collected comparable data

Continued

*The author extends appreciation to Mary Coleman, whose coverage of iron metabolism in the prior editions provided the foundation for this chapter.

CASE STUDY—cont'd

After studying the material in this chapter, the reader will be able to respond to the following case study:

from nondonors. Of the donors, 10 women and 6 men took a dietary supplement providing approximately 20 mg of iron per day. In addition, mean dietary iron intake was 18 mg/day for the women and 20 mg/day for the men. Over the period of the study, mean iron stores in women donors decreased from 12.53 to 1.14 mg/kg of body weight. Mean iron stores in male donors declined from 12.45 to 1.92 mg/kg. Nondonors' iron stores remained unchanged. Based on hemoglobin and hematocrit results, no donors became anemic. As iron stores decreased,

the calculated iron absorption rose to 3.55 mg/day for the women and 4.10 mg/day for the men—more than double the normal rate for both women and men.
1. Why did the donors' iron stores decrease?
2. Why did the donors' iron absorption rate rise? Explain using the names of all proteins involved.
3. Name the laboratory test(s) performed in the study used to evaluate directly the iron storage compartment?
4. What is the diagnostic value of the % transferrin saturation? What iron compartment does it assess?

Among the metals that are required for metabolic processes, none is more important than iron. It is critical to energy production in all cells, being at the center of the cytochromes of mitochondria. Oxygen needed for energy production is carried attached to iron by the hemoglobin molecule in red blood cells. Iron is so critical to the body that there is no mechanism for active excretion, just minimal daily loss with exfoliated skin and hair and intestinal epithelia. Iron is even recycled to conserve as much as possible in the body. To insure against times when iron may be scarce in the diet, the body stores iron as well.

The largest percentage of body iron, nearly 65% of it, is held within hemoglobin in red blood cells of various stages (Table 11-1) while about 25% of body iron is in storage, mostly within macrophages and hepatocytes.[2] The remaining 10% is divided among the muscles, the plasma, the cytochromes of cells, and various iron-containing enzymes within cells. A more functional approach to thinking about body iron distribution conceives of the iron as distributed in three compartments (Table 11-1). The *functional compartment* contains all iron that is functioning within cells. Though most of this is the iron in hemoglobin, the iron in myoglobin (in muscles) and cytochromes (in all cells) is part of the functional compartment. The *storage compartment* is the iron that is not currently functioning but is available when needed. The major sources of this stored iron are the macrophages and hepatocytes, but every cell, except mature red blood cells, stores some iron. The third compartment is the *transport compartment* of iron that is in transit from one body site to another in the plasma.

Although the reactivity of iron ions makes them central to energy production processes, it also makes them dangerous to the stability

of cells. Thus the body regulates iron carefully at the level of the whole body and also within individual cells, maintaining levels that are necessary for critical metabolic processes, while avoiding the dangers of excess iron accumulation. The conditions that develop when this balance is perturbed are described in Chapter 20. The routine tests used to assess body iron status are discussed here.

IRON CHEMISTRY

The metabolic functions of iron depend on its ability to change its valence state from reduced ferrous (Fe^{+2}) iron to the oxidized ferric (Fe^{+3}) state. Thus it is involved in oxidation and reduction reactions such as the electron transport within mitochondrial cytochromes. In cells, ferrous iron can react with peroxide via the Fenton reaction, forming highly reactive oxygen molecules.

$$Fe^{+2} + H_2O_2 = Fe^{+3} + OH^- + OH\cdot$$

The resulting hydroxyl radical ($OH\cdot$), also known as a free radical, is especially reactive as a short-lived but potent oxidizing agent, able to damage proteins, lipids, and nucleic acids. As will be described in the section on iron kinetics, there are various mechanisms within cells to reduce the potential for this type of damage.

IRON KINETICS

Systemic Body Iron Regulation

Figure 11-1 provides an overview of systemic body iron regulation that can be a reference throughout the section on iron

TABLE 11-1 Iron Compartments in Normal Humans

Compartment	Form and Anatomical Site	Percent of Total Body Iron	Typical Iron Content (g)
Functional	Hemoglobin iron in the blood	~68	2.400
	Myoglobin iron in muscles	~10	0.360
	Peroxidase, catalase, cytochromes, riboflavin enzymes in all cells	~3	0.120
Storage	Ferritin and hemosiderin mostly in macrophages and hepatocytes; small amounts in all cells except mature red blood cells	~18	0.667
Transport	Transferrin in plasma	<1	0.001

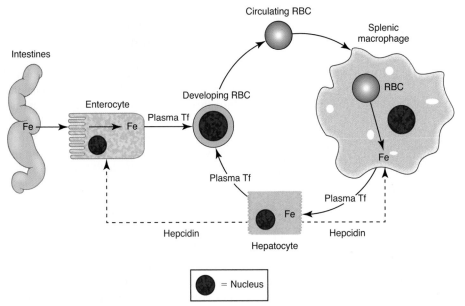

Figure 11-1 Overview of the iron cycle regulating systemic body iron. Iron is absorbed through the enterocyte of the duodenum and into the plasma via the portal circulation. There it binds to apotransferrin for transport to cells, such as the developing red blood cells. In red blood cells, the iron is used in hemoglobin that circulates with the cell until it becomes aged and is ingested by a macrophage. There the iron is removed from the hemoglobin and can be recycled into the plasma for use by other cells. The level of stored and circulating body iron is detected by the hepatocyte, which is able to produce a protein, hepcidin, when iron levels get too high. Hepcidin will inactivate the absorption and recycling of iron by acting on enterocytes, macrophages, and hepatocytes. When body iron decreases, hepcidin will also decrease so that absorption and recycling are again activated. (From Doig K: Iron: the body's most precious metal. Denver, 2013, Colorado Association for Continuing Medical Laboratory Education, Inc., p. 1.)

kinetics. The total amount of iron available to all body cells, systemic body iron, is regulated by absorption into the body because there is no mechanism for excretion. Ferrous iron in the lumen of the small intestine is carried across the luminal side of the enterocyte by divalent metal transporter 1 (DMT1) (Figure 11-2). Once iron has been absorbed into enterocytes, it requires another transporter, ferroportin, to carry it across the basolaminal enterocyte membrane into the bloodstream, thus truly absorbing it into the body. Ferroportin is the only known protein that exports iron across cell membranes. When the body has adequate stores of iron, the hepatocytes sense that and will increase production of hepcidin, a protein able to bind to ferroportin, leading to its inactivation. As a result, iron absorption into the body decreases. When the body iron begins to drop, the liver senses that change and decreases hepcidin production. As a result, ferroportin is once again active and able to transport iron into the blood. Thus homeostasis of iron is maintained by modest fluctuations in liver hepcidin production in response to body iron status. The regulation of systemic body iron is summarized in Figure 11-3.

The mechanism by which the hepatocytes are able to sense iron levels and produce hepcidin is highly complex, with multiple stimulatory pathways likely involved. Although this system is not yet fully elucidated, a number of critical molecules have been identified. One postulated system for the interaction of these molecules is modeled in Figure 11-4. The proteins involved include, at least, the hemochromatosis receptor (HFE), transferrin receptor 2, hemojuvelin, bone morphogenic protein (BMP) and its receptor (BMPR), and

sons of mothers against decapentaplegic (SMAD).[3] Table 11-2 lists their functions. The importance of these various molecules to iron kinetics has been demonstrated via mutations, both natural in humans and induced in mice, that lead to either iron overload or iron deficiency. Testing for these mutations is increasing in molecular diagnostic laboratories. The diseases associated with the known human mutations are described in Chapter 20.

Iron Transport

Iron exported from the enterocyte into the blood is ferrous and must be converted to the ferric form for transport in the blood. Hephaestin, a protein on the basolaminal enterocyte membrane, is able to oxidize iron as it exits the enterocyte. Once oxidized, the iron is ready for plasma transport, carried by a specific protein, apotransferrin (ApoTf). Once iron binds, the molecule is known as transferrin (Tf). Apotransferrin binds two molecules of ferric iron.

Cellular Iron Absorption and Disposition

Individual cells regulate the amount of iron they absorb to minimize the adverse effects of free radicals. This is accomplished by relying on an iron-specific carrier to move it into the cell by a process called *receptor-mediated endocytosis* (Figure 11-5). Cell membranes possess a receptor for transferrin, transferrin receptor 1 (TfR1). TfR1 has the highest affinity for diferric Tf at the physiologic pH of the plasma and extracellular fluid. When the TfR1 molecules bind Tf, they move and cluster together in the membrane. Once a critical mass accumulates, the membrane begins to invaginate, progressing

GI lumen

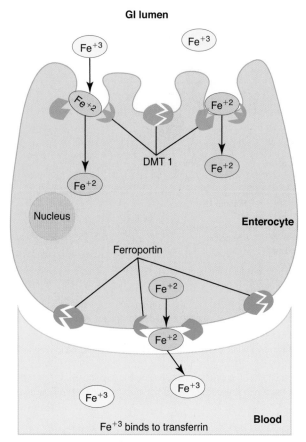

Figure 11-2 Absorption of ionic iron in the small intestine. Ferric iron in the intestinal lumen is reduced prior to transport across the luminal membrane of the enterocyte by divalent metal transporter 1 (DMT1). It is carried across the opposite membrane into the blood by ferroportin. It is reoxidized by hephaestin (not shown) as it exits for transport in the blood. (From Doig K: Iron: the body's most precious metal. Denver, 2013, Colorado Association for Continuing Medical Laboratory Education, Inc., p. 6.)

until the invagination pinches off a vesicle inside the cytoplasm called an *endosome*. Hydrogen ions are pumped into the vesicle. The resulting drop in pH changes the affinity of transferrin for iron, so the iron releases. Simultaneously, the affinity of TfR1 for apotransferrin at that pH increases so the apotransferrin remains bound to the receptor. The iron is exported from the vesicle into the cytoplasm of the cell by divalent metal transporter 1 (DMT1). Cytoplasmic trafficking is still not fully understood. However, some of the iron finds its way to storage. Other molecules of iron are transferred into the mitochondria,[4] where they are incorporated into cytochromes, or in the case of red blood cells, into heme for the production of hemoglobin. Meanwhile, the endosome returns to the cell membrane, where the endosome membrane fuses with the cell membrane, opening the endosome and essentially reversing its formation. At the pH of the extracellular fluid, TfR1 has a very low affinity for apotransferrin, so the apotransferrin releases into the plasma, available to bind iron once again. The TfR1 is also available again to carry new molecules of Tf-bound iron into the cell.

Cells are able to store iron so they have a reserve if supplies of new iron decline. Although all cells store iron, those cells that

are central to regulating systemic body iron, macrophages and hepatocytes, typically contain the most. Ferric iron is stored in a cage-like protein called apoferritin. Once iron binds, it is known as *ferritin*. One ferritin molecule can bind more than 4000 iron ions.[5] Ferritin iron can be mobilized for use during times of iron need by lysosomal degradation of the protein.[6] Partially degraded ferritin is known as hemosiderin and is considered to be less metabolically available than ferritin, though greater understanding of ferritin chemistry may revise this view.

In order to regulate the amount of iron inside the cell and avoid free radicals, cells are able to control the amount of TfR1 on their surface. The process depends on an elegant system of iron-sensitive cytoplasmic proteins that are able to affect the posttranscriptional function of the mRNA for TfR1.[7] The result is that when iron stores inside the cell are sufficient, production of TfR1 declines. Conversely, when iron stores inside the cell are low, TfR1 production increases. This is useful diagnostically to detect iron deficiency because a truncated form of the TfR1 is sloughed from cells and is measurable in serum as *soluble transferrin receptor* (sTfR).[8] The serum sTfR levels reflect the number of TfRs expressed on cells. So increases in sTfR can indicate increases in membrane TfR that result from low intracellular iron as seen in iron deficiency anemia.

Red blood cells deserve special mention in regard to cellular iron regulation. Because production of hemoglobin requires them to acquire far more iron than other cells, special mechanisms exist that allow them to circumvent the usual limitations on iron accumulation. The complete understanding of these processes has yet to be developed, but hypotheses suggest that the iron may bypass the cytoplasmic iron-sensing system, moving directly into the mitochondria from the endosome.[9]

Iron Recycling

When cells die, their iron is recycled. Multiple mechanisms salvage iron from dying cells. The largest percentage of recycled iron comes from red blood cells. Senescent (aging) red blood cells are ingested by macrophages in the spleen. The hemoglobin is degraded, with the iron being held by the macrophages as ferritin. Like enterocytes, macrophages possess ferroportin in their membranes.[10] This allows macrophages to be iron exporters so that the salvaged iron can be used by other cells. The exported iron is bound to plasma apotransferrin, just as if it were newly absorbed from the intestine.

Haptoglobin and hemopexin are plasma proteins able to salvage free hemoglobin or heme, respectively, preventing them from urinary loss at the glomerulus and returning the iron to the liver. Like macrophages, hepatocytes are important to iron salvage. They also possess ferroportin so that the salvaged iron can be exported to transferrin and ultimately to other body cells.[11] These salvage pathways are described in greater detail in Chapter 23.

DIETARY IRON, BIOAVAILABILITY, AND DEMAND

Under normal circumstances, the only source of iron for the body is from the diet. Foods containing high levels of iron

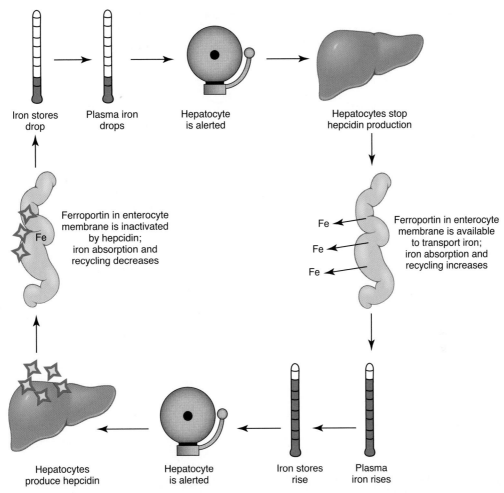

Figure 11-3 Summary of body iron regulation. When body iron stores drop sufficiently low that plasma iron also drops, the liver's iron-sensing system is activated and hepcidin production is decreased. As a result, ferroportin in the enterocyte and macrophage membranes will transport iron into the circulation. Plasma iron will rise and body stores will be restored. The hepatocyte iron-sensing system recognizes this and produces hepcidin. Hepcidin inactivates ferroportin in the enterocyte and macrophage membranes so that less iron is absorbed and recirculated. The resulting drop in iron stores and plasma iron is detected by the liver, repeating the cycle. (From Doig K: Iron: the body's most precious metal. Denver, 2013, Colorado Association for Continuing Medical Laboratory Education, Inc., p. 18.)

include red meats, legumes, and dark green leafy vegetables.[12] Although some foods may be high in iron, that iron may not be readily absorbed and thus is not bioavailable. Iron can be absorbed as either ionic iron or nonionic iron in the form of heme. Ionic iron must be in the ferrous (Fe^{+2}) form for absorption into the enterocyte via the luminal membrane carrier, divalent metal transporter (DMT1). However, most dietary iron is ferric, especially from plant sources. As a result, it is not readily absorbed. Furthermore, other dietary compounds can bind iron and inhibit its absorption. These include oxalates, phytates, phosphates, and calcium.[12] Release from these binders and reduction to the ferrous form are enhanced by gastric acid, acidic foods (e.g., citrus), and an enterocyte luminal membrane protein, duodenal cytochrome B (DcytB). Thus, although the U.S. diet contains on the order of 10 to 20 mg of iron/day, only 1 to 2 mg is absorbed.[12] This amount is adequate for most men, but menstruating women, pregnant and lactating women, and growing children usually need additional iron supplementation to meet their increased need for iron. Chapter 20 discusses this further.

Heme with its bound iron is more readily absorbed than ionic iron.[13] Thus meat, with heme in both myoglobin of muscle and hemoglobin of blood, is the most bioavailable source of dietary iron. The means by which heme is absorbed by enterocytes is not entirely clear. Although one carrier has been identified, it is actually more efficient at carrying folic acid.[14,15] So the primary heme carrier protein is still being sought.

LABORATORY ASSESSMENT OF BODY IRON STATUS

Disease occurs when body iron levels are either too low or too high (Chapter 20). The tests used to assess body iron status are able to detect both conditions. They include the traditional or classic iron studies: serum iron (SI), total iron-binding capacity (TIBC), percent transferrin saturation, and Prussian blue staining of tissues. More recently, ferritin assays have been included among the routine tests. For special circumstances

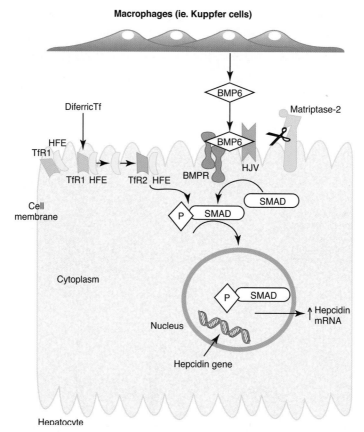

Figure 11-4 Hepatic iron-sensing systems leading to hepcidin production. One system of iron sensing by hepatocytes involves the release of the hemochromatosis receptor (HFE) from transferrin receptor 1(TfR1) when the latter binds transferrin (Tf). The freed HFE then binds to transferrin receptor 2 (TfR2), initiating a membrane signal that phosphorylates sons of mothers against decapentaplegic (SMAD) proteins that move to the nucleus and upregulate hepcidin gene expression. A second system activated when body iron is high in secretion of bone morphogenic protein 6 (BMP6) by liver macrophages. BMP6 binds with its receptor, BMPR, and coreceptor, hemojuvelin (HJV), to phosphorylate SMAD and ultimately increase hepcidin production. Matriptase 2 can inactivate HJV and is an important mechanism to reduce hepcidin production when body iron is low. (From Camaschella C, Silvestri L: Molecular mechanisms regulating hepcidin revealed by hepcidin disorders. The Scientific World 11: 1357-1366, 2011 and Doig K: Iron: the body's most precious metal. Denver, 2013, Colorado Association for Continuing Medical Laboratory Education, Inc., p. 17.)

when the results of routine assays are equivocal or too invasive, newer assays include the soluble transferrin receptor (sTfR) and hemoglobin content of reticulocytes. The results of these measured parameters can be combined to calculate an sTfR/log ferritin ratio or graph a Thomas plot. Finally, zinc protoporphyrin is another assay with special application in sideroblastic anemia. Diagnostically, the tests can be organized to assess each of the iron compartments as indicated in Table 11-3.

Serum Iron (SI)

Serum iron can be measured colorimetrically using any of several reagents such as ferrozine. The iron is first released from transferrin by acid, and then the reagent is allowed to react with the freed iron, forming a colored complex that can be detected spectrophotometrically. Reference intervals are reported separately for men, women, and children, and will vary from laboratory to laboratory and from method to method. The serum iron level has limited utility on its own because of its high within-day and between-day variability; it also increases after recent ingestion of iron-containing foods

and supplements. To avoid the apparent diurnal variation, the standard practice has been to collect the specimen fasting and early in the morning when levels are expected to be highest. However, this practice has recently been questioned.[16] A diurnal variation in hepcidin has been detected that may explain some of the serum iron variability and may still support the early-morning phlebotomy practice.[17] A typical reference interval is provided in Table 11-3.

Total Iron-Binding Capacity (TIBC)

The amount of iron in plasma or serum will be limited by the amount of transferrin that is available to carry it. To assess this, transferrin is maximally saturated by addition of excess ferric iron to the specimen. Any unbound iron is removed by precipitation with magnesium carbonate powder. Then the basic iron method as described above is performed on the absorbed serum, beginning with the release of the iron from transferrin. The amount of iron detected represents all the binding sites available on transferrin—that is, the total iron-binding capacity (TIBC). It is expressed as an iron value, although it is actually an indirect measure of transferrin. A typical reference interval is provided in Table 11-3.

TABLE 11-2 Functions and Locations of Proteins Involved in Body Iron Sensing and Hepcidin Production

Protein	Location	Function
Hemochromatosis protein (HFE)	Hepatocyte membrane	A protein that is bound to transferrin receptor 1 (TfR1) until released by the binding of transferrin to TfR1
Transferrin receptor 2 (TfR2)	Hepatocyte membrane	A hepatocyte transferrin receptor that is able to bind freed HFE to initiate an internal cell signal for hepcidin production
Bone morphogenic protein (BMP)	Secreted product of macrophages	The ligand secreted by macrophages that initiates signal transduction when it binds to its receptor in a cell membrane
Bone morphogenic protein receptor (BMPR)	Hepatocyte (and other cells) membrane	A common membrane receptor initiating signal transduction within a cell when its ligand (BMP) binds
Hemojuvelin (HJV)	Hepatocyte membrane	A coreceptor acting with BMPR for signal transduction, leading to hepcidin production
Sons of mothers against decapentaplegic (SMAD)	Hepatocyte (and other cells) cytoplasm	A second messenger of signal transduction activated by BMPR-HJV complex, able to migrate to the nucleus and upregulate hepcidin gene expression

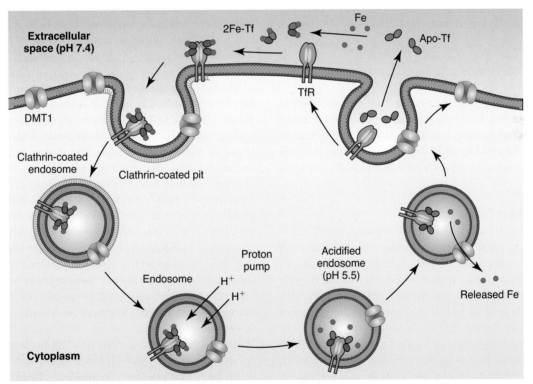

Figure 11-5 Cellular iron regulation. A critical mass of transferrin receptor 1 (TfR) with bound transferrin (Tf) will initiate an invagination of the membrane that ultimately fuses to form an endosome. Hydrogen ion (H$^+$) inside the endosome releases the iron from Tf, and once reduced, it is transported into the cytosol by divalent mental transporter 1 (DMT1). In the cytosol, iron may be stored as ferritin or transferred to the mitochondria, where it is transported across the membrane by mitoferrin (not shown). The TfR with apotransferrin is returned to the cell membrane, where the ApoTf releases and the TfR is available to bind more Tf for iron transport into the cell. (From http://walz.med.harvard.edu/Research/Iron_Transport/Tfr-Tf-Figure-1.gif)

TABLE 11-3 Assessment of Body Iron Status

Laboratory Assay	Typical Adult Male Reference Interval	Diagnostic Use and Compartment Assessed
Serum iron level	50–160 µg/dL	Indicator of available transport iron
Serum transferrin level (TIBC)	250–400 µg/dL	Indirect indicator of iron stores
Transferrin saturation	20%–55%	Indirect indicator of iron stores with transport iron
Serum ferritin level	40–400 ng/mL	Indicator of iron stores
Bone marrow or liver biopsy with Prussian blue staining	Normal iron stores visualized	Visual qualitative assessment of tissue iron stores
Soluble transferrin receptor (sTfR) level	1.15–2.75 mg/L	Indicator of functional iron available in cells
sTfR/log ferritin index	0.63–1.8	Indicator of functional iron available in cells
RBC zinc protoporphyrin level	<80 µg/dL of RBCs	Indicator of functional iron available in red blood cells
Hemoglobin content of reticulocytes	27–34 pg/cell	Indicator of functional iron available in developing red blood cells

RBC, Red blood cell; *TIBC,* total iron-binding capacity.

Percent Transferrin Saturation

Since the TIBC represents the total number of sites for iron binding and the SI represents the number bound with iron, the degree to which the available sites are occupied by iron can be calculated. The percent of transferrin saturated with iron is calculated as:

$$SI/TIBC \times 100\% = \% \text{ transferrin saturation}$$

It is important that both the SI and TIBC be expressed in the same units, but it does not matter which units are used in the calculation. A typical reference interval is provided in Table 11-3. A convenient rule of thumb evident from the table is that about one third ($^1/_3$) of transferrin is typically saturated with iron.

Prussian Blue Staining

Prussian blue is actually a chemical compound with the formula $Fe_7(CN)_{18}$.[18] The compound forms during the staining process, which uses acidic potassium ferrocyanide as the reagent/stain. The ferric iron in the tissue reacts with the reagent, forming the Prussian blue compound that is readily seen microscopically as dark blue dots. Tissues can be graded or scored semiquantitatively by the amount of stain that is observed. Prussian blue stain is considered the gold standard for assessment of body iron. Staining is conducted routinely when bone marrow or liver biopsies are taken for other purposes. Although ferric iron reacts with the reagent, ferritin is not detected, likely due to the intact protein cage. However, hemosiderin stains readily.

Ferritin

As mentioned above, until the development of serum ferritin assays, the only way to truly assess body iron stores was to take a sample of bone marrow and stain it with Prussian blue. Such an invasive procedure prevented regular assessment of body iron. The development of the serum immunoassay for ferritin provided a convenient assessment of body iron stores. Though ferritin is an intracellular protein, it is secreted by macrophages into plasma for reasons that are not yet understood.[19] The level of serum ferritin has been shown to correlate highly with stored iron as indicated by Prussian blue stains of bone marrow.[20] Typical reference intervals are provided in Table 11-3.

There is a significant drawback in the interpretation of serum ferritin results. Ferritin is an acute phase protein or acute phase reactant (APR).[21] The APRs are proteins that are produced, mostly by the liver, during the acute (i.e., initial) phase of inflammation, especially during infections. They include cytokines that are nonspecific, but also other proteins with the apparent intent to suppress bacteria. Since bacteria need iron, the body's production of ferritin during the acute phase seems to be an attempt to sequester the iron away from the bacteria. Thus increases in ferritin can be induced without an increase in the amount of systemic body iron. These rises may not be outside the reference interval but still high enough to elevate a patient's ferritin above what it would otherwise be. Ferritin values between 20 and 100 ng/mL are most equivocal, making it difficult to recognize true iron deficiency when an inflammatory condition is also present.[22] Therefore, the predictive value of a ferritin result within the reference interval is weak. However, only a decreased level of stored body iron can lower ferritin levels below the reference interval, so the predictive value of a low ferritin result is high for iron deficiency.

Soluble Transferrin Receptor (sTfR)

As described above, cells regulate the amount of TfR on their membrane based on the amount of intracellular iron. When the latter drops, the cell expresses more TfR on the membrane. A truncated form of the receptor is shed into the plasma and can be detected with immunoassay.[8] Thus increases in the sTfR reflect either increases in the amounts of TfR on individual cells, as in iron deficiency, or an increase in the number of cells each with a normal number of TfRs. The latter occurs during instances of rapid erythropoiesis, such as a response to hemolytic anemia. Typical reference intervals are provided in Table 11-3.

Hemoglobin Content of Reticulocytes

Chapter 15 describes how some hematology instruments are able to report a value for the amount of hemoglobin in reticulocytes; it is analogous to the mean cell hemoglobin (MCH), but just for reticulocytes. Because, under normal conditions, the number of circulating reticulocytes represents the status of erythropoiesis in the prior 24-hour period, the amount of hemoglobin in reticulocytes provides a near real-time assessment of iron available for hemoglobin production.[23] The hemoglobin content of reticulocytes will drop when iron for erythropoiesis is restricted. A representative adult reference interval is provided in Table 11-3. Separate reference intervals may be provided for children and infants.

Soluble Transferrin Receptor/Log Ferritin

Although ferritin and sTfR values alone can point to iron deficiency, the ratio of sTfR to ferritin or sTfR to log ferritin improves the identification of iron deficiency when values are equivocal.[24,25] Because the sTfR rises in iron deficiency and the ferritin (and its log) drops, these ratios are especially useful when one of the parameters has changed but is not outside the reference interval. A typical reference interval is provided in Table 11-3.

Thomas Plot

Thomas and Thomas[26] demonstrated that when the sTfR/log ferritin is plotted against the hemoglobin content of reticulocytes, a four-quadrant plot results that can improve the identification of iron deficiency (Figure 11-6).[27] In instances where there is *true iron deficiency*, the sTfR will rise and the ferritin will drop so that the sTfR/log ferritin will be high and the hemoglobin content of reticulocytes will be low; patient results will plot to the lower right quadrant. In instances where the ferritin may be falsely elevated by inflammation, the sTfR/log ferritin will be normal despite reduced availability of iron for hemoglobin production—thus a low hemoglobin content in reticulocytes. In this instance, patient values will plot to the lower left quadrant called *functional iron deficiency* because the systemic body stores are adequate but not available for transport and use by cells. As iron deficiency develops, other cells

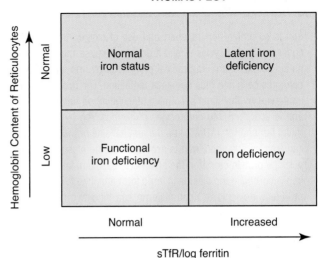

Figure 11-6 Thomas plot. Plotting the ratio of soluble transferrin receptor to log ferritin (sTfR/log ferritin) against the hemoglobin content of reticulocytes produces a graph with four quadrants. Patients with values within the reference intervals for each assay will cluster in the upper left quadrant. Those with functional iron deficiency, like the anemia of chronic inflammation, will cluster at the lower left. Latent iron deficiency, before anemia develops, will cluster to the upper right with frank iron deficiency in the lower right quadrant. (Modified from Doig K: Iron: the body's most precious metal. Denver, 2013, Colorado Association for Continuing Medical Laboratory Education, Inc., p. 24.)

are starved before erythrocytes; production of hemoglobin in reticulocytes remains at a normal level for as long as possible. However, the body's other iron-starved cells will increase sTfR production and systemic iron stores of ferritin will be depleted, thus elevating the sTfR/log ferritin value. These early iron-deficient patients' results will plot to the upper right quadrant called *latent iron deficiency*. By incorporating several different assessments of iron status, the use of the *Thomas plot*, as it is called, can improve the identification of iron deficiency in instances when other tests are equivocal. Chapter 20 will elucidate further the impact of various diseases on the parameters of the Thomas plot.

Zinc Protoporphyrin

Zinc protoporphyrin (ZPP) accumulates in red blood cells when iron is not incorporated into heme and zinc binds instead to protoporphyrin IX. It is easily detected by fluorescence. Although ZPP will rise during iron-deficient erythropoiesis, the value of this test is greatest when the activity of the ferrochelatase is impaired, as in lead poisoning (Chapter 20).

SUMMARY

- Iron is so critical for transport and use of oxygen that the body conserves and recycles it, and it does not have a mechanism for its active excretion. Free radical production by iron ions severely damages cells and thus demands regulation. The body adjusts its iron levels by intestinal absorption, depending on need.
- Iron is absorbed into enterocytes as ferrous iron by the divalent metal transporter 1 (DMT1) on the luminal side of the cells. Heme can also be absorbed. Iron is exported into the plasma via ferroportin, a protein carrier in the enterocyte basolaminal membrane.
- Iron is carried in the plasma in ferric form attached to apotransferrin. Each molecule of apotransferrin can bind two molecules of iron. Apotransferrin with bound iron is called transferrin.
- Individual cells absorb iron when diferric transferrin binds to transferrin receptor 1 (TfR1) on their surfaces. Bound receptors cluster and invaginate the membrane to form an endosome. Iron released by acid within the endosome is exported into the plasma and ultimately into the mitochondria for incorporation into cytochromes and heme. Alternatively, it can also be stored as ferritin in the cytosol. The iron-depleted endosome fuses with the cell membrane, releasing the apotransferrin and thus allowing the TfR1 on the cell membrane to bind more diferric transferrin.
- Macrophages ingest dying red blood cells. They salvage and store the iron derived from heme.
- Hepatocytes sense body iron status through the interaction of the hemochromatosis receptor, transferrin receptor 2, hemojuvelin, bone morphogenic protein, and SMAD.
- When the hepatocyte iron-sensing system detects that body iron levels are high, the hepatocyte secretes hepcidin. Hepcidin inactivates ferroportin in enterocyte, macrophage, and hepatocyte membranes, reducing the absorption of new iron and the release of stored iron. When the hepatocyte senses low body iron, hepcidin secretion is reduced, and ferroportin is active for intestinal iron

absorption and macrophage and hepatocyte iron export into the plasma.
- Individual cells adjust the number of transferrin receptors on their surface to regulate the amount of iron they absorb; receptor numbers rise when the cell needs additional iron but decrease when the iron in the cell is adequate. Truncated soluble transferrin receptors are also shed into the plasma in proportion to their number on cells.
- Cells store iron as ferritin when they have an excess. Iron can be released from ferritin when needed by degradation of the protein by lysosomes. Partially degraded ferritin can be detected in cells as stainable hemosiderin. Ferritin is secreted into the plasma by macrophages in proportion to the amount of iron that is in storage. Ferritin is elevated in plasma by the acute phase response, unrelated to amounts of stored iron.
- Dietary iron is most bioavailable as heme from meat sources. Plant sources typically supply ferric iron that must be released from iron-binding compounds and reduced before absorption.
- Most body iron is found in hemoglobin or stored as ferritin. Less than 10% of all body iron is found in muscles, plasma, cytochromes, and iron-dependent enzymes throughout body cells.
- Laboratory tests for assessment of iron status include total serum iron, total iron-binding capacity, percent transferrin saturation, serum ferritin, soluble transferrin receptor, tissue staining for hemosiderin, zinc protoporphyrin, and the hemoglobin content of reticulocytes. Additional parameters derived from these, the Thomas plot and sTfR/log ferritin, are particularly useful for the recognition of iron deficiency when other test results are equivocal.

Now that you have completed this chapter, go back and read again the case study at the beginning and respond to the questions presented.

REVIEW QUESTIONS

Answers can be found in the Appendix.

1. Iron is transported in plasma via:
   a. Hemosiderin
   b. Ferritin
   c. Transferrin
   d. Hemoglobin

2. What is the major metabolically available storage form of iron in the body?
   a. Hemosiderin
   b. Ferritin
   c. Transferrin
   d. Hemoglobin

3. The total iron-binding capacity (TIBC) of the serum is an indirect measure of which iron-related protein?
   a. Hemosiderin
   b. Ferritin
   c. Transferrin
   d. Hemoglobin

4. For a patient with classic iron study values that are equivocal for iron deficiency, which of the following tests would be most helpful in determining whether iron deficiency is present or not?
   a. Zinc protoporphyrin
   b. Peripheral blood sideroblast assessment
   c. Soluble transferrin receptor
   d. Mean cell hemoglobin

5. What membrane-associated protein in enterocytes transports iron from the intestinal lumen into the enterocyte?
   a. Transferrin
   b. Ferroportin
   c. DMT1
   d. Ferrochelatase

6. Iron is transported out of macrophages, hepatocytes, and enterocytes by what membrane protein?
   a. Transferrin
   b. Ferroportin
   c. DMT1
   d. Ferrochelatase

7. Below are several of the many steps in the process from absorption and transport of iron to incorporation into heme. Place them in proper order.
   i. Transferrin picks up ferric iron.
   ii. Iron is transferred to the mitochondria.
   iii. DMT1 transports ferrous iron into the enterocyte.
   iv. Ferroportin transports iron from enterocyte to plasma.
   v. The transferrin receptor transports iron into the cell.
       a. v, iv, i, ii, iii
       b. iii, ii, iv, i, v
       c. ii, i, v, iii, iv
       d. iii, iv, i, v, ii

8. What is the fate of the transferrin receptor when it has completed its role in the delivery of iron to a cell?
   a. It is recycled to the plasma membrane and released into the plasma.
   b. It is recycled to the plasma membrane, where it can bind its ligand again.
   c. It is catabolized and the amino acids are returned to the metabolic pool.
   d. It is retained in the endosome for the life span of the cell.

9. The transfer of iron from the enterocyte into the plasma is REGULATED by:
   a. Transferrin
   b. Ferroportin
   c. Hephaestin
   d. Hepcidin

10. What is the percent transferrin saturation for a patient with total serum iron of 63 μg/dL and TIBC of 420 μg/dL ?
    a. 6.7%
    b. 12%
    c. 15%
    d. 80%

11. Referring to Figure 11-6, into which quadrant of a Thomas plot would a patient's results fall with the following test results:
    Soluble transferrin receptor: increased above reference interval
    Ferritin: decreased below reference interval
    Hemoglobin content of reticulocytes: within the reference interval
    a. Normal iron status
    b. Latent iron deficiency
    c. Functional iron deficiency
    d. Iron deficiency

12. A physician is concerned that a patient is developing iron deficiency from chronic intestinal bleeding due to aspirin use for rheumatoid arthritis. The iron studies on the patient show the following results:

Laboratory Assay	Adult Reference Intervals	Patient Values
Serum ferritin level	12–400 ng/mL	25 ng /mL
Serum iron level	50–160 μg/dL	45 μg/dL
Total iron-binding capacity (TIBC)	250–400 μg/dL	405 μg/dL
Transferrin saturation	20%–55%	CALCULATE IT

How would these results be interpreted?
   a. Latent iron deficiency
   b. Functional iron deficiency
   c. Iron deficiency
   d. Equivocal for iron deficiency

REFERENCES

1. Garry, P. J., Koehler, K. M., & Simon, T. L. (1995). Iron stores and iron absorption: effects of repeated blood donations. *Am J Clin Nutr, 62*(3), 611–620.
2. Sharma, N., Butterworth, J., Cooper, B. T., et al. (2005). The emerging role of the liver in iron metabolism. *Am J Gastroenterol, 100*, 201–206.
3. Camaschella, C., & Silvestri, L. (2011). Molecular mechanisms regulating hepcidin revealed by hepcidin disorders. *Scientific World Journal, 11*, 1357–1366.
4. Shaw, G. C., Cope, J. J., Li, L., et al. (2006). Mitoferrin is essential for erythroid iron assimilation. *Nature, 440*(2), 96–100.
5. Theil, E. C. (1990). The ferritin family of iron storage proteins. *Adv Enzymol Relat Areas Mol Biol, 63*, 421–449.
6. Zhang, Y., Mikhael, M., Xu, D., et al. (2010). Lysosomal proteolysis is the primary degradation pathway for cytosolic ferritin and cytosolic ferritin degradation is necessary for iron exit. *Antioxid Redox Signal, 13*(7), 999–1009.
7. Thomson, A. M., Rogers, J. T., & Leedman, P. J. (1999). Iron-regulatory proteins, iron-responsive elements and ferritin mRNA translation. *Int J Biochem Cell Biol, 31*(10), 1139–1152.
8. Shih, Y. J., Baynes, R. D., Hudson, B. G., et al. (1990). Serum transferrin receptor is a truncated form of tissue receptor. *J Biol Chem, 265*, 19077–19081.

9. Richardson, D. R., Lane, D. J. R., Becker, E. M., et al. (2010). Mitochondrial iron trafficking and the integration of iron metabolism between the mitochondrion and cytosol. *PNAS, 107*(24), 10775–10782.

10. Abboud, S., & Haile, D. J. (2000). A novel mammalian iron-regulated protein involved in intracellular iron metabolism. *J Biolog Chem, 275*, 19906–19912.

11. Donovan, A., Brownlie, A., Zhou, Y., et al. (2000). Positional cloning of zebrafish ferroportin1 identifies a conserved vertebrate iron exporter. *Nature, 403*, 776–781.

12. Hallberg, L. (1981). Bioavailability of dietary iron in man. *Annu Rev Nutr, 1*, 123–147.

13. Layrisse, M., Cook, J. D., Martinez, C., et al. (1969). Food iron absorption: a comparison of vegetable and animal foods. *Blood, 33*, 430–443.

14. Le Blanc, S., Garrick, M. D., & Arredondo, M. (2012). Heme carrier protein 1 transports heme and is involved in heme-Fe metabolism. *Am J Physiol Cell Physiol, 302*, C1780–C1785.

15. Laftah, A. H., Latunde-Dada, G. O., Fakih, S., et al. (2009). Haem and folate transport by proton-coupled folate transporter/haem carrier protein 1 (SLC46A1). *Br J Nutr, 101*(8), 1150–1156.

16. Dale, J. C., Burritt, M. F., & Zinsmeister, A. R. (2002). Diurnal variation of serum iron, iron-binding capacity, transferrin saturation, and ferritin levels. *Am J Clin Pathol, 117*, 802–808.

17. Schaap, C. C., Hendriks, J. C., Kortman, G. A., et al. (2013). Diurnal rhythm rather than dietary iron mediates daily hepcidin variations. *Clin Chem Mar, 59*(3), 527–535.

18. Ellis, R. *Perls Prussian Blue Staining Protocol.* Available at: http://www.ihcworld.com/_protocols/special_stains/perls_prussian_blue_ellis.htm. Accessed 01.09.14.

19. Cohen, L. A., Gutierrez, L., Weiss, A., et al. (2010). Serum ferritin is derived primarily from macrophages through a non-classical secretory pathway. *Blood, 116*(9), 1574–1584.

20. Lipschitz, D. A., Cook, J. D., & Finch, C. A. (1974). A clinical evaluation of serum ferritin as an index of iron stores. *N Engl J Med, 290*(22), 1213–1216.

21. Konijn, A. M., & Hershko, C. (1977). Ferritin synthesis in inflammation. I. Pathogenesis of impaired iron release. *Br J Haematol, 37*(1), 7–16.

22. Castel, R., Tax, M. G., Droogendijk, J., et al. (2012). The transferrin/log(ferritin) ratio: a new tool for the diagnosis of iron deficiency anemia. *Clin Chem Lab Med, 50*(8), 1343–1349.

23. Brugnara, C., Zurakowski, D., DiCanzio, J., et al. (1999). Reticulocyte hemoglobin content to diagnose iron deficiency in children. *JAMA, 281*(23), 2225–2230.

24. Punnonen, K., Irjala, K., & Rajamaki, A. (1997). Serum transferrin receptor and its ratio to serum ferritin in the diagnosis of iron deficiency. *Blood, 89*(3), 1052–1057.

25. Castel, R., Tax, M. G., Droogendijk, J., et al. (2012). The transferrin/log(ferritin) ratio: a new tool for the diagnosis of iron deficiency anemia. *Clin Chem Lab Med, 50*(8), 1343–1349.

26. Thomas, C., & Thomas, L. (2002). Biochemical markers and hematologic indices in the diagnosis of functional iron deficiency. *Clin Chem, 48*(7), 1066–1076.

27. Leers, M. P. G., Keuren, J. F. W., & Oosterhuis, W. P. (2010). The value of the Thomas-plot in the diagnostic work up of anemic patients referred by general practitioners. *Int J Lab Hemat, 32*, 572–581.

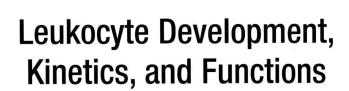

Leukocyte Development, Kinetics, and Functions

12

Woodlyne Roquiz, Sameer Al Diffalha, Ameet R. Kini*

OBJECTIVES

After completion of this chapter, the reader will be able to:

1. Describe the pathways and progenitor cells involved in the derivation of leukocytes from the hematopoietic stem cell to mature forms.
2. Name the different stages of neutrophil, eosinophil, and basophil development and describe the morphology of each stage.
3. Discuss the important functions of neutrophils, eosinophils, and basophils.
4. Describe the morphology of promonocytes, monocytes, macrophages, T and B lymphocytes, and immature B cells (hematogones).
5. Discuss the functions of monocytes, macrophages, T cells, B cells, and natural killer cells in the immune response.
6. Compare the kinetics of neutrophils and monocytes.
7. Discuss in general terms how the various types of lymphocytes are produced.

CASE STUDY

After studying the material in this chapter, the reader should be able to respond to the following case study:

A 5-year-old girl presents with shortness of breath and wheezing. The patient gives a history of similar symptoms in the last 6 months. After the patient was given albuterol to control her acute symptoms, long-term control of her disease was achieved through the use of corticosteroids, along with monoclonal antibodies to IL-5.

1. Which leukocytes are important in mediating the clinical symptoms in this patient?
2. A complete blood count with differential was performed on this patient. What are the typical findings in such patients?
3. How did monoclonal antibodies to IL-5 help in controlling her disease?

Leukocytes (also known as *white blood cells,* or *WBCs*) are so named because they are relatively colorless compared to red blood cells. The number of different types of leukocytes varies depending on whether they are being viewed with a light microscope after staining with a Romanowsky stain (5 or 6 types) or are identified according to their surface antigens using flow cytometry (at least 10 different types). For the purposes of this chapter, the classic, light microscope classification of leukocytes will be used.

Granulocytes are a group of leukocytes whose cytoplasm is filled with granules with differing staining characteristics and whose nuclei are segmented or lobulated. Individually, they include *eosinophils,* with granules containing basic proteins that stain with acid stains such as eosin; *basophils,* with granules that are acidic and stain with basic stains such as methylene blue; and *neutrophils,* with granules that react with both acid and basic stains, which gives them a pink to lavender color. Because nuclear segmentation is quite prominent in mature neutrophils, they have also been called *polymorphonuclear cells,* or *PMNs.*

Mononuclear cells are categorized into *monocytes* and *lymphocytes.* These cells have nuclei that are not segmented but are round, oval, indented, or folded. Leukocytes develop from hematopoietic stem cells (HSCs) in the bone marrow, where most undergo differentiation and maturation (Figure 12-1), and then are released into the circulation. The number of circulating leukocytes varies with sex, age, activity, time of day, and ethnicity; it

---

*The authors acknowledge the contributions of Anne Stiene-Martin, author of this chapter in the previous edition.

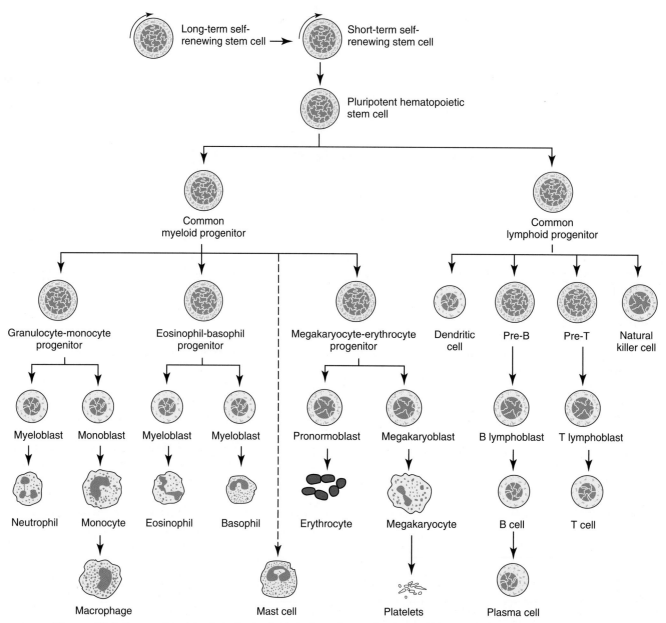

Figure 12-1 Diagram of hematopoiesis showing the derivation pathways of each type of blood cell from a hematopoietic stem cell.

also differs according to whether or not the leukocytes are reacting to stress, being consumed, or being destroyed, and whether or not they are being produced by the bone marrow in sufficient numbers.[1] Reference intervals for total leukocyte counts vary among laboratories, depending on the patient population and the type of instrumentation being used, but a typical reference interval is 4.5×10^9/L to 11.5×10^9/L for adults.

The overall function of leukocytes is in mediating *immunity,* either innate (nonspecific), as in phagocytosis by neutrophils, or specific (adaptive), as in the production of antibodies by lymphocytes and plasma cells. The term *kinetics* refers to the movement of cells through developmental stages, into the circulation, and from the circulation to the tissues and includes the time spent in each phase of the cell's life. As each cell type is discussed in this chapter, developmental stages, kinetics, and specific functions will be addressed.

GRANULOCYTES

Neutrophils

Neutrophils are present in the peripheral blood in two forms according to whether the nucleus is segmented or still in a band shape. Segmented neutrophils make up the vast majority of circulating leukocytes.

Neutrophil Development

Neutrophil development occurs in the bone marrow. Neutrophils share a common progenitor with monocytes, known as the granulocyte-monocyte progenitor (GMP). The major cytokine responsible for the stimulation of neutrophil production is granulocyte colony-stimulating factor, or G-CSF.[2,3]

There are three pools of developing neutrophils in the bone marrow (Figure 12-2): the stem cell pool, the proliferation

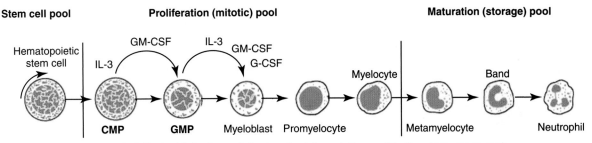

Figure 12-2 Neutrophil development showing stimulating cytokines and the three bone marrow pools.

pool, and the maturation pool.[4-7] The stem cell pool consists of hematopoietic stem cells (HSCs) that are capable of self-renewal and differentiation.[8] The proliferation (mitotic) pool consists of cells that are dividing and includes (listed in the order of maturation) common myeloid progenitors (CMPs), also known as colony-forming units–granulocyte, erythrocyte, monocyte, and megakaryocyte (CFU-GEMMs); granulocyte-macrophage progenitors (GMPs); myeloblasts; promyelocytes; and myelocytes. The third marrow pool is the maturation (storage) pool consisting of cells undergoing nuclear maturation that form the marrow reserve and are available for release: metamyelocytes, band neutrophils, and segmented neutrophils.

HSCs, CMPs, and GMPs are not distinguishable with the light microscope and Romanowsky staining and may resemble early type I myeloblasts or lymphoid cells. They can, however, be identified through surface antigen detection by flow cytometry.

Myeloblasts make up 0% to 3% of the nucleated cells in the bone marrow and measure 14 to 20 μm in diameter. They are frequently subdivided into type I, type II, and type III myeloblasts. The type I myeloblast has a high nucleus-to-cytoplasm (N:C) ratio of 8:1 to 4:1 (the nucleus occupies most of the cell, with very little cytoplasm), slightly basophilic cytoplasm, fine nuclear chromatin, and two to four visible nucleoli. Type 1 blasts have no visible granules when observed under light microscopy with Romanowsky stains. The type II myeloblast shows the presence of dispersed *primary (azurophilic) granules* in the cytoplasm; the number of granules does not exceed 20 per cell (Figure 12-3). Type III myeloblasts have a darker chromatin and a more purple cytoplasm, and they contain more than 20 granules that do not obscure the nucleus. Type III myeloblasts are rare in normal bone marrows, but they can be seen in certain types of acute myeloid leukemias. Recently, Mufti and colleagues[9] proposed combining type II and type III blasts into a single category of "granular blasts" due to the difficulty in distinguishing type II blasts from type III blasts.

Promyelocytes comprise 1% to 5% of the nucleated cells in the bone marrow. They are relatively larger than the myeloblast cells and measure 16 to 25 μm in diameter. The nucleus is round to oval and is often eccentric. A paranuclear halo or "hof" is usually seen in normal promyelocytes but not in the malignant promyelocytes of acute promyelocytic leukemia (described in Chapter 35). The cytoplasm is evenly basophilic and full of primary (azurophilic) granules. These granules are the first in a series of granules to be produced during neutrophil maturation (Box 12-1).[10] The nucleus is similar to that described earlier for myeloblasts except that chromatin clumping

(heterochromatin) may be visible, especially around the edges of the nucleus. One to three nucleoli can be seen but may be obscured by the granules (Figure 12-4).

Neutrophil myelocytes make up 6% to 17% of the nucleated cells in the bone marrow and are the final stage in which cell division (mitosis) occurs. During this stage, the production of primary granules ceases, and the cell begins to manufacture secondary (specific) neutrophil granules. This stage of neutrophil development is sometimes divided into early and late myelocytes. Early myelocytes may look very similar to the promyelocytes (described earlier) in size and nuclear characteristics except that patches of grainy pale pink cytoplasm representing secondary granules begin to be evident in the area of the Golgi apparatus. This has been referred to as the *dawn of neutrophilia.* Secondary neutrophilic granules slowly spread through the cell until its cytoplasm is more lavender-pink than blue. As the cell divides, the number of primary granules per cell is decreased, and their membrane chemistry changes so that they are much less visible. Late myelocytes are somewhat smaller than promyelocytes (15 to 18 μm), and the nucleus has considerably more heterochromatin. Nucleoli are difficult to see by light microscopy (Figure 12-5).

Neutrophil metamyelocytes constitute 3% to 20% of nucleated marrow cells. From this stage forward, the cells are no longer capable of division, and the major morphologic change is in the shape of the nucleus. The nucleus is indented (kidney bean shaped or peanut shaped), and the chromatin is increasingly clumped. Nucleoli are absent. Synthesis of tertiary granules (also known as *gelatinase granules*) may begin during this stage. The size of the metamyelocyte is slightly smaller than that of the myelocyte (14 to 16 μm). The cytoplasm contains very little residual ribonucleic acid (RNA) and therefore little or no basophilia (Figure 12-6).

Neutrophil bands make up 9% to 32% of nucleated marrow cells and 0% to 5% of the nucleated peripheral blood cells. All evidence of RNA (cytoplasmic basophilia) is absent, and tertiary granules continue to be formed during this stage. Secretory granules (also known as *secretory vesicles*) may begin to be formed during this stage. The nucleus is highly clumped, and the nuclear indentation that began in the metamyelocyte stage now exceeds one half the diameter of the nucleus, but actual segmentation has not yet occurred (Figure 12-7). Over the past 70 years, there has been considerable controversy over the definition of a band and the differentiation between bands and segmented forms. There have been three schools of thought concerning identification of bands, from the most

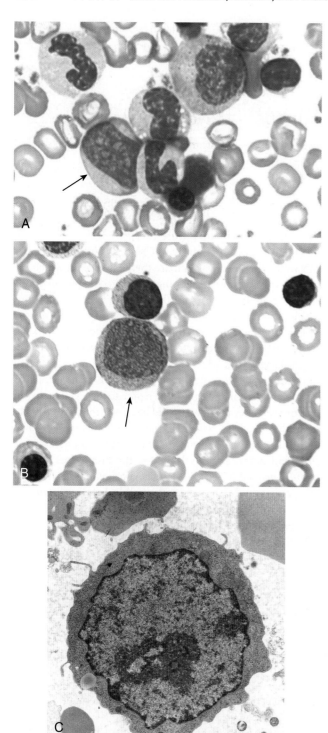

Figure 12-3 A, Type I myeloblast (*arrow*). Note that no granules are visible in the cytoplasm. **B,** Type II myeloblast (*arrow*) with a few azure granules in the cytoplasm. **C,** Electron micrograph of a myeloblast. (**C** from Rodak BF, Carr JH: Clinical hematology atlas, ed 4, St. Louis, 2013, Saunders, Elsevier.)

BOX 12-1 Neutrophil Granules

Primary (Azurophilic) Granules
Formed during the promyelocyte stage
Last to be released (exocytosis)
Contain:

- Myeloperoxidase
- Acid β-glycerophosphatase
- Cathepsins
- Defensins
- Elastase
- Proteinase-3
- Others

Secondary (Specific) Granules
Formed during myelocyte and metamyelocyte stages
Third to be released
Contain:

- β_2-Microglobulin
- Collagenase
- Gelatinase
- Lactoferrin
- Neutrophil gelatinase-associated lipocalin
- Transcobalamin I
- Others

Tertiary Granules
Formed during metamyelocyte and band stages
Second to be released
Contain:

- Gelatinase
- Collagenase
- Lysozyme
- Acetyltransferase
- β_2-Microglobulin

Secretory Granules (Secretory Vesicles)
Formed during band and segmented neutrophil stages
First to be released (fuse to plasma membrane)
Contain (attached to membrane):

- CD11b/CD18
- Alkaline phosphatase
- Vesicle-associated membrane-2
- CD10, CD13, CD14, CD16
- Cytochrome b_{558}
- Complement 1q receptor
- Complement receptor-1

---

conservative—holding that the nucleus in a band must have the same diameter throughout its length—to the most liberal—requiring that a filament between segments be visible before a band becomes a segmented neutrophil. The middle ground states that when doubt exists, the cell should be called a segmented neutrophil. An elevated band count was thought to be useful in the diagnosis of patients with infection. However, the clinical utility of band counts has been called into question,[11] and most laboratories no longer perform routine band counts. The Clinical and Laboratory Standards Institute (CLSI) recommends that bands should be included within the neutrophil counts and not reported as a separate

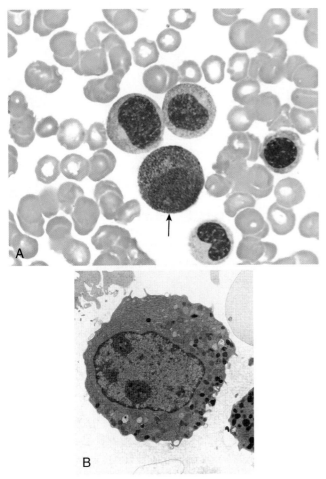

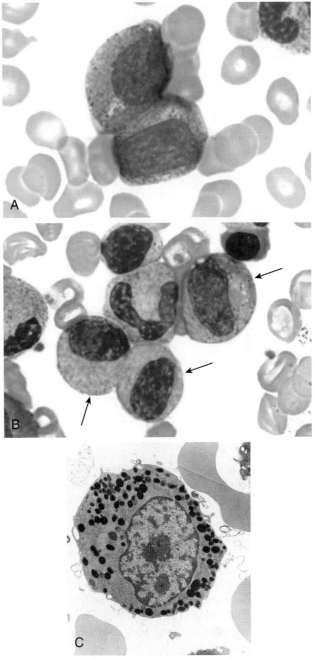

Figure 12-4 A, Promyelocyte. Note the large number of azure granules and the presence of nucleoli. **B,** Electron micrograph of a promyelocyte. (**B** from Rodak BF, Carr JH: Clinical hematology atlas, ed 4, St. Louis, 2013, Saunders, Elsevier.)

Figure 12-5 A, Two early neutrophil myelocytes. Note that they are very similar to the promyelocyte except for several light areas in their cytoplasm where specific granules are beginning to appear. **B,** Arrows are pointing to three late myelocytes in the field. Their cytoplasm has few if any primary granules, and the lavender secondary granules are easily seen. **C,** Electron micrograph of a late neutrophil myelocyte. (**C** from Rodak BF, Carr JH: Clinical hematology atlas, ed 4, St. Louis, 2013, Saunders, Elsevier.)

category, due to the difficulty in reliably distinguishing bands from segmented neutrophils.[12]

Segmented neutrophils make up 7% to 30% of nucleated cells in the bone marrow. Secretory granules continue to be formed during this stage. The only morphologic difference between segmented neutrophils and bands is the presence of between two and five nuclear lobes connected by threadlike filaments (Figure 12-8). Segmented neutrophils are present in the highest numbers in the peripheral blood of adults (50% to 70% of leukocytes in relative numbers and 2.3 to 8.1 $\times$ 10^9/L in absolute terms). As can be seen from the table on the inside front cover, pediatric values are quite different; relative percentages can be as low as 18% of leukocytes in the first few months of life and do not begin to climb to adult values until after 4 to 7 years of age.

Neutrophil Kinetics

Neutrophil kinetics involves the movement of neutrophils and neutrophil precursors between the different pools in the bone marrow, the peripheral blood, and tissues. Neutrophil production has been calculated to be on the order of between 0.9 and 1.0 $\times$ 10^9 cells/kg per day.[13]

The proliferative pool contains approximately 2.1 $\times$ 10^9 cells/kg, whereas the maturation pool contains roughly 5.6 $\times$ 10^9 cells/kg or a 5-day supply.[13] The transit time from the HSC to the myeloblast has not been measured. The transit time from myeloblast through myelocyte has been estimated to be roughly 6 days, and the transit time through the maturation pool is approximately 4 to 6 days.[4,13,14] Granulocyte release from the bone marrow is stimulated by G-CSF.[2,3]

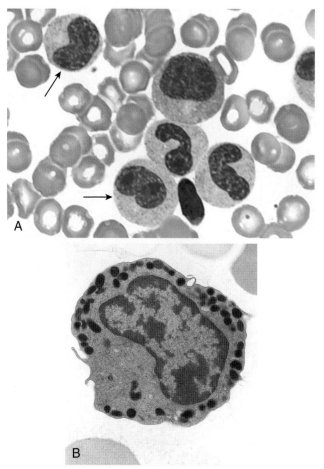

Figure 12-6 A, Two neutrophil metamyelocytes (*arrows*). Note that there is no remaining basophilia in the cytoplasm, and the nucleus is indented. **B,** Electron micrograph of a neutrophil metamyelocyte. (**B** from Rodak BF, Carr JH: Clinical hematology atlas, ed 4, St. Louis, 2013, Saunders, Elsevier.)

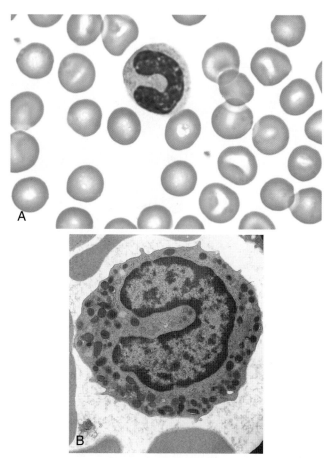

Figure 12-7 A, Neutrophil band; note the nucleus is indented more than 50% of the width of the nucleus. **B,** Electron micrograph of a band neutrophil. (**B** from Rodak BF, Carr JH: Clinical hematology atlas, ed 4, St. Louis, 2013, Saunders, Elsevier.)

Once in the peripheral blood, neutrophils are divided randomly into a circulating neutrophil pool (CNP) and a marginated neutrophil pool (MNP). The neutrophils in the MNP are loosely localized to the walls of capillaries in tissues such as the liver, spleen, and lung. There does not appear to be any functional differences between neutrophils of either the CNP or the MNP, and cells move freely between the two peripheral pools.[15] The ratio of these two pools is roughly equal overall;[4,16] however, marginated neutrophils in the capillaries of the lungs make up a considerably larger portion of peripheral neutrophils.[17] The half-life of neutrophils in the blood is relatively short at approximately 7 hours.[4,18]

Integrins and selectins are of significant importance in allowing neutrophils to marginate as well as exit the blood and enter the tissues by a process known as *diapedesis*.[19,20] Those neutrophils that do not migrate into the tissues eventually undergo programmed cell death or apoptosis and are removed by macrophages in the spleen.[21]

Once neutrophils are in the tissues, their life span is variable, depending on whether or not they are responding to infectious or inflammatory agents. In the absence of infectious or inflammatory agents, the neutrophil's life span is measured in hours. Some products of inflammation and infection tend to

prolong the neutrophil's life span through anti-apoptotic signals, whereas others such as MAC-1 trigger the death and phagocytosis of neutrophils.[20]

Neutrophil Functions

Neutrophils are part of the innate immune system. Characteristics of innate immunity include destruction of foreign organisms that is not antigen specific; no protection against reexposure to the same pathogen; reliance on the barriers provided by skin and mucous membranes, as well as phagocytes such as neutrophils and monocytes; and inclusion of a humoral component known as the *complement system.*

The major function of neutrophils is phagocytosis and destruction of foreign material and microorganisms. The process involves seeking (chemotaxis, motility, and diapedesis) and destruction (phagocytosis and digestion).

Neutrophil recruitment to an inflammatory site begins when chemotactic agents bind to neutrophil receptors. Chemotactic agents may be produced by microorganisms, by damaged cells, or by other leukocytes such as lymphocytes or other phagocytes. The first neutrophil response is to roll along endothelial cells of the blood vessels using stronger adhesive molecules than those used by nonstimulated marginated neutrophils. Rolling consists of transient adhesive

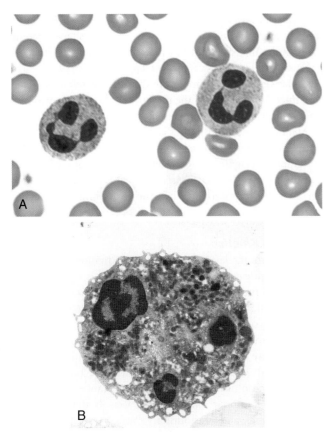

Figure 12-8 A, Segmented neutrophil (also known as a *polymorphonuclear cell* or *PMN*). **B,** Electron micrograph of a segmented neutrophil. (**B** from Rodak BF, Carr JH: Clinical hematology atlas, ed 4, St. Louis, 2013, Saunders, Elsevier.)

BOX 12-2 Phagocytosis

Recognition and Attachment
Phagocyte receptors recognize and bind to certain foreign molecular patterns and opsonins such as antibodies and complement components.

Ingestion
Pseudopodia are extended around the foreign particle and enclose it within a "phagosome" (engulfment).

The phagosome is pulled toward the center of the cell by polymerization of actin and myosin and by microtubules.

Killing and Digestion
Oxygen Dependent
Respiratory burst through the activation of NADPH oxidase. H_2O_2 and hypochlorite are produced.

Oxygen Independent
The pH within the phagosome becomes alkaline and then neutral, the pH at which digestive enzymes work.

Primary and secondary lysosomes (granules) fuse to the phagosome and empty hydrolytic enzymes and other bactericidal molecules into the phagosome.

Formation of Neutrophil Extracellular Traps
Nuclear and organelle membranes dissolve, and activated cytoplasmic enzymes attach to DNA.

The cytoplasmic membrane ruptures, and DNA with attached enzymes is expelled so that the bacteria are digested in the external environment.

NADPH, Nicotinamide adenine dinucleotide phosphate (reduced form).

---

contacts between neutrophil selectins and adhesive molecules on the surface of endothelial cells. At the same time, secretory granules containing additional adhesive molecules are fused to the neutrophil's plasma membrane. β_2 integrins such as CD11b/CD18 from secretory granules contribute to tight stationary binding between neutrophils and endothelial cells. This is followed by diapedesis or transmigration of neutrophils either between or through endothelial cells—a process that is also mediated by integrins and integrin-associated proteins. Tertiary granules containing gelatinase and collagenase are released by transmigrating neutrophils. Gelatinase degrades denatured collagen as well as types IV and V collagen and activates chemokines such as interleukin-8 (IL-8).[22] Neutrophils then migrate in a directional manner toward the area of greatest concentration of chemotactic agents.

Once at the site of infection or inflammation, neutrophils begin the process of phagocytosis (Box 12-2). They utilize their enormous inventory of surface receptors either to directly recognize the pathogen, apoptotic cell, or particle, or to recognize opsonic molecules attached to the foreign particle such as antibodies or complement components. With recognition comes attachment and engulfment, in which cytoplasmic pseudopodia surround the particle, forming a phagosome within the neutrophil cytoplasm.[23] Formation of the phagosome allows the reduced nicotinamide adenine dinucleotide (NADH) oxidase complex within the phagosome membrane to assemble; this leads to the generation of reactive oxygen species such as hydrogen peroxide, which is converted to hypochlorite by myeloperoxidase. Likewise, a series of metabolic changes culminate in the fusion of primary and/or secondary granules to the phagosome and the release of numerous bactericidal molecules into the phagosome.[24] This combination of reactive oxygen species and non-oxygen-dependent mechanisms is generally able to destroy most pathogens.

In addition to emptying their contents into phagosomes, secondary and primary granules may fuse to the plasma membrane, which results in release of their contents into the extracellular matrix. These molecules can then act as chemotactic agents for additional neutrophils and as stimulating agents for macrophages to phagocytize dead neutrophils, as well as inflammatory agents that may cause tissue damage.

A second function of neutrophils is the generation of neutrophil extracellular traps, or NETs.[25,26] NETs are extracellular threadlike structures believed to represent chains of nucleosomes from unfolded nuclear chromatin material (DNA). These structures have enzymes from neutrophil granules attached to them and have been shown to be able to trap and kill gram-positive and gram-negative bacteria as well as fungi.

NETs are generated at the time that neutrophils die as a result of antibacterial activity. The term *NETosis* has been used to describe this unique form of neutrophil cell death that results in the release of NETs.

A third and final function of neutrophils is their secretory function. Neutrophils are a source of transcobalamin I or R binder protein, which is necessary for the proper absorption of vitamin B_{12}. In addition, they are a source of a variety of cytokines.

Eosinophils

Eosinophils make up 1% to 3% of nucleated cells in the bone marrow. Of these, slightly more than a third are mature, a quarter are eosinophilic metamyelocytes, and the remainder are eosinophilic promyelocytes or eosinophilic myelocytes. Eosinophils account for 1% to 3% of peripheral blood leukocytes, with an absolute number of up to 0.4×10^9/L in the peripheral blood.

Eosinophil Development

Eosinophil development is similar to that described earlier for neutrophils, and evidence indicates that eosinophils arise from the common myeloid progenitor (CMP).[27,28] Eosinophil lineage is established through the interaction between the cytokines IL-3, IL-5, and GM-CSF and three transcription factors (GATA-1, PU.1, and c/EBP). IL-5 is critical for eosinophil growth and survival.[29] Whether or not there exist myeloblasts that are committed to the eosinophil line has not been established. Eosinophilic promyelocytes can be identified cytochemically due to the presence of Charcot-Leyden crystal protein in their primary granules. The first maturation phase that can be identified as eosinophilic using light microscopy and Romanowsky staining is the early myelocyte.

Eosinophil myelocytes are characterized by the presence of large (resolvable at the light microscope level), pale, reddish-orange secondary granules, along with azure granules in blue cytoplasm. The nucleus is similar to that described for neutrophil myelocytes. Transmission electron micrographs of eosinophils reveal that many secondary eosinophil granules contain an electron-dense crystalline core (Figure 12-9).[30]

Eosinophil metamyelocytes and bands resemble their neutrophil counterparts with respect to their nuclear shape. Secondary granules increase in number, and a third type of granule is generated called the *secretory granule* or *secretory vesicle*. The secondary granules become more distinct and refractory. Electron microscopy indicates the presence of two other organelles: lipid bodies and small granules (Box 12-3).[31]

Mature eosinophils usually display a bilobed nucleus. Their cytoplasm contains characteristic refractile, orange-red secondary granules (Figure 12-10). Electron microscopy of mature eosinophils reveals extensive secretory vesicles, and their number increases considerably when the eosinophil is stimulated or activated.[30]

Eosinophil Kinetics

The time from the last myelocyte mitotic division to the emergence of mature eosinophils from the marrow is about 3.5 days. The mean turnover of eosinophils is approximately 2.2×10^8 cells/kg per day. There is a large storage pool of eosinophils in the marrow consisting of between 9 and 14×10^8 cells/kg.[31]

Once in the circulation, eosinophils have a circulating half-life of roughly 18 hours;[32] however, the half-life of eosinophils is prolonged when eosinophilia occurs. The tissue destinations of eosinophils under normal circumstances appear to be underlying columnar epithelial surfaces in the respiratory, gastrointestinal, and genitourinary tracts. Survival time of eosinophils in human tissues ranges from 2 to 5 days.[33]

Eosinophil Functions

Eosinophils have multiple functions. Eosinophil granules are full of a large number of previously synthesized proteins, including cytokines, chemokines, growth factors, and cationic proteins. There is more than one way for eosinophils to degranulate. By classical exocytosis, granules move to the plasma membrane, fuse with the plasma membrane, and empty their contents into the extracellular space. Compound exocytosis is a second mechanism in which granules fuse together within the eosinophil prior to fusing with the plasma membrane. A third method is known as *piecemeal degranulation*, in which secretory vesicles remove specific proteins from the secondary granules.

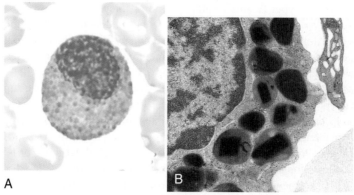

Figure 12-9 A, Eosinophil myelocyte. Note the rounded nucleus and the cytoplasm in which there are numerous large, pale eosinophil granules. **B,** Electron micrograph of eosinophil granules showing the central crystalline core in some of the granules. (**A, B** from Rodak BF, Carr JH: Clinical hematology atlas, ed 4, St. Louis, 2013, Saunders, Elsevier.).

BOX 12-3 Eosinophil Granules

Primary Granules
Formed during promyelocyte stage
Contain:
- Charcot-Leyden crystal protein

Secondary Granules
Formed throughout remaining maturation
Contain:
- Major basic protein (core)
- Eosinophil cationic protein (matrix)
- Eosinophil-derived neurotoxin (matrix)
- Eosinophil peroxidase (matrix)
- Lysozyme (matrix)
- Catalase (core and matrix)
- β-Glucuronidase (core and matrix)
- Cathepsin D (core and matrix)
- Interleukins 2, 4, and 5 (core)
- Interleukin-6 (matrix)
- Granulocyte-macrophage colony-stimulating factor (core)
- Others

Small Lysosomal Granules
Acid phosphatase
Arylsulfatase B
Catalase
Cytochrome b_{558}
Elastase
Eosinophil cationic protein

Lipid Bodies
Cyclooxygenase
5-Lipoxygenase
15-Lipoxygenase
Leukotriene C_4 synthase
Eosinophil peroxidase
Esterase

Storage Vesicles
Carry proteins from secondary granules to be released into the extracellular medium

---

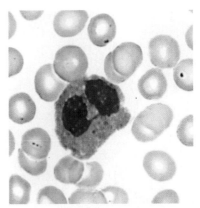

Figure 12-10 Mature eosinophil. Note that the nucleus has only two segments, which is usual for these cells. The background cytoplasm is colorless and filled with eosinophil secondary granules. (From Carr JH, Rodak BF: Clinical hematology atlas, ed 4, St. Louis, 2013, Saunders.)

well as cytokine production, and they also produce nerve growth factor that promotes mast cell survival and activation.

Eosinophil production is increased in infection by parasitic helminths, and in vitro studies have shown that the eosinophil is capable of destroying tissue-invading helminths through the secretion of major basic protein and eosinophil cationic protein as well as the production of reactive oxygen species.[35] There is also a suggestion that eosinophils play a role in preventing reinfection.[37]

Finally, eosinophilia is a hallmark of allergic disorders, of which asthma has been the best studied. The number of eosinophils in blood and sputum correlates with disease severity. This has led to the suggestion that the eosinophil is one of the causes of airway inflammation and mucosal cell damage through secretion or production of a combination of basic proteins, lipid mediators, reactive oxygen species, and cytokines such as IL-5.[35] Eosinophils have also been implicated in airway remodeling (increase in thickness of the airway wall) through eosinophil-derived fibrogenic growth factors.[38] Treatment with an anti-IL-5 monoclonal antibody has been shown to reduce exacerbations in certain asthmatic patients.[39] Eosinophil accumulation in the gastrointestinal tract occurs in allergic disorders such as food allergy, allergic colitis, and inflammatory bowel disease such as Crohn's disease and ulcerative colitis.[40,41]

Basophils

Basophils and mast cells are two cells with morphologic and functional similarities; however, basophils are true leukocytes because they mature in the bone marrow and circulate in the blood as mature cells with granules, whereas mast cell precursors leave the bone marrow and use the blood as a transit system to gain access to the tissues where they mature. Basophils are discussed first. Basophils are the least numerous of the WBCs, making up between 0% and 2% of circulating leukocytes and less than 1% of nucleated cells in the bone marrow.

Basophil Development

Basophils are derived from progenitors in the bone marrow, where they differentiate under the influence of a number of

These vesicles then migrate to the plasma membrane and fuse to empty the specific proteins into the extracellular space.[30]

Eosinophils play important roles in immune regulation. They transmigrate into the thymus of the newborn and are believed to be involved in the deletion of double-positive thymocytes.[34] Eosinophils are capable of acting as antigen-presenting cells and promoting the proliferation of effector T cells.[35] They are also implicated in the initiation of either type 1 or type 2 immune responses due to their ability to rapidly secrete preformed cytokines in a stimulus-specific manner.[36] Eosinophils regulate mast cell function through the release of *major basic protein* (MBP) that causes mast cell degranulation as

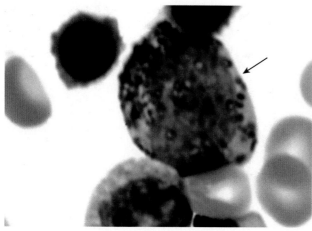

Figure 12-11 Immature basophil (*arrow*). Note that the background cytoplasm is deeply basophilic with few large basophilic granules and there appears to be a nucleolus.

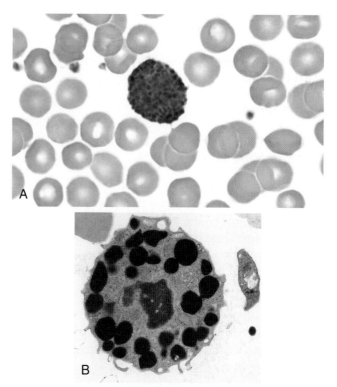

Figure 12-12 A, Mature basophil. Note that granules tend to obscure the nucleus and the background cytoplasm is only slightly basophilic. **B,** Electron micrograph of a basophil. (**B** from Rodak BF, Carr JH: Clinical hematology atlas, ed 4, St. Louis, 2013, Saunders, Elsevier.)

cytokines, including IL-3.[42,43] Due to their very small numbers, the stages of basophil maturation are very difficult to observe and have not been well characterized. Basophils will therefore be described simply as immature basophils and mature basophils.

Immature basophils have round to somewhat lobulated nuclei with only slightly condensed chromatin. Nucleoli may or may not be apparent. The cytoplasm is blue and contains large blue-black secondary granules (Figure 12-11). Primary azure granules may or may not be seen. Basophil granules are water soluble and therefore may be dissolved if the blood film is washed too much during the staining process.

Mature basophils contain a lobulated nucleus that is often obscured by its granules. The chromatin pattern, if visible, is clumped. Actual nuclear segmentation with visible filaments occurs rarely. The cytoplasm is colorless and contains large numbers of the characteristic large blue-black granules. If any granules have been dissolved during the staining process, they often leave a reddish-purple rim surrounding what appears to be a vacuole (Figure 12-12).

Basophil Kinetics

Basophil kinetics is poorly understood because of their very small numbers. According to a recent study, the life span of a mature basophil is 60 hours.[44] This life span of basophils is relatively longer than that of the other granulocytes. This has been attributed to the fact that when they are activated by the cytokine IL-3, anti-apoptotic pathways are initiated that cause the prolongation of the basophil life span.[45]

Basophil Functions

Basophil functions are also poorly understood because of the small numbers of these cells and the lack of animal models such as basophil-deficient animals. However, the recent development of a conditional basophil-deficient mouse model promises to enhance the understanding of basophil function.[46] In the past, basophils have been regarded as the "poor relatives" of mast cells and minor players in allergic inflammation because, like mast cells, they have immunoglobulin E (IgE) receptors on their

surface membranes that, when cross-linked by antigen, result in granule release.[47] Today, something of a reawakening has occurred regarding basophils and their functions in both innate and adaptive immunity. Basophils are capable of releasing large quantities of subtype 2 helper T cell (T_H2) cytokines such as IL-4 and IL-13 that regulate the T_H2 immune response.[48,49] Basophils also induce B cells to synthesize IgE.[50] Whereas mast cells are the effectors of IgE-mediated chronic allergic inflammation, basophils function as *initiators* of the allergic inflammation through the release of preformed cytokines.[47] Basophil activation is not restricted to antigen-specific IgE cross-linking, but it can be triggered in nonsensitized individuals by a growing list of parasitic antigens, lectins, and viral superantigens binding to nonspecific IgE antibodies.[51]

The contents of basophil granules are not well known. Box 12-4 provides a short list of some of the substances released by activated basophils. Moreover, mature basophils are evidently capable of synthesizing granule proteins based on activation signals. For example, basophils can be induced to produce a mediator of allergic inflammation known as *granzyme B*.[52] Mast cells can induce basophils to produce and release retinoic acid, a regulator of immune and resident cells in allergic diseases.[53] Basophils also play a role in angiogenesis through the expression of vascular endothelial growth factor (VEGF) and its receptors.[54]

Along with eosinophils, basophils are involved in the control of helminth infections. They promote eosinophilia, are associated with the differentiation of alternatively activated

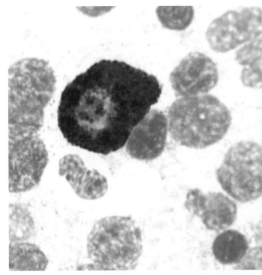

Figure 12-13 Tissue mast cell in bone marrow. Note that the nucleus is rounded and the cell is packed with large basophilic granules. Mast cells tend to be a little larger than basophils (12 to 25 μm). (From Rodak BF, Carr JH: *Clinical hematology atlas*, ed 4, Philadelphia, 2013, Saunders, Elsevier.)

macrophages in the lung, and contribute to efficient worm expulsion.[44] Finally, data from the basophil-deficient mouse model indicate that basophils play a nonredundant role in mediating acquired immunity against ticks.[46]

Mast Cells

Mast cells are not considered to be leukocytes. They are tissue effector cells of allergic responses and inflammatory reactions. A brief description of their development and function is included here because (1) their precursors circulate in the peripheral blood for a brief period on their way to their tissue destinations,[55] and (2) mast cells have several phenotypic and functional similarities with both basophils and eosinophils.[56]

Mast cell progenitors (MCPs) originate from the bone marrow and spleen.[55] The progenitors are then released to the blood before finally reaching tissues such as the intestine and lung, where they mediate their actions.[55] The major cytokine responsible for mast cell maturation and differentiation is KIT ligand (stem cell factor).[57] Once the MCP reaches its tissue destination, complete maturation into mature mast cells occurs under the control of the local microenvironment (Figure 12-13).[58]

Mast cells function as effector cells in allergic reactions through the release of a wide variety of lipid mediators, proteases, proteoglycans, and cytokines as a result of cross-linking of IgE on the mast cell surface by specific allergens. Mast cells can also be activated independently of IgE, which leads to inflammatory reactions. Mast cells can function as antigen-presenting cells to induce the differentiation of T_H2 cells;[59] therefore, mast cells act in both innate and adaptive immunity.[60] In addition, mast cells can have anti-inflammatory and immunosuppressive functions, and thus they can both enhance and suppress features of the immune response.[61]

MONONUCLEAR CELLS

Monocytes

Monocytes make up between 2% and 11% of circulating leukocytes, with an absolute number of up to $1.3 \times 10^9/L$.

Monocyte Development

Monocyte development is similar to neutrophil development because both cell types are derived from the granulocyte-monocyte progenitor (GMP) (see Figure 12-1). Macrophage colony-stimulating factor (M-CSF) is the major cytokine responsible for the growth and differentiation of monocytes. The morphologic stages of monocyte development are monoblasts, promonocytes, and monocytes. Monoblasts in normal bone marrow are very rare and are difficult to distinguish from myeloblasts based on morphology. Malignant monoblasts in acute monoblastic leukemia are described in Chapter 35. Therefore, only promonocytes and monocytes are described here.

Promonocytes are 12 to 18 μm in diameter, and their nucleus is slightly indented or folded. The chromatin pattern is delicate, and at least one nucleolus is apparent. The cytoplasm is blue and contains scattered azure granules that are fewer and smaller than those seen in promyelocytes (Figure 12-14).

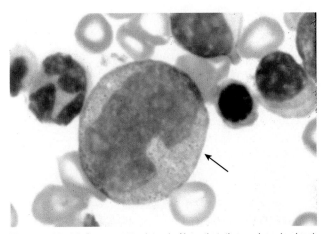

Figure 12-14 Promonocyte (*arrow*). Note that the nucleus is deeply indented and should not be confused with a neutrophil band form (compare the chromatin patterns of the two). The cytoplasm is basophilic with azure granules that are much smaller than those seen in promyelocytes. The azure granules in this cell are hard to see and give the cytoplasm a slightly grainy appearance.

Electron microscopic and cytochemical studies have shown that monocyte azure granules are heterogeneous with regard to their content of lysosomal enzymes, peroxidase, nonspecific esterases, and lysozyme.[62]

Monocytes appear to be larger than neutrophils (diameter of 15 to 20 μm) because they tend to stick to and spread out on glass or plastic. Monocytes are slightly immature cells whose ultimate goal is to enter the tissues and mature into macrophages, osteoclasts, or dendritic cells.

The nucleus may be round, oval, or kidney shaped, but more frequently is deeply indented (horseshoe shaped) or folded on itself. The chromatin pattern is looser than in the other leukocytes and has sometimes been described as lacelike or stringy. Nucleoli are generally not seen with the light microscope; however, electron microscopy reveals nucleoli in roughly half of circulating monocytes. Their cytoplasm is blue-gray, with fine azure granules often referred to as *azure dust* or a ground-glass appearance. Small cytoplasmic pseudopods or blebs may be seen. Cytoplasmic and nuclear vacuoles may also be present (Figure 12-15). Based on flow cytometry immunophenotyping, three subsets of human monocytes have been described: the classical, intermediate, and nonclassical monocytes.[63] The roles of these monocyte subsets in health and disease are currently being characterized.

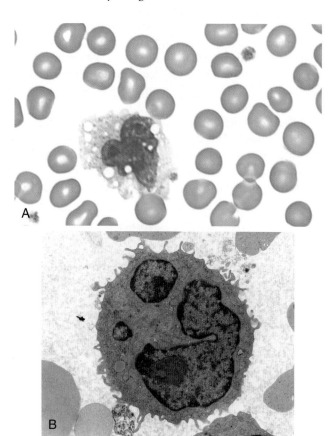

Figure 12-15 A, Typical monocyte. Note the vacuolated cytoplasm, a contorted nucleus that folds on itself, loose or lacelike chromatin pattern, and very fine azure granules. **B,** Electron micrograph of a monocyte. Note that the villi on the surface are much greater in number than is seen on neutrophils. (**B** from Rodak BF, Carr JH: Clinical hematology atlas, ed 4, St. Louis, 2013, Saunders, Elsevier.)

Monocyte/Macrophage Kinetics

The promonocyte pool consists of approximately 6×10^8 cells/kg, and they produce 7×10^6 monocytes/kg per hour. Under normal circumstances, promonocytes undergo two mitotic divisions in 60 hours to produce a total of four monocytes. Under conditions of increased demand for monocytes, promonocytes undergo four divisions to yield a total of 16 monocytes in 60 hours. There is no storage pool of mature monocytes in the bone marrow,[64] and unlike neutrophils, monocytes are released immediately into the circulation upon maturation. Therefore, when the bone marrow recovers from marrow failure, monocytes are seen in the peripheral blood before neutrophils and a relative monocytosis may occur. There is recent evidence, however, that a relatively large reservoir of immature monocytes resides in the subcapsular red pulp of the spleen. Monocytes in this splenic reservoir appear to respond to tissue injury such as myocardial infarction by migrating to the site of tissue injury to participate in wound healing.[65]

Like neutrophils, monocytes in the peripheral blood can be found in a marginal pool and a circulating pool. Unlike with neutrophils, the marginal pool of monocytes is 3.5 times the circulating pool.[66] Monocytes remain in the circulation approximately 3 days.[67] Monocytes with different patterns of chemokine receptors have different target tissues and different functions. Box 12-5 contains a list of the various tissue destinations of monocytes.[68] Once in the tissues, monocytes differentiate into macrophages, osteoclasts (Figure 12-16), or dendritic cells, depending on the microenvironment of the local tissues. Macrophages can be as large as 40 to 50 μm in diameter. They usually have an oval nucleus with a netlike (reticulated) chromatin pattern. Their cytoplasm is pale, frequently vacuolated, and often filled with debris of phagocytized cells or organisms.

The life span of macrophages in the tissues depends on whether they are responding to inflammation or infection, or are "resident" macrophages such as Kupffer cells or alveolar macrophages. Resident macrophages survive far longer than tissue neutrophils. For example, Kupffer cells have a life span of approximately 21 days.[69] Inflammatory macrophages, on the other hand, have a life span measured in hours.

Monocyte/Macrophage Functions

Functions of monocytes/macrophages are numerous and varied. They can be subdivided into innate immunity, adaptive immunity, and housekeeping functions.

- *Innate immunity:* Monocytes/macrophages recognize a wide range of bacterial pathogens by means of pattern recognition receptors (toll-like receptors) that stimulate inflammatory cytokine production and phagocytosis. Macrophages can synthesize nitric oxide, which is cytotoxic against viruses, bacteria, fungi, protozoa, helminths, and tumor cells.[24] Monocytes and macrophages also have Fc receptors and complement receptors. Hence, they can phagocytize foreign organisms or materials that have been coated with antibodies or complement components.

- *Adaptive immunity:* Both macrophages and dendritic cells degrade antigen and present antigen fragments on their surfaces

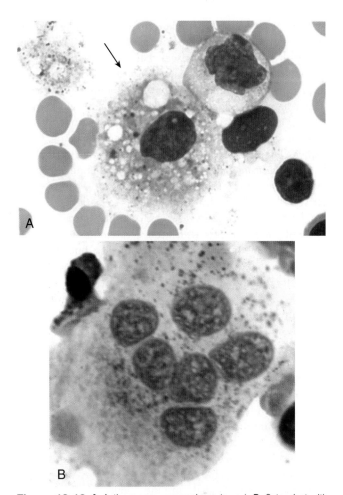

Figure 12-16 A, Active marrow macrophage (*arrow*). **B,** Osteoclast with 6 nuclei. Both of these cells are derived from monocytes.

(antigen-presenting cells). Because of this, they interact with and activate both T lymphocytes and B lymphocytes to initiate the adaptive immune response. Dendritic cells are the most efficient and potent of the antigen-presenting cells.

- *Housekeeping functions:* These include removal of debris and dead cells at sites of infection or tissue damage, destruction of senescent red blood cells and maintenance of a storage pool of iron for erythropoiesis, and synthesis of a wide variety of proteins, including coagulation factors, complement components, interleukins, growth factors, and enzymes.[70]

Lymphocytes

Lymphocytes are divided into three major groups: T cells, B cells, and natural killer (NK) cells. T and B cells are major players in adaptive immunity. NK cells make up a small percentage of lymphocytes and are part of innate immunity. Adaptive immunity has three characteristics: it relies on an enormous number of distinct lymphocytes, each having surface receptors for a different specific molecular structure on a foreign antigen; after an encounter with a particular antigen, memory cells are produced that will react faster and more vigorously to that same antigen upon reexposure; and self-antigens are "ignored" under normal circumstances (referred to as *tolerance*).

Lymphocytes can be subdivided into two major categories: those that participate in humoral immunity by producing antibodies and those that participate in cellular immunity by attacking foreign organisms or cells directly. Antibody-producing lymphocytes are called *B lymphocytes* or simply *B cells* because they develop in the bone marrow. Cellular immunity is accomplished by two types of lymphocytes: T cells, so named because they develop in the thymus, and NK cells, which develop in both the bone marrow and the thymus.[71-73]

Lymphocytes are different from the other leukocytes in several ways, including the following:

1. Lymphocytes are not end cells. They are resting cells, and when stimulated, they undergo mitosis to produce both memory and effector cells.

2. Unlike other leukocytes, lymphocytes recirculate from the blood to the tissues and back to the blood.

3. B and T lymphocytes are capable of rearranging antigen receptor gene segments to produce a wide variety of antibodies and surface receptors.

4. Although early lymphocyte progenitors such as the common lymphoid progenitor originate in the bone marrow, T and NK lymphocytes develop and mature outside of the bone marrow.

For these reasons, lymphocyte kinetics is extremely complicated, not well understood, and beyond the scope of this chapter.

Lymphocytes make up between 18% and 42% of circulating leukocytes with an absolute number of 0.8 to 4.8×10^9/L.

Lymphocyte Development

For both B and T cells, development can be subdivided into antigen-independent and antigen-dependent phases. Antigen-independent lymphocyte development occurs in the bone marrow and thymus (sometimes referred to as *central* or *primary lymphatic organs*), whereas antigen-dependent lymphocyte development occurs in the spleen, lymph nodes, tonsils, and mucosa-associated lymphoid tissue such as the Peyer's patches in the intestinal wall (sometimes referred to as *peripheral* or *secondary lymphatic organs*).

B lymphocytes develop initially in the bone marrow and go through three stages known as *pro-B, pre-B,* and *immature B cells.* It is during these stages that immunoglobulin gene rearrangement occurs so that each B cell produces a unique immunoglobulin antigen receptor. The immature B cells, which have not yet been exposed to antigen (*antigen-naive B cells*), leave the bone marrow to migrate to secondary lymphatic organs, where they take up residence in specific zones such as lymph node follicles. These immature B cells, also known as *hematogones,*[74] have a homogeneous nuclear chromatin pattern and extremely scanty cytoplasm (Figure 12-17). These cells are normally seen in newborn peripheral blood and bone marrow and in regenerative bone marrows. Leukemic cells from patients with acute lymphoblastic leukemia (ALL) can sometimes resemble hematogones, but the leukemic cells can be distinguished from hematogones by flow cytometry immunophenotyping.[75]

It is in the secondary lymphatic organs or in the blood where B cells may come in contact with antigen, which results in cell division and the production of memory cells as well as effector cells. Effector B cells are antibody-producing cells known as *plasma cells* and *plasmacytoid lymphocytes* (Figure 12-18).

Approximately 3% to 21% of circulating lymphocytes are B cells. Resting B lymphocytes cannot be distinguished morphologically from resting T lymphocytes. Resting lymphocytes are small (around 9 μm in diameter), and the N:C ratio ranges from 5:1 to 2:1. The chromatin is arranged in blocks, and the nucleolus is rarely seen, although it is present (Figure 12-19).

T lymphocytes develop initially in the thymus—a lymphoepithelial organ located in the upper mediastinum.[76] Lymphoid progenitor cells migrate from the bone marrow to the thymic cortex, where, under the regulation of cytokines produced by thymic epithelial cells, they progress through stages known as *pro-T, pre-T,* and *immature T cells.* During these phases they undergo antigen receptor gene rearrangement to produce T cell receptors that are unique to each T cell. T cells whose receptors react with self-antigens are allowed to undergo apoptosis.[77] In addition, T cells are subdivided into two major categories, depending on whether or not they have CD4 or

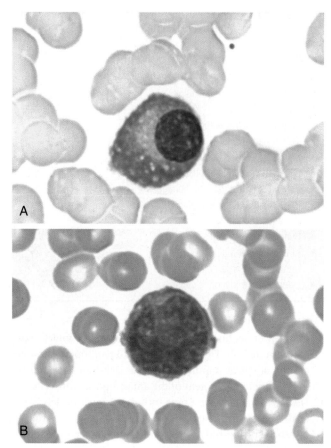

Figure 12-18 A, Plasma cell. **B,** Plasmacytoid lymphocyte. These are effector cells of the B lymphocyte lineage.

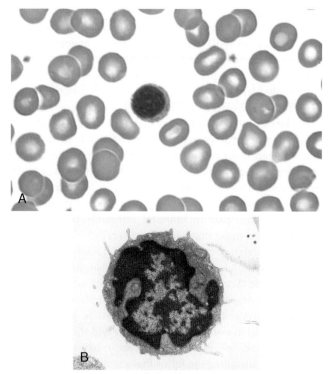

Figure 12-19 A, Small resting lymphocyte. **B,** Electron micrograph of a small lymphocyte. (**B** from Rodak BF, Carr JH: Clinical hematology atlas, ed 4, St. Louis, 2013, Saunders, Elsevier.)

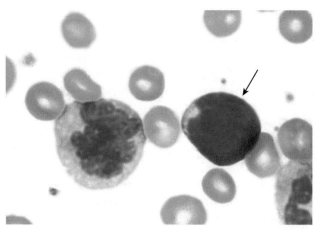

Figure 12-17 Immature B lymphocyte or hematogone (*arrow*). Note the extremely scanty cytoplasm. This was taken from the bone marrow of a newborn infant.

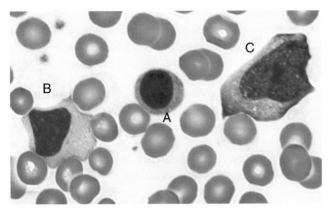

Figure 12-20 Three cells representing lymphocyte activation. A small resting lymphocyte (**A**) is stimulated by antigen and begins to enlarge to form a medium to large lymphocyte (**B**). The nucleus reverts from a clumped to a delicate chromatin pattern with nucleoli (**C**). The cell is capable of dividing to form effector cells or memory cells.

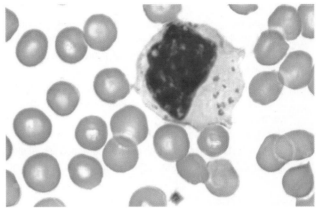

Figure 12-21 A large granular lymphocyte that could be either a cytotoxic T lymphocyte or a natural killer lymphocyte.

CD8 antigen on their surfaces. Immature T cells then proceed to the thymic medulla, where further apoptosis of self-reactive T cells occurs. The remaining immature T cells (or *antigen-naive T cells*) then leave the thymus and migrate to secondary lymphatic organs, where they take up residence in specific zones such as the paracortical areas. T cells comprise 51% to 88% of circulating lymphocytes.

T cells in secondary lymphatic organs or in the circulating blood eventually come in contact with antigen. This results in cell activation and the production of either memory cells or effector T cells, or both (Figure 12-20). The transformation of resting lymphocytes into activated forms is the source of so-called medium and large lymphocytes that have increased amounts of cytoplasm and usually make up only about 10% of circulating lymphocytes. The morphology of effector T cells varies with the subtype of T cell involved, and they are often referred to as *reactive* or *variant lymphocytes*.

NK cells are a heterogeneous group of cells with respect to their surface antigens. The majority are CD56⁺CD16⁺CD3⁻CD7⁺ large granular lymphocytes. (Figure 12-21).[78] The mature NK cell is relatively large compared with other resting lymphocytes because of an increased amount of cytoplasm. Its cytoplasm contains azurophilic granules that are peroxidase negative. Approximately 4% to 29% of circulating lymphocytes are NK cells.

Lymphocyte Functions

Functions can be addressed according to the type of lymphocyte. *B lymphocytes* are essential for antibody production. In addition, they have a role in antigen presentation to T cells and may be necessary for optimal CD4 activation. B cells also produce cytokines that regulate a variety of T cell and antigen-presenting cell functions.[79]

T lymphocytes can be divided into CD4⁺ T cells and CD8⁺ T cells. CD4⁺ effector lymphocytes are further subdivided into T_H1, T_H2, T_H17, and T_{reg} (CD4⁺CD25⁺ regulatory T) cells. T_H1 cells mediate immune responses against intracellular pathogens. T_H2 cells mediate host defense against extracellular parasites, including helminths. They are also important in the induction of asthma and other allergic diseases. T_H17 cells are involved in the immune responses against extracellular bacteria and fungi. T_{reg} cells play a role in maintaining self-tolerance by regulating immune responses.[80,81]

CD8⁺ effector lymphocytes are capable of killing target cells by secreting granules containing granzyme and perforin or by activating apoptotic pathways in the target cell.[82] These cells are sometimes referred to as *cytotoxic T lymphocytes*.

NK lymphocytes function as part of innate immunity and are capable of killing certain tumor cells and virus-infected cells without prior sensitization. In addition, NK cells modulate the functions of other cells, including macrophages and T cells.[83]

SUMMARY

- Granulocytes are classified according to their staining characteristics and the shape of their nuclei. Neutrophils are a major component of innate immunity as phagocytes; eosinophils are involved in allergic reactions and helminth destruction; and basophils function as initiators of allergic reactions, helminth destruction, and immunity against ticks.
- Neutrophil development can be subdivided into specific stages, with cells at each stage having specific morphologic characteristics

(myeloblast, promyelocyte, myelocyte, metamyelocyte, band, and segmented neutrophil). Various granule types are produced during neutrophil development, each with specific contents.
- Eosinophil development can also be subdivided into specific stages, although eosinophilic myeloblasts are not recognizable and eosinophil promyelocytes are rare.
- Basophil development is difficult to describe, and basophils have been divided simply into immature and mature basophils.

- Mononuclear cells consist of monocytes and lymphocytes. Monocytes are precursors to tissue cells such as osteoclasts, macrophages, and dendritic cells. As a group, they perform several functions as phagocytes.
- Monocyte development can be subdivided into the promonocyte, monocyte, and macrophage stages, each with specific morphologic characteristics.
- The majority of lymphocytes are involved in adaptive immunity. B lymphocytes and plasma cells produce antibodies against foreign organisms or cells, and T lymphocytes mediate the immune response against intracellular and extracellular invaders. Both B and T lymphocytes produce memory cells for specific antigens so that the immune response is faster if the same antigen is encountered again.
- Lymphocyte development is complex, and morphologic divisions are not practical because a large number of lymphocytes develop in the thymus. Benign B-lymphocyte precursors (hematogones) as well as B-lymphocyte effector cells (plasma cells and plasmacytoid lymphocytes) have been described. NK lymphocytes and cytotoxic T cells also have a distinct and similar morphology.

REVIEW QUESTIONS

Answers can be found in the Appendix.

1. Neutrophils and monocytes are direct descendants of a common progenitor known as:
   a. CLP
   b. GMP
   c. MEP
   d. HSC

2. The stage in neutrophilic development in which the nucleus is indented in a kidney bean shape and the cytoplasm has secondary granules that are lavender in color is the:
   a. Band
   b. Myelocyte
   c. Promyelocyte
   d. Metamyelocyte

3. Type II myeloblasts are characterized by:
   a. Presence of fewer than 20 primary granules per cell
   b. Basophilic cytoplasm with many secondary granules
   c. Absence of granules
   d. Presence of a folded nucleus

4. Which one of the following is a function of neutrophils?
   a. Presentation of antigen to T and B lymphocytes
   b. Protection against reexposure by same antigen
   c. Nonspecific destruction of foreign organisms
   d. Initiation of delayed hypersensitivity response

5. Which of the following cells are important in immune regulation, allergic inflammation, and destruction of tissue invading helminths?
   a. Neutrophils and monocytes
   b. Eosinophils and basophils
   c. T and B lymphocytes
   d. Macrophages and dendritic cells

6. Basophils and mast cells have high-affinity surface receptors for which immunoglobulin?
   a. A
   b. D
   c. E
   d. G

7. Which of the following cell types is capable of differentiating into osteoclasts, macrophages, or dendritic cells?
   a. Neutrophils
   b. Lymphocytes
   c. Monocytes
   d. Eosinophils

8. Macrophages aid in adaptive immunity by:
   a. Degrading antigen and presenting it to lymphocytes
   b. Ingesting and digesting organisms that neutrophils cannot
   c. Synthesizing complement components
   d. Storing iron from senescent red cells

9. Which of the following is the final stage of B cell maturation after activation by antigen?
   a. Large, granular lymphocyte
   b. Plasma cell
   c. Reactive lymphocyte
   d. Immunoblast

10. The following is unique to *both* B and T lymphocytes and occurs during their early development:
    a. Expression of surface antigens CD4 and CD8
    b. Maturation in the thymus
    c. Synthesis of immunoglobulins
    d. Rearrangement of antigen receptor genes

REFERENCES

1. von Vietinghoff, S., & Ley, K. (2008) Homeostatic regulation of blood neutrophil counts. *J Immunol, 181*(8), 5183–5188.
2. Price, T. H., Chatta, G. S., & Dale, D. C. (1996). Effect of recombinant granulocyte colony-stimulating factor on neutrophil kinetics in normal young and elderly humans. *Blood, 88*(1), 335–340.
3. Chaiworapongsa, T., Romero, R., Berry, S. M., et al. (2011). The role of granulocyte colony-stimulating factor in the neutrophilia observed in the fetal inflammatory response syndrome. *J Perinat Med, 39*(6), 653–666.
4. Summers, C., Rankin, S. M., Condliffe, A. M., et al. (2010). Neutrophil kinetics in health and disease. *Trends Immunol, 31*(8), 318–324.
5. Iwasaki, H., & Akashi, K. (2007). Hematopoietic developmental pathways: on cellular basis. *Oncogene, 26*(47), 6687–6696.
6. Terstappen, L. W., Huang, S., Safford, M., et al. (1991). Sequential generations of hematopoietic colonies derived from single nonlineage-committed CD34+CD38– progenitor cells. *Blood, 77*(6), 1218–1227.
7. Manz, M. G., Miyamoto, T., Akashi, K., & Weissman, I. L. (2002). Prospective isolation of human clonogenic common myeloid progenitors. *Proc Natl Acad Sci U S A, 99*(18), 11872–11877.
8. Adams, G. B., & Scadden, D. T. (2006). The hematopoietic stem cell in its place. *Nat Immunol, 7*(4), 333–337.
9. Mufti, G. J., Bennett, J. M., Goasguen, J., et al. (2008). Diagnosis and classification of myelodysplastic syndrome: International Working Group on Morphology of Myelodysplastic Syndrome (IWGM-MDS) consensus proposals for the definition and enumeration of myeloblasts and ring sideroblasts. *Haematologica, 93*(11), 1712–1717.
10. Faurschou, M., & Borregaard, N. (2003). Neutrophil granules and secretory vesicles in inflammation. *Microbes Infect, 5*(14), 1317–1327.
11. Cornbleet, P. J. (2002). Clinical utility of the band count. *Clin Lab Med, 22*(1), 101–136.
12. *Reference leukocyte (WBC) differential count (proportional) and evaluation of instrumental methods; approved standard-Second Edition. (H20-A2).* Vol 27(4): Clinical and Laboratory Standards Institute (CLSI); 2007.
13. Dancey, J. T., Deubelbeiss, K. A., Harker, L. A., & Finch, C. A. (1976). Neutrophil kinetics in man. *J Clin Invest, 58*(3), 705–715.
14. Athens, J. W., Haab, O. P., Raab, S. O., et al. (1961). Leukokinetic studies. IV. The total blood, circulating and marginal granulocyte pools and the granulocyte turnover rate in normal subjects. *J Clin Invest, 40*, 989–995.
15. Hetherington, S. V., & Quie, P. G. (1985). Human polymorphonuclear leukocytes of the bone marrow, circulation, and marginated pool: function and granule protein content. *Am J Hematol, 20*(3), 235–246.
16. Cartwright, G. E., Athens, J. W., & Wintrobe, M. M. (1964). The kinetics of granulopoiesis in normal man. *Blood, 24*, 780–803.
17. Cowburn, A. S., Condliffe, A. M., Farahi, N., et al. (2008). Advances in neutrophil biology: clinical implications. *Chest, 134*(3), 606–612.
18. Saverymuttu, S. H., Peters, A. M., Keshavarzian, A., et al. (1985). The kinetics of 111indium distribution following injection of 111indium labelled autologous granulocytes in man. *Br J Haematol, 61*(4), 675–685.
19. Zarbock, A., Ley, K., McEver, R. P., & Hidalgo, A. (2011). Leukocyte ligands for endothelial selectins: specialized glycoconjugates that mediate rolling and signaling under flow. *Blood, 118*(26), 6743–6751.
20. Ley, K., Laudanna, C., Cybulsky, M. I., & Nourshargh, S. (2007). Getting to the site of inflammation: the leukocyte adhesion cascade updated. *Nat Rev Immunol, 7*(9), 678–689.
21. Mayadas, T. N., & Cullere, X. (2005). Neutrophil beta2 integrins: moderators of life or death decisions. *Trends Immunol, 26*(7), 388–395.
22. Burg, N. D., & Pillinger, M. H. (2001). The neutrophil: function and regulation in innate and humoral immunity. *Clin Immunol, 99*(1), 7–17.
23. Stuart, L. M., & Ezekowitz, R. A. (2005). Phagocytosis: elegant complexity. *Immunity, 22*(5), 539–550.
24. Dale, D. C., Boxer, L., & Liles, W. C. (2008). The phagocytes: neutrophils and monocytes. *Blood, 112*(4), 935–945.
25. Brinkmann, V., & Zychlinsky, A. (2007). Beneficial suicide: why neutrophils die to make NETs. *Nat Rev Microbiol, 5*(8), 577–582.
26. Brinkmann, V., & Zychlinsky, A. (2012). Neutrophil extracellular traps: is immunity the second function of chromatin? *J Cell Biol, 198*(5), 773–783.
27. Mori, Y., Iwasaki, H., Kohno, K., et al. (2009). Identification of the human eosinophil lineage-committed progenitor: revision of phenotypic definition of the human common myeloid progenitor. *J Exp Med, 206*(1), 183–193.
28. Uhm, T. G., Kim, B. S., & Chung, I. Y. (2012). Eosinophil development, regulation of eosinophil-specific genes, and role of eosinophils in the pathogenesis of asthma. *Allergy Asthma Immunol Res, 4*(2), 68–79.
29. Takatsu, K., & Nakajima, H. (2008). IL-5 and eosinophilia. *Curr Opin Immunol, 20*(3), 288–294.
30. Melo, R. C., Spencer, L. A., Perez, S. A., et al. (2009). Vesicle-mediated secretion of human eosinophil granule-derived major basic protein. *Lab Invest, 89*(7), 769–781.
31. Giembycz, M. A., & Lindsay, M. A. (1999). Pharmacology of the eosinophil. *Pharmacol Rev, 51*(2), 213–340.
32. Steinbach, K. H., Schick, P., Trepel, F., et al. (1979). Estimation of kinetic parameters of neutrophilic, eosinophilic, and basophilic granulocytes in human blood. *Blut, 39*(1), 27–38.
33. Park, Y. M., & Bochner, B. S. (2010). Eosinophil survival and apoptosis in health and disease. *Allergy Asthma Immunol Res, 2*(2), 87–101.
34. Throsby, M., Herbelin, A., Pleau, J. M., & Dardenne, M. (2000). CD11c+ eosinophils in the murine thymus: developmental regulation and recruitment upon MHC class I-restricted thymocyte deletion. *J Immunol, 165*(4), 1965–1975.
35. Hogan, S. P., Rosenberg, H. F., Moqbel, R., et al. (2008). Eosinophils: biological properties and role in health and disease. *Clin Exp Allergy, 38*(5), 709–750.
36. Spencer, L. A., Szela, C. T., Perez, S. A., et al. (2009). Human eosinophils constitutively express multiple Th1, Th2, and immunoregulatory cytokines that are secreted rapidly and differentially. *J Leukoc Biol, 85*(1), 117–123.
37. Hagan, P., Wilkins, H. A., Blumenthal, U. J., Hayes, R. J., & Greenwood, B. M. (1985). Eosinophilia and resistance to *Schistosoma haematobium* in man. *Parasite Immunol, 7*(6), 625–632.
38. Phipps, S., Benyahia, F., Ou, T. T., et al. (2004). Acute allergen-induced airway remodeling in atopic asthma. *Am J Respir Cell Mol Biol, 31*(6), 626–632.
39. Robinson, D. S. (2013). Mepolizumab for severe eosinophilic asthma. *Expert Rev Respir Med, 7*(1), 13–17.
40. Walsh, R. E., & Gaginella, T. S. (1991). The eosinophil in inflammatory bowel disease. *Scand J Gastroenterol, 26*(12), 1217–1224.
41. Hogan, S. P., Waddell, A., & Fulkerson, P. C. (2013). Eosinophils in infection and intestinal immunity. *Curr Opin Gastroenterol, 29*(1), 7–14.
42. Min, B., Brown, M. A., & Legros, G. (2012). Understanding the roles of basophils: breaking dawn. *Immunology, 135*(3), 192–197.

43. Ohmori, K., Luo, Y., Jia, Y., et al. (2009). IL-3 induces basophil expansion in vivo by directing granulocyte-monocyte progenitors to differentiate into basophil lineage-restricted progenitors in the bone marrow and by increasing the number of basophil/mast cell progenitors in the spleen. *J Immunol, 182*(5), 2835–2841.

44. Ohnmacht, C., & Voehringer, D. (2009). Basophil effector function and homeostasis during helminth infection. *Blood, 113*(12), 2816–2825.

45. Didichenko, S. A., Spiegl, N., Brunner, T., & Dahinden, C. A. (2008). IL-3 induces a Pim1-dependent antiapoptotic pathway in primary human basophils. *Blood, 112*(10), 3949–3958.

46. Wada, T., Ishiwata, K., Koseki, H., et al. (2010). Selective ablation of basophils in mice reveals their nonredundant role in acquired immunity against ticks. *J Clin Invest, 120*(8), 2867–2875.

47. Obata, K., Mukai, K., Tsujimura, Y., et al. (2007). Basophils are essential initiators of a novel type of chronic allergic inflammation. *Blood, 110*(3), 913–920.

48. Sullivan, B. M., & Locksley, R. M. (2009). Basophils: a nonredundant contributor to host immunity. *Immunity, 30*(1), 12–20.

49. Schroeder, J. T., MacGlashan, D. W., Jr., & Lichtenstein, L. M. (2001). Human basophils: mediator release and cytokine production. *Adv Immunol, 77*, 93–122.

50. Gauchat, J. F., Henchoz, S., Mazzei, G., et al. (1993). Induction of human IgE synthesis in B cells by mast cells and basophils. *Nature, 365*(6444), 340–343.

51. Falcone, F. H., Zillikens, D., & Gibbs, B. F. (2006). The 21st century renaissance of the basophil? Current insights into its role in allergic responses and innate immunity. *Exp Dermatol, 15*(11), 855–864.

52. Tschopp, C. M., Spiegl, N., Didichenko, S., et al. (2006). Granzyme B, a novel mediator of allergic inflammation: its induction and release in blood basophils and human asthma. *Blood, 108*(7), 2290–2299.

53. Spiegl, N., Didichenko, S., McCaffery, P., et al. (2008). Human basophils activated by mast cell-derived IL-3 express retinaldehyde dehydrogenase-II and produce the immunoregulatory mediator retinoic acid. *Blood, 112*(9), 3762–3771.

54. de Paulis, A., Prevete, N., Fiorentino, I., et al. (2006). Expression and functions of the vascular endothelial growth factors and their receptors in human basophils. *J Immunol, 177*(10), 7322–7331.

55. Hallgren, J., & Gurish, M. F. (2011). Mast cell progenitor trafficking and maturation. *Adv Exp Med Biol, 716*, 14–28.

56. Valent, P. (1994). The phenotype of human eosinophils, basophils, and mast cells. *J Allergy Clin Immunol, 94*(6 Pt 2), 1177–1183.

57. Valent, P., Spanblochl, E., Sperr, W. R., et al. (1992). Induction of differentiation of human mast cells from bone marrow and peripheral blood mononuclear cells by recombinant human stem cell factor/kit-ligand in long-term culture. *Blood, 80*(9), 2237–2245.

58. Kambe, N., Hiramatsu, H., Shimonaka, M., et al. (2004). Development of both human connective tissue-type and mucosal-type mast cells in mice from hematopoietic stem cells with identical distribution pattern to human body. *Blood, 103*(3), 860–867.

59. Nakano, N., Nishiyama, C., Yagita, H., et al. (2009). Notch signaling confers antigen-presenting cell functions on mast cells. *J Allergy Clin Immunol, 123*(1), 74–81, e71.

60. Heib, V., Becker, M., Taube, C., & Stassen, M. (2008). Advances in the understanding of mast cell function. *Br J Haematol, 142*(5), 683–694.

61. Galli, S. J., Grimbaldeston, M., & Tsai, M. (2008). Immunomodulatory mast cells: negative, as well as positive, regulators of immunity. *Nat Rev Immunol, 8*(6), 478–486.

62. Nichols, B. A., Bainton, D. F., & Farquhar, M. G. (1971). Differentiation of monocytes. Origin, nature, and fate of their azurophil granules. *J Cell Biol, 50*(2), 498–515.

63. Ziegler-Heitbrock, L., Ancuta, P., Crowe, S., et al. (2010). Nomenclature of monocytes and dendritic cells in blood. *Blood, 116*(16), e74–80.

64. Meuret, G., Bammert, J., & Hoffmann, G. (1974). Kinetics of human monocytopoiesis. *Blood, 44*(6), 801–816.

65. Swirski, F. K., Nahrendorf, M., Etzrodt, M., et al. (2009). Identification of splenic reservoir monocytes and their deployment to inflammatory sites. *Science, 325*(5940), 612–616.

66. Meuret, G., Batara, E., & Furste, H. O. (1975). Monocytopoiesis in normal man: pool size, proliferation activity and DNA synthesis time of promonocytes. *Acta Haematol, 54*(5), 261–270.

67. Whitelaw, D. M. (1972). Observations on human monocyte kinetics after pulse labeling. *Cell Tissue Kinet, 5*(4), 311–317.

68. Kumar, S., & Jack, R. (2006). Origin of monocytes and their differentiation to macrophages and dendritic cells. *J Endotoxin Res, 12*(5), 278–284.

69. Crofton, R. W., Diesselhoff-den Dulk, M. M., & van Furth, R. (1978). The origin, kinetics, and characteristics of the Kupffer cells in the normal steady state. *J Exp Med, 148*(1), 1–17.

70. Nathan, C. F. (1987). Secretory products of macrophages. *J Clin Invest, 79*(2), 319–326.

71. Lotzova, E., Savary, C. A., Champlin, R. E. (1993). Genesis of human oncolytic natural killer cells from primitive CD34+CD33− bone marrow progenitors. *J Immunol, 150*(12), 5263–5269.

72. Res, P., Martinez-Caceres, E., Cristina Jaleco, A., et al. (1996). CD34+CD38dim cells in the human thymus can differentiate into T, natural killer, and dendritic cells but are distinct from pluripotent stem cells. *Blood, 87*(12), 5196–5206.

73. Di Santo, J. P., & Vosshenrich, C. A. (2006). Bone marrow versus thymic pathways of natural killer cell development. *Immunol Rev, 214*, 35–46.

74. Sevilla, D. W., Colovai, A. I., Emmons, F. N., et al. (2010). Hematogones: a review and update. *Leuk Lymphoma, 51*(1), 10–19.

75. McKenna, R. W., Washington, L. T., Aquino, D. B., et al. (2001). Immunophenotypic analysis of hematogones (B-lymphocyte precursors) in 662 consecutive bone marrow specimens by 4-color flow cytometry. *Blood, 98*(8), 2498–2507.

76. Haynes, B. F. (1984). The human thymic microenvironment. *Adv Immunol, 36*, 87–142.

77. von Boehmer, H., The, H. S., & Kisielow, P. (1989). The thymus selects the useful, neglects the useless and destroys the harmful. *Immunol Today, 10*(2), 57–61.

78. Grossi, C. E., Cadoni, A., Zicca, A., et al. (1982). Large granular lymphocytes in human peripheral blood: ultrastructural and cytochemical characterization of the granules. *Blood, 59*(2), 277–283.

79. LeBien, T. W., & Tedder, T. F. (2008). B lymphocytes: how they develop and function. *Blood, 112*(5), 1570–1580.

80. Zhu, J., & Paul, W. E. (2008). CD4 T cells: fates, functions, and faults. *Blood, 112*(5), 1557–1569.

81. Vignali, D. A., Collison, L. W., & Workman, C. J. (2008). How regulatory T cells work. *Nat Rev Immunol, 8*(7), 523–532.

82. Rufer, N., Zippelius, A., Batard, P., et al. (2003). Ex vivo characterization of human CD8+ T subsets with distinct replicative history and partial effector functions. *Blood, 102*(5), 1779–1787.

83. Vivier, E., Tomasello, E., Baratin, M., et al. (2008). Functions of natural killer cells. *Nat Immunol, 9*(5), 503–510.

Platelet Production, Structure, and Function

13

George A. Fritsma

OBJECTIVES

After completion of this chapter, the reader will be able to:

1. Diagram megakaryocyte localization in bone marrow.
2. List the transcription products that trigger and control megakaryocytopoiesis and endomitosis.
3. Diagram terminal megakaryocyte differentiation, the proplatelet process, and thrombocytopoiesis.
4. Describe the ultrastructure of resting platelets in the circulation, including the plasma membrane, tubules, microfibrils, and granules.

5. List the important platelet receptors and their ligands.
6. Recount platelet function, including adhesion, aggregation, and secretion.
7. Reproduce the biochemical pathways of platelet activation, including integrins, G proteins, the eicosanoid, and the diacylglycerol-inositol triphosphate pathway.

CASE STUDY

After studying this chapter, the reader should be able to respond to the following case study:

A 35-year-old woman noticed multiple pinpoint red spots and bruises on her arms and legs. The hematologist confirmed the presence of petechiae, purpura, and ecchymoses on her extremities and ordered a complete blood count, prothrombin time, and partial thromboplastin time. The platelet count was 35×10^9/L, the mean platelet volume was 13.2 fL, and the diameter of platelets on the Wright-stained peripheral blood film appeared to exceed 6 μm. Other complete blood count parameters and the coagulation parameters were within normal limits. A Wright-stained bone marrow aspirate smear revealed 10 to 12 small unlobulated megakaryocytes per low-power microscopic field.

1. Do these signs and symptoms indicate systemic (mucocutaneous) or anatomical (soft tissue) bleeding?
2. What is the probable cause of the bleeding?
3. Is the thrombocytopenia the result of inadequate bone marrow production?
4. List the growth factors involved in recruiting megakaryocyte progenitors.

MEGAKARYOCYTOPOIESIS

Platelets are nonnucleated blood cells that circulate at 150 to 400×10^9/L, with average platelet counts slightly higher in women than in men and slightly lower in both sexes when over 65 years old.[1] Platelets trigger primary hemostasis upon exposure to subendothelial collagen or endothelial cell inflammatory proteins at the time of blood vessel injury. On a Wright-stained wedge-preparation blood film, platelets are distributed throughout the red blood cell monolayer at 7 to 21 cells per 100× field. On the blood film they have an average diameter of 2.5 μm, corresponding to a mean platelet volume (MPV) of 8 to 10 fL when measured by impedance in a buffered isotonic suspension, as determined using laboratory profiling instruments.[2] Their internal structure, although complex, is granular but scarcely visible using light microscopy.

Platelets arise from unique bone marrow cells called *megakaryocytes*. Megakaryocytes are the largest cells in the bone marrow and are polyploid, possessing multiple chromosome copies. On a Wright-stained bone marrow aspirate smear, each megakaryocyte is 30 to 50 μm in diameter with a multilobulated nucleus and abundant granular cytoplasm. Megakaryocytes account for less than 0.5% of all bone marrow cells, and on a normal Wright-stained bone marrow aspirate smear the microscopist may identify two to four megakaryocytes per 10× low-power field (Chapter 7).[3]

In healthy intact bone marrow tissue, megakaryocytes, under the influence of an array of stromal cell cytokines, cluster with hematopoietic stem cells in vascular niches adjacent to venous sinusoid endothelial cells (Figure 13-1).[4] Responding to the growth factor thrombopoietin (TPO), megakaryocyte progenitors are recruited from *common myeloid progenitors* (Chapter 7) and subsequently differentiate through several maturation stages. They extend proplatelet processes, projections that resemble strings of beads, through or between the endothelial cells and into the venous sinuses, releasing platelets from the tips of the processes into the circulation. Megakaryocytes are also found in the lungs.[5]

Megakaryocyte Differentiation and Progenitors

Megakaryocyte progenitors arise from the common myeloid progenitor under the influence of the transcription gene product, GATA-1, regulated by cofactor FOG1 (Box 13-1).[4] Megakaryocyte differentiation is suppressed by another transcription gene product, MYB, so GATA-1 and MYB act in opposition to balance megakaryocytopoiesis in one arm with differentiation to the red blood cell line in another arm, called erythropoiesis. From the common myeloid progenitor there arise three megakaryocyte lineage-committed progenitor

---

BOX 13-1 Endomitosis

Endomitosis is no longer a mystery to the molecular biologists who mapped its translational control genes, but it may seem mysterious to those of us who do not work daily with gene, gene product, and mutation abbreviations. The abbreviations have antecedents—for instance, GATA-1 stands for "globin transcription factor-1," a protein product of the X chromosome gene *GATA1*. FOG1 stands for "friend of GATA," a product of the *ZFPM1* (zinc finger protein multitype 1) gene. Laboratory scientists rarely refer to gene names, only their abbreviations, though they are familiar with their characteristics and functions. The abbreviations have moved rapidly into clinical laboratory jargon, as they are becoming key diagnostic markers. In this chapter we use gene product abbreviations without reference to their antecedents.

---

stages, defined by their in vitro culture colony characteristics (Figure 7-13). In order of differentiation, these are the least mature *burst-forming unit* (BFU-Meg), the intermediate *colony-forming unit* (CFU-Meg), and the more mature progenitor, the *light-density CFU* (LD-CFU-Meg).[6] All three progenitor stages resemble lymphocytes and cannot be distinguished by Wright-stained light microscopy. The BFU-Meg and CFU-Meg are diploid and participate in normal mitosis, maintaining a viable pool of megakaryocyte progenitors. Their proliferative properties are reflected in their ability to form hundreds (BFU-Megs) or scores (CFU-Megs) of colonies in culture (Figure 13-2).[7] The third stage, LD-CFU-Meg, loses its capacity to divide but retains its DNA replication and cytoplasmic maturation, a partially characterized form of mitosis unique to megakaryocytes known as *endomitosis*.

Endomitosis

Endomitosis is a form of mitosis that lacks telophase and cytokinesis (separation into daughter cells). As GATA-1 and

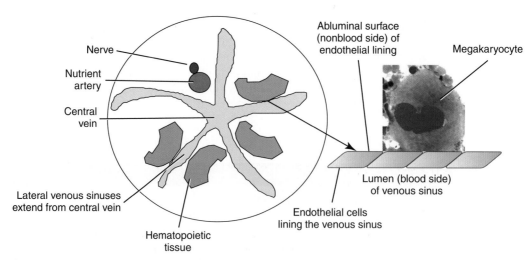

Figure 13-1 Cross section of bone marrow hematopoietic tissue. The nerve, artery, and vein run longitudinally through the center of the marrow. Venous sinuses extend laterally from the central vein throughout the hematopoietic tissue. Differentiating and mature megakaryocytes localize to the abluminal (non-blood) surface of sinusoid-lining endothelial cells.

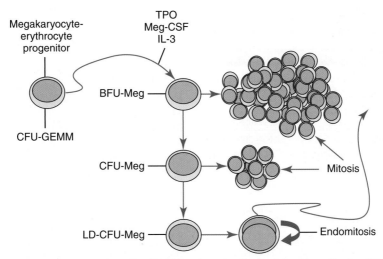

Figure 13-2 Three stages of megakaryocyte progenitors. The BFU-Meg clones hundreds of daughter cells, the CFU-Meg clones scores of daughter cells, and the LD-CFU-Meg undergoes the first stage of endomitosis. *BFU-Meg,* Burst-forming unit megakaryocyte; *CFU-Meg,* colony-forming unit megakaryocyte; *CFU-GEMM,* colony-forming unit, granulocyte, erythrocyte, monocyte, megakaryocyte, *LD-CFU-Meg,* low-density CFU-Meg; *TPO,* thrombopoietin; *Meg-CSF,* megakaryocyte colony stimulating factor; *IL-3,* interleukin-3.

FOG1 transcription slows, another transcription factor, RUNX1, mediates the switch from mitosis to endomitosis by suppressing the Rho/ROCK signaling pathway, which suppresses the assembly of the actin cytoskeleton.[8] In response to the reduced Rho/ROCK signal, inadequate levels of actin and myosin (muscle fiber–like molecules) assemble in the cytoplasmic constrictions where separation would otherwise occur, preventing cytokinesis. Subsequently, under the influence of yet another transcription factor, NF-E2, DNA replication proceeds to the production of 8N, 16N, or even 32N ploidy with duplicated chromosome sets.[4] Some megakaryocyte nuclei replicate five times, reaching 128N; this level of ploidy is unusual, however, and may signal hematologic disease.

Megakaryocytes employ their multiple DNA copies to synthesize abundant cytoplasm, which differentiates into platelets. A single megakaryocyte may shed 2000 to 4000 platelets,

a process called thrombopoiesis or *thrombocytopoiesis.* In an average-size healthy human there are 10^8 megakaryocytes producing 10^{11} platelets per day, a total turnover rate of 8 to 9 days. In instances of high platelet consumption, such as immune thrombocytopenic purpura, platelet production rises by as much as tenfold.

Terminal Megakaryocyte Differentiation

As endomitosis proceeds, megakaryocyte progenitors leave the proliferative phase and enter *terminal differentiation,* a series of stages in which microscopists become able to recognize their unique Wright-stained morphology in bone marrow aspirate films (Figure 13-3) or hematoxylin and eosin–stained bone marrow biopsy sections (Table 13-1).

Morphologists call the least differentiated megakaryocyte precursor the *MK-I stage* or *megakaryoblast.* Although they no

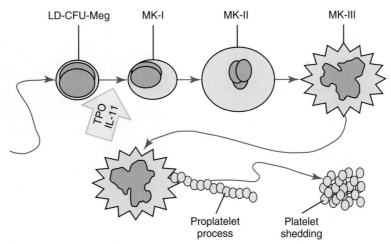

Figure 13-3 Morphologically identifiable megakaryocytes of the terminal megakaryocyte differentiation compartment. *LD-CFU-Meg,* Low-density colony forming unit megakaryocyte; *MK-I,* megakaryocyte I or megakaryoblast; *MK-II,* megakaryocyte II or promegakaryocyte; *MK-III,* megakaryocyte III or megakaryocyte; *TPO,* thrombopoietin; *IL-11,* interleukin 11.

TABLE 13-1 Features of the Three Terminal Megakaryocyte Differentiation Stages

	MK-I	MK-II	MK-III
% of precursors	20	25	55
Diameter	14—18 μm	15—40 μm	30—50 μm
Nucleus	Round	Indented	Multilobed
Nucleoli	2—6	Variable	Not visible
Chromatin	Homogeneous	Moderately condensed	Deeply and variably condensed
Nucleus-to-cytoplasm ratio	3:1	1:2	1:4
Mitosis	Absent	Absent	Absent
Endomitosis	Present	Ends	Absent
Cytoplasm	Basophilic	Basophilic and granular	Azurophilic and granular
α-Granules	Present	Present	Present
Dense granules	Present	Present	Present
Demarcation system	Present	Present	Present

MK-I, Megakaryoblast; *MK-II,* promegakaryocyte; *MK-III,* megakaryocyte.

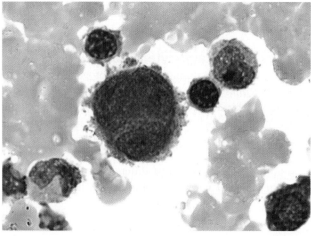

Figure 13-4 The megakaryoblast (MK-I) resembles the myeloblast and pronormoblast (rubriblasts); identification by morphology alone is inadvisable. This megakaryoblast has cytoplasmic "blebs" that resemble platelets.

longer look like lymphocytes, megakaryoblasts cannot be reliably distinguished from bone marrow myeloblasts or pronormoblasts (also named rubriblasts) using light microscopy (Figure 13-4). The morphologist may occasionally see a vague clue: plasma membrane *blebs,* blunt projections from the margin that resemble platelets. The megakaryoblast begins to develop most of its cytoplasmic ultrastructure, including procoagulant-laden α-granules, dense granules (dense bodies), and the demarcation system (DMS).[9]

The contents and functions of α-granules and dense granules are described in the subsequent sections on mature platelet ultrastructure and function. The DMS is a series of membrane-lined channels that invade from the plasma membrane and grow inward to subdivide the entire cytoplasm. The DMS is biologically identical to the megakaryocyte plasma membrane and ultimately delineates the individual platelets during thrombocytopoiesis.

Nuclear lobularity first becomes apparent as an indentation at the 4N replication stage, rendering the cell identifiable as an *MK-II* stage, or *promegakaryocyte,* by light microscopy. The morphologist seldom makes the effort to distinguish MK-I, MK-II, and MK-III stages during a routine examination of a bone marrow aspirate smear.

The promegakaryocyte reaches its full ploidy level by the end of the MK-II stage. At the most abundant *MK-III* stage, the megakaryocyte is easily recognized at 10× magnification on the basis of its 30- to 50-μm diameter (Figures 13-5 and 13-6). The nucleus is intensely indented or lobulated, and the degree of lobulation is imprecisely proportional to ploidy.

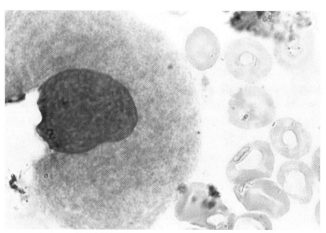

Figure 13-5 Promegakaryocyte (MK II). Cytoplasm is abundant, and nucleus shows minimal lobularity.

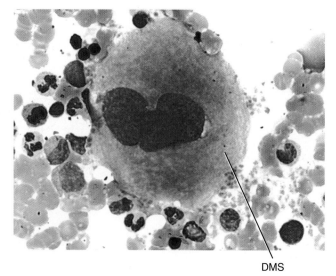

DMS

Figure 13-6 Megakaryocyte. The nucleus is lobulated with basophilic chromatin. The cytoplasm is azurophilic and granular, with evidence of the demarcation system (DMS).

When necessary, ploidy levels are measured using *mepacrine*, a nucleic acid dye in megakaryocyte flow cytometry.[10] The chromatin is variably condensed with light and dark patches. The cytoplasm is azurophilic (lavender), granular, and platelet-like because of the spread of the DMS and α-granules. At full maturation, platelet shedding, or thrombocytopoiesis, proceeds.

Megakaryocyte Membrane Receptors and Markers

In specialty and tertiary care laboratories, scientists and technicians employ immunostaining of fixed tissue, flow cytometry with immunologic probes, and fluorescent in situ hybridization (FISH) with genetic probes to identify visually indistinguishable megakaryocyte progenitors in hematologic disease. There are several flow cytometric megakaryocyte membrane markers, including MPL, which is the TPO receptor site present at all maturation stages, and the stem cell and common myeloid progenitor marker CD34. The CD34 marker disappears as differentiation proceeds. The platelet membrane glycoprotein IIb/IIIa (CD41, a marker located on the IIb portion) first appears on megakaryocyte progenitors and remains present throughout maturation, along with immunologic markers CD36, CD42, CD61, and CD62. Cytoplasmic coagulation factor VIII, von Willebrand factor (VWF), and fibrinogen, may be detected by immunostaining in the fully developed megakaryocyte (Table 13-2).[11-13]

Thrombocytopoiesis (Platelet Shedding)

Figure 13-7 shows platelet shedding, termed *thrombocytopoiesis*. One cannot find reliable evidence for platelet budding or shedding simply by examining megakaryocytes in situ, even in well-structured bone marrow biopsy preparations. However, in megakaryocyte cultures examined by transmission electron microscopy, the DMS dilates, longitudinal bundles of tubules form, proplatelet processes develop, and transverse constrictions appear throughout the proplatelet processes. In the bone marrow environment, processes are believed to pierce through or between sinusoid-lining endothelial cells, extend into the venous blood, and shed platelets (Figure 13-8). Thrombocytopoiesis leaves behind naked megakaryocyte nuclei to be consumed by marrow macrophages.[14]

Hormones and Cytokines of Megakaryocytopoiesis

The growth factor TPO is a 70,000 Dalton molecule that possesses 23% homology with the red blood cell–producing hormone erythropoietin (Table 13-3).[15] Messenger ribonucleic acid (mRNA) for TPO has been found in the kidney, liver, stromal cells, and smooth muscle cells, though the liver has the most copies and is considered the primary source. TPO circulates as a hormone in plasma and is the ligand that binds the megakaryocyte and platelet membrane receptor protein identified above, MPL, named for v-mpl, a viral oncogene associated with murine myeloproliferative leukemia. The plasma concentration of TPO is inversely proportional to platelet and megakaryocyte mass, implying that membrane binding and consequent removal of TPO by platelets is the primary platelet count control mechanism.[16] Investigators have used both in vitro and in vivo experiments to show that TPO, in synergy with other cytokines, induces stem cells to differentiate into megakaryocyte progenitors and that it further induces the differentiation of megakaryocyte progenitors into megakaryoblasts and megakaryocytes. TPO also induces the proliferation and maturation of megakaryocytes and induces thrombocytopoiesis, or platelet release (Table 13-3). Synthetic TPO mimetics (analogues) elevate the platelet count in patients being treated for a variety of cancers, including acute leukemia. One commercial MPL receptor agonist, romiplostim (NPlate™, Amgen Inc., Thousand Oaks, CA, FDA cleared in 2008), is a nonimmunogenic oligopeptide that is also effective in raising the platelet count in immune thrombocytopenic purpura.[17] A second nonpeptide MPL receptor agonist, eltrombopag (Promacta® and Revolade®, Glaxo Smith

TABLE 13-2 Markers at Each Stage of Megakaryocyte Maturation Detected by Flow Cytometry, Immunostaining, Fluorescence In Situ Hybridization, or Cytochemical Stain

	BFU-Meg	CFU-Meg	LD-CFU-Meg	MK-I	MK-II	MK-III	PLTs
MPL, TPO receptor by FCM	←——————————————————————————————————→						
CD34; stem cell marker by FCM	←———————————————→						
CD41: β3 portion of αIIbβ3; peroxidase by TEM cytochemical stain	←—————————————————————————————→						
• **CD42;** GP Ib portion of VWF receptor, by FCM • **PF4** by FCM • **VWF** by immunostaining	←——————————————→						
Fibrinogen							←——→

The arrows indicate at which stage of differentiation the marker appears and at which stage it disappears. *BFU-Meg*, Burst-forming unit–megakaryocyte; *CFU-Meg*, colony-forming unit–megakaryocyte; *LD-CFU-Meg*, low-density colony-forming unit–megakaryocyte; *MK-I*, megakaryoblast; *MK-II*, promegakaryocyte; *MK-III*, megakaryocyte; *FCM*, flow cytometry; *TEM*, transmission electron microscopy; *GP*, glycoprotein; *PF4*, platelet factor 4; *TPO*, thrombopoietin; *VWF*, von Willebrand factor

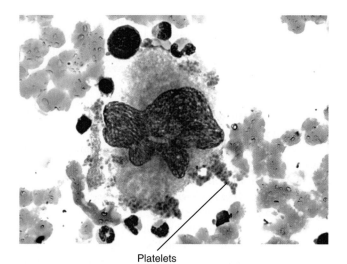

Figure 13-7 This image illustrates a terminal megakaryocyte shedding platelets.

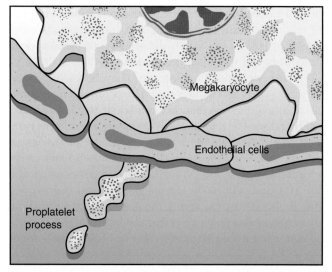

Figure 13-8 Megakaryocyte is adjacent to the abluminal (nonblood) membrane of the sinusoid-lining endothelial cell and extends a proplatelet process through or between the endothelial cells into the vascular sinus. (Modified from Powers LW: Diagnostic hematology: clinical and technical principles, St. Louis, 1989, Mosby.)

Kline, Inc., Philadelphia, PA, FDA cleared in 2011), binds and activates an MPL site separate from romiplostim. They may have additive effects.[18]

Other cytokines that function with TPO to stimulate megakaryocytopoiesis include interleukin-3 (IL-3), IL-6, and IL-11. IL-3 seems to act in synergy with TPO to induce the early differentiation of stem cells, whereas IL-6 and IL-11 act in the presence of TPO to enhance the later phenomena of endomitosis, megakaryocyte maturation, and thrombocytopoiesis. An IL-11 polypeptide mimetic, oprelvekin (Neumega®, Wyeth Ayerst Genetics Institute, Cambridge, MA, FDA cleared in 1997), stimulates platelet production in patients with chemotherapy-induced thrombocytopenia.[19] Other cytokines and hormones that participate synergistically with TPO and the interleukins are *stem cell factor,* also called *kit ligand* or *mast cell growth factor;* granulocyte-macrophage colony-stimulating factor (GM-CSF); granulocyte colony-stimulating factor (G-CSF); and *acetylcholinesterase-derived megakaryocyte growth stimulating peptide.* The list continues to grow.[20]

Platelet factor 4 (PF4), β-thromboglobulin, neutrophil-activating peptide 2, IL-8, and other factors inhibit in vitro megakaryocyte growth, which indicates that they may have a role in the control of megakaryocytopoiesis in vivo. Internally, reduction in the transcription factors FOG1, GATA-1, and NF-E2 diminish megakaryocytopoiesis at the progenitor, endomitosis, and terminal maturation phases.[21]

PLATELETS

The proplatelet process sheds platelets, cells consisting of granular cytoplasm with a membrane but no nuclear material, into the venous sinus of the bone marrow. Their diameter in the monolayer of a Wright-stained peripheral blood wedge film averages 2.5 μm. MPV, as measured in a buffered isotonic suspension flowing through the impedance-based detector cell of a clinical profiling instrument, ranges from 8 to 10 fL (Figure 1-1). A frequency distribution of platelet volume is log-normal, however, which indicates a subpopulation of large platelets (Figure 15-14). Heterogeneity in the MPV of normal healthy humans reflects random variation in platelet release volume and is not a function of platelet age or vitality, as many authors claim.[22]

TABLE 13-3 Hormones and Cytokines That Control Megakaryocytopoiesis

Cytokine/ Hormone	Differentiation to Progenitors	Differentiation to Megakaryocytes	Late Maturation	Thrombocytopoiesis	Clinical Use
TPO	+	+	+	0	Available
IL-3	+	+	0	—	—
IL-6	0	0	+	+	—
IL-11	0	+	+	+	Available

Cytokines and hormones that have been shown to interact synergistically with TPO and IL-3 include IL-6 and IL-11; stem cell factor, also called *kit ligand* or *mast cell growth factor;* granulocyte-macrophage colony–stimulating factor; granulocyte colony–stimulating factor; and erythropoietin.
Substances that inhibit megakaryocyte production include platelet factor 4, β-thromboglobulin, neutrophil-activating peptide 2, and IL-8.
IL, Interleukin; *TPO,* thrombopoietin.

Circulating, resting platelets are biconvex, although the platelets in blood collected using the anticoagulant ethylenediaminetetraacetic acid (EDTA, lavender closure tubes) tend to "round up." On a Wright-stained wedge-preparation blood film, platelets appear circular to irregular, lavender, and granular, although their small size makes them hard to examine for internal structure.[23] In the blood, their surface is even, and they flow smoothly through veins, arteries, and capillaries. In contrast to leukocytes, which tend to roll along the vascular endothelium, platelets cluster with the erythrocytes near the center of the blood vessel. Unlike erythrocytes, however, platelets move back and forth with the leukocytes from venules into the white pulp of the spleen, where both become sequestered in dynamic equilibrium.

The normal peripheral blood platelet count is 150 to 400 × 10^9/L. The count decreases after 65 years old to 122 to 350 × 10^9/L in men and 140 to 379 × 10^9/L in women. This count represents only two thirds of available platelets because the spleen sequesters an additional one third. Sequestered platelets are immediately available in times of demand—for example, in acute inflammation or after an injury, after major surgery, or during plateletpheresis. In hypersplenism or splenomegaly, increased sequestration may cause a relative thrombocytopenia. Under conditions of hemostatic need, platelets answer cellular and humoral stimuli by becoming irregular and sticky, extending pseudopods, and adhering to neighboring structures or aggregating with one another.

Reticulated platelets, sometimes known as *stress platelets*, appear in compensation for thrombocytopenia (Figure 13-9).[22] Reticulated platelets are markedly larger than ordinary mature circulating platelets; their diameter in peripheral blood films exceeds 6 μm, and their MPV reaches 12 to 14 fL.[23] Like ordinary platelets, they round up in EDTA, but in *citrated* (blue-closure tubes) whole blood, reticulated platelets are cylindrical and beaded, resembling fragments of megakaryocyte proplatelet processes. Reticulated platelets carry free ribosomes and

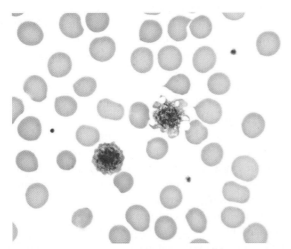

Figure 13-9 A "stress" or "reticulated" platelet. The stress platelet may appear in compensation for thrombocytopenia, which produces early and rapid proplatelet extension and release. The diameter of reticulated platelets exceeds 6 μm. Reticulated platelets carry free ribosomes and fragments of rough endoplasmic reticulum, detectable in flow cytometry using nucleic acid dyes.

fragments of rough endoplasmic reticulum, analogous to red blood cell reticulocytes, which triggers speculation that they arise from early and rapid proplatelet extension and release. Nucleic acid dyes such as thiazole orange bind the RNA of the endoplasmic reticulum. This property is exploited by profiling instruments to provide a quantitative evaluation of reticulated platelet production under stress, a measurement that may be more useful than the MPV.[24] Platelet dense granules, however, may interfere with this measurement, falsely raising the reticulated platelet count by taking up nucleic acid dyes. Reticulated platelets are potentially prothrombotic, and may be associated with increased risk of cardiovascular disease.[25-29]

PLATELET ULTRASTRUCTURE

Platelets, although anucleate, are strikingly complex and are metabolically active. Their ultrastructure has been studied using scanning and transmission electron microscopy, flow cytometry, and molecular sequencing.

Resting Platelet Plasma Membrane

The platelet *plasma membrane* resembles any biological membrane: a bilayer composed of proteins and lipids, as diagrammed in Figure 13-10. The predominant lipids are phospholipids, which form the basic structure, and cholesterol, which distributes asymmetrically throughout the phospholipids. The phospholipids form a bilayer with their polar heads oriented toward aqueous environments—toward the plasma externally and the cytoplasm internally. Their fatty acid chains, esterified to carbons 1 and 2 of the phospholipid triglyceride backbone, orient toward each other, perpendicular to the plane of the membrane, to form a hydrophobic barrier sandwiched within the hydrophilic layers.

The neutral phospholipids phosphatidylcholine and sphingomyelin predominate in the plasma layer; the anionic or polar phospholipids phosphatidylinositol, phosphatidylethanolamine, and phosphatidylserine predominate in the inner, cytoplasmic layer. These phospholipids, especially phosphatidylinositol, support platelet activation by supplying arachidonic acid, an unsaturated fatty acid that becomes converted to the eicosanoids prostaglandin and thromboxane A_2 during platelet activation. Phosphatidylserine flips to the outer surface upon activation and is the charged phospholipid surface on which the coagulation enzymes, especially coagulation factor complex VIII and IX and coagulation factor complex X and V, assemble.[30,31]

Esterified cholesterol moves freely throughout the hydrophobic internal layer, exchanging with unesterified cholesterol from the surrounding plasma. Cholesterol stabilizes the membrane, maintains fluidity, and helps control the transmembranous passage of materials.

Anchored within the membrane are glycoproteins and proteoglycans; these support surface glycosaminoglycans, oligosaccharides, and glycolipids. The platelet membrane surface, called the *glycocalyx*, also absorbs albumin, fibrinogen, and other plasma proteins, in many instances transporting them to storage organelles within using a process called *endocytosis*.

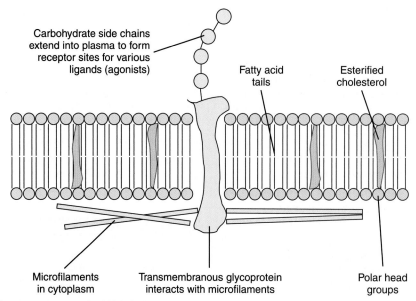

Figure 13-10 The platelet possesses a standard biological membrane composed of a phospholipid bilayer with polar head groups oriented toward the aqueous plasma and cytoplasm and nonpolar fatty acid tails that orient toward the center. The phospholipid backbone is interspersed with esterified cholesterol. A series of transmembranous proteins communicate with microfilaments, G proteins, and enzymes. The transmembranous proteins support carbohydrate side chains that extend into the plasma.

At 20 to 30 nm, the platelet glycocalyx is thicker than the analogous surface layer of leukocytes or erythrocytes. This thick layer is adhesive and responds readily to hemostatic demands. The platelet carries its functional environment with it, meanwhile maintaining a negative surface charge that repels other platelets, other blood cells, and the endothelial cells that line the blood vessels.

The plasma membrane is selectively permeable, and the membrane bilayer provides phospholipids that support platelet activation internally and plasma coagulation externally. The anchored glycoproteins support essential plasma surface–oriented glycosylated receptors that respond to cellular and humoral stimuli, called *ligands* or *agonists,* transmitting their stimulus through the membrane to internal activation organelles.

Surface-Connected Canalicular System

The plasma membrane invades the platelet interior, producing its unique surface-connected canalicular system (SCCS; Figures 13-11 and 13-12). The SCCS twists spongelike throughout the platelet, enabling the platelet to store additional quantities of the same hemostatic proteins found on the glycocalyx and raising its capacity manyfold. The SCCS also allows for enhanced interaction of the platelet with its environment, increasing access to the platelet interior as well as increasing egress of platelet release products. The glycocalyx is less developed in the SCCS and lacks some of the glycoprotein receptors present on the platelet surface. However, the SCCS is the route for endocytosis and for secretion of α-granule contents upon platelet activation.

Dense Tubular System

Parallel and closely aligned to the SCCS is the dense tubular system (DTS), a condensed remnant of the rough endoplasmic reticulum (Figures 13-11 and 13-12). Having abandoned its usual protein production function upon platelet release, the DTS sequesters Ca^{2+} and bears a series of enzymes that support platelet activation. These enzymes include phospholipase A_2, cyclooxygenase, and thromboxane synthetase, which support the eicosanoid synthesis pathway that produces thromboxane A_2, and phospholipase C, which supports production of inositol triphosphate (IP_3) and diacylglycerol (DAG). The DTS is the "control center" for platelet activation.

Platelet Plasma Membrane Receptors That Provide for Adhesion

The platelet membrane supports more than 50 categories of receptors, including members of the cell adhesion molecule (CAM) *integrin* family, the CAM *leucine-rich repeat* family, the CAM *immunoglobulin gene* family, the CAM *selectin* family, the *seven-transmembrane receptor* (STR) family, and some miscellaneous receptors.[32] Table 13-4 lists the receptors that support the initial phases of platelet adhesion and aggregation.

Several *integrins* bind collagen, enabling the platelet to adhere to the injured blood vessel lining. Integrins are heterodimeric (composed of two dissimilar proteins) CAMs that integrate their ligands, which they bind on the outside of the cell, with the internal cytoskeleton, triggering activation. GP Ia/IIa, or, using integrin terminology, $\alpha_2\beta_1$, is an integrin that binds the subendothelial collagen that becomes uncovered in the damaged blood vessel wall, promoting adhesion of the platelet to the vessel wall (Figures 13-11 and 13-12). Likewise, $\alpha_5\beta_1$ and $\alpha_6\beta_1$ bind the adhesive endothelial cell proteins *laminin* and *fibronectin,* which further promotes platelet adhesion. Another collagen-binding receptor is GP VI, a member of the *immunoglobulin gene* family, so named because the genes of its members have multiple immunoglobulin-like domains. The

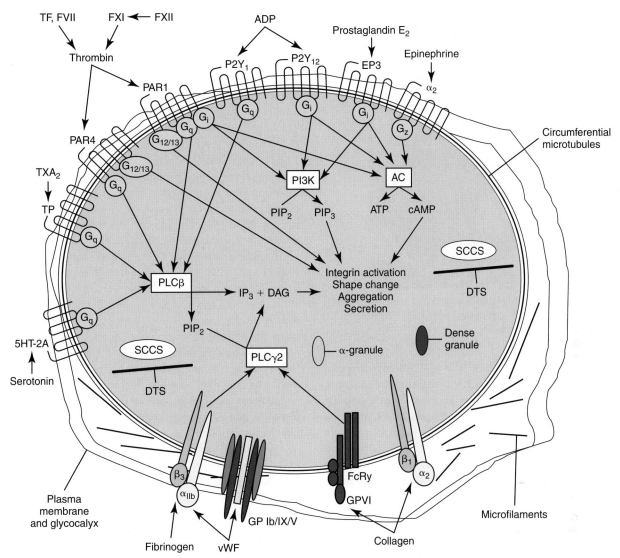

Figure 13-11 Circulating nonactivated platelet illustrating membrane receptors and activation pathways. The STR receptors include the serotonin receptor 5HT-2A, TXA$_2$ receptor TP, thrombin receptors PAR1 and PAR4, ADP receptors P2Y$_1$ and P2Y$_{12}$, prostaglandin E$_2$ receptor EP3, and epinephrine receptor, α_2. Integrins include collagen receptor $\beta_1\alpha_2$ and fibrinogen/VWF receptor $\beta_3\alpha_{IIb}$. The key collagen receptor is GPVI, and the key VWF receptor is GP Ib/IX/V. The STR receptors are coupled to G-proteins, which become stimulated when agonists bind their respective receptors to subsequently activate enzymes PLCβ, PI3K, and AC. The activated enzymes in turn activate the PIP$_2$ pathway to produce IP$_3$ and DAG and the eicosanoid synthesis pathway (not shown) to produce TXA$_2$ and cAMP. The integrins and GPs activate PLCγ2 that also activates the PIP$_2$ pathway. These generate shape change, secretion, and aggregation. *DTS*, Dense tubular system; *SCCS*, surface-connected canalicular system; *TF*, tissue factor; *TXA$_2$*, thromboxane A$_2$; *TP*, TXA$_2$ receptor; *PAR1* and *PAR4*, protease activated receptors that are activated by thrombin; *GPVI*, glycoprotein VI collagen receptor; *GP Ib/IX/V*, complex of glycoproteins Ib, IX, and V, which is the VWF receptor; *VWF*, von Willebrand factor; *PLCγ2, phospholipase Cγ2; PLCβ, phospholipase Cβ; PI3K*, phosphoinositide-3-kinase; *AC*, adenyl cyclase; *PIP2*, phosphotidylinositol-4-5 bisphosphate; *PIP3*, phosphotidylinositol-4-5 triphosphate; *IP3*, inositol-1-4-5-triphosphate; *DAG*, diacyl glycerol.

unclassified platelet receptor GP IV is a key collagen receptor that also binds the adhesive protein *thrombospondin*.[33]

Another adhesion receptor is GP Ib/IX/V, a *leucine-rich-repeat* family CAM, named for its members' multiple leucine-rich domains. GP Ib/IX/V arises from the genes *GP1BA, GP1BB, GP5*, and *GP9*. It is composed of two molecules each of GP Ibα, GP Ibβ, and GP IX, and one molecule of GP V. These total seven noncovalently bound subunits. The two copies of subunit GP Ibα bind VWF and support platelet *tethering* (deceleration), necessary in capillaries and arterioles where blood flow shear rates exceed 1000 s^{-1}. The accompanying GP Ibβ molecules cross the platelet membrane and interact with

actin-binding protein to provide "outside-in" signaling. Two molecules of GP IX and one of GP V help assemble the four GP Ib molecules. Mutations in GP Ibα, GP Ibβ, or GP IX (but not GP V) are associated with a moderate-to-severe mucocutaneous bleeding disorder, Bernard-Soulier syndrome (Chapter 41). Additionally, VWF deficiency is the basis for the most common inherited bleeding disorder, von Willebrand disease (VWD). VWD also is associated with mucocutaneous bleeding, although the disorder is technically a plasma protein (VWF) deficiency, not a platelet abnormality.[34]

The subunits of the integrin GP IIb/IIIa ($\alpha_{IIb}\beta_3$), are separate and inactive (α_{IIb} and β_3) as they are distributed across the

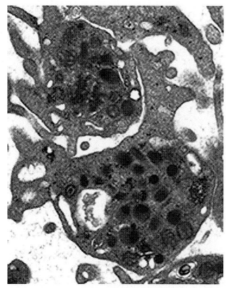

Figure 13-12 Transmission electron micrograph of a circulating nonactivated platelet. Visible are α-granules, vacuoles, and fragments of the surface-connected canalicular system.

plasma membrane, the SCCS, and the internal layer of α-granule membranes. These form their active heterodimer, $\alpha_{IIb}\beta_3$, only when they encounter an "inside-out" signaling mechanism triggered by collagen binding to GP VI. Although various agonists may activate the platelet, $\alpha_{IIb}\beta_3$ is a physiologic requisite because it binds fibrinogen, generating interplatelet cohesion, called platelet aggregation. Mutations in α_{IIb} or β_3 cause a severe inherited mucocutaneous bleeding disorder, Glanzmann thrombasthenia (Chapter 41). The $\alpha_{IIb}\beta_3$ integrin also binds VWF, vitronectin, and fibronectin, all adhesive proteins that share the target *arginine-glycine-aspartate* (RGD) amino acid sequence with fibrinogen.[35,36]

The Seven-Transmembrane Repeat Receptors

Thrombin, thrombin receptor activation peptide (TRAP), adenosine diphosphate (ADP), epinephrine, and the eicosanoid synthesis pathway (also called the prostaglandin or the cyclooxygenase pathway) product thromboxane A_2 (TXA_2) all function individually or together to activate platelets (Figures 13-11 and 13-12). These platelet "agonists" are ligands for the seven-transmembrane repeat receptors (STRs), so named for their unique membrane-anchoring structure. The STRs have seven hydrophobic anchoring domains supporting an external binding site and an internal terminus that interacts with G proteins for outside-in platelet signaling. The STRs are listed in Table 13-5.[37]

Thrombin *cleaves* two STRs, protease-activated receptor 1 (PAR1) and PAR4, that together have a total of 1800 membrane copies on an average platelet. Thrombin cleavage of either of these two receptors activates the platelet through G-proteins that in turn activate at least two internal physiologic pathways, described subsequently. Thrombin also interacts with platelets by binding or digesting two CAMs in the leucine-rich repeat family, GP Ibα and GP V, both of which are parts of the GP Ib/IX/V VWF adhesion receptor.[37]

There are about 600 copies of the high-affinity ADP receptors P2Y$_1$ and P2Y$_{12}$ per platelet. These STRs also activate the platelet through the G-protein signaling pathways.[38]

TPα and TPβ bind TXA_2. This interaction produces more TXA_2 from the platelet, a G-protein based autocrine (self-perpetuating) system that activates neighboring platelets. Epinephrine binds α_2-adrenergic sites that also couple to G-proteins and open up membrane calcium channels. The

TABLE 13-4 Glycoprotein Platelet Membrane Receptors That Participate in Adhesion and the Initiation of Aggregation by Binding Specific Ligands

Electrophoresis Nomenclature	Current Nomenclature	Ligand	Cluster Designation	Comments
GP Ia/IIa	Integrin: $\alpha_2\beta_1$	Collagen	CD29, CD49b	Avidity is upregulated via "inside-out" activation that depends on collagen binding to GP VI.
	Integrin: $\alpha_v\beta_1$	Vitronectin		
	Integrin: $\alpha_5\beta_1$	Laminin	CD29, CD49e	
	Integrin: $\alpha_6\beta_1$	Fibronectin	CD29, CD49f	
GP VI	CAM of the immunoglobulin gene family	Collagen		Key collagen receptor, triggers activation, release of agonists that increase the avidity of integrins $\alpha_2\beta_1$ and $\alpha_{IIb}\beta_3$.
GP Ib/IX/V	CAM of the leucine-rich repeat family	VWF and thrombin bind GP Ibα; thrombin cleaves a site on GP V	CD42a, CD42b, CD42c, CD42d	GP Ib/IX/V is a 2:2:2:1 complex of GP Ibα and Ibβ, GP IX, and GP V. There are 25,000 copies on the resting platelet membrane surface, 5% to 10% on the α-granule membrane, but few on the SCCS membrane. GP Ibα is the VWF-specific site. Fifty percent of GP Ibα/Ibβ is cleared from the membrane on activation. Bernard-Soulier syndrome mutations are identified for all but GP V. Bound to subsurface actin-binding protein.
GP IIb/IIIa	Integrin: $\alpha_{IIb}\beta_3$	Fibrinogen, VWF	CD41, CD61	GP IIb and IIIa are distributed on the surface membrane, SCCS, and α-granule membranes (30%). Heterodimer forms on activation.

CAM, Cell adhesion molecule; *GP,* glycoprotein; *SCCS,* surface-connected canalicular system; *VWF,* von Willebrand factor.

TABLE 13-5 Platelet STR Receptor-Ligand Interaction Coupled to Signaling

Receptor	Ligand	G Proteins
PAR1	Thrombin	Coupled to G_i protein that reduces cAMP; coupled to G_q and G_{12} proteins that increase IP_3 and DAG
PAR4	Thrombin	Coupled to G_q and G_{12} proteins that increase IP_3 and DAG
P2Y$_1$	ADP	Coupled to G_q protein that increases IP_3 and DAG
P2Y$_{12}$	ADP	Coupled to G_i protein that reduces cAMP
TPα and TPβ	TXA$_2$	Coupled to G_q protein that increases IP_3 and DAG
α$_2$-adrenergic	Epinephrine	Coupled to G_i protein that reduces cAMP; potentiates effects of ADP, thrombin, and TXA$_2$
IP	PGI$_2$	Coupled to G_s protein that increases cAMP to inhibit activation

STRs are named for their peculiar sevenfold membrane anchorage. These receptors mediate "outside-in" platelet activation by transmitting signals initiated by external ligand binding to internal G proteins.
ADP, Adenosine diphosphate; *cAMP,* cyclic adenosine monophosphate; *DAG,* diacylglycerol; *IP$_3$,* inositol triphosphate; *PAR,* protease-activated receptor; *PGI$_2$,* prostaglandin I$_2$ (prostacyclin); *STR,* seven-transmembrane receptor; *TXA$_2$,* thromboxane A$_2$; *P2Y$_1$* and *P2Y$_{12}$,* ADP receptors; *TPα* and *TPβ,* thromboxane receptors; *IP,* PGI$_2$ receptor.

α$_2$-adrenergic sites function similarly to those located on heart muscle. Finally, the receptor site IP binds *prostacyclin* (prostaglandin I$_2$, PGI$_2$), a prostaglandin produced from endothelial cells. Prostacyclin enters the platelet and raises the internal cyclic adenosine monophosphate (cAMP) concentration of the platelet, thus blocking platelet activation. The platelet membrane also presents STRs for serotonin, platelet-activating factor, prostaglandin E$_2$, PF4, and β-thromboglobulin.[39]

Additional Platelet Membrane Receptors

About 15 clinically relevant receptors were discussed in the preceding paragraphs. The platelet supports many additional receptors. The CAM immunoglobulin family includes the ICAMs (CD50, CD54, CD102), which play a role in inflammation and the immune reaction; PECAM (CD31), which mediates platelet–to–white blood cell and platelet–to–endothelial cell adhesion; and FcγIIA (CD32), a low-affinity receptor for the immunoglobulin Fc portion that plays a role in a dangerous condition called heparin-induced thrombocytopenia (Chapter 39).[40] P-selectin (CD62) is an integrin that facilitates platelet binding to endothelial cells, leukocytes, and one another.[41] P-selectin is found on the α-granule membranes of the resting platelet but migrates via the SCCS to the surface of activated platelets. P-selectin or CD62 quantification by flow cytometry is a successful clinical means for measuring in vivo platelet activation.

Platelet Cytoskeleton: Microfilaments and Microtubules

A thick circumferential bundle of microtubules maintains the platelet's discoid shape. The *circumferential microtubules*

(Figures 13-11 and 13-12) parallel the plane of the outer surface of the platelet and reside just within, although not touching, the plasma membrane. There are 8 to 20 tubules composed of multiple subunits of tubulin that disassemble at refrigerator temperature or when treated with colchicine. When microtubules disassemble in the cold, platelets become round, but upon warming to 37° C, they recover their original disc shape. On cross section, microtubules are cylindrical, with a diameter of 25 nm. The circumferential microtubules could be a single spiral tubule.[42] Besides maintaining the platelet shape, microtubules move inward on activation to enable the expression of α-granule contents. They also reassemble in long parallel bundles during platelet shape change to provide rigidity to pseudopods.

In the narrow area between the microtubules and the membrane lies a thick meshwork of microfilaments composed of actin (Figures 13-11 and 13-12). Actin is contractile in platelets (as in muscle) and anchors the plasma membrane glycoproteins and proteoglycans. Actin also is present throughout the platelet cytoplasm, constituting 20% to 30% of platelet protein. In the resting platelet, actin is globular and amorphous, but as the cytoplasmic calcium concentration rises, actin becomes filamentous and contractile.

The cytoplasm also contains intermediate filaments, ropelike polymers 8 to 12 nm in diameter, of *desmin* and *vimentin.* The intermediate filaments connect with actin and the tubules, maintaining the platelet shape. Microtubules, actin microfilaments, and intermediate microfilaments control platelet shape change, extension of pseudopods, and secretion of granule contents.

Platelet Granules: α-Granules, Dense Granules, and Lysosomes

There are 50 to 80 α-granules in each platelet. Unlike the nearly opaque dense granules, α-granules stain medium gray in osmium-dye transmission electron microscopy preparations (Figures 13-11 and 13-12). The α-granules are filled with proteins, some endocytosed, some synthesized within the megakaryocyte and stored in platelets (Table 13-6). Several α-granule proteins are membrane bound. As the platelet becomes activated, α-granule membranes fuse with the SCCS. Their contents flow to the nearby microenvironment, where they participate in platelet adhesion and aggregation and support plasma coagulation.[43]

There are two to seven dense granules per platelet. Also called dense bodies, these granules appear later than α-granules in megakaryocyte differentiation and stain black (opaque) when treated with osmium in transmission electron microscopy (Figures 13-11 and 13-12). Small molecules are probably endocytosed and are stored in the dense granules; these are listed in Table 13-7. In contrast to the α-granules, which employ the SCCS, dense granules migrate to the plasma membrane and release their contents directly into the plasma upon platelet activation. Membranes of dense granules support the same integral proteins as the α-granules—P-selectin, α$_{IIb}$β$_3$, and GP Ib/IX/V, for instance—which implies a common source for the membranes of both types of granules.[44]

TABLE 13-6 Representative Platelet α-Granule Proteins

	Coagulation Proteins	Noncoagulation Proteins
Proteins Present in Platelet Cytoplasm and α-Granules		
Endocytosed	Fibronectin	Albumin
	Fibrinogen	Immunoglobulins
Megakaryocyte-synthesized	Factor V	—
	Thrombospondin	—
	VWF	—
Proteins Present in α-Granules but Not Cytoplasm		
Megakaryocyte-Synthesized	β-thromboglobulin	EGF
	HMWK	Multimerin
	PAI-1	PDC1
	Plasminogen	PDGF
	PF4	TGF-β
	Protein C inhibitor	VEGF/VPF
Platelet Membrane-Bound Proteins		
Restricted to α-granule membrane	P-selectin	GMP33
	—	Osteonectin
In α-granule and plasma membrane	GP IIb/IIIa	cap1
	GP IV	CD9
	GP Ib/IX/V	PECAM-1

EGF, Endothelial growth factor; *GMP,* guanidine monophosphate; *GP,* glycoprotein; *HMWK,* high-molecular-weight kininogen; *Ig,* immunoglobulin; *PAI-1,* plasminogen activator inhibitor-1; *PDCI,* platelet-derived collagenase inhibitor; *PDGF,* platelet-derived growth factor; *PECAM-1,* platelet–endothelial cell adhesion molecule-1; *PF4,* platelet factor 4; *TGF-β,* transforming growth factor-*β;* *VEGF/VPF,* vascular endothelial growth factor/vascular permeability factor; *VWF,* von Willebrand factor; *cap1,* adenyl cyclase–associated protein.

TABLE 13-7 Dense Granule (Dense Body) Contents

Small Molecule	Comment
ADP	Nonmetabolic, supports neighboring platelet aggregation by binding to ADP receptors P2Y$_1$, P2Y$_{12}$
ATP	Function unknown, but ATP release is detectable upon platelet activation
Serotonin	Vasoconstrictor that binds endothelial cells and platelet membranes
Ca^{2+} and Mg^{2+}	Divalent cations support platelet activation and coagulation

ADP, Adenosine diphosphate; *ATP,* adenosine triphosphate; *P2Y$_1$ and P2Y$_{12}$,* members of the purigenic receptor family (receptors that bind purines).

Platelets also have a few lysosomes, similar to those in neutrophils, 300-nm-diameter granules that stain positive for arylsulfatase, β-glucuronidase, acid phosphatase, and catalase. The lysosomes probably digest vessel wall matrix components during in vivo aggregation and may also digest autophagic debris.

PLATELET ACTIVATION

Although the following discussion seems to imply a linear and stepwise process, adhesion, aggregation, and secretion are often simultaneous.[45,46]

Adhesion: Platelets Bind Elements of the Vascular Matrix

As blood flows, vessel walls create stress, or shear force, measured in units labeled s^{-1}. Shear forces range from 500 s^{-1} in venules and veins to 5000 s^{-1} in arterioles and capillaries and up to 40,000 s^{-1} in stenosed (hardened) arteries (Figure 13-13). In vessels where the shear rate is over 1000 s^{-1}, platelet adhesion and aggregation require a defined sequence of events that involves collagen, tissue factor, phospholipid, VWF, and a number of platelet CAMs, ligands, and activators (Figure 13-14).[47]

Injury to the blood vessel wall disrupts the collagen of the extracellular matrix (ECM).[48] Damaged endothelial cells release VWF from cytoplasmic storage organelles (Figure 13-15).[49] VWF, whose molecular weight ranges from 800,000 to 2,000,000 Daltons "unrolls" like a carpet and adheres to the injured site. Though VWF circulates as a globular protein, it become fibrillar as it unrolls and exposes sites that partially bind the GPIbα portion of the platelet membrane GP Ib/IX/V leucine-rich receptor. This is a reversible binding process that "tethers" or decelerates the platelet. Platelet and VWF interactions remain localized by a liver-secreted plasma enzyme, ADAMTS-13, also called *VWF-cleaving protease,* that digests "unused" VWF.

At high shear rates, the VWF-GP Ibα tethering reaction is temporary, and the platelet rolls along the surface unless GP VI comes in contact with the exposed ECM collagen.[50] When type I fibrillar collagen binds platelet GP VI, the receptor, which is anchored in the membrane by an Fc receptor–like molecule, triggers internal platelet activation pathways, releasing TXA$_2$ and ADP, an "outside-in" reaction.[51] These agonists attach to their respective receptors: TPα and TPβ for TXA$_2$, and P2Y$_1$ and P2Y$_{12}$ for ADP, triggering an "inside-out" reaction that raises the affinity of integrin α$_2$β$_1$ for collagen. The combined effect of GP Ib/IX/V, GP VI, and α$_2$β$_1$ causes the platelet to become firmly affixed to the damaged surface, where it subsequently loses its discoid shape and spreads.[52]

The internal platelet activators TXA$_2$ and ADP are also secreted from the platelet to the microenvironment, where they activate neighboring platelets through their respective receptors. Further, they provide inside-out activation of integrin α$_{IIb}$β$_3$, the key receptor site for fibrinogen, which assists in platelet aggregation.

Aggregation: Platelets Irreversibly Cohere

In addition to collagen exposure and VWF secretion, blood vessel injury releases constitutive (integral) *tissue factor* from endothelial cells. Tissue factor triggers the production of thrombin, which reacts with platelet STRs PAR1 and PAR4. This further activation generates the "collagen and thrombin activated" or *COAT* platelet, integral to the cell-based coagulation model

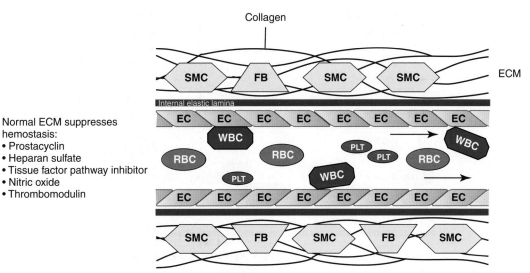

Figure 13-13 Normal blood flow in intact vessels. RBCs and platelets flow near the center, and WBCs marginate and roll. Endothelial cells and the ECM provide several properties that suppress hemostasis. *EC,* Endothelial cell; *ECM,* extracellular matrix; *FB,* fibroblast; *PLT,* platelet; *RBC,* red blood cell; *SMC,* smooth muscle cell; *WBC,* white blood cell.

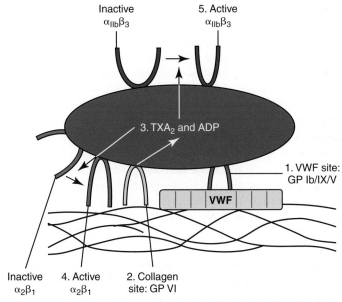

Figure 13-14 Initial platelet activation leading to platelet adhesion. The glycoprotein (GP) 1bα portion of the GP Ib/IX/V von Willebrand factor (VWF) receptor site binds VWF (1) and GP VI binds collagen (2). The bound GP VI initiates the release of thromboxane A$_2$ (TXA$_2$) and adenosine diphosphate (ADP, 3), which activate α$_2$β$_1$, an additional collagen receptor (4), stabilizing platelet adhesion, and α$_{IIb}$β$_3$, the arginine-glycine-aspartate (RGD) receptor site (5) that binds fibrinogen and VWF to support platelet aggregation.

described in Chapter 37 (Figure 13-16). Meanwhile, integrin α$_{IIb}$β$_3$ assembles from its resting membrane units α$_{IIb}$ and β$_3$, binding RGD sequences of fibrinogen and VWF and supports platelet-to-platelet aggregation. P-selectin from the α-granule membranes moves to the surface membrane to further promote aggregation. Platelets lose their shape and extend pseudopods. Membrane phospholipids redeploy with the more polar molecules, especially phosphatidylserine, flipping to the outer layer, establishing a surface for the assembly of coagulation

factor complexes. As platelet aggregation continues, membrane integrity is lost, and a syncytium of platelet cytoplasm forms as the platelets exhaust internal energy sources.

Platelet aggregation is a key part of primary hemostasis, which in arteries may end with the formation of a "white clot," a clot composed primarily of platelets and VWF (Figure 13-17). Although aggregation is a normal part of vessel repair, white clots often imply inappropriate platelet activation in seemingly uninjured arterioles and arteries and are the pathological basis for arterial thrombotic events, such as acute myocardial infarction, peripheral artery disease, and strokes. The risk of these cardiovascular events rises in proportion to the numbers and avidity of platelet membrane α$_2$β$_1$ and GP VI.[53]

The combination of polar phospholipid exposure on activated platelets, platelet fragmentation with cellular microparticle dispersion, and secretion of the platelet's α-granule and dense granule contents triggers secondary hemostasis, called *coagulation* (see Chapter 37). Fibrin and red blood cells deposit around and within the platelet syncytium, forming a bulky "red clot" (Figure 13-18). The red clot is essential to wound repair, but it may also be characteristic of inappropriate coagulation in venules and veins, resulting in deep vein thrombosis and pulmonary emboli.

Secretion: Activated Platelets Release Granular Contents

Outside-in platelet activation through ligand (agonist) binding to integrins, STRs (such as ADP binding to P2Y$_{12}$), and the immunoglobulin gene product GP VI triggers actin microfilament contraction. Intermediate filaments also contract, moving the circumferential microtubules inward and compressing the granules. Contents of α-granules and lysosomes flow through the SCCS, while dense granules migrate to the plasma membrane, where their contents are secreted (Figure 13-11). The dense granule contents are vasoconstrictors and platelet agonists that amplify primary hemostasis; most of the α-granule

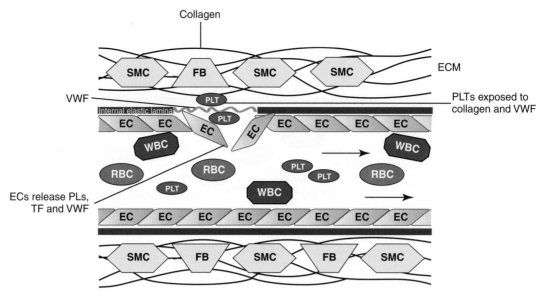

Figure 13-15 Trauma to the blood vessel wall exposes collagen and tissue factor, triggering platelet adhesion and aggregation. *EC,* Endothelial cell; *ECM,* extracellular matrix; *FB,* fibroblast; *PL,* phospholipid; *PLT,* platelet; *RBC,* red blood cell; *SMC,* smooth muscle cell; *TF,* tissue factor; *VWF,* von Willebrand factor; *WBC,* white blood cell.

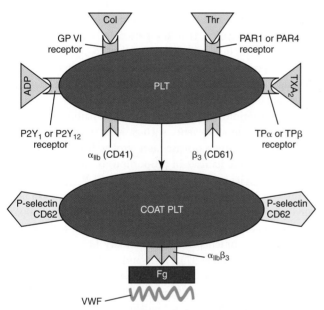

Figure 13-16 Further activation yields the "collagen and thrombin activated (COAT)" platelet (PLT) leading to aggregation. Platelets become activated by agonists—for example, adenosine diphosphate (ADP), thromboxane A_2 (TXA$_2$), collagen (Col), or thrombin (Thr). P-selectin (CD 62) moves from the α-granules to the platelet membrane to support adhesion. The inactive α_{IIb} and β_3 units assemble to form the active arginine-glycine-aspartate (RGD) receptor $\alpha_{IIb}\beta_3$, which binds fibrinogen (Fg) and von Willebrand factor (VWF).

contents are coagulation proteins that participate in secondary hemostasis (Tables 13-6 and 13-7).

By presenting polar phospholipids on their membrane surfaces, platelets provide a localized cellular milieu that supports coagulation. Phosphatidylserine is the polar phospholipid on which two coagulation pathway complexes assemble: *factor*

IX/VIII (*tenase*) and factor *X/V* (*prothrombinase*), both supported by ionic calcium secreted by the dense granules. The α-granule contents fibrinogen, factors V and VIII, and VWF (which binds and stabilizes factor VIII) are secreted and increase the localized concentrations of these essential coagulation proteins. Their presence further supports the action of tenase and prothrombinase. Platelet secretions provide for cell-based, controlled, localized coagulation. Table 13-8 lists some additional α-granule secretion products that, although not proteins of the coagulation pathway, indirectly support hemostasis. The lists in Tables 13-6, 13-7, and 13-8 are not exhaustive because more and more platelet granule contents continue to be identified through platelet research activities.

PLATELET ACTIVATION PATHWAYS

G Proteins

G proteins control cellular activation for all cells (not just platelets) at the inner membrane surface (Figure 13-19). G proteins are $\alpha\beta\gamma$ heterotrimers (proteins composed of three dissimilar peptides) that bind guanosine diphosphate (GDP) when inactive. Membrane receptor-ligand (agonist) binding promotes GDP release and its replacement with guanosine triphosphate (GTP). The Gα portion of the three-part G molecule briefly disassociates, exerts enzymatic guanosine triphosphatase activity, and hydrolyzes the bound GTP to GDP, releasing a phosphate radical. The G protein resumes its resting state, but the hydrolysis step provides the necessary phosphorylation trigger to energize the eicosanoid synthesis or the IP$_3$-DAG pathway (Table 13-9).

Eicosanoid Synthesis

The *eicosanoid synthesis* pathway, alternatively called the *prostaglandin, cyclooxygenase,* or *thromboxane* pathway, is one of two essential platelet activation pathways triggered by G proteins

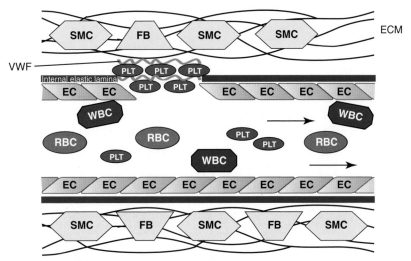

Figure 13-17 In arteries and arterioles, the "white clot" consists of platelets and von Willebrand factor. Though primarily a protective mechanism, the white clot may occlude the vessel, causing acute myocardial infarction, stroke, or peripheral artery disease. *EC,* Endothelial cell; *ECM,* extracellular matrix; *SMC,* smooth muscle cell; *FB,* fibroblast; *PLT,* platelet; *RBC,* red blood cell; *WBC,* white blood cell; *VWF,* von Willebrand factor; *lines* indicate collagen.

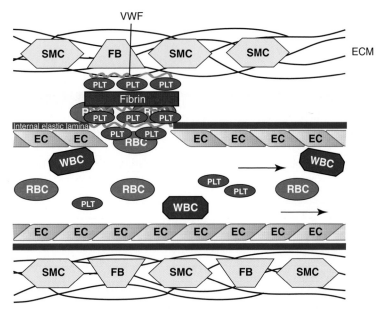

Figure 13-18 In veins and venules, the bulky "red clot" consists of platelets, von Willebrand factor, fibrin, and RBCs. Though a protective mechanism, the red clot may occlude the vessel, causing venous thromboembolic disease. *EC,* Endothelial cell; *ECM,* extracellular matrix; *SMC,* smooth muscle cell; *FB,* fibroblast; *PLT,* platelet; *RBC,* red blood cell; *WBC,* white blood cell; *VWF,* von Willebrand factor; *lines* indicate collagen.

TABLE 13-8   Selected α-Granule Proteins and Their Properties

α-Granule Protein	Properties
Platelet-derived growth factor	Supports mitosis of vascular fibroblasts and smooth muscle cells
Endothelial growth factor	Supports mitosis of vascular fibroblasts and smooth muscle cells
Transforming growth factor-β	Supports mitosis of vascular fibroblasts and smooth muscle cells
Fibronectin	Adhesion molecule
Thrombospondin	Adhesion molecule
Platelet factor 4	Heparin neutralization, suppresses megakaryocytopoiesis
β-thromboglobulin	Found nowhere but platelet α-granules
Plasminogen	Fibrinolysis promotion
Plasminogen activator inhibitor-1	Fibrinolysis control
α$_2$-Antiplasmin	Fibrinolysis control
Protein C inhibitor	Coagulation control

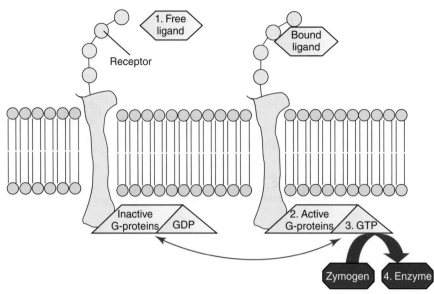

Figure 13-19 G-protein mechanism. (1) A ligand (agonist) binds its corresponding receptor; (2) G-protein swaps GDP for GTP; (3) GTP donates a high energy phosphate radical to a zymogen, remains attached to the G-protein as GDP; (4) the zymogen is activated. The G-protein returns to a resting state bound to GDP. *GDP,* Guanosine diphosphate.

TABLE 13-9 G Proteins in Platelets and Their Functions

G Protein	Coupled to Receptor	Agonist (Ligand)	Action	Outcome
G_1	PAR1	Thrombin	Decelerates adenylate cyclase	Reduce cAMP concentration
	$P2Y_{12}$	ADP		
	α_2-adrenergic	Epinephrine		
G_q	PAR1	Thrombin	Activates phospholipase C	Increase IP_3-DAG
	PAR4	Thrombin		
	$P2Y_1$	ADP		
	TPα and TPβ	TXA_2		
G_{12}	PAR1	Thrombin	Activates protein kinase C	Activate pleckstrin, actin microfilaments
	PAR4	Thrombin		
	$P2Y_1$	ADP		
	TPα and TPβ	TXA_2		
G_s	IP	Prostacyclin	Accelerates adenylate cyclase	Increase cAMP concentration

ADP, Adenosine diphosphate; *cAMP,* cyclic adenosine monophosphate; *DAG,* diacylglycerol; *IP₃,* inositol triphosphate; *PAR,* protease-activated receptor; *TXA₂,* thromboxane A₂; *P2Y₁ and P2Y₁₂,* ADP receptors; *TPα and TPβ,* thromboxane receptors; *IP,* PGI₂ receptor.

(Figure 13-20). The platelet membrane's inner leaflet is rich in phosphatidylinositol, a phospholipid whose number 2 carbon binds numerous types of unsaturated fatty acids, but especially 5,8,11,14-eicosatetraenoic acid, commonly called *arachidonic acid.* Membrane receptor-ligand binding and the consequent G-protein activation triggers phospholipase A_2, a membrane enzyme that cleaves the ester bond connecting the number 2 carbon of the triglyceride backbone with arachidonic acid. Cleavage releases arachidonic acid to the cytoplasm, where it becomes the substrate for *cyclooxygenase,* anchored in the DTS. Cyclooxygenase converts arachidonic acid to prostaglandin G_2 and prostaglandin H_2, and then thromboxane synthetase acts on prostaglandin H_2 to produce TXA_2. TXA_2 binds membrane receptors TPα or TPβ, decelerating adenylate cyclase activity

and reducing cAMP concentrations, which mobilizes ionic calcium from the DTS (Figure 13-21). The rising cytoplasmic calcium level causes contraction of actin microfilaments and platelet activation.

The cyclooxygenase pathway in endothelial cells incorporates the enzyme prostacyclin synthetase in place of the thromboxane synthetase in platelets. The eicosanoid pathway end point for the endothelial cell is prostaglandin I_2, or prostacyclin, which infiltrates the platelet and binds its IP receptor site. Prostacyclin binding accelerates adenylate cyclase, increasing cAMP, and sequesters ionic calcium to the DTS. The endothelial cell pathway suppresses platelet activation in the intact blood vessel through this mechanism, creating a dynamic equilibrium.

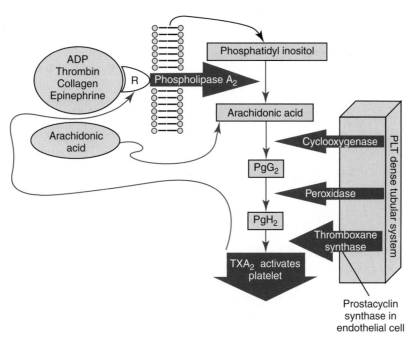

Figure 13-20 Eicosanoid synthesis. Ligands (agonists) ADP, thrombin, collagen, or epinephrine bind their respective membrane receptors. The combination activates phospholipase A_2 through the G-protein mechanism described in Figure 13-19. Phospholipase A_2 releases arachidonic acid from membrane phosphatidyl inositol. Arachidonic acid is acted upon by cyclooxygenase, peroxidase, and thromboxane synthase to produce TXA_2, which activates the platelet through adenylate cyclase, as shown in Figure 13-21. When reagent arachidonic acid is used as an agonist, it bypasses the membrane and directly enters the eicosanoid synthesis pathway. In the endothelial cell, the eicosanoid pathway is nearly identical, except that prostacyclin synthase replaces thromboxane synthase. *ADP,* Adenosine diphosphate; *PgG2,* prostaglandin G_2; *PgH2,* prostaglandin H_2; *TXA2,* thromboxane A_2.

TXA_2 has a half-life of 30 seconds, diffuses from the platelet, and becomes spontaneously reduced to thromboxane B_2, a stable, measurable plasma metabolite. Efforts to produce a clinical assay for plasma thromboxane B_2 have been unsuccessful, because special specimen management is required to prevent ex vivo platelet activation with unregulated release of thromboxane B_2 subsequent to collection. Thromboxane B_2 is acted on by a variety of liver enzymes to produce an array of soluble urine metabolites, including 11-dehydrothromboxane B_2, which is stable and measurable.[54,55]

Inositol Triphosphate–Diacylglycerol Activation Pathway

The IP_3-DAG pathway is the second G protein–dependent platelet activation pathway (Figure 13-22). G-protein activation triggers the enzyme phospholipase C. Phospholipase C

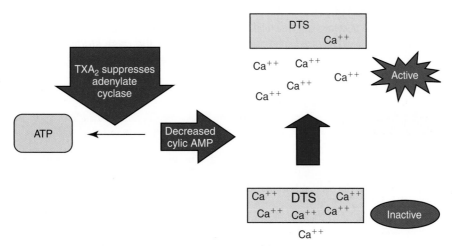

Figure 13-21 The second messenger system. In the platelet, TXA_2 suppresses adenylate cyclase and reduces cyclic AMP concentration. This allows the release of ionic calcium from the DTS. Ionic calcium supports the contraction of actin microfilaments, activating the platelet. In the endothelial cell, prostacyclin (not pictured) has the opposite effect upon adenylate cyclase, raising cyclic AMP and sequestering ionic calcium in the DTS. *ATP,* Adenosine triphosphate; *AMP,* adenosine monophosphate; *DTS,* dense tubular system; *TXA2,* thromboxane A_2.

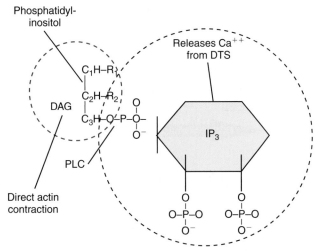

Figure 13-22 PLC is activated by the G-protein mechanism and cleaves the phosphodiester bond from carbon 3 of phosphatidylinositol. One product is DAG, which directly generates actin microfilament contraction. The other product is IP3, which releases ionic calcium from the DTS. *DAG,* Diacylglycerol; *DTS,* dense tubular system; *IP3,* inositol triphosphate; *PLC,* phospholipase C; *R1,* saturated fatty acid remains attached to carbon 1; *R2,* unsaturated fatty acid remains attached to carbon 2. (Courtesy of Larry D. Brace, PhD, Edward Hospital, Naperville, IL.)

cleaves membrane phosphatidylinositol 4,5-bisphosphate to form IP_3 and DAG, both second messengers for intracellular activation. IP_3 promotes release of ionic calcium from the DTS, which triggers actin microfilament contraction. IP_3 may also activate phospholipase A_2. DAG triggers a multistep process: activation of phosphokinase C, which triggers phosphorylation of the protein pleckstrin, which regulates actin microfilament contraction.

Internal platelet activation pathways, like internal pathways of all metabolically active cells, are often called *second messengers* because they are triggered by a primary ligand-receptor binding event. Second messengers include G proteins, the eicosanoid synthesis pathway, the IP_3-DAG pathway, adenylate cyclase, cAMP, and intracellular ionic calcium. This discussion has been limited to activation pathways whose aberrations cause hemostatic disease. The reader is referred to cell physiology texts for a comprehensive discussion of cellular activation pathways.

SUMMARY

- Platelets arise from bone marrow megakaryocytes, which reside adjacent to the venous sinusoid. Megakaryocyte progenitors are recruited by IL-3, IL-6, IL-11, and TPO and mature via endomitosis.
- Platelets are released into the bone marrow through shedding from megakaryocyte proplatelet processes, a process called *thrombocytopoiesis.*
- Circulating platelets are complex anucleate cells with a thick surface glycocalyx bearing an assortment of coagulation factors and plasma proteins.
- Platelets' SCCS and closely aligned DTS facilitate the storage and release of hemostatic proteins, Ca^{+2}, and enzymes.
- In platelet cytoplasm resides a system of cytoplasmic microfibrils and microtubules that accomplish platelet contraction and pseudopod extension.

- Also within platelet cytoplasm are platelet α-granules and dense granules that store and secrete coagulation factors and vasoactive molecules.
- The platelet membrane supports an array of receptor sites that control platelet activation upon binding their respective ligands.
- Platelets adhere to exposed collagen, aggregate with each other, and secrete the substances stored within their granules.
- Platelet activation is managed internally through G proteins, the eicosanoid synthesis pathway, and the IP_3-DAG pathway.

Now that you have completed this chapter, go back and read again the case study at the beginning and respond to the questions presented.

REVIEW QUESTIONS

Answers can be found in the Appendix.

1. The megakaryocyte progenitor that undergoes endomitosis is:
   a. MK-I
   b. BFU-Meg
   c. CFU-Meg
   d. LD-CFU-Meg

2. The growth factor that is produced in the kidney and induces growth and differentiation of committed megakaryocyte progenitors is:
   a. IL-3
   b. IL-6
   c. IL-11
   d. TPO

3. What platelet organelle sequesters ionic calcium and binds a series of enzymes of the eicosanoid pathway?
   a. G protein
   b. Dense granules
   c. DTS
   d. SCCS

4. What platelet membrane receptor binds fibrinogen and supports platelet aggregation?
   a. GP Ib/IX/V
   b. GP IIb/IIIa
   c. GP Ia/IIa
   d. $P2Y_1$

5. What platelet membrane phospholipid flips from the inner surface to the plasma surface on activation and serves as the assembly point for coagulation factors?
   a. Phosphatidylethanolamine
   b. Phosphatidylinositol
   c. Phosphatidylcholine
   d. Phosphatidylserine

6. What is the name of the eicosanoid metabolite produced from endothelial cells that suppresses platelet activity?
   a. TXA_2
   b. Arachidonic acid
   c. Cyclooxygenase
   d. Prostacyclin

7. Which of the following molecules is stored in platelet dense granules?
   a. Serotonin
   b. Fibrinogen
   c. PF4
   d. Platelet-derived growth factor

8. What plasma protein is essential to platelet adhesion?
   a. VWF
   b. Factor VIII
   c. Fibrinogen
   d. P-selectin

9. Reticulated platelets can be enumerated in peripheral blood to detect:
   a. Impaired production in disease states
   b. Abnormal organelles associated with diseases such as leukemia
   c. Increased platelet production in response to need
   d. Inadequate rates of membrane cholesterol exchange with the plasma

10. Platelet adhesion refers to platelets:
    a. Sticking to other platelets
    b. Releasing platelet granule constituents
    c. Providing the surface for assembly of coagulation factors
    d. Sticking to surfaces such as subendothelial collagen

REFERENCES

1. Butkiewicz, A. M., Kemona, H., Dymicka-Piekarska, V., et al. (2006). Platelet count, mean platelet volume and thrombocytopoietic indices in healthy women and men. *Thromb Res, 118*, 199–204.
2. Lance, M. D., Sloep, M., Henskens, Y. M., & Marcus, M. A. (2012). Mean platelet volume as a diagnostic marker for cardiovascular disease: drawbacks of preanalytical conditions and measuring techniques. *Clin Appl Thromb Hemost, 18*, 561–568.
3. Reddy, V., Marques, M. B., & Fritsma, G. A. (2013). *Quick Guide to Hematology Testing.* (2nd Ed.). Washington, DC: AACC Press.
4. Deutsch, V. R., & Tomer, A. (2013). Advances in megakaryocytopoiesis and thrombopoiesis: from bench to bedside. *Br J Haematol, 161*, 778–793.
5. Kosaki, G. (2005). In vivo platelet production from mature megakaryocytes: does platelet release occur via proplatelets? *Int J Hematol, 81*, 208–219.
6. Chang, Y., Bluteau, D., Bebili, N., et al. (2007). From hematopoietic stem cells to platelets. *J Thrombos Haemostas, 5*(Suppl. 1), 318–327.
7. Italiano, J. E. Jr., & Hartwig, J. H. (2012). Megakaryocyte structure and platelet biogenesis. In Marder, V. J., Aird, W. C., Bennett, J. S., Schulman, S., & White, G. C. (Eds.), *Hemostasis and Thrombosis: Basic Principles and Clinical Practice.* (6th ed., pp. 365–372). Philadelphia: Lippincott Williams & Wilkins.
8. Lordier, L., Jalil, A., Aurade, F., et al. (2008). Megakaryocyte endomitosis is a failure of late cytokinesis related to defects in the contractile ring and Rho/Rock signaling. *Blood, 112*, 3164–74.
9. Italiano, J. E., & Hartwig, J. H. (2013). Megakaryocyte and platelet structure. In Hoffman, R., Benz, E. J., Silbestein, L. E., Heslop, H. E., Weitz, J. I., Anastasi, J. (Eds.), *Hematology: Basic Principles and Practice.* (6th ed., pp. 1797–1808). St. Louis: Elsevier.

10. Ramstrom, A. S., Fagerberg, I. H., & Lindahl, T. L. (1999). A flow cytometric assay for the study of dense granule storage and release in human platelets. *Platelets, 10*, 153–158.
11. Della Porta, M. G., Lanza, F., Del Vecchio, L., & Italian Society of Cytometry (GIC). (2011). Flow cytometry immunophenotyping for the evaluation of bone marrow dysplasia. *Cytometry B Clin Cytom, 80*, 201–211.
12. Berndt, M. C., & Andrews, R. K. (2012).Major platelet glycoproteins: platelet glycoprotein Ib-IX-V. In Marder, V. J., Aird, W. C., Bennett, J. S., Schulman, S., & White, G. C. (Eds.), *Hemostasis and Thrombosis: Basic Principles and Clinical Practice.* (6th ed., pp. 382–385). Philadelphia: Lippincott Williams & Wilkins.
13. Yee, F., & Ginsberg, M. H. (2012). Major platelet glycoproteins: Integrin $\alpha_{IIb}\beta_3$ (GP IIb-IIIa). In Marder, V. J., Aird, W. C., Bennett, J. S., Schulman, S., & White, G. C. (Eds.), *Hemostasis and Thrombosis: Basic Principles and Clinical Practice.* (6th ed., pp. 386–392). Philadelphia: Lippincott Williams & Wilkins.
14. Junt, T., Schulze, H., Chen, Z., et al. (2007). Dynamic visualization of thrombopoiesis within bone marrow. *Science, 317*, 1767–1770.
15. Kuter, D. J. (2010). Biology and chemistry of thrombopoietic agents. *Semin Hematol, 47*, 243–248.
16. Kaushansky, K. (2005). The molecular mechanisms that control thrombopoiesis. *J Clin Invest, 115*, 3339–3347.
17. Neunert, C., Lim, W., Crowther, M., et al. (2011). The American Society of Hematology 2011 evidence-based practice guideline for immune thrombocytopenia. *Blood, 117*, 4190–4207.
18. Bussel, J. B., & Pinheiro, M. P. (2011). Eltrombopag. *Cancer Treatment and Research, 157*, 289–303.

19. Sitaraman, S. V., & Gewirtz, A. T. (2001). Oprelvekin. Genetics Institute. *Curr Opin Investig Drugs, 2*, 1395–1400.

20. Stasi, R. (2009). Therapeutic strategies for hepatitis- and other infection-related immune thrombocytopenias. *Semin Hematol, 46*(Suppl. 2), S15–S25.

21. Yu, M, & Cantor, A. B. (2012). Megakaryopoiesis and thrombopoiesis: an update on cytokines and lineage surface markers. *Methods Mol Biol, 788*, 291-303.

22. Leader, A., Pereg, D., & Lishner, M. Are platelet volume indices of clinical use? A multidisciplinary review. *Ann Med, 44*, 805–816.

23. Rodak, B. F., & Carr, J. H. (2013). *Clinical Hematology Atlas*. (4th ed.). St. Louis: Elsevier.

24. Michur, H., Maślanka, K., Szczepiński, A., & Mariańska, B. (2008). Reticulated platelets as a marker of platelet recovery after allogeneic stem cell transplantation. *Int J Lab Hematol, 30*, 519–525.

25. Tsiara, S., Elisaf, M., Jagroop, I. A., et al. (2003). Platelets as predictors of vascular risk: is there a practical index of platelet activity? *Clin Appl Thromb Hemost, 9*, 177–190.

26. Briggs, C., Harrison, P., & Machin, S. J. (2007). Continuing developments with the automated platelet count. *Int J Lab Hematol, 29*, 77–91.

27. Abe, Y., Wada, H., Sakakura, M., et al. (2005). Usefulness of fully automated measurement of reticulated platelets using whole blood. *Clin Appl Thromb Hemost, 11*, 263–270.

28. Briggs, C., Kunka, S., Hart, D., et al. (2004). Assessment of an immature platelet fraction (IPF) in peripheral thrombocytopenia. *Br J Haematol, 126*, 93–99.

29. Cesari, F., Marcucci, R., Gori, A. M., et al. (2013). Reticulated platelets predict cardiovascular death in acute coronary syndrome patients. Insights from the AMI-Florence 2 Study. *Thromb Haemost, 109*, 846–853.

30. Kunicki, T. J., & Nugent, D. J. (2012). Platelet glycoprotein polymorphisms and relationship to function, immunogenicity, and disease. In Marder, V. J., Aird, W. C., Bennett, J. S., Schulman, S., White, G. C, (Eds.), *Hemostasis and Thrombosis: Basic Principles and Clinical Practice*. (6th ed., pp. 393–399), Philadelphia: Lippincott Williams & Wilkins.

31. Zieseniss, S., Zahler, S., Muller, I., et al. (2001). Modified phosphatidylethanolamine as the active component of oxidized low density lipoprotein promoting platelet prothrombinase activity. *J Biol Chem, 276*, 19828–19835.

32. Savage, B., & Ruggeri, Z. V. (2012). The basis for platelet adhesion. In Marder, V. J., Aird, W. C., Bennett, J. S., Schulman, S., & White, G. C. (Eds.), *Hemostasis and Thrombosis: Basic Principles and Clinical Practice*. (6th ed., pp. 400–449), Philadelphia: Lippincott Williams & Wilkins.

33. Tandon, N. N., Kraslisz, U., & Jamieson, G. A. (1989). Identification of glycoprotein IV (CD36) as a primary receptor for platelet-collagen adhesion. *J Biol Chem, 264*, 7576–7583.

34. Rivera, J., Lozano, M. L., Corral, J., et al. (2000). Platelet GP Ib/IX/V complex: physiological role. *J Physiol Biochem, 56*, 355–365.

35. Jobe, S., & Di Paola, J. (2013). Congenital and acquired disorders of platelet function and number. In Kitchens, C. S., Kessler, C. M,. & Konkle, B. A. (Eds.), *Consultative Hemostasis and Thrombosis*. (3rd ed., pp. 132–149). St. Louis: Elsevier.

36. Granada, J. F., & Kleiman, N. S. (2004). Therapeutic use of intravenous eptifibatide in patients undergoing percutaneous coronary intervention: acute coronary syndromes and elective stenting. *Am J Cardiovasc Drugs, 4*, 31–41.

37. Jackson, S. P., Nesbitt, W. S., & Kulkarni, S. Signaling events underlying thrombus formation. *J Thromb Haemost, 1*, 1602–1612.

38. Moliterno, D. J. (2008). Advances in antiplatelet therapy for ACS and PCI. *J Interven Cardiol, 21*(Suppl. 1), S18–S24.

39. Israels, S. J., & Rand, M. L. (2013). What we have learned from inherited platelet disorders. *Pediatr Blood Cancer, 60*(Suppl. 1), S2–S7.

40. Walenga, J. M., Jeske, W. P., Prechel, M. M., et al. (2004). Newer insights on the mechanism of heparin-induced thrombocytopenia. *Semin Thromb Hemost, 30*(Suppl. 1), 57–67.

41. Keating, F. K., Dauerman, H. L., Whitaker, D. A., et al. (2006). Increased expression of platelet P-selectin and formation of platelet-leukocyte aggregates in blood from patients treated with unfractionated heparin plus eptifibatide compared with bivalirudin. *Thromb Res, 118*, 361–369.

42. White, J. G., & Rao, G. H. (1998). Microtubule coils versus the surface membrane cytoskeleton in maintenance and restoration of platelet discoid shape. *Am J Pathol, 152*, 597–609.

43. Blair, P., & Flaumenhaft, R. (2009). Platelet alpha-granules: basic biology and clinical correlates. *Blood Rev, 23*, 177–189.

44. Abrams, C. S., & Plow, E. F. (2013). Molecular basis for platelet function. In Hoffman, R. H., Benz, E. J., Silberstein, L. E., et al, (Eds.), *Hematology: Basic Principles and Practice*. (6th ed., pp. 1809–1820). St. Louis: Elsevier.

45. Ye, S., & Whiteheart, S. W. (2012). Molecular basis for platelet secretion. In Marder, V. J., Aird, W. C., Bennett, J. S., Schulman, S., & White, G. C. (Eds.), *Hemostasis and Thrombosis: Basic Principles and Clinical Practice*. (6th ed., pp. 441–449). Philadelphia: Lippincott Williams & Wilkins.

46. Abrams, C. S. (2005). Intracellular signaling in platelets. *Curr Opin Hematol, 12*, 401–405.

47. Stegner, D., & Nieswantdt, B. (2011). Platelet receptor signaling in thrombus formation. *J Mol Med, 89*, 109–121.

48. Tailor, A., Cooper, D., & Granger, D. N. (2005.) Platelet-vessel wall interactions in the microcirculation. *Microcirculation, 12*, 275–285.

49. Zhou, Z., Nguyen, T. C., Guchhait, P., & Dong, J. F. (2010). Von Willebrand factor, ADAMTS-13, and thrombotic thrombocytopenic purpura. *Semin Thromb Hemost, 36*, 71–81.

50. Nieswandt, B., & Watson, S. P. (2003). Platelet-collagen interaction: is GPVI the central receptor? *Blood, 102*, 449–461.

51. Varga-Szabo, D., Pleines, I., & Nieswandt, B. (2008). Cell adhesion mechanisms in platelets. *Arterioscler Thromb Vasc Biol, 28*, 403–412.

52. Jung, S. M., Moroi, M., Soejima, K., et al. (2012). Constitutive dimerization of glycoprotein VI (GPVI) in resting platelets is essential for binding to collagen and activation in flowing blood. *J Biol Chemistry, 287*, 30000–30013.

53. Furihata, K., Nugent, D. J., & Kunicki, T. J. (2002). Influence of platelet collagen receptor polymorphisms on risk for arterial thrombosis. *Arch Pathol Lab Med, 126*, 305–309.

54. Fritsma, G. A., Ens, G. E., Alvord, M. A., et al. (2001). Monitoring the antiplatelet action of aspirin. *JAAPA, 14*, 57–62.

55. Eikelboom, J. W., & Hankey, G. J. (2004). Failure of aspirin to prevent atherothrombosis: potential mechanisms and implications for clinical practice. *Am J Cardiovasc Drugs, 4*, 57–67.

Manual, Semiautomated, and Point-of-Care Testing in Hematology

14

Karen S. Clark and Teresa G. Hippel

OBJECTIVES

After completion of this chapter, the reader will be able to:

1. State the dimensions of the counting area of a Neubauer ruled hemacytometer.
2. Describe the performance of manual cell counts for white blood cells, red blood cells, and platelets, including types of diluting fluids, typical dilutions, and typical areas counted in the hemacytometer.
3. Calculate dilutions for cell counts when given appropriate data.
4. Calculate hemacytometer cell counts when given numbers of cells, area counted, and dilution.
5. Correct white blood cell counts for the presence of nucleated red blood cells.
6. Describe the principle of the cyanmethemoglobin assay for determination of hemoglobin.
7. Calculate the values for a standard curve for cyanmethemoglobin determination when given the appropriate data, describe how the standard curve is constructed, and use the standard curve to determine hemoglobin values.
8. Describe the procedure for performing a microhematocrit.
9. Identify sources of error in routine manual procedures discussed in this chapter and recognize written scenarios describing such errors.
10. Compare red blood cell count, hemoglobin, and hematocrit values using the rule of three.

11. Calculate red blood cell indices (mean cell volume, mean cell hemoglobin, and mean cell hemoglobin concentration) when given appropriate data, and interpret the results relative to the volume and hemoglobin content and concentration in the red blood cells.
12. Describe the principle and procedure for performing a manual reticulocyte count and the clinical value of the test.
13. Given the appropriate data, calculate the relative, absolute, and corrected reticulocyte counts and the reticulocyte production index; interpret results to determine the adequacy of the bone marrow erythropoietic response in an anemia.
14. Describe the procedure for performing the Westergren erythrocyte sedimentation rate and state its clinical utility.
15. Describe the aspects of establishing a point-of-care testing program, including quality management and selection of instrumentation.
16. Discuss the advantages and disadvantages of point-of-care testing as they apply to hematology tests.
17. Describe the principles of common instruments used for point-of-care testing for hemoglobin level, hematocrit, white blood cell counts, and platelet counts.

CASE STUDIES

After studying the material in this chapter, the reader should be able to respond to the following case studies:

Case 1

The following results are obtained for a patient with normocytic, normochromic red blood cells on a peripheral blood film:

RBC count = 4.63×10^{12}/L

HGB = 15 g/dL

HCT = 40% (0.40 L/L)

Continued

1. Using the rule of three, given the hemoglobin concentration above, what is the expected value for the hematoctrit?
2. What could cause the hemoglobin to be falsely elevated or the hematocrit to be falsely low?
3. What would you do to correct for the interferences you listed in question 2?

Case 2

For another patient, the following results are obtained:
RBC count = 3.20×10^{12}/L
HGB = 5.8 g/dL
HCT = 18.9% (0.19 L/L)
1. Calculate the red blood cell indices.
2. How would you describe the red blood cell volume and hemoglobin concentration based on these indices?
3. How should you verify this?

Case 3

The following results are obtained for a patient using a point-of-care device that employs the conductivity method to measure the hematocrit:

Sodium = 160 mmol/L (Reference interval: 135 to 145 mmol/L)

Potassium = 3.6 mmol/L (Reference interval: 3.5 to 5.5 mmol/L)

HCT = 17.0% (0.17 L/L)

HGB = 6.0 g/dL

1. Which electrolyte concentration could affect the hematocrit?
2. Would this electrolyte concentration falsely decrease or increase the hematocrit value?
3. What other factors can decrease the hematocrit value using this point-of-care device?

Clinical laboratory hematology has evolved from simple observation and description of blood and its components to a highly automated, extremely technical science, including examination at the molecular level. However, some of the more basic tests have not changed dramatically over the years. This chapter provides an overview of these basic tests and presents the manual and semiautomated methods that can be used in lieu of automated instrumentation. Included in this chapter is a discussion of point-of-care testing in hematology.

MANUAL CELL COUNTS

Although most routine cell-counting procedures in the hematology laboratory are automated, it may be necessary to use manual methods when counts exceed the linearity of an instrument, when an instrument is nonfunctional and there is no backup, in remote laboratories in Third World countries, or in a disaster situation when testing is done in the field. Although the discussion in this chapter concerns whole blood, body fluid cell counts are also often performed using manual methods. Chapter 18 discusses the specific diluents and dilutions used for body fluid cell counts. Chapter 15 discusses automated cell-counting instrumentation in detail.

Manual cell counts are performed using a hemacytometer, or counting chamber, and manual dilutions made with calibrated, automated pipettes and diluents (commercially available or laboratory prepared). The principle for the performance of cell counts is essentially the same for white blood cells (WBCs), red blood cells (RBCs), and platelets; only the dilution, diluting fluid, and area counted vary. Any particle (e.g., sperm) can be counted using this system.

Equipment

Hemacytometer

The manual cell count uses a hemacytometer, or counting chamber. The most common one is the Levy chamber with improved Neubauer ruling. It is composed of two raised surfaces, each with a 3 mm × 3 mm square counting area or grid (total area 9 mm²), separated by an H-shaped moat. As shown in Figure 14-1, this grid is made up of nine 1 mm × 1 mm squares. Each of the four corner (WBC) squares is subdivided further into 16 squares, and the center square subdivided into 25 smaller squares. Each of these smallest squares is 0.2 mm × 0.2 mm which is $^1/_{25}$ of the center square or 0.04 mm². A coverslip is placed on top of the counting surfaces. The distance between each counting surface and the coverslip is 0.1 mm; thus the total *volume* of one entire grid or counting area on one side of the hemacytometer is 0.9 mm³. Hemacytometers and coverslips must meet the specifications of the National Bureau of Standards, as indicated by the initials "NBS" on the chamber. When the dimensions of the hemacytometer are thoroughly understood, the area counted can be changed to facilitate the counting of samples with extremely low or high counts.

Calculations

The general formula for manual cell counts is as follows and can be used to calculate any type of cell count:

$$\text{Total count} = \frac{\text{cells counted} \times \text{dilution factor}}{\text{area (mm}^2） \times \text{depth (0.1)}}$$

Or

$$\text{Total count} = \frac{\text{cells counted} \times \text{dilution factor} \times 10^*}{\text{area (mm}^2）}$$

*Reciprocal of depth.

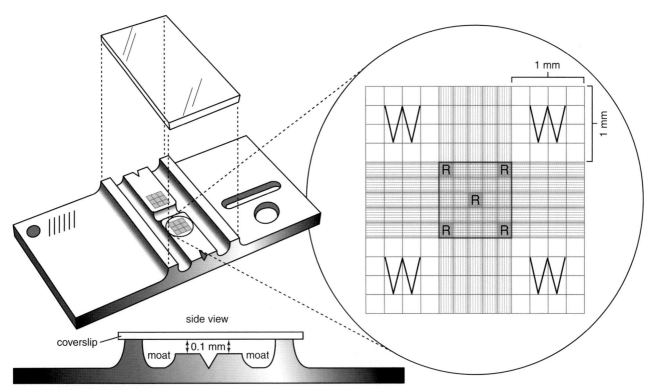

Figure 14-1 Hemacytometer and a close-up view of the counting areas as seen under the microscope. The areas for the standard white blood cell count are labeled *W*, and the areas for the standard red blood cell count are labeled *R*. The entire center square, outlined in blue, is used for counting platelets. The side view of the hemacytometer shows a depth of 0.1 mm from the surface of the counting grid to the coverslip.

The calculation yields the number of cells per mm³. One mm³ is equivalent to one microliter (μL). The count per μL is converted to the count per liter (L) by multiplying by a factor of 10^6.

White Blood Cell Count

The WBC or leukocyte count is the number of WBCs in 1 liter (L) or 1 microliter (μL) of blood. Whole blood anticoagulated with ethylenediaminetetraacetic acid (EDTA) or blood from a skin puncture is diluted with 1% buffered ammonium oxalate or a weak acid solution (3% acetic acid or 1% hydrochloric acid). The diluting fluid lyses the nonnucleated red blood cells in the sample to prevent their interference in the count. The typical dilution of blood for the WBC count is 1:20. A hemacytometer is charged (filled) with the well-mixed dilution and placed under a microscope and the number of cells in the 4 large corner squares (4 mm²) is counted.

PROCEDURE

1. Clean the hemacytometer and coverslip with alcohol and dry thoroughly with a lint-free tissue. Place the coverslip on the hemacytometer.
2. Make a 1:20 dilution by placing 25 μL of well-mixed blood into 475 μL of WBC diluting fluid in a small test tube.
3. Cover the tube and mix by inversion.
4. Allow the dilution to sit for 10 minutes to ensure that the red blood cells have lysed. The solution will be clear once lysis has occurred. WBC counts should be performed within 3 hours of dilution.
5. Mix again by inversion and fill a plain microhematocrit tube.
6. Charge both sides of the hemacytometer by holding the microhematocrit tube at a 45-degree angle and touching the tip to the coverslip edge where it meets the chamber floor.
7. After charging the hemacytometer, place it in a moist chamber (Box 14-1) for 10 minutes before counting the cells to give them time to settle. Care should be taken not to disturb the coverslip.
8. While keeping the hemacytometer in a horizontal position, place it on the microscope stage.
9. Lower the condenser on the microscope and focus by using the low-power (10×) objective lens (100× total magnification). The cells should be distributed evenly in all of the squares.
10. For a 1:20 dilution, count all of the cells in the four corner squares, starting with the square in the upper left-hand corner (Figure 14-1). Cells that touch the top and left lines should be counted; cells that touch the bottom and right lines should be ignored (Figure 14-2). See Figure 14-3 for the appearance of WBCs in the hemacytometer using the low-power objective lens of a microscope.

BOX 14-1 How to Make a Moist Chamber

A moist chamber may be made by placing a piece of damp filter paper in the bottom of a Petri dish. An applicator stick broken in half can serve as a support for the hemacytometer.

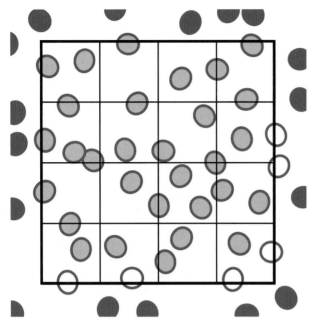

Figure 14-2 One large corner square of a hemacytometer indicating which cells to count. Cells touching the left and top lines (*solid circles*) are counted. Cells touching bottom and right (*open circles*) are not counted.

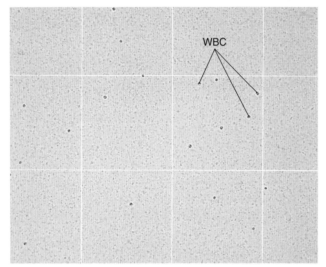

Figure 14-3 White blood cells as seen in the hemacytometer under low power (10× objective) 100× total magnification.

11. Repeat the count on the other side of the counting chamber. The difference between the total cells counted on each side should be less than 10%. A greater variation could indicate an uneven distribution, which requires that the procedure be repeated.
12. Average the number of WBCs counted on the two sides. Using the average, calculate the WBC count using one of the equations given earlier.

Example Using the First Equation

When a 1:20 dilution is used, the four large squares on one side of the chamber yield counts of 23, 26, 22, and 21. The total count is 92. The four large squares on the other side of

the chamber yield counts of 28, 24, 22, and 26. The total count is 100. The difference between sides is less than 10%.

The average number of cells of the two sides of the chamber is 96. Using the average in the formula:

$$\text{WBC count} = \frac{\text{cells counted} \times \text{dilution factor}}{\text{area counted (mm}^2) \times \text{depth}}$$
$$= \frac{96 \times 20}{4 \times 0.1}$$
$$= 4800/\text{mm}^3 \text{ or } 4800/\mu L \text{ or}$$
$$4.8 \times 10^3/\mu L \text{ or } 4.8 \times 10^9/L$$

Alternately, a 1:100 dilution may be used counting the number of cells in the entire counting area (9 large squares, 9 mm²) on both sides of the chamber (Table 14-1). As an example, if an average of 54 cells were counted in the entire counting area on both sides of the chamber:

$$\text{WBC count} = \frac{\text{cells counted} \times \text{dilution factor}}{\text{area counted (mm}^2) \times \text{depth}}$$
$$= \frac{54 \times 100}{9 \times 0.1}$$
$$= 6000/\text{mm}^3 \text{ or } 6000/\mu L \text{ or}$$
$$6.0 \times 10^3/\mu L \text{ or } 6.0 \times 10^9/L$$

General reference intervals for males and females in different age groups can be found on the inside front cover of this text. *Reference intervals may vary slightly according to the population tested and should be established for each laboratory.*

Sources of Error and Comments

1. The hemacytometer and coverslip should be cleaned properly before they are used. Dust and fingerprints may cause difficulty in distinguishing the cells.
2. The diluting fluid should be free of contaminants.

TABLE 14-1 Manual Cell Counts with Most Common Dilutions, Counting Areas

Cells Counted	Diluting Fluid	Dilution	Objective	Area Counted
White blood cells	1% ammonium oxalate or 3% acetic acid or 1% hydrochloric acid	1:20 1:100	10× 10×	4 mm² 9 mm²
Red blood cells	Isotonic saline	1:100	40×	0.2 mm² (5 small squares of center square)
Platelets	1% ammonium oxalate	1:100	40× phase	1 mm²

3. If the count is low, a greater area may be counted (e.g., 9 mm²) to improve accuracy.

4. The chamber must be charged properly to ensure an accurate count. Uneven flow of the diluted blood into the chamber results in an irregular distribution of cells. If the chamber is overfilled or underfilled, the chamber must be cleaned and recharged.

5. After the chamber is filled, allow the cells to settle for 10 minutes before counting.

6. Any nucleated red blood cells (NRBCs) present in the sample are not lysed by the diluting fluid. The NRBCs are counted as WBCs because they are indistinguishable when seen on the hemacytometer. If five or more NRBCs per 100 WBCs are observed on the differential count on a stained peripheral blood film, the WBC count must be corrected for these cells. This is accomplished by using the following formula:

$$\frac{\text{Uncorrected WBC count} \times 100}{\text{Number of NRBCs per 100 WBCs} + 100}$$

Report the result as the "corrected" WBC count.

7. The accuracy of the manual WBC count can be assessed by performing a WBC estimate on a Wright-stained peripheral blood film made from the same specimen (Chapter 16).

Platelet Count

A platelet count is the number of platelets in 1 liter (L) or 1 microliter (μL) of whole blood. Platelets adhere to foreign objects and to each other, which makes them difficult to count. They also are small and can be confused easily with dirt or debris. In this procedure, whole blood, with EDTA as the anticoagulant, is diluted 1:100 with 1% ammonium oxalate to lyse the nonnucleated red blood cells. The platelets are counted in the 25 small squares in the large center square (1 mm²) of the hemacytometer using a phase-contrast microscope in the reference method described by Brecher and Cronkite.[1] A light microscope can also be used, but visualizing the platelets may be more difficult.

PROCEDURE

1. Make a 1:100 dilution by placing 20 μL of well-mixed blood into 1980 μL of 1% ammonium oxalate in a small test tube.

2. Mix the dilution thoroughly and charge the chamber. (NOTE: A special thin, flat-bottomed counting chamber is used for phase-microscopy platelet counts.)

3. Place the charged hemacytometer in a moist chamber (Box 14-1) for 15 minutes to allow the platelets to settle.

4. Platelets are counted using the 40× objective lens (400× total magnification). The platelets have a diameter of 2 to 4 μm and appear round or oval, displaying a light purple sheen when phase-contrast microscopy is used. The shape and color help distinguish the platelets from highly refractile dirt and debris. "Ghost" RBCs often are seen in the background.

5. Count the number of platelets in the 25 small squares in the center square of the grid (Figure 14-1). The area of this center square is 1 mm². Platelets should be counted on each side of the hemacytometer, and the difference between the totals should be less than 10%.

6. Calculate the platelet count by using one of the equations given earlier. Using the first equation as an example, if 200 platelets were counted in the entire center square,

$$\frac{200 \times 100}{1 \times 0.1}$$
$$= 200{,}000/\text{mm}^3 \text{ or } 200{,}000/\mu\text{L}$$
$$\text{or } 200 \times 10^3/\mu\text{L or } 200 \times 10^9/\text{L}$$

7. The accuracy of the manual platelet count should be verified by performing a platelet estimate on a Wright-stained peripheral blood film made from the same specimen (Chapter 16).

General reference intervals for males and females according to age groups can be found on the inside front cover of this text.

Sources of Error and Comments

1. Inadequate mixing and poor collection of the specimen can cause the platelets to clump on the hemacytometer. If the problem persists after redilution, a new specimen is needed. A skin puncture specimen is less desirable because of the tendency of the platelets to aggregate or form clumps.

2. Dirt in the pipette, hemacytometer, or diluting fluid may cause the counts to be inaccurate.

3. If fewer than 50 platelets are counted on each side, the procedure should be repeated by diluting the blood to 1:20. If more than 500 platelets are counted on each side, a 1:200 dilution should be made. The appropriate dilution factor should be used in calculating the results.

4. If the patient has a normal platelet count, the 5 small, red blood cell squares (Figure 14-1) may be counted. Then, the area is 0.2 mm² on each side.

5. The phenomenon of "platelet satellitosis" may occur when EDTA anticoagulant is used. This refers to the adherence of platelets around neutrophils, producing a ring or satellite effect (Figure 16-1). Using sodium citrate as the anticoagulant should correct this problem. Because of the dilution in the citrate evacuated tubes, it is necessary to multiply the obtained platelet count by 1.1 for accuracy (Chapter 16).

Red Blood Cell Count

Manual RBC counts are rarely performed because of the inaccuracy of the count and questionable necessity. Use of other, more accurate manual RBC procedures, such as the microhematocrit and hemoglobin concentration, is desirable when automation is not available.

Table 14-1 contains information on performing manual WBC, platelet, and RBC counts.

Disposable Blood Cell Count Dilution Systems

Capillary pipette and diluent reservoir systems are commercially available for WBC and platelet counts. One such system is LeukoChek™ (Biomedical Polymers, Inc., Gardner, MA). It consists of a capillary pipette (calibrated to accept 20 μL of blood) that fits into a plastic reservoir containing 1.98 mL of 1% buffered ammonium oxalate (Figure 14-4). Blood from a well-mixed EDTA-anticoagulated specimen or from a skin puncture is allowed to enter the pipette by capillary action to the fill volume. The blood is added to the reservoir making a 1:100 dilution. After mixing the reservoir and allowing 10 minutes for lysis of the red blood cells, the reverse end of the capillary pipette is placed in the reservoir cap making a dropper. The first 3 or 4 drops of the diluted sample is discarded, and the capillary pipette is used to charge the hemacytometer.

Both WBC and platelet counts can be done from the same diluted sample. WBCs are counted in all 9 large squares (9 mm²) using low power (100× total magnification). Platelets are counted in the 25 small squares in the center square (1 mm²) using high power (400× total magnification). The standard formula is used to calculate the cell counts.

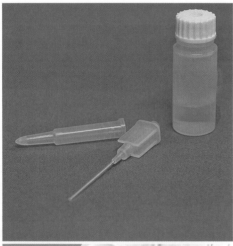

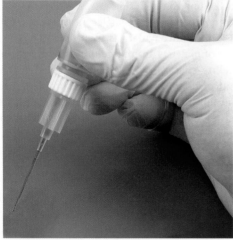

Figure 14-4 LeukoChek™ blood diluting system for manual white blood cell and platelet counts. It consists of a 20 μL capillary pipette and plastic reservoir containing 1.98 mL of 1% buffered ammonium oxalate that makes a 1:100 dilution of whole blood. (Courtesy Biomedical Polymers, Inc., Gardner, MA.)

Body Fluid Cell Counts

Body fluid cell counts are discussed in detail in Chapter 18.

HEMOGLOBIN DETERMINATION

The primary function of hemoglobin within the red blood cell is to carry oxygen to and carbon dioxide from the tissues. The cyanmethemoglobin (hemoglobincyanide) method for hemoglobin determination is the reference method approved by the Clinical and Laboratory Standards Institute.[2]

Principle

In the cyanmethemoglobin method, blood is diluted in an alkaline Drabkin solution of potassium ferricyanide, potassium cyanide, sodium bicarbonate, and a surfactant. The hemoglobin is oxidized to methemoglobin (Fe^{3+}) by the potassium ferricyanide, $K_3Fe(CN)_6$. The potassium cyanide (KCN) then converts the methemoglobin to cyanmethemoglobin:

$$\text{Hemoglobin (Fe}^{2+}) + K_3Fe(CN)_6 \rightarrow \text{methemoglobin (Fe}^{3+}) + KCN \rightarrow \text{cyanmethemoglobin}$$

The absorbance of the cyanmethemoglobin at 540 nm is directly proportional to the hemoglobin concentration. Sulfhemoglobin is not converted to cyanmethemoglobin; it cannot be measured by this method. Sulfhemoglobin fractions of more than 0.05 g/dL are seldom encountered in clinical practice, however.[3]

PROCEDURE

1. Create a standard curve, using a commercially available cyanmethemoglobin standard.
   a. When a standard containing 80 mg/dL of hemoglobin is used, the following dilutions should be made:

Hemoglobin Concentration (g/dL)	Blank	5	10	15	20
Cyanmethemoglobin standard (mL)	0	1.5	3	4.5	6
Cyanmethemoglobin reagent (mL)	6	4.5	3	1.5	0

   b. Transfer the dilutions to cuvettes. Set the wavelength on the spectrophotometer to 540 nm and use the blank to set to 100% transmittance.
   c. Using semilogarithmic paper, plot percent transmittance on the *y*-axis and the hemoglobin concentration on the *x*-axis. The hemoglobin concentrations of the control and patient samples can be read from this standard curve (Figure 14-5).
   d. A standard curve should be set up with each new lot of reagents. It also should be checked when alterations are made to the spectrophotometer (e.g., bulb change).
2. Controls should be run with each batch of samples. Commercial controls are available.

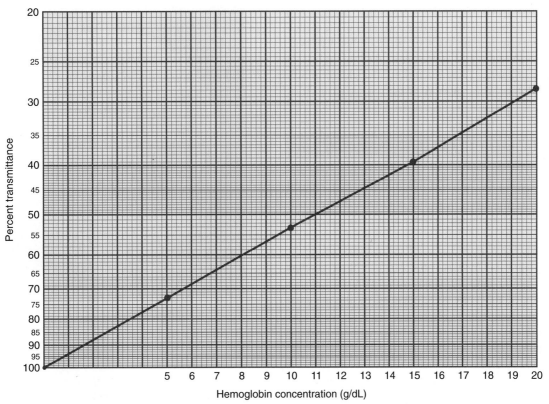

Figure 14-5 Standard curve obtained when a cyanmethemoglobin standard of 80 mg/dL is used. A blank (100% transmittance) and four dilutions were made: 5 g/dL (72.9% transmittance), 10 g/dL (53.2% transmittance), 15 g/dL (39.1% transmittance), and 20 g/dL (28.7% transmittance).

3. Using the patient's whole blood anticoagulated with EDTA or heparin or blood from a capillary puncture, make a 1:251 dilution by adding 0.02 mL (20 μL) of blood to 5 mL of cyanmethemoglobin reagent. The pipette should be rinsed thoroughly with the reagent to ensure that no blood remains. Follow the same procedure for the control samples.
4. Cover and mix well by inversion or use a vortex mixer. Let stand for 10 minutes at room temperature to allow full conversion of hemoglobin to cyanmethemoglobin.
5. Transfer all of the solutions to cuvettes. Set the spectrophotometer to 100% transmittance at the wavelength of 540 nm, using cyanmethemoglobin reagent as a blank.
6. Using a matched cuvette, continue reading the % transmittance of the patient samples and record the values.
7. Determine the hemoglobin concentration of the control samples and the patient samples from the standard curve.
General reference intervals can be found on the inside cover of this text.

Sources of Error and Comments

1. Cyanmethemoglobin reagent is sensitive to light. It should be stored in a brown bottle or in a dark place.
2. A high WBC count (greater than 20×10^9/L) or a high platelet count (greater than 700×10^9/L) can cause turbidity and a falsely high result. In this case, the reagent-sample solution can be centrifuged and the supernatant measured.
3. Lipemia also can cause turbidity and a falsely high result. It can be corrected by adding 0.01 mL of the patient's plasma to 5 mL of the cyanmethemoglobin reagent and using this solution as the reagent blank.

4. Cells containing Hb S and Hb C may be resistant to hemolysis, causing turbidity; this can be corrected by making a 1:2 dilution with distilled water (1 part diluted sample plus 1 part water) and multiplying the results from the standard curve by 2.
5. Abnormal globulins, such as those found in patients with plasma cell myeloma or Waldenström macroglobulinemia, may precipitate in the reagent. If this occurs, add 0.1 g of potassium carbonate to the cyanmethemoglobin reagent. Commercially available cyanmethemoglobin reagent has been modified to contain KH_2PO_4 salt, so this problem is not likely to occur.
6. Carboxyhemoglobin takes 1 hour to convert to cyanmethemoglobin and theoretically could cause erroneous results in samples from heavy smokers. The degree of error is probably not clinically significant, however.
7. Because the hemoglobin reagent contains cyanide, it is highly toxic and must be used cautiously. Consult the safety data sheet (Chapter 2) supplied by the manufacturer. Acidification of cyanide in the reagent releases highly toxic hydrogen cyanide gas. A licensed waste disposal service should be contracted to discard the reagent; reagent-sample solutions should not be discarded into sinks.
8. Commercial absorbance standards kits are available to calibrate spectrophotometers.
9. Handheld systems are commercially available to measure the hemoglobin concentration. An example is the HemoCue[4,5] (HemoCue, Inc., Brea, CA) (Figure 14-19) in which hemoglobin is converted to azidemethemoglobin and is read photometrically at two wavelengths (570 nm and 880 nm).

This method avoids the necessity of sample dilution and interference from turbidity. It is discussed later in the section on point-of-care testing. Another method that has been used in some automated instruments involves the use of sodium lauryl sulfate (SLS) to convert hemoglobin to SLS-methemoglobin. This method does not generate toxic wastes.[6-9]

MICROHEMATOCRIT

The hematocrit is the volume of packed red blood cells that occupies a given volume of whole blood. This is often referred to as the *packed cell volume* (PCV). It is reported either as a percentage (e.g., 36%) or in liters per liter (0.36 L/L).

PROCEDURE

1. Fill two plain capillary tubes approximately three quarters full with blood anticoagulated with EDTA or heparin. Mylar-wrapped tubes are recommended by the National Institute for Occupational Safety and Health to reduce the risk of capillary tube injuries.[10] Alternatively, blood may be collected into heparinized capillary tubes by skin puncture. Wipe any excess blood from the outside of the tube.
2. Seal the end of the tube with the colored ring using nonabsorbent clay. Hold the filled tube horizontally and seal by placing the dry end into the tray with sealing compound at a 90-degree angle. Rotate the tube slightly and remove it from the tray. The plug should be at least 4 mm long.[10]
3. Balance the tubes in a microhematocrit centrifuge with the clay ends facing the outside away from the center, touching the rubber gasket.
4. Tighten the head cover on the centrifuge and close the top. Centrifuge the tubes at 10,000 *g* to 15,000 *g* for the time that has been determined to obtain maximum packing of red blood cells, as detailed in Box 14-2. Do not use the brake to stop the centrifuge.
5. Determine the hematocrit by using a microhematocrit reading device (Figure 14-6). Read the level of red blood cell packing; do not include the buffy coat (WBCs and platelets) when taking the reading (Figure 14-7).
6. The values of the duplicate hematocrits should agree within 1% (0.01 L/L).[10]

BOX 14-2 Determining Maximum Packing Time for Microhematocrit

The time to obtain maximum packing of red blood cells should be determined for each centrifuge. Duplicate microhematocrit determinations should be made using fresh, well-mixed blood anticoagulated with ethylenediaminetetraacetic acid (EDTA). Two specimens should be used, with one of the specimens having a known hematocrit of 50% or higher. Starting at 2 minutes, centrifuge duplicates at 30-second intervals and record results. When the hematocrit has remained at the same value for two consecutive readings, optimum packing has been achieved, and the second time interval should be used for microhematocrit determinations.[10]

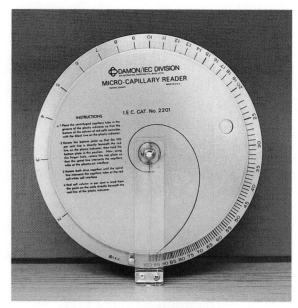

Figure 14-6 Microhematocrit reader.

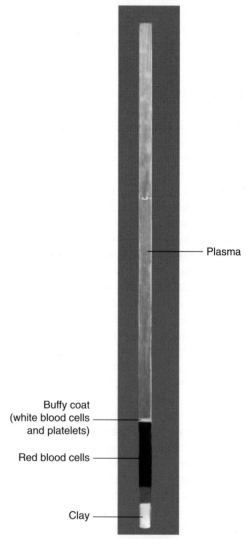

Plasma

Buffy coat (white blood cells and platelets)

Red blood cells

Clay

Figure 14-7 Capillary tube with anticoagulated whole blood after it has been centrifuged. Notice the layers containing plasma, the buffy coat (white blood cells and platelets), and the red blood cells.

General reference intervals according to sex and age can be found on the inside front cover of this text.

Sources of Error and Comments

1. Improper sealing of the capillary tube causes a decreased hematocrit reading as a result of leakage of blood during centrifugation. A higher number of red blood cells are lost compared with plasma due to the packing of the cells in the lower part of the tube during centrifugation.

2. An increased concentration of anticoagulant (short draw in an evacuated tube) decreases the hematocrit reading as a result of red blood cell shrinkage.

3. A decreased or increased result may occur if the specimen was not mixed properly.

4. The time and speed of the centrifugation and the time when the results are read are important. Insufficient centrifugation or a delay in reading results after centrifugation causes hematocrit readings to increase. Time for complete packing should be determined for each centrifuge and rechecked at regular intervals. When the microhematocrit centrifuge is calibrated, one of the samples used must have a hematocrit of 50% or higher.[10]

5. The buffy coat of the sample should not be included in the hematocrit reading because this falsely elevates the result.

6. A decrease or increase in the readings may be seen if the microhematocrit reader is not used properly.

7. Many disorders, such as sickle cell anemia, macrocytic anemias, hypochromic anemias, spherocytosis, and thalassemia, may cause plasma to be trapped in the red blood cell layer even if the procedure is performed properly. The trapping of the plasma causes the microhematocrit to be 1% to 3% (0.01 to 0.03 L/L) higher than the value obtained using automated instruments that calculate or directly measure the hematocrit and are unaffected by the trapped plasma.

8. A temporarily low hematocrit reading may result immediately after a blood loss because plasma is replaced faster than are the red blood cells.

9. The fluid loss associated with dehydration causes a decrease in plasma volume and falsely increases the hematocrit reading.

10. Proper specimen collection is an important consideration. The introduction of interstitial fluid from a skin puncture or the improper flushing of an intravenous catheter causes decreased hematocrit readings.

The READACRIT centrifuge (Becton, Dickinson and Company, Franklin Lakes, NJ) uses precalibrated capillary tubes and has built-in hematocrit scales, which eliminates the need for separate reading devices (Figure 14-8). The use of SUREPREP Capillary Tubes (Becton, Dickinson) eliminates the use of sealants. They have a factory-inserted plug that seals automatically when the blood touches the plug.[11]

RULE OF THREE

When samples are analyzed by automated or manual methods, a quick visual check of the results of the hemoglobin and

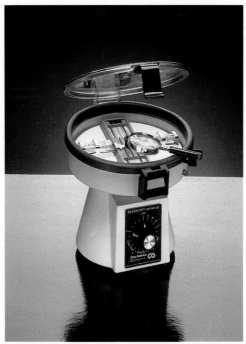

Figure 14-8 READACRIT centrifuge with built-in capillary tube compartments and hematocrit scales. (Courtesy and © Becton, Dickinson and Company, Franklin Lakes, NJ.)

hematocrit can be done by applying the "rule of three." This rule applies only to samples that have normocytic normochromic red blood cells. The value of the hematocrit should be three times the value of the hemoglobin plus or minus 3: HGB × 3 = HCT ± 3 (0.03 L/L). It should become habit for the analyst to multiply the hemoglobin by 3 mentally for every sample; a value discrepant with this rule may indicate abnormal red blood cells, or it may be the first indication of error.

For example, the following results are obtained from patients:

Case 1

    HGB = 12 g/dL
    HCT = 36% (0.36 L/L)
    According to the rule of three,

$$HGB\ (12) \times 3 = HCT\ (36)$$

An acceptable range for the hematocrit would be 33% to 39%. These values conform to the rule of three.

Case 2

    HGB = 9 g/dL
    HCT = 32%
    According to the rule of three,

$$HGB\ (9.0) \times 3 = HCT\ (27\ versus\ actual\ value\ of\ 32)$$

An acceptable range for hematocrit would be 24% to 30%, so these values do not conform to the rule of three.

Case 3
   HGB = 15 g/dL
   HCT = 36%
   According to the rule of three,

   HGB (15) × 3 = HCT (45 versus obtained value of 36)

An acceptable range for hematocrit would be 42% to 48%, so these values do not conform to the rule of three.

If values do not agree, the blood film should be examined for abnormal red blood cells; causes of false increases and decreases in the hemoglobin and/or hematocrit values should also be investigated. In the second example, the blood film reveals red blood cells that are low in hemoglobin concentration (hypochromic) and are smaller in volume (microcytic), so the rule of three cannot be applied. If red blood cells do appear normal, possible causes of a falsely low hemoglobin concentration or a falsely elevated hematocrit should be investigated. In the third example, the specimen is determined to have lipemic plasma causing a falsely elevated hemoglobin concentration, and a correction must be made to obtain an accurate hemoglobin value. (See Hemoglobin Determination in this chapter.)

When an unexplained discrepancy is found, the sample processed before and after the sample in question should be checked to determine whether they conform to the rule. If they do not conform, further investigation should be done to find the problem. A control sample should be run when such a discrepancy is found. If the instrument produces appropriate results for the control, random error may have occurred (Chapter 5).

RED BLOOD CELL INDICES

The mean cell volume (MCV), mean cell hemoglobin (MCH), and mean cell hemoglobin concentration (MCHC) are the RBC indices. These are calculated to determine the average volume and hemoglobin content and concentration of the red blood cells in the sample. In addition to serving as a quality control check, the indices may be used for initial classification of anemias. Table 14-2 provides a summary of the RBC indices, morphology, and correlation with various anemias. The morphologic classification of anemia on the basis of MCV is discussed in detail in Chapter 19.

Mean Cell Volume

The MCV is the average volume of the red blood cell, expressed in femtoliters (fL), or 10^{-15} L:

$$MCV = \frac{HCT\ (\%) \times 10}{RBC\ count\ (\times\ 10^{12}/L)}$$

For example, if the HCT = 45% and the RBC count = 5×10^{12}/L, the MCV = 90 fL.

The reference interval for MCV is 80 to 100 fL. RBCs with an MCV of less than 80 fL are microcytic; those with an MCV of more than 100 fL are macrocytic.

Mean Cell Hemoglobin

The MCH is the average weight of hemoglobin in a red blood cell, expressed in picograms (pg), or 10^{-12} g:

$$MCH = \frac{HGB\ (g/dL) \times 10}{RBC\ count\ (\times\ 10^{12}/L)}$$

For example, if the hemoglobin = 16 g/dL and the RBC count = 5×10^{12}/L, the MCH = 32 pg.

The reference interval for adults is 26 to 32 pg. The MCH generally is not considered in the classification of anemias.

Mean Cell Hemoglobin Concentration

The MCHC is the average concentration of hemoglobin in each individual red blood cell. The units used are grams per deciliter (formerly given as a percentage):

$$MCHC = \frac{HGB\ (g/dL) \times 100}{HCT\ (\%)}$$

For example, if the HGB = 16 g/dL and the HCT = 48%, the MCHC = 33.3 g/dL.

Values of normochromic red blood cells range from 32 to 36 g/dL; values of hypochromic cells are less than 32 g/dL, and values of "hyperchromic" cells are greater than 36 g/dL. Hypochromic red blood cells occur in thalassemias, iron deficiency, and other conditions listed in Table 14-2. The term *hyperchromic* is a misnomer: a cell does not really contain more than 36 g/dL of hemoglobin, but its shape may have become spherocytic, which makes the cell appear full. An MCHC between 36 and 38 g/dL should be checked for spherocytes. An MCHC

TABLE 14-2 Red Blood Cell Indices, Red Blood Cell Morphology, and Disease States

MCV (fL)	MCHC (g/dL)	Red Blood Cell Morphology	Found in
<80	<32	Microcytic; hypochromic	Iron deficiency anemia, anemia of inflammation, thalassemia, Hb E disease and trait, sideroblastic anemia
80–100	32–36	Normocytic; normochromic	Hemolytic anemia, myelophthisic anemia, bone marrow failure, chronic renal disease
>100	32–36	Macrocytic; normochromic	Megaloblastic anemia, chronic liver disease, bone marrow failure, myelodysplastic syndrome

Hb, Hemoglobin; *MCHC,* mean cell hemoglobin concentration; *MCV,* mean cell volume.

greater than 38 g/dL should be investigated for an error in hemoglobin value (see Sources of Error and Comments in the section on hemoglobin determination). Another cause for a markedly increased MCHC could be the presence of a cold agglutinin. Incubating the specimen at 37° C for 15 minutes before analysis usually produces accurate results. Cold agglutinin disease is discussed in more detail in Chapter 26.

RETICULOCYTE COUNT

The reticulocyte is the last immature red blood cell stage. Normally, a reticulocyte spends 2 days in the bone marrow and 1 day in the peripheral blood before developing into a mature red blood cell. The reticulocyte contains remnant cytoplasmic ribonucleic acid (RNA) and organelles such as the mitochondria and ribosomes (Chapter 8). The reticulocyte count is used to assess the erythropoietic activity of the bone marrow.

Principle

Whole blood, anticoagulated with EDTA, is stained with a supravital stain, such as new methylene blue. Any nonnucleated red blood cell that contains two or more particles of blue-stained granulofilamentous material after new methylene blue staining is defined as a *reticulocyte* (Figure 14-9).

PROCEDURE

1. Mix equal amounts of blood and new methylene blue stain (2 to 3 drops, or approximately 50 µL each), and allow to incubate at room temperature for 3 to 10 minutes.[12]
2. Remix the preparation.
3. Prepare two wedge films (Chapter 16).
4. In an area in which cells are close together but not touching, count 1000 RBCs under the oil immersion objective lens (1000× total magnification). Reticulocytes are included in the total RBC count (i.e., a reticulocyte counts as both an RBC and a reticulocyte).

5. To improve accuracy, have another laboratorian count the other film; counts should agree within 20%.
6. Calculate the % reticulocyte count:

$$\text{Reticulocytes (\%)} = \frac{\text{number of reticulocytes} \times 100}{1000 \text{ (RBCs counted)}}$$

For example, if 15 reticulocytes are counted,

$$\text{Reticulocytes (\%)} = \frac{15 \times 100}{1000} = 1.5\%$$

Or the number of reticulocytes counted can be multiplied by 0.1 (100/1000) to obtain the result.

Miller Disc

Because large numbers of red blood cells should be counted to obtain a more precise reticulocyte count, the Miller disc was designed to reduce this labor-intensive process. The disc is composed of two squares, with the area of the smaller square measuring $^1/_9$ the area of the larger square. The disc is inserted into the eyepiece of the microscope and the grid in Figure 14-10 is seen. RBCs are counted in the smaller square, and reticulocytes are counted in the larger square. Selection of the counting area is the same as described earlier. A minimum of 112 cells should be counted in the small square, because this is equivalent to 1008 red cells in the large square and satisfies the College of American Pathologists (CAP) hematology standard for a manual reticulocyte count based on at least 1000 red cells.[13] The calculation formula for percent reticulocytes is

$$\text{Reticulocytes \%} = \frac{\begin{array}{c}\text{no. reticulocytes in square A}\\\text{(large square)} \times 100\end{array}}{\text{no. RBCs in square B (small square)} \times 9}$$

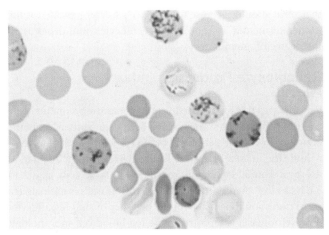

Figure 14-9 Reticulocytes with new methylene blue vital stain (peripheral blood ×1000). Reticulocytes are nonnucleated red blood cells with two or more blue-stained filaments or particles.

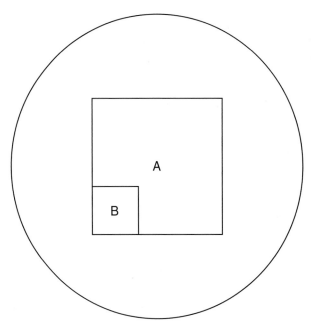

Figure 14-10 Miller ocular disc counting grid as viewed through a microscope. The area of square B is 1/9 the area of square A. Alternatively, square B may be in the center of square A.

For example, if 15 reticulocytes are counted in the large square and 112 red blood cells are counted in the small square,

$$\text{Reticulocytes \%} = \frac{15 \times 100}{112 \times 9} = 1.5\%$$

Equation Reference Interval

General reference intervals can be found on the inside front cover of this text.

Sources of Error and Comments

1. If a patient is very anemic or polycythemic, the proportion of dye to blood should be adjusted accordingly.
2. An error may occur if the blood and stain are not mixed before the films are made. The specific gravity of the reticulocytes is lower than that of mature red blood cells, and reticulocytes settle at the top of the mixture during incubation.
3. Moisture in the air, poor drying of the slide, or both may cause areas of the slide to appear refractile, and these areas could be confused with reticulocytes. The RNA remnants in a reticulocyte are not refractile.
4. Other red blood cell inclusions that stain supravitally include Heinz, Howell-Jolly, and Pappenheimer bodies (Table 19-3). Heinz bodies are precipitated hemoglobin, usually appear round or oval, and tend to adhere to the cell membrane (Figure 14-11). Howell-Jolly bodies are round nuclear fragments and are usually singular. Pappenheimer bodies are iron in the mitochondria whose presence can be confirmed with an iron stain, such as Prussian blue. This stain is discussed in Chapter 17.
5. If a Miller disc is used, it is important to heed the "edge rule" as described in the WBC count procedure and illustrated in Figure 14-2. A significant bias is observed if the rule is ignored.[12]

Absolute Reticulocyte Count
Principle

The absolute reticulocyte count (ARC) is the actual number of reticulocytes in 1 liter (L) or 1 microliter (μL) of blood.

Calculations

$$ARC = \frac{\text{reticulocytes (\%)} \times \text{RBC count } (\times 10^{12}/L)}{100}$$

For example, if a patient's reticulocyte count is 2% and the RBC count is $2.20 \times 10^{12}/L$, the ARC is calculated as follows (note that the calculated result has to be converted from $10^{12}/L$ to $10^9/L$):

$$ARC = \frac{2 \times (2.20 \times 10^{12}/L)}{100} = 44 \times 10^9/L$$

The absolute reticulocyte count can also be reported as the number of cells per μL. Using the example above, the RBC count in μL ($2.20 \times 10^6/\mu L$) is used in the formula, and the ARC result is $44 \times 10^3/\mu L$.

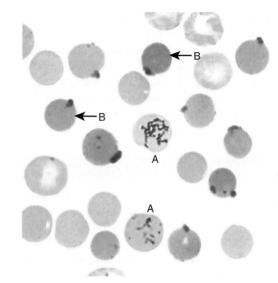

Figure 14-11 Reticulocytes (A) and Heinz bodies (B) stained with supravital stain (peripheral blood ×1000).

Reference Interval

Values between $20 \times 10^9/L$ and $115 \times 10^9/L$ are within the reference interval for most populations.[14]

Corrected Reticulocyte Count
Principle

In specimens with a low hematocrit, the percentage of reticulocytes may be falsely elevated because the whole blood contains fewer red blood cells. A correction factor is used, with the average normal hematocrit considered to be 45%.

Calculation

$$\text{Corrected reticulocyte count (\%)} =$$
$$\text{reticulocyte (\%)} \times \frac{\text{patient HCT (\%)}}{45}$$

Reference Interval

Patients with a hematocrit of 35% should have an elevated corrected reticulocyte count of 2% to 3% to compensate for the mild anemia. In patients with a hematocrit of less than 25%, the count should increase to 3% to 5% to compensate for the moderate anemia. The corrected reticulocyte count depends on the degree of anemia.

Reticulocyte Production Index
Principle

Reticulocytes that are released from the marrow prematurely are called *shift reticulocytes*. These reticulocytes are "shifted" from the bone marrow to the peripheral blood earlier than usual to compensate for anemia. Instead of losing their reticulum in 1 day, as do most normal circulating reticulocytes, these cells take 2 to 3 days to lose their reticula. When erythropoiesis is evaluated, a correction should be made for the presence of shift reticulocytes if polychromasia is reported in the red blood cell morphology. Most normal (nonshift) reticulocytes become mature red blood cells within 1 day after entering the bloodstream and thus represent 1 day's production of red blood cells in the bone marrow.

Cells shifted to the peripheral blood prematurely stay longer as reticulocytes and contribute to the reticulocyte count for more than 1 day. For this reason, the reticulocyte count is falsely increased when polychromasia is present, because the count no longer represents the cells maturing in just 1 day. On many automated instruments, this mathematical adjustment of the reticulocyte count has been replaced by the measurement of immature reticulocyte fraction (Chapter 15).[12]

The patient's hematocrit is used to determine the appropriate correction factor (reticulocyte maturation time in days):

Patient's Hematocrit Value (%)	Correction Factor (Maturation Time, Days)
40–45	1
35–39	1.5
25–34	2
15–24	2.5
<15	3

Calculation

The reticulocyte production index (RPI) is calculated as follows:

$$RPI = \frac{\text{reticulocyte (\%)} \times [\text{HCT (\%)}/45]}{\text{maturation time}}$$

Or

$$RPI = \frac{\text{corrected reticulocyte count}}{\text{maturation time}}$$

For example, for a patient with a reticulocyte count of 7.8% and a HCT of 30%, and with polychromasia noted, the previous table indicates a maturation time of 2 days. Thus

$$RPI = \frac{7.8 \times [30/45]}{2}$$
$$RPI = 2.6$$

Reference Interval

An adequate bone marrow response usually is indicated by an RPI that is greater than 3. An inadequate erythropoietic response is seen when the RPI is less than 2.[14]

Reticulocyte Control

Several commercial controls are now available for monitoring manual and automated reticulocyte counts [e.g., Retic-Chex II, Streck Laboratories, Omaha, NE; Liquichek Reticulocyte Control (A), Bio-Rad Laboratories, Hercules, CA]. Most of the controls are available at three levels. The control samples are treated in the same manner as the patient samples. The control can be used to verify the laboratorian's accuracy and precision when manual counts are performed.

Automated Reticulocyte Counts

The major instrument manufacturers offer are analyzers that perform automated reticulocyte counts. All of the analyzers evaluate reticulocytes using optical scatter or fluorescence after the red blood cells are treated with fluorescent dyes or nucleic acid stains to stain residual RNA in the reticulocytes. The percentage and the absolute count are provided. These results are statistically more valid because of the large number of cells counted. Other reticulocyte parameters that are offered on some automated instruments include a maturation index/immature reticulocyte fraction or IRF (reflecting the proportion of the more immature reticulocytes in the sample), the reticulocyte hemoglobin concentration, and reticulocyte indices (such as the mean reticulocyte volume and distribution width). The IRF may be especially useful in detecting early erythropoietic activity after chemotherapy or hematopoietic stem cell transplantation. The reticulocyte hemoglobin is useful to detect early iron deficiency (Chapter 20). Automated reticulocyte counting is discussed in Chapter 15.

ERYTHROCYTE SEDIMENTATION RATE

The erythrocyte sedimentation rate (ESR) is ordered with other tests to detect and monitor the course of inflammatory conditions such as, rheumatoid arthritis, infections, or certain malignancies. It is also useful in the diagnosis of temporal arteritis and polymyalgia rheumatica.[15] The ESR, however, is not a specific test for inflammatory diseases and is elevated in many other conditions such as plasma cell myeloma, pregnancy, anemia, and older age. It is also prone to technical errors that can falsely elevate or decrease the sedimentation rate. Because of its low specificity and sensitivity, the ESR is not recommended as a screening test to detect inflammatory conditions in asymptomatic individuals.[15] Other tests for inflammation, such as the C-reactive protein level, may be a more predictable and reliable alternative to monitor inflammation.[16]

Principle

When anticoagulated blood is allowed to stand at room temperature undisturbed for a period of time, the red blood cells settle toward the bottom of the tube. The ESR is the distance in millimeters that the red blood cells fall in 1 hour. The ESR is affected by red blood cell, plasma, and mechanical and technical factors. Red blood cells have a net negative surface charge and tend to repel one another. The repulsive forces are partially or totally counteracted if there are increased quantities of positively charged plasma proteins. Under these conditions the red blood cells settle more rapidly as a result of the formation of rouleaux (stacking of red blood cells). Examples of macromolecules that can produce this reaction are fibrinogen, β-globulins, and pathologic immunoglobulins.[17,18]

Normal red blood cells have a relatively small mass and settle slowly. Certain diseases can cause rouleaux formation, in which the plasma fibrinogen and globulins are altered. This alteration changes the red blood cell surface, which leads to stacking of the red blood cells, increased red blood cell mass, and a more rapid ESR. The ESR is directly proportional to the red blood cell mass and inversely proportional to plasma viscosity. Several methods, both manual and automated, are available for measuring the ESR. Only the most commonly used methods are discussed here.

Modified Westergren Erythrocyte Sedimentation Rate

The most commonly used method today is the modified Westergren method. One advantage of this method is that the taller column height allows the detection of highly elevated ESRs. It is the method recommended by the International Council for Standardization in Hematology and the Clinical and Laboratory Standards Institute.[15,19]

PROCEDURE

1. Use well-mixed blood collected in EDTA and dilute at four parts blood to one part 3.8% sodium citrate or 0.85% sodium chloride (e.g., 2 mL blood and 0.5 mL diluent). Alternatively, blood can be collected directly into special sedimentation test tubes containing sodium citrate. Standard coagulation test tubes are not acceptable, because the dilution is nine parts blood to one part sodium citrate.[15]
2. Place the diluted sample in a 200-mm column with an internal diameter of 2.55 mm or more.
3. Place the column into the rack and allow to stand undisturbed for 60 minutes at room temperature (18 to 25° C). Ensure that the rack is level.
4. Record the number of millimeters the red blood cells have fallen in 1 hour. The buffy coat should not be included in the reading. Read the tube from the bottom of the plasma layer to the top of the sedimented red blood cells (Figure 14-12). Report the result as the ESR, 1 hour = x mm.[15]

Wintrobe Erythrocyte Sedimentation Rate

When the Wintrobe method was first introduced, the specimen used was oxalate-anticoagulated whole blood. This was placed in a 100-mm column. Today, EDTA-treated or citrated whole blood is used with the shorter column. The shorter column height allows a somewhat increased sensitivity in detecting mildly elevated ESRs.

PROCEDURE

1. Use fresh blood collected in EDTA anticoagulant. A minimum of 2 mL of whole blood is needed.
2. After mixing the blood thoroughly, fill a Pasteur pipette using a rubber pipette bulb.
3. Place the filled pipette into the Wintrobe tube until the tip reaches the bottom of the tube.
4. Carefully squeeze the bulb and expel the blood into the Wintrobe tube while pulling the Pasteur pipette up from the bottom of the tube. There must be steady, even pressure on the bulb to expel blood into the tube as well as continuous movement of the pipette up the tube to prevent the introduction of air bubbles into the column of blood.
5. Fill the Wintrobe tube to the 0 mark.
6. Place the tube into a Wintrobe rack (tube holder) and allow to stand undisturbed for 1 hour at room temperature. The rack must be perfectly level and placed in a draft-free room.
7. Record the number of millimeters the red blood cells have fallen. Read the tube from the bottom of the plasma meniscus

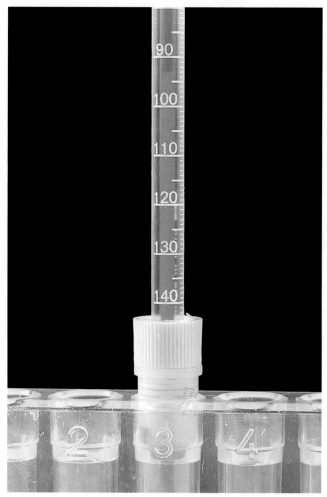

Figure 14-12 Erythrocyte sedimentation rate (ESR), 1 hour = 93 mm, which is elevated above the reference intervals.

to the top of the sedimented red cells. The result is reported in millimeters per hour.

Reference Interval

Reference intervals according to sex and age can be found on the inside front cover of this text. Table 14-3 lists some of the factors that influence the ESR.

Sources of Error and Comments

1. If the concentration of anticoagulant is increased, the ESR will be falsely low as a result of sphering of the RBCs, which inhibits rouleaux formation.
2. The anticoagulants sodium or potassium oxalate and heparin cause the red blood cells to shrink and falsely elevate the ESR.
3. A significant change in the temperature of the room alters the ESR.
4. Even a slight tilt of the pipette causes the ESR to increase.
5. Blood specimens must be analyzed within 4 hours of collection if kept at room temperature (18 to 25° C).[15] If the specimen is allowed to sit at room temperature for more than 4 hours, the red blood cells start to become

TABLE 14-3 Factors Affecting the Erythrocyte Sedimentation Rate (ESR)

Category	Increased ESR	Decreased ESR
Blood proteins and lipids	Hypercholesterolemia	Hyperalbuminemia
	Hyperfibrinogenemia	Hyperglycemia
	Hypergammaglobulinemia	Hypofibrinogenemia
	Hypoalbuminemia	Hypogammaglobulinemia
		Increased bile salts
		Increased phospholipids
Red blood cells	Anemia	Acanthocytosis
	Macrocytosis	Anisocytosis (marked)
		Hemoglobin C
		Microcytosis
		Polycythemia
		Sickle cells
		Spherocytosis
		Thalassemia
White blood cells	Leukemia	Leukocytosis (marked)
Drugs	Dextran	Adrenocorticotropic hormone (corticotropin)
	Heparin	Cortisone
	Penicillamine	Ethambutol
	Procainamide	Quinine
	Theophylline	Salicylates
	Vitamin A	
Clinical conditions	Acute heavy metal poisoning	Cachexia
	Acute bacterial infections	Congestive heart failure
	Collagen vascular diseases	Newborn status
	Diabetes mellitus	
	End-stage renal failure	
	Gout	
	Malignancy	
	Menstruation	
	Multiple myeloma	
	Myocardial infarction	
	Pregnancy	
	Rheumatic fever	
	Rheumatoid arthritis	
	Syphilis	
	Temporal arteritis	
Specimen handling	Refrigerated sample not returned to room temperature	Clotted blood sample
		Delay in testing
Technique	High room temperature	Bubbles in ESR column
	Tilted ESR tube	Low room temperature
	Vibration	Narrow ESR column diameter

From American Society for Clinical Pathology/American Proficiency Institute: 2006 2nd Test Event—Educational Commentary—The Erythrocyte Sedimentation Rate and Its Clinical Utility. API is the proficiency testing group that provides testing materials to the American Society for Clinical Pathology. The educational commentary itself is written by ASCP. This reference can also be accessed at: http://www.api-pt.com/Reference/Commentary/2006Bcoag.pdf. Accessed November 5, 2014.

spherical, which may inhibit the formation of rouleaux. Blood specimens may be stored at 4° C up to 24 hours prior to testing, but must be rewarmed by holding the specimen at ambient room temperature for at least 15 minutes prior to testing.[15]

6. Bubbles in the column of blood invalidate the test results.

7. The blood must be filled properly to the zero mark at the beginning of the test.

8. A clotted specimen cannot be used.

9. The tubes must not be subjected to vibrations on the lab bench which can falsely increase the ESR.

10. Hematologic disorders that prevent the formation of rouleaux (e.g., the presence of sickle cells and spherocytes) decrease the ESR.

11. The ESR of patients with severe anemia is of little diagnostic value, because it will be falsely elevated.

Disposable Kits

Disposable commercial kits are available for ESR testing (Figure 14-13). Several kits include safety caps for the columns that allow the blood to fill precisely to the zero mark. This safety cap makes the column a closed system and eliminates the error involved in manually setting the blood to the zero mark.

Automated Erythrocyte Sedimentation Rate

There are several automated ESR systems available using the traditional Westergren and Wintrobe methods, as well as alternate methods such as centrifugation. The Ves-Matic system (Diesse, Inc., Hialeah, FL) is a bench-top analyzer designed to determine ESR by use of an optoelectronic sensor, which measures the change in opacity of a column of blood as sedimentation of blood progresses. Blood is collected in special Ves-Tec or Vacu-Tec tubes, which contain sodium citrate and are compatible with the Vacutainer system. These tubes are used directly in the instrument (Figure 14-14). Acceleration of sedimentation is achieved by positioning the tubes at an 18-degree angle in relation to the vertical axis. Results comparable with Westergren 1-hour values are obtained in 20 minutes.[20]

Another automated ESR analyzer is the Sedimat 15 (Polymedco, Cortlandt Manor, NY), which uses the principle of infrared measurement. It is capable of testing one to eight samples randomly or simultaneously and provides results in 15 minutes (Figure 14-15).

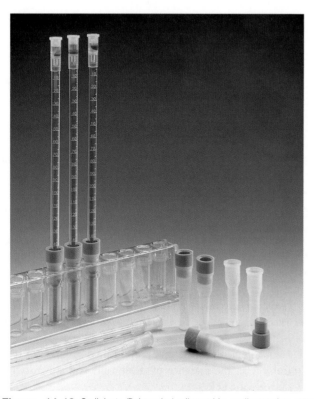

Figure 14-13 Sediplast (Polymedco) disposable sedimentation rate system. (Courtesy Polymedco, Cortlandt Manor, NY.)

The ESR STAT PLUS system (HemaTechnologies, Lebanon, NJ) is based on centrifugation. The advantages of this method are a smaller required sample volume and shorter testing time, which makes it more suitable for a pediatric patient population. The disadvantage of this method is the number of exacting preanalytical steps that must be strictly followed to prevent erroneous results. Compliance with these steps may be difficult to achieve consistently in a busy hematology laboratory.[21]

ADDITIONAL METHODS

Additional manual and semi-automated methods are included in other chapters that are relevant to their clinical application. Examples include: Chapter 24 for the osmotic fragility test and qualitative and quantitative assays for glucose-6-phosphate dehydrogenase and pyruvate kinase activity; Chapter 27 for the solubility test for Hb S, hemoglobin electrophoresis (alkaline and acid pH), and unstable hemoglobin test; and Chapter 28 for the vital stain for hemoglobin H and the Kleihauer-Betke acid elution test for Hb F distribution in the RBCs.

POINT-OF-CARE TESTING

Point-of-care testing offers the ability to produce rapid and accurate results that help facilitate faster treatment, which can decrease patient length of stay. This testing is rarely performed by trained laboratory personnel; most often, it is carried out by nurses. Manufacturers have created analyzers with nonlaboratory operators in mind, but results obtained using these systems are still affected by preanalytic and analytical variables. The laboratory's partnership with nursing is the key to success in any hospital's point-of-care program.

Point-of-care testing is defined as diagnostic testing at or near the site of patient care. The Clinical Laboratory Improvement Amendments of 1988 (CLIA) introduced the concept of "testing site neutrality," which means that regardless of where the diagnostic testing is performed or who performs the test, all testing sites must follow the same regulatory requirements based on the "complexity" of the test. Under CLIA, point-of-care testing (including physician-performed microscopy) is classified as "waived" or "moderately complex." Tests are classified as waived if they are determined to be "simple tests with an insignificant risk of an erroneous result." Point-of-care testing is commonly performed in hospital inpatient units, outpatient clinics, surgery centers, emergency departments, long-term care facilities, and dialysis units. For waived point-of-care testing, facilities are required to obtain a certificate of waiver, pay the appropriate fees, and follow the manufacturers' testing instructions.[22] For any point-of-care program to be successful, certain key elements must be present. Clear administrative responsibility, well-written procedures, a training program, quality control, proficiency testing, and equipment maintenance are essential for success. The first step is appointing a laboratory point-of-care testing coordinator. This person

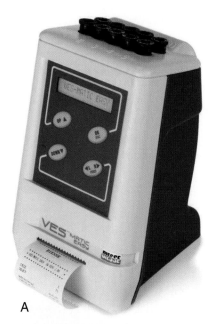
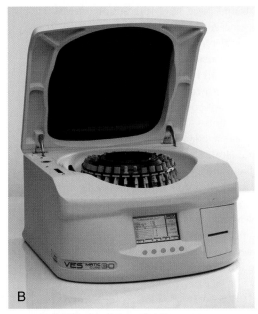

A   B

Figure 14-14 Two models of the Ves-Matic instruments for sedimentation rates: The Ves-Matic Easy **(A)** for up to 10 specimens (requiring special tubes) and the Ves-Matic Cube 30 **(B)** for up to 30 specimens, determining the ESR directly from EDTA tubes. Products with up to 190-specimen capacity are also available. (Courtesy Diesse Inc., Hialeah, FL.)

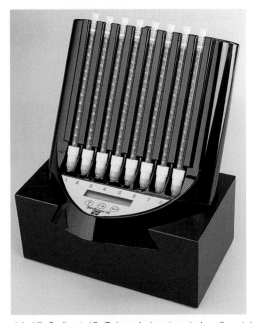

Figure 14-15 Sedimat 15 (Polymedco) automated sedimentation rate system. (Courtesy Polymedco, Cortlandt Manor, NY.)

not only is the "go-to" person but is also an important liaison between the laboratory and nursing staff. The second step to ensuring a successful program is to create a multidisciplinary team with authority to impact all aspects of the POC program. This committee would have the authority to oversee the integrity and quality of the existing POC program and institute changes or new testing as needed. It is also important to have administrative support to help remove barriers.

A point-of-care testing program must incorporate all of the following. A written policy should be developed that defines

the program. This policy should outline who is responsible for each part of the program. The policy should also indicate where the testing is to be performed and who is going to perform the testing. Testing procedures should be written that clearly state how to perform the tests and that address how to handle critical values and/or any discrepant results. The program must be monitored. An ongoing evaluation of the point-of-care testing is vital for success.

When the instrument to be used in the point-of-care testing program is being selected, it is helpful to invite the vendors to demonstrate their equipment. An equipment display that is available for hands-on use by the operators can be very helpful in selection of the appropriate instrumentation. Patient correlation studies are very useful in choosing equipment that best covers the patient population for that particular institution. Point-of-care operators need handheld analyzers that are lightweight, accurate, fast, and that require little specimen material. The point-of-care testing system should also address the following laboratory concerns:

- What is the range of measurement?
- How well does the test system correlate with laboratory instrumentation?
- Can it be interfaced to the laboratory information system?
- Does it give reliable results?
- Does the company supply excellent technical support?
- Is it affordable?

Paramount to point-of-care testing is patient safety. It is important to maintain good practices, and with waived testing, this often comes down to the basics. Such basics include proper and appropriate specimen collection, proper identification of the patient and specimen, proper storage of reagents, and good documentation of patient test results (use of point-of-care interfaces is beneficial), as well as proper performance of any necessary instrument maintenance. Laboratory oversight is sometimes absent, and basic safety precautions necessary for waived tests can be easily overlooked, often due to a lack of understanding, lack of training, and high personnel turnover rates.[23] Patient safety, risk management, and error reduction are primary goals of all health care facilities. All testing personnel should be properly trained in best practices to avoid exposure. The individual responsible for oversight—whether laboratory or nonlaboratory—must avoid taking safety for granted. All applicable standards (including those of the Occupation Safety and Health Administration, Centers for Disease Control and Prevention, The Joint Commission, CAP, CLIA, and so forth) should be implemented and easily accessible. Because the number of waived tests has grown significantly since waived tests were first defined by CLIA, it is paramount that standard safety precautions and the basic steps outlined earlier be implemented to ensure that patient safety is not sacrificed in the unique situation of CLIA-waived testing.

Point-of-Care Tests

Various point-of-care instruments are available to measure parameters such as hemoglobin level and hematocrit, and some perform a complete blood count.

Hematocrit

The most common methods for determining the hematocrit include the microhematocrit centrifuge, conductometric methods, and calculation by automated cell counters (Chapter 15).

Centrifuge-based microhematocrit systems have been available for years, and the results obtained correlate well with the results produced by standard cell counters. Nonlaboratorians and inexperienced operators, however, may be unaware of the error that can be introduced by insufficient centrifugation time and inaccurate reading of the microhematocrit tube (see comments in the Microhematocrit section). Examples of centrifuge-based devices are the Hematastat II (Separation Technology, Inc., Altamonte Springs, FL) and STAT Crit (Wampole Laboratories, Cranbury, NJ).

The i-STAT 1 (Abbott Laboratories, Abbott Park, IL)[24] (Figure 14-16) and the Epoc (Epocal, Inc., Ottawa, ON) (Figure 14-17)[25] use the conductivity method to determine the hematocrit. Plasma conducts electrical current, whereas WBCs act as insulators. In the i-STAT system, before the measured sample conductance is converted into the hematocrit value, corrections are applied for the temperature of the sample, the size of the fluid segment being measured, and the relative conductivity of the plasma component. The first two corrections are determined from the measured value of the calibrant conductance and the last correction from the measured concentrations of sodium and potassium in the sample.[24]

Sources of Error and Comments.   Conductivity of a whole blood sample is dependent on the amount of electrolytes in the plasma portion. Conductivity does not distinguish red blood cells from other nonconductive elements such as proteins, lipids, and WBCs that may be present in the sample. A low total protein level will falsely decrease the hematocrit. The presence of lipids can interfere with the hematocrit

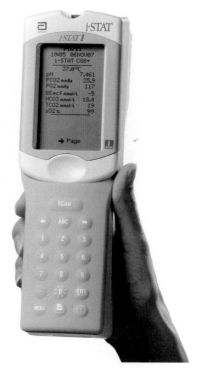

Figure 14-16 i-STAT instrument for measuring hematocrit. (Courtesy Abbott Laboratories, Abbott Park, IL.)

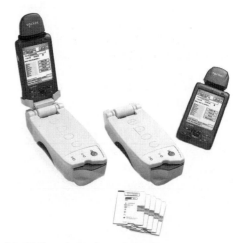

Figure 14-17 Epoc device for measuring hematocrit. (Courtesy Epocal, Inc., Ottawa, Ontario, Canada.)

measurement. An increased WBC count will falsely increase the hematocrit. The presence of cold agglutinins can falsely decrease the hematocrit.[24]

Other Instruments.   Other instruments that measure the hematocrit include the following:
- ABL 77 (Radiometer, Westlake, OH)
- IRMA (ITC, a subsidiary of Thoratec Corporation, Edison, NJ)
- Gem Premier (Instrumentation Laboratory Company, Lexington, MA) (Figure 14-18)

Hemoglobin Concentration

In point-of-care testing, hemoglobin concentration is measured by modified hemoglobinometers or by oximeters integrated

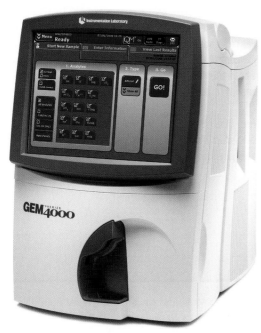

Figure 14-18 Gem Premier instrument for measuring hematocrit. (Courtesy Instrumentation Laboratory Company, Lexington, MA.)

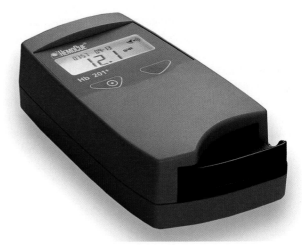

Figure 14-19 The HemoCue ® Hb 201+ System for measuring hemoglobin. (Courtesy HemoCue, Inc., Brea, CA.)

with a blood gas analyzer. The HemoCue hemoglobinometer (HemoCue, Inc., Brea, CA) uses a small cuvette that contains a lysing agent and reagents to form a hemoglobin azide, which is measured by a photometer at two wavelengths (570 nm and 880 nm) (Figure 14-19).[6] This eliminates interference from turbidity in the sample. Results obtained with the instrument compare well with those produced by reference methods, but a major source of error is mixture of blood with tissue fluid during skin puncture collection. The AVOX 1000E (ITC) measures total hemoglobin by a spectrophotometric method. The STAT-Site MHbg Meter (Stanbio Laboratory, Boerne, TX) uses the azidemethemoglobin principle and reflectance photometry to measure reflected light in the test area. The test card is composed of molded plastic with a fluid well that contains numerous pads impregnated with specific chemical reagents. A drop of whole blood is applied to the center of the well and reacts with the chemicals in the pad to produce a specific color that is measured from the bottom of the card.[26]

Cell and Platelet Counts

Traditional cell-counting methods can be employed at the point of care for the analysis of WBCs, RBCs, and platelets. The Ichor Hematology Analyzer (Helena Laboratories, Beaumont, TX) performs a complete blood count along with platelet aggregation. Another option for cell quantitation and differentiation employs a buffy coat analysis method. Quantitative buffy coat analysis (QBC STAR, manufactured by QBC Diagnostics, Inc., Philipsburg, PA) involves centrifugation in specialized capillary tubes designed to expand the buffy coat layer. The components (platelets, mononuclear cells, and granulocytes) can be measured with the assistance of fluorescent dyes and a measuring device.[27]

SUMMARY

- Although most laboratories are highly automated, the manual tests discussed in this chapter, such as the cyanmethemoglobin method of hemoglobin determination and centrifuge-based measurement of the microhematocrit, are used as a part of many laboratories' quality control and backup methods of analysis.
- The hemacytometer allows counts of any type of cell or particle (e.g., WBCs or platelets) to be performed.
- The reference method for hemoglobin determination is based on the absorbance of cyanmethemoglobin at 540 nm. When a spectrophotometer is used, a standard curve is employed to obtain the results.
- The microhematocrit is a measure of packed red blood cell volume.
- The rule of three specifies that the value of the hematocrit should be three times the value of the hemoglobin plus or minus 3 (%) or

0.03 (L/L). A value discrepant with this rule may indicate abnormal red blood cells or it may be the first indication of error.
- RBC indices—the mean cell volume (MCV), mean cell hemoglobin (MCH), and mean cell hemoglobin concentration (MCHC)—are calculated to determine the average volume, hemoglobin content, and hemoglobin concentration of red blood cells. The indices give an indication of possible causes of an anemia.
- The reticulocyte count, which is used to assess the erythropoietic activity of the bone marrow, is accomplished through the use of supravital stains (e.g., new methylene blue) or by flow cytometric methods.
- The erythrocyte sedimentation rate (ESR), a measure of the settling of red blood cells in a 1-hour period, depends on the red blood cells' ability to form rouleaux. It is used to detect and monitor conditions

with inflammation such as rheumatoid arthritis, infections, and some malignancies. It is subject to many physiologic and technical errors.
- Point-of-care testing is often performed by nonlaboratory personnel. It is defined as diagnostic laboratory testing at or near the site of patient care.
- CLIA introduced the concept of "testing site neutrality," which means that it does not matter where diagnostic testing is performed or who performs the test; all testing sites must follow the same regulatory requirements based on the "complexity" of the test.
- Tests are classified as waived if they are determined to be "simple tests with an insignificant risk of an erroneous result." Most, but not all, point-of-care testing is waived.

- For a point-of-care testing program to be successful, key elements such as clear administrative responsibility, well-written procedures, quality control, proficiency testing, and equipment maintenance must be present.
- Paramount to point-of-care testing is patient safety.

Now that you have completed this chapter, read again the case studies at the beginning and respond to the questions presented.

REVIEW QUESTIONS

1. A 1:20 dilution of blood is made with 3% glacial acetic acid as the diluent. The four large corner squares on both sides of the hemacytometer are counted, for a total of 100 cells. What is the total WBC count ($\times 10^9$/L)?
   a. 0.25
   b. 2.5
   c. 5
   d. 10

2. The total WBC count is 20×10^9/L. Twenty-five NRBCs per 100 WBCs are observed on the peripheral blood film. What is the corrected WBC count ($\times 10^9$/L)?
   a. 0.8
   b. 8
   c. 16
   d. 19

3. If potassium cyanide and potassium ferricyanide are used in the manual method for hemoglobin determination, the final product is:
   a. Methemoglobin
   b. Azide methemoglobin
   c. Cyanmethemoglobin
   d. Myoglobin

4. Which of the following would *not* interfere with the result when hemoglobin determination is performed by the cyanmethemoglobin method?
   a. Increased lipids
   b. Elevated WBC count
   c. Lyse-resistant RBCs
   d. Fetal hemoglobin

5. A patient has a hemoglobin level of 8.0 g/dL. According to the rule of three, what is the expected range for the hematocrit?
   a. 21% to 24%
   b. 23.7% to 24.3%
   c. 24% to 27%
   d. 21% to 27%

6. Calculate the MCV and MCHC for the following values:
   RBCs = 5.00×10^{12}/L
   HGB = 9 g/dL
   HCT = 30%

	MCV (fL)	MCHC (g/dL)
a.	30	18
b.	60	30
c.	65	33
d.	85	35

7. What does the reticulocyte count assess?
   a. Inflammation
   b. Response to infection
   c. Erythropoietic activity of the bone marrow
   d. Ability of red blood cells to form rouleaux

8. For a patient with the following test results, which measure of bone marrow red blood cell production provides the most accurate information?
   Observed reticulocyte count = 5.3%
   HCT = 35%
   Morphology—moderate polychromasia
   a. Observed reticulocyte count
   b. Corrected reticulocyte count
   c. RPI
   d. ARC

9. Given the following values, calculate the RPI:
   Observed reticulocyte count = 6%
   HCT = 30%
   a. 2
   b. 3
   c. 4
   d. 5

10. Which of the following would be associated with an elevated ESR value?
   a. Microcytosis
   b. Polycythemia
   c. Decreased globulins
   d. Inflammation

REFERENCES

1. Brecher, G., & Cronkite, E. P. (1950). Morphology and enumeration of human blood platelets. *J Appl Physiol, 3,* 365–377.
2. Clinical and Laboratory Standards Institute (CLSI). (2000). Reference and selected procedures for the quantitative determination of hemoglobin in blood: approved standard. (3rd ed.), CLSI Document H15–A3, Wayne, PA: CLSI.
3. Zwart, A., van Assendelft, O. W., Bull, B. S., et al. (1996). Recommendations for reference method for haemoglobinometry in human blood (ICSH Standard 1995) and specifications for international haemiglobincyanide reference preparation (4th ed.) *J Clin Pathol, 49,* 271–274.
4. von Schenck H, Falkensson M, & Lundberg B. (1986). Evaluation of "HemoCue," a new device for determining hemoglobin. *Clin Chem, 32,* 526–529.
5. HemoCue. Retrieved from http://www.hemocue.com/. Accessed 11.05.14.
6. MacLaren, I. A., Conn, D. M., & Wadsworth, L. D. (1991). Comparison of two automated hemoglobin methods using Sysmex SULFOLYSER and STROMATOLYSER. *Sysmex J Int, 1,* 59–61.
7. Karsan, A., MacLaren, I., Conn, D., et al. (1993). An evaluation of hemoglobin determination using sodium lauryl sulfate. *Am J Clin Pathol, 100,* 123–126.
8. Matsubara, T., Mimura, T. (1990). Reaction mechanism of SLS-Hb Method. *Sysmex J (Japan), 13,* 206–211.
9. Fujiwara, C., Hamaguchi, Y., Toda, S., et al. (1990). The reagent SULFOLYSER for hemoglobin measurement by hematology analyzers. *Sysmex J (Japan), 13,* 212–219.
10. Clinical and Laboratory Standards Institute (CLSI). (2000). Procedure for determining packed cell volume by the microhematocrit method: approved standard. (3rd ed.), NCCLS document H7–A3, Wayne, PA: CLSI.
11. Becton Dickinson Primary Care Diagnostics. (1998). *Clay Adams brand SUREPREP capillary tubes,* Sparks, MD: Becton Dickinson Primary Care Diagnostics (product brochure).
12. Clinical and Laboratory Standards Institute (CLSI). (2004). Methods for reticulocyte counting (automated blood cell counters, flow cytometry, and supravital dyes): approved guideline. (2nd ed.), CLSI document H44–A2, Wayne, PA: CLSI.
13. College of American Pathologists. (2001). Q & A Miller disk clarification. *CAP Today, 95.* Retrieved from http://www.cap.org. Accessed 03.06.13.
14. Koepke, J. F., & Koepke, J. A. (1986). Reticulocytes. *Clin Lab Haematol, 8,* 169–179.
15. Clinical and Laboratory Standards Institute (CLSI). (2011). Procedures for the erythrocyte sedimentation rate (ESR) test: approved standard. (5th ed.), CLSI document H2–A5, Wayne, PA: CLSI.
16. Colombet, I., Pouchot, J., Kronz, V., et al. (2010). Agreement between the erythrocyte sedimentation rate and C-reactive protein in hospital practice. *Am J Med, 123,* 863.e7–863.e13.
17. Perkins, S.L. (2009). Examination of the blood and bone marrow. In Greer, J. P., Foerster, J. L., Rodgers, G. M., et al, (Eds.), *Wintrobe's Clinical Hematology.* (12th ed., pp. 1–20). Philadelphia: Wolters Kluwer Health/Lippincott Williams & Wilkins.
18. Mims, M. P., & Prchal, J. T. (2010). Hematology during pregnancy. In Lichtman, M. A., Kipps, T. J., Seligsohn, U., et al, (Eds.), *Williams Hematology.* (8th ed.). New York: McGraw-Hill.
19. Jou, J. M., Lewis, S. M., Briggs, C., et al. (2011). International Council for Standardization in Haematology: ICSH review of the measurement of the erythrocyte sedimentation rate. *Int J Lab Hematol, 33,* 125–32.
20. DIESSE. *Ves-Matic line.* Retrieved from http://www.diesse.it/. Accessed 11.05.14.
21. Shelat, S., Chacosky, D., & Shibutani, S. (2008). Differences in erythrocyte sedimentation rates using the Westergren method and a centrifugation method. *Am J Clin Pathol, 130*(1), 127–130.
22. Centers for Medicare and Medicaid Services. Clinical laboratory improvement amendments (CLIA 1988): overview. Retrieved from http://www.cms.hhs.gov/clia/. Accessed 11.05.14.
23. Good laboratory practices. (12.17.2002). Retrieved from http://www.cms.hhs.gov/CLIA/downloads/wgoodlab.pdf. Accessed 11.05.14.
24. Abbott Point of Care Cartridge and Hematocrit/HCT and Calculated Hemoglobin/HB information sheets, in i-STAT 1 system manual (revised June 11, 2008). Abbott Park, Ill, Abbott Laboratories.
25. Theory of operation, in Epocal system manual, rev 01, Ottawa, Ont, Canada: Epocal, Inc., pp. 11–17. Retrieved from http://www.epocal.com/system.html. Accessed 29.05.13.
26. Wu, J., Peterson., Mohammad, A., et al. (March 2003). Point-of-care hemoglobin measurements by Stat-Site MHgb Reflectance Meter. *Point of Care,* 8–11.
27. QBC operator's service manual, rev B. (2006). Philipsburg, PA: QBC Diagnostics, Inc., pp. 1–2.

ADDITIONAL RESOURCES

College of American Pathologists, http://www.cap.org.
Howerton D, Anderson N, Bosse D, et al: Good laboratory practices for waived testing sites. Available at: http://www.cdc.gov/mmWR/PDF/rr/rr5413.pdf.
Centers for Disease Control and Prevention: Health disparities experienced by black or African Americans—United States. (2005). *MMWR Morb Mortal Wkly Rep, 54,* 1–37.
The Joint Commission, http://www.jcaho.org.

Point of Care.net, http://www.pointofcare.net.
http://us.instrumentationlaboratory.com
www.abbottpointofcare.com
www.hemocue.com
www.itcmed.com
www.radiometer.com
www.stanbio.com
www.Helena.com

15 Automated Blood Cell Analysis

Sharral Longanbach and Martha K. Miers

OBJECTIVES

After completion of this chapter, the reader will be able to:

1. Explain the different principles of automated blood cell counting and analysis.
2. Describe how the general principles are implemented on different instruments.
3. Identify the parameters directly measured on the four analyzers discussed.
4. Explain the derivation of calculated or indirectly measured parameters for the same four analyzers.
5. Explain the derivation of the white blood cell differential count on the different instruments discussed.
6. Interpret and compare patient data, including white blood cell, red blood cell, and platelet histograms or cytograms or both, obtained from the four major hematology instruments.
7. Explain the general principles of automated reticulocyte counting.
8. Identify sources of error in automated cell counting and determine appropriate corrective action.

Since the 1980s, automated blood cell analysis has virtually replaced manual hemoglobin, hematocrit, and cell counting, due to its greater accuracy and precision, with the possible exception of phase platelet counting in certain circumstances. Hematology analyzers are marketed by multiple instrument manufacturers. These analyzers typically provide the eight standard hematology parameters (complete blood count [CBC]), plus a three-part, five-part, or six-part differential leukocyte count in less than 1 minute on 200 μL or less of whole blood. Automation allows more efficient workload management and more timely diagnosis and treatment of disease.

GENERAL PRINCIPLES OF AUTOMATED BLOOD CELL ANALYSIS

Despite the number of hematology analyzers available from different manufacturers and their varying levels of sophistication and complexity, most rely on only two basic principles of operation: electronic impedance (resistance) and optical scatter. *Electronic impedance*, or low-voltage direct current (DC) resistance, was developed by Coulter in the 1950s[1,2] and is the most common methodology used. *Radiofrequency* (RF), or alternating current resistance, is a modification sometimes used in conjunction with DC electronic impedance. Technicon Instruments Corporation (Tarrytown, NY) introduced darkfield optical scanning in the 1960s, and Ortho Clinical Diagnostics, Inc. (Raritan, NJ), followed with a laser-based optical instrument in the 1970s.[3] *Optical scatter*, using both laser and nonlaser light, is frequently employed in today's hematology instrumentation.

Electronic Impedance

The impedance principle of cell counting is based on the detection and measurement of changes in electrical resistance produced by cells as they traverse a small aperture. Cells suspended in an electrically conductive diluent such as saline are pulled through an aperture (orifice) in a glass tube. In the counting chamber, or transducer assembly, low-frequency electrical current is applied between an external electrode (suspended in the cell dilution) and an internal electrode (housed inside the aperture tube). Electrical resistance between the two electrodes, or impedance in the current, occurs as the cells pass through the sensing aperture, causing voltage pulses that are measurable (Figure 15-1).[4,5] Oscilloscope screens on some instruments display the pulses that are generated by the cells as they interrupt the current. The number of pulses is proportional to the number of cells counted. The height of the voltage pulse is directly proportional to the volume of the cell, which allows discrimination and counting of cells of specific volumes through the use of threshold circuits. Pulses are collected and sorted (channelized) according to their amplitude by pulse height analyzers. The data are plotted on a frequency distribution graph, or *volume distribution histogram*, with relative number on the *y*-axis and volume (channel number equivalent to a specific volume) on the *x*-axis. The histogram produced depicts the volume distribution of the cells counted. Figure 15-2 illustrates the construction of a frequency distribution graph. Volume thresholds separate the cell populations on the histogram, and the count is the cells enumerated between the lower and upper set thresholds for each population. Volume distribution histograms may be used for the evaluation of one cell population or subgroups within a population.[5] The use of proprietary lytic reagents to control shrinkage and lysis of specific cell types, as in the older Coulter S-Plus IV, STKR, and Sysmex E-5000 models, allows separation and quantitation of white blood cells (WBCs) into three populations (lymphocytes, mononuclear cells, and granulocytes) for the *three-part differential* on one volume distribution histogram.[6-8]

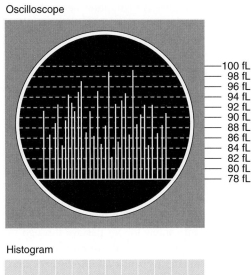

Oscilloscope

— 100 fL
— 98 fL
— 96 fL
— 94 fL
— 92 fL
— 90 fL
— 88 fL
— 86 fL
— 84 fL
— 82 fL
— 80 fL
— 78 fL

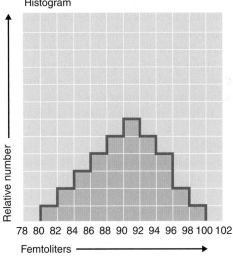

Histogram

78 80 82 84 86 88 90 92 94 96 98 100 102
Femtoliters ⟶

Figure 15-2 Oscilloscope display and histogram showing the construction of a frequency distribution graph. (Modified from Coulter Electronics: Significant advances in hematology: hematology education series, PN 4206115A, Hialeah, FL, 1983, Coulter Electronics.)

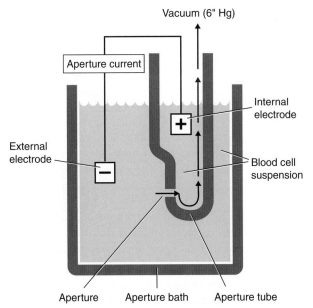

Vacuum (6" Hg)

Aperture current

External electrode

Internal electrode

Blood cell suspension

Aperture   Aperture bath   Aperture tube

Figure 15-1 Coulter principle of cell counting. (From Coulter Electronics: Coulter STKR product reference manual, PN 4235547E, Hialeah, FL, 1988, Coulter Electronics.)

Several factors may affect volume measurements in impedance or volume displacement instruments. Aperture diameter is crucial, and the red blood cell (RBC)/platelet aperture is smaller than the WBC aperture to increase platelet counting sensitivity. On earlier systems, protein buildup occurred, decreasing the diameter of the orifice, slowing the flow of cells, and increasing their relative electrical resistance. Protein buildup results in lower cell counts, which result in falsely elevated cell volumes. Impedance instruments once required frequent manual aperture cleaning, but current instruments incorporate *burn circuits* or other internal cleaning systems to prevent or slow protein buildup.[6-9] Carryover of cells from one sample to the next also is minimized by these internal cleaning systems. Coincident passage of more than one cell at a time through the orifice causes artificially large pulses, which results in falsely increased cell volumes and falsely decreased cell counts. This count reduction, or *coincident passage loss,* is statistically predictable (and mathematically correctable) because of its direct relationship to cell concentration and the effective volume of the aperture.[7-9] Coincidence correction typically is completed by the analyzer computer before final printout of cell counts from the instrument. Other factors affecting pulse height include orientation of the cell in the center of the aperture and deformability of the RBC, which may be altered by decreased hemoglobin content.[10,11] Recirculation of cells back into the sensing zone creates erroneous pulses and falsely elevates cell counts. A backwash or sweep-flow mechanism prevents recirculation of cells back into the sensing zone, and anomalously shaped pulses are edited out electronically.[6,7,9]

The use of hydrodynamic focusing avoids many of the potential problems inherent in a rigid aperture system. The *sample stream* is surrounded by a sheath fluid as it passes through the central axis of the aperture. Laminar flow allows the central sample stream to narrow sufficiently to separate and align the cells into single file for passage through the sensing zone.[12-14] The outer sheath fluid minimizes protein buildup and plugs, eliminates recirculation of cells back into the sensing zone with generation of spurious pulses, and reduces pulse height irregularity because off-center cell passage is prevented and better resolution of the blood cells is obtained. Coincident passage loss also is reduced because blood cells line up one after another in the direction of the flow.[15] Laminar flow and hydrodynamic focusing are discussed further in Chapter 32.

Radiofrequency

Low-voltage DC impedance, as described previously, may be used in conjunction with RF resistance, or resistance to a high-voltage electromagnetic current flowing between both electrodes simultaneously. Although the total volume of the cell is proportional to the change in DC, the cell interior density is proportional to pulse height or change in the RF signal. *Conductivity*, as measured by this high-frequency electromagnetic probe, is attenuated by nucleus-to-cytoplasm ratio, nuclear density, and cytoplasmic granulation. DC and RF voltage changes may be detected simultaneously and separated by two different pulse processing circuits.[15,16] Figure 15-3 illustrates the simultaneous use of DC and RF current.

Two different cell properties, such as low-voltage DC impedance and RF resistance, can be plotted against each other to create a *two-dimensional distribution cytogram* or *scatterplot* (Figure 15-4). Such plots display the cell populations as clusters, with the number of dots in each cluster representing the concentration of that cell type. Computer cluster analysis can determine absolute counts for specific cell populations. The use of multiple methods by a given instrument for the determination of at least two cell properties allows the separation of WBCs into a five-part differential (neutrophils, lymphocytes, monocytes, eosinophils, and basophils). DC and RF detection are two methods used by the Sysmex analyzers to perform WBC differentials.[15,16]

Optical Scatter

Optical scatter may be used as the primary methodology or in combination with other methods. In optical scatter systems (flow cytometers), a hydrodynamically focused sample stream is directed through a quartz flow cell past a focused light source (Figure 32-3). The light source is generally a tungsten-halogen lamp or a helium-neon *laser* (*l*ight *a*mplification by *s*timulated *e*mission of *r*adiation). Laser light, termed *monochromatic light* because it is emitted at a single wavelength, differs from brightfield light in its intensity, its coherence (i.e., it travels in phase), and its low divergence or spread. These characteristics allow for the detection of interference in the laser beam and enable enumeration and differentiation of cell types.[12,17] Optical scatter may be used to study RBCs, WBCs, and platelets.

As the cells pass through the sensing zone and interrupt the beam, light is scattered in all directions. Light scatter results from the interaction between the processes of absorption, diffraction (bending around corners or the surface of a cell),

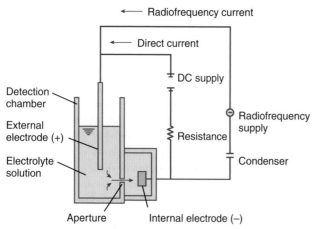

Figure 15-3 Radiofrequency/direct current (RF/DC) detection method, showing simultaneous use of DC and RF in one measurement system on the Sysmex SE-9500. (From TOA Medical Electronics Company: Sysmex SE-9500 operator's manual [CN 461-2464-2], Kobe, Japan, 1997, TOA Medical Electronics Co.)

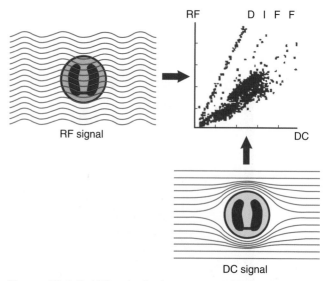

Figure 15-4 Illustration of cell volume measurement with direct current (DC) voltage change versus measurement of cell nuclear volume/complexity with change in the radiofrequency (RF) signal. The two measurements can be plotted against each other to form a two-dimensional distribution scatterplot. (From TOA Medical Electronics Company: Sysmex SE-9500 operator's manual [CN 461-2464-2], Kobe, Japan, 1997, TOA Medical Electronics Co.)

refraction (bending because of a change in speed), and reflection (backward scatter of rays caused by an obstruction).[18] The detection of scattered rays and their conversion into electrical signals is accomplished by photodetectors (photodiodes and photomultiplier tubes) at specific angles. Lenses fitted with *blocker bars* to prevent nonscattered light from entering the detector are used to collect the scattered light. A series of filters and mirrors separate the varying wavelengths and present them to the photodetectors. Photodiodes convert light photons to electronic signals proportional in magnitude to the amount of light collected. Photomultiplier tubes are used to collect the weaker signals produced at a 90-degree angle and multiply the photoelectrons into stronger, useful signals. Analogue-to-digital converters change the electronic pulses to digital signals for computer analysis.[12,17]

Forward-angle light scatter (0 degrees) correlates with cell volume, primarily because of diffraction of light. Orthogonal light scatter (90 degrees), or side scatter, results from refraction and reflection of light from larger structures inside the cell and correlates with degree of internal complexity. Forward low-angle scatter (2 to 3 degrees) and forward high-angle scatter (5 to 15 degrees) also correlate with cell volume and refractive index or with internal complexity.[17,19] Differential scatter is the combination of this low-angle and high-angle forward light scatter and is primarily used on Siemens systems for cellular analysis. The angles of light scatter measured by the different flow cytometers are manufacturer and method specific.

Scatter properties at different angles may be plotted against each other to generate two-dimensional cytograms or scatterplots, as on the Abbott CELL-DYN instruments.[20,21] Optical scatter may also be plotted against absorption, as on the Siemens systems,[22,23] or against volume, as on the larger Beckman Coulter systems.[9] Computer cluster analysis of the cytograms may yield quantitative and qualitative information.

PRINCIPAL INSTRUMENTS

Overview

Hematology blood cell analyzers are produced by multiple manufacturers, including, but not limited to, Abbott Laboratories (Abbott Park, IL);[24] HORIBA Medical (Irvine, CA);[25] Siemens Healthcare Diagnostics, Inc. (Deerfield, IL);[26] Beckman Coulter, Inc. (Brea, CA);[27] and Sysmex Corporation (Kobe, Japan).[28] The following discussion is limited to instrumentation produced by four of these suppliers. Emphasis is not placed on sample size or handling, speed, level of automation, or comparison of instruments or manufacturers. Likewise, technology continues to improve, and the newest (or most recent) models produced by a manufacturer may not be mentioned. Instead, a detailed description of primary methods used by these manufacturers is given to show the application of, and clarify further, the principles presented earlier and to enable the medical laboratory scientist or technician to interpret patient data, including instrument-generated histograms and cytograms. Table 15-1 summarizes methods used for the hemogram, reticulocyte,

nucleated red blood cell, and WBC differential count determination on four major hematology instruments.

Hematology analyzers have some common basic components, including hydraulics, pneumatics, and electrical systems. The hydraulics system includes an aspirating unit, dispensers, diluters, mixing chambers, aperture baths or flow cells or both, and a hemoglobinometer. The pneumatics system generates the vacuums and pressures required for operating the valves and moving the sample through the hydraulics system. The electrical system controls operational sequences of the total system and includes electronic analyzers and computing circuitry for processing the data generated. Some older-model instruments have oscilloscope screens that display the electrical pulses in real time as the cells are counted. A data display unit receives information from the analyzer and prints results, histograms, or cytograms.

Specimen handling varies from instrument to instrument based on degree of automation, and systems range from discrete analyzers to walkaway systems with *front-end load* capability. Computer functions also vary, with the larger instruments having extensive microprocessor and data management capabilities. Computer software capabilities include automatic start-up and shutdown, with internal diagnostic self-checks and some maintenance; quality control, with automatic review of quality control data, calculations, graphs, moving averages, and storage of quality control files; patient data storage and retrieval, with δ checks (Chapter 5), critical value flagging, and automatic verification of patient results based on user-defined algorithms; host query with the laboratory or hospital information system to allow random access discrete testing capability; analysis of animal specimens; and even analysis of body fluids.

Beckman Coulter Instrumentation

Beckman Coulter, Inc., manufactures an extensive line of hematology analyzers, including the smaller Ac-T series that provide complete RBC, platelet, and WBC analysis with a five-part differential. The LH 780 system, part of the LH 700 series, provides a fully automated online reticulocyte analysis.[27] The LH series also has the capability to perform CD4 and CD8 counts.[29] Coulter instruments typically have two measurement channels in the hydraulics system for determining the hemogram data. The RBC and WBC counts and hemoglobin are considered to be measured directly. The aspirated whole-blood sample is divided into two aliquots, and each is mixed with an isotonic diluent. The first dilution is delivered to the RBC aperture chamber, and the second is delivered to the WBC aperture chamber. In the RBC chamber, RBCs and platelets are counted and discriminated by electrical impedance as the cells are pulled through each of three sensing apertures (50 μm in diameter, 60 μm in length). Particles 2 to 20 fL are counted as platelets, and particles greater than 36 fL are counted as RBCs. In the WBC chamber, a reagent to lyse RBCs and release hemoglobin is added before WBCs are counted simultaneously by impedance in each of three sensing apertures (100 μm in diameter, 75 μm in length). Alternatively, some models employ consecutive counts in the same RBC or WBC aperture. After

TABLE 15-1 Methods for Hemogram, Reticulocyte, Nucleated RBC, and WBC Differential Counts on Four Major Hematology Instruments

Parameter	Beckman Coulter UniCel DxH 800	Sysmex XN Series	Abbott CELL-DYN Sapphire	Siemens ADVIA 2120i
WBC	Impedance volume and conductivity and five-angle light scatter measurement	Fluorescent staining; forward light scatter and side fluorescent light detection	Light scatter (primary count), impedance (secondary count)	Light scatter and absorption
RBC	Impedance	Impedance	Impedance	Low-angle and high-angle laser light scatter
HGB	Modified cyanmethemoglobin (525 nm)	Sodium lauryl sulfate-HGB (555 nm)	Modified cyanmethemoglobin (540 nm)	Modified cyanmethemoglobin (546 nm)
HCT	(RBC × MCV)/10	Cumulative RBC pulse height detection	(RBC × MCV)/10	(RBC × MCV)/10
MCV	Mean of RBC volume distribution histogram	(HCT/RBC) × 10	Mean of RBC volume distribution histogram	Mean of RBC volume distribution histogram
MCH	(HGB/RBC) × 10	(HGB/RBC) × 10	(HGB/RBC) × 10	(HGB/RBC) × 10
MCHC	(HGB/HCT) × 100	(HGB/HCT) × 100	(HGB/HCT) × 100	(HGB/HCT) × 100
Platelet count	Impedance volume and conductivity and five-angle light scatter measurement	Impedance; light scatter; fluorescent staining, forward light scatter, and side fluorescent light detection	Dual angle light scatter analysis; impedance count for verification; optional CD61 monoclonal antibody count	Low-angle and high-angle light scatter; refractive index
RDW	RDW as CV (%) of RBC histogram or RDW-SD (fL)	RDW-SD (fL) or RDW-CV (%)	Relative value, equivalent to CV	CV (%) of RBC histogram
Reticulocyte count	Supravital staining; impedance volume and conductivity and light scatter measurement	Fluorescent staining; forward light scatter and side fluorescent light detection	Fluorescent staining; low-angle scatter, and fluorescent light detection	Supravital staining (oxazine 750); low-angle and high-angle light scatter and absorbance
NRBC*	Impedance volume and conductivity and five-angle light scatter measurement	Fluorescent staining; forward light scatter and side fluorescent light detection	Red fluorescent dye staining; forward light scatter and fluorescent light detection	Multi-angle light scatter measurements in the two WBC differential channels
WBC differential	Impedance volume and conductivity and five-angle light scatter measurement	Fluorescent staining; forward and side light scatter, and side fluorescent light detection	Multi-angle polarized scatter separation (MAPSS) and three-color fluorescence detection	Peroxidase staining, light scatter and absorption; for basos, differential lysis, low-angle and high-angle laser light scatter

CV, Coefficient of variation; *DC*, direct current; *HCT*, hematocrit; *HGB*, hemoglobin; *MCH*, mean cell hemoglobin; *MCHC*, mean cell hemoglobin concentration; *MCV*, mean cell volume; *NRBC*, nucleated red blood cell count; *RBC*, red blood cell (or count); *RDW*, RBC distribution width; *SD*, standard deviation; *VCS*, volume, conductivity, scatter; *WBC*, white blood cell (or count).
*Instruments auto-correct the WBC count for the presence of nucleated RBCs.

counting cycles are completed, the WBC dilution is passed to the hemoglobinometer for determination of hemoglobin concentration (light transmittance read at a wavelength of 525 nm). Electrical pulses generated in the counting cycles are sent to the analyzer for editing, coincidence correction, and digital conversion. Two of the three counts obtained in the RBC and the WBC baths must match within specified limits for the counts to be accepted by the instrument.[5,9] This multiple counting procedure prevents data errors resulting from aperture obstructions or statistical outliers and allows for excellent reproducibility on the Beckman Coulter instruments.

Pulse height is measured and categorized by pulse height analyzers; 256 channels are used for WBC and RBC analysis, and 64 channels are used for platelet analysis. Volume-distribution histograms of WBC, RBC, and platelet populations are generated. The RBC mean cell volume (MCV) is the average volume of the RBCs taken from the volume distribution data. The hematocrit (HCT), mean cell hemoglobin (MCH), and mean cell hemoglobin concentration (MCHC) are calculated from measured and derived values. The RBC distribution width (RDW) is calculated directly from the histogram as the coefficient of variation (CV) of the RBC volume distribution, with a reference interval of 11.5% to 14.5%.[5] The RDW is an index of anisocytosis, but it may be falsely skewed because it reflects the ratio of the standard deviation (SD) to MCV. That is, an RBC distribution histogram with normal divergence but a decreased

MCV may imply a high RDW, falsely indicating increased anisocytosis. MCV and RDW are used by the instrument to flag possible anisocytosis, microcytosis, and macrocytosis.[9]

Platelets are counted within the range of 2 to 20 fL, and a volume-distribution histogram is constructed. If the platelet volume distribution meets specified criteria, a statistical least-squares method is applied to the raw data to fit the data to a log-normal curve. The curve is extrapolated from 0 to 70 fL, and the final count is derived from this extended curve. This fitting procedure eliminates interference from particles in the noise region, such as debris, and in the larger region, such as small RBCs. The mean platelet volume (MPV), analogous to the RBC MCV, also is derived from the platelet histogram. The reference interval for the MPV is about 6.8 to 10.2 fL. The MPV increases slightly with storage of the specimen in ethylenediaminetetraacetic acid (EDTA).[5]

Many older-model Beckman Coulter instruments, such as the STKR, and the newer, smaller models, such as the Ac-T series, provide three-part leukocyte subpopulation analysis, which differentiates WBCs into lymphocytes, mononuclear cells, and granulocytes. In the WBC channel, a special lysing reagent causes *differential shrinkage* of the leukocytes, which allows the different cells to be counted and volumetrically sized based on their impedance. A WBC histogram is constructed from the channelized data. Particles between approximately 35 and 90 fL are considered lymphocytes; particles between 90 and 160 fL are considered *mononuclears* (monocytes, blasts,

immature granulocytes, and reactive lymphocytes); and particles between 160 and 450 fL are considered granulocytes. This allows the calculation of relative and absolute numbers for these three populations (Figure 15-5).[6] Proprietary computerized algorithms further allow flagging for increased eosinophils or basophils or both and interpretation of the histogram differential, including flagging for abnormal cells, such as reactive lymphocytes and blasts.[7] When cell populations overlap or a distinct separation of populations does not exist, a region alarm (R flag) may be triggered that indicates the area of interference on the volume-distribution histogram. An R1 flag represents excess signals at the lower threshold region of the WBC histogram and a questionable WBC count. This interference is visualized as a *high takeoff* of the curve and may indicate the presence of nucleated RBCs, clumped platelets, unlysed RBCs, or electronic noise.[6,7]

More recent Beckman Coulter instruments, the LH 700 Series and UniCel DxH series, generate hemogram data (including the WBC count) as before but use Coulter's proprietary *VCS (volume, conductivity, scatter) technology* in a separate channel to evaluate WBCs for the determination of a five-part differential. The VCS technology includes the volumetric sizing of cells by impedance, conductivity measurements of cells, and laser light scatter, all performed simultaneously for each cell. After RBCs are lysed and WBCs are treated with a stabilizing reagent to maintain them in a near-native state, a hydrodynamically focused sample stream is directed through the flow

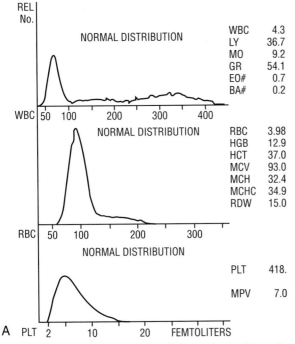
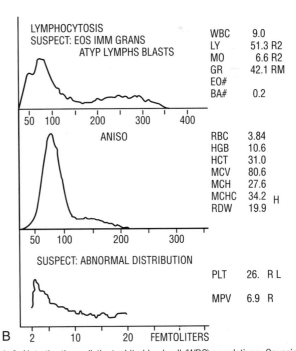

Figure 15-5 Printouts from the Coulter STKR showing the interpretive differential. **A,** Note the three distinct white blood cell (WBC) populations, Gaussian or normal distribution of red blood cells (RBCs), and right-skewed or log-normal distribution of platelets. **B,** Note the left shift in the WBC histogram with possible interference at the lower threshold region. R2 flag indicates interference and loss of valley owing to overlap or insufficient separation between the lymphocyte and mononuclear populations at the 90-fL region. RM flag indicates interference at more than one region. Eosinophil data have been suppressed. Also note the abnormal platelet volume distribution with a low platelet count. Manual 200-cell differential counts on the same samples: **A,** 52.5% neutrophils (47% segmented neutrophils, 5.5% bands), 41.5% lymphocytes, 4.0% monocytes, 1% basophils, 0.5% metamyelocytes, 0.5% reactive lymphocytes; **B,** 51% neutrophils (23% segmented neutrophils, 28% bands), 12% lymphocytes, 9.5% monocytes, 1% metamyelocytes, 1.5% myelocytes, 25% reactive lymphocytes, and 17 nucleated RBCs/100 WBCs.

cell past the sensing zone. Low-frequency DC measures cell volume, whereas a high-frequency electromagnetic probe measures conductivity, an indicator of cellular internal content. The conductivity signal is corrected for cellular volume, which yields a unique measurement called *opacity*. Each cell also is scanned with monochromatic laser light that reveals information about the cell surface, such as structure, shape, and reflectivity. Beckman Coulter's unique rotated light scatter detection method, which covers a 10-degree to 70-degree range, allows for separation of cells with similar volume but different scatter characteristics.[27] Beckman Coulter's newest analyzer, the UniCel DxH 800, uses volume and conductivity as well as five additional parameters: axial light loss (AL2), low-angle light scatter (LALS), median-angle light scatter (MALS), lower median–angle light scatter (LMALS), and upper median–angle light scatter (UMALS).[30,31] Using the data collected by the parameters listed above, the instrument applies *data transformation*, the process by which populations of cells are separated, allowing the determination of major populations as well as the enhancement of subpopulations of cells. Once those populations are established, a technique called the *watershed concept* searches for those populations and aids in determining counts as well as flagging based on all the populations found for that sample.[30,31]

This combination of technologies provides a three-dimensional plot or cytograph of the WBC populations, which are separated by computer cluster analysis. Two-dimensional scatterplots of the measurements represent different views of the cytograph. The scatterplot of volume (*y*-axis) versus light scatter (*x*-axis) shows clear separation of lymphocytes, monocytes, neutrophils, and eosinophils. Basophils are hidden behind the lymphocytes but are separated by conductivity owing to their cytoplasmic granulation. Single-parameter histograms of volume, conductivity, and light scatter also are available.[9]

Two types of WBC flags (alarms or indicators of abnormality) are generated on all hematology analyzers that provide a WBC differential count: (1) user defined, primarily set for distributional abnormalities, such as eosinophilia or lymphocytopenia (based on absolute eosinophil or lymphocyte counts); and (2) instrument specific, primarily suspect flags for morphologic abnormalities. For *distributional flags*, the user establishes reference intervals and programs the instrument to flag each parameter as high or low. *Suspect flags* indicating the possible presence of abnormal cells are triggered when cell populations fall outside expected regions or when specific statistical limitations are exceeded. Instrument-specific *suspect* flags on the Coulter UniCel DxH 800 system and LH 700 series include immature granulocytes/bands, blasts, variant lymphocytes, nucleated RBCs, and platelet clumps. The UniCel DxH 800 also utilizes the International Society for Laboratory Hematology (ISLH) consensus rules in addition to the user defined and system defined flags for complete data analysis.[32,33] In addition to the flags listed above, inadequate separation of cell populations may disallow reporting of differential results by the instrument and may elicit a *review slide* message.[9,33,34]

The UniCel DxH 800 system utilizes VCS as well as digital signal processing from five light scatter angles for clear cellular resolution. On the LH 700 series, Coulter utilizes an *IntelliKinetics* application. This application is used to ensure consistency with the kinetic reactions. It provides the instrument the best signals for analysis independent of laboratory environment variations. Compared with earlier models Coulter IntelliKinetics provides better separation of cell populations for WBCs and reticulocytes, which enables better analysis by the system algorithms.[33,34]

The UniCel DxH 800 also includes the number of nucleated RBCs as part of the standard CBC report. They are identified, counted, and subtracted from the white blood cell count using volume, conductivity, and the same five light scatter measurement described above. The AL2 measurement (which reflects the amount of light absorbed as it passes through the flow cell) initially separates the nucleated RBCs from the WBCs. Algorithms are applied using the scatter from the other angles to electronically separate and count the nucleated RBCs. Two scatterplots display the nucleated RBC data by plotting axial light loss (AL2) on the *x*-axis against low-angle light scatter (RLALS) and upper-median angle light scatter (RUMALS) on *y*-axis.

Figure 15-6 represents a standard patient printout from the Beckman Coulter UniCel DxH 800.

Sysmex Instrumentation

Sysmex Corporation, formerly TOA Medical Electronics Company, Ltd., manufactures a full line of hematology analyzers that provide complete RBC, platelet, and WBC analysis with three-part differential; the larger XT-1800i (SF-3000 and SE-9000) that performs a CBC with five-part differential; and the XE series and the newest XN series that also provide a fully automated reticulocyte count.[28,33] The newest XN series is modular. The series is scalable, and multiple modules can be combined onto one platform. Each module contains the XN-CBC and XN-DIFF with other options available, including XN-BF, the body fluid application. Included standard on the CBC and DIFF modules are NRBCs, RET-He (reticulocyte hemoglobin), and IRF (immature reticulocyte fraction). The platelet analysis on the XN also utilizes a fluorescent count, in addition to the impedance count and optical count, called the PLT-F, performed by optical measurement.[35-38] The PLT-F can be performed on each sample or set up as a reflex based on the laboratory's PLT criteria. The method uses a fluorocell fluorescent dye (oxazine) combined with an extended PLT counting volume and time. The PLTs can be differentiated from other cells based on differences in intensity of the fluorescence combined with forward scattered light.[35] The WBC, RBC, platelet counts, hemoglobin, and hematocrit are considered to be measured directly. Three hydraulic subsystems are used for determining the hemogram: the WBC channel, the RBC/platelet channel, and a separate hemoglobin channel. In the WBC and RBC transducer chambers, diluted WBC and RBC samples are aspirated through the different apertures and counted using the impedance (DC detection) method for counting and volumetrically sizing cells. Two unique features enhance the impedance technology: in the RBC/platelet channel, a sheathed stream with hydrodynamic focusing is used to direct cells through the aperture, which reduces coincident

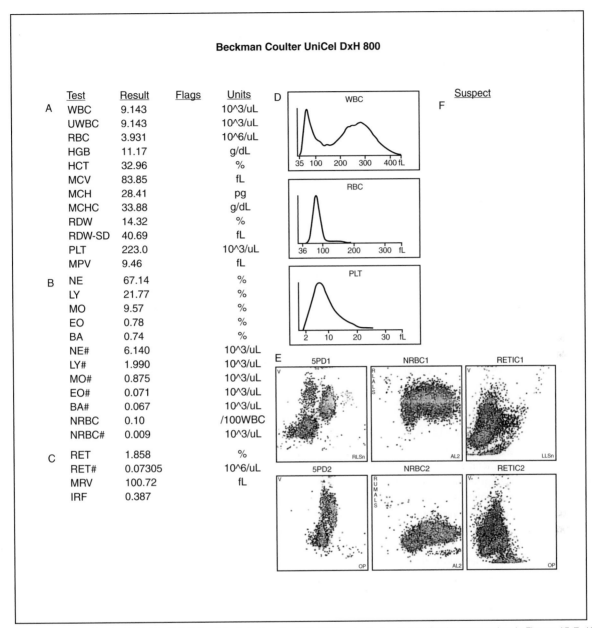

Figure 15-6 Coulter UniCel DxH 800. The DxH 800 printout displays the CBC, DIFF and reticulocyte data for the same patient in Figures 15-7, 15-9, and 15-12. **A,** CBC data; **B,** Differential with the nucleated red blood cells (NRBCs); **C,** Reticulocyte data, including the IRF (immature reticulocyte fraction); **D,** Impedance histograms for the WBC, RBC, and PLT; **E,** Advanced two-dimensional optical scatterplots for WBCs, NRBCs, and reticulocytes; **F,** *Suspect* area in which any sample or system flags will display.

passage, particle volume distortion, and recirculation of blood cells around the aperture; and in the WBC and RBC/platelet channels, *floating thresholds* are used to discriminate each cell population.[8,15,16]

As cells pass through the apertures, signals are transmitted in sequence to the analogue circuit and particle volume distribution analysis circuits for conversion to cumulative cell volume distribution data. Particle volume distribution curves are constructed, and optimal position of the *autodiscrimination level* (i.e., threshold) is set by the microprocessor for each cell population. The lower platelet threshold is automatically adjusted in the 2- to 6-fL volume range, and the upper threshold is adjusted in the 12- to 30-fL range, based on particle volume

distribution. Likewise, the RBC lower and upper thresholds may be set in the 25- to 75-fL and 200- to 250-fL volume ranges. This floating threshold circuitry allows for discrimination of cell populations on a sample-by-sample basis. Cell counts are based on pulses between the lower and upper autodiscriminator levels, with dilution ratio, volume counted, and coincident passage error accounted for in the final computer-generated numbers. In the RBC channel, the floating discriminator is particularly useful in separating platelets from small RBCs. The hematocrit also is determined from the RBC/platelet channel, based on the principle that the pulse height generated by the RBC is proportional to cell volume. The hematocrit is the RBC cumulative pulse height and is considered a true relative percentage volume of erythrocytes.[8,15] In the hemoglobin flow cell, hemoglobin is oxidized and binds to sodium lauryl sulfate (SLS) forming a stable SLS–hemoglobin complex, which is measured photometrically at 555 nm.[16]

The following indices are calculated in the microprocessor using directly measured or derived parameters: MCV, MCH, MCHC, RDW-SD, RDW-CV, MPV, and plateletcrit. RDW-SD is the RBC arithmetic distribution width measured at 20% of the height of the RBC curve, reported in femtoliters, with a reference interval of 37 to 54 fL. RDW-CV is the RDW reported as a CV. Plateletcrit is the platelet volume ratio, analogous to the hematocrit. MPV is calculated from the plateletcrit and platelet count just as erythrocyte MCV is calculated from the hematocrit and RBC count. The proportion of platelets greater than 12 fL in the total platelet count may be an indicator of possible platelet clumping, giant platelets, or cell fragments.[8,15,16] The XE series has the capability to run the platelet counting in the optical mode, which eliminates common interferences found with impedance counting. In the optical mode, the, immature platelet fraction or IPF, can be measured to provide additional information concerning platelet kinetics in cases of thrombocytopenia.[39]

The SE-9000/9500 uses four detection chambers to analyze WBCs and obtain a five-part differential: the DIFF, IMI (immature myeloid information), EO, and BASO chambers. The high-end instrumentation such as the XE-series and the XN series has a six-part differential: neutrophils, lymphocytes, monocytes, eosinophils, basophils, and immature granulocytes. Every differential performed generates a percentage and absolute number for immature granulocytes, thus providing valuable information about the complete differential.[28] In the DIFF detection chamber, RBCs are hemolyzed and WBCs are analyzed simultaneously by low-frequency DC and high-frequency current (*DC/RF detection method*). A scattergram of RF detection signals (*y*-axis) versus DC detection signals (*x*-axis) allows separation of the WBCs into lymphocytes, monocytes, and granulocytes. Floating discriminators determine the optimal separation between these populations. Granulocytes are analyzed further in the IMI detection chamber to determine immature myeloid information. RBCs are lysed, and WBCs other than immature granulocytes are selectively shrunk by temperature and chemically controlled reactions. Analysis of the treated sample using the DC/RF detection method allows separation of immature cells on the IMI scattergram. A similar differential shrinkage and lysis method is also used in the EO and BASO chambers. That is, eosinophils and basophils are counted by impedance (DC detection) in separate chambers in which the RBCs are lysed, and WBCs other than eosinophils or basophils are selectively shrunk by temperature and chemically controlled reactions. Eosinophils and basophils are subtracted from the granulocyte count derived from the DIFF scattergram analysis to determine the neutrophil count. User-defined distributional flags may be set, and instrument-specific suspect flags, similar to those described for the Beckman Coulter LH 700 series, are triggered for the possible presence of morphologic abnormalities.[15,16] A POSITIVE or NEGATIVE interpretive message is displayed.

In the XN-1000, fluorescent flow cytometry is used for the WBC count, WBC differential, and enumeration of nucleated RBCs. In the *WDF channel*, RBCs are lysed, WBC membranes are perforated, and the DNA and RNA in the WBCs are stained with a fluorescent dye. Plotting side scatter on the *x*-axis and side fluorescent light on the *y*-axis enables separation and enumeration of neutrophils, eosinophils, lymphocytes, monocytes, and immature granulocytes. In the *WNR channel*, the RBCs are lysed including nucleated RBCs, and WBC membranes are perforated. A fluorescent polymethine dye stains the nucleus and organelles of the WBCs with high fluorescence intensity and stains the released nuclei of the nucleated RBCs with low intensity. Plotting side fluorescent light on the *x*-axis and forward scatter on the *y*-axis enables separation and enumeration of the total WBC count, basophils, and nucleated RBCs. The WBC count is automatically corrected when nucleated RBCs are present in the sample. A *WPC channel* detects blasts and abnormal lymphocytes in a similar manner using a lysing agent and fluorescent dye and plotting side scatter on the *x*-axis and side fluorescent light on the *y*-axis. Figure 15-7 shows a patient report from the Sysmex XN-1000 analyzing the same patient specimen for which data are given in Figure 15-6.

Abbott Instrumentation

Instruments offered by Abbott Laboratories include the smaller CELL-DYN Emerald, which provides complete RBC, platelet, and WBC analysis with three-part differential, and the larger CELL-DYN Sapphire and the midrange CELL-DYN Ruby, both of which provide a CBC with five-part differential and random fully automated reticulocyte analysis.[33] The CELL-DYN 4000 system has three independent measurement channels for determining the hemogram and differential: an optical channel for WBC count and differential data, an impedance channel for RBC and platelet data, and a hemoglobin channel for hemoglobin determination.[20,21] The WBC, RBC, hemoglobin, and platelet parameters are considered to be measured directly. A 60- to 70-μm aperture is used in the RBC/platelet transducer assembly for counting and volumetrically sizing of RBCs and platelets by the electronic impedance method.

A unique von Behrens plate is located in the RBC/platelet counting chamber to minimize the effect of recirculating cells. Pulses are collected and sorted in 256 channels according to their amplitudes: particles between 1 and 35 fL are included in the initial platelet data, and particles greater than 35 fL are counted as RBCs. Floating thresholds are used to determine the best separation of the platelet population and to eliminate interference, such as noise, debris, or small RBCs, from the count. Coincident passage loss is corrected for in the final RBC and platelet counts. RBC pulse editing is applied before MCV derivation to compensate for aberrant pulses produced by nonaxial passage of RBCs through the aperture. The MCV is the average volume of the RBCs derived from RBC volume distribution data. Hemoglobin is measured directly using a modified hemiglobincyanide method that measures absorbance at 540 nm. Hematocrit, MCH, and MCHC are calculated from the directly measured or derived parameters. The RDW, equivalent to CV, is a relative value, derived from the RBC histogram by using the

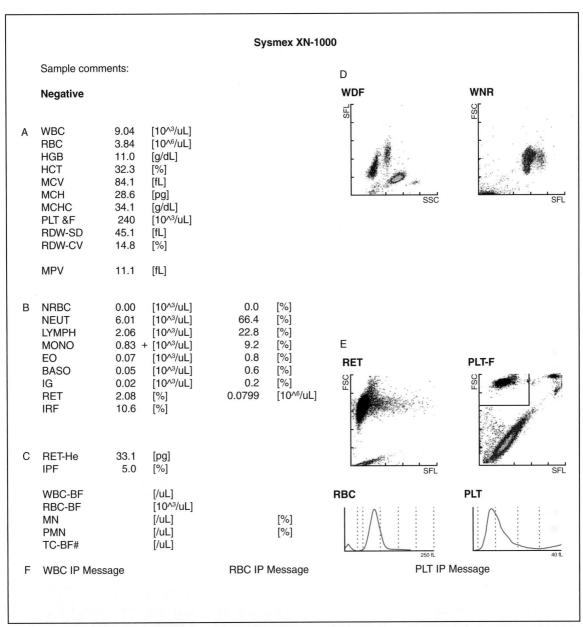

Sysmex XN-1000

Sample comments:

Negative

A	WBC	9.04	[10^3/uL]			
	RBC	3.84	[10^6/uL]			
	HGB	11.0	[g/dL]			
	HCT	32.3	[%]			
	MCV	84.1	[fL]			
	MCH	28.6	[pg]			
	MCHC	34.1	[g/dL]			
	PLT &F	240	[10^3/uL]			
	RDW-SD	45.1	[fL]			
	RDW-CV	14.8	[%]			
	MPV	11.1	[fL]			

B	NRBC	0.00	[10^3/uL]	0.0	[%]	
	NEUT	6.01	[10^3/uL]	66.4	[%]	
	LYMPH	2.06	[10^3/uL]	22.8	[%]	
	MONO	0.83 +	[10^3/uL]	9.2	[%]	
	EO	0.07	[10^3/uL]	0.8	[%]	
	BASO	0.05	[10^3/uL]	0.6	[%]	
	IG	0.02	[10^3/uL]	0.2	[%]	
	RET	2.08	[%]	0.0799	[10^6/uL]	
	IRF	10.6	[%]			

C	RET-He	33.1	[pg]		
	IPF	5.0	[%]		
	WBC-BF		[/uL]		
	RBC-BF		[10^3/uL]		
	MN		[/uL]	[%]	
	PMN		[/uL]	[%]	
	TC-BF#		[/uL]		

F WBC IP Message   RBC IP Message

D

WDF   WNR

E

RET   PLT-F

RBC   PLT
              250 fL   40 fL

PLT IP Message

Figure 15-7   Sysmex XN-1000. The XN-1000 printout displays the CBC, DIFF, and reticulocyte data for the same patient in Figures 15-6, 15-9, and 15-12. **A,** CBC data; note the "&F" to indicate the fluorescent platelet count result; **B,** Nucleated red blood cells (NRBCs), six-part differential, including the IG (immature granulocyte), reticulocyte count (RET), and immature reticulocyte fraction (IRF); **C,** Reticulocyte hemoglobin (RET-He), immature platelet fraction (IPF), and body fluid counts, if done; **D,** Two scatterplots, WDF (lymphocytes, monocytes, neutrophils, eosinophils, and immature granulocytes) and WNR (WBC count, basophils, and nucleated RBCs); **E,** Reticulocyte (RET) and platelet (PLT-F) scatterplots, and RBC and PLT impedance histograms; **F,** Sample-related flags are listed at the bottom of the printout, if any are generated.

20th and 80th percentiles. The platelet analysis is based on a two-dimensional optical platelet count using fluorescent technology, the same technology used for direct nucleated RBC counting by adding a red fluorescence to the sample to stain nucleated red cells.[40] Further analysis of platelets and platelet aggregates can be performed by using an automated CD61 monoclonal antibody to generate an immunoplatelet count.[41-43] Other indices available include MPV and plateletcrit.[20,21]

The WBC count and differential are derived from the optical channel using CELL-DYN's patented multiangle polarized scatter separation (MAPSS) technology with three-color fluorescent technology. A hydrodynamically focused sample stream is directed through a quartz flow cell past a focused light source, an argon ion laser. Scattered light is measured at multiple angles: 0-degree forward light scatter measurement is used for determination of cell volume, 90-degree orthogonal light scatter measurement is used for determination of cellular lobularity, 7-degree narrow-angle scatter measurement is used to correlate with cellular complexity, and 90-degree depolarized light scatter measurement is used for evaluation of cellular granularity. Orthogonal light scatter is split, with one portion directed to a 90-degree photomultiplier tube and the other portion directed through a polarizer to the 90-degree depolarized photomultiplier tube. Light that has changed polarization (depolarized) is the only light that can be detected by the 90-degree depolarized photomultiplier tube. Various combinations of these four measurements are used to differentiate and quantify the five major WBC subpopulations: neutrophils, lymphocytes, monocytes, eosinophils, and basophils.[20,40,44] Figure 15-8 illustrates CELL-DYN's MAPSS technology.

The light scatter signals are converted into electrical signals, sorted into 256 channels on the basis of amplitude for each angle of light measured, and graphically presented as scatterplots. Scatter information from the different angles is plotted in various combinations: 90 degrees/7 degrees, or lobularity versus complexity; 0 degrees/7 degrees, volume versus complexity; and 90 degrees depolarized/90 degrees, granularity versus lobularity. Lobularity or 90-degree scatter (*y*-axis) plotted against complexity or 7-degree scatter (*x*-axis) yields separation of mononuclear and segmented (polymorphonuclear neutrophil) subpopulations. Basophils cluster with the mononuclears in this analysis, because the basophil granules dissolve in the sheath reagent, and the degranulated basophil is a less complex cell. Each cell in the two clusters

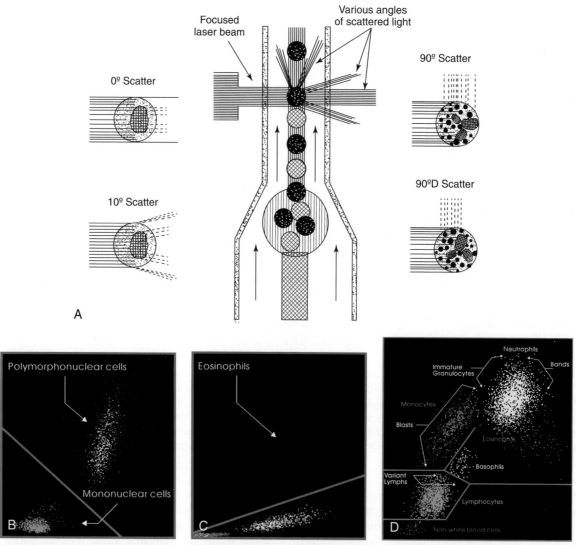

Figure 15-8 A, Multiangle polarized scatter separation (MAPSS) technology. Cells are measured and characterized by plotting light scatter from four different angles. **B,** Mononuclear and polymorphonuclear scatter with MAPPS technology. It plots 10 degree scatter (complexity) on the *x*-axis and 90 degree scatter (lobularity) on the *y*-axis. The system uses algorithms to further separate the two populations, displaying mononuclear on the lower left and polymorphonuclear on the upper right. **C,** Separation and plotting of the polymorphonuclear cells into neutrophils and eosinophils based on MAPPS technology. It plots 90 degree scatter (lobularity) on the *x*-axis and 90 degree depolarized (90 D) scatter on the *y*-axis. The system uses algorithms to further separate the two populations of cells. **D,** Scatter of all WBC populations by MAPPS technology plotting 10 degree scatter (complexity) on the *x*-axis and 0 degree scatter (size or volume) on the *y*-axis. On the newer instruments, a 7-degree angle for complexity is now used instead of the 10-degree angle. The change reflects use of the midrange of the angle instead of the end range; however, it still provides the same information. (From Abbott Laboratories: CELL-DYN 3700 system operator's manual [914032C], Abbott Park, IL, 2000.)

is identified as a mononuclear or segmented neutrophil for further evaluation.

The mononuclear subpopulation is plotted on a 0-degree/ 7-degree scatterplot, with volume on the *y*-axis and complexity on the *x*-axis. Three populations (lymphocytes, monocytes, and basophils) are seen clearly on this display. Nucleated RBCs, unlysed RBCs, giant platelets, and platelet clumps fall below the lymphocyte cluster on this scatterplot and are excluded from the WBC count and differential. Information from the WBC impedance channel also is used in discriminating these particles.[21]

The segmented neutrophil subpopulation is plotted on a 90-degree depolarized/90-degree scatterplot, with granularity or 90-degree depolarized scatter on the *y*-axis and lobularity or 90-degree scatter on the *x*-axis. Because of the unique nature of eosinophil granules, eosinophils scatter more 90-degree depolarized light, which allows clear separation of eosinophils and neutrophils on this display. Dynamic thresholds are used for best separation of the different populations in the various scatterplots. Each cell type is identified with a distinct color, so that after all classifications are made and volume (0-degree scatter) is plotted on the *y*-axis against complexity (7-degree scatter) on the *x*-axis, each cell population can be visualized easily by the operator on the data terminal screen. Other scatterplots (90 degrees/0 degrees, 90 degrees depolarized/0 degrees, 90 degrees depolarized/7 degrees) are available and may be displayed at operator request. On earlier instruments, the 7-degree angle measurement for complexity was referred to as the 10-degree angle. The change reflects use of the midrange of the angle instead of the end range; however, it still provides the same information.[45-46] As on the previously described instruments, user-defined distributional flags may be set, and instrument-specific suspect flags may alert the operator to the presence of abnormal cells.[20,45] Figure 15-9 represents a patient printout from the CELL-DYN Sapphire analyzing the same patient specimen for which data are given in Figures 15-6 and 15-7.

Siemens Healthcare Diagnostics Instrumentation

Siemens Healthcare Diagnostics Inc. manufactures the ADVIA 2120 and 2120i, the next generation of the ADVIA 120.[26,33,47] Siemens has simplified the hydraulics and operations of the analyzer by replacing multiple complex hydraulic systems with a unified fluids circuit assembly, or *Unifluidics technology*. The ADVIA 2120, 2120i, and 120 provide a complete hemogram and WBC differential, while also providing a fully automated reticulocyte count.[22,23]

Four independent measurement channels are used in determining the hemogram and differential: RBC/platelet channel, hemoglobin channel, and peroxidase (PEROX) and basophil-lobularity (BASO) channels for WBC and differential data. WBC, RBC, hemoglobin, and platelets are measured directly. Hemoglobin is determined using a modified cyanmethemoglobin method that measures absorbance in a colorimeter flow cuvette at approximately 546 nm. The RBC/platelet method uses flow cytometric light scattering measurements determined

as cells, in a sheath-stream, pass through a flow cell by a laser optical assembly (laser diode light source). RBCs and platelets are isovolumetrically sphered before entering the flow cell to eliminate optical orientation noise. Laser light scattered at two different angular intervals—low angle (2 to 3 degrees), correlating with cell volume, and high angle (5 to 15 degrees), correlating with internal complexity (i.e., refractive index or hemoglobin concentration)—is measured simultaneously (Figure 15-10). This *differential scatter technique*, in combination with isovolumetric sphering, eliminates the adverse effect of variation in cellular hemoglobin concentration on the determination of RBC volume (as seen by differences in cellular deformability affecting the pulse height generated on impedance instruments).[10,48] The Mie theory of light scatter of dielectric spheres[18] is applied to plot scatter-intensity signals from the two angles against each other for a cell-by-cell RBC volume (*y*-axis) versus hemoglobin concentration (*x*-axis) cytogram or RBC map (Figure 15-11).[19]

Independent histograms of RBC volume and hemoglobin concentration also are plotted. On the ADVIA 2120 and 120 platelets are counted and volumetrically sized using a two-dimensional (low-angle and high-angle) platelet analysis, which allows better discrimination of platelets from interfering particles, such as RBC fragments and small RBCs.[22] Larger platelets can be included in the platelet count.[23,47]

Several parameters and indices are derived from the measurements described in the previous paragraph. MCV and MPV are the mean of the RBC volume histogram and the platelet volume histogram. Hematocrit, MCH, and MCHC are mathematically computed using RBC, hemoglobin, and MCV values. RDW is calculated as the CV of the RBC volume histogram, whereas hemoglobin distribution width (HDW), an analogous index, is calculated as the SD of the RBC hemoglobin concentration histogram. The reference interval for HDW is 2.2 to 3.2 g/dL. Cell hemoglobin concentration mean (CHCM), analogous to MCHC, is derived from cell-by-cell direct measures of hemoglobin concentration. Interferences with the hemoglobin colorimetric method, such as lipemia or icterus, affect the calculated MCHC but do not alter measured CHCM. CHCM generally is not reported as a patient result but is used by the instrument as an internal check for the MCHC and is available to the operator for calculating the cellular hemoglobin if interferences are present. Unique RBC flags derived from CHCM include hemoglobin concentration variance (HC VAR), hypochromia (HYPO), and hyperchromia (HYPER).[22,23]

Siemens hematology analyzers determine WBC count and a six-part WBC differential (neutrophils, lymphocytes, monocytes, eosinophils, basophils, and large unstained cells [LUCs]) by cytochemistry and optical flow cytometry, using the PEROX and BASO channels. LUCs include reactive or variant lymphocytes and blasts.

Peroxidase (PEROX) Channel

In the PEROX channel, RBCs are lysed, and WBCs are stained for their peroxidase activity. The following reaction is catalyzed by cellular peroxidase, which converts the substrate to a dark

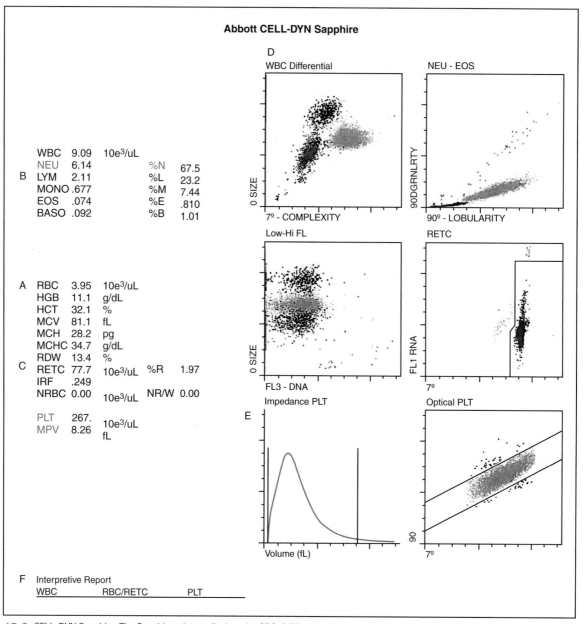

Abbott CELL-DYN Sapphire

	WBC	9.09	10e³/uL	
	NEU	6.14	%N	67.5
B	LYM	2.11	%L	23.2
	MONO	.677	%M	7.44
	EOS	.074	%E	.810
	BASO	.092	%B	1.01

A	RBC	3.95	10e³/uL	
	HGB	11.1	g/dL	
	HCT	32.1	%	
	MCV	81.1	fL	
	MCH	28.2	pg	
	MCHC	34.7	g/dL	
	RDW	13.4	%	
C	RETC	77.7	10e³/uL	%R 1.97
	IRF	.249		
	NRBC	0.00	10e³/uL	NR/W 0.00
	PLT	267.	10e³/uL	
	MPV	8.26	fL	

Figure 15-9 CELL-DYN Sapphire. The Sapphire printout displays the CBC, DIFF, and reticulocyte data for the same patient in Figures 15-6, 15-7, and 15-12. **A,** CBC data; **B,** Differential count data. Note that the WBC is listed with the differential instead of the CBC data; **C,** Reticulocyte and nucleated RBC data displayed under the CBC data but before the PLT data; **D,** Two scattergrams for the differential; both 7-degree scatter (complexity) vs 0-degree scatter (size or volume) and 90-degree scatter (lobularity) vs 90-degree depolarized (90D) scatter (granularity) are plotted for the WBCs; two histograms are also plotted for the nucleated RBC and reticulocyte data; **E,** Impedance histogram and optical platelet scatterplot side by side; **F,** At the bottom where the interpretative report flags display if there are any for the sample.

precipitate in peroxidase-containing cells (neutrophils, monocytes, and eosinophils):

$$H_2O_2 + 4\text{-chloro-1-naphthol} \xrightarrow{\text{cellular peroxidase}} \text{dark precipitate}$$

A portion of the cell suspension is fed to a sheath-stream flow cell where a tungsten-halogen darkfield optics system is used to measure absorbance (proportional to the amount of peroxidase in each cell) and forward scatter (proportional to the volume of each cell). Absorbance is plotted on the *x*-axis of the cytogram, and scatter is plotted on the *y*-axis.[22,23] A total WBC count (WBC-PEROX) is obtained from the optical

signals in this channel and is used as an internal check of the primary WBC count obtained in the basophil-lobularity channel (WBC-BASO). If significant interference occurs in the WBC-BASO count, the instrument substitutes the WBC-PEROX value.[23]

Computerized cluster analysis allows classification of the different cell populations, including abnormal clusters such as nucleated RBCs and platelet clumps. Nucleated RBCs are analyzed for every sample using four counting algorithms, which permits the system to choose the most accurate count based on internal rules and conditions. Neutrophils and eosinophils contain the most peroxidase and cluster to the right on

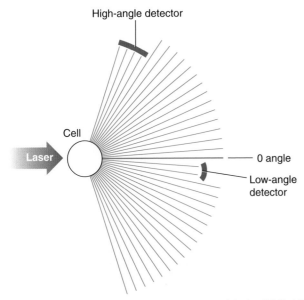

Figure 15-10 Differential scatter detection as used in the ADVIA 120. Forward high-angle scatter (5 to 15 degrees) and forward low-angle scatter (2 to 3 degrees) are detected for analysis of red and white blood cells. (From Miles: Technicon H systems training guide, Tarrytown, NY, 1993, Miles.)

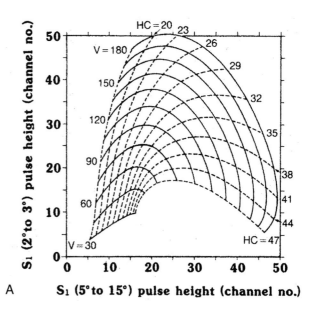

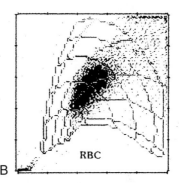

Figure 15-11 Cytograms or red blood cell (RBC) maps derived using the Mie theory of light scatter of dielectric spheres. **A,** Transformation between scatter angles (2 to 3 degrees and 5 to 15 degrees) and RBC volume (V) and hemoglobin concentration (HC). **B,** RBC map for a patient sample. (From Groner W: New developments in flow cytochemistry technology. In Simson E, editor: Proceedings of Technicon H-1 hematology symposium, October 11, 1985, Tarrytown, NY, 1986, Technicon Instruments Corp, p. 5.)

the cytogram. Monocytes stain weakly and cluster in the midregion of the cytogram. Lymphocytes, basophils, and LUCs (including variant or reactive lymphs and blasts) contain no peroxidase and appear on the left of the cytogram, with LUCs appearing above the lymphocyte area. Basophils cluster with the small lymphocytes and require further analysis for classification.[22,23,49]

Basophil-Lobularity (BASO) Channel

In the BASO channel, cells are treated with a reagent containing a nonionic surfactant in an acidic solution. Basophils are particularly resistant to lysis in this temperature-controlled reaction, whereas RBCs and platelets lyse and other leukocytes (nonbasophils) are stripped of their cytoplasm. Laser optics, using the same two-angle (2 to 3 degrees and 5 to 15 degrees) forward scattering system of the RBC/platelet channel, is used to analyze the treated cells. High-angle scatter (proportional to nuclear complexity) is plotted on the x-axis, and low-angle scatter (proportional to cell volume) is plotted on the y-axis. Cluster analysis allows for identification and quantification of the individual cellular populations. The intact basophils are identifiable by their large low-angle scatter. The remaining nuclei are classified as mononuclear, segmented, and blast cell nuclei based on their nuclear complexity (shape and cell density) and high-angle scatter.[22,23]

Basophils fall above a horizontal threshold on the cytogram. The stripped nuclei fall below the basophils, with segmented cells to the right and mononuclear cells to the left along the x-axis. Blast cells uniquely cluster below the mononuclear cells. Lack of distinct separation between the segmented and mononuclear clusters indicates WBC immaturity

or suspected left shift. As indicated earlier, this channel provides the primary WBC count, the WBC-BASO. Relative differential results (in percent) are computed by dividing absolute numbers of the different cell classifications by the total WBC count.[22,23]

The nucleated RBC method is based on the physical characteristics of volume and density of the nucleated RBC nuclei. These characteristics allow counting in both WBC channels on the ADVIA 2120, and algorithms are applied to determine the absolute number and percentage of nucleated RBCs. Information from the PEROX and BASO channels is used to generate differential morphology flags indicating the possible presence of reactive lymphocytes, blasts, left shift, immature granulocytes, nucleated RBCs, or large platelets or platelet clumps.[22,23,49] Figure 15-12 shows a patient printout from the ADVIA 2120i analyzing the same patient specimen for which data are given in Figures 15-6, 15-7, and 15-9.

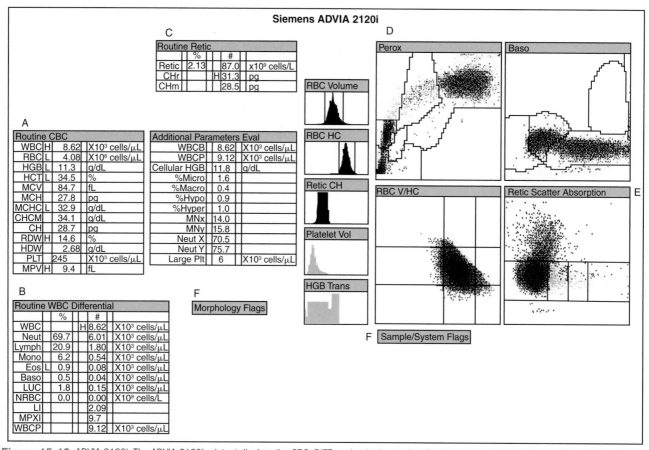

Figure 15-12 ADVIA 2120i. The ADVIA 2120i printout displays the CBC, DIFF, and reticulocyte data for the same patient in Figures 15-6, 15-7, and 15-9. **A,** CBC data; **B,** Six-part differential, including large unstained cells (LUCs); nucleated RBCs; **C,** Reticulocyte information includes the CHr (cellular hemoglobin reticulocyte). **D,** Cytograms for the differential, both the perox and baso channels, on the right; **E,** Scattergram for the reticulocyte and RBC counts; **F,** Morphology flags and Sample/System Flags where flags are displayed.

AUTOMATED RETICULOCYTE COUNTING

Reticulocyte counting is the last of the manual cell-counting procedures to be automated and has been a primary focus of hematology analyzer advancement in recent years. The imprecision and inaccuracy in manual reticulocyte counting are due to multiple factors, including stain variability, slide distribution error, statistical sampling error, and interobserver error.[50] All of these potential errors, with the possible exception of stain variability, are correctable with automated reticulocyte counting. Increasing the number of RBCs counted produces increased precision.[51] This was evidenced in the 1993 College of American Pathologists pilot reticulocyte proficiency survey (Set RT-A, Sample RT-01) on which the CV for the reported manual results was 35% compared with 8.3% for results obtained using flow cytometry.[52] Precision of automated methods has continued to improve. The manual reticulocyte results for one specimen in the 2000 Reticulocyte Survey Set RT/RT2-A showed a CV of 28.7%, whereas the CV was 2.8% for results obtained using one of the automated methods.[53] Automated reticulocyte analyzers may count 32,000 RBCs compared with 1000 cells in the routine manual procedure.[54]

Available automated reticulocyte analyzers include flow cytometry systems such as the FACS system from Becton, Dickinson and Company (Franklin Lakes, NJ) or the Coulter EPICS system; the Sysmex R-3500, R-500, XE-2100, XE-5000, and XN-series systems; the CELL-DYN 3500R, 3700, and 4000 systems; the Coulter LH 750 systems and the UniCel DxH800; and the Siemens ADVIA 2120, 2120i, and 120. All of these analyzers evaluate reticulocytes based on optical scatter or fluorescence after the RBCs are treated with fluorescent dyes or nucleic acid stains to stain residual RNA in the reticulocytes. Because neither the FACS nor EPICS system is generally available in the routine hematology laboratory, the discussion here is limited to the other analyzers.

The Sysmex R-3000/3500 is a stand-alone reticulocyte analyzer that uses auramine O, a supravital fluorescent dye, and measures forward scatter and side fluorescence as the cells, in a sheath-stream, pass through a flow cell by an argon laser. The signals are plotted on a scattergram with forward scatter intensity, which correlates with volume, plotted against fluorescence intensity, which is proportional to RNA content. Automatic discrimination separates the populations into mature RBCs and reticulocytes. The reticulocytes fall into low-fluorescence, middle-fluorescence, or high-fluorescence regions, with the less mature reticulocytes showing higher fluorescence. The *immature reticulocyte fraction* (IRF) is the sum of the middle-fluorescence and high-fluorescence ratios and indicates the ratio of immature reticulocytes to total reticulocytes in a sample. The XE-5000, the XT-2000i and the XN series also determines the reticulocyte count and IRF by measuring forward scatter and side fluorescence. They also have a parameter called *RET-He* (reticulocyte hemoglobin equivalent) that measures the hemoglobin content of the reticulocytes.[55] It uses a proprietary polymethine dye to fluorescently stain the reticulocyte nucleic acids. This is similar to the reticulocyte hemoglobin content (CHr) parameter on the ADVIA 2120i (discussed below). Platelets, which also are counted, fall below a lower discriminator line.[56] The Sysmex SE-9500/9000+RAM-1 module uses the same flow cytometry methodology for reticulocyte counting as the R-3500.[16] Off-line sample preparation is not required. The smaller Sysmex R-500 uses flow cytometry with a semiconductor laser as the light source and polymethine supravital fluorescent dye to provide automated reticulocyte counts.[28]

The CELL-DYN 3500R performs reticulocyte analysis by measuring 10-degree and 90-degree scatter in the optical channel (MAPSS technology) after the cells have been isovolumetrically sphered to eliminate optical orientation noise. The RBCs are stained with the thiazine dye new methylene blue N in an off-line sample preparation before the sample is introduced to the instrument. The operator simply must change computer functions on the instrument before aspiration of the reticulocyte preparation.[45] The CELL-DYN Sapphire also uses MAPSS technology but adds fluorescence detection to allow fully automated, random access reticulocyte testing.[24,46] The RBCs are stained with a proprietary membrane-permeable fluorescent dye (CD4K530) that binds stoichiometrically to nucleic acid and emits green light as the cells, in a sheath-stream, pass through a flow cell by an argon ion laser. Platelets and reticulocytes are separated based on intensity of green fluorescence (scatter measured at 7 degrees and 90 degrees), and the reticulocyte count along with the IRF is determined.[46]

Beckman Coulter also has incorporated reticulocyte methods into its primary cell-counting instruments: LH 700 series systems and the UniCel DxH800. The Coulter method uses a new methylene blue stain and the VCS technology described earlier. Volume is plotted against light scatter (DF 5 scatterplot) and against conductivity (DF 6 scatterplot), which correlates with opacity of the RBC. Stained reticulocytes show greater optical scatter and greater opacity than mature RBCs. Relative and absolute reticulocyte counts are reported, along with mean reticulocyte volume and maturation index or IRF.[54]

The Siemens ADVIA 2120, 2120i, and 120 systems enumerate reticulocytes in the same laser optics flow cell used in the RBC/platelet and BASO channels described earlier. The reticulocyte reagent isovolumetrically spheres the RBCs and stains the reticulocytes with oxazine 750, a nucleic acid–binding dye. Three detectors measure low-angle scatter (2 to 3 degrees), high-angle scatter (5 to 15 degrees), and absorbance simultaneously as the cells pass through the flow cell. Three cytograms are generated: high-angle scatter versus absorption, low-angle scatter versus high-angle scatter (Mie cytogram or RBC map), and volume versus hemoglobin concentration. The absorption cytogram allows separation and quantitation of reticulocytes, with additional subdivision into low-absorbing, medium-absorbing, and high-absorbing cells based on amount of staining. The sum of the medium-absorbing and high-absorbing cells reflects the IRF. Volume and hemoglobin concentration for each cell are derived from the RBC map by applying Mie scattering theory.[26,57] Unique reticulocyte indices (MCVr, CHCMr, RDWr, HDWr, CHr, and CHDWr) are provided. The CHr or reticulocyte hemoglobin content of each cell is calculated as the product of the cell volume and the cell hemoglobin concentration. A single-parameter histogram of CHr is constructed, with a corresponding distribution width (CHDWr) calculated.[22,23] These reticulocyte indices are not reported on the routine patient printout but are available to the operator. Figure 15-13 is a reticulocyte printout from an ADVIA 120, showing the cytograms and reticulocyte indices.

Automation of reticulocyte counting has allowed increased precision and accuracy and has greatly expanded the analysis of immature RBCs, providing new parameters and indices that may be useful in the diagnosis and treatment of anemias. The IRF, first introduced to indicate immature reticulocytes, shows an early indication of erythropoiesis. The IRF and the absolute reticulocyte count can be used to distinguish types of anemias. Anemias with increased marrow erythropoiesis, such as hemolytic anemia, have a high total reticulocyte count and increased IRF, while chronic renal disease has decreased absolute count and an IRF indicating decreased marrow erythropoiesis.[57,58] An increased IRF and normal to decreased absolute reticulocyte count indicates an early response to therapy in nutritional anemias.[58] Utilization of both tests is a reliable indicator of changes in erythropoietic activity and may prove to be a valuable therapeutic monitoring tool in patients.[58] The reticulocyte maturity measurements also may be useful in evaluating bone marrow suppression during chemotherapy, monitoring hematopoietic regeneration after bone marrow or stem cell transplantation, monitoring renal transplant engraftment, and assessing efficacy of anemia therapy.[57-61] The reticulocyte hemoglobin content, CHr (Advia) and Ret-He (Sysmex), provides an assessment of the availability of iron for erythropoiesis (Chapters 11 and 20). The additional reticulocyte indices derived on the ADVIA 2120 and 120 are valuable in following the response to erythropoietin therapy, and the CHr in particular has proved useful in the early detection and diagnosis of iron deficient erythropoiesis in children.[61,62] The National Kidney Foundation KDOQI (Kidney Disease Outcomes Quality Initiative) recommends the addition of the reticulocyte hemoglobin content to the CBC, in addition to the reticulocyte count and ferritin level to assess the iron status in patients with chronic kidney disease.[63] Widespread use of the new parameters may be limited by the availability of instrumentation.

ADVIA 120

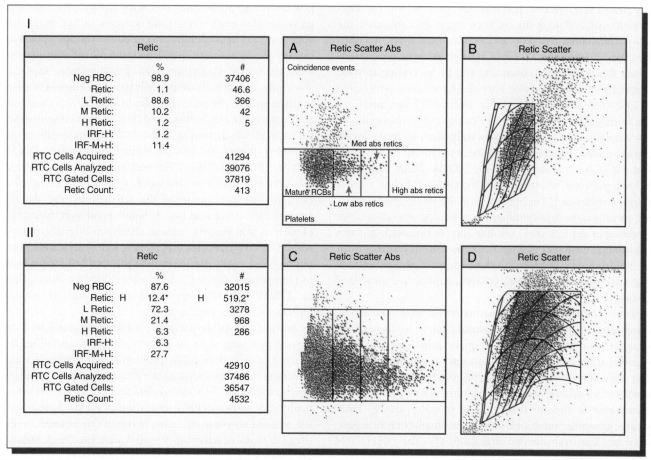

Figure 15-13 Composite cytograms obtained from the ADVIA 120. **I,** Normal reticulocyte count. **II,** High reticulocyte count with a large immature reticulocyte fraction (IRF). **I-A** and **II-C,** Reticulocyte scatter/absorption cytograms show high-angle (5- to 15-degree) scatter on the *y*-axis versus absorption on the *x*-axis, which allows separation of low-absorbing, medium-absorbing, and high-absorbing cells based on the amount of staining with nucleic acid–binding dye (oxazine 750). **I-B** and **II-D,** Reticulocyte scatter cytograms show low-angle (2- to 3-degree) scatter on the *y*-axis versus high-angle (5- to 15-degree) scatter on the *x*-axis (red blood cell [RBC] map). Because the RBCs are evaluated by the instrument on a cell-by-cell basis, unique reticulocyte indices can be derived.

LIMITATIONS AND INTERFERENCES

Implementing automation in the hematology laboratory requires critical evaluation of the instrument's methods and limitations, and the performance goals for the individual laboratory. The Clinical and Laboratory Standards Institute (CLSI) has approved a standard for validation, verification, and quality assurance of automated hematology analyzers.[64] This standard provides guidelines for instrument calibration and assessment of performance criteria, including accuracy, precision, linearity, sensitivity, and specificity. The clinical accuracy (sensitivity and specificity) of the methods should be such that the instrument appropriately identifies patients who have disease and patients who do not have disease.[65] Quality control systems should reflect the laboratory's established performance goals and provide a high level of assurance that the instrument is working within its specified limits.

Calibration

Calibration is crucial in defining the accuracy of the data produced (Chapter 5). Calibration, or the process of electronically correcting an instrument for analytical bias (numerical difference from the "true" value), may be accomplished by appropriate use of reference methods, reference materials, or commercially prepared calibrators.[64] Because few instruments are precalibrated by the manufacturer, calibration must be performed at initial installation and verified at least every 6 months under the requirements of the Clinical Laboratory Improvement Act of 1988.[66] Periodic recalibration may be required after major instrument repair requiring optical alignment or part replacement.

Whole-blood calibration using fresh whole-blood specimens requires the use of reference methods, materials, and procedures to determine "true" values.[1,67,68] The International Committee for Standardization in Haematology has established guidelines for selecting a reference blood cell counter for this purpose,[1] but the cyanmethemoglobin method remains the only standard available in hematology for calibration and quality control.[69] Whole-blood calibration, which historically has been considered the preferred method for calibration of multichannel hematology analyzers, has been almost completely replaced by the use of commercial calibrators assayed using reference methods. Calibration bias is possible with the use of these calibrators because of inherent differences in stabilized and preserved cell suspensions.[70] It is essential that calibrations be carried out properly and verified by comparison with reference methods or review of quality control data after calibration and by external comparison studies such as proficiency testing.[1]

Instrument Limitations

The continual improvement of automated technologies has resulted in greater sensitivity and specificity of instrument flagging with detection of possible interferences in the data. The parallel improvement in instrument walk-away capabilities has increased the importance of the operator's awareness and understanding of instrument limitations, however, and of his or her ability to recognize factors that may interfere and cause erroneous laboratory results. Limitations and interferences may be related to methodology or to inherent problems in the blood specimen.

Each instrument has limitations related to methodology that are defined in instrument operation manuals and in the literature. A common limitation of impedance methods is an instrument's inability to distinguish cells reliably from other particles or cell fragments of the same volume. Cell fragments may be counted as platelets in specimens from chemotherapy-treated patients with increased WBC fragility.[1] Likewise, schistocytes or small RBCs may interfere with the platelet count. Larger platelet clumps may be counted as WBCs, which results in a falsely decreased platelet count and potentially increases the WBC count. Micromegakaryocytes may be counted as nucleated RBCs or WBCs. RBCs containing variant hemoglobins such as Hb S or Hb C are often resistant to lysis, and the unlysed cells can be falsely counted as nucleated RBCs or WBCs and interfere in the hemoglobin reaction.[71] This phenomenon has become more apparent with the use of milder diluent and lysing reagents in the analyzers with automated WBC differential technology. Non-lysis also may be seen in specimens from patients with severe liver disease, those undergoing chemotherapy treatment, and neonates (due to increased levels of Hb F) on the older Sysmex instruments.[15] The ADVIA 2120 and 120 reports the WBC-BASO as the primary WBC count.[23] An extended lyse cycle may be used on the CELL-DYN 3500, and the newer instruments are able to provide a correct WBC impedance count when lyse-resistant RBCs are present.[21] The Sysmex SE-9000 and Sysmex SE-9500 also have an additional WBC impedance channel.[28]

Suppression of automated data, particularly WBC differential data, may occur when internal instrument checks fail or cast doubt on the validity of the data. Instruments from some manufacturers release results with specific error codes or flagging for further review. The suppression of automated differential data ensures that a manual differential count is performed, whereas the release of data with appropriate flagging mandates the need for careful review of the data and possibly a blood film examination. This suggests a difference in philosophy among the manufacturers and affects the work flow in different ways.[72] More importantly, each laboratory must establish its own criteria for directed blood film review based on established performance goals, instrument flagging, and inherent instrument limitations.

Specimen Limitations

Limitations resulting from inherent specimen problems include those related to the presence of cold agglutinins, icterus, and lipemia. Cold agglutinins manifest as a classic pattern of increased MCV (frequently greater than 130 fL), markedly decreased RBC count, and increased MCHC (frequently greater than 40 g/dL). Careful examination of the histograms or cytograms from the instruments may yield clues to this abnormality.[73] Icterus and lipemia directly affect hemoglobin measurements and related indices.[71] Table 15-2 summarizes conditions that cause interference on some hematology analyzers and offers suggestions for manually obtaining correct patient results. As instrumentation advances, instrumentation software can adjust or correct for some of the conditions listed. Historically, a nucleated RBC flag required examination of a blood film to enumerate the nucleated RBCs and correct the WBC. All four major vendors offer online nucleated RBC enumeration and WBC correction, although the laboratory must validate the results. Lipemia interferes with the hemoglobin reading by falsely elevating the hemoglobin and associated indices. The Siemens technology uses direct measurement of the CHCM parameter, which allows back-calculation of the hemoglobin unaffected by lipemia and thus eliminates the need for the manual method of saline replacement in lipemic specimens. These two examples involving nucleated RBCs and lipemia illustrate instrument advances, and continued future improvements in technology will eliminate or decrease the need for manual intervention to obtain accurate results.

Specimen age and improper specimen handling can have profound effects on the reliability of hematology test results. These factors have even greater significance as hospitals move toward greater use of off-site testing by large reference laboratories. Specific problems with older specimens include increased WBC fragility, swelling and possible lysis of RBCs, and the deterioration of platelets.[15] Stability studies should be performed before an instrument is used, and specific guidelines should be established for specimen handling and rejection.

CLINICAL UTILITY OF AUTOMATED BLOOD CELL ANALYSIS

The use of automated hematology analyzers has directly affected the availability, accuracy, and clinical usefulness of the CBC and WBC differential count. Some parameters that are available on hematology analyzers, but cannot be derived manually, have provided further insight into various clinical conditions. The RDW, a quantitative estimate of erythrocyte anisocytosis, can be used with the MCV for initial classification of an anemia.[74,75] Although the classification scheme is not absolute, a low MCV with a high RDW suggests iron deficiency, while a high MCV and high RDW suggests a folate/vitamin B_{12} deficiency or myelodysplasia (Chapter 19). The immature reticulocyte fraction and the immature platelet fraction provide an early indication of engraftment success after hematopoietic stem cell transplant.[76] The reticulocyte hemoglobin content (Chr and Ret-He) provides an assessment of the iron available for hemoglobin synthesis. It is useful in the early diagnosis of

TABLE 15-2 Conditions That Cause Interference on Most Hematology Analyzers

Condition	Parameters Affected*	Rationale	Instrument Indicators	Corrective Action
Cold agglutinins	RBC ↓, MCV ↑, MCHC ↑, grainy appearance	Agglutination of RBCs	Dual RBC population on RBC map, or right shift on RBC histogram	Warm specimen to 37° C and rerun
Lipemia, icterus	HGB ↑, MCH ↑	↑ Turbidity affects spectrophotometric reading for HGB	HGB × 3 ≠ HCT ± 3, abnormal histogram/cytogram[†]	Plasma replacement[‡]
Hemolysis	RBC ↓, HCT ↓	RBCs lysed and not counted	HGB × 3 ≠ HCT ± 3, may show lipemia pattern on histogram/cytogram[†]	Request new specimen
Lysis-resistant RBCs with abnormal hemoglobins	WBC ↑, HGB ↑	RBCs with hemoglobin S, C, or F may fail to lyse; will be counted as WBCs	Interference at noise-WBC interface on histogram/cytogram	Perform manual dilutions, allow incubation time for lysis
Microcytes or schistocytes	RBC ↓, PLT ↑	Volume of RBCs or RBC fragments less than lower RBC threshold, and/or within PLT threshold	Left shift on RBC histogram, MCV flagged if below limits; abnormal PLT histogram may be flagged	Review blood film
Nucleated RBCs, megakaryocyte fragments, or micromegakaryoblasts	WBC ↑ (older instruments)	Nucleated RBCs or micromegakaryoblasts counted as WBCs	Nucleated RBC flag resulting from interference at noise-lymphocyte interface on histogram/cytogram	Newer instruments eliminate this error and count nucleated RBCs and correct the WBC count; count micromegakaryoblasts per 100 WBCs and correct
Platelet clumps	PLT ↓, WBC ↑	Large clumps counted as WBCs and not platelets	Platelet clumps/N flag, interference at noise-lymphocyte interface on histogram/cytogram	Redraw specimen in sodium citrate, multiply result by 1.1
WBC > 100,000/μL	HGB ↑, RBC ↑, HCT incorrect	↑ Turbidity affects spectrophotometric reading for HGB, WBCs counted with RBC count	HGB × 3 ≠ HCT ± 3, WBC count may be above linearity	Manual HCT; perform manual HGB (spin/read supernatant),[‡] correct RBC count, recalculate indices; if above linearity, dilute for correct WBC count
Leukemia, especially with chemotherapy	WBC ↓, PLT ↑	Fragile WBCs, fragments counted as platelets	Platelet count inconsistent with previous results	Review film, perform phase platelet count or CD61 count
Old specimen	MCV ↑, MPV ↑, PLT ↓, automated differential may be incorrect	RBCs swell as specimen ages, platelets swell and degenerate, WBCs affected by prolonged exposure to EDTA	Abnormal clustering on WBC histogram/cytogram	Establish stability and specimen rejection criteria

↑, Increased; ↓, decreased; *EDTA,* ethylenediaminetetraacetic acid; *HGB,* hemoglobin; *HCT,* hematocrit; *MCH,* mean cell hemoglobin; *MCHC,* mean cell hemoglobin concentration; *MCV,* mean cell volume; *MPV,* mean platelet volume; *PLT,* platelet count; *RBC,* red blood cell (or count); *WBC,* white blood cell (or count).
*Manufacturer's labeling.
[†]Lipemia shows signature pattern on Siemens ADVIA 120 H cytograms.
[‡]HGB can be back-calculated from directly measured MCHC on Siemens ADVIA 120 cytograms.

iron deficiency, functional iron deficiency, as well as an early indicator of recovery after iron therapy.[61,62,77] The MPV may be useful in distinguishing thrombocytopenia due to idiopathic thrombocytopenia purpura (high MPV), inherited macrothrombocytopenia (higher MPV), or bone marrow suppression (low MPV).[78,79] High MPV values are also associated with higher-risk cardiovascular disease and may have use in assessing a patient's risk of thrombosis.[79,80] However the use of the MPV in these conditions has been hampered by the varying ability of instruments

to accurately measure MPV in patients with macroplatelets (they are underestimated in impedance methods), the lack of standardization of MPV cut-off values in various conditions, and the lack of well-controlled prospective studies to prove clinical utility.[79] In addition to method variations, anticoagulation and storage time also influence the MPV, which further impacts the reliability and clinical utility of MPV results.[81]

Automation of the WBC differential has had a significant impact on the laboratory work flow because of the labor-intensive nature of the manual differential count. The three-part differential available on earlier instruments generally proved suitable as a screening leukocyte differential count to identify specimens that required further workup or a manual differential count.[82-84] Partial differential counts, however, do not substitute for a complete differential count in populations with abnormalities.[85-87] The five-part or six-part automated differentials available on the larger instruments have been evaluated extensively and have acceptable clinical sensitivity and specificity for detection of distributional and morphologic abnormalities.[42,43,88-94] Abnormal cells such as blasts and nucleated RBCs in low concentrations may not be detected by the instruments but likewise may be missed by the routine 100-cell manual/visual differential count.[93-96] The CELL-DYN Sapphire, with its added fluorescent detection technology, has been shown to have high sensitivity and specificity for flagging nucleated RBCs and platelet clumps.[24,48,97] As technology continues to improve, blood film review to confirm the presence of platelet clumps or nucleated RBCs and to correct leukocyte counts for interference from platelet clumps or nucleated RBCs is becoming unnecessary, especially for nucleated RBCs, because the four major vendors now count and correct the WBC for nucleated RBCs on their high-end analyzers.[43,97,98]

Instrument evaluations based on the Clinical and Laboratory Standards Institute H20-A2 standard on reference leukocyte differential counting[99] using an 800-cell or 400-cell manual leukocyte differential count as the reference method have shown acceptable correlation coefficients for all WBC types, with the possible exception of monocytes.[43,72,93,94,100-102] However, further studies using monoclonal antibodies as the reference method for counting monocytes suggest that automated analyzers yield a more accurate assessment of monocytosis than do manual methods.[103,104]

Histograms and cytograms, along with instrument flagging, provide valuable information in the diagnosis and treatment of RBC and WBC disorders. Multiple reports indicate the usefulness of histograms and cytograms in the characterization of various abnormal conditions, including RBC disorders such as cold agglutination and WBC diseases such as leukemias and myelodysplastic disorders.[33,73,93,94]

Manufacturers are developing integrated hematology workstations for the greatest automation and laboratory efficiency. The Beckman Coulter LH 1500 Automation Series is Beckman's solution to integrated hematology. The line can be customized to have two to four LH analyzers as well as SlideMakers and SlideStainers based on the laboratory's needs for efficiency and automation.[33] The Sysmex Total Hematology Automation System (HST series) robotically links the SE-9000, R-3500 (automated reticulocyte analyzer), and SP-100 (automatic slide maker/stainer). The HST line links two XE-2100 units and one SP-100 instrument for complete automation or systemization of hematology testing. The SE-Alpha is a smaller version that links the SE-9000 and SP-100.[28] The Siemens ADVIA LabCell links the ADVIA 2120i to the track, and the Autoslide (automatic slide maker/stainer) links to the ADVIA 2120i. Finally, as a result of increasing customer needs, manufacturers have added body fluid counting to their high-end instrumentation. The Beckman Coulter UniCel DxH 800 system, the LH 780, and the Sysmex XN series and XE-5000 count WBCs and RBCs in body fluids; the ADVIA 2120i/120 counts WBCs and RBCs in body fluids and, in addition to cerebrospinal fluid WBC and RBC cell counts, performs a differential count on cerebrospinal fluid.[33,105,106]

Selection of a hematology analyzer for an individual laboratory requires careful evaluation of the laboratory's needs and close scrutiny of several important instrument issues, including instrument specifications and system requirements, methods used, training requirements, maintenance needs, reagent usage, data management capabilities, staff response, and short-term and long-term expenditures.[107] All instruments claim to improve laboratory efficiency through increased automation that results in improved work flow and faster turnaround time or through the addition of new parameters that may have clinical efficacy. All four major vendors offer a slide maker/stainer that can be connected directly to their high-end analyzers. The slide makers/stainers can be programmed to make blood films for every specimen or to make films based on the laboratory's internal criteria for a film review. This reduces, but does not completely eliminate, the use of manual peripheral blood film review. Automated slide makers/stainers connect only to high-end analyzers and as such are not suitable for some laboratories. Each laboratory must assess its own efficiency needs to determine if a slidemaker and stainer is a value-added instrument to the laboratory.[108] The instrument selected should suit the workload and patient population and should have a positive effect on patient outcomes.[109] The instrument selected for a cancer center may be different from that chosen for a community hospital.[110] Ultimately, however, the instrument decision may be swayed by individual preferences.

SUMMARY

- Automated cell counting provides greater accuracy and precision compared to manual cell-counting methods.
- The primary principles of operation, electronic impedance and optical scatter, are used by most automated hematology analyzers. Radiofrequency (RF) is sometimes used in conjunction with electronic impedance.
- The electronic impedance method detects and measures changes in electrical resistance between two electrodes as cells pass through a sensing aperture. The measurable voltage changes are plotted on frequency distribution graphs, or histograms, that allow the evaluation of cell populations based on cell volume.
- RF resistance uses high-voltage electromagnetic current. Measurable changes in the RF signal are proportional to cell interior density, or conductivity. Impedance and conductivity can be plotted against each other on a two-dimensional distribution cytogram

or scatterplot, which allows the evaluation of cell populations using cluster analysis.

- Optical scatter systems (flow cytometers) use detection of interference in a laser beam or light source to differentiate and enumerate cell types.

- Major manufacturers of hematology instrumentation include Beckman Coulter, Inc.; Sysmex Corporation; Abbott Diagnostics; and Siemens Healthcare Diagnostics, Inc. Table 15-1 summarizes the methods used for the hemogram, and reticulocyte, nucleated RBC, and WBC differential counts in the newer instruments.

- Reticulocyte analysis has been incorporated into the primary cell-counting instruments of all major manufacturers. All use either fluorescent or other dyes that stain nucleic acid in reticulocytes before the cells are counted using fluorescence or absorbance and light scatter.

- Each instrument has limitations related to methodology that may result in instrument flagging of specific results or suppression of automated data. Likewise, inherent specimen problems may result in instrument flagging that indicates possible rejection of automated results.

- Automated hematology analyzers have had a significant impact on laboratory work flow, particularly automation of the WBC differential. In addition, newer parameters that can now be measured, such as the immature reticulocyte fraction (IRF) and the reticulocyte hemoglobin concentration (RET-He and CHr), have documented clinical utility.

REVIEW QUESTIONS

Answers can be found in the Appendix.

Examine the histograms/scatterplots obtained from four major instruments for the same patient specimen (Figure 15-14, A-D). Compare the results, and respond to questions 1 to 4 based on the results.

1. Which printout lets the end user know at a glance that the results are acceptable and no manual work needs to be performed?
   a. CELL-DYN Sapphire
   b. UniCel DxH 800
   c. ADVIA 2120i
   d. Sysmex XN-series

2. Which instrument printout has a system flag on the platelet count?
   a. CELL-DYN Sapphire
   b. UniCel DxH 800
   c. ADVIA 2120i
   d. XN-series

3. What do you suspect is the cause of the variation in platelet counting among the four instruments?
   a. Different instruments have different levels of sensitivity.
   b. All instruments use the same principle for counting platelets.
   c. Some instruments are susceptible to false-positive platelet flagging under certain conditions.
   d. Different instruments use different thresholds to capture and count platelets.

4. Based on the overall flagging for this specimen on each instrument, should a manual differential count be performed for this patient?
   a. Yes, because immature granulocytes are present in the sample.
   b. Yes, because the WBC scatterplots are abnormal.
   c. No, because each differential count is complete with no system or morphology flags.

5. A patient peripheral blood film demonstrates agglutinated RBCs, and the CBC shows an elevated MCHC. What other parameters will be affected by the agglutination of the RBCs?
   a. MCV will be decreased and the RBC count will be increased.
   b. MCV will be decreased and the RBC count will be decreased.
   c. MCV will be increased and the RBC count will be decreased.
   d. MCV will be increased and the RBC count will be increased.

6. Match the cell-counting methods listed with the appropriate definition:

   ___ Impedance   a. Uses diffraction, reflection, and refraction of light waves

   ___ RF   b. Uses high-voltage electrical waves to measure the internal complexity of cells

   ___ Optical scatter c. Involves detection and measurement of changes in electrical current between two electrodes

7. Low-voltage DC is used to measure:
   a. Cell nuclear volume
   b. Total cell volume
   c. Cellular complexity in the nucleus
   d. Cellular complexity in the cytoplasm

8. Orthogonal light scatter is used to measure:
   a. Cell volume
   b. Internal complexity of the cell
   c. Cellular granularity
   d. Nuclear density

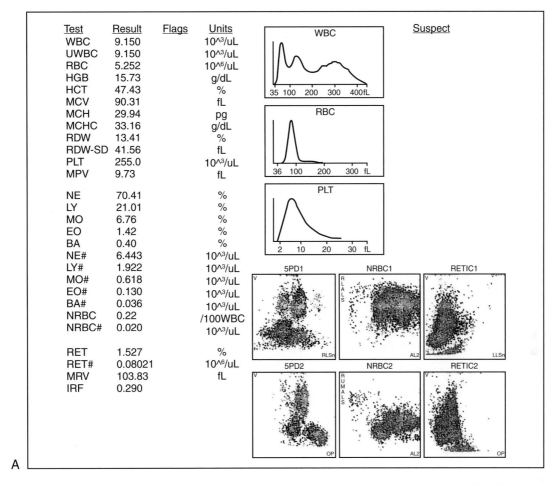

Test	Result	Flags	Units
WBC	9.150		10^3/uL
UWBC	9.150		10^3/uL
RBC	5.252		10^6/uL
HGB	15.73		g/dL
HCT	47.43		%
MCV	90.31		fL
MCH	29.94		pg
MCHC	33.16		g/dL
RDW	13.41		%
RDW-SD	41.56		fL
PLT	255.0		10^3/uL
MPV	9.73		fL
NE	70.41		%
LY	21.01		%
MO	6.76		%
EO	1.42		%
BA	0.40		%
NE#	6.443		10^3/uL
LY#	1.922		10^3/uL
MO#	0.618		10^3/uL
EO#	0.130		10^3/uL
BA#	0.036		10^3/uL
NRBC	0.22		/100WBC
NRBC#	0.020		10^3/uL
RET	1.527		%
RET#	0.08021		10^6/uL
MRV	103.83		fL
IRF	0.290		

A

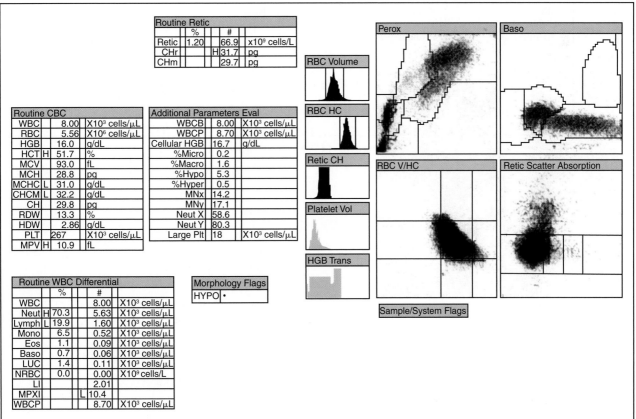

Routine Retic	%		#	
Retic	1.20		66.9	x10^9 cells/L
CHr		H	31.7	pg
CHm			29.7	pg

Routine CBC		
WBC	8.00	X10^3 cells/µL
RBC	5.56	X10^6 cells/µL
HGB	16.0	g/dL
HCT H	51.7	%
MCV	93.0	fL
MCH	28.8	pg
MCHC L	31.0	g/dL
CHCM L	32.2	g/dL
CH	29.8	pg
RDW	13.3	%
HDW	2.86	g/dL
PLT	267	X10^3 cells/µL
MPV H	10.9	fL

Additional Parameters Eval		
WBCB	8.00	X10^3 cells/µL
WBCP	8.70	X10^3 cells/µL
Cellular HGB	16.7	g/dL
%Micro	0.2	
%Macro	1.6	
%Hypo	5.3	
%Hyper	0.5	
MNx	14.2	
MNy	17.1	
Neut X	58.6	
Neut Y	80.3	
Large Plt	18	X10^3 cells/µL

Routine WBC Differential		%		#	
WBC				8.00	X10^3 cells/µL
Neut	H	70.3		5.63	X10^3 cells/µL
Lymph	L	19.9		1.60	X10^3 cells/µL
Mono		6.5		0.52	X10^3 cells/µL
Eos		1.1		0.09	X10^3 cells/µL
Baso		0.7		0.06	X10^3 cells/µL
LUC		1.4		0.11	X10^3 cells/µL
NRBC		0.0		0.00	X10^9 cells/L
LI				2.01	
MPXI			L	10.4	
WBCP				8.70	X10^3 cells/µL

Morphology Flags	
HYPO	•

RBC Volume

RBC HC

Retic CH

Platelet Vol

HGB Trans

Perox

Baso

RBC V/HC

Retic Scatter Absorption

Sample/System Flags

B

Figure 15-14 Composite scatterplots/histograms obtained from four major instruments. **A,** Coulter UniCel DxH 800; **B,** ADVIA 2120i;

Continued

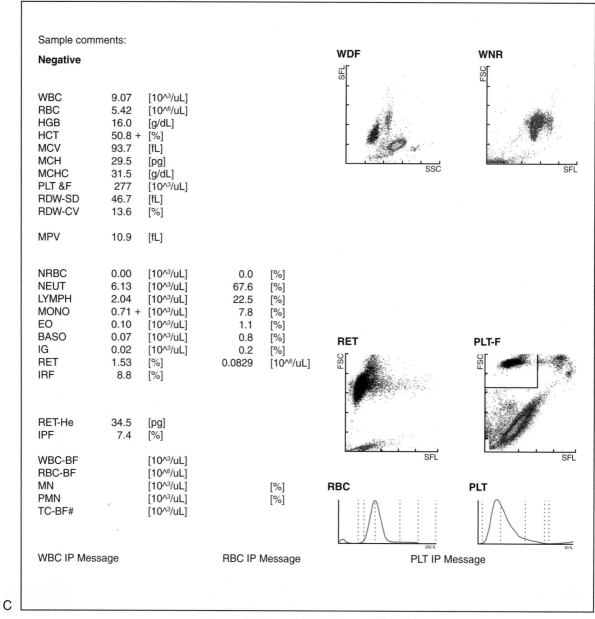

Sample comments:

Negative

WBC	9.07	[10^3/uL]
RBC	5.42	[10^6/uL]
HGB	16.0	[g/dL]
HCT	50.8 +	[%]
MCV	93.7	[fL]
MCH	29.5	[pg]
MCHC	31.5	[g/dL]
PLT &F	277	[10^3/uL]
RDW-SD	46.7	[fL]
RDW-CV	13.6	[%]
MPV	10.9	[fL]

NRBC	0.00	[10^3/uL]	0.0	[%]
NEUT	6.13	[10^3/uL]	67.6	[%]
LYMPH	2.04	[10^3/uL]	22.5	[%]
MONO	0.71 +	[10^3/uL]	7.8	[%]
EO	0.10	[10^3/uL]	1.1	[%]
BASO	0.07	[10^3/uL]	0.8	[%]
IG	0.02	[10^3/uL]	0.2	[%]
RET	1.53	[%]	0.0829	[10^6/uL]
IRF	8.8	[%]		

RET-He	34.5	[pg]
IPF	7.4	[%]
WBC-BF		[10^3/uL]
RBC-BF		[10^6/uL]
MN		[10^3/uL] [%]
PMN		[10^3/uL] [%]
TC-BF#		[10^3/uL]

WBC IP Message   RBC IP Message   PLT IP Message

Figure 15-14, cont'd   **C,** Sysmex XN-1000;

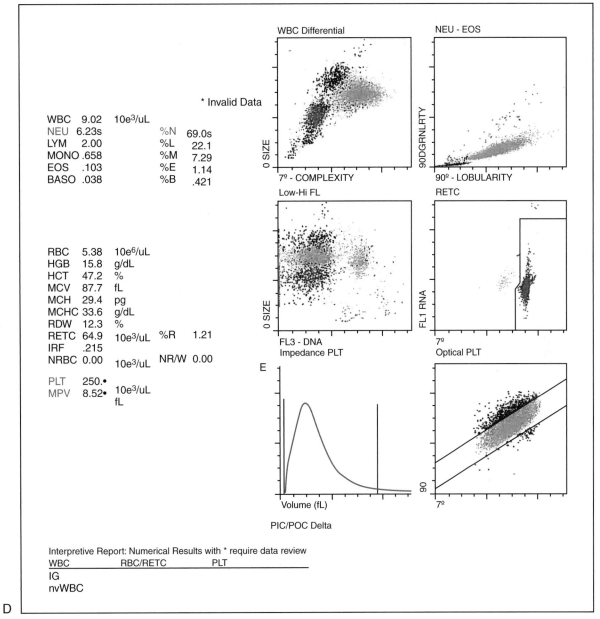

Figure 15-14, cont'd   D, CELL-DYN Sapphire.

9. On the Beckman Coulter instruments, hematocrit is a calculated value. Which of the following directly measured parameters is used in the calculation of this value?
   a. RDW
   b. Hemoglobin
   c. MCV
   d. MCHC

10. Match each instrument listed with the technology it uses to determine WBC differential counts.

____ Abbott CELL-DYN Sapphire	a. Volume, conductivity, and five angles of light scatter
____ Siemens ADVIA 2120i	b. MAPSS technology and three-color fluorescence
____ Sysmex XN-1000	c. Peroxidase-staining absorbance and light scatter
____ Beckman Coulter UniCel DxH 800	d. Detection of forward and side scattered light and fluorescence

REFERENCES

1. Koepke, J. A. (1991). Quantitative blood cell counting. In Koepke, J. A. (Ed.), *Practical Laboratory Hematology* (pp. 43–60). New York: Churchill Livingstone.
2. Rappaport, E. S., Helbert, B., & Beissner, R. S. (1988). Automated hematology: where we stand. *South Med J, 81*, 365–370.
3. Dotson, M. A. (1998). Multiparameter hematology instruments. In Stiene-Martin, E. A., Lotspeich-Steininger, C. A., & Koepke, J. A. (Eds.), *Clinical Hematology: Principles, Procedures, Correlations* (pp. 519–551). Philadelphia: Lippincott-Raven Publishers.
4. Coulter, W. H. (1956). High speed automatic blood cell counter and cell size analyzer. *Proc Natl Electron Conf, 12*, 1034.
5. Coulter Electronics. (1983). *Significant Advances in Hematology: Hematology Education Series*, PN 4206115 A, Hialeah (Fla): Coulter Electronics.
6. Coulter Electronics. (1983). *Coulter Counter Model S-Plus IV with Three-Population Differential: Product Reference Manual*, PN 423560B, Hialeah (Fla): Coulter Electronics.
7. Coulter Electronics. (1988). *Coulter STKR Product Reference Manual*, PN 4235547E, Hialeah (Fla): Coulter Electronics.
8. TOA Medical Electronics Company. (1985). *Sysmex Model E-5000 Operator's Manual* (CN 461-2104-2), Kobe, Japan: TOA Medical Electronics Co.
9. Coulter Corporation. (1992). *Coulter STKS Operator's Guide*, PN 423592811, Hialeah (Fla): Coulter Corporation.
10. Mohandas, N., Clark, M. R., Kissinger, S., et al. (1980). Inaccuracies associated with the automated measurement of mean cell hemoglobin concentration in dehydrated cells. *Blood, 56*, 125–128.
11. Arnfred, T., Kristensen, S. D., & Munck, V. (1981). Coulter counter model S and model S-plus measurements of mean erythrocyte volume (MCV) are influenced by the mean erythrocyte haemoglobin concentration (MCHC). *Scand J Clin Lab Invest, 41*, 717–721.
12. Johnson, K. L. (1992). Basics of flow cytometry. *Clin Lab Sci, 5*, 22–24.
13. Scott, R., Sethu, P., & Harnett, C. K. (2008). Three-dimensional hydrodynamic focusing in a microfluidic Coulter counter. *Rev Sci Instrum, 79*, 046104.
14. Rodriquez-Trujillo, R., Mills, C. A., Samitier, J., et al. (2007). Low cost micro-Coulter counter with hydrodynamic focusing. *Microfluid Nanofluid, 3*, 171–176.
15. TOA Medical Electronics Company. (1990). *Sysmex NE-8000 Operator's Manual* (CN 461-2326-5), Kobe, Japan: TOA Medical Electronics Co.
16. Sysmex Corporation. (1999). *Sysmex XE-2100 Operator's Manual*, Kobe, Japan: Sysmex Corp.
17. Sun, T. (2008). Principles of flow cytometry. In *Flow Cytometry and Immunohistochemistry for Hematologic Neoplasms* (pp. 4–14). Philadelphia: Wolters Kluwer/Lippincott Williams & Wilkins.
18. Jovin, T. M., Morris, S. J., Striker, G., et al. (1976). Automatic sizing and separation of particles by ratios of light scattering intensities. *J Histochem Cytochem, 24*, 269–283.
19. Ryan, D. H. (2010). Chapter 2. Examination of blood cells. In Lichtman, M. A., Kipps, T. J., Seligsohn, U., Kaushansky, K., Prchal, J. T. (Eds.), *Williams Hematology* (8th ed., pp. 11–24). New York: McGraw-Hill. http://accessmedicine.mhmedical.com.libproxy2.umdnj.edu/content.aspx?bookid=358&Sectionid=39835815. Accessed 02.03.14.
20. Abbott Laboratories. (1993). *CELL-DYN 3000 System Operator's Manual* (LN 92420-92401), Abbott Park (Ill): Abbott Laboratories.
21. Abbott Laboratories. (1996). *CELL-DYN 3500 System Operator's Manual* (LN 92722-92705), Abbott Park (Ill): Abbott Laboratories.
22. Siemens Healthcare Diagnostics. (2009). *ADVIA 120 Operator's Guide*, V 3.01.00, Tarrytown (NY): Siemens Healthcare Diagnostics.
23. Siemens Healthcare Diagnostics. (2008). *ADVIA 2120/2120i Operator's Guide*, V4.00.00, Tarrytown (NY): Siemens Healthcare Diagnostics.
24. Abbott Diagnostics. *Diagnostic Products*. Retrieved from http://www.abbottdiagnostics.com/Products/Instruments_by_Platform/yl.cfm?syscat_id=4. Accessed 28.02.14.
25. Horiba Medical. *ABX Hematology: the Product Line*. Retrieved from http://www.horiba.com. Accessed 28.02.14.
26. Siemens Healthcare Diagnostics. *Laboratory Diagnostics*. Retrieved from http://www.healthcare.siemens.com/laboratory-diagnostics. Accessed 28.02.14.
27. Beckman Coulter. *Hematology Systems*. Retrieved from https://www.beckmancoulter.com/wsrportal/wsr/diagnostics/index.htm. Accessed 28.02.14.
28. Sysmex Corporation. *Hematology Products*. Retrieved from https://www.sysmex.com/us/en/Products/Hematology/Pages/Sysmex-Hematology-Overview.aspx. Accessed 28.02.14.
29. Beckman Coulter. *LH750*. Retrieved from https://www.beckmancoulter.com/wsrportal/wsr/diagnostics/clinical-products/hematology/coulter-lh-750-hematology-analyzer/index.htm. Accessed 28.02.14.
30. Beckman Coulter. *UniCel DxH 800 Coulter Cellular Analysis System. Advancements in Technology CBC Methodology*. Retrieved from www.beckman.com/wsrportal/wsr/diagnostics/clinical-products/hematology/unicel-dxh-800-coulter-celluarl-analysis-system/index.htm. Accessed 10.01.14.
31. Beckman Coulter. *UniCel DxH 800 Coulter Cellular Analysis System. WBC Differential Methodology*. Retrieved from www.beckman.com/wsrportal/wsr/diagnostics/clinical-products/hematology/unicel-dxh-800-coulter-celluarl-analysis-system/index.htm. Accessed 10.01.14.
32. Barnes, P. W., McFadden, S. L., Machin, S. J., et al. (2005). The international consensus group for hematology review: suggested criteria for action following automated CBC and WBC differential analysis. *Lab Hematol, 11*, 83–90.
33. CAP Today. (2012, December). *Hematology Analyzers* (pp. 20–36). Retrieved from www.captodayonline.com/productguides/instruments/hematology-analyzers-2012.html. Accessed 06.12.13.
34. Beckman Coulter. (2003). *Coulter LH 700 Series Operator's Guide*, Fullerton, Calif: Beckman Coulter.
35. Schoorl, M., Schoorl, M., Oomes, J., et al. (2013). New fluorescent method (PLT-F) on Sysmex XN 2000 Hematology Analyzers achieved higher accuracy in low platelet counting. *Am J Clin Pathol, 140*, 495–499.
36. Sysmex. *XP 300 Automated Hematology Analyzer Brochure*. Retrieved from www.sysmex.com/us/en/Brochures/XP-300%20brochure-MKT-10-1195_07-2013pdf. Accessed 06.12.13.
37. Sysmex. *Reshaping compact automation. XN Series Automated Hematology Systems*. Retrieved from www.sysmex.com/us/en/Brochures/XN_compact_automation_MKT-10-1175.pdf. Accessed 06.12.13.
38. Sysmex. *Reshaping scalable automation. XN-9000 Automated Hematology Systems*. Retrieved from www.sysmex.com/us/en/Brochures/XN-Series-mainBrochure_MKT-10-1174.pdf. Accessed 06.12.13.
39. Abe, Y., Wada, H., Tomatsu, H., et al. (2006). A simple technique to determine thrombopoiesis level using immature platelet fraction (IPF). *Thromb Res, 118*, 463–469.
40. Abbott Diagnostics. *CELL-DYN Sapphire*. Retrieved from www.abbottdiagnostics.com.au/products/instruments_by_platform/default/default.cfm?sys_id=155. Accessed 10.01.14.
41. Matzdorff, A. C., Kühnel, G., Scott, S., et al. (1998). Comparison of flow cytometry and the automated blood analyzer system CELL-DYN 4000 for platelet analysis. *Lab Hematol, 4*, 163–168.

42. Bowden, K. L., Procopio, N., Wystepek, E., et al. (1998). Platelet clumps, nucleated red cells, and leukocyte counts: a comparison between the Abbott CELL-DYN 4000 and Coulter STKS. *Lab Hematol, 4*, 7–16.

43. Jones, R. G., Faust, A., Glazier, J., et al. (1998). CELL-DYN 4000: utility within the core laboratory structure and preliminary comparison of its expanded differential with the 400-cell manual differential count. *Lab Hematol, 4*, 34–44.

44. Abbott Diagnostics. (1992). *CELL-DYN Rainbow Classification Program*, PN 97-9427/R3-20, Abbott Park (Ill): September, Abbott Diagnostics.

45. Abbott Laboratories. (1999). *CELL-DYN 3500 System Operator's Manual: Reticulocyte Package*, (9140293D). Abbott Park (Ill): Abbott Laboratories.

46. Abbott Laboratories. (1997). *CELL-DYN 4000 Operator's Manual*, Santa Clara, Calif: Abbott Laboratories.

47. Bayer Healthcare. (2005). *Bayer ADVIA 2120 Operator's Guide*, Tarrytown (NY): Bayer Healthcare.

48. Mohandas, N., Kim, Y. R., Tycko, D. H., et al. (1986). Accurate and independent measurement of volume and hemoglobin concentration of individual red cells by laser light scattering. *Blood, 68*, 506–513.

49. Harris, N., Jou, J. M., Devoto, G., et al. (2005). Performance evaluation of the ADVIA 2120 hematology analyzer: an international multicenter clinical trial. *Lab Hematol, 11*, 62–70.

50. Koepke, J. (1993). Current limitations in reticulocyte counting: implications for clinical laboratories. In Porstmann, B. (Ed.), *The emerging importance of accurate reticulocyte counting* (pp. 18–22). New York: Caduceus Medical.

51. Clinical and Laboratory Standards Institute. (2004). *Methods for Reticulocyte Counting (Flow Cytometry and Supravital Dyes): approved guideline*, CLSI document H44-A-2, Wayne (Pa): Clinical and Laboratory Standards Institute.

52. College of American Pathologists. (1993). *CAP surveys: reticulocyte (pilot) survey set RT-A*, Northfield (Ill): College of American Pathologists.

53. College of American Pathologists. (2000). *CAP surveys: reticulocyte survey set RT/RT2-A*, Northfield (Ill): College of American Pathologists.

54. Coulter Corporation. (1993). *Introducing a New Reticulocyte Methodology using Coulter VCS Technology on Coulter STKS and MAXM Hematology Systems*, product brochure TC93003201, Miami (Fla): Coulter Corp.

55. Sysmex America. *DaVita Study Demonstrates Clinical Application of Sysmex Reticulocyte Hemoglobin Equivalent (RET-He) Parameter*. https://www.sysmex.com/us/en/Company/News/Pages/DaVita-Study-Demonstrates-Clinical-Application-of-Sysmex-Reticulocyte-Hemoglobin-Equivalent-%28RET-He%29-Parameter.aspx. Accessed 28.02.14.

56. TOA Medical Electronics Company. (1991). *Sysmex R-3000 Automated Reticulocyte Analyzer*, product brochure literature No. SP-9620, Los Alamitos, Calif: TOA Medical Electronics Co.

57. Davis, B. H., Bigelow, N. C., van Hove, L., et al. (1998). Evaluation of automated reticulocyte analysis with immature reticulocyte fraction as a potential outcomes indicator of anemia in chronic renal failure patients. *Lab Hematol, 4*, 169–175.

58. Buttarello, M., & Plebani, M. (2008). Automated blood cell counts. *Am J Clin Pathol, 130*, 104–116.

59. Fourcade, C., Jary, L., & Belaouni, H. (1999). Reticulocyte analysis provided by the Coulter GEN-S: significance and interpretation in regenerative and non-regenerative hematologic conditions. *Lab Hematol, 5*, 153–158.

60. Davis, B. H., & Bigelow, N. C. (1994). Automated reticulocyte analysis: clinical practice and associated new parameters. *Hematol Oncol Clin North Am, 8*, 617–630.

61. Brugnara, C., Zurakowski, D., DiCanzio, J., et al. (1999). Reticulocyte hemoglobin content to diagnose iron deficiency in children. *JAMA, 281*, 2225–2230.

62. Ullrich, C., Wu, A., Armbsy, C., et al. (2005). Screening healthy infants for iron deficiency using reticulocyte hemoglobin content. *JAMA, 294*, 924–930.

63. National Kidney Foundation. (2006). KDOQI Clinical practice guidelines and clinical practice recommendations for anemia in chronic kidney disease. *Evaluation of Anemia in CKD*. Retrieved from http://www.kidney.org/professionals/KDOQI/guidelines_anemia/cpr12.htm. Accessed 30.12.13.

64. Clinical and Laboratory Standards Institute. (2010). *Validation, verification, and quality assurance of automated hematology analyzers; approved standard-second edition*, CLSI publication H26-A2, Wayne, (PA): Clinical and Laboratory Standards Institute.

65. Clinical and Laboratory Standards Institute. (2011). *Assessment of the Diagnostic Accuracy of Laboratory Tests using Receiver Operating Characteristic Curves; Approved Guideline*. (2nd ed.). CLSI document EP24-A2, Wayne (Pa): Clinical and Laboratory Standards Institute.

66. Calibration and calibration verification. *Clinical Laboratory Improvement Amendments Brochure No. 3*. Retrieved from https://www.cms.gov/CLIA/downloads/6065bk.pdf. Accessed 28.02.13.

67. Gilmer, P. R., Williams, U., Koepke, J. A., et al. (1977). Calibration methods for automated hematology instruments. *Am J Clin Pathol, 68*, 185–190.

68. Koepke, J. A. (1977). The calibration of automated instruments for accuracy in hemoglobinometry. *Am J Clin Pathol, 68*, 180–184.

69. International Committee for Standardization in Haematology. (1996). Recommendations for reference method for haemoglobinometry in human blood (ICSH Standard 1995) and specifications for international haemiglobincyanide standard. (4th ed.). *J Clin Pathol, 49*, 271–274.

70. Savage, R. A. (1985). Calibration bias and imprecision for automated hematology analyzers: an evaluation of the significance of short-term bias resulting from calibration of an analyzer with S Cal. *Am J Clin Pathol, 84*, 186–190.

71. Cornbleet, J. (1983). Spurious results from automated hematology cell counters. *Lab Med 14*, 509–514.

72. Bentley, S. A., Johnson, A., & Bishop, C. A. (1993). A parallel evaluation of four automated hematology analyzers. *Am J Clin Pathol, 100*, 626–632.

73. Strobel, S. L., Panke, T. W., & Bills, G. L. (1993). Cold erythrocyte agglutination and infectious mononucleosis. *Lab Med, 24*, 219–221.

74. Bessman, J. D., Gilmer, P. R., & Gardner, F. H. (1983). Improved classification of anemia by MCV and RDW. *Am J Clin Pathol, 80*, 322–326.

75. Marks, P. W. (2013). Approach to anemia in the adult and child. In Hoffman, R., Benz E. J. Jr, Silberstein, L. E., et al. (Eds.), *Hematology: Basic Principles and Practice*. (6th ed., pp. 418–426). Philadelphia: Elsevier, Saunders.

76. Gonçalo, A. P., Barbosa, I. L., Campilho, F., et al. (2011). Predictive value of immature reticulocyte and platelet fractions in hematopoietic recovery of allograft patients. *Transplant Proc, 43*, 241–243.

77. Brugnara, C., Schiller, B., & Moran, J. (2006). Reticulocyte hemoglobin equivalent (Ret He) and assessment of iron deficient states. *Clin Lab Haem, 29*, 303–306.

78. Noris, P., Klersy, C., & Gresele, P. (2013). Platelet size for distinguishing between inherited thrombocytopenias and immune thrombocytopenia: a multicentric, real life study. *Br J Haematol, 162*, 112–119.

79. Leader, A., Pereg, D., & Lishner, M. (2012). Are platelet volume indices of clinical use? A multidisciplinary review. *Ann Med, 44*, 805–816.

80. Chu, S. G., Becker, R. C., & Berger, P. B. (2010). Mean platelet volume as a predictor of cardiovascular risk: a systematic review and meta-analysis. *J Thromb Haemost, 8*, 148–156.

81. Reardon, D. M., Hutchinson, D., Preston, F. E., et al. (1985). The routine measurement of platelet volume: a comparison of aperture-impedance and flow cytometric systems. *Clin Lab Haematol, 7,* 251–257.

82. Allen, J. K., & Batjer, I. D. (1985). Evaluation of an automated method for leukocyte differential counts based on electronic volume analysis. *Arch Pathol Lab Med, 109,* 534–539.

83. Pierre, R. V., Payne, B. A., Lee, W. K., et al. (1987). Comparison of four leukocyte differential methods with the National Committee for Clinical Laboratory Standards (NCCLS) reference method. *Am J Clin Pathol, 87,* 201–209.

84. Payne, B. A., Pierre, R. V., & Lee, W. K. (1987). Evaluation of the TOA E-5000 automated hematology analyzer. *Am J Clin Pathol, 88,* 51–57.

85. Ross, D. W., Watson, J. S., Davis, P. H., et al. (1985). Evaluation of the Coulter three-part differential screen. *Am J Clin Pathol, 84,* 481–484.

86. Cornbleet, J., & Kessinger, S. (1985). Evaluation of Coulter S-Plus three-part differential in a population with a high prevalence of abnormalities. *Am J Clin Pathol, 84,* 620–626.

87. Miers, M. K., Fogo, A. B., Federspiel, C. F., et al. (1987). Evaluation of the Coulter S-Plus IV differential as a screening tool in a tertiary care hospital. *Am J Clin Pathol, 87,* 745–751.

88. Warner, B. A., & Reardon, D. M. (1991). A field evaluation of the Coulter STKS. *Am J Clin Pathol, 95,* 207–217.

89. Hallawell, R., O'Malley, C., Hussein, S., et al. (1991). An evaluation of the Sysmex NE-8000 hematology analyzer. *Am J Clin Pathol, 96,* 594–601.

90. Cornbleet, P. J., Myrick, D., Judkins, S., et al. (1992). Evaluation of the CELL-DYN 3000 differential. *Am J Clin Pathol, 98,* 603–614.

91. Cornbleet, P. J., Myrick, D., & Levy, R. (1993). Evaluation of the Coulter STKS five-part differential. *Am J Clin Pathol, 99,* 72–81.

92. Brigden, M. L., Page, N. E., & Graydon, C. (1993). Evaluation of the Sysmex NE-8000 automated hematology analyzer in a high-volume outpatient laboratory. *Am J Clin Pathol, 100,* 618–625.

93. Meintker, L., Ringwald, J., Rauh, M., et al. (2013). Comparison of automated differential blood cell counts from Abbott Sapphire, Siemens Advia 120, Beckman Coulter DxH 800, and Sysmex XE-2100 in normal and pathologic samples. *Am J Clin Pathol, 139,* 641–650.

94. Hotton, J., Broothaers, J., Swaelens, C., et al. (2013). Performance and abnormal cell flagging comparisons of three automated blood cell counters: Cell-Dyn Sapphire, DxH-800, and XN-2000. *Am J Clin Pathol, 140,* 845–852.

95. Rumke, C. L. (1978). The statistically expected variability in differential leukocyte counting. In Koepke, J. A. (Ed.), *Differential leukocyte counting,* Skokie (Ill): College of American Pathologists.

96. Koepke, J. A., Dotson, M. A., & Shifman, M. A. (1985). A critical evaluation of the manual/visual differential leukocyte counting method. *Blood Cells, 11,* 173–181.

97. Paterakis, G., Kossivas, L., Kendall, R., et al. (1998). Comparative evaluation of the erythroblast count generated by three-color fluorescence flow cytometry, the Abbott CELL-DYN 4000 hematology analyzer, and microscopy. *Lab Hematol, 4,* 64–70.

98. Bowen, K. L., Glazier, J., & Mattson, J. C. (1998). Abbott CELL-DYN 4000 automated red blood cell analysis compared with routine red blood cell morphology by smear review. *Lab Hematol, 4,* 45–47.

99. Clinical Laboratory and Standards Institute. (2007). *Reference Leukocyte (WBC) Differential Count (Proportional) and Evaluation of Instrumental Methods: Approved Standard.* (2nd ed.). CLSI document H20-A2, Wayne, Pa: Clinical Laboratory and Standards Institute.

100. Warner, B. A., Reardon, D. M., & Marshall, D. P. (1990). Automated haematology analysers: a four-way comparison. *Med Lab Sci, 47,* 285–296.

101. Swaim, W. R. (1991). Laboratory and clinical evaluation of white blood cell differential counts: comparison of the Coulter VCS, Technicon H-1, and 800-cell manual method. *Am J Clin Pathol, 95,* 381–388.

102. Buttarello, M., Gadotti, M., Lorenz, C., et al. (1992). Evaluation of four automated hematology analyzers: a comparative study of differential counts (imprecision and inaccuracy). *Am J Clin Pathol, 97,* 345–352.

103. Goossens, W., Hove, L. V., & Verwilghen, R. L. (1991). Monocyte counting: discrepancies in results obtained with different automated instruments. *J Clin Pathol, 44,* 224–227.

104. Seaberg, R., & Cuomo, J. (1993). Assessment of monocyte counts derived from automated instrumentation. *Lab Med, 24,* 222–224.

105. Harris, N., Kunicka, J., & Kratz, A. (2005). The ADVIA 2120 hematology system: flow cytometry-based analysis of blood and body fluids in the routine hematology laboratory. *Lab Hematol, 11,* 47–61.

106. de Jonge, R., Brouwer, R., de Graaf, M. T., et al. (2010). Evaluation of the new body fluid mode on the Sysmex XE-5000 for counting leukocytes and erythrocytes in cerebrospinal fluid and other body fluids. *Clin Chem Lab Med, 48,* 665–675.

107. Camden, T. L. (1993). How to select the ideal hematology analyzer. *MLO Med Lab Obs, 25,* 29–33.

108. Dabkowski B. (2012, December). New fixes, configurations in automation solutions. CAP TODAY. Retrieved from www.cap.org/apps.portal?_nfpb=true&cntvwrptlt_action. Accessed 06.11.13.

109. van Hove, L. (1998). Guest editorial: which hematology analyzer do you need? *Lab Hematol 4,* 32–33.

110. Albitar, M., Dong, Q., Saunder, D., et al. (1999). Evaluation of automated leukocyte differential counts in a cancer center. *Lab Hematol, 5,* 10–14.

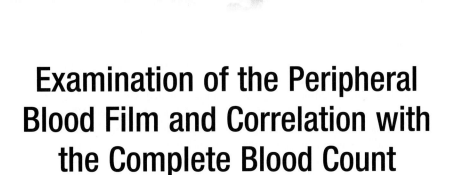

Examination of the Peripheral Blood Film and Correlation with the Complete Blood Count

16

Lynn B. Maedel and Kathryn Doig

OBJECTIVES

After completion of this chapter, the reader will be able to:

1. List the specimen sources and collection processes that are acceptable for blood film preparation.
2. Describe the techniques for making peripheral blood films.
3. Describe the appearance of a well-prepared peripheral blood film, recognize a description of a slide that is consistent or inconsistent with that appearance, and troubleshoot problems with poorly prepared films.
4. Explain the principle, purpose, and basic method of Wright staining of blood films.
5. Identify and troubleshoot problems that cause poorly stained blood films.
6. Describe the proper examination of a peripheral blood film, including selection of the correct area, sequence of examination, and observations to be made at each magnification. Recognize deviations from this protocol.
7. Given the number of cells observed per field and the magnification of the objective, apply formulas to estimate white blood cell (WBC) counts and platelet counts.
8. Explain the effect that platelet satellitosis and clumping may have on automated complete blood count (CBC) results. Recognize examples of results that would be consistent with these effects.
9. Follow the appropriate course of action to recognize and correct ethylenediaminetetraacetic acid–induced pseudothrombocytopenia and pseudoleukocytosis.
10. Implement a systematic approach to interpretation of CBC data that results in a verbal summary of the numerical data and communicates the blood picture succinctly.
11. Calculate absolute WBC differential counts.

CASE STUDY

After studying the material in this chapter, the reader should be able to respond to the following case study:

A healthy-looking 56-year-old man had an automated CBC performed as part of a preoperative evaluation. Results are shown here. Refer to reference intervals provided on the inside front cover of this book.

WBC—15.8 × 10⁹/L
RBC—4.93 × 10¹²/L
HGB—14.8 g/dL
HCT—45.1%
MCV—91.5 fL
MCH—30 pg
MCHC—32.8 g/dL
RDW—14.2%
PLT—34 × 10⁹/L
MPV—6.6 fL

The peripheral blood film was examined, and the only abnormal finding was "platelets in clumps."

1. Describe the blood picture succinctly, using proper terminology for red blood cells, white blood cells, and platelets.
2. What automated results should be questioned?
3. What is the best course of action to handle this problem?

A well-made, well-stained, and carefully examined peripheral blood film can provide valuable information regarding a patient's health. More can be learned from this test than from many other routinely performed hematologic tests. White blood cell (WBC) and platelet count estimates can be achieved, relative proportions of the different types of WBCs can be obtained, and the morphology of all three cell lines can be evaluated for abnormalities. Although routine work is now handled by the sophisticated automated instruments found in most hematology laboratories, skilled and talented laboratory professionals are still essential to the reporting of reliable test results. Accurate peripheral film evaluation is quite likely to be needed for some time.

The peripheral film evaluation is the capstone of a panel of tests called the *complete blood count* (CBC) or *hemogram*. The CBC includes enumeration of cellular elements, quantitation of hemoglobin, and statistical analyses that provide a snapshot of cell appearances. These results can be derived using the manual methods and calculations described in Chapter 14 or using the automated instruments described in Chapter 15. Regardless of method, the numerical values should be consistent with the assessment derived by examining the cells microscopically. Careful examination of the data in a systematic way ensures that all relevant results are noted and taken into consideration in the diagnosis.

This chapter begins with a discussion of the preparation and assessment of the blood film, followed by a systematic approach to review of the CBC, including blood film evaluation. Such an evaluation can be applied in the hematology chapters that follow.

PERIPHERAL BLOOD FILMS

Specimen Collection

Sources of Specimens

Essentially all specimens received for routine testing in the hematology section of the laboratory have been collected in lavender (purple)–topped tubes (Chapter 3). These tubes contain disodium or tripotassium ethylenediaminetetraacetic acid (EDTA), which anticoagulates the blood by chelating the calcium that is essential for coagulation. Liquid tripotassium EDTA is often preferred to the powdered form because it mixes more easily with blood. High-quality blood films can be made from the blood in the EDTA tube, provided that they are made within 2 to 3 hours of drawing the specimen.[1] Blood films from EDTA tubes that remain at room temperature for more than 5 hours often have unacceptable blood cell artifacts (echinocytic red blood cells [RBCs], spherocytes, necrobiotic leukocytes, and vacuolated neutrophils). Vacuolization of monocytes normally occurs almost immediately with EDTA but causes no evaluation problems.

The main advantages of making films from blood in the EDTA tube are that multiple slides can be made if necessary and they do not have to be prepared immediately after the blood is drawn. In addition, EDTA generally prevents platelets from clumping on the glass slide, which makes the platelet estimate more accurate during film evaluation. There are purists, however, who believe that anticoagulant-free blood is still the specimen of choice for evaluation of blood cell morphology.[2] Although some artifacts can be avoided in this way, samples made from unanticoagulated blood pose other problems.

Under certain conditions, use of a different anticoagulant or no anticoagulant may be helpful. Some patients' blood undergoes an in vitro phenomenon called *platelet satellitosis*[3] when anticoagulated with EDTA. The platelets surround or adhere to neutrophils, which potentially causes pseudothrombocytopenia when counting is done by automated methods (Figure 16-1).[3,4] In addition, spuriously low platelet counts and falsely increased WBC counts (pseudoleukocytosis) can result from EDTA-induced platelet clumping.[5] Pseudoleukocytosis occurs when platelet agglutinates are similar in size to WBCs and automated analyzers cannot distinguish the two. The platelet clumps are counted as WBCs instead of platelets. Platelet-specific autoantibodies that react best at room temperature are one of the mechanisms known to cause this phenomenon.[6] In these circumstances, the examination of a blood film becomes an important quality control strategy, identifying these phenomena so that they can be corrected before the results are reported to the patient's chart or health care provider.

Problems such as these can be eliminated by recollecting specimens in sodium citrate tubes (light blue top) and ensuring that the proper ratio of nine parts blood to one part anticoagulant is observed (a properly filled tube). These new specimens can be analyzed in the usual way by automated instruments. Platelet counts and WBC counts from sodium citrate specimens must be corrected for the dilution of blood with the anticoagulant, however. In a full-draw tube, the blood is nine tenths of the total tube volume (2.7 mL of blood and 0.3 mL of sodium citrate). The "dilution factor" is the reciprocal of the dilution (i.e., 10/9 or 1.1). The WBC and platelet counts are multiplied by 1.1 to obtain accurate counts. All other CBC parameters should be reported from the original EDTA tube specimen and slide.

Another source of blood for films is from finger and heel punctures. In general, the films are made immediately at the patient's side. There are, however, a few limitations to this procedure. First, some platelet clumping must be expected if

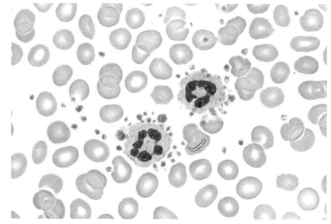

Figure 16-1 Photomicrograph of platelet satellitosis.

films are made directly from a drop of finger-stick or heel-stick blood or if blood is collected in heparinized microhematocrit tubes. Generally, this clumping is not enough to interfere with platelet estimates if the films are made promptly before clotting begins in earnest. Second, only a few films can be made directly from blood from a skin puncture before the site stops bleeding. If slides are made quickly and correctly, however, cell distribution and morphology should be adequate. These problems with finger and heel sticks can be eliminated with the use of EDTA microcollection tubes, such as Microtainer® Tubes (Becton, Dickinson and Company, Franklin Lakes, NJ) (Chapter 3).

Peripheral Film Preparation
Types of Films

Manual Wedge Technique. The wedge film technique is probably the easiest to master. It is the most convenient and commonly used method for making peripheral blood films. This technique requires at least two 3-inch × 1-inch (75-mm × 25-mm) clean glass slides. High-quality, beveled-edge microscopic slides with chamfered (beveled) corners for good lateral borders are recommended. A few more slides may be kept handy in case a good-quality film is not made immediately. One slide serves as the film slide, and the other is the pusher or spreader slide. They can then be reversed. It is also possible to make good wedge films by using a hemacytometer coverslip attached to a handle (pinch clip or tongue depressor) as the spreader.

A drop of blood (about 2 to 3 mm in diameter) from a finger, heel, or microhematocrit tube (nonheparinized for EDTA-anticoagulated blood or heparinized for capillary blood) is placed at one end of the slide. The drop also may be delivered using a Diff-Safe dispenser (Alpha Scientific Corporation, Malvern, PA). The Diff-Safe dispenser is inserted through the rubber stopper of the EDTA tube, which eliminates the need to remove the stopper.[7] The size of the drop of blood is important: too large a drop creates a long or thick film, and too small a drop often makes a short or thin blood film. The pusher slide, held securely in the dominant hand at about a 30- to 45-degree angle (Figure 16-2, *A*), is drawn back into the drop of blood, and the blood is allowed to spread across the width of the slide (Figure 16-2, *B*). It is then quickly and smoothly pushed forward to the end of the slide to create a wedge film (Figure 16-2, *C*). It is important that the whole drop be picked up and spread. Moving the pusher slide forward too slowly accentuates poor leukocyte distribution by pushing larger cells, such as monocytes and granulocytes, to the very end and sides of the film. Maintaining an even, gentle pressure on the slide is essential. It is also crucial to keep the same angle all the way to the end of the film. When the hematocrit is higher than normal (i.e., >60%), as is found in patients with polycythemia or in newborns, the angle should be lowered (i.e., 25 degrees) so the film is not too short and thick. For extremely low hematocrits, the angle may need to be raised. If two or three films are made, the best one is chosen for staining, and the others are disposed of properly. Some laboratories require two good films and save one unstained in case another slide is required.

The procedure just described is for a push-type wedge preparation. It is called *push* because the spreader slide is

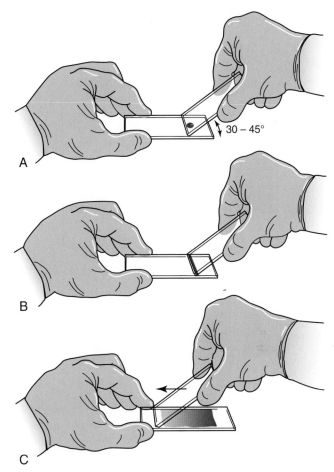

Figure 16-2 **A-C,** Wedge technique of making a peripheral blood film.

pulled into the drop of blood, and the film is made by pushing the blood along the slide. The same procedure can be modified to produce a *pulled* film. In this procedure, the spreader slide is pushed into the drop of blood and pulled along the length of the slide to make the film. Although this method is much less commonly used, it also provides a satisfactory wedge preparation and may be easier for some individuals to perform. Other variations on the wedge technique include using the 3-inch side of the slide as the spreader slide or balancing the spreader slide on the fingers to avoid placing too much pressure on it. Learning to make consistently good blood films takes a lot of practice but can be accomplished if one is patient and persistent.

Features of a well-made wedge peripheral blood film
1. The film is two thirds to three fourths the length of the slide (Figure 16-3).
2. The film is finger shaped, very slightly rounded at the feather edge, not bullet shaped; this provides the widest area for examination.
3. The lateral edges of the film are visible.
4. The film is smooth without irregularities, holes, or streaks.
5. When the slide is held up to the light, the thin portion (feather edge) of the film has a "rainbow" appearance.
6. The whole drop of blood is picked up and spread. Figure 16-4, *A-H*, shows unacceptable films.

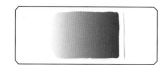

Figure 16-3 Well-made peripheral blood film.

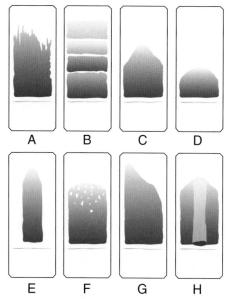

Figure 16-4 Unacceptable peripheral blood films. Slide appearances associated with the most common errors are shown, but note that a combination of causes may be responsible for unacceptable films. **A,** Chipped or rough edge on spreader slide. **B,** Hesitation in forward motion of spreader slide. **C,** Spreader slide pushed too quickly. **D,** Drop of blood too small. **E,** Drop of blood not allowed to spread across the width of the slide. **F,** Dirt or grease on the slide; may also be due to elevated lipids in the blood specimen. **G,** Uneven pressure on the spreader slide. **H,** Time delay; drop of blood began to dry.

Automated Slide Making and Staining. The Sysmex SP-10 (Sysmex Corporation of America, Mundelein, IL) is an automated slide-making and -staining system (Figure 16-5). After the instrument has performed a CBC for a specimen, a conveyor moves the racked tube to the SP-10, where the bar code is read. User-definable, onboard rules built into the system determine whether a slide is required. Criteria for a

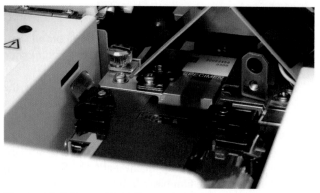

Figure 16-5 Sysmex SP-10 (Sysmex America, Inc., Lincolnshire, IL) is an automated slide making and staining system.

manual slide review are determined by each laboratory based on its patient population. Based on the hematocrit reading, the system adjusts the size of the drop of blood used and the angle and speed of the spreader slide in making a wedge preparation. After each blood film is prepared, the spreader slide is automatically cleaned and is ready for the next blood film to be made. Films can be produced approximately every 30 seconds. Patient identification information, such as name, number, and date for the specimen, is printed on the slide. The slide is dried, loaded into a cassette, and moved to the staining position. Based on the laboratory's desired stain protocol, stain and then buffer and rinse are added at designated times. When staining is complete, the slide is moved to a dry position, then to a collection area where it can be picked up for microscopic evaluation. Films made off-line, such as bone marrow smears and cytospin preparations, may be stained using this system as well. Other blood analyzer manufacturers, such as Beckman Coulter (Brea, CA), also have automated slide making and staining instruments.

Drying of Films
Regardless of film preparation method, before staining, all blood films and bone marrow smears should be dried as quickly as possible to avoid drying artifact. In some laboratories, a small fan is used to facilitate drying. Blowing breath on a slide is counterproductive because the moisture in breath causes RBCs to become echinocytic (crenated) or to develop water artifact (also called *drying artifact*).

Staining of Peripheral Blood Films
Pure Wright stain or a Wright-Giemsa stain (Romanowsky stain)[8] is used for staining peripheral blood films and bone marrow smears. These are considered polychrome stains because they contain both eosin and methylene blue. Giemsa stains also contain methylene blue azure. The purpose of staining blood films is simply to make the cells more visible and to allow their morphology to be evaluated. Consistent day-to-day staining quality is essential.

Methanol in the stain fixes the cells to the slide. Actual staining of cells or cellular components does not occur until the buffer is added. The oxidized methylene blue and eosin form a thiazine-eosinate complex, which stains neutral components. Because staining reactions are pH dependent, the buffer that is added to the stain should be 0.05 M sodium phosphate (pH 6.4) or aged distilled water (distilled water placed in a glass bottle for at least 24 hours; pH 6.4 to 6.8). Free methylene blue is basic and stains acidic (and basophilic) cellular components, such as ribonucleic acid (RNA). Free eosin is acidic and stains basic (and eosinophilic) components, such as hemoglobin and eosinophilic granules. Neutrophils are so named because they have cytoplasmic granules that have a neutral pH and pick up some staining characteristics from both stains. The slides must be completely dry before staining or the thick part of the blood film may come off the slide in the staining process.

Water or drying artifact has long been a nuisance to hematology laboratories. It has several appearances. It can give a moth-eaten look to the RBCs, or it may appear as a heavily demarcated central pallor. It also may appear as refractive (shiny) blotches on the RBCs. Other times, it manifests simply as echinocytes (crenation) seen in the areas of the slide that dried most slowly.

Multiple factors contribute to this problem. Humidity in the air as the slide dries may add to the punched-out, moth-eaten, or echinocytic appearance of the RBCs. It is difficult to avoid drying artifact on films from extremely anemic patients because of the very high ratio of plasma to RBCs. Water absorbed from the air into the alcohol-based stain also can contribute. Drying the slide as quickly as possible helps, and keeping a stopper tightly on the stain bottle keeps moisture out. In some laboratories, slides are fixed in pure, anhydrous methanol before staining to help reduce water artifact. More recently, stain manufacturers have used 10% volume-to-volume methanol to minimize water or drying artifact.

Wright Staining Methods

Manual Technique. Traditionally, Wright staining has been performed over a sink or pan with a staining rack. Slides are placed on the rack, film side facing upward. The Wright stain may be filtered before use or poured directly from the bottle through a filter onto the slide. It is important to flood the slide completely. The stain should remain on the slide at least 1 to 3 minutes to fix the cells to the glass. Then an approximately equal amount of buffer is added to the slide. Surface tension allows very little of the buffer to run off. A metallic sheen (or green "scum") should appear on the slide if mixing is correct (Figure 16-6). More buffer can be added if necessary. The mixture is allowed to remain on the slide for 3 minutes or more (bone marrow smears take longer to stain than peripheral blood films). The timing may be adjusted to produce the best staining characteristics. When staining is complete, the slide is rinsed with a steady but gentle stream of neutral-pH water, the back of the slide is wiped to remove any stain residue, and the slide is air-dried in a vertical position.

Use of the manual Wright staining technique is desirable for staining peripheral blood films containing very high WBC counts, such as the films from leukemic patients. As with bone marrow smears, the time can be easily lengthened to enhance the staining required by the increased numbers of cells. Understaining is common when a leukemia slide is placed on an automated slide stainer. The main disadvantages of the manual technique are the increased risk of spilling the stain and the longer time required to complete the procedure. This technique is best suited for low-volume laboratories.

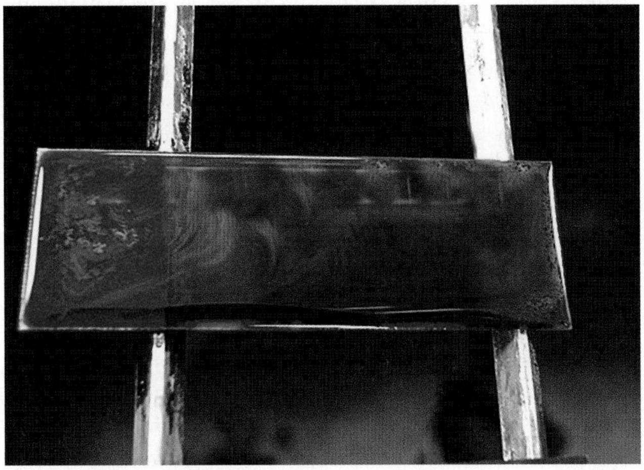

Automated Slide Stainers. Numerous automated slide stainers are commercially available. For high-volume laboratories, these instruments are essential. Once they are set up and loaded with slides, staining proceeds without operator attention. In general, it takes about 5 to 10 minutes to stain a batch of slides. The processes of fixing/staining and buffering are similar in practice to those of the manual method. The slides may be automatically dipped in stain and then in buffer and a series of rinses (Midas III, EM Science, Gibbstown, NJ) (Figure 16-7) or propelled along a platen surface by two conveyor spirals (Hema-Tek, Siemens Healthcare Diagnostics, Inc., Deerfield, IL) (Figure 16-8). In the Hema-Tek device, stain, buffer, and rinse are pumped through holes in the platen surface, flooding the slide at the appropriate time. Film quality and color consistency are usually good with any of these

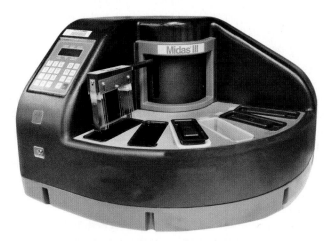

Figure 16-7 Midas III slide stainer. (Courtesy EM Science, Gibbstown, NJ.)

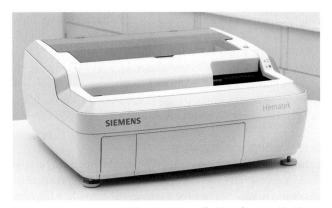

Figure 16-8 Hematek 3000 slide stainer. (© 2014 Siemens Healthcare Diagnostics, Inc. Photo courtesy Siemens Healthcare Diagnostics.)

Figure 16-6 Manual Wright staining of slides. Note metallic sheen of stain indicating proper mixing.

instruments. Some commercially prepared stain, buffer, and rinse packages do vary from lot to lot or manufacturer to manufacturer, so testing is recommended. Some disadvantages of the dip-type batch stainers are (1) stat slides cannot be added to the batch once the staining process has begun, and (2) working or aqueous solutions of stain are stable for only 3 to 6 hours and need to be made often. Stat slides can be added at any time to the Hema-Tek stainer, and stain packages are stable for about 6 months.

Quick Stains. Quick stains, as the name implies, are fast and easy. The whole process takes about 1 minute. The stain is purchased in a bottle as a modified Wright or Wright-Giemsa stain. The required quantity can be filtered into a Coplin jar or a staining dish, depending on the quantity of slides to be stained. Aged, distilled water is used as the buffer. Stained slides are given a final rinse under a gentle stream of tap water and allowed to air-dry. It is helpful to wipe off the back of the slide with alcohol to remove any excess stain. Quick stains are convenient and cost effective for low-volume laboratories, such as clinics and physician office laboratories, or whenever rapid turnaround time is essential. Quality is often a concern with quick stains. With a little time and patience in adjusting the staining and buffering times, however, color quality can be acceptable.

Features of a Well-Stained Peripheral Blood Film. Properly staining a peripheral blood film is just as important as making a good film. Macroscopically, a well-stained blood film should be pink to purple. Microscopically, the RBCs should appear orange to salmon pink, and WBC nuclei should be purple to blue. The cytoplasm of neutrophils should be pink to tan with violet or lilac granules. Eosinophils should have bright orange refractile granules. Faulty staining can be troublesome for reading the films, causing problems ranging from minor shifts in color to the inability to identify cells and assess morphology. Trying to interpret a poorly prepared or poorly stained blood film is extremely frustrating. If possible, a newly stained film should be studied. Hints for troubleshooting poorly stained blood films are provided in Box 16-1.

The best staining results are obtained on fresh slides because the blood itself acts as a buffer in the staining process. Slides stained after 1 week or longer turn out too blue. In addition, specimens that have increased levels of proteins (i.e., globulins) produce bluer-staining blood films, even when freshly stained.

Peripheral Film Examination

Microscopic blood film review is essential whenever instrument analysis indicates that specimen abnormalities exist. The laboratory professional evaluates the platelet and WBC count and differential, along with WBC, RBC, and platelet morphology.

Macroscopic Examination

Examining the film before placing it on the microscope stage sometimes can give the evaluator an indication of abnormalities or test results that need rechecking. For example, a film that is bluer overall than normal may indicate that the patient has increased blood proteins, as in plasma cell myeloma, and that

---

BOX 16-1 Troubleshooting Poorly Stained Blood Films

First Scenario
Problems
RBCs appear gray.
WBCs are too dark.
Eosinophil granules are gray, not orange.

Causes
Stain or buffer too alkaline (most common)
Inadequate rinsing
Prolonged staining
Heparinized blood sample

Second Scenario
Problems
RBCs are too pale or are red.
WBCs are barely visible.

Causes
Stain or buffer too acidic (most common)
Underbuffering (too short)
Over-rinsing

RBC, Red blood cell; *WBC*, white blood cell.

---

rouleaux may be seen on the film. A grainy appearance to the film may indicate RBC agglutination, as found in cold hemagglutinin diseases. In addition, holes all over the film could mean that the patient has increased lipid levels, and some of the automated CBC parameters should be rechecked for interferences from lipemia. Markedly increased WBC counts and platelet counts can be detected from the blue specks out at the feather edge. Valuable information might be obtained before the evaluator looks through the microscope.

Microscopic Examination

The microscope should be adjusted correctly for blood film evaluation. The light from the illuminator should be properly centered, the condenser should be almost all the way up and adjusted correctly for the magnification used, and the iris diaphragm should be opened to allow a comfortable amount of light to the eye. Many individuals prefer to use a neutral density filter over the illuminator to create a whiter light from a tungsten light source. If the microscope has been adjusted for Koehler illumination, all these conditions should have been met (Chapter 4).

10× Objective Examination. Blood film evaluation begins using the 10× or low-power objective lens (total magnification = 100×). Not much time needs to be spent at this magnification. However, it is a common error to omit this step altogether and go directly to the higher-power oil immersion lens. At the low-power magnification, overall film quality, color, and distribution of cells can be assessed. The feather edge and lateral edges should be checked quickly for WBC distribution. The presence of more than four times the number of cells per field at the edges or feather compared with the monolayer area of the film indicates that the film is unacceptable (i.e., a "snowplow" effect), and the film should be remade. Under the 10× objective, it is possible to check for the presence of fibrin strands; if they are present, the sample should be rejected, and another one should be collected. RBC distribution can be noted as well. Rouleaux formation or RBC agglutination is easy to recognize at this power. The film can be scanned quickly for any large abnormal cells, such as blasts, reactive lymphocytes, or even unexpected parasites. Finally, the area available for suitable examination can be assessed.

40× High-Dry or 50× Oil Immersion Objective Examination.   The next step is using the 40× high-dry objective lens (total magnification = 400×) or, as many laboratories now use, a 50× oil immersion objective instead. At either of these magnifications, it is easy to select the correct area of the film in which to begin the differential count and to evaluate cellular morphology. The WBC estimate also can be performed at these powers. To perform a WBC estimate, the evaluator selects an area in which the RBCs are separated from one another with minimal overlapping (where only two or three RBCs can overlap). Depending on which lens is used (40× or 50×), the procedure is the same; only the multiplication factor changes. Count the WBCs in 10 fields and find the average number of WBCs/field. The average number of WBCs per high-power field (40×) is multiplied by 2000 (if a 50× oil lens is used, multiply by 3000) to get an approximation of the WBC count per μL of blood. For example, when using a 50× oil objective, if after 10 fields are scanned it is determined that there are four to five WBCs per field, this would yield a WBC estimate of 12,000 to 15,000/μL or mm³ (12 to 15 × 10⁹/L). Box 16-2 contains a summary of the procedure for the WBC count estimate. This technique can be helpful for internal quality control, although there are inherent errors in the process. Using an area of the

film that is too thick (toward the origin of the film) or too thin (toward the feather edge) affects the estimates. In addition, field diameters may vary among microscope manufacturers and models, so validation of the estimation multiplication factor should be performed first (Box 16-3). Checking for a discrepancy between the estimate and the instrument WBC count makes it easier to discover problems such as a film made using the wrong patient's blood sample or a mislabeled film. In many laboratories, WBC estimates are performed on a routine basis; in others, these estimates are performed only as needed to confirm instrument values.

100× Oil Immersion Objective Examination.   The 100× oil immersion objective provides the highest magnification on most standard binocular microscopes (10× eyepiece × 100× objective lens = 1000× magnification). The WBC differential count generally is performed using the 100× oil immersion objective. Performing the differential normally includes counting and classifying 100 WBCs to obtain percentages of WBC types. The RBC, WBC, and platelet morphology evaluation and the platelet estimate also are executed under the 100×

BOX 16-2 **Performing a White Blood Cell Estimate**

1. Select an area of the blood film in which most RBCs are separated from one another with minimal overlapping of RBCs.
2. Using the 40× high-dry or 50× oil immersion objective, count the number of WBCs in 10 consecutive fields, and calculate the average number of WBCs per field.
3. To obtain the WBC estimate per μL of blood, multiply the average number of WBCs per field by 2000* (if using the 40× high-dry objective) or 3000* (if using the 50× oil immersion objective).
4. Compare the instrument WBC count with the WBC estimate from the blood film.

Example: If an average of three WBCs were observed per field:
Using a 40× high-dry objective, the WBC estimate is 6000/μL or mm³ or 6.0 × 10⁹/L.
Using a 50× oil immersion objective, the WBC estimate is 9000/μL or mm³ or 9.0 × 10⁹/L.

BOX 16-3 **Validation of the White Blood Cell and Platelet Estimation Factor**

1. Perform automated white blood cell (WBC) and platelet (PLT) counts on 30 consecutive fresh patient blood specimens. Make sure the counts are in control.
2. Prepare and stain one peripheral blood film for each specimen.
3. Using the 40× high-dry or 50× oil immersion objective for the WBC estimate and the 100× oil immersion objective for the PLT estimate, select an area of the blood film in which most RBCs are separated from one another with minimal overlapping of RBCs.
4. Count the number of WBCs or PLTs in 10 consecutive fields using the magnification specified in step 3, and calculate the average number of WBCs and PLTs per field.
5. For each of the 30 specimens, divide the automated WBC count by the average number of WBCs per field (40× or 50×); divide the automated PLT count by the average number of PLTs per field (100×).
6. Add the numbers obtained in step 5 for the WBCs, and divide by 30 (the number of observations in this analysis) to obtain the average ratio of the WBC count-to-WBCs per 40× or 50× field; add the numbers obtained in step 5 for the PLTs, and divide by 30 (the number of observations in this analysis) to obtain the average ratio of the PLT count-to-PLTs per 100× field.
7. Round the number calculated in step 6 to the nearest whole number to obtain an estimation factor for WBCs and PLTs at the specified magnification.

NOTE: Because of the variation in the field diameter among different microscopes, an estimation factor should be determined for each microscope in use, and that number should be used to obtain the WBC and PLT estimates when using that microscope.

Modified from Terrell JC: Laboratory evaluation of leukocytes. In Stiene-Martin EA, Lotspeich-Steininger CA, Koepke JA, editors: *Clinical hematology—principles, procedures, correlations*, ed 2, Philadelphia, 1998, Lippincott-Raven Publishers, p. 337.

---

* WBC estimation factors of 2000 (40× objective) and 3000 (50× objective) are provided as general guidelines. A WBC estimation factor should be determined and validated for each microscope in use (Box 16-3).

oil immersion objective lens. At this magnification segmented neutrophils can be readily differentiated from bands. RBC inclusions, such as Howell-Jolly bodies, and WBC inclusions, such as Döhle bodies, can be seen easily if present. Reactive or abnormal cells are enumerated under the 100× objective as well. If present, nucleated RBCs (NRBCs) are counted and reported as NRBCs per 100 WBCs (Chapter 14).

50× Oil Immersion Objective Examination. The WBC differential and morphology examinations described for the 100× oil immersion objective also can be accomplished by experienced morphologists using a 50× oil immersion objective. The larger field of view allows more cells to be evaluated faster. Examination at this power is especially efficient for validating or verifying instrument values when a total microscopic assessment of the film is not needed. Particular cell features that may require higher magnification can be assessed by moving the parfocal 100× objective into place and then returning to the 50× objective to continue the differential. As previously mentioned, the WBC estimate also can be performed with the 50× objective, but the multiplication factor is 3000. The observer should conform to the estimation protocol of the particular laboratory.

Optimal Assessment Area. The tasks described, especially for the 100×, 40×, and 50× objectives, need to be performed in the best possible area of the peripheral blood film. That occurs between the thick area, or "heel," where the drop of blood was initially placed and spread, and the very thin feather edge. In the ideal area, microscopically, the RBCs are uniformly and singly distributed, with few touching or overlapping, and have their normal biconcave appearance (central pallor) (Figure 16-9, *A*). An area that is too thin, in which there are holes in the film or the RBCs look flat, large, and distorted, is unacceptable (Figure 16-9, *B*). A too-thick area also distorts the RBCs by piling them on top of one another like rouleaux (Figure 16-9, *C*). WBCs are similarly distorted, which makes morphologic evaluation more difficult and classification potentially incorrect. When the correct area of a specimen from a patient with a normal RBC count is viewed, there are generally about 200 to 250 RBCs per 100× oil immersion field.

Although already discussed in Chapter 4, a common problem encountered with the oil immersion objective lens is worth mentioning again. If the blood film was in focus under the 10× and 40× objectives but is impossible to bring into focus under the 100× objective, the slide is probably upside down. The 100× objective does not have sufficient depth of field to focus through the slide. The oil must be completely removed before the film is put on the stage right-side up.

Performance of the White Blood Cell Differential. Fewer manual differentials are performed today because of the superior accuracy of automated differentials and because of cost and time constraints. When indicated, however, the manual differential always should be performed in a systematic manner. When the correct area has been selected, use of a back-and-forth serpentine, or "battlement," track pattern is preferred to minimize distribution errors (Figure 16-10)[9] and

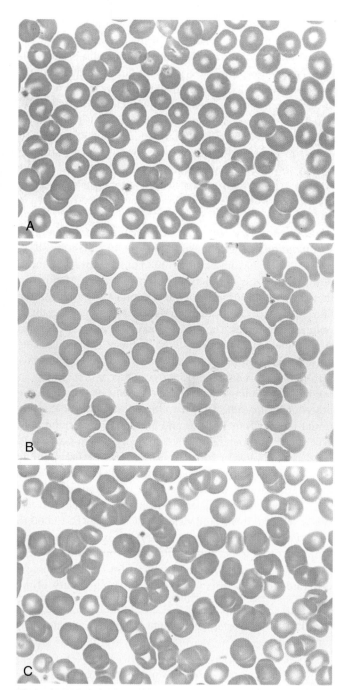

Figure 16-9 **A,** Photomicrograph of good area of peripheral blood film. Photomicrographs of peripheral blood film with areas too thin **(B)** and too thick **(C)** to read.

ensure that each cell is counted only once. One hundred WBCs are counted and classified through the use of push-down button counters (Figure 16-11, *A*) or newer computer-interfaced key pads (Figure 16-11, *B*). To increase accuracy, it is advisable to count at least 200 cells when the WBC count is higher than $40 \times 10^9/L$. If the WBC count is $100 \times 10^9/L$ or greater, it would be more precise and accurate to count 300 or 400 cells. Results are reported as percentages—for example, 54% segmented neutrophils, 6% bands, 28% lymphocytes, 9% monocytes, 3% eosinophils. The evaluator always should check to ensure that the sum of the percentages is 100.

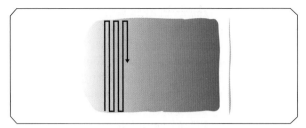

Figure 16-10 "Battlement" pattern for performing a differential count.

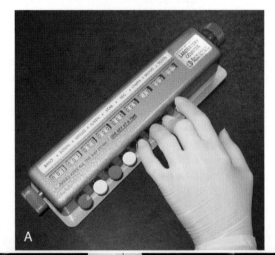

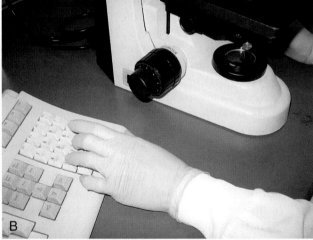

Figure 16-11 A, Laboratory differential tally counter. **B,** Computer interfaced key pad counter.

Performing 100-cell differentials on extremely low WBC counts can become tedious and time consuming, even when the 50× oil immersion objective is used. In some laboratories, the WBCs are concentrated by centrifugation, and buffy coat smears are made. This practice is helpful for examining the morphology of the cells; however, it is not recommended for performing differentials because of possible errors in cell distribution from centrifugation. In other laboratories evaluators may perform a 50-cell differential and multiply the results by 2 to get a percentage. The accuracy of this practice is questionable, and it should be avoided if possible. In some laboratories the buffy coat smear is examined for the presence of blasts, but no differential is performed. It is essential to include the side margins of the blood

film in any differential so that the larger cells, such as monocytes, reactive lymphocytes, and immature cells, are not missed.

In addition to counting the cells, the evaluator assesses their appearance. If present, WBC abnormalities such as toxic granulation, Döhle bodies, reactive lymphocytes, and Auer rods (Chapters 29 and 35) are evaluated and reported. Unfortunately, the exact method by which these are reported varies from laboratory to laboratory. Reactive lymphocytes may be reported as a separate percentage of the 100 cells, as a percentage of the total number of lymphocytes, or semiquantitatively ("occasional" to "many"). Toxic granulation generally is reported as "present" or is sometimes reported semiquantitatively ("slight" to "marked," or 1+ to 3+). Standardization of this process has been difficult, but laboratorians must look to simplify blood film morphology reports to help ensure better accuracy, consistency, and clinical relevance. Simply reporting "present" is becoming preferable to the older "semiquantitative" reporting of morphology abnormalities. Regardless of reporting format, each laboratory should establish criteria for reporting microscopic cell morphology.

Because the differential alone provides only partial information, reported in relative percentages, the absolute cell counts are calculated for each cell type in some laboratories. Automated differentials already include this information.

Automation has also been applied to the processes of microscopic cell location and identification. These automated systems are especially dependent on the quality and consistency of the blood film and stain in order for the digital systems to recognize and identify the cells. Once cells are located, a digital image is made and the cell is classified using sophisticated computerized visual recognition systems. Digital images of the classified cells are presented to the operator, who can override the instrument's identification, if needed, or add identifications for cells that the instrument could not classify (Figure 16-12).

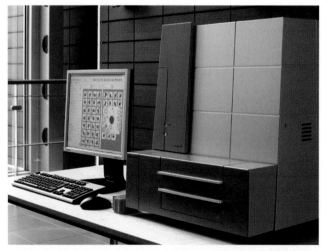

Figure 16-12 CellaVision DM96. CellaVision is an example of an automated system for differential counting that locates blood cells on a stained peripheral blood film, takes digital images, classifies the cells, and presents the cells in the 100-cell differential count to the operator on a computer screen. The operator can override the instrument's classification and identify cells that the instrument could not classify. (Courtesy of Cellavision AB, Lund, Sweden.)

Red Blood Cell Morphology.   Evaluation of RBC morphology is an important part of the blood film examination and includes an assessment of cell size (microcytosis, macrocytosis), variability in size (anisocytosis), cell color (hypochromia), cell shape (poikilocytosis), and cellular inclusions (Chapter 19). Some laboratories use specific terminology for reporting the degree of abnormal morphology, such as "slight," "moderate," or "marked," or use a scale from 1+ to 3+. Other laboratories more recently have gone to a more simple report, using the term *present* for morphologic abnormalities that are clinically significant. Still other laboratories provide a summary statement regarding the overall RBC morphology that is consistent with the RBC indices and histogram. The latter methods are becoming more popular with the increased computer interfacing in most laboratories. Regardless of the reporting method used, the microscopic RBC morphology assessment should be congruent with the information given by the automated hematology analyzer. If not, further investigation is needed.

Platelet Estimate.   As previously mentioned, the platelet estimate is performed under the 100× oil immersion objective lens. In an area of the film where the RBCs barely touch, with a few overlapping, the number of platelets in 10 oil immersion fields is counted. The average number of platelets per oil immersion field times 20,000 approximates the platelet count per µL or mm³. For example, 12 to 16 platelets per oil immersion field equals about 280,000 platelets/µL or mm³ (280×10^9/L) and is considered adequate. Box 16-4 contains a summary of the procedure for the platelet estimate. In situations in which the patient is anemic or has erythrocytosis, however, the relative proportion of platelets to RBCs is altered. In these instances, a more involved formula for platelet estimates may be used:

$$\frac{\text{Average no. of platelets/field} \times \text{total RBC count}}{200 \text{ RBCs/field}}$$

BOX 16-4 **Performing a Platelet Estimate**

1. Select an area of the blood film in which most RBCs are separated from one another with minimal overlapping of RBCs.
2. Using the 100× oil immersion objective, count the number of platelets in 10 consecutive fields, and calculate the average number of platelets per field.
3. To obtain the platelet estimate per µL of blood, multiply the average number of platelets per field by 20,000*.
4. Compare the instrument platelet count with the platelet estimate from the blood film.

Example: If an average of 20 platelets were observed per 100× oil immersion field, the platelet estimate is 400,000/µL or mm³ (400×10^9/L).

In instances of significant anemia or erythrocytosis, use the following formula for the platelet estimate:

$$\frac{\text{Average no. of platelets/field} \times \text{total RBC count}}{200 \text{ RBCs/field}}$$

---

*A platelet estimation factor of 20,000 is provided as a general guideline. A platelet estimation factor should be determined and validated for each microscope in use (Box 16-3).

(200 is the average number of RBCs per oil immersion field in the optimal assessment area)

Regardless of whether or not an "official" estimate is made, verification of the instrument platelet count should be included in the overall examination for internal quality control purposes. Blood film examination also includes an assessment of the morphology of the platelets, including size as well as granularity and overall appearance.

As mentioned in Chapter 4, and worth mentioning again, immersion oils with different viscosities do not mix well. If slides are taken to another microscope for review, oil should be wiped off first.

SUMMARIZING COMPLETE BLOOD COUNT

To this point, this chapter has focused on slide preparation and performance of a differential cell count. The differential is only the capstone, however, of a panel of tests collectively called the complete blood count, or *CBC*, that includes many of the routine tests described in Chapter 14. Now that the testing for the component parts has been described, interpretation of the results for the total panel can be discussed.

The CBC has evolved over time to the typical test panel reported today, including assessment of WBCs, RBCs, and platelets. The CBC provides information about the hematopoietic system, but because abnormalities of blood cells can be caused by diseases of other organ systems, the CBC also plays a role in screening of those organs for disease. The CBC provides such valuable information about a patient's health status that it is among the most frequently ordered laboratory tests performed by medical laboratory scientists and laboratory technicians.

The process of interpreting the CBC test results has two phases. In phase 1, the numbers and descriptions generated by the testing are summarized using appropriate terminology. This summary provides a verbal picture of the numbers that is easy to communicate to the physician, other health care provider, or another laboratorian. It is much more convenient to be able to say, "The patient has a microcytic anemia" than to say, "The hemoglobin was low, and the mean cell volume was also low." Phase 2 of interpretation is to recognize a pattern of results consistent with various diseases and to be able to narrow the diagnosis for the given patient or perhaps even to pinpoint it so that appropriate follow-up testing or treatment can be recommended.

The following discussion focuses on phase 1 of CBC interpretation—how to collect the pertinent information and summarize it. Phase 2 of the interpretation is the essence of the remaining chapters of this book on various hematologic conditions or other metabolic conditions that have an impact on the hematologic system.

Organization of Complete Blood Count Results

Today, most laboratorians perform CBCs using sophisticated automated analyzers as described in Chapter 15, but the component tests can be performed using the manual methods described in Chapter 14. The blood film assessment described in this chapter is also part of a CBC. As previously mentioned, the CBC "panel" is essentially divided into WBC, RBC, and platelet parameters.

For phase 2 interpretation, it is sometimes important to look at all three groupings of the CBC results; at other times, only one or two may be of interest. If a patient has an infection, the WBC parameters may be the only ones of interest. If the patient has anemia, all three sets—WBCs, RBCs, and platelets—may require assessment. Generally, all the parameters interpreted together provide the best information, so a complete summary of the results should be generated.

Assessing Hematology Results Relative to Reference Intervals

Proper performance of the phase 1 summary of test results requires comparison of the patient values with the reference intervals. The table of reference intervals for the CBC on the inside cover of this text shows that there are different reference intervals for men and women, particularly for the RBC parameters. There also are different intervals for children of different ages, with the WBC changes the most notable. It is important to select the appropriate set of reference intervals in hematology for the gender and age of the patient.

CBC results can be reported in standard international (SI) units or in common units. For example the following results in SI units (WBC count = 7.2×10^9/L, RBC count = 4.20×10^{12}/L, HGB = 128 g/L, HCT = 0.41 L/L, and PLT = 237×10^9/L) are equivalent to the following results in common units (WBC count = 7.2×10^3/μL, RBC count = 4.20×10^6/μL, HGB = 12.8 g/dL, HCT = 41%, and PLT = 237×10^3/μL). The older mm^3 for cell count units is equivalent to μL (Chapter 14). Since either system may be used on laboratory reports, the laboratorian should be able to easily interconvert CBC results between the systems. SI units are used for the cell counts in this chapter.

Several strategies can help in determining the significance of the results. First, if the results are very far from the reference interval, it is more likely that they are truly outside the interval and represent a pathologic process. Second, if two or more diagnostically related parameters are slightly or moderately outside the interval in the same direction (both high or both low), this suggests that the results are clinically significant and associated with some pathologic process. Because some healthy individuals always have results slightly outside the reference interval, the best comparison for their results is not the reference interval but their own results from a prior time when they were known to be healthy.

Summarizing White Blood Cell Parameters

The WBC-related parameters of a routine CBC include the following:
1. Total WBC count (WBCs $\times 10^9$/L)
2. WBC differential count values expressed as percentages, called *relative counts*
3. WBC differential count values expressed as the actual number of each type of cell (e.g., neutrophils $\times 10^9$/L), called *absolute counts*
4. WBC morphology

Step 1

Start by ensuring that there is an accurate WBC count. Compare the WBC histogram and/or scatterplot to the respective cell counts to make sure they correlate with one another. Today's automated instruments are able to eliminate nucleated RBCs that falsely increase the WBC count. However, manual WBC results must be corrected mathematically to eliminate the contribution of the NRBCs (Chapter 14).

Step 2

Look at the total WBC count. When the count is elevated, it is called *leukocytosis*. When the WBC count is low, it is called *leukopenia*. As described later, increases and decreases of WBCs are associated with infections and conditions such as leukemias. Because there is more than one type of WBC, increases and decreases in the total count are usually due to changes in one of the subtypes—for example, neutrophils or lymphocytes. Determining which one is the next step.

Step 3

Examine the relative differential counts for a preliminary assessment of which cell lines are affected. The relative differential count is reported in percentages. The proportion of each cell type can be described by its relative number (i.e., percent) and compared with its reference interval. Then it is described using appropriate terminology, such as a relative neutrophilia, which is an increase in neutrophils, or a relative lymphopenia, which is a decrease in lymphocytes. The terms used for increases and decreases of each cell type are provided in Table 16-1.

If the total WBC count or any of the relative values are outside the reference interval, further analysis of the WBC differential is needed. If the proportion of one of the cell types increases, then the proportion of others must decrease because the proportions are relative to one another. The second cell type may not have changed in actual number at all, however. The way to assess this accurately is with absolute differential counts.

Step 4

If not reported by the instrument, absolute counts can be calculated easily using the total WBC count and the relative differential. Multiply each relative cell count (i.e., percentage) by the total WBC count and by so doing determine the absolute count for each cell lineage.

TABLE 16-1 Terminology for Increases and Decreases in White Blood Cells

Cell Type	Increases	Decreases
Neutrophil	Neutrophilia	Neutropenia
Eosinophil	Eosinophilia	N/A
Basophil	Basophilia	N/A
Lymphocyte	Lymphocytosis	Lymphopenia (lymphocytopenia)
Monocyte	Monocytosis	Monocytopenia

N/A, Not applicable because the reference interval begins at or near zero.

TABLE 16-2 Comparison of Relative and Absolute White Blood Cell Counts

Complete Blood Count Parameter	Patient Value	Reference Interval	Interpretation Relative to Reference Interval	Description/ Summary
White blood cell count	13.6	4.3–10.8 × 10⁹/L	Elevated	Leukocytosis
Relative Differential				
Neutrophils	67	48%–70%	WRI	
Lymphocytes	26	18%–42%	WRI	
Monocytes	3	1%–10%	WRI	
Eosinophils	3	1%–4%	WRI	
Basophils	1	0%–2%	WRI	
Absolute Differential				
Absolute neutrophils	9.1	2.4-8.2 × 10⁹/L	Elevated	Absolute neutrophilia
Absolute lymphocytes	3.5	1.4-4 × 10⁹/L	WRI	
Absolute monocytes	0.4	0.1-1.2 × 10⁹/L	WRI	

WRI, Within reference interval.

Examine the set of WBC parameters from a CBC shown in Table 16-2. On first inspection, one may look at the WBC count and recognize that a leukocytosis is present, but it is important to determine what cell line is causing the increased count. In this case, the cells are all within reference intervals relative to one another. There is no indication as to which cell line could be causing the increase in total numbers of WBCs.

When each relative number (e.g., neutrophils at 0.67 or 67%) is multiplied by the total WBC count (13.6×10^9/L), the absolute numbers indicate that the neutrophils are elevated (9.1×10^9/L compared with the reference interval provided). The acronym for absolute neutrophil count is *ANC*. The ANC is a very useful parameter for assessing neutropenia and neutrophilia. The absolute lymphocyte count (3.5×10^9/L) is still within the reference interval. Given this information, these results can be described as showing a leukocytosis with only an absolute neutrophilia, and the overall increase in the WBC count is due to an increase only in neutrophils. This description provides a concise summary of the WBC counts without the need to refer to every type of cell. Box 16-5 extends this concept to a convention used to describe the neutrophilic cells, and Box 16-6 addresses the clinical utility of reporting % bands as a separate category.

When the absolute numbers of each of the individual cell types are totaled, the sum equals the WBC count (slight differences may occur due to rounding, as in the example). This is a method for checking whether the absolute calculations are correct. Absolute counts may be obtained directly from automated analyzers, which count actual numbers (i.e., produce absolute counts) and calculate relative values. Some laboratories do not report the absolute counts, so being able to calculate them is important.

As will be evident in later chapters, the findings in this particular example point toward a bacterial infection. Had there been an absolute lymphocytosis, a viral infection would be likely.

BOX 16-5 Summarizing Neutrophilia When Young Cells Are Present

A subtle convention in assessing the differential counts has to do with the presence of young cells of the neutrophilic series (e.g., bands). They typically are grouped together with the mature neutrophils in judging whether neutrophilia is present. For example, look at the following differential and the reference intervals provided in parentheses:

White blood cells—10.8 × 10⁹/L
Neutrophils (also called segmented neutrophils)—65 (48% to 70%)
Bands—18 (0% to 10%)
Lymphocytes—13 (18% to 42%)
Monocytes—3 (1% to 10%)
Eosinophils—1 (1% to 4%)
Basophils—0 (0% to 2%)

Although the mature neutrophils are within the reference interval, the bands exceed their reference interval. The total of the two, 83 (65% + 18%), exceeds the upper limit of neutrophilic cells even when the two intervals are combined, 80 (70% + 10%), so these results would be described as a neutrophilia even though the neutrophil value itself is within the reference interval. See steps 4 and 5 under Summarizing White Blood Cell Parameters for how to communicate the increase in bands.

Step 5

Each cell line should be examined for immature cells. Young WBCs are not normally seen in the peripheral blood, and they may indicate infections or malignancies such as leukemia. For neutrophilic cells, there is a unique term that refers to the presence of increased numbers of bands or cells younger than bands in the peripheral blood: *left shift* or *shift to the left* (Box 16-7).

When young lymphocytic or monocytic cells are present, they can be reported in the differential as prolymphocytes, lymphoblasts, promonocytes, or monoblasts. When observed, young eosinophils and basophils are typically just called *immature* and are not specifically staged. For example, *eosinophilic metamyelocytes* are counted as eosinophils.

Step 6

Any abnormalities of appearance are reported in the morphology section of the report. For WBCs, abnormal morphologic features that would be noted include changes in overall cellular appearance, such as cytoplasmic toxic granulation and nuclear abnormalities such as hypersegmentation. The clinical significance of these types of changes is discussed in Chapter 29.

To summarize the WBC parameters, begin with an accurate total WBC count, followed by the relative differential, or preferably the absolute counts, noting whether any abnormal young cells are present in the blood. Finally, note the presence of any abnormal morphology or inclusions.

Summarizing Red Blood Cell Parameters

RBC parameters are as follows:
1. RBC count (RBCs $\times 10^{12}$/L)
2. HGB (g/dL)
3. HCT (% or L/L)
4. Mean cell volume (MCV, fL)
5. Mean cell hemoglobin (MCH, pg)
6. Mean cell hemoglobin concentration (MCHC, g/dL)
7. RBC distribution width (RDW, %)
8. Morphology

Step 1

Examine the hemoglobin (or hematocrit) for anemia or polycythemia. Anemia is the more common condition. If the RBC morphology is relatively normal, three times the hemoglobin approximates the hematocrit; this is called the *rule of three* (Chapter 14). If the rule of three holds, the expectation is that the following assessments will find normal RBC parameters. If the rule of three fails and all test results are reliable, further assessment should uncover some patient RBC abnormalities. Remember that the rule of three only holds true when overall red blood cell morphology is normocytic and normochromic.

Hemoglobin concentration (HGB) is a more reliable indicator of anemia than is the hematocrit, because the hematocrit can be influenced by the size of the RBCs. Hemoglobin concentration is a more direct indicator of the ability of the blood to carry oxygen.

Step 2

When the hemoglobin and hematocrit values have been inspected and the rule of three applied, the next RBC parameter that should be evaluated is the MCV (Chapter 14). This value provides the average RBC volume. The MCV should be correlated with the RBC histogram from the instrument and morphologic appearance of the cells using the classification first introduced by Wintrobe a century ago (Table 16-3).

The MCV is expected to be within the established reference interval (approximately 80 to 100 fL), and the RBC histogram and morphology are expected to be normal (normocytic). For a patient with anemia, classifying the anemia morphologically by the MCV narrows the range of possible causes to microcytic, normocytic, or macrocytic anemias (Chapter 19).

Step 3

Examine the MCHC to evaluate how well the cells are filled with hemoglobin. Remember that MCHC is a concentration and takes into consideration the volume of the red blood cells when considering decreased or normal color. If the MCHC is within the reference interval, the cells are considered normal or *normochromic* and display typical central pallor of one third the volume of the cell. If the MCHC is below the reference interval, the cells are called *hypochromic*, which literally means "too little color." This correlates with a larger central pallor (hypochromia) when the cells are examined on a Wright-stained blood film.

It is possible for the MCHC to be elevated in two situations, but this does not correlate with hyperchromia. In fact, the term *hyperchromia* is never used. A slight elevation may be seen when

TABLE 16-3 Interpretation of Mean Cell Volume Values Using the Wintrobe Terminology

Mean Cell Volume Value	Wintrobe Description
Within reference interval (80–100 fL)	Normocytic
Lower than reference interval (<80 fL)	Microcytic
Higher than reference interval (>100 fL)	Macrocytic

cells are spherocytic (MCHC over 36 g/dL). They retain roughly normal volume but have decreased surface area. So the hemoglobin is slightly more concentrated than usual, and the cells look darker with no central pallor. A more dramatic increase in MCHC (values even as high as 60) can be caused by analytical problems, often associated with patient sample problems that falsely elevate hemoglobin measurement. Common problems of this type include interference from lipemia, icterus, or grossly elevated WBC counts. Each of these interferes with the spectrophotometric measurement of hemoglobin, thus falsely elevating the hemoglobin and affecting the calculation of the MCHC (Chapter 14). It is worth noting that the MCHC is often best used as an internal quality control parameter.

Step 4

The RDW is determined from the histogram of RBC volumes. Briefly, when the volumes of the RBCs are about the same, the histogram is narrow (Figure 16-13, *A*). If the volumes are variable (more small cells, more large cells, or both), the histogram becomes wider. The width of the histogram, the RDW, is reflected statistically as a coefficient of variation (CV) or a standard deviation (SD). Most analyzer manufacturers provide a CV and an SD, and the operator can select which to report. Figure 16-13, *A-D*, depicts RBC histograms demonstrating normal, microcytosis, macrocytosis, anisocytosis, and dimorphic red cell populations.

Therefore, the RDW provides information about the presence and degree of anisocytosis (variation in RBC volume). What is important is increased values only, not decreased values. If an RDW-CV reference interval is 11.5% to 14.5% and a patient has an RDW-CV of 20.6%, the patient has a more heterogeneous RBC population with more variation in cell volume (anisocytosis). If the RDW is elevated, a notation about anisocytosis is expected in the morphologic evaluation of the blood film. Using the MCV along with the RDW provides the most helpful information (Chapter 19).

Step 5

Examine the morphology for pertinent abnormalities. Whenever anemia is indicated by the RBC parameters reported by the analyzer, and potential abnormal RBC morphology is suggested by the indices and the rule of three, a Wright-stained peripheral blood film must be reviewed. Abnormalities include abnormal volume, abnormal shape, inclusions, immature RBCs, abnormal color, and abnormal arrangement (Chapter 19). The blood film also serves as quality control, because the morphologic characteristics seen through the microscope (e.g., microcytosis, anisocytosis) should be congruent with the results provided by the analyzer. When they do not agree, further investigation is necessary.

If everything in the morphology is normal, by convention, no notation regarding morphology is included. Therefore, any notation in the morphology section requires scrutiny. All RBC-related abnormal morphologic findings should be noted, including specific poikilocytosis (abnormal shape) and the presence of RBC inclusions, such as Howell-Jolly bodies. One of the major challenges is in determining when

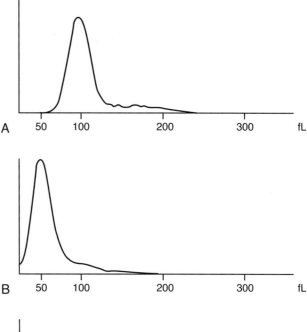

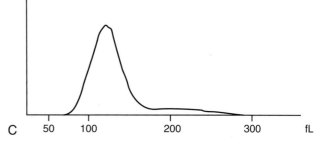

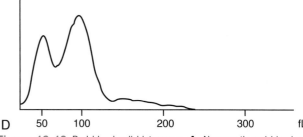

Figure 16-13 Red blood cell histograms. **A,** Normocytic red blood cell population with MCV of 96.8 fL and RDW(CV) of 14.1%; **B,** Microcytosis with MCV of 54.6 fL and RDW(CV) of 13.2%; **C,** Macrocytosis and anisocytosis with MCV of 119.2 fL and RDW(CV) of 23.9%; **D,** Dimorphic red blood cells with MCV of 80.2 fL and RDW(CV) of 37.2%. Note the microcytic and the normocytic red blood cell populations. Reference intervals: MCV, 80-100 fL; RDW(CV), 11.5%-14.5%. *MCV,* Mean cell volume; *RDW(CV),* red blood cell distribution width, coefficient of variation.

the amount or degree of an abnormality is worth noting at all (i.e., when it should be reported). Laboratories strive for standardization of reporting. All laboratories must have good standardized morphology criteria and competent staff whose evaluations are consistent with one another and with the standardized criteria used in that facility. Generally a semiquantitative method is used that employs terms such as *slight, moderate,* and *marked* or the numbers 1+, 2+, and 3+. Numerical ranges representing the reporting unit are defined; for example, three to six spherocytes per oil immersion field might be reported as 2+ spherocytes. Although this practice has been followed for many years, this semiquantitative method may not best serve the needs of medical staff, and many laboratories are moving toward simplifying their reports to state *present* for morphologic abnormalities.

The presence of immature RBCs suggests that the bone marrow is attempting to respond to an anemia. Polychromasia on the peripheral blood film indicates bone marrow response. This is manifested by the bluer color of reticulocytes that have entered the bloodstream earlier than usual in the body's attempt to improve oxygen-carrying capacity. If the anemia is severe, NRBCs also may be present. As noted earlier, it is also important to recognize NRBCs because they may falsely elevate the WBC count and may be an indication of an underlying disease process.

A better way to assess replacement erythropoiesis is with the reticulocyte count and subsequent calculation of the reticulocyte production index, if appropriate. The reticulocyte count is not normally part of the CBC, although it is now performed on the same analyzers. If the reticulocyte count is available with the CBC, its interpretation can improve the assessment of young RBCs (Chapter 14).

Step 6

Examine the RBC count and MCH. On a practical level, the RBC count is not the parameter used to judge anemia, because there are some types of anemia, such as the thalassemias (Chapter 28), in which the RBC count is normal or even elevated. Thus the assessment of anemia would be missed by relying only on the RBC count. However, this inconsistency (low hemoglobin and high RBC count) is often helpful diagnostically.

The MCH follows the MCV; that is, smaller cells necessarily hold less hemoglobin, whereas larger cells can hold more. For this reason it is less often used than the MCV and MCHC. In the instances in which the MCH does *not* follow the MCV, the MCHC detects the discrepancy between size and hemoglobin content of the cell. The MCH is not crucial to the assessment of anemia when the other parameters are provided. In summary, when evaluating the RBC parameters of the CBC, examine the hemoglobin first, then the MCV, RDW, and MCHC. Finally, take note of any abnormal morphology.

Summarizing Platelet Parameters

The platelet parameters of the CBC are as follows:
1. Platelet count (platelets $\times 10^9$/L)
2. Mean platelet volume (MPV, fL)
3. Morphology

Step 1

The platelet count should be examined for increases (thrombocytosis) or decreases (thrombocytopenia) outside the established reference interval. A patient who has unexplained bruising or bleeding may have a decreased platelet count. The platelet count should be assessed along with the WBC count and hemoglobin to determine whether all three are decreased (pancytopenia) or increased (pancytosis). Pancytopenia is clinically significant

because it can indicate a possible developing acute leukemia (Chapter 35) or aplastic anemia (Chapter 22). Pancytosis frequently is associated with a diagnosis of polycythemia vera (Chapter 33).

Step 2

Compare the instrument-generated MPV with the MPV reference interval, 6.9 to 10.2 fL, and with the platelet diameter observed on the peripheral blood film. An elevated MPV should correspond with increased platelet diameter, just as an elevated MCV reflects macrocytosis. In platelet consumption disorders such as immune thrombocytopenic purpura, an elevated MPV, accompanied by platelets 6 μm or larger in diameter (giant platelets), reflects bone marrow release of early "stress" or "reticulated" platelets, evidence for bone marrow compensation (Chapter 13 and Figure 13-9).[10,11] Comparing platelet diameter by visual inspection with MPV is a recommended quality control step; however, the MPV has a wide percent CV, which reflects interindividual variation and platelet swelling in EDTA and reduces its clinical effectiveness.[12] Some instruments identify and record a reticulated platelet count using nucleic acid dye, analogous to a reticulocyte count. Figure 16-14 demonstrates platelet histograms with a normal platelet population (A) and one with giant platelets (B).

Step 3

Examine platelet morphology and platelet arrangement. Although the MPV can recognize abnormally large platelets, the morphologic evaluation also notes this. Some laboratories distinguish between large platelets (two times normal size) and giant platelets (more than twice as large as normal) or compare platelet size to RBC size.

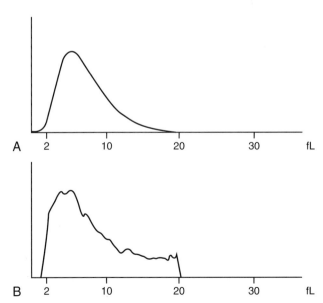

Figure 16-14 Platelet histograms. **A,** Normal with MPV of 8.0 fL; **B,** Platelet population with abnormal histogram and MPV of 9.1 fL. Although the MPV is within the reference interval, the histogram shows an increase in the number of platelets with a volume between 10 and 20 fL (curve above baseline) representing giant platelets. Reference interval for MPV: 6.8-10.2 fL. *MPV,* Mean platelet volume.

Additional morphologic descriptors include terms for reporting granularity, which is most important if missing, and in this case the platelets are described as "hypogranular" or "agranular." Sometimes the abnormalities are too variable to classify, and the platelets are described simply as "bizarre" or dysplastic. In some cases, platelets can be clumped or adherent to WBCs, and these arrangements should be noted. As described previously, corrective actions can be taken to derive accurate platelet and WBC counts when these arrangements are observed on the film. Summarizing platelet parameters includes reporting total number, platelet size by either instrument MPV or morphologic evaluation, and platelet appearance.

Box 16-8 gives an example of how the entire CBC can be summarized using the steps described. When results of the CBC are properly summarized and no information has been overlooked, there is confidence that the phase 2 interpretation of the results will be reliable. Adopting a methodical approach to examining each parameter ensures that the myriad information available from the CBC can be used effectively and efficiently in patient care. Box 16-9 summarizes the systematic approach to CBC interpretation.

BOX 16-8 Applying a Systematic Approach to Complete Blood Count Summarization

A specimen from an adult male patient yields the following CBC results (refer to the reference intervals inside the front cover of this book):

WBCs—3.20×10^9/L
RBCs—2.10×10^{12}/L
HGB—8.5 g/dL
HCT—26.3%
MCV—125 fL
MCH—40.5 pg
MCHC—32.3 g/dL
RDW—20.6%
PLT—115×10^9/L
Differential in percentages:
Neutrophils—43
Bands—2
Lymphocytes—45
Monocytes—10
Morphology: hypersegmentation of neutrophils, anisocytosis, macrocytes, oval macrocytes, occasional teardrop, Howell-Jolly bodies, and basophilic stippling

The step-by-step assessment of the WBCs indicates that the WBC count is accurate and can be interpreted as leukopenia. Although the relative differential values are all within the reference intervals, calculation of absolute counts indicates an absolute neutropenia and lymphopenia. No unexpected young WBCs are noted, but the morphology indicates hypersegmentation of neutrophils. For the RBCs, the hemoglobin concentration (8.5) indicates that this person is anemic. Inspection of the MCV indicates macrocytosis because the MCV is increased to more than 100 fL, the upper limit of the reference interval. Examination of the MCHC shows it to be normal, so for these results, the RBC morphology would be described as macrocytic, normochromic. The elevated RDW indicates substantial anisocytosis. There is no mention of polychromasia, so no young RBCs are seen. The morphologic description supports the interpretation of the RDW with mention of anisocytosis due to macrocytosis and poikilocytosis characterized by oval macrocytes and occasional teardrop cells. Howell-Jolly bodies and basophilic stippling are significant RBC inclusions. The platelet count indicates thrombocytopenia. Although MPV is not reported, the platelets are of normal size and show no morphologic abnormalities because there are no notations in the morphologic descriptions.

CBC, Complete blood count; *HCT,* hematocrit; *HGB,* hemoglobin; *MCH,* mean cell hemoglobin; *MCHC,* mean cell hemoglobin concentration; *MCV,* mean cell volume; *MPV,* mean platelet volume; *RBC,* red blood cell; *RDW,* RBC distribution width; *WBC,* white blood cell.

BOX 16-9 Systematic Approach to Complete Blood Count Interpretation

White Blood Cells

Step 1: Ensure that the WBC count is accurate. Review WBC histogram and/or scatterplot and correlate with counts. The presence of nucleated RBCs may require correction of the WBC count.

Step 2: Compare the patient's WBC count with the laboratory's established reference interval.

Steps 3 and 4: Examine the differential information (relative and absolute) on variations in the distribution of WBCs.

Step 5: Make note of immature cells in any cell line reported in the differential that should not appear in normal peripheral blood.

Step 6: Make note of any morphologic abnormalities and correlate film findings with the numerical values.

Red Blood Cells

Step 1: Examine the HGB concentration first to assess anemia.

Step 2: Examine the MCV to assess cell volume.

Step 3: Examine the MCHC to assess cell HGB concentration in RBC.

Step 4: Examine the RDW to assess anisocytosis. (Correlate both MCV and RDW with RBC histogram.)

Step 5: Examine the morphologic description and correlate with the numerical values. Look for evidence of a reticulocyte response.

Step 6: Review remaining information.

Platelets

Step 1: Examine the total platelet count.

Step 2: Examine the MPV to assess platelet size.

Step 3: Examine platelet morphology and correlate with the numerical values.

HGB, Hemoglobin; *MCHC,* mean cell hemoglobin concentration; *MCV,* mean cell volume; *MPV,* mean platelet volume; *RBC,* red blood cell; *RDW,* RBC distribution width; *WBC,* white blood cell.

SUMMARY

- Although fewer manual peripheral blood film evaluations are performed today, much valuable information still can be obtained from a well-made and well-stained film.
- The specimen of choice for routine hematology testing is whole blood collected in a lavender/purple topped tube. The tube additive is EDTA, which anticoagulates the blood by chelating plasma calcium.
- Only rarely does EDTA create problems in analyzing certain individuals' blood. EDTA-induced platelet clumping or satellitosis causes automated analyzers to report falsely decreased platelet counts (pseudothrombocytopenia) and falsely increased WBC counts (pseudoleukocytosis). This problem must be recognized through blood film examinations and the proper course of action followed to produce accurate results.
- Several methods exist for making peripheral blood films; however, the manual wedge film technique is used most frequently.
- Learning to make consistently good blood films takes practice. The basic technique can be modified as needed to accommodate specimens from patients with very high or very low hematocrits.
- The stain used routinely in hematology is Wright or Wright-Giemsa stain. Staining of all cellular elements occurs when the pH-specific buffer is added to the stain already on the slide. Staining reactions depend on the pH of the cellular components.
- Wright staining is done manually, by automated techniques, or by quick stains, depending on the laboratory and the number of slides to be processed.
- Peripheral blood films and bone marrow smears always should be evaluated in a systematic manner, beginning with the 10× objective lens and finishing with the 100× oil immersion objective lens. Leukocyte differential and morphologic evaluation, RBC and platelet morphologic evaluation, and platelet number estimate all are included.
- Use of a systematic approach to CBC interpretation ensures that all valuable information is assessed and nothing is overlooked. The systematic approach to CBC interpretation is summarized in Box 16-9.

Now that you have completed this chapter, go back and read again the case study at the beginning and respond to the questions presented.

REVIEW QUESTIONS

Answers can be found in the Appendix.

1. A laboratory science student consistently makes wedge-technique blood films that are too long and thin. What change in technique would improve the films?
   a. Increasing the downward pressure on the pusher slide
   b. Decreasing the acute angle of the pusher slide
   c. Placing the drop of blood closer to the center of the slide
   d. Increasing the acute angle of the pusher slide

2. When a blood film is viewed through the microscope, the RBCs appear redder than normal, the neutrophils are barely visible, and the eosinophils are bright orange. What is the most likely cause?
   a. The slide was overstained.
   b. The stain was too alkaline.
   c. The buffer was too acidic.
   d. The slide was not rinsed adequately.

3. A stained blood film is held up to the light and observed to be bluer than normal. What microscopic abnormality might be expected on this film?
   a. Rouleaux
   b. Spherocytosis
   c. Reactive lymphocytosis
   d. Toxic granulation

4. A laboratorian using the 40× objective lens sees the following numbers of WBCs in 10 fields: 8, 4, 7, 5, 4, 7, 8, 6, 4, 6. Which of the following WBC counts most closely correlates with the estimate?
   a. $1.5 \times 10^9/L$
   b. $5.9 \times 10^9/L$
   c. $11.8 \times 10^9/L$
   d. $24 \times 10^9/L$

5. A blood film for a very anemic patient with an RBC count of $1.25 \times 10^{12}/L$ shows an average of seven platelets per oil immersion field. Which of the following values most closely correlates with the estimate per microliter?
   a. 14,000
   b. 44,000
   c. 140,000
   d. 280,000

6. A blood film for a patient with a normal RBC count has an average of 10 platelets per oil immersion field. Which of the following values best correlates with the estimate per microliter?
   a. 20,000
   b. 100,000
   c. 200,000
   d. 400,000

7. What is the absolute count ($\times 10^9$/L) for the lymphocytes if the total WBC count is 9.5×10^9/L and there are 37% lymphocytes?
   a. 3.5
   b. 6.5
   c. 13
   d. 37

8. Which of the following blood film findings indicates EDTA-induced pseudothrombocytopenia?
   a. The platelets are pushed to the feathered end.
   b. The platelets are adhering to WBCs.
   c. No platelets at all are seen on the film.
   d. The slide has a bluish discoloration when examined macroscopically.

9. Which of the following is the best area to review or perform a differential on a stained blood film?
   a. Red blood cells are all overlapped in groups of three or more.
   b. Red blood cells are mostly separated, with a few overlapping.
   c. Red blood cells look flattened, with none touching.
   d. Red blood cells are separated and holes appear among the cells.

10. Use the reference intervals provided inside the front cover of this text. Given the following data, summarize the following blood picture:
    WBC: 86.3×10^9/L
    HGB: 9.7 g/dL
    HCT: 24.2%
    MCV: 87.8 fL
    MCHC: 33.5%
    PLT: 106×10^9/L
    a. Leukocytosis, normocytic-normochromic anemia, thrombocytopenia
    b. Microcytic-hypochromic anemia, thrombocytopenia
    c. Neutrophilia, macrocytic anemia, thrombocytosis
    d. Leukocytosis, thrombocytopenia

REFERENCES

1. Kennedy, J. B., Maehara, K. T., & Baker, A. M. (1981). Cell and platelet stability in disodium and tripotassium EDTA. *Am J Med Technol, 47*, 89–93.
2. Perkins, S. L. (2009). Examination of the blood and bone marrow. In Greer, J. P., Foerster, J., Rodgers, G. M., et al. (Eds.), *Wintrobe's Clinical Hematology.* (12th ed., pp. 1–20). Philadelphia: Wolters Kluwer Health/Lippincott Williams & Wilkins.
3. Shahab, N., & Evans, M. L. (1998). Platelet satellitism. *N Engl J Med, 338*, 591.
4. Bartels, P. C., Schoorl, M., & Lombarts, A. J. (1997). Screening for EDTA-dependent deviations in platelet counts and abnormalities in platelet distribution histograms in pseudothrombocytopenia. *Scand J Clin Lab Invest, 57*, 629–636.
5. Lombarts, A., & deKieviet, W. (1988). Recognition and prevention of pseudothrombocytopenia and concomitant pseudoleukocytosis. *Am J Clin Pathol, 89*, 634–639.
6. De Caterina, M., Fratellanza, G., Grimaldi, E., et al. (1993). Evidence of a cold immunoglobulin M autoantibody against 78 kD platelet gp in a case of EDTA-dependent pseudothrombocytopenia. *Am J Clin Pathol, 99*, 163–167.
7. Alpha Scientific Corp. *Diff-safe blood dispenser.* Retrieved from http://www.alpha-scientific.com/Diff-safe.html. Accessed 11.04.14.
8. Power, K. T. (1982). The Romanowsky stains: a review. *Am J Med Technol, 48*, 519–523.
9. MacGregor, R. G., Scott, R. W., & Loh, G. L. (1940). The differential leukocyte count. *J Pathol Bacteriol, 51*, 337–368.
10. Briggs, C., Harrison, P., & Machin, S. J. (2007). Continuing developments with the automated platelet count. *Int J Lab Hematol, 29*, 77–91.
11. Abe, Y., Wada, H., Sakakura, M., et al. (2005). Usefulness of fully automated measurement of reticulated platelets using whole blood. *Clin Appl Thromb Hemost, 11*, 263–270.
12. Ryan, D. H. (2011). Examination of the blood. In Lichtman, M. A., Beutler, E., Kipps, T. J., et al. (Eds.), *Williams Hematology.* (8th ed.). New York: McGraw-Hill, Ch. 2.
13. Cornbleet, P. J. (2002). Clinical utility of the band count. *Clin Lab Med. Mar, 22*(1), 101–136.
14. Clinical and Laboratory Standards Institute. (2007). *Reference leukocyte (WBC) differential count (proportional) and evaluation of instrumental methods; approved standard.* (2nd ed.). (H20-A2). Vol 27(4): Clinical and Laboratory Standards Institute (CLSI).

Bone Marrow Examination 17

*George A. Fritsma**

OBJECTIVES

After completion of this chapter, the reader will be able to:

1. Diagram bone marrow architecture and locate hematopoietic tissue.
2. List indications for bone marrow examinations.
3. Specify sites for bone marrow aspirate and biopsy.
4. Assemble supplies for performing and assisting in bone marrow specimen collection.
5. Assist the physician with bone marrow sample preparation subsequent to collection.
6. List the information gained from bone marrow aspirates and biopsy specimens.
7. Perform a bone marrow aspirate smear and core biopsy specimen examination.
8. List the normal hematopoietic and stromal cells of the bone marrow and their anticipated distribution.
9. Perform a bone marrow differential count and compute the myeloid-to-erythroid ratio.
10. Characterize features of hematopoietic and metastatic tumor cells.
11. Prepare specimens for and assist in performing specialized confirmatory bone marrow studies.
12. Prepare a systematic written bone marrow examination report.

CASE STUDY

After studying the material in this chapter, the reader should be able to respond to the following case study:

A patient came for treatment complaining of weakness, fatigue, and malaise. Complete blood count results were as follows:

HGB concentration: 7.5 gm/dL
HCT: 21%
RBC count: 2.5×10^{12}/L
WBC count: 30×10^9/L
Platelet count: 540×10^9/L

Segmented neutrophils: 21×10^9/L (70%)
Immature neutrophils: 6×10^9/L (20%)
Basophils: 1.5×10^9/L (5%)
Eosinophils: 0.3×10^9/L (1%)

Bone marrow was hypercellular with 90% myeloid precursors and 10% erythroid precursors. There were 15 megakaryocytes per 10× microscopic objective field.

1. What bone marrow finding provides information on blood cell production?
2. What is the myeloid-to-erythroid ratio in this patient, and what does it indicate?
3. What megakaryocyte distribution is normally seen in a bone marrow aspirate?

*The author thanks Lynne Shaw, MT (ASCP), director of the University of Alabama at Birmingham Hospital Laboratory of Bone Marrow Pathology, for substantive contribution to this chapter.

BONE MARROW ANATOMY AND ARCHITECTURE

In adults, bone marrow accounts for 3.4% to 5.9% of body weight, contributes 1600 to 3700 g or a volume of 30 to 50 mL/kg, and produces roughly 6 billion blood cells per kilogram per day in a process called *hematopoiesis.*[1] At birth, nearly all the bones contain red hematopoietic marrow (Chapter 7). In the fifth to seventh year, *adipocytes* (fat cells) begin to replace red marrow in the long bones of the hands, feet, legs, and arms, producing *yellow marrow,* and by late adolescence hematopoietic marrow is limited to the lower skull, vertebrae, shoulder, pelvic girdle, ribs, and sternum (Figure 7-2). Although the percentage of bony space devoted to hematopoiesis is considerably reduced, the overall volume remains constant as the individual matures.[2] Yellow marrow reverts to hematopoiesis, increasing red marrow volume, in conditions such as chronic blood loss or hemolytic anemia that raise demand.

The arrangement of red marrow and its relationship to the central venous sinus are illustrated in Figure 7-3. Hematopoietic tissue is enmeshed in spongy *trabeculae* (bony tissue) surrounding a network of sinuses that originate at the *endosteum* (vascular layer just within the bone) and terminate in collecting venules.[3] Adipocytes occupy approximately 50% of red hematopoietic marrow space in a 30- to 70-year-old adult, and fatty metamorphosis increases approximately 10% per decade after age 70.[4]

INDICATIONS FOR BONE MARROW EXAMINATION

Because the procedure is invasive, the decision to collect and examine a bone marrow specimen requires clinical judgment and the application of *inclusion criteria.* With the development of cytogenetic chromosome studies, flow cytometry, immunohistochemistry, and molecular diagnostics, peripheral blood may often provide information historically available only from bone marrow, reducing the demand for marrow specimens. On the other hand, these advanced techniques also augment bone marrow–based diagnosis and thus potentially raise the demand for bone marrow examinations in assessment of conditions not previously diagnosed through bone marrow examination.

Table 17-1 summarizes indications for bone marrow examination.[5] Bone marrow examinations may be used to diagnose and stage hematologic and nonhematologic *neoplasia,* to determine the cause of cytopenias, and to confirm or exclude metabolic or infectious conditions suspected on the basis of clinical symptoms and peripheral blood findings.[6]

Each bone marrow procedure is ordered after thorough consideration of clinical and laboratory information. For instance, bone marrow examination is most likely unnecessary in anemia when the cause is apparent from red blood cell (RBC) indices, serum iron and ferritin levels, or vitamin B_{12} and folate

TABLE 17-1 Indications for Bone Marrow Examination

Indication	Examples
Neoplasia diagnosis	Acute leukemias
	Myeloproliferative neoplasms such as chronic leukemias, myelofibrosis
	Myelodysplastic neoplasms such as refractory anemia
	Lymphoproliferative disorders such as acute lymphoblastic leukemia
	Immunoglobulin disorders such as plasma cell myeloma, macroglobulinemia
	Metastatic tumors
Neoplasia diagnosis and staging	Hodgkin and non-Hodgkin lymphoma
Marrow failure: cytopenias	Hypoplastic or aplastic anemia
	Pure red cell aplasia
	Idiosyncratic drug-induced marrow suppression
	Myelodysplastic syndromes such as refractory anemia
	Marrow necrosis secondary to tumor
	Marrow necrosis secondary to severe infection such as parvovirus B19 infection
	Immune versus amegakaryocytic thrombocytopenia
	Sickle cell crisis
	Differentiation of megaloblastic, iron deficiency, sideroblastic, hemolytic, and blood loss anemia
	Estimation of storage iron to assess for iron deficiency
	Infiltrative processes or fibrosis
Metabolic disorders	Gaucher disease
	Mast cell disease
Infections	Granulomatous disease
	Miliary tuberculosis
	Fungal infections
	Hemophagocytic syndromes
Monitoring of treatment	After chemotherapy or radiation therapy to assess minimal residual disease
	After stem cell transplantation to assess engraftment

levels. Multilineage abnormalities, circulating blasts in adults, and unexpected pancytopenia usually prompt marrow examination. Bone marrow puncture is prohibited in patients with coagulopathies such as hemophilia or vitamin K deficiency, although *thrombocytopenia* (low platelet count) is not an absolute contraindication. Special precautions such as bridging therapy may be necessary to prevent uncontrolled bleeding when a bone marrow procedure is performed on a patient receiving antithrombotic therapy, for instance, Coumadin or heparin.

BONE MARROW SPECIMEN COLLECTION SITES

Bone marrow specimen collection is a collaboration between a medical laboratory scientist and a skilled specialty physician, often a pathologist or hematologist.[7] Prior to bone marrow collection, a medical laboratory practitioner or phlebotomist collects peripheral blood for a complete blood count with blood film examination. During bone marrow collection, the laboratory scientist assists the physician by managing the specimens and producing initial preparations for examination.

Red marrow is gelatinous and amenable to sampling. Most bone marrow specimens consist of an *aspirate* (obtained by bone marrow aspiration) and a *core biopsy* specimen (obtained by trephine biopsy), both examined with light microscopy using 100× and 500× magnification. The aspirate is examined to identify the types and proportions of hematologic cells and to look for morphologic variance. The core biopsy specimen demonstrates bone marrow architecture: the spatial relationship of hematologic cells to fat, connective tissue, and bony stroma. The core biopsy specimen is also used to estimate cellularity.

The core biopsy specimen is particularly important for evaluating diseases that characteristically produce focal lesions, rather than diffuse involvement of the marrow. *Hodgkin lymphoma, non-Hodgkin lymphoma, multiple myeloma, metastatic tumors, amyloid,* and *granulomas* produce predominantly focal lesions. Granulomas, or granulomatous lesions, are cell accumulations that contain *Langerhans cells*—large, activated granular macrophages that look like epithelial cells. Granulomas signal chronic infection. The biopsy specimen also allows for morphologic evaluation of bony spicules, which may reveal changes associated with *hyperparathyroidism* or *Paget disease.*[8]

Bone marrow collection sites include the following:
- *Posterior superior iliac crest* (spine) of the pelvis (Figure 17-1). In both adults and children, this site provides adequate red marrow that is isolated from anatomical structures that are subject to injury. This site is used for both aspiration and core biopsy.
- *Anterior superior iliac crest* (spine) of the pelvis. This site has the same advantages as the posterior superior iliac crest, but the cortical bone is thicker. This site may be preferred for a patient who can only lie supine.
- *Sternum,* below the angle of Lewis at the second intercostal space. In adults, the sternum provides ample material for aspiration but is only 1 cm thick and cannot be used for core biopsy. It is possible for the physician to accidentally

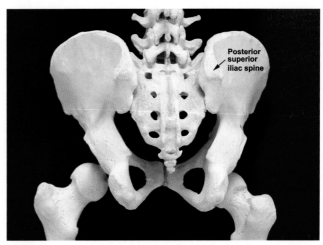

Figure 17-1 The posterior superior iliac crest is the favored site for obtaining the bone marrow aspirate and core biopsy specimen because it provides ample marrow and is isolated from structures that could be damaged by accidental puncture. (Courtesy Indiana Pathology Images, Indianapolis, IN.)

transfix the sternum and enter the pericardium within, damaging the heart or great vessels.
- *Anterior medial surface of the tibia* in children younger than age 2. This site may be used only for aspiration.
- *Spinous process of the vertebrae, ribs,* or other red marrow–containing bones. These locations are available but are rarely used unless one is the site of a suspicious lesion discovered on a radiograph.

Adverse outcomes are seen in less than 0.05% of marrow collections. Infections and reactions to anesthetics may occur, but the most common side effect is hemorrhage associated with platelet function disorder or thrombocytopenia.

BONE MARROW ASPIRATION AND BIOPSY

Preparation

Less than 24 hours prior to bone marrow collection, the medical laboratory scientist or phlebotomist collects venous peripheral blood for a complete blood count and blood film examination using a standard collection procedure. Peripheral blood collection is often accomplished immediately before bone marrow specimen collection. The peripheral blood specimen is seldom collected after bone marrow collection to avoid stress-related white blood cell (WBC) count elevation.

Most institutions purchase or assemble disposable sterile bone marrow specimen collection trays that provide the following:
- Surgical gloves.
- Shaving equipment.
- Antiseptic solution and alcohol pads.
- Drape material.
- Local anesthetic injection, usually 1% lidocaine, not to exceed 20 mL per patient.
- No. 11 scalpel blade for skin incision.

- Disposable Jamshidi biopsy needle (Care Fusion, McGaw Park, IL; Figure 17-2) or Westerman-Jensen needle (Becton, Dickinson and Company, Franklin Lakes, NJ; Figure 17-3). Both provide an obturator, core biopsy tool, and stylet. A Snarecoil biopsy needle also is available (Kendall Company, Mansfield, MA). The Snarecoil has a coil mechanism at the needle tip that allows for capture of the bone marrow specimen without needle redirection (Figure 17-4).
- Disposable 14- to 18-gauge aspiration needle with obturator. Alternatively, the University of Illinois aspiration needle may be used for sternal puncture. The University of Illinois needle provides a flange that prevents penetration of the sternum to the pericardium.

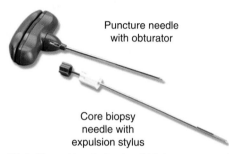

Puncture needle with obturator

Core biopsy needle with expulsion stylus

Figure 17-2 Disposable sterile Jamshidi bone marrow biopsy and aspiration needle. The outer puncture cannula is advanced to the medulla with the obturator in place to prevent bone coring. The physician removes the obturator and slides the core biopsy needle through the cannula and into the medulla with the expulsion stylus removed. The core biopsy needle is removed from the puncture needle with the specimen in place. The specimen is expelled using the stylus. (Courtesy Care Fusion, McGaw Park, IL.)

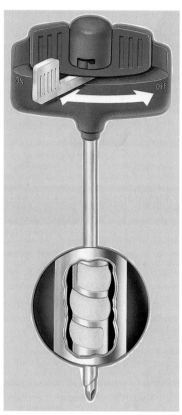

Figure 17-4 Snarecoil bone marrow biopsy needle. The coil mechanism resides within the biopsy needle as illustrated in the magnified image. The coil is turned to draw the marrow specimen into the needle. (Courtesy Tyco Healthcare/Kendall, Mansfield, MA.)

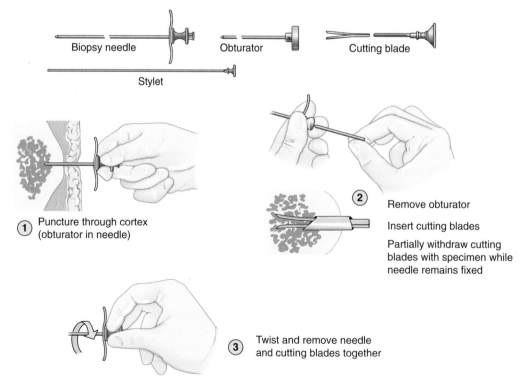

Biopsy needle   Obturator   Cutting blade

Stylet

① Puncture through cortex (obturator in needle)

② Remove obturator
Insert cutting blades
Partially withdraw cutting blades with specimen while needle remains fixed

③ Twist and remove needle and cutting blades together

Figure 17-3 Bone marrow biopsy technique using the Westerman-Jensen needle.

- Microscope slides or coverslips washed in 70% ethanol.
- Petri dishes or shallow circular watch glasses.
- Vials or test tubes with closures.
- Wintrobe hematocrit tubes.
- Anticoagulant liquid tripotassium ethylenediaminetetraacetic acid (K$_3$EDTA).
- Zenker fixative: potassium dichromate, mercuric chloride, sodium sulfate, and glacial acetic acid; B5 fixative: aqueous mercuric chloride and sodium acetate, or 10% neutral formalin. *Because Zenker fixative and B5 contain toxic mercury, controlled disposal is required.*
- Gauze dressings.

The patient is asked to lie supine, prone, or in the right or left lateral *decubitus* position (lying on the right or left side). With attention to standard precautions, the skin is shaved if necessary, disinfected, and draped. The physician infiltrates the skin, dermis, and subcutaneous tissue with a local anesthetic solution, such as 1% or 2% lidocaine or procaine, through a 25-gauge needle, producing a 0.5- to 1.0-cm papule (bubble). The 25-gauge needle is replaced with a 21-gauge needle, which is inserted through the papule to the *periosteum* (bone surface). With the point of the needle on the periosteum, the physician injects approximately 2 mL of anesthetic over a dime-sized area while rotating the needle, then withdraws the anesthesia needle. Next, the physician makes a 3-mm skin incision over the puncture site with a No. 11 scalpel blade to prevent skin coring during insertion of the needle.

Core Biopsy

The biopsy specimen is usually collected first, because aspiration may destroy marrow architecture. After the incision is made, the physician inserts a Jamshidi outer cannula with the obturator in place through the skin and cortex of the bone. The obturator prevents coring of skin or bone. Reciprocating rotation promotes the forward advancement of the cannula until the resistance weakens, which indicates penetration through the cortex to the medullary cavity of the bone. The physician removes the obturator, inserts the biopsy needle through the cannula and slowly advances the needle 2 to 3 cm with continuous reciprocating rotation along the long axis. The physician changes the needle angle slightly to separate the core cylinder specimen from its marrow cavity attachments, and withdraws the biopsy needle and cannula from the bone, taking the core cylinder with them. The core cylinder is 1 to 1.5 cm long and 1 to 2 mm in diameter and weighs about 150 mg. The biopsy needle is placed over an ethanol-cleaned slide and the stylus is pushed through to dislodge the core cylinder onto the slide. Using sterile forceps, the laboratory scientist prepares imprints (touch preparations) and transfers the core cylinder to the chosen fixative, Zenker, B5, or formalin.

When the Westerman-Jensen needle is used, the physician removes the obturator, inserts the cutting blades through the cannula, and advances the blades into the medullary cavity. The cutting blades are pressed into the medullary bone, with the outer cannula held firmly in a stationary position. The physician slowly withdraws the blades so that the cannula entraps the tissue, then withdraws the entire unit. The core cylinder is removed by inserting the probe through the cutting tip and extruding the specimen through the hub of the needle to the selected slide and fixative-containing receptacles.

Aspiration

In a separate location from the biopsy, the physician inserts a 14- to 18-gauge aspiration needle such as the University of Illinois needle, with obturator, through the skin and cortex of the bone. The obturator is removed, and a 10- to 20-mL syringe is attached. The physician withdraws the plunger to create negative pressure and aspirates 1.0 to 1.5 mL of marrow into the syringe. Collecting more than 1.5 mL dilutes the hematopoietic marrow with sinusoidal (peripheral) blood. The physician detaches the syringe and passes it *immediately* to the laboratory scientist, who expels the material onto a series of clean and sterile microscopic slides or coverslips. The physician may attach a second syringe to aspirate an additional specimen for *cytogenetic analysis, molecular diagnosis,* or *immunophenotyping* using flow cytometry. The needle is then withdrawn, and pressure is applied to the wound.

If no marrow is obtained, the physician returns the obturator to the needle, advances the needle, attaches a fresh syringe, and tries again. The syringe and needle are retracted slightly and the process is repeated. If this attempt is unsuccessful, the physician removes the needle and syringe, applies pressure, and begins the procedure at a new site. If the marrow is fibrotic, acellular, or packed with leukemic cells, the first and second aspiration may be unsuccessful, known as a *dry tap*. In this case, a biopsy is necessary, and the laboratory scientist may observe cell morphology using a slide imprint, or touch preparation.

Patient Care

Subsequent to bone marrow biopsy or aspiration, the physician applies a pressure dressing and advises the patient to remain in the same position for 60 minutes to prevent bleeding.

MANAGING THE BONE MARROW SPECIMEN

Direct Aspirate Smears

The medical laboratory scientist receives the aspirate syringe from the physician at the bedside and immediately transfers drops of the marrow specimen onto six to eight ethanol-washed microscope slides. Marrow clots rapidly, so good organization is essential. Using spreader slides, the scientist spreads the drop into a wedge-shaped smear $^1/_2$ to $^3/_4$ the length of the slide, similar to a peripheral blood film. Bony spicules 0.5 to 1.0 mm in diameter and larger fat globules follow behind the spreader and become deposited on the slide. In the direct smear preparation the scientist avoids crushing the spicules. The scientist may lightly fan the smears to promote rapid drying in an effort to preserve cell morphology.

In the syringe, the specimen consists of peripheral blood with suspended light-colored bony spicules and fat globules. The scientist evaluates the syringe blood for spicules: more spicules mean a specimen with more cells to identify and categorize. If the specimen has few fat globules or spicules, the scientist may alert the physician to collect an additional specimen.

Anticoagulated Aspirate Smears

Anticoagulated specimens are a more leisurely alternative to direct aspirate smears. The scientist expresses the aspirate from the syringe into a vial containing K_3EDTA and subsequently pipettes the anticoagulated aspirate to clean glass slides, spreading the aspirate using the same approach as in direct smear preparation. All anticoagulants distort cell morphology, but K_3EDTA generates the least distortion.

Crush Smears

To prepare crush smears, the medical laboratory scientist expels a portion of the aspirate to a Petri dish or watch glass covered with a few milliliters of K_3EDTA solution and spreads the aspirate over the surface with a sterile applicator. Individual bony spicules are transferred using applicators, forceps, or micropipettes (preferred) to several ethanol-washed glass slides. The scientists places additional glass slides directly over the specimens at right angles and presses gently to crush the spicules. The slides are separated laterally to create two rectangular smears, which the scientist may fan to encourage rapid drying.

Some scientists prefer to transfer aspirate directly to the slide, subsequently tilting the slide to drain off peripheral blood while retaining spicules. Once drained, the spicules are then crushed with a second slide as described earlier.

The scientist may add one drop of 22% albumin to the EDTA solution, particularly if the specimen is suspected to contain prolymphocytes or lymphoblasts, which tend to rupture. The albumin reduces the occurrence of "smudge" or "basket" cells often seen in lymphoid marrow lesions.

The crush preparation procedure may also be performed using ethanol-washed coverslips in place of slides. The coverslip method demands adroit manipulation but may yield better morphologic information, because the smaller coverslips generate less cell rupture during separation. Use of glass slides offers the opportunity for automated staining, whereas coverslip preparations must first be affixed smear side up to slides and then stained manually (Chapter 16).

Imprints (Touch Preparations)

Core biopsy specimens and clotted marrow may be held in forceps and repeatedly touched to a washed glass slide or coverslip so that cells attach and rapidly dry. The scientist lifts directly upward to prevent cell distortion. Imprints are valuable when the specimen has clotted or there is a dry tap: the cell morphology may closely replicate aspirate morphology, although few spicules are transferred.

Concentrate (Buffy Coat) Smears

Buffy coat smears are useful when there are sparse nucleated cells in the direct marrow smear or when the number of nucleated cells is anticipated to be small, as in aplastic anemia. The scientist transfers approximately 1.5 mL of K_3EDTA-anticoagulated marrow specimen to a narrow-bore glass or plastic tube such as a *Wintrobe hematocrit* tube. The tube is centrifuged at 2500 *g* for 10 minutes and examined for four layers.

The top layer is yellowish fat and normally occupies 1% to 3% of the column. The second layer, plasma, varies in volume, depending on the amount of peripheral blood in the specimen. The third layer consists of nucleated cells and is called the *myeloid-erythroid* (ME) layer. The ME layer is normally 5% to 8% of the total column. The bottom layer is RBCs, and its volume, like that of the plasma layer, depends on the amount of peripheral blood present. The scientist records the ratio of the fat and ME layers using millimeter gradations on the tube.

Once the column is examined, the scientist aspirates a portion of the ME layer with a portion of plasma and transfers the suspension to a Petri dish or watch glass. Marrow smears are subsequently prepared using the crush smear technique.

The concentrated buffy coat smear compensates for hypocellular marrow and allows for examination of large numbers of nucleated cells without interference from fat or RBCs. On the other hand, cell distribution is distorted by the procedure. Therefore, the scientist does not estimate numbers of different cell types or maturation stages on a buffy coat smear.

Histologic Sections (Cell Block)

After the scientist has prepared aspirate smears and has distributed aliquots of marrow for cytogenetic, molecular, and immunophenotypic studies, the remaining core biopsy specimen, spicules, or clotted specimen is submitted for histologic examination. The specimen is suspended in 10% formalin, Zenker glacial acetic acid, or B5 fixative for approximately 2 hours.

The fixed specimen is subsequently centrifuged, and the pellet is decalcified and wrapped in an embedding bag or lens paper and placed in a paraffin-embedding cassette. A histotechnologist sections the embedded specimen, applies hematoxylin and eosin (H&E) dye, and examines the section.

Marrow Smear Dyes

Marrow aspirate smears are stained with Wright or Wright-Giemsa dyes using the same protocols as for peripheral blood film staining. Some laboratory managers increase staining time to compensate for the relative thickness of marrow smears compared with peripheral blood films.

Marrow aspirate smears and core biopsy specimens may also be stained using a ferric ferricyanide (*Prussian blue*) solution to detect and estimate marrow storage iron or iron metabolism abnormalities (Chapter 20). Further, a number of *cytochemical* dyes may be used for cell identification or differentiation (Table 17-2).

EXAMINING BONE MARROW ASPIRATE OR IMPRINT

Box 17-1 describes the uses of low- and high-power objectives in examining bone marrow aspirate direct smears or imprints.

Low-Power (100×) Examination

Once the bone marrow aspirate direct smear or imprint is prepared and stained, the scientist or pathologist begins the microscopic examination using the low-power (10×) dry lens, which, when linked with 10× oculars, provides a total 100× magnification. Most bone marrow examinations are

TABLE 17-2 Cytochemical Dyes Used to Identify Bone Marrow Cells and Maturation Stages

Cytochemical Dye	Application
Myeloperoxidase (MPO)	Detects myelocytic cells by staining cytoplasmic granular contents
Sudan black B (SBB)	Detects myelocytic cells by staining cytoplasmic granular contents
Periodic acid–Schiff (PAS)	Detects lymphocytic cells and certain abnormal erythrocytic cells by staining of cytoplasmic glycogen
Esterases	Distinguish myelocytic from monocytic maturation stages (several esterase substrates)
Tartrate-resistant acid phosphatase (TRAP)	Detects tartrate-resistant acid phosphatase granules in hairy cell leukemia

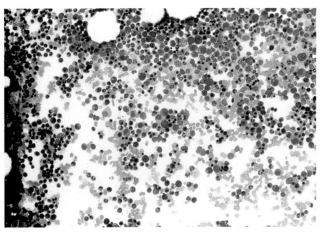

Figure 17-5 Bone marrow aspirate specimen illustrating intact, contiguous cells and adipocytes. This is a good site for morphologic evaluation and cell counting (Wright stain, 100×).

BOX 17-1 Bone Marrow Aspirate Microscopic Smear Examination: Low and High Power

Low Power: 10x Objective (100x total magnification)
- Assess peripheral blood dilution
- Find bony spicules and areas of clear cell morphology
- Observe fat-to-marrow ratio, estimate cellularity
- Search for tumor cells in clusters
- Examine and estimate megakaryocytes

High Power: 50x and 100x objective (500x and 1000x total magnification)
- Observe myelocytic and erythrocytic maturation
- Distinguish abnormal distribution of cells or cell maturation stages
- Perform differential count on 300 to 1000 cells
- Compute myeloid-to-erythroid ratio

---

performed using a teaching report format that employs projection or multiheaded microscopes to allow observation by residents, fellows, medical laboratory students, and attending staff. The microscopist locates the bony spicules, aggregations of bone and hematopoietic cells, which stain dark blue (Figure 17-5). In imprints, spicules are sparse or absent, and the search is for hematopoietic cells in the absence of spicules. Within these areas the microscopist selects intact and nearly contiguous nucleated cells for examination, avoiding areas of distorted morphology or areas diluted with sinusoidal blood.

Near the spicules, cellularity is estimated by observing the proportion of hematopoietic cells to adipocytes (clear fat areas).[9] For anterior or posterior iliac crest marrow, 50% cellularity is normal for patients aged 30 to 70 years. In childhood, cellularity is 80%, and after age 70, cellularity becomes reduced. For those older than age 70, a rule of thumb is to subtract patient age from 100% and add ±10%. Thus, for a 75-year-old, the anticipated cellularity is 15% to 35%. By comparing with the age-related normal cellularity values, the microscopist classifies the observed area as *hypocellular, normocellular,* or *hypercellular.* If a core biopsy specimen was collected, it provides a more accurate estimate of cellularity than an aspirate smear, because in aspirates there is always some dilution of hematopoietic tissue with peripheral blood. In the absence of leukemia, lymphocytes should total fewer than 30% of nucleated cells; if more are present, the marrow specimen has been substantially diluted and should not be used to estimate cellularity.[10]

Using the 10× objective, the microscopist searches for abnormal, often molded, cell clusters (syncytia) of *metastatic tumor cells or lymphoblasts.* Tumor cell nuclei often stain darkly (hyperchromatic), and vacuoles are seen in the cytoplasm. Tumor cell clusters are often found near the edges of the smear.

Although myelocytic cells and erythrocytic cells are best examined using 500× magnification, they may be more easily distinguished from each other using the 10× objective. The erythrocytic maturation stages stain more intensely, and their margins are more sharply defined, features more easily distinguished at lower magnification.

The microscopist evaluates *megakaryocytes* using low power (Figure 17-6). Megakaryocytes are the largest cells in the bone marrow, 30 to 50 μm in diameter, with multilobed nuclei (Chapter 13). Although in special circumstances microscopists may differentiate three megakaryocyte maturation stages—*megakaryoblast, promegakaryocyte,* and *megakaryocyte* (MK-I to MK-III)—a total megakaryocyte estimate is generally satisfactory. In a well-prepared aspirate or biopsy specimen, the microscopist observes 2 to 10 megakaryocytes per low-power field. Deviations yield important information and are reported as decreased or increased megakaryocytes. Bone marrow megakaryocyte estimates are essential to the evaluation of peripheral blood thrombocytopenia and thrombocytosis; for instance, in immune thrombocytopenia, marrow megakaryocytes proliferate markedly.

Abnormal megakaryocytes may be small, lack granularity, or have poorly lobulated or hyperlobulated nuclei. Indications of abnormality may be visible using low power; however, conclusive descriptions require 500× or even 1000× total magnification.

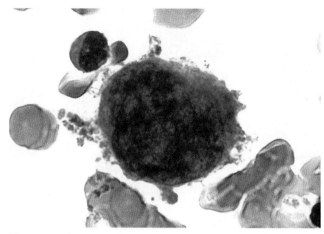

Figure 17-6 Bone marrow aspirate smear showing megakaryocyte with budding platelets at the plasma membrane (Wright stain, 1000×). Megakaryocytes are counted at 100× magnification, but if there is abnormal morphology, cells are examined at 500× or 1000×.

High-Power (500×) Examination

Having located a suitable examination area, the microscopist places a drop of immersion oil on the specimen and switches to the 50× objective, providing 500× total magnification. All of the nucleated cells are reviewed for morphology and normal maturation. Besides megakaryocytes, cells of the myelocytic (Figures 17-7 through 17-10) and erythrocytic (rubricytic, normoblastic; Figure 17-11) series should be present, along with eosinophils, basophils, lymphocytes, plasma cells, monocytes, and histiocytes. Chapters 7, 8, and 12 provide detailed cell and cell maturation stage descriptions. Table 17-3 names all normal marrow cells and provides their expected percentages.

The microscopist searches for maturation gaps, misdistribution of maturation stages, and abnormal morphology. Although the specimen is customarily reviewed using the 50× oil immersion objective, the 100× oil immersion objective is frequently employed to detect small but significant morphologic abnormalities in the nuclei and cytoplasm of suspect cells.

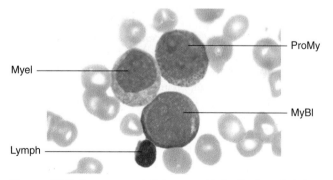

Figure 17-7 Bone marrow aspirate smear. Myelocytic stages include a myeloblast (MyBl), promyelocyte (ProMy), and myelocyte (Myel). The lymphocyte (Lymph) diameter illustrates its size relative to the myelocytic stages. The source of the lymphocyte is sinus blood (Wright stain, 1000×).

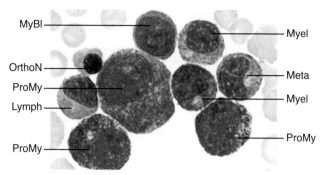

Figure 17-8 Bone marrow aspirate smear. Myelocytic stages include a myeloblast (MyBl), promyelocytes (ProMy), a myelocyte (Myel), and metamyelocyte (Meta). One orthochromic normoblast (OrthoN) and one lymphocyte (Lymph) are present (Wright stain, 1000×).

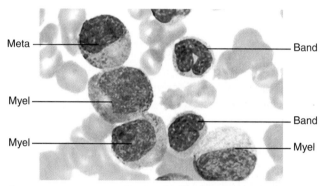

Figure 17-9 Bone marrow aspirate smear. Myelocytic stages include myelocytes (Myel), a metamyelocyte (Meta), and neutrophilic bands (Wright stain, 1000×).

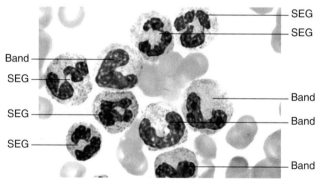

Figure 17-10 Bone marrow aspirate smear illustrating neutrophilic bands and segmented neutrophils (SEGs) (Wright stain, 1000×).

Many laboratory directors require a differential count of 300 to 1000 nucleated cells. These seemingly large totals are rapidly reached in a well-prepared bone marrow smear at 500× magnification and compensate statistically for the anticipated uneven distribution of spicules and hematopoietic cells. The microscopist counts cells and maturation stages surrounding several spicules to maximize the opportunity for

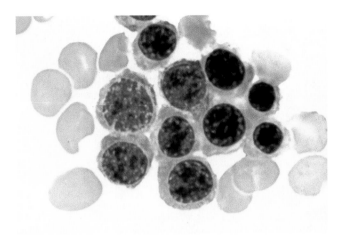

Figure 17-11 Bone marrow aspirate smear showing an island of erythrocytic precursors with polychromatophilic and orthochromic normoblasts (Wright stain, 1000×).

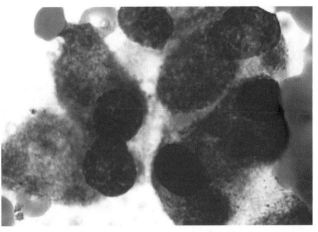

Figure 17-12 Bone marrow aspirate smear showing a cluster of osteoblasts that superficially resemble plasma cells. Osteoblasts have round to oval eccentric nuclei and mottled blue cytoplasm that is devoid of secretory granules. They may have a clear area within the cytoplasm but lack the well-defined central Golgi complex of the plasma cell (Wright stain, 1000×).

detecting disease-related cells. Some laboratory directors eschew the differential in favor of a thorough examination of the smear.

Many microscopists choose not to differentiate the four nucleated erythrocytic maturation stages, and others may combine three of the four—*basophilic, polychromatophilic,* and *orthochromic normoblasts*—in a single total, counting only pronormoblasts separately. In normal marrow, most erythrocytic precursors are either polychromatophilic or orthochromic normoblasts, and differentiation yields little additional information. On the other hand, differentiation may be helpful in megaloblastic, iron deficiency, or refractory anemias.

The microscopist may infrequently find *osteoblasts* and *osteoclasts* (Figure 17-12). Osteoblasts are responsible for bone formation and remodeling, and they derive from *endosteal* (inner lining) cells. Osteoblasts resemble plasma cells with eccentric round to oval nuclei and abundant blue, mottled cytoplasm, but

they lack the prominent Golgi apparatus characteristic of plasma cells. Osteoblasts are usually found in clusters resembling myeloma cell clusters. Their presence in marrow aspirates and core biopsy specimens is incidental; they do not signal disease, but they may create confusion.

Osteoclasts are nearly the diameter of megakaryocytes, but their multiple, evenly spaced nuclei distinguish them from multilobed megakaryocyte nuclei (Figure 17-13). Osteoclasts appear to derive from myeloid progenitor cells and are responsible for bone resorption, acting in concert with osteoblasts. Osteoclasts are recognized more often in core biopsy specimens than in aspirates.

Adipocytes, endothelial cells that line blood vessels, and fibroblast-like *reticular cells* complete the bone marrow stroma (Chapter 7). Stromal cells and their extracellular matrix provide

TABLE 17-3 Anticipated Distribution of Cells and Cell Maturation Stages in Aspirates or Imprints

Cell or Cell Maturation Stage	Distribution	Cell or Cell Maturation Stage	Distribution
Myeloblasts	0%–3%	Pronormoblasts/rubriblasts	0%–1%
Promyelocytes	1%–5%	Basophilic normoblasts/ prorubricytes	1%–4%
Myelocytes	6%–17%	Polychromatophilic normoblasts/rubricytes	10%–20%
Metamyelocytes	3%–20%	Orthochromic normoblasts/ metarubricytes	6%–10%
Neutrophilic bands	9%–32%	Lymphocytes	5%–18%
Segmented neutrophils	7%–30%	Plasma cells	0%–1%
Eosinophils and eosinophilic precursors	0%–3%	Monocytes	0%–1%
Basophils and mast cells	0%–1%	Histiocytes	0%–1%
Megakaryocytes	2–10 visible per low-power field	Myeloid-to-erythroid ratio	1.5:1–3.3 : 1

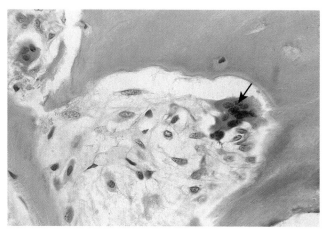

Figure 17-13 Bone marrow core biopsy section from a patient with hyperparathyroidism. The large multinucleated cell near the endosteal surface is an osteoclast, a cell that reabsorbs bone. The spindle-shaped cells are fibroblasts (hematoxylin and eosin stain, 500×).

the suitable microenvironment for the maturation and proliferation of hematopoietic cells but are seldom examined for diagnosis of hematologic or systemic disease. Finally, *Langerhans cells*, giant cells with "palisade" nuclei found in granulomas, signal chronic inflammation.

Once the differential is completed, the *myeloid-to-erythroid* (M:E) ratio is computed from the total of myeloid to the total of nucleated erythroid cell stages. Excluded from the M:E ratio are lymphocytes, plasma cells, monocytes, histiocytes, nonnucleated erythrocytes, and nonhematopoietic stromal cells.

Prussian Blue Iron Stain Examination

A Prussian blue (ferric ferricyanide) iron stain is commonly used on the aspirate smear. Figure 17-14 illustrates normal iron, absence of iron, and increased iron stores in aspirate smears. The iron stain may be used for core biopsy specimens, but decalcifying agents used to soften the biopsy specimen during processing may leach iron, which gives a false impression of decreased or absent iron stores. For this reason, the aspirate is favored for the iron stain if sufficient spicules are present.

EXAMINING THE BONE MARROW CORE BIOPSY SPECIMEN

The standard dye for the core biopsy specimen is H&E. Other dyes and their purposes are listed in Table 17-4. Bone marrow core biopsy specimen and imprint (touch preparation) examinations are essential when the aspiration procedure yields a dry tap, which may be the result of hypoplastic or aplastic anemia, fibrosis, or tight packing of the marrow cavity with leukemic cells. The key advantage of the core biopsy specimen is preservation of bone marrow architecture so that cells, tumor clusters (Figure 17-15), and maturation stages may be examined relative to stromal elements. The disadvantage is that individual hematopoietic cell morphology is obscured.

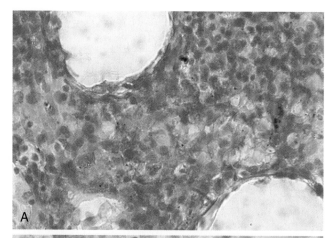

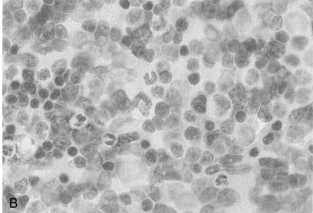

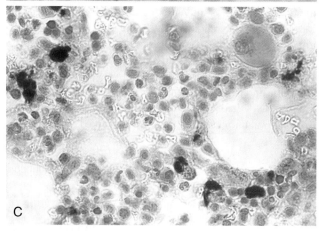

Figure 17-14 Prussian blue dye on bone marrow aspirate smears (500×). **A,** Normal iron stores. **B,** Absence of iron stores. **C,** Increased iron stores.

The microscopist first examines the core biopsy specimen preparation using the 10× objective (100× total magnification) to assess cellularity. Because the sample is larger, the core biopsy specimen provides a more accurate estimate of cellularity than the aspirate. The microscopist compares cellular areas with the clear-appearing adipocytes, using a method identical to that employed in examination of aspirate smears to assess cellularity. All fields are examined because cells distribute unevenly. Examples of hypocellular and hypercellular core biopsy

TABLE 17-4 Dyes Used in Examination of Bone Marrow Core Biopsy Specimens

Dye	Application
Hematoxylin and eosin (H&E)	Evaluate cellularity and hematopoietic cell distribution, locate abnormal cell clusters.
Prussian blue (ferric ferricyanide) iron stain	Evaluate iron stores for deficiency or excess iron. Decalcification may remove iron from fixed specimens; thus ethylenediaminetetraacetic acid chelation or the aspirate smear is preferred for iron store estimation.
Reticulin and trichrome dyes	Examine for marrow fibrosis.
Acid-fast stains	Examine for acid-fast bacilli, fungi, or bacteria in granulomatous disease.
Gram stain	Examine for acid-fast bacilli, fungi, or bacteria in granulomatous disease.
Immunohistochemical dyes	Establish the identity of malignant cells with dye-tagged monoclonal antibodies specific for tumor surface markers
Wright or Wright-Giemsa dyes	Observe hematopoietic cell structure. Cell identification is less accurate in a biopsy specimen than in an aspirate smear.

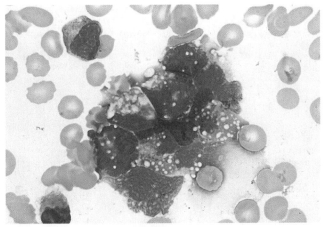

Figure 17-15 Bone marrow aspirate smear showing a cluster or syncytia of tumor cells. Nuclei are irregular and hyperchromatic, and cytoplasm is vacuolated. Cytoplasmic margins are poorly delineated (Wright stain, 500×).

sections are provided for comparison with normocellular marrow in Figure 17-16.

Megakaryocytes are easily recognized by their outsized diameter and even distribution throughout the biopsy. They exhibit the characteristic lobulated nucleus, although nuclei of the more mature megakaryocytes are smaller and more darkly stained in H&E preparations than on a Wright-stained aspirate. Their cytoplasm varies from light pink in younger cells to dark pink in older cells (Figure 17-17). Owing to the greater sample volume, microscopists assess megakaryocyte numbers more accurately by examining a core biopsy section than an aspirate smear. Normally there are 2 to 10 megakaryocytes per 10× field, the same as in an aspirate smear or imprint.

Using the 50× oil immersion objective, the microscopist next observes cell distribution relative to bone marrow stroma. For instance, in people older than age 70, normal lymphocytes may form small aggregates in nonparatrabecular regions, whereas *malignant lymphoma cell clusters* are often paratrabecular. In addition, normal lymphocytes remain as discrete cells, whereas lymphoma cells are pleomorphic and syncytial.

If no aspirate or imprint smears could be prepared, the core biopsy specimen may be stained using Wright, Giemsa, or Wright-Giemsa dyes to make limited observations of cellular morphology. In Wright- or Giemsa-stained biopsy sections, myeloblasts and promyelocytes have oval or round nuclei with cytoplasm that stains blue (Figure 17-18). Neutrophilic myelocytes and metamyelocytes have light pink cytoplasm. Mature segmented neutrophils (SEGs) and neutrophilic bands (BANDs) are recognized by their smaller diameter and darkly stained C-shaped nuclei (BANDs) or nuclear segments (SEGs). The cytoplasm of BANDs and SEGs may be light pink or may seem unstained (Figure 17-19).

The cytoplasm of eosinophils stains red or orange, which makes them the most brightly stained cells of the marrow. Basophils cannot be recognized on marrow biopsy specimens fixed with Zenker glacial acetic acid solution.

The microscopist may find it difficult to differentiate myelocytic cells from erythrocytic cells in biopsy specimens other than to observe that the latter tend to cluster with more mature normoblasts and often surround histiocytes. Polychromatophilic and orthochromic normoblasts, the two most common erythrocytic maturation stages, have centrally placed, round nuclei that stain intensely (Figure 17-20). Their cytoplasm is not appreciably stained, but the plasma membrane margin is clearly discerned, which gives the cells of these stages a "fried egg" appearance. Because erythrocytic cells have a tendency to cluster in small groups, they are more easily recognized using the 10× objective, although their individual morphology cannot be seen.

Lymphocytes are among the most difficult cells to recognize in the core biopsy specimen, unless they occur in clusters. Mature lymphocytes exhibit speckled nuclear chromatin in a small, round nucleus, along with a scant amount of blue cytoplasm (Figure 17-21). Immature lymphocytes (prolymphocytes) have larger round or lobulated nuclei but still only a small rim of blue cytoplasm.

Plasma cells are difficult to distinguish from myelocytes in H&E-stained sections but are recognized using Wright-Giemsa dye as cells with eccentric dark nuclei and blue cytoplasm and a prominent pale central Golgi apparatus (Figure 17-22). Characteristically, plasma cells are located adjacent to blood vessels.

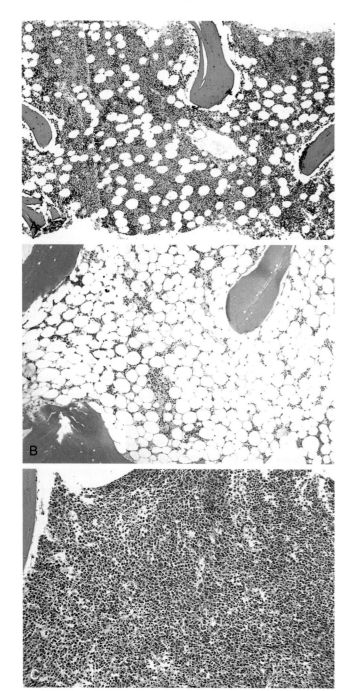

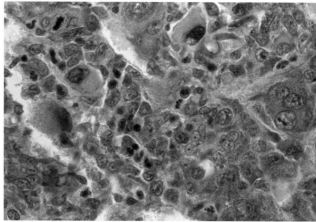

Figure 17-17 Core biopsy section containing many large lobulated megakaryocytes and increased blasts (Giemsa stain, 400×).

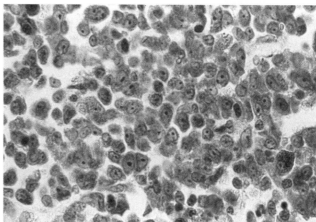

Figure 17-18 Core biopsy section infiltrated by blasts with blue cytoplasm and a few myelocytes with pink cytoplasm (Giemsa, 400×).

Figure 17-16 A, Representative core biopsy section showing normal cellularity, approximately 50% fat and 50% hematopoietic cells (hematoxylin and eosin, 50×). **B,** Hypocellular core biopsy specimen with only fat and connective tissue cells from a patient with aplastic anemia (hematoxylin and eosin stain, 100×). **C,** Hypercellular core biopsy specimen from a patient with chronic myelogenous leukemia. There is virtually 100% cellularity with no fat visible (hematoxylin and eosin stain, 100×). (**B** courtesy Dennis P. O'Malley, MD, director, Immunohistochemistry Laboratory, Indiana University School of Medicine, Indianapolis, IN.)

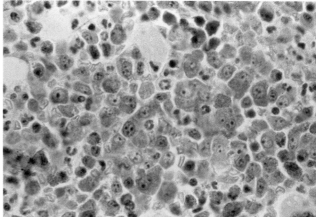

Figure 17-19 Core biopsy section showing myelocytes, metamyelocytes, bands, segmented neutrophils, and bright red-orange eosinophils (Giemsa stain, 400×).

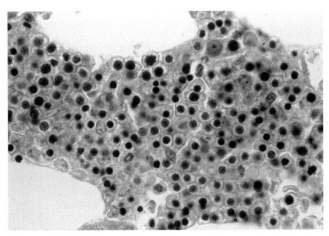

Figure 17-20 Erythrocytic island in a core biopsy section. Late-stage normoblasts often have a "fried egg" appearance (Giemsa stain, 400×).

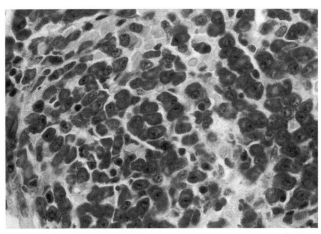

Figure 17-22 Plasma cells in a core biopsy section. Nuclei are eccentric, cytoplasm is blue with a prominent central unstained Golgi apparatus (Giemsa stain, 400×).

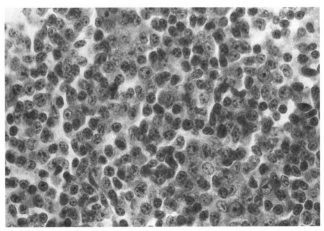

Figure 17-21 Core biopsy section showing small mature lymphocytes. A few are immature with larger nuclei containing a single prominent nucleolus (Giemsa, 400×).

DEFINITIVE BONE MARROW STUDIES

Although in many cases the aspirate smear and biopsy specimen are diagnostic, additional studies may be needed. Such studies and their applications are given in Table 17-5. These studies require additional bone marrow volume and specialized specimen collection. Information on Prussian blue iron stains and cytochemistry was provided earlier. Each study is described in the chapter referenced in Table 17-5.

BONE MARROW EXAMINATION REPORTS

The components of a bone marrow report should be generated systematically and are given in Table 17-6. An example of a bone marrow examination report is provided in Figure 17-23.

TABLE 17-5 Definitive Studies Performed on Selected Bone Marrow Specimens

Bone Marrow Study	Application	Specimen	Chapter
Iron stain	Identification of iron deficiency, iron overload	Fresh marrow aspirate	20
Cytochemical studies	Diagnosis of leukemias and lymphomas	Fresh marrow aspirate	29, 33, 35, 36
Cytogenetic studies	Diagnosis of acute leukemias via deletions, translocations, and polysomy; remission studies	1 mL marrow in heparin	30
Molecular studies	Polymerase chain reaction for diagnostic point mutations; minimal residual disease studies	1 mL marrow in EDTA	31
Fluorescence in situ hybridization	Staining for diagnostic mutations; minimal residual disease studies	Fresh marrow aspirate	31
Flow cytometry	Immunophenotyping, usually of malignant hematopoietic cells, clonality; minimal residual disease studies	1 mL marrow in heparin, EDTA, or ACD	32

ACD, Acid-citrate dextrose; *EDTA,* ethylenediaminetetraacetic acid.

Laboratory of Bone Marrow Pathology Report

Name		Room number and Unit	Patient number		Specimen number
Date		Age	Sex		Race

Address

City, State, Zip

Site	Aspirate	Biopsy	Markers	Cytogenetics and Molecular Studies

Attending Physician		Pathologist

Clinical Diagnosis

Acute leukemia

Pathology Diagnosis

Acute myelomonocytic leukemia (FAB M4) with mild eosinophilia. M98613, M47150, D 40800

Differential

Date	PB	Marrow	Marrow Range (percent)		PB	Marrow	Marrow Range (percent)
Blast, unclassified	4	77	0-2	Normal lymphocytes	50	2	3-24
Myeloblasts			3-5	Reactive lymphocytes			
Promyelocytes			1-8	Lymphoblasts			
Myelocytes		4	5-21	Prolymphocytes			
Metamyelocytes			6-22	Monocytes	3		0-3
Band neutrophils			6-22	Plasma cells			0-2
Segmented neutrophils	40	4	9-27	Rubriblasts			0-4
Eosinophils	3	4		Prorubricytes			1-6
Basophils				Rubricytes			5-25
Other				Metarubricytes			1-21
Other				Erythroid		8	10-30

WBC	PLT	MPV	HGB	HCT	MCHC
2,300	89,000	8	8.1	23	110

Peripheral blood film: Leukopenia, few blasts, myelocytes, neutrophils. Relative lymphocytosis. RBCs normochromic, macrocytes, mild anisocytosis. Rare teardrop cells. Normal platelet morphology.
Bone marrow aspirate: Few spicules, blasts 70-90% with large nuclei with fine chromatin and delicate creases. Moderate gray cytoplasm. Few blasts with high N/C ratio and large cells with cytoplasmic "blebs." Few mature myeloid precursors. Erythroid precursors markedly decreased, with rare binucleate rubricytes. Few eosinophil precursors noted. Dysmorphic megakaryocytes with increased nuclear lobulation.
Bone marrow imprint: Significant blast increase, most have myelomonocytic morphology. Few mature myeloid precursors, erythroid precursors markedly decreased.
Bone marrow biopsy: Hypercellular, 50-80%. Most cells are blasts, few mature myeloid precursors. Erythroid and megakaryocytic precursors markedly reduced.
Iron stain: Stainable iron in macrophages. Sideroblasts and rare ringed sideroblasts.
Flow cytometry: Bright CD15, HLA-DR, CD33, CD56, and CD11c. CD14 minimally expressed. Bright CD15 and CD11c consistent with monocytic differentiation.

AMML with eosinophilia (FAB M4e) cannot be ruled out, chromosome analysis pending. Rare ringed sideroblasts suggest transformation from preexisting myelodysplastic syndrome.

Figure 17-23 Example of a bone marrow examination report, including reference intervals, peripheral blood complete blood count results, marrow differential, and narrative. *PB,* Peripheral blood; **BMA,** bone marrow aspirate; **BMBX,** bone marrow biopsy specimen; **DX,** diagnosis.

TABLE 17-6 Components of a Bone Marrow Examination Report

Component	Description
Patient history	Patient identity and age, narration of symptoms, physical findings, findings in kindred, treatment
Complete blood count (CBC)	Peripheral blood CBC collected no more than 24 hours before the bone marrow puncture, includes hemogram and peripheral blood film examination
Cellularity	Hypocellular, normocellular, or hypercellular classification based on ratio of hematopoietic cells to adipocytes
Megakaryocytes	Estimate using 10× objective (100× magnification), compare with reference interval and comment on morphology
Maturation	Narrative characterizing the maturation of the myelocytic and erythrocytic (normoblastic, rubricytic) series
Additional hematologic cells	Narrative describing numbers and morphology of eosinophils, basophils, mast cells, lymphocytes, plasma cells, monocytes, and histiocytes if appropriate, with reference intervals
Stromal cells	Narrative describing numbers and morphology of osteoblasts, osteoclasts, bony trabeculae, fibroblasts, adipocytes, and endothelial cells; appearance of sinuses; presence of amyloid, granulomas, fibrosis, necrosis
Differential count	Numbers of all cells and cell stages observed after performing a differential count on 300 to 1000 cells and comparing results with reference intervals
Myeloid-to-erythroid ratio	Computed from nucleated hematologic cells less lymphocytes, plasma cells, monocytes, and histiocytes
Iron stores	Categorization of findings as increased, normal, or decreased iron stores
Diagnostic narrative	Summary of the recorded findings and additional laboratory chemical, microbiologic, and immunoassay tests

SUMMARY

- Adult hematopoietic tissue is located in the flat bones and the ends of the long bones. Hematopoiesis occurs within the spongy trabeculae of the bone adjacent to vascular sinuses.
- Bone marrow collection is a safe but invasive procedure performed by a pathologist or hematologist in collaboration with a medical laboratory scientist to obtain specimens used to diagnose hematologic and systemic disease and to monitor treatment.
- The necessity for a bone marrow examination should be evaluated in light of all clinical and laboratory information. In anemias for which the cause is apparent from the RBC indices, a bone marrow examination is not required. Examples of indications for bone marrow examination include multilineage abnormalities in the peripheral blood, pancytopenia, circulating blasts, and staging of lymphomas and carcinomas.
- A peripheral blood specimen is collected for a complete blood count no more than 24 hours before the bone marrow is collected, and the results of the CBC are reported with the bone marrow examination results.
- Bone marrow may be collected from the posterior or anterior iliac crest or sternum using sterile disposable biopsy and aspiration needles and cannulas. The site and equipment depend on how old the patient is and whether both an aspirate and a biopsy specimen are desired.

- The medical laboratory scientist receives the bone marrow specimen and prepares aspirate smears, crush preparations, imprints, anticoagulated bone marrow smears, and fixed biopsy sections, and specimens for confirmatory studies.
- The medical laboratory scientist and pathologist collaborate with residents, fellows, attending physicians, and medical laboratory science students to stain and review bone marrow aspirate smears, biopsy sections, and confirmatory procedure results.
- Confirmatory procedures include cytochemistry, cytogenetics, and immunophenotyping by flow cytometry; fluorescence in situ hybridization; and molecular diagnostics.
- The medical laboratory scientist and pathologist determine cellularity and megakaryocyte distribution, then perform a differential count of 300 to 1000 bone marrow hematopoietic cells and compute the M:E ratio, comparing the results with reference intervals.
- The pathologist characterizes features of hematopoietic disease, metastatic tumor cells, and abnormalities of the bone marrow stroma and prepares a systematic written bone marrow examination report including a diagnostic narrative.

Now that you have completed this chapter, go back and read again the case study at the beginning and respond to the questions presented.

REVIEW QUESTIONS

Answers can be found in the Appendix.

1. Where is most hematopoietic tissue found in adults?
   a. Liver
   b. Lungs
   c. Spleen
   d. Long bones

2. What is the preferred bone marrow collection site in adults?
   a. Second intercostal space on the sternum
   b. Anterior or posterior iliac crest
   c. Any of the thoracic vertebrae
   d. Anterior head of the femur

3. The aspirate should be examined under low power to assess all of the following *except:*
   a. Cellularity
   b. Megakaryocyte numbers
   c. Morphology of abnormal cells
   d. Presence of tumor cell clusters

4. What is the normal M:E ratio range in adults?
   a. 1.5:1 to 3.3:1
   b. 5.1:1 to 6.2:1
   c. 8.6:1 to 10.2:1
   d. 10:1 to 12:1

5. Which are the most common erythrocytic stages found in normal marrow?
   a. Pronormoblasts
   b. Pronormoblasts and basophilic normoblasts
   c. Basophilic and polychromatophilic normoblasts
   d. Polychromatophilic and orthochromic normoblasts

6. What cells, occasionally seen in bone marrow biopsy specimens, are responsible for the formation of bone?
   a. Macrophages
   b. Plasma cells
   c. Osteoblasts
   d. Osteoclasts

7. What is the largest hematopoietic cell found in a normal bone marrow aspirate?
   a. Osteoblast
   b. Myeloblast
   c. Pronormoblast
   d. Megakaryocyte

8. Which of the following is *not* an indication for a bone marrow examination?
   a. Pancytopenia (reduced numbers of RBCs, WBCs, and platelets in the peripheral blood)
   b. Anemia with RBC indices corresponding to low serum iron and low ferritin levels
   c. Detection of blasts in the peripheral blood
   d. Need for staging of Hodgkin lymphoma

9. In a bone marrow biopsy specimen, the RBC precursors were estimated to account for 40% of the cells in the marrow, and the other 60% were granulocyte precursors. What is the M:E ratio?
   a. 4:6
   b. 1.5:1
   c. 1:1.5
   d. 3:1

10. On a bone marrow core biopsy sample, several large cells with multiple nuclei were noted. They were located close to the endosteum, and their nuclei were evenly spaced throughout the cell. What are these cells?
    a. Megakaryocytes
    b. Osteoclasts
    c. Adipocytes
    d. Fibroblasts

11. The advantage of a core biopsy bone marrow sample over an aspirate is that the core biopsy specimen:
    a. Can be acquired by a less invasive collection technique
    b. Permits assessment of the architecture and cellular arrangement
    c. Retains the staining qualities of basophils owing to the use of Zenker fixative
    d. Is better for the assessment of bone marrow iron stores with Prussian blue stain

REFERENCES

1. Koury, M. J., & Lichtman, M. A. (2010). Structure of the marrow and the hematopoietic microenvironment. In Kaushansky, K., Lichtman, M., Beutler, E., et al. *Williams Hematology.* (8th ed., pp. 41–74). New York: McGraw Hill.
2. Farhi, D. C. (2008). *Pathology of Bone Marrow and Blood Cells.* (2nd ed.). Philadelphia: Lippincott Williams & Wilkins.
3. Foucar, K., Reichard, K., & Czuchlewski, D. (2010). *Bone Marrow Pathology.* (3rd ed.). Chicago: ASCP Press.
4. Silberstein, L., & Scadden, D. (2013). Hematopoietic microenvironment. In Hoffman, R., Benz, E. J., Silberstein, L., et al. (Eds.), *Hematology Basic Principles and Practice.* (6th ed.). St. Louis: Elsevier.
5. Reddy, V., Marques, M. B., & Fritsma, G. A. (2013). *Quick Guide to Hematology Testing.* (2nd ed.). Washington, DC: AACC Press.
6. Perkins, S. L. (2013). Examination of the blood and bone marrow. In Greer, J. P., Arber, D. A., Glader, B., et al. *Wintrobe's Clinical Hematology.* (13th ed.). Philadelphia: Wolters Kluwer Health/Lippincott Williams & Wilkins.
7. Ryan, D. H. (2010). Examination of the marrow. In Kaushansky, K., Lichtman, M., Beutler, E., et al. *Williams Hematology.* (8th ed.). New York: McGraw Hill.
8. Krause, J. R. (1981). *Bone Marrow Biopsy,* New York: Churchill Livingstone.
9. Hartsock, R. J., Smith, E. B., & Pett, C. S. (1965). Normal variations with aging of the amount of hemopoietic tissue in bone marrow from the anterior iliac crest. *Am J Clin Pathol, 43,* 326–331.
10. Abrahamson, J. F., Lund-Johansen, F., Laerum, O. D., et al. (1995). Flow cytometric assessment of peripheral blood contamination and proliferative activity of human bone marrow cell populations. *Cytometry, 19,* 77–85.

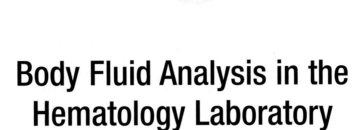

Body Fluid Analysis in the Hematology Laboratory

18

Bernadette F. Rodak*

OUTLINE

OBJECTIVES

After completion of this chapter, the reader will be able to:

1. Describe the method for performing cell counts on body fluids.
2. Given a description of a body fluid for cell counting, choose the appropriate diluting fluid, select a counting area, and calculate and correct (if necessary) the counts.
3. Using the proper terminology, discuss the gross appearance of body fluids, including its significance and its practical use in determining cell count dilutions.
4. Discuss the advantages and disadvantages of cytocentrifuge preparations.
5. Differentiate between traumatic spinal tap and cerebral hemorrhage on the basis of cell counts and the appearance of uncentrifuged and centrifuged specimens.

6. Identify from written descriptions normal cells found in cerebrospinal, serous, and synovial fluids.
7. Describe the characteristics of benign versus malignant cells in body fluids, and recognize written descriptions of each.
8. Differentiate exudates and transudates based on formation (cause), specific gravity, protein concentration, appearance, and cell concentration.
9. Identify crystals in synovial fluids from written descriptions, including polarization characteristics.
10. Describe the process of obtaining bronchoalveolar lavage (BAL) samples, including safety precautions for analysis; state the purpose of BAL; and recognize types of cells that normally would be found in BAL specimens.

CASE STUDY

After studying the material in this chapter, the reader should be able to respond to the following case study:

A 33-year-old semiconscious woman was brought to the emergency department by her husband. The previous day she had complained of a headache and had left work early. When she got home, she took aspirin and took a brief nap, and she reported she felt better that evening. Her husband stated that the next morning "she couldn't talk," so he brought her to the emergency department. A spinal tap was performed. The fluid that arrived in the laboratory was cloudy. The WBC count was 10.6×10^9/L. Most of the cells seen on the cytocentrifuge slide were neutrophils.

1. When multiple tubes of CSF are obtained, which tube should be used for cell counts?
2. What dilution should be made to obtain a satisfactory cytocentrifuge slide?
3. What should you look for on the cytocentrifuge slide?
4. What is the most likely diagnosis for this patient?

The author would like to acknowledge Leilani Collins for her work on this chapter in the previous edition.

The analysis of body fluids, including nucleated blood cell count and differential count, can provide valuable diagnostic information. This chapter is not intended as a comprehensive treatment of all body fluids, but it covers cell counting and morphologic hematology. The fluids discussed in this chapter include cerebrospinal fluid (CSF), serous or body cavity fluids (pleural, pericardial, and peritoneal fluids), and synovial (joint) fluids. Bronchoalveolar lavage (BAL) specimens are discussed briefly.

PERFORMING CELL COUNTS ON BODY FLUIDS

Examination of all fluids should include observation of color and turbidity, determination of cell counts, and white blood cell (WBC) evaluation. Blood cell counts should be performed and cytocentrifuge slides should be prepared as quickly as possible after collection of the specimen, because WBCs begin to deteriorate within 30 minutes after collection.[1] It is important to mix the specimen gently but thoroughly before every manipulation (i.e., counting cells, preparing any dilution, and preparing cytocentrifuge slides). Cell counts on fluids usually are performed using a hemacytometer (Chapter 14); however, many automated instruments now are capable of performing blood cell counts on fluids. Even specimens with low counts can be reported as long as the WBC count is above the limits of linearity of the instrument and no cellular interference flags are noted.[2-5] Each instrument manufacturer should provide a statement of intended use that defines which body fluids have been approved by a regulatory agency for testing on the instrument.[2,4] Care should be taken to observe the operating limits of these instruments—that is, the analytical measurement range (AMR) and the volume limits for the fluid received. Red blood cell (RBC) counts on serous and synovial fluids have little clinical value;[6] relevant clinical information is obtained merely from the appearance of the fluid (grossly bloody, bloody, slightly bloody).

Cell counts are performed with undiluted fluid if the fluid is clear. If the fluid is hazy or bloody, appropriate dilutions should be made to permit accurate counts of WBCs and RBCs. The smallest reasonable dilution should be made. The diluting fluid for RBCs is isotonic saline. Diluting fluids for WBCs include glacial acetic acid to lyse the RBCs, or Türk solution, which contains glacial acetic acid and methylene blue to stain the nuclei of the WBCs. Acetic acid cannot be used for synovial fluids because synovial fluid contains hyaluronic acid, which coagulates in acetic acid. A small amount of hyaluronidase powder (a pinch, or what can be picked up between two wooden sticks) or one drop of 0.05% hyaluronidase in phosphate buffer per milliliter of fluid should be added to the synovial fluid sample to liquefy it before performing cell counts or preparing cytocentrifuge slides. Dilutions should be based on the turbidity of the fluid or on the number of cells seen on the hemacytometer when using an undiluted sample.

A WBC count of approximately 200/μL or an RBC count of approximately 400/μL[3] causes a fluid to be slightly hazy. If the fluid is blood-tinged to slightly bloody, the RBCs can be counted using undiluted fluid, but it is advisable to use a small (1:2) dilution with Türk solution (or similar) to lyse the RBCs and provide an accurate WBC or nucleated cell count. If the fluid is bloody, a 1:200 dilution with isotonic saline for RBCs and either a 1:2 or a 1:20 dilution with Türk solution for nucleated cells should be used to obtain an accurate count. When performing dilutions for blood cell counts, a calibrated pipette should be used, such as MLA pipettes or the Ovation BioNatural pipettes (VistaLab Technologies, Inc. Brewster, NY).

The number of squares to be counted on the hemacytometer should be determined on the basis of the number of cells present. In general, all nine squares on both sides of the hemacytometer should be counted. If the number of cells is high, however, fewer squares may be counted.[7] Each square equals 1 mm². The formula for calculating the number of cells (Chapter 14) is:

$$\frac{\text{Cells counted} \times \text{depth factor} \times \text{dilution factor}}{\text{Area counted (mm}^2)}$$

Guidelines for counting are summarized in Table 18-1.

PREPARING CYTOCENTRIFUGE SLIDES

The cytocentrifuge enhances the ability to identify the types of cells present in a fluid. This centrifuge spins at a low speed, which minimizes distortion of the cellular elements and provides a "button" of cells that are concentrated into a small area. The cytocentrifuge assembly consists of a cytofunnel, filter paper to absorb excess fluid, and a glass slide. These three components are fastened together in a clip assembly, a few drops of well-mixed specimen are dispensed into the cytofunnel, and the entire assembly is centrifuged slowly. The cells are deposited onto the slide, and excess fluid is absorbed into the filter paper, which produces a monolayer of cells in a small button (Figure 18-1).

Although there is some cell loss into the filter paper, this is not selective, and an accurate representation of the types of cells present in a fluid is provided. There also may be some distortion of cells as a result of the centrifugation process or crowding of cells when high cell counts are present. To minimize distortion resulting from overcrowding of cells, appropriate dilutions should be made with normal saline before centrifugation. The basis for this dilution should be the WBC count or the nucleated cell count. A nucleated cell count of 200/μL or fewer provides a good basis for the differential. If the RBC count is extremely elevated, a larger dilution may be necessary; however, an RBC count of 5000/μL would not cause significant nucleated cell distortion. If a fluid has a nucleated cell count of 2000/μL and an RBC count of 10,000/μL, a 1:10 dilution should be made, which produces a nucleated cell count of 200/μL and an RBC count of 1000/μL for the cytocentrifuge slide. If the RBC count of a fluid is greater than 1 million/μL[3], it is best to make a "push" slide to perform the differential. In this case, the differential should be performed on the cells "pushed out" on the end of the smear instead of in the body of the

TABLE 18-1 Guidelines for Counting Fluids

Test	Clear	Hazy	Blood-Tinged	Cloudy	Bloody
			GROSS APPEARANCE		
WBCs	0–200/μL	>200/μL	Unknown	High	Unknown
Dilution for counting cells	None	1:2 Türk	1:2 Türk	1:20 in Türk solution	1:2 in Türk solution
No. squares to count on hemacytometer	9	9	9	9 or 4	9 or 4
RBCs	0–400/μL	Unknown	>400/μL	Unknown	>6000/μL
Dilution for counting cells	None	None	None	None	1:200 in isotonic saline
No. squares to count on hemacytometer	9 large	9 large	9 or 4 large	4 large or 5 small	5 small
Cytospin dilution (0.25 mL [5 drops] of fluid)*	Undiluted	Dilute with saline to 100–200/μL nucleated cell count	Straight or by nucleated cell count	Dilute with saline to 100–200/μL nucleated cell count	Dilute by nucleated cell count; if RBC count >1 million/μL, make a push smear and differentiate cells that are pushed out on the end

RBC, Red blood cell; *WBC*, white blood cell.
*Expected cell yield (WBC count for number of cells recovered on slide): 0/μL for 0–70, 1-2/μL for 12–100, >3/μL for >100.

smear, because that is where the larger, and possibly more significant, cells would be deposited.

If a consistent amount of fluid is used when cytocentrifuge slides are prepared, a consistent yield of cells can be expected; this can be used to confirm the WBC or nucleated cell count. For example, if five drops of fluid (undiluted or diluted) are always used to prepare cytocentrifuge slides, a 100-cell differential count should be obtainable if the WBC or nucleated cell count is equal to or greater than $3/\mu L^3$. In all cases, the entire cell button should be scanned before the differential count is performed to ensure that significant clumps of cells are not overlooked. The area of the cell button that is used for performing the differential

count is not important, but if the number of nucleated cells present is small, use of a "systematic meander" starting at one side of the button and working toward the other side is best. In case the number of cells recovered is small, the area around the cell button should be marked on the back of the slide with a wax pencil, or premarked slides should be used to prepare cytocentrifuge slides (Figure 18-1).

CEREBROSPINAL FLUID

CSF is the only fluid that exists in quantities sufficient to sample in healthy individuals. CSF is present in volumes of 100 to 150 mL in adults, 60 to 100 mL in children, and 10 to 60 mL in newborns.[8,9] This fluid bathes the brain and spinal column and serves as a cushion to protect the brain, as a circulating nutrient medium, as an excretory channel for nervous tissue metabolism, and as lubrication for the central nervous system. CSF is collected by lumbar puncture using either the L3-4 or L4-5 interspace (Figure 18-2).[6]

Gross Examination

Normal CSF is nonviscous, clear, and colorless. A cloudy or hazy appearance may indicate the presence of WBCs (greater than 200/μL), RBCs (greater than 400/μL), or microorganisms.[8,9] Bloody fluid may be caused by a traumatic tap, in which blood is acquired as the puncture is performed, or by a pathologic hemorrhage within the central nervous system. If more than one tube is received, the tubes can be observed for clearing from tube to tube. If the first tube contains blood but the remaining tubes are clear or progressively clearer, the blood is the result of a traumatic puncture. If all tubes are uniformly bloody, the probable cause is a subarachnoid hemorrhage. When a bloody sample is received, an aliquot should be centrifuged, and the color of the supernatant should be observed and reported. A clear, colorless supernatant indicates a traumatic

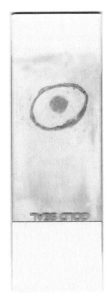

Figure 18-1 Wright-stained cytocentrifuge slide showing a concentrated button of cells within a marked circle. (Rodak BF, Carr JH: *Clinical hematology atlas*, ed 4, St. Louis, 2013, Saunders.)

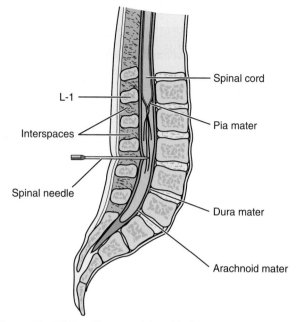

Figure 18-2 Schematic representation of lumbar puncture procedure with spinal needle placed between vertebrae L4-5. (From Brunzel NA: *Fundamentals of urine and body fluid analysis*, ed 4, St. Louis, 2013, Saunders.)

tap, whereas a yellowish or pinkish yellow tinge may indicate a subarachnoid hemorrhage. This yellowish color sometimes is referred to as *xanthochromia*, but because not all xanthochromia is pathologic, the Clinical and Laboratory Standards Institute recommends avoiding the term and simply reporting the actual color of the supernatant (Figure 18-3 and Table 18-2).[7]

Cell Counts

When multiple tubes of spinal fluid are collected, the cell count is generally performed on tube 3, or the tube with the lowest possibility of peripheral blood contamination. Tube 1 is used for chemistry and immunology, and tube 2 is used for microbiology. Normal cell counts in CSF are 0 to 5 WBCs/μL and 0 RBCs/μL in adults, and 0 to 30 WBCs/μL and 0 RBCs/μL in neonates. If a high RBC count is obtained, one may determine whether the source of WBCs is peripheral blood contamination by using the peripheral blood ratio of 1 WBC per 500 to 900 RBCs. If peripheral blood cell counts are known, the number of blood WBCs added to the CSF sample can be calculated using the following formula:

$$WBC_B \times \frac{RBC_{CSF}}{RBC_B} = WBCs \text{ added by traumatic puncture}$$

where WBC_B is the WBC count for peripheral blood, RBC_{CSF} is the RBC count for CSF, and RBC_B is the RBC count for peripheral blood. The corrected or true CSF WBC count (WBC_{CSF}) is calculated as follows:[7]

$$\text{True } WBC_{CSF} = \text{CSF WBC hemacytometer count} - \text{WBCs added}$$

Some laboratories have questioned the value of an RBC count on CSF and report only the WBC count.

A high WBC count may be found in fluid from patients with infective processes, such as meningitis. In general, WBC counts are much higher (in the thousands) in patients with

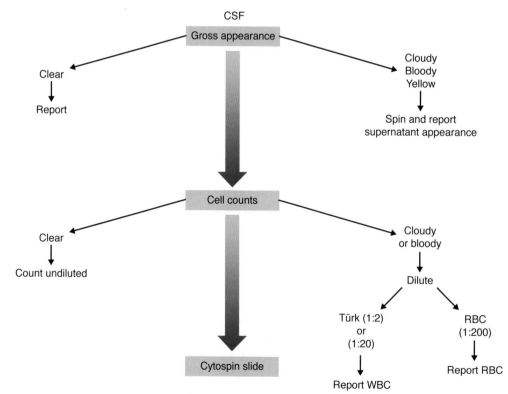

Figure 18-3 Flowchart for examination of cerebrospinal fluid (CSF). *RBC*, Red blood cell; *WBC*, white blood cell. (Modified from Kjeldsberg CR, Knight JA: *Body fluids*, ed 3, Chicago, 1993, ASCP Press; reprinted with permission.)

TABLE 18-2 Characteristics of Cerebrospinal Fluid

Traumatic Tap	Pathologic Hemorrhage
Clear supernatant	Colored or hemolyzed supernatant
Clearing from tube to tube	Same appearance in all tubes
Bone marrow contamination	Erythrophages
Cartilage cells	Siderophages (may have bilirubin crystals)

bacterial meningitis than in patients with viral meningitis (in the hundreds).[10-12] The predominant cell type present on the cytocentrifuge slide (neutrophils or lymphocytes), however, is a better indicator of the type of meningitis—bacterial or viral. Elevated WBC or nucleated cell counts also may be obtained in patients with inflammatory processes and malignancies.

Differential Cell Counts

The cells normally seen in CSF are lymphocytes and monocytes (Figure 18-4). In adults, the predominant cells are lymphocytes, and in newborns, the predominant cells are monocytes.[8,9] Neutrophils are not normal in CSF but may be seen in small numbers because of concentration techniques. When the WBC count is elevated and large numbers of neutrophils are seen, a thorough and careful search should be made for bacteria because organisms may be present in very small numbers early in bacterial meningitis (Figure 18-5). In viral meningitis, the predominant cells seen are lymphocytes, including reactive or viral lymphocytes and plasmacytoid lymphocytes (Figure 18-6). However, early in the course of the illness, neutrophils may predominate.[10-12] Eosinophils and basophils may be seen in response to the presence of foreign materials such as shunts, in parasitic infections, or in allergic reactions (Figure 18-7).[8,9] When nucleated RBCs are seen, bone marrow contamination resulting from accidental puncture of the vertebral body during spinal tap should be suspected and reported. In the case of bone marrow contamination, other immature neutrophils and megakaryocytes also may be seen. When there is obvious bone

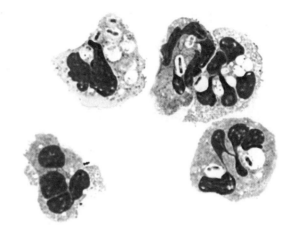

Figure 18-5 Neutrophils with bacteria in cerebrospinal fluid from a patient with bacterial meningitis (Wright stain, ×1000). (From Rodak BF, Carr JH: *Clinical hematology atlas*, ed 4, St. Louis, 2013, Saunders.)

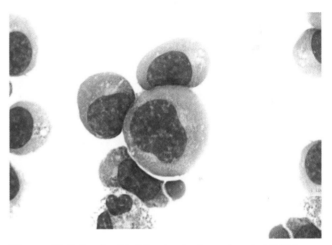

Figure 18-6 Reactive (viral) lymphocytes in cerebrospinal fluid from a patient with viral meningitis (×1000).

marrow contamination, the WBC differential is likely to be equivalent to that of the bone marrow and not that of the CSF.

Ependymal and choroid plexus cells, lining cells of the central nervous system, may be seen. These are large cells with abundant cytoplasm that stains lavender with Wright stain. They most often appear in clumps, and although they are not diagnostically significant, it is important not to confuse them with malignant cells (Figure 18-8).

Cartilage cells may be seen if the vertebral body is accidentally punctured. These cells usually occur singly, are medium to large, and have cytoplasm that stains wine red with a deep wine red nucleus with Wright stain (Figure 18-9).

Siderophages are macrophages (i.e., monocytes or histiocytes) that have ingested RBCs and, as a result of the breakdown of the RBCs, contain hemosiderin. Hemosiderin appears as large, rough-shaped, dark blue or black granules in the cytoplasm of the macrophage. These cells also may contain bilirubin or hematoidin crystals, which are golden yellow and are a result of further breakdown of the ingested RBCs. The presence of siderophages indicates a pathologic

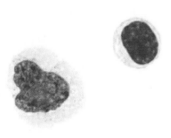

Figure 18-4 Monocyte *(left)* and lymphocyte *(right)* seen in normal cerebrospinal fluid (×1000).

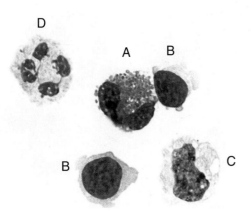

Figure 18-7 Eosinophil **(A)**, lymphocytes **(B)**, monocyte **(C)**, and neutrophil **(D)** in cerebrospinal fluid from a patient with a shunt (×1000).

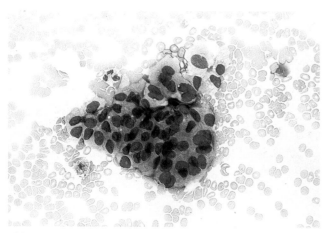

Figure 18-8 Clump of ependymal cells in cerebrospinal fluid (×200).

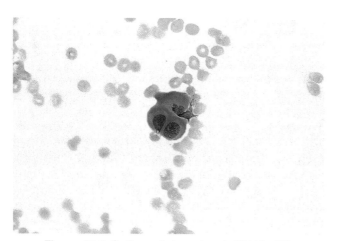

Figure 18-9 Cartilage cells in cerebrospinal fluid (×400).

hemorrhage. Siderophages appear approximately 48 hours after hemorrhage and may persist for 2 to 8 weeks after the hemorrhage has occurred (Figure 18-10).

A high percentage of patients with acute lymphoblastic leukemia or acute myeloid leukemia have central nervous system involvement.[8,9] It is always important to look carefully for

leukemic cells (i.e., blast forms) in the CSF of patients with leukemia. Patients with lymphoma, myeloma, and chronic myelogenous leukemia in blast crisis also may have blast cells in the CSF. These blast cells have the characteristics of blast forms in the peripheral blood, including a high nucleus-to-cytoplasm ratio, a fine stippled nuclear chromatin pattern, and prominent nucleoli. They are usually large cells that stain basophilic with Wright stain and have a fairly uniform appearance (Figure 18-11). If a traumatic tap has occurred and the patient has a high blast count in the peripheral blood, the blasts seen in the CSF may be the result of peripheral blood contamination and not central nervous system involvement. The possibility of peripheral blood contamination should be reported and the tap should be repeated in a few days.

Malignant cells resulting from metastases to the central nervous system may be found. The most common primary tumors that metastasize to the central nervous system in adults are breast, lung, and gastrointestinal tract tumors and melanoma.[8,9] In children, metastases to the central nervous system are related to Wilms tumor, Ewing sarcoma, neuroblastoma, and embryonal rhabdomyosarcoma.[9] Malignant cells are usually large with a high nucleus-to-cytoplasm ratio and

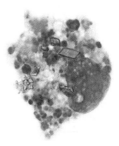

Figure 18-10 Siderophage with bilirubin crystals (hematoidin) in cerebrospinal fluid (×400).

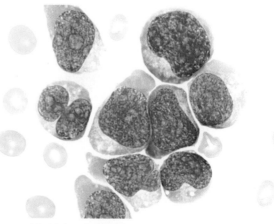

Figure 18-11 Lymphoblasts in cerebrospinal fluid (×1000). (From Rodak BF, Carr JH: *Clinical hematology atlas*, ed 4, St. Louis, 2013, Saunders.)

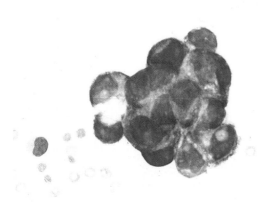

Figure 18-12 Clump of breast tumor cells in cerebrospinal fluid (×400).

are often basophilic or hyperchromic. They often occur in clumps but may occur singly. Within clumps of malignant cells, there is dissimilarity between cells, and in multinucleated cells, there may be variation in nuclear size. Clumps of malignant cells may appear three-dimensional, requiring up-and-down focusing to see the cells on different planes, and there are usually no "windows" (clear spaces) between the cells. The nuclei of these cells are usually large, often with abnormal distribution of chromatin, and they may have an indistinct or jagged border, or there may be "blebbing" at the border. Increased mitosis may be shown by the presence of several mitotic figures in the cell button. Malignant cells frequently have a pleomorphic appearance (Figure 18-12 and Table 18-3).

SEROUS FLUID

Serous fluids, including pleural, pericardial, and peritoneal fluids, normally exist in very small quantities and serve as lubricant

between the membranes of an organ and the sac in which it is housed. Pleural fluid is found in the space between the lungs and the pleural sac; pericardial fluid, in the space between the heart and the pericardial sac; and peritoneal fluid, between the intestine and the peritoneal sac (Figure 18-13). An accumulation of fluid in a cavity is termed an *effusion*. When an effusion is in the peritoneal cavity, it also may be referred to as *ascites* or *ascitic fluid*.[6] It would be difficult to remove these fluids from a healthy individual; the presence of these fluids in detectable amounts indicates a disease state.

Transudates Versus Exudates

As noted, the accumulation of a large amount of fluid in a cavity is called an *effusion*. Effusions are subdivided further into *transudates* and *exudates* to distinguish whether disease is present within or outside the body cavity. In general, transudates develop as part of systemic disease processes, such as congestive heart failure, whereas exudates indicate disorders associated with bacterial or viral infections, malignancy, pulmonary embolism, or systemic lupus erythematosus. Several parameters can be measured to determine whether an effusion is a transudate or an exudate (Table 18-4).

Gross Examination

Transudates should appear straw-colored and clear. A cloudy or hazy fluid may indicate an exudate from an infectious process; a bloody fluid, trauma, or malignancy; and a milky fluid, effused chyle in the pleural cavity.

Differential Cell Counts

The cells found in normal serous fluid are lymphocytes, histiocytes (macrophages), and mesothelial cells. Neutrophils commonly are seen in the fluid sent to the laboratory for analysis but would not be present in normal fluid. When neutrophils are seen, they have more segments and longer filaments than in peripheral blood (Figure 18-14).

TABLE 18-3 Characteristics of Benign and Malignant Cells

Benign	Malignant
Occasional large cells	Many cells may be very large.
Light to dark staining	May be very basophilic.
Rare mitotic figures	May have several mitotic figures.
Round to oval nucleus; nuclei are uniform in size with varying amounts of cytoplasm.	May have irregular or jagged nuclear shape.
Nuclear edge is smooth.	Edges of nucleus may be indistinct and irregular.
Nucleus is intact.	Nucleus may be disintegrated at edges.
Nucleoli are small, if present.	Nucleoli may be large and prominent.
In multinuclear cells (mesothelial), all nuclei have similar appearance (size and shape).	Multinuclear cells have varying sizes and shapes of nuclei.
Moderate to small N:C ratio	May have high N:C ratio.
Clumps of cells have similar appearance among cells, are in the same plane of focus, and may have "windows" between cells.	Clumps of cells contain cells of varying sizes and shapes, are "three-dimensional" (require focusing up and down to see all cells), and have dark-staining borders.

N:C, Nucleus-to-cytoplasm.

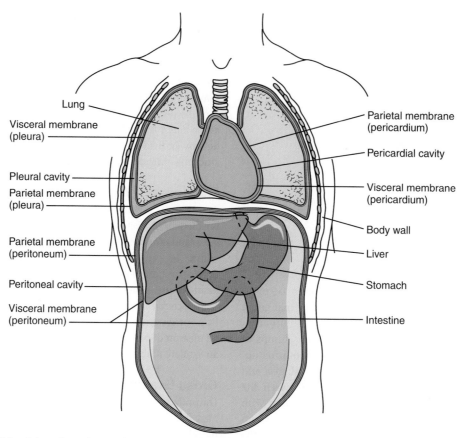

Figure 18-13 Parietal and visceral membranes of the pleural, pericardial, and peritoneal cavities. Parietal membranes line the body wall, whereas visceral membranes enclose organs. The two membranes are actually one continuous membrane. The space between opposing surfaces is identified as the body cavity (i.e., pleural, pericardial, and peritoneal cavities). (From Brunzel NA: *Fundamentals of urine and body fluid analysis,* ed 3, St. Louis, 2013, Saunders.)

TABLE 18-4 Serous Fluid: Transudates Versus Exudates

Characteristic	Transudates	Exudates
Specific gravity	<1.016	>1.016
Protein	<3 g/dL	>3 g/dL
Lactate dehydrogenase	<200 IU	>200 IU
White blood cells	<1000/μL (predominant cell type mononuclear)	>1000/μL
Protein: fluid-to-serum ratio	<0.5	>0.5
Lactate dehydrogenase: fluid-to-serum ratio	<0.6	>0.6
Color	Clear or straw-colored	Cloudy or yellow, amber, or grossly bloody
Volume	—	Extremely large

Mesothelial cells are the lining cells of body cavities and are shed into these cavities constantly. These are large (12- to 30-μm) cells and have a "fried egg" appearance with basophilic cytoplasm, oval nucleus with smooth nuclear borders, stippled nuclear chromatin pattern, and one to three nucleoli.[8,9] Mesothelial cells may vary in size, may be multinucleated (including giant cells with 20 to 25 nuclei), and may have frayed cytoplasmic borders, cytoplasmic vacuoles, or both. They may occur singly, in small or large clumps, or in sheets. When they occur in clumps, there are usually "windows" between the cells. The nucleus-to-cytoplasm ratio is 1:2 to 1:3, and this is generally consistent despite the variability in cell size.[6] They tend to have a similar appearance to each other on a slide. Mesothelial cells are seen in most effusions, and their numbers are increased in sterile inflammations and decreased in tuberculous pleurisy and bacterial infections (Figure 18-15).[8]

Macrophages appear as monocytes or histiocytes in serous fluids and may contain RBCs (erythrophages) or siderotic granules (siderophages), or they may appear as signet ring cells when lipid has been ingested and the resulting large vacuole pushes the nucleus to the periphery of the cell (Figure 18-16).

Eosinophils and basophils are not normally seen. These may be present in large numbers, however, as a result of allergic reaction or sensitivity to foreign material.

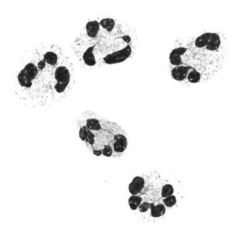

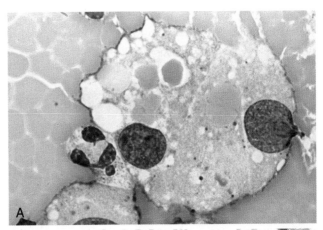

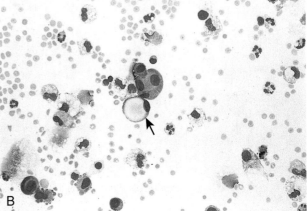

Figure 18-14 Hypersegmented neutrophil with prominent filaments. Normal appearance of neutrophils in body fluids (×1000). (From Rodak BF, Carr JH: *Clinical hematology atlas,* ed 4, St. Louis, 2013, Saunders.)

Figure 18-16 **A,** Erythrophage in peritoneal fluid (×1000). **B,** Signet ring cell (*arrow*) in peritoneal fluid (×200).

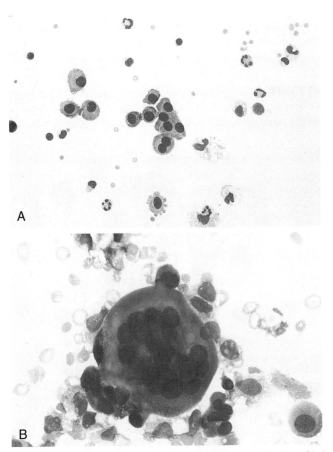

Figure 18-15 **A,** Mesothelial cells in peritoneal fluid (×200). Note "fried egg" appearance. **B,** Mesothelial cell with 21 nuclei in pleural fluid (×400).

TABLE 18-5 Gram-Stained Organisms Most Commonly Seen in Body Fluids

Fluid	Organism
Cerebrospinal	Gram-negative diplococci
	Gram-positive cocci
	Gram-negative coccobacilli
	Yeast—stains gram-positive
	Cryptococcus—look for capsule
Serous (peritoneal, pleural, or pericardial)	Gram-positive cocci
	Gram-negative bacilli
	Gram-positive bacilli
	Yeast—stains gram-positive
Synovial (joint)	Gram-positive cocci
	Gram-negative bacilli
	Gram-negative diplococci
	Gram-negative coccobacilli

Note: If the Gram-stained organisms seen in a fluid are not listed above for that fluid, do not report Gram stain results. Save the slide for review.

When large numbers of neutrophils are seen, a thorough search should be made for bacteria. If possible, Gram staining should be performed on a second cytocentrifuge slide to aid in rapid identification if bacteria are found. Table 18-5 lists Gram-stained organisms most commonly seen in body fluids.

Lupus erythematosus cells may be seen in serous fluids of patients with systemic lupus erythematosus, because all the factors necessary for the formation of these cells—presence of the lupus erythematosus factor, incubation, and trauma to the cells—exist in vivo. A lupus erythematosus cell is an intact neutrophil that has engulfed a homogeneous mass of degenerated nuclear material, which displaces the normal nucleus. Lupus erythematosus cells can form in vivo and in vitro in serous and synovial fluids and should be reported (Figure 18-17).

Malignant cells are seen in serous fluids from primary or metastatic tumors. They have the characteristics of malignant cells found in CSF (Figure 18-18). Figure 18-19 presents a flow chart for examination of serous fluids.

SYNOVIAL FLUID

Gross Examination

Synovial fluid is normally present in very small amounts in the synovial cavity surrounding joints. When fluid is present in

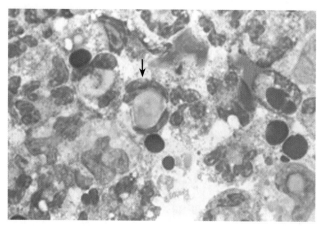

Figure 18-17 Lupus erythematosus cell (*arrow*) in pleural fluid (×1000).

amounts large enough to aspirate, there is a disease process in the joint. Figure 18-20 demonstrates placement of the needle for synovial fluid collection from a knee. Normally this fluid is straw-colored and clear. Synovial fluid contains hyaluronic acid, which makes it very viscous. A small amount (pinch) of hyaluronidase powder should be added to all joint fluids to liquefy them before cell counts are performed or cytocentrifuge slides are prepared. If a crystal analysis is to be performed, an aliquot of fluid should be removed for this purpose *before* the hyaluronidase is added.

Differential Cell Counts

Cells found in normal synovial fluid are lymphocytes, monocytes/histiocytes, and synovial cells. Synovial cells line the synovial cavity and are shed into the cavity. They resemble mesothelial cells but are usually present in smaller numbers (Figure 18-21).

Lupus erythematosus cells may be present in synovial fluid just as in serous fluid. Malignant cells are rarely seen in synovial fluid, but when present resemble tumor cells seen in serous fluids or CSF.

Many neutrophils are present in synovial fluid in acute inflammation of joints. As always, a careful search should be made for bacteria when many neutrophils are seen.

Crystals

Intracellular and extracellular crystals may be present in synovial fluid. Crystal examination may be performed by placing a drop of

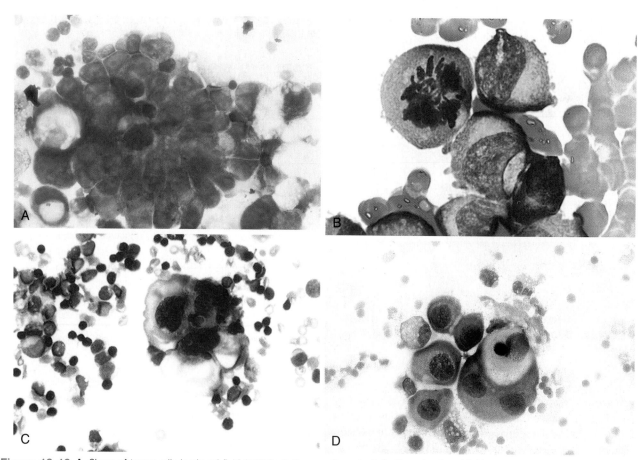

Figure 18-18 A, Clump of tumor cells in pleural fluid (×200). **B,** Tumor cells and mitotic figure in pleural fluid (×1000). **C,** Adenocarcinoma cells in pleural fluid (×200). **D,** Tumor cells in peritoneal fluid (×200). Note cannibalism.

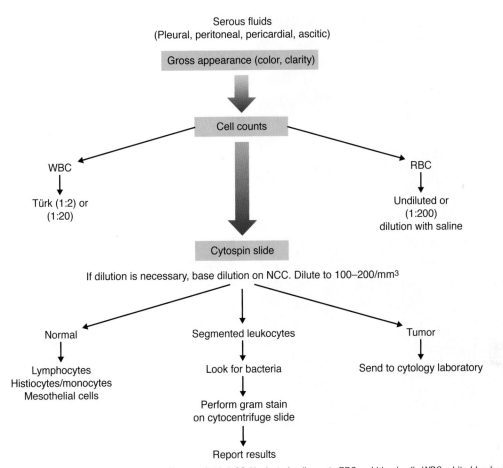

Figure 18-19 Flowchart for examination of serous fluid. *NCC,* Nucleated cell count; *RBC,* red blood cell; *WBC,* white blood cell.

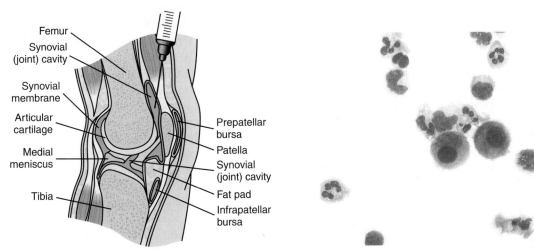

Figure 18-20 Schematic of knee demonstrating placement of the needle for synovial fluid aspiration. (From Applegate E: The anatomy and physiology learning system, ed 4, Philadlephia, 2011, Saunders.)

Figure 18-21 Synovial cells in synovial fluid (×400). Note similarity to mesothelial cells.

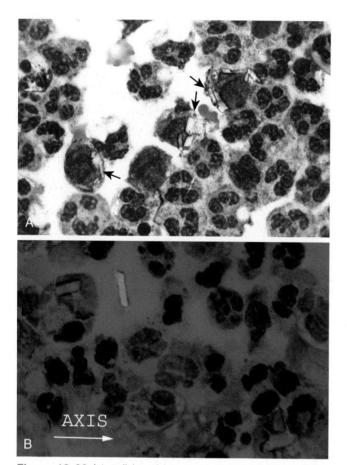

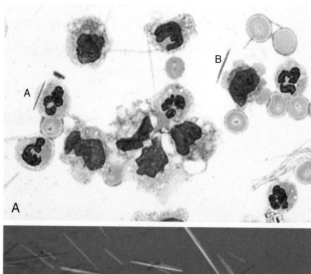

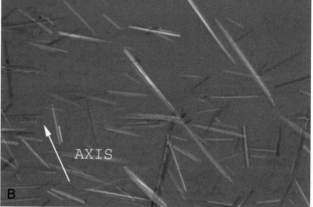

Figure 18-22 Intracellular calcium pyrophosphate crystals in synovial fluid (×1000). **A,** Wright stain. **B,** Polarized with red compensator. (**B** courtesy of George Girgis, MT[ASCP], Indiana University Health, Indianapolis, IN.)

Figure 18-23 Intracellular (**A**) and extracellular (**B**) monosodium urate crystals in synovial fluid (×1000). **A,** Wright stain. **B,** Polarized with red compensator. (**A** from Rodak BF, Carr JH: *Clinical hematology atlas*, ed 4, St. Louis, 2013, Saunders. **B** courtesy of George Girgis, MT[ASCP], Indiana University Health, Indianapolis, IN.)

fluid on a slide and adding a coverslip or by examining a cytocentrifuge preparation. However, the specimen should be fresh, without hyaluronidase added. All synovial fluids should be examined carefully for crystals using a polarizing microscope with a red compensator. The crystals most commonly seen in synovial fluids are cholesterol, calcium pyrophosphate, and monosodium urate.

Cholesterol crystals are large, flat, extracellular crystals with a notched corner.[13] They are seen in patients with chronic effusions, particularly patients with rheumatoid arthritis.

Calcium pyrophosphate crystals are seen in pseudogout. These crystals are intracellular and are small rhomboid, platelike, or rodlike crystals.[13] The crystals are weakly birefringent when polarized (i.e., they do not appear bright when polarized). When the red compensator is used, calcium pyrophosphate crystals appear blue when the longitudinal axis of the crystal is parallel to the γ-axis (Figure 18-22).[13]

Monosodium urate crystals are seen in gout. They are large needlelike crystals that may be intracellular or extracellular. These crystals are strongly birefringent when polarized. When the red compensator is used, monosodium urate crystals appear yellow when the longitudinal axis of the crystal is parallel to the γ-axis (Figure 18-23).[13] Figure 18-24 presents a flowchart for synovial fluid analysis.

BRONCHOALVEOLAR LAVAGE SPECIMENS

Procedure and Precautions

BAL specimens are not naturally occurring fluids; they are produced when the BAL procedure is performed. The procedure consists of introducing warmed saline into the lungs in 50-mL aliquots and then withdrawing it. The specimen received in the laboratory is the withdrawn fluid. The purpose of the procedure is to determine types of organisms and cells that are present in areas of the lung that are otherwise inaccessible. This procedure is performed on patients with severe lung dysfunction. The specimen should always undergo an extensive microbiologic workup and often cytologic examination. It is common to see bacteria, yeast, or both on cytocentrifuge slides prepared from these specimens. Because samples are obtained from the interior of the lung and may contain airborne organisms, care should be taken to avoid aerosol production. Samples should be mixed and containers opened under a biologic safety hood, and a mask should be worn when performing cell counts. Because the risk of performing cell counts and preparing cytocentrifuge slides on BAL specimens outweighs the clinical relevance of the information obtained, some

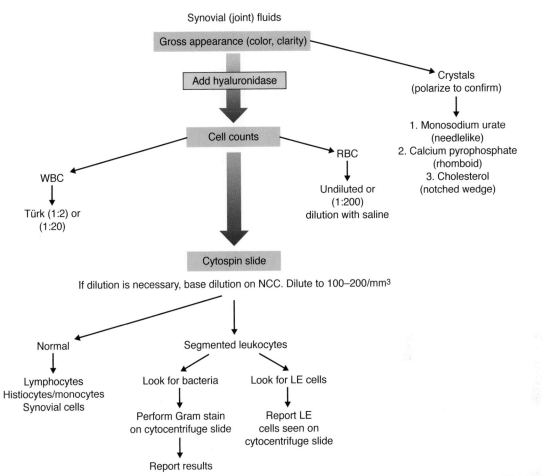

Figure 18-24 Flowchart for examination of synovial (joint) fluid. *LE,* Lupus erythematosus; *NCC,* nucleated cell count; *RBC,* red blood cell; *WBC,* white blood cell.

hematology laboratories no longer perform this procedure and defer to information reported from the microbiology laboratory.

Cell counts and cytocentrifuge preparations are performed as with any body fluid. Significant cell deterioration occurs within 30 minutes of collection, with the neutrophils disintegrating most rapidly.

Differential Cell Counts

The cell types most commonly seen in BAL specimens are neutrophils, monohistiocytes (macrophages), and lymphocytes. Mesothelial cells are not seen in BAL specimens because these cells line the body cavities and not the interior of the lung. Pneumocytes, which can resemble mesothelial cells or adenocarcinoma, may be seen in patients with adult respiratory distress syndrome.

Ciliated epithelial cells can be seen and should be reported because they indicate that the sample was obtained from the upper respiratory tract instead of deeper in the lung. These are columnar cells, with the nucleus at one end of the cell, elongated cytoplasm, and cilia at the opposite end of the cell from the nucleus. They can occur in clusters. If the sample is not aged when the cell count is performed, these cells are in motion in the hemacytometer, because they can be propelled by their cilia (Figure 18-25).

Histiocytes laden with carbonaceous material are seen in patients who use tobacco. These cells resemble siderophages in other fluids, but the carbonaceous material is black, brown, or blue-black and is more dropletlike (Figure 18-26).

Pneumocystis jiroveci (formerly *Pneumocystis carinii*) may be seen in specimens from patients infected with human immunodeficiency virus. The *P. jiroveci* organisms appear as clumps of amorphous material. Close examination of the clumps may reveal cysts (Figure 18-27).

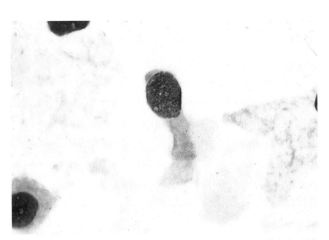

Figure 18-25 Ciliated epithelial cells in bronchoalveolar lavage fluid (×100).

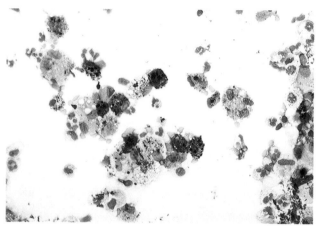

Figure 18-26 Histiocytes with carbonaceous material in bronchoalveolar lavage fluid (×40).

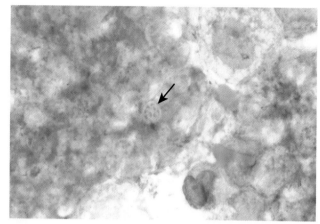

Figure 18-27 Cyst of *Pneumocystis jiroveci* (formerly *Pneumocystis carinii*) in bronchoalveolar lavage fluid (×100).

SUMMARY

- Cell counts and differential counts performed on body fluid specimens are valuable diagnostic tools.
- Calibrated methods must be used when performing cell counts to provide accurate counts.
- To optimize cell morphologic features, specimens should not be overdiluted or underdiluted when cytocentrifuge slides are prepared.
- Normal cell types in any fluid are lymphocytes, macrophages (monocytes, histiocytes), and lining cells (ependymal cells in CSF, mesothelial cells in serous fluids, synovial cells in joint fluids).

- Bacteria and yeast may be seen in any fluid.
- Malignant cells may be seen in any fluid but are rare in synovial fluid.
- Synovial fluid should be examined for crystals using a compensated polarizing microscope.
- BAL specimens are not a true body fluid, but examination of cells present may provide diagnostic information.

Now that you have completed this chapter, go back and read again the case study at the beginning and respond to the questions presented.

REVIEW QUESTIONS

Answers can be found in the Appendix.

Refer to the following scenario to answer questions 1 and 2: A spinal fluid specimen is diluted 1:2 with Türk solution to perform the nucleated cell count. A total of 6 nucleated cells are counted on both sides of the hemacytometer, with all nine squares counted on both sides. Undiluted fluid is used to perform the RBC count. A total of 105 RBCs is counted on both sides of the hemacytometer, with four large squares on both sides counted.

1. The nucleated cell count is ___/μL.
   a. 3
   b. 7
   c. 13
   d. 66

2. The RBC count is ___/μL.
   a. 131
   b. 263
   c. 1050
   d. 5830

3. Based on the cell counts, the appearance of the fluid is:
   a. Turbid
   b. Hemolyzed
   c. Clear
   d. Cloudy

4. All of the following cells are normally seen in CSF, serous fluids, and synovial fluids *except:*
   a. Lining cells
   b. Neutrophils
   c. Lymphocytes
   d. Monocytes/histiocytes (macrophages)

5. Spinal fluid was obtained from a 56-year-old woman. On receipt in the laboratory, the fluid was noted to be slightly bloody. When a portion of the fluid was centrifuged, the supernatant was clear. The cell counts were 5200 RBCs/μL^3 and 24 WBCs/μL. On the cytocentrifuge preparation, several nucleated RBCs were seen. The differential was 52% lymphocytes, 20% neutrophils, 22% monocytes, 4% myelocytes, and 2% blasts. What is the most likely explanation for these results?
   a. Bone marrow contamination
   b. Bacterial meningitis
   c. Peripheral blood contamination
   d. Leukemic infiltration in the central nervous system

6. A 34-year-old woman with a history of breast cancer developed a pleural effusion. The fluid obtained was bloody and had a nucleated cell count of 284/μL. On the cytocentrifuge preparation, there were several neutrophils and a few monocytes/histiocytes. There were also several clusters of large, dark-staining cells. These cell clumps appeared "three-dimensional" and contained some mitotic figures. What is the most likely identification of the cells in clusters?
   a. Mesothelial cells
   b. Metastatic tumor cells
   c. Cartilage cells
   d. Pneumocytes

7. A serous fluid with a clear appearance, specific gravity of 1.010, protein concentration of 1.5 g/dL, and fewer than 500 mononuclear cells/μL would be considered:
   a. Infectious
   b. An exudate
   c. A transudate
   d. Sterile

8. On the cytocentrifuge slide prepared from a peritoneal fluid sample, many large cells are seen, singly and in clumps. The cells have a "fried egg" appearance and basophilic cytoplasm, and some are multinucleated. These cells should be reported as:
   a. Suspicious for malignancy
   b. Macrophages
   c. Large lymphocytes
   d. Mesothelial cells

Refer to the following scenario to answer questions 9 and 10: A 56-year-old man came to the physician's office with complaints of pain and swelling in his left big toe. Fluid aspirated from the toe was straw-colored and cloudy. The WBC count was 2543/μL. The differential consisted mainly of neutrophils and monocytes/histiocytes. Intracellular and extracellular crystals were seen on the cytocentrifuge slide. The crystals were needle-shaped and, when polarized with the use of the red compensator, appeared yellow on the *y*-axis.

9. The crystals are:
   a. Cholesterol
   b. Hyaluronidase
   c. Monosodium urate
   d. Calcium pyrophosphate

10. This patient's painful toe was caused by:
   a. Gout
   b. Infection
   c. Inflammation
   d. Pseudogout

REFERENCES

1. Glasser, L. (1981). Cells in cerebrospinal fluid. *Diagn Med, 4,* 33–50.
2. Brown, W., Keeney, M., Chin-Yee, I., et al. (2003). Validation of body fluid analysis on the Coulter LH 750. *Lab Hematol, 9,* 155–159.
3. Perné, A., Hainfellner, J. A., Womastek, I., Haushofer, A., Szekeres, T., & Schwarzinger, I. (2012). Performance evaluation of the Sysmex XE-5000 hematology analyzer for white blood cell analysis in cerebrospinal fluid. *Arch Pathol Lab Med, 136,* 194–198.
4. Yang, D., Zhou, Y., & Chen, B. (2013). Performance evaluation and result comparison of the automated hematology analyzers Abbott CD3700, Sysmex XE 2100 and Coulter LH 750 for cell counts in serous fluids. *Clinic Chimica Acta, 419,* 113–118.
5. Boer, K., Deufel, T., & Reinhoefer, M. (2009). Evaluation of the XE-5000 for the automated analysis of blood cells in cerebrospinal fluid. *Clin Biochem, 42,* 684–691.
6. Brunzel, N. A. (2013). *Fundamentals of urine and body fluid analysis.* (3rd ed.). St Louis: Saunders.
7. Clinical and Laboratory Standards Institute (CLSI). (2006). *Body fluid analysis for cellular composition: proposed guideline.* Wayne, PA: CLSI. CLSI document H56-A, vol. 26, no. 26.
8. Kjeldsberg, C., & Knight, J. (1993). *Body fluids.* (3rd ed.). Chicago: ASCP Press.
9. Galagan, K., Blomberg, D., Cornbleet, P. J., et al. (2006). *Color atlas of body fluids,* Northfield, Ill.: College of American Pathologists.
10. Bartt, R. (2012). Acute bacterial and viral meningitis. *Continuum Lifelong Learning Neurol, 18,* 1255–1270.
11. Rotbart, H. A. (2000). Viral meningitis. *Semin Neurol, 20,* 277–292.
12. Spanos, A., Harrell, F. E., & Durack, D. T. (1989). Differential diagnosis of acute meningitis. *JAMA, 262,* 2700–2707.
13. Strasinger, S. K., & DiLorenzo, M. S. (2008). *Urinalysis and body fluids.* (5th ed.). Philadelphia: FA Davis.

19 Anemias: Red Blood Cell Morphology and Approach to Diagnosis

*Naveen Manchanda**

OUTLINE

OBJECTIVES

After completion of this chapter, the reader will be able to:

1. Define anemia and recognize laboratory results consistent with anemia.
2. Describe clinical findings in anemia.
3. Discuss the importance of the history and the physical examination in the diagnosis of anemia.
4. Explain how the body adapts to anemia and the symptoms experienced by the patient.
5. Distinguish among effective, ineffective, and insufficient erythropoiesis when given examples.
6. List laboratory procedures that are initially performed for the diagnosis of anemia.
7. Discuss the importance of the reticulocyte count in the evaluation of anemia.
8. Explain the importance of examining the peripheral blood film when investigating the cause of an anemia and distinguish the important findings.
9. Describe variations in red blood cell morphology such as inclusions and changes in shape, volume, or color.
10. Use an algorithm incorporating the absolute reticulocyte count to specify three groups of anemias involving decreased or ineffective red blood cell production and give one example of each.
11. Use an algorithm incorporating the mean cell volume to narrow the differential diagnosis of anemia.

CASE STUDY

After studying the material in this chapter, the reader should be able to respond to the following case study:

A 45-year-old female phoned her physician and complained of fatigue, shortness of breath on exertion, and general malaise. She requested "B_{12} shots" to make her feel better. The physician asked the patient to schedule an appointment so that she could determine the cause of the symptoms before offering treatment. A point-of-care hemoglobin determination performed in the office was 9.0 g/dL. The physician then requested additional laboratory tests, including a CBC with a peripheral blood film examination and a reticulocyte count.

1. Why did the physician want the patient to come to the office before she prescribed therapy?
2. How do the mean cell volume and reticulocyte count help determine the classification of the anemia?
3. Why is the examination of the peripheral blood film important in the investigation of an anemia?

---

*Ann Bell and Dr. Rakesh Mehta have contributed to the admirable framework and contents of this chapter.

R ed blood cells (RBCs) perform the vital physiologic function of oxygen delivery to tissues. Hemoglobin within the RBCs has the remarkable capacity to bind oxygen in the lungs and then release it appropriately in the tissues.[1] The term *anemia* is derived from the Greek word *anaimia,* meaning "without blood."[2] A decrease in hemoglobin concentration or number of RBCs results in decreased oxygen delivery to tissue, resulting in tissue hypoxia. Anemia is a common condition affecting an estimated 1.62 billion people worldwide.[3] Anemia should not be thought of as a disease but rather as a manifestation of an underlying disease or deficiency.[4,5] Therefore, causes of anemia should be thoroughly investigated. This chapter provides an overview of the mechanisms, diagnosis, and classification of anemia. In the following chapters, each anemia is discussed in detail.

DEFINITION OF ANEMIA

A functional definition of *anemia* is a decrease in the oxygen-carrying capacity of the blood. It can arise if there is insufficient hemoglobin or the hemoglobin has impaired function. The former is the more frequent cause.

Anemia is defined operationally as a reduction in the hemoglobin content of blood that can be caused by a decrease in RBCs, hemoglobin, and hematocrit below the reference interval for healthy individuals of similar age, sex, and race, under similar environmental conditions.[4-8] The reference intervals are derived from large pools of "healthy" individuals; however, the definition of *healthy* is different for each of these groups. Thus these pools of "healthy" individuals may lack the heterogeneity required to be universally applied to any one of these populations of individuals.[6] This fact has led to the development of different reference intervals for individuals of different sex, age, and race.

Examples of hematologic reference intervals for the adult and pediatric populations are included on the inside cover of this text. They are listed according to age and sex, but race, environmental, and laboratory factors can also influence the values. Each laboratory must determine its own reference intervals based on its particular instrumentation, the methods used, and the demographics and environment of its patient population. For the purpose of the discussion in this chapter, a patient is considered anemic if the hemoglobin value falls below those listed in these tables.

PATIENT HISTORY AND CLINICAL FINDINGS

The history and physical examination are important components in making a clinical diagnosis of anemia. A decrease in oxygen delivery to tissues decreases the energy available to individuals to perform day-to-day activities. This gives rise to the classic symptoms associated with anemia, fatigue and shortness of breath. To elucidate the reason for a patient's anemia, one starts by obtaining a good history that requires carefully questioning the patient, particularly with regard to diet, drug ingestion, exposure to chemicals, occupation, hobbies, travel, bleeding history, race or ethnic group, family history of disease, neurologic symptoms, previous medication, previous episodes of jaundice, and various underlying disease processes that

result in anemia.[4,7-9] Therefore, a thorough discussion is required to elicit any potential cause of the anemia. For example, iron deficiency can lead to an interesting symptom called *pica.*[10] Patients with pica have cravings for unusual substances such as ice (pagophagia), cornstarch, or clay. Alternatively, individuals with anemia may be asymptomatic, as can be seen in mild or slowly progressive anemias.

Certain features should be evaluated closely during the physical examination to provide clues to hematologic disorders, such as skin (for petechiae), eyes (for pallor, jaundice, and hemorrhage), and mouth (for mucosal bleeding). The examination should also search for sternal tenderness, lymphadenopathy, cardiac murmurs, splenomegaly, and hepatomegaly.[4,11] Jaundice is important for the assessment of anemia, because it may be due to increased RBC destruction, which suggests a hemolytic component to the anemia. Measuring vital signs is also a crucial component of the physical evaluation. Patients experiencing a rapid fall in hemoglobin concentration typically have tachycardia (fast heart rate), whereas if the anemia is long-standing, the heart rate may be normal due to the body's ability to compensate for the anemia (discussed below).

Moderate anemias (hemoglobin concentration of 7 to 10 g/dL) may cause pallor of conjunctivae and nail beds but may not produce clinical symptoms if the onset of anemia is slow.[4] However, depending on the patient's age and cardiovascular state, symptoms such as dyspnea, vertigo, headache, muscle weakness, and lethargy can occur.[4,8] Severe anemias (hemoglobin concentration of less than 7 g/dL) usually produce tachycardia, hypotension, and other symptoms of volume loss, in addition to the symptoms listed earlier. Thus, severity of the anemia is gauged by the degree of reduction in hemoglobin, cardiopulmonary adaptation, and the rapidity of progression of the anemia.[4]

PHYSIOLOGIC ADAPTATIONS

Anemia resulting from acute blood loss, such as with severe hemorrhage, can lead to profound changes in physiological processes that ensure adequate perfusion of vital organs and maintenance of homeostasis. In cases of severe blood loss, such as in trauma, blood volume decreases and hypotension develops, resulting in decreased blood supply to the brain and heart. As an immediate adaptation, there is sympathetic overdrive that results in increasing heart rate, respiratory rate, and cardiac output.[4,7,8] In severe anemia, blood is preferentially shunted to organs that are key to survival, including the brain, muscle, and heart.[4,7,8] This results in oxygen being preferentially supplied to vital organs even in the presence of reduced oxygen-carrying capacity. In addition, tissue hypoxia triggers an increase in RBC 2,3-bisphosphoglycerate that shifts the oxygen dissociation curve to the right (decreased oxygen affinity of hemoglobin) and results in increased delivery of oxygen to tissues (Chapter 10).[8,12] This is also a significant mechanism in chronic anemias that enables patients with low levels of hemoglobin to remain relatively asymptomatic. Thus with persistent anemia, the body develops physiologic adaptations to increase the oxygen-carrying capacity of a reduced amount of hemoglobin, which improves oxygen delivery to tissue. With persistent

---

BOX 19-1 Human Body Adaptations to Anemia

Anemia Caused by Sudden Loss of Blood Volume
The following adaptations occur in minutes to hours:
- Increase in heart rate, respiratory rate, and cardiac output
- Redistribution of blood flow from skin and viscera to heart, brain, and muscle

Anemia Caused by Slow Loss of Blood
The following adaptations occur over days to weeks:
- Decrease in hemoglobin-oxygen affinity by increasing the production of 2,3-bisphosphoglycerate
- Increase in erythropoietin production by kidneys

---

and severe anemia, however, the strain on the heart can ultimately lead to cardiac failure.

Reduced delivery of oxygen to tissues caused by reduced hemoglobin concentration elicits an increase in erythropoietin secretion by the kidneys. Erythropoietin stimulates the RBC precursors in the bone marrow, which leads to the release of more RBCs into the circulation[7,8] (Chapter 8).

It should be noted that with rapid blood loss, the hemoglobin and hematocrit may be initially unchanged because there is balanced loss of plasma and cells. However, as the drop in blood volume is compensated for by movement of fluid from the extravascular to the intravascular compartment or by administration of resuscitation fluid, there will be a dilution of RBCs and anemia. Box 19-1 summarizes the body's physiologic adaptations to anemia.

MECHANISMS OF ANEMIA

The life span of the RBC in the circulation is about 120 days. In a healthy individual with no anemia, each day, approximately 1% of the RBCs are removed from circulation due to senescence, but the bone marrow continuously produces RBCs to replace those lost. Hematopoietic stem cells differentiate into erythroid (RBC) precursor cells, and the bone marrow releases reticulocytes (immature anucleated RBCs) that mature into RBCs in the peripheral circulation. Adequate RBC production requires several nutritional factors such as iron, vitamin B_{12}, and folate. Globin (polypeptide chain) synthesis must also function normally. In conditions with excessive bleeding or hemolysis, the bone marrow must increase RBC production to compensate for the increased RBC loss. Therefore, the maintenance of a stable hemoglobin concentration requires the production of functionally normal RBCs in sufficient numbers to replace the amount lost.[4]

Ineffective and Insufficient Erythropoiesis

Erythropoiesis is the term used for marrow erythroid proliferative activity. Normal erythropoiesis occurs in the bone marrow and is under the control of the hormone *erythropoietin* (produced by the kidney) and other growth factors and cytokines (Chapters 7 and 8).[7,8] When erythropoiesis is effective, the bone marrow is able to produce functional RBCs that replace the daily loss of RBCs.

Ineffective erythropoiesis refers to the production of erythroid precursor cells that are defective. These defective precursors often undergo apoptosis (programmed cell death) in the bone marrow before they have a chance to mature to the reticulocyte stage and be released into the peripheral circulation. Several conditions, such as megaloblastic anemia (deficient DNA synthesis due to vitamin B_{12} or folate deficiency), thalassemia (deficient globin chain synthesis), and sideroblastic anemia (deficient protoporphyrin synthesis) involve ineffective erythropoiesis as a mechanism of anemia. In these anemias, the peripheral blood hemoglobin is low, which triggers an increase in erythropoietin leading to increased erythropoietic activity. Although the RBC production rate is high, it is ineffective in that many of the defective RBC precursors undergo destruction in the bone marrow. The end result is a decreased number of circulating RBCs resulting in anemia.[4,11]

Insufficient erythropoiesis refers to a decrease in the number of erythroid precursors in the bone marrow, resulting in decreased RBC production and anemia. Many factors can lead to the decreased RBC production, including a deficiency of iron (inadequate intake, malabsorption, excessive loss from chronic bleeding); a deficiency of erythropoietin (renal disease); or loss of the erythroid precursors due to an autoimmune reaction (aplastic anemia, acquired pure red cell aplasia) or infection (parvovirus B19). Infiltration of the bone marrow with granulomas (sarcoidosis) or malignant cells (acute leukemia) can also suppress erythropoiesis.[4,7]

Blood Loss and Hemolysis

Anemia can also develop as a result of acute blood loss (such as a traumatic injury) or chronic blood loss (such as an intermittently bleeding colonic polyp). Increased hemolysis results in a shortened RBC life span, thus increasing the risk for anemia. Chronic blood loss induces iron deficiency as a cause of anemia. With acute blood loss and excessive hemolysis, the bone marrow takes a few days to increase production of RBCs.[4,7,8] This response may be inadequate to compensate for a sudden excessive RBC loss as in traumatic hemorrhage or in conditions with a high rate of hemolysis and shortened RBC survival. Numerous causes of hemolysis exist, including intrinsic defects in the RBC membrane, enzyme systems, or hemoglobin, or extrinsic causes such as antibody-mediated processes, mechanical fragmentation, or infection-related destruction.[4,7,8]

LABORATORY DIAGNOSIS OF ANEMIA

Complete Blood Count with Red Blood Cell Indices

To detect the presence of anemia, the medical laboratory professional performs a complete blood count (CBC) using an automated hematology analyzer to determine the RBC count, hemoglobin concentration, hematocrit, RBC indices, white blood cell count, and platelet count. The RBC indices include the mean cell volume (MCV), mean cell hemoglobin (MCH), and mean cell hemoglobin concentration (MCHC) (Chapter 14).[13] The most important of these indices is the

MCV, a measure of the average RBC volume in femtoliters (fL). Reference intervals for these determinations are listed on the inside front cover of the text. Automated hematology analyzers also provide the red cell distribution width (RDW), an index of variation of cell volume in a red blood cell population (discussed below). A reticulocyte count should be performed for every patient with anemia. As with RBCs, automated analyzers provide accurate measurements of reticulocyte counts.

The RBC histogram provided by the automated analyzer is an RBC volume frequency distribution curve with the relative number of cells plotted on the ordinate and RBC volume (fL) on the abscissa. In healthy individuals, the distribution is approximately Gaussian. Abnormalities include a shift in the curve to the left (population of smaller cells or microcytosis) or to the right (larger cell population or macrocytosis). A widening of the curve caused by a greater variation of RBC volume about the mean can occur due to a population of RBCs with different volumes (anisocytosis). The histogram complements the peripheral blood film examination in identifying variable RBC populations. A discussion of histograms with examples can be found in Chapters 15 and 16.

The RDW is the coefficient of variation of RBC volume expressed as a percentage.[13] It indicates the variation in RBC volume within the population measured and an increased RDW correlates with anisocytosis on the peripheral blood film. Automated analyzers calculate the RDW by dividing the standard deviation of the RBC volume by the MCV and then multiplying by 100 to convert to a percentage. The usefulness of the RDW is discussed later.

Reticulocyte Count

The reticulocyte count serves as an important tool to assess the bone marrow's ability to increase RBC production in response to an anemia. Reticulocytes are young RBCs that lack a nucleus but still contain residual ribonucleic acid (RNA) to complete the production of hemoglobin. Normally, they circulate peripherally for only 1 day while completing their development. The adult reference interval for the reticulocyte count is 0.5% to 2.5% expressed as a percentage of the total number of RBCs.[13] The newborn reference interval is 1.5% to 6.0%, but these values change to approximately those of an adult within a few weeks after birth.[13] An absolute reticulocyte count is determined by multiplying the percent reticulocytes by the RBC count. The reference interval for the absolute reticulocyte count

is 20 to 115 $\times$ 10^9/L, based on an adult RBC count within the reference interval.[4,7] A patient with a severe anemia may seem to be producing increased numbers of reticulocytes if only the percentage is considered. For example, an adult patient with 1.5 $\times$ 10^{12}/L RBCs and 3% reticulocytes has an absolute reticulocyte count of 45 $\times$ 10^9/L. The percentage of reticulocytes is above the reference interval, but the absolute reticulocyte count is within the reference interval. For the degree of anemia, however, both of these results are inappropriately low. In other words, production of reticulocytes within the reference interval is inadequate to compensate for an RBC count that is approximately one third of normal.

Two successive corrections are made to the reticulocyte count to obtain a better representation of RBC production. First, to obtain a corrected reticulocyte count, one corrects for the degree of anemia by multiplying the reticulocyte percentage by the patient's hematocrit and dividing the result by 45 (the average normal hematocrit). If the reticulocytes are released prematurely from the bone marrow and remain in the circulation 2 to 3 days (instead of 1 day), the corrected reticulocyte count must be divided by maturation time to determine the reticulocyte production index (RPI) (Table 19-1). The RPI is a better indication of the rate of RBC production than is the corrected reticulocyte count.[4] The reticulocyte count and derivation of RPI is discussed in Chapter 14.

In addition, state-of-the-art automated hematology analyzers determine the fraction of immature reticulocytes among the total circulating reticulocytes, called the *immature reticulocyte fraction* (IRF). The IRF is helpful in assessing early bone marrow response after treatment for anemia and is covered in Chapter 15.

Analysis of the reticulocyte count plays a crucial role in determining whether an anemia is due to an RBC production defect or to premature hemolysis and shortened survival defect. If there is shortened RBC survival, as in the hemolytic anemias, the bone marrow tries to compensate by increasing RBC production to release more reticulocytes into the peripheral circulation. Although an increased reticulocyte count is a hallmark of the hemolytic anemias, it can also be observed over time in acute blood loss.[4,7,8] Chronic blood loss, on the other hand, does *not* lead to an appropriate increase in the reticulocyte count, but rather leads to iron deficiency and a subsequent low reticulocyte count. Thus an inappropriately low reticulocyte count results from decreased production of normal RBCs, due to either insufficient or ineffective erythropoiesis.

TABLE 19-1 Formulas for Reticulocyte Counts and Red Blood Cell Indices

Test	Formula	Adult Reference Interval
Absolute reticulocyte count ($\times$ 10^9/L)	= [reticulocytes (%)/100] $\times$ RBC count ($\times$ 10^{12}/L)	20–115 $\times$ 10^9/L
Corrected reticulocyte count (%)	= reticulocytes (%) $\times$ patient's HCT (%)/45	—
Reticulocyte production index (RPI)	= corrected reticulocyte count/maturation time	In anemic patients, RPI should be >3
Mean cell volume (MCV) (fL)	= HCT (%) $\times$ 10/RBC count ($\times$ 10^{12}/L)	80–100 fL
Mean cell hemoglobin (MCH) (pg)	= HGB (g/dL) $\times$ 10/RBC count ($\times$ 10^{12}/L)	26–32 pg
Mean cell hemoglobin concentration (MCHC) (g/dL)	= HGB (g/dL) $\times$ 100/HCT (%)	32–36 g/dL

HGB, Hemoglobin; *HCT*, hematocrit; *RBC*, red blood cell.

Peripheral Blood Film Examination

An important component in the evaluation of an anemia is examination of the peripheral blood film, with particular attention to RBC diameter, shape, color, and inclusions. The peripheral blood film also serves as a quality control to verify the results produced by automated analyzers. Normal RBCs on a Wright-stained blood film are nearly uniform, ranging from 6 to 8 μm in diameter. Small or microcytic cells are less than 6 μm in diameter, and large or macrocytic RBCs are greater than 8 μm in diameter. Certain shape abnormalities of diagnostic value (such as sickle cells, spherocytes, schistocytes, and oval macrocytes) and RBC inclusions (such as malarial parasites, basophilic stippling, and Howell-Jolly bodies) can be detected only by studying the RBCs on a peripheral blood film (Tables 19-2 and 19-3). Examples of abnormal shapes and inclusions are provided in Figure 19-1.

Finally, a review of the white blood cells and platelets may help show that a more generalized bone marrow problem is leading to the anemia. For example, hypersegmented neutrophils can be seen in vitamin B_{12} or folate deficiency, whereas blast cells and decreased platelets may be an indication of acute leukemia. Chapter 16 contains a complete discussion of

TABLE 19-2 Description of Red Blood Cell (RBC) Abnormalities and Commonly Associated Disease States

RBC Abnormality	Cell Description	Commonly Associated Disease States
Anisocytosis	Abnormal variation in RBC volume or diameter	Hemolytic, megaloblastic, iron deficiency anemia
Macrocyte	Large RBC (>8 μm in diameter), MCV >100 fL	Megaloblastic anemia
		Myelodysplastic syndrome
		Chronic liver disease
		Bone marrow failure
		Reticulocytosis
Oval macrocyte	Large oval RBC	Megaloblastic anemia
Microcyte	Small RBC (<6 μm in diameter), MCV <80 fL	Iron deficiency anemia
		Anemia of chronic inflammation
		Sideroblastic anemia
		Thalassemia/Hb E disease and trait
Poikilocytosis	Abnormal variation in RBC shape	Severe anemia; certain shapes helpful diagnostically
Spherocyte	Small, round, dense RBC with no central pallor	Hereditary spherocytosis
		Immune hemolytic anemia
		Extensive burns (along with schistocytes)
Elliptocyte, ovalocyte	Elliptical (cigar-shaped), oval (egg-shaped), RBC	Hereditary elliptocytosis or ovalocytosis
		Iron deficiency anemia
		Thalassemia major
		Myelophthisic anemias
Stomatocyte	RBC with slit-like area of central pallor	Hereditary stomatocytosis
		Rh deficiency syndrome
		Acquired stomatocytosis (liver disease, alcoholism)
		Artifact
Sickle cell	Thin, dense, elongated RBC pointed at each end; may be curved	Sickle cell anemia
		Sickle cell–β-thalassemia
Hb C crystal	Hexagonal crystal of dense hemoglobin formed within the RBC membrane	Hb C disease
Hb SC crystal	Fingerlike or quartz-like crystal of dense hemoglobin protruding from the RBC membrane	Hb SC disease
Target cell (codocyte)	RBC with hemoglobin concentrated in the center and around the periphery resembling a target	Liver disease
		Hemoglobinopathies
		Thalassemia
Schistocyte (schizocyte)	Fragmented RBC due to rupture in the peripheral circulation	Microangiopathic hemolytic anemia* (along with microspherocytes)
		Macroangiopathic hemolytic anemia**
		Extensive burns (along with microspherocytes)
Helmet cell (keratocyte)	RBC fragment in shape of a helmet	Same as schistocyte
Folded cell	RBC with membrane folded over	Hb C disease
		Hb SC disease
Acanthocyte (spur cell)	Small, dense RBC with few irregularly spaced projections of varying length	Severe liver disease (spur cell anemia)
		Neuroacanthocytosis (abetalipoproteinemia, McLeod syndrome)

TABLE 19-2 Description of Red Blood Cell (RBC) Abnormalities and Commonly Associated Disease States—cont'd

RBC Abnormality	Cell Description	Commonly Associated Disease States
Burr cell (echinocyte)	RBC with blunt or pointed, short projections that are usually evenly spaced over the surface of cell; present in all fields of blood film but in variable numbers per field[†]	Uremia Pyruvate kinase deficiency
Teardrop cell (dacryocyte)	RBC with a single pointed extension resembling a teardrop or pear	Primary myelofibrosis Myelophthisic anemia Thalassemia Megaloblastic anemia

Hb, Hemoglobin; *MCV,* mean cell volume.
*Such as thrombotic thrombocytopenic purpura, hemolytic uremic syndrome, disseminated intravascular coagulation.
**Such as traumatic cardiac hemolysis.
[†]Cells with similar morphology that are unevenly distributed in a blood film (not present in all fields) are likely due to a drying artifact in blood film preparation; these artifacts are sometimes called *crenated RBCs.*

TABLE 19-3 Erythrocyte Inclusions: Description, Composition, and Some Commonly Associated Disease States*

Inclusion	Appearance in Supravital Stain**	Appearance in Wright Stain	Inclusion Composed of	Associated Diseases/Conditions
Diffuse basophilia	Dark blue granules and filaments in cytoplasm (seen in reticulocytes)	Bluish tinge throughout cytoplasm; also called *polychromasia* (seen in polychromatic erythrocytes)	RNA	Hemolytic anemia After treatment for iron, vitamin B_{12}, or folate deficiency
Basophilic stippling	Dark blue-purple, fine or coarse punctate granules distributed throughout cytoplasm	Dark blue-purple, fine or coarse punctate granules distributed throughout cytoplasm	Precipitated RNA	Lead poisoning Thalassemia Hemoglobinopathies Megaloblastic anemia Myelodysplastic syndrome
Howell-Jolly body	Dark blue-purple dense, round granule; usually one per cell; occasionally multiple	Dark blue-purple dense, round granule; usually one per cell; occasionally multiple	DNA (nuclear fragment)	Hyposplenism Postsplenectomy Megaloblastic anemia Hemolytic anemia Thalassemia Myelodysplastic syndrome
Heinz body	Round, dark blue-purple granule attached to inner RBC membrane	Not visible	Denatured hemoglobin	Glucose-6-phosphate dehydrogenase deficiency Unstable hemoglobins Oxidant drugs/chemicals
Pappenheimer bodies***	Irregular clusters of small, light to dark blue granules, often near periphery of cell	Irregular clusters of small, light to dark blue granules, often near periphery of cell	Iron	Sideroblastic anemia Hemoglobinopathies Thalassemias Megaloblastic anemia Myelodysplastic syndrome Hyposplenism Post-splenectomy
Cabot ring	Rings or figure-eights	Blue rings or figure-eights	Remnant of mitotic spindle	Megaloblastic anemia Myelodysplastic syndromes
Hb H	Fine, evenly dispersed, dark blue granules; imparts "golf ball" appearance to RBCs	Not visible	Precipitate of β-globin chains of hemoglobin	Hb H disease

Hb, Hemoglobin.
*Inclusions of hemoglobin crystals (Hb S, Hb C, Hb SC) are covered in Table 19-2.
**Such as new methylene blue.
***Stain dark blue and are called *siderotic* granules when observed in Prussian blue stain.

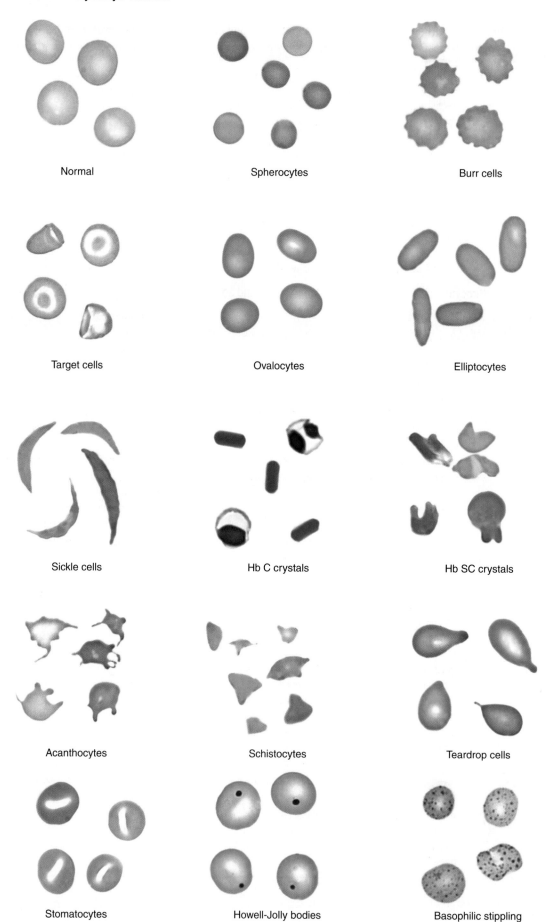

Normal

Spherocytes

Burr cells

Target cells

Ovalocytes

Elliptocytes

Sickle cells

Hb C crystals

Hb SC crystals

Acanthocytes

Schistocytes

Teardrop cells

Stomatocytes

Howell-Jolly bodies

Basophilic stippling

Figure 19-1 Red blood cells (RBCs): varied RBC shapes and inclusions. *Hb,* Hemoglobin. (Modified from Rodak BF, Carr JH: *Clinical hematology atlas,* ed 4, St Louis, 2013, Elsevier, Saunders.)

the peripheral blood film evaluation. Information from the blood film examination always complements the data from the automated hematology analyzer.

Bone Marrow Examination

The cause of many anemias can be determined from the history, physical examination, and results of laboratory tests on peripheral blood. When the cause cannot be determined, however, or the differential diagnosis remains broad, a bone marrow aspiration and biopsy may help in establishing the cause of anemia.[4,8] A bone marrow examination is indicated for a patient with an unexplained anemia associated with or without other cytopenias, fever of unknown origin, or suspected hematologic malignancy. A bone marrow examination evaluates hematopoiesis and can determine if there is an infiltration of abnormal cells into the bone marrow. Important findings in the bone marrow that can point to the underlying cause of the anemia include abnormal cellularity (e.g., hypocellularity in aplastic anemia); evidence of ineffective erythropoiesis and megaloblastic changes (e.g., folate/vitamin B_{12} deficiency or myelodysplastic syndrome); lack of iron on iron stains of the bone marrow (the gold standard for diagnosis of iron deficiency); and the presence of granulomata, fibrosis, infectious agents, and tumor cells that may be inhibiting normal erythropoiesis. Chapter 17 discusses bone marrow procedures and bone marrow examination in detail.

Other tests that can assist in the diagnosis of anemia can be performed on the bone marrow sample as well, including immunophenotyping of membrane antigens by flow cytometry (Chapter 32), cytogenetic studies (Chapter 30), and molecular analysis to detect specific genetic mutations and chromosome abnormalities in leukemia cells (Chapter 31).

Other Laboratory Tests

Other laboratory tests that can assist in establishing the cause of anemia include routine urinalysis (to detect hemoglobinuria or an increase in urobilinogen) with a microscopic examination (to detect hematuria or hemosiderin) and analysis of stool (to detect occult blood or intestinal parasites). Also, certain chemistry studies are very useful, such as serum haptoglobin, lactate dehydrogenase, and unconjugated bilirubin (to detect excessive hemolysis) and renal and hepatic function tests. With more patients having undergone gastric bypass surgery for obesity, certain rare deficiencies such as insufficient copper have become more common as another nutritional deficiency that can cause anemia.[14]

After the hematologic laboratory studies are completed, the anemia may be classified based on reticulocyte count, MCV, and peripheral blood film findings. Iron studies (including serum iron, total iron-binding capacity, transferrin saturation, and serum ferritin) are valuable if an inappropriately low reticulocyte count and a microcytic anemia are present. Serum vitamin B_{12} and serum folate assays are helpful in investigating a macrocytic anemia with a low reticulocyte count, whereas a direct antiglobulin test can differentiate autoimmune hemolytic anemias from hemolytic anemias due to other causes. Because of the numerous potential etiologies of anemia, the specific cause needs to be determined to initiate appropriate therapy.[11]

APPROACH TO EVALUATING ANEMIAS

The approach to the patient with anemia begins with taking a complete history and performing a physical examination.[4,7] For example, new-onset fatigue and shortness of breath suggest an acute drop in the hemoglobin concentration, whereas minimal or lack of symptoms suggests a long-standing condition where adaptive mechanisms have compensated for the drop in hemoglobin. A strict vegetarian may not be getting enough vitamin B_{12} in the diet, whereas an individual with alcoholism may not be getting enough folate. A large spleen may be an indication of hereditary spherocytosis, whereas a stool positive for occult blood may indicate iron deficiency. Thus a complete history and physical examination can yield information to narrow the possible cause or causes of the anemia and thus lead to a more rational and cost-effective approach to ordering the appropriate diagnostic tests.

The first step in the laboratory diagnosis of anemia is detecting its presence by the accurate measurement of the hemoglobin, hematocrit, MCV and RBC count and comparison of these values with the reference interval for healthy individuals of the same age, sex, race, and environment. Knowledge of previous hematologic values is valuable as a reduction of 10% or more in these values may be the first clue that an abnormal condition may be present.[4,6,15]

There are numerous causes of anemia, so a rational algorithm to initially evaluate this condition utilizing the above-mentioned tests is required. A reticulocyte count and a peripheral blood film examination are of paramount importance in evaluating anemia.

The remainder of this chapter discusses the importance of individual RBC measurements, the MCV, reticulocyte count, and RDW, and how they assist in classifying anemias so as to arrive at a specific diagnosis. Two widely used classification schemes for anemias relate to the morphology of red cells and the pathophysiological condition responsible for the patient's anemia.

Morphologic Classification of Anemia Based on Mean Cell Volume

The MCV is an extremely important tool and is key in the *morphologic classification* of anemia. *Microcytic anemia* is characterized by an MCV of less than 80 fL with small RBCs (less than 6 μm in diameter). Microcytosis is often associated with hypochromia, characterized by an increased central pallor in the RBCs and an MCHC of less than 32 g/dL. Microcytic anemias are caused by conditions that result in reduced hemoglobin synthesis. Heme synthesis is diminished in iron deficiency, iron sequestration (chronic inflammatory states), and defective protoporphyrin synthesis (sideroblastic anemia, lead poisoning). Globin chain synthesis is defective in thalassemia and in Hb E disease. Iron deficiency is the most common cause of microcytic anemia; the low iron level is insufficient for maintaining normal erythropoiesis. Although iron deficiency anemia is characterized by abnormal iron studies, the early stages of iron deficiency do not result in microcytosis or anemia and are manifested only by reduced iron stores. The causes of iron deficiency vary in infants, children, adolescents, and adults, and it is imperative to find the cause before beginning treatment (Chapter 20).

Macrocytic anemia is characterized by an MCV greater than 100 fL with large RBCs (greater than 8 μm in diameter). Macrocytic anemias arise from conditions that result in megaloblastic or nonmegaloblastic red cell development in the bone marrow. Megaloblastic anemias are caused by conditions that impair synthesis of deoxyribonucleic acid (DNA), such as vitamin B_{12} and folate deficiency or myelodysplasia. Nuclear maturation lags behind cytoplasmic development as a result of the impaired DNA synthesis. This asynchrony between nuclear and cytoplasmic development results in larger cells. All cells of the body are ultimately affected by the defective production of DNA (Chapter 21). Pernicious anemia is one cause of vitamin B_{12} deficiency, whereas malabsorption secondary to inflammatory bowel disease is one cause of folate deficiency. A megaloblastic anemia is characterized by oval macrocytes and hypersegmented neutrophils in the peripheral blood and by megaloblasts or large nucleated RBC precursors in the bone marrow. The MCV in megaloblastic anemia can be markedly increased (up to 150 fL), but modest increases (100 to 115 fL) occur as well.

Nonmegaloblastic forms of macrocytic anemias are also characterized by large RBCs, but in contrast to megaloblastic anemias, they are typically related to membrane changes owing to disruption of the cholesterol-to-phospholipid ratio. These macrocytic cells are mostly round, and the marrow nucleated RBCs do not display megaloblastic maturation changes. Macrocytic anemias are often seen in patients with chronic liver disease, alcohol abuse, and bone marrow failure. It is rare for the MCV to be greater than 115 fL in these nonmegaloblastic anemias.

Normocytic anemia is characterized by an MCV in the range of 80 to 100 fL. The RBC morphology on the peripheral blood film must be examined to rule out a dimorphic population of microcytes and macrocytes that can yield a normal MCV. The presence of a dimorphic population can also be verified by observing a bimodal distribution on the RBC histogram produced by an automated hematology analyzer (Chapters 15 and 16). Some normocytic anemias develop due to the premature destruction and shortened survival of RBCs (*hemolytic anemias*), and they are characterized by an elevated reticulocyte count. The hemolytic anemias can be further divided into those due to intrinsic causes (membrane defects, hemoglobinopathies, and enzyme deficiencies) and those due to extrinsic causes (immune and nonimmune RBC injury). A direct antiglobulin test helps differentiate immune-mediated destruction from the other causes. In the other hemolytic anemias, reviewing the peripheral blood film is vital for determining the cause of the hemolysis (Table 19-2, Table 19-3, and Figure 19-1). Hemolytic anemias are discussed in Chapters 23 to 26.

Other normocytic anemias develop due to a decreased production of RBCs and are characterized by a decreased reticulocyte count. Figure 19-2 presents an algorithm for initial morphologic classification of anemia based on the MCV.

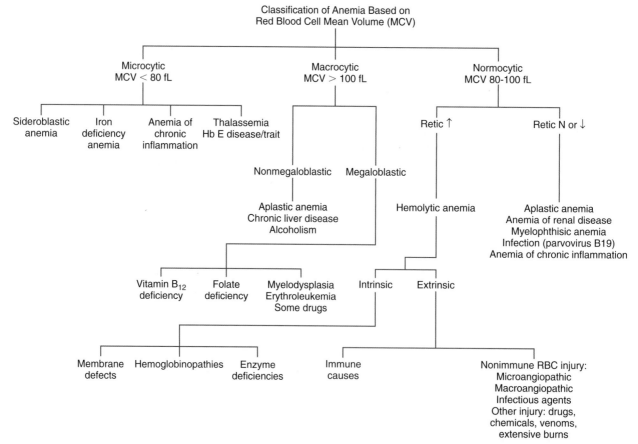

Figure 19-2 Algorithm for morphologic classification of anemia based on mean cell volume (MCV). Anemia of chronic liver disease is multifactorial and can be normocytic. ↑, Increased; ↓, decreased; *Hb,* hemoglobin; *N,* normal; *retic,* absolute reticulocyte count.

Morphologic Classification of Anemias and the Reticulocyte Count

The absolute reticulocyte count is useful in initially classifying anemias into the categories of decreased or ineffective RBC production (decreased reticulocyte count) and excessive RBC loss (increased reticulocyte count). Using the *morphologic classification* in the first category, when the reticulocyte count is decreased, the MCV can further classify the anemia into three subgroups: normocytic anemias, microcytic anemias, and macrocytic anemias. The excessive RBC loss category includes acute hemorrhage and the hemolytic anemias with shortened RBC survival. Figure 19-3 presents an algorithm that illustrates how anemias can be classified based on the absolute reticulocyte count and MCV.[4,7]

Morphologic Classification and the Red Blood Cell Distribution Width

The RDW can help determine the cause of an anemia when used in conjunction with the MCV. Each of the three MCV categories mentioned previously (normocytic, microcytic, macrocytic) can also be subclassified by the RDW as homogeneous (normal RDW) or heterogeneous (increased or high RDW), according to Bessman and colleagues.[7,16] For example, a decreased MCV with an increased RDW is suggestive of iron deficiency (Table 19-4). This classification is not absolute, however, because there can be an overlap of RDW values among some of the conditions in each MCV category.

Pathophysiologic Classification of Anemias and the Reticulocyte Count

In a *pathophysiologic classification* of anemia, related conditions are grouped by the mechanism causing the anemia. In this classification scheme, the anemias caused by decreased RBC production have inappropriately low reticulocyte counts (e.g., disorders of DNA synthesis and aplastic anemia) and are distinguished from other anemias caused by increased RBC destruction (intrinsic and extrinsic abnormalities of RBCs) or blood loss, which have increased reticulocyte counts. Some anemias have more than one pathophysiologic mechanism. Box 19-2 presents a pathophysiologic classification of anemia based on the causes of the abnormality and gives one or more examples of an anemia in each classification.

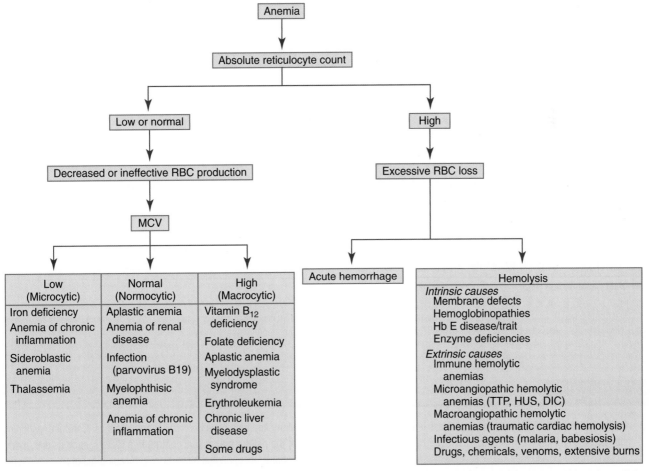

Figure 19-3 Algorithm for evaluating causes of anemia based on absolute reticulocyte count and mean cell volume (MCV). The list of anemias contains examples; there are numerous other causes not listed. Anemia of chronic liver disease is multifactorial and can be normocytic. *DIC,* Disseminated intravascular coagulation; *Hb,* hemoglobin; *HUS,* hemolytic uremic syndrome; *RBC,* red blood cell; *TTP,* thrombotic thrombocytopenic purpura.

TABLE 19-4 Morphologic Classification of Anemia Based on Red Blood Cell Mean Volume (MCV) and Red Blood Cell Distribution Width (RDW)*

	MEAN CELL VOLUME		
	Decreased	**Normal**	**Increased**
RDW Normal	α- or β-thalassemia trait	Anemia of chronic inflammation	Aplastic anemia
	Anemia of chronic inflammation	Anemia of renal disease	Chronic liver disease
	Hb E disease/trait	Acute hemorrhage	Alcoholism
		Hereditary spherocytosis	Chemotherapy
RDW Increased	Iron deficiency	Early iron, folate, or vitamin B_{12} deficiency	Folate or vitamin B_{12} deficiency
	Sickle cell–β-thalassemia	Mixed deficiency of iron + vitamin B_{12} or folate	Myelodysplastic syndrome
		Sickle cell anemia	Cold agglutinin disease
		Hb SC disease	Chronic liver disease
		Myelodysplastic syndrome	Chemotherapy

Hb, hemoglobin; *MCV*, mean cell volume; *RDW*, red blood cell distribution width.
*This classification scheme is not absolute because there can be overlap of RDW values among some of the conditions in each MCV category.
Modified from Bessman JD, Gilmer PR, Gardner FH: Improved classification of anemias by MCV and RDW, *Am J Clin Pathol* 80:324, 1983; and Marks PW: Approach to anemia in the adult and child. In Hoffman R, Benz EJ, Silberstein LE, et al, editors. *Hematology: basic principles and practice,* ed 6, Philadelphia, 2013, Elsevier, Saunders, p. 423.

BOX 19-2 Pathophysiologic Classification of Anemias

Anemia Caused by Decreased Production of Red Blood Cells
Hematopoietic stem cell failure: acquired and inherited aplastic anemia
Functional impairment of erythroid precursors:
- Disturbance of DNA synthesis: megaloblastic anemia
- Disturbance of hemoglobin synthesis: iron deficiency anemia, thalassemia, sideroblastic anemia, anemia of chronic inflammation
- Disturbance of proliferation and differentiation of erythroid precursors: anemia of renal failure, anemia associated with marrow infiltration

Anemia Caused by Increased Red Blood Cell Destruction or Loss
Intrinsic abnormality
- Membrane defect: hereditary spherocytosis, hereditary elliptocytosis, pyropoikilocytosis, paroxysmal nocturnal hemoglobinuria
- Enzyme deficiency: glucose-6-phosphate dehydrogenase deficiency, pyruvate kinase deficiency
- Globin abnormality: sickle cell anemia, other hemoglobinopathies
Extrinsic abnormality
- Immune causes: warm-type autoimmune hemolytic anemia, cold agglutinin disease, paroxysmal cold hemoglobinuria, hemolytic transfusion reaction, hemolytic disease of the fetus and newborn
- Nonimmune red blood cell injury: microangiopathic hemolytic anemia (thrombotic thrombocytopenic purpura, hemolytic uremic syndrome, HELLP syndrome, disseminated intravascular coagulation), macroangiopathic hemolytic anemia (traumatic cardiac hemolysis), infectious agents (malaria, babesiosis, bartonellosis, clostridial sepsis), other injury (chemicals, drugs, venoms, extensive burns)
- Blood loss: acute blood loss anemia

HELLP, Hemolysis, elevated liver enzymes, and low platelets syndrome.
The list of anemias is not all-inclusive; numerous other conditions are not listed.
Modified from Prchal JT: Clinical manifestations and classification of erythrocyte disorders. In Prchal JT, Kaushansky K, Lichtman MA, et al, editors: *Williams hematology,* ed 8, New York, 2010, McGraw-Hill. Available at: 6108487. Accessed September 28, 2013.

SUMMARY

- *Anemia* is defined conventionally as a decrease in RBCs, hemoglobin, and hematocrit below the reference interval for healthy individuals of the same age, sex, and race, under similar environmental conditions.
- Diagnosis of anemia is based on history, physical examination, symptoms, and laboratory test results.

- Many anemias have common manifestations. Careful questioning of the patient may reveal contributing factors, such as diet, medications, occupational hazards, and bleeding history.
- A thorough physical examination is valuable in determining the cause of anemia. Some of the areas that should be evaluated are

skin, nail beds, eyes, mucosa, lymph nodes, heart, and size of the spleen and liver.

- Moderate anemias (hemoglobin concentration between 7 and 10 g/dL) may not manifest clinical symptoms if the onset is slow. Severe anemias (hemoglobin concentration of less than 7 g/dL) usually produce pallor, dyspnea, vertigo, headache, weakness, lethargy, hypotension, and tachycardia.
- Laboratory procedures helpful in the initial diagnosis of anemia include the complete blood count (CBC) with RBC indices and the red blood cell distribution width (RDW), reticulocyte count, and examination of the peripheral blood film with emphasis on RBC morphology. Examination of a peripheral blood film is very important in the diagnosis of hemolytic anemias.
- Bone marrow examination is not usually required for diagnosis of anemia but is indicated in cases of unexplained anemia, fever of unknown origin, or suspected hematologic malignancy. Other tests are indicated based on the RBC indices, history, and physical examination, such as serum iron, total iron-binding capacity,

and serum ferritin (for microcytic anemias), and serum folate and vitamin B_{12} (for macrocytic anemias).

- The reticulocyte count and mean cell volume (MCV) play crucial roles in investigation of the cause of an anemia.
- The morphologic classification of anemias is based on the MCV and includes normocytic, microcytic, and macrocytic anemias. The MCV, when combined with the reticulocyte count and the RDW, also can aid in classification of anemia.
- Major subgroups of the pathophysiologic classification include anemias caused by decreased RBC production and those caused by increased RBC destruction or loss. Anemias may have more than one pathophysiologic cause.
- The cause of anemia should be determined before treatment is initiated.

Now that you have completed this chapter, go back and read again the case study at the beginning and respond to the questions presented.

REVIEW QUESTIONS

Answers can be found in the Appendix.

1. Which of the following patients would be considered anemic with a hemoglobin value of 14.5 g/dL? Refer to reference intervals inside the front cover of this text.
   a. An adult man
   b. An adult woman
   c. A newborn boy
   d. A 10-year-old girl

2. Common clinical symptoms of anemia include:
   a. Splenomegaly
   b. Shortness of breath and fatigue
   c. Chills and fever
   d. Jaundice and enlarged lymph nodes

3. Which of the following are important to consider in the in the patient's history when investigating the cause of an anemia?
   a. Diet and medications
   b. Occupation, hobbies, and travel
   c. Bleeding episodes in the patient or in his or her family members
   d. All of the above

4. Which one of the following is reduced as an adaptation to long-standing anemia?
   a. Heart rate
   b. Respiratory rate
   c. Oxygen affinity of hemoglobin
   d. Volume of blood ejected from the heart with each contraction

5. An autoimmune reaction destroys the hematopoietic stem cells in the bone marrow of a young adult patient, and the amount of active bone marrow, including RBC precursors, is diminished. The RBC precursors that are present are normal in appearance, but there are too few to meet the demand for circulating red blood cells, and anemia develops. The reticulocyte count is low. The mechanism of the anemia would be described as:
   a. Effective erythropoiesis
   b. Ineffective erythropoiesis
   c. Insufficient erythropoiesis

6. What are the *initial* laboratory tests that are performed for the diagnosis of anemia?
   a. CBC, iron studies, and reticulocyte count
   b. CBC, reticulocyte count, and peripheral blood film examination
   c. Reticulocyte count and serum iron, vitamin B_{12}, and folate assays
   d. Bone marrow study, iron studies, and peripheral blood film examination

7. An increase in which one of the following suggests a shortened life span of RBCs and hemolytic anemia?
   a. Hemoglobin
   b. Hematocrit
   c. Reticulocyte count
   d. Red cell distribution width

8. Which of the following is detectable only by examination of a peripheral blood film?
   a. Microcytosis
   b. Anisocytosis
   c. Hypochromia
   d. Poikilocytosis

9. Schistocytes, ovalocytes, and acanthocytes are examples of abnormal changes in RBC:
   a. Volume
   b. Shape
   c. Inclusions
   d. Hemoglobin concentration

10. Refer to Figure 19-3 to determine which one of the following conditions would be included in the differential diagnosis of an anemic adult patient with an absolute reticulocyte count of 20×10^9/L and an MCV of 65 fL.
    a. Aplastic anemia
    b. Sickle cell anemia
    c. Iron deficiency
    d. Folate deficiency

11. Which one of the following conditions would be included in the differential diagnosis of an anemic adult patient with an MCV of 125 fL and an RDW of 20% (reference interval 11.5% to 14.5%)? Refer to Table 19-4.
    a. Aplastic anemia
    b. Sickle cell anemia
    c. Iron deficiency
    d. Vitamin B_{12} deficiency

REFERENCES

1. Schecther, A. N. (2008). Hemoglobin research and the origins of molecular medicine. *Blood, 112*, 3927–3938.
2. *The American Heritage dictionary of the English language.* (4th ed.). (2001). Boston: Houghton Mifflin.
3. de Benoist, B., McLean, E., Egli, I., et al. (2008). *Worldwide prevalence of anaemia 1993-2005: WHO global database on anaemia*, Geneva, WHO Press. Retrieved from http://whqlibdoc.who.int/publications/2008/9789241596657_eng.pdf. Accessed 28.09.13.
4. Means, R. T., Jr., & Glader, B. (2009). Anemia: general considerations. In Greer, J. P., Foerster, J., Rodgers, G. M., et al. (Eds.), *Wintrobe's clinical hematology.* (12th ed., pp. 779–809). Philadelphia: Wolters Kluwer Health/Lippincott Williams & Wilkins.
5. Tefferi, A. (2003). Anemia in adults: a contemporary approach to diagnosis. *Mayo Clin Proc, 78*, 1274–1280.
6. Beutler, E., & Waalen, J. (2006). The definition of anemia: what is the lower limit of normal of the blood hemoglobin concentration? *Blood, 107*, 1747–1750.
7. Marks, P. W. (2013). Approach to anemia in the adult and child. In Hoffman, R., Benz, E. J., Jr., Silberstein, L. E., et al. (Eds.), *Hematology: basic principles and practice.* (6th ed., pp. 418–426). Philadelphia: Elsevier, Saunders.
8. Bunn, H. F. (2012). Approach to anemias. In Goldman, L., & Schafer, A. I. (Eds.), *Goldman's Cecil medicine.* (24th ed., pp. 1031–1039). Philadelphia: Elsevier, Saunders.
9. Irwin, J. J., & Kirchner, J. T. (2001). Anemia in children. *Am Fam Physician, 64*, 1379–1386.
10. Kettaneh, A., Eclache, V., Fain, O., et al. (2005). Pica and food craving in patients with iron-deficiency anemia: a case-control study in France. *Am J Med, 118*, 185–188.
11. Adamson, J. W., & Longo, D. L. (2012). Anemia and polycythemia. In Longo, D. L., Fauci, A. S., Kasper, D. L., et al. (Eds.), *Harrison's principles of internal medicine.* (18th ed.). New York: McGraw-Hill. http://www.accessmedicine.com/content.aspx?aID=9113377. Accessed 28.09.13.
12. Prchal, J. T. (2010). Chapter 33. Clinical manifestations and classification of erythrocyte disorders. In Prchal, J. T., Kaushansky, K., Lichtman, M. A., Kipps, T. J., & Seligsohn, U. (Eds.), *Williams Hematology.* (8th ed.). New York: McGraw-Hill. http://www.accessmedicine.com.libproxy2.umdnj.edu/content.aspx?aID=6108487. Accessed 14.11.13.
13. Perkins, S. L. (2009). Examination of the blood and bone marrow. In Greer, J. P., Foerster, J., Rodgers, G. M., et al. (Eds.), *Wintrobe's clinical hematology.* (12th ed., pp. 1–20). Philadelphia: Wolters Kluwer Health/Lippincott Williams & Wilkins.
14. Halfdanarson, T. R., Kumarm, N., Li, C. Y., et al. (2008). Hematologic manifestations of copper deficiency: a retrospective review. *Eur J Haemotol, 80*, 523–531.
15. Brill, J. R., & Baumgardner, D. J. (2000). Normocytic anemia. *Am Fam Physician, 62*, 2255–2263.
16. Bessman, J. D., Gilmer, P. R., & Gardner, F. H. (1983). Improved classification of anemia by MCV and RDW. *Am J Clin Pathol, 80*, 322–326.

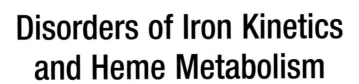

Disorders of Iron Kinetics and Heme Metabolism

20

Kathryn Doig

OBJECTIVES

After completion of this chapter, the reader should be able to:

1. Recognize complete blood count (CBC) results consistent with iron deficiency anemia, anemia of chronic inflammation, and sideroblastic anemias.
2. Given the results of classical iron studies, as well as free erythrocyte protoporphyrin (FEP), soluble transferrin receptor, hemoglobin content of reticulocytes, sTfR/log ferritin, and Thomas plots, distinguish findings consistent with iron deficiency anemia, latent iron deficiency, anemia of chronic inflammation, sideroblastic anemias, and iron overload conditions.
3. Recognize individuals at risk for iron deficiency anemia by virtue of age, gender, diet, physiologic circumstance such as pregnancy and menstruation, or pathologic conditions such as chronic gastrointestinal bleeding.
4. Given a description of a Wright-stained bone marrow smear and the appearance of bone marrow stained with Prussian blue stain, recognize results consistent with iron deficiency anemia, anemia of chronic inflammation, or a sideroblastic anemia.

5. Recognize clinical conditions that can predispose a patient to develop anemia of chronic inflammation.
6. Recognize predisposing factors for sideroblastic anemias or conditions in which sideroblastic anemias may develop.
7. Discuss the clinical significance of increased levels of FEP.
8. Describe the pathogenesis of iron deficiency anemia, anemia of chronic inflammation, sideroblastic anemia secondary to lead poisoning, and hemochromatosis, generically.
9. Discuss the differences in disease etiology, diagnosis, and treatment between iron overload resulting from hereditary forms of hemochromatosis and transfusion-related hemosiderosis.
10. Describe the etiology of the erythropoietic porphyrias, expected CBC picture, diagnostic metabolites, and clinical presentation.

CASE STUDY

After studying the material in this chapter, the reader should be able to respond to the following case study:

An 85-year-old slender, frail white woman was hospitalized for diagnosis and treatment of anemia suspected during a routine examination by her physician. The physician noted that she appeared pale and inquired about fatigue and tiredness. Although the patient generally felt well, she admitted to feeling slightly tired when climbing stairs. A point-of-care hemoglobin performed in the physician's office showed a dangerously low value of 3.5 g/dL, so the patient was hospitalized for further evaluation. Her hospital CBC results are as follows:

	Patient Value	Reference Intervals
WBCs ($\times 10^9$/L)	8.5	4.5–11
RBCs ($\times 10^{12}$/L)	1.66	4.3–5.9
HGB (g/dL)	3.0	13.9–16.3
HCT (%)	11.0	39–55

	Patient Value	Reference Intervals
MCV (fL)	66.3	80–100
MCH (pg)	18.1	26–32
MCHC (g/dL)	27.3	32–36
RDW (%)	20	11.5–14.5
Platelets ($\times 10^9$/L)	165.0	150–450
WBC differential	Unremarkable	
RBC morphology	Marked anisocytosis, marked poikilocytosis, marked hypochromia, marked microcytosis	

1. Using the systematic approach to interpretation of a CBC described in Chapters 16 and 19, describe the patient's blood picture.

Continued

GENERAL CONCEPTS IN ANEMIA

Anemia may result whenever red blood cell (RBC) production is impaired, RBC life span is shortened, or there is frank loss of cells. The anemias associated with iron and heme typically are categorized as anemias of impaired production resulting from the lack of raw materials for hemoglobin assembly. Depending on the cause, lack of available iron results in iron deficiency anemia or the anemia of chronic inflammation. Inadequate production of protoporphyrin leads to diminished production of heme and thus hemoglobin, but with a relative excess of iron. The result is sideroblastic anemia. These causes are discussed in this chapter. Inadequate globin production results in the thalassemias, which are discussed separately in Chapter 28.

As described more extensively in Chapter 11, iron is absorbed from the diet in the small intestine, carried by transferrin to a cell in need, and brought into the cell, where it is held as ferritin until incorporated into its final functional molecule. That functional molecule may be a heme-based cytochrome, muscle myoglobin, or, in the case of developing RBCs, hemoglobin. Iron may be unavailable for incorporation into heme because of inadequate stores of body iron or impaired mobilization. The anemia associated with inadequate stores is termed *iron deficiency anemia*, whereas the anemia resulting from impaired iron mobilization is known as *anemia of chronic inflammation* because of its association with chronic inflammatory conditions, such as rheumatoid arthritis. When the iron supply is adequate and mobilization is unimpaired but an RBC defect or impairment prevents production of protoporphyrin or incorporation of iron into it, the resulting anemia is termed *sideroblastic*, which refers to the presence of nonheme iron in the developing RBCs. One other form of anemia develops when the porphyrin component of hemoglobin is in short supply as with several of the porphyrias, diseases of impaired porphyrin production. Tests of body iron status are critical in diagnosis of these conditions, so the reader is referred to Chapter 11, where these tests are described in detail.

IRON DEFICIENCY ANEMIA

Etiology

Iron deficiency anemia develops when the intake of iron is inadequate to meet a standard level of demand, when the need for iron expands without compensated intake, when there is impaired absorption, or when there is chronic loss of hemoglobin from the body.

Inadequate Intake

Iron deficiency anemia can develop when the erythron is slowly starved for iron. Each day, approximately 1 mg of iron is lost from the body, mainly in the mitochondria of desquamated skin and sloughed intestinal epithelium.[1] Because the body tenaciously conserves all other iron from senescent cells, including RBCs, daily replacement of 1 mg of iron from the diet maintains iron balance and supplies the body's need for RBC production as long as there is no other source of loss. When the iron in the diet is consistently inadequate, over time the body's stores of iron become depleted. Ultimately, RBC production slows as a result of the inability to produce hemoglobin. With approximately 1% of cells dying naturally each day, the anemia becomes apparent when the production rate is insufficient for replacement of lost cells.

Increased Need

Iron deficiency can also develop when the level of iron intake is inadequate to meet the needs of an expanding erythron. This is the case in periods of rapid growth, such as infancy (especially in prematurity), childhood, and adolescence. For example, although both infants and adult men need about 1 mg/day of iron, that corresponds to a much higher amount per kilogram of body weight for the infant. Pregnancy and nursing place similar demands on the mother's body to provide iron for the developing fetus or nursing infant in addition to her own iron needs. In each of these instances, what had previously been an adequate intake of iron for the individual becomes inadequate as the need for iron increases.

Impaired Absorption

Even when the diet is adequate in iron, the inability to absorb that iron through the enterocyte into the blood over time will result in a deficiency of iron in the body. The impairments may be pathologic, as with malabsorption due to celiac disease. Others may be inherited mutations of iron regulatory proteins, like the mutations of the matriptase 2 protein (Chapter 11) that lead to a persistent production of hepcidin, causing ferroportin in the enterocyte to be inactivated, thus preventing iron absorption in the intestine.[2] In addition, diseases that decrease stomach acidity impair iron absorption by decreasing the capacity to reduce dietary ferric iron to the absorbable ferrous form. Some loss of acidity accompanies normal aging, but gastrectomy or bariatric surgeries can impair iron absorption dramatically. Medications such as antacids can inhibit absorption, and others may even bind the iron in the intestine, preventing its absorption.

Chronic Blood Loss

A fourth way iron deficiency develops is with chronic hemorrhage or hemolysis that results in the loss of small amounts of heme iron from the body over a prolonged period of time. Eventually anemia develops when the iron loss continually exceeds iron intake and the storage iron is exhausted. Excessive heme iron can be lost through chronic gastrointestinal bleeding from ulcers, gastritis due to alcohol or aspirin ingestion, tumors, parasitosis, diverticulitis, ulcerative colitis, or hemorrhoids. In women, prolonged menorrhagia (heavy menstrual bleeding) or conditions such as fibroid tumors or uterine malignancies can also lead to heme iron loss. Heme iron can also be lost excessively through the urinary tract with kidney stones, tumors, or chronic infections. Individuals with chronic intravascular hemolytic processes, such as paroxysmal nocturnal hemoglobinuria, can develop iron deficiency due to the loss of iron in hemoglobin passed into the urine.

Pathogenesis

Iron deficiency anemia develops slowly, progressing through stages that physiologically blend into one another but are useful delineations for understanding disease progression.[3] As shown in Figure 20-1, iron is distributed among three compartments: the storage compartment, principally as ferritin in the bone marrow macrophages and liver cells; the transport compartment of serum transferrin; and the functional compartment of hemoglobin, myoglobin, and cytochromes. Hemoglobin and intracellular ferritin and hemosiderin constitute nearly 90% of the total distribution of iron (Table 11-1).

For a period of time as an increase in demand or increased loss of iron exceeds iron intake, essentially normal iron status continues. The body strives to maintain iron balance by accelerating absorption of iron from the intestine through a decrease in the production of hepcidin in the liver. This state of declining body iron with increased absorption is not apparent in routine laboratory test results or patient symptoms. The individual appears healthy. As the negative iron balance continues, however, a stage of iron depletion develops.

Stage 1

Stage 1 of iron deficiency is characterized by a progressive loss of storage iron. RBC development is normal, however, because the body's reserve of iron is sufficient to maintain the transport and functional compartments through this phase. There is no evidence of iron deficiency in the peripheral blood because RBCs survive 120 days, and the patient does not experience symptoms of anemia. Serum ferritin levels are low, however, which indicates the decline in stored iron, and this also could

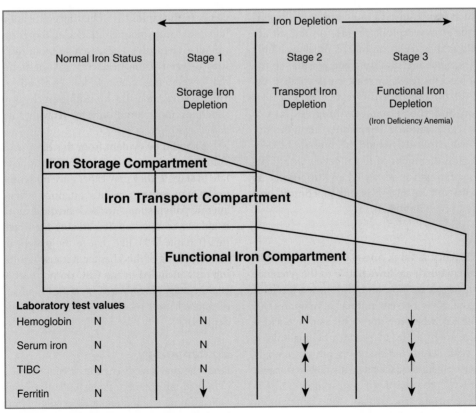

Figure 20-1 Development of iron deficiency anemia. ↑ Increased; ↓, decreased; *N*, normal; *TIBC*, total iron-binding capacity. (Adapted from Suominen P, Punnonen K, Rajamäki A, et al: Serum transferrin receptor and transferrin receptor–ferritin index identify healthy subjects with subclinical iron deficits, Blood 92:2934–2939, 1998; reprinted with permission.)

be detected in an iron stain of the bone marrow. Without evidence of anemia, however, these tests would not be performed because individuals appear healthy. The prevalence of stage 1 iron deficiency in the United States has been estimated at 14.4% for 1- to 2-year-olds, 3.7% for 3- to 5-year-olds, 9.3% for 12- to 19-year-old females, and 9.2% for 20- to 49-year-old females.[4] This stage is sometimes called latent or subclinical iron deficiency because the iron stores are inadequate but the hemoglobin value remains normal, and thus the deficiency is unlikely to be recognized.

Stage 2

Stage 2 of iron deficiency is defined by the exhaustion of the storage pool of iron (Figure 20-1). For a time, RBC production continues as normal, relying on the iron available in the transport compartment. Quickly the hemoglobin content of reticulocytes begins to decrease, which reflects the onset of iron deficient erythropoiesis, but because the bulk of the circulating RBCs were produced during the period of adequate iron availability, the overall hemoglobin measurement is still normal. Thus anemia is still not evident, although an individual's hemoglobin may begin dropping, and the RBC distribution width (RDW) may begin increasing as some smaller RBCs are released from the bone marrow. Other iron-dependent tissues, such as muscles, may begin to be affected, although the symptoms may be nonspecific. The serum iron and serum ferritin levels decrease, whereas total iron-binding capacity (TIBC), an indirect measure of transferrin, increases. Free erythrocyte protoporphyrin (FEP), the porphyrin into which iron is inserted to form heme, begins to accumulate. Transferrin receptors increase on the surface of iron-starved cells as they try to capture as much available iron as possible. They also are shed into the plasma, so the soluble transferrin receptor levels increase measurably. Prussian blue stain of the bone marrow in stage 2 shows essentially no stored iron, and iron deficient erythropoiesis is evident (subsequent description). Hepcidin, though not commonly measured clinically, would be measurably decreased. The hemoglobin content of reticulocytes would begin to drop, demonstrating iron-restricted erythropoiesis. As in stage 1, iron deficiency in stage 2 is still subclinical, and testing is not likely to be undertaken.

Stage 3

Stage 3 of iron deficiency is frank anemia. The hemoglobin concentration and hematocrit are low relative to the reference intervals. Depletion of storage iron and diminished levels of transport iron (Figure 20-1) prevent normal development of RBC precursors. The RBCs become microcytic and hypochromic (Figure 20-2) as their ability to produce hemoglobin is restricted. As expected, serum ferritin levels are exceedingly low. Results of other iron studies (see later) are also abnormal, and the free erythrocyte protoporphyrin and soluble transferrin receptor levels continue to increase. The hemoglobin content of reticulocytes will continue to drop. If measured, erythropoietin would be elevated, while hepcidin would be decreased.

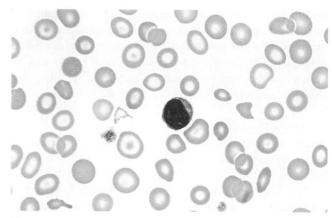

Figure 20-2 Peripheral blood film from a patient with hypochromic, microcytic anemia. Note the variation in red blood cell (RBC) diameters compared to the lymphocyte's nuclear diameter. Variation in RBC diameters is termed *anisocytosis* and corresponds to an elevated RBC distribution width (RDW), a measure of variation in RBC volume. Hypochromia, microcytosis, and an elevated RDW may indicate iron deficiency anemia. Several target cells are seen.

In this phase, the patient experiences the nonspecific symptoms of anemia, typically fatigue, weakness, and shortness of breath, especially with exertion. Pallor is evident in light-skinned individuals but also can be noted in the conjunctivae, mucous membranes, or palmar creases of dark-skinned individuals. More severe signs are not seen as often in the United States[5] but include a sore tongue (glossitis) due to iron deficiency in the rapidly proliferating epithelial cells of the alimentary tract and inflamed cracks at the corners of the mouth (angular cheilosis). Koilonychia (spooning of the fingernails) may be seen if the deficiency is long-standing. Patients also may experience cravings for nonfood items, called *pica*. The cravings may be for things such as dirt, clay, laundry starch, or, most commonly, ice (craving for the latter is called *pagophagia*).[5]

As should be evident from this discussion, numerous individuals may be iron deficient while appearing healthy. Until late in stage 2, they may experience no symptoms at all and are unlikely to come to medical attention. Even in stage 3, frankly anemic patients may not seek medical care, because the body is able to compensate remarkably for slowly developing anemia (Chapter 19), like that in the patient in the case study at the beginning of this chapter. Because results of routine screening tests included in the CBC do not become abnormal until late in stage 2 or early in stage 3, most patients are not diagnosed until relatively late in the progression of the iron depletion.

Epidemiology

From the previous discussion, it is apparent that certain groups of individuals are more prone to develop iron deficiency anemia. Menstruating women are at especially high risk. Their monthly loss of blood increases their routine need for iron, which often is not met with the standard U.S. diet.[5] For adolescent girls, this is compounded by increased iron needs associated with growth. If women of childbearing age do not receive proper iron supplementation, pregnancy and nursing can lead to a loss of nearly 900 mg of iron,[6] which further depletes iron stores. Succeeding pregnancies can exacerbate the problem, leading to iron deficient fetuses.[6]

Growing children also are at high risk. Growth requires iron for the cytochromes of all new cells, myoglobin for new muscle cells, and hemoglobin in the additional RBCs needed to supply oxygen for a larger body. The increasing need for iron as the child grows can be coupled with dietary inadequacies, especially in circumstances of poverty or neglect. Cow's milk is not a good source of iron, and infants need to be placed on iron-supplemented formula by about age 6 months, when their fetal stores of iron become depleted.[5] This assumes that the infants were able to establish adequate iron stores by drawing iron from their mothers in utero. Even though breast milk is a better source of iron than cow's milk,[7] it is not a consistent source.[8] Therefore, iron supplementation is also recommended for breastfed infants after 6 months of age.[5]

Iron deficiency is relatively rare in men and postmenopausal women because the body conserves iron so tenaciously, and these individuals lose only about 1 mg/day. Gastrointestinal disease, such as ulcers, tumors, or hemorrhoids, should be suspected in iron deficient patients in either of these groups if the diet is known to be adequate in iron. Regular aspirin ingestion and alcohol consumption can lead to gastritis and chronic bleeding. Elderly individuals, particularly those living alone, may not eat a balanced diet, so pure dietary deficiency is seen among these individuals. In some elderly individuals, the loss of gastric acidity with age can impair iron absorption. Iron deficiency is associated with infection by hookworms, *Necator americanus* and *Ancylostoma duodenale*. The worm attaches to the intestinal wall and literally sucks blood from the gastric vessels. Iron deficiency is also associated with infection with other parasites, such as *Trichuris trichiura*, *Schistosoma mansoni*, and *Schistosoma haematobium*, in which the heme iron is lost from the body due to intestinal or urinary bleeding.

Soldiers subjected to prolonged maneuvers and long-distance runners also can develop iron deficiency. Exercise-induced hemoglobinuria, also called march hemoglobinuria, develops when RBCs are hemolyzed by foot-pounding trauma and iron is lost as hemoglobin in the urine.[9] The amount lost in the urine can be so little that it is not apparent on visual inspection of the urine. Nevertheless, in rare cases, the cumulative iron loss can lead to anemia if the foot-pounding trauma is recurrent and especially severe.

Laboratory Diagnosis

Iron deficiency can be readily diagnosed in later stages using routine tests. Detection in the early stages requires sophisticated tests, but individuals are unlikely to be referred for such studies because there is virtually no physiologic evidence of the declining iron state. Nevertheless, early iron deficiency might be suspected in an individual in a high-risk group, and appropriate testing can be ordered.[9] The tests for iron deficiency can be grouped into three general categories: screening, diagnostic,

and specialized. The principles are discussed in more detail in Chapter 11.

Screening for Iron Deficiency Anemia

When iron deficient erythropoiesis is under way, the CBC results begin to show evidence of anisocytosis, microcytosis, and hypochromia (Figure 20-2). The classic picture of iron deficiency anemia in stage 3 includes a decreased hemoglobin level. An RDW greater than 15% is expected and may precede the decrease in hemoglobin.[10] For patients in high-risk groups, the elevated RDW can be an early and sensitive indicator of iron deficiency that is provided in a routine CBC.[11] As the hemoglobin level continues to fall, microcytosis and hypochromia become more prominent, with progressively declining values for mean cell volume (MCV), mean cell hemoglobin (MCH), and mean cell hemoglobin concentration (MCHC). The RBC count ultimately becomes decreased, as does the hematocrit. Polychromasia may be apparent early, although it is not a prominent finding. A low absolute reticulocyte count confirms a diminished rate of effective erythropoiesis because this is a nonregenerative anemia.[12] Poikilocytosis, including occasional target cells and elliptocytes, may be present, although no particular shape is characteristic or predominant. Thrombocytosis may be present, particularly if the iron deficiency results from chronic bleeding, but this is not a diagnostic parameter. White blood cells (WBCs) are typically normal in number and appearance. Iron deficiency should be suspected when the CBC findings show a hypochromic, microcytic anemia with an elevated RDW but no consistent shape changes to the RBCs.

Diagnosis of Iron Deficiency

Iron studies remain the backbone for diagnosis of iron deficiency. They include assays of serum iron, total iron-binding capacity (TIBC), transferrin saturation, and serum ferritin; Chapter 11 covers the principle of each assay and technical considerations affecting test performance and interpretation. Serum iron is a measure of the amount of iron bound to transferrin (transport protein) in the serum. TIBC is an indirect measure of transferrin and the available binding sites for iron in the plasma. The percent of transferrin saturated with iron can be calculated from the total iron and the TIBC:

$$\text{Transferrin saturation (\% sat)} = \frac{\text{serum iron (μg/dL)} \times 100}{\text{TIBC (μg/dL)}}$$

Ferritin is not truly an extracellular protein because it provides an intracellular storage repository for metabolically active iron. However, ferritin is present in serum, and serum levels reflect the levels of iron stored within cells. Serum ferritin is an easily accessible surrogate for stainable bone marrow iron. The iron studies are used collectively to assess the iron status of an individual. Table 20-1 shows that, as expected, serum ferritin and serum iron values are decreased in iron deficiency anemia, a state called sideropenia. Transferrin levels increase when the hepatocytes detect low iron levels, and research shows that this is a transcriptional and posttranslational response to low iron levels.[13] The result is a decline in the iron

TABLE 20-1 Results of Iron Studies in Microcytic, Hypochromic Anemias

	Iron Deficiency	Thalassemia Minor	Anemia of Chronic Inflammation	Sideroblastic Anemia	Lead Poisoning
Serum ferritin	↓	↑/N	↑/N	↑	N
Serum iron	↓/N	↑/N	↓	↑	Variable
TIBC	↑	N	↓	↓/N	N
Transferrin saturation	↓	↑/N	↓/N	↑	↑
FEP/ZPP	↑	N	↑	↑	↑ (marked)
BM iron (Prussian blue reaction)	No stainable iron	↑/N	↑/N	↑	N
Sideroblasts in BM	None	N	None/very few	↑ (ring)	N (ring)
Other special tests		↑ Hb A₂ (β-thalassemia minor)	Specific tests for inflammatory disorders or cancer		↑ ALA in urine ↑ Whole-blood lead levels

↑, Increased; ↓, decreased; *ALA*, aminolevulinic acid; *BM*, bone marrow; *FEP/ZPP*, free erythrocyte protoporphyrin/zinc protoporphyrin; *Hb*, hemoglobin; *N*, normal.

saturation of transferrin that is more dramatic than might be expected simply from the decrease in serum iron level.

The amount of hemoglobin in reticulocytes can be assessed on some automated hematology analyzers (Chapter 15).[14] The hemoglobin content of reticulocytes is analogous to the MCH, but for reticulocytes only. The MCH is the average weight of hemoglobin per cell across the entire RBC population. Some of the RBCs are nearly 120 days old, whereas others are just 1 to 2 days old. If iron deficiency is developing, the MCH does not change until a substantial proportion of the cells are iron deficient, and the diagnosis is effectively delayed for weeks or months after iron deficient erythropoiesis begins. Measuring the hemoglobin content of reticulocytes enables detection of iron-restricted erythropoiesis within days as the first iron deficient cells leave the bone marrow. It is a sensitive indicator of iron deficiency. Even in stage 2 of iron deficiency, before anemia is apparent, the hemoglobin content of reticulocytes will be low.[14]

Specialized Tests

Other tests, although not commonly used for the diagnosis of iron deficiency, show abnormalities that become important in the differential diagnosis of similar conditions. Test results for the accumulated porphyrin precursors to heme are elevated (Table 20-1). Free erythrocyte protoporphyrin accumulates when iron is unavailable. In the absence of iron, free erythrocyte protoporphyrin may be preferentially chelated with zinc to form zinc protoporphyrin (ZPP).[15] The FEP and zinc chelate can be assayed fluorometrically, although they are not particularly valuable in the diagnosis of iron deficiency. Soluble transferrin receptors (sTfR) also can be assayed using immunoassay. Levels increase as the disease progresses, and individual cells seek to take in as much iron as possible.[16]

A bone marrow assessment is not indicated for suspected uncomplicated iron deficiency. A therapeutic trial of iron (see Response to Treatment) provides a less invasive and less expensive diagnostic assessment. However, marrow examination for iron is routinely performed when a bone marrow sample is indicated for other reasons. With routine stains, the iron deficient bone marrow appears hyperplastic early in the progression of the disease, with a decreased myeloid-to-erythroid ratio as a result of increased erythropoiesis.[5] As the disease progresses, hyperplasia subsides, and the profound deficiency of iron leads to slowed RBC production. Polychromatic normoblasts (i.e., rubricytes) show the most dramatic morphologic changes (Figure 20-3). Nuclear-cytoplasmic asynchrony is evident, with cytoplasmic maturation lagging behind nuclear maturation. Without the pink provided by hemoglobin, the cytoplasm remains bluish after the nucleus has begun to condense. The cell membranes appear irregular and are usually described as "shaggy."

Treatment and Its Effects
Treatment

The first therapy for iron deficiency is to treat any underlying contributing cause, such as hookworms, tumors, or ulcers. As in the treatment of simple nutritional deficiencies or increased need, dietary supplementation is necessary to replenish the body's iron stores. Oral supplements of ferrous sulfate (3 tablets/day

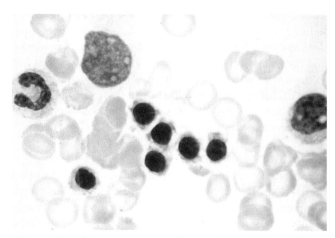

Figure 20-3 Bone marrow smear from a patient with iron deficiency anemia. The late-nucleated red blood cells show the characteristic "shaggy" blue cytoplasm due to asynchrony in maturation (×1000). (Courtesy Ann Bell, University of Tennessee, Memphis.)

containing 65 mg of elemental iron) are the standard prescription.[5] The supplements should be taken on an empty stomach to maximize absorption. Many patients experience side effects such as nausea and constipation, however, which leads to poor patient compliance. Vigilance on the part of the health care providers is important to ensure that patients complete the course of iron replacement, which usually lasts 6 months or longer.[17] In rare cases in which intestinal absorption of iron is impaired (for example, in conditions like gastric achlorhydria, celiac disease, or with mutations like those in matriptase-2) parenteral administration of iron dextrans can be used, although the side effects of this therapy are notable.[5] Because of the risks associated with red blood cell transfusions, they are rarely warranted for the correction of uncomplicated iron deficiency unless the patient's hemoglobin level has become dangerously low, like the patient in this chapter's case study.

Response to Treatment

When optimal treatment with iron is initiated, the effects are quickly evident. Reticulocyte hemoglobin content will correct within 2 days.[14] Reticulocyte counts (relative and absolute) begin to increase within 5 to 10 days.[17] The anticipated rise in hemoglobin appears in 2 to 3 weeks, and levels should return to normal for the individual by about 2 months after the initiation of adequate treatment.[18] The peripheral blood film and indices still reflect the microcytic RBC population for several months, with a biphasic population including the younger normocytic cells. The normocytic population eventually predominates. Iron therapy must continue for another 3 to 4 months to replenish the storage pool and prevent a relapse.

It is common and reasonable for care providers to assume that iron deficiency is due to dietary deficiency because that is the case in most instances of iron deficiency. Thus supplementation should correct it. If the patient has been adherent to the therapeutic regimen, the failure to respond to iron treatment points to the need for further investigation. The patient may be experiencing continued occult loss of blood or inadequate absorption, justifying additional diagnostics. Alternatively, causes of hypochromic, microcytic anemia unrelated to iron deficiency, such as thalassemia, should be considered.

ANEMIA OF CHRONIC INFLAMMATION

Anemia is commonly associated with systemic diseases, including chronic inflammatory conditions such as rheumatoid arthritis, chronic infections such as tuberculosis or human immunodeficiency virus infection, and malignancies. Cartwright[19] was the first to suggest that although the underlying diseases seem quite disparate, the associated anemia may be from a single cause, proposing the concept of anemia of chronic disease. This anemia represents the most common anemia among hospitalized patients.[20]

Etiology

Although the anemia associated with chronic systemic disorders was originally called *anemia of chronic disease*, chronic blood loss is not among the conditions leading to the anemia of chronic disease. Chronic blood loss results in clear-cut iron deficiency. Anemia of chronic disease is more correctly termed *anemia of chronic inflammation* (ACI), because inflammation is the unifying factor among the three aforementioned general types of conditions in which this anemia is seen. The central feature of anemia of chronic inflammation is sideropenia in the face of abundant iron stores. The cause is now understood to be largely impaired ferrokinetics.

The apparent inconsistency of decreased serum iron but abundant iron stores is explained by the role of hepcidin in regulation of body iron (Chapter 11). Hepcidin is a hormone produced by hepatocytes to regulate body iron levels, particularly absorption of iron in the intestine and release of iron from macrophages. Hepcidin interacts with and causes the degradation of the transmembrane protein ferroportin, which exports iron from enterocytes into the plasma, reducing the amount of iron absorbed into the blood from the intestine.[21] Macrophages and hepatocytes also use ferroportin to export iron into plasma and are affected by hepcidin.[21,22] When systemic body iron levels decrease, hepcidin production by hepatocytes decreases,[23] and enterocytes export more iron into the plasma. Macrophage and hepatocyte release of iron also increases. When systemic iron levels are high, hepcidin increases, enterocytes export less iron into the plasma, and macrophages and hepatocytes retain iron.

Hepcidin is an acute phase reactant.[24] During inflammation, the liver increases the synthesis of hepcidin in response to interleukin-6 produced by activated macrophages. This increase occurs regardless of systemic iron levels in the body. As a result, during inflammation, there is a decrease in iron absorption from the intestine and iron release from macrophages and hepatocytes (Figure 20-4). Although there is plenty of iron in the body, it is unavailable to developing RBCs because it is sequestered in the macrophages and hepatocytes.

This response of hepcidin during inflammation is likely a nonspecific defense against invading bacteria. If the body can sequester iron, it reduces the amount of iron available to bacteria and contributes to their demise. Although this response of hepcidin is not harmful during disorders of short duration, chronically high levels of hepcidin sequester iron for long periods, which leads to diminished production of RBCs.

A second acute phase reactant seems to contribute to anemia of chronic inflammation, although probably to a much smaller extent than hepcidin. Lactoferrin is an iron-binding protein in the granules of neutrophils. Its avidity for iron is greater than that of transferrin. Lactoferrin is important intracellularly for phagocytes to prevent phagocytized bacteria from using intracellular iron for their metabolic processes.[25] During infection and inflammation, however, neutrophil lactoferrin also is released into the plasma. There it scavenges available iron, at the expense of transferrin. When it is carrying iron, the lactoferrin becomes bound to macrophages and liver cells that salvage the iron. RBCs are deprived of this source of plasma iron, however, because they do not have lactoferrin receptors.

Finally, a third acute phase reactant, ferritin, contributes to the anemia of chronic inflammation. Increased levels of

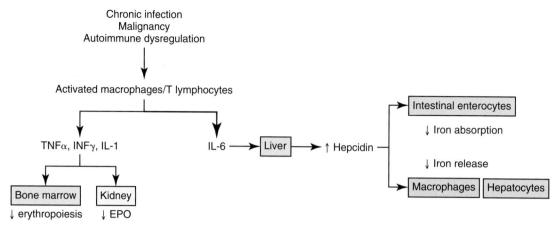

Figure 20-4 Mechanisms of anemia in chronic inflammatory conditions. Chronic infections (bacterial, viral, parasitic, or fungal), malignancy, or autoimmune dysregulation result in the release of inflammatory cytokines from activated macrophages and T lymphocytes. Interleukin-6 (IL-6) promotes liver production of hepcidin, an acute phase reactant that impairs iron absorption in intestinal enterocytes and iron release from macrophages and hepatocytes. Inflammatory cytokines, such as tumor necrosis factor-α (TNF-α), interleukin-1 (IL-1), and interferon-γ (INF-γ), also inhibit erythropoiesis and decrease erythropoietin (EPO) production by the kidney. Although these latter mechanisms contribute to the anemia of chronic inflammation, the hepcidin-induced inhibition of intestinal iron absorption and iron release from storage sites in macrophages and hepatocytes is the more significant cause of the anemia. (Adapted from Weiss G, Goodnough LT. Anemia of chronic disease. N Eng J Med 352, 2005, p. 1013.)

ferritin in the plasma also bind some iron. Because developing RBCs do not have a ferritin receptor, this iron is also unavailable for incorporation into hemoglobin.

The result of these effects is that although iron is present in abundance in bone marrow macrophages, its release to developing erythrocytes is slowed. This can be seen histologically with iron stains that show iron in macrophages but not in erythroblasts (Figure 17-14, *C*).[26] The effect on the developing RBCs is essentially no different from that in mild iron deficiency because they are effectively deprived of the iron. Like iron deficiency anemia, this is iron-restricted erythropoiesis.

Production of inflammatory cytokines (such as tissue necrosis factor-α and interleukin-1 from activated macrophages and interferon-γ from activated T-cells) also impairs proliferation of erythroid progenitor cells, diminishes their response to erythropoietin, and decreases production of erythropoietin by the kidney (Figure 20-4).[27] Although these mechanisms contribute to the anemia of chronic inflammation, the impaired ferrokinetics is the more significant cause of the anemia.

Laboratory Diagnosis

The peripheral blood picture in anemia of chronic inflammation is that of a mild anemia, with hemoglobin concentration usually 8 to 10 g/dL and without reticulocytosis. The cells are usually normocytic and normochromic, although microcytosis and hypochromia develop in about one third of patients and may represent coexistent iron deficiency.[28] The inflammatory condition leading to the anemia also may cause leukocytosis, thrombocytosis, or both. Iron studies (Table 20-1) show low serum iron and TIBC values. Because hepatocyte production of transferrin is regulated by intracellular iron levels, the low TIBC (an indirect measure of transferrin) reflects the abundant iron stores in the body. The transferrin saturation may be normal or low. The serum ferritin level is usually

increased beyond the value that would be expected for the same patient in the absence of the inflammatory condition. It may not be outside the reference interval, but it is nevertheless increased. The failure to incorporate iron into heme results in elevation of free erythrocyte protoporphyrin, although this test typically is not used diagnostically. The hemoglobin content of reticulocytes will be decreased, reflecting the iron restricted hematopoiesis, but the soluble transferrin receptor will be normal, reflecting normal intracellular iron. The bone marrow shows hypoproliferation of the RBCs, consistent with the lack of reticulocytes in the peripheral blood. Prussian blue stain of the bone marrow confirms abundant stores of iron in macrophages, although not in RBC precursors, but bone marrow examination is not usually required in the diagnostic evaluation.

Patients with iron deficiency anemia who have an inflammatory condition present a special diagnostic dilemma. The iron deficiency may be missed because of the increase in serum ferritin levels associated with the inflammation. Serum ferritin values generally in the 30 to 100 ng/mL range are most equivocal.[27] Iron deficiency anemia and anemia of chronic inflammation may be distinguished in such situations, or their coexistence can be verified, by measuring soluble transferrin receptors (sTfRs) in the serum.[29] These receptors are sloughed from cells into the plasma. As noted earlier, levels increase during iron deficiency anemia but remain essentially normal during anemia of chronic inflammation.

Additional modifications to the use of the sTfR have been developed to better distinguish iron deficiency, latent iron deficiency, and ACI. The principles of these assays and calculations are discussed in Chapter 11 and the measurement of the hemoglobin content of reticulocytes is discussed in Chapter 15. It is expected that the sTfR/log ferritin will rise most dramatically in iron deficiency as the numerator rises and the denominator falls; in ACI, both remain essentially normal, and thus a normal

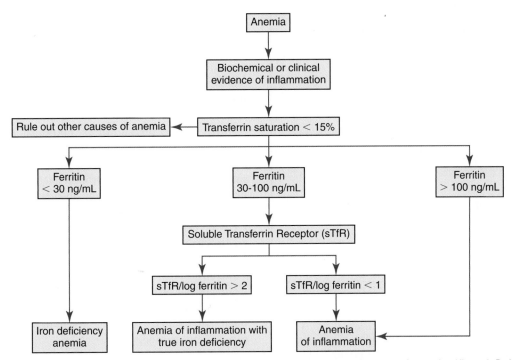

Figure 20-5 Algorithm for diagnosis and differentiation of iron deficiency anemia and the anemia of chronic inflammation (disease). Patients with iron deficiency may exhibit normal ferritin levels in the range of 30 to 100 ng/mL when there is a rise of ferritin due to coexistent anemia of chronic inflammation (disease). Use of the soluble transferrin receptor assay in conjunction with ferritin can help distinguish these conditions or establish their coexistence. *sTfR*, Soluble transferrin receptor in mg/L. (Adapted from Weiss G, Goodnough LT. Anemia of chronic disease. N Eng J Med 352, 2005, p. 1020.)

ratio results (Figure 20-5).[30] The hemoglobin content of reticulocytes will be reduced in both iron deficiency and ACI. However, when graphed against the sTfR/log ferritin in a Thomas plot (Figure 11-6), the two conditions may be distinguished, sometimes better than with the sTfR/log ferritin alone (Chapter 11).[31,32] Additional research should help resolve this diagnostic dilemma.

Treatment

Therapeutic administration of erythropoietin can correct anemia of chronic inflammation,[33] but iron must be administered concurrently because stored body iron remains sequestered and unavailable.[34] The anemia is typically not severe, however, and this costly treatment is warranted only in select patients. The best course of treatment is effective control or alleviation of the underlying condition.

SIDEROBLASTIC ANEMIAS

Just as anemia can result from inadequate supplies of iron for production of hemoglobin, diseases that interfere with the production of adequate amounts of protoporphyrin also can produce anemia. (Chapter 10 covers heme synthesis.) As in iron deficiency, the anemia may be microcytic and hypochromic. In contrast to iron deficiency, however, iron is abundant in the bone marrow. A Prussian blue stain of the bone marrow shows normoblasts with iron deposits in the mitochondria surrounding the nucleus. Its presence in the mitochondria shows that the iron is awaiting incorporation into heme. These

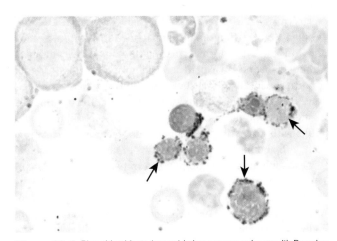

Figure 20-6   Ring sideroblasts (*arrows*) in bone marrow shown with Prussian blue stain (×1000).

ring sideroblasts are the hallmark of the sideroblastic anemias (Figure 20-6).

The sideroblastic anemias are a diverse group of diseases that include hereditary and acquired conditions (Box 20-1). Among the hereditary forms, X-linked and autosomal varieties of this condition are known. Some patients experience at least modest improvement of anemia with pharmacologic doses of pyridoxine to stimulate heme synthesis.[35] Pyridoxine is a cofactor in the first step of porphyrin synthesis (Figure 10-5) in which glycine is condensed with succinyl coenzyme A to form aminolevulinic acid.

> **BOX 20-1** Disorders Included in Sideroblastic Anemias
>
> **Hereditary**
> X-linked
> Autosomal
>
> **Acquired**
> Primary sideroblastic anemia (refractory)
> Secondary sideroblastic anemias caused by drugs and bone marrow toxins
> - Antitubercular drugs
> - Chloramphenicol
> - Alcohol
> - Lead
> - Chemotherapeutic agents

Lead Poisoning

The acquired conditions leading to sideroblastic anemia constitute a diverse group in themselves. Certain drugs, such as chloramphenicol or isoniazid, can induce sideroblastic anemia.[36] Other toxins, including heavy metals, also have been implicated. Among these, lead is a significant public health concern. Adults may be exposed at work to leaded compounds. Adults and children living in older homes can be exposed to lead from paints produced before the 1970s. They are at risk if dust is created during renovations or paint is permitted to peel. Toddlers and crawling infants are at special risk from getting dust on their hands and placing them in their mouths. Although anyone can experience lead poisoning, it is of special concern in children because the metal affects the central nervous system and the hematologic system, leading to impaired mental development as well as anemia.[37] In children and adults with lead poisoning, a peripheral neuropathy[38] can be seen with abdominal cramping and vomiting or seizures.

Lead interferes with porphyrin synthesis at several steps. The most critical are as follows (Figure 10-5):

1. The conversion of aminolevulinic acid (ALA) to porphobilinogen (PBG) by ALA dehydratase (also called *PBG synthase*); the result is the accumulation of aminolevulinic acid.
2. The incorporation of iron into protoporphyrin IX by ferrochelatase (also called *heme synthase*); the result is accumulation of iron and protoporphyrin.[39]

Accumulated aminolevulinic acid is measurable in the urine, and protoporphyrin is measurable in an extract of RBCs as free erythrocyte protoporphyrin or zinc protoporphyrin. Chapter 11 covers the principles of these assays.

Anemia, when present in lead poisoning, is most often normocytic and normochromic; however, with chronic exposure to lead, a microcytic, hypochromic clinical picture may be seen. The degree of anemia in adults may not be dramatic, but in children it may be more profound. The reticulocyte count in acute poisoning may be quite elevated, which suggests that the anemia has a hemolytic component. The presence of a hemolytic component is supported by studies showing impairment of the pentose-phosphate shunt by lead,[40] which makes the cells sensitive to oxidant stress as in glucose-6-phosphate dehydrogenase deficiency (Chapter 24). Although the bone marrow may show erythroid hyperplasia, consistent with the elevated reticulocyte count, in some patients it may be hypoplastic.[41] Basophilic stippling is a classic finding associated with lead toxicity. Lead inhibits pyrimidine 5′-nucleotidase, an enzyme involved in the breakdown of ribosomal ribonucleic acid (RNA) in reticulocytes.[42] This causes undegraded ribosomes to aggregate, forming basophilic stippling. The size of the aggregates in lead poisoning is typically large, so the stippling is heavier than that seen in many anemias and thus represents truly punctate basophilia. Because basophilic stippling is also seen in other anemias, this is not a pathognomonic finding but an expected finding, and whenever basophilic stippling is seen, lead poisoning should be under consideration.

Removal of the drug or toxin is usually successful for the treatment of acquired sideroblastic anemias. In the case of lead, salts of ethylenediaminetetraacetic acid (EDTA) are often used to chelate the lead present in the body so it can be excreted in the urine.[41]

Porphyrias

Lead poisoning is an example not only of an acquired sideroblastic anemia but also of an acquired porphyria. The porphyrias are diseases characterized by impaired production of the porphyrin component of heme. The impairments to heme synthesis may be acquired, as with lead poisoning, or hereditary. The term *porphyria* is most often used to refer to the hereditary conditions that impair production of protoporphyrin. Among the inherited disorders, single deficiencies of most enzymes in the synthetic pathway for heme have been identified (Figure 10-5). Although even the autosomal dominant conditions are relatively rare, the disease has been influential historically. The intermarrying European monarchies of past centuries were plagued with some variants of the porphyrias in which psychosis is a prominent clinical feature.

When an enzyme in heme synthesis is missing, the products from earlier stages in the pathway accumulate in cells that actively produce heme, such as erythrocytes and hepatocytes. The excess porphyrins leak from the cells as they age or die, and may be excreted in urine or feces, which allows diagnosis. The accumulated products also deposit in body tissues. Some of the accumulated products are fluorescent. Their deposition in skin can lead to photosensitivity with severe burns upon exposure to sunlight. Accumulation during childhood leads to fluorescence of developing teeth and bones. Only three of the porphyrias have hematologic manifestations; the others have a greater effect on liver cells. Even in those with hematologic effects, the hematologic impact is relatively minimal, and photosensitivity is a greater clinical problem. The fluorescence of some accumulated compounds can be used diagnostically—for example, to measure free erythrocyte protoporphyrin (Chapter 11). In a sample of bone marrow, the erythroblasts will be bright red under a fluorescent microscope. Table 20-2 summarizes the deficient enzymes, affected genes, inheritance, and clinical and

TABLE 20-2 Erythropoietic Porphyrias

		Congenital Erythropoietic Porphyria (CEP)	Erythropoietic Protoporphyria (EPP)	X-linked Erythropoietic Protoporphyria (XLEPP)
Enzyme affected		Uroporphyrinogen III synthase deficiency	Ferrochelatase deficiency	ALA-synthase 2 (gain of function)
Affected gene		*UROS*	*FECH*	*ALAS2*
Inheritance		Autosomal recessive	Autosomal dominant	X-linked dominant
Clinical features		Photosensitivity, hemolytic anemia	Photosensitivity; anemia is mild if present	Photosensitivity; mild microcytic, hypochromic anemia with reticulocyte response is possible
Laboratory features				
Red blood cells	Protoporphyrin	N	↑↑↑	↑
	Uroporphyrin	↑↑↑	N	N
	Coproporphyrin	↑↑	N	N
Urine	Porphobilinogen	N	N	N
	Uroporphyrin	↑↑↑	N	N
	Coproporphyrin	↑↑	N	N
Feces	Protoporphyrin	N	↑↑	N or ↑
	Coproporphyrin	↑	N	N
Confirmatory tests		↓↓↓ Uroporphyrinogen III synthase activity Genetic testing	↓↓ Ferrochelatase activity Genetic testing	↑↑ ALA-synthase activity; ↑↑ free erythrocyte protoporphyrin and zinc protoporphyrin

↑, Minimally increased levels; ↑↑, moderately increased levels; ↑↑↑, markedly increased levels; ↓↓, moderately decreased levels; ↓↓↓, markedly decreased levels.
Adapted from Desnick RJ, Balwani M: The porphyrias. In Longo DL, Fauci AS, Kasper DL, et al., eds: *Harrison's principles of internal medicine*, 18th ed., New York, 2012, McGraw Hill, chap. 358. Available at: http://www.accessmedicine.com.proxy1.cl.msu.edu/content.aspx?aid=9144015. Accessed November 24, 2013.

laboratory features that can be used in the diagnosis of the hematologically significant porphyrias.

IRON OVERLOAD

Chapter 11 describes the body's tenacity in conserving iron. For some individuals, this tenacity becomes the basis for disease related to excess iron accumulations in nearly all cells. Iron overload may be primary, as in hereditary hemochromatosis, or secondary to chronic anemias and their treatments. In both cases, the toxic effects of excess iron lead to serious health problems as lipids, proteins, and heme iron become oxidized.

Etiology

Excess accumulation of iron results from acquired or hereditary conditions in which the body's rate of iron acquisition exceeds the rate of loss, which is usually about 1 mg/day. Regardless of the source of the iron, the body's first reaction is to store excess iron in the form of ferritin and, ultimately, hemosiderin within cells. Eventually the storage system is overwhelmed, and, as described later, parenchymal cells are damaged in organs such as the liver, heart, and pancreas.

Accumulation of excess iron may be an acquired condition. It occurs when there is a need for repeated transfusions, as in the treatment of anemias such as sickle cell anemia and β-thalassemia major (Chapters 27 and 28). The iron present in the transfused RBCs exceeds the usual 1 mg/day of iron typically added to the body's stores by a healthy diet. This is sometimes called *transfusion-related hemosiderosis*.

Hemochromatosis may develop as a result of mutations to genes for the proteins of iron metabolism (Table 11-2) so that the feedback regulation of iron is impaired and the body continues to absorb iron, even when stores are full. An autosomal recessive disease was recognized for many years before modern methods allowed a molecular investigation of its cause. In the mid-1990s, a mutation was identified affecting the hereditary hemochromatosis (HFE) protein,[43] and shortly after that, additional mutations of the same gene were identified.[44,45] With reliable and specific molecular tests, individuals with the phenotypic disease (i.e., excess iron deposition in tissues) were soon discovered who did not have the HFE mutations. Trying to explain their diseases led to discovery of the other proteins that we now know are involved in iron metabolism. What has emerged is a picture of hereditary hemochromatosis as a general phenotype that can be produced by various genotypes when a gene for an iron regulatory protein is mutated (Table 20-3). The biologic default is to absorb and store iron, and the regulatory mechanisms typically dampen that process. Failure of normal regulation due to mutations leads to excessive absorption and storage, causing the diseases collectively known as the *hereditary hemochromatoses*. Although substantial understanding of the proteins involved in iron kinetics has emerged in the past 2 decades, likely more remains to be discovered.

TABLE 20-3 Known Mutations Producing Hemochromatosis Phenotypes

Feature	Hemochromatosis, Type 1 (*HFE*-Associated Hereditary Hemochromatosis)	Hemochromatosis, Type 2A Juvenile (*HFE2*-Related Juvenile Hemochromatosis)	Hemochromatosis, Type 2B Juvenile (*HAMP*-Related Juvenile Hemochromatosis)	Hemochromatosis, Type 3 (*TFR2*-Related Hereditary Hemochromatosis)	Hemachromatosis, Type 4 (Ferroportin-Related Iron Overload)	Hemachromatosis, Type 5
Affected gene	*HFE*	*HFE2 (HJV)*	*HAMP*	*TFR2*	*SLC40A1*	*FTH1*
Mutated protein	Hereditary hemochromatosis protein	Hemojuvelin	Hepcidin	Transferrin receptor protein 2	Solute carrier family 40 member 1 (Ferroportin-1)	Ferritin heavy chain
Normal function of affected protein	Inhibits TfR1-mediated iron uptake; regulates hepcidin expression	Regulates hepcidin expression	Downregulates ferroportin-mediated iron transport in macrophages and enterocytes	Provides hepatocyte iron uptake; regulates hepcidin expression	Transports iron out of enterocytes and macrophages	Iron storage
Age of onset of symptoms (yr)	30–40	Teens–20	Teens–20	20–40, mild	30–40	*

TfR1, Transferrin receptor 1; *TfR2*, transferrin receptor 2.
* Found in three members of a Japanese family.
Names of hemochromatosis types from Online Mendelian Inheritance of Man: http://omim.org/entry/235200?search5HFE&highlight5hfe. Accessed December 31, 2013.
Approved gene symbols from The Human Genome Organization (HUGO) Gene Nomenclature Committee (HGNC): http://www.genenames.org.
Approved protein names from Uni Prot KB, 2002–2014 UniProt Consortium: http://www.uniprot.org.

Table 20-3 describes each of the known forms of hemochromatosis, its mutated protein, age of onset, and the nature of the mutation and its effect. As mutations of HFE remain the most common, that form of the disease will be discussed here with some references to differences seen in other forms of the disease. However, in general, all the hereditary hemochromatoses involve mutated proteins that impair hepcidin regulation of ferroportin activity.

Homozygous hereditary hemochromatosis involving the *HFE* gene occurs in approximately 5 of 1000 northern Europeans.[46] Heterozygosity approaches 13%.[46] The first two mutations known to produce the hereditary hemochromatosis phenotype involve *HFE*, a gene on the short arm of chromosome 6 that encodes an HLA class I–like molecule that is closely linked to HLA-A.[43] The most common of the two mutations substitutes tyrosine for cysteine at position 282 (Cys282Tyr or C282Y), while the other substitutes aspartate for histidine at position 63 (His63Asp or H63D).[44] Other mutations are now known.[45] The normal HFE protein binds β_2-microglobulin intracellularly.[44] This binding is necessary for the HFE to appear on the cell surface, where it interacts with transferrin receptor 1 (TfR1). HFE is bound to TfR1 until TfR1 binds transferrin, and then the HFE is released. It subsequently binds to transferrin receptor 2 (TfR2), which initiates a signal for hepcidin production, ultimately reducing iron absorption. The mutated HFE molecule either does not bind β_2-microglobulin and thus does not reach the cell surface or it does not bind TfR1 or TfR2 if it does reach the cell surface.[47] In either case, the result is that when HFE protein is mutated, the TfR2-mediated signal

to produce hepcidin is diminished. Without hepcidin, ferroportin in the intestinal enterocyte membrane is continually active and absorbing iron, even when the body stores are replete.

Pathogenesis

The processes described previously lead to increased amounts of iron in parenchymal cells throughout the body. The first cellular reaction to excess iron is to form ferritin and ultimately hemosiderin, essentially a degenerate and non–metabolically active form of ferritin. When cells exhaust the capacity to store iron as hemosiderin, free iron (ferrous) accumulates intracellularly. In the presence of oxygen, ferrous iron initiates the generation of superoxide and other free radicals, which results in the peroxidation of membrane lipids (Chapter 11).[48] The membranes affected include not only the cell membranes but also mitochondrial, nuclear, and lysosomal membranes. Cell respiration is compromised, and lysosomal enzymes are released intracellularly. Vitamins E and C can act to moderate the effects and interrupt the chain reaction, but in iron overload, even these protective mechanisms are overwhelmed. The ultimate result is cell death due to irreversible membrane damage.

Because all cells except mature RBCs require iron and have the cellular machinery for iron acquisition, most cells have the potential for iron damage. The tissues most obviously affected are the skin, where deposition of hemosiderin gives the skin a golden color; the liver, where cirrhosis-induced jaundice and subsequent cancer develop; and the pancreas, where damage results in diabetes mellitus. Hence the traditional characterization of hemochromatosis is "bronzed diabetes." The heart muscle also is especially vulnerable to excessive iron deposition, which leads to congestive heart failure. Early diagnosis and treatment (see later) can prevent the development of these secondary effects of iron overload. Hepatocellular carcinoma occurs more frequently in patients with hemochromatosis. Mutations of the *p53* tumor suppressor gene seem to contribute to the pathogenesis of the carcinoma,[49] and there is some evidence that the free radicals produced by the iron cause the mutations in the *p53* gene.[50]

The disease (i.e., hemochromatosis phenotype) is rarer than the C282Y gene frequency predicts, so the penetrance of the genes is not heavy.[46] Other factors also affect the development of clinical disease, including the particular mutation, zygosity, presence of other physiologic conditions, diet, and other environmental influences.

In classic hereditary hemochromatosis (*HFE* mutations), individuals usually harbor 20 to 30 g of iron by the time their disease becomes clinically evident at the age of 40 to 60 years.[51] This is more than 10 times the amount of stored iron in normal individuals and represents just 1 to 2 mg/day of excess iron absorbed over many years.[52] In the juvenile forms of the disease associated with mutations to the hepcidin or hemojuvelin genes, the process of iron accumulation is accelerated, so these effects may appear as early as the teenage years.

In the slower-developing diseases, phenotypic expression of the tissue damage in hereditary hemochromatosis is more common in men, although the gene frequency of HFE mutations is not higher in men. This is because the blood loss associated with menstruation and childbirth forestalls the effects of excess iron in affected women, and they usually develop clinical symptoms later in life than affected men. In each sex, homozygous individuals develop disease faster than heterozygotes.

The amount of iron available in the diet for absorption affects the rate at which disease can develop. Substances that can promote iron absorption even in normal individuals, such as ascorbic acid and alcohol, also affect absorption in individuals with hemochromatosis. In transfusion-related hemosiderosis, the frequency of transfusions over time affects the rate of development of clinical disease.

Laboratory Diagnosis

Laboratory testing in hemochromatosis serves four purposes. It can be used to screen for the condition, diagnose the cause of organ damage, pinpoint the mutation for family genetic counseling, and monitor treatment. Elevations of transferrin saturation or serum ferritin can be used as a screening test for hereditary hemochromatosis.[53] Although screening was estimated to be performed cost-effectively in populations with a disease prevalence of at least 3 per 1000,[54] large-scale screening programs remain controversial, even in Europe, where the incidence of the disease is high.[55]

Individuals with undiagnosed hereditary hemochromatosis may come to medical attention because of organ function problems leading to nonspecific physical complaints (e.g., abdominal pain), or the disease may be discovered incidentally with routine laboratory testing. Abnormal results on common tests of liver function (e.g., elevated alanine transaminase levels) may be among the first laboratory findings that lead a physician to order further testing to identify the cause. Because inflammation is minimal, however, a finding of diminished levels of the liver's synthetic products, such as albumin, may be more helpful. If hereditary hemochromatosis is among the disorders being considered to explain organ dysfunction, serum iron, transferrin saturation, and serum ferritin testing are warranted because elevations in these values are among the earliest findings in most forms of hemochromatosis. Genetic testing for known mutations provides confirmation of the diagnosis for most patients with hereditary hemochromatosis. It is especially valuable for testing nonaffected family members who can be counseled in lifestyle changes to prevent the phenotype from developing or for whom early treatment interventions can prevent organ damage.

Whether hemochromatosis is acquired or hereditary, the serum ferritin level provides an assessment of the degree of iron overload and can be monitored after treatment is initiated to reduce iron stores. Hemoglobin concentration and hematocrit are inexpensive tests that can also be used to monitor treatment, as described later.

Determination of the actual extent of tissue damage is beyond the scope of the clinical laboratory. Liver biopsy with assessment of iron staining and degree of scarring in liver specimens is essential to determining the degree of organ damage.

Treatment

The treatment of secondary tissue damage, such as liver cirrhosis and heart failure, follows standard protocols. Treatment of the underlying condition leading to excess iron accumulation is also needed. Hereditary hemochromatosis and transfusion-related hemosiderosis require different treatment approaches. In forms of hereditary hemochromatosis, withdrawal of blood by phlebotomy provides a simple, inexpensive, and effective means of removing iron from the body. The regimen calls for weekly phlebotomy early in treatment to remove about 500 mL of blood per treatment. Maintenance phlebotomies are required about every 3 months for life.[56] Hemoglobin levels are monitored, and a mild anemia is sought and maintained. Such monitoring is an easy and inexpensive substitute for iron studies because, as explained in the discussion of iron deficiency, iron stores must be exhausted before anemia develops.

Individuals who rely on transfusions to maintain hemoglobin levels and prevent anemia cannot be treated with phlebotomy. Instead, iron-chelating drugs are used to bind excess iron in the body for excretion. Desferrioxamine is the classic treatment, although it is not without side effects.[57] The drug typically is injected subcutaneously to maximize exposure time for iron binding. When absorbed into the bloodstream with its bound iron, it is readily excreted in the urine. Recently, oral iron chelators have been developed.[58,59] Although they also have side effects, the convenience of oral administration with the potential for improved patient outcomes may lead to a greater reliance on this form of treatment.

SUMMARY

- Impaired iron kinetics or heme metabolism can result in microcytic, hypochromic anemias.

- Three conditions affecting iron kinetics can result in microcytic, hypochromic anemias: iron deficiency, anemia of chronic inflammation, and sideroblastic anemias, especially lead poisoning. The RBCs in thalassemias also may be microcytic and hypochromic, and this condition must be differentiated from the anemias of disordered iron metabolism.

- Iron deficiency results from inadequate iron intake, increased need, decreased absorption, or excessive loss. All four of these situations create a relative deficit of body iron that over time results in a microcytic, hypochromic anemia.

- Infants, children, and women of childbearing age are at greatest risk for iron deficiency anemia. If iron deficiency anemia is present in men and postmenopausal women, the possibility of gastrointestinal bleeding should be investigated because it is the primary, although not the only, cause of iron loss.

- Iron deficiency is suspected when the CBC shows microcytic, hypochromic RBCs and elevated RDW but no consistent morphologic abnormality. The diagnosis is confirmed with iron studies showing low levels of serum iron and serum ferritin, elevated TIBC, and decreased transferrin saturation.

- Inadequate dietary iron is treated by oral supplementation, and with good patient adherence, the anemia should be corrected within 3 months. Gastrointestinal distress resulting from iron supplements can make patient adherence a significant concern. Other causes of iron deficiency must be treated by eliminating the underlying cause or with intravascular iron administration.

- The anemia of chronic inflammation (ACI) is associated with chronic infections such as tuberculosis, chronic inflammatory conditions such as rheumatoid arthritis, and tumors. It may be a microcytic, hypochromic anemia, but most often it is a mild normocytic, normochromic anemia.

- In ACI, increased levels of hepcidin, an acute phase reactant, decrease iron absorption in the intestines and sequester iron in macrophages and hepatocytes. Bone marrow macrophages show abundant stainable iron, whereas developing RBCs show inadequate iron. Inflammatory cellular products also impair the production and action of erythropoietin.

- Iron studies in the anemia of chronic inflammation show decreased serum iron level, decreased TIBC, decreased or normal transferrin saturation, and normal or increased ferritin level.

- Sideroblastic anemias develop when the synthesis of protoporphyrin or the incorporation of iron into protoporphyrin is blocked. The result is accumulation of iron in the mitochondria of developing RBCs. When stained using Prussian blue, the iron appears in deposits around the nucleus of the developing cells in the bone marrow. These cells are called *ring sideroblasts.*

- Protoporphyrin synthesis and iron incorporation into protoporphyrin can be blocked when any of the enzymes of the heme synthetic pathway are deficient or impaired. Deficiencies of these enzymes may be hereditary, as in the porphyrias, or acquired, as in heavy metal poisoning. The most common of the latter conditions is lead poisoning.

- Iron studies in sideroblastic anemias show elevated levels of serum iron and serum ferritin, decreased or normal TIBC, and increased transferrin saturation. Test values for the accumulating products of the heme synthetic pathway, such as zinc protoporphyrin (ZPP) or free erythrocyte protoporphyrin (FEP), are also elevated.

- Lead interferes with several steps in heme synthesis, preventing iron incorporation into heme and resulting in a normocytic, normochromic anemia, although with long-term exposure it can be microcytic and hypochromic. Lead also impairs glucose-6-phosphate dehydrogenase, which adds a hemolytic component to the anemia.

- Children are especially vulnerable to the effects of lead on the central nervous system, which may result in irreversible brain damage. Treatment consists of removing the source of lead from the patient's environment and, if necessary, chelating drug therapy to facilitate excretion of lead in the urine.

- Because the body has no mechanism for iron excretion, iron overload can occur when transfusions are used to sustain patients with chronic anemias such as β-thalassemia major (called *transfusion-related hemosiderosis*).

- A defective *HFE* gene can lead to hereditary hemochromatosis by decreased hepcidin production. Affected men develop symptoms earlier in life than women; homozygotes develop more severe disease than heterozygotes.

- Mutations of other genes affecting iron regulation can produce a phenotype similar to that of hereditary hemochromatosis. When the hepcidin or hemojuvelin gene is mutated, the disease develops early in life, affecting even teenagers.

- Free iron becomes available in cells when ferritin and hemosiderin become saturated. Free iron causes tissue damage by creating free radicals that lead to cell membrane damage and perhaps mutations. The liver, pancreas, skin, and heart muscle are especially damaged by excess iron deposition.

- Elevated transferrin saturation can be an indicator of hemochromatosis that can be diagnosed fully using genetic testing to identify mutated genes.

- Hereditary hemochromatosis and similar diseases are treated by lifelong periodic phlebotomy to induce a mild iron deficiency anemia and keep body iron levels low. Transfusion-related hemosiderosis must be treated with iron-chelating drugs.

Now that you have completed this chapter, go back and read again the case study at the beginning and respond to the questions presented.

Answers can be found in the Appendix.

1. The mother of a 4-month-old infant who is being breastfed sees her physician for a routine postpartum visit. She expresses concern that she may be experiencing postpartum depression because she does not seem to have any energy. Although the physician is sympathetic to the patient's concern, she orders a CBC and iron studies seeking an organic explanation for the patient's symptoms. The results are as follows:
   CBC: all results within reference intervals except
   RDW = 15%
   Serum iron: decreased
   TIBC: increased
   % transferrin saturation: decreased
   Serum ferritin: decreased
   Correlate the patient's laboratory and clinical findings. What can you conclude?
   a. The results of the iron studies reveal findings consistent with a thalassemia that was apparently previously undiagnosed.
   b. The patient is in stage 2 of iron deficiency, before frank anemia develops.
   c. The results of the iron studies are inconsistent with the CBC results, and a laboratory error should be suspected.
   d. There is no evidence of a hematologic explanation for the patient's symptoms.

2. A bone marrow biopsy was performed as part of the cancer staging protocol for a patient with Hodgkin lymphoma. Although no evidence of spread of the tumor was apparent in the marrow, other abnormal findings were noted, including a slightly elevated myeloid-to-erythroid ratio. WBC and RBC morphology appeared normal, however. The Prussian blue stain showed abundant stainable iron in the marrow macrophages. The patient's CBC revealed a hemoglobin of 10.8 g/dL, but RBC indices were within reference intervals. RBC morphology was unremarkable. These findings would be consistent with:
   a. Anemia of chronic inflammation
   b. Sideroblastic anemia
   c. Thalassemia
   d. Iron deficiency anemia

3. Predict the iron study results for the patient with Hodgkin lymphoma described in question 2.

	Serum Iron Level	TIBC	% Transferrin Saturation	Serum Ferritin Level
a.	Decreased	Increased	Decreased	Decreased
b.	Increased	Normal	Increased	Normal
c.	Increased	Increased	Normal	Increased
d.	Decreased	Decreased	Normal	Normal

4. A 35-year-old white woman went to her physician complaining of headaches, dizziness, and nausea. The headaches had been increasing in severity over the past 6 months. This was coincident with her move into an older house built about 1900. She had been renovating the house, including stripping paint from the woodwork. Her CBC results showed a mild hypochromic, microcytic anemia, with polychromasia and basophilic stippling noted. Which of the following tests would be most useful in confirming the cause of her anemia?
   a. Serum lead level
   b. Serum iron level and TIBC
   c. Absolute reticulocyte count
   d. Prussian blue staining of the bone marrow to detect iron stores in macrophages

5. In men and postmenopausal women whose diets are adequate, iron deficiency anemia most often results from:
   a. Increased need associated with aging
   b. Impaired absorption in the gastric mucosa
   c. Chronic gastrointestinal bleeding
   d. Diminished resistance to hookworm infections

6. Which one of the following individuals is at greatest risk for the development of iron deficiency anemia?
   a. A 15-year-old boy who eats mainly fast food and junk food
   b. A 37-year-old woman who has never been pregnant and has amenorrhea
   c. A 63-year-old man with reactivation of tuberculosis from his childhood
   d. A 40-year-old man who lost blood during surgery to repair a fractured leg

7. Which of the following individuals is at the greatest risk for the development of anemia of chronic inflammation?
   a. A 15-year-old girl with asthma
   b. A 40-year-old woman with type 2 diabetes mellitus
   c. A 65-year-old man with hypertension
   d. A 30-year-old man with severe rheumatoid arthritis

8. In what situation will increased levels of free erythrocyte protoporphyrin be present?
   a. Gain of function mutation to one of the enzymes in the heme synthesis pathway
   b. A mutation that prevents heme attachment to globin so that protoporphyrin remains free
   c. Any condition that prevents iron incorporation into protoporphyrin IX
   d. When red blood cells lyse, freeing their contents into the plasma

9. In the pathogenesis of the anemia of chronic inflammation, hepcidin levels:
   a. Decrease during inflammation and reduce iron absorption from enterocytes
   b. Increase during inflammation and reduce iron absorption from enterocytes
   c. Increase during inflammation and increase iron absorption from enterocytes
   d. Decrease during inflammation and increase iron absorption from enterocytes

10. Sideroblastic anemias result from:
    a. Sequestration of iron in hepatocytes
    b. Inability to incorporate heme into apohemoglobin
    c. Sequestration of iron in myeloblasts
    d. Failure to incorporate iron into protoporphyrin IX

11. In general, the hereditary hemochromatoses result from mutations that impair:
    a. The manner in which developing red cells acquire and manage iron
    b. The hepcidin-ferroportin iron regulatory system
    c. The TfR-Tf endocytic iron acquisition process for body cells other than blood cells
    d. The function of divalent metal transporter in enterocytes and macrophages

12. In the erythropoietic porphyrias, mild anemia may be accompanied by what distinctive clinical finding?
    a. Gallstones
    b. Impaired night vision
    c. Unintentional nighttime leg movements
    d. Heightened propensity for sunburn

Also review Chapter 11, questions 4 and 12 to 14 pertinent to the diagnostic value of various tests of iron status.

REFERENCES

1. Hallberg, L. (1981). Bioavailability of dietary iron in man. *Annu Rev Nutr, 1,* 123–147.
2. Silvestri, L., Guillem, F., Pagani, A., et al. (2009). Molecular mechanisms of the defective hepcidin inhibition in TMPRSS6 mutations associated with iron-refractory iron deficiency anemia. *Blood, 113*(22), 5605–5608.
3. Suominen, P., Punnonen, K., Rajamaki, A., et al. (1998). Serum transferrin receptor and transferrin receptor–ferritin index identify healthy subjects with subclinical iron deficits. *Blood, 92,* 2934–2939.
4. Cogswell, M. E., Looker, A. C., Pfeiffer, C. M., et al. (2009). Assessment of iron deficiency in US preschool children and nonpregnant females of childbearing age: National Health and Nutrition Examination Survey 2003-2006. *Am J Clin Nutr, 89,* 1334–1342.
5. Goodnough, L. T., & Nemeth, E. (2014). Chapter 23. Iron deficiency and related disorders. In Greer, J. P., Arber, D. A., Glader, D., List, A. F., Means, R. T., Paraskevas, F., Rodgers, G. M., & Foerster, J. (Eds.), *Wintrobe's Clinical Hematology.* (13th ed.). Philadelphia: Lippincott Williams & Wilkins. Accessed 03.01.14.
6. Green, R., Charlton, R., Seftel, H., et al. (1968). Body iron excretion in man: a collaborative study. *Am J Med, 45,* 336–353.
7. Saarinen, U. M., Siimes, M. A., & Dallman, P. R. (1977). Iron absorption in infants: high bioavailability of breast milk iron as indicated by the extrinsic tag method of iron absorption and by the concentration of serum ferritin. *J Pediatr, 91,* 36–39.
8. Siimes, M. A., Vuori, E., & Kuitunen, P. (1979). Breast milk iron: a declining concentration during the course of lactation. *Acta Paediatr Scand, 68,* 29–31.
9. Yoshimura, H. (1970). Anemia during physical training (sports anemia). *Nutri Rev, 28,* 251–276.
10. Thompson, W. G., Meola, T., Lipkin, M., Jr., et al. (1988). Red cell distribution width, mean corpuscular volume, and transferrin saturation in the diagnosis of iron deficiency. *Arch Intern Med, 148,* 2128–2130.
11. McClure, S., Custer, E., & Bessman, J. D. (1985). Improved detection of early iron deficiency in nonanemic subjects. *JAMA, 253,* 1021–1023.
12. Charlton, R. W., & Bothwell, T. H. (1982). Definition, prevalence and prevention of iron deficiency. *Clin Haematol, 11,* 309–325.
13. Cox, L. A., & Adrian, G. S. (1993). Postranscriptional regulation of chimeric human transferrin genes by iron. *Biochemistry, 32,* 4738–4745.
14. Brugnara, C., Schiller, B., & Moran, J. (2006). Reticulocyte hemoglobin equivalent (Ret He) and assessment of iron deficient states. *Clin Lab Haem, 29,* 303–306.
15. Lamola, A. A., Joselow, M., & Yamane, T. (1975). Zinc protoporphyrin (ZPP): a simple, sensitive fluorometric screening test for lead poisoning. *Clin Chem, 21,* 93–97.
16. Huebers, H. A., Beguin, Y., Pootrakul, P., et al. (1990). Intact transferrin receptors in human plasma and their relation to erythropoiesis. *Blood, 75,* 102–107.
17. O'Sullivan, D. J., Higgins, P. G., & Wilkinson, J. F. (1955). Oral iron compounds: a therapeutic comparison. *Lancet, 2,* 482–485.
18. Swan, H. T., & Jowett, G. H. (1959). Treatment of iron deficiency with ferrous fumarate: assessment by a statistically accurate method. *BMJ, 2,* 782–787.
19. Cartwright, G. E. (1966). The anemia of chronic disorders. *Semin Hematol, 3,* 351–375.
20. Sears, D. A. (1992). Anemia of chronic disease. *Med Clin North Am, 76,* 567–579.
21. Nemeth, E., Tuttle, M. S., Powelson, J., et al. (2004). Hepcidin regulates iron efflux by binding to ferroportin and inducing its internalization. *Science, 306,* 2090–2093.
22. Rivera, S., Liu, L., Nemeth, E., et al. (2005). Hepcidin excess induces the sequestration of iron and exacerbates tumor-associated anemia. *Blood, 105,* 1797–1802.
23. Nicolas, G., Bennoun, M., Devaux, I., et al. (2001). Lack of hepcidin gene expression and severe tissue iron overload in upstream stimulatory factor 2 (USF2) knockout mice. *Proc Natl Acad Sci U S A, 98,* 8780–8785.
24. Nicolas, G., Chauvet, C., Viatte, L., et al. (2002). The gene encoding the iron regulatory peptide hepcidin is regulated by anemia, hypoxia, and inflammation. *J Clin Invest, 110,* 1037–1044.
25. Masson, P. L., Heremans, J. F., & Schonne, E. (1969). Lactoferrin: an iron binding protein in neutrophilic leukocytes. *J Exp Med, 130,* 643–658.
26. Ganz, T. (2003). Hepcidin, a key regulator of iron metabolism and mediator of anemia in inflammation. *Blood, 102,* 783–788.
27. Weiss, G., & Goodnough, L. T. (2005). Anemia of chronic disease. *N Engl J Med, 352,* 1011–1023.

28. Means, R. T. (2014). Chapter 41. Anemias secondary to chronic disease and systemic disorders. In Greer, J. P., Arber, D. A., Glader, D., List, A. F., Means, R. T., Paraskevas, F., Rodgers, G. M., & Foerster, J. (Eds.), *Wintrobe's Clinical Hematology*. (13th ed.). Philadelphia: Lippincott Williams & Wilkins. Accessed 03.01.14.

29. Castel, R., Tax, M. G., Droogendijk, J., et al. (2012). The transferrin/log(ferritin) ratio: a new tool for the diagnosis of iron deficiency anemia. *Clin Chem Lab Med, 50,* 1343-1349.

30. Mast, A. E., Blinder, M. A., Gronowski, A. M., et al. (1998). Clinical utility of the soluble transferrin receptor and comparison with serum ferritin in several populations. *Clin Chem, 44,* 45–51.

31. Thomas, C., & Thomas, L. (2002). Biochemical markers and hematologic indices in the diagnosis of functional iron deficiency. *Clin Chem, 48,* 1066–1076.

32. Leers, M. P. G., Keuren, J. F. W., & Oosterhuis, W. P. (2010). The value of the Thomas-plot in the diagnostic work up of anemic patients referred by general practitioners. *Int J Lab Hemat, 32,* 572–581.

33. Pincus, T., Olsen, N. J., Russell, I. J., et al. (1990). Multicenter study of recombinant human erythropoietin in correction of anemia in rheumatoid arthritis. *Am J Med, 89,* 161–168.

34. Arndt, U., Kaltwasser, J. P., Gottschalk, R., et al. (2005). Correction of iron-deficient erythropoiesis in the treatment of anemia of chronic disease with recombinant human erythropoietin. *Ann Hematol, 84,* 159–166.

35. Horrigan, D. L., & Harris, J. W. (1964). Pyridoxine responsive anemia: analysis of 62 cases. *Adv Intern Med, 12,* 103–174.

36. Verwilghen, R., Reybrouck, G., Callens, L., et al. (1965). Antituberculosis drugs and sideroblastic anemia. *Br J Haematol, 11,* 92–98.

37. Benson, P. (1965). Lead poisoning in children. *Dev Med Child Neurol, 7,* 569–571.

38. Campbell, A. M., & Williams, E. R. (1968). Chronic lead intoxication mimicking motor neurone disease. *BMJ, 4,* 582.

39. Granick, S., Sassa, S., Granick, J. L., et al. (1972). Assays for porphyrins, delta-aminolevulinic acid dehydratase, and porphyrinogen synthetase in microliter samples of blood: application to metabolic defects involving the heme pathway. *Proc Natl Acad Sci U S A, 69,* 2381–2385.

40. Lachant, N. A., Tomoda, A., & Tanaka, K. R. (1984). Inhibition of the pentose phosphate shunt by lead: a potential mechanism for hemolysis in lead poisoning. *Blood, 63,* 518–524.

41. Bottomley, S. S. (2014). Chapter 24. Sideroblastic anemias. In Greer, J. P., Arber, D. A., Glader, D., List, A. F., Means, R. T., Paraskevas, F., Rodgers, G. M., Foerster, J. (Eds.), *Wintrobe's Clinical Hematology*. (13th ed.). Philadelphia: Lippincott Williams & Wilkins. Accessed 03.01.14.

42. Valentine, W. N., Paglia, D. E., Fink, K., et al. (1976). Lead poisoning. Association with hemolytic anemia, basophilic stippling, erythrocyte pyrimidine 5′-nucleotidase deficiency, and intraerythrocytic accumulation of pyrimidines. *J Clin Invest, 58,* 926–932.

43. Feder, J. N., Gnirke, A., Thomas, W., et al. (1996). A novel MHC class I-like gene is mutated in patients with hereditary haemochromatosis. *Nat Genet, 13,* 399–408.

44. Waheed, A., Parkkila, S., Zhou, X. Y., et al. (1997). Hereditary hemochromatosis: effect of C282Y and H63D mutations on association with β_2-microglobulin, intracellular processing, and cell surface expression of the HFE protein in COS-7 cells. *Proc Natl Acad Sci U S A, 94,* 12384–12389.

45. Brissot, P., Bardou-Jacquet, E., Troadec, M. B., et al. (2010). Molecular diagnosis of genetic iron-overload disorders. *Expert Rev Mol Diagn, 10,* 755–763.

46. Beutler, E. (2003). The HFE Cys282Tyr mutation as a necessary but not sufficient cause of clinical hereditary hemochromatosis. *Blood, 101,* 3347–3350.

47. Lebron, J. A., & Bjorkman, P. J. (1999). The transferrin receptor binding site on HFE, the class I MHC-related protein mutated in hereditary hemochromatosis. *J Mol Biol, 289,* 1109–1118.

48. McCord, J. M. (1998). Iron, free radicals, and oxidative injury. *Semin Hematol, 35,* 5–12.

49. Vautier, G., Bomford, A. B., Portmann, B. C., et al. (1999). p53 mutations in British patients with hepatocellular carcinoma: clustering in genetic hemochromatosis. *Gastroenterology, 117,* 154–160.

50. Hussain, S. P., Raja, K., Amstad, P. A., et al. (2000). Increased p53 mutation load in nontumorous human liver of Wilson disease and hemochromatosis: oxyradical overload diseases. *Proc Natl Acad Sci U S A, 97,* 12770–12775.

51. Niederau, C., Strohmeyer, G., & Stremmel, W. (1996). Long term survival in patients with hereditary hemochromatosis. *Gastroenterology, 110,* 1107–1119.

52. Bothwell, T. H., & MacPhail, A. P. (1998). Hereditary hemochromatosis: etiologic, pathologic, and clinical aspects. *Semin Hematol, 35,* 55–71.

53. Nadakkavukaran, I. M., Gan, E. K., & Olynyk, J. K. (2012). Screening for hereditary haemochromatosis. *Pathology, 44,* 148–152.

54. Phatak, P. D., Guzman, G., Woll, J. E., et al. (1994). Cost effectiveness of screening for hemochromatosis. *Arch Intern Med, 154,* 769–776.

55. Rogowski, W. H. (2009). The cost-effectiveness of screening for hereditary hemochromatosis in Germany: a remodeling study. *Med Decis Making, 29,* 224–38.

56. Edwards, C. Q., & Barton, J. C. (2014). Chapter 25. Hemochromatosis. In Greer, J. P., Arber, D. A., Glader, D., List, A. F., Means, R. T., Paraskevas, F., Rodgers, G. M., & Foerster, J. (Eds.), *Wintrobe's Clinical Hematology*. (13th ed.). Philadelphia: Lippincott Williams & Wilkins. Accessed 3.01.14.

57. Borgna-Pignatti, C., & Galanello, R. (2014). Thalassemias and related disorders: Quantitative disorders of hemoglobin synthesis. In Greer, J. P., Arber, D. A., Glader, D., List, A. F., Means, R. T., Paraskevas, F., Rodgers, G. M., Foerster, J. (Eds.). *Wintrobe's Clinical Hematology*. (13th ed.). Philadelphia: Lippincott Williams & Wilkins. Accessed 03.01.14.

58. Cappellini, M. D., & Pattoneri, P. (2009). Oral iron chelators. *Annu Rev Med, 60,* 25–38.

59. Imran, F., & Phatak, P. (2009). Pharmacoeconomic benefits of deferasirox in the management of iron overload syndromes. *Expert Rev Pharmacoecon Outcomes Res, 9,* 297–304.

21

Anemias Caused by Defects of DNA Metabolism

Linda H. Goossen

OBJECTIVES

After completion of this chapter, the reader will be able to:

1. Discuss the relationships among macrocytic anemia, megaloblastic anemia, and pernicious anemia, and classify anemias appropriately within these categories.
2. Discuss the physiologic roles of folate and vitamin B₁₂ in DNA production and the general metabolic pathways in which they act.
3. Describe the absorption and distribution of vitamin B₁₂, including carrier proteins and the biologic activity of various vitamin-carrier complexes.
4. Describe the biochemical basis for development of anemia with deficiencies of vitamin B₁₂ and folate, and explain the cause of the accompanying megaloblastosis.
5. Recognize individuals at risk for megaloblastic anemia by virtue of age, dietary habits, or physiologic circumstance such as pregnancy, drug regimens, or pathologic conditions.
6. Recognize complete blood count, reticulocyte count, red and white blood cell morphologies, and bone marrow findings consistent with megaloblastic anemia.
7. Given the results of tests measuring levels of serum vitamin B₁₂, serum methylmalonic acid, serum folate, plasma or serum homocysteine, and antibodies to intrinsic factor, determine the likely cause of a patient's deficiency.
8. Recognize results of bilirubin and lactate dehydrogenase tests that are consistent with megaloblastic anemia and explain why the test values are elevated in this condition.

CASE STUDY

After studying the material in this chapter, the reader should be able to respond to the following case study:

During a holiday visit, the children of a 76-year-old man noticed that he seemed more forgetful than usual and that he had difficulty walking. Concerned about the possibility of a mild stroke, the children insisted that he see his physician. The physician diagnosed a peripheral neuropathy affecting the father's ability to walk. In addition, the physician noted that he was pale and slightly jaundiced and ordered routine hematologic studies. The results were as follows:

	Patient Value	Reference Interval
WBCs (×10⁹/L)	3.2	4.5–11.0
RBCs (×10¹²/L)	2.22	4.60–6.00
HGB (g/dL)	8.5	14.0–18.0

	Patient Value	Reference Interval
HCT (%)	27.0	40–54
MCV (fL)	121.6	80–100
MCH (pg)	38.3	26–32
MCHC (g/dL)	31.5	32–36
RDW (%)	18	11.5–14.5
Platelets (×10⁹/L)	115	150–450
Reticulocytes (%)	1.8	0.5–2.5

WBC differential: unremarkable with the exception of hypersegmentation of neutrophils
RBC morphology: moderate anisocytosis, moderate poikilocytosis, macrocytes, oval macrocytes, few teardrop cells

CASE STUDY—cont'd

After studying the material in this chapter, the reader should be able to respond to the following case study:

Because of these findings, additional tests were ordered, with the following results:
- Serum vitamin B_{12}: decreased
- Serum folate: within reference interval
- Serum methylmalonic acid: increased
    1. Which of the CBC findings led the physician to order the vitamin assays?

2. Is the patient's reticulocyte response adequate to compensate for the anemia?
3. Based on the available test results, what can you conclude about the cause of the patient's anemia?
4. What additional testing would be helpful to diagnose the specific cause of this patient's anemia?

Impaired deoxyribonucleic acid (DNA) metabolism causes systemic effects by impairing production of all rapidly dividing cells of the body. These are chiefly the cells of the skin, the epithelium of the gastrointestinal tract, and the hematopoietic tissues. Because these all must be replenished throughout life, any impairment of cell production is evident in these tissues first. Patients may experience symptoms in any of these systems, but the blood provides a ready tissue for analysis. The hematologic effects, especially megaloblastic anemia, have come to be recognized as the hallmark of the diseases affecting DNA metabolism.

ETIOLOGY

The root cause of megaloblastic anemia is impaired DNA synthesis. The anemia is named for the very large cells of the bone marrow that develop a distinctive morphology (see section on laboratory diagnosis) due to a reduction in the number of cell divisions. Megaloblastic anemia is one example of a macrocytic anemia. Box 21-1 shows the classification of macrocytic anemias. Understanding the etiology of megaloblastic anemia requires a review of DNA synthesis with particular attention to the roles of vitamin B_{12} (cobalamin) and folic acid (folate).

Physiologic Roles of Vitamin B_{12} and Folate

Vitamin B_{12} (cobalamin) is an essential nutrient consisting of a tetrapyrrole (corrin) ring containing cobalt that is attached to 5,6-dimethylbenzimidazolyl ribonucleotide (Figure 21-1). Vitamin B_{12} is a coenzyme in two biochemical reactions in humans. One is isomerization of methylmalonyl coenzyme A (CoA) to succinyl CoA, which requires vitamin B_{12} (in the adenosylcobalamin form) as a cofactor and is catalyzed by the enzyme methylmalonyl CoA mutase (Figure 21-2). In the absence of vitamin B_{12}, the impaired activity of methylmalonyl CoA mutase leads to a high level of serum methylmalonic acid (MMA), which is useful for the diagnosis of vitamin B_{12} deficiency (discussed in the section on laboratory diagnosis). The second reaction is the transfer of a methyl group from 5-methyltetrahydrofolate (5-methyl THF) to homocysteine, which thereby generates methionine. This reaction is catalyzed by the enzyme methionine synthase and uses vitamin B_{12}

BOX 21-1 Classification of Macrocytic Anemias by Cause

Megaloblastic anemia
    Folate deficiency
        Inadequate intake
        Increased need
        Impaired absorption (e.g., inflammatory bowel disease)
        Impaired use due to drugs
        Excessive loss with renal dialysis
    Vitamin B_{12} deficiency
        Inadequate intake
        Increased need
        Impaired absorption
            Failure to split from food
            Failure to split from haptocorrin
            Lack of intrinsic factor
                Pernicious anemia
                Helicobacter pylori infection
                Gastrectomy
                Hereditary intrinsic factor deficiency
            General malabsorption (e.g., inflammatory bowel disease)
            Inherited errors in absorption or transport
                Imerslund-Gräsbeck syndrome
                Transcobalamin deficiency
            Competition for the vitamin
                Diphyllobothrium latum (fish tapeworm) infection
                Blind loop syndrome
    Other causes of megaloblastosis
        Myelodysplastic syndrome
        Acute erythroid leukemia
        Congenital dyserythropoietic anemia
        Reverse transcriptase inhibitors
Macrocytic, nonmegaloblastic anemias
    Normal newborn status
    Reticulocytosis
    Liver disease
    Chronic alcoholism
    Bone marrow failure

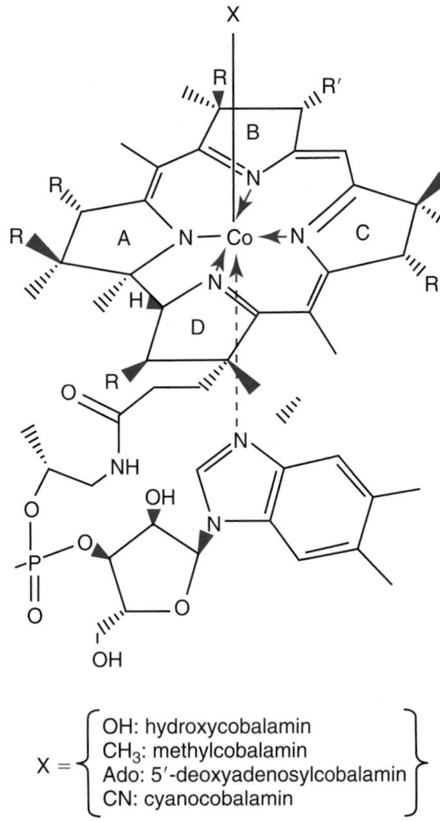

$$X = \begin{cases} \text{OH: hydroxycobalamin} \\ \text{CH}_3\text{: methylcobalamin} \\ \text{Ado: 5'-deoxyadenosylcobalamin} \\ \text{CN: cyanocobalamin} \end{cases}$$

Figure 21-1 Structure of vitamin B_{12} (cobalamin) and its analogs, hydroxycobalamin and cyanocobalamin (forms often found in food and supplements) and methylcobalamin and 5'-deoxyadenosylcobalamin (coenzyme forms). The basic structure of cobalamin includes a tetrapyrrole (corrin) ring with a central cobalt atom linked to 5,6-dimethylbenzimidazolyl ribonucleotide. (From Scott JM, Browne P: Megaloblastic anemia. In Caballero B, Allen L, Prentice A, editors: Encyclopedia of human nutrition, ed 2, Oxford, 2006, Academic Press, p 113.)

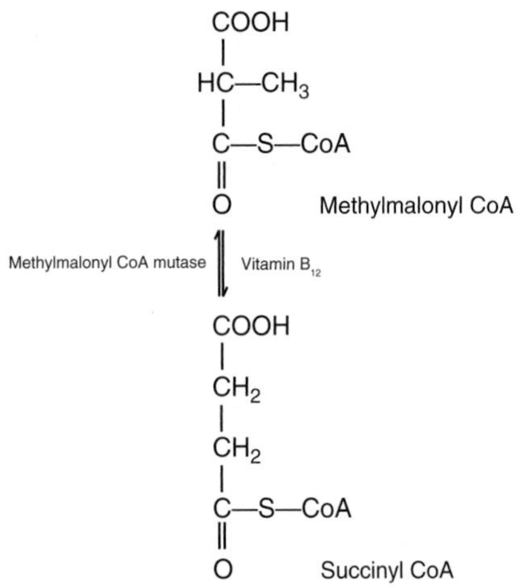

Figure 21-2 Role of vitamin B_{12} in the metabolism of methylmalonyl coenzyme A (CoA). Vitamin B_{12}, in the 5'-deoxyadenosylcobalamin form, is a coenzyme in the isomerization of methylmalonyl CoA to succinyl CoA. The reaction is catalyzed by the enzyme methylmalonyl CoA mutase.

(in the methylcobalamin form) as a coenzyme (discussed later in this section). Methylcobalamin is synthesized through reduction and methylation of vitamin B_{12}. This reaction represents the link between folate and vitamin B_{12} coenzymes and appears to account for the requirement for both vitamins in normal erythropoiesis.[1,2]

Folate is the general term used for any form of the vitamin folic acid. Folic acid is the synthetic form in supplements and fortified food. Folates consist of a pteridine ring attached to para-aminobenzoate with one or more glutamate residues (Figure 21-3). The function of folate is to transfer carbon units in the form of methyl groups from donors to receptors. In this capacity, folate plays an important role in the metabolism of amino acids and nucleotides. Deficiency of the vitamin leads to impaired cell replication and other metabolic alterations.

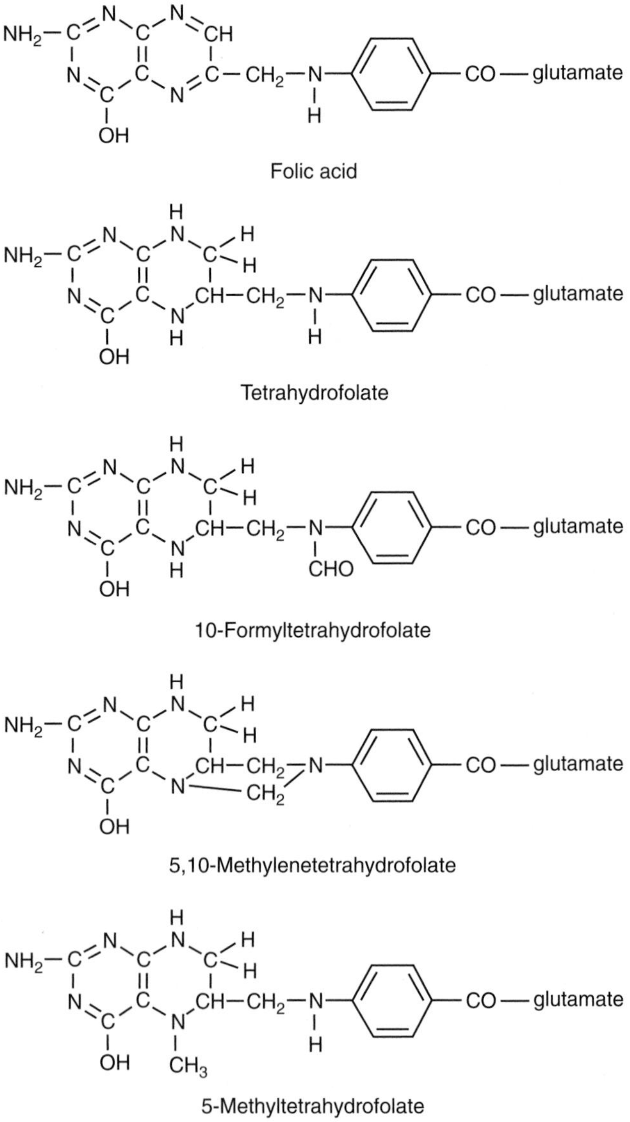

Figure 21-3 Structure of synthetic folic acid and the naturally occurring forms of the vitamin. (From Scott JM, Browne P: Megaloblastic anemia. In Caballero B, Allen L, Prentice A, editors: Encyclopedia of human nutrition, ed 2, Oxford, 2006, Academic Press, p 114.)

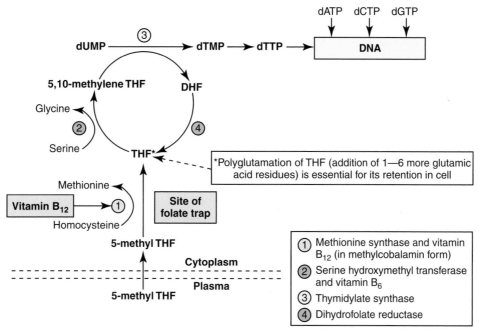

Figure 21-4 Role of folate and vitamin B_{12} in DNA synthesis. Folate enters the cell as 5-methyltetrahydrofolate (5-methyl THF). In the cell, a methyl group is transferred from 5-methyl THF to homocysteine, converting it to methionine and generating tetrahydrofolate (THF). This reaction is catalyzed by methionine synthase and requires vitamin B_{12} as a cofactor. THF is then converted to 5,10-methylene THF by the donation of a methyl group from serine. The methyl group of 5,10-methylene THF is then transferred to deoxyuridine monophosphate (dUMP), which converts it to deoxythymidine monophosphate (dTMP) and converts 5,10-methylene THF to dihydrofolate (DHF). This reaction is catalyzed by thymidylate synthase. dTMP is a precursor of deoxythymidine triphosphate (dTTP), which is used to synthesize DNA. THF is regenerated by the conversion of DHF to THF by the enzyme dihydrofolate reductase. A deficiency of vitamin B_{12} prevents the production of THF from 5-methyl THF; as a result, folate becomes metabolically trapped as 5-methyl THF. This constitutes the "folate trap."

Folate circulates in the blood predominantly as 5-methyl THF.[3] 5-Methyl THF is metabolically inactive until it is demethylated to tetrahydrofolate (THF), whereupon folate-dependent reactions may take place.

Folate has an important role in DNA synthesis. As seen in Figure 21-4, within the cytoplasm of the cell, a methyl group is transferred from 5-methyl THF to homocysteine, which converts it to methionine and generates THF. This reaction is catalyzed by the enzyme methionine synthase and requires vitamin B_{12} in the form of methylcobalamin as a cofactor. THF is then converted to 5,10-methylenetetrahydrofolate (5,10-methylene THF); the methyl group for this reaction comes from serine as it is converted to glycine. The methyl group of 5,10-methylene THF is then transferred to deoxyuridine monophosphate (dUMP), which converts it to deoxythymidine monophosphate (dTMP). This reaction is catalyzed by thymidylate synthase and results in the conversion of 5,10-methylene THF to dihydrofolate (DHF). Deoxythymidine monophosphate is a precursor to deoxythymidine triphosphate (dTTP), which, like the other nucleotide triphosphates, is a building block of the DNA molecule. THF is regenerated by the conversion of DHF to THF by the enzyme dihydrofolate reductase. Because some of the folate is catabolized during the cycle, the regeneration of THF also requires additional 5-methyl THF from the plasma. Once in the cell, folate is rapidly polyglutamated by the addition of one to six glutamic acid residues. This conjugation is required for

retention of THF in the cell, and it also promotes attachment of folate to enzymes.[4]

Defect in Megaloblastic Anemia Due to Deficiency in Folate and Vitamin B_{12}

When either folate or vitamin B_{12} is missing, thymidine nucleotide production for DNA synthesis is impaired. Folate deficiency has the more direct effect, ultimately preventing the methylation of dUMP. The effect of vitamin B_{12} deficiency is more indirect, preventing the production of THF from 5-methyl THF. When vitamin B_{12} is deficient, progressively more and more of the folate becomes metabolically trapped as 5-methyl THF. This constitutes what has been called the *folate trap* as 5-methyl THF accumulates and is unable to supply the folate cycle with THF. Some 5-methyl THF also leaks out of the cell if it is not readily polyglutamated. This results in a decrease in intracellular folate.[5] In addition, when either folate or vitamin B_{12} is deficient, homocysteine accumulates because methionine synthase is unable to convert it to methionine without vitamin B_{12} as a cofactor (see Figure 21-4).

In this state of diminished thymidine availability, uridine is incorporated into DNA.[6,7] The DNA repair process can remove the uridine, but without available thymidine, the repair process is unsuccessful. Although the DNA can unwind and replication can begin, at any point where a thymidine nucleotide is needed, there is essentially an empty space in the replicated DNA sequence, which results in many single-strand breaks.

When excisions at opposing DNA strand sites coincide, double-strand breaks occur. Repeated DNA strand breaks lead to fragmentation of the DNA strand.[4] The resulting DNA is nonfunctional, and the DNA replication process is incomplete. Cell division is halted, resulting in either cell lysis or apoptosis[8] of many erythroid progenitor cells within the bone marrow. Cells that survive continue the abnormal maturation with a fewer number of red blood cells (RBCs) released into the circulation. This abnormal blood cell development is called *ineffective hematopoiesis*. The dependency of DNA production on folate has been used in cancer chemotherapy (Box 21-2).

In addition to the increased apoptosis of erythroid progenitor cells in the bone marrow discussed above, the remaining erythroid cells are larger than normally seen during the final stages of erythropoiesis, and their nuclei are immature-appearing compared with the cytoplasm. In contrast to the normally dense chromatin of comparable normoblasts, the nuclei of megaloblastic erythroid precursors have an open, finely stippled, reticular pattern.[5] The nuclear changes seen in the megaloblastic cells are related to cell cycle delay, prolonged resting phase, and arrest in nuclear maturation. Electron microscopy has revealed that reduced synthesis of histones is also responsible for morphologic changes in the chromatin of megaloblastic erythroid precursors.[9] Ribonucleic acid (RNA) function is not affected by vitamin B_{12} or folate deficiency because RNA contains uracil instead of thymidine nucleotides, so cytoplasmic development progresses normally. The slower maturation rate of the nucleus compared with the cytoplasm is called *nuclear-cytoplasmic asynchrony*. Together, the accumulation of cells with nuclei at earlier stages of development and cells with increased size and immaturity result in the appearance of erythroid cells in the bone marrow that are pathognomonic of megaloblastic anemia.[8] Because ineffective hematopoiesis affects all three blood cell lineages, pancytopenia is also evident,

with certain distinctive cellular changes (see section on laboratory diagnosis).

Other Causes of Megaloblastosis

Vitamin B_{12} and folate deficiency are not the only causes of megaloblastic erythrocytes. Dysplastic erythroid cells in myelodysplastic syndrome (MDS) can also have megaloblastoid features (Chapter 34). In MDS, however, the macrocytic erythrocytes and their progenitors characteristically show delayed cytoplasmic and nuclear maturation, including cytoplasmic vacuole formation, nuclear budding, multinucleation, and nuclear fragmentation, and thus may be distinguished from the megaloblastic RBCs seen in the vitamin deficiencies. In addition, nuclear-cytoplasmic asynchrony and megaloblastic RBCs may be seen in congenital dyserythropoietic anemia (CDA) types I and III (Chapter 22). The CDAs are rare conditions that usually manifest in childhood and may be distinguished from the acquired causes of megaloblastosis by clinical history and morphologic differences. In CDA I, internuclear chromatin bridging of erythroid cells or binucleated forms are observed, and in CDA III, giant multinucleated erythroblasts are present. Another rare condition in which RBC precursors have a megaloblastic appearance is acute erythroid leukemia, previously classified as FAB M6 (Chapter 35). In this condition, the cells are macrocytic, and the immature appearance of the nuclear chromatin is similar to the more open appearance of the chromatin in megaloblasts. There are usually other aberrant findings in erythroid leukemia, including an increase of myeloblasts in the bone marrow; however, an experienced morphologist can discern the subtle differences. Reverse transcriptase inhibitors, used to treat human immunodeficiency virus (HIV) infections, interfere with DNA production and may also lead to megaloblastic changes.[10]

Although the conditions described in this section are characterized by megaloblastic morphology, they are due to acquired or inherited mutations in progenitor cells or interference with DNA synthesis and are refractory to therapy with vitamin B_{12} or folic acid.

SYSTEMIC MANIFESTATIONS OF FOLATE AND VITAMIN B_{12} DEFICIENCY

When DNA synthesis and subsequent cell division are impaired by lack of folate or vitamin B_{12}, megaloblastic anemia and its systemic manifestations develop. With either vitamin deficiency, patients may experience general symptoms related to the anemia (fatigue, weakness, and shortness of breath) and symptoms related to the alimentary tract. The loss of epithelium on the tongue results in a smooth surface and soreness (glossitis). Loss of epithelium along the gastrointestinal tract can result in gastritis, nausea, or constipation.

Although the blood pictures seen with the two vitamin deficiencies are indistinguishable, the clinical presentations vary. In vitamin B_{12} deficiency, neurologic symptoms may be pronounced and may even occur in the absence of anemia.[5] These include memory loss, numbness and tingling in toes and fingers, loss of balance, and further impairment of walking by

---

BOX 21-2 Disruption of the Folate Cycle in Cancer Chemotherapy

Folate has a complex relationship with cancer. Folate deficiency leads to DNA strand breaks, which leave the DNA vulnerable to mutation. In this way, folate deficiency is a risk factor for the initiation of cancer. The central role of folate in cell division also makes it a target for chemotherapeutic drugs used to treat cancer. Folate analogues can be used to compete for folate in DNA production and result in impaired cell division. The cells in the cell cycle, such as cancer cells and other normally rapidly dividing cells such as epithelium and blood cells, are most susceptible to the drug interference. Methotrexate, used in the treatment of leukemia and arthritis, is an example of a folate antimetabolite drug. Methotrexate has a higher affinity for dihydrofolate reductase than does tetrahydrofolate. Thus methotrexate enters the folate cycle in preference to tetrahydrofolate, and the folate cycle is blocked by the drug. Methotrexate treatment typically is followed by what is known as *leucovorin rescue*. Leucovorin is a folic acid derivative that can be administered to counteract the effects of methotrexate or other folate antagonists.

loss of vibratory sense, especially in the lower limbs.[11] Neuropsychiatric symptoms may also be present, including personality changes and psychosis. These symptoms seem to be the result of demyelinization of the spinal cord and peripheral nerves, but the relationship of this demyelinization to vitamin B_{12} deficiency is unclear. The roles of increases in tumor necrosis factor-α, a neurotoxic agent, and decreases in epidermal growth factor, a neurotrophic agent, in the development of neurologic symptoms in vitamin B_{12}-deficient patients are being researched.[12,13]

At one time, folate deficiency was believed to be more benign clinically than vitamin B_{12} deficiency. Later research suggested that low levels of folate and the resulting high homocysteine levels were risk factors for cardiovascular disease.[14] More recent research has provided mixed results, with studies both refuting this association[15,16] as well as substantiating the association between high circulating homocysteine levels and the risk of cardiovascular disease.[17] Several studies suggest that high folate levels provide a cardioprotective effect in diabetic patients and certain ethnic populations.[15,18,19] The evidence at this time is unclear as to whether persistent suboptimal folate status may have a significant long-term health impact. In addition, there is evidence of depression, peripheral neuropathy, and psychosis related to folate deficiency.[20-22] Folate levels appear to influence the effectiveness of treatments for depression.[23] Folate deficiency during pregnancy can result in impaired formation of the fetal nervous system, resulting in neural tube defects such as spina bifida,[24] despite the fact that the fetus accumulates folate at the expense of the mother. Pregnancy requires a considerable increase in folate to fulfill the requirements related to rapid fetal growth, uterine expansion, placental maturation, and expanded blood volume.[3] Insuring adequate folate levels in women of childbearing age is particularly important because many women are likely to be unaware of their pregnancy during the first crucial weeks of fetal development. Fortification of the U.S. food supply with folic acid in grain and cereal products was mandated by the Food and Drug Administration in 1998 to lower the risk of neural tube defects in the unborn.

CAUSES OF VITAMIN DEFICIENCIES

In general, vitamin deficiencies may arise because the vitamin is in relatively short supply, because use of the vitamin is impaired, or because of excessive loss. Folate deficiency can be caused by all of these mechanisms.

Folate Deficiency
Inadequate Intake
Folate is synthesized by microorganisms and higher plants. Folate is ubiquitous in foods, but a generally poor diet can result in deficiency. Good sources of folate include leafy green vegetables, dried beans, liver, beef, fortified breakfast cereals, and some fruits, especially oranges.[3,25] Folates are heat labile, and overcooking of foods can diminish their nutritional value.[3]

Increased Need
Increased need for folate occurs during pregnancy and lactation when the mother must supply her own needs plus those of the fetus or infant. Infants and children also have increased need for folate during growth.[3]

Impaired Absorption
Food folates must be hydrolyzed in the gut before absorption in the small intestine; however, only 50% of what is ingested is available for absorption.[3] A rare autosomal recessive deficiency of a folate transporter protein (PCFT) severely decreases intestinal absorption of folate.[5,26] Once across the intestinal cell, most folate is transported in the plasma as 5-methyl THF unbound to any specific carrier.[11] Its entry into cells, however, is carrier mediated.[27]

Folate absorption may also be impaired by intestinal disease, especially sprue and celiac disease. Sprue is characterized by weakness, weight loss, and steatorrhea (fat in the feces), which is evidence that the intestine is not absorbing food properly. It is seen in the tropics (tropical sprue), where its cause is generally considered to be overgrowth of enteric pathogens.[28] Celiac disease (nontropical sprue) has been traced to intolerance of the gluten in some grains[28] (gluten-induced enteropathy) and can be controlled by eliminating wheat, barley, and rye products from the diet. Surgical resection of the small intestine and inflammatory bowel disease can also decrease folate absorption.

Impaired Use of Folate
Numerous drugs impair folate metabolism (Box 21-3).[29,30] Antiepileptic drugs are particularly known for this,[31] and the result is macrocytosis with frank megaloblastic anemia. In most instances, folic acid supplementation is sufficient to override the impairment and allow the patient to continue therapy.[32] Because folate deficiency results in inhibition of cell replication, several anticancer drugs, including methotrexate, are folate inhibitors.[3]

Excessive Loss of Folate
Physiologic loss of folate occurs through the kidney. The amount is small and not a cause of deficiency. Patients undergoing renal dialysis lose folate in the dialysate, however; thus supplemental folic acid is routinely provided to these individuals to prevent megaloblastic anemia.[11]

BOX 21-3 Some Drugs That May Lead to Impaired Use of Folate

Impair Folate Metabolism
- Methotrexate (Trexall): antiarthritic, chemotherapeutic
- 5-Fluorouracil (Adrucil): chemotherapeutic
- Hydroxyurea (Hydrea): antimetabolite
- Pyrimethamine (Daraprim): antibacterial
- Pentamidine (Pentam): antimicrobial
- Phenytoin (Dilantin): anticonvulsant
- Trimethoprim (Primsol): antimicrobial

Impair Folate Absorption
- Metformin (Glucophage): oral antidiabetic
- Cholestyramine (Questran): cholesterol lowering

Vitamin B₁₂ Deficiency

Inadequate Intake

While true dietary deficiency of vitamin B_{12} is rare, this condition is possible for strict vegetarians (vegans) who do not eat meat, eggs, or dairy products. Although it is an essential vitamin for animals, plants cannot synthesize vitamin B_{12}, and it is not available from vegetable sources. The best dietary sources are animal products such as liver, dairy products, fish, shellfish, and eggs.[33] In contrast to the heat-labile folate, vitamin B_{12} is not destroyed by cooking.

Increased Need

Increased need for vitamin B_{12} occurs during pregnancy, lactation, and growth. Due to the vigorous cell replication, what would otherwise be a diet adequate in vitamin B_{12} can become inadequate during these periods.

Impaired Absorption

Vitamin B_{12} in food is released from food proteins primarily in the acid environment of the stomach, aided by pepsin, and is subsequently bound by a specific salivary protein, haptocorrin, also known as *R protein* or *transcobalamin I* (Figure 21-5). In the

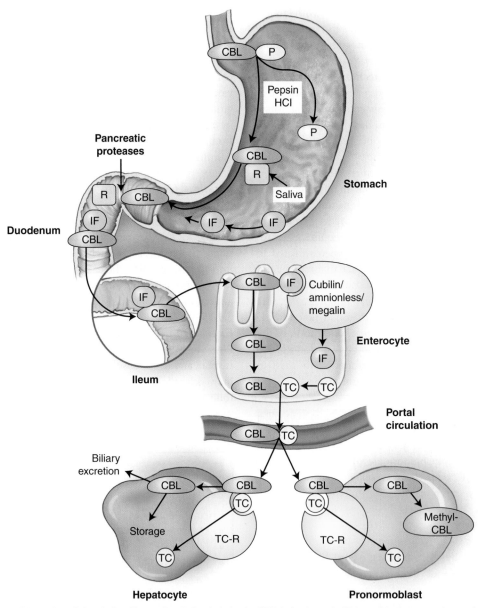

Figure 21-5 Normal absorption of vitamin B_{12}. Dietary vitamin B_{12} (cobalamin, CBL) is food protein (P) bound. In the stomach, pepsin and hydrochloric acid (HCl) secreted by parietal cells release CBL from P. CBL then binds haptocorrin (R protein, R), released from salivary glands, and remains bound until intestinal pancreatic proteases, including trypsin, catalyze its release. Parietal cells secrete intrinsic factor (IF), which binds CBL in the duodenum. Cubilin-amnionless (cubam) and megalin receptors in ileal enterocytes bind CBL-IF and release the CBL. Enterocytes produce transcobalamin (TC), which binds CBL and transports it through the portal circulation. Bone marrow pronormoblast membrane TC receptors (TC-R) bind CBL-TC and release the CBL, which is converted to methylcobalamin (methyl-CBL). Methyl-CBL is a coenzyme that supports homocysteine-methionine conversion. Hepatocyte TC-R receptors bind CBL-TC and release the CBL, which is moved to storage organelles or excreted through the biliary system.

small intestine, vitamin B_{12} is released from haptocorrin by the action of pancreatic proteases, including trypsin. It is then bound by intrinsic factor, which is produced by the gastric parietal cells. Vitamin B_{12} binding to intrinsic factor is required for absorption by ileal enterocytes that possess receptors for the complex. These receptors are cubilin-amnionless complex, collectively known as *cubam*, which binds the vitamin B_{12}–intrinsic factor complex, and megalin, a membrane transport protein.[5,33-36] Once in the enterocyte, the vitamin B_{12} is then freed from intrinsic factor and bound to transcobalamin (previously called *transcobalamin II*) and released into the circulation. In the plasma, only 10% to 30% of the vitamin B_{12} is bound to transcobalamin; the remaining 75% is bound to transcobalamin I and III, referred to as the *haptocorrins*.[33,37] The vitamin B_{12}–transcobalamin complex, termed *holotranscobalamin* (holoTC), is the metabolically active form of vitamin B_{12}. Holotranscobalamin binds to specific receptors on the surfaces of many different types of cells and enters the cells by endocytosis, with subsequent release of vitamin B_{12} from the carrier.[38] The body maintains a substantial reserve of absorbed vitamin B_{12} in hepatocytes.[4]

The absorption of vitamin B_{12} can be impaired by (1) failure to separate vitamin B_{12} from food proteins in the stomach, (2) failure to separate vitamin B_{12} from haptocorrin in the intestine, (3) lack of intrinsic factor, (4) malabsorption, and (5) competition for available vitamin B_{12}.

Failure to Separate Vitamin B_{12} from Food Proteins. A condition known as *food-cobalamin malabsorption* is characterized by hypochlorhydria and the resulting inability of the body to release vitamin B_{12} from food or intestinal transport proteins for subsequent binding to intrinsic factor. Food-cobalamin malabsorption is caused primarily by atrophic gastritis or atrophy of the stomach lining that often occurs with increasing age.[39] Because histamine 2 receptor blockers and proton pump inhibitors lower gastric acidity, the long-term use of these drugs for the treatment of ulcers and gastroesophageal reflux disease, and gastric bypass surgery also induce food-cobalamin malabsorption.[39]

Failure to Separate Vitamin B_{12} from Haptocorrin. Lack of gastric acidity or lack of trypsin as a result of chronic pancreatic disease can prevent vitamin B_{12} absorption because the vitamin remains bound to haptocorrin in the intestine and unavailable to intrinsic factor.[11]

Lack of Intrinsic Factor. Lack of intrinsic factor constitutes a significant cause of impaired vitamin B_{12} absorption. It is most commonly due to autoimmune disease, as in pernicious anemia, but can also result from the loss of parietal cells with *Helicobacter pylori* infection, total or partial gastrectomy, or hereditary intrinsic factor deficiency.

Pernicious anemia. Pernicious anemia is an autoimmune disorder characterized by impaired absorption of vitamin B_{12} due to a lack of intrinsic factor.[40] This condition is called *pernicious anemia* because the disease was fatal before its cause was discovered. The incidence per year is roughly 25 new cases per 100,000 persons older than 40 years of age.[5] Pernicious anemia most often manifests in the sixth decade or later, but can also be

found in children. Patients with pernicious anemia have an increased risk of developing gastric tumors.[4]

In pernicious anemia, autoimmune lymphocyte-mediated destruction of gastric parietal cells severely reduces the amount of intrinsic factor secreted in the stomach. Pathologic CD4 T cells inappropriately recognize and initiate an autoimmune response against the H^+/K^+–adenosine triphosphatase embedded in the membrane of the parietal cells.[41] A chronic inflammatory infiltration follows, which extends into the wall of the stomach.[40] Over a period of years and even decades, there is progressive development of atrophic gastritis resulting in the loss of the parietal cells with their secretory products, H^+ and intrinsic factor. The loss of H^+ production in the stomach constitutes achlorhydria. Low gastric acidity was previously an important diagnostic criterion for pernicious anemia. Serum gastrin levels can be markedly elevated due to the gastric achlorhydria.[4] The absence of intrinsic factor can also be detected using the Schilling test. However, because the test requires a 24-hour urine collection and the use of radioactive cobalt in vitamin B_{12} to trace absorption, safer diagnostic tests are currently used (see section on laboratory diagnosis).

Another feature of the autoimmune response in pernicious anemia is the production of antibodies to intrinsic factor[42] and gastric parietal cells[43] that are detectable in serum. The most common antibody to intrinsic factor blocks the site on intrinsic factor where vitamin B_{12} binds,[40] which inhibits the formation of the intrinsic factor–vitamin B_{12} complex and prevents the absorption of the vitamin. These blocking antibodies are present in serum or gastric fluid in about 90% of patients with pernicious anemia.[5] Parietal cell antibodies are detectable in the serum of about 90% of patients with pernicious anemia.[5,40]

Other causes of lack of intrinsic factor. A lack of intrinsic factor may also be related to *H. pylori* infection. Left untreated, colonization of the gastric mucosa with *H. pylori* progresses until the parietal cells are entirely destroyed, a process involving both local and systemic immune processes.[44,45] In addition, partial or total gastrectomy, which results in removal of intrinsic factor–producing parietal cells, invariably leads to vitamin B_{12} deficiency.

Impaired absorption of vitamin B_{12} can also be caused by hereditary intrinsic factor deficiency. This is a rare autosomal recessive disorder characterized by the absence or nonfunctionality of intrinsic factor. In contrast to the acquired forms of pernicious anemia, histology and gastric acidity are normal.[35]

Malabsorption. General malabsorption of vitamin B_{12} can be caused by the same conditions interfering with folate absorption, such as celiac disease, tropical sprue, and inflammatory bowel disease.

Inherited Errors of Vitamin B_{12} Absorption and Transport. Imerslund-Gräsbeck syndrome is a rare autosomal recessive condition caused by mutations in the genes for either cubilin or amnionless. This defect results in decreased endocytosis of the intrinsic factor–vitamin B_{12} complex by ileal enterocytes. Transcobalamin deficiency is another rare autosomal recessive condition resulting in a deficiency of physiologically available vitamin B_{12}.[35,46]

Competition for Vitamin B₁₂. Competition for available vitamin B_{12} in the intestine may come from intestinal organisms. The fish tapeworm *Diphyllobothrium latum* is able to split vitamin B_{12} from intrinsic factor,[47] rendering the vitamin unavailable for host absorption. Also, *blind loops*, portions of the intestines that are stenotic as a result of surgery or inflammation, can become overgrown with intestinal bacteria that compete effectively with the host for available vitamin B_{12}.[11] In both of these cases, the host is unable to absorb sufficient vitamin B_{12}, and megaloblastic anemia results.

LABORATORY DIAGNOSIS

The tests used in the diagnosis of megaloblastic anemia include screening tests and specific diagnostic tests to identify the specific vitamin deficiency and perhaps its cause.

Screening Tests

Five tests used to screen for megaloblastic anemia are the complete blood count (CBC), reticulocyte count, white blood cell (WBC) manual differential, serum bilirubin, and lactate dehydrogenase.

Complete Blood Count and Reticulocyte Count

Slight macrocytosis often is the earliest sign of megaloblastic anemia. Patients with uncomplicated megaloblastic anemia are expected to have decreased hemoglobin and hematocrit values, pancytopenia, and reticulocytopenia. Megaloblastic anemia develops slowly, and the degree of anemia is often severe when first detected. Hemoglobin values of less than 7 or 8 g/dL are not unusual.[4] When the hematocrit is less than 20%, erythroblasts with megaloblastic nuclei, including an occasional promegaloblast, may appear in the peripheral blood. The mean cell volume (MCV) is usually 100 to 150 fL and commonly is greater than 120 fL, although coexisting iron deficiency, thalassemia trait, or inflammation can prevent macrocytosis. The mean cell hemoglobin (MCH) is elevated by the increased volume of the cells, but the mean cell hemoglobin concentration (MCHC) is usually within the reference interval because hemoglobin production is unaffected. The red blood cell distribution width (RDW) is also elevated.

The characteristic morphologic findings of megaloblastic anemia in the peripheral blood include oval macrocytes (enlarged oval RBCs) (Figure 21-6) and hypersegmented neutrophils with six or more lobes (Figure 21-7).[48] Impaired cell production results in a low absolute reticulocyte count, especially in light of the severity of the anemia, and polychromasia is not observed on the peripheral blood film. Additional morphologic changes may include the presence of teardrop cells, RBC fragments, and microspherocytes. These smaller cells further increase the RDW. The presence of schistocytes sometimes leads to a paradoxically lower mean cell volume (MCV) than is seen in less severe cases. These erythrocyte changes reflect the severity of the dyserythropoiesis and should not be taken as evidence of microangiopathic hemolysis. Nucleated RBCs, Howell-Jolly bodies, basophilic stippling, and Cabot rings may also be observed.

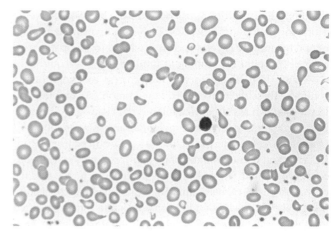

Figure 21-6 Oval macrocytes, teardrop cells (dacryocytes), other red blood cell abnormalities, and a small lymphocyte for size comparison in megaloblastic anemia (peripheral blood, ×500).

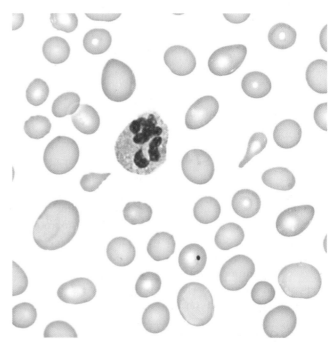

Figure 21-7 Hypersegmented neutrophil, oval macrocytes, and a Howell-Jolly body in megaloblastic anemia (peripheral blood, ×500). (From Rodak BF, Carr JH: Clinical hematology atlas, ed 4, St. Louis, 2013, Elsevier, Saunders.)

White Blood Cell Manual Differential

Hypersegmentation of neutrophils is essentially pathognomonic for megaloblastic anemia. It appears early in the course of the disease[49] and may persist for up to 2 weeks after treatment is initiated.[5] Hypersegmented neutrophils noted in the WBC differential report are a significant finding and require a reporting rule that can be applied consistently because even healthy individuals may have an occasional one. One such rule is to report hypersegmentation when there are at least 5 five-lobed neutrophils per 100 WBCs or at least 1 six-lobed neutrophil is noted.[11] Some laboratories perform a lobe count on 100 neutrophils and then calculate the mean. In megaloblastic anemia, the mean lobe count should be greater than 3.4.[11] The cause of the hypersegmentation is not understood, despite considerable investigation.[50] More recent advances in the understanding of growth factors and their impact on transcription factors may yet solve this mystery. Nevertheless, a search for neutrophil hypersegmentation on a peripheral blood film constitutes an inexpensive yet sensitive screening test for megaloblastic anemia.

Bilirubin and Lactate Dehydrogenase Levels

Although generally considered a nutritional anemia, megaloblastic anemia is in one sense a hemolytic anemia. Because many RBC precursors die during division in the bone marrow, many RBCs never enter the circulation (ineffective hematopoiesis), so a decrease in reticulocytes occurs in the peripheral blood. The usual signs of hemolysis are evident in the serum, including an elevation in the levels of total and indirect bilirubin and lactate dehydrogenase (predominantly RBC derived).

The constellation of findings including macrocytic anemia, moderate to marked pancytopenia, reticulocytopenia, oval macrocytes, hypersegmented neutrophils, plus increased levels of total and indirect bilirubin and lactate dehydrogenase justifies further testing to confirm a diagnosis of megaloblastic anemia and determine its cause. Occasionally, the classic findings may be obscured by coexisting conditions such as iron deficiency, which makes the diagnosis more challenging. Most hematologic aberrations do not appear until vitamin deficiency is fairly well advanced (Box 21-4).[51]

Specific Diagnostic Tests

Bone Marrow Examination

Modern tests for vitamin deficiencies and autoimmune antibodies have made bone marrow examination an infrequently used diagnostic test for megaloblastic anemia. Nevertheless, it remains the reference confirmatory test to identify the megaloblastic appearance of the developing RBCs.

Megaloblastic, in contrast to *macrocytic*, anemia refers to specific morphologic changes in the developing RBCs. The cells are characterized by a nuclear-cytoplasmic asynchrony in which the cytoplasm matures as expected with increasing pinkness as hemoglobin accumulates. The nucleus lags behind, however, appearing younger than expected for the degree of maturity of the cytoplasm (Figure 21-8). This asynchrony is most striking at the stage of the polychromatic normoblast. The cytoplasm appears pinkish-blue as expected for that stage, but the nuclear chromatin remains more open than expected, similar to that in the nucleus of a basophilic normoblast. Overall, the marrow is hypercellular, with a myeloid-to-erythroid

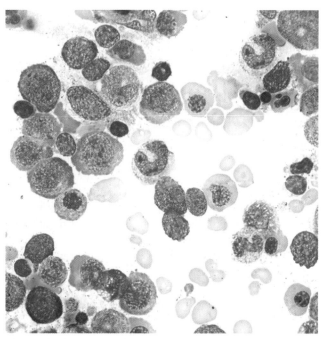

Figure 21-8 Erythroid precursors in megaloblastic anemia. Note nuclear-cytoplasmic asynchrony (bone marrow, ×500). (From Rodak BF, Carr JH: Clinical hematology atlas, ed 4, St. Louis, 2013, Elsevier, Saunders.)

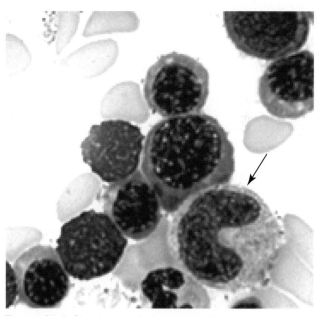

Figure 21-9 Giant band (early) in megaloblastic anemia (bone marrow, original magnification ×1000).

ratio of about 1:1 by virtue of the increased erythropoietic activity. The hematopoiesis is ineffective, however, and although cell production in the bone marrow is increased, the apoptosis of cells in the marrow results in peripheral pancytopenia.

The WBCs are also affected in megaloblastic anemia and appear larger than normal. This is most evident in metamyelocytes and bands, because in the usual development of neutrophils, the cells should be getting smaller at these stages. The effect creates "giant" metamyelocytes and bands (Figure 21-9).

BOX 21-4 Sequence of Development of Megaloblastic Anemias

1. Decrease in vitamin levels
2. Hypersegmentation of neutrophils in peripheral blood
3. Oval macrocytes in peripheral blood
4. Megaloblastosis in bone marrow
5. Anemia

Megakaryocytes do not show consistent changes in megaloblastic anemia. They may be either increased or decreased in number and may show diminished lobulation. The latter finding is not consistently seen, however, and even when present, it is difficult to assess.

Assays for Folate, Vitamin B₁₂, Methylmalonic Acid, and Homocysteine

Although bone marrow aspiration is confirmatory for megaloblastosis, the invasiveness of the procedure and its expense mean that other testing is performed more often than a bone marrow examination. Furthermore, the confirmation of megaloblastic morphology in the marrow does not identify its cause. Tests for serum levels of folate and vitamin B_{12} are readily available using immunoassay; serum vitamin B_{12} may also be assayed by competitive binding chemiluminescence.[52] However, there are a number of interferences with these assays that can cause false increased and decreased results[5,52] (Box 21-5); reflexive testing to methylmalonic acid and homocysteine (covered below) can increase diagnostic accuracy. RBC folate levels may also be measured. Unlike serum folate levels, which fluctuate with diet, RBC folate values are stable and may be a more accurate reflection of true folate status[53]; however, current RBC folate tests have less than optimal sensitivity and specificity and have not been validated in actual patients with normal and deficient folate levels. Thus the serum folate level is preferred over RBC folate level in the United States as the initial test for evaluation of folate deficiency.[5]

Some laboratories conduct a reflexive assay for methylmalonic acid if vitamin B_{12} levels are low. As indicated previously, in addition to playing a role in folate metabolism, vitamin B_{12} is a cofactor in the conversion of methylmalonyl CoA to succinyl CoA by the enzyme methylmalonyl CoA mutase (Figure 21-2). If vitamin B_{12} is deficient, methylmalonyl CoA accumulates. Some of it hydrolyzes to methylmalonic acid, and the increase can be detected in serum and urine. Because methylmalonic acid is also elevated in patients with impaired renal function, the test is not specific, and thus increased levels cannot be definitively related to vitamin B_{12} deficiency.[3] Methylmalonic acid is assayed by gas chromatography–tandem mass spectrometry.

Homocysteine levels are affected by deficiencies in either folate or vitamin B_{12}. 5-Methyl THF donates a methyl group to homocysteine in the generation of methionine. This reaction uses vitamin B_{12} as a coenzyme (Figure 21-4). Thus a deficiency in either folate or vitamin B_{12} results in elevated levels of homocysteine. Total homocysteine can be measured in either plasma or serum. Homocysteine may be assayed by gas chromatography–mass spectrometry, high-performance liquid chromatography, or fluorescence polarization immunoassay. Homocysteine levels are also elevated in patients with renal failure and dehydration. Figure 21-10 presents an algorithm of the analysis of these analytes in the diagnosis of vitamin B_{12} and folate deficiency.

Gastric Analysis and Serum Gastrin

Gastric analysis may be used to confirm achlorhydria, an expected finding in pernicious anemia. Achlorhydria occurs in other conditions, however, including natural aging. When other causes of vitamin B_{12} deficiency have been eliminated, a finding of achlorhydria is supportive, although not diagnostic, of pernicious anemia. The H^+ concentration is determined by pH measurement.

As a result of the gastric achlorhydria, serum gastrin levels can be markedly elevated.[4] Serum gastrin is measured by immunoassay, including chemiluminescent immunometric assays.

Antibody Assays

Antibodies to intrinsic factor and parietal cells can be detected in the serum of most patients with pernicious anemia. Various immunoassays can detect intrinsic factor–blocking antibodies; parietal cell antibodies can be detected by indirect fluorescent antibody techniques or enzyme-linked immunosorbent assays. Anti-IF antibodies are highly specific and confirmatory for pernicious anemia, but their absence does not rule out the condition. The test for parietal cell antibodies is nonspecific and not clinically useful for the diagnosis of pernicious anemia.[5]

Figure 21-11 presents an algorithm for the diagnosis of pernicious anemia using tests for serum vitamin B_{12}, methylmalonic

---

BOX 21-5 Causes of False Increases and Decreases of Vitamin B_{12} and Folate Assays[5,52]

False Increases in Vitamin B_{12} Assay Results
Assay technical failure
Occult malignancy
Alcoholic liver disease
Renal disease
Increased transcobalamin I and II binders (e.g., myeloproliferative states, hepatomas, and fibrolamellar hepatic tumors)
Activated transcobalamin II–producing macrophages (e.g., autoimmune diseases, monoblastic leukemias, and lymphomas)
Release of cobalamin from hepatocytes (e.g., active liver disease)
High serum anti–intrinsic factor antibody titer

False Decreases in Vitamin B_{12} Assay Results
Haptocorrin deficiency
Folate deficiency
Plasma cell myeloma
Human immunodeficiency virus
Pregnancy
Plasma cell myeloma
Transcobalamin I deficiency
Megadose vitamin C therapy

False Increases in Folate Assay Results
Recent meal
Alcoholism

False Decreases in Folate Assay Results
Severe anorexia requiring hospitalization
Acute alcohol consumption
Normal pregnancy
Anticonvulsant therapy

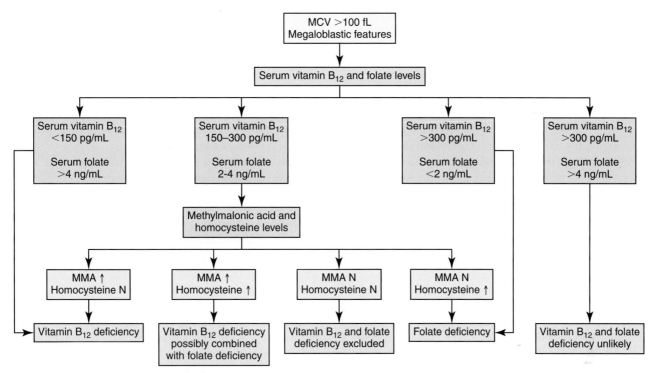

Figure 21-10 Algorithm for the use of assays for serum folate, vitamin B$_{12}$, methylmalonic acid, and homocysteine in the diagnosis of vitamin B$_{12}$ and folate deficiency.[5,44] ↑, Increased; *MCV*, mean cell volume; *MMA*, methylmalonic acid; *N*, within reference interval.

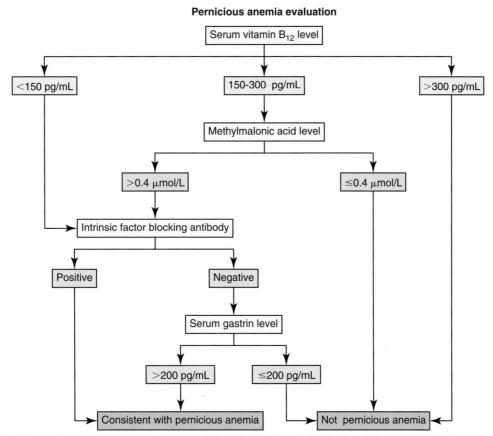

Figure 21-11 Algorithm for the diagnosis of pernicious anemia. (Adapted from Klee GG. Cobalamin and folate evaluation: Measurement of methylmalonic acid and homocysteine vs vitamin B$_{12}$ and folate. Clin Chem 2000;46, p. 1281.)

acid, intrinsic factor blocking antibody, and serum gastrin levels.

Holotranscobalamin Assay

Holotranscobalamin is the metabolically active form of vitamin B_{12}. Until recently, methods for measuring holotranscobalamin were manual and not suitable for use in clinical laboratories. Newer, more rapid immunoassays using monoclonal antibodies specific for holotranscobalamin have been developed in the past several years that are both sensitive and specific.[54,55] Recent studies suggest the specificity of holotranscobalamin to detect vitamin B_{12} deficiency is low; thus the adoption of holotranscobalamin in routine clinical testing is not supported.[53]

Deoxyuridine Suppression Test

The principle of the deoxyuridine suppression test is that the preincubation of normal bone marrow with deoxyuridine will suppress the subsequent incorporation of labeled thymidine into DNA because the normal cells can successfully methylate the uridine into thymidine. However, in patients with either a vitamin B_{12} or a folate deficiency, this suppression is abnormally low. By adding either vitamin B_{12} or folate to the test cells, one can determine whether the inadequate suppression is caused by

vitamin B_{12} or folate deficiency.[56-58] Although micromethods have been developed, the necessity of using bone marrow tissue and the complexity of the test make it impractical for clinical testing.

Stool Analysis for Parasites

When vitamin B_{12} is found to be deficient, a stool analysis for eggs or proglottids of the fish tapeworm D. latum may be part of the diagnostic workup.

Table 21-1 contains a summary of laboratory tests used to diagnose vitamin B_{12} and folate deficiency.

MACROCYTIC NONMEGALOBLASTIC ANEMIAS

The macrocytic nonmegaloblastic anemias are macrocytic anemias in which DNA synthesis is unimpaired. The macrocytosis tends to be mild; the MCV usually ranges from 100 to 110 fL and rarely exceeds 120 fL. Patients with nonmegaloblastic, macrocytic anemia lack hypersegmented neutrophils and oval macrocytes in the peripheral blood and megaloblasts in the bone marrow. Macrocytosis may be physiologically normal, as in the newborn (Chapter 45), or the result of pathology, as in liver disease, chronic alcoholism, or bone marrow failure. Reticulocytosis is a

TABLE 21-1 Laboratory Tests Used to Diagnose Vitamin B_{12} and Folate Deficiency

		Folate Deficiency	Vitamin B_{12} Deficiency
Screening tests	Complete blood count	↓ HGB, HCT, RBCs, WBCs, PLTs ↑ MCV, MCH	Same as Folate Deficiency
	Manual differential count	Hypersegmented neutrophils, oval macrocytes, anisocytosis, poikilocytosis, RBC inclusions	Same as Folate Deficiency
	Absolute reticulocyte count	↓	↓
	Serum total and indirect bilirubin	↑	↑
	Serum lactate dehydrogenase	↑	↑
Specific diagnostic tests	Bone marrow examination*	Erythroid hyperplasia (ineffective) Presence of megaloblasts	Same as Folate Deficiency
	Serum vitamin B_{12}	N	↓
	Serum folate	↓	N or ↑[†]
	RBC folate	↓	N or ↓[†]
	Serum methylmalonic acid	N	↑
	Serum/plasma homocysteine	↑	↑
	Antibodies to intrinsic factor and gastric parietal cells	Absent	Present in pernicious anemia
	Serum gastrin	N	Can be markedly elevated in pernicious anemia
	Gastric analysis*	N	Achlorhydria in pernicious anemia
	Holotranscobalamin assay[‡]	N	↓
	Stool analysis for parasites	Negative	Diphyllobothrium latum may be the cause of deficiency

↑, Increased; ↓, decreased; HGB, hemoglobin; HCT, hematocrit; MCH, mean cell hemoglobin; MCV, mean cell volume; N, within reference interval; PLT, platelet; RBC, red blood cell; WBC, white blood cell.
*Bone marrow examination and gastric analysis are not usually required for diagnosis.
[†]Without vitamin B_{12}, the cell is unable to produce intracellular polyglutamated tetrahydrofolate; therefore, 5-methyltetrahydrofolate leaks out of the cell, which results in a decreased level of intracellular folate.
[‡]Holotranscobalamin level is also decreased in transcobalamin deficiency.

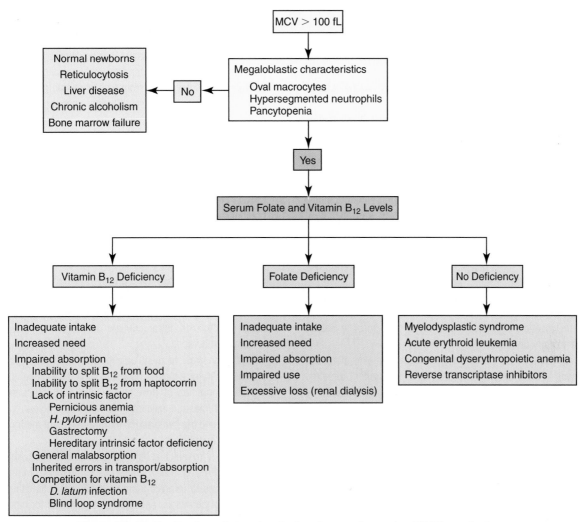

Figure 21-12 Algorithm for preliminary investigation of macrocytic anemias. *MCV,* Mean cell volume.

common cause of macrocytosis. Figure 21-12 presents an algorithm for the preliminary investigation of macrocytic anemias.

TREATMENT

Treatment should be directed at the specific vitamin deficiency established by the diagnostic tests and should include addressing the cause of the deficiency (e.g., better nutrition, treatment for *D. latum*), if possible. Vitamin B$_{12}$ is administered intramuscularly to treat pernicious anemia to bypass the need for intrinsic factor. High-dose oral vitamin B$_{12}$ treatment is increasingly popular in the treatment of pernicious anemia.[39,59,60] Regardless of the treatment modality, those with pernicious anemia or malabsorption must have lifelong vitamin replacement therapy. Folic acid can be administered orally. The inappropriate treatment of vitamin B$_{12}$ deficiency with folic acid improves the anemia but does not correct or stop the progress of the neurologic damage, which may advance to an irreversible state.[3] Thus proper diagnosis prior to treatment is important. Iron is often supplemented concurrently to support the rapid cell production that accompanies effective treatment.

When proper treatment is initiated, the body's response is prompt and brisk and can be used to confirm the accuracy of the diagnosis. The bone marrow morphology will begin to revert to a normoblastic appearance within a few hours of treatment. A substantial reticulocyte response is apparent at about 1 week, with hemoglobin increasing toward normal levels in about 3 weeks.[11] Hypersegmented neutrophils disappear from the peripheral blood within 2 weeks of initiation of treatment.[5] Thus with proper treatment, hematologic parameters may return to normal within 3 to 6 weeks.

SUMMARY

- Impaired DNA synthesis affects all rapidly dividing cells of the body, including the skin, gastrointestinal tract, and bone marrow. The effect on hematologic cells results in megaloblastic anemia.
- Vitamin B_{12} and folate are needed for the production of thymidine nucleotides for DNA synthesis. Deficiencies of either vitamin impair DNA replication, halt cell division, and increase apoptosis, which results in ineffective hematopoiesis and megaloblastic morphology of erythrocyte precursors.
- Vitamin B_{12} deficiency is associated with peripheral neuropathies and neuropsychiatric abnormalities as a result of demyelinization of nerves in the peripheral and central nervous system. Peripheral neuropathy and depression also may accompany folate deficiency. Folate deficiency in early pregnancy can lead to neural tube defects in the fetus.
- Lack of vitamin B_{12} leads to the accumulation of methylmalonic acid (MMA) and homocysteine. Folate deficiency, in particular, leads to elevation of homocysteine levels and possible risk of coronary artery disease.
- Folate deficiency may result from inadequate intake, increased need with growth or pregnancy, impaired absorption, impaired use, or excessive loss. The action of folate can be impaired by drugs such as those used to treat epilepsy or cancer. Renal dialysis patients experience significant folate loss to the dialysate.
- Vitamin B_{12} deficiency arises from inadequate intake, increased need, or inadequate absorption. Inadequate intake of vitamin B_{12}, although possible, is uncommon because vitamin B_{12} is ubiquitous in animal products. Pregnancy, lactation, and growth create increased need for vitamin B_{12}.
- Absorption of vitamin B_{12} depends on production of intrinsic factor by parietal cells of the stomach. Vitamin B_{12} bound to transcobalamin— holotranscobalamin—is the metabolically active form of the vitamin in the circulation.
- Impaired absorption of vitamin B_{12} can be caused by several mechanisms. Decrease in gastric acid production or lack of trypsin in the intestine causes vitamin B_{12} to be excreted in the stool rather than absorbed. Malabsorption can be caused by intestinal diseases, such as sprue, celiac disease, and inflammatory bowel

disease. Competition for vitamin B_{12} can develop from an intestinal parasite (*D. latum*) or bacteria in intestinal blind loops. Lack of intrinsic factor may result from loss of gastric parietal cells with pernicious anemia, *H. pylori* infection, gastrectomy, or inherited intrinsic factor deficiency.
- Pernicious anemia is vitamin B_{12} deficiency resulting from an autoimmune disease that causes destruction of gastric parietal cells. H^+ and intrinsic factor secretion is lost. Antibodies to parietal cells or intrinsic factor, or both, are detectable in the serum.
- Classic CBC findings in megaloblastic anemia include decreased hemoglobin, hematocrit, and RBC count; leukopenia; thrombocytopenia; decreased absolute reticulocyte count; elevated MCV (usually greater than 120 fL); elevated RDW and MCH; MCHC within the reference interval; and oval macrocytes and hypersegmented neutrophils observed on the peripheral blood film. Additional abnormal laboratory test findings may include elevated levels of total and indirect serum bilirubin and lactate dehydrogenase due to the intramedullary hemolysis of megaloblastic erythroid precursors.
- The bone marrow in megaloblastic anemia is hyperplastic with increased erythropoiesis; however, it is ineffective due to increased apoptosis of developing cells. RBC precursors show nuclear-cytoplasmic asynchrony, with the nuclear maturation lagging behind the cytoplasmic maturation. Giant metamyelocytes and bands are evident.
- The cause of megaloblastic anemia is determined using specific immunoassays for serum folate and vitamin B_{12}. Immunoassays for antibodies to intrinsic factor and parietal cells can aid in the diagnosis of pernicious anemia. Additional tests for gastrointestinal disease or parasites may be needed.
- Treatment of megaloblastic anemia is directed at correcting the cause of the deficiency and supplementing the missing vitamin.
- For pernicious anemia, lifelong supplementation with vitamin B_{12} is necessary.

Now that you have completed this chapter, go back and read again the case study at the beginning and respond to the questions presented.

REVIEW QUESTIONS

Answers can be found in the Appendix.

1. Which of the following findings is consistent with a diagnosis of megaloblastic anemia?
   a. Hyposegmentation of neutrophils
   b. Decreased serum lactate dehydrogenase level
   c. Absolute increase in reticulocytes
   d. Increased MCV

2. A patient has a clinical picture of megaloblastic anemia. The serum folate level is decreased, and the serum vitamin B_{12} level is 600 pg/mL (reference interval is 200–900 pg/mL). What is the expected value for the methylmalonic acid assay?
   a. Increased
   b. Decreased
   c. Within the reference interval

3. Which one of the following statements characterizes the relationships among macrocytic anemia, megaloblastic anemia, and pernicious anemia?
   a. Macrocytic anemias are megaloblastic.
   b. Macrocytic anemia is pernicious anemia.
   c. Megaloblastic anemia is macrocytic.
   d. Megaloblastic anemia is pernicious anemia.

4. Which of the following CBC findings is most suggestive of a megaloblastic anemia?
   a. MCV of 103 fL
   b. Hypersegmentation of neutrophils
   c. RDW of 16%
   d. Hemoglobin concentration of 9.1 g/dL

5. In the following description of a bone marrow smear, find the statement that is *inconsistent* with the expected picture in megaloblastic anemia.

   "The marrow appears hypercellular with a myeloid-to-erythroid ratio of 1:1 due to prominent erythroid hyperplasia. Megakaryocytes appear normal in number and appearance. The WBC elements appear larger than normal, with especially large metamyelocytes, although they otherwise appear morphologically normal. The RBC precursors also appear large. There is nuclear-cytoplasmic asynchrony, with the nucleus appearing more mature than expected for the color of the cytoplasm."
   a. Erythroid nuclei that are more mature than cytoplasm
   b. Larger than normal WBC elements
   c. Larger than normal RBCs
   d. Normal appearance of megakaryocytes

6. Which one of the following findings would be *inconsistent* with elevated titers of intrinsic factor blocking antibodies?
   a. Hypersegmentation of neutrophils
   b. Low levels of methylmalonic acid
   c. Macrocytic RBCs
   d. Low levels of vitamin B_{12}

7. Which of the following is the most metabolically active form of absorbed vitamin B_{12}?
   a. Transcobalamin
   b. Intrinsic factor–vitamin B_{12} complex
   c. Holotranscobalamin
   d. Haptocorrin–vitamin B_{12} complex

8. Folate and vitamin B_{12} work together in the production of:
   a. Amino acids
   b. RNA
   c. Phospholipids
   d. DNA

9. The macrocytosis associated with megaloblastic anemia results from:
   a. Reduced numbers of cell divisions with normal cytoplasmic development
   b. Activation of a gene that is typically active only in megakaryocytes
   c. Reduced concentration of hemoglobin in the cells so that larger cells are needed to provide the same oxygen-carrying capacity
   d. Increased production of reticulocytes in an attempt to compensate for the anemia

10. Which one of the following groups has the highest risk for pernicious anemia?
   a. Malnourished infants
   b. Children during growth periods
   c. Persons older than 60 years of age
   d. Pregnant women

REFERENCES

1. Scott, J. M. (1999). Folate and vitamin B_{12}. *Proc Nutr Soc, 58,* 441–448.
2. Wickramasinghe, S. N. (1999). The wide spectrum and unresolved issues of megaloblastic anemia. *Semin Hematol, 36,* 3–18.
3. Miller, J. W. (2013). Folic acid. In Caballero, B. (Ed.), *Encyclopedia of human nutrition* (3rd ed., pp. 262–269). Amsterdam: Elsevier/Academic Press.
4. Carmel, R. (2009). Megaloblastic anemias: disorders of impaired DNA synthesis. In Greer, J. P., Foerster, J., Rodgers, G. M., et al. (Eds.), *Wintrobe's Clinical Hematology.* (12th ed., pp. 1143–1172). Philadelphia: Wolters Kluwer Health/Lippincott Williams & Wilkins.
5. Antony, A. C. (2013). Megaloblastic anemias. In Hoffman, R., Benz, E. J., Silberstein, L. E., et al. (Eds.), *Hematology: basic principles and practice.* (6th ed., pp. 473–504). Philadelphia: Churchill Livingstone.
6. Goulian, M., Bleile, B., & Tseng, B. Y. (1980). Methotrexate-induced misincorporation of uracil into DNA. *Proc Natl Acad Sci U S A, 77,* 1956–1960.
7. Wickramasinghe, S. N., & Fida, S. (1994). Bone marrow cells from vitamin B_{12}- and folate-deficient patients misincorporate uracil into DNA. *Blood, 83,* 1656–1661.
8. Koury, M. J., Horne, D. W., Brown, Z. A., et al. (1997). Apoptosis of late stage erythroblasts in megaloblastic anemia: association with DNA damage and macrocyte production. *Blood, 89,* 4617–4623.
9. Das, K. C., Das, M., Mohanty, D., et al. (2006). Megaloblastosis: from morphos to molecules. *Med Princ Pract, 14,* 2–14.
10. Geené, D., Sudre, P., Anwar, D., et al. (2000). Causes of macrocytosis in HIV-infected patients not treated with zidovudine. Swiss HIV Cohort Study. *J Infect, 40,* 160–163.
11. Carmel, R., & Rosenblatt, D. S. (2003). Disorders of cobalamin and folate metabolism. In Handin, R. I., Lux, S. E., & Stossel, T. P. (Eds.), *Blood: principles and practice of hematology.* (2nd ed., pp. 1361–1398). Philadelphia: Lippincott Williams & Wilkins.
12. Solomon, L. R. (2007). Disorders of cobalamin (vitamin B_{12}) metabolism: emerging concepts in pathophysiology, diagnosis and treatment. *Blood Rev, 21,* 113–130.

13. Scalabrino, G., & Peracchi, M. (2006). New insights into the pathophysiology of cobalamin deficiency. *Trends Mol Med, 12,* 247–254.
14. Morrison, H. I., Schaubel, D., Desmeules, M., et al. (1996). Serum folate and risk of fatal coronary heart disease. *JAMA, 275,* 1893–1896.
15. Voutilainen, S., Virtanen, J. K., Rissanen, T. H., et al. (2004). Serum folate and homocysteine and the incidence of acute coronary events: the Kuopio Ischaemic Heart Disease Risk Factor Study. *Am J Clin Nutr, 80,* 317–323.
16. de Bree, A., Verschuren, W. M., Blom, H. J., et al. (2003). Coronary heart disease mortality, plasma homocysteine, and B-vitamins: a prospective study. *Atherosclerosis, 166,* 369–377.
17. Blom, H. J., & Smulders, Y. (2011). Overview of homocysteine and folate metabolism. With special references to cardiovascular disease and neural tube defects. *J Inherit Metab Dis, 346,* 75–81.
18. Soinio, M., Marniemi, J., Laakso, M., et al. (2004). Elevated plasma homocysteine level is an independent predictor of coronary heart disease events in patients with type 2 diabetes mellitus. *Ann Intern Med, 140,* 94–100.
19. Lindeman, R. D., Romero, L. J, Yau, C. L., et al. (2003). Serum homocysteine concentrations and their relation to serum folate and vitamin B_{12} concentrations and coronary artery disease prevalence in an urban, bi-ethnic community. *Ethn Dis, 13,* 178–185.
20. Bottiglieri, T., Laundry, M., Crellin, R., et al. (2000). Homocysteine, folate, methylation, and monoamine metabolism in depression. *J Neurol Neurosurg Psychiatry, 69,* 228–232.
21. Kronenberg, G., Colla, M., & Endres, M. (2009). Folic acid, neurodegenerative and neuropsychiatric disease. *Curr Mol Med, 9,* 315–323.
22. Reynolds, E. H., Rothfeld, P., & Pincus, J. H. (1973). Neurological disease associated with folate deficiency. *BMJ, 2,* 398–400.
23. Alpert, J. E., Mischoulon, D., Nierenberg, A. A., et al. (2000). Nutrition and depression: focus on folate. *Nutrition, 16,* 544–546.
24. Blom, H. J., Shaw, G. M., den Heijer, M., et al. (2006). Neural tube defects and folate: case far from closed. *Nat Rev Neurosci, 7,* 724–731.
25. Gallagher, M. L. (2004). Vitamins. In Mahan, L. K., & Escott-Stump, S. (Eds.), *Krause's food, nutrition, and diet therapy.* (11th ed., pp. 74–119). Philadelphia: Saunders.
26. Qui, A., Jansen, M., Sakaris, A., et al. (2006). Identification of an intestinal folate transporter and the molecular basis for hereditary folate malabsorption. *Cell, 127,* 917–928.
27. Dixon, K. H., Lanpher, B. C., Chiu, J., et al. (1994). A novel cDNA restores reduced folate carrier activity and methotrexate sensitivity to transport deficient cells. *J Biol Chem, 269*(1), 17–20.
28. Nath, S. K. (2005). Tropical sprue. *Curr Gastroenterol Rep, 7,* 343–349.
29. Waxman, S., Metz, J., & Herbert, V. (1969). Defective DNA synthesis in human megaloblastic bone marrow: effects of homocysteine and methionine. *J Clin Invest 48,* 284–289.
30. Moran, R. G., & Keyomarsi, K. (1987). Biochemical rationale for the synergism of 5-fluorouracil and folinic acid. *NCI Monogr, 5,* 159–163.
31. Kishi, T., Fujita, N., Eguchi, T., et al. (1997). Mechanism for reduction of serum folate by antiepileptic drugs during prolonged therapy. *J Neurol Sci, 145,* 109–112.
32. Froscher, W., Maier, V., Laage, M., et al. (1995). Folate deficiency, anticonvulsant drugs, and psychiatric morbidity. *Clin Neuropharmacol, 18,* 165–182.
33. Green, R. (2013). Vitamin B_{12} physiology, dietary sources, and requirements. In Caballero, B. (Ed.), *Encyclopedia of human nutrition.* (3rd ed., pp. 351–356). Amsterdam: Elsevier/Academic Press.
34. He, Q., Madsen, M., Kilkenney, A., et al. (2005). Amnionless function is required for cubilin brush-border expression and intrinsic factor-cobalamin (vitamin B_{12}) absorption in vivo. *Blood, 106,* 1447–1453.
35. Morel, C. F., & Rosenblatt, D. S. (2009). In Sarafoglou, K., Hoffman, G. F., & Roth, K. S. (Eds.), *Pediatric endocrinology and inborn errors of metabolism.* (pp. 195–210). New York: McGraw-Hill.
36. Fyfe, J. C., Madsen, M., Hojrup, P., et al. (2004). The functional cobalamin (vitamin B_{12})–intrinsic factor receptor is a novel complex of cubilin and amnionless. *Blood, 103,* 1573–1579.
37. Afman, L. A., Van Der Put, N. M. J., Thomas, C. M. G., et al. (2001). Reduced vitamin B_{12} binding by transcobalamin II increases the risk of neural tube defects. *QJM 94,* 159–166.
38. Seetharam, B., Bose, S., & Li, N. (1999). Cellular import of cobalamin (vitamin B-12). *J Nutr, 129,* 1761–1764.
39. Dali-Youcef, N., & Andres, E. (2009). An update on cobalamin deficiency in adults. *QJM, 102,* 17–28.
40. Toh, B. H., van Driel, I. R., & Gleeson, P. A. (1997). Pernicious anemia. *N Engl J Med, 337,* 1441–1448.
41. Karlsson, F. A., Burman, P., Loof, L., et al. (1988). Major parietal cell antigen in autoimmune gastritis with pernicious anemia in the acid-producing H^+,K^+-adenosine triphosphatase of the stomach. *J Clin Invest, 81,* 475–479.
42. Bardhan, K. D., Hall, J. R., Spray, G. H., et al. (1968). Blocking and binding autoantibody to intrinsic factor. *Lancet 1,* 62–64.
43. Strickland, R. G., & Hooper, B. (1972). The parietal cell heteroantibody in human sera: prevalence in a normal population and relationship to parietal cell autoantibody. *Pathology, 4,* 259–263.
44. Kaferle, J., & Strzoda, C. E. (2009). Evaluation of macrocytosis. *Am Fam Physician, 79*(3), 203–208.
45. Kaptan, K., Beyan, C., Ural, A. U., et al. (2000). *Helicobacter pylori*—is it a novel causative agent in vitamin B_{12} deficiency? *Arch Intern Med, 160,* 1349–1353.
46. Morel, C. F., Watkins, D., Scott, P., et al. (2005). Prenatal diagnosis for methylmalonic acidemia and inborn errors of vitamin B_{12} metabolism and transport. *Mol Genet Metab, 86,* 160–171.
47. Nyberg, W., Gräsbeck, R., Saarni, M., et al. (1961). Serum vitamin B_{12} levels and incidence of tape worm anemia in a population heavily infected with *Diphyllobothrium latum. Am J Clin Nutr, 9,* 606–612.
48. Zittoun, J., & Zittoun, R. (1999). Modern clinical testing strategies in cobalamin and folate deficiency. *Semin Hematol, 36,* 35–46.
49. Herbert, V. (1962). Experimental nutritional folate deficiency in man. *Trans Assoc Am Physicians, 75,* 307–320.
50. Wickramasinghe, S. N. (1999). The wide spectrum and unresolved issues in megaloblastic anemia. *Semin Hematol, 36,* 3–18.
51. Carmel, R. (1999). Introduction: beyond megaloblastic anemia. *Semin Hematol, 36,* 1–2.
52. Oberley, M. J., & Yang, D. T. (2013). Laboratory testing for cobalamin deficiency in megaloblastic anemia. *Am J Hematol, 88,* 522–526.
53. Piyathilake, C. J., Robinson, C. B., & Cornwell, P. (2007). A practical approach to red blood cell folate analysis. *Anal Chem Insights, 2,* 107–110.
54. Brady, J., Wilson, L., McGregor, L., et al. (2008). Active B_{12}: a rapid, automated assay for holotranscobalamin on the Abbott AxSYM analyzer. *Clin Chem, 54*(3), 567–573.
55. Ulleland, M., Eilertsen, I., Quadros, E. V., et al. (2002). Direct assay for cobalamin bound to transcobalamin (holotranscobalamin) in serum. *Clin Chem, 48*(3), 526–532.
56. Metz, J. (1984). The deoxyuridine suppression test. *CRC Crit Rev Clin Lab Sci, 20,* 205–241.
57. Wickramasinghe, S. N., & Matthew, J. H. (1988). Deoxyuridine suppress: biochemical basis and diagnostic applications. *Blood Rev, 2,* 168–177.
58. Carmel, R., Bedros, A. A., Mace, J. W., et al. (1980). Congenital methylmalonic aciduria—homocystinuria with megaloblastic anemia: observation on response to hydroxycobalamin and on the effect of homocysteine and methionine on the deoxyuridine suppression test. *Blood, 55,* 570–579.
59. Butler, C. C., Vidal-Alaball, J., & Cannings-John, R., et al. (2006). Oral vitamin B_{12} versus intramuscular vitamin B_{12} for vitamin B_{12} deficiency: a systematic review of randomized controlled trials. *Fam Pract, 23,* 279–285.
60. Stabler, S. P. (2013). Clinical practice. Vitamin B_{12} deficiency. *N Engl J Med, 368,* 149–160.

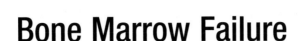

Bone Marrow Failure

22

Clara Lo, Bertil Glader, and Kathleen M. Sakamoto*

OUTLINE

OBJECTIVES

After completion of this chapter, the reader will be able to:

1. Describe the clinical consequences of bone marrow failure.
2. Describe the etiology of acquired and inherited aplastic anemias.
3. Discuss the pathophysiologic mechanisms of acquired and inherited aplastic anemias.
4. Describe the characteristic peripheral blood and bone marrow features in aplastic anemia.
5. Classify aplastic anemia as nonsevere, severe, or very severe based on laboratory tests.
6. Discuss treatment modalities for acquired and inherited aplastic anemia and the patients for whom each is most appropriate.
7. Differentiate among causes of pancytopenia based on laboratory tests and clinical findings.
8. Discuss the possible relationship between defects in the telomerase complex and bone marrow failure in acquired and inherited aplastic anemia.
9. Compare and contrast the pathophysiology, clinical picture, and laboratory findings in inherited aplastic anemia, transient erythroblastopenia of childhood, Diamond-Blackfan anemia, and congenital dyserythropoietic anemia.
10. Describe the mechanisms causing cytopenia in myelophthisic anemia and anemia of chronic kidney disease.

CASE STUDY

After studying the material in this chapter, the reader should be able to respond to the following case study:

A 16-year-old female presented to her pediatrician with jaundice. Her pediatrician checked liver enzyme and bilirubin levels, which were elevated. Hepatitis A, B, and C serologies were all negative. She was referred to a gastroenterologist, who diagnosed her with autoimmune hepatitis. With immunomodulatory treatment, her hepatitis improved. However, over the next several months, she noticed increasing fatigue and bruising. She also developed heavier menses, with menstrual cycles lasting up to 2 weeks in duration. Physical examination revealed pallor and scattered ecchymoses with petechiae on her chest and shoulders with no other abnormalities. Complete blood count results were as follows:

	Patient	Reference Interval
WBCs (×10⁹/L)	2.0	4.5–11.0
HGB (g/dL)	7.9	12.0–15.0
MCV (fL)	104	80–100
Platelets (×10⁹/L)	15	150–450
Reticulocytes (%)	0.6	0.5–2.5
Reticulocytes (×10⁹/L)	16	20–115
Neutrophils (×10⁹/L)	0.5	2.3–8.1
Lymphocytes (×10⁹/L)	0.4	0.8–4.8

Serum vitamin B_{12} and folate levels were within reference intervals. Bone marrow aspirate revealed mild dyserythropoiesis but normal myelopoiesis and megakaryopoiesis. Iron stain revealed normal stores. A bone marrow biopsy specimen was moderately hypocellular (15%) with a reduction in all three cell lines. There was no increase in reticulin or blasts. Cytogenetic testing revealed a normal karyotype, and results of flow cytometry for paroxysmal nocturnal hemoglobinuria (PNH) cells was negative.

1. What term is used to describe a decrease in all cell lines in the peripheral blood?
2. Which anemia of bone marrow failure should be considered?
3. How would an increase in either reticulin or blasts alter the preliminary diagnosis?
4. How would the severity of this patient's condition be classified?
5. What treatment modality would be considered for this patient?

---

*The authors acknowledge the contributions of Elaine M. Keohane, author of this chapter in the previous edition

PATHOPHYSIOLOGY OF BONE MARROW FAILURE

Bone marrow failure is the reduction or cessation of blood cell production affecting one or more cell lines. Pancytopenia—or decreased numbers of circulating red blood cells (RBCs), white blood cells (WBCs), and platelets—is seen in most cases of bone marrow failure, particularly in severe or advanced stages.

The pathophysiology of bone marrow failure includes (1) the destruction of hematopoietic stem cells due to injury by drugs, chemicals, radiation, viruses, or autoimmune mechanisms; (2) premature senescence and apoptosis of hematopoietic stem cells due to genetic mutations; (3) ineffective hematopoiesis due to stem cell mutations or vitamin B_{12} or folate deficiency; (4) disruption of the bone marrow microenvironment that supports hematopoiesis; (5) decreased production of hematopoietic growth factors or related hormones; and (6) the loss of normal hematopoietic tissue due to infiltration of the marrow space with abnormal cells.

The clinical consequences of bone marrow failure vary, depending on the extent and duration of the cytopenias. Severe pancytopenia can be rapidly fatal if untreated. Some patients may initially be asymptomatic, and their cytopenia may be detected during a routine blood examination. Thrombocytopenia can result in bleeding and increased bruising. Decreased RBCs and hemoglobin can result in fatigue, pallor, and cardiovascular complications. Sustained neutropenia increases the risk of life-threatening bacterial or fungal infections.

This chapter focuses on aplastic anemia, a bone marrow failure syndrome resulting from damaged or defective stem cells (mechanisms 1 and 2 listed earlier). Bone marrow failure resulting from other mechanisms may present similarly to aplastic anemia, and differentiation is discussed later. Because there are many mechanisms involved in the various bone marrow failure syndromes, accurate diagnosis is essential to ensure appropriate treatment.

APLASTIC ANEMIA

Aplastic anemia is a rare but potentially fatal bone marrow failure syndrome. In 1888, Ehrlich provided the first case report of aplastic anemia involving a patient with severe anemia, neutropenia, and a hypocellular marrow on postmortem examination.[1] The name *aplastic anemia* was given to the disease by Vaquez and Aubertin in 1904.[2] The characteristic features of aplastic anemia include pancytopenia, reticulocytopenia, bone marrow hypocellularity, and depletion of hematopoietic stem cells (Box 22-1). Approximately 80% to 85% of aplastic anemia cases are acquired, whereas 15% to 20% are inherited.[3] Box 22-2 provides etiologic classifications.[3-5]

Acquired Aplastic Anemia

Acquired aplastic anemia is classified into two major categories: idiopathic and secondary. Idiopathic acquired aplastic anemia has no known cause. Secondary acquired aplastic anemia is associated with an identified cause. Approximately 70% of all aplastic anemia cases are idiopathic, whereas 10% to 15% are secondary.[3] Idiopathic and secondary acquired aplastic anemia have similar clinical and laboratory findings. Patients may initially present with macrocytic or normocytic anemia and reticulocytopenia. Pancytopenia may develop slowly or progress at a rapid rate, with complete cessation of hematopoiesis.

Incidence

In North America and Europe, the annual incidence is approximately 1 in 500,000.[6] In Asia and East Asia, the incidence is two to three times higher than in North America or Europe, which may be due to environmental and/or genetic differences.[7] Aplastic anemia can occur at any age, with peak incidence at 15 to 25 years and the second highest frequency at greater than 60 years.[4,6,8] There is no gender predisposition.[6]

BOX 22-1   Characteristic Features of Aplastic Anemia

Pancytopenia
Reticulocytopenia
Bone marrow hypocellularity
Depletion of hematopoietic stem cells

BOX 22-2   Etiologic Classification of Aplastic Anemia

Acquired (80% to 85% of cases)
Idiopathic (70% of cases)
Secondary (10% to 15% of cases)
    Dose dependent/predictable
        Cytotoxic drugs
        Benzene
        Radiation
    Idiosyncratic
        Drugs (Box 22-3)
        Chemicals
            Insecticides
            Cutting/lubricating oils
    Viruses
        Epstein-Barr virus
        Hepatitis virus (non-A, non-B, non-C, non-G)
        Human immunodeficiency virus
    Miscellaneous conditions
        Paroxysmal nocturnal hemoglobinuria
        Autoimmune diseases
        Pregnancy

Inherited (15% to 20% of cases)
Fanconi anemia
Dyskeratosis congenita
Shwachman-Bodian-Diamond syndrome

Etiology

As the name indicates, the cause of idiopathic aplastic anemia is unknown. Secondary aplastic anemia is associated with exposure to certain drugs, chemicals, radiation, or infections. Cytotoxic drugs, radiation, and benzenes are responsible for 10% of secondary aplastic anemia cases and suppress the bone marrow in a predictable, dose-dependent manner.[4,5] Depending on the dose and exposure duration, the bone marrow generally recovers after withdrawal of the agent. Alternatively, approximately 70% of cases of secondary aplastic anemia occur due to idiosyncratic reactions to drugs or chemicals. In idiosyncratic reactions, the bone marrow failure is unpredictable and unrelated to dose.[4] Documentation of a responsible factor or agent in these cases is difficult, because evidence is primarily circumstantial and symptoms may occur months or years after exposure. Some drugs associated with idiosyncratic secondary aplastic anemia are listed in Box 22-3.[4,8]

Generally, idiosyncratic secondary aplastic anemia is a rare event and is likely due to a combination of genetic and environmental factors in susceptible individuals. Currently, there are no readily available tests that predict individual susceptibility to these idiosyncratic reactions. However, genetic variations in immune response pathways or metabolic enzymes may play a role.[4] There is an approximately twofold higher incidence of HLA-DR2 and its major serologic split, HLA-DR15, in aplastic anemia patients compared to the general population, but the relationship of this finding to disease pathophysiology has not been elucidated.[9,10] There are also reports that genetic polymorphisms in enzymes that metabolize benzene increase susceptibility to toxicity, even at low exposure levels.[4,11] These include polymorphisms in glutathione S-transferase (GST) enzymes (GSTT1 and GSTM1), myeloperoxidase, nicotinamide adenine dinucleotide phosphate (reduced form, NADPH), quinine oxidoreductase 1, and cytochrome oxidase P450 2E1.[11] A deficiency in GST due to the GSTT1 null genotype is overrepresented in whites, Hispanics, and Asians with aplastic anemia, with a frequency of 30%, 28%, and 75%, respectively.[12] White patients with aplastic anemia also have a higher frequency (22%) of the GSTM1/GSTT1 null genotype than the general population.[12] GST is important for metabolism and neutralization of chemical toxins, and deficiencies of this enzyme may increase the risk of aplastic anemia. Further study is required to assess how these genetic variations, and other yet undiscovered factors, contribute to aplastic anemia.

Acquired aplastic anemia occurs occasionally as a complication of infection with Epstein-Barr virus, human immunodeficiency virus (HIV), hepatitis virus, and human parvovirus B19.[4] A history of acute non-A, non-B, or non-C hepatitis 1 to 3 months before the onset of pancytopenia is found in 2% to 10% of patients with acquired aplastic anemia.[13] The acquired aplastic anemia in these cases may be mediated by such mechanisms as interferon gamma and cytokine release.[13]

Aplastic anemia associated with pregnancy is a rare occurrence, with fewer than 100 cases reported in the literature.[14]

BOX 22-3 Selected Drugs Reported to Have a Rare Association with Idiosyncratic Secondary Aplastic Anemia

Antiarthritics
Gold compounds
Penicillamine

Antibiotics
Chloramphenicol
Sulfonamides

Anticonvulsants
Carbamazepine
Hydantoins
Phenacemide

Antidepressants
Dothiepin
Phenothiazine

Antidiabetic Agents
Chlorpropamide
Tolbutamide
Carbutamide

Anti-inflammatories (nonsteroidal)
Diclofenac
Fenbufen
Fenoprofen
Ibuprofen
Indomethacin
Naproxen
Phenylbutazone
Piroxicam
Sulindac

Antiprotozoals
Chloroquine
Quinacrine

Antithyroidals
Methimazole
Methylthiouracil

Carbonic Anhydrase Inhibitors
Methazolamide
Mesalazine
Acetazolamide

Approximately 10% of individuals with acquired aplastic anemia have a concomitant autoimmune disease,[15] and approximately 10% develop hemolytic or thrombotic manifestations of paroxysmal nocturnal hemoglobinuria (PNH).[16] The overlap between acquired aplastic anemia and PNH is discussed later.

Pathophysiology

The primary lesion in acquired aplastic anemia is a quantitative and qualitative deficiency of hematopoietic stem cells. Stem cells of patients with acquired aplastic anemia have diminished colony formation in methylcellulose cultures.[17] The hematopoietic stem and early progenitor cell compartment is identified by expression of CD34 surface antigens. The CD34[+] cell population in the bone marrow of patients with acquired aplastic anemia can be 10% or lower than that seen in healthy individuals.[17] In addition, these CD34[+] cells have increased expression of Fas receptors that mediate apoptosis and increased expression of apoptosis-related genes.[18-20]

The bone marrow stromal cells are functionally normal in acquired aplastic anemia. They produce normal or even increased quantities of growth factors and are able to support the growth of CD34[+] cells from healthy donors in culture and in vivo after transplantation.[4,21] Individuals with aplastic anemia also have elevated serum levels of erythropoietin, thrombopoietin, granulocyte colony-stimulating factor (G-CSF), and granulocyte-macrophage colony-stimulating factor (GM-CSF).[22] In addition, serum levels of FLT3 ligand, a growth factor that stimulates proliferation of stem and progenitor cells, is up to 200 times higher in patients with severe aplastic anemia compared to healthy controls.[22,23] However, despite their elevated levels, growth factors are generally unsuccessful in correcting the cytopenias found in acquired aplastic anemia.

The severe depletion of hematopoietic stem and progenitor cells from the bone marrow may be due to direct damage to stem cells, immune damage to stem cells, or other unknown mechanisms. Direct damage to stem and progenitor cells results from DNA injury following exposure to cytotoxic drugs, chemicals, radiation, or viruses.[4]

Immune damage to stem cells results from exposure to drugs, chemicals, viruses, or other agents that cause an autoimmune cytotoxic T-lymphocytic destruction of stem and progenitor cells.[24] An autoimmune pathophysiology was first suggested in the 1970s when aplastic anemia patients undergoing pretransplant immunosuppressive conditioning had an improvement in cell counts.[25] Further evidence supporting an autoimmune pathophysiology include (1) elevated blood and bone marrow cytotoxic (CD8[+]) T lymphocytes with an oligoclonal expansion of specific T-cell clones[26]; (2) increased T cell production of such cytokines as interferon-γ (IFN-γ) and tumor necrosis factor-α (TNF-α), which inhibit hematopoiesis and induce apoptosis[27-29]; (3) upregulation of T-bet, a transcription factor that binds to the promoter of the IFN-γ gene[30]; (4) increased TNF-α receptors on CD34[+] cells[31]; and (5) improvement in cytopenias after immunosuppressive therapy (IST).[4,24] Approximately two thirds of patients with acquired aplastic anemia respond to IST.[32] The nonresponders may have a severely depleted stem cell compartment or other pathophysiologic factors contributing to their cytopenias.[32]

Possible autoimmune mechanisms include mutation of stem cell antigens and disruption of immune regulation. Young and co-workers showed that environmental exposures may alter self-proteins, induce expression of abnormal or novel antigens, or induce an immune response that cross-reacts with self-antigens.[24,28] Solomou and co-workers demonstrated that CD4[+]CD25[+]FOXP3[+] regulatory T cells are decreased in aplastic anemia.[33] These regulatory T cells normally suppress autoreactive T cells, and a deficit of these cells may facilitate an autoimmune reaction. Furthermore, a number of individuals with aplastic anemia have single nucleotide polymorphisms in IFN-γ/[+]874 TT, TNF-α/−308 AA, transforming growth factor-β1/−509 TT, and interleukin-6/−174 GG.[34] These polymorphisms result in cytokine overproduction and may impart a genetic susceptibility to aplastic anemia as well as contribute to its severity.[34]

The specific antigens responsible for triggering and sustaining the autoimmune attack on stem cells are unknown. Candidate antigens have been identified from aplastic anemia patient sera, including kinectin,[35] diazepam-binding inhibitor-related protein 1,[36] and moesin.[37] These proteins are expressed in hematopoietic progenitor cells, but their role in the pathogenesis of aplastic anemia requires further investigation.

Approximately one third of patients with acquired aplastic anemia have shortened telomeres in their peripheral blood granulocytes compared with age-matched controls.[38,39] Telomeres protect the ends of chromosomes from damage and erosion, and cells with abnormally short telomeres undergo proliferation arrest and premature apoptosis. Telomerase is an enzyme complex that repairs and maintains the telomeres. Approximately 10% of patients with acquired aplastic anemia and shortened telomeres have a mutation in the telomerase complex gene for either the ribonucleic acid (RNA) template (*TERC*) or the reverse transcriptase (*TERT*).[39-41] The cause for shortened telomeres in the other 90% of patients may be due to stress hematopoiesis or other yet unidentified mutations.[39] In stress hematopoiesis, there is an increase in progenitor cell turnover, and the telomeres become shorter with each cell division.

Approximately 4% of patients with acquired aplastic anemia and shortened telomeres have mutations in the Shwachman-Bodian-Diamond syndrome (*SBDS*) gene.[42] The *SBDS* gene product is involved in ribosome biogenesis, and its relationship to telomere maintenance is currently unknown.[42] *TERT/TERC* and *SBDS* mutations also occur in the inherited aplastic anemias, dyskeratosis congenita (DKC) and SBDS, respectively, and some patients diagnosed with acquired aplastic anemia who have these mutations may actually have DKC or SBDS.[3,4] Correct differentiation between acquired and inherited aplastic anemia has important implications for appropriate treatment and prognosis. Immunosuppressive therapy is not nearly as effective in inherited aplastic anemia as it is in acquired aplastic anemia. Furthermore, hematopoietic stem cell transplantation (HSCT), the only known curative treatment for DKC and SBDS and a treatment option for acquired aplastic anemia, should not be performed with human leukocyte antigen (HLA)–matched siblings who test positive for the same genetic mutation.[39] Brummerndorf and colleagues reported that shortened telomeres occur more often in patients whose pancytopenia does not respond to immunosuppressive therapy.[43] Defective telomere maintenance may be another pathophysiologic mechanism of stem cell injury, imparting susceptibility to aplastic anemia after an environmental insult.[39,41]

Clinical Findings

Symptoms vary in acquired aplastic anemia, ranging from asymptomatic to severe. Patients usually present with symptoms of insidious-onset anemia, with pallor, fatigue, and weakness. Severe and prolonged anemia can result in serious cardiovascular complications, including tachycardia, hypotension, cardiac failure, and death. Symptoms of thrombocytopenia are also varied and include petechiae, bruising, epistaxis, mucosal bleeding, menorrhagia, retinal hemorrhages, intestinal bleeding, and intracranial hemorrhage. Fever and bacterial or fungal infections are unusual at initial presentation but may occur after prolonged periods of neutropenia. Splenomegaly and hepatomegaly are typically absent.

Laboratory Findings

Pancytopenia is typical, although initially only one or two cell lines may be decreased. The absolute neutrophil count is decreased, and the absolute lymphocyte count may be normal or decreased. The hemoglobin is usually less than 10 g/dL, the mean cell volume (MCV) is increased or normal, and the percent and absolute reticulocyte counts are decreased. Table 22-1 lists the diagnostic criteria for aplastic anemia by degree of severity.[6,8,44,45]

Neutrophils, monocytes, and platelets are decreased in the peripheral blood, and the red blood cells are macrocytic or normocytic (Figure 22-1). Toxic granulation may be observed in the neutrophils, but the RBCs and platelets are usually normal in appearance. Leukemic blasts and other immature blood cells are characteristically absent. The serum iron level and percent transferrin saturation are increased, which reflects decreased iron use for erythropoiesis. Liver function test results may be abnormal in cases of hepatitis-associated aplastic anemia.

Approximately two thirds of patients have small numbers (less than 25%) of PNH clones in the peripheral blood,[46] but only 10% of patients develop a sufficient number of PNH cells to have the clinical and biochemical manifestations of PNH disease.[16] PNH is characterized by an acquired stem cell mutation resulting in lack of the glycosylphosphatidylinositol

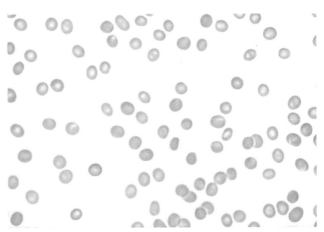

Figure 22-1 Peripheral blood film for a patient with aplastic anemia (×500). Note occasional macrocytes and absence of white blood cells and platelets.

(GPI)-linked proteins CD55 and CD59. The absence of CD55 and CD59 on the surface of the RBCs renders them more susceptible to complement-mediated cell lysis. It is important to test for PNH in acquired aplastic anemia because of the increased risk of hemolytic and/or thrombotic complications (Chapter 24). Historically, PNH diagnosis depended on the Ham acid hemolysis test: patients' cells were placed in acidified serum, and a positive result demonstrated lysis of RBCs. However, this test was poorly sensitive, because complement-mediated hemolysis was detected only in the presence of large numbers of circulating PNH cells. Currently, flow cytometric analysis for CD59 on RBCs and CD24 and CD14 on granulocytes and monocytes is used as a more sensitive diagnostic method and has replaced the Ham test in nearly all laboratories (Chapter 24).[8,46,47]

Bone marrow aspirate and biopsy specimens have prominent fat cells with areas of patchy marrow cellularity. Biopsy samples are required for accurate quantitative assessment of marrow cellularity, and severe hypocellularity is a characteristic feature of aplastic anemia (Figure 22-2). Erythroid, granulocytic, and megakaryocytic cells are decreased or absent. Dyserythropoiesis may be present, but there is typically no dysplasia of the granulocyte or platelet cell lines. Blasts and other abnormal cell infiltrates are characteristically absent. Reticulin staining is usually normal.

In patients receiving immunosuppressive therapy, the risk of developing an abnormal karyotype is 14% at 5 years and

TABLE 22-1 Diagnostic Criteria for Aplastic Anemia

	MAA	SAA	VSAA
Bone marrow	Hypocellular bone marrow plus at least two of the following:	Bone marrow cellularity <25%* plus at least two of the following:	Same as SAA
Neutrophils (×10⁹/L)	0.5–1.5	0.2–0.5	<0.2
Platelets (×10⁹/L)	20–50	<20	Same as SAA
Other	HGB ≤10 g/dL plus reticulocytes <30 × 10⁹/L	Reticulocytes <20 × 10⁹/L or <1% corrected for HCT	Same as SAA

HGB, Hemoglobin; *HCT*, hematocrit; *MAA*, moderate aplastic anemia; *SAA*, severe aplastic anemia; *VSAA*, very severe aplastic anemia; *g*, grams; *dL*, deciliter; *L*, liter.
*Or 25% to 50% cellularity with <30% residual hematopoietic cells.

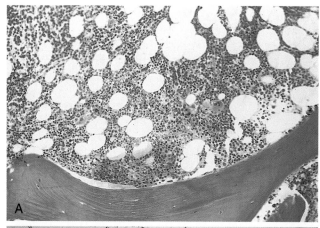

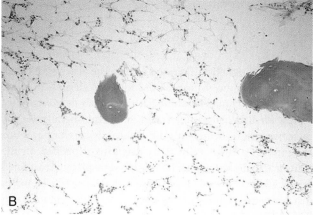

Figure 22-2 A, Normal bone marrow tissue section (hematoxylin and eosin stain). **B,** Hypoplastic bone marrow tissue section from a patient with aplastic anemia (hematoxylin and eosin stain). (Courtesy Ann Bell, University of Tennessee, Memphis.)

20% at 10 years.[48] Monosomy 7 and trisomy 8 are the most common cytogenetic abnormalities.[47,48] Cytogenetic analysis using conventional culture techniques often underestimates the incidence of karyotype abnormalities because of bone marrow hypocellularity and scarcity of cells in metaphase.[49] Alternatively, interphase fluorescence in situ hybridization (FISH) using deoxyribonucleic acid (DNA) probes for specific chromosome abnormalities may be used. In comparison to conventional cytogenetic analysis, FISH has greater sensitivity in the detection of chromosome abnormalities and can also be performed using nondividing cells.[49] In a study performed by Kearns and colleagues, FISH detected monosomy 7 or trisomy 8 in 26% of aplastic anemia patients who had a normal karyotype by conventional cytogenetic testing.[49]

Patients with inherited aplastic anemia may be misdiagnosed with acquired aplastic anemia if symptoms manifest in late adolescence or adulthood or if the patients lack the typical clinical and physical characteristics of an inherited marrow failure syndrome (e.g., abnormal thumbs, short stature).[3,4] Consideration of inherited aplastic anemia syndromes in the differential diagnosis of acquired aplastic anemia is essential, because these conditions require a different therapeutic

approach. The inherited aplastic anemia syndromes are discussed later in the chapter.

Treatment and Prognosis

Severe acquired aplastic anemia requires immediate attention to prevent serious complications. If a causative agent is identified, its use should be discontinued. Blood product replacement should be given judiciously to avoid alloimmunization.[8] Platelets should not be transfused at levels greater than 10,000/μL, unless the patient is bleeding.[8]

One of the most important early decisions is determining whether the patient is a candidate for hematopoietic stem cell transplantation (HSCT). HSCT is the treatment of choice for patients with severe aplastic anemia who are younger than 40 years of age and have a human leukocyte antigen (HLA)-identical sibling.[4,8] Unfortunately, only 20% to 30% of patients meet these criteria.[4] Therefore, IST, consisting of antithymocyte globulin and cyclosporine, is used for patients older than 40 years of age and for patients without an HLA-identical sibling.[8,16] Antithymocyte globulin decreases the number of activated T cells, and cyclosporine inhibits T-cell function, thereby suppressing the autoimmune reaction against the stem cells. Approximately two thirds of patients initially respond to IST; unfortunately, 30% to 40% relapse.[16,32] For patients with severe acquired aplastic anemia who are not responsive to IST, a second course of IST or an HSCT from an HLA-matched unrelated donor is an option, but survival is not as high as with HSCT from an HLA-identical sibling.[8,50] The response rate for a second course of IST is approximately 65% for those who experienced relapse and 30% for those whose disorder was initially refractory to IST.[51] Individuals with PNH cells (CD55⁻ CD59⁻) are almost twice as likely to respond to IST than are those who lack these cells.[46] In addition, the presence of both PNH cells and HLA-DR2 increases the likelihood of response by 3.5-fold.[52] Granulocyte colony-stimulating factor (G-CSF), other hematopoietic growth factors, and steroids do not increase overall survival or improve the response rate; therefore, they are not recommended for routine use.[8,53,54]

Other supportive therapy includes antibiotic and antifungal prophylaxis in cases of prolonged neutropenia. Patients with mild to moderate aplastic anemia may not require treatment but must be monitored periodically for pancytopenia and abnormal cells.

The overall outcome for patients with acquired aplastic anemia has dramatically improved in the past 2 decades. Among patients who receive an HSCT from an HLA-identical sibling, 91% of children and 74% of adults achieve 10-year overall survival.[50] Those percentages decrease slightly to 75% of children and 63% of adults when the bone marrow transplant is from an HLA-matched unrelated donor.[50] In patients treated with IST, 75% of children and 63% of adults achieve 10-year survival.[50] Additional outcomes in the IST-treated patients include a 10-year risk of developing hemolytic or thrombotic PNH and a 10% to 20% risk of myelodysplastic syndrome (MDS) or leukemia.[16,47] Development of monosomy 7 predicts poor outcome, with a greater likelihood of unresponsiveness to IST and progression to MDS or leukemia.[48]

Inherited Aplastic Anemia

In comparison with acquired aplastic anemia, patients with inherited aplastic anemia present at an earlier age and may have characteristic physical stigmata. The three inherited diseases for which bone marrow failure and pancytopenia are a consistent feature are Fanconi anemia, dyskeratosis congenita, and Shwachman-Bodian-Diamond syndrome.

Fanconi Anemia

Fanconi anemia (FA) is a chromosome instability disorder characterized by aplastic anemia, physical abnormalities, and cancer susceptibility. In 1927, Dr. Guido Fanconi first described this syndrome in three brothers with skin pigmentation, short stature, and hypogonadism.[55] FA has a prevalence of 1 to 5 cases per million.[56] The carrier rate is 1 in 300 in the United States and Europe, with a threefold higher prevalence in Ashkenazi Jews and South African Africaners.[57] FA is the most common of the inherited aplastic anemias.

Clinical Findings. Patients with FA have variable features and symptoms. Physical malformations may be present at birth, though hematologic abnormalities may not appear until older childhood or adulthood. Furthermore, only two thirds of patients have physical malformations.[3,58] These anomalies vary considerably, though there is a higher frequency of skeletal abnormalities (thumb malformations, radial hypoplasia, microcephaly, hip dislocation, and scoliosis); skin pigmentation (hyperpigmentation, hypopigmentation, café-au-lait lesions); short stature; and abnormalities of the eyes, kidneys, and genitals.[56-58] Low birth weight and developmental delay are also common.

The symptoms associated with pancytopenia usually become apparent at 5 to 10 years of age, though some patients may not present until adulthood.[3,57] Individuals with FA also have an increased cancer risk. This includes an increased incidence of leukemia in childhood and solid tumors (e.g., oral, esophageal, anogenital, cervical) in adulthood.[59] In approximately 5% of cases, a malignancy is diagnosed before the FA is recognized.[59]

Genetics and Pathophysiology. There are currently 15 reported genes associated with FA: *FANCA, FANCB, FANCC, FANCD1* (also called *BRCA2*), *FANCD2, FANCE, FANCF, FANCG* (also called *XRCC9*), *FANCI, FANCJ* (also called *BRIP1/BACH1*), *FANCL, FANCM, FANCN* (also called *PALB2*), *FANCO* (also called *RAD51C*), and *FANCP* (also called *SLX4*).[56] Patients with FA typically have biallelic mutations or deletions in one of these genes. The mode of inheritance is autosomal recessive except for *FANCB*, which is X-linked recessive. Mutations in the *FANCA* gene occur with the highest frequency.[3,58] The relationship between mutations in the FA genes and disease pathology is not clear. Cells are highly susceptible to chromosome breakage after exposure to DNA cross-linking agents. FA cells may also have accelerated telomere shortening

and apoptosis, a late S-phase cell cycle delay, hypersensitivity to oxidants, and cytokine dysregulation.[3,56,58,60]

The range of FA protein function is not completely known, but these proteins participate in a highly elaborate DNA damage response pathway. The FA pathway consists of a nuclear core complex, a protein ID complex, and effector proteins.[58,60] The FA proteins A, B, C, E, F, G, L, and M form the nuclear core complex; proteins D2 and I form the ID complex; and the effector proteins are D1, J, N, O, and P.[56,58,60] The core complex facilitates the monoubiquitylation and activation of the ID complex. The ID complex then localizes with effector DNA repair proteins at foci of DNA damage to effect DNA repair.[58,60]

Laboratory Findings. Laboratory results are similar to those in acquired aplastic anemia, with pancytopenia, reticulocytopenia, and a hypocellular bone marrow. Macrocytic RBCs are often the first detected abnormality, and thrombocytopenia usually precedes the development of the other cytopenias.[56] Fetal hemoglobin (Hb F) may be strikingly elevated, and α-fetoprotein is also increased.[56]

Chromosomal breakage analysis is the diagnostic test for Fanconi anemia.[56] Patients' peripheral blood lymphocytes are cultured with the DNA cross-linking agents diepoxybutane (DEB) or mitomycin C (MMC). Compared to normal lymphocytes, FA cells have a greater number of characteristic chromosome breaks and ring chromosomes, indicating increased fragility.[3,56] Caution must be made in interpreting peripheral blood results, because they may be negative in the 10% to 15% of FA patients who have somatic mosaicism due to a reversion of one abnormal allele to the normal type.[3,56] To confirm the diagnosis in these cases, chromosome breakage studies can be performed on cultured skin fibroblasts from a skin biopsy specimen.[56,61]

Treatment and Prognosis. More than 90% of FA patients develop bone marrow failure by 40 years of age.[59] Furthermore, one third of patients develop MDS and/or acute myeloid leukemia (AML) by a median age of 14 years, and 25% develop solid tumors by a median age of 26 years.[59,62] Squamous cell carcinomas of the head and neck, anogenital region, and skin are the most common solid tumors, followed by tumors of the liver, brain, and kidney.[59] Patients with FA have an increased risk of developing vulvar cancer (4300-fold), esophageal cancer (2300-fold), AML (800-fold), and head/neck cancer (700-fold) compared with the general population.[63] Approximately 3% of patients develop more than one type of malignancy.[62] Left untreated, death by 20 years of age secondary to bone marrow failure or malignancy is common. Patients with mutations in the *FANCC* gene experience bone marrow failure at a particularly young age and have the poorest survival.[62] Increased telomere shortening in FA cells is associated with more severe pancytopenia and a higher risk of malignancy. However, the precise role of telomere shortening in the evolution of bone marrow failure and cancer is currently unclear.[64]

Supportive treatment for cytopenia includes transfusions and administration of cytokines (G-CSF and GM-CSF).[56,57] The only curative treatment is HSCT, preferably from an HLA-identical sibling. It is important to screen donor siblings for FA prior to transplant. Patients should also have decreased intensity pretransplant conditioning because of their underlying chromosomal instability.[56,62] Gene therapy has been attempted in clinical trials but has not been successful.

Dyskeratosis Congenita

Dyskeratosis congenita (DKC) is a rare inherited bone marrow failure syndrome with fewer than 600 known cases worldwide.[56,65]

Clinical Findings. DKC is characterized by mucocutaneous abnormalities, bone marrow failure, and pancytopenia. The typical clinical presentation involves a triad of abnormal skin pigmentation, dystrophic nails, and oral leukoplakia. Skin and nail findings usually appear before 10 years of age.[3,56] Median age of diagnosis is 15 years.[66] By 30 years of age, 80% to 90% of patients have bone marrow abnormalities.[3] Patients can also manifest a wide range of multisystem abnormalities, including pulmonary fibrosis, liver disease, developmental delay, short stature, microcephaly, prematurely gray hair or hair loss, immunodeficiency, dental caries, and periodontal disease.[66] Patients have a 40% risk of cancer by 50 years of age, most commonly AML, MDS, and epithelial malignancies.[65]

Genetics and Pathophysiology. DKC chromosomes have very short telomeres, and inherited defects in the telomerase complex are implicated in the pathophysiology.[66] The telomerase complex synthesizes telomere repeats to elongate chromosome ends, maintaining the telomere length needed for cell survival.

There are currently eight different genes implicated in DKC, and it can be inherited in three different patterns: X-linked recessive, autosomal dominant, and autosomal recessive.[3,56,66] The best-characterized form results from one or more mutations on the long arm of the X-chromosome on the *DKC1* gene dyskerin. Dyskerin is a ribonucleoprotein involved in RNA processing, and it associates with TERC (telomerase RNA component) in the telomerase complex. The autosomal dominant form is due to mutations in the genes that encode TERC, TERT (telomerase enzyme), or TINF2 (component of the shelterin complex that regulates telomere length).[66] In the autosomal recessive form, mutations in *TERT, NHP2, NOP10, WRAP53*, and *CTC1* have been identified.[66] The proteins encoded by these genes are also involved in telomere maintenance. Although the exact pathophysiologic mechanisms are still unknown, the shortened telomeres in DKC cause premature death in the rapidly dividing cells in the bone marrow and epithelium and likely lead to genomic instability and a predisposition to cancer.[3,56,67]

Laboratory Findings. Pancytopenia and macrocytic RBCs are typical peripheral blood findings. The fetal hemoglobin level

may also be increased. Only about 40% of patients have an identified mutation in one of the eight known telomerase complex genes.[67] A new flow fluorescence in situ hybridization (FISH) test for detection of very short telomeres in WBC subsets has been proposed as a diagnostic test for those with suspected DKC who lack mutations in known genes.[67] Patients with FA, SBDS, and acquired aplastic anemia may also have cells with shortened telomeres, though they are not found in multiple WBC subsets.[67] In contrast, DKC cells often have shortened telomeres in several WBC subsets, including naive T cells and B cells.

Treatment and Prognosis. Median survival for patients with DKC is 42 years.[65] Approximately 60% to 70% of deaths are due to bone marrow failure complications. Ten percent to 15% of deaths result from severe pulmonary disease, and 10% of deaths result from malignancies.[3,56] Treatment with bone marrow transplantation has not been optimal because of the high incidence of fatal pulmonary fibrosis and vascular complications.[3,66] Although androgen therapy produces a transient response in 50% to 70% of patients, it does not halt the progression of the bone marrow failure.[3]

Shwachman-Bodian-Diamond Syndrome

Shwachman-Bodian-Diamond syndrome (SBDS) is an inherited multisystem disorder characterized by pancreatic insufficiency, cytopenia, skeletal abnormalities, and a predisposition for hematologic malignancies. The incidence has been estimated to be approximately 8.5 cases per 1 million live births.[56]

Clinical Findings. Patients with SBDS have peripheral blood cytopenia and decreased pancreatic enzyme secretion.[45] The pancreatic insufficiency causes gastrointestinal malabsorption, which typically presents in early infancy.[3] Patients have neutropenia and immune dysfunction and are at increased risk of severe infections and sepsis.[45,68] Nearly all SBDS patients have delayed bone maturation, and approximately 50% have failure to thrive and short stature.[45,69]

Genetics and Pathophysiology. SBDS is an autosomal recessive disorder, and 90% of patients have biallelic mutations in the *SBDS* gene.[3,45,68] The *SBDS* gene is involved in ribosome metabolism and mitotic spindle stability,[70] but its relationship to the disease manifestations is currently unknown. There are quantitative and qualitative deficiencies in CD34+ cells, dysfunctional bone marrow stromal cells, increased apoptosis and mitotic spindle destabilization in hematopoietic cells, and short telomeres in peripheral blood granulocytes.[3,45,68,70]

Laboratory Findings. Nearly all patients with SBDS have neutropenia (less than 1.5×10^9 neutrophils/L).[71] Half of the patients also develop anemia or thrombocytopenia, and one fourth develop pancytopenia.[71] The RBCs are usually normocytic but can be macrocytic, and approximately two thirds of patients have elevated Hb F.[45,71] The bone marrow is usually hypocellular but can be normal or even hypercellular. Due to the pancreatic insufficiency, 72-hour fecal fat testing shows increased fat excretion, and serum trypsinogen and isoamylase levels are decreased compared with age-related reference intervals.[68] In comparison to cystic fibrosis, which can have a similar malabsorption presentation, patients with SBDS have normal sweat chloride tests. Testing for the *SBDS* gene mutation is commercially available and should be done in suspected patients and their parents.

Treatment and Prognosis. In some cases no treatment of hematologic features is required. However, if needed, treatment consists of G-CSF for neutropenia, transfusion support for anemia and thrombocytopenia, and enzyme replacement for pancreatic insufficiency. The risk of AML and MDS is approximately 19% at 20 years and 36% at 30 years.[72] Allogeneic bone marrow transplantation is recommended in cases of severe pancytopenia, AML, or MDS. Unfortunately, despite supportive care and attempted curative therapy, 5-year overall survival is 60% to 65%, with many deaths occurring from severe infections and malignancy.[45,68] Poor outcomes after

HSCT occur due to graft failure, transplant-related toxicities, and recurrent leukemia.[68]

Differential Diagnosis

A distinction must be made between acquired aplastic anemia, inherited aplastic anemia, and other causes of pancytopenia, including PNH, MDS, megaloblastic anemia, and leukemia. The importance of a correct diagnosis is clear, as diagnostic conclusions dictate therapeutic management and prognosis. The distinguishing features of these conditions are listed in Tables 22-2 and 22-3.[3,8]

Alternative diagnoses include lymphoma, myelofibrosis, and mycobacterial infections, which also may present with pancytopenia. However, these diagnoses often can be distinguished with a careful history, physical exam, and laboratory testing. Review of a peripheral blood film by an experienced morphologist is important. If needed, bone marrow evaluation and molecular testing for chromosome abnormalities and gene mutations can further distinguish these diagnoses. Anorexia nervosa also may present with pancytopenia. In these cases, the bone marrow is hypocellular and has a decreased number of fat cells.[8] The cytopenias revert with correction of the underlying disease.

TABLE 22-2   Differentiation of Aplastic Anemia from Other Causes of Pancytopenia

Condition	Peripheral Blood	Bone Marrow	Laboratory Test Results	Clinical Findings
Failure of Bone Marrow to Produce Blood Cells				
Aplastic anemia	No immature WBCs or RBCs; ↓ reticulocytes; MCV ↑ or normal	Hypocellular; blasts and abnormal cells absent; reticulin normal; RBC dyspoiesis may be present; WBC and platelet dyspoiesis absent	Acquired: PNH cells* may be present; chromosome abnormalities may be present Inherited: Table 22-3	Splenomegaly absent
Increased Destruction of Blood Cells				
PNH	Reticulocytes ↑; MCV normal or ↑; nucleated RBCs present or absent	Erythroid hyperplasia; may be hypocellular	PNH cells* present; hemoglobinuria +/−; chromosome abnormalities may be present	Splenomegaly absent; thrombosis may be present
Ineffective Hematopoiesis				
Myelodysplastic syndrome	Variable pancytopenia; reticulocytes ↓; MCV normal or ↑; blasts and abnormal WBCs, RBCs, and platelets may be present	Hypercellular; 20% of cases hypocellular; dyspoiesis in one or more cell lines present; blasts and immature cells present; reticulin ↑	Chromosome abnormalities usually present	Splenomegaly uncommon
Megaloblastic anemias	MCV ↑; oval macrocytes; hypersegmented neutrophils	Hypercellular with megaloblastic features	Serum vitamin B_{12} or folate or both ↓	Splenomegaly absent
Bone Marrow Infiltration				
Acute leukemia	Blasts present	Hypercellular; blasts ↑; reticulin ↑	Chromosome abnormalities may be present	Splenomegaly may be present
Hairy cell leukemia	Hairy cells present; monocytes ↓	Hairy cells and fibrosis present; reticulin ↑	Hairy cells† present; TRAP +	Splenomegaly present (60–70% of cases)

↑, Increased; ↓, decreased; +, positive result; +/−, positive or negative result; *MCV*, mean cell volume; *PNH*, paroxysmal nocturnal hemoglobinuria; *RBC*, red blood cell; *TRAP*, tartrate-resistant acid phosphatase; *WBC*, white blood cell.
*PNH erythrocytes are detected by flow cytometry by their lack of expression of CD59; PNH granulocytes and monocytes lack expression of CD24, CD16, and CD14 (Chapter 24).
†Hairy cells are detected by flow cytometry by their expression of CD19, CD20, CD22, CD11c, CD25, CD103, and FMC7.

TABLE 22-3 Key Characteristics of Inherited/Congenital Bone Marrow Failure Anemias

Condition	Genetics*	Peripheral Blood	Bone Marrow	Laboratory Test Results	Clinical Findings
Due to Bone Marrow Hypoplasia					
FA	AR, XLR 15 genes	Pancytopenia; reticulocytes ↓; MCV ↑	Hypocellular with ↓ in all cell lines	Chromosome breakage with DEB/MMC; Hb F may be ↑	Physical malformations may be present; risk of cancers, leukemia, myelodysplastic syndrome
DKC	AR, XLR, AD 8 genes	Pancytopenia; reticulocytes ↓; MCV ↑	Hypocellular with ↓ in all cell lines	75% have mutations in *TERC, TERT, DKC1, TINF2, NHP2, NOP10, WRAP53,* or *CTC1*; Hb F may be ↑; very short telomeres in lymphocyte subsets	Physical malformations may be present; pulmonary disease; risk of cancers, leukemia, myelodysplastic syndrome
SBDS	AR 1 gene	Neutropenia; pancytopenia (25% of cases); reticulocytes ↓; MCV normal or ↑	Hypocellular, normocellular, or hypercellular	90% have mutations in *SBDS* gene; serum trypsinogen and isoamylase ↓ for age; Hb F may be ↑	Pancreatic insufficiency; physical malformations may be present; risk of infections, leukemia, myelodysplastic syndrome
DBA	AD (50% of cases) 9 genes	Anemia; reticulocytes ↓; MCV ↑	Erythroid hypoplasia	Erythrocyte adenosine deaminase ↑; Hb F may be ↑; 25% have mutations in *RPS19* gene; another 25% have mutations in *RPS7, RPS10, RPS17, RPS24, RPS26, RPL5, RPL11,* or *RPL35A*	Physical malformations may be present; risk of cancers, leukemia, myelodysplastic syndrome
Due to Ineffective Hematopoiesis					
CDA I	AR 1 gene	Anemia; reticulocytes ↓; MCV ↑; poik, baso stipp, Cabot rings	Hypercellular; RBC precursors megaloblastoid with internuclear chromatin bridges and <5% binucleated forms	Mutations in *CDAN1* gene; spongy, "Swiss cheese" heterochromatin in erythroblasts by electron microscopy	Physical malformations may be present; iron overload; splenomegaly; hepatomegaly
CDA II	AR 1 gene	Anemia; reticulocytes ↓; MCV normal; poik, baso stipp	Hypercellular; RBC precursors normoblastic with 10% to 35% binucleated forms	Mutations in *SEC23B* gene; positive Ham test result (rarely done)	Physical malformations may be present; iron overload; jaundice; gallstones; splenomegaly
CDA III	AD 1 gene	Mild anemia; reticulocytes ↓; MCV ↑; poik, baso stipp	Hypercellular; RBC precursors megaloblastoid with giant multinucleated forms with up to 12 nuclei	Mutations in *KIF23* gene	Treatment usually not needed

↑, Increased; ↓, decreased; *AR,* autosomal recessive; *AD,* autosomal dominant; *XLR,* X-linked recessive; *baso stipp,* basophilic stippling; *CDA,* congenital dyserythropoietic anemia; *DBA,* Diamond-Blackfan anemia; *DKC,* dyskeratosis congenita; *DEB,* diepoxybutane; *FA,* Fanconi anemia; *MCV,* mean cell volume; *MMC,* mitomycin C; *poik,* poikilocytosis; *RBC,* red blood cell; *SBDS,* Shwachman-Bodian-Diamond syndrome; *SDS-PAGE,* sodium dodecyl sulfate polyacrylamide gel electrophoresis; *Hb F,* fetal hemoglobin.
*Genes identified as of 2013; genetic discovery is ongoing.

OTHER FORMS OF BONE MARROW FAILURE

Pure Red Cell Aplasia

Pure red cell aplasia (PRCA) is a rare disorder of erythropoiesis characterized by a selective and severe decrease in erythrocyte precursors in an otherwise normal bone marrow. Patients have severe anemia (usually normocytic), reticulocytopenia, and normal WBC and platelet counts. PRCA may be acquired or congenital. It is important to distinguish between acquired and congenital forms, as they require different therapeutic approaches.

Acquired Pure Red Cell Aplasia

Acquired PRCA may occur in children or adults and can be acute or chronic. Primary PRCA may be idiopathic or autoimmune-related. Secondary PRCA may occur in association with an underlying thymoma, hematologic malignancy, solid tumor, infection, chronic hemolytic anemia, collagen vascular disease, or exposure to drugs or chemicals.[73,74] Therapy is first directed at treatment of the underlying condition, but immunosuppressive therapy may be considered if the PRCA is not responsive. Cyclosporine is associated with a higher response rate (65% to 87%) than corticosteroids (30% to 62%) and is better suited for long-term maintenance if needed.[74]

The acquired form of PRCA in young children is also known as *transient erythroblastopenia of childhood* (TEC). A history of viral infection is found in half of patients, which is thought to trigger an immune mechanism that targets red cell production.[75] The anemia is typically normocytic, and Hb F and erythrocyte adenosine deaminase levels usually are normal.[73,75] Red cell transfusion support is the mainstay of therapy if the child is symptomatic from anemia. Normalization of erythropoiesis occurs within weeks in the vast majority patients.[75] There may be a genetic predisposition to TEC in some families.[75]

Congenital Pure Red Cell Aplasia: Diamond-Blackfan Anemia

Diamond-Blackfan anemia (DBA) is a congenital erythroid hypoplastic disorder of early infancy with an estimated incidence of 7 to 10 cases per million live births.[56] Mutations have been identified in nine genes that encode structural ribosome proteins: *RPS7, RPS10, RPS17, RPS19, RPS24,* and *RPS26* in the 40S subunit and *RPL5, RPL11,* and *RPL35A* in the 60S subunit.[76] Approximately 25% of patients have a mutation in the *RPS19* gene, and mutations in the other eight genes account for another 25% of cases.[76,77] Many mutations are still unidentified, and it is of interest that an additional 15% to 20% of cases can be accounted for by haplo-deletions of these same RPS genes.[78] Mutations in these ribosomal proteins disrupt ribosome biogenesis in DBA, but the pathophysiologic mechanisms leading to the clinical manifestations are currently unknown. Nearly 50% of DBA cases are linked to an autosomal dominant inheritance pattern, but sporadic mutations have also been reported.[76]

Over 90% of patients show signs of the disorder during the first year of life, with a median age of 8 weeks; however, some patients with DBA are asymptomatic until adulthood.[79] Approximately half of patients have characteristic physical anomalies, including craniofacial dysmorphisms, short stature, and neck and thumb malformations.[56,79]

The characteristic peripheral blood finding is a severe macrocytic anemia with reticulocytopenia.[56] The WBC count is normal or slightly decreased, and the platelet count is normal or slightly increased. Bone marrow examination distinguishes DBA from the hypocellular marrow in aplastic anemia, because there is normal cellularity of myeloid cells and megakaryocytes and hypoplasia of erythroid cells. The karyotype in DBA is normal. In most cases, Hb F and erythrocyte adenosine deaminase are increased; these findings distinguish DBA from TEC, in which these levels are normal.[56,76] Other features distinguishing DBA from TEC are detailed in Table 22-4.

TABLE 22-4 Distinguishing Characteristics of Diamond-Blackfan Anemia and Transient Erythroblastopenia of Childhood.

Test Result	DBA*	TEC*
Erythrocyte ADA increased at diagnosis	85%	5%
MCV increased at diagnosis	80%	5%
MCV increased in remission	80%	0%
Hb F increased at diagnosis	50%–85%	1%–2%
Hb F increased in remission	50%–85%	0%

DBA, Diamond-Blackfan anemia; *TEC,* transient erythroblastopenia of childhood; *ADA,* adenosine deaminase; *MCV,* mean corpuscular volume; *Hb F,* fetal hemoglobin.
*Percent of patients displaying the test results.
Modified from D'Andrea AD, Dahl N, Guinan EC, Shimamura A: Marrow failure. Hematology Am Soc Hematol Educ Program, 58-72, 2002.

Therapy includes RBC transfusions and corticosteroids. Although 50% to 75% of patients respond to corticosteroid therapy, side effects are severe with long-term use, including immunosuppression and growth delay.[56,76] Overall survival is 75% at 40 years.[79] Bone marrow transplantation improves outcomes, with greater than 90% overall survival in patients younger than 10 years old transplanted with a matched-related donor, and 80% in those with a matched unrelated donor.[76]

Congenital Dyserythropoietic Anemia

The congenital dyserythropoietic anemias (CDAs) are a heterogeneous group of rare disorders characterized by refractory anemia, reticulocytopenia, hypercellular bone marrow with markedly ineffective erythropoiesis, and distinctive dysplastic changes in bone marrow erythroblasts. Megaloblastoid development occurs in some types, but it is not related to vitamin B_{12} or folate deficiency. Granulopoiesis and thrombopoiesis are normal. The anemia varies from mild to moderate, even among affected siblings. Secondary hemosiderosis arises from chronic intramedullary and extramedullary hemolysis, as well as increased iron absorption associated with ineffective erythropoiesis. Iron overload develops even in the absence of blood transfusions. Jaundice, cholelithiasis, and splenomegaly are also common findings. CDAs do not progress to aplastic anemia or hematologic malignancies.[80]

Symptoms of CDA usually occur in childhood or adolescence but may first appear in adulthood.[56] CDA is classified into three major types: CDA I, CDA II, and CDA III. There are rare variants that do not fall into these categories, and they have been assigned to four other groups: CDA IV through CDA VII.[56,80] Whether CDA types IV through VII actually are separate entities is a matter of some controversy. This merely may be a reflection of the insensitive tests to classify CDA disorders. Further gene mutation studies should clarify this issue.

CDA I is inherited in an autosomal recessive pattern and is characterized by a mild to severe chronic anemia. Over 150 cases have been reported.[81] CDA I is caused by mutations in the *CDAN1* gene on chromosome 15, which encodes codanin-1, a cell-cycle regulated nuclear protein.[82,83] The exact role of codanin-1 in the pathophysiology of CDA I is unknown. Malformations of fingers or toes, brown skin pigmentation, and neurologic defects are found more frequently in CDA I than in the other CDA subtypes. The hemoglobin usually ranges from 6.5 g/dL to 11.5 g/dL, with a mean of 9.5 g/dL.[80] RBCs are macrocytic and may exhibit marked poikilocytosis, basophilic stippling, and Cabot rings. The erythroblasts are megaloblastoid and characteristically have internuclear chromatin bridges or nuclear stranding (Figure 22-3). There are less than 5% binucleated erythroblasts. The characteristic feature of the CDA I erythroblast is a spongy heterochromatin with a "Swiss cheese" appearance.[80] Treatment includes interferon-α and iron chelation.[56,81]

CDA II is the most common subtype and is inherited in an autosomal recessive pattern. More than 300 cases have been reported.[81] It results from mutations in the *SEC23B* gene on chromosome 20.[84] *SEC23B* encodes a component of the coat protein complex (COPII) that forms vesicles for transport of secretory proteins from the endoplasmic reticulum to the Golgi apparatus.[85] Its exact role in the pathophysiology of CDA II is unknown. The anemia in CDA II is mild to moderate, with hemoglobins ranging from 9 g/dL to 12 g/dL and a mean hemoglobin of 11 g/dL.[80] On peripheral blood film, RBCs are normocytic with anisocytosis, poikilocytosis, and basophilic stippling. The bone marrow has normoblastic erythropoiesis, with 10% to 35% binucleated forms and rare multinucleated forms.[80] Occasional pseudo-Gaucher cells are also evident.[80] Circulating RBCs hemolyze with the Ham acidified serum test but not with the sucrose hemolysis test.[56] For this reason, CDA II is also known as *HEMPAS* (*h*ereditary *e*rythroblastic *m*ultinuclearity with *p*ositive *a*cidified *s*erum).[56] The Ham test is no longer routinely used for CDA II confirmation, given the difficulty of appropriate quality control and the relative lack of testing availability in most laboratories.[80] RBCs also agglutinate with anti antisera and show abnormal migration of band 3 using sodium dodecyl sulfate polyacrylamide gel electrophoresis.[80] Treatment includes splenectomy and iron chelation.[56,81]

CDA III is the least common of the CDA subtypes, with about 60 cases reported in the literature, the majority being from one Swedish family.[86] This familial autosomal dominant form is associated with mutations in the *KIF23* gene, which codes for a protein involved in cytokinesis.[86, 87] The nonfamilial or sporadic form is extremely rare, with fewer than 20 cases reported.[81,86] The anemia is mild, and the hemoglobin is usually in the range of 8 to 14 g/dL, with a mean of 12 g/dL.[80] RBCs are macrocytic, and poikilocytosis and basophilic stippling are evident. The bone marrow has megaloblastic changes, and giant erythroblasts with up to 12 nuclei are a characteristic feature. Patients rarely require RBC transfusions, and iron overload is not observed.

Myelophthisic Anemia

Myelophthisic anemia is due to the infiltration of abnormal cells into the bone marrow and subsequent destruction and replacement of normal hematopoietic cells. Metastatic solid tumor cells (particularly from lung, breast, and prostate), leukemic cells, fibroblasts, and inflammatory cells (found in miliary tuberculosis and fungal infections) have been implicated.[88,89] Cytopenia results from the release of substances such as cytokines and growth factors that suppress hematopoiesis and destroy stem, progenitor, and stromal cells.[89] With disruption of normal bone marrow architecture by the infiltrating cells, the marrow releases immature hematopoietic cells. Furthermore, because of the unfavorable bone marrow environment, stem and progenitor cells migrate to the spleen and liver and establish extramedullary hematopoietic sites.[89] Since blood cell production in the liver and spleen is inefficient, these extramedullary sites also release immature cells into the circulation.[88]

The severity of anemia is mild to moderate, with normocytic erythrocytes and reticulocytopenia. Peripheral blood findings include teardrop erythrocytes and nucleated RBCs, as well as immature myeloid cells and megakaryocyte fragments (Figure 22-4).[88] The infiltrating abnormal cells are detected in a bone marrow aspirate or biopsy specimen.

Anemia of Chronic Kidney Disease

Anemia is a common complication of chronic kidney disease (CKD), with a positive correlation between anemia and renal disease severity.[90,91] Coresh and colleagues reported that between 1999 and 2004, approximately 26 million adults over

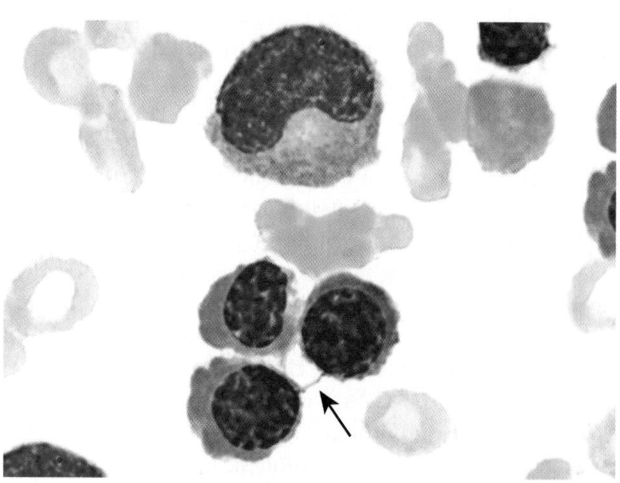

Figure 22-3 Erythrocyte precursors with nuclear bridging indicating dyserythropoiesis (bone marrow, ×1000). (Modified from Rodak BF, Carr JH: *Clinical hematology atlas*, ed 4, St. Louis, 2013, Elsevier, Saunders.)

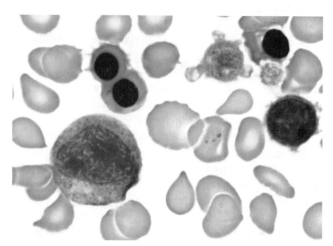

Figure 22-4 Myelophthisic anemia showing a leukoerythroblastic blood picture with a myelocyte, three orthochromic normoblasts, teardrop erythrocytes, a giant platelet with abnormal morphology, and a micromegakaryocyte (peripheral blood, ×1000).

20 years of age in the United States had CKD.[92] The primary cause of anemia in CKD is inadequate renal production of erythropoietin.[90,91] Without erythropoietin, the bone marrow lacks adequate stimulation to produce RBCs. Another contributor to the anemia of CKD is uremia, which inhibits erythropoiesis and increases RBC fragility.[93,94] Furthermore, patients experience chronic blood loss and iron deficiency from hemodialysis and frequent blood draws. Chronic inflammation and a restricted diet may also limit the iron available for erythropoiesis.[90,91] Anemia of CKD is normocytic and normochromic with reticulocytopenia. Burr cells are common peripheral blood film findings in cases complicated by uremia.[90]

Anemia in CKD can lead to cardiovascular complications, kidney failure, and suboptimal quality of life.[90] The Kidney Disease Outcomes Quality Initiative of the National Kidney Foundation recommends annual hemoglobin testing in patients with CKD and investigation of the anemia if the hemoglobin is less than 13.5 g/dL in adult men and less than 12 g/dL in adult women.[90] Treatment includes recombinant human erythropoietin or other erythropoiesis-stimulating agents (ESAs), with a goal hemoglobin range of 11 g/dL to 12 g/dL.[90,95] Maintaining the hemoglobin above 13 g/dL is not recommended because of the increased risk of cardiovascular and thromboembolic complications.[90,95] Successful ESA therapy requires adequate iron stores, so plasma ferritin level and percent transferrin saturation should also be monitored. Iron is administered with ESA therapy to maintain the transferrin saturation above 20% and the plasma ferritin level above 100 ng/mL for non-dialysis-dependent patients and above 200 ng/mL for hemodialysis-dependent patients.[90] Iron therapy is not routinely recommended for ferritin levels above 500 ng/mL.[90]

Patients may become hyporesponsive to ESA therapy because of functional iron deficiency (FID). In FID, the bone marrow is unable to release iron rapidly enough to accommodate the accelerated erythropoiesis. The transferrin saturation remains below 20%, but the serum ferritin level is normal or increased, indicating adequate iron stores.[96] Patients with FID are unable to reach or maintain the target hemoglobin, even with high ESA doses. However, patients are able to reach the target hemoglobin after intravenous iron therapy.[96] Researchers have proposed diagnostic criteria for FID in CKD: decreased reticulocyte hemoglobin content, increased soluble transferrin receptor, and greater than 10% hypochromic RBCs in the peripheral blood.[96,97] Other causes of ESA hyporesponsiveness include chronic inflammatory disease, infection, malignancy, aplastic anemia, antibody-mediated pure red cell aplasia, thalassemia, multiple myeloma, and the presence of hemoglobin H or hemoglobin S variants.[90]

SUMMARY

- Bone marrow failure is the reduction or cessation of blood cell production affecting one or more cell lines. Pancytopenia (decreased RBCs, WBCs, and platelets) is a common finding. Sequelae of pancytopenia include weakness and fatigue, infections, and bleeding.
- Aplastic anemia may be acquired or inherited. Acquired aplastic anemia may be idiopathic or secondary to drugs, chemical exposures, radiation, or viruses. Acquired aplastic anemia may also occur with conditions such as paroxysmal nocturnal hemoglobinuria, autoimmune diseases, and pregnancy.
- Bone marrow failure in acquired aplastic anemia occurs from destruction of hematopoietic stem cells by direct toxic effects of a drug, autoimmune T-cell targeting of stem cells, or other unknown mechanisms. The autoimmune reactions are rare adverse events after exposure to drugs, chemicals, or viruses. They are *idiosyncratic* in that they are unpredictable, and severity is unrelated to the dose or duration of exposure.
- Aplastic anemia is classified as nonsevere, severe, or very severe, based on bone marrow hypocellularity, absolute neutrophil count, platelet count, hemoglobin level, and reticulocyte count (Table 22-1). The severity classification helps to guide treatment decisions.
- Preferred treatment for severe and very severe acquired aplastic anemia is hematopoietic stem cell transplant (HSCT) for younger patients with an HLA-identical sibling. For those without a matched sibling donor and for those who are not HSCT candidates, immunosuppressive therapy with antithymocyte globulin and cyclosporine is recommended.
- Fanconi anemia (FA), dyskeratosis congenita (DKC), and Shwachman-Bodian-Diamond syndrome (SBDS) are inherited forms of aplastic anemia with progressive bone marrow failure, and patients may present with characteristic physical malformations. FA is inherited in an autosomal recessive or X-linked pattern, and mutations in 15 genes have been identified. A positive chromosome breakage study with diepoxybutane is diagnostic. DKC can be X-linked, autosomal dominant, or autosomal recessive, and mutations in eight genes have been identified. SBDS is autosomal recessive and is associated with mutations in the *SBDS* gene.
- Telomerase complex defects play a role in the pathophysiology of inherited aplastic anemias and some acquired aplastic anemias. The defects result in the inability of telomerase to elongate telomeres at the ends of chromosomes, which leads to premature hematopoietic stem cell senescence and apoptosis.
- Pure red cell aplasia is a disorder of erythrocyte production. Acquired transient erythroblastopenia of childhood (TEC) and Diamond-Blackfan anemia (DBA) are disparate subtypes with distinct etiologies, clinical features, and courses (Table 22-4). Mutations in nine different ribosomal protein genes have been identified in DBA.
- Patients with congenital dyserythropoietic anemia (CDA) exhibit refractory anemia, reticulocytopenia, secondary hemosiderosis, and distinct abnormalities of erythroid precursors. Three major subtypes are recognized: CDA I, CDA II, and CDA III.
- Myelophthisic anemia results from the replacement of normal bone marrow with abnormal cells. The main cause of anemia of chronic kidney disease is inadequate production of erythropoietin by the kidneys.

Now that you have completed this chapter, go back and read again the case study at the beginning and respond to the questions presented.

REVIEW QUESTIONS

Answers can be found in the Appendix.

1. The clinical consequences of pancytopenia include:
   a. Pallor and thrombosis
   b. Kidney failure and fever
   c. Fatigue, infection, and bleeding
   d. Weakness, hemolysis, and infection

2. Idiopathic acquired aplastic anemia is due to a(n):
   a. Drug reaction
   b. Benzene exposure
   c. Inherited mutation in stem cells
   d. Unknown cause

3. The pathophysiologic mechanism in acquired idiosyncratic aplastic anemia is:
   a. Replacement of bone marrow by abnormal cells
   b. Destruction of stem cells by autoimmune T cells
   c. Defective production of hematopoietic growth factors
   d. Inability of bone marrow stroma to support stem cells

4. Based on the criteria in Table 22-1, what is the aplastic anemia classification of a 15-year-old female with a bone marrow cellularity of 10%, hemoglobin of 7 g/dL, absolute neutrophil count of 0.1×10^9/L, and platelet count of 10×10^9/L?
   a. Nonsevere
   b. Moderate
   c. Severe
   d. Very severe

5. The most consistent peripheral blood findings in severe aplastic anemia are:
   a. Hairy cells, monocytopenia, and neutropenia
   b. Macrocytosis, thrombocytopenia, and neutropenia
   c. Blasts, immature granulocytes, and thrombocytopenia
   d. Polychromasia, nucleated RBCs, and hypersegmented neutrophils

6. The treatment that has shown the best success rate in young patients with severe aplastic anemia is:
   a. Immunosuppressive therapy
   b. Long-term red blood cell and platelet transfusions
   c. Administration of hematopoietic growth factors and androgens
   d. Stem cell transplant with an HLA-identical sibling

7. The test that is most useful in differentiating FA from other causes of pancytopenia is:
   a. Bone marrow biopsy
   b. Ham acidified serum test
   c. Diepoxybutane-induced chromosome breakage
   d. Flow cytometric analysis of CD55 and CD59 cells

8. Mutations in genes that code for the telomerase complex may induce bone marrow failure by causing which one of the following?
   a. Resistance of stem cells to normal apoptosis
   b. Autoimmune reaction against telomeres in stem cells
   c. Decreased production of hematopoietic growth factors
   d. Premature death of hematopoietic stem cells

9. Diamond-Blackfan anemia differs from inherited aplastic anemia in that in the former:
   a. Reticulocyte count is increased
   b. Fetal hemoglobin is decreased
   c. Only erythropoiesis is affected
   d. Congenital malformations are absent

10. Which anemia should be suspected in a patient with refractory anemia, reticulocytopenia, hemosiderosis, and binucleated erythrocyte precursors in the bone marrow?
    a. Fanconi anemia
    b. Dyskeratosis congenita
    c. Acquired aplastic anemia
    d. Congenital dyserythropoietic anemia

11. The primary pathophysiologic mechanism of anemia associated with chronic kidney disease is:
    a. Inadequate production of erythropoietin
    b. Excessive hemolysis
    c. Hematopoietic stem cell mutation
    d. Toxic destruction of stem cells

REFERENCES

1. Ehrlich, P. (1888). Über einen Fall von Anämie mit Bemerkungen über regenerative Veränderungen des Knochenmarks. *Charite Annal, 13,* 301.
2. Vaquez, M. H., & Aubertin, C. (1904). L'anémie pernicieuse d'après les conceptions actuelles. *Bull Soc Med Hop Paris, 21,* 288–297.
3. Dokal, I., & Vulliamy, T. (2008). Inherited aplastic anaemias/bone marrow failure syndromes. *Blood Rev, 22,* 141–153.
4. Young, N. S., & Maciejewski, J. P. (2013). Aplastic anemia. In Hoffman, R., Benz, E. J., Silberstein, S. E., et al., (Eds.), *Hematology: basic principles and practice.* (6th ed., pp. 350–372). Philadelphia: Saunders, Elsevier.
5. Muir, K. R., Chilvers, C. E. D., Harriss, C., et al. (2003). The role of occupational and environmental exposures in the aetiology of acquired severe aplastic anaemia: a case control investigation. *Br J Haematol, 123,* 906–914.

6. International Agranulocytosis and Aplastic Anemia Study. (1987). Incidence of aplastic anemia: the relevance of diagnostic criteria. *Blood, 70,* 1718–1721.

7. Kojima, S. (2002). Aplastic anemia in the Orient. *Int J Hematol, 76*(suppl 2),173–174.

8. Scheinberg, P. and Young, N. (2012). How I treat acquired aplastic anemia. *Blood, 102,* 1185–1196.

9. Nimer, S. D., Ireland, P., Meshkinpour, A., et al. (1994). An increased HLA DR2 frequency is seen in aplastic anemia patients. *Blood, 84,* 923–927.

10. Saunthararajah, Y., Nakamura, R., Nam, J. M., et al. (2002). HLA-DR15 (DR2) is overrepresented in myelodysplastic syndrome and aplastic anemia and predicts a response to immunosuppression in myelodysplastic syndrome. *Blood, 100,* 1570–1574.

11. Dougherty, D., Garte, S., Barchowsky, A., et al. (2008). NQO1, MPO, CYP2E1, GSTT1 and GSTM1 polymorphisms and biological effects of benzene exposure—a literature review. *Toxicol Lett, 182,* 7–17.

12. Sutton, J. F., Stacey, M., Kearns, W. G., et al. (2004). Increased risk for aplastic anemia and myelodysplastic syndrome in individuals lacking glutathione *S*-transferase genes. *Pediatr Blood Cancer, 42,* 122–126.

13. Gonzalez-Casas, R., Garcia-Buey, L., Jones, E. A., et al. Systematic review: hepatitis-associated aplastic anaemia—a syndrome associated with abnormal immunological function. *Aliment Pharmacol Ther, 30,* 6–43, 2009.

14. Choudhry, V. P., Gupta, S., Gupta, M., et al. (2002). Pregnancy associated aplastic anemia—a series of 10 cases with review of literature. *Hematol, 7,* 233–238.

15. Stalder, M. P., Rovó, A., Halter, J., et al. (2009). Aplastic anemia and concomitant autoimmune diseases. *Ann Hematol, 88,* 659–665.

16. Frickhofen, N., Heimpel, H., Kaltwasser, J. P., et al. (2003). Antithymocyte globulin with or without cyclosporin A: 11-year follow-up of a randomized trial comparing treatments of aplastic anemia. *Blood, 101,* 1236–1242.

17. Maciejewski, J. P., Selleri, C., Sato, T., et al. (1996). A severe and consistent deficit in marrow and circulating primitive hematopoietic cells (long-term culture-initiating cells) in acquired aplastic anemia. *Blood, 88,* 1983–1991.

18. Philpott, N. J., Scopes, J., Marsh, J. C. W., et al. (1995). Increased apoptosis in aplastic anemia bone marrow progenitor cells: possible pathophysiologic significance. *Exp Hematol, 23,* 1642–1648.

19. Maciejewski, J. P., Selleri, C., Sato, T., et al. (1995). Increased expression of Fas antigen on bone marrow CD34 sup^+ cells of patients with aplastic anaemia. *Br J Haematol, 91,* 245–252.

20. Zeng, W., Chen, G., Kajigaya, S., et al. (2004). Gene expression profiling in CD34 cells to identify differences between aplastic anemia patients and healthy volunteers. *Blood, 103,* 325–332.

21. Novitzky, N., & Jacobs, P. (1995). Immunosuppressive therapy in bone marrow aplasia: the stroma functions normally to support hematopoiesis. *Exp Hematol, 23,* 1472–1477.

22. Koijima, S. (1998). Hematopoietic growth factors and marrow stroma in aplastic anemia. *Int J Hematol, 68,* 19–28.

23. Wodnar-Filipowicz, A., Lyman, S. D., Gratwohl, A., et al. (1996). Flt3 ligand level reflects hematopoietic progenitor cell function in aplastic anemia and chemotherapy-induced bone marrow aplasia. *Blood, 88,* 4493–4499.

24. Young, N. S., & Maciejewski, J. (1997). The pathophysiology of acquired aplastic anemia. *N Engl J Med, 336,* 1365–1372.

25. Mathe, G., Amiel, J. L., Schwarzenberg, L., et al. (1970). Bone marrow graft in man after conditioning by antilymphocytic serum. *Br Med J, 2,* 131–136.

26. Risitano, A. M., Maciejewski, J. P., Green, S., et al. (2004). In-vivo dominant immune responses in aplastic anaemia: molecular tracking of putatively pathogenic T-cell clones by TCR-(-CDR3 sequencing. *Lancet, 364,* 355–364.

27. Hara, T., Ando, K., Tsurumi, H., et al. (2004). Excessive production of tumor necrosis factor-alpha by bone marrow T lymphocytes is essential in causing bone marrow failure in patients with aplastic anemia. *Eur J Haematol, 73,* 10–16.

28. Young, N. S. (2000). Hematopoietic cell destruction by immune mechanisms in acquired aplastic anemia. *Semin Hematol, 37,* 3–14.

29. Selleri, C., Sato, T., Anderson, S., et al. (1995). Interferon-gamma and tumor necrosis factor-alpha suppress both early and late stages of hematopoiesis and induce programmed cell death. *J Cell Physiol, 165,* 538–546.

30. Solomou, E. E., Keyvanfar, K., & Young, N. S. (2006). T-bet, a Th1 transcription factor, is up-regulated in T cells from patients with aplastic anemia. *Blood, 107,* 3983–3991.

31. Kasahara, S., Hara, T., Itoh, H., et al. (2002). Hypoplastic myelodysplastic syndromes can be distinguished from acquired aplastic anaemia by bone marrow stem cell expression of the tumour necrosis factor receptor. *Br J Haematol, 118,* 181–188.

32. Young, N. S., Calado, R. T., & Scheinberg, P. (2006). Current concepts in the pathophysiology and treatment of aplastic anemia. *Blood, 108,* 2509–2519.

33. Solomou, E. E., Rezvani, K., Mielke, S., et al. (2007). Deficient CD4^+ CD25^+ FOXP3^+ T regulatory cells in acquired aplastic anemia. *Blood, 110,* 1603–1606.

34. Gidvani, V., Ramkissoon, S., Sloand, E. M., et al. (2007). Cytokine gene polymorphisms in acquired bone marrow failure. *Am J Hematol, 82,* 721–724.

35. Hirano, N., Butler, M. O., von Bergwelt-Baildon, M. S., et al. (2003). Autoantibodies frequently detected in patients with aplastic anemia. *Blood, 102,* 4567–4575.

36. Feng, X., Chuhjo, T., Sugimori, C., et al. (2004). Diazepam-binding inhibitor-related protein 1: a candidate autoantigen in acquired aplastic anemia patients harboring a minor population of paroxysmal nocturnal hemoglobinuria-type cells. *Blood, 104,* 2425–2431.

37. Takamatsu, H., Feng, X., Chuhjo, T., et al. (2007). Specific antibodies to moesin, a membrane-cytoskeleton linker protein, are frequently detected in patients with acquired aplastic anemia. *Blood, 109,* 2514–2520.

38. Ball, S. E., Gibson, F. M., Rizzo, S., et al. (1998). Progressive telomere shortening in aplastic anemia. *Blood, 91,* 3582–3592.

39. Calado, R. T., & Young, N. S. (2008). Telomere maintenance and human bone marrow failure. *Blood, 111,* 4446–4455.

40. Xin, Z-T., Beauchamp, A. D., Calado, R. T., et al. (2007). Functional characterization of natural telomerase mutations found in patients with hematologic disorders. *Blood, 109,* 524–532.

41. Yamaguchi, H., Calado, R. T., Ly, H., et al. (2005). Mutations in *TERT*, the gene for telomerase reverse transcriptase, in aplastic anemia. *N Engl J Med, 352,* 1413–1424.

42. Calado, R. T., Graf, S. A., Wilkerson, K. L., et al. (2007). Mutations in the *SBDS* gene in acquired aplastic anemia. *Blood, 110,* 1141–1146.

43. Brummendorf, T. H., Maciejewski, J. P., Mak, J., et al. (2001). Telomere length in leukocyte subpopulations of patients with aplastic anemia. *Blood, 97,* 895–900.

44. Camitta, B. M., Thomas, E. D., Nathan, D. G., et al. (1976). Severe aplastic anemia: a prospective study of the effect of early marrow transplantation on acute mortality. *Blood, 48,* 63–70.

45. Bacigalupo, A., Hows, J., Gluckman, E., et al. (1988). Bone marrow transplantation (BMT) versus immunosuppression for the treatment of severe aplastic anaemia (SAA): a report of the EMBT SAA working party. *Br J Haematol, 70,* 177–182.

46. Sugimori, C., Chuhjo, T., Feng, X., et al. (2006). Minor population of CD55⁻CD59⁻ blood cells predicts response to immunosuppressive therapy and prognosis in patients with aplastic anemia. *Blood, 107,* 1308–1314.

47. Socie, G., Rosenfeld, S., Frickhofen, N., et al. (2000). Late clonal diseases of treated aplastic anemia. *Semin Hematol, 37,* 91–101.

48. Maciejewski, J. P., Risitano, A., Sloand, E., et al. (2002). Distinct clinical outcomes for cytogenetic abnormalities evolving from aplastic anemia. *Blood, 99,* 3129–3135.

49. Kearns, W. G., Sutton, J. F., Maciejewski, J. P., et al. (2004). Genomic instability in bone marrow failure syndromes. *Am J Hematol, 76,* 220–224.

50. Locasciulli, A., Oneto, R., Bacigalupo, A., et al. (2007). Outcome of patients with acquired aplastic anemia given first line bone marrow transplantation or immunosuppressive treatment in the last decade: a report from the European group for blood and marrow transplantation. *Haematologica, 92,* 11–18.

51. Scheinberg, P., Nunez, O., & Young, N. S. (2006). Retreatment with rabbit anti-thymocyte globulin and ciclosporin for patients with relapsed or refractory severe aplastic anaemia. *Br J Haematol, 133,* 622–627.

52. Maciejewski, J. P., Follmann, D., Nakamura, R., et al. (2001). Increased frequency of HLA-DR2 in patients with paroxysmal nocturnal hemoglobinuria and the PNH/aplastic anemia syndrome. *Blood, 98,* 3513–3519.

53. Socie, G., Mary, J-Y., Schrezenmeier, H., et al. (2007). Granulocyte-stimulating factor and severe aplastic anemia: a survey by the European group for blood and marrow transplant (EBMT). *Blood, 109,* 2794–2796.

54. Gurion, R., Gafter-Gvili, A., Paul, M., et al. (2009). Hematopoietic growth factors in aplastic anemia patients treated with immunosuppressive therapy—systematic review and meta-analysis. *Hematologica, 94,* 712–719.

55. Fanconi, G. (1927). Familiaere infantile perniziosaartige Anaemie (pernizioeses Blutbild und Konstitution). *Jahrbuch Kinderheil, 117,* 257–280.

56. Dror, Y., & Freedman, M. H. (2013). Inherited forms of bone marrow failure. In Hoffman, R., Benz, E. J., Silberstein, L. E., et al., (Eds.), *Hematology: basic principles and practice.* (6th ed., pp. 307–349). Philadelphia: Saunders Elsevier.

57. Tischkowitz, M. D., & Hodgson, S. V. (2003). Fanconi anaemia. *J Med Genet, 40,* 1–10.

58. Green, A. M., & Kupfer, G. M. (2009). Fanconi anemia. *Hematol Oncol Clin North Am, 23,* 193–214.

59. Alter, B. P. (2003). Cancer in Fanconi anemia, 1927-2001. *Cancer, 97,* 425–440.

60. Levitus, M., Joenje, H., & de Winter, J. P. (2006). The Fanconi anemia pathway of genomic maintenance. *Cell Oncol, 28,* 3–19.

61. Pinto, F. O., Leblanc, T., Chamousset, D., et al. (2009). Diagnosis of Fanconi anemia patients with bone marrow failure. *Haematologica, 94,* 487–495.

62. Kutler, D. I., Singh, B., Satagopan, J., et al. (2003). A 20-year perspective on the International Fanconi Anemia Registry (IFAR). *Blood, 101,* 1249–1256.

63. Rosenberg, P. S., Greene, M. H., & Alter, B. P. (2003). Cancer incidence in persons with Fanconi anemia. *Blood, 101,* 822–826.

64. Li, X., Leteurtre, F., Rocha, V., et al. (2003). Abnormal telomere metabolism in Fanconi's anaemia correlates with genomic instability and the probability of developing severe aplastic anaemia. *Br J Haematol, 120,* 836–845.

65. Alter, B. P., Giri, N., Savage, S. A., et al. (2009). Cancer in dyskeratosis congenita. *Blood, 113,* 6549–6557.

66. Savage, S. A., & Alter, B. P. (2009). Dyskeratosis congenita. *Hematol Oncol Clin North Am, 23,* 215–231.

67. Alter, B. P., Baerlocher, G. M., Savage, S. A., et al. (2007). Very short telomere length by flow fluorescence in situ hybridization identifies patients with dyskeratosis congenita. *Blood, 110,* 1439–1447.

68. Burroughs, L., Woolfrey, A., & Shimamura, A. (2009). Shwachman-Diamond syndrome: a review of the clinical presentation, molecular pathogenesis, diagnosis, and treatment. *Hematol Oncol Clin North Am, 23,* 233–248.

69. Myers, K. C., Rose, S. R., Rutter, M. M., et al. (2013). Endocrine evaluation of children with and without Shwachman-Bodian-Diamond syndrome gene mutations and Shwachman-Diamond syndrome. *J Pediatr, 162,* 1235–1240.

70. Austin, K. M., Gupta M. L. Jr., Coats, S. A., et al. (2008). Mitotic spindle destabilization and genomic instability in Shwachman-Diamond syndrome. *J Clin Invest, 118,* 1511–1518.

71. Dror, Y., & Freedman, M. H. (2002). Shwachman-Diamond syndrome. *Br J Haematol, 118,* 701–713.

72. Donadieu, J., Leblanc, T., Meunier, B. B., et al. (2005). Analysis of risk factors for myelodysplasias, leukemias and death from infection among patients with congenital neutropenia. Experience of the French Severe Chronic Neutropenia Study Group. *Hematologica, 90,* 45–53.

73. Maciejewski, J. P., & Tiu, R. V. (2013). Acquired disorders of red cell and white cell production. In Hoffman, R., Benz, E. J., Silberstein, L. E., et al., (Eds.), *Hematology: basic principles and practice.* (6th ed., pp. 383–404). Philadelphia: Saunders Elsevier.

74. Sawada, K., Hirokawa, M., & Fujishima, N. (2009). Diagnosis and management of acquired pure red cell aplasia. *Hematol Oncol Clin North Am, 23,* 249–259.

75. Shaw, J., & Meeder, R. (2007). Transient erythroblastopenia of childhood in siblings: case report and review of the literature. *J Pediatr Hematol Oncol, 29,* 659–660.

76. Lipton, J. M., & Ellis, S. R. (2009). Diamond-Blackfan anemia: diagnosis, treatment, and molecular pathogenesis. *Hematol Oncol Clin North Am, 23,* 261–282.

77. Boria, I., Garelli, E., Gazda, H. T., et al. (2010). The ribosomal basis of Diamond-Blackfan anemia: mutation and database update. *Hum Mutat, 12,* 1269–1279.

78. Farrar, J. E., Vlachos, A., Atsidaftos, E., et al. (2011). Ribosomal protein gene deletions in Diamond-Blackfan anemia. *Blood, 118,* 6943–6951.

79. Lipton, J. M., Atsidaftos, E., Zyskind, I., et al. (2006). Improving clinical care and elucidating the pathophysiology of Diamond Blackfan anemia: an update from the Diamond Blackfan anemia registry. *Pediatr Blood Cancer, 46,* 558–564.

80. Renella, R., & Wood, W. G. (2009). The congenital dyserythropoietic anemias. *Hematol Oncol Clin North Am, 23,* 283–306.

81. Heimpel, H. (2004). Congenital dyserythropoietic anemias: epidemiology, clinical significance, and progress in understanding their pathogenesis. *Ann Hematol, 83,* 613–621.

82. Dgany, O., Avidan, N., Delaunay, J., et al. (2002). Congenital dyserythropoietic anemia type I is caused by mutations in codanin-1. *Am J Hum Genet, 71,* 1467–1474.

83. Noy-Lotan, S., Dgany, O., Lahmi, R., et al. (2009). Codanin-1, the protein encoded by the gene mutated in congenital dyserythropoietic anemia type I (*CDAN1*), is cell cycle-regulated. *Haematologica, 94,* 629–637.

84. Schwarz, K., Iolascon, A., Verissimo, F., et al. (2009). Mutations affecting secretory COPII coat component SEC23B cause congenital dyserythropoietic anemia type II. *Nat Genet 41,* 936–940.

85. Kirchhausen, T. (2007). Making COPII coats. *Cell, 129,* 1325–1336.

86. Liljeholm, M., Irvine, A. F., Vikberg, A. L., et al. (2013). Congenital dyserythropoietic anemia type III (CDA III) is caused by a mutation in kinesin family member, KIF23. *Blood, 121,* 4791–4799.

87. Iolascon, A., Heimpel, H., Wahlin, A., & Tamary, H. (2013). Congenital dyserythropoietic anemias: molecular insights and diagnostic approach. *Blood, 122,* 2162–2166.

88. Agarwal, A. M., & Prchal, J. T. (2010). Anemia associated with marrow infiltration. In Prchal, J. T., Kaushansky, K., Lichtman, M. A., et al., (Eds.), *Williams Hematology*. (8th ed.). New York: McGraw-Hill. http://www.accessmedicine.com.libproxy2.umdnj.edu/content.aspx?aID=6109833. Accessed 19.09.13.

89. Makoni, S. N., & Laber, D. A. (2004). Clinical spectrum of myelophthisis in cancer patients. *Am J Hematol, 76,* 92–93.

90. National Kidney Foundation. (2006). KDOQI clinical practice guidelines and clinical practice recommendations for anemia in chronic kidney disease. *Am J Kidney Dis, 47*(Suppl. 3), S1–146.

91. Marks, P. W., Rosovsky, R., & Benz, E. J. Jr. (2013). Hematologic manifestations of systemic disease: renal disease. In Hoffman, R., Benz, E. J., Silberstein, L. E., et al., (Eds.), *Hematology: basic principles and practice.* (6th ed., pp. 2173–2175). Philadelphia: Saunders-Elsevier.

92. Coresh, J., Selvin, E., Stevens, L. A., et al. Prevalence of chronic kidney disease in the United States. *JAMA, 298,* 2038–2047.

93. Macdougall, I. C. (2001). Role of uremic toxins in exacerbating anemia in renal failure. *Kidney Int 59*(Suppl. 78), S67–S72.

94. Caro, J., & Outschoorn, U. M. (2010). Anemia of chronic renal disease. In Prchal, J. T., Kaushansky, K., Lichtman, M. A., et al., (Eds.), *Williams Hematology*, (8th ed.). New York: McGraw-Hill. http://www.accessmedicine.com.libproxy2.umdnj.edu/content.aspx?aID=6108595. Accessed 19.09.13.

95. National Kidney Foundation. (2007). KDOQI clinical practice guideline and clinical practice recommendations for anemia in chronic kidney disease: 2007 update of hemoglobin target. *Am J Kidney Dis, 50,* 479–512.

96. Wish, J. B. (2006). Assessing iron status: beyond serum ferritin and transferrin saturation. *Clin J Am Soc Nephrol, 1,* S4–S8.

97. Bovy, C., Gothot, A., Delanaye, P., et al. (2007). Mature erythrocyte parameters as new markers of functional iron deficiency in haemodialysis: sensitivity and specificity. *Nephrol Dial Transplant, 22,* 1156–1162.

23

Introduction to Increased Destruction of Erythrocytes

Kathryn Doig

OBJECTIVES

After completion of this chapter, the reader will be able to:

1. Define *hemolysis* and recognize its hallmark clinical findings.
2. Differentiate a hemolytic disorder from hemolytic anemia by definition and recognition of laboratory findings.
3. Discuss methods of classifying hemolytic anemias and apply the classification to an unfamiliar anemia.
4. Describe the processes of fragmentation (intravascular) and macrophage-mediated (extravascular) hemolysis, including sites of hemolysis, catabolic products, and time frame for the appearance of those products after hemolysis.
5. Describe protoporphyrin catabolism (bilirubin production), including metabolites and their sites of production and excretion.
6. Describe the mechanisms that salvage hemoglobin and heme during fragmentation hemolysis.
7. Describe changes to bilirubin metabolism and iron salvage systems that occur when the rate of fragmentation or macrophage-mediated hemolysis increases.
8. Identify, explain the diagnostic value, and interpret the results of laboratory tests that indicate increased hemolysis and erythropoiesis.
9. Differentiate between hemolytic anemias and other causes of increased erythropoiesis given laboratory or clinical information.
10. Differentiate between hemolytic anemias and other causes of bilirubinemia given laboratory or clinical information.

CASE STUDY

After studying the material in this chapter, the reader should be able to respond to the following case study:

A 34-year-old woman was admitted to the hospital for a vaginal hysterectomy. Except for excessive menstrual bleeding, she was in otherwise good health, and all of her preoperative laboratory test results were within their respective reference intervals. There was no excessive blood loss during or after surgery, and recovery was uneventful except for some expected pain, for which the patient received ibuprofen.

Three days after surgery, the patient began to experience abdominal pain and passed "root beer"-colored urine. A CBC at that time revealed a hemoglobin level of 5.8 g/dL.

1. What process is indicated by the root beer–colored urine?
2. What laboratory tests can be used to differentiate the cause of the hemolysis?
3. Based on the patient's clinical presentation, predict the results expected for each test listed for question 2.

This chapter presents an overview of the hemolytic process and provides a foundation that is applicable in the following chapters on red blood cell (RBC) disorders. The term *hemolysis* or *hemolytic disorder* refers to increased rate of destruction (i.e., lysis) of RBCs, shortening their life span. The reduced number of cells results in reduced tissue oxygenation and increased erythropoietin production by the kidney. When the patient is otherwise healthy, the bone marrow responds by accelerating erythrocyte production, which leads to reticulocytosis. A hemolytic process is present without anemia if the bone marrow is able to compensate by accelerating RBC production sufficiently to replace the RBCs lost through hemolysis. Healthy bone marrow can increase its production of RBCs by six to eight times normal;[1] therefore, significant RBC destruction must occur before an anemia develops. A *hemolytic anemia* results when the rate of RBC destruction exceeds the increased rate of RBC production.

CLASSIFICATION

Many anemias have a hemolytic component, including the anemia associated with vitamin B_{12} or folate deficiency and the anemia of chronic inflammation, renal disease, and iron deficiency. In these conditions, the hemolysis alone does not cause anemia, and so they are not typically classified as hemolytic disorders. Rather, these anemias develop as a result of the inability of the bone marrow to increase production of RBCs. Because hemolysis is not the primary underlying cause, these disorders are considered anemias with a secondary hemolytic component.

When hemolysis is the primary feature, the anemias can be classified as follows:
- Acute versus chronic
- Inherited versus acquired
- Intrinsic versus extrinsic
- Intravascular versus extravascular
- Fragmentation versus macrophage-mediated

Every hemolytic condition can be classified according to each of these descriptors. Table 23-1 shows this and provides a noncomprehensive list of hemolytic anemias. This chapter focuses on the mechanism of hemolysis—that is, the distinction between fragmentation and macrophage-mediated hemolytic conditions. The other classifying schemes are summarized here briefly for application in the chapters that follow.

Acute versus chronic hemolysis delineates the clinical presentation. Acute hemolysis has a rapid onset and is isolated (sudden), episodic, or paroxysmal, as in *paroxysmal cold hemoglobinuria* or *paroxysmal nocturnal hemoglobinuria*. Patients with paroxysmal cold hemoglobinuria experience hemolysis after exposure to cold, and patients with paroxysmal nocturnal hemoglobinuria may experience intermittent episodes of hemolysis. A hemolytic transfusion reaction is an example of a single acute incident. Whatever the cause, acute hemolysis either disappears or subsides between episodes, during which time the patient's condition may return to normal.

Chronic hemolysis may not be evident if the bone marrow is able to compensate, but it may be punctuated over time with hemolytic *crises* that cause anemia. Glucose-6-phosphate dehydrogenase deficiency is such a condition. RBC life span is chronically shortened, but bone marrow compensation prevents anemia. When the cells are challenged with oxidizing agents such as antimalarial drugs, a dramatic acute hemolytic event occurs. When the drug is withdrawn, compensation returns.

Other chronic conditions result in anemia that is so severe that the bone marrow cannot generate cells fast enough to compensate for the anemia. Thalassemia is an example of such a condition. Although red blood cell production is brisk, each cell possesses an inadequate complement of one type of globin chain, and functional hemoglobin production is decreased

TABLE 23-1 Classification of Selected Hemolytic Anemias by Primary Cause and Type of Hemolysis

	Predominantly Fragmentation (Intravascular) Hemolysis	Predominantly Macrophage-Mediated (Extravascular) Hemolysis	
Extrinsic defects	**Agents from Outside the RBC**		**Acquired conditions**
	Immune hemolysis: cold antibody Microangiopathic hemolysis Infectious agents, as in malaria Thermal injury Chemicals/drugs Venoms Prosthetic heart valve	Immune hemolysis: warm antibody Drugs	
	Membrane Abnormalities		
Intrinsic defects	Spur cell anemia of severe liver disease Paroxysmal nocturnal hemoglobinuria	Hereditary membrane defects	**Hereditary conditions**
	Abnormalities of the RBC Interior		
	Enzyme defects such as G6PD deficiency Globin abnormalities such as sickle cell, thalassemia		

Green text indicates acute or episodic hemolysis.
Red text indicates chronic hemolysis.
Some conditions may exhibit mixed presentations under certain circumstances. It is evident that most hereditary conditions lead to chronic hemolysis, whereas acquired conditions are more often acute. Furthermore, the intrinsic red blood cell defects typically are due to hereditary conditions, whereas extrinsic factors typically lead to acquired hemolytic disorders.
G6PD, Glucose-6-phosphate dehydrogenase; *RBC,* red blood cell.

overall. As a result, the oxygen-carrying capacity of the blood is chronically low. Cells lyse in thalassemia because excess normal globin chains precipitate inside the erythroid cells, which leads to hemolysis and exacerbates chronically reduced hemoglobin production.

Inherited hemolytic conditions, such as thalassemia, are passed to offspring by mutant genes from the parents. *Acquired* hemolytic disorders develop in individuals who were previously hematologically normal but acquire an agent or condition that lyses RBCs. Infectious diseases such as malaria are an example.

The hemolytic disorders are also classified as involving *intrinsic* or *extrinsic* RBC defects, with the latter caused by the action of external agents. This is the classification scheme used for subsequent chapters in this book. Examples of *intrinsic* hemolytic disorders are abnormalities of the RBC membrane, enzymatic pathways, or the hemoglobin molecule. With intrinsic defects, if the RBCs of the affected patient were to be transfused into a healthy individual, they would still have a shortened life span because the defect is in the RBC. If normal RBCs are transfused into a patient who has an intrinsic defect, the transfused cells have a normal life span because the transfused cells are normal.

Extrinsic hemolytic conditions are those that arise from outside the RBC, typically substances in the plasma or conditions affecting the anatomy of the circulatory system. Even though malaria protozoa and other infectious agents are within the RBC, they are classified as extrinsic because the RBC was normal until it was invaded by an outside agent. An antibody against RBC antigens and a prosthetic heart valve are examples of noninfectious extrinsic agents that can damage RBCs. In extrinsic hemolysis, cross-transfusion studies have shown that the patient's RBCs have a normal life span in the bloodstream of a healthy individual, but normal cells are lysed more rapidly in the patient's circulation. These studies confirm that something outside the RBCs is causing the hemolysis. (Of course, in the case of intracellular parasites, the cross-transfusion study is not applicable.) Most intrinsic defects are inherited; most extrinsic ones are acquired (Table 23-1). A few exceptions exist, such as paroxysmal nocturnal hemoglobinuria, an acquired disorder involving an intrinsic defect (Chapter 24).

Intrinsic disorders are subclassified as membrane defects, enzyme defects, and hemoglobinopathies. Extrinsic hemolysis may be immunohemolytic, traumatic, or microangiopathic, or may be caused by infectious agents, chemical agents (drugs and venoms), or physical agents (Table 23-1).

Another classification scheme is based on the site of hemolysis and related to the general mechanism of lysis. *Intravascular* hemolysis occurs by *fragmentation*. Although this takes place most often within the bloodstream, RBCs can lyse by fragmentation in the spleen and bone marrow as well. *Macrophage-mediated* hemolysis occurs when RBCs are engulfed by macrophages and lysed by their digestive enzymes. The designation *extravascular*, meaning outside the vessels, can refer either to lysis within the macrophage and not in the bloodstream or to the fact that most of the macrophages are in tissues, chiefly the spleen and the liver, and thus are outside the vasculature. Commonly the terms *fragmentation* and *intravascular* are used interchangeably, as are *macrophage-mediated* and *extravascular*.

The mechanistic classifying scheme is useful because screening laboratory tests rely on the differences in the hemolytic processes. However, the exact cause of the hemolysis must still be determined by targeted testing for appropriate treatment to be implemented.

HEMOLYSIS

Normal Bilirubin Metabolism

Detection of hemolysis depends partly on detection of RBC breakdown products. A prominent product is bilirubin. The process of normal bilirubin production is described to clarify the relationship between hemolysis and increased bilirubin levels.

The story of bilirubin production is, in part, a story of iron salvage. The body salvages and recycles iron like a precious metal. There is also a process for recycling the amino acids of the globin chains to build new proteins. The protoporphyrin component, however, is catabolized and excreted but facilitates dietary fat absorption in the process. Bilirubin is the excretory product derived from the protoporphyrin component of heme.

RBCs live approximately 120 days. During this time, they undergo various metabolic and chemical changes, which result in a loss of deformability. Under normal circumstances, macrophages of the mononuclear phagocyte system (or reticuloendothelial system) recognize these changes and phagocytize the aged erythrocytes (Chapter 8), creating a macrophage-mediated hemolytic process. The organs involved include the spleen, bone marrow, liver, lymph nodes, and circulating monocytes, but it is primarily the macrophages in spleen and liver that process senescent RBCs.

The majority of RBC degradation occurs inside macrophages as enzymes of the macrophage granules lyse the phagocytized erythrocytes (Figure 23-1). Hemoglobin is hydrolyzed into heme and globin; the latter is further degraded into amino acids that return to the amino acid pool. Iron is released from the heme, returned to the plasma via ferroportin, bound to its protein carrier molecule (transferrin), and recycled to needy cells. The remaining protoporphyrin is degraded through a series of biochemical reactions in different tissues and organs.

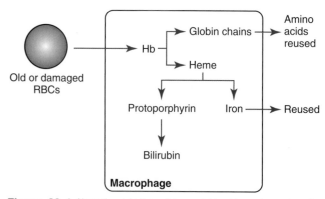

Figure 23-1 Normal catabolism of hemoglobin. Macrophages lyse ingested red blood cells (*RBCs*) and separate hemoglobin (*Hb*) into globin chains and heme components. The amino acids from the globin chains are reused. Heme is degraded to iron and protoporphyrin. Iron is returned to the plasma to be reused. Protoporphyrin is degraded to bilirubin.

Figure 23-2 illustrates protoporphyrin catabolism. While protoporphyrin is inside the macrophage, heme oxygenase acts on it, breaking the protoporphyrin ring to yield a linear molecule, biliverdin. The lungs excrete a by-product of that reaction, carbon monoxide. The green biliverdin is reduced to bilirubin, a nonpolar yellow molecule that is secreted into the plasma (Box 23-1). This form of bilirubin is called unconjugated for reasons that will be evident shortly. Because it is hydrophobic, this form of bilirubin must bind to albumin to be transported in plasma to the liver. In the liver sinusoid, the bilirubin dissociates from the albumin. The bilirubin is then transported across the hepatocyte membrane by a process that is not yet clear. It may be carrier independent or involve organic anion transporter (OAT) proteins.[2,3] Once inside the hepatocyte, the unconjugated bilirubin is joined (i.e., conjugated) with two molecules of glucuronic acid by glucuronyl transferase to form bilirubin diglucuronide. The addition of the two sugar acid

---

BOX 23-1 Visualizing the Color Changes of Hemoglobin Degradation

The degradation of heme can be seen in bruises in fair-skinned individuals or in the sclera of the eye after a vascular bleed. The same process that macrophages facilitate can occur in tissues. At first, the extravasated but deoxygenated blood gives the injury the purple-red appearance of hemoglobin. As the hemoglobin is degraded, the color changes to a greenish hue due to biliverdin, but ultimately it becomes yellow due to bilirubin.

---

molecules makes the molecule polar and water soluble. Bilirubin diglucuronide is also called *conjugated* bilirubin or *direct* bilirubin (Box 23-2). Thus the bilirubin originally released from macrophages that lacks these sugars is termed *unconjugated bilirubin* or *indirect* bilirubin (Box 23-2).

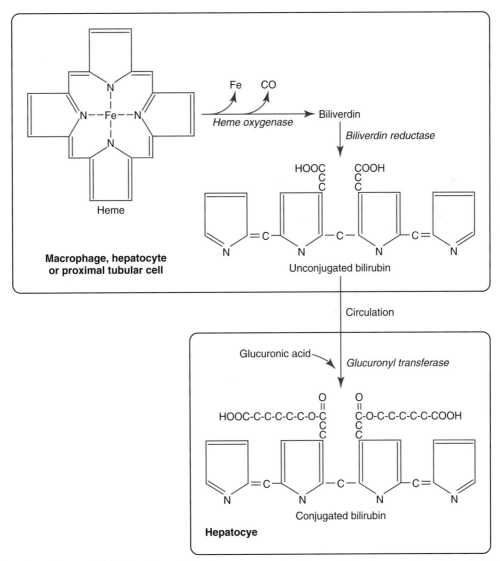

Figure 23-2 Catabolism of heme to bilirubin. In cells containing heme oxygenase, iron is removed from heme, and the protoporphyrin ring is opened up to form an intermediate, biliverdin. Biliverdin is converted to unconjugated bilirubin by biliverdin reductase. The unconjugated bilirubin is secreted into the plasma and binds to albumin for transport to the liver. When unconjugated bilirubin enters the hepatocyte, glucuronyl transferase adds two molecules of glucuronic acid to form bilirubin diglucuronide, also called conjugated bilirubin.

BOX 23-2 Laboratory Testing for Serum Bilirubin

Because bilirubin occurs in two forms, conjugated and unconjugated, the total bilirubin level in serum is the total of the two forms: total serum bilirubin = unconjugated serum bilirubin + conjugated serum bilirubin (each expressed in mg/dL).

Normally, there is relatively little total bilirubin, and most of it is composed of the unconjugated form in transit from the macrophages, where it was produced, to the liver. The small amount of direct bilirubin in the plasma has been absorbed from the intestine by the portal circulation.

Typical reference intervals are as follows:

Total serum bilirubin level = 0.5–1.0 mg/dL

Direct (conjugated) serum bilirubin level = 0–0.2 mg/dL

Indirect (unconjugated) serum bilirubin level = 0–0.8 mg/dL

Conjugated bilirubin is a polar molecule and reacts well in the water-based spectrophotometric assay that uses diazotized sulfanilic acid. Unconjugated bilirubin does not react well in this system unless alcohol is added to promote its solubility in water. Conjugated bilirubin also is called *direct bilirubin* because it reacts directly with the reagent, and unconjugated bilirubin is called *indirect* because it has to be solubilized first.* When alcohol is added to the test system, however, both the direct and indirect forms react. In practice, the total bilirubin level is measured by adding a solubilizing reagent. In a separate test, the direct bilirubin is measured alone without addition of the solubilizing agent. The indirect bilirubin level is calculated by subtracting the direct value from the total value: total serum bilirubin − direct serum bilirubin = indirect serum bilirubin.

---

*Van den Bergh AA, Muller P: Über eine direkte und eine indirekte diazoreaktion aus bilirubin, *Biochem Z* 77:90, 1916; and Hutchinson DW, Johnson B, Knell AJ: The reaction between bilirubin and aromatic diazo compounds, *Biochem J* 127:907-908, 1972.

Conjugated bilirubin is excreted into the hepatic bile duct, continues down the common bile duct, and goes into the intestines (Figure 23-3). There it assists with the emulsification of fats for absorption from the diet. Conjugated bilirubin is oxidized by gut bacteria into various water-soluble compounds, collectively called *urobilinogen.* Most urobilinogen is oxidized further to stercobilin and similar compounds that give the brown color to stool, which is the ultimate route for excretion of protoporphyrin.

Because they are water soluble, some conjugated bilirubin and urobilinogen molecules are absorbed from the intestines

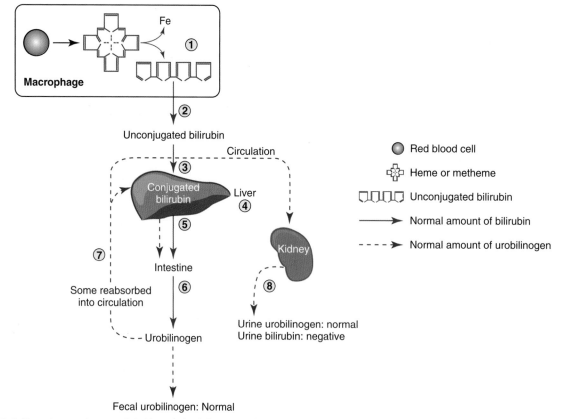

Figure 23-3 Normal macrophage-mediated hemolysis. **1,** In a macrophage, hemoglobin is degraded to heme, the iron is released, and the protoporphyrin ring is converted to unconjugated bilirubin. **2,** Macrophages release unconjugated bilirubin into the plasma, where it binds to albumin for transport to the liver. **3,** Unconjugated bilirubin enters the hepatocyte. **4,** The hepatocyte converts unconjugated bilirubin to conjugated bilirubin. **5,** Conjugated bilirubin leaves the liver in the bile and enters the small intestine. **6,** Bacteria convert conjugated bilirubin to urobilinogen, most of which is excreted in the stool. **7,** Some of the water-soluble urobilinogen is reabsorbed in the portal circulation, and most is recycled through the liver for excretion. **8,** A small component of the reabsorbed urobilinogen is filtered and excreted in the urine. (Adapted from Brunzel NA. Fundamentals of Urine and Body Fluid Analysis. 3e. St. Louis, Elsevier, 2013.)

into the plasma by osmosis (Figure 23-3). The portal circulation (the blood vessels that surround the intestines to absorb nutrients) collects these bile products. The portal circulation carries blood directly to the liver, so most of the absorbed conjugated bilirubin and urobilinogen is recycled directly into the bile again. Some remains in the plasma, however, and is filtered by the renal glomerulus and excreted in the urine. Conjugated bilirubin is virtually undetectable in urine, but a measurable amount of urobilinogen can be expected normally. The yellow color of urine is not due to the urobilinogen, which is colorless. It is due to urobilin, a derivative of urobilinogen that is also water-soluble.

Normal Plasma Hemoglobin Salvage During Fragmentation Hemolysis

Fragmentation hemolysis is the result of trauma to the RBC membrane that causes a breach sufficient for the cell contents, chiefly hemoglobin, to spill directly into plasma (Box 23-3). Approximately 10% to 20% of normal RBC destruction is via fragmentation,[4] secondary to turbulence and anatomic restrictions in the vasculature.

Because hemoglobin is filtered by the kidney, some iron could be lost daily with even normal amounts of fragmentation hemolysis. In addition, free hemoglobin, and especially free heme, can cause oxidative damage to cells. Several mechanisms exist to salvage hemoglobin iron and prevent oxidation reactions (Box 23-4) and are collectively called the *haptoglobin-hemopexin-methemalbumin system* (Figure 23-4).

BOX 23-3 Laboratory Impact of Significant Hemoglobinemia

The results of a routine complete blood count are unreliable for patients with significant hemoglobinemia. Under normal circumstances, the measured hemoglobin represents the hemoglobin present inside the red blood cells. For individuals with hemoglobinemia, the intracellular hemoglobin and the plasma hemoglobin both are measured. The hemoglobin value therefore is falsely elevated. An unrealistically high value for mean cell hemoglobin concentration may provide a clue to this problem, which can be remedied in several ways (Chapters 14 and 15).

BOX 23-4 Therapeutic Applications of Haptoglobin and Hemopexin

During severe fragmentation hemolysis, the oxidizing capabilities of hemoglobin and heme cause serious tissue damage. Both readily transfer into extravascular spaces, damaging cells and causing organ dysfunction, such as renal failure. When hemoglobin binds to haptoglobin and heme binds to hemopexin, they are retained in the vasculature, diminishing tissue damage. As a result, the two proteins are gaining serious consideration as therapeutic agents that could be used during instances of fragmentation hemolysis to reduce organ damage. Haptoglobin has been used in Japan since 1985. Hemopexin has not yet been used clinically, but Schaer and colleagues report that both salvage proteins are under investigation by U.S. and European pharmaceutical firms.[5]

When free in the plasma, hemoglobin exists mostly as α/β dimers[5] that rapidly complex to a liver-produced plasma protein called *haptoglobin*. This is the first mechanism of hemoglobin iron salvage. By binding to haptoglobin, hemoglobin avoids filtration at the glomerulus, and the iron is saved from urinary loss. Haptoglobin binds a hemoglobin dimer in a conformation that is very similar to the complementary dimer in the native hemoglobin structure, so the conformation of the complex has been termed a *pseudotetramer*.[6,7] In this complex, the hemes are sequestered, as they are in intact hemoglobin, so that cells are protected from their oxidative properties.[6] As the plasma is carried to various tissues, the complex is taken up by macrophages, principally those in the liver, spleen, bone marrow, and lung.[8] In these tissues, the macrophages express CD163, the haptoglobin scavenger receptor, on their membranes. Once the hemoglobin-haptoglobin complex binds to CD163, the entire complex is internalized into the macrophage in a lysosome.[8,9] Inside the lysosome, iron is salvaged, the globin is catabolized, and the protoporphyrin is converted to unconjugated bilirubin, just as though an intact RBC had been ingested by the macrophage. The haptoglobin is also degraded within the lysosome.

The level of haptoglobin in plasma is typically adequate to salvage only the small amount of plasma hemoglobin generated each day. If hemolysis is accelerated, haptoglobin is depleted because the liver's production does not increase in response to the increased consumption of haptoglobin. See Excessive Fragmentation (Intravascular) Hemolysis below.

A secondary mechanism of iron salvage and oxidation prevention involves *hemopexin* (Figure 23-4). The iron in free plasma hemoglobin rapidly becomes oxidized, forming methemoglobin. The heme molecule (actually *metheme* or *hemin*) dissociates from the globin and binds to another liver-produced plasma protein, hemopexin.[10,11] This binding also saves the iron from urinary loss and prevents oxidant injury to cells and tissues. Hemopexin-metheme binds to hepatocyte CD91 receptors, the lipoprotein receptor-related protein (LRP1),[12] and is internalized.[13] The fate of the internalized heme remains an area of research because some studies suggest that intact heme can be incorporated into needed proteins within the hepatocyte, like cytochromes, and others suggest it is broken down to bilirubin with reuse of the iron.[13] It appears that under normal circumstances, the bulk of the hemopexin is recycled to the plasma from the hepatocyte.[14]

A third mechanism of iron salvage is the metheme-albumin system. Albumin acts as a carrier for many molecules, including metheme. This is just a temporary holding state for the metheme, merely by virtue of the high concentration of albumin in plasma. But metheme is rapidly transferred to hemopexin, which has a higher binding affinity for metheme than does albumin.[15] The hemopexin-metheme complex then travels to the liver for processing.

If the previous systems are overloaded, the excess (met) hemoglobin and metheme will be filtered into the urine. Normally, this is a negligible amount so that the kidney is not significantly involved in normal iron salvage. Yet, it has been known for some time that the proximal tubular cells can reabsorb iron, since iron staining of tubular cells in urinary sediment

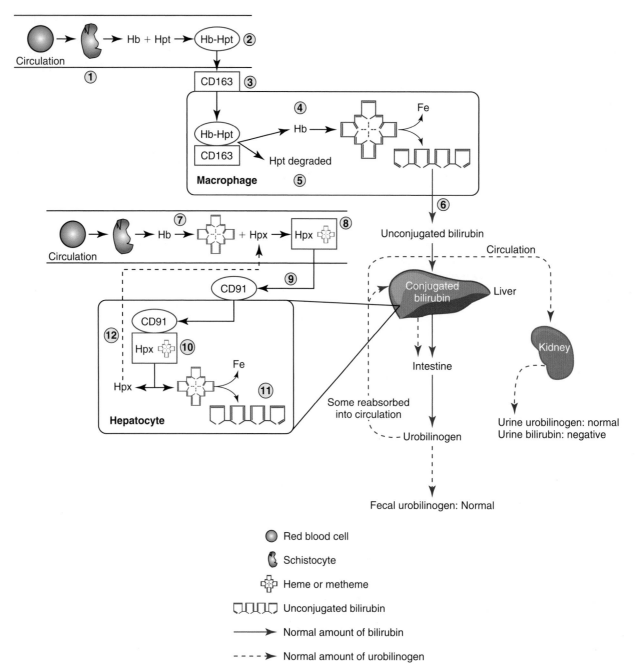

Figure 23-4 Normal fragmentation hemolysis. **1,** Normally a small number of red blood cells lyse within the circulation, forming schistocytes and releasing hemoglobin (*Hb*) into the plasma, mostly as αβ dimers. **2,** The plasma protein haptoglobin (*Hpt*) binds a hemoglobin dimer in a complex. **3,** The hemoglobin-haptoglobin complex binds to CD163 on the surface of macrophages in various organs. **4,** The complex is internalized into the macrophage, where the hemoglobin dimer is released. The hemoglobin dimer is degraded to heme, the iron is released, and the protoporphyrin ring is converted to unconjugated bilirubin. **5,** The haptoglobin is degraded. **6,** The unconjugated bilirubin released into the plasma is bound to albumin and processed through the liver as in Figure 23-3 (steps 2-8). **7,** When free hemoglobin is released into the plasma with fragmentation, the iron is rapidly oxidized, forming methemoglobin, and the heme (met-heme) molecule dissociates from the globin. **8,** The plasma protein hemopexin (*Hpx*) binds free metheme into a complex. **9,** The hemopexin-metheme complex binds to CD91 on the surface of hepatocytes. **10,** The complex is internalized into the hepatocyte. **11,** The iron is released from the metheme, and the proto-porphyrin ring is converted to unconjugated bilirubin, ready for conjugation and further processing, as in Figure 23-3 (steps 4-8). **12,** Hemopexin is recycled to the plasma. Note that metheme can also bind to albumin, forming metheme-albumin (not shown), but this complex is temporary because metheme is rapidly transferred to hemopexin. (Adapted from Brunzel NA. Fundamentals of Urine and Body Fluid Analysis. 3e. St. Louis, Elsevier, 2013.)

during periods of excessive hemolysis demonstrates the presence of hemosiderin. The full picture of renal handling of iron and related proteins is an area of active research yet to be fully eluci-dated. However, an emerging picture suggests that under normal circumstances, a small amount of filtered transferrin is salvaged by transferrin receptor on the apical surface of proximal tubular cells.[16] This may be the normal source of iron for those cells' metabolic needs. Ferroportin has been identified on the basolat-eral membrane of proximal tubular cells, suggesting that renal cells are then able to transfer additional salvaged iron back into the plasma.[17] Once again, these systems evolved to manage the amount and "form" of iron present in normal urinary filtrate. During excessive fragmentation hemolysis, other forms of iron are presented to and processed by the kidney.

EXCESSIVE MACROPHAGE-MEDIATED (EXTRAVASCULAR) HEMOLYSIS

Many hemolytic anemias are a result of increased macrophage-mediated hemolysis (Figure 23-5), during which more than the usual number of RBCs are removed from the circulation daily. Under normal circumstances, senescent RBCs display surface markers that identify them to macrophages as aged cells requiring removal (Chapter 8). Pathologic processes also lead to expression of the same markers, so cells are recognized and removed. If the number of affected cells increases beyond the quantity normally removed each day due to senescence, and if the bone marrow cannot compensate, then anemia develops. As an example, Heinz bodies, aggregates of denatured hemoglobin formed in various

anemias, bind to the inner surface of the RBC membrane, producing changes to the exterior of the membrane that can be detected by macrophages. When excessive oxidation of hemoglobin causes increased formation of Heinz bodies, the cells are removed from the circulation prematurely by macrophages. A similar process occurs when intracellular parasites are present or when complement or immunoglobulins are on the surface of the RBC.

When an RBC is ingested by a macrophage, it is lysed within a phagolysosome, and the contents are processed entirely within the macrophage as described previously. The contents of the RBC are not detected in plasma because it is lysed inside the macrophage, and the contents are degraded there—hence the designation *extravascular hemolysis*. Since defective cells display markers like those of senescent RBCs, macrophage-mediated hemolysis of defective cells occurs most often in the spleen and liver, where the macrophages possess receptors for those markers.

Sometimes the macrophage ingests a portion of the membrane, leaving the remainder to reseal. Little, if any, cytoplasmic volume is lost, but with less membrane, the cell becomes a

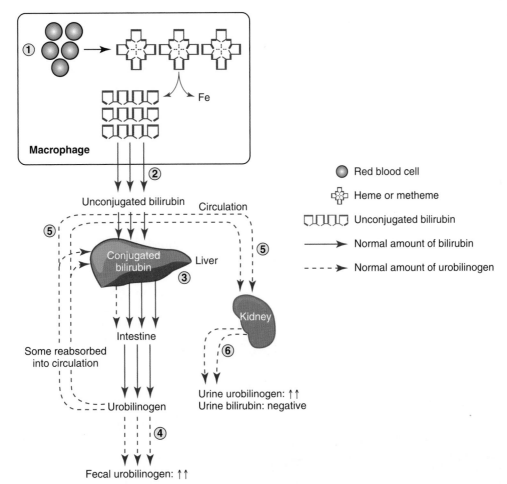

Figure 23-5 Excess macrophage-mediated hemolysis. **1,** More than the usual number of red blood cells are ingested each day by macrophages. **2,** An increased amount of unconjugated bilirubin is produced, released into the plasma, and binds to albumin. **3,** When increased unconjugated bilirubin is presented to the liver, an increased amount of conjugated bilirubin is made and excreted into the intestine. **4,** When an increased amount of conjugated bilirubin is present in the intestine, an increased amount of urobilinogen is formed and excreted in the stool. **5,** Increased urobilinogen in the intestine results in increased urobilinogen reabsorbed into the plasma. **6,** Increased urobilinogen in the plasma results in increased urobilinogen filtered and excreted in the urine. (Adapted from Brunzel NA. Fundamentals of Urine and Body Fluid Analysis. 3e. St. Louis, Elsevier, 2013.)

TABLE 23-2 Comparison of Laboratory Findings Indicating Accelerated Red Blood Cell Destruction in Fragmentation Versus Macrophage-Mediated Hemolysis

Test Specimen	Result	Fragmentation	Macrophage-Mediated
Serum	Total bilirubin	↑	↑
	Indirect (unconjugated) bilirubin	↑	↑
	Direct (conjugated) bilirubin	WRI	WRI
	Lactate dehydrogenase activity (RBC fraction)	↑	sl ↑
	Haptoglobin	↓	sl ↓
	Free hemoglobin	↑	sl ↑
	Hemopexin	↓	sl ↓
Urine	Urobilinogen	↑	↑
	Free hemoglobin	Positive	Negative
	Methemoglobin	Positive	Negative
	Prussian blue staining of urine sediment	Positive	Negative
Anticoagulated whole blood	Hemoglobin, hematocrit, RBC count	↓	↓
	Schistocytes	Often present	
	Spherocytes		Often present
	Glycated hemoglobin	↓	↓
Special tests	Endogenous carbon monoxide	↑	↑
	Erythrocyte life span	↓	↓

↑, Typically increased; *sl* ↑, typically only slightly increased, minor component; ↓, typically decreased; *RBC*, red blood cell; *WRI*, within the reference interval.

spherocyte, the characteristic shape change associated with macrophage-mediated hemolysis. Although the spherocyte may enter the circulation, its survival is shortened because of its rigidity and inability to traverse the splenic sieve during subsequent passages through the red pulp. It may become trapped against the basement membrane of the splenic sinus and be fully ingested by a macrophage, or it may lyse mechanically due to its rigidity and in so doing contribute a fragmentation component to what is otherwise a macrophage-mediated process.

In macrophage-mediated hemolytic anemias, the total plasma bilirubin level rises as RBCs lyse prematurely. The rise of the total bilirubin is due to the increase of the unconjugated fraction (Figure 23-5). As long as the liver is healthy, it processes the increased load of unconjugated bilirubin, producing more than the usual amount of conjugated bilirubin that enters the intestine. Increased urobilinogen forms in the intestines and is subsequently absorbed by the portal circulation and excreted by the kidney. As a result, increased urobilinogen is detectable in the urine. Although there is an increase in unconjugated bilirubin in the plasma, none of it appears in the urine because it is bound to albumin and cannot pass through the glomerulus. These findings are summarized in Table 23-2.

EXCESSIVE FRAGMENTATION (INTRAVASCULAR) HEMOLYSIS

Although fragmentation hemolysis is a minor component of normal RBC destruction, it can be a major feature of pathologic processes. Dramatic examples of fragmentation hemolysis are the traumatic, physical lysis of RBCs caused by prosthetic heart valves and the exit of mature intracellular RBC parasites, such as malaria protozoa, by bursting out of the cell. In these instances, the fragmentation destruction of RBCs can cause profound anemias.

Excessive fragmentation hemolysis is characterized by the appearance in the plasma of the contents of the red blood cell, chiefly hemoglobin, and thus the development of (met) hemoglobinemia. As a result, the salvage proteins form complexes with their ligands (Figure 23-6, *A, B*), and hemoglobin-haptoglobin, metheme-hemopexin, and metheme-albumin are detectable, if measured. The levels of free haptoglobin will drop, since more than the usual amounts of the complex will form and be taken up by macrophages (Table 23-2). The endocytosed protein is not recycled to the plasma and there is no compensatory increase in production, so the plasma is depleted of haptoglobin. The levels of free hemopexin can also decrease even though it is normally recycled. It appears that the hepatic recycling system can become saturated when there are high levels of metheme to be salvaged.[12] During these circumstances, hemopexin then gets degraded within the hepatocyte, and plasma levels fall. Still the drop in hemopexin is not as dramatic as the decline of haptoglobin,[4] since some recycling continues.

In roughly the same time frame that hemoglobin appears in the plasma, it can also appear in the urine (hemoglobinuria) (Table 23-2) if the amount of liberated hemoglobin and heme exceeds the salvage capacity of the plasma proteins. Increased amounts of iron-containing proteins are then absorbed into the proximal tubular cells (Figure 23-6, *C*).

The mechanisms by which renal cells are able to reabsorb more than usual amounts of iron, heme, or iron-containing proteins are still emerging. At least one mechanism is the megalin-cubilin receptor endocytosis system.[18] These receptors are not specific for heme/iron-containing compounds. They

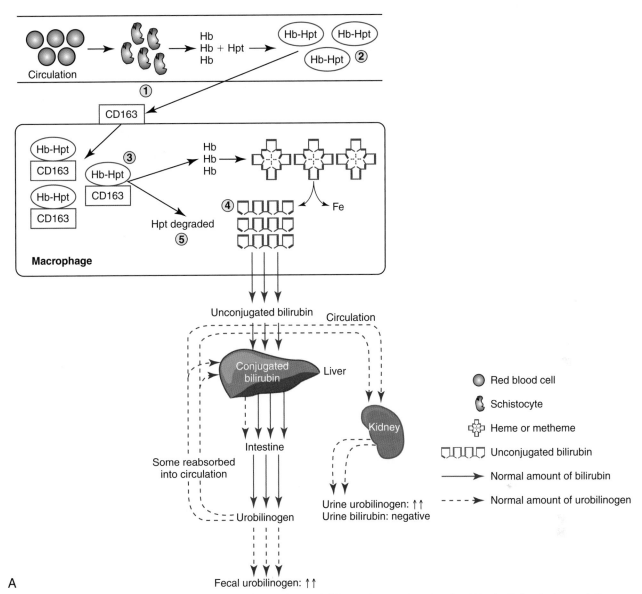

A

Figure 23-6 A, Excess fragmentation hemolysis: the role of macrophages. **1,** When an increased number of red blood cells lyse by fragmentation, more than the usual amount of hemoglobin (*Hb*) is released into the plasma, mostly as αβ dimers. **2,** Haptoglobin (*Hpt*) binds the increased hemoglobin dimers, forming more than usual numbers of complexes. **3,** The hemoglobin-haptoglobin complexes are taken up by macrophages bearing the CD163 receptor in various organs. **4,** An increased amount of hemoglobin dimers is released from the complexes. The hemoglobin is degraded to heme, the iron is released, and the protoporphyrin ring is converted to unconjugated bilirubin. The increased amount of unconjugated bilirubin is then transported to the liver and processed as with excess macrophage mediated hemolysis (Figure 23-5, steps 2-6). **5,** Degradation of haptoglobin is accelerated as compared to normal.

Continued

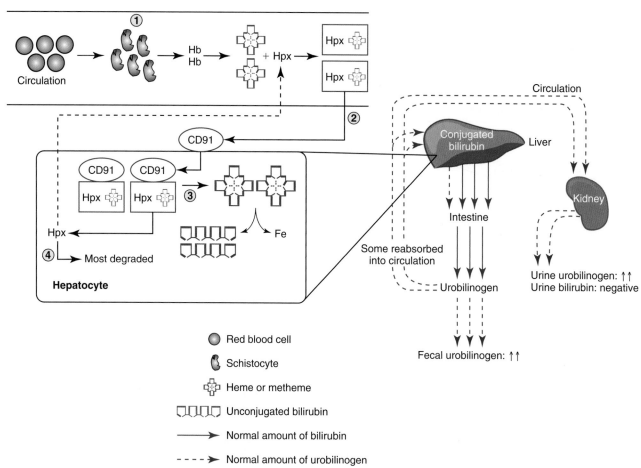

Circulation

CD91

Hepatocyte

- 🔴 Red blood cell
- 🦠 Schistocyte
- ⬦ Heme or metheme
- ⬜⬜⬜⬜ Unconjugated bilirubin
- ⟶ Normal amount of bilirubin

B

- ⤑ Normal amount of urobilinogen

Figure 23-6, cont'd **B,** Excess fragmentation hemolysis: the role of the liver. **1,** If the amount of hemoglobin released from lysing red blood cells exceeds the capacity of haptoglobin, the unbound free hemoglobin is rapidly oxidized, forming methemoglobin, and the metheme molecule dissociates from the globin. **2,** Hemopexin binds to metheme, and the complex is captured by the CD91 receptor on hepatocytes. **3,** The complex is internalized by the hepatocyte, the iron is released from the metheme, and the protoporphyrin ring is converted to unconjugated bilirubin and ultimately to conjugated bilirubin to be processed, as in Figure 23-5, steps 3-6. **4,** Although a small of amount of hemopexin is recycled to the plasma, most is degraded. Metheme can also temporarily bind to albumin, forming metheme-albumin (not shown), but metheme is rapidly transferred to hemopexin

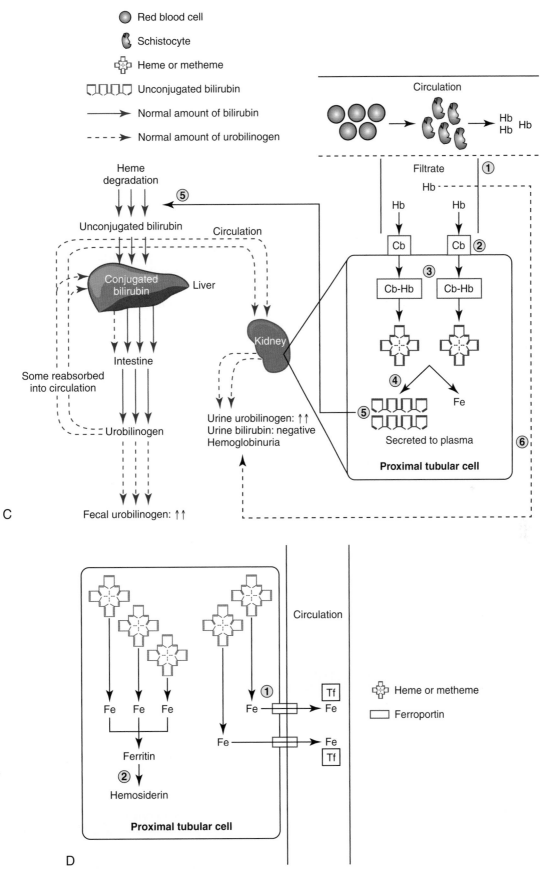

Figure 23-6, cont'd
For legend see next page

Figure 23-6, cont'd C, Excess fragmentation hemolysis: the role of the kidney. **1,** When excess red blood cells lyse by fragmentation and other systems are saturated, free (met)hemoglobin enters the urinary filtrate. **2,** Cubilin (*Cb*) on the luminal side of the proximal tubular cells binds proteins for reabsorption, including hemoglobin. **3,** Cubilin carries hemoglobin into the proximal tubular cells. **4,** The hemoglobin is degraded to heme, the iron is released, and the protoporphyrin ring is converted to unconjugated bilirubin and secreted into the plasma **(5)** in the same manner as in the macrophages (Figure 23-1). **6,** When the amount of hemoglobin exceeds the capacity of the proximal tubular cells to absorb it from the filtrate, hemoglobinuria occurs. **D,** Fate of iron removed from salvaged hemoglobin in the kidney. **1,** Iron (Fe) salvaged from absorbed hemoglobin can be transported into the circulation by ferroportin on the basolaminal side of the tubular cell. In the plasma it will be bound to transferrin (Tf) for transport. **2,** Iron in excess of what can be transported into the circulation is stored as ferritin, and some is converted to hemosiderin. If the tubular cell is sloughed into the filtrate and appears in the urine sediment, the hemosiderin can be detected using the Prussian blue stain. (**A-C,** Adapted from Brunzel NA. Fundamentals of Urine and Body Fluid Analysis. 3e. St. Louis, Elsevier, 2013.)

---

are responsible for nonspecific but very efficient reabsorption of proteins from the urinary filtrate in the proximal tubule. Each has been shown to bind hemoglobin and myoglobin.[18] Additionally, megalin can bind lactoferrin, and cubilin can bind transferrin.[18] The kinetics of such nonspecific competitive reabsorption favors the iron-containing proteins when they are present in high concentrations. A mechanism for reabsorption of free (met)heme has not been clearly identified. Proximal tubular cells are able to dismantle heme from hemoglobin via heme-oxygenase-1,[19] contributing to elevations of unconjugated bilirubin in plasma and thus freeing the iron for export to the plasma by ferroportin. It is reasonable to expect that a specific heme receptor in the kidney may yet be identified.

Proximal tubular cell iron in excess of what can be transported into the circulation is stored as ferritin, and some is converted to hemosiderin (Figure 23-6, *D*). If the tubular cell is sloughed into the filtrate and appears in the urine sediment, the hemosiderin can be detected using the Prussian blue stain. This provides evidence that hemoglobin has been salvaged from the filtrate.

Elevated levels of plasma indirect bilirubin and urinary urobilinogen are also measurable, although not immediately, because time is needed to produce these products. The time course of these findings assists with the differential diagnosis. Following an acute onset, a rise in reticulocytes several days later would also be seen.

CLINICAL FEATURES

The clinical findings typical of hemolysis may be prominent if the hemolytic process is the primary cause of anemia. For patients in whom hemolysis is secondary, however, other clinical features may be more noticeable. If hemolysis is sufficient to result in anemia, patients experience the general symptoms of fatigue, dyspnea, and dizziness to a degree that is consistent with the severity and rate of development of the anemia. The associated signs of pallor and tachycardia can be expected.

Increase in plasma bilirubin gives a yellow tinge, not only to the plasma but also to body tissues. It is readily evident in the sclera of the eyes and the skin of fair-skinned individuals. *Jaundice* refers to the yellow color of the skin and sclera, whereas *icterus* describes plasma and tissues. An increase in plasma bilirubin and subsequent jaundice can occur in other conditions besides hemolysis, such as hepatitis or gallstones. If the jaundice is the result of hemolysis, it is called *hemolytic jaundice* or *prehepatic jaundice,* which reflects the predominance of unconjugated bilirubin in plasma. The lipid solubility of unconjugated bilirubin also leads to deposition in the brain when hemolysis affects newborns (Chapter 26), since the blood-brain barrier is not fully developed. This can lead to a type of brain damage called *kernicterus,* which refers to the yellow coloring (icterus) of the brain tissue.

The frequency or constancy of jaundice provides clues to the cause. In glucose-6-phosphate dehydrogenase deficiency, for example, jaundice is periodic, appearing following a crisis. In thalassemia, jaundice is chronic. Jaundice may not be present at all if hemolysis is minimal and the liver is able to process the additional bilirubin, as is often the case in hereditary elliptocytosis.

Some signs differentiate chronic from acute hemolysis. Splenomegaly can develop, particularly with chronic macrophage-mediated hemolytic processes. Gallstones (cholelithiasis) can occur whenever hemolysis is chronic; the constantly increased amount of bilirubin in the bile leads to the formation of the stones.[20] When hemolysis is chronic in children, the persistent compensatory bone marrow hyperplasia can lead to bone deformities because the bones are still forming (Figure 28-3). For patients in whom an acquired, acute hemolytic process develops, the associated malaise, aches, vomiting, and possible fever may cause it to be confused with an acute infectious process. Profound prostration and shock may develop, particularly with acute fragmentation hemolysis. Flank pain, oliguria, or anuria develops, which leads to acute renal failure.

Other clinical features may offer a clue as to whether hemolysis is macrophage-mediated or due to fragmentation. In particular, brown urine, associated with (met)hemoglobinuria, points to a fragmentation hemolytic process.

LABORATORY FINDINGS

In patients with the clinical features of hemolytic anemia, laboratory tests typically show evidence of increased erythrocyte destruction and the compensatory increase in the rate of erythropoiesis. Other tests that are specific to a particular diagnosis also may be indicated.

Tests of Accelerated Red Blood Cell Destruction

Visual examination of the plasma and urine may suggest fragmentation hemolysis. The presence of methemoglobin, methemalbumin and hemopexin-heme impart a coffee-brown color to plasma, strongly suggestive of fragmentation hemolysis. When these compounds are present in urine, the color is more often described as root beer- or beer-colored. In a properly collected blood specimen, the normal physiologic fragmentation hemolysis produces a plasma hemoglobin level of less than 1 mg/dL.[21] Plasma does not become visibly red/brown until the plasma hemoglobin level is at 50 mg/dL.[21] Typical values during hemolytic processes may be as low as 15 mg/dL, so an increase in plasma hemoglobin may not always be visible.[22]

Hemoglobin/heme from fragmentation hemolysis can be detected in urine when the capacity of the plasma salvage systems is exceeded and the hemoglobin/heme is filtered into the urine. The urinalysis test strip for blood can be positive even when the hemoglobin is not present in a high enough concentration to change the color of the urine significantly. Since the product entering the urine is free hemoglobin/heme, the sediment will be negative for red blood cells. However, renal tubular cells sloughed into the filtrate during the period of hemoglobinuria can demonstrate deposits of hemosiderin (iron), resulting from absorbed hemoglobin, when stained with Prussian blue stain.

For a patient with a hemolytic process, a complete blood count (CBC) may provide clues to the cause. Spherocytes can be expected to be seen with macrophage-mediated hemolysis (Table 23-2), whereas fragmented cells, or schistocytes, are noted with fragmentation hemolysis. Other clues to the particular cause of the hemolysis may be present in the morphology, such as ring forms in malaria, sickle cells in sickle cell anemia, target cells and microcytes in thalassemia, and spherocytes in hereditary spherocytosis or immune-related hemolysis.

In either fragmentation or macrophage-mediated hemolysis, the increased rate of hemoglobin catabolism results in increased amounts of plasma unconjugated bilirubin and carbon monoxide. If liver function is normal, conjugated bilirubin is formed and excreted as urobilinogen in the stool, and the serum level of conjugated bilirubin remains within the reference interval. No bilirubin is detected in the urine because unconjugated bilirubin is bound to albumin and the complex is not filtered by the glomerulus. The urinary urobilinogen level may be increased, however, because there is increased urobilinogen in the stool, and more than usual amounts are absorbed by the portal circulation. In some patients, serum indirect (unconjugated) bilirubin values can be misleadingly low because the amount of bilirubin in the blood depends on the rate of RBC catabolism as well as hepatic function. If the rate of hemolysis is low and liver function is normal, the total serum bilirubin level can be within the reference interval. Quantitative measurements of fecal urobilinogen, however, would demonstrate an increase.

A substantial decline in the serum haptoglobin level indicates fragmentation hemolysis. In what is mostly a macrophage-mediated hemolysis, there can still be a minor component of fragmentation lysis involving spherical cells that are fragile, so a modest decline in haptoglobin level can be seen. In short, whenever the level of hemoglobin in the plasma increases, the haptoglobin level declines. In one study, a low haptoglobin level indicated an 87% probability of hemolytic disease.[23] Haptoglobin measurement is, however, prone to both false-positive and false-negative results. Low values suggest hemolysis but may be due instead to impaired synthesis of haptoglobin caused by liver disease. Alternatively, a patient with hemolysis may have a relatively normal haptoglobin level if there is also a complicating infection or inflammation, because haptoglobin is an acute phase reactant. Although quantitation of hemopexin may also demonstrate a low value, it is not often measured, relying instead on the more dramatic haptoglobin decline to detect fragmentation hemolysis.

Tests to determine the rate of endogenous carbon monoxide production have been developed, because carbon monoxide is produced in the first step of heme breakdown by heme oxygenase. Values of 2 to 10 times the normal rate have been detected in some patients with hemolytic anemia,[24] but testing for carbon monoxide production is not typically required for clinical diagnosis.

Other laboratory test results are incidentally abnormal. Serum lactate dehydrogenase activity is often increased in patients with fragmentation hemolysis due to the release of the enzyme from ruptured RBCs, but other conditions, such as myocardial infarction or liver disease, also can cause increases. Although enzyme isoform fractionation could be used to identify lactate dehydrogenase of RBC origin, this test is generally not needed. Rather, when other results point to fragmentation hemolysis, one should expect an increase in the level of serum lactate dehydrogenase and other RBC enzymes and should not be misled into assuming that there is liver damage (Table 23-2).

General evidence of reduced RBC survival can be gleaned by measuring glycated hemoglobin (by the Hb A_{1c} test).[25] Glycated hemoglobin increases over the life of a cell as it is exposed to plasma glucose. Glycated hemoglobin level is usually decreased in chronic hemolytic disease because the cells have less exposure to plasma glucose before lysis. The mean reference interval for glycated hemoglobin in one report was 6.7%; in a hemolytic process, the mean value decreased to 3.9%.[25] The magnitude of the decrease is related to the magnitude of the hemolytic process over the previous 4- to 8-week period. Glycated hemoglobin level is not a reliable indicator of shortened RBC survival in patients with diabetes mellitus because of the increased rate of glycation with elevated blood glucose levels. Thus glycated hemoglobin measurement is more useful for diagnosis or monitoring blood glucose control in diabetic patients, rather than detection of hemolysis.

A more exact RBC survival assay uses random labeling of blood with chromium radioisotope. This is the reference method for RBC survival studies published by the International Committee for Standardization in Haematology.[26] A sample of blood is collected, mixed with the isotope, and returned to the patient. The labeled cells are of all ages, reflecting normal peripheral blood. This method differs from cohort labeling in which RBCs are labeled with radioactive iron or heavy nitrogen as they are produced in the bone marrow, so the labeled cells are generally of the same age. In both methods, the disappearance of the label from the blood is measured over time. As measured using the random chromium labeling technique, the normal half-time of chromium is 25 to 32 days.[26] A half-time of 20 to 25 days suggests mild hemolysis; 15 to 20 days, moderate hemolysis; and less than 15 days, severe hemolysis.[26] There are clinical instances when an estimation of red cell survival would be useful for assessing erythropoietin treatment.[27] However, both cohort and random techniques have significant limitations,[28] in addition to being time consuming, expensive, and requiring the use of radioactive isotopes. Therefore, these methods are not often used clinically but are used for research, particularly in the search for improved methods of determining red blood cell survival.

Tests of Increased Erythropoiesis

If the bone marrow is healthy, the hypoxia associated with hemolysis leads to increased erythropoiesis. Recognition of this increase may be a first clue to the presence of a hemolytic process. Laboratory findings indicating increased erythropoiesis include an increase in circulating reticulocytes and, in severe cases, nucleated red blood cells (Table 23-3). These findings are persistently present in chronic hemolytic disease and are evident within 3 to 6 days after an acute hemolytic episode. Increased erythropoiesis is not unique to hemolytic anemias and is not diagnostic. Similar results are expected after hemorrhage and with successful specific therapy for anemia caused by iron, folate, or vitamin B_{12} deficiency. An assessment of erythropoiesis can determine the effectiveness of the bone marrow response, however, and should be factored into the differential diagnosis (see Differential Diagnosis).

Complete Blood Count and Morphologic Features

Peripheral blood film evaluation is crucial. An increase in polychromatic RBCs (reticulocytes) and nucleated RBCs represents bone marrow compensation for hemolysis or blood loss. Schistocytes are expected with excessive fragmentation hemolysis, while spherocytes may be seen with macrophage-mediated processes. Additional morphologic changes to red blood cells may point toward the etiology of the hemolysis (see below).

An increase in the mean cell volume (MCV) is usually seen with extreme compensatory reticulocytosis resulting from the larger, prematurely released "shift" reticulocytes. The increase

must be assessed by comparison with the value seen early in hemolysis, before the shift reticulocytes have emerged. The MCV may not increase above the reference interval but rather may be above the baseline value for that patient. Exceptions occur if the hemolytic condition itself involves smaller cells that counter the increased volume of the reticulocytes. In hereditary spherocytosis, microspherocytes are the cause of the anemia, and the MCV may be within the reference interval even when larger shift reticulocytes are generated—hence the importance of a baseline value for comparison. In other circumstances, such as severe burns, numerous schistocytes or microspherocytes may outnumber the reticulocytes so that the MCV remains low.

Leukocytosis and thrombocytosis may accompany acute hemolytic anemia and are considered reactions to the hemolytic process. Conversely, conditions that directly cause leukocytosis, such as sepsis, might cause hemolysis. Low platelet counts in association with other signs of hemolysis may indicate a platelet-consuming microangiopathic process, such as disseminated intravascular coagulopathy.

Reticulocyte Count

The reticulocyte count is the most commonly used test to detect accelerated erythropoiesis and is expected to rise during hemolysis or hemorrhage. Assuming the bone marrow is healthy and there are adequate raw materials, all measures of reticuloycyte production should rise: absolute reticulocyte count, relative reticulocyte count, reticulocyte production index, and the immature reticulocyte fraction. The association of reticulocytosis with hemolysis is so strong that if an anemic patient has an elevated reticulocyte count and hemorrhage is ruled out, a cause of hemolysis should be investigated. The reticulocyte increase usually correlates well with the severity of the hemolysis. Exceptions occur during aplastic crises of some hemolytic anemias and in some immunohemolytic anemias with hypoplastic marrow, which suggests that the autoantibodies were directed against the bone marrow RBC precursors and circulating erythrocytes.[21] Chapters 14 and 19 describe the interpretation of reticulocyte indices in patients with anemia.

Bone Marrow Examination

Bone marrow examination is usually not necessary to diagnose hemolytic anemia. If conducted, however, bone marrow examination will reveal erythroid hyperplasia that results in peripheral blood reticulocytosis. As the erythroid component (the denominator) of the myeloid-to-erythroid ratio increases, the overall ratio decreases. (The myeloid-to-erythroid ratio is defined in Chapter 17.) As always, the cellularity of the bone marrow should be determined on a core biopsy specimen, rather than an aspirated specimen, for a more accurate judgment.

Laboratory Tests to Determine Specific Hemolytic Processes

As noted above, the appearance of spherocytes or schistocytes on a peripheral blood film can point to a hemolytic cause for anemia. Other abnormalities found on the film,

TABLE 23-3 Hematologic Findings Indicating Accelerated Red Blood Cell Production

Specimen	Findings
Anticoagulated peripheral blood	Increased absolute reticulocyte count, immature reticulocyte fraction, reticulocyte production index
	Rising mean cell volume (compared with baseline)
	Polychromasia, nucleated RBCs
Bone marrow	Erythroid hyperplasia

RBC, Red blood cell.

TABLE 23-4 Morphologic Abnormalities Associated with Hemolytic Anemia

RBC Morphology	Hemolytic Disorders
Spherocytes	Hereditary spherocytosis, IgG-mediated immune hemolytic anemia, thermal injury to RBCs
Elliptocytes (ovalocytes)	Hereditary elliptocytosis
Acanthocytes	Abetalipoproteinemia, severe liver disease (spur cell anemia)
Burr cells	Pyruvate kinase deficiency, uremia
Schistocytes	Microangiopathic hemolytic anemia, macroangiopathic (traumatic cardiac hemolytic anemia), IgM-mediated immune hemolytic anemia
Erythrophagocytosis	Damage to RBC surface, especially due to complement-fixing antibodies
RBC agglutination	Cold agglutinins, immunohemolytic disease

RBC, Red blood cell.

such as elliptocytes, acanthocytes, burr cells, sickle cells, target cells, agglutination, erythrophagocytosis, or parasites, may help reveal the specific disorder causing the hemolysis (Table 23-4).

Other tests dealing with specific types of hemolytic anemia are discussed in subsequent chapters. They include the direct antiglobulin test, osmotic fragility test, eosin-5′-maleimide binding test, Heinz body test, RBC enzyme studies, serologic tests, and immunophenotyping.

DIFFERENTIAL DIAGNOSIS

The differential diagnosis of hemolytic anemias incorporates several intersecting lines of deduction. The first is to establish the hemolytic nature of the anemia. A rapid decrease in hemoglobin concentration (e.g., 1 g/dL per week) from levels previously within the reference interval can signal hemolysis when hemorrhage and hemodilution have been ruled out. Jaundice and reticulocytosis provide additional confirmation of a hemolytic cause for an anemia of at least several days' duration. When only the indirect (unconjugated) fraction of the total serum bilirubin is elevated, hemolytic jaundice is confirmed. An elevated urinary urobilinogen level strengthens the conclusion.

The rapid decrease in hemoglobin during an acute hemolytic episode, however, usually is apparent before reticulocytosis and bilirubinemia develop. For acute hemolysis, hemoglobinemia and hemoglobinuria are expected with fragmentation causes; therefore, their absence suggests a macrophage-mediated cause. RBC morphology and haptoglobin levels can assist in differentiating fragmentation from a macrophage-mediated cause. Figure 23-7 is a graphic representation of the general time line of the events in acute fragmentation and macrophage-mediated hemolysis. In chronic hemolysis, persistence of hemoglobinemia, hemoglobinuria, decreased serum haptoglobin level, indirect bilirubinemia,

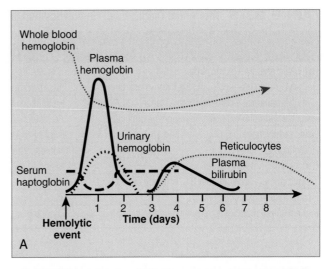

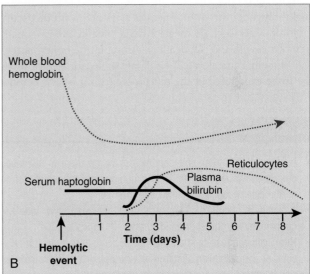

Figure 23-7 A, Fragmentation (intravascular) hemolysis time line. During fragmentation hemolysis, hemoglobin is detectable in plasma and urine for a period of time very soon after the hemolysis occurs. Haptoglobin levels will drop as the plasma hemoglobin rises. When hemolysis ends, the hemoglobin will disappear from plasma and urine as the haptoglobin returns to normal. However, the protoporphyrin of salvaged hemoglobin will be processed to bilirubin that will rise after the hemolytic event. Assuming the hemolysis has resulted in anemia, reticulocyte indices will also rise several days after the hemolytic event. **B,** Macrophage-mediated (extravascular) hemolysis time line. With macrophage-mediated hemolysis, the contents of the red blood cells do not enter the plasma, so evidence of hemolysis is delayed until bilirubin and reticulocytes rise.

and reticulocytosis can be expected, depending on the mechanism of the hemolysis.

Hemolytic anemias must be differentiated from other anemias associated with bilirubinemia, reticulocytosis, or both. Anemia with reticulocytosis but without bilirubinemia is expected during recovery from hemorrhage not treated with transfusion or with effective treatment of deficiencies such as iron deficiency. Anemia that results from hemorrhage into a body cavity is characterized by reticulocytosis during recovery and bilirubinemia due to catabolism of the hemoglobin in the

TABLE 23-5 Differential Diagnosis of Hemolytic Anemias Versus Other Causes of Indirect Bilirubinemia and Reticulocytosis

	Hemoglobin Level	Indirect Bilirubinemia	Reticulocytosis	Spherocytes or Schistocytes
Hemolytic anemia—acute, fragmentation	Rapidly dropping	Delayed	Delayed	Schistocytes
Hemolytic anemia—acute, macrophage-mediated	Rapidly dropping	Delayed	Delayed	Spherocytes
Hemolytic anemia—chronic, fragmentation	Persistently low	Persistent	Persistent	Schistocytes
Hemolytic anemia—chronic, macrophage-mediated	Persistently low	Persistent	Persistent	Spherocytes
Acute hemorrhage	Rapidly dropping	Absent	Absent	Absent
Hemodilution	Rapidly dropping	Absent	Absent	Absent
Recovery from hemorrhage	Rising	Absent	Present	Absent
Treated anemia (iron, vitamin B$_{12}$, or folate deficiency)	Rising	Absent	Present	Absent
Hemorrhage into a body cavity	Rapidly dropping	Delayed	Delayed	Absent
Ineffective erythropoiesis (e.g., megaloblastic anemia)	Dropping	Persistent	Absent	Absent

hemorrhaged cells. The RBC morphology should remain normal throughout the event. Anemias associated with ineffective erythropoiesis, such as megaloblastic anemia, are essentially hemolytic, with the cell death occurring in the bone marrow. Bilirubinemia and elevated serum lactate dehydrogenase levels are to be expected, but the reticulocyte count is low. Because most of the RBCs never reach the periphery, such anemias are typically classified as anemias of diminished production rather than as hemolytic anemias. As summarized in Table 23-5, the differential diagnosis in each of these instances may rely on negative results of tests for increased cell destruction or accelerated production.

SUMMARY

- A hemolytic disorder is a condition in which there is increased destruction of erythrocytes and a compensatory acceleration in erythrocyte production by the bone marrow.
- A hemolytic anemia develops when the bone marrow is unable to compensate for the shortened survival of the RBCs.
- Hemolytic anemias can be classified as acute or chronic, intravascular or extravascular, acquired or inherited, intrinsic or extrinsic, and fragmentation or macrophage-mediated.
- Normally, most erythrocyte death occurs via macrophages of the spleen and liver. A small amount occurs by fragmentation due to mechanical trauma.
- Hemoglobin from the RBCs is converted to heme and globin within macrophages. Heme is further degraded to iron, carbon monoxide, and unconjugated bilirubin. The bilirubin is secreted into the plasma, where it binds to albumin and is transported to the liver. In the liver, the bilirubin is conjugated with glucuronic acid, excreted as bile into the intestines, and converted to urobilinogen. Some urobilinogen is reabsorbed into the portal circulation and reexcreted through the liver. A small amount of urobilinogen remains in the plasma, and it is excreted by the kidney into the urine.
- In macrophage-mediated (extravascular) hemolytic anemia, there is a delayed increase in unconjugated bilirubin in the plasma and an increase in urobilinogen in the stool and urine. Spherocytes may be seen on the blood film.
- Signs of fragmentation (intravascular) hemolysis include (met)hemoglobinemia, (met)hemoglobinuria, and hemosiderinuria. Serum

haptoglobin is markedly decreased or absent. Schistocytes may be seen on the blood film.
- Jaundice can result from increased serum unconjugated bilirubin during any hemolytic anemia.
- The major clinical features of chronic inherited hemolytic anemia are varying degrees of anemia, jaundice, splenomegaly, and the development of cholelithiasis. In children, bone abnormalities may develop as a result of accelerated erythropoiesis.
- Laboratory studies providing evidence of hemolytic anemia include tests for increased erythrocyte destruction and compensatory increase in the rate of erythropoiesis. Elevated serum indirect bilirubin level with a normal serum direct bilirubin level suggests accelerated RBC destruction. A moderate to marked decrease in serum haptoglobin level suggests a fragmentation cause of hemolysis. The reticulocyte count is the most commonly used laboratory test to identify accelerated erythropoiesis, including an elevation of the immature reticulocyte fraction. Other tests that are specific to a particular diagnosis also may be needed.
- Hemolytic anemias must be differentiated from other anemias with reticulocytosis, including the post-acute hemorrhage state and recovery from iron, vitamin B$_{12}$, or folate deficiency, and from those with bilirubinemia, such as with internal bleeding.

Now that you have completed this chapter, go back and read again the case study at the beginning and respond to the questions presented.

REVIEW QUESTIONS

Answers can be found in the Appendix.

1. The term *hemolytic disorder* in general refers to a disorder in which there is:
   a. Increased destruction of RBCs after they enter the bloodstream
   b. Excessive loss of RBCs from the body
   c. Inadequate RBC production by the bone marrow
   d. Increased plasma volume with unchanged red cell mass

2. RBC destruction that occurs when macrophages ingest and destroy RBCs is termed:
   a. Extracellular
   b. Macrophage-mediated
   c. Intra-organ
   d. Extrahematopoietic

3. A sign of hemolysis that is typically associated with both fragmentation and macrophage-mediated hemolysis is:
   a. Hemoglobinuria
   b. Hemosiderinuria
   c. Hemoglobinemia
   d. Elevated urinary urobilinogen level

4. An elderly white woman is evaluated for worsening anemia, with a decrease of approximately 0.5 mg/dL of hemoglobin each week. The patient is pale, and her skin and eyes are slightly yellow. She complains of extreme fatigue and is unable to complete the tasks of daily living without napping in midmorning and midafternoon. She also tires with exertion, finding it difficult to climb even five stairs. Which of the features of this description points to a hemolytic cause for her anemia?
   a. Pallor
   b. Yellow skin and eyes
   c. Need for naps
   d. Tiredness on exertion

5. Which of the following tests provides a good indication of accelerated erythropoiesis?
   a. Urine urobilinogen level
   b. Hemosiderin level
   c. Reticulocyte count
   d. Glycated hemoglobin level

6. A 5-year-old girl was seen by her physician several days prior to this visit and was diagnosed with pneumonia. Her mother has brought her to the physician again because the girl's urine began to darken after the first visit and now is alarmingly dark. The girl has no history of anemia, and there is no family history of any hematologic disorder. The CBC shows a mild anemia, polychromasia, and a few schistocytes. This anemia could be categorized as:
   a. Acquired, fragmentation
   b. Acquired, macrophage-mediated
   c. Hereditary, fragmentation
   d. Hereditary, macrophage-mediated

7. A patient has a personal and family history of a mild hemolytic anemia. The patient has consistently elevated levels of total and indirect serum bilirubin and urinary urobilinogen. The serum haptoglobin level is consistently decreased, whereas the reticulocyte count is elevated. The latter can be seen as polychromasia on the patient's blood film, along with spherocytes. Which of the findings reported for this patient is *inconsistent* with a classical diagnosis of fragmentation hemolysis?
   a. Elevated total and indirect serum bilirubin
   b. Elevated urinary urobilinogen
   c. Decreased haptoglobin
   d. Spherocytes on the peripheral film

8. Select the statement that is *true* about bilirubin metabolism.
   a. Indirect bilirubin is formed in the liver by the addition of two sugar molecules to direct bilirubin.
   b. Macrophages of the spleen liberate bilirubin during hemoglobin catabolism.
   c. Urobilinogen is not water soluble and is not excreted in the urine.
   d. Normally, the major fraction of bilirubin in the blood is the direct (conjugated) form released from macrophages.

9. A patient has anemia that has been worsening over the last several months. The hemoglobin level has been declining slowly, with a drop of 1.5 g/dL of hemoglobin over about 6 weeks. Polychromasia and anisocytosis are seen on the blood film, consistent with the elevated reticulocyte count and RBC distribution width (RDW). Serum levels of total bilirubin and indirect fractions are normal. Urinary urobilinogen level also is normal. When these findings are evaluated, the conclusion is drawn that the anemia does not have a hemolytic component. Based on the data given here, why was hemolysis ruled out as the cause of the anemia?
   a. The decline in hemoglobin is too gradual to be associated with hemolysis.
   b. The elevation of the reticulocyte count suggests a malignant cause.
   c. Evidence of increased protoporphyrin catabolism is lacking.
   d. Elevated RDW points to an anemia of decreased production.

10. Which of the following sets of test results is typically expected with chronic fragmentation hemolysis?

	Serum Haptoglobin	Urine Hemoglobin	Urine Sediment Prussian Blue Stain
a.	Increased	Positive	Positive
b.	Decreased	Negative	Negative
c.	Decreased	Positive	Positive
d.	Increased	Positive	Negative

REFERENCES

1. Crosby, W. H., & Akeroyd, J. H. (1952). The limit of hemoglobin synthesis in hereditary hemolytic anemia. *Am J Med, 13,* 273–283.
2. McDonagh, A. F. (2010). Controversies in bilirubin biochemistry and their clinical relevance. *Sem Fetal Neonatal Med, 15,* 141–147.
3. Cui, Y., Konig, J., Leier, I., et al. (2001). Hepatic uptake of bilirubin and its conjugates by the human organic anion transporter SLC21A6. *J Biol Chem, 276,* 9626–9630.
4. Quigley, J. G., Means, R. T., & Glader, B. (2014). The birth, life, and death of red blood cells: erythropoiesis, the mature red blood cell, and cell destruction. In Greer, J. P., Arber, D. A., Glader, B., et al. (Eds.). *Wintrobe's Clinical Hematology.* (13th ed.). Philadelphia: Wolters Kluwer Health/Lippincott Williams & Wilkins. Accessed 05.01.14.
5. Schaer, D. J., Buehler, P. W., Alayash, A. I., et al. (2013). Hemolysis and free hemoglobin revisited: exploring hemoglobin and hemin scavengers as a novel class of therapeutic proteins. *Blood, 121,* 1276–1284.
6. Andersen, C. B. F., Torvund-Jensen, M., Nielsen, M. J., et al. (2012). Structure of the haptoglobin-haemoglobin complex. *Nature, 489,* 456–460.
7. Ratanasopa, K., Chakane, S., Ilyas, M., et al. (2013). Trapping of human hemoglobin by haptoglobin: molecular mechanisms and clinical applications. *Antiox Redox Signal, 18,* 2364–2374.
8. Etzerodt, A., & Moestrup, S. (2013). CD163 and Inflammation: biological, diagnostic and therapeutic aspects. *Antioxid Redox Signal, 18,* 2352–2363.
9. Kristiansen, M., Graversen, J. H., Jacobsen, C., et al. (2001). Identification of the haemoglobin scavenger receptor. *Nature, 409,* 198–201.
10. Tolosano, E., & Altruda, F. (2002). Hemopexin: structure, function, and regulation. *DNA Cell Biol, 21,* 297–306.
11. Delanghe, J. R., & Langlois, M. R. (2001). Hemopexin: a review of biological aspects and the role in laboratory medicine. *Clin Chim Acta, 312,* 13–23.
12. Hvidberg, V., Maniecki, M. B., Jacobsen, C., et al. (2005). Identification of the receptor scavenging hemopexin-heme complexes. *Blood, 106,* 2572–2579.
13. Tolosano, E., Fagoonee, S., Morello, N., et al. (2010). Heme scavenging and the other facets of hemopexin. *Antioxid Redox Signal, 12,* 305–320.
14. Smith, A., & Morgan, W. T. (1979). Haem transport to the liver by haemopexin. *Biochem J, 182,* 47–54.
15. Morgan, W. T., Liem, H. H., Sutor, R. P., et al. (1976). Transfer of heme from heme-albumin to hemopexin. *Biochem Biophys Acta, 444,* 435–445.
16. Zhang, D., Meyron-Holtz, E., & Rouault, T. A. (2007). Renal iron metabolism: transferrin iron delivery and the role of iron regulatory proteins. *J Am Soc Nephrol, 18,* 401–406.
17. Wolff, N., Liu, W., Fenton, R. A., et al. (2011). Ferroportin 1 is expressed basolaterally in rat kidney proximal tubule cells and iron excess increases its membrane trafficking. *J Cell Mol Med, 15,* 209–219.
18. Christiansen, E. I., Verroust, P. J., & Nielsen, R. (2009). Receptor-mediated endocytosis in renal proximal tubule. *Pfulgers Arch-Eur J Physiol, 458,* 1039–1048.
19. Ferenbach, D. A., Kluth, D. C., & Hughes, J. (2010). Hemeoxygenase-1 and renal ischaemia-reperfusion injury. *Exp Nephrol, 115,* e33–e37.
20. Trotman, B. W. (1991). Pigment gallstone disease. *Gastroenterol Clin North Am, 20,* 111–126.
21. Means, R. T. Jr., & Glader, B. (2014). Anemia: general considerations. In Greer, J. P., Arber, D. A., Glader, B., et al. (Eds.). *Wintrobe's Clinical Hematology.* (13th ed.). Philadelphia: Wolters Kluwer Health/Lippincott Williams & Wilkins. Accessed 05.01.14.
22. Crosby, W. H., & Dameshek, W. (1951). The significance of hemoglobinemia and associated hemosiderinuria, with particular reference to various types of hemolytic anemia. *J Lab Clin Med, 38,* 829–841.
23. Marchand, A., Galen, R. S., Van Lente, F. (1980). The predictive value of serum haptoglobin in hemolytic disease. *JAMA, 243,* 1909–1911.
24. Coburn, R. F. (1970). Endogenous carbon monoxide production in man. *N Engl J Med, 282,* 207–209.
25. Panzer, S., Kronik, G., Lechner, K., et al. (1982). Glycosylated hemoglobin (GHb): an index of red cell survival. *Blood, 59,* 1348–1350.
26. International Committee for Standardization in Haematology. (1980). Recommended method for radioisotope red cell survival studies. *Br J Haematol, 45,* 659–666.
27. Uehlinger, D. E., Gotch, F. A., & Sheiner, L. B. (1992). A pharmacodynamics model of erythropoietin therapy for uremic anemia. *Clin Pharmacol Ther, 51,* 76–89.
28. Korell, J., Coulter, C. V., & Duffull, S. B. (2011). Evaluation of red blood cell labeling methods based on a statistical model for red blood cell survival. *J Theor Biol, 291,* 88–98.

Intrinsic Defects Leading to Increased Erythrocyte Destruction

24

Elaine M. Keohane

OBJECTIVES

After completion of this chapter, the reader will be able to:

1. Describe the intrinsic cell properties that affect red blood cell (RBC) deformability.
2. Explain how defects in vertical and horizontal membrane protein interactions can result in a hemolytic anemia.
3. Compare and contrast the inheritance pattern, membrane proteins mutated, mechanism of hemolysis, typical RBC morphology, and clinical and laboratory findings of hereditary spherocytosis, hereditary elliptocytosis, and hereditary ovalocytosis.
4. Compare and contrast the RBC morphology and laboratory findings of hereditary spherocytosis and immune-associated hemolytic anemias.
5. Explain the principle, interpretation, and limitations of the osmotic fragility and eosin-5′-maleimide (EMA) binding tests in the diagnosis of hereditary spherocytosis.
6. Describe the causes, pathophysiology, RBC morphology, and clinical and laboratory findings of hemolytic anemias characterized by stomatocytosis.
7. Describe the causes and pathophysiology of hereditary and acquired conditions characterized by acanthocytosis.
8. Describe the cause, pathophysiology, clinical manifestations, laboratory findings, and treatment for paroxysmal nocturnal hemoglobinuria.
9. Compare and contrast the inheritance pattern, pathophysiology, clinical symptoms, and typical laboratory findings of glucose-6-phosphate dehydrogenase deficiency and pyruvate kinase deficiency.
10. Given the history, symptoms, laboratory findings, and a representative microscopic field from a peripheral blood film for a patient with a suspected intrinsic hemolytic anemia, discuss possible causes of the anemia and indicate the data that support these conclusions.

CASE STUDY

After studying the material in this chapter, the reader should be able to respond to the following case study:

A 45-year-old man sought medical attention for the onset of chest pain. Physical examination revealed slight jaundice and splenomegaly. The medical history included gallstones, and there was a family history of anemia. A CBC yielded the following results:

	Patient Results	Reference Interval
WBCs ($\times 10^9$/L)	13.4	3.6–10.6
RBCs ($\times 10^{12}$/L)	4.20	4.60–6.00
HGB (g/dL)	11.9	14.0–18.0
HCT (%)	32.4	40–54
MCV (fL)	77.1	80–100
MCH (pg)	28.3	26–32
MCHC (g/dL)	36.7	32–36
RDW (%)	22.9	11.5–14.5
Platelets ($\times 10^9$/L)	290	150–450

Continued

The peripheral blood film revealed anisocytosis, polychromasia, and spherocytes (Figure 24-1).

1. From the data given, what is a likely cause of the anemia?
2. What additional laboratory tests would be of value in establishing the diagnosis, and what abnormalities in the results of these tests would be expected to confirm your impression?
3. What is the cause of this type of anemia?

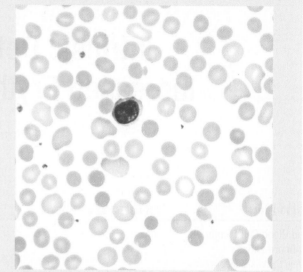

Figure 24-1 Peripheral blood film for the patient in the case study (×500). (From Carr JH, Rodak BF: *Clinical hematology atlas,* ed 3, Philadelphia, 2009, Saunders.)

Intrinsic hemolytic anemias comprise a large group of disorders in which defects in the red blood cells (RBCs) themselves result in premature hemolysis and anemia. Intrinsic disorders can be divided into abnormalities of the RBC membrane, metabolic enzymes, or hemoglobin. Most of these defects are hereditary. This chapter covers defects in the RBC membrane and enzymes causing hemolytic anemia. Chapter 27 covers qualitative hemoglobin disorders, and Chapter 28 covers quantitative hemoglobin disorders.

RED BLOOD CELL MEMBRANE ABNORMALITIES

Red Blood Cell Membrane Structure and Function

The RBC maintains a biconcave discoid shape that is essential for normal function and survival for 120 days in the peripheral circulation. The key to maintaining this shape is the plasma membrane, a lipid bilayer embedded with proteins and connected to an underlying protein cytoskeleton (Figure 9-2). The insoluble lipid portion serves as a barrier to separate the vastly different ion and metabolite concentrations of the interior of the RBC from its external environment, the blood plasma. The concentration of the constituents in the cytoplasm is tightly regulated by proteins embedded in the membrane that serve as pumps and channels for movement of ions and other material between the RBC's interior and the blood plasma. Various membrane proteins also act as receptors, RBC antigens, enzymes, and support for the surface carbohydrates to form a protective glycocalyx with the surface glycolipids. The lipid bilayer remains intact because transmembrane proteins embedded in the membrane anchor it to a two-dimensional protein lattice (cytoskeleton) immediately beneath its surface.[1] Together, the transmembrane proteins and underlying cytoskeleton provide structural integrity, cohesion, and mechanical stability to the cell.

In a normal life span of 120 days, RBCs must repeatedly maneuver through very narrow capillaries and squeeze through the splenic sieve (narrow slits or fenestrations in the endothelial cell lining of the splenic sinuses) as they move from the splenic cords to the sinuses. To accomplish this without premature lysis, the RBCs must have *deformability,* or the ability to repeatedly bend, stretch, distort, and then return to the normal discoid, biconcave shape.[2] The cellular properties that enable RBC deformability include the RBC's biconcave, discoid geometry; the elasticity (pliancy) of its membrane; and its cytoplasmic viscosity (Chapter 9).[3,4]

The biconcave, discoid geometry of the RBC is dependent on vertical and horizontal interactions between the transmembrane and cytoskeletal proteins (listed in Tables 9-5 and 9-6).[3] Two transmembrane protein complexes, the ankyrin complex and protein 4.1 complex, provide *vertical* structural integrity to the cell by anchoring the lipid bilayer to the underlying spectrin cytoskeleton.[3,5,6] In the ankyrin complex, ankyrin and protein 4.2 link transmembrane proteins, band 3 and RhAG (the Rh-associated glycoprotein) to the cytoskeleton.[6-8] In the protein 4.1 complex, protein 4.1 links transmembrane proteins, glycophorin C, XK, Rh, and Duffy to the cytoskeleton, and adducin and dematin link with transmembrane proteins, band 3 and glucose transport (glut 1) (Figure 9-2).[6,9] These interactions are called *vertical* because they are perpendicular to the plane of the cytoskeleton. They prevent loss of membrane and the resultant decrease in the surface area–to–volume ratio of the

RBC.[5] Two major cytoskeletal proteins, α-spectrin and β-spectrin, interact laterally with each other to form antiparallel heterodimers, which link with other spectrin heterodimers to form tetramers. The spectrin heterodimers also form a spectrin–actin–protein 4.1 junctional complex with accessory proteins (tropomyosin, tropomodulin, dematin, and adducin), thus linking the spectrin tetramers in a two-dimensional lattice.[10,11] These proteins provide *horizontal* mechanical stability, which prevents the membrane from fragmenting in response to mechanical stress.[3,5]

Factors that impact the elasticity of the cell are not as clear. Interactions between the spectrin dimers and their junctional complexes are flexible and allow for movement as the RBCs stretch and bend (Figure 9-4).[11] In addition, the ability of spectrin repeats to unfold and refold is likely to be one of the determinants of membrane elasticity.[11,12]

The cytoplasmic viscosity depends on the concentration of hemoglobin, as well as the maintenance of the proper cell volume by the normal functioning of various channels and pumps that allow the passage of ions, water, and macromolecules in and out of the cell.[3]

A defect in the RBCs that changes the membrane geometry, its elasticity, or the viscosity of the cytoplasm affects RBC deformability and can result in premature hemolysis and anemia.[3] The RBC membrane is discussed in more detail in Chapter 9; the reader is encouraged to review that chapter when studying defects in the membrane.

Hereditary Red Blood Cell Membrane Abnormalities

Most defects in the RBC membrane that can cause hemolytic anemia are hereditary; however, acquired defects also exist. Hereditary RBC membrane defects have historically been classified by morphologic features. The major disorders are hereditary spherocytosis, characterized by spherocytes, and hereditary elliptocytosis, characterized by elliptical RBCs. Hereditary pyropoikilocytosis, a variant of hereditary elliptocytosis, is characterized by marked poikilocytosis and heat sensitivity. Other less common membrane disorders include hereditary ovalocytosis, overhydrated hereditary stomatocytosis, and dehydrated hereditary stomatocytosis (also called hereditary xerocytosis). Hereditary membrane defects can also be classified as those that affect membrane structure (and alter geometry and elasticity) and those that affect membrane transport (and alter cytoplasmic viscosity) (Box 24-1).[11] The membrane structural defects can be further divided into those that affect vertical membrane protein interactions and those that affect horizontal membrane protein interactions.[5,11] The major hereditary membrane defects are described in Table 24-1.

Mutations That Alter Membrane Structure

Hereditary Spherocytosis. Hereditary spherocytosis (HS) is a heterogeneous group of hemolytic anemias caused by defects in proteins that disrupt the vertical interactions between transmembrane proteins and the underlying protein cytoskeleton. HS has worldwide distribution and affects 1 in 2000 to 3000 individuals of northern European ancestry.[6,11,13] In 75% of families, it is inherited as an autosomal dominant

---

> ### BOX 24-1 Classification of Major Hereditary Membrane Defects Causing Hemolytic Anemia
>
> **Mutations That Alter Membrane Structure**
> Hereditary spherocytosis
> Hereditary elliptocytosis/pyropoikilocytosis
> Hereditary ovalocytosis (Southeast Asian ovalocytosis)
>
> **Mutations That Alter Membrane Transport Proteins**
> Overhydrated hereditary stomatocytosis
> Dehydrated hereditary stomatocytosis or hereditary xerocytosis

---

trait and is expressed in heterozygotes who have one affected parent.[6] Homozygotes are rare; such patients present with severe hemolytic anemia but have asymptomatic parents.[13] In approximately 25% of cases, the inheritance is nondominant, with some autosomal recessive cases.[11,13]

Pathophysiology. HS results from gene mutations in which the defective proteins disrupt the vertical linkages between the lipid bilayer and the cytoskeletal network.[5] Various mutations in five known genes can result in the HS phenotype (Table 24-1). Mutations can occur in genes for (1) cytoskeletal proteins, including *ANK1*, which codes for ankyrin (40% to 65% of cases in the United States and Europe; 5% to 10% of cases in Japan); *SPTA1*, which codes for α-spectrin (fewer than 5% of cases); *SPTB*, which codes for β-spectrin (15% to 30% of cases); and *EPB42*, which codes for protein 4.2 (fewer than 5% of cases in the United States and Europe; 45% to 50% of cases in Japan); and (2) transmembrane protein, *SLC4A1*, which codes for band 3 (20% to 35% of cases).[6,11] Less than 10% of cases involve de novo mutations, with most affecting the ankyrin gene.[13] A mutation database for hereditary spherocytosis lists 130 different mutations (*ANK1*, 52; *SCL4A1*, 49; *SPTA1*, 2; *SPTB*, 19; and *EPB42*, 8).[14] Because of the vertical interactions of the transmembrane proteins and cytoskeletal protein lattice, a primary mutation in one gene may have a secondary effect on another protein in the membrane. For example, primary mutations in *ANK1* result in both ankyrin and spectrin deficiencies in the RBC membrane.[13,15,16] In approximately 10% of patients, no mutation is identified.[11]

The defects in vertical membrane protein interactions cause RBCs to lose unsupported lipid membrane over time because of local disconnections of the lipid bilayer and underlying cytoskeleton. Essentially, small portions of the membrane form vesicles; the vesicles are released with little loss of cell volume.[13] The RBCs acquire a decreased surface area–to–volume ratio, and the cells become spherical. These cells do not have the deformability of normal biconcave discoid RBCs, and their survival in the spleen is decreased.[4,13,15] As the spherocytes attempt to move through the narrow, elliptical fenestrations of the endothelial cells lining the splenic sinusoids, they acquire further membrane loss or become trapped and are rapidly removed by the macrophages of the red pulp of the spleen.[4,13] In addition, as the RBCs are sequestered in the spleen, the

TABLE 24-1 Characteristics of Major Hemolytic Anemias Caused by Hereditary Membrane Defects

Condition	Inheritance Pattern	Deficient Protein (Mutated Gene)	Pathophysiology	Typical RBC Morphology	Clinical Findings/Comments
Hereditary spherocytosis	75% autosomal dominant 25% nondominant	Ankyrin (*ANK1*) Band 3 (*SLC4A1*) α-Spectrin (*SPTA1*) β-Spectrin (*SPTB*) Protein 4.2 (*EPB42*)	Defect in protein(s) that disrupts vertical membrane interactions between transmembrane proteins and underlying cytoskeleton; loss of membrane and decreased surface area–to–volume ratio	Spherocytes, polychromasia	Varies from asymptomatic to severe Typical features: splenomegaly, jaundice, anemia
Hereditary elliptocytosis	Autosomal dominant	α-Spectrin (*SPTA1*) β-Spectrin (*SPTB*) Protein 4.1 (*EPB41*)	Defect in proteins that disrupt the horizontal linkages in the protein cytoskeleton; loss of mechanical stability of membrane	Few to 100% elliptocytes; schistocytes in severe cases	90% of cases asymptomatic; 10% of cases show moderate to severe anemia
Hereditary pyropoikilocytosis (rare subtype of hereditary elliptocytosis)	Autosomal recessive	α-Spectrin (*SPTA1*) β-Spectrin (*SPTB*) Homozygous or compound heterozygous	Severe defect in spectrin that disrupts horizontal linkages in protein cytoskeleton; severe RBC fragmentation	Elliptocytes, schistocytes, microspherocytes	Severe anemia
Southeast Asian ovalocytosis	Autosomal dominant	Band 3 (*SLC4A1*); only one known mutation	Defect in band 3 causing increased membrane rigidity; only exists in heterozygous state	30% oval cells with one or two transverse ridges	Asymptomatic or mild hemolysis; resistant to malaria; prevalent in some areas of Southeast Asia
Overhydrated hereditary stomatocytosis	Autosomal dominant	Rh-associated protein (*RHAG*) Others unknown	Increased membrane permeability to sodium and potassium; increased intracellular sodium causing influx of water, increase in cell volume, and decreased cytoplasmic viscosity	Stomatocytes (5%–50%), macrocytes	Moderate to severe hemolytic anemia; splenectomy is contraindicated due to thrombotic risk
Dehydrated hereditary stomatocytosis (Hereditary xerocytosis)	Autosomal dominant	Piezo-type mechanosensitive ion channel component 1 (*PIEZO1*)	Increased membrane permeability to potassium; decreased intracellular potassium, resulting in loss of water from cell, decrease in cell volume, and increased cytoplasmic viscosity	Target cells, burr cells, stomatocytes (<10%), RBCs with "puddled" hemoglobin at periphery, desiccated cells with spicules	Mild to moderate anemia, splenomegaly; may lead to fetal loss, hydrops fetalis; may be accompanied by pseudohyperkalemia

RBC, Red blood cell.

membrane can acquire yet more damage, lose more lipid membrane, and become more spherical due to splenic conditioning.[4,13,15] The conditioning may be enhanced by the acidic conditions in the spleen and the prolonged contact of the RBCs with macrophages.[13,15] Low levels of adenosine triphosphate (ATP) and glucose, and phagocyte-produced free radicals, which cause oxidative damage, may also play a role (Figure 24-2).[13,15]

In HS, RBC membranes also have abnormal permeability to cations, particularly sodium and potassium, which is likely due to disruption of the integrity of the protein cytoskeleton.[4,17] The cells become dehydrated, but the exact mechanism is not clear. Overactivity of the Na$^+$-K$^+$ ATPase may cause a reduction in intracellular cations, causing more

water to diffuse out of the cell.[4,13] This results in an increase in viscosity and cellular dehydration.[13] The abnormality is not related to defects in cation transport proteins, and dehydration occurs regardless of the type of primary mutation causing the HS.[17]

Clinical and Laboratory Findings. Symptomatic HS has three key clinical manifestations: anemia, jaundice, and splenomegaly. Symptoms of HS may first appear in infancy, childhood, or adulthood, or even at an advanced age.[16] There is wide variation in symptoms. Silent carriers are clinically asymptomatic with normal laboratory findings and usually are identified only if they are the parents of a child with recessively inherited HS.[4,13,16] Approximately 20% to 30% of patients have

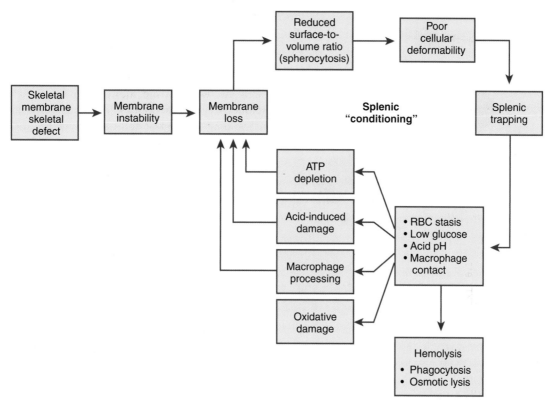

Figure 24-2 Pathophysiology of splenic trapping and destruction of spherocytes. *ATP,* Adenosine triphosphate; *RBC,* red blood cell. (Modified from Becker PS, Lux SE: Disorders of the red cell membrane. In Nathan DG, Oski FA, editors: *Hematology of infancy and childhood,* ed 4, Philadelphia, 1993, Saunders, pp. 529-633.)

mild HS and are asymptomatic because an increase in erythropoiesis compensates for the RBC loss.[4,6] They usually have normal hemoglobin levels but may show subtle signs of HS, with a slight increase in serum bilirubin in the range of 1.0 to 2.0 mg/dL, an increased reticulocyte count of up to 6%, and a few spherocytes on the peripheral blood film.[4,6,16] Mild HS may first become evident during pregnancy, during illnesses that cause splenomegaly (such as infectious mononucleosis), or in aging, when the rate of erythropoiesis starts to decline.[13,16] Approximately 60% of patients have moderate HS with incompletely compensated hemolytic anemia, hemoglobin levels greater than 8 g/dL, serum bilirubin over 2 mg/dL, reticulocyte counts in the range of 6% to 10%, and spherocytes on the peripheral blood film.[4,6,16] Jaundice is seen at some time in about half of these patients, usually during viral infections. About 5% to 10% of patients have moderate to severe HS, with hemoglobin levels usually in the range of 6 to 8 g/dL, serum bilirubin between 2 to 3 mg/dL, and reticulocyte counts greater than 10%.[4,6,16] About 3% to 5% of patients have severe HS, with hemoglobin levels below 6 g/dL, serum bilirubin over 3 mg/dL, and reticulocyte counts greater than 10%.[4,6,15] Patients with severe HS are usually homozygous for HS mutations and require regular transfusions.[13] Splenomegaly is found in about half of young children and in 75% to 95% of older children and adults with HS.[4]

The hallmark of HS is spherocytes on the peripheral blood film. When present in patients with childhood hemolytic anemia and a family history of similar abnormalities, the uniform spherocytes are highly suggestive of HS. Some of these are microspherocytes—small, round, dense RBCs that are filled with hemoglobin and lack a central pallor (Figure 24-3). Normal-appearing RBCs, along with polychromasia and varying degrees of anisocytosis and poikilocytosis, are present. In addition to spherocytes, occasionally other RBC morphologic variants may be observed in some types of mutations: acanthocytes in some β-spectrin mutations,[18] pincered or mushroom-shaped cells in some cases of band 3 deficiency in patients without splenectomy,[19] and ovalostomatocytes in homozygous *EPB4.2* mutations.[20] Note that spherocytes are not specific for HS and can be seen in other hereditary and acquired conditions.

Because of the spherocytosis, HS patients have an increase in the mean cell hemoglobin concentration (MCHC) to between 35 and 38 mg/dL and an increase in the red cell distribution width (RDW) to greater than 14%.[4,16,21] The mean cell volume is variable, ranging from within the reference interval to slightly below.[6,13] Using laser-based automated analyzers, there is an increase in hyperchromic or hyperdense RBCs representing cells with an MCHC over 41 g/dL.[6,13] A cutoff of greater than 4% hyperchromic cells has been proposed to screen patients for HS.[6,22] Biochemical evidence of extravascular hemolysis may be present in moderate to severe forms of HS, and the extent is dependent on the severity of the hemolysis. This includes a decrease in serum haptoglobin level and an increase in levels of serum indirect bilirubin and lactate dehydrogenase (Chapter 23). The bone marrow shows erythroid

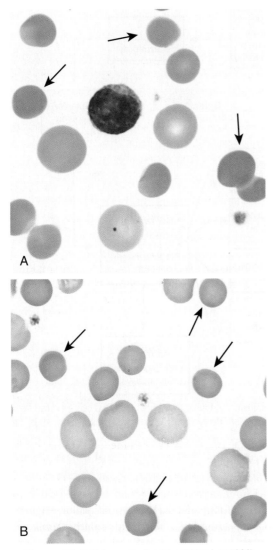

Figure 24-3 Spherocytes (peripheral blood, ×1000).

hyperplasia due to the increased demand for RBCs to replace the circulating spherocytes that are prematurely destroyed, but bone marrow analysis is not required for diagnosis.

Additional tests. In patients with a family history of HS, splenomegaly, an increased MCHC and reticulocyte count, and spherocytes on the peripheral blood film, no further special testing is needed for the diagnosis of HS.[16] In cases in which HS is suspected, but the family history and mode of inheritance are not clear, or there are atypical clinical and/or laboratory findings, further special testing is needed to confirm a diagnosis.[16] No one method will detect all cases of HS, so a combination of methods is needed for definitive diagnosis.

Osmotic fragility. The osmotic fragility test demonstrates increased RBC fragility in blood specimens in which the RBCs have decreased surface area–to–volume ratios. Blood is added to a series of tubes with increasingly hypotonic sodium chloride (NaCl) solutions. In each tube, water enters and leaves the RBCs until equilibrium is achieved. In 0.85% NaCl, the amount of water entering the cell is equivalent to the water

leaving the cell because the intracellular and extracellular osmolarity is the same. In a hypotonic solution, more water will enter the cell to dilute the intracellular contents until equilibrium is reached between the cytoplasm and the hypotonic extracellular solution. As this phenomenon occurs, the cells swell. As the RBCs are subjected to increasingly hypotonic solutions, even more water will enter the RBCs until the internal volume is too great and lysis occurs. Because spherocytes already have a decreased surface area–to–volume ratio, they lyse in less hypotonic solutions than normal-shaped, biconcave RBCs and thus have increased osmotic fragility.

In the procedure, a standard volume of fresh, heparinized blood is mixed with NaCl solutions ranging from 0.85% (isotonic saline) to 0.0% (distilled water) in 0.05% to 0.1% increments.[23] After a 30-minute incubation at room temperature, the tubes are centrifuged and the absorbance of the supernatant is measured spectrophotometrically at 540 nm.[23] The percent hemolysis is calculated for each tube as follows:[23]

$$\% \text{ hemolysis} = \frac{A_{x\%} - A_{0.85\%}}{A_{0.0\%} - A_{0.85\%}} \times 100$$

$A_{x\%}$ is the absorbance in the tube being measured, $A_{0.85\%}$ is the absorbance in the 0.85% NaCl tube (representing 0% hemolysis), and $A_{0.0\%}$ is the absorbance in the 0.0% NaCl tube (representing 100% hemolysis). The % hemolysis for each % NaCl concentration is plotted, and an osmotic fragility curve is drawn (Figure 24-4). Normal biconcave RBCs show initial hemolysis at 0.45% NaCl, and 100% or complete hemolysis generally occurs between 0.35% and 0.30% NaCl. If the curve is shifted to the left, the patient's RBCs have increased osmotic fragility, and in this case, initial hemolysis begins at an NaCl concentration greater than 0.5%. Conversely, if the curve is shifted to the right, the RBCs have decreased osmotic fragility.

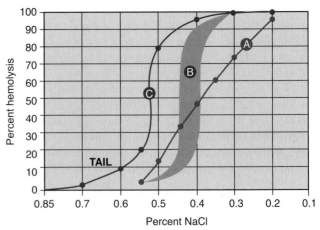

Figure 24-4 Erythrocyte osmotic fragility curve. **A,** Curve in thalassemia showing two cell populations: one with increased fragility (*lower left of curve*) and one with decreased fragility (*upper right of curve*). **B,** Normal curve. **C,** Curve indicating increased fragility, as in hereditary spherocytosis.

Decreased osmotic fragility is found in conditions characterized by numerous target cells, such as thalassemia.

The existence of a distinct subpopulation of the most fragile cells, those most conditioned by the spleen, is reflected by the presence of a "tail" on the osmotic fragility curve (Figure 24-4).[13] After splenectomy is performed, the osmotic fragility improves, and this subpopulation of conditioned cells disappears.[13]

Incubating the blood at 37° C for 24 hours before performing the test (called the *incubated osmotic fragility test*) allows HS cells to become more spherical and is often needed to detect mild cases. Patients who have increased osmotic fragility only when their blood is incubated tend to have mild disease and a low number of spherocytes in the total RBC population. The osmotic fragility test is time-consuming, and it requires a fresh heparinized blood specimen collected without trauma (to avoid hemolysis) and accurately made NaCl solutions. Specimens are stable for 2 hours at room temperature or 6 hours if the specimen is refrigerated.[23] A major drawback of the osmotic fragility test is its lack of sensitivity.[16] In a 2011 study of 150 HS patients by Bianchi and colleagues, the sensitivity for the unincubated test was 68%, with only a modest increase in sensitivity to 81% with the incubated test.[24] In nonsplenectomized HS patients with compensated anemia, those sensitivity figures dropped to only 53% and 64%, respectively.[24] The osmotic fragility test is also nonspecific. A result indicating increased fragility does not differentiate between HS and spherocytosis caused by other conditions, such as burns, immune hemolytic anemias, and other acquired disorders.[13,16] These disadvantages have led some not to recommend this test for routine use.[16]

Eosin-5′-maleimide (EMA) binding test. The eosin-5′-maleimide (EMA) binding test has been proposed as a more sensitive alternative for confirmation of HS.[16] EMA is a fluorescent dye that binds to transmembrane proteins band 3, Rh, RhAg, and CD47 in the RBC membrane.[25] When measured in a flow cytometer, specimens from HS patients show a lower mean fluorescence intensity (MFI) than RBCs from normal controls and from patients with spherocytes due to immune-mediated hemolysis.[25] The result is reported in % decrease in MFI when the patient specimen is compared to normal controls.[6] The sensitivity and specificity of the EMA-binding assay varies from 93% to 96% and 94% to 99%, respectively.[6,24,26] Positive tests can also occur with congenital dyserythropoietic anemia type II, Southeast Asian ovalocytosis, and hereditary pyropoikilocytosis, but these are rare conditions.[6,24,27] The EMA binding test offers advantages in that it is suitable for low-volume pediatric specimens, it can be performed within 3 hours, specimens are acceptable for analysis up to 7 days after collection, and gating can be used to eliminate the interference from transfused or fragmented RBCs.[6] However, there is disagreement among laboratories on the % MFI decrease cutoff value for HS, and standardization is needed across laboratories.[6,27]

Other tests. In atypical HS cases, additional tests may be required to identify the defective proteins.[16] Sodium dodecyl sulfate-polyacrylamide gel electrophoresis (SDS-PAGE) can be used to identify membrane protein deficiencies by electrophoretic separation of the various proteins in solubilized RBC membranes with quantitation of the proteins by densitometry.[13,16] Membrane proteins can also be quantitated by radioimmunoassay.[13] Variation in membrane surface area and cell water content can be determined by osmotic gradient ektacytometry.[28] The ektacytometer is a laser-diffraction viscometer that records the laser diffraction pattern of a suspension of RBCs exposed to constant shear stress in solutions of varying osmolality from hypotonic to hypertonic. An RBC osmotic deformability index is calculated and plotted against the osmolality of the suspending solution to generate an osmotic gradient deformability profile.[28] This method, however, is available only in specialized laboratories.[6,13]

Several other tests have been used for diagnosis of HS, but they are cumbersome to perform; lack sensitivity and specificity, or both; and are not widely used in the United States.[4,13] The acidified glycerol lysis test measures the amount of hemolysis after patient RBCs are incubated with a buffered glycerol solution at an acid pH. The test has a sensitivity of 95% but is not specific in that other conditions with spherocytes will yield a positive result, including autoimmune hemolytic anemias.[24,29] In the autohemolysis test, patient's RBCs and serum are incubated for 48 hours, with and without glucose. Normal controls generally have less than 5.0% hemolysis at the end of the 48-hour incubation period, and they have less than 1.0% hemolysis if glucose is added. Glucose catabolism (anaerobic glycolysis) provides the ATP to drive the cation pumps to help maintain the osmotic balance in the RBCs. In HS, the hemolysis is 10% to 50%, which corrects considerably but not to the reference interval when glucose is added. The test has a sensitivity similar to that of the incubated osmotic fragility test.[4,13] The hypertonic cryohemolysis test is based on the fact that cells from HS patients are particularly sensitive to cooling at 0° C in hypertonic solutions.[30] The percent hemolysis is calculated after the patient's RBCs are incubated in buffered 0.7 mol/L sucrose, first at 37° C for 10 minutes and then at 0° C for 10 minutes. Normal cells show 3% to 15% hemolysis, whereas RBCs in HS have greater than 20% hemolysis.[30] Increased hemolysis can also occur in Southeast Asian ovalocytosis, some types of hereditary elliptocytosis, and congenital dyserythropoietic anemia type II.[16,30]

Molecular techniques for detection of genetic mutations are not usually required.[13,16] The polymerase chain reaction procedure followed by single-strand conformational polymorphism analysis can identify potential regions in HS genes that may contain a mutation.[13,16] Once a region has been identified, nucleic acid sequencing can be performed to identify the specific mutation.[13] Genetic diagnosis is likely to become more important in the future.

Complications. Although most patients with HS have a well-compensated hemolytic anemia and are rarely symptomatic, complications may occur that require medical intervention. Patients may experience various crises, classified as hemolytic, aplastic, and megaloblastic.[13] Hemolytic crises are rare and usually associated with viral syndromes. In aplastic crises there is a dramatic decrease in hemoglobin level and reticulocyte count. The crisis usually occurs in conjunction with parvovirus

B19 infection, which suppresses erythropoiesis, and patients can become rapidly and severely anemic, often requiring transfusion.[16] This complication is more common in children, but it can occur in adults.[13,16] Patients with moderate and severe HS can also develop folic acid deficiency resulting from increased folate utilization to support the chronic erythroid hyperplasia in the bone marrow.[13] This phenomenon is termed *megaloblastic crisis* and is particularly acute during pregnancy and during recovery from an aplastic crisis. Providing folic acid supplementation to patients with moderate and severe HS avoids this complication.[16] About half of patients, even those with mild disease, also experience cholelithiasis (bilirubin stones in the gallbladder or bile ducts) due to the chronic hemolysis.[13] Chronic ulceration or dermatitis of the legs is a rare complication.[13]

Treatment.   Mild HS usually requires no treatment.[16] Splenectomy is reserved for moderate to severe cases, and laparoscopy is the recommended method.[16] Splenectomy results in longer RBC survival in the peripheral blood and helps prevent gallstones by decreasing the amount of hemolysis and thus the amount of bilirubin produced.[13,16] The major drawbacks of splenectomy are the lifelong risk of overwhelming sepsis and death from encapsulated bacteria and an increased risk of cardiovascular disease with age.[13,16] Prior to splenectomy, patients receive vaccines for pneumococcus, meningococcus, and *H. influenza* type b, and postsplenectomy antibiotics may be recommended.[13] Because infants and young children are especially susceptible to postsplenectomy sepsis, splenectomy is usually postponed until after the age of 6 years.[16] In a nationwide sample of 1657 children (aged 5 to 12 years) with HS who underwent splenectomy, there were no cases of postoperative sepsis and no fatalities from any cause during hospitalization for the surgery.[31] Partial splenectomy has been performed in young children with severe HS, but further evaluation of the risks and benefits of this procedure is needed.[13,16]

After splenectomy, spherocytes are still apparent on the blood film, and all of the typical changes in RBC morphology seen after splenectomy also are observed, including Howell-Jolly bodies, target cells, and Pappenheimer bodies (Figure 24-5).

Reticulocyte counts decrease to high-normal levels, and the anemia is usually corrected. Leukocytosis and thrombocytosis are present. Bilirubin levels decrease but may remain in the high-reference interval.

Occasionally, a patient does not improve because of an accessory spleen missed during surgery or the accidental autotransplantation of splenic tissue during splenectomy. In these cases hemolysis may resume years later.[13] The resumption of splenic function can be ascertained from liver or spleen scans.[13] Patients with severe HS usually require regular transfusions. Transfusions are rarely needed in the less severe forms of HS.[13,15,16]

Differential diagnosis.   HS must be distinguished from immune-related hemolytic anemia with spherocytes. Family history and evaluation of family members, including parents, siblings, and children of the patient, help differentiate the hereditary disease from the acquired disorder. The immune disorders with spherocytes are usually characterized by a positive result on the direct antiglobulin test (DAT), whereas the results are negative in HS. The eosin-5′-maleimide (EMA) binding test shows decreased fluorescence typical of HS. Increased osmotic fragility is not diagnostic of HS, because the cells in acquired hemolytic anemia with spherocytes also show increased osmotic fragility. The typical clinical and laboratory findings in HS are summarized in Table 24-2.

Hereditary Elliptocytosis.   Hereditary elliptocytosis (HE) is a heterogeneous group of hemolytic anemias caused by defects in proteins that disrupt the horizontal or lateral interactions in the protein cytoskeleton. It reportedly exists in all of its forms in 1 in 2000 to 1 in 4000 individuals, but because the majority of cases are asymptomatic, the actual prevalence is not known.[13,32] The disease is more common in Africa and Mediterranean regions, where there is a high prevalence of malaria. The prevalence in West Africa of certain spectrin mutations associated with HE is between 0.6% and 1.6%.[13,33] The molecular basis for the association of spherocytosis and malaria is unknown. The inheritance pattern in HE is mainly autosomal dominant, with a small number of autosomal recessive cases.[11,13]

Pathophysiology.   HE results from gene mutations in which the defective proteins disrupt the horizontal linkages in the protein cytoskeleton and weaken the mechanical stability of the membrane.[4,5] The HE phenotype can result from various mutations in at least three genes: *SPTA1*, which codes for α-spectrin (65% of cases); *SPTB*, which codes for β-spectrin (30% of cases); and *EPB41*, which codes for protein 4.1 (5% of cases) (Table 24-1).[11,32] A mutation database for hereditary elliptocytosis is available and lists 46 different mutations.[14] The spectrin mutations disrupt spectrin dimer interactions and the *EPB41* mutations result in weakened spectrin–actin–protein 4.1 junctional complexes.[6,11] RBCs are biconcave and discoid at first, but become elliptical over time after repeated exposure to the shear stresses in the peripheral circulation.[13] The extent of the disruption of the spectrin dimer interactions seems to be associated with the severity of the clinical manifestations.[11] In severe cases, the protein cytoskeleton is weakened

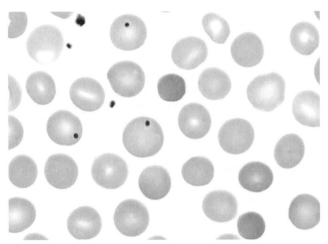

Figure 24-5 Red blood cell morphology in hereditary spherocytosis after splenectomy. Howell-Jolly bodies and spherocytes are seen (peripheral blood, ×1000).

TABLE 24-2 Typical Clinical and Laboratory Findings in Hereditary Spherocytosis (HS)[13,16]

Clinical manifestations	Splenomegaly
	Anemia*
	Jaundice (can be intermittent)
Mode of inheritance	75% autosomal dominant
	25% nondominant
Complete blood count results	↓ Hemoglobin*
	↑ Mean cell hemoglobin concentration
	↑ Red cell distribution width
	↑ Reticulocyte count*
	↑ Hyperchromic (hyperdense) RBCs**
Peripheral blood film findings†	Spherocytes
	Polychromasia
Direct antiglobulin test result	Negative
Indicators of hemolysis	↓ Serum haptoglobin
	↑ Serum lactate dehydrogenase
	↑ Serum indirect bilirubin
Selected additional tests for atypical cases	Not required for diagnosis of HS with the typical features listed above
	↓ Fluorescence in eosin-5′-maleimide binding test by flow cytometry‡
	↑ Osmotic fragility and incubated osmotic fragility tests‡
	SDS-PAGE analysis of membrane proteins

*Varies with severity of HS and ability of the bone marrow to compensate for the hemolysis.
**As measured on some automated blood cell analyzers.
†With some rare mutations, acanthocytes, pincered cells, stomatocytes, or ovalocytes may be seen in addition to spherocytes.
‡A result within the reference interval does not rule out HS; similar results can be observed in conditions other than HS.
↑, Increased; ↓, decreased; *SDS-PAGE*, sodium dodecyl sulfate-polyacrylamide gel electrophoresis.

to such a point that cell fragmentation occurs. As a result, there is membrane loss and a decrease in surface area–to–volume ratio that reduces the deformability of the RBCs. The damaged RBCs become trapped or acquire further damage in the spleen, which results in extravascular hemolysis and anemia. In general, patients who are heterozygous for a mutation are asymptomatic, and their RBCs have a normal life span; those who are homozygous for a mutation or compound heterozygous for two mutations can have moderate to severe anemia that can be life-threatening.[6,11]

The RBCs in HE patients all show some degree of decreased thermal stability. Cases in which the RBCs show marked RBC fragmentation upon heating were previously classified as hereditary pyropoikilocytosis (HPP). HPP is now considered a severe form of HE that exists in either the homozygous or compound heterozygous state.[11,13]

Patients with the Leach phenotype lack the Gerbich antigens and glycoprotein C (GPC).[4] The phenotype is due to a mutation in the genes for GPC and results in the absence of the glycoprotein in the RBC membrane.[34] The Gerbich antigens are normally expressed on the extracellular domains of GPC and thus are absent in this condition. Heterozygotes have normal RBC morphology, and homozygotes have mild elliptocytosis but no anemia.[4] The reason for the elliptocyte morphology may be a defect in the interaction between GPC and protein 4.1 in the junctional complex.[4]

Clinical and laboratory findings. The vast majority of patients with HE are asymptomatic, and only about 10% have moderate to severe anemia.[11] Some may have a mild compensated hemolytic anemia as evidenced by a slight increase in the reticulocyte count and a decrease in haptoglobin level, or develop transient hemolysis in response to other conditions such as viral infections, pregnancy, hypersplenism, or vitamin B_{12} deficiency.[13] Often an asymptomatic patient is diagnosed after a peripheral blood film is examined for another condition. Rarely, heterozygous parents with undiagnosed, asymptomatic HE have offspring who are homozygous or compound heterozygous for their mutation(s) and have moderate to very severe hemolysis. Some of these asymptomatic parents have normal RBC morphology and laboratory tests.[13]

The characteristic finding in HE is elliptical or cigar-shaped RBCs on the peripheral blood film in numbers that can vary from a few to 100%[4] (Figure 24-6). The number of elliptocytes does not correlate with disease severity.[4] Investigation of elliptocytosis begins by taking a thorough patient and family history and performing a physical examination, and examining the peripheral blood films of the parents.[4] Other laboratory tests may be needed to rule out other conditions in which elliptocytes may be present, such as iron deficiency anemia, thalassemia, megaloblastic anemia, myelodysplastic syndrome, and primary myelofibrosis.[4] In these cases, the elliptocytes

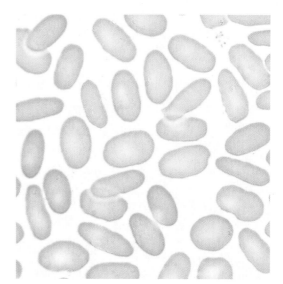

Figure 24-6 Red blood cell morphology in hereditary elliptocytosis (peripheral blood, ×1000). (From Carr JH, Rodak BF: *Clinical hematology atlas*, ed 3, Philadelphia, 2009, Saunders.)

usually comprise less than one third of the RBCs.[35] An acquired defect in the gene for 4.1 may be found in myelodysplastic syndrome.[36] In the homozygous or compound heterozygous states, the anemia is moderate to severe, the osmotic fragility is increased, and biochemical evidence of excessive hemolysis is present. The peripheral blood film in patients with the HPP phenotype shows extreme poikilocytosis with fragmentation, microspherocytosis, and elliptocytosis similar to that in patients with thermal burns (Figure 24-7, *A*). The mean cell volume (MCV) is very low (50 to 65 fL) because of the RBC fragments.[4,35] RBCs in the HPP phenotype show marked thermal sensitivity. After incubation of a blood sample at 41° C to 45° C, the RBCs fragment (Figure 24-7, *B*).[13] Normal RBCs do not fragment until reaching a temperature of 49° C. Thermal sensitivity is not specific for HPP, however; it also occurs in cases of HE with spectrin mutations.[4,13] RBCs with the HPP phenotype show a lower fluorescence than RBCs in HS when incubated with eosin-5′-maleimide and analyzed by flow cytometry (see earlier section on special tests for HS).[37] Mutation screening using molecular tests or quantitation of membrane proteins by SDS-PAGE may be also be performed.

As in HS, patients with moderate or severe hemolytic anemia due to HE can develop cholelithiasis due to bilirubin gallstones, and hemolytic, aplastic, and megaloblastic crises can occur (see earlier section on HS complications).

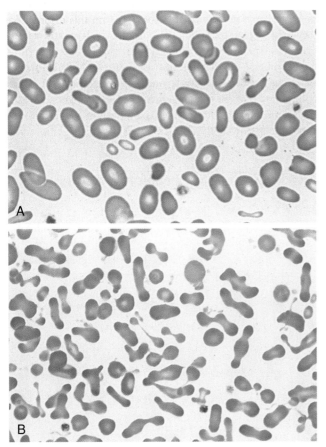

Figure 24-7 A, Morphology of red blood cells in hereditary pyropoikilocytosis before incubation. **B,** Morphology after 1 hour at 45° C (peripheral blood, ×500).

Treatment. Asymptomatic HE patients require no treatment. All HE patients who are significantly anemic and show signs of hemolysis respond well to splenectomy.[4] Transfusions are occasionally needed for life-threatening anemia.

Hereditary Ovalocytosis (Southeast Asian Ovalocytosis).

Hereditary ovalocytosis or Southeast Asian ovalocytosis (SAO) is a condition caused by a mutation in the gene for band 3 that results in increased rigidity of the membrane and resistance to invasion by malaria.[3,4] It is common in the malaria belt of Southeast Asia, where its prevalence can reach 30%.[13,38] The inheritance pattern is autosomal dominant, and all patients identified are heterozygous.[3,4]

Pathophysiology. SAO is the result of one mutation, a deletion of 27 base pairs in *SLC4A1*, the gene that codes for band 3.[39] Deletion occurs at the interface between the transmembrane and cytoplasmic domains.[4,40] The mutation causes an increase in membrane rigidity that may be due to tighter binding of band 3 to ankyrin or decreased lateral mobility of band 3 in the membrane.[4,13,38] RBC membranes also have decreased elasticity as measured by ektacytometry and micropipette aspiration.[3,38] The molecular mechanism responsible for the increased membrane rigidity that results from the band 3 mutation has not yet been elucidated.[3,4]

Clinical and laboratory findings. In patients with SAO, hemolysis is mild or absent. On a peripheral blood film, typical cells of SAO are oval RBCs with one to two transverse bars or ridges and usually comprise about 30% of the RBCs.[3,13] No treatment is required for this condition.

Mutations That Alter Membrane Transport Proteins

RBC volume is regulated by various membrane proteins that serve as passive transporters, active transporters, and ion channels. When RBCs lose the ability to regulate volume, the cells are prematurely hemolyzed. Cell volume is determined by the intracellular concentration of cations, particularly sodium.[11] If the total cation content is increased, water enters the cell and increases the cell volume, forming a stomatocyte. If the total cation content is decreased, water leaves the cell, which decreases the cell volume and produces a dehydrated RBC, also called a *xerocyte.*

Hereditary stomatocytosis comprises a group of heterogeneous conditions in which the RBC membrane leaks monovalent cations. The two major categories are overhydrated hereditary stomatocytosis and dehydrated hereditary stomatocytosis or hereditary xerocytosis. Molecular characterization of these conditions is ongoing and should provide a better means of classification and clearer understanding of their pathophysiology.

Overhydrated Hereditary Stomatocytosis. Overhydrated hereditary stomatocytosis (OHS) is a very rare hemolytic anemia due to a defect in membrane cation permeability that causes the RBCs to be overhydrated.[3,6] It is inherited in an autosomal dominant pattern.[11,13]

Pathophysiology. In OHS, the RBC membrane is excessively permeable to sodium and potassium at 37° C.[41] There is an influx of sodium into the cell that exceeds the loss of potassium, which results in a net increase in the intracellular cation concentration. As a result, more water enters the cell, and the cell swells and becomes stomatocytic. Because of the water influx, the cytoplasm has decreased density and viscosity. The increase in cell volume without an increase in membrane surface area causes premature hemolysis in the spleen.[3] The exact molecular defect is unknown, but mutations in the *RHAG* gene that codes for RhAG protein, along with a deficiency of the RhAG protein in the membrane, has been found in some patients with OHS.[41,42] Most patients also have a secondary deficiency of stomatin, a transmembrane protein, but its gene is not mutated.[6,41,42] Stomatin may participate in regulation of ion channels, but its role in OHS is unclear.[41] The RhAG is a transmembrane protein and a component of the ankyrin complex.

Clinical and laboratory findings. OHS can cause moderate to severe hemolytic anemia. The diagnostic features include 5% to 50% stomatocytes on the peripheral blood film (Figure 24-8), macrocytes (MCV of 110 to 150 fL), decreased MCHC (24 to 30 g/dL), reticulocytosis, reduced erythrocyte potassium concentration, elevated erythrocyte sodium concentration, and increased net cation content in the erythrocytes.[3,6] Because of the increased cell volume, the RBCs have increased osmotic fragility due to a decreased surface area–to–volume ratio.[11] Splenectomy should be carefully considered in OHS because it is associated with an increased risk of thromboembolic complications.[3]

Dehydrated Hereditary Stomatocytosis or Hereditary Xerocytosis.
Dehydrated hereditary stomatocytosis (DHS) or hereditary xerocytosis (HX) is an autosomal dominant hemolytic anemia due to a defect in membrane cation permeability that causes the RBCs to be dehydrated.[3,4] It is the most common form of stomatocytosis.[4]

Pathophysiology. In DHS/HX, the RBC membrane is excessively permeable to potassium. The potassium leaks out of the cell, but this is not balanced by an increase in sodium. Because of the reduced intracellular cation concentration, water is lost from the cell.[3,4] It is due to mutations in the *PIEZO1* gene that codes for the Piezo-type mechanosensitive

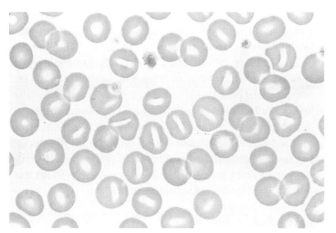

Figure 24-8 Red blood cell morphology in hereditary stomatocytosis (peripheral blood, ×1000).

ion channel component 1 protein in the RBC membrane.[43,44] Two mutations have been identified to date.[44] The PIEZO1 protein combines with other proteins to form a pore in a channel to mediate cation transport.[43] The mutations result in an increase in ion channel activity and an increase in cation transport.[45]

Clinical and laboratory findings. Patients with DHS/HX generally have mild to moderate anemia, reticulocytosis, jaundice, and mild to moderate splenomegaly.[4,11] Fetal loss, hydrops fetalis, and neonatal hepatitis can also be features of DHS/HX.[4] The RBCs are dehydrated, as evidenced by the elevated MCHC and decreased osmotic fragility.[4,11] The RBC morphology includes stomatocytes (usually fewer than 10%), target cells, burr cells, desiccated cells with spicules, and RBCs in which the hemoglobin appears to be puddled in discrete areas on the cell periphery.[4,11] Most patients with DHS/HX do not require treatment. Splenectomy does not improve the anemia and is contraindicated because it increases the risk of thromboembolic complications.[3,4]

Other Hereditary Membrane Defects with Stomatocytes
Familial Pseudohyperkalemia.
Familial pseudohyperkalemia (FP) is a rare disorder in which excessive potassium leaks out of the RBCs at room temperature in vitro but not at body temperature in vivo.[6] CBC parameters are near the reference intervals, although some patients have a mild anemia.[6,29] Occasional stomatocytes may be observed on the peripheral blood film.[6] The gene defect associated with this disorder has not yet been identified.

Cryohydrocytosis.
Cryohydrocytosis (CHC) is another rare disorder that manifests as a mild to moderate hemolytic anemia with leakage of sodium and potassium from the RBCs and stomatocytosis.[6] The RBCs have marked cell swelling and hemolysis when stored at 4° C for 24 to 48 hours.[29] Mutations in band 3 have been identified in some patients, which cause it to leak cations out of the RBCs, while other patients have a deficiency in membrane stomatin.[4,6,29]

Rh Deficiency Syndrome.
Rh deficiency syndrome comprises a group of rare hereditary conditions in which the expression of Rh membrane proteins is absent (Rh-null) or decreased (Rh-mod).[4,13] Cases of the syndrome can be genetically divided into the amorph type (caused by mutations in Rh proteins) and the regulatory type (caused by mutations in a protein that regulates Rh gene expression).[4,13] Patients with Rh deficiency syndrome present with mild to moderate hemolytic anemia. Stomatocytes and occasional spherocytes may be observed on the peripheral blood film. Symptomatic patients may be treated by splenectomy, which improves the anemia.

Other Hereditary Membrane Defects with Acanthocytes
Acanthocytes (spur cells) are small, dense RBCs with a few irregular projections that vary in width, length, and surface distribution (Figure 24-9). These are distinct from burr cells (echinocytes), which typically have small, uniform projections

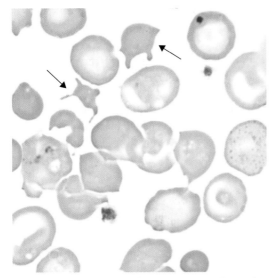

Figure 24-9 Two acanthocytes (*arrows*). Note that cells are dense with irregularly spaced projections of varying length (peripheral blood, ×1000).

evenly distributed on the surface of the RBC (Chapter 19). The differentiation is easier to make on scanning electron micrographs and on wet preparations than on dried blood films.[35,36] A small number of burr cells (less than 3% of RBCs) can be present on the peripheral blood films of healthy individuals, while increased numbers of burr cells are observed in uremia and pyruvate kinase deficiency.[13,35] Acanthocytes, however, are not present on peripheral blood films of healthy individuals but can be found in hereditary neuroacanthocytosis (including abetalipoproteinemia), and acquired conditions such as spur cell anemia in severe liver disease (discussed below), myelodysplasia, malnutrition, and hypothyroidism.[13]

Neuroacanthocytosis. *Neuroacanthocytosis* is a term used to describe a group of rare inherited disorders characterized by neurologic impairment and acanthocytes on the peripheral blood film. Three disorders are provided as examples in this group: abetalipoproteinemia, McLeod syndrome, and chorea acanthocytosis.[46]

Abetalipoproteinemia (ABL) is a rare autosomal recessive disorder characterized by fat malabsorption, progressive ataxia, neuropathy, retinitis pigmentosa, and acanthocytosis.[46] ABL can first manifest with steatorrhea and failure to thrive in young children (due to fat malabsorption) or as ataxia and neuropathy in young adults (due to decreased absorption of fat-soluble vitamin E).[46] ABL is caused by mutations in the *MTP* (microsomal triglyceride transfer protein) gene; MTP is needed to transfer and assemble lipids onto apolipoprotein B.[46] The mutations result in an absence in the plasma of chylomicrons, very low-density lipoproteins (which transport triglycerides), and low-density lipoproteins (which transport cholesterol).[13,46] Consequently, triglycerides and cholesterol are decreased, but sphingomyelin is increased in the plasma.[13] Because RBC membrane lipids are in equilibrium with plasma lipids, the RBC membrane acquires increased sphingomyelin, which decreases the fluidity of the RBC membrane and results in the

shape change. The shape defect is not present in developing nucleated RBCs or reticulocytes but progresses as RBCs age in the circulation.[13] Other unknown mechanisms may also contribute to the formation of acanthocytes in ABL. Usually, 50% to 90% of the RBCs are acanthocytes.[4,13] Affected individuals have a mild hemolytic anemia, normal RBC indices, and normal to slightly elevated reticulocyte counts.[13] Early treatment with high doses of vitamins A and E can reduce the neuropathy and retinopathy.[13] Patients with other related disorders, such as hypobetalipoproteinemia due to mutations in the *APOB* gene, also may have acanthocytosis and neurologic disease.[4,46]

The *McLeod syndrome* (MLS) is an X-linked disorder caused by mutations in the *KX* gene.[47] *KX* codes for the Kx protein, a membrane precursor of the Kell blood group antigens.[46] Men who lack Kx on their RBCs have reduced expression of Kell antigens, reduced RBC deformability, and shortened RBC survival.[46] Patients with MLS have variable acanthocytosis (up to 85%), mild anemia, and late-onset (aged 40 to 60 years), slowly progressive chorea (movement disorders), peripheral neuropathy, myopathy, and neuropsychiatric manifestations.[46,47] Some female heterozygote carriers may have acanthocytes, but neurologic symptoms are rare. Clinical manifestations in females depend on the proportion of RBCs with the normal X chromosome inactivated versus those with the mutant X chromosome inactivated.[13,47]

Chorea acanthocytosis (ChAc) is a rare autosomal recessive disorder characterized by chorea, hyperkinesia, cognitive impairments, and neuropsychiatric symptoms.[46] The mean age of onset of the neurologic symptoms is 35 years.[46] In patients with ChAc, 5% to 50% of RBCs on the peripheral blood film are acanthocytes.[46] ChAc is caused by mutations in *VPS13A*, a gene that codes for chorein, a protein with uncertain cellular functions.[47] Chorein may be involved in trafficking proteins to the cell membrane; consequently, a deficiency of chorein may lead to abnormal membrane protein structure and acanthocyte formation.[46]

Acquired Red Blood Cell Membrane Abnormalities

Acquired Stomatocytosis

Stomatocytosis occurs frequently as a drying artifact on Wright-stained peripheral blood films. A medical laboratory professional should examine many areas on several films before categorizing the result as stomatocytosis, because in true stomatocytosis such cells should be found in all areas of the blood film. In normal individuals, 3% to 5% of RBCs may be stomatocytes.[4] In wet preparations in which RBCs are diluted in their own plasma and examined under phase microscopy, stomatocytes tend to be bowl shaped or uniconcave, rather than the normal biconcave shape. This technique can eliminate some of the artifactual stomatocytosis, but target cells also may appear bowl shaped in solution. Acute alcoholism and a wide variety of other conditions (such as malignancies and cardiovascular disease) and medications have been associated with acquired stomatocytosis.[4,13]

Spur Cell Anemia

A small percentage of patients with severe liver disease develop a hemolytic anemia with acanthocytosis called *spur cell anemia*.

The acanthocytes are due to a defect in the lipid component of the membrane. In severe liver disease, there is excess free cholesterol because of the presence of abnormal plasma lipoproteins. An equilibrium is sought between free cholesterol in the plasma and the RBC membrane cholesterol, and cholesterol preferentially accumulates in the outer leaflet of the membrane.[4,13] The spleen remodels the membrane into the acanthocyte shape.[13] Acanthocytes have long, rigid projections and become entrapped and hemolyzed in the spleen, which results in a rapidly progressive anemia of moderate severity, splenomegaly, and jaundice.[4,13] Spur cell anemia in end-stage liver disease has a poor prognosis. The anemia may resolve, however, if the patient is able to undergo liver transplantation.[4]

Paroxysmal Nocturnal Hemoglobinuria

Paroxysmal nocturnal hemoglobinuria (PNH) is a rare chronic intravascular hemolytic anemia caused by an acquired clonal hematopoietic stem cell mutation that results in circulating blood cells that lack glycosylphosphatidylinositol (GPI)–anchored proteins, such as CD55 and CD59.[48] The absence of CD55 and CD59 on the surface of the RBCs renders them susceptible to spontaneous lysis by complement. Because the mutation occurs in a hematopoietic stem cell, the defect is also found in platelets, granulocytes, monocytes, and lymphocytes.[49] PNH is uncommon, with an annual incidence of two to five new cases per million persons in the United States.[50]

Pathophysiology of the Hemolytic Anemia.   The GPI anchor consists of a phosphatidylinositol (PI) molecule and a glycan core. The phosphatidylinositol is incorporated in the outer leaflet of the lipid bilayer. The glycan core consists of glucosamine, three mannose residues, and ethanolamine phosphate. At least 24 genes code for enzymes and proteins involved in the biosynthesis of the GPI anchor.[50] GPI-anchored proteins attach to the ethanolamine in the glycan core by an amide bond at their C-termini (Figure 24-10).

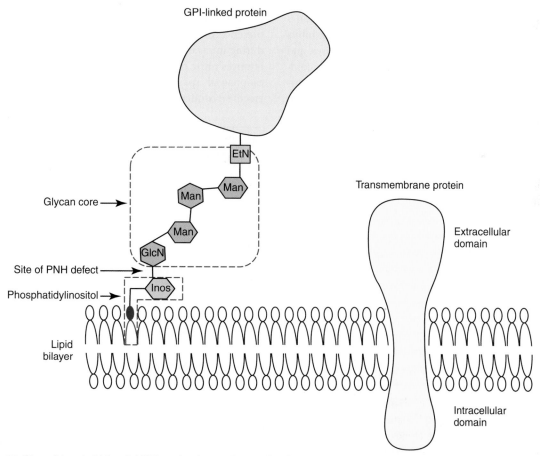

Figure 24-10 Glycosylphosphatidylinositol (GPI) anchor for attachment of surface proteins to the cell membrane. *Left:* The structure of a GPI-anchored protein. The GPI anchor consists of phosphatidylinositol in the outer leaflet of the lipid bilayer, which is connected to a glycan core consisting of glucosamine (*GlcN*), three mannose (*Man*) residues, and ethanolamine phosphate (*EtN*). The protein is linked to the anchor at its C-terminus by an amide bond. The result is a surface protein with a fluid and mobile attachment to the cell surface. The GPI anchor and GPI-linked protein is extracellular. In paroxysmal nocturnal hemoglobinuria (*PNH*), a mutation occurs in the *PIGA* gene coding for phosphatidylinositol glycan class A (PIG-A), one of seven subunits of a glycosyl transferase enzyme needed to add *N*-acetylglucosamine to the inositol (*Inos*) component of the phosphatidylinositol molecule (see arrow for location of the PNH defect). The mutated PIG-A enzyme subunit inhibits or prevents the first step in the biosynthesis of the GPI anchor. *Right:* In contrast, a transmembrane protein has an extracellular domain, a short transmembrane domain, and an intracellular domain. (Adapted from Ware RE, Rosse WF: Autoimmune hemolytic anemia. In Nathan DG, Orkin SH, editors: *Nathan and Oski's hematology of infancy and childhood,* ed 5, Philadelphia, 1998, Saunders, p. 514.)

In PNH, a hematopoietic stem cell acquires a mutation in the *PIGA* gene that codes for phosphatidylinositol glycan class A (PIG-A), also known as phosphatidylinositol *N*-acetylglucosaminyltransferase subunit A.[51] It is one of seven subunits of a glycosyl transferase enzyme needed to add *N*-acetylglucosamine to phosphatidylinositol.[48-50] This is the first step in the biosynthesis of the GPI anchor in the endoplasmic reticulum membrane. The *PIGA* gene is located on the X chromosome, and over 180 different mutations have been identified.[49] Without a fully functional glycosyl transferase enzyme, the hematopoietic stem cell is unable to effectively synthesize the glycan core on phosphatidylinositol in the membrane; therefore, the cell is deficient in membrane GPI anchors. Without GPI anchors, all the progeny of the mutated stem cell are unable to express any of the approximately 16 currently known GPI-anchored proteins found on normal hematopoietic cells.[49] The GPI-anchored proteins are complement regulators, enzymes, adhesion molecules, blood group antigens, or receptors.[49-50] Relevant to the expression of the hemolysis in PNH, two GPI-anchored proteins are absent or deficient on the RBC membrane: decay-accelerating factor (DAF, or CD55) and membrane inhibitor of reactive lysis (MIRL, or CD59).[50] CD55 and CD59 are complement-inhibiting proteins. CD55 inhibits the complement alternate pathway C3 and C5 convertases, and CD59 prevents the formation of the membrane attack complex.[48] When CD55 and CD59 are absent from the RBC surface, the cell is unable to prevent the activation of complement, and spontaneous and chronic intravascular hemolysis occurs. Out of all the genes needed for GPI anchor synthesis, *PIGA* is the only one located on the X chromosome. Therefore, only one acquired mutation in a stem cell is needed for the PNH phenotype (males have only one X chromosome, and in females one of the X chromosomes is inactivated).[48]

The *PIGA* mutant clone coexists with normal hematopoietic stem cells and progenitors, which results in a population of RBCs that is GPI-deficient and a population that is normal.[48] Some patients have a greater expansion of the mutant clone, a higher percentage of circulating GPI-deficient RBCs, and a more severe chronic hemolytic anemia.[48] On the other hand, other patients have minimal expansion of the mutant clone and have a lower percentage of circulating GPI-deficient RBCs. These patients may be asymptomatic and may not require any treatment. It is unclear why there is a greater expansion of the GPI-deficient clone and chronic hemolysis in some patients and not others.

Patients with PNH also display *phenotypic mosaicism*.[48,50] The mosaicism results when a single patient is able to harbor normal clones as well as mutant clones with different *PIGA* mutations. Those different mutations result in variable expression of CD55 and CD59 on the RBCs within an individual patient, giving rise to three RBC phenotypes: type I, type II, and type III.[48,49] Type I RBCs are phenotypically normal, express normal amounts of CD55 and CD59, and undergo little or no complement-mediated hemolysis. Type II RBCs are the result of a *PIGA* mutation that causes only a partial deficiency of CD55 and CD59, and these cells are relatively resistant to complement-mediated hemolysis. Type III RBCs are the result

of a *PIGA* mutation that causes a complete deficiency of the GPI anchor, and therefore no CD55 and CD59 proteins are anchored to the RBC surface. Type III RBCs are highly sensitive to spontaneous lysis by complement. The most common RBC phenotype in PNH is a combination of type I and type III cells, while the second most common has all three types.[48] When the severity of the hemolysis in PNH is being assessed, both the relative amount and the type of circulating RBCs are considered.

In addition to hemolysis, patients with PNH may have bone marrow dysfunction that contributes to the severity of the anemia. Many patients have a history of bone marrow failure caused by acquired aplastic anemia or myelodysplastic syndrome that precedes or coincides with the onset of PNH.[52]

Clinical Manifestations.   The onset of PNH most frequently occurs in the third or fourth decade, but it can occur in childhood and advanced age.[48-50] The major clinical manifestations and complications of PNH are those associated with hemolytic anemia, thrombosis, and bone marrow failure (Box 24-2).[49] Anemia is mild to severe, depending on the predominant type of RBC, the degree of hemolysis, and the presence of bone marrow failure. Free hemoglobin released during intravascular hemolytic episodes rapidly scavenges and removes nitric oxide (NO). The decreased NO can manifest as esophageal spasms and dysphagia (difficulty swallowing), erectile dysfunction, abdominal pain, or platelet activation and

---

BOX 24-2 **Major Clinical Manifestations and Complications of Paroxysmal Nocturnal Hemoglobinuria**

Related to Intravascular Hemolysis
- Anemia
- Hemoglobinuria
- Chronic renal failure
- Cholelithiasis
- Esophageal spasm, erectile dysfunction

Related to Thrombosis
- Venous thrombosis
  - Abdominal vein thrombosis: hepatic (Budd-Chiari syndrome), splenic, renal veins
  - Portal hypertension
  - Cerebral vein thrombosis
  - Retinal vein thrombosis and loss of vision
  - Deep vein thrombosis, pulmonary emboli
- Arterial thrombosis (less common)
  - Stroke
  - Myocardial infarction

Related to Bone Marrow Failure
- Pancytopenia: fatigue, infections, bleeding
- Myelodysplastic syndrome

Adapted from Bessler M, Hiken J: The pathophysiology of disease in patients with paroxysmal nocturnal hemoglobinuria, *Hematology Am Soc Hematol Educ Program*, pp. 104-110, 2008.

thrombosis.[49,50] The most common thrombotic manifestation is hepatic vein thrombosis, which obstructs venous outflow from the liver (Budd-Chiari syndrome), a serious, often fatal complication.[50]

Laboratory Findings. Biochemical evidence of intravascular hemolysis includes hemoglobinemia, hemoglobinuria, decreased level of serum haptoglobin, increased levels of serum indirect bilirubin and lactate dehydrogenase, and hemosiderinuria (Chapter 23). Hemolysis can be exacerbated by conditions such as infections, strenuous exercise, and surgery.[50] Hemoglobinuria is present in only 25% of patients at diagnosis, but it will occur in most patients during the course of the illness.[52] Very few patients report periodic hemoglobinuria at night, a symptom for which the condition was originally named.[50] Hemosiderinuria due to chronic intravascular hemolysis (Chapter 23) may be detected with Prussian blue staining of the urine sediment.

Reticulocyte counts are mildly to moderately increased, with less elevation than would be expected in other hemolytic anemias of comparable severity. The MCV may be slightly elevated due to the reticulocytosis. The direct antiglobulin test (DAT) is negative. If the patient does not receive transfusions, iron deficiency develops due to the loss of hemoglobin iron in the urine, and the RBCs become microcytic and hypochromic. Serum iron studies (serum iron, total iron-binding capacity, and serum ferritin) are performed to detect iron deficiency (Chapter 20). Folate deficiency often occurs if there is chronic erythroid hyperplasia and a greater need for folate, which leads to secondary macrocytosis. Pancytopenia may occur if there is concomitant bone marrow failure.

The bone marrow aspirate and biopsy specimen are examined for evidence of an underlying bone marrow failure syndrome, abnormal cells, and cytogenetic abnormalities.[52] The bone marrow may be normocellular to hypercellular with erythroid hyperplasia in response to the hemolysis, or it may be hypocellular in concomitant bone marrow failure.[50] A finding of dysplasia or certain chromosome abnormalities is helpful in diagnosis of a myelodysplastic syndrome (Chapter 34). An abnormal karyotype is found in 20% of patients with PNH.[50]

Confirmation of PNH requires demonstration of GPI-deficient cells in the peripheral blood. Flow cytometric analysis (Chapter 32) of RBCs with fluorescence-labeled anti-CD59 determines the proportion of types I, II, and III RBCs, and thus can provide an assessment of the severity of the hemolysis (Figure 24-11, and Figure 32-17).[48,50] Type I cells with normal expression of CD59 show the highest intensity level of fluorescence; type II cells with a partial deficiency of CD59 show moderate fluorescence; and type III cells with no CD59 are negative for fluorescence. Patients with a greater proportion of type III cells (complete deficiency of GPI-anchored proteins) are expected to have a high-grade hemolysis.[48,52] Patients with a high percentage of type II cells (partial deficiency of GPI-anchored proteins) and a low percentage of type III cells may have only modest hemolysis.[48-52] A high-sensitivity two-parameter flow cytometry method using labeled anti-CD59 and anti-CD235a (anti-glycophorin A) was able to detect

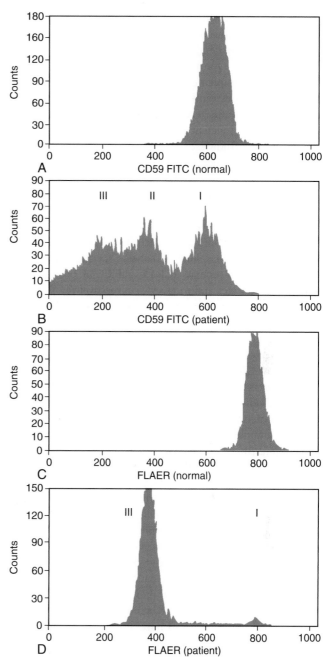

Figure 24-11 Flow cytometric analysis of peripheral blood cells from a patient with paroxysmal nocturnal hemoglobinuria (PNH). **A,** Fluorescence intensity of erythrocytes from a healthy control participant after staining with anti-CD59. **B,** Fluorescence intensity of erythrocytes from an untransfused PNH patient after staining with anti-CD59. Type II cells are "blended" between the type I (normal) and type III cells. **C,** Fluorescence intensity of granulocytes from a healthy control participant stained with FLAER. **D,** Fluorescence intensity of granulocytes from the same PNH patient as in **B** after staining with FLAER. Note that the granulocytes are almost exclusively type III cells. A small population of type I granulocytes is present. *FITC,* Fluorescein isothiocyanate; *FLAER,* fluorescein-labeled proaerolysin variant. (From Brodsky RA: Paroxysmal nocturnal hemoglobinuria. In Hoffman R, Benz EJ, Jr., Silberstein LE, et al, editors: *Hematology: basic principles and practice,* ed 6, Philadelphia, 2013, Saunders, an imprint of Elsevier. Figure 29-2, p. 375.)

type III PNH RBCs with a sensitivity of 0.002% (1 in 50,000 normal cells).[53] However, flow cytometry methods to detect PNH RBCs have two major disadvantages. They underestimate the percentage of type III cells because RBCs lacking CD59 undergo rapid complement lysis in the circulation.[52] In addition, these methods cannot accurately determine the percentage of PNH RBCs after recent transfusion.

Because of the inherent problems with flow cytometry methods to detect PNH RBCs, diagnosis of PNH is accomplished by detection of the absence of GPI-anchored proteins on WBCs using multiparameter flow cytometry. The absence of at least two GPI-anchored proteins in two WBC lineages (usually granulocytes and monocytes) is recommended for greater diagnostic accuracy.[50,53] Methods typically use fluorescent monoclonal antibodies to GPI-anchored proteins (such as CD59, CD55, CD24, CD16, CD66b, CD14), along with lineage-specific antibodies to non-GPI-anchored proteins (CD15 and CD33 or CD64) to identify granulocytes and monocytes, respectively.[50,53,54] An alternative flow cytometric method uses a fluorescein-labeled proaerolysin variant (FLAER).[53-55] FLAER binds directly to the glycan core of the GPI anchor with a high signal-to-noise ratio. The absence of binding on granulocytes and/or monocytes is indicative of GPI deficiency (Figure 24-11).[53-55] Using multiparameter flow cytometry with FLAER in combination with monoclonal antibodies to GPI-anchored antigens and lineage-specific antigens increases sensitivity and specificity for detection of GPI-deficient granulocytes and monocytes.[53,54] A high-sensitivity four-color protocol using FLAER, CD24, CD15, and CD45 for granulocytes and FLAER, CD14, CD64, and CD45 for monocytes was able to detect GPI-deficient granulocytes and monocytes with a sensitivity of 0.01% (1 in 10,000) and 0.04% (1 in 2500), respectively.[53] The results are not affected by recent transfusions, since donor neutrophils and monocytes have a short life span in stored blood; therefore, it can reliably be used to estimate the percentage of GPI-deficient granulocytes and monocytes in recently transfused patients.[50] The high sensitivity is also important for posttherapy monitoring of PNH clones.

The sugar water test (sucrose hemolysis test) and the Ham test (acidified serum lysis test) have insufficient sensitivity for diagnosis of PNH and have been replaced by flow cytometric techniques.

Classification.   The International PNH Interest Group proposed three subcategories of PNH: classic PNH, PNH in the setting of another specified bone marrow disorder, and subclinical PNH.[48,52] In classic PNH, there is clinical and biochemical evidence of intravascular hemolysis, reticulocytosis, a cellular bone marrow with erythroid hyperplasia and normal morphology, and a normal karyotype. In addition, more than 50% of the circulating neutrophils are GPI-deficient.[52] In PNH in the setting of another bone marrow disorder, patients have evidence of hemolysis but have a history of or concomitant aplastic anemia, myeloproliferative disorder, or other myelopathy. The number of GPI-deficient neutrophils is variable but is usually less than 30% of the total neutrophils. In subclinical PNH, patients have no clinical or biochemical evidence of hemolysis but have a small subpopulation of GPI-deficient neutrophils that comprise less than 1% of the total circulating neutrophils.[52] This subcategory is found in association with bone marrow failure syndromes. Features of each subgroup are summarized in Table 24-3.

Treatment.   In 2007, the U.S. Food and Drug Administration approved eculizumab (Soliris®) for the treatment of hemolysis in PNH.[56] Eculizumab is a humanized monoclonal antibody that binds to complement C5, prevents its cleavage to C5a and C5b, and thus inhibits the formation of the membrane attack unit.[56] Eculizumab is the treatment of choice for patients with classic PNH. It results in an improvement of the anemia and a decrease in transfusion requirements.[56,57] There is also a reduction in the lactate dehydrogenase level in the serum, reflecting a reduction in hemolysis.[56,57] In a study by Hillman and colleagues (2013) of 195 patients taking eculizumab for a duration of 30 to 66 months, 96.4% of patients did not have an episode of thrombosis, and in 93%, markers of their chronic kidney disease stabilized or even improved.[57] Because of the inhibition of the complement system, patients taking eculizumab have an increased risk for infections with *Neisseria meningitidis* and need to be vaccinated prior to administration of the drug.[56] Patients continue to have a mild to moderate anemia and reticulocytosis likely due to extravascular hemolysis of RBCs sensitized with C3 (eculizumab does not inhibit complement C3).[48,58] To address this issue, research is under way to identify therapies that target the

TABLE 24-3 Classification of Paroxysmal Nocturnal Hemoglobinuria (PNH)

Subcategory	Rate of Intravascular Hemolysis	Bone Marrow	% GPI-AP Deficient Neutrophils
Classic PNH*	Marked; visible hemoglobinuria frequent	Normocellular to hypercellular with erythroid hyperplasia and normal or near-normal morphology	>50%
PNH in the setting of another specified bone marrow disorder†	Mild to moderate; visible hemoglobinuria is intermittent or absent	Evidence of a concomitant bone marrow failure syndrome†	Variable; usually <30%
Subclinical PNH	No clinical or biochemical evidence of intravascular hemolysis	Evidence of a concomitant bone marrow failure syndrome†	<1%‡

*Subclassification proposed by the International PNH Interest Group.[48,52]
†Bone marrow failure syndromes include aplastic anemia, refractory anemia/myelodysplastic syndrome, and other myelopathy (e.g., myelofibrosis).
‡Determined by high-sensitivity flow cytometric analysis.

early events of complement activation, including monoclonal antibodies to C3, but a universal inhibition of C3 may increase the patient's susceptibility to infections and immune complex disease.[58] A promising new therapy under investigation is a novel recombinant fusion protein (TT30) designed to prevent the formation of C3 convertase only on the membranes of GPI-deficient RBCs.[58]

Eculizumab is not curative and does not address the bone marrow failure complications of PNH. Other treatments for PNH are mainly supportive. Iron therapy is given to help alleviate the iron deficiency caused by the urinary loss of hemoglobin, and folate supplementation is given to replace the folate consumed in accelerated erythropoiesis. Administration of androgens and glucocorticoids to ameliorate anemia is not universally accepted.[48] Anticoagulants are used in the treatment of thrombotic complications. In suitable patients with severe intravascular hemolysis, hematopoietic stem cell transplantation with an HLA-matched sibling donor may be an option and can be a curative therapy, but with an overall survival of only 50% to 60%.[48]

PNH is a disease with significant morbidity and mortality. Prior to eculizumab, thrombosis was the major cause of death, and the median survival after diagnosis was approximately 10 years.[48] Long-term studies of patients on eculizumab therapy are in progress, and early results show a decrease in the debilitating complications and an increase in survival of patients with PNH.[57]

RED BLOOD CELL ENZYMOPATHIES

The major function of the RBCs is to transport oxygen to the tissues over their life span of 120 days. For the RBCs to do that effectively, they need functional enzymes to maintain glycolysis, preserve the shape and deformability of the cell membrane, keep hemoglobin iron in a reduced state, protect hemoglobin and other cellular proteins from oxidative denaturation, and degrade and salvage nucleotides. Deficiencies in RBC enzymes may impair these functions to varying degrees and decrease the life span of the cell. The most important metabolic pathways are the Embden-Meyerhof pathway (anaerobic glycolysis) and the hexose monophosphate (pentose) shunt[59] (Figure 9-1). The most commonly encountered enzymopathies are deficiencies of glucose-6-phosphate dehydrogenase and pyruvate kinase. Other RBC enzymopathies are rare.[59]

Glucose-6-Phosphate Dehydrogenase Deficiency

RBCs normally produce free oxygen radicals (O_2^-) and hydrogen peroxide (H_2O_2) during metabolism and oxygen transport, but they have multiple mechanisms to detoxify these oxidants (Chapter 9). Occasionally RBCs are subjected to an increased level of oxidants (*oxidant stress*) due to exposure to certain oxidizing drugs, foods, chemicals, herbal supplements, and even through reactive oxygen molecules produced in the body during infections. If allowed to accumulate in the RBCs, these reactive oxygen species would oxidize and denature hemoglobin, membrane proteins and lipids, and ultimately cause

premature hemolysis. Therefore, the RBCs' capacity to detoxify oxidants, especially during oxidant stress, is critical to maintain their normal life span.

Glucose-6-phosphate dehydrogenase (G6PD) is one of the important intracellular enzymes needed to protect hemoglobin and other cellular proteins and lipids from oxidative denaturation. G6PD catalyzes the first step in a series of reactions that detoxify hydrogen peroxide formed from oxygen radicals (Figure 24-12). In the hexose monophosphate shunt (Chapter 9), G6PD generates reduced nicotinamide adenine dinucleotide phosphate (NADPH) by converting glucose-6-phosphate to 6-phosphogluconate. In the next step, glutathione reductase uses the NADPH to reduce oxidized glutathione (GSSG) to reduced glutathione (GSH) and NADP. In the final reaction, glutathione peroxidase uses the GSH generated in the previous step to detoxify hydrogen peroxide to water (H_2O).[59-61] GSSG is formed in the reaction and is rapidly transported out of the cell. During oxidant stress, RBCs with normal G6PD activity are able to readily detoxify hydrogen peroxide to prevent cellular damage and safeguard hemoglobin. G6PD is especially critical to the cell because it provides the only means of generating NADPH. Consequently, G6PD-deficient RBCs are particularly vulnerable to oxidative damage and subsequent hemolysis during oxidant stress.[59-61]

The *G6PD* gene is located on the X chromosome. It codes for the G6PD enzyme, which assembles into a dimer and tetramer in its functional configuration.[59] With the X-linked inheritance pattern, men can be normal hemizygotes (have the normal allele) or deficient hemizygotes (have a mutant allele). Women can be normal homozygotes (both alleles normal), deficient homozygotes (both alleles have same mutation), compound heterozygotes (each allele has a different mutation), or heterozygotes (have one normal allele and one mutant allele). The G6PD enzyme activity in female heterozygotes lies between normal and deficient due to the random inactivation of one of the X chromosomes in each cell (lyonization).[59-61] Therefore, the RBCs of female heterozygotes are a mosaic, with some cells

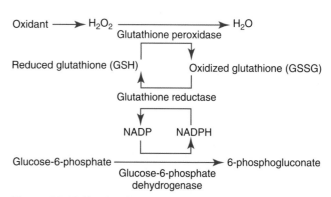

Figure 24-12 Function of glucose-6-phosphate dehydrogenase (G6PD) in generating the reduced form of nicotinamide adenine dinucleotide phosphate (NADPH) and reduced glutathione. G6PD converts glucose-6-phosphate (from the Embden-Meyerhof pathway) to 6-phosphogluconate. In the reaction, oxidized NADP is reduced to NADPH. Glutathione reductase uses the NADPH to reduce oxidized glutathione (GSSG) to reduced glutathione (GSH). Glutathione peroxidase uses the GSH to detoxify hydrogen peroxide to water.

having normal G6PD activity and some cells having deficient G6PD activity. Because the X inactivation is random, the proportion of normal to G6PD-deficient RBCs varies among different heterozygous women.[61] Some heterozygous women experience acute hemolytic episodes after exposure to oxidants if they have a high proportion of G6PD-deficient RBCs.

G6PD deficiency is the most common RBC enzyme defect, with a prevalence of 5% of the global population, or approximately 400 million people worldwide.[62] The prevalence of G6PD deficiency varies by geographic location: sub-Saharan Africa (7.5%), the Middle East (6.0%), Asia (4.7%), Europe (3.9%), and the Americas (3.4%).[62] In the United States, the prevalence of G6PD deficiency in African American males is approximately 10%.[59] G6PD deficiency has the highest prevalence in geographic areas in which malaria is endemic because of the selective pressure of malaria.[63] Studies in Africa show that G6PD deficiency (A− variant) in hemizygous males confers protection against life-threatening *Plasmodium falciparum* malaria.[64] This protective effect is not observed in heterozygous females because of their mosaicism of normal and G6PD-deficient RBCs.[64] In a 2010 case-control study in Pakistan, G6PD deficiency (Mediterranean variant) conferred protection against *Plasmodium vivax* infection, also with a greater protective effect in hemizygous males.[65] This protective effect may be due to parasite susceptibility to excess free oxygen radicals produced in G6PD-deficient RBCs.[66] In addition, significant oxidative damage may occur to the RBCs early after parasite invasion so that these early-infected cells are more readily phagocytized with elimination of the parasite.[67]

A mutation database published in 2012 reported 186 known mutations in the *G6PD* gene, with over 85% of them being single missense mutations.[68] An amino acid substitution changes the structure of the enzyme and thus affects its function, stability, or both. In addition, more than 400 variant isoenzymes have been identified.[61] The normal or wildtype G6PD variant is designated G6PD-B.[59,61] Some G6PD variants have significantly reduced enzyme activity, while others have mild or moderately reduced activity or normal activity. The different variants of G6PD have been divided into classes by the World Health Organization, based on clinical symptoms and amount of enzyme activity (Table 24-4).[68,69]

Pathophysiology

G6PD-deficient RBCs cannot generate sufficient NADPH to reduce glutathione and thus cannot effectively detoxify the hydrogen peroxide produced upon exposure to oxidative stress. Oxidative damage to cellular proteins and lipids occurs, particularly affecting hemoglobin and the cell membrane. Oxidation converts hemoglobin to methemoglobin and forms sulfhydryl groups and disulfide bridges in hemoglobin polypeptides. This leads to decreased hemoglobin solubility and precipitation as Heinz bodies.[59] Heinz bodies adhere to the inner RBC membrane, causing irreversible membrane damage (Figure 14-11). Because of the membrane damage and loss of deformability, RBCs with Heinz bodies are rapidly removed from the circulation by intravascular and extravascular hemolysis.[61] Reticulocytes have approximately five times more G6PD activity than older RBCs, because enzyme activity decreases as the cells age. Therefore, during exposure to oxidants, the older RBCs with less G6PD are preferentially hemolyzed.[63]

Clinical Manifestations

The vast majority of individuals with G6PD deficiency are asymptomatic throughout their lives. However, some patients have clinical manifestations. The clinical syndromes are acute hemolytic anemia, neonatal jaundice (hyperbilirubinemia), and chronic hereditary nonspherocytic hemolytic anemia (HNSHA).[63]

Acute Hemolytic Anemia. *Oxidative stress* can precipitate a hemolytic episode, and the main triggers are certain oxidizing drugs or chemicals, infections, and ingestion of fava beans. Hemolysis secondary to drug exposure is the classic manifestation of G6PD deficiency. The actual discovery of

---

TABLE 24-4 Classification of Glucose-6-Phosphate Dehydrogenase Variants by the World Health Organization

Class	G6PD Enzyme Activity	Clinical Manifestations	Examples of Variants
I	Severely deficient: <1% activity or not detectable	Chronic, hereditary nonspherocytic hemolytic anemia; severity is variable; rare	G6PD-Serres G6PD-Madrid
II	Severely deficient: <10% activity	Severe, episodic acute hemolytic anemia associated with infections, certain drugs, and fava beans; not self-limited and may require transfusions during hemolytic episodes	G6PD-Mediterranean G6PD-Chatham
III	Mild to moderately deficient: 10%–60% activity	Episodic, acute hemolytic anemia associated with infections and certain drugs; self-limited	G6PD-A− G6PD-Canton
IV	Mildly deficient to normal: 60%–150% activity	None	G6PD-B (wildtype) G6PD-A+ (may also manifest as class III)
V	Increased: >150% activity	None	

From Beutler E, Gaetani G, der Kaloustian V et al. World Health Organization (WHO) Working Group. Glucose-6-phosphate dehydrogenase deficiency. *Bull World Health Organ* 67:601-611, 1989; and Minucci A, Moradkhani K, Hwang MJ, et al. Glucose-6-phosphate dehydrogenase (G6PD) mutations database: Review of the "old" and update of the new mutations. *Blood Cells Mol Dis* 48:154-165, 2012.

G6PD deficiency in the 1950s was a direct consequence of investigations into the development of hemolysis in certain individuals after ingestion of the antimalarial agent primaquine.[59] Box 24-3 lists drugs that show strong evidence-based association with hemolysis in G6PD-deficient individuals or have been reported in well-documented case reports.[70,71] The degree of hemolysis can vary, depending on the dosage, coexisting infection, concomitant use of other drugs, or type of mutation.[70] Exposure to naphthalene in mothballs and some herbal supplements have also been associated with hemolysis in some G6PD-deficient individuals.[59]

Individuals with classes II and III G6PD deficiency are clinically and hematologically normal until the offending drug is taken. Clinical hemolysis can begin abruptly within hours or occur gradually 1 to 3 days after the drug is taken.[61,63] Typical symptoms include chills, fever, headache, nausea, and back pain.[59] A rapid drop in hemoglobin may occur, and the anemia can range from mild to very severe. Hemoglobinuria is a usual finding and indicates that the hemolysis is intravascular, although some extravascular hemolysis occurs. Reticulocytes increase within 4 to 6 days.[61] Generally, with class III variants such as G6PD-A⁻, the hemolytic episode is self-limiting because the newly formed reticulocytes have higher G6PD activity. With class II variants such as G6PD-Mediterranean, the RBCs are severely G6PD-deficient, so the hemolytic episode may be longer and the hemolysis is not self-limiting.[61]

Infection is probably the most common cause of hemolysis in individuals with G6PD deficiency. During the episode, the hemoglobin can drop 3 to 4 g/dL if reticulocyte production is suppressed by the infection.[59] The hemolysis resolves after recovery from the infection.[61] The mechanism of hemolysis induced by acute and subacute infection is poorly understood, but the generation of hydrogen peroxide by phagocytizing leukocytes may play a role.[61] Diminished liver function may contribute further to the oxidant stress by allowing the accumulation of oxidizing metabolites. Infectious agents implicated in hemolytic episodes include bacteria, viruses, and rickettsia.

Favism is a rare, severe hemolytic episode that occurs in some G6PD-deficient individuals after ingestion of fava beans. Favism can initially manifest with a sudden onset of acute intravascular hemolysis within hours of ingesting fava beans, or hemolysis can occur gradually over a period of 24 to 48 hours.[61] Hemoglobinuria is one of the first signs. Specific patient factors may affect the severity of the hemolysis, including the type of mutation, presence of underlying disorders, and the amount of fava beans ingested. Only a small percentage of G6PD-deficient individuals manifest favism, and most of these have the G6PD-Mediterranean variant.

Neonatal Hyperbilirubinemia.   *Neonatal hyperbilirubinemia* is associated with G6PD deficiency. Jaundice generally appears 2 to 3 days after birth without concomitant anemia.[63] The jaundice is mainly attributed to inefficient conjugation of indirect bilirubin by the liver rather than to excessive hemolysis.[72] These neonates must be closely monitored because the hyperbilirubinemia can be severe and cause bilirubin encephalopathy (kernicterus) and permanent brain damage.[61] Severe hyperbilirubinemia occurs more often in infants who, in addition to a mutated *G6PD* gene, are homozygous for a mutation in the promoter region of the bilirubin-uridine diphosphoglucuronate glucuronosyltransferase 1 (*UGT1A1*) gene, which impairs their ability to conjugate and excrete indirect bilirubin.[61] In addition, the particular G6PD variant and environmental factors (such as drugs given to the mother or infant, the presence of infection, and gestational age) probably play an important role in the occurrence of neonatal hyperbilirubinemia, because a wide variation exists in frequency and severity in different populations with G6PD deficiency.

Chronic Hereditary Nonspherocytic Hemolytic Anemia.
A small percentage of G6PD-deficient patients have chronic HNSHA, as evidenced by persistent hyperbilirubinemia, decreased serum haptoglobin level, and increased serum lactate dehydrogenase level. Most of these patients are diagnosed at birth as having neonatal hyperbilirubinemia, and the hemolysis continues into adulthood. They usually do not have hemoglobinuria, which suggests that the ongoing hemolysis is extravascular as opposed to intravascular. The RBC morphology is unremarkable. These patients also are vulnerable to acute oxidative stress from the same agents as those affecting other G6PD-deficient individuals and may have acute episodes of hemoglobinuria. The severity of HNSHA is extremely variable, likely related to the type of mutation in the *G6PD* gene.

Laboratory Findings
General Tests for Hemolytic Anemia.   The anemia occurring during a hemolytic crisis may range from moderate to extremely severe and is usually normocytic and normochromic. The morphology of G6PD-deficient RBCs is normal except during a hemolytic episode. The degree of change in morphology during a hemolytic episode varies, depending on

---

BOX 24-3   Drugs Causing Predictable Hemolysis in Glucose-6-Phosphate Dehydrogenase Deficiency

Drugs with strong evidence-based support for an association with drug-induced hemolysis:[1]

   Dapsone
   Methylthioninium chloride (methylene blue)
   Nitrofurantoin
   Phenazopyridine
   Primaquine
   Rasburicase
   Tolonium chloride (toluidine blue)

Drugs with well-documented case reports for an association with drug-induced hemolysis:[2]

   Cotrimoxazole
   Quinolones
   Sulfadiazine

[1]Youngster I, Arcavi L, Schechmaster R, et al: Medications and glucose-6-phosphate dehydrogenase deficiency: an evidence-based review, *Drug Saf* 33:713-726, 2010.
[2]Luzzatto L, Seneca E. G6PD deficiency: a classic example of pharmacogenetics with on-going clinical implications. *Br J Haematol* 164:469-480, 2014.

the severity of the hemolysis. In some patients, the change is not striking, but in other individuals with severe variants, marked anisocytosis, poikilocytosis, spherocytosis, and schistocytosis may occur.[61] Bite cells (RBCs in which the margin appears indented and the hemoglobin is concentrated) may be observed in rare cases of drug-induced hemolysis but should not be considered a specific feature of G6PD deficiency.[61,73] Bite cells are absent in acute and chronic hemolytic states associated with common G6PD-deficient variants, and they can also be found in other conditions.[61,73] Heinz bodies cannot be detected with Wright staining. They can be visualized with supravital stains, such as crystal violet, as dark purple inclusions attached to the inner RBC membrane (Figure 14-11). The reticulocyte count is increased and may reach 30% of RBCs. Consistent with intravascular hemolysis, the serum haptoglobin level is severely decreased, the serum lactate dehydrogenase activity is elevated, and there is hemoglobinemia and hemoglobinuria. The indirect bilirubin level is also elevated. The white blood cell (WBC) count is moderately elevated, and the platelet count varies. Importantly, the direct antiglobulin test (DAT) is negative, indicating that an immune cause of the hemolysis is unlikely (Chapter 26). Table 24-5 contains a summary of the clinical and laboratory findings in G6PD deficiency during an acute hemolytic episode.

Tests for G6PD Deficiency.

The two major categories of tests for G6PD deficiency are quantitative and qualitative biochemical assays for G6PD activity (phenotypic assays) and DNA-based molecular tests for mutation detection (genotypic assays). Quantitative spectrophotometric assays are the gold standard to determine G6PD activity, make a definitive diagnosis, and assess the severity of the deficiency.[59,74] The assays are based on the direct measurement of NADPH generated by the patient's G6PD in the reaction shown in Figure 24-13. The assays require venous blood collected in heparin or ethylenediaminetetraacetic acid (EDTA) anticoagulant. A hemolysate is prepared and incubated with the substrate/cofactor (glucose-6-phosphate/NADP) reagent. The rate of NADPH formation is proportional to G6PD activity and is measured as an increase in absorbance at 340 nm using a spectrophotometer.[59,74] The activity is typically reported as a ratio of the units of G6PD activity per gram of hemoglobin (IU/g Hb), so a standard hemoglobin assay must be done on the same specimen used for the G6PD assay. Cutoff points to determine G6PD deficiency are usually set at less than 20% of normal activity (usually less than 4.0 IU/g Hb), but this varies by method, laboratory, and population screened.[71]

Qualitative tests are designed as rapid screening tools to distinguish normal from G6PD-deficient patients. G6PD deficiency is defined by various methods as less than 20% to 50% of normal G6PD activity.[71,74,75] Similar to quantitative assays, these tests also incubate a lysate of heparin or EDTA-anticoagulated blood with a glucose-6-phosphate/NADP reagent to generate NADPH (Figure 24-13). The endpoint in qualitative tests, however, is visually observed, and the results are reported as "G6PD-deficient" or "normal." Qualitative tests with deficient or intermediate results are

TABLE 24-5 Typical Clinical and Laboratory Findings in Glucose-6-Phosphate Dehydrogenase Deficiency During Acute Hemolytic Episode

History	Recent infection, administration of drugs associated with hemolysis, or ingestion of fava beans
Clinical manifestations	Chills, fever, headache, nausea, back pain, abdominal pain
	Jaundice
	Dark urine
Complete blood count results	↓ Hemoglobin (moderate to severe)
	↑ Reticulocyte count
Peripheral blood film findings	Polychromasia
	RBC morphology varies from normal to marked anisocytosis, poikilocytosis, spherocytosis, or schistocytosis, depending on severity
Direct antiglobulin test result	Negative
Indicators of hemolysis	↓ Serum haptoglobin (severe)
	↑ Serum lactate dehydrogenase
	↑ Serum indirect bilirubin
	Hemoglobinemia
	Hemoglobinuria
Selected additional tests	↓ G6PD activity (mild to severe); may be falsely normal due to reticulocytosis, leukocytosis, thrombocytosis, and in individuals with mild deficiencies
	DNA-based mutation detection usually needed to identify heterozygous females
	Heinz bodies observed on supravital stain

↓, Decreased; ↑, increased; *G6PD*, glucose-6-phosphate dehydrogenase; *RBC*, red blood cell.

reflexed to the quantitative assay for verification of the G6PD deficiency.

The fluorescent spot test is based on the principle that the NADPH generated in the reaction is fluorescent, while the NADP in the reagent is not fluorescent. Blood and glucose-6-phosphate/NADP reagent are incubated and spotted on filter paper in timed intervals. Specimens with normal G6PD activity appear as moderate to strong fluorescent spots under long-wave ultraviolet (UV) light; specimens with decreased or no activity do not fluoresce or display weak fluorescence compared to a normal control.

Dye-reduction qualitative assays use the same G6PD enzymatic reaction but have a second step in which the NADPH reduces a dye, giving a visually observed color change. An example is BinaxNOW® (Alere/Inverness Medical, Waltham, MA), which is a handheld device that uses the enzyme chromographic test (ECT) method.[76] Hemolysate is applied to one section of a lateral flow test strip in the device. The specimen migrates to the reaction pad of the strip containing the glucose-6-phosphate/NADP substrate/cofactor and a nitroblue

$$\text{Glucose-6-phosphate} + \text{NADP} \xrightarrow{\text{G6PD}} \text{6-Phosphogluconate} + \text{NADPH}$$
$$\text{Not fluorescent} \qquad\qquad\qquad \text{Fluorescent;}$$
$$\uparrow \text{absorbance at 340 nm}$$

Figure 24-13 Principle of the glucose-6-phosphate dehydrogenase (G6PD) activity assay. G6PD (in patient's hemolysate) converts glucose-6-phosphate to 6-phosphogluconate with the conversion of oxidized nicotinamide adenine dinucleotide phosphate (NADP) (not fluorescent) to the reduced form of nicotinamide adenine dinucleotide phosphate (NADPH) (fluorescent). In the quantitative assay, the rate of production of NADPH is proportional to G6PD activity and is measured as an increase in absorbance at 340 nm using a spectrophotometer. In the qualitative assay, the appearance of a fluorescent spot under ultraviolet light when the reaction mixture is spotted on filter paper indicates normal G6PD activity.

tetrazolium dye.[76] If the specimen has normal G6PD activity, the NADPH generated reduces the dye to a formazan product that is visually observed as a brown-black color on the reaction pad.[76] This method has a sensitivity of 98% in detecting deficient specimens with G6PD activity less than 4.0 U/g Hb.[76] In another formazan-based test, the NADPH reduces a tetrazolium monosodium salt (WST-8) substrate, forming a formazan orange-colored product.[75] The dye-reduction methods have an advantage, since they do not need a UV light for visualization. A disadvantage of the BinaxNOW® method, however, is its higher cost compared to other assays. Rapid, point-of-care screening methods that do not require a venipuncture specimen are in development.

Biochemical qualitative screening tests are reliable to identify hemizygous males and homozygous or compound heterozygous mutant females with severe deficiency (less than 20% of normal activity), but lack the sensitivity to detect mild and moderate deficiencies found in some class III G6PD deficiency and in heterozygous females. They also have subjective endpoints that may affect test reproducibility and accuracy.

Phenotypic assays for G6PD activity have several additional limitations. As covered earlier in the chapter, reticulocytes have higher G6PD activity compared to mature RBCs. Reticulocytosis typically occurs as a response to an acute hemolytic episode and will falsely increase the patient's G6PD activity over baseline values.[59,74] Patients who are not G6PD deficient are expected to have high G6PD activity during hemolytic episodes. When a patient with reticulocytosis has an unexpectedly normal G6PD activity result, G6PD deficiency should be suspected. To avoid falsely elevated or falsely normal results, biochemical assays for G6PD activity should not be performed during acute hemolysis. The testing should be performed after the reticulocyte and total RBC counts have returned to baseline, which may take 2 weeks to 2 months after the hemolytic episode.[71,74]

Another limitation of phenotypic assays is that testing cannot be done after recent transfusion because the mixture of donor and patient RBCs does not reflect the patient's true G6PD activity. WBCs and platelets also contain G6PD activity. In cases of severe anemia, or in severe leukocytosis or thrombocytosis, the buffy coat should be removed from the specimen before preparing the hemolysate for testing.[74]

DNA-based mutation detection (genotyping) is available in larger hospital and reference laboratories. Typically, the DNA is extracted from WBCs isolated from whole blood. Since the vast majority of G6PD mutations involve single nucleotide substitutions, molecular testing is straightforward. Although there are approximately 186 known mutations, rapid PCR-based methods can be used that target specific mutations with high prevalence in a particular geographic area, racial group, or ethnic group.[74] If targeted mutation testing is negative, whole gene DNA sequencing is required.[74]

DNA-based testing is best suited for prenatal testing, family studies, and identification of heterozygous females who typically have indeterminate or normal biochemical (phenotypic) tests owing to their mosaicism of normal and G6PD-deficient cells.[59,74] DNA-based methods can be done on patients who were recently transfused because donor WBCs have a short half-life in stored blood and will not interfere with the test. In addition, DNA-based tests are not affected by reticulocytosis and can be done during an acute hemolytic episode.

The disadvantage of DNA-based methods is the requirement for technical expertise and specialized equipment. In addition, knowing the genotype of heterozygous females does not predict the clinical phenotype in terms of the proportion of normal and G6PD-deficient cells.[71]

An additional application of tests for G6PD deficiency is screening asymptomatic patients prior to prescribing the drugs listed in Box 24-3. Screening is recommended for patients with a family history of G6PD deficiency or for those who are members of ethnic/racial groups with a high prevalence of G6PD variants.

Treatment

Treatment for G6PD-deficient patients with acute hemolysis begins with discontinuing drugs associated with hemolysis. Most hemolytic episodes, especially in individuals with G6PD-A⁻, are self-limited. In patients with more severe types, such as G6PD-Mediterranean, RBC transfusions may be required. Screening is important in populations that have a high incidence of G6PD deficiency. The prevention of acute hemolytic anemia is difficult because multiple causes exist; however, some cases of acute hemolytic anemia are easily preventable, such as by avoidance of fava bean consumption in families in which this sensitivity exists. Neonates in high risk populations should be screened for hyperbilirubinemia associated with G6PD deficiency, and treated immediately to prevent kernicterus and permanent brain damage.

Favism is a relatively dangerous manifestation and potentially fatal in individuals who do not have access to appropriate medical facilities and a transfusion service. Prevention of drug-induced disease is possible by choosing alternate drugs when possible. In cases in which the offending drugs must be used, especially in individuals with G6PD-A⁻, the dosage can be lowered to decrease the hemolysis to a manageable level. Infection-induced hemolysis is more difficult to prevent but can be detected early in the course of the episode and treated if necessary. Most episodes resolve without treatment but may be severe enough to warrant RBC transfusion. In patients with hemoglobin levels greater than 9 g/dL with persistent hemoglobinuria, close monitoring is important. Neonates with moderate hyperbilirubinemia and jaundice secondary to G6PD deficiency can be treated with phototherapy, but those with severe hyperbilirubinemia may require exchange transfusion.[59]

Pyruvate Kinase Deficiency

Pyruvate kinase (PK) is a rate-limiting key enzyme of the glycolytic pathway of RBCs. It catalyzes the conversion of phosphoenolpyruvate to pyruvate, forming ATP (Figure 9-1). PK deficiency is an autosomal recessive disorder, with an estimated prevalence of 1 per 20,000 in the white population.[77] It is the most common form of hereditary nonspherocytic hemolytic anemia and is found worldwide.[59,61] PK deficiency is due to a mutation in the *PKLR* gene that codes for PK in red blood cells and hepatocytes. Over 180 mutations (predominantly missense) have been reported.[78] Symptomatic hemolytic anemia occurs in homozygotes or compound heterozygotes. Certain mutations are more common in the United States, parts of Europe, and Asia.[59] There is a high prevalence of PK-deficient homozygotes with the same point mutations in two isolated, consanguineous communities in the United States: 27 Amish kindred in Pennsylvania (1436G>A) and 6 children born into polygamist families in a small town in the Midwest (1529G>A).[79,80]

Pathophysiology

The mechanisms causing hemolysis and premature destruction of PK-deficient cells are not completely known. The metabolic consequence of PK deficiency is a depletion of cellular ATP and an increase in 2,3-bisphosphoglycerate (2,3-BPG).[81,82] The increase in 2,3-BPG shifts the hemoglobin-oxygen dissociation curve to the right and decreases the oxygen affinity of hemoglobin[81] (Chapter 10). This promotes greater release of oxygen to the tissues and enables affected individuals to tolerate lower levels of hemoglobin.[59,81,82] ATP depletion also affects the ability of the cell to maintain its shape and membrane integrity.

Clinical Manifestations

Individuals with PK deficiency have a wide range of clinical presentations, varying from severe neonatal anemia and hyperbilirubinemia requiring exchange or multiple transfusions to a fully compensated hemolytic process in apparently healthy adults.[81] Most patients, however, have manifestations of chronic hemolysis, including anemia, jaundice, splenomegaly, and increased incidence of gallstones (due to the production of excessive bilirubin).[59] Rarely, folate deficiency (due to accelerated erythropoiesis), bone marrow aplasia (usually due to parvovirus B19 infection), and skin ulcers can occur.[73,82] Pregnancy carries the risk of fetal loss and exacerbation of the anemia in the mother.[79] There is an increased risk of iron

overload and organ damage that occurs with age, even in the absence of transfusions.[79,82,83] The mechanism of dysregulation of iron homeostasis is not clear but may be related to a decrease in or lack of response to hepcidin, the major iron-regulating protein.[79]

Laboratory Findings

The hemoglobin level is variable, depending on the extent of the hemolysis. Reticulocytosis is usually present, but not in proportion to the severity of the anemia, because the reticulocytes are preferentially destroyed in the spleen.[59,82] After splenectomy, the number of circulating reticulocytes can increase fivefold.[82] In addition to showing anisocytosis, poikilocytosis, and polychromasia, the peripheral blood film reveals a variable number of burr cells, or echinocytes (in the range of 3% to 30%), which increase in number after splenectomy.[82] The postsplenectomy peripheral blood film may also show Howell-Jolly bodies, Pappenheimer bodies, and target cells. The WBC and platelet counts are normal or slightly increased. Patients usually have the characteristic laboratory findings of chronic hemolysis, including an increased serum indirect bilirubin level, a decreased serum haptoglobin level, and increased urinary urobilinogen. The osmotic fragility is usually normal, and the direct antiglobulin test is negative.

Tests for PK deficiency include quantitative and qualitative biochemical assays for PK activity (phenotypic assays) and DNA-based molecular tests for mutation detection (genotypic assays). In the quantitative PK assay, a hemolysate is prepared from patient's anticoagulated blood after careful removal of the WBCs. WBCs have a very high PK level, and contamination of the hemolysate with WBCs falsely increases the result (i.e., in a PK deficiency, the result could be falsely normal).[82] The reagents include phosphoenolpyruvate, adenosine diphosphate (ADP), lactate dehydrogenase, and the reduced form of nicotinamide adenine dinucleotide (NADH). In the first step of the reaction, the patient's PK converts phosphoenolpyruvate to pyruvic acid, and a phosphate is transferred to ADP, forming adenosine triphosphate (ATP). In the second step, lactate dehydrogenase converts the pyruvic acid to lactic acid, and the NADH is converted to its oxidized form, NAD (Figure 24-14). The rate of NAD formation is proportional to PK activity and is measured as a decrease in absorbance at 340 nm using a spectrophotometer. The activity is typically reported as a ratio of the units of PK activity per gram of hemoglobin (IU/g Hb). More complex techniques may be necessary when some variant forms of PK are suspected.[82]

Qualitative tests for PK deficiency are used for screening and are based on the same principle as that described earlier, except the hemolysate and reagents are incubated and spotted onto filter paper. The loss of fluorescence is visually evaluated to determine the oxidation of NADH to NAD (Figure 24-14).[84]

Mutation detection (genotypic testing) can be accomplished by sequencing the exons, flanking regions, and promoter region of the *PKLR* gene.[82] Molecular diagnosis is superior in sensitivity and specificity, is applicable for use in prenatal testing, and enables correlation of certain mutations with disease severity.[59,79,82]

The enzyme pyruvate kinase catalyzes the following reaction:

1. $\text{ADP} + \text{Phosphoenolpyruvic acid} \xrightarrow[\text{kinase}]{\text{Pyruvate}} \text{ATP} + \text{Pyruvic acid}$

The pyruvic acid formed then takes part in the following reaction:

2. $\text{Pyruvic acid} + \underset{\text{Fluorescent}}{\text{NADH}} \xrightarrow[\text{dehydrogenase}]{\text{Lactate}} \underset{\substack{\text{Not fluorescent;}\\ \downarrow \text{absorbance at}\\ 340 \text{ mn}}}{\text{Lactic acid} + \text{NAD}}$

Figure 24-14 Principle of the pyruvate kinase (PK) activity test. The reagent contains adenosine diphosphate (ADP), phosphoenolpyruvic acid, lactate dehydrogenase, and the reduced form of nicotinamide adenine dinucleotide (NADH). In the first step, PK (in patient's hemolysate) converts phosphoenolpyruvic acid to pyruvic acid, and a phosphate is transferred to ADP, forming adenosine triphosphate (ATP). In the second step, lactate dehydrogenase converts pyruvic acid to lactic acid with the conversion of NADH (fluorescent) to the oxidized form of nicotinamide adenine dinucleotide (NAD) (not fluorescent). In the quantitative assay, the rate of production of NAD is proportional to PK activity and is measured as a decrease in absorbance at 340 nm using a spectrophotometer. In the qualitative assay, the disappearance of fluorescence under ultraviolet light when the reaction mixture is spotted on filter paper indicates normal PK activity.

Treatment

No specific therapy is available for PK deficiency except supportive treatment and RBC transfusion as necessary. Splenectomy is beneficial in severe cases, and after this procedure the hemoglobin level usually increases enough to reduce or eliminate the need for transfusion.[73] Splenectomy, however, results in a lifelong increased risk of sepsis by encapsulated bacteria. Hematopoietic stem cell transplant may be curative for children with severe hemolytic disease who have an unaffected HLA-identical sibling for a donor.[79]

Other Enzymopathies

Pyrimidine 5′-nucleotidase type 1 (P5′NT-1) is an enzyme needed for the degradation and elimination of ribosomal ribonucleic acid (RNA) in reticulocytes. P5′NT-1 removes the phosphate from pyrimidine 5′ ribonucleoside monophosphate to form ribonucleoside and inorganic phosphate. These degradation products are then able to diffuse out of the cell.[59] P5′NT-1 deficiency is inherited in an autosomal recessive manner.[59,85] It is the third most common RBC enzyme deficiency that causes hereditary nonspherocytic hemolytic anemia (after G6PD and PK).[59,85] The NT5C3A gene codes for P5′NT-1, and over 20 different mutations have been reported.[85]

Patients who are homozygotes or compound heterozygotes for NT5C3A mutations develop chronic hemolytic anemia. The P5′NT-1-deficient RBCs accumulate pyrimidine ribonucleoside monophosphates, which precipitate and appear as very coarse basophilic stippling in the cell.[59,85] These RBCs ultimately undergo premature hemolysis. Most patients have a mild to moderate anemia with reticulocytosis, jaundice, and splenomegaly.[85] Mental retardation has been reported in some patients.[61,85] Diagnostic tests include measurement of P5′NT-1 activity and the concentration of intracellular pyrimidine nucleotides in RBCs and DNA-based testing for mutations.[85] Therapy consists of RBC transfusion as needed.

Other RBC enzymopathies are rarely encountered. In addition to PK deficiency, deficiencies of other enzymes of the RBC Embden-Meyerhof pathway that cause hereditary nonspherocytic hemolytic anemia have been described, including hexokinase, glucose-6-phosphate isomerase, 6-phosphofructokinase, fructose-bisphosphate aldolase, triosephosphate isomerase, and phosphoglycerate kinase.[61] All of these deficiencies are autosomal recessive conditions, except for phosphoglycerate kinase deficiency, which is X-linked. Mutations in enolase are rare, and their association with hemolytic anemia is uncertain.[61] Deficiencies in glyceraldehyde-3-phosphate dehydrogenase and lactate dehydrogenase are not associated with hemolytic anemia.[61] Phosphoglycerate mutase deficiency results in a depletion of 2,3-bisphosphoglycerate. This causes a shift in the hemoglobin-oxygen dissociation curve to the left and an increased affinity of hemoglobin for oxygen. The resulting tissue hypoxia manifests as a mild erythrocytosis.[61]

SUMMARY

- The RBC membrane must have deformability for the RBC to maneuver through the microcirculation and the splenic sieve over its life span of 120 days. The cellular properties that enable deformability are the biconcave, discoid shape of the cell; the viscoelasticity of the membrane; and cytoplasmic viscosity.
- Two transmembrane protein complexes, the ankyrin complex and protein 4.1 complex, provide vertical structural integrity to the cell by anchoring the lipid bilayer to the underlying spectrin skeleton. α-Spectrin, β-spectrin, and their accessory proteins form a two-dimensional lattice to provide horizontal mechanical stability to the membrane.
- Hereditary spherocytosis (HS) is caused by mutations that disrupt the vertical membrane protein interactions, which results in loss of membrane, decrease in surface area–to–volume ratio, and formation of spherocytes that are destroyed in the spleen. Patients

with HS have anemia, splenomegaly, jaundice, an increased MCHC, a negative DAT result, biochemical evidence of hemolysis, and spherocytes and polychromasia on the peripheral blood film. RBCs in HS show decreased fluorescence in the eosin-5′-maleimide binding test when measured by flow cytometry, and the osmotic fragility test usually shows increased fragility.
- Hereditary elliptocytosis (HE) and hereditary pyropoikilocytosis (HPP) are caused by mutations that disrupt the horizontal interactions in the protein cytoskeleton, which results in loss of mechanical stability of the membrane. Elliptocytes are present on the peripheral blood film. Only 10% of HE patients have moderate or severe anemia. HPP is a severe thermal-sensitive form of HE in which extreme poikilocytosis along with schistocytes, microspherocytes, and elliptocytes are seen on the peripheral blood film.

- Hereditary ovalocytosis, also called Southeast Asian ovalocytosis (SAO), is caused by a mutation in band 3 that increases membrane rigidity. The prevalence is high in Southeast Asia, and hemolysis is mild or absent; typical cells are oval with one to two transverse bars or ridges.
- Hereditary stomatocytosis is a group of disorders characterized by an RBC membrane that leaks cations. In overhydrated hereditary stomatocytosis (OHS), the RBCs have decreased cytoplasmic viscosity and stomatocytes are observed on the peripheral blood film. In dehydrated hereditary stomatocytosis (DHS) or hereditary xerocytosis (HX), the RBCs have increased cytoplasmic viscosity, and the peripheral blood film shows burr cells, target cells, few stomatocytes, and cells with puddled hemoglobin at the periphery. Stomatocytosis may also occur in Rh deficiency syndrome and in a variety of acquired conditions.
- Neuroacanthocytosis comprises a group of inherited disorders characterized by neurologic impairment and the presence of acanthocytes on the peripheral blood film. Major disorders in this group include abetalipoproteinemia, McLeod syndrome, and chorea acanthocytosis. Acquired acanthocytosis can occur in severe liver disease (spur cell anemia).
- Paroxysmal nocturnal hemoglobinuria (PNH) is due to an acquired hematopoietic stem cell mutation that results in the lack of GPI-anchored proteins on blood cell surfaces. CD55 and CD59, complement-regulating proteins, are partially or completely deficient on RBCs, which makes the RBCs susceptible to spontaneous complement lysis. Flow cytometry is a sensitive method to detect the absence of GPI-anchored proteins on cell surfaces. The rate of hemolysis in classic PNH improves after treatment with eculizumab, a complement C5 inhibitor.
- Glucose-6-phosphate dehydrogenase (G6PD) deficiency is the most common RBC enzymopathy, but the vast majority of patients are asymptomatic. Patients with classes II and III G6PD variants may develop acute hemolytic anemia after infections or after ingestion of certain drugs or fava beans. A small percentage of patients have class I G6PD variant and chronic hereditary nonspherocytic hemolytic anemia (HNSHA).
- Most patients with pyruvate kinase (PK) deficiency have symptoms of hemolysis. Burr cells are commonly observed on the peripheral blood film. PK deficiency is the most common cause of HNSHA.

Now that you have completed this chapter, go back and read again the case study at the beginning and respond to the questions presented.

REVIEW QUESTIONS

Answers can be found in the Appendix.

1. In HS a characteristic abnormality in the CBC results is:
   a. Increased MCV
   b. Increased MCHC
   c. Decreased MCH
   d. Decreased platelet and WBC counts

2. The altered shape of the spherocyte in HS is due to:
   a. An abnormal RBC membrane protein affecting vertical protein interactions
   b. Defective RNA synthesis
   c. An extrinsic factor in the plasma
   d. Abnormality in the globin composition of the hemoglobin molecule

3. Which of the following results are consistent with HS?
   a. Increased osmotic fragility, negative DAT result
   b. Decreased osmotic fragility, positive DAT result
   c. Increased osmotic fragility, positive DAT result
   d. Decreased osmotic fragility, negative DAT result

4. The RBCs in HE are abnormally shaped and have unstable cell membranes as a result of:
   a. Abnormal shear stresses in the circulation
   b. Defects in horizontal membrane protein interactions
   c. Mutations in ankyrin
   d. Lack of all Rh antigens in the RBC membrane

5. The peripheral blood film for patients with mild HE is characterized by:
   a. Elliptical RBCs
   b. Oval RBCs with one or two transverse ridges
   c. Overhydrated RBCs with oval central pallor
   d. Densely stained RBCs with a few irregular projections

6. Laboratory test results for patients with HPP include all of the following *except:*
   a. RBCs that show marked thermal sensitivity at 41° C to 45° C
   b. Marked poikilocytosis with elliptocytes, RBC fragments, and microspherocytes
   c. Low fluorescence when incubated with eosin-5′-maleimide
   d. Increased MCV and normal RDW

7. Acanthocytes are found in association with:
   a. Abetalipoproteinemia
   b. G6PD deficiency
   c. Rh deficiency syndrome
   d. Vitamin B_{12} deficiency

8. The most common manifestation of G6PD deficiency is:
   a. Chronic hemolytic anemia caused by cell shape change
   b. Acute hemolytic anemia caused by drug exposure or infections
   c. Mild compensated hemolysis caused by ATP deficiency
   d. Chronic hemolytic anemia caused by intravascular RBC lysis

9. A patient experiences an episode of acute intravascular hemolysis after taking primaquine for the first time. The physician suspects that the patient may have G6PD deficiency and orders an RBC G6PD assay 2 days after the hemolytic episode begins. How will this affect the test result?
   a. No effect
   b. False increase due to reticulocytosis
   c. False decrease due to hemoglobinemia
   d. Absence of enzyme activity

10. The most common defect or deficiency in the anaerobic glycolytic pathway that causes chronic HNSHA is:
    a. Pyruvate kinase deficiency
    b. Lactate dehydrogenase deficiency
    c. Glucose-6-phosphate dehydrogenase deficiency
    d. Methemoglobin reductase deficiency

11. Which of the following laboratory tests would be best to confirm PNH?
    a. Acidified serum test (Ham test)
    b. Osmotic fragility test
    c. Flow cytometry for detection of eosin-5′-maleimide binding on erythrocytes
    d. Flow cytometry for detection of CD55, CD59, and FLAER binding on neutrophils and monocytes

REFERENCES

1. Mohandas, N., & Evans, E. (1994). Mechanical properties of the red cell membrane in relation to molecular structure and genetic defects. *Annu Rev Biophys Biomol Struct, 23,* 787–818.
2. Mohandas, N., & Chasis, J. A. (1993). Red blood cell deformability, membrane material properties and shape: regulation by transmembrane, skeletal and cytosolic proteins and lipids. *Semin Hematol, 30,* 171–192.
3. Mohandas, N., & Gallagher, P. G. (2008). Red cell membrane: past, present, future. *Blood, 112,* 3939–3948.
4. Gallagher, P. G. (2010). The red blood cell membrane and its disorders: hereditary spherocytosis, elliptocytosis, and related diseases. In Lichtman, M. A., Kipps, T. J., Seligsohn, U., et al. (Eds.), *Williams Hematology.* (8th ed.). New York: McGraw-Hill.
5. Palek, J., & Jarolim, P. (1993). Clinical expression and laboratory detection of red blood cell membrane protein mutations. *Semin Hematol, 30,* 249–283.
6. Da Costa, L., Galimand, J., Fenneteau, et al. (2013). Hereditary spherocytosis, elliptocytosis, and other red cell membrane disorders. *Blood Rev, 27,* 167–178.
7. Bennett, V. (1983). Proteins involved in membrane-cytoskeleton association in human erythrocytes: spectrin, ankyrin, and band 3. *Methods Enzymol, 96,* 313–324.
8. Nicolas, V., Le Van Kim, C., Gane, P., et al. (2003). Rh-RhAG/ankyrin-R, a new interaction site between the membrane bilayer and the red cell skeleton, is impaired by Rh$_{null}$-associated mutation. *J Biol Chem, 278,* 25526–25533.
9. Salomao, M., Zhang, X., Yang, Y., et al. (2008). Protein 4.1R-dependent multiprotein complex: new insights into the structural organization of the red blood cell membrane. *Proc Natl Acad Sci U S A, 105,* 8026–8031.
10. An, X., Debnath, G., Guo, X., et al. (2005). Identification and functional characterization of protein 4.1R and actin-binding sites in erythrocyte beta-spectrin: regulation of the interactions by phosphatidylinositol-4,5-bisphosphate. *Biochemistry, 44,* 10681–10688.
11. An, X., Mohandas, N. (2008). Disorders of red cell membrane. *Br J Haematol, 141,* 367–375.
12. An, X., Guo, X., Zhang, X., et al (2006). Conformational stabilities of the structural repeats of erythroid spectrin and their functional implications. *J Biol Chem, 281,* 10527–10532.
13. Gallagher, P. G. (2013). Red blood cell membrane disorders. In Hoffman, R., Benz, E. J. Jr, Silberstein, L. E., et al. (Eds.), *Hematology: Basic Principles and Practice.* (6th ed.). Philadelphia: Saunders, an imprint of Elsevier.
14. National Human Genome Research Institute. *Red Cell Membrane Disorder Mutations Database.* http://research.nhgri.nih.gov/RBCmembrane/. Accessed 08.03.14.
15. Perrotta, S., Gallagher, P. G., & Mohandas, N. (2008). Hereditary spherocytosis. *Lancet, 372,* 1411–1426.
16. Bolton-Maggs, P. H. B., Langer, J. C., Iolascon, A., et al. (2011). Guidelines for the diagnosis and management of hereditary spherocytosis—2011 update. *Br J Haematol, 156,* 37–49.
17. De Franceschi, L., Olivieri, O., Miraglia del Giudice, E., et al. (1997). Membrane cation and anion transport activities in erythrocytes of hereditary spherocytosis: effects of different membrane protein defects. *Am J Hematol, 55,* 121–128.
18. Hassoun, H., Vassiliadis, J. N., Murray, J., et al. (1997). Characterization of the underlying molecular defect in hereditary spherocytosis associated with spectrin deficiency. *Blood, 90,* 398–406.
19. Dhermy, D., Galand, C., Bournier, O., et al. (1997). Heterogenous band 3 deficiency in hereditary spherocytosis related to different band 3 gene defects. *Br J Haematol, 98,* 32–40.
20. Bouhassira, E. E., Schwartz, R. S., Yawata, Y., et al. (1992). An alanine-to-threonine substitution in protein 4.2 cDNA is associated with a Japanese form of hereditary hemolytic anemia (protein 4.2^{NIPPON}). *Blood, 79,* 1846–1854.
21. Michaels, L. A., Cohen, A. R., Zhao, H. J., et al. (1997). Screening for hereditary spherocytosis by use of automated erythrocyte indexes. *J Pediatr, 130,* 957–960.
22. Cynober, T., Mohandas, N., & Tchernia, G. (1996). Red cell abnormalities in hereditary spherocytosis: relevance to diagnosis and understanding of the variable expression of clinical severity. *J Lab Clin Med, 128,* 259–269.
23. Hansen, D. M. (1998). Hereditary anemias of increased destruction. In Steine-Martin, E. A., Lotspeich-Steininger, C. A., & Koepke, J. A., (Eds.), *Clinical Hematology: Principles, Procedures, Correlations.* (2nd ed., pp. 255–256). Philadelphia: Lippincott.
24. Bianchi, P., Fermo, E., Vercellati, C., et al. (2012). Diagnostic power of laboratory tests for hereditary spherocytosis: a comparison study in 150 patients groups according to molecular and clinical characteristics. *Haematologica, 97,* 516–523.
25. King, M-J., Smythe, J., & Mushens, R. (2004). Eosin-5-maleimide binding to band 3 and Rh-related proteins forms the basis of a screening test for hereditary spherocytosis. *Br J Haematol, 124,* 106–113.
26. Kar, R., Mishra, P., & Pati, H. P. (2008). Evaluaiton of eosin-5-maleimide flow cytometric test in diagnosis of hereditary spherocytosis. *Int J Lab Hematol, 32,* 8–16.

27. Mackiewicz, G., Bailly, F., Favre, B., et al. (2012). Flow cytometry test for hereditary spherocytosis. *Haematologica, 97*, e47.

28. Clark, M. R., Mohandas, N., & Shohet, S. B. (1983). Osmotic gradient ektacytometry: comprehensive characterization of red cell volume and surface maintenance. *Blood, 61*, 899–910.

29. King, M. J., & Zanella, A. (2013). Hereditary red cell membrane disorders and laboratory diagnostic testing. *Int J Lab Hem, 35*, 237–243.

30. Streichman, S., & Gescheidt, Y. (1998). Cryohemolysis for the detection of hereditary spherocytosis: correlation studies with osmotic fragility and autohemolysis. *Am J Hematol, 58*, 206–212.

31. Abdullah, F., Zhang, Y., Camp, M., et al. (2009). Splenectomy in hereditary spherocytosis: review of 1,657 patients and application of the pediatric quality indicators. *Pediatr Blood Cancer, 52*, 834–837.

32. Gallagher, P. G. (2004). Hereditary elliptocytosis: spectrin and protein 4.1R. *Semin Hematol 41*, 142–164.

33. Dhermy, D., Schrevel, J., & Lecomte, M-C. (2007). Spectrin-based skeleton in red blood cells and malaria. *Curr Opin Hematol, 14*, 198–202.

34. Winardi, R., Reid, M., Conboy, J., et al: (1993). Molecular analysis of glycophorin C deficiency in human erythrocytes. *Blood, 81*, 2799–2803.

35. Gallagher, P. G. (2013). Abnormalities of the erythrocyte membrane. *Pediatr Clin N Am, 60*, 1349–1362.

36. Ideguchi, H., Yamada, Y., Kondo, S., et al. (1993). Abnormal erythrocyte band 4.1 protein in myelodysplastic syndrome with elliptocytosis. *Br J Haematol, 85*, 387–392.

37. King, M-J., Telfer, P., MacKinnon, H., et al. (2008). Using the eosin-5-maleimide binding test in the differential diagnosis of hereditary spherocytosis and hereditary pyropoikilocytosis. *Cytometry B Clin Cytom, 74B*, 244–250.

38. Mohandas, N., Winardi, R., Knowles, D., et al. (1992). Molecular basis for membrane rigidity of hereditary ovalocytosis. A novel mechanism involving the cytoplasmic domain of band 3. *J Clin Invest, 89*, 686–692.

39. Liu, S-C., Zhai, S., Palek, J., et al. (1990). Molecular defect of the band 3 protein in Southeast Asian ovalocytosis. *N Engl J Med, 323*, 1530–1538.

40. Schofield, A. E., Tanner, M. J. A., Pinder, J. C., et al. (1992). Basis of unique red cell membrane properties in hereditary ovalocytosis. *J Mol Biol, 223*, 949–958.

41. Bruce, L. J. (2009). Hereditary stomatocytosis and cation leaky red cells—recent developments. *Blood Cells Mol Dis, 42*, 216–222.

42. Bruce, L. J., Guizouarn, H., Burton, N. M., et al. (2009). The monovalent cation leak in overhydrated stomatocytic red blood cells results from amino acid substitutions in the Rh-associated glycoprotein. *Blood, 113*, 1350–1357.

43. Zarychanski, R., Schulz, V. P., Houston, B. L., et al. (2012). Mutations in the mechanotransduction protein PIEZO1 are associated with hereditary xerocytosis. *Blood, 120*, 1908–1915.

44. Bae, C., Gnanasambandam, R., Nicolai, C., et al. (2013). Xerocytosis is caused by mutations that alter the kinetics of the mechanosensitive channel PIEZO1. *Proc Natl Acad Sci U S A, 110*, E1162–E1168.

45. Andolfo, I., Alper, S. L., De Franceschi, L., et al. (2013). Multiple clinical forms of dehydrated hereditary stomatocytosis arise from mutations in PIEZO1. *Blood, 121*, 3925–3935.

46. Rampoldi, L., Danek, A., & Monaco, A. P. (2002). Clinical features and molecular bases of neuroacanthocytosis. *J Mol Med, 80*, 475–491.

47. Walker, R. H., Jung, H. H., Dobson-Stone, C., et al. (2007). Neurologic phenotypes associated with acanthocytosis. *Neurology, 68*, 92–98.

48. Parker, C. J. (2010). Paroxysmal nocturnal hemoglobinuria. In Lichtman, M. A., Kipps, T. J., Seligsohn, U., et al. (Eds.), *Williams Hematology*. (8th ed.). New York: McGraw-Hill. http://accessmedicine.mhmedical.com.libproxy2.umdnj.edu/content.aspx?bookid=358&Sectionid=39835858. Accessed 09.03.14.

49. Besslar, M., & Hiken, J. (2008). The pathophysiology of disease in patients with paroxysmal nocturnal hemoglobinuria. *Hematology Am Soc Hematol Educ Program*, 104–110.

50. Brodsky, R. A. (2013). Paroxysmal nocturnal hemoglobinuria. In Hoffman, R., Benz, E. J. Jr, Silberstein, L. E., et al. (Eds.), *Hematology: Basic Principles and Practice*. (6th ed.). Philadelphia: Saunders, an imprint of Elsevier.

51. Takeda, J., Miyata, T., Kawagoe, K., et al. (1993). Deficiency of the GPI anchor caused by a somatic mutation of the *PIG-A* gene in paroxysmal nocturnal hemoglobinuria. *Cell, 73*, 703–711.

52. Parker, C., Omine, M., Richards, S., et al. (2005). Diagnosis and management of paroxysmal nocturnal hemoglobinuria. *Blood, 106*, 3699–3709.

53. Sutherland, R. D., Keeney, M., & Illingworth, A. (2012). Practical guidelines for the high-sensitivity detection and monitoring of paroxysmal nocturnal hemoglobinuria clones by flow cytometry. *Cytometry Part B, 82B*, 195–208.

54. Preis, M., & Lowrey, C. H. (2014). Laboratory tests for paroxysmal nocturnal hemoglobinuria. *Am J Hematol, 89*, 339–341.

55. Sutherland, D. R., Kuek, N., Azcona-Olivera, J., et al. (2009). Use of FLAER-based WBC assay in the primary screening of PNH clones. *Am J Clin Pathol, 132*, 564–572.

56. Dmytrijuk, A., Robie-Suh, K., Cohen, M. H., et al. (2008). FDA report: eculizumab (Soliris) for the treatment of patients with paroxysmal nocturnal hemoglobinuria. *Oncologist, 13*, 993–1000.

57. Hillmen, P., Muus, P., Röth, A., et al. (2013). Long-term safety and efficacy of sustained eculizumab treatment in patients with paroxysmal nocturnal hemoglobinuria. *Br J Haematol, 162*, 62–73.

58. Risitano, A. M., Notaro, R., Pascariello, C., et al. (2012). The complement receptor 2/factor H fusion protein TT30 protects paroxysmal nocturnal hemoglobinuria erythrocytes from complement-mediated hemolysis and C3 fragment opsonization. *Blood, 119*, 6307–6316.

59. Price, E. A., Otis, S., & Schrier, S. L. (2013). Red blood cell enzymopathies. In Hoffman, R., Benz, E. J. Jr, Silberstein, L. E., et al. (Eds.), *Hematology: Basic Principles and Practice*. (6th ed.). Philadelphia: Saunders, an imprint of Elsevier.

60. Cappellini, M. D., & Fiorelli, G. (2008). Glucose-6-phosphate dehydrogenase deficiency. *Lancet, 371*, 64–74.

61. van Solinge, W. W., & van Wijk, R. (2010). Disorders of red cells resulting from enzyme abnormalities. In Lichtman, M. A., Kipps, T. J., Seligsohn, U., Kaushansky, K., & Prchal, J. T. (Eds.), *Williams Hematology*. (8th ed.). New York: McGraw-Hill. http://accessmedicine.mhmedical.com.libproxy2.umdnj.edu/content.aspx?bookid=358&Sectionid=39835864. Accessed 31.03.14.

62. Nkhoma, E. T., Poole, C., Vannappagari, V., et al. (2009). The global prevalence of glucose-6-phosphate dehydrogenase deficiency: a systematic review and meta-analysis. *Blood Cells Mol Dis, 42*, 267–278.

63. Luzzatto, L. (2006). Glucose 6-phosphate dehydrogenase deficiency: from genotype to phenotype. *Hematologica, 91*, 1303–1306.

64. Guindo, A., Fairhurst, R. M., Doumbo, O. K., et al. (2007). X-linked G6PD deficiency protects hemizygous males but not heterozygous females against severe malaria. *PLoS, 4*(3), e66.

65. Leslie, T., Briceno, M., Mayan, I., et al. (2010). The impact of phenotypic and genotypic G6PD deficiency on risk of *Plasmodium vivax* infection: a case-control study amongst Afghan refugees in Pakistan. *PLoS, 7*(5), e1000283.

66. Clark, I. A., & Hunt, N. H. (1983). Evidence for reactive oxygen intermediates causing hemolysis and parasite death in malaria. *Infect Immun, 39*, 1–6.

67. Cappadoro, M., Giribaldi, G., O'Brien, E., et al. (1998). Early phagocytosis of glucose-6-phosphate dehydrogenase (G6PD)-deficient erythrocytes parasitized by *Plasmodium falciparum* may explain malaria protection in G6PD deficiency. *Blood, 92,* 2527–2534.

68. Minucci, A., Moradkhani, K., Hwang, M. J., et al. (2012). Glucose-6-phosphate dehydrogenase (*G6PD*) mutations database: review of the "old" and update of the new mutations. *Blood Cells Mol Dis, 48,* 154–165.

69. Beutler, E., Gaetani, G., der Kaloustian, V., et al. (1989). World Health Organization (WHO) Working Group. Glucose-6-phosphate dehydrogenase deficiency. *Bull World Health Organ, 67,* 601–611.

70. Youngster, I., Arcavi, L., Schechmaster, R., et al. (2010). Medications and glucose-6-phosphate dehydrogenase deficiency: an evidence-based review. *Drug Saf, 33,* 713–726.

71. Luzzatto, L., & Seneca, E. (2014). G6PD deficiency: a classic example of pharmacogenetics with on-going clinical implications. *Br J Haematol, 164,* 469–480.

72. Kaplan, M., Muraca, M., Vreman, H. J., et al. (2005). Neonatal bilirubin production-conjugation imbalance: effect of glucose-6-phosphate dehydrogenase deficiency and borderline prematurity. *Arch Dis Child Fetal Neonatal Ed, 90,* F123–F127.

73. Prchal, J. T., & Gregg, X. T: (2005). Red cell enzymes. *Hematol Am Soc Hematol Educ Program,* pp. 19–23.

74. Minucci, A., Giardina, B., & Zuppi, C., et al. (2009). Glucose-6-phosphate dehydrogenase laboratory assay: how, when, and why? *IUBMB Life, 61,* 27–34.

75. Tantular, I. S., & Kawamoto, F. (2003). An improved simple screening method for detection of glucose-6-phosphate dehydrogenase deficiency. *Trop Med Int Health, 8,* 569–574.

76. Tinley, K. E., Loughlin, A. M., Jepson, A., et al. (2010). Evaluation of a rapid qualitative enzyme chromatographic test for glucose-6-phosphate dehydrogenase deficiency. *Am J Trop Med Hyg, 82,* 210–214.

77. Beutler, E., & Gelbart, T. (2000). Estimating the prevalence of pyruvate kinase deficiency from the gene frequency in the general white population. *Blood, 95,* 3585–3588.

78. Zanella, A., Bianchi, P., Fermo, E., et al. (2007). Pyruvate kinase deficiency. *Hematologica, 92,* 721–722.

79. Rider, N. L., Strauss, K. A., Brown, K., et al. (2011). Erythrocyte pyruvate kinase deficiency in an old-order Amish cohort: longitudinal risk and disease management. *Am J Hematol, 86,* 827–834.

80. Christensen, R. D., Yaish, H. M., Johnson, C. B., et al. (2011). Six children with pyruvate kinase deficiency in one small town: Molecular characterization of the PK-LR gene. *J Pediatr, 159,* 695–697.

81. Van Wijk, R., & van Solinge, W. W. (2005). The energy-less red blood cell is lost: erythrocyte enzyme abnormalities of glycolysis. *Blood, 106,* 4034–4042.

82. Zanella, A., Fermo, E., Bianchi, P., et al. (2005). Red cell pyruvate kinase deficiency: molecular and clinical aspects. *Br J Haematol, 130,* 11–25.

83. Andersen, F. D., d'Amore, F., Nielsen, F. C., et al. (2004). Unexpectedly high but still asymptomatic iron overload in a patient with pyruvate kinase deficiency. *Hematol J, 5,* 543–545.

84. Tsang, S. S., & Feng, C. S. (1993). A modified screening procedure to detect pyruvate kinase deficiency. *Am J Clin Pathol, 99,* 128–131.

85. Zanella, A., Bianchi, P., Fermo, E., et al. (2006). Hereditary pyrimidine 5'-nucleotidase deficiency: from genetics to clinical manifestations. *Br J Haematol, 133,* 113–123.

25

Extrinsic Defects Leading to Increased Erythrocyte Destruction— Nonimmune Causes

Elaine M. Keohane

OBJECTIVES

After completion of this chapter, the reader will be able to:

1. Describe the general pathophysiology and clinical laboratory findings in microangiopathic hemolytic anemia, including the characteristic red blood cell morphology.
2. Compare and contrast the pathophysiology, clinical symptoms, and typical laboratory findings in thrombotic thrombocytopenic purpura, hemolytic uremic syndrome, HELLP (*h*emolysis, *e*levated *l*iver enzymes, and *l*ow *p*latelet count) syndrome, and disseminated intravascular coagulation.
3. Explain the pathophysiology and typical laboratory features of traumatic cardiac hemolytic anemia and exercise-induced hemoglobinuria.
4. Describe the life cycle of *Plasmodium,* including the hepatic and erythrocytic cycles, and the insect vector.
5. Explain the pathophysiologic mechanisms in *P. falciparum* infection that lead to anemia and neurologic manifestations.

6. Differentiate the five *Plasmodium* species affecting humans based on the geographic distribution, characteristic morphology on a peripheral blood film, the extent of parasitemia, and the length of the erythrocytic cycle.
7. Describe the proper specimen collection and procedure for performing a thin and thick blood film examination.
8. Compare and contrast *Babesia* species and *Plasmodium* species in terms of geographic distribution, clinical symptoms of infection, and morphology.
9. Describe the pathophysiology, laboratory findings, and peripheral blood morphology in hemolytic anemia due to clostridial sepsis, bartonellosis, drugs, chemicals, venoms, and extensive burns.
10. Given the history, symptoms, laboratory findings, and a representative microscopic field from a peripheral blood film of a patient with suspected extrinsic, nonimmune hemolytic anemia, discuss possible causes of the anemia and indicate the data that support the conclusions.

CASE STUDY

After studying the material in this chapter, the reader should be able to respond to the following case study:

A 24-year-old woman was brought to the emergency department with a 2-day history of fever, chills, excessive sweating, nausea, and general malaise. Because she had recently returned from a 3-week family trip to Ghana in Western Africa, the treating physician ordered a CBC and examination of thin and thick peripheral blood films. The following are the patient's laboratory results:

	Patient Results	Reference Interval
WBCs ($\times 10^9$/L)	11.0	4.5–11.0
HGB (g/dL)	8.7	12.0–15.0
HCT (%)	25	35–49
MCV (fL)	92	80–100
Platelets ($\times 10^9$/L)	176	150–450

After studying the material in this chapter, the reader should be able to respond to the following case study:

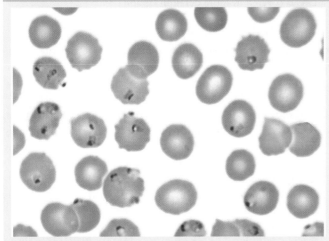

Figure 25-1 Thin peripheral blood film for the patient in the case study (×1000).

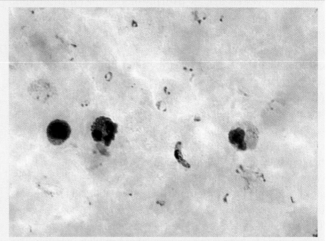

Figure 25-2 Thick peripheral blood film for the patient in the case study (×1000). (Courtesy Linda Marler, Indiana Pathology Images.)

Inclusions were noted on the thin and thick peripheral blood films (Figures 25-1 and 25-2).

Based on the results of the CBC and peripheral blood films, the patient was treated with oral quinine sulfate and doxycycline.

1. Identify the inclusions present on the thin and thick peripheral blood films.

2. What is the likely diagnosis for this patient?
3. What clues in the history support this diagnosis?
4. What other forms might be found on the peripheral blood films in this disease?
5. What are the pathophysiologic mechanisms for the anemia in this disease?

Extrinsic hemolytic anemias comprise a diverse group of disorders in which red blood cells (RBCs) are structurally and functionally normal, but a condition outside of the RBCs causes premature hemolysis. The extrinsic hemolytic anemias can be divided into conditions with nonimmune and immune causes. A common feature in the nonimmune extrinsic hemolytic anemias is the presence of a condition that causes physical or mechanical injury to the RBCs. This injury can be caused by abnormalities in the microvasculature (microangiopathic) or the heart and large blood vessels (macroangiopathic), infectious agents, chemicals, drugs, venoms, or extensive burns. The nonimmune disorders causing hemolytic anemia are discussed in this chapter and are summarized in Box 25-1. In immune hemolytic anemia, hemolysis is mediated by antibodies, complement, or both, and these conditions are covered in Chapter 26. Examination of a peripheral blood film is important in suspected extrinsic hemolytic anemias, because observation of abnormal RBC morphology, such as schistocytes, spherocytes, or the presence of intracellular organisms, provides an important clue to the diagnosis.

MICROANGIOPATHIC HEMOLYTIC ANEMIA

Microangiopathic hemolytic anemias (MAHAs) are a group of potentially life-threatening disorders characterized by RBC

BOX 25-1 Extrinsic Conditions Causing Nonimmune Red Blood Cell Injury and Hemolytic Anemia

Microangiopathic hemolytic anemia
  Thrombotic thrombocytopenic purpura
  Hemolytic uremic syndrome
  HELLP syndrome
  Disseminated intravascular coagulation
Macroangiopathic hemolytic anemia
  Traumatic cardiac hemolytic anemia
  Exercise-induced hemoglobinuria
Infection
  Malaria
  Babesiosis
  Clostridial sepsis
  Bartonellosis
RBC injury due to other causes
  Chemicals
  Drugs
  Venoms
  Extensive burns

HELLP, Hemolysis, elevated liver enzymes, and low platelet count; *RBC,* red blood cell.

fragmentation and thrombocytopenia. The RBC fragmentation occurs intravascularly by the mechanical shearing of RBC membranes as the cells rapidly pass through turbulent areas of small blood vessels that are partially blocked by microthrombi or damaged endothelium.[1,2] Upon shearing, RBC membranes quickly reseal with minimal escape of hemoglobin, but the resulting fragments (called *schistocytes*) are distorted and become rigid.[1] The spleen clears the rigid RBC fragments from the circulation through the extravascular hemolytic process (Chapter 23).[1] Laboratory evidence of the hemolytic anemia includes a decreased hemoglobin level, increased reticulocyte count, increased serum indirect (unconjugated) bilirubin, increased serum lactate dehydrogenase activity, decreased serum haptoglobin level, and increased urine urobilinogen. In some cases, the fragmentation is so severe that intravascular hemolysis occurs with varying amounts of hemoglobinemia, hemoglobinuria, and markedly decreased levels of serum haptoglobin.[1] The presence of schistocytes on the peripheral blood film is a characteristic feature of microangiopathic hemolytic anemia. The RBC shearing may also produce helmet cells and, occasionally, microspherocytes. Polychromasia and nucleated RBCs may also be present on the blood film, depending on the severity of the anemia.

Thrombocytopenia is also a feature of microangiopathic hemolytic anemia; it is due to the consumption of platelets in thrombi that form in the microvasculature.[3] Thus these disorders are sometimes called *thrombotic microangiopathies*.[4,5]

The major microangiopathic hemolytic anemias include thrombotic thrombocytopenic purpura (TTP), hemolytic uremic syndrome (HUS), HELLP (*h*emolysis, *e*levated *l*iver enzymes, *l*ow *p*latelet count) syndrome, and disseminated intravascular coagulation (DIC).[1,4,5] TTP and HUS can be difficult to differentiate because they have overlapping clinical and laboratory findings (Box 25-2). Definitive diagnosis, however, is critical because

they have different etiologies and require different treatments.[3] This chapter provides an overview of these conditions. TTP, HUS, and HELLP syndrome are covered in more detail in Chapter 40. DIC is covered in more detail in Chapter 39.

Thrombotic Thrombocytopenic Purpura

Thrombotic thrombocytopenic purpura is a rare, life-threatening disorder characterized by the abrupt appearance of microangiopathic hemolytic anemia, severe thrombocytopenia, and markedly elevated serum lactate dehydrogenase activity.[2,6] Neurologic dysfunction, fever, and renal failure may also occur, but they are not consistently present.[2,6] TTP is most commonly found in adults in their fourth decade, but it can present at any age.[5,6] There is a higher incidence in females than in males.[5]

TTP is caused by a deficiency of the von Willebrand factor-cleaving protease known as a *disintegrin and metalloproteinase with a thrombospondin type 1 motif, member 13* (ADAMTS-13).[6-9] ADAMTS-13 regulates the size of circulating von Willebrand factor (VWF) by cleaving ultra-long VWF multimers (ULVWF) into shorter segments that have less hemostatic potential.[6,10] VWF multimers circulate in a folded conformation so that their cleavage sites for ADAMTS-13 (in the A2 domain) and binding sites for platelets (GP Ibα receptor in the A1 domain) are hidden.[5,6,10] These sites normally become accessible only when the ULVWF multimer is "unrolled or stretched out," which occurs (1) during its release from endothelial cells, (2) during passage through small blood vessels with very high shear forces, or (3) after binding to collagen in the subendothelium after vascular injury (Chapter 37).[5,6,10] Once unrolled, ADAMTS-13 binds to the cleavage sites on the ULVWFs and cuts them into smaller multimers.[6,10] Thus ADAMTS-13 serves an important antithrombotic function by preventing VWF from excessively binding and activating platelets.[6]

When ADAMTS-13 is deficient, however, the hyperreactive ULVWF multimers adhere to the endothelial cells of the microvasculature, where they readily unroll as a result of hydrodynamic shear forces.[5-7,10] Platelets are then able to bind to the A1 domains of the ULVWF multimers, and platelet aggregation is triggered.[5,6] The platelet-VWF microthrombi accumulate in and block small blood vessels, leading to severe thrombocytopenia; ischemia in the brain, kidney, and other organs; and hemolytic anemia due to RBC rupture as they pass through blood vessels partially blocked by microthrombi.[2,3,7] The intravascular hemolysis along with the extensive tissue ischemia result in a striking increase in serum lactate dehydrogenase activity that is characteristic of TTP.[5]

TTP can be idiopathic, secondary, or inherited. Idiopathic TTP has no known precipitating event.[5,6] In idiopathic TTP, autoantibodies to ADAMTS-13 inhibit its activity, causing a severe deficiency.[5,8,9] These autoantibodies are usually of the IgG class but can be IgM or IgA.

Secondary TTP can be triggered by infections, pregnancy, surgery, trauma, inflammation, and disseminated malignancy, possibly by depressing the synthesis of ADAMTS-13.[3,5] Other conditions may induce an inhibitory reaction to ADAMTS-13, including hematopoietic stem cell transplantation; autoimmune disorders; human immunodeficiency virus (HIV); and

---

BOX 25-2   **Typical Laboratory Findings in TTP and HUS**

Hematologic
   Decreased hemoglobin
   Decreased platelets
   Increased reticulocyte count
Peripheral blood film
   Schistocytes
   Polychromasia
   Nucleated red blood cells (severe cases)
Biochemical
   Markedly increased lactate dehydrogenase activity*
   Increased serum total and indirect bilirubin
   Decreased serum haptoglobin level
   Hemoglobinemia
   Hemoglobinuria
   Proteinuria, hematuria, casts†

HUS, Hemolytic uremic syndrome; *TTP*, thrombotic thrombocytopenic purpura.
*From systemic ischemia and hemolysis; more commonly found in TTP.
†From acute renal failure; more commonly found in HUS.

certain drugs, such as quinine, ticlopidine, and trimethoprim. [3-6,11] Secondary TTP is very heterogeneous, and the mechanisms that trigger the TTP pathophysiology are not completely clear.[3]

Inherited TTP, also called *Upshaw-Schülman syndrome,* is a severe ADAMTS-13 deficiency caused by mutations in the *ADAMTS13* gene.[5,6,12] Over 75 different mutations have been identified, and symptomatic individuals are either homozygous for one of the mutations or compound heterozygous for two different mutations.[5,12,13] Inherited TTP may present in infancy or childhood with recurrent episodes throughout life; however, some patients may not be symptomatic until adulthood after their system is stressed by pregnancy or a severe infection.

Typical initial laboratory findings in all types of TTP include a hemoglobin level of 8 to 10 g/dL, a platelet count of 10 to 30 × 10⁹/L, and schistocytes on the peripheral blood film (Figure 25-3).[6] After the bone marrow begins to respond to the anemia, polychromasia and nucleated RBCs may also be present on the blood film. The white blood cell count is often increased, and immature granulocytes may appear. The bone marrow shows erythroid hyperplasia and a normal number of megakaryocytes. Hemoglobinuria occurs when there is extensive intravascular hemolysis. Various amounts of protein, RBCs, and urinary casts may also be present in the urine, depending on the extent of the renal damage. Results of coagulation tests are usually within the reference interval, which differentiates TTP from DIC (covered below). An elevation of the serum indirect bilirubin level does not occur for several days after an acute onset of hemolysis, but the serum lactate dehydrogenase activity will be markedly elevated and the serum haptoglobin level will be reduced.

In idiopathic and inherited TTP, the ADAMTS-13 activity is usually severely reduced to less than 5% to 10% of normal.[4,6,7] In secondary TTP, the ADAMTS-13 deficiency is not as severe. ADAMTS-13 autoantibodies can be detected in idiopathic TTP but are absent in inherited TTP.[6]

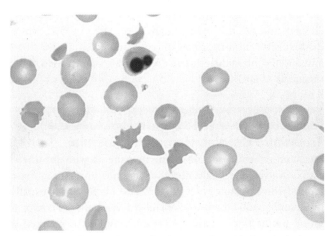

Figure 25-3 Peripheral blood film from a patient with thrombotic thrombocytopenic purpura. Note the schistocytes and a nucleated red blood cell (×1000).

Approximately 80% to 90% of patients with idiopathic TTP respond favorably to plasma exchange therapy due to the removal of the offending ADAMTS-13 autoantibody and infusion of replacement ADAMTS-13 enzyme from donor plasma.[6,11] Therefore, it is important that this type of TTP be recognized and quickly treated with plasma exchange therapy to avoid a fatal outcome. Corticosteroids are also administered to suppress the autoimmune response.[5,6] Approximately one third of patients who respond to plasma exchange experience recurrent episodes of TTP.[4] Rituximab (anti-CD20) is effective in suppressing an autoantibody response in some patients with relapsing TTP.[6] Patients with secondary TTP generally do not respond well to plasma exchange, and the prognosis in these cases is poor, except when the TTP is related to autoimmune disease, pregnancy, or ticlopidine use.[11,13] Plasma exchange is not required in inherited TTP, which is treated by infusion of fresh frozen plasma to supply the deficient ADAMTS-13 enzyme.[3,4,6]

Hemolytic Uremic Syndrome

HUS is characterized by microangiopathic hemolytic anemia, thrombocytopenia, and acute renal failure from damage to endothelial cells in the glomerular microvasculature.[3,5] There are two general types: typical and atypical HUS. Typical HUS (Shiga toxin-associated HUS or stx-HUS) is caused by bacteria that produce Shiga toxin and is preceded by an episode of acute gastroenteritis, often with bloody diarrhea.[5] Atypical HUS (aHUS) is caused by unregulated activation of the alternative complement pathway.[3,5] Patients with HUS have the typical laboratory findings of microangiopathic hemolytic anemia discussed previously. However, the platelet count is only mildly to moderately decreased, and evidence of renal failure is usually present, including an elevated level of serum creatinine, proteinuria, hematuria, and the presence of hyaline, granular, and RBC casts in the urine (Box 25-2).

The stx-HUS type comprises 90% of cases of HUS.[5,14] The most common cause is infection with Shiga toxin-producing *Escherichia coli* (STEC), such as serotype O157:H7, but strains of toxin-producing *Shigella* have also been implicated.[4,5] Stx-HUS occurs most often in young children but can be found in patients of all ages. Patients initially have acute gastroenteritis, often with bloody diarrhea, and after approximately 5 to 13 days develop oliguria and other symptoms of renal damage.[5] About one fourth of patients also develop neurologic manifestations.[5,14]

E. coli and *Shigella* serotypes implicated in HUS release Shiga toxins (Stx-1 and Stx-2, also called *verotoxins*) that are absorbed from the intestines into the plasma. The toxins have an affinity for the Gb3 glycolipid receptors (CD77) on endothelial cells, particularly those in the glomerulus and brain.[4,5,15] The toxin is transported into the endothelial cells, where it inhibits protein synthesis and causes endothelial cell injury and eventual apoptosis.[5,15] The Shiga toxin, together with many cytokines secreted as a result of the infection, also induces changes in endothelial cells that are prothrombotic, including expression of tissue factor, adhesion molecules, and secretion of increased amounts of ULVWF multimers.[4,5,15] The endothelial cell damage can cause stenosis (narrowing) of small blood vessels which can be exacerbated by activation of platelets and formation platelet-fibrin thrombi.[3,5,15] The resultant blockages in the microvasculature of the glomeruli results in acute renal failure.[3,15] Endothelial damage and microthrombi can also occur in the microvasculature of the brain and other organs.[3,5] There is no specific treatment for stx-HUS, but patients are provided supportive care as needed, including hydration, dialysis, and transfusions.[14,15] The symptoms usually resolve spontaneously in 1 to 3 weeks, and the prognosis is favorable for most patients.[14]

Atypical HUS comprises about 10% of cases of HUS and can first present in infancy, childhood, or adulthood.[5,16] The characteristic feature is uncontrolled activation of the alternative complement system, which causes endothelial cell injury, activation of platelets and coagulation factors, and formation of platelet-fibrin thrombi that obstruct the microvasculature in the glomerulus and other organs.[3,5] Approximately 50% to 70% of aHUS patients have inherited mutations in genes that code for components of the alternative complement pathway or its regulatory proteins.[5,16] Inactivating mutations have been identified in genes for complement regulatory proteins, including complement factor H, complement factor I, membrane cofactor protein, and thrombomodulin.[3,5,16] Activating mutations have been identified in the genes for complement factor B and C3.[3,5,16] An acquired form of aHUS is associated with autoantibodies against complement factor H and accounts for approximately 5% to 10% of cases.[5] In the remaining cases, no mutation or autoantibodies have been identified.[5] aHUS may be triggered by hematopoietic stem cell therapy, pregnancy, infection, inflammation, surgery, or trauma.[3] Plasma exchange and plasma infusion have limited efficacy in aHUS.[5,16] In recent studies, therapy with eculizumab (antibody to C5) has improved platelet counts and renal function in aHUS patients and may become the therapy of choice.[16]

Differential diagnosis of aHUS and TTP is difficult due to the similarities in their clinical presentation and initial laboratory findings. Both are life-threatening disorders that require rapid action to prevent a fatal outcome, with plasma exchange most beneficial for TTP, and eculizumab more likely to benefit patients with aHUS.[5,16] Assays for ADAMTS-13 activity currently lack sufficient sensitivity and specificity and are not available in all laboratories.[16] DNA analysis for complement system gene mutations is available in specialized laboratories but the results are not timely enough to be used in initial therapy decisions.[16] More sensitive, specific, and rapid tests are needed for definitive diagnosis of these two conditions.

HELLP Syndrome

HELLP syndrome is a serious complication in pregnancy and is named for its characteristic presentation of *h*emolysis, *e*levated *l*iver enzymes, and *l*ow *p*latelet count. It occurs in less than 1% of all pregnancies but develops in approximately 10% to 20% of pregnancies with severe preeclampsia, most often in the third trimester.[17] The exact pathogenesis is not known. In preeclampsia, abnormalities in the development of placental vasculature result in poor perfusion and hypoxia. As a result,

antiangiogenic proteins are released from the placenta that block the action of placental growth factors, including vascular endothelial growth factor.[18] Continued vascular insufficiency of the placenta results in maternal endothelial cell dysfunction, which leads to platelet activation and fibrin deposition in the microvasculature, particularly in the liver.[18]

Anemia, biochemical evidence of hemolysis, and schistocytes on the peripheral blood film are found as in the other microangiopathies. The platelet count is less than $100 \times 10^9/L$; counts falling below $50 \times 10^9/L$ indicate a worse prognosis.[18,19] The serum lactate dehydrogenase activity is elevated, which reflects the hepatic necrosis as well as the hemolysis. The serum aspartate aminotransferase activity can be markedly elevated due to the severe hepatocyte injury. The low platelet count and increased serum lactate dehydrogenase and aspartate aminotransferase activity are major diagnostic criteria for the HELLP syndrome and are used to assess the severity of the disease.[17,18] The prothrombin time and the partial thromboplastin time are within the reference interval, which distinguishes the HELLP syndrome from DIC. Therapy includes delivery of the fetus and placenta as soon as possible, along with supportive care to control seizures, hypertension, and fluid balance. The mortality rate is 3% to 5% for the mother and 9% to 24% for the fetus.[18]

Disseminated Intravascular Coagulation

Disseminated intravascular coagulation (DIC) is characterized by the widespread activation of the hemostatic system, resulting in fibrin thrombi formation throughout the microvasculature. The major clinical manifestations are organ damage due to obstruction of the microvasculature and bleeding due to the consumption of platelets and coagulation factors and secondary activation of fibrinolysis. DIC is a complication of many disorders, such as metastatic cancers, acute leukemias, infections, obstetric complications, crush or brain injuries, acute hemolytic transfusion reactions, extensive burns, snake or spider envenomation, and chronic inflammation (Table 39-14).

Thrombocytopenia of varying degrees is a consistent finding. Only about half of the patients have schistocytes on the peripheral blood film.[20] The prothrombin time and partial thromboplastin time are prolonged, the fibrinogen level is decreased, and the level of D-dimer is increased in DIC, which distinguish it from the other microangiopathies. Tables 39-15 and 39-16 contain the primary and specialized tests used in the diagnosis of DIC.

MACROANGIOPATHIC HEMOLYTIC ANEMIA

Traumatic Cardiac Hemolytic Anemia

Mechanical hemolysis can occur in patients with prosthetic cardiac valves due to the turbulent blood flow through and around the implanted devices.[18,21] The hemolysis is usually mild, and anemia does not generally develop due to compensation by the bone marrow.[21] Severe hemolysis is rare and is usually due to paravalvular leaks in prosthetic cardiac valves.[21] Hemolysis can also occur in patients with cardiac valve disease prior to corrective surgery.[18] The anemia that occurs in severe cases is usually normocytic but can be microcytic if iron deficiency develops due to chronic urinary hemoglobin loss.

Depending on the severity of the hemolysis and the ability of the bone marrow to compensate for the reduced RBC life span, patients can be asymptomatic or present with pallor, fatigue, and even heart failure.[21] On the peripheral blood film, schistocytes are a characteristic feature due to the mechanical fragmentation of the RBCs (Figure 25-4). The reticulocyte count is increased, but the platelet count is within the reference interval. Serum lactate dehydrogenase activity and levels of serum indirect bilirubin and plasma hemoglobin are elevated, and the serum haptoglobin level is decreased. Hemoglobinuria may be observed in severe hemolysis. Hemosiderinuria and a decreased level of serum ferritin occur with chronic hemoglobinuria due to the urinary loss of iron.

Surgical repair or replacement of the prothesis may be required if the anemia is severe enough to require transfusions. For patients with hemoglobinuria, iron supplementation is provided to replace urinary iron loss. Folic acid may also be required, because deficiencies can occur due to the increased erythropoietic activity in the bone marrow.[21]

Exercise-Induced Hemoglobinuria

RBC lysis, with an increase in free plasma hemoglobin and a decrease in serum haptoglobin level, has been demonstrated in some individuals after long-distance running and to a lesser extent after intensive cycling and swimming,[1,22-24] but frank hemoglobinuria after exercise is a rare occurrence.[25] Exercise-induced hemoglobinuria has been reported mainly in endurance runners but has also been observed after strenuous hand drumming.[22,26] Various causes have been proposed, including mechanical trauma from the forceful, repeated impact of the feet or hands on hard surfaces;[22,23,26] increased RBC susceptibility to oxidative stress;[27] and exercise-induced alterations in membrane cytoskeletal proteins.[28,29]

Exercise-induced hemoglobinuria does not usually cause anemia unless the hemoglobinuria is particularly severe and recurrent.[1,25] Laboratory findings include a decreased level of serum haptoglobin, an elevated level of free plasma hemoglobin, and hemoglobinuria observed after strenuous exercise.

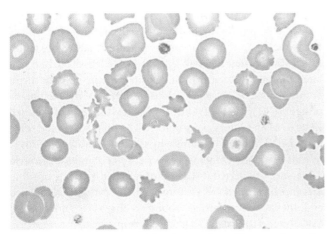

Figure 25-4 Peripheral blood film for a patient with traumatic cardiac hemolytic anemia. Note the presence of schistocytes (×1000).

Patients also have a slight increase in mean cell volume (MCV) and reticulocyte count. Schistocytes are not present on the peripheral blood film except in rare cases.[25,26] Exercise-induced hemoglobinuria is a diagnosis of exclusion, and other possible causes of hemolysis and hemoglobinuria should be investigated and ruled out.[25] There is no treatment for the disorder other than minimizing the physical impact on the feet with padding in shoes, running on softer terrain, or, if hemolysis is severe, discontinuing the activity.

HEMOLYTIC ANEMIA CAUSED BY INFECTIOUS AGENTS

Malaria

Malaria is a potentially fatal condition caused by infection of RBCs with protozoan parasites of the genus *Plasmodium*. Most human infections are caused by *P. falciparum* and *P. vivax*, but *P. ovale*, *P. malariae*, and a fifth species, *P. knowlesi*, also infect humans. *P. knowlesi*, a natural parasite of macaque monkeys, is easily misdiagnosed as *P. malariae* by microscopy, because the organisms are difficult to distinguish morphologically. Since 2004, hundreds of microscopically identified cases of *P. malariae* infection in Malaysia were actually found to be caused by *P. knowlesi* when polymerase chain reaction (PCR) assays were used, including tests on archival blood films from 1996.[30-32] With the use of molecular techniques, *P. knowlesi* malaria is now known to be widespread in Malaysia, and cases have been reported in other areas of Southeast Asia.[30-32]

Prevalence

Approximately 3.4 billion people live in areas in which malaria is endemic and are at risk for the disease.[33] Worldwide in 2012, there were an estimated 207 million cases of malaria, with 627,000 deaths, mostly in children younger than 5 years of age.[33] The majority of deaths were in Africa (90%), followed by Southeast Asia (7%) and the Eastern Mediterranean region (3%).[33] The World Health Organization is coordinating a major global effort to control and eliminate malaria. These efforts include implementation of indoor chemical spraying, distribution of millions of insecticide-treated sleeping nets in high-risk areas, and promotion of policies for appropriate treatment in regions of endemic disease.[33] An estimated 42% reduction in mortality rates from malaria occurred worldwide between 2000 and 2012, and the goal is to reduce mortality rates by 75% by 2015.[33]

In 2011, 1925 cases of malaria were diagnosed in the United States, and almost all of the cases were associated with travel to a malaria-endemic country.[34] *P. falciparum* and *P. vivax* cause most of the infections seen in the United States.

Plasmodium Life Cycle

Malaria is transmitted to humans by the bite of an infected female *Anopheles* mosquito. During a blood meal, sporozoites from the salivary gland of the mosquito are injected into the skin and migrate into the bloodstream of the human host. The sporozoites rapidly leave the circulating blood and invade hepatic parenchymal cells to begin *exoerythrocytic schizogony*, the parasite's asexual cycle. After 5 to 16 days (depending on the species), hepatic cells rupture, with each cell releasing tens of thousands of merozoites into the bloodstream to invade circulating RBCs, thus beginning erythrocytic schizogony.[35] Inside the erythrocyte, the merozoite grows and metabolizes the hemoglobin. The merozoite becomes a ring form, which grows into a mature trophozoite, then into an immature schizont (chromatin dividing), and finally into a mature schizont that contains merozoites. The merozoites are released from the erythrocytes into the bloodstream and invade other RBCs to continue the asexual cycle. As the infection continues, the cycles often recur at regular intervals as all the individual parasitic cycles become synchronous; this produces paroxysms of fever and chills at a frequency that varies according to malaria species. Resting stages of *P. vivax* and *P. ovale*, called *hypnozoites*, can remain dormant in the liver and produce a relapse months or years later.[36,37]

Some merozoites enter RBCs and form male and female gametocytes (sexual stages). Gametocytes are ingested by an *Anopheles* mosquito when it takes in a blood meal. The female gamete is fertilized by the male gamete in the mosquito gut to produce a zygote, which becomes an ookinete that migrates to the outer wall of the mosquito midgut and develops into an oocyst. The oocyst produces sporozoites that are released into the hemocele and migrate to the salivary glands of the mosquito. When the mosquito takes in a blood meal, the sporozoites are inoculated into the human host.

Other modes of transmission include congenital infection and transmission by blood transfusion, organ transplantation, or sharing of syringes and needles, but malaria acquired by these routes and local mosquito-transmitted malaria occur infrequently in the United States.[34]

Pathogenesis

If an individual is bitten by infected mosquitos, the clinical outcome may be (1) no infection, (2) *asymptomatic parasitemia* (the patient has no symptoms, but parasites are present in the blood), (3) *uncomplicated malaria* (the patient has symptoms and parasitemia but no organ dysfunction), or (4) *severe malaria* (the patient has symptoms, parasitemia, and major organ dysfunction).[33,36] The clinical outcome depends on parasite factors (species, number of sporozoites injected, multiplication rate, virulence, drug resistance), host factors (age, pregnancy status, immune status, previous exposure, genetic polymorphisms, nutrition status, coinfection with other pathogens, and duration of infection), geographic and social factors (endemicity, poverty, and availability of prompt and effective treatment), and other as yet unknown factors.[35,36,38] In areas of high *Plasmodium* transmission, most individuals develop immunity, and the major risk groups for severe malaria are children younger than 5 years of age and women in their first pregnancy.[39] Even in these risk groups, severe malaria is infrequent.[36] On the other hand, immunity is low or nonexistent in individuals living in regions with low *Plasmodium* transmission and in travelers to regions where malaria is endemic, so all age groups are at risk for severe malaria.[39] Most cases of severe malaria are due to *P. falciparum*; however, *P. vivax* and

P. knowlesi can also cause severe disease.[31,35] Infection with *P. malariae* or *P. ovale*, however, is usually uncomplicated and benign. *Hyperparasitemia*, defined as greater than 2% to 5% of the total RBCs parasitized, is usually present in severe malaria.[39] Major complications of severe malaria include respiratory distress syndrome, metabolic acidosis, circulatory shock, renal failure, hepatic failure, hypoglycemia, severe anemia (defined as a hemoglobin level below 5 g/dL),[39] poor pregnancy outcome, and cerebral malaria.[35] Even with treatment, the fatality rate of severe malaria is 10% to 20%.[39]

The causes of anemia in malaria include direct lysis of infected RBCs during schizogony, immune destruction of infected and noninfected RBCs in the spleen, and inhibition of erythropoiesis and ineffective erythropoiesis.[37,38] The destruction of noninfected RBCs contributes significantly to the anemia. In the invasion process, parasites shed proteins that bind to infected as well as noninfected RBCs.[40] These proteins may change the RBC membrane in noninfected cells, allowing adherence of immunoglobulins and complement and thus enhancing their removal by the spleen.[40,41] In addition, parasite proteins may also cause oxidative damage, resulting in decreased RBC survival.[42]

Malaria parasites metabolize hemoglobin, forming toxic *hemozoin* or malaria pigment. When RBCs lyse in schizogony, the hemozoin and other toxic metabolites are released, which results in an inflammatory response and cytokine imbalance.[40] Abnormal levels of tumor necrosis factor-α and interferon-γ result in inhibition of erythropoiesis as well as ineffective erythropoiesis; increased levels of interleukin-6 stimulate hepcidin production in the liver, which decreases the iron available to developing RBCs (Chapter 20).[40] In areas where malaria is endemic, poor nutrition and coinfection with hookworm or HIV contribute to the anemia, inflammation, and cytokine imbalance.[38,40]

P. falciparum is unique and particularly lethal in that infected RBCs adhere to endothelial cells in the microvasculature of internal organs, including the brain, heart, lung, liver, kidney, dermis, and placenta.[35,36] This contributes to the pathogenesis by obstructing the microvasculature and decreasing oxygen delivery to organs and by protecting the parasite from clearance by the spleen.[35,36] In the placental microvasculature, adherence of infected RBCs to endothelial cells results in local inflammation that can cause severe maternal anemia, decreased fetal growth, premature delivery, and increased risk of fetal loss.[35,36] In the brain microvasculature, adherence of infected RBCs to endothelial cells can cause lethal cerebral malaria. Infected RBCs express a parasite protein on their membranes, called *Plasmodium falciparum* erythrocyte membrane protein 1 (PfEMP1). PfEMP1 mediates binding of infected RBCs to cell receptors, particularly CD36 on platelets and some endothelial cells.[35,43] Reasons why some strains are more likely to cause severe cerebral malaria is a subject of intense research. Adherence of infected RBCs in the brain has been attributed to a complex formed by VWF released by cytokine-stimulated endothelial cells, platelets bound to the VWF, and infected RBCs bound to platelet CD36.[44] A recent mechanism was proposed whereby a specific variant of PfEMP1, expressed on the surface of RBCs infected with certain strains of *P. falciparum*, specifically binds to endothelial protein C receptor (EPCR) on endothelial cells lining the microvessels in the brain.[45] This binding prevents the activation of protein C (an inhibitor of activated factors V and VIII), creating a local hypercoagulable state in the brain. The result is fibrin deposition and parasite sequestration in the brain microvasculature and symptoms of severe cerebral malaria.[45]

The ability of the parasite to invade RBCs affects the extent of the parasitemia and the severity of the disease. *P. vivax* and *P. ovale* can only invade reticulocytes, and *P. malariae* can only invade older RBCs. On the other hand, *P. falciparum* and *P. knowlesi* are able to invade RBCs of all ages and thus can lead to very high levels of parasitemia.[35,37] *P. vivax* requires Duffy antigens on RBCs for invasion, so individuals lacking Duffy antigens are resistant to infection with *P. vivax*. The expansion of the Duffy-negative population in West Africa seems to be an effective genetic adaptation because *P. vivax* infection is almost nonexistent in West Africa.[35]

Polymorphisms in genes for the α and β hemoglobin chains (Hb S, Hb C, Hb E, and α- and β-thalassemia) and for glucose-6-phosphate dehydrogenase (G6PD) protect individuals from developing severe *falciparum* malaria. Although individuals with these polymorphisms become infected, they do not develop serious complications.[36] The reason for this protection has not been completely elucidated. Enhanced phagocytosis of ring forms (sickle cell trait, β-thalassemia trait, and G6PD deficiency),[46] decreased expression of *Pf*EMP1 on infected erythrocytes causing reduced endothelial adherence (sickle cell trait, Hb C disease and trait),[47,48] and decreased RBC invasion (Hb E trait)[49] may contribute to this protective effect. Over thousands of years, the evolutionary pressure of *P. falciparum* has resulted in a higher frequency of these polymorphisms in populations located in high-prevalence malaria regions, including sub-Saharan Africa, the Middle East, and Southeast Asia (Figure 27-3). Polymorphisms in cytokines and cellular receptors are also being investigated as modulators of malaria severity.[35]

Clinical and Laboratory Findings

The clinical symptoms of malaria are variable and can include fever, chills, rigors, sweating, headache, muscle pain, nausea, and diarrhea. In severe malaria, jaundice, splenomegaly, hepatomegaly, shock, prostration, bleeding, seizures, or coma may occur.[39] In patients with chronic malaria or with repeated malarial infections, the spleen may be massively enlarged.

During fevers, the WBC count is normal to slightly increased, but neutropenia may develop during chills and rigors. In chronic malaria with anemia, the reticulocyte count is decreased due to the negative effect of the inflammation on erythropoiesis. In severe malaria, one or more of the following laboratory features are found: metabolic acidosis, decreased serum glucose (less than 40 mg/dL), increased serum lactate, increased serum creatinine, decreased hemoglobin level (less than 5 g/dL), hemoglobinuria, and hyperparasitemia.[39]

Microscopic Examination

Malarial infection can be diagnosed microscopically by demonstration of the parasites in the peripheral blood. Optimally, blood should be collected before treatment is initiated.[37,50] At least two thick and two thin peripheral blood films should be made as soon as possible after collection of venous blood in ethylenediaminetetraacetic acid (EDTA) anticoagulant.[50] Alternatively, blood films can be made directly from a capillary puncture. Wright-Giemsa stain is used for visualization of the parasites.[37] Thick blood films concentrate the parasites and are ideal for initial screening of peripheral blood. They are stained with a water-based Wright-Giemsa stain without methanol fixation to lyse the RBCs (Box 25-3). Thin blood films are used for species identification and determination of the percent parasitemia; they are stained after methanol fixation. The percent parasitemia is determined by counting the number of parasitized RBCs (asexual stages) among 500 to 2000 RBCs on a thin peripheral blood film and converting to a percentage.[51] At least 300 fields on the thick and thin blood films should be examined with the 100× objective before a negative result is reported.[37,51] Multiple samples taken at 8- to 12-hour intervals may be needed because the number of circulating parasites may vary with the timing of the erythrocytic schizogony.[50] Microscopy can detect 5 to 20 parasites per microliter of blood, or 0.0001% parasitemia.[37] A negative result for a single set of thick and thin peripheral blood films does not rule out a diagnosis of malaria.[37] Malarial parasite detection and species identification require experienced laboratory personnel. A platelet lying on top of an erythrocyte in a thin blood film may be confused with a malarial parasite by an inexperienced observer (Figure 25-5).

BOX 25-3 **Thick Film Preparation for Malaria**

To make a thick film, place three small drops of blood close together near one end of the slide. With one corner of a clean slide, stir the blood for about 30 seconds to mix the three drops over an area approximately 1 to 2 cm in diameter. Allow the film to dry thoroughly. Stain the film using a water-based Giemsa stain. (The water-based stain lyses the red blood cells. Thin blood films are fixed in methyl alcohol to preserve the red blood cells so they do not lyse.) In a thick film, more parasites are seen in each field.

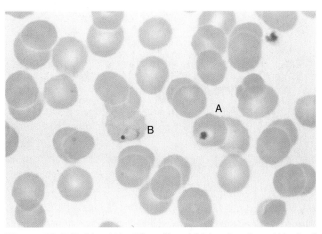

Figure 25-5 Peripheral blood film with a platelet on top of a red blood cell (**A**) compared with an intraerythrocytic *Plasmodium vivax* ring form (**B**) (×1000).

Plasmodium vivax. *P. vivax* is widely distributed and causes 40% of human malaria cases worldwide.[39] It is the predominant species in Asia and South and Central America, but also occurs in Southeast Asia, Oceania, and the Middle East.[52] It is rare in Africa and virtually absent in West Africa.[52] The early ring forms are delicate with a red chromatin dot and blue-staining cytoplasm. As the trophozoite grows, the RBC becomes enlarged. Schüffner stippling appears in all stages except the early ring forms. The growing trophozoite is ameboid in appearance and has fine light brown hemozoin pigment. The mature trophozoite almost fills the RBC (Figure 25-6). In an immature schizont, red chromatin begins to divide into two or more dots, and the mature schizont has 12 to 24 merozoites (Figure 25-7). Gametocytes are round with blue cytoplasm and light brown pigment; they have either centrally located (microgametocyte) or eccentrically located (macrogametocyte) red chromatin. The length of the erythrocytic cycle is 44 to 48 hours.[37] *P. vivax* is difficult to eradicate because the hypnozoite forms remain dormant in the liver and may cause a relapse.

Plasmodium ovale. *P. ovale* is found mainly in West Africa and India.[52] The young ring forms are larger and more ameboid than those of *P. vivax*, and as the trophozoite grows, the RBCs become enlarged, oval, and fringed (Figure 25-8). Schüffner stippling is present in all stages, including early ring forms. In the schizont stage, the RBCs are oval, and the parasite is round and compact. The mature schizont has 8 to 12 merozoites. Gametocytes are smaller than those of *P. vivax* but have a similar appearance. The length of the erythrocytic cycle is 48 hours.[37]

Plasmodium malariae. *P. malariae* is found worldwide but at low frequency. The highest prevalence is in East Africa and India.[52] The ring stage is often smaller and wider than that of *P. vivax*, although the two may be indistinguishable. In growing trophozoites, the cytoplasm forms a characteristic narrow band across the cell and contains dark brown pigment (Figure 25-9). RBCs do not become enlarged, and there is no stippling. The mature schizont has 6 to 12 merozoites and often forms a rosette around clumped pigment. Gametocytes

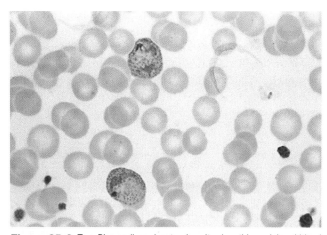

Figure 25-6 Two *Plasmodium vivax* trophozoites in a thin peripheral blood film. Note that the infected red blood cells are enlarged and contain Schüffner stippling, and the trophozoites are large and ameboid in appearance.

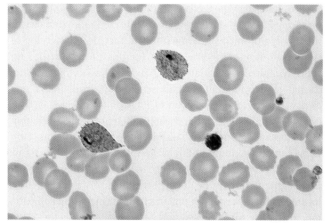

Figure 25-8 Two *Plasmodium ovale* trophozoites in a thin peripheral blood film. Note that the infected cells are enlarged, are oval, have fringed edges, and contain Schüffner stippling. (Courtesy Linda Marler, Indiana Pathology Images.)

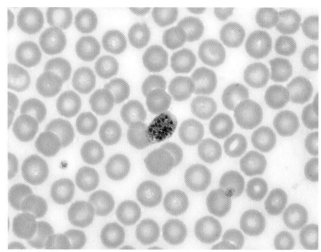

Figure 25-7 *Plasmodium vivax* schizont in a thin peripheral blood film. Note the number of merozoites and the presence of brown hemozoin pigment. (Courtesy Linda Marler, Indiana Pathology Images.)

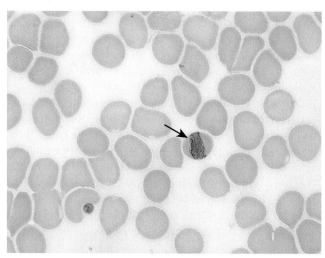

Figure 25-9 *Plasmodium malariae* band form in a thin peripheral blood film. (Courtesy Linda Marler, Indiana Pathology Images.)

are similar to those of *P. vivax* but are smaller. The length of the erythrocytic cycle is 72 hours.[37]

Plasmodium falciparum. *P. falciparum* is the predominant species in sub-Saharan Africa, Saudi Arabia, Haiti, and the Dominican Republic.[52] It is also found in Asia, Southeast Asia, the Philippines, Indonesia, and South America.[52] *P. falciparum* can produce high parasitemia (greater than 50% of RBCs infected) due to its ability to invade RBCs of all ages. Only ring forms and crescent- or banana-shaped gametocytes are observed in the peripheral blood. RBCs with trophozoites and schizonts adhere to the endothelial cells in various organs and do not circulate. Ring forms are small and can be easily missed. One or more rings may occupy a given cell, with some rings located at the cell periphery (Figure 25-1). The crescent-shaped gametocytes have deep blue cytoplasm with brownish pigment and red chromatin near the center and are easily recognized on blood films (Figure 25-10). The length of the erythrocytic cycle is 36 to 48 hours.[37]

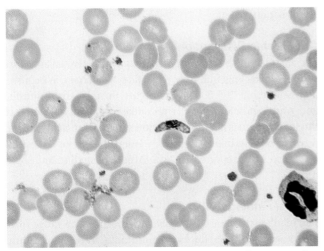

Figure 25-10 *Plasmodium falciparum* crescent-shaped gametocyte in a thin peripheral blood film (×1000). (Courtesy Linda Marler, Indiana Pathology Images.)

Plasmodium knowlesi. *P. knowlesi* is widespread in Malaysia, and cases have been reported in Myanmar, the Philippines, and Thailand.[52] In the early trophozoite stage, it can look similar to *P. falciparum* with high parasitemia and multiple ring forms in one cell. In the growing trophozoite, the cytoplasm forms a band across the cell, similar to *P. malariae* (Figure 25-11). Mature schizonts have an average of 16 merozoites and do not form rosettes.[37] The length of the erythrocytic cycle is only 24 hours, so infected patients can rapidly develop a high level of parasitemia and severe malaria; thus prompt diagnosis and treatment are critical.[31] Molecular methods may be required for definitive diagnosis. Figure 25-12 illustrates four species of *Plasmodium*.

Other Tests for Diagnosis

Fluorescent dyes may be used to stain *Plasmodium* species; they are sensitive for parasite detection but are not useful for speciation.[37] Molecular-based tests (such as PCR) can be used for detection and speciation of malarial parasites and are especially helpful in cases of mixed infections, low parasitemia, and infection with *P. knowlesi*. A rapid antigen test, the BinaxNOW® Malaria Test, has been approved by the Food and Drug Administration for use in the United States.[53] It is based on the detection of *P. falciparum* histidine-rich protein II and generic *Plasmodium* aldolase.[53] The sensitivity of the test is low when there are fewer than 100 parasites per microliter of blood.[37,53] Therefore, thick and thin blood film microscopy should be done with the antigen test.[53]

Treatment

Chloroquine or hydroxychloroquine is used for treatment of all malaria, except for disease caused by strains of *P. falciparum* and *P. vivax* acquired from areas known to harbor chloroquine-resistant organisms.[54] For infection with the chloroquine-resistant strains, combination therapy (use of two drugs with different mechanisms of action) is recommended, including atovaquone-proguanil, quinine sulfate plus doxycycline or tetracycline, or

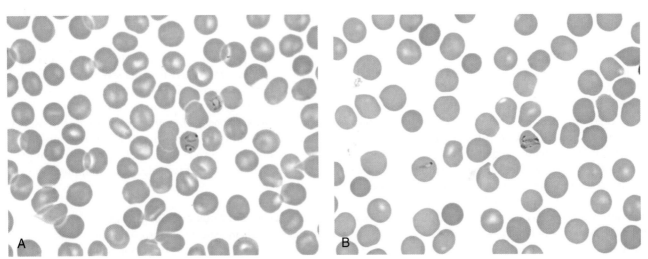

Figure 25-11 *Plasmodium knowlesi* ring forms **(A)** and a ring form and trophozoite **(B)** in a thin peripheral blood film (×1000). (Courtesy Wadsworth Center Laboratories, New York State Department of Health, New York, NY.)

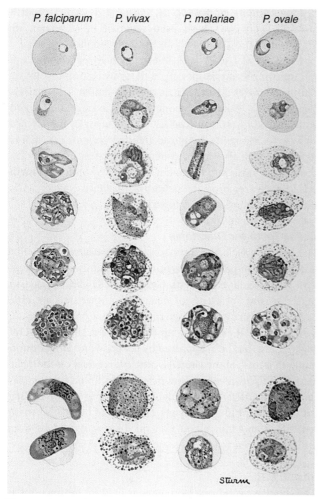

P. falciparum   P. vivax   P. malariae   P. ovale

Sturm

Figure 25-12 Malarial parasites from four species of *Plasmodium.* (From Diggs LW, Sturm D, Bell A: Morphology of human blood cells, ed 5, Abbott Park, Ill, 1985, Abbott Laboratories. Permission has been granted with approval of Abbott Laboratories, all rights reserved by Abbott Laboratories, Inc.)

mefloquine.[54] Another choice for resistant *P. falciparum* is artemether-lumefantrine.[54] Primaquine is also administered in *P. vivax* and *P. ovale* infections to eradicate the hypnozoites in the liver and prevent relapse.[39,54] Prior to administration of primaquine, testing for G6PD deficiency is recommended because patients with moderate to severe deficiency can develop hemolytic anemia after primaquine treatment (Chapter 24).[39,54] There is growing concern about the widespread resistance of *P. falciparum* to chloroquine, the increase in chloroquine-resistant *P. vivax* strains, and the possible emergence and spread of resistance to other antimalarial drugs.[39] Transfusion therapy is used for severe anemia, including exchange transfusion for patients with a level of parasitemia greater than 10% infected RBCs. Because infections with *P. falciparum* or *P. knowlesi* have the potential for a rapid, fatal course, patients must be treated without delay after confirmation of the diagnosis. Intensive research is under way to develop an effective vaccine.

Babesiosis

Babesiosis is a tick-transmitted disease caused by intraerythrocytic protozoan parasites of the genus *Babesia.* There are hundreds of species of *Babesia,* but only a few are known to cause disease in humans. *B. microti* is the most common cause of babesiosis in the United States, where it was originally called *Nantucket fever* because the first cluster of cases was found on Nantucket Island, off Massachusetts, in 1969 and the early 1970s.[55,56] The sexual cycle of *B. microti* occurs in the tick, *Ixodes scapularis,* whereas its asexual cycle primarily occurs in the white-footed mouse, the reservoir host in the United States.[57] Humans are incidental hosts and become infected after injection of sporozoites during a blood meal by infected ticks. Other *Babesia* species, such as *B. duncani* and *B. divergens,* can be found sporadically in humans.[56,57] Babesia may also be transmitted by transfusion of RBCs from asymptomatic donors. Between 1979 and 2009, 159 cases of transfusion-transmitted babesiosis were identified.[58] Congenitally acquired babesiosis has been reported, but it is rare.[57,59]

Geographic Distribution

The areas in which *B. microti* is endemic in the United States are southern New England, New York State, New Jersey, Wisconsin, and Minnesota.[56,57] *B. duncani* occurs in northern California and Washington State; *B. divergens*–like organisms are found in Missouri, Kentucky, and Washington state; and *B. divergens* and *B. venatorum* occur in Europe.[56,60] Isolated cases of babesiosis have also been reported in Asia, Africa, Australia, and South America.[56,60]

Clinical Findings

The incubation period for *B. microti* infection can range from 1 to 9 weeks.[56] Infection is asymptomatic in perhaps a third of individuals, so the exact prevalence is unknown.[56,61] In other individuals, *B. microti* causes a mild to severe hemolytic anemia.[56,57] The patient usually experiences fever and nonrespiratory flu-like symptoms, including chills, headache, sweats, nausea, arthralgias, myalgia, anorexia, and fatigue, that last from several weeks to months. Jaundice, splenomegaly, or hepatomegaly may be present. Some individuals progress to severe, life-threatening disease due to acute respiratory failure, congestive heart failure, renal shutdown, liver failure, central nervous system involvement, or disseminated intravascular coagulation. Severe disease may occur at any age, but it is more common in individuals over 50 years of age.[1,56] Immune deficiency due to asplenia, malignancy, immunosuppressive drugs, or HIV infection increases the risk of severe disease.[1,56,57] The overall mortality rate is less than 10% but is likely higher in immunocompromised individuals.[56,62]

Laboratory Findings and Diagnosis

Evidence of hemolytic anemia is usually present in symptomatic infection, including decreased hemoglobin level, increased reticulocyte count, decreased serum haptoglobin level, and bilirubinemia. Leukopenia, thrombocytopenia, hemoglobinuria, and proteinuria may also be present, along with abnormal results on renal and liver function tests.[56]

The diagnosis of babesiosis is made by demonstration of the parasite on Wright-Giemsa–stained thin peripheral blood films. Babesia appear as tiny rings or occasionally as tetrads inside the RBCs. The ring forms may be round, oval, or ameboid; they have a dark purple chromatin dot and a minimal amount of blue cytoplasm surrounding a vacuole. Multiple rings can be found in one RBC (Figures 25-13 and 25-14). Tetrads may also appear in a "Maltese cross" formation. Babesia can be distinguished from *P. falciparum* by the pleomorphism of their ring forms, absence of hemozoin pigment and gametocytes, and occurrence of extraerythrocytic forms. Parasitemia may be low (fewer than 1% of RBCs affected) in early infections, but as many as 80% of RBCs may be infected in asplenic patients.[63] In cases of low parasitemia, babesiosis can be diagnosed by detection of IgG and IgM antibodies to

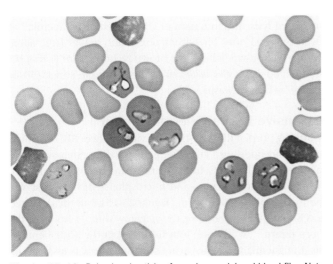

Figure 25-13 *Babesia microti* ring forms in a peripheral blood film. Note the varying appearance of the ring forms and the presence of multiple ring forms in individual red blood cells (×1000).

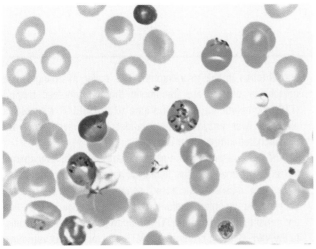

Figure 25-14 *Babesia microti* ring and tetrad forms in a peripheral blood film (×1000).

B. microti by indirect immunofluorescent antibody assay.[57] The sensitivity of the assay ranges from 88% to 96%.[64] Definitive species identification requires PCR-based methods.[56,57]

Treatment

Babesiosis is treated with combination therapy using azithromycin/atovaquone or clindamycin/quinine.[56,57] Exchange transfusion is used when greater than 10% of RBCs are infected or when there is evidence of major organ failure.[56] Asymptomatic infections usually require no treatment.[56,57]

Clostridial Sepsis

Sepsis with massive intravascular hemolysis, which is often fatal, is a rare complication of infection with *Clostridium perfringens*, an anaerobic gram-positive bacillus. *C. perfringens* grows very rapidly (7-minute doubling time) and produces an α-toxin with phospholipase C and sphingomyelinase activity that hydrolyzes RBC membrane phospholipids.[65,66] The RBCs become spherical and extremely susceptible to osmotic lysis, which results in sudden, massive hemolysis and dark red plasma and urine.[1,65,67] The hematocrit may drop to below 10%.[1,67] The intravascular hemolysis can trigger DIC and renal failure. Spherocytes, microspherocytes, and toxic changes to neutrophils can be observed on a peripheral blood film.[1,65,67] Some conditions that increase the risk of clostridial sepsis and hemolytic anemia include malignancies (genitourinary, gastrointestinal, and hematologic), solid organ transplantation, postpartum or postabortion infections, biliary surgery, acute cholecystitis, and deep wounds.[1,65,68] Rapid therapy with transfusions, antibiotics, and fluid management is required. The prognosis is grave, and many patients die despite intensive treatment.

Bartonellosis

Human bartonellosis (Carrión disease) is transmitted by the bite of a female sandfly and is endemic in certain regions of Peru, Ecuador, and Colombia.[69,70] It is caused by *Bartonella bacilliformis*, a small, pleomorphic, intracellular coccobacillus that adheres to RBCs and causes hemolysis.[1,71] The bacteria produce a protein called *deformin* that forms pits or invaginations in the RBC membrane.[1,71] There are two clinical stages: the first stage is characterized by acute hemolytic anemia (called *Oroya fever* after a city in the Peruvian Andes); the second or chronic verruga stage is characterized by the eruption of skin lesions and warts on the extremities, face, and trunk. The acute phase begins with fever, malaise, headache, and chills, followed by pallor, jaundice, general lymphadenopathy, and, less commonly, hepatosplenomegaly.[69-71] Over several days, there is rapid hemolysis, with the hematocrit dropping below 20% in two thirds of patients.[69,71] Polychromasia, nucleated RBCs, and mild leukocytosis with a left shift are observed on the peripheral blood film. The mortality rate is approximately 10% for hospitalized patients and 90% for those who are untreated.[69,70] Diagnosis is made by blood culture and observation of bacilli or coccobacilli on the erythrocytes on a Wright-Giemsa–stained peripheral blood film. During the acute phase, 80% of the RBCs can be involved.[1] Serologic diagnosis with indirect immunofluorescent antibody or immunoblotting has a sensitivity of 89%.[70] The acute stage is treated with transfusions and ciprofloxacin or chloramphenicol.[70]

Carrión disease was named for a Peruvian medical student, Daniel Alcides Carrión, who in 1885 inoculated himself with fluid from a wart of a patient in the chronic stage of infection. He subsequently developed fatal hemolytic anemia similar to that in Oroya fever, which linked the two stages of the disease to the same agent.[71,72]

HEMOLYTIC ANEMIA CAUSED BY OTHER RED BLOOD CELL INJURY

Drugs and Chemicals

Hemolytic anemia of varying severity may result from drugs or chemicals that cause the oxidative denaturation of hemoglobin, leading to the formation of methemoglobin and Heinz bodies.[1] Examples of agents that can cause hemolytic anemia in individuals with normal RBCs include dapsone, a drug used to treat leprosy and dermatitis herpetiformis,[1,73] and naphthalene, a chemical found in mothballs.[74] Individuals deficient in G6PD are particularly sensitive to the effects of oxidative agents. For example, primaquine can cause hemolytic anemia in G6PD-deficient individuals (Chapter 24).[39]

The typical laboratory findings include a decrease in hemoglobin level, increase in the reticulocyte count, increase in serum indirect bilirubin, and decrease in serum haptoglobin level. In severe drug- or chemical-induced hemolytic anemia, Heinz bodies (denatured hemoglobin) may be observed in RBCs. Heinz bodies can only be visualized with a supravital stain, and they appear as round, blue granules attached to the inner RBC membrane (Figure 14-11). Exposure to high levels of arsine hydride, copper, and lead can also cause hemolysis.[1,75]

Venoms

Envenomation from contact with snakes, spiders, bees, or wasps can induce hemolytic anemia in some individuals. The hemolysis can occur acutely or be delayed 1 or more days after a bite or sting.[1,75] The severity of the hemolysis depends on the amount of venom injected, and in severe cases, renal failure and death can result. Some mechanisms by which venoms can

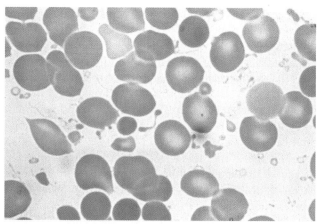

Figure 25-15 Peripheral blood film for a patient with extensive burns. Note the presence of schistocytes, microspherocytes, and spherocytes (×1000).

induce hemolysis are direct disruption of the RBC membrane, alteration of the RBC membrane that results in complement-mediated lysis, and initiation of DIC.[75] Hemolytic anemia has been reported after bites from poisonous snakes (e.g., some cobras and pit vipers) and the brown recluse spider (*Loxosceles reclusa* and *Loxosceles laeta*), and after multiple stings (50 or more) by bees or wasps.[1,75-79]

Extensive Burns (Thermal Injury)

Warming normal RBCs to 49° C in vitro induces RBC fragmentation and budding.[1] Likewise, patients with extensive burns manifest similar RBC injury with acute hemolytic anemia. Schistocytes, spherocytes, and microspherocytes are observed on the peripheral blood film (Figure 25-15), but the damaged RBCs are usually cleared by the spleen within 24 hours of the burn injury.[75] In addition to resulting from the acute hemolysis, the anemia associated with extensive burns is also caused by blood loss during surgical excision and grafting of the burn wounds, nutritional deficiency, impaired metabolism, and anemia of chronic inflammation.[80] Overheating blood in malfunctioning blood warmers prior to transfusion can also result in RBC fragmentation and hemolysis of the donor RBCs.[1]

SUMMARY

- A common feature of the nonimmune extrinsic hemolytic anemias is the presence of a condition that causes physical or mechanical injury to the RBCs. These conditions include microangiopathic hemolytic anemia; macroangiopathic hemolytic anemia; some infections; exposure to certain drugs, chemicals, or venoms; and extensive burns.

- Microangiopathic hemolytic anemia is characterized by the shearing of RBCs as they pass through small blood vessels partially blocked by microthrombi. Fragmented RBCs (called *schistocytes*) are formed, and the premature RBC destruction results in hemolytic anemia. Ischemic injury to the brain, kidney, and other organs also occurs. Thrombocytopenia also occurs as a result of

consumption in the microthrombi. The major microangiopathic hemolytic anemias are thrombotic thrombocytopenic purpura (TTP), hemolytic uremic syndrome (HUS), HELLP (hemolysis, elevated liver enzymes, low platelet count) syndrome, and disseminated intravascular coagulation (DIC).

- TTP is a rare disorder found predominantly in adults and characterized by microangiopathic hemolytic anemia, severe thrombocytopenia, a markedly increased serum lactate dehydrogenase activity, and variable symptoms of fever, neurologic dysfunction, and renal failure. Idiopathic TTP is due to autoimmune antibodies to the VWF-cleaving protease ADAMTS-13 causing a severe functional deficiency. Secondary TTP is associated with stem cell transplantation, disseminated cancer, pregnancy, and use of certain drugs. Inherited TTP is due to mutations in the *ADAMTS13* gene.

- HUS is characterized by microangiopathic hemolytic anemia, thrombocytopenia, and acute renal failure. Typical HUS (stx-HUS) comprise 90% of cases, is found predominantly in young children, and is caused by toxin-producing strains of *E. coli.* Atypical HUS (aHUS) is due to inherited mutations in genes coding for complement components and regulators or autoantibodies to complement factor H. It also occurs secondary to organ transplantation, cancer, pregnancy, HIV infection, and some drugs.
- HELLP syndrome is a serious complication of pregnancy presenting with microangiopathic hemolytic anemia, thrombocytopenia, and elevated levels of liver enzymes.
- DIC is due to the widespread intravascular activation of the hemostatic system and formation of fibrin thrombi; coagulation factors and platelets are consumed in the thrombi, and secondary fibrinolysis occurs. Schistocytes are found in about half of the cases.
- Macroangiopathic hemolytic anemia is caused by traumatic cardiac hemolysis (RBC fragmentation from damaged or prosthetic cardiac valves) or exercise-induced hemolysis (mechanical trauma from forceful impact on feet or hands or from strenuous exercise).

The platelet count is normal in both conditions; schistocytes are seen only in traumatic cardiac hemolysis.

- Infections associated with hemolytic anemia due to invasion of RBCs include malaria and babesiosis. Hemolysis in bartonellosis is due to attachment of the bacteria to red blood cells and production of a lytic protein. Hemolysis in clostridial sepsis is due to the production of α-toxin.
- In malaria, severe anemia is due to direct lysis of infected RBCs, immune destruction of infected and uninfected RBCs in the spleen, and inhibition of erythropoiesis.
- *Plasmodium* (five species) and *Babesia* organisms are identified by the morphology of their intraerythrocytic stages on a Wright-Giemsa–stained peripheral blood film. *Plasmodium* species are transmitted to humans by mosquitoes, whereas a tick is the vector for *Babesia*.
- Hemolytic anemia can also be caused by injury to RBCs by drugs, chemicals, venoms, and extensive burns (thermal injury). In patients with extensive burns, schistocytes, spherocytes, and microspherocytes are observed on the peripheral blood film.

Now that you have completed this chapter, go back and read again the case study at the beginning and respond to the questions presented.

REVIEW QUESTIONS

Answers can be found in the Appendix.

1. Which one of the following is a feature found in *all* microangiopathic hemolytic anemias?
   a. Pancytopenia
   b. Thrombocytosis
   c. Intravascular RBC fragmentation
   d. Prolonged prothrombin time and partial thromboplastin time

2. Typical laboratory findings in TTP and HUS include:
   a. Schistocytosis and thrombocytopenia
   b. Anemia and reticulocytopenia
   c. Reduced levels of lactate dehydrogenase and aspartate aminotransferase
   d. Increased levels of free plasma hemoglobin and serum haptoglobin

3. The pathophysiology of idiopathic TTP involves:
   a. Shiga toxin damage to endothelial cells and obstruction of small blood vessels in glomeruli
   b. Formation of platelet-VWF thrombi due to autoantibody inhibition of ADAMTS-13
   c. Overactivation of the complement system and endothelial cell damage due to loss of regulatory function
   d. Activation of the coagulation and fibrinolytic systems with fibrin clots throughout the microvasculature

4. Which of the following tests yields results that are abnormal in DIC but are usually within the reference interval or just slightly abnormal in TTP and HUS?
   a. Indirect serum bilirubin and serum haptoglobin
   b. Prothrombin time and partial thromboplastin time
   c. Lactate dehydrogenase and aspartate aminotransferase
   d. Serum creatinine and serum total protein

5. Which one of the following laboratory results may be seen in BOTH traumatic cardiac hemolytic anemia and exercise-induced hemoglobinuria?
   a. Schistocytes on the peripheral blood film
   b. Thrombocytopenia
   c. Decreased serum haptoglobin
   d. Hemosiderinuria

6. Which of the following species of *Plasmodium* produce hypnozoites that can remain dormant in the liver and cause a relapse months or years later?
   a. *P. falciparum*
   b. *P. vivax*
   c. *P. knowlesi*
   d. *P. malariae*

7. Which one of the following is *not* a mechanism causing anemia in *P. falciparum* infections?
   a. Inhibition of erythropoiesis
   b. Lysis of infected RBCs during schizogony
   c. Competition for vitamin B_{12} in the erythrocyte
   d. Immune destruction of noninfected RBCs in the spleen

8. Which *Plasmodium* species is widespread in Malaysia, has RBCs with multiple ring forms, has band-shaped early trophozoites, shows a 24-hour erythrocytic cycle, and can cause severe disease and high parasitemia?
   a. *P. falciparum*
   b. *P. vivax*
   c. *P. knowlesi*
   d. *P. malariae*

9. One week after returning from a vacation in Rhode Island, a 60-year-old man experienced fever, chills, nausea, muscle aches, and fatigue of 2 days' duration. A complete blood count (CBC) showed a WBC count of 4.5×10^9/L, hemoglobin level of 10.5 g/dL, a platelet count of 134×10^9/L, and a reticulocyte count of 2.7%. The medical laboratory scientist noticed tiny ameboid ring forms in some of the RBCs and some tetrad forms in others. These findings suggest:
   a. Bartonellosis
   b. Malaria
   c. Babesiosis
   d. Clostridial sepsis

10. What RBC morphology is characteristically found within the first 24 hours following extensive burn injury?
    a. Macrocytosis and polychromasia
    b. Burr cells and crenated cells
    c. Howell-Jolly bodies and bite cells
    d. Schistocytes and microspherocytes

11. A 36-year-old woman was brought to the emergency department by her husband because she had experienced a seizure. He reported that she had been well until that morning, when she complained of a sudden headache and malaise. She was not taking any medications and had no history of previous surgery or pregnancy. Laboratory studies showed a WBC count of 15×10^9/L, hemoglobin level of 7.8 g/dL, a platelet count of 18×10^9/L, and schistocytes and helmet cells on the peripheral blood film. Chemistry test results included markedly elevated serum lactate dehydrogenase activity and a slight increase in the level of total and indirect serum bilirubin. The urinalysis results were positive for protein and blood, but there were no RBCs in the urine sediment. Prothrombin time and partial thromboplastin time were within the reference interval. When the entire clinical and laboratory picture is considered, which of the following is the most likely diagnosis?
    a. HUS
    b. HELLP syndrome
    c. TTP
    d. Exercise-induced hemoglobinuria

REFERENCES

1. Price, E. A., & Schrier, S. S. (2013). Extrinsic nonimmune hemolytic anemias. In Hoffman, R., Benz, E. J. Jr, Silberstein, L. E., et al. (Eds.), *Hematology: Basic Principles and Practice.* (6th ed., pp. 628–637). Philadelphia: Saunders, an imprint of Elsevier.
2. Moake, J. L. (2002). Thrombotic microangiopathies. *N Engl J Med, 347*, 589–600.
3. Tsai H-M. (2013). Thrombotic thrombocytopenic purpura and the atypical hemolytic uremic syndrome. *Hematol Oncol Clin N Am, 27*, 565–584.
4. Moake, J. (2009). Thrombotic microangiopathies: multimers, metalloprotease, and beyond. *Clin Transl Sci, 2*, 366–373.
5. McCrae, K. R., Sadler, J. E., & Cines, D. B. (2013). Thrombotic thrombocytopenic purpura and the hemolytic uremic syndrome. In Hoffman, R., Benz, E. J. Jr, Silberstein, L. E., et al. (Eds.), *Hematology: Basic Principles and Practice.* (6th ed., pp. 1925–1939). Philadelphia: Saunders, an imprint of Elsevier.
6. Crawley, J. T. B., & Scully, M. A. (2013). Thrombotic thrombocytopenic purpura: basic pathophysiology and therapeutic strategies. *Hematology Am Soc Hematol Educ Program*, 292–299.
7. Moake, J. L., Rudy, C. K., Troll, J. H., et al. (1982). Unusually large plasma factor VIII: von Willebrand factor multimers in chronic relapsing thrombotic thrombocytopenic purpura. *N Engl J Med, 307*, 1432–1435.
8. Furlan, M., Robles, R., Galbusera, M., et al. (1998). Von Willebrand factor–cleaving protease in thrombotic thrombocytopenic purpura and the hemolytic-uremic syndrome. *N Engl J Med, 339*, 1578–1584.
9. Tsai, H-M., & Lian, E C-Y. (1998). Antibodies to von Willebrand factor–cleaving protease in acute thrombotic thrombocytopenic purpura. *N Engl J Med, 339*, 1585–1594.
10. Zhang, Q., Zhou, Y. F., Zhang, C. Z., et al. (2009). Structural specializations of A2, a force-sensing domain in the ultralarge vascular protein von Willebrand factor. *Proc Natl Acad Sci U S A, 106*, 9226–9231.
11. Kremer Hovinga JA, Vesely SK, Terrell DR, et al. (2010). Survival and relapse in patients with thrombotic thrombocytopenic purpura. *Blood, 115*, 1500–1511.
12. Lotta, L. A., Garagiola, I., Palla, R., et al. (2010). *ADAMTS13* mutations and polymorphisms in congenital thrombotic thrombocytopenic purpura. *Hum Mutat, 31*, 11–19.
13. Verbeke, L., Delforge, M., & Dierickx, D. (2010). Current insight into thrombotic thrombocytopenic purpura. *Blood Coagul Fibrinolysis, 21*, 3–10.
14. Scheiring, J., Rosales, A., & Zimmerhackl, L. B. (2010). Clinical practice: today's understanding of the haemolytic uraemic syndrome. *Eur J Pediatr, 169*, 7–13.
15. Petruzziello, T. N., Mawji, I. A., Khan, M., et al. (2009). Verotoxin biology: molecular events in vascular endothelial injury. *Kidney Int, 75*, S17–S19.
16. Cataland, S. R., & Wu, H. F. (2014). Diagnosis and management of complement mediated thrombotic microangiopathies. *Blood Reviews, 28*, 67–74.
17. Haram, K., Svendsen, E., & Abildgaard, U. (2009). The HELLP syndrome: clinical issues and management. *BMC Pregnancy Childbirth, 9*, 1–15.
18. Baker, K. R., & Moake, J. (2010). Hemolytic anemia resulting from physical injury to red cells. In Lichtman, M. A., Kipps, T. J., Seligsohn, U., Kaushansky, K., & Prchal, J. T. (Eds.), *Williams Hematology.* (8th ed.). New York: McGraw-Hill. http://accessmedicine.mhmedical.com.libproxy2.umdnj

.edu/content.aspx?bookid=358&Sectionid=39835868. Accessed 16.04.14.

19. Mihu, D., Costin, N., Mihu, C. M., et al. (2007). HELLP syndrome—a multisystemic disorder. *J Gastrointest Liver Dis, 16,* 419–424.

20. Labelle, C. A., & Kitchens, C. S. (2005). Disseminated intravascular coagulation: treat the cause, not the lab values. *Cleve Clin J Med, 72,* 377–397.

21. Shapira, Y., Vaturi, M., & Sagie, A. (2009). Hemolysis associated with prosthetic heart valves. a review. *Cardiol Rev, 17,* 121–124.

22. Davidson, R. J. L. (1964). Exertional haemoglobinuria: a report on three cases with studies on the haemolytic mechanism. *J Clin Pathol, 17,* 536–540.

23. Telford, R. D., Sly, G. J., Hahn, A. G., et al. (2003). Footstrike is the major cause of hemolysis during running. *J Appl Physiol, 94,* 38–42.

24. Selby, G. B., & Eichner, E. R. (1986). Endurance swimming, intravascular hemolysis, anemia, and iron depletion. New perspective on athlete's anemia. *Am J Med, 81,* 791–794.

25. Shaskey, D. J., & Green, G. A. (2000). Sports haematology. *Sports Med, 29,* 27–38.

26. Tobal, D., Olascoaga, A., Moreira, G., et al. (2008). Rust urine after intense hand drumming is caused by extracorpuscular hemolysis. *Clin J Am Soc Nephrol, 3,* 1022–1027.

27. Smith, J. A., Kolbuch-Braddon, M., Gillam, I., et al. (1995). Changes in the susceptibility of red blood cells to oxidative and osmotic stress following submaximal exercise. *Eur J Appl Physiol, 70,* 427–436.

28. Beneke R, Bihn D, Hütler M, et al. (2005). Haemolysis caused by alterations of α- and β-spectrin after 10 to 35 min of severe exercise. *Eur J Appl Physiol, 95,* 307–312.

29. Yusof, A., Leithauser, R. M., Roth, H. J., et al. (2007). Exercise-induced hemolysis is caused by protein modification and most evident during the early phase of an ultraendurance race. *J Appl Physiol, 102,* 582–586.

30. Singh, B., Lee, K. S., Matusop, A., et al. (2004). A large focus of naturally acquired *Plasmodium knowlesi* infections in human beings. *Lancet, 363,* 1017–1024.

31. Cox-Singh, J., Davis, T. M. E., Lee, K. S., et al. (2008). *Plasmodium knowlesi* malaria in humans is widely distributed and potentially life-threatening. *Clin Infect Dis, 46,* 165–171.

32. Lee, K. S., Cox-Singh, J., Brooke, G., et al. (2009). *Plasmodium knowlesi* from archival blood films: further evidence that human infections are widely distributed and not newly emergent in Malaysian Borneo. *Int J Parasitol, 39,* 1125–1128.

33. World Health Organization. (2013). *World malaria report 2013.* Geneva: WHO Press. http://www.who.int/malaria/publications/world_malaria_report_2013/report/en/. Accessed 19.04.14.

34. Centers for Disease Control and Prevention. (2014). *Malaria facts.* Retrieved from http://www.cdc.gov/malaria/about/facts.html. Accessed 20.04.14.

35. Miller, L. H., Baruch, D. I., Marsh, K., et al. (2002). The pathogenic basis of malaria. *Nature, 415,* 673–679.

36. Wellems, T. E., Hayton, K., & Fairhurst, R. M. (2009). The impact of malaria parasitism: from corpuscles to communities. *J Clin Invest, 119,* 2496–2505.

37. Garcia, L. S. (2010). Malaria. *Clin Lab Med, 30,* 93–129.

38. Ekvall, H. (2003). Malaria and anemia. *Curr Opin Hematol, 10,* 108–114.

39. World Health Organization. (2010). *Guidelines for treatment of malaria.* (2nd ed). Geneva: WHO Press.

40. Haldar, K., & Mohandas, N. (2009). Malaria, erythrocytic infection, and anemia. *Hematology Am Soc Hematol Educ Program,* 87–93.

41. Waitumbi, J. N., Opollo, M. O., Muga, R. O., et al. (2000). Red cell surface changes and erythrophagocytosis in children with severe *Plasmodium falciparum* anemia. *Blood, 95,* 1481–1486.

42. Griffiths, M. J., Ndungu, F., Baird, K. L., et al. (2001). Oxidative stress and erythrocyte damage in Kenyan children with severe *Plasmodium falciparum* malaria. *Br J Haematol, 113,* 486–491.

43. Craig, A., & Scherf, A. (2001). Molecules on the surface of the *Plasmodium falciparum* infected erythrocyte and their role in malaria pathogenesis and immune evasion. *Mol Biochem Parasitol, 115,* 129–143.

44. Bridges, D. J., Bunn, J., van Mourik, J. A., et al. (2010). Rapid activation of endothelial cells enables *Plasmodium falciparum* adhesion to platelet-decorated von Willebrand factor strings. *Blood, 115,* 1472–1474.

45. Aird, W. C., Mosnier, L. O., & Fairhurst, R. M. (2014). *Plasmodium falciparum* picks (on) EPCR. *Blood, 123,* 163–167.

46. Ayi, K., Turrini, F., Piga, A., et al. (2004). Enhanced phagocytosis of ring-parasitized mutant erythrocytes: a common mechanism that may explain protection against *falciparum* malaria in sickle trait and beta-thalassemia trait. *Blood, 104,* 3364–3371.

47. Fairhurst, R. M., Baruch, D. I., Brittain, N. J., et al. (2005). Abnormal display of PfEMP-1 on erythrocytes carrying haemoglobin C may protect against malaria. *Nature, 435,* 1117–1121.

48. Cholera, R., Brittain, N. J., Gillrie, M. R., et al. (2008). Impaired cytoadherence of *Plasmodium falciparum*–infected erythrocytes containing sickle hemoglobin. *Proc Natl Acad Sci U S A, 105,* 991–996.

49. Chotivanich, K., Udomsangpetch, R., Pattanapanyasat, K., et al. (2002). Hemoglobin E: a balanced polymorphism protective against high parasitemias and thus severe *P. falciparum* malaria. *Blood, 100,* 1172–1176.

50. Centers for Disease Control and Prevention. *Diagnostic procedures—blood specimens: specimen collection.* Retrieved from http://www.cdc.gov/dpdx/diagnosticProcedures/blood/specimencoll.html. Accessed 20.04.14.

51. Centers for Disease Control and Prevention. *Diagnostic procedures—blood specimens: microscopic examination.* Retrieved from http://www.cdc.gov/dpdx/diagnosticProcedures/blood/microexam.html. Accessed 20.04.14.

52. Centers for Disease Control and Prevention. *Malaria map.* Retrieved from http://cdc-malaria.ncsa.uiuc.edu. Accessed 20.04.14.

53. Centers for Disease Control and Prevention. *Diagnostic procedures—blood specimens: detection of parasite antigens.* Retrieved from http://www.cdc.gov/dpdx/diagnosticProcedures/blood/antigendetection.html. Accessed 20.04.14.

54. Centers for Disease Control and Prevention (2013, July 1). *Guidelines for treatment of malaria in the United States.* Retrieved from http://www.cdc.gov/malaria/resources/pdf/treatmenttable.pdf. Accessed 20.04.14.

55. Ruebush, T. K., II, Juranek, D. D., Spielman, A., et al. (1981). Epidemiology of human babesiosis on Nantucket Island. *Am J Trop Med Hyg, 30,* 937–941.

56. Vannier, E., & Krause, P. J. (2009). Update on babesiosis. *Interdiscip Perspect Infect Dis, 2009,* 984568.

57. Centers for Disease Control and Prevention. *Babesiosis.* Retrieved from http://www.cdc.gov/babesiosis/. Accessed 20.04.14.

58. Centers for Disease Control and Prevention. *Babesiosis and the U.S. blood supply.* http://www.cdc.gov/parasites/babesiosis/resources/babesiosis_policy_brief.pdf. Accessed 20.04.14.

59. Sethi, S., Alcid, D., Kesarwala, H., et al. (2009). Probable congenital babesiosis in infant, New Jersey, USA. *Emerg Infect Dis, 15,* 788–791.

60. Hildebrandt, A., Gray, J. S., & Hunfeld, K. P. (2013). Human babesiosis in Europe: what clinicians need to know. *Infection, 41,* 1057–1072.

61. Krause, P. J., McKay, K., Gadbaw, J., et al. (2003). Increasing health burden of human babesiosis in endemic sites. *Am J Trop Med Hyg, 68,* 431–436.

62. Meldrum, S. C., Birkhead, G. S., White, D. J., et al. (1992). Human babesiosis in New York State: an epidemiological description of 136 cases. *Clin Infect Dis, 15,* 1019–1023.

63. Blevins, S. M., Greenfield, R. A., & Bronze, M. S. (2008). Blood smear analysis in babesiosis, ehrlichiosis, relapsing fever, malaria, and Chagas disease. *Cleve Clin J Med, 75,* 521–530.

64. Krause, P. J., Telford, S. R. 3rd., Ryan, R., et al. (1994). Diagnosis of babesiosis: evaluation of a serologic test for the detection of *B. microti* antibody. *J Infect Dis, 169,* 923–926.

65. Kapoor, J. R., Montiero, B., Tanoue, L., et al. (2007). Massive intravascular hemolysis and a rapid fatal outcome. *Chest, 132,* 2016–2019.

66. Urbina, P., Flores-Díaz, M., Alape-Girón, A., et al. (2009). Phospholipase C and sphingomyelinase activities of the *Clostridium perfringens* (α-toxin. *Chem Phys Lipids, 159,* 51–57.

67. Merino, A., Pereira, A., & Castro, P. (2009). Massive intravascular haemolysis during *Clostridium perfringens* sepsis of hepatic origin. *Eur J Haematol, 84,* 278–279.

68. Barrett, J. P., Whiteside, J. L., & Boardman, L. A. (2002). Fatal clostridial sepsis after spontaneous abortion. *Obstet Gynecol, 99,* 899–901.

69. Maguina, C., & Gotuzzo, E. (2000). Bartonellosis new and old. *Infect Dis Clin North Am, 14,* 1–22.

70. Huarcaya, E., Maguina, C., Torres, R., et al. (2004). Bartonellosis (Carrion's disease) in the pediatric population of Peru: an overview and update. *Braz J Infect Dis, 8,* 331–339.

71. Lichtman, M. A. (2010). Hemolytic anemia resulting from infections with microorganisms. In Lichtman, M. A., Kipps, T. J., Seligsohn, U., Kaushansky, K., Prchal, J. T. (Eds.), *Williams Hematology.* (8th ed.). New York: McGraw-Hill. http://accessmedicine .mhmedical.com.libproxy2.umdnj.edu/content.aspx?bookid= 358&Sectionid=39835870. Accessed 16.04.14.

72. Garcia-Caceres, U., & Garcia, F. U. (1991). Bartonellosis. An immunodepressive disease and the life of Daniel Alcides Carrion. *Am J Clin Pathol, 95,* S58–S66.

73. Ranawaka, R. R., Mendis, S., & Weerakoon, H. S. (2008). Dapsone-induced haemolytic anemia, hepatitis and agranulocytosis in a leprosy patient with normal glucose-6-phosphate-dehydrogenase activity. *Lepr Rev, 79,* 436–440.

74. Lim, H. C., Poulose, V., & Tan, H. H. (2009). Acute naphthalene poisoning following the non-accidental ingestion of mothballs. *Singapore Med J, 50,* e298–e301.

75. Bull, B. S., & Herrmann, P. C. (2010). Hemolytic anemia resulting from chemical and physical agents. In. Lichtman, M. A., Kipps, T. J., Seligsohn, U., Kaushansky, K., & Prchal, J. T. (Eds.), *Williams Hematology.* (8th ed.). New York: McGraw-Hill. http:// accessmedicine.mhmedical.com.libproxy2.umdnj.edu/content .aspx?bookid=358&Sectionid=39835869. Accessed 16.04.14.

76. Athappan, G., Balaji, M. V., Navaneethan, U., et al. (2008). Acute renal failure in snake envenomation: a large prospective study. *Saudi J Kidney Dis Transpl, 19,* 404–410.

77. McDade, J., Aygun, B., & Ware, R. E. (2010). Brown recluse spider (*Loxosceles reclusa*) envenomation leading to acute hemolytic anemia in six adolescents. *J Pediatr, 156,* 155–157.

78. Kolecki, P. (1999). Delayed toxic reaction following massive bee envenomation. *Ann Emerg Med, 33,* 114–116.

79. Paudel, B., & Paudel, K. (2009). A study of wasp bites in a tertiary hospital of western Nepal. *Nepal Med Coll J, 11,* 52–56.

80. Posluszny, J. A., & Gamelli, R. L. (2010). Anemia of thermal injury: combined acute blood loss anemia and anemia of critical illness. *J Burn Care Res, 31,* 229–242.

Extrinsic Defects Leading to Increased Erythrocyte Destruction—Immune Causes

26

Kim A. Przekop *

OUTLINE

OBJECTIVES

After completion of this chapter, the reader will be able to:

1. Define immune hemolytic anemia and indicate the types of antibodies involved.
2. Compare and contrast the mechanisms of immune hemolysis mediated by immunoglobulin M (IgM) and IgG antibodies.
3. Describe typical laboratory findings in immune hemolytic anemia and the importance of the direct antiglobulin test (DAT).
4. Compare and contrast four types of autoimmune hemolytic anemia in terms of the immunoglobulin class involved, the temperature for optimal reactivity of the autoantibody, the proteins detected by the DAT on the patient's red blood cells, the presence or absence of complement activation, the type and site of hemolysis, and the specificity of the autoantibody.
5. Relate results of the DAT to the pathophysiology and clinical findings in autoimmune hemolytic anemia.
6. Describe three mechanisms of drug-induced immune hemolysis.
7. Compare and contrast the pathophysiology of immune hemolysis due to drug-dependent and drug-independent antibodies, including the related laboratory findings.
8. Describe two types of hemolytic transfusion reactions, the usual immunoglobulin class involved, the typical site of hemolysis, and important laboratory findings.
9. Describe the cause, pathophysiology, and laboratory findings in Rh and ABO hemolytic disease of the fetus and newborn (HDFN).
10. Given a patient history and results of a complete blood count, peripheral blood film examination, pertinent biochemical tests on serum and urine, and the direct and indirect antiglobulin tests, determine the type of immune hemolysis.

CASE STUDY

After studying the material in this chapter, the reader should be able to respond to the following case study:

A 37-year-old man sought medical attention from his general practitioner for malaise, shortness of breath, and difficulty concentrating for the past five days. Physical examination revealed an otherwise healthy adult with tachycardia (faster than normal heart rate). There was no significant past medical history and the patient was not taking any medications. The physician ordered a complete blood count (CBC), urinalysis, comprehensive metabolic panel (CMP), and electrocardiogram (EKG). The following are the patient's key laboratory results:

	Patient Results	Reference Interval
WBC ($\times 10^9$/L)	12.4 (corrected)	3.6–10.6
HGB (g/dL)	7.1	14.0–18.0

Continued

*The author acknowledges the contributions to the framework and content of the chapter by Elaine M. Keohane, author of this chapter in the previous edition.

CASE STUDY—cont'd

After studying the material in this chapter, the reader should be able to respond to the following case study:

	Patient Results	Reference Interval
MCV (fL)	105.4	80.0–100.0
MCHC (g/dL)	36.3	32.0–36.0
RDW (%)	17.3	11.5–14.5
PLT (×10⁹/L)	325	150–450
Reticulocytes (%)	18.1	0.5–2.5
Neutrophils (%)	72	50–70
Bands (%)	10	0–5

The EKG was normal. The CBC instrument printout flagged for nucleated red blood cells (and corrected the WBC for them), 3+ anisocytosis, and reticulocytosis. The peripheral blood film had moderate spherocytes, moderate polychromasia, few macrocytes, 3+ anisocytosis, and 15 nucleated red blood cells/100 WBCs (Figure 26-1). Occasional schistocytes and neutrophilia with a slight left shift were also observed on the blood film (not shown in figure). The urinalysis report included 2+ protein, 2+ blood, increased urobilinogen, with 0 to 5 RBCs seen on the microscopic exam. The patient's serum was moderately icteric, and the total serum bilirubin was increased. The patient was admitted for further testing. The serum haptoglobin was decreased, the serum indirect (unconjugated) bilirubin and lactate dehydrogenase (LD) were elevated, and urine hemosiderin was positive.

A type and screen was ordered. The antibody screen was negative at the immediate spin and 37° C incubation phase but showed 3+ agglutination in the antihuman globulin (AHG) phase for all panel cells and the autocontrol. The direct antiglobulin test (DAT) showed 3+ agglutination with polyspecific AHG and monospecific anti-IgG but was negative with monospecific anti-C3b/C3d (complement). An acid elution was performed on the patient's RBCs, and the eluate showed 2+ reactions with all panel cells and autocontrol at the AHG phase. The patient was diagnosed with warm autoimmune

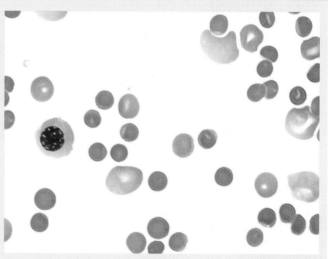

Figure 26-1 Wright-stained peripheral blood film from the patient in the case study (×1000).

hemolytic anemia (WAIHA) and started on 1 mg/kg/d prednisone until the hemoglobin reached 10.0 g/dL (2 weeks of treatment). The patient was continued on prednisone for 4 months with slowly decreasing levels of the drug. He also received bisphosphonates, vitamin D, and calcium to combat the ill effects of prednisone. At 3 weeks postdiagnosis, the spherocytes disappeared, the urinalysis was normal, and the DAT was negative.

1. Explain why the WBC count, MCV, RDW, and reticulocyte count results were elevated.
2. Describe the immune mechanism that caused the spherocytosis, and explain why spherocytes have a shortened life span.
3. Relate the chemistry, urinalysis, and blood bank results with the pathophysiology of the patient's anemia.
4. Explain why the treatment was effective, and explain if the patient's WAIHA was acute or chronic.

OVERVIEW OF IMMUNE HEMOLYTIC ANEMIAS

Immune hemolytic anemia and nonimmune hemolytic anemia are the two broad categories comprising the extrinsic hemolytic anemias, disorders in which red blood cells (RBCs) are structurally and functionally normal, but a condition outside of the RBCs causes premature hemolysis. The nonimmune extrinsic hemolytic anemias are the result of physical or mechanical injury to the RBCs and are covered in Chapter 25. The immune hemolytic anemias are conditions in which RBC survival is shortened due to an antibody-mediated mechanism. The antibody may be an *autoantibody* (directed against a self RBC antigen), an *alloantibody* (directed against an RBC antigen

of another person), or an antibody directed against a drug (or its metabolite) taken by the patient. Some antibodies are able to activate the classical complement pathway, which results in the attachment of activated complement proteins to the RBC membrane. RBCs with bound antibody or complement are prematurely removed from the circulation extravascularly by macrophages (due to their receptors for complement and the Fc component of antibody), intravascularly by complement-mediated hemolysis, or by a combination of both mechanisms.[1] Anemia develops when the amount of hemolysis exceeds the ability of the bone marrow to replace the RBCs that are destroyed. The degree of anemia varies from asymptomatic and mild to severe and life-threatening.

The immune hemolytic anemias may be classified into the following groups: autoimmune hemolytic anemia, drug-induced immune hemolytic anemia, and alloimmune hemolytic anemia (Box 26-1).[1,2] It is important to determine the cause of an immune hemolytic anemia so that the appropriate therapy can be administered to the patient.

Pathophysiology of Immune Hemolysis

In immune hemolysis an antibody binds to an antigen on the surface of RBCs, which signals premature removal of those cells from the circulation through extravascular or intravascular hemolysis (Chapter 23). The two classes or isotypes of antibodies involved in most immune hemolytic anemias are immunoglobulin G (IgG) and M (IgM). IgG is a monomer in a Y-like structure with two identical heavy chains (γ H chains) and two identical light chains (either κ or λ) connected by disulfide bonds.[3] At the top of the Y-like structure are two antigen-binding (Fab) domains, each formed from the N-terminus of the variable domain of one light and one heavy chain. IgG has one Fc domain (the stem of the Y) consisting of the C-terminus of the two heavy chains (Figure 26-2). IgM is a pentamer consisting of five monomeric units connected by disulfide linkages at the C-termini of their heavy chains (μ H chains).[3,4] Because the composition, structure, and size of IgG and IgM are different, their properties and mechanisms in mediating hemolysis are also different.

The classical complement pathway is an important mediator of immune hemolysis. The major proteins of the classical complement pathway are designated C1 through C9, and their components or fragments are designated with lowercase suffixes. The first protein, C1, has three components: C1q, C1r, and C1s. After an antibody binds to an antigen on the RBC surface, C1q must bind to two adjacent Fc domains to activate the pathway.[4] Theoretically only one IgM molecule is needed for complement activation due to its larger pentameric structure with five Fc domains; however, at least two molecules of monomeric IgG in close proximity are required for C1q attachment.[4] Therefore, IgM antibodies are highly effective in activating complement, whereas IgG antibodies are unable to activate the pathway unless there is a sufficient number of IgG molecules on the RBC surface.[4,5] In addition, subclasses IgG1 and IgG3 have high binding affinity for C1q, while subclasses IgG2 and IgG4 have minimal ability to bind complement.[4,5]

The binding of C1q to adjacent Fc domains requires calcium and magnesium ions and activates C1r, which then activates C1s. This activated C1q-C1r-C1s complex is an enzyme that cleaves C4 and then C2, which results in the binding of a small number of C4bC2a complexes to the RBC membrane. The C4bC2a complex is an active C3 convertase enzyme that cleaves C3 in plasma; the result is the binding of many C3b molecules to C4bC2a on the RBC surface. The last phase of the classical pathway occurs when C4bC2aC3b converts C5 to C5b, which combines with C6, C7, C8, and multiple C9s to form the membrane attack complex (MAC). The MAC resembles a cylinder that inserts into the lipid bilayer of the membrane, forming a pore that allows water and small ions to enter the cell, causing lysis (Figure 26-3).[3] Negative regulators inhibit various complement proteins and complexes in the pathway to prevent uncontrolled activation and excessive hemolysis.[1,3,4]

Hemolysis mediated by IgM antibodies requires complement and can result in both extravascular and intravascular hemolysis.[5] When IgM molecules attach to the RBC surface in relatively low density, complement activation results in C3b binding to the membrane, but complement inhibitors prevent full activation of the pathway to the terminal membrane attack complex.[1,5] C3b-sensitized RBCs are destroyed by extravascular hemolysis, predominantly by macrophages (Kupffer cells) in the liver, which have C3b receptors. Some of the C3b on the RBCs can be cleaved, however, which leaves the C3d fragment on the cell. RBCs sensitized with only C3d are not prematurely removed from circulation because macrophages lack a C3d receptor.[5] In severe cases of immune hemolysis involving heavy sensitization of RBCs with IgM antibody, significantly more complement is activated, which overwhelms the complement inhibitors. In these cases, complement activation proceeds from C1 to C9 and results in rapid intravascular hemolysis.[5]

Hemolysis mediated by IgG antibodies occurs with or without complement and predominantly by extravascular mechanisms.[5] RBCs sensitized with IgG are removed from circulation by macrophages in the spleen, which have receptors for the Fc

---

BOX 26-1   Classification of Immune Hemolytic Anemias

Autoimmune hemolytic anemia
  Warm autoimmune hemolytic anemia (WAIHA)
    Idiopathic
    Secondary
      Lymphoproliferative disorders
      Nonlymphoid neoplasms
      Collagen-vascular disease
      Immunodeficiency disorders
      Viral infections
  Cold agglutinin disease (CAD)
    Idiopathic
    Secondary
      Acute: infections (*Mycoplasma pneumoniae*, infectious mononucleosis, other viruses)
      Chronic: lymphoproliferative disorders
  Paroxysmal cold hemoglobinuria (PCH)
    Idiopathic
    Secondary
      Viral infections
      Syphilis
  Mixed-type autoimmune hemolytic anemia
Drug-induced immune hemolytic anemia (DIIHA)
  Drug dependent
  Drug independent
Alloimmune hemolytic anemias
  Hemolytic transfusion reaction (HTR)
  Hemolytic disease of the fetus and newborn (HDFN)

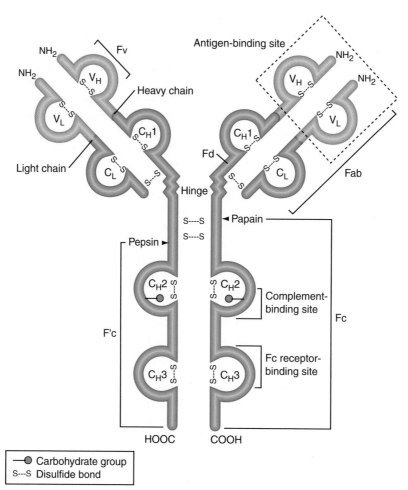

Figure 26-2 Schematic of an IgG molecule consisting of two heavy chains and two light chains. Note the antigen binding sites at the amino (NH₂) end formed by the variable region (Fv) of one heavy chain and one light chain. Note the Fc region at the carboxyl (COOH) end of the heavy chains. The chains are held together by disulfide linkages. (From McPherson RA, Massey HD. Laboratory Evaluation of Immunoglobulin Function and Humoral Immunity. In Henry's Clinical Diagnosis and Management by Laboratory Methods, ed 22. Philadelphia, 2011, Saunders, an imprint of Elsevier.)

component of IgG1 and IgG3.[1,5] IgG antibodies are not efficient in activating complement, and intravascular hemolysis by full activation of complement from C1 to C9 is rare (except with anti-P in paroxysmal cold hemoglobinuria).[5] However, if there is a high density of IgG1 or IgG3 bound to antigens on the RBCs, some complement is activated and C3b binds to the membrane. If both IgG and C3b are on the RBC membrane, there is faster clearance from the circulation by macrophages in both the spleen and the liver.[1,5] Often, IgG-sensitized RBCs are only partially phagocytized by macrophages, which results in the removal of some membrane. Spherocytes are the result of this process, and they are the characteristic cell of IgG-mediated hemolysis.[5] The spherocytes are eventually removed from circulation by entrapment in the red pulp of the spleen (splenic cords), where they are rapidly phagocytized by macrophages (Chapter 8).[5] The mechanisms of immune hemolysis are summarized in Table 26-1.

Laboratory Findings in Immune Hemolytic Anemia

Laboratory findings in immune hemolytic anemia are similar to the findings in other hemolytic anemias and include decreased hemoglobin; increased reticulocyte count; increased levels of indirect serum bilirubin and lactate dehydrogenase; and decreased serum haptoglobin level. If the hemolysis is predominantly intravascular, or the extravascular hemolysis is severe, the haptoglobin level will be moderately to severely decreased, plasma hemoglobin will be increased, and the patient may have hemoglobinuria or even hemosiderinuria (in cases of chronic hemolysis) (Chapter 23). The mean cell volume (MCV) may be increased due to the reticulocytosis and RBC agglutination (if present). Leukocytosis and thrombocytosis may occur along with the increased erythroid proliferation in the bone marrow.[1] Findings on the peripheral blood film include polychromasia (due to the reticulocytosis), spherocytes (due to IgG-mediated membrane damage by macrophages), and occasionally RBC agglutination.[5] Nucleated RBCs, fragmented RBCs or schistocytes, and erythrophagocytosis (phagocytes engulfing RBCs) may also be observed on the peripheral blood film.[1]

To determine if the hemolysis is due to an immune mechanism, a *direct antiglobulin test* (DAT) is performed. The DAT detects in vivo sensitization of the RBC surface by IgG, C3b, or

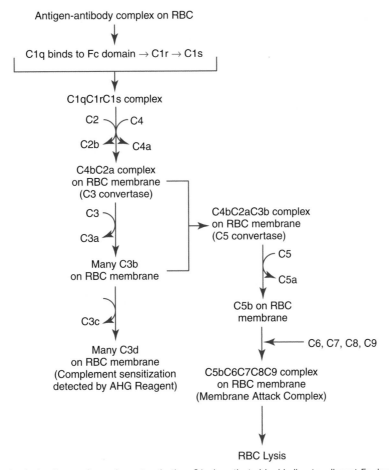

Figure 26-3 Diagram of the classical pathway of complement activation. C1q is activated by binding to adjacent Fc domains of immunoglobulin bound to RBC antigen. C1q activates C1r; C1r activates C1s which forms the complex, C1qC1rC1s. The complex activates C2 and C4 to form the C4bC2a complex (C3 convertase) on the membrane. The complex converts C3 to many C3b molecules on the membrane. If there is no further activation, C3b will degrade to C3d on the membrane, which can be detected by polyspecific antihuman globulin (AHG). C3b can also form the complex C4bC2aC3b or C5 convertase, which converts C5 to C5b on the membrane. C5b forms the membrane attack complex, C5bC6C7C8C9, which inserts into the bilipid layer, causing lysis.

TABLE 26-1 Major Mechanisms of Immune Hemolysis

	IgM Mediated	IgG Mediated
Extravascular hemolysis	IgM activation of classical complement pathway from C1 to C3b only; clearance of C3b-sensitized RBCs by macrophages mainly in liver	Clearance of IgG-sensitized RBCs by macrophages mainly in spleen Formation of spherocytes by partial phagocytosis of IgG-sensitized RBCs; spherocytes cleared by macrophages after entrapment in spleen IgG* activation of classical complement pathway from C1 to C3b only; requires high-density IgG on RBC surface; clearance of IgG- and C3b-sensitized RBCs by macrophages in spleen and liver
Intravascular hemolysis	Full IgM activation of classical complement pathway from C1 to C9 and direct RBC lysis; requires high-density IgM on RBCs to overcome complement inhibitors	Full IgG activation of classical complement pathway from C1 to C9 and direct RBC lysis; requires very high-density IgG on RBCs for activation and to overcome complement inhibitors; uncommon

Ig, Immunoglobulin; *RBC*, red blood cell.
*IgG3 and IgG1 are most efficient in complement activation.

C3d.[2] In the DAT procedure, polyspecific antihuman globulin (AHG) is added to saline-washed patient RBCs. Polyspecific AHG has specificity for the Fc portion of human IgG and complement components C3b and C3d; agglutination will occur if a critical number of any of these molecules is present on the RBC surface (Figure 26-4).[2] If the DAT result is positive with polyspecific AHG, then the cells are tested with monospecific anti-IgG and anti-C3b/C3d to identify the type of sensitization. If IgG is detected on the RBCs, elution procedures are used to remove the antibody from the RBCs for identification.

The specificity of the IgG antibody may be determined by assessing the reaction of the eluate with screening and panel

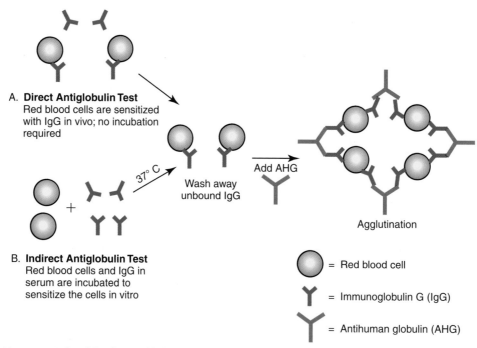

Figure 26-4 Graphic representation of the direct and indirect antihuman globulin reaction. **A,** The direct antiglobulin test (DAT) detects IgG antibodies that are bound to corresponding antigens on the patient's red blood cells in vivo. It does not require an incubation step. **B,** The indirect antiglobulin test (IAT) requires a 37° C incubation step to bind IgG antibodies (from patient's serum or from typing reagents) to corresponding antigens on red blood cells in vitro. Polyspecific antihuman globulin (AHG) is a mixture of antibodies to IgG and complement components C3d/C3b. The anti-IgG produces agglutination by binding to the Fc domain of immunoglobulin G (IgG) antibodies that are bound to antigens on the red blood cell membranes. Similarly, the anti-C3d/C3b produces agglutination by binding to the respective complement components if present on the red blood cell membranes (reaction not shown). Monospecific AHG has specificity for either IgG or C3b/C3d. Although AHG is depicted as an IgG antibody in the figure above, in some reagents it can be an IgM isotype.

reagent RBCs (RBCs genotyped for the major RBC antigens) using the *indirect antiglobulin test* (IAT) (Figure 26-4). Identification of any circulating alloantibodies or autoantibodies by the indirect antiglobulin test is also important in the investigation.[2] The DAT result may be negative in patients with some immune hemolytic anemias.[2] In addition, other disorders beside immune hemolytic anemia can cause a positive DAT finding.[2] Therefore, diagnosis of immune hemolytic anemia cannot rely solely on the DAT and must take into account the patient history; symptoms; recent medications; previous transfusions; coexisting conditions, including pregnancy; and the results of the applicable hematologic, biochemical, and serologic tests.[2,5]

AUTOIMMUNE HEMOLYTIC ANEMIA

Autoimmune hemolytic anemia (AIHA) is a rare disorder characterized by premature RBC destruction and anemia caused by autoantibodies that bind the RBC surface with or without complement activation. AIHA can affect both children and adults, and its annual incidence is estimated to be between 1 and 3 per 100,000 individuals.[6] In children, more males are affected, but in adults, more females are affected.[6] Autoantibodies may arise as a result of immune system dysregulation and loss of immune tolerance, exposure to an antigen similar to an autoantigen, B-lymphocyte neoplasm, or other unknown reason.[1,6] The type, amount, and duration of antigen exposure

and genetic and environmental factors may also contribute to the development of autoantibodies.[5] The anemia can be mild or severe, and the onset can be acute or gradual. The severity of the anemia depends on the autoantibody characteristics (titer, ability to react at 37° C, ability to activate complement, and specificity and affinity for the autoantigen), antigen characteristics (density on RBCs, immunogenicity), as well as patient factors (age, ability of the bone marrow to compensate for the hemolysis, function of macrophages, complement proteins and regulators, and underlying conditions).[1,6]

The autoimmune hemolytic anemias may be divided into four major categories based on the characteristics of the autoantibody and the mechanism of hemolysis: warm autoimmune hemolytic anemia, cold agglutinin disease, paroxysmal cold hemoglobinuria, and mixed-type autoimmune hemolytic anemia (Table 26-2).[2,5,6]

Warm Autoimmune Hemolytic Anemia

Warm autoimmune hemolytic anemia (WAIHA) is the most commonly encountered autoimmune hemolytic anemia, comprising up to 70% of cases.[5] The autoantibodies causing WAIHA react optimally at 37° C, and the vast majority of them are IgG.[1] WAIHA may be classified as idiopathic or secondary. In patients with idiopathic WAIHA, the etiology is unknown. Secondary WAIHA may occur in many conditions such as lymphoproliferative diseases (chronic lymphocytic leukemia, B-lymphocytic lymphomas, and Waldenström macroglobulinemia), nonlymphoid

TABLE 26-2 Characteristics of Autoimmune Hemolytic Anemias

	Warm Autoimmune Hemolytic Anemia	Cold Agglutinin Disease	Paroxysmal Cold Hemoglobinuria	Mixed-Type Autoimmune Hemolytic Anemia
Immunoglobulin class	IgG (rarely IgM, IgA)	IgM	IgG	IgG, IgM
Optimum reactivity temperature of autoantibody	37° C	4° C; reactivity extends to >30° C	4° C	4°–37° C
Sensitization detected by direct antiglobulin test	IgG or IgG + C3d; only C3d uncommon	C3d	C3d	IgG and C3d
Complement activation	Variable	Yes	Yes	Yes
Hemolysis	Extravascular primarily	Extravascular; rarely intravascular	Intravascular	Extravascular and intravascular
Autoantibody specificity	Panreactive or Rh complex; rarely specific Rh or other antigen	I (most), i (some), Pr (rare)	P	Panreactive; unclear specificity

Ig, Immunoglobulin.

neoplasms (thymoma and cancers of the colon, kidney, lung, and ovary), autoimmune disorders (rheumatoid arthritis, scleroderma, polyarteritis nodosa, Sjögren syndrome, and systemic lupus erythematosus), immunodeficiency disorders, and viral infections.[1,5]

The onset of WAIHA is usually insidious, with symptoms of anemia (fatigue, dizziness, dyspnea), but some cases can be acute and life-threatening with fever, jaundice, splenomegaly, and hepatomegaly, especially in children with WAIHA secondary to viral infections.[1,5] Massive splenomegaly, lymphadenopathy, fever, petechiae, ecchymosis, or renal failure in adults suggests an underlying lymphoproliferative disorder.[1,5]

Although most autoantibodies that cause WAIHA are IgG, rare cases involving IgA autoantibodies as well as cases with fatal outcomes caused by warm-reacting IgM antibodies have been reported.[1,2] Hemolysis is predominantly extravascular in WAIHA, and cases of fulminant intravascular hemolysis are rare.[5]

The result of the DAT is positive in over 95% of patients, with approximately 85% of patients having IgG alone or both IgG and C3d on their RBCs, and 10% to 14% having C3d only.[1,2,5] Between 1% and 4% of patients have a negative DAT result caused by IgA or IgM autoantibodies that are not detected by the polyspecific AHG; IgG or C3d in an amount below the reagent detection limit; dissociation of IgG antibodies with low avidity during the washing phase of the DAT; or by various technical errors.[1,2,5] Therefore, a negative DAT result does not rule out autoimmune hemolytic anemia.

Warm autoantibodies are usually panreactive; that is, they will agglutinate all screening and panel cells, donor RBCs, and the patient's own RBCs, so the specificity of the autoantibody is not apparent.[2,5] In some cases Rh complex specificity can be demonstrated.[2,5] Rarely, a specific autoantibody to an antigen in the Rh blood group system is identified. Autoantibodies to other antigens (such as LW, Jk, K, Di, Ge, Lu, M, N, S, U, En^a, and Wr^b) are occasionally identified.[2,5] For most patients (approximately 80%) the autoantibody can be detected in the serum. Because the autoantibody is panreactive, it may mask reactions of alloantibodies with RBC panel cells. If an RBC transfusion is necessary, it is crucial to perform tests to determine if clinically significant *allo*antibodies are also present.[5]

Anemia in WAIHA can be mild or severe, with RBC life span sometimes reduced to 5 days or less.[1] Laboratory findings for serum and urine reflect the predominantly extravascular hemolysis that occurs in IgG-mediated immune hemolysis. Polychromasia and spherocytes are the typical findings on the peripheral blood film (Figure 26-1). Occasionally the WAIHA is accompanied by immune thrombocytopenic purpura and a decreased platelet count, a condition known as *Evans syndrome,* which occurs primarily in children.[6,7]

In symptomatic but non-life-threatening WAIHA, a glucocorticosteroid such as prednisone is the initial treatment of choice.[1,2,8] Approximately 70% to 80% of patients show improvement with prednisone, but many adult patients need to be on a long-term maintenance dosage to remain asymptomatic.[1,8] Osteoporosis, osteonecrosis, and bone fracture, particularly of the lumbar spine, are serious side effects of long-term steroid use and occur in approximately 30% to 50% of patients.[1] The highest loss of bone density occurs early in treatment, even at smaller steroid doses, and the risk of fracture increases by 75% during the first months of treatment.[1] Patients should also receive bisphosphonates, vitamin D, and calcium according to the recommendation of the American College of Rheumatology.[9]

Splenectomy is an option in patients with chronic WAIHA who are refractory to prednisone therapy or require long-term, high-dose prednisone therapy; a favorable response is achieved in 50% to 75% of patients.[1] Immunosuppressive drugs, such as cyclophosphamide or azathioprine, are used for refractory WAIHA, but the side effects may be severe.[1,6,8] Rituximab, a monoclonal anti-CD20 antibody that binds to the corresponding antigen found on B cells, has also been used extensively. It causes minimal side effects and produces a response rate of 17% to 100%, according to various published case reports.[1,8] Hematopoietic stem cell transplantation (HSCT) has been used for severe, life-threatening autoimmune syndromes, including hemolytic anemia and Evans syndrome. Sources of the stem cells have been autologous, HLA-matched sibling, and cord blood, all of which carry lethal risks. In secondary WAIHA, successful management of the underlying condition often controls the hemolysis and anemia. WAIHA with a critically low hemoglobin level requires RBC transfusion. If the autoantibody has broad specificity, all RBC units may be incompatible with the autoantibody.[1,2,5] In such cases a minimum volume of RBCs is given, and the patient is carefully monitored during the transfusion.

Cold Agglutinin Disease

Cold agglutinins are autoantibodies of the IgM class that react optimally at 4° C and are commonly found in healthy individuals. These nonpathologic cold agglutinins are polyclonal, occur in low titers (less than 1:64 at 4° C), and have no reactivity above 30° C.[1,5] Most pathologic cold agglutinins are monoclonal, occur at high titers (greater than 1:1000 at 4° C), and are capable of reacting at temperatures greater than 30° C.[2] Because pathologic cold agglutinins can react at body temperature, they may induce cold agglutinin disease (CAD). Cold agglutinins that are able to bind RBC antigens near or at 37° C (high thermal amplitude) cause more severe symptoms.[1,10,11] CAD has recently been recognized as a clonal lymphoproliferative B cell disorder.[6,10] It comprises approximately 15% to 20% of the cases of autoimmune hemolytic anemia.[6]

In CAD, the IgM autoantibody binds to RBCs after exposure to the cold, particularly in the peripheral circulation and the vessels of the skin, where temperatures can drop to 30° C.[11] During the brief transit through these colder areas, IgM autoantibodies activate the classical complement pathway.[10] When the RBCs return to the central circulation, the IgM antibody dissociates, but C3b components remain on the cell.[2,10] Hemolysis is predominantly extravascular by hepatic macrophages, which have receptors for C3b.[1,10] However, if the autoantibody has a high thermal amplitude or there is a deficiency in complement regulatory proteins, full complement activation and intravascular hemolysis can occur.[2,12]

Acute CAD occurs secondary to *Mycoplasma pneumoniae* infection, infectious mononucleosis, and other viral infections. These cold agglutinins are polyclonal IgM, with a normal distribution of κ and λ light chains.[2,5] Chronic CAD is a rare hemolytic anemia that typically occurs in middle-aged and elderly individuals, and the autoantibody is usually monoclonal IgM with κ light chains.[6,10,11] In a study of 86 patients with chronic CAD by Berentsen and colleagues, the median age at onset was 67 years, with the median age at death reported to be 82 years.[10] Chronic CAD can be idiopathic, with no known cause, or secondary due to lymphoproliferative neoplasms such as B-lymphocytic lymphomas, Waldenström macroglobulinemia, or chronic lymphocytic leukemia.[10]

Clinical manifestations are variable in chronic CAD. Most patients have a mild anemia with a hemoglobin result ranging from 9 to 12 g/dL, but others can develop life-threatening anemia with hemoglobin levels falling below 5 g/dL, especially after exposure to cold temperatures.[5,11,13] Individuals often experience fluctuations between mild and severe symptoms, and approximately half of those affected require transfusions over the course of the disease.[10] Symptoms include fatigue, weakness, dyspnea, pallor (due to the anemia), and acrocyanosis.[11] *Acrocyanosis* is a bluish discoloration of the extremities (fingers,

toes, feet, earlobes, nose) due to RBC autoagglutination, which causes local capillary stasis.[1,2,11] Some patients also have episodes of hemoglobinuria, especially after exposure to cold temperatures.[2,11] In contrast, patients with acute CAD may have mild to severe hemolysis that appears abruptly within 2 to 3 weeks after the onset of infectious mononucleosis, other viral infection, or *M. pneumoniae* infection, but it resolves spontaneously within days to a few weeks.[11]

The DAT result is positive with polyspecific AHG because of the presence of C3d on the RBC surface. The specificity of the cold agglutinin is most often anti-I but can be anti-i or, very rarely, anti-Pr.[2,12] Virtually all adult RBCs are positive for the I antigen, so anti-I will agglutinate all screening and panel cells, donor RBCs, and the patient's own RBCs at room temperature and higher, depending on the thermal amplitude of the autoantibody. Anti-I will show weaker or negative reactions with cord RBCs (cord cells are negative for I antigen but positive for i antigen).[2]

A cold agglutinin method is used to determine the titer of the antibody at 4° C. Pathologic cold agglutinins can reach titers of 1:10,000 to 1:1,000,000 at 4° C.[1,5] Blood specimens for cold agglutinin testing must be maintained at 37° C after collection to prevent the binding of the autoantibody to the patient's own RBCs, which can falsely decrease the antibody titer in the serum. Alternatively, a sample anticoagulated with EDTA can be warmed for 15 minutes at 37° C to dissociate autoabsorbed antibody prior to determining the titer.

When a high-titer cold agglutinin is present, an EDTA-anticoagulated blood specimen can show visible agglutinates in the tube at room temperature or below.[1] The agglutination can also be observed on a peripheral blood film (Figure 26-5). Blood specimens from patients with cold agglutinins must be warmed to 37° C for 15 minutes before complete blood count analysis by automated hematology analyzers. RBC agglutination grossly elevates the mean cell volume, reduces the RBC count, and has unpredictable effects on other indices (Chapter 15). When the sample is warmed to 37° C, the antibody dissociates from the RBCs, and agglutination usually disappears. If not, a new specimen is collected and maintained at 37° C for

Figure 26-5 Wright-stained peripheral blood film showing red blood cell agglutination (×500).

the entire time before testing. To avoid agglutination on a peripheral blood film, the slide can also be warmed to 37° C prior to the application of blood. Cold agglutinins can also interfere with ABO typing.[2]

Acute CAD associated with infections is self-limiting, and the cold agglutinin titers are usually less than 1:4000.[11] If the hemolysis is mild, no treatment is required; however, patients with severe hemolysis require transfusion and supportive care.[11] Patients with chronic CAD and mild anemia are regularly monitored and advised to avoid cold temperatures.[1] In chronic CAD with moderate to severe symptoms, rituximab produces partial remission in about half of patients due to its targeting and ultimate destruction of the B-lymphocytes containing the CD-20 antigen, but median remission is less than a year.[14] In a 2010 study by Berentsen and colleagues, a combination of rituximab with fludarabine resulted in a better response rate (76%) and median duration of remission (66 months); however, hematologic toxicity was reported in almost half of the patients.[13] Even with the occasional severe side effects, rituximab is currently the best second-line treatment for CAD and primary AIHA, it can be given multiple times, and children tolerate it well. Plasmapheresis may be used in severe cases but provides only temporary benefit.[1] Corticosteroid therapy and immunosuppressive therapy with cyclophosphamide and chlorambucil are not effective for most patients.[11,12] Splenectomy is also not effective because C3b-sensitized RBCs in IgM-mediated autoimmune hemolysis are cleared primarily by the liver.[1,5,11]

RBC transfusion is reserved for patients with life-threatening anemia or cardiovascular or cerebrovascular symptoms.[1] If transfusion is needed, the presence of clinically significant alloantibodies must be ruled out.[2] In CAD cases involving an autoantibody with wide thermal amplitude, detection of coexisting warm-reactive alloantibodies can be time-consuming and difficult. During transfusion, the patient is kept warm, small amounts of blood are given while the patient is observed for symptoms of a hemolytic transfusion reaction, and a blood warmer is used to minimize the in vivo reactivity of the cold autoantibody.[1]

Paroxysmal Cold Hemoglobinuria

Paroxysmal cold hemoglobinuria (PCH) is an acute form of cold-reactive hemolytic anemia. PCH can be idiopathic or secondary. Historically, secondary PCH was associated with late-stage syphilis, but now it is most commonly seen in young children after a viral respiratory infection.[1,2,11] PCH is rare in adults. The prevalence of PCH has been reported to be as high as 32% to 40% of children with autoimmune hemolytic anemia, with a median age at presentation of 5 years.[15,16]

The anti-P autoantibody, also called the *Donath-Landsteiner antibody*, is a complement-binding IgG hemolysin with specificity for the P antigen on RBCs. The anti-P autoantibody is biphasic in that at cold temperatures it binds to the P antigen on RBCs and partially activates complement (C1 to C4), but full complement activation (C3 through C9) and hemolysis occur only upon warming to 37° C.[17] Exposure to cold temperatures is not required for the hemolytic manifestations in vivo, however, and the reasons for this have yet to be explained.[2] The anti-P autoantibody binds RBC antigen optimally at 4° C and

has a thermal amplitude of less than 20° C. At warmer temperatures, the anti-P autoantibody dissociates from the RBCs; the titer is usually less than 1:64.[11]

Children typically present with acute fever; malaise; and back, leg, and/or abdominal pain 1 to 2 weeks after an upper respiratory tract infection.[11] Pallor, jaundice, and dark urine due to hemoglobinuria are frequently present.[11] The abrupt onset of hemolysis causes a rapidly progressing and severe anemia, with hemoglobin levels often dropping below 5 gm/dL.[11]

Reticulocytosis is typical but can be preceded by reticulocytopenia.[11] The peripheral blood film shows polychromasia and spherocytes, but schistocytes, nucleated RBCs, anisocytosis, poikilocytosis, and erythrophagocytosis can also be observed.[11] At first, leukopenia may be present; later, leukocytosis occurs.[11] In addition, laboratory findings typical for intravascular hemolysis are found. Because the anti-P autoantibody is dissociated from the RBCs at body temperature, the DAT result is usually positive for C3d only.[2,15]

The classic Donath-Landsteiner test for anti-P is done by collecting blood samples in two tubes, one for the patient test and the other for the patient control.[16] The patient test sample is incubated first at 4° C for 30 minutes (to allow anti-P binding to the P antigen and partial complement activation on the RBCs) and then at 37° C for 30 minutes (to allow full activation of the complement pathway to lysis). The patient control tube is kept at 37° C for both incubations (and a total of 60 minutes). After centrifugation the supernatant is examined for hemolysis. A positive test result for anti-P is indicated by hemolysis in the patient test sample incubated first at 4° C and then at 37° C and no hemolysis in the patient control sample kept at 37° C. In the control tube, the anti-P is not able to bind to antigen at 37° C, so complement is not activated and hemolysis does not occur.[16] Initial test results may be falsely negative due to low complement and/or anti-P levels in the patient sample because of the brisk hemolysis in vivo.[16] Incubating patient serum with complement and papain-treated compatible group O RBCs increases the sensitivity of the test in detecting anti-P. The enzyme treatment provides greater exposure of the P antigen on the RBC surface for antibody binding.[16]

PCH is severe but self-limiting and resolves in several days to a few weeks, with an excellent prognosis.[1,11,15] In most patients, the anemia is severe and can be life-threatening, so transfusion is usually needed until the symptoms resolve. Because the anti-P autoantibody reacts only at lower temperatures and P antigen–negative blood is very rare, P-positive blood can be transfused.[2]

Mixed-Type Autoimmune Hemolytic Anemia

Mixed-type autoimmune hemolytic anemia occurs very infrequently.[18] In this condition, the patient simultaneously develops an IgG autoantibody with optimum reactivity at 37° C (WAIHA) and a pathologic IgM autoantibody that reacts optimally at 0° C to 10° C but has a thermal amplitude of greater than 30° C (CAD).[18] Patients with WAIHA and a nonpathogenic cold agglutinin (i.e., an agglutinin that does not react at a temperature greater than 20° C) should not be classified as having a mixed-type autoimmune hemolytic anemia because the cold agglutinin is not clinically significant.[11]

The hemolysis results from a combination of extravascular and intravascular mechanisms. The disease course appears to be chronic, with intermittent episodes of severe anemia.[5,11] The DAT results can be positive with IgG only, C3d only, or IgG and C3d.[2] The warm autoantibody is typically panreactive with unclear specificity, whereas the cold-reacting antibody usually has anti-I specificity.[5] Treatment is the same as that described for WAIHA.[5]

DRUG-INDUCED IMMUNE HEMOLYTIC ANEMIA

Drug-induced immune hemolytic anemia (DIIHA) is very rare, with an estimated annual incidence of about 1 per million persons.[19] This condition is suspected when there is a sudden decrease in hemoglobin after administration of a drug, clinical and biochemical evidence of extravascular or intravascular hemolysis, and a positive DAT result.[20] Over 125 drugs have been reported to cause DIIHA, with the most common drug categories being antimicrobial, antiinflammatory, and antineoplastic drugs.[21,22] The most common drugs implicated in DIIHA in the last 10 years are cefotetan, ceftriaxone, trimethoprim, and piperacillin. Severe, even fatal, cases have been reported.[19,22-24]

Mechanisms of Drug-Induced Immune Hemolysis

Various theories have been proposed to explain the mechanisms of DIIHA.[19,24] Three generally accepted mechanisms involve an antibody produced by the patient as a result of exposure to the drug and include drug adsorption, drug–RBC membrane protein immunogenic complex, and RBC autoantibody induction. A fourth mechanism, drug-induced nonimmunologic protein adsorption (NIPA), can result in a positive DAT result, but no drug or RBC antibody is produced by the patient. This mechanism is discussed at the end of this section.

1. *Drug adsorption:* The patient produces an IgG antibody to a drug. When the drug is taken by the patient, the drug binds strongly to the patient's RBCs (see paragraph below on unifying theory). The IgG drug antibody binds to the drug attached to the RBCs, usually without complement activation. Because the offending antibody is IgG and is strongly attached to the RBCs via the drug, hemolysis is extravascular by splenic macrophages, which remove the antibody- and drug-coated RBCs from the circulation.
2. *Drug–RBC membrane protein immunogenic complex:* A drug binds loosely to an RBC membrane protein to form a drug–RBC protein immunogenic complex or epitope. The patient produces an IgM and/or IgG antibody that binds to the complex on the RBCs, and complement is fully activated, which causes acute intravascular hemolysis.
3. *RBC autoantibody induction:* A drug induces the patient to produce IgG warm-reactive autoantibodies against RBC self-antigens. These autoantibodies react at 37° C, and the laboratory findings are indistinguishable from those in WAIHA. Hemolysis is extravascular and is mediated by macrophages predominantly in the spleen.

Several authors have suggested that all drug-induced immune hemolysis is explained by a single mechanism, known as the *unifying theory.* This theory proposes that a drug interacts with the RBC membrane and generates multiple immunogenic epitopes that can elicit an immune response to the drug alone, to the drug–RBC membrane protein combination, or to an RBC membrane protein alone.[2,21,25] Diagnosis of DIIHA can only be made if the antibody screen is positive and the RBC eluate contains an antibody.[1]

Antibody Characteristics

Antibodies implicated in DIIHA can be divided into two general types: drug-dependent (most common) and drug-independent antibodies.[2,21] Some drugs are able to induce a combination of both types of antibodies.[19,24,25]

Drug-Dependent Antibodies

Drug-dependent antibodies only react in vitro when the suspected drug or its metabolite is present.[2,21] There are two types of drug-dependent antibodies:

1. *Antibodies that react only with drug-treated cells:*[2] These are IgG drug antibodies that bind to the drug when it is strongly associated with the RBC surface (drug adsorption mechanism). Because they have bound IgG, the RBCs are cleared from the circulation extravascularly by macrophages in the spleen, and a hemolytic anemia gradually develops. Complement is not usually activated. If the DIIHA is not recognized, the patient may continue to take the drug to a point in which life-threatening anemia develops.[2,19] Examples of drugs that elicit antibodies in this category are penicillin and cyclosporin.[2,21] Laboratory features include a positive DAT reaction with anti-IgG, whereas the reaction with anti-C3b/C3d is usually negative. In the indirect antiglobulin test, the patient's serum and an eluate of the patient's cells react only with drug-treated RBCs and not with untreated RBCs.[2]
2. *Antibodies that react only in the presence of the drug:*[2] These IgG and/or IgM antibodies bind to the drug or its metabolite only when it is weakly associated in a drug–RBC membrane protein complex (drug–RBC membrane protein immunogenic complex mechanism). The antibodies activate complement and trigger acute intravascular hemolysis that may progress to renal failure.[2] Hemolysis occurs abruptly after short periods of drug exposure or upon readministration of the drug.[19] Examples of drugs that elicit antibodies in this category are phenacetin, trimethoprim, quinine, and ciprofloxacin.[2,19,22,23] Laboratory features include a positive DAT reaction with anti-C3b/C3d and occasionally with anti-IgG. In the indirect antiglobulin test, the patient's serum reacts with untreated, normal RBCs only in the presence of the drug.

Drug-Independent Antibodies

Drug-independent antibodies are IgG, warm-reactive, RBC autoantibodies induced by the drug (RBC autoantibody induction mechanism). These autoantibodies have the same serologic reactivity as those causing WAIHA, and they do not require the presence of the drug for in vitro reactivity. Hemolysis is extravascular, mediated by macrophages predominantly in the spleen, usually with a gradual onset of anemia. Examples of drugs that elicit antibodies in this category are fludarabine, methyldopa, and procainamide.[2,19,21] Laboratory features include a positive DAT reaction with anti-IgG. In the indirect antiglobulin test, the patient's serum and an eluate of the patient's cells generally react at 37° C with all screening and panel RBCs and with the patient's own RBCs.[2]

Nonimmune Drug-Induced Hemolysis

In *drug-induced nonimmunologic protein adsorption*, the patient does not produce an antibody to the drug or to RBCs. The mechanism is also called the *membrane modification method*, because certain drugs such as high-dose clavulanate and cisplatin can alter the RBC membrane so that numerous proteins, including IgG and complement, adsorb onto the RBC surface.[21,24] This phenomenon results in a positive DAT finding, but only rarely has hemolysis been reported. The indirect antiglobulin test on the patient's serum and an eluate of the patient's RBCs yield negative results.[2]

Treatment

After a DIIHA is recognized and confirmed, the first treatment is to discontinue the drug. Most patients will gradually show improvement within a few days to several weeks.[19] In cases in which a warm-reacting autoimmune antibody is present, the positive DAT result may persist for months after a hematologic recovery. If the anemia is severe, the patient may require RBC transfusion or plasma exchange.[19] Regardless of mechanism, future episodes of DIIHA are prevented by avoidance of the drug.

ALLOIMMUNE HEMOLYTIC ANEMIAS

Hemolytic Transfusion Reaction

One of the most severe and potentially life-threatening complications of blood transfusion is a hemolytic transfusion reaction (HTR) due to immune-mediated destruction of donor cells by an antibody in the recipient. The offending antibody in the recipient may be IgM or IgG, complement may be partially or fully activated or not activated at all, and the hemolysis may be intravascular or extravascular, depending on the characteristics of the antibody. HTRs can have an acute or delayed onset.[2]

Acute Hemolytic Transfusion Reaction

Acute hemolytic transfusion reactions (AHTRs) occur within minutes to hours of the initiation of a transfusion.[26] The most common cause of AHTR is the accidental transfusion of ABO-incompatible donor red blood cells into a recipient. An example is the transfusion of group A red blood cells into a group O recipient. The recipient has preformed, non-RBC stimulated anti-A (IgM) that is capable of fully activating complement to C9 upon binding to the A antigen on donor red blood cells. There is rapid, complement-mediated intravascular hemolysis and activation of the coagulation system. ABO-incompatible transfusions are usually due to clerical error and have been estimated to occur in approximately 1 in 38,000 to 1 in 70,000 RBC transfusions.[26] The severity of AHTR is variable and is affected by the infusion rate and volume of blood transfused.[2,27] AHTR carries an estimated mortality rate of 2%.[26] AHTRs can occur due to incompatibilities involving other blood group systems, but these are rare.[26]

Symptoms of severe intravascular hemolysis found in ABO-related AHTRs begin within minutes or hours and may include chills, fever, urticaria, tachycardia, nausea and vomiting, chest and back pain, shock, anaphylaxis, pulmonary edema, congestive heart failure, and bleeding due to disseminated intravascular coagulation (DIC). The transfusion should be immediately terminated upon first appearance of symptoms. Treatment is urgent and includes an effort to prevent or correct shock, maintain renal circulation, and control the DIC.[27]

The immediate investigation of a suspected HTR includes a clerical check for errors, an examination of a posttransfusion blood specimen for hemolysis, and performance of the DAT on the RBCs in a posttransfusion specimen.[26] If an AHTR occurred, hemoglobinemia and hemoglobinuria are detectable, and the DAT result is positive. DAT findings may be negative, however, if all the donor cells are lysed.[26] The hemoglobin and serum haptoglobin levels decrease, but the serum indirect bilirubin will not begin to rise until 2 to 3 days after the episode. The ABO and Rh typing, antibody screen, and cross-matching are repeated on the recipient and the donor blood to identify the blood group incompatibility. Coagulation tests such as D-dimer, fibrinogen, factors V and VIII, and platelet count can help reveal and assess the risk of DIC.[2]

Delayed Hemolytic Transfusion Reaction

A delayed hemolytic transfusion reaction (DHTR) may occur days to weeks after transfusion as the titer of alloantibodies increases.[2,27] Often, the patient has been alloimmunized by a pregnancy or previous transfusion, but the antibody titer was below the level of serologic detection at the time of transfusion. The second exposure to the antigen results in an increase in titer (anamnestic response). The antibody is usually IgG, is reactive at 37° C, and may or may not be able to partially or fully activate complement. The antibodies most often implicated in DHTRs are directed against antigens in the Duffy and Kidd blood groups.[26,27] The patient's antibody binds to the transfused RBCs, which leads to extravascular hemolysis, with or without complement activation. The principal signs are an inadequate posttransfusion hemoglobin increase, positive DAT results for IgG and/or C3d, morphologic evidence of hemolysis, and an increase in serum indirect bilirubin.[25,26] Management of DHTR includes monitoring of kidney function, especially in acutely ill patients.[26]

Hemolytic Disease of the Fetus and Newborn

Hemolytic disease of the fetus and newborn (HDFN) occurs when an IgG alloantibody produced by the mother crosses the placenta into the fetal circulation and binds to fetal RBCs that are positive for the corresponding antigen. The IgG-sensitized fetal RBCs are cleared from the circulation by macrophages in the fetal spleen (extravascular hemolysis), and an anemia gradually develops. There is erythroid hyperplasia in the fetal bone marrow and extramedullary erythropoiesis in the fetal spleen, liver, kidneys, and adrenal glands.[28] Many nucleated

RBCs are released into the fetal circulation. If the anemia is severe in utero, it can lead to generalized edema, ascites, and a condition called *hydrops fetalis*, which is fatal if untreated.[2,28] Anti-Kell antibodies are an exception because they also cause anemia by suppressing fetal erythropoiesis.[28]

In Rh HDFN, which causes the highest number of fetal fatalities, an Rh (D)-negative mother has preformed anti-D antibodies (IgG, reactive at 37° C) from exposure to the D antigen either through immunization in a previous pregnancy with a D-positive baby or from previous transfusion of blood products with D-positive RBCs. In subsequent pregnancies, the anti-D crosses the placenta, and if the fetus is D positive, the anti-D binds to D antigen sites on the fetal RBCs. These anti-D–sensitized fetal RBCs are cleared from the circulation by macrophages in the fetal spleen, and anemia and hyperbilirubinemia develop. Amniocentesis is accurate at predicting severe fetal anemia, but it is an invasive procedure and carries some risk of fetal loss.[28] If severe fetal anemia and HDFN due to anti-D is suspected, a percutaneous umbilical fetal blood sample can be obtained and tested for the hemoglobin level to determine the severity of the anemia; more recently, a noninvasive assessment of anemia can be done by ultrasound measurement of fetal cerebral flow.[2,28]

Laboratory Findings

ABO, Rh typing, and an antibody screen are performed on the mother when the fetus is between 10 and 16 weeks' gestation, and again at 28 weeks' gestation.[28] The antibody screen during pregnancy detects antibodies other than those caused by ABO incompatibility.[2] If the antibody screen is positive, an RBC panel is performed to identify the specificity of the antibody. Mothers with initial positive antibody screens are retested for an antibody screen every month until 28 weeks, then every two weeks thereafter; antibody titers are reported from each sample. Titration of the antibody does not predict the severity of HDFN; rather, it helps determine when to monitor for HDFN by additional methods, such as spectrophotometric analysis of amniotic fluid bilirubin.[2,28] After the first affected pregnancy, the antibody titer is no longer useful, and other means of monitoring the fetus are used, such as amniocentesis and ultrasonography.[28]

An unimmunized D-negative mother receives antenatal Rh immune globulin (RhIG) at 28 weeks' gestation and again within 72 hours of delivery of a D-positive infant to prevent alloimmunization to the D antigen.[2] Even one antenatal dose of 200 μg RhIG will reduce by half the risk of the mother developing anti-D antibodies and having a child with HDFN in the next pregnancy.[29] Rh-negative women who experience spontaneous or induced abortion also receive Rh immune globulin.

At delivery, newborn testing is performed on umbilical cord blood. Neonates with Rh HDFN have a decreased hemoglobin level, increased reticulocyte count, and increased level of serum indirect bilirubin. The peripheral blood film shows polychromasia and many nucleated RBCs. ABO (only forward typing), Rh typing, and the DAT are also performed. The DAT result is positive for IgG, and anti-D can be demonstrated in an eluate of the infant's RBCs.[28]

Treatment for the Affected Infant

Treatment for a fetus affected by HDFN may include intrauterine transfusion, whereby pooled hemolyzed blood is removed via amniocentesis from the fetal abdomen and replaced with a small amount of fresh red blood cells. This procedure can be used to correct fetal anemia and prevent hydrops fetalis.[30] Cordocentesis is also utilized, whereby fresh red blood cells are injected into the umbilical vein. The survival rates of fetuses receiving transfusions are 85% to 90%; the risk of premature death from these procedures varies from 1% to 3%.[30] After delivery, the neonate may need exchange transfusions and phototherapy to reduce the level of serum indirect bilirubin and prevent kernicterus (bilirubin accumulation in the brain).[28] Prolonged postnatal anemia can be due to a slow decrease of maternal antibody in the newborn's circulation; rare cases of prolonged anemia are documented in infants who received intrauterine transfusions.[31,32]

Hemolytic Disease of the Fetus and Newborn Caused by Other Blood Group Antigens

ABO HDFN is more common than Rh disease and may occur during the first pregnancy. Unlike Rh disease, ABO disease is asymptomatic or produces mild hyperbilirubinemia and anemia. ABO HDFN is seen in some type A or B infants born to type O mothers who produce IgG anti-A and anti-B which are capable of crossing the placenta. The disease is milder than Rh HDFN likely because A and B antigens are poorly developed on fetal and newborn RBCs, and other cells and tissues express A and B antigens which reduces the amount of maternal antibody directed against fetal RBCs. The DAT result for the newborn with ABO HDFN is only weakly positive and may be negative. Spherocytes and polychromasia on the peripheral blood film are typical.[2] Table 26-3 presents a comparison of HDFN caused by ABO and Rh incompatibility.

HDFN can be caused by other IgG antibodies, particularly antibodies to the K, c, and Fy[a] antigens.[2] HDFN due to other blood group antibodies is rare.[28,33-36] Antibody screening in the first trimester can assist in identifying rare antibodies that can cause HDFN.[37] Varying degrees of anemia, jaundice, and kernicterus are the adverse clinical outcomes in all forms of HDFN.

TABLE 26-3 Characteristics of Rh and ABO Hemolytic Disease of the Fetus and Newborn

	Rh	ABO
Blood Groups		
Mother	Rh (D) negative	O
Child	Rh (D) positive	A or B
Severity of disease	Severe	Mild
Jaundice	Severe	Mild
Spherocytes on peripheral blood film	Rare	Usually present
Anemia	Severe	If present, mild
Direct antiglobulin test result	Positive	Negative or weakly positive

SUMMARY

- The immune hemolytic anemias are classified into autoimmune hemolytic anemia, drug-induced immune hemolytic anemia, and alloimmune hemolytic anemia.
- Hemolysis mediated by IgM requires complement; hemolysis may be extravascular (mainly in the liver) if complement is partially activated to C3b, or intravascular if complement is fully activated to C9.
- Hemolysis mediated by IgG occurs with or without complement activation; IgG-sensitized RBCs are removed from the circulation by macrophages in the spleen; partial phagocytosis produces spherocytes, which are prematurely trapped in the spleen and phagocytized; IgG- and C3b-sensitized RBCs are removed by macrophages in the spleen and liver.
- Laboratory findings in immune hemolytic anemia include decreased hemoglobin level, increased reticulocyte count, increased levels of serum indirect bilirubin and lactate dehydrogenase, and decreased serum haptoglobin level. The peripheral blood film may show polychromasia, spherocytes (IgG-mediated hemolysis), or RBC agglutination (cold agglutinins). The DAT detects in vivo sensitization of RBCs by IgG and/or C3b/C3d.
- The classification of autoimmune hemolytic anemia includes warm autoimmune hemolytic anemia (WAIHA), cold agglutinin disease (CAD), paroxysmal cold hemoglobinuria (PCH), and mixed-type autoimmune hemolytic anemia.
- WAIHA is the most common form of autoimmune hemolytic anemia and involves IgG autoantibodies with optimum reactivity at 37° C. The anemia varies from mild to severe, and characteristic morphologic features on the peripheral blood film are polychromasia and spherocytes.
- CAD is caused by an IgM autoantibody with optimum reactivity at 4° C and a thermal amplitude of greater than 30° C. RBC agglutination may be observed on a peripheral blood film, and agglutinates may cause interference with the complete blood count analysis on automated hematology analyzers.

- Paroxysmal cold hemoglobinuria (PCH) is due to a biphasic IgG autoantibody with anti-P specificity. The antibody binds to the P antigen on the RBCs and partially activates complement at 4° C; complete complement activation and hemolysis occur upon warming the sample to 37° C.
- In drug-induced immune hemolytic anemia (DIIHA), the patient produces antibodies to (1) a drug only, (2) a complex of a drug loosely bound to an RBC membrane protein, or (3) an RBC membrane protein only. In vitro reactions of antibodies in DIIHA may be drug-dependent or drug-independent.
- Acute hemolytic transfusion reactions (AHTRs) occur within minutes to hours after the start of an RBC transfusion and most often involve transfusion of ABO-incompatible blood; the hemolysis is predominantly intravascular. Delayed hemolytic transfusion reactions (DHTRs) may occur days or weeks after the transfusion and represent an anamnestic response to a donor red blood cell antigen; the hemolysis is usually extravascular.
- Hemolytic disease of the fetus and newborn (HDFN) occurs when an IgG alloantibody produced by the mother crosses the placenta into the fetal circulation and binds to fetal RBCs that are positive for the corresponding antigen. The IgG-sensitized fetal RBCs are cleared from the circulation by macrophages in the fetal spleen, and an anemia gradually develops; the usual laboratory findings in the neonate are anemia, hyperbilirubinemia, and a positive direct antiglobulin test (DAT) result.
- ABO HDFN is more common than Rh HDFN and produces no symptoms or mild anemia. Rh HDFN due to anti-D results in severe anemia. Antenatal administration of Rh immune globulin to a D-negative mother when the fetus is at 28 weeks' gestation and within 72 hours after delivery of a D-positive baby prevents immunization to the D antigen.

Now that you have completed this chapter, go back and read again the case study at the beginning and respond to the questions presented.

REVIEW QUESTIONS

Answers can be found in the Appendix.

1. Immune hemolytic anemia is due to a(n):
   a. Structural defect in the RBC membrane
   b. Allo- or autoantibody against an RBC antigen
   c. T cell immune response against an RBC antigen
   d. Obstruction of blood flow by intravascular thrombi

2. The pathophysiology of immune hemolysis with IgM antibodies always involves:
   a. Complement
   b. Autoantibodies
   c. Abnormal hemoglobin molecules
   d. Alloantibodies

3. In hemolysis mediated by IgG antibodies, which abnormal RBC morphology is typically observed on the peripheral blood film?
   a. Spherocytes
   b. Nucleated RBCs
   c. RBC agglutination
   d. Macrocytes

4. The most important finding in the diagnostic investigation of a suspected autoimmune hemolytic anemia is:
   a. Detection of a low hemoglobin and hematocrit
   b. Observation of hemoglobinemia in a specimen
   c. Recognition of a low reticulocyte count
   d. Demonstration of IgG and/or C3d on the RBC surface

5. In autoimmune hemolytic anemia, a positive DAT is evidence that an:
   a. IgM antibody is in the patient's serum
   b. IgG antibody is in the patient's serum
   c. IgM antibody is sensitizing the patient's red blood cells
   d. IgG antibody is sensitizing the patient's red blood cells

6. Which of the following is NOT a mechanism of drug-induced hemolytic anemia?
   a. Drug adsorption on red blood cell membrane
   b. Drug–RBC membrane protein immunogenic complex
   c. RBC autoantibody induction
   d. IgM autoantibody sensitization of RBCs after exposure to the cold

7. Which of the following describes a penicillin-induced AIHA?
   a. Extravascular hemolysis, positive DAT with IgG, gradual anemia
   b. Intravascular, possible renal failure, positive DAT with C3d
   c. Rare hemolysis, positive DAT with IgG
   d. Intravascular hemolysis, positive DAT with IgG

8. Which one of the following statements is *true* about DHTR:
   a. It is usually due to an ABO incompatibility
   b. Hemoglobinemia and hemoglobinuria frequently occur
   c. It is due to an anamnestic response after repeat exposure to a blood group antigen
   d. The DAT yields a positive result for C3d only

9. Chronic secondary CAD is most often associated with:
   a. Antibiotic therapy
   b. *M. pneumoniae* infection
   c. B cell malignancies
   d. Infectious mononucleosis

10. A 63-year-old man is being evaluated because of a decrease in hemoglobin of 5 gm/dL after a second cycle of fludarabine for treatment of chronic lymphocytic leukemia. The patient's DAT result is strongly positive for IgG only, and antibody testing on his serum and an eluate of his RBCs yield positive results with all panel cells and the patient's own cells. This suggests which mechanism of immune hemolysis for this patient?
    a. Drug-RBC membrane protein complex
    b. Drug adsorption
    c. RBC autoantibody induction
    d. Drug-induced nonimmunologic protein adsorption

11. A Group A Rh-negative mother gave birth to a Group O Rh-positive baby. The baby is at risk for HDFN if:
    a. This was the mother's first pregnancy
    b. The mother has IgG ABO antibodies
    c. The mother was previously immunized to the D antigen
    d. The mother received Rh immune globulin prior to delivery

REFERENCES

1. Jäger, U., & Lechner, K. (2013). Autoimmune hemolytic anemia. In Hoffman, R., Benz, E. Jr, Silberstein, L., et al (Eds.), *Hoffman: Hematology: Basic Principles and Practice.* (6th ed.). Philadelphia: Saunders, an imprint of Elsevier. Accessed 23.03.13.
2. Leger, R. (2011). The positive direct antiglobulin test and immune-mediated hemolysis. In Roback, J., Combs, M., Grossman, B., et al. (Eds.), *Technical Manual.* (17th ed.). Bethesda, MD: American Association of Blood Banks.
3. Mandle, R., Barrington, R., & Carroll, M. (2013). Complement and immunoglobulin biology. In Hoffman, R., Benz, E. Jr, Silberstein, L., et al. (Eds.), *Hoffman: Hematology: Basic Principles and Practice.* (6th ed.). Philadelphia: Saunders, an imprint of Elsevier. Accessed 23.03.13.
4. Prodinger, W., Würzner, R., Stoiber, H., et al. (2008). Complement. In Paul, W., (Ed.), *Fundamental Immunology.* (6th ed.). Philadelphia: Lippincott Williams & Wilkins.
5. Friedberg, R., & Johari, V. (2009). Autoimmune hemolytic anemia. In Greer, J., Foerster, J., Rodgers, G., et al. (Eds.), *Wintrobe's Clinical Hematology.* (12th ed.). Philadelphia: Lippincott Williams & Wilkins.
6. Michel, M. (2011). Classification and therapeutic approaches in autoimmune hemolytic anemia: an update. *Expert Rev Hematol, 4,* 607–618.
7. Dhingra, K., Jain, D., Mandal, S., et al. (2008). Evans syndrome: a study of six cases with review of literature. *Hematology, 13,* 356–360.
8. Liu, B., & Gu, W. (2013). Immunotherapy treatments of warm autoimmune hemolytic anemia. *Clin Dev Immunol, 2013,* 561852. doi: 10.1155/2013/561852. Epub 2013 Sep 11.
9. Lechner, K., & Jäger, U. (2010). How I treat autoimmune hemolytic anemia. *Blood, 116,* 1831–1838.
10. Berentsen, S., Beiske, K., & Tjonnfjord, G. (2007). Primary chronic cold agglutinin disease: an update on pathogenesis, clinical features and therapy. *Hematology, 12,* 361–370.
11. Petz, L. (2008). Cold antibody autoimmune hemolytic anemias. *Blood Rev, 22,* 1–15.
12. Berentsen, S., Ulvestad, E., Langholm, R., et al. (2006). Primary chronic cold agglutinin disease: a population based clinical study of 86 patients. *Haematologica, 91,* 460–466.
13. Berentsen, S., Randen, U., Vagan, A., et al. (2010). High response rate and durable remissions following fludarabine and rituximab combination therapy for chronic cold agglutinin disease. *Blood, 116,* 3180–3184.
14. Schöllkopf, C., Kjeldsen, L., Bjerrum, O. W., et al. (2006). Rituximab in chronic cold agglutinin disease: a prospective study of 20 patients. *Leuk Lymphoma, 47,* 253–260.
15. Karafin, M., Shirey, S., Ness, P., et al. (2012). A case study of a child with chronic hemolytic anemia due to a Donath-Landsteiner positive, IgM anti-I autoantibody. *Pediatr Blood Cancer, 59,* 953–955.
16. Gertz, M. (2007). Management of cold haemolytic syndrome. *Br J Haematol, 138,* 422–429.

17. Sokol, R., Hewitt, S., & Stamps, B. (1981). Autoimmune haemolysis: an 18 year study of 865 cases referred to a regional transfusion centre. *Br Med J, 282*, 2023–2027.

18. Mayer, B., Yurek, S., Kiesewetter, H., et al. (2008). Mixed-type autoimmune hemolytic anemia: differential diagnosis and critical review of reported cases. *Transfusion, 48*, 2229–2234.

19. Garratty, G. (2010). Immune hemolytic anemia associated with drug therapy. *Blood Rev, 24*, 143–150.

20. Johnson, S., Fueger, J., & Gottschall, J. (2007). One center's experience: the serology and drugs associated with drug-induced hemolytic anemia—a new paradigm. *Transfusion, 47*, 697–702.

21. Garratty, G. (2009). Drug-induced immune hemolytic anemia. *Hematology Am Soc Hematol Educ Program*, 73–79.

22. Garratty, G., & Arndt, P. (2007). An update on drug-induced immune hemolytic anemia. *Immunohematology, 23*, 105–119.

23. Gupta, S., Piefer, C., Fueger, J., et al. (2010). Trimethoprim-induced immune hemolytic anemia in a pediatric oncology patient presenting as an acute hemolytic transfusion reaction. *Pediatr Blood Cancer, 55*, 1201–1203.

24. Arndt, P., Garratty, G., Isaak, E., et al. (2009). Positive direct and indirect antiglobulin tests associated with oxaliplatin can be due to drug antibody and/or drug-induced nonimmunologic protein adsorption. *Transfusion, 49*, 711–718.

25. Salama, A. (2009). Drug-induced immune hemolytic anemia. *Expert Opin Drug Saf, 8*, 73–79.

26. Lerner, N. B., Refaai, M. A., & Blumberg, N. (2010). Red cell transfusion. In Lichtman, M. A., Kipps, T. J., Seligsohn, U., et al. (Eds.), *Williams Hematology*. (8th ed.). New York: McGraw-Hill. http://accessmedicine.mhmedical.com.libproxy2.umdnj.edu/content.aspx?bookid=358&Sectionid=39835965. Accessed 28.02.14.

27. Eder, A., & Chambers, L. (2007). Noninfectious complications of blood transfusion. *Arch Pathol Lab Med, 131*, 708–718.

28. Ramasethu, J., & Luban, N. C. (2010). Alloimmune hemolytic disease of the fetus and newborn. In Lichtman, M. A., Kipps, T. J., Seligsohn, U., et al. (Eds.), *Williams Hematology*. (8th ed.). New York: McGraw-Hill. http://accessmedicine.mhmedical.com.libproxy2.umdnj.edu/content.aspx?bookid=358&Sectionid=39835872. Accessed 28.02.14.

29. Koelewijn, J., Haas, M., Vrijkotte, T., et al. (2008). One single dose of 200 µg of antenatal RhIG halves the risk of anti-D immunization and hemolytic disease of the fetus and newborn in the next pregnancy. *Transfusion, 48*, 1721–1729.

30. Dodd, J. M., Windrim, R. C., & van Kamp, I. L. (2012). Techniques of intrauterine fetal transfusion for women with red-cell isoimmunisation for improving health outcomes. *Cochrane Database Syst Rev Sept 12*, 9:CD007096.

31. Patel, L. L., Myers, J. C., Palma, J. P., et al. (2013). Anti-Ge3 causes late-onset hemolytic disease of the newborn: the fourth case in three Hispanic families. *Transfusion, 53*, 2152–2157.

32. Dorn, I., Schlenke, P., & Hartel, C. (2010). Prolonged anemia in an intrauterine-transfused neonate with Rh-negative hemolytic disease: no evidence for anti-D-related suppression of erythropoiesis in vitro. *Transfusion, 50*, 1064–1070.

33. Michalewska, B., Wielgos, M., Zupanska, B., et al. (2008). Anti-Coª implicated in severe haemolytic disease of the foetus and newborn. *Transfus Med, 18*, 71–73.

34. Dohmen, S., Muit, J., Ligthart, P., et al. (2008). Anti-e found in a case of hemolytic disease of the fetus and newborn makes use of the IGHV3 superspecies genes. *Transfusion, 48*, 194–194.

35. van Gammeren, A. J., Overbeeke, M. A., Idema, R. N., et al. (2008). Haemolytic disease of the newborn because of rare anti-Vel. *Transfus Med, 18*, 197–198.

36. Li, B. J., Jiang, Y. J., Yuan, F., et al. (2010). Exchange transfusion of least incompatible blood for severe hemolytic disease of the newborn due to anti-Rh17. *Transfus Med, 20*, 66–69.

37. Koelewijn, J. M., Vrijkotte, T. G., van der Schoot, C. E., et al. (2008). Effect of screening for red cell antibodies, other than anti-D, to detect hemolytic disease of the fetus and newborn: a population study in the Netherlands. *Transfusion, 48*, 941–952.

27 Hemoglobinopathies (Structural Defects in Hemoglobin)

Tim R. Randolph

OUTLINE

Structure of Globin Genes
Hemoglobin Development
Genetic Mutations
Zygosity
Pathophysiology
Nomenclature
Hemoglobin S
- *Sickle Cell Anemia*
- *Sickle Cell Trait*

Hemoglobin C
- *Prevalence, Etiology, and Pathophysiology*

Hemoglobin C-Harlem (Hemoglobin C-Georgetown)
Hemoglobin E
- *Prevalence, Etiology, and Pathophysiology*
- *Clinical Features*

Hemoglobin O-Arab
Hemoglobin D and Hemoglobin G
Compound Heterozygosity with Hemoglobin S and Another β-Globin Gene Mutation
- *Hemoglobin SC*
- *Hemoglobin S–β-Thalassemia*
- *Hemoglobin SD and Hemoglobin SG-Philadelphia*
- *Hemoglobin S/O-Arab and HbS/D-Punjab*
- *Hemoglobin S-Korle Bu*

Concomitant Cis Mutations with Hemoglobin S
- *Hemoglobin C-Harlem*
- *Hemoglobin S-Antilles and Hemoglobin S-Oman*

Hemoglobin M
Unstable Hemoglobin Variants
- *Clinical Features*
- *Treatment and Prognosis*

OBJECTIVES

After completion of this chapter, the reader will be able to:

1. Explain the difference between structural hemoglobin disorders and thalassemias, and describe the types of mutations found in the structural disorders.
2. Describe globin gene structure and the development of normal human hemoglobins throughout prenatal and postnatal life.
3. Differentiate between homozygous and heterozygous states and the terms "disease" and "trait" as they relate to the hemoglobinopathies.
4. Given the hemoglobin genotypes of parents involving common β chain variants, determine the possible genotypes of their children using a Punnett square.
5. Describe the general geographic distribution of common hemoglobin variants and the relationship of that distribution with the prevalence of malaria and glucose-6-phosphate dehydrogenase deficiency.
6. For disorders involving Hb S and Hb C, describe the genetic mutation, the effect of the mutation on the hemoglobin molecule, the inheritance pattern, pathophysiology, symptoms, clinical findings, peripheral blood findings, laboratory diagnosis, and genetic counseling and treatment considerations.
7. Describe the genetic mutation, clinical findings, and laboratory diagnosis for disorders involving Hb C-Harlem, Hb E, Hb O-Arab, Hb D, and Hb G.
8. Describe the clinical and laboratory findings for the compound heterozygous disorders of Hb S with Hb C, β-thalassemia, Hb D, Hb O-Arab, Hb Korle Bu, and Hb C-Harlem.
9. Describe the electrophoretic mobility of Hb A, Hb F, Hb S, and Hb C at an alkaline pH, and explain how other methods (including the Hb S solubility test, citrate agar electrophoresis at acid pH, and high-performance liquid chromatography) are used to distinguish Hb S and Hb C from other hemoglobins with the same mobility.
10. Describe the genetic mutations, inheritance patterns, pathophysiology, and clinical and laboratory findings in hemoglobin variants that result in methemoglobinemia.
11. Describe the inheritance patterns, causes, and clinical and laboratory findings of unstable hemoglobin variants.
12. Discuss the pathophysiology of hemoglobin variants with increased and decreased oxygen affinities, and explain how they differ from unstable hemoglobins.
13. Given a case history and clinical and laboratory findings, interpret test results to identify the hemoglobin variants present in the patient.

CASE STUDY

After studying the material in this chapter, the reader should be able to respond to the following case study:

An 18-year-old African-American woman was seen in the emergency department for fever and abdominal pain. The following results were obtained on a complete blood count:

	Patient Results	Reference Interval
WBCs ($\times 10^9$/L)	11.9	3.6–10.6
RBCs ($\times 10^{12}$/L)	3.67	4.00–5.40
HGB (g/dL)	10.9	12.0–15.0
HCT (%)	32.5	35–49
RDW (%)	19.5	11.5–14.5
Platelets ($\times 10^9$/L)	410	150–450
Segmented neutrophils (%)	75	50–70
Lymphocytes (%)	18	18–42
Monocytes (%)	3	2–11

CASE STUDY—cont'd

After studying the material in this chapter, the reader should be able to respond to the following case study:

	Patient Results	Reference Interval
Eosinophils (%)	3	1–3
Basophils (%)	1	0–2
Reticulocytes (%)	3.1	0.5–2.5

A typical field in the patient's peripheral blood film is shown in Figure 27-1. Electrophoresis on cellulose acetate at alkaline pH showed 50.9% Hb S and 49.1% Hb C.

1. Select confirmatory tests that should be performed and describe the expected results.
2. Describe the characteristic red blood cell morphology on the peripheral blood film.
3. Based on the electrophoresis and red blood cell morphology results, what diagnosis is suggested?
4. If this patient were to marry a person of genotype Hb AS, what would be the expected frequency of genotypes for each of four children?

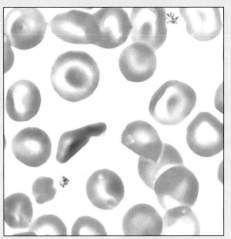

Figure 27-1 Peripheral blood film for the patient in the case study (×1000). (Courtesy Ann Bell, University of Tennessee, Memphis.)

Hemoglobinopathy refers to a disease state (*opathy*) involving the hemoglobin (Hb) molecule. Hemoglobinopathies are the most common genetic diseases, affecting approximately 7% of the world's population.[1] Approximately 300,000 children are born each year with some form of inherited hemoglobin disorder.[2] All hemoglobinopathies result from a genetic mutation in one or more genes that affect hemoglobin synthesis. The genes that are mutated can code for either the proteins that make up the hemoglobin molecule (globin or polypeptide chains) or the proteins involved in synthesizing or regulating synthesis of the globin chains. Regardless of the mutation encountered, all hemoglobinopathies affect hemoglobin synthesis in one of two ways: qualitatively or quantitatively. In qualitative hemoglobinopathies, hemoglobin synthesis occurs at a normal or near-normal rate, but the hemoglobin molecule has an altered amino acid sequence within the globin chains. This change in amino acid sequence alters the structure of the hemoglobin molecule (structural defect) and its function (qualitative defect). In contrast, thalassemias result in a reduced rate of hemoglobin synthesis (quantitative) but do not affect the amino acid sequence of the globin chains. A reduction in the amount of hemoglobin synthesized produces an anemia and stimulates the production of other hemoglobins not affected by the mutation in an attempt to compensate for the anemia. Based on this distinction, hematologists divide hemoglobinopathies into two categories: structural defects (qualitative) and thalassemias (quantitative). To add confusion to the classification scheme, many hematologists also refer to *only* the structural defects as hemoglobinopathies. This chapter describes the structural or qualitative defects that are referred to as *hemoglobinopathies*; the quantitative defects (thalassemias) are described in Chapter 28.

STRUCTURE OF GLOBIN GENES

As discussed in Chapter 10, there are six functional human globin genes located on two different chromosomes. Two of the globin genes, α and ζ, are located on chromosome 16 and are referred to as *α-like genes*. The remaining four globin genes, β, γ, δ, and ϵ, are located on chromosome 11 and are referred to as *β-like genes*. In the human genome, there is one copy of each globin gene per chromatid, for a total of two genes per diploid nucleus, with the exception of α and γ. There are two copies of the α and γ genes per chromatid, for a total of four genes per diploid nucleus. Each globin gene codes for the corresponding globin chain: the α-globin genes (*HBA1* and *HBA2*) are used as the template to synthesize the α-globin chains, the β-globin gene (*HBB*) codes for the β-globin chain, the γ-globin genes (*HBG1* and *HBG2*) code for the γ-globin chains, and the δ-globin gene (*HBD*) codes for the δ-globin chain.

HEMOGLOBIN DEVELOPMENT

Each human hemoglobin molecule is composed of four globin chains: a pair of α-like chains and a pair of β-like chains. During the first 3 months of embryonic life, only one α-like gene (ζ) and one β-like gene (ϵ) are activated, which results in the production of ζ and ϵ globin chains that pair to form hemoglobin Gower-1 ($\zeta_2\epsilon_2$). Shortly thereafter, α and γ chain synthesis begins, which leads to the production of Hb Gower-2 ($\alpha_2\epsilon_2$) and Hb Portland ($\zeta_2\gamma_2$). Later in fetal development, ζ and ϵ synthesis ceases; this leaves α and γ chains, which pair to produce Hb F ($\alpha_2\gamma_2$), also known as *fetal hemoglobin*. During the 6 months after birth, γ chain synthesis gradually decreases and is replaced by β chain synthesis so that Hb A ($\alpha_2\beta_2$), also known as *adult hemoglobin,* is produced. Recent evidence suggests BCL11A and KLF1, zinc-finger transcriptional repressors, are necessary to silence the γ-globin gene and mutations in the gene that codes for either factor results in elevated HbF levels.[3] The remaining globin gene, δ, becomes activated around birth, producing δ chains at low levels that pair with α chains to produce the second adult hemoglobin, Hb A$_2$ (α$_2$δ$_2$). Normal adults produce Hb A (95%), Hb A$_2$ (less than 3.5%), and Hb F (less than 1% to 2%).

GENETIC MUTATIONS

More than 1000 structural hemoglobin variants (hemoglobinopathies) are known to exist throughout the world, and more are being discovered regularly (Table 27-1).[4,5] Each of these hemoglobin variants results from one or more genetic mutations that alter the amino acid sequence. Some of these changes alter the molecular structure of the hemoglobin molecule, ultimately affecting hemoglobin function. The types of genetic mutations that occur in the hemoglobinopathies include point mutations, deletions, insertions, and fusions involving one or more of the adult globin genes—α, β, γ, and δ.[5]

Point mutation is the most common type of genetic mutation occurring in the hemoglobinopathies. Point mutation is the replacement of one original nucleotide in the normal gene with a different nucleotide. Because one nucleotide is replaced by one nucleotide, the codon triplet remains intact, and the reading frame is unaltered. This results in the substitution of one amino acid in the globin chain product at the position corresponding to the location of the original point mutation. As can be seen in Table 27-1, 1109 of the 1181 known hemoglobin variants result from a point mutation that causes an amino acid substitution. It also is possible to have two point mutations occurring in the same globin gene, which results in two amino acid substitutions within the same globin chain. Over 35 mutations occur by this mechanism.[5]

Deletions involve the removal of one or more nucleotides, whereas insertions result in the addition of one or more nucleotides. Usually deletions and insertions are not divisible by three and disrupt the reading frame, which leads to the nullification of synthesis of the corresponding globin chain. This is the case for the quantitative thalassemias (Chapter 28). In hemoglobinopathies, the reading frame usually remains intact, however; the result is the addition or deletion of one or more amino acids in the globin chain product, which sometimes affects the structure and function of the hemoglobin molecule. Of the 1181 variants described in Table 27-1, 72 variants result from deletions or insertions, or both.[5]

Chain extensions occur when the stop codon is mutated so that translation continues beyond the typical last codon. Amino acids continue to be added until a stop codon is reached by chance. This process produces globin chains that are longer than normal. Significant globin chain extensions usually result in degradation of the globin chain and a quantitative defect. If the extension of the globin chain is insufficient to produce significant degradation, however, the defect is qualitative and is classified as a hemoglobinopathy. Hemoglobin molecules with extended globin chains fold inappropriately, which affects hemoglobin structure and function.

Gene fusions occur when two normal genes break between nucleotides, switch positions, and anneal to the opposite gene. For example, if a β-globin gene and a δ-globin gene break in similar locations, switch positions, and reanneal, the resultant genes would be βδ and δβ fusion genes in which the head of the fusion gene is from one original gene and the tail is from the other. As long as the reading frames are not disrupted and the globin chain lengths are similar, the genes are transcribed and translated into hybrid globin chains. The fusion chains fold differently, however, and affect the corresponding hemoglobin function. Nine fusion globin chains have been identified (see Table 27-1).

ZYGOSITY

Zygosity refers to the association between the number of gene mutations and the level of severity of the resultant genetic defect. Generally, there is a level of severity associated with each gene that is normally used to synthesize the globin chain product. For the normal adult globin genes, there are four copies of the α and γ genes and two copies of the β and δ genes. In theory, this could result in four levels of severity for α and γ gene mutations and two levels of severity for the β and δ gene mutations. Expressed another way, if all things were equal, it would require twice as many mutations within the α and γ genes to produce the same physiologic effect as mutations within the β and δ genes. Because the γ and δ genes are transcribed and translated at such low levels in adults, however, mutations of either gene would have little impact on overall hemoglobin function. In addition, because the dominant hemoglobin in adults, Hb A, is composed of α and β chains, β gene mutations would affect overall hemoglobin function to a greater extent than the same number of α gene mutations. This partially explains the greater number of identified β chain

TABLE 27-1 Molecular Abnormalities of Hemoglobin Variants

| | NUMBER OF VARIANTS BY GLOBIN CHAIN | | | | |
	α	β	δ	γ	**Total**
Amino acid substitution	413	535	65	96	1109
Deletions or insertions	22	48	1	1	72
Total	435	583	66	97	1181
Fusions	—	—	—	—	9*

*Seven fusions involve the β and δ chains; two fusions involve the β and γ chains.
Data from Patrinos GP, Giardine B, Riemer W, et al: Improvements in the HbVar database of human hemoglobin variants and thalassemia mutations for population and sequence variation studies, *Nucl Acids Res* 32(database issue):D537-541, 2004. Available at: http://globin.cse.psu.edu/hbvar/menu.html. Accessed November 29, 2013.
The table is designed to provide a relative distribution of mutation types and just includes structural variants. Fifty-one of the variants are also categorized as thalassemias. Mutations are being added regularly.

variants compared with α chain variants, because a single β gene mutation would be more likely to create a clinical condition than would a single α gene mutation.

The inheritance pattern of β chain variants is referred to as *heterozygous* when only one β gene is mutated and *homozygous* when both β genes are mutated. The terms *disease* and *trait* are also commonly used to refer to the homozygous (disease) and heterozygous (trait) states.

PATHOPHYSIOLOGY

Pathophysiology refers to the manner in which a disorder translates into clinical symptoms. The impact of point mutations on hemoglobin function depends on the chemical nature of the substituted amino acid, where it is located in the globin chain, and the number of genes mutated (zygosity). The charge and size of the substituted amino acid may alter the manner in which the globin chain folds. A change in charge affects the interaction of the substituted amino acid with adjacent amino acids. In addition, the size of the substituted amino acid makes the globin chain either more or less bulky. Therefore, the charge and the size of the substituted amino acid determine its impact on hemoglobin structure by potentially altering the tertiary structure of the globin chain and the quaternary structure of the hemoglobin molecule. Changes in hemoglobin structure usually affect function. Location of the substitution within the globin chain also has an impact on the degree of structural alteration and hemoglobin function based on its positioning within the molecule and the interactions with the surrounding amino acids. In the case of the sickle cell mutation, one amino acid substitution results in hemoglobin polymerization, leading to the formation of long hemoglobin crystals that stretch the red blood cell (RBC) membrane and produce the characteristic crescent moon or sickle cell shape.

Zygosity also affects the pathophysiology of the disease. In β-hemoglobinopathies, zygosity predicts two severities of disease. In homozygous β-hemoglobinopathies, in which both β genes are mutated, the variant hemoglobin becomes the dominant hemoglobin type, and normal hemoglobin (Hb A) is absent. Examples are sickle cell disease (SCD, Hb SS) and Hb C disease (Hb CC). In heterozygous β-hemoglobinopathies, one β gene is mutated and the other is normal, which suggests a 50/50 distribution. In an attempt to minimize the impact of the abnormal hemoglobin, however, the variant hemoglobin is usually present in lesser amounts than Hb A. Nevertheless, in some cases they may be present in equal amounts. Examples are Hb S trait (Hb AS) and Hb C trait (Hb AC). Patients with homozygous sickle cell disease (Hb SS) inherit a severe form of the disease that occurs less frequently but requires lifelong medical intervention, which must begin early in life, whereas heterozygotes (Hb AS) are much more common but rarely experience symptoms.

Fishleder and Hoffman[6] divided the structural hemoglobins into four groups: abnormal hemoglobins that result in hemolytic anemia, such as Hb S and the unstable hemoglobins; abnormal hemoglobins that result in methemoglobinemia, such as Hb M; hemoglobins with either increased or decreased oxygen affinity; and abnormal hemoglobins with no clinical or functional effect. Imbalanced chain production also may be associated in rare instances with a structurally abnormal chain, such as Hb Lepore,[4] because of the reduced production of the abnormal chain. The functional classification of selected hemoglobin variants is summarized in Box 27-1.

Many of the variants are clinically insignificant because they do not show any physiologic effect. As discussed previously, most clinical abnormalities are associated with the β chain followed by the α chain. Involvement of the γ and δ chains does occur, but because of the small amount of hemoglobin involved, it is rarely detected and is usually of no consequence. Box 27-2 lists clinically significant abnormal hemoglobins. The most frequently occurring of the abnormal hemoglobins and the most severe is Hb S.

NOMENCLATURE

As hemoglobins were reported in the literature, they were designated by letters of the alphabet. Normal adult hemoglobin and fetal hemoglobin were called *Hb A* and *Hb F*. By the time the middle of the alphabet was reached, however, it became apparent that the alphabet would be exhausted before all mutations were named. Currently, some abnormal hemoglobins are assigned a common designation and a scientific designation. The common name is selected by the discoverer and usually represents the geographic area where the hemoglobin was identified. A single capital letter is used to indicate a special characteristic of the hemoglobin variants, such as hemoglobins demonstrating identical electrophoretic mobility but containing different amino acid substitutions, as in Hb G-Philadelphia, Hb G-Copenhagen, and Hb C-Harlem. The variant description also can involve scientific designations that indicate the variant chain, the sequential and the helical number of the abnormal amino acid, and the nature of the substitution. The designation [β$_6$ (A$_3$) Glu→Val] for the Hb S mutation indicates the substitution of valine for glutamic acid in the A helix in the β chain at position 6.[4]

HEMOGLOBIN S

Sickle Cell Anemia
History
Although the origin of sickle cell anemia has not been identified, symptoms of the disease have been traced in one Ghanaian family back to 1670.[7] Sickle cell anemia was first reported by a Chicago cardiologist, Herrick, in 1910 in a West Indian student with severe anemia. In 1917, Emmel recorded that sickling occurred in nonanemic patients and in patients who were severely anemic. In 1927, Hahn and Gillespie described the pathologic basis of the disorder and its relationship to the hemoglobin molecule. These investigators showed that sickling occurred when a solution of RBCs was deficient in oxygen and that the shape of the RBCs was reversible when that solution was oxygenated again.[4,8] In 1946, Beet reported that malarial parasites were present less frequently in blood films from patients with SCD than in individuals without SCD.[9] It was determined that the sickle cell trait confers a resistance against infection with *Plasmodium falciparum*

BOX 27-1 Functional Classification of Selected Hemoglobin (Hb) Variants

I. Homozygous: Hemoglobin Polymorphisms: The Variants That Are Most Common

Hb S: $\alpha_2\beta_2^{6Val}$—severe hemolytic anemia; sickling

Hb C: $\alpha_2\beta_2^{6Lys}$—mild hemolytic anemia

Hb D-Punjab: $\alpha_2\beta_2^{121Gln}$—no anemia

Hb E: $\alpha_2\beta_2^{26Lys}$—mild microcytic anemia

II. Heterozygous: Hemoglobin Variants Causing Functional Aberrations or Hemolytic Anemia in the Heterozygous State

A. Hemoglobins Associated with Methemoglobinemia and Cyanosis

1. Hb M-Boston: $\alpha_2^{58Tyr}\beta_2$
2. Hb M-Iwate: $\alpha_2^{87Tyr}\beta_2$
3. Hb Auckland: $\alpha_2^{87Asn}\beta_2$
4. Hb Chile: $\alpha_2\beta_2^{28Met}$
5. Hb M-Saskatoon: $\alpha_2\beta_2^{63Tyr}$
6. Hb M-Milwaukee-1: $\alpha_2\beta_2^{67Glu}$
7. Hb M-Milwaukee-2: $\alpha_2\beta_2^{92Tyr}$
8. Hb F-M-Osaka: $\alpha_2\gamma_2^{63Tyr}$
9. Hb F-M-Fort Ripley: $\alpha_2\gamma_2^{92Tyr}$

B. Hemoglobins Associated with Altered Oxygen Affinity

1. Increased affinity and erythrocytosis
   a. Hb Chesapeake: $\alpha_2^{92Leu}\beta_2$
   b. Hb J-Capetown: $\alpha_2^{92Gln}\beta_2$
   c. Hb Malmo: $\alpha_2\beta_2^{97Gln}$
   d. Hb Yakima: $\alpha_2\beta_2^{99His}$
   e. Hb Kempsey: $\alpha_2\beta_2^{99Asn}$
   f. Hb Ypsi (Ypsilanti): $\alpha_2\beta_2^{99Tyr}$
   g. Hb Hiroshima: $\alpha_2\beta_2^{146Asp}$
   h. Hb Rainier: $\alpha_2\beta_2^{145Cys}$
   i. Hb Bethesda: $\alpha_2\beta_2^{145His}$
2. Decreased affinity—may have mild anemia or cyanosis
   a. Hb Kansas: $\alpha_2\beta_2^{102Thr}$
   b. Hb Titusville: $\alpha_2^{94Asn}\beta_2$

   c. Hb Providence: $\alpha_2\beta_2^{82Asn}$
   d. Hb Agenogi: $\alpha_2\beta_2^{90Lys}$
   e. Hb Beth Israel: $\alpha_2\beta_2^{102Ser}$
   f. Hb Yoshizuka: $\alpha_2\beta_2^{108Asp}$

C. Unstable Hemoglobins

1. Hemoglobin may precipitate as Heinz bodies after splenectomy (congenital Heinz body anemia)
   a. Severe hemolysis: no improvement after splenectomy
      Hb Bibba: $\alpha_2^{136Pro}\beta_2$
      Hb Hammersmith: $\alpha_2\beta_2^{42Ser}$
      Hb Bristol-Alesha: $\alpha_2\beta_2^{67Asp \text{ or } 67Met}$
      Hb Olmsted: $\alpha_2\beta_2^{141Arg}$
   b. Severe hemolysis: improvement after splenectomy
      Hb Torino: $\alpha_2^{43Val}\beta_2$
      Hb Ann Arbor: $\alpha_2^{80Arg}\beta_2$
      Hb Genova: $\alpha_2\beta_2^{28Pro}$
      Hb Shepherds Bush: $\alpha_2\beta_2^{74Asp}$
      Hb Köln: $\alpha_2\beta_2^{98Met}$
      Hb Wien: $\alpha_2\beta_2^{130Asp}$
   c. Mild hemolysis: intermittent exacerbations
      Hb Hasharon: $\alpha_2^{47His}\beta_2$
      Hb Leiden: $\alpha_2\beta_2^{6 \text{ or } 7}$ (Glu deleted)
      Hb Freiburg: $\alpha_2\beta_2^{23}$ (Val deleted)
      Hb Seattle: $\alpha_2\beta_2^{70Asp}$
      Hb Louisville: $\alpha_2\beta_2^{42Leu}$
      Hb Zurich: $\alpha_2\beta_2^{63Arg}$
      Hb Gun Hill: $\alpha_2\beta_2^{91-95}$ (5 amino acids deleted)
   d. No disease
      Hb Etobicoke: $\alpha_2^{84Arg}\beta_2$
      Hb Sogn: $\alpha_2\beta_2^{14Arg}$
      Hb Tacoma: $\alpha_2\beta_2^{30Ser}$
2. Tetramers of normal chains; appear in thalassemias
   Hb Bart: γ_4
   Hb H: β_4

From Elghetany MT, Banki K: Erythrocyte disorders. In McPherson RA, Pincus MR: *Henry's clinical diagnosis and management by laboratory methods,* ed 22, Philadelphia, 2011, Elsevier, Saunders, p. 578. Originally modified from Winslow RM, Anderson WF: The hemoglobinopathies. In Stanbury JB, Wyngaarden JB, Fredrickson DS, et al, editors: *The metabolic basis of inherited disease,* ed 5, New York, 1983, McGraw-Hill, pp. 2281-2317. Updated from Patrinos GP, Giardine B, Riemer C, et al: Improvements in the HbVar database of human hemoglobin variants and thalassemia mutations for population and sequence variation studies, *Nucl Acids Res* 32 (database issue):D537-541, 2004. Available at: http://globin.cse.psu.edu/hbvar/menu.html. Accessed November 30, 2013.

Arg, Arginine; *Asn,* asparagine; *Asp,* aspartic acid; *Cys,* cysteine; *Gln,* glutamine; *Glu,* glutamic acid; *His,* histidine; *Leu,* leucine; *Lys,* lysine; *Met,* methionine; *Pro,* proline; *Ser* serine; *Thr,* threonine; *Tyr,* tyrosine; *Val,* valine.

---

occurring early in childhood between the time that passively acquired immunity dissipates and active immunity develops.[10] In 1949, Pauling showed that when Hb S is subjected to electrophoresis, it migrates differently than does Hb A. This difference was shown to be caused by an amino acid substitution in the globin chain. Pauling and coworkers defined the genetics of the disorder and clearly distinguished heterozygous sickle trait (Hb AS) from the homozygous state (Hb SS).[4]

The term *sickle cell diseases* is used to describe a group of symptomatic hemoglobinopathies that have in common sickle cell formation and the associated crises. Patients with SCD are either homozygous for Hb S (SS) or are compound heterozygotes expressing Hb S in combination with another hemoglobin β chain mutation like Hb C or β-thalassemia. SCDs are the most common form of hemoglobinopathy, with Hb SS and the variants Hb SC and Hb S–β-thalassemia (Hb S–β-thal) occurring most frequently.

BOX 27-2 **Clinically Important Hemoglobin (Hb) Variants**

I. Sickle syndromes
   A. Sickle cell trait (AS)
   B. Sickle cell disease
      1. SS
      2. SC
      3. SD-Punjab (Los Angeles)
      4. SO-Arab
      5. S–β-Thalassemia
      6. S–hereditary persistence of fetal hemoglobin
      7. SE
II. Unstable hemoglobins→congenital Heinz body anemia (>140 variants)
III. Hemoglobins with abnormal oxygen affinity
   A. High affinity→familial erythrocytosis (>90 variants)
   B. Low affinity→familial cyanosis (Hbs Kansas, Beth Israel, Yoshizuka, Agenogi, Titusville, Providence)
IV. M hemoglobins→familial cyanosis (9 variants): Hb M-Boston, Hb M-Iwate, Hb Auckland, Hb Chile, Hb M-Saskatoon, Hb M-Milwaukee-1, Hb M-Milwaukee-2 (Hyde Park), Hb FM-Osaka, Hb FM-Fort Ripley
V. Structural variants that result in a thalassemic phenotype
   A. β-Thalassemia phenotype
      1. Hb Lepore (δβ fusion)
      2. Hb E
      3. Hb-Indianapolis, Hb-Showa-Yakushiji, Hb-Geneva
   B. α-Thalassemia phenotype chain termination mutants (e.g., Hb Constant Spring)

Modified from Lukens JN: Abnormal hemoglobins: general principles (chap 39); Wong WC: Sickle cell anemia and other sickling syndromes (chap 40); Lukens JN: Unstable hemoglobin disease (chap 41). In Greer JP, Foerster J, Lukens JN, et al, editors: *Wintrobe's clinical hematology*, ed 11, Philadelphia, 2004, Lippincott Williams & Wilkins. Updated from Patrinos GP, Giardine B, Riemer C, et al: Improvements in the HbVar database of human hemoglobin variants and thalassemia mutations for population and sequence variation studies, *Nucl Acids Res* 32(database issue):D537-541, 2004. Available at: http://globin.cse.psu.edu/hbvar/menu.html. Accessed November 30, 2013.

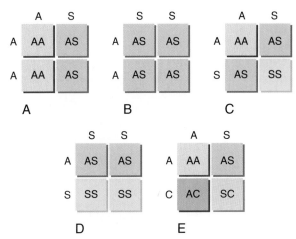

Figure 27-2 Punnett square illustrating the standard method for predicting the inheritance of abnormal hemoglobins. Each parent contributes one gene.

Inheritance Pattern

As stated earlier, the genes that code for the globin chains are located at specific loci on chromosomes 16 and 11. The α-like genes (α and ζ) are located on the short arm of chromosome 16, whereas the β-like genes (β, γ, δ, and ε) are located on the short arm of chromosome 11. With the exception of the γ genes, which have four loci, each β-like gene has two loci. β-hemoglobin variants are inherited as autosomal codominants, with one gene inherited from each parent.[4]

Patients with SCD (Hb SS), Hb SC, or Hb S–β-thal have inherited a sickle (S) gene from one parent and an S, C, or β-thalassemia gene from the other. Among patients with SCD, individuals who are homozygotes (Hb SS) have more severe disease than individuals who are compound heterozygotes for Hb S (Hb SC or Hb S–β-thal). Heterozygotes (Hb AS) are generally asymptomatic. Using Hb S and Hb C as examples,

Figure 27-2 illustrates the inheritance of abnormal hemoglobins involving mutations in the β gene.

Prevalence

The highest frequency of the sickle cell gene is found in sub-Saharan Africa, where each year approximately 230,000 babies are born with sickle cell disease (Hb SS), representing 0.74% of all live births occurring in this area.[11] In contrast, approximately 2600 babies are born annually with sickle cell disease in North America and 1300 in Europe.[11] Globally, the sickle cell gene occurs at the highest frequency in five geographic areas: sub-Saharan Africa, Arab-India, the Americas, Eurasia, and Southeast Asia. In 2010, these five geographic areas accounted for 64.4%, 22.7%, 7.4%, 5.4%, and 0.1%, respectively, of all neonates born globally with sickle cell trait, and 75.5%, 16.9%, 4.6%, 3.0%, and 0%, respectively, of all neonates born globally with sickle cell disease. Three countries accounted for approximately 50% of neonates with SS and AS genotypes: Nigeria, India, and DR Congo.[12] Although in the United States, SCD is found mostly in individuals of African descent, it also has been found in individuals from the Middle East, India, and the Mediterranean area (Figure 27-3). SCD can also be found in individuals from the Caribbean and Central and South America.[13] The sickle cell mutation is becoming more prominent in southern India, particularly in certain tribes.[14] It is estimated that 25,000 babies are born annually with sickle cell anemia in India.[2]

Etiology and Pathophysiology

Hb S is defined by the structural formula $\alpha_2\beta_2^{6Glu \rightarrow Val}$, which indicates that on the β chain at position 6, glutamic acid is replaced by valine. The mutation occurs in nucleotide 17, where thymine is changed to adenine, resulting in a change in codon 6 and the substitution of valine for glutamic acid at amino acid position 6.[11] Glutamic acid has a net charge of (−1), whereas valine has a net charge of (0). This amino acid substitution produces a change in charge of (+1), which affects the electrophoretic mobility of the hemoglobin molecule. This amino acid substitution also affects the way the hemoglobin molecules interact with one another within the erythrocyte

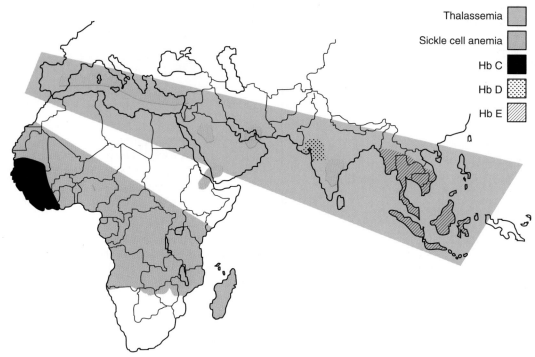

Figure 27-3 Geographic distribution of common inherited structural hemoglobin variants and the thalassemias. (From Hoffbrand AV, Pettit JE: *Essential haematology*, ed 3, Oxford, 1993, Blackwell Scientific.)

cytosol. The nonpolar (hydrophobic) valine amino acid has been placed in the position that the polar glutamic acid once held. Because glutamic acid is polar, the β chain folds in such a way that glutamic acid extends outward from the surface of the hemoglobin tetramer to bind water and contribute to hemoglobin solubility in the cytosol. Therefore, the hydrophobic valine is also extended outward, but instead of binding water, it seeks a hydrophobic niche with which to bind. When Hb S is fully oxygenated, the quaternary structure of the molecule does not produce a hydrophobic pocket for valine to bind to, which allows the hemoglobin molecules to remain soluble in the erythrocyte cytosol like Hb A and maintains the normal biconcave disc shape of the RBCs. However, the natural allosteric change that occurs upon deoxygenation creates a hydrophobic pocket in the area of phenylalanine 85 and leucine 88, which allows the valine from an adjacent hemoglobin molecule to bind. This hemoglobin pairing creates an orientation that helps other hemoglobin molecules to form electrostatic bonds between amino acids and becomes the seed for polymer formation. Other hemoglobin pairs polymerize, forming a hemoglobin core composed of four hemoglobin molecules that elongate in a helical formation. An outer layer of 10 hemoglobin molecules forms around the 4-hemoglobin-molecule core, creating the long, slender Hb S polymer.[15-18] Hb S molecules within the RBCs become less soluble, forming tactoids or liquid crystals of Hb S polymers that grow in length beyond the diameter of the RBC, causing sickling. In homozygotes, the sickling process begins when oxygen saturation decreases to less than 85%. In heterozygotes, sickling does not occur unless the oxygen saturation of hemoglobin is reduced to less than 40%.[19] The blood becomes more viscous when polymers are formed and sickle cells are created.[19] Increased blood viscosity

and sickle cell formation slow blood flow. In addition to a decrease in oxygen tension, there is a reduction in the pH and an increase in 2,3-bisphosphoglycerate. Reduced blood flow prolongs the exposure of Hb S-containing erythrocytes to a hypoxic environment, and the lower tissue pH decreases the oxygen affinity, which further promotes sickling. The end result is occlusion of capillaries and arterioles by sickled RBCs and infarction of surrounding tissue.

Sickle cells occur in two forms: reversible sickle cells and irreversible sickle cells.[20] Reversible sickle cells are Hb S–containing erythrocytes that change shape in response to oxygen tension. Reversible sickle cells circulate as normal biconcave discs when fully oxygenated but undergo hemoglobin polymerization, show increased viscosity, and change shape on deoxygenation. The vasoocclusive complications of SCD are thought to be due to reversible sickle cells that are able to travel into the microvasculature in the biconcave disk conformation due to their normal rheologic properties when oxygenated and then become distorted and viscous as they become deoxygenated, converting to the sickle cell configuration in the vessel.

In contrast, irreversible sickle cells do not change their shape regardless of the change in oxygen tension or degree of hemoglobin polymerization. These cells are seen on the peripheral blood film as elongated sickle cells with a point at each end. It is thought that irreversible sickle cells are recognized as abnormal by the spleen and removed from circulation, which prevents them from entering the microcirculation and causing vasoocclusion.

Not only the oxygen tension but also the level of intracellular hydration affects the sickling process. When RBCs containing Hb S are exposed to a low oxygen tension, hemoglobin polymerization occurs. Polymerized deoxyhemoglobin S activates a membrane channel called P_{sickle} that is otherwise inactive in normal RBCs. These membrane channels open when the blood partial pressure of oxygen decreases to less than 50 mm Hg. Open P_{sickle} channels allow the influx of Ca^{2+}, raising the intracellular calcium levels and activating a second membrane channel called the *Gardos channel*. An activated Gardos channel causes the efflux of K^+, which stimulates the efflux of Cl^- through another membrane channel to maintain charge equilibrium across the RBC membrane. The efflux of these ions leads to water efflux and intracellular dehydration, effectively increasing the intracellular concentration of Hb S and intensifying polymerization. Another contributor to K^+ and Cl^- efflux and the resultant dehydration is the K^+/Cl^- cotransporter system. Ironically, this system is activated by dehydration and positively charged hemoglobins such as Hb S and Hb C. The K^+/Cl^- cotransporter pathway is also activated by the low pH encountered in the spleen and kidneys. One potential explanation for the altered function of the membrane channels is oxidative damage triggered by Hb S polymerization. Injury to the RBC membrane induces adherence to endothelial surfaces, which causes RBC aggregation, produces ischemia, and exacerbates Hb S polymerization.[10]

Another important factor in the pathophysiology of SCD involves the redistribution of phospholipids in the RBC membrane, which contributes to hemolysis, vasoocclusive crisis, stroke, and acute chest syndrome. In the bilayer membranes of normal RBCs, choline phospholipids like sphingomyelin and phosphatidylcholine are located on the outer plasma layer, whereas aminophospholipids like phosphatidylserine (PS) and phosphatidylethanolamine are primarily on the inner cytoplasmic layer of the membrane. This asymmetrical distribution of membrane phospholipids is accomplished by adenosine triphosphate–dependent enzymes called *translocases* or *flippases*. Inhibition of flippases and activation of an enzyme called *scramblase* cause a more random distribution of membrane phospholipids, which increases the number of choline phospholipids on the interior half of the membrane and the number of aminophospholipids on the exterior membrane surface. The sickle cells of homozygotes (Hb SS) express 2.1% PS on erythrocyte exterior surfaces compared with 0.2% for normal Hb AA controls.[21,22] It is hypothesized that Hb S polymerization may produce microparticles and iron complexes that adhere to the RBC membrane and generate reactive oxygen species, which, along with increased intracellular calcium or protein kinase C activation, may contribute to flippase inhibition and scramblase activation.[23,24] PS on the exterior surface of RBCs binds thrombospondin on vascular endothelial cells,[25] enhancing adherence between RBCs and the vessel wall and contributing to vasoocclusive crisis, activation of coagulation, and decreased RBC survival.[26,27] In addition, RBCs with PS on the external membrane surface are vulnerable to hydrolysis by secretory phospholipase A_2 ($sPLA_2$), which generates lysophospholipids and fatty acids like lysophosphatidic acid. This results in vascular damage that contributes to acute chest syndrome.[28,29]

Clinical Features

The clinical manifestations of SCD can vary from no symptoms to a potentially lethal state. Symptoms also vary between ethnic groups with Indian patients expressing a much milder disease than their African counterparts.[14] People with SCD can develop a variety of symptoms as listed in Box 27-3. Over a

---

BOX 27-3 Clinical Features of Sickle Cell Disease

I. Vasoocclusion
  A. Causes:
    Acidosis
    Hypoxia
    Dehydration
    Infection
    Fever
    Extreme cold
  B. Clinical manifestations
    1. Bones:
      Pain
      Hand-foot dactylitis
      Infection (osteomyelitis)
    2. Lungs:
      Pneumonia
      Acute chest syndrome
    3. Liver:
      Hepatomegaly
      Jaundice
    4. Spleen:
      Sequestration splenomegaly
      Autosplenectomy

    5. Penis:
      Priapism
    6. Eyes:
      Retinal hemorrhage
    7. Central nervous system
    8. Urinary tract:
      Renal papillary necrosis
    9. Leg ulcers
II. Bacterial infections
  A. Sepsis
  B. Pneumonia
  C. Osteomyelitis
III. Hematologic defects
  A. Chronic hemolytic anemia
  B. Megaloblastic episodes
  C. Aplastic episodes
IV. Cardiac defects
  A. Enlarged heart
  B. Heart murmurs
V. Other clinical features
  A. Stunted growth
  B. High-risk pregnancy

thousand hemoglobin variants are known; however, only eight genotypes cause severe disease: Hb SS, Hb S–β⁰-thal, severe Hb S–β⁺-thal, Hb SD-Punjab, Hb SO-Arab, Hb SC-Harlem, Hb CS-Antilles, and Hb S-Quebec-CHORI. These eight clinically significant forms are listed in the order of severity and can have high morbidity and mortality rates. Three additional genotypes produce moderate disease: Hb SC, moderate Hb S-β⁺-thal, and Hb AS-Oman. Three produce mild disease: mild Hb S-β^silent-thal, Hb SE, and Hb SA-Jamaica Plain. Two produce very mild disease: Hb S-HPFH and Hb S with a variety of mild variants.[11] Symptom variability in patients with sickle cell disease and across the genotypes listed above are largely due to the intracellular ratio of Hb S to Hb F, as well as factors that affect vessel tone and cellular activation.[30] Individuals affected with SCD are characteristically symptom free until the second half of the first year of life because of the protective effect of Hb F.[31] Toward the end of the first 6 months of life, mutated β chains begin to be produced and gradually replace normal γ chains, which causes Hb S levels to increase and Hb F levels to decrease. Erythrocytes containing Hb S become susceptible to hemolysis, and a progressive hemolytic anemia and splenomegaly may become evident.

Many individuals with SCD undergo episodes of recurring pain termed *crises*. Sickle cell crises were described by Diggs as "any new syndrome that develops rapidly in patients with SCD owing to the inherited abnormality."[32] The pathogenesis of the acute painful episode first described by Diggs is not fully understood. Various crises may occur: vasoocclusive or "painful," aplastic, megaloblastic, sequestration, and chronic hemolytic.

The hallmark of SCD is vasoocclusive crisis (VOC), which accounts for most hospital and emergency department visits. This acute, painful aspect of SCD occurs with great predictability and severity in many individuals and can be triggered by acidosis, hypoxia, dehydration, infection and fever, and exposure to extreme cold. Painful episodes manifest most often in the bones, lungs, liver, spleen, penis, eyes, central nervous system, and urinary tract.

The pathogenesis of vasoocclusion in SCD is not fully understood, but Hb S polymerization and sickling of RBCs play a major role, with other factors also affecting this process. Most VOC events occur in capillaries and postcapillary venules.[6,33] The list of possible risk factors includes polymerization, decreased deformability, sickle cell–endothelial cell adherence, endothelial cell activation, white blood cell (WBC) and platelet activation, hemostatic activation, and altered vascular tone.[33] The interrelationships among these risk factors is shown in Figure 27-4. Vasoocclusion can be triggered by any of these factors under various circumstances. During inflammation, increased WBCs interacting with endothelium, platelet activation causing elevation of thrombospondin level, or clinical dehydration resulting in an increase in von Willebrand factor can trigger RBC adherence to endothelium, precipitating vascular obstruction. Another mechanism of obstruction can be dense cells, which are less deformable and are at greatest risk for intracellular polymerization because of their higher Hb S concentration.[34,35] Vasoocclusive episodes gradually consume

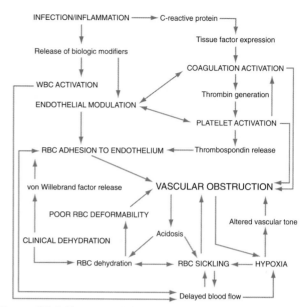

Figure 27-4 Numerous risk factors for vasoocclusion are highly interrelated physiologically, as shown here. *RBC*, Red blood cell; *WBC*, white blood cell. (From Embury SH, Hebbel RP, Mohandas N, et al: *Sickle cell disease: basic principles and clinical practice*, Philadelphia, 1994, Lippincott Williams & Wilkins, p. 322.)

the patient organ by organ, through the destructive and debilitative effects of cumulative infarcts. Approximately 8% to 10% of SCD patients develop cutaneous manifestations in the form of ulcers or sores on the lower leg.[11]

The abnormal interaction between sickle cells and vascular endothelium seems to have a great impact on the vasoocclusive event. Endothelial adherence correlates significantly with the severity of painful episodes. In addition, sickle cell adherence to vascular endothelium results in intimal hyperplasia that can slow blood flow.[36] Cells of patients with Hb SC disease produce less sickling with fewer adherent RBCs.[8,37]

The frequency of painful episodes varies from none to six per year.[8] On average, each episode persists for 4 to 5 days, although protracted episodes may last for weeks. Repeated splenic infarcts produce scarring resulting in diminished splenic tissue and abnormal function. Splenic sequestration is characterized by a sudden trapping of blood in the spleen, which leads to a rapid decline in hemoglobin, often to less than 6 g/dL.[37] This phenomenon occurs most often in infants and young children whose spleens are chronically enlarged. Children experiencing splenic sequestration episodes may have earlier onset of splenomegaly and a lower level of Hb F at 6 months of age.[8] Crises are often associated with respiratory tract infections. Gradual loss of splenic function is referred to as *autosplenectomy* and is evidenced by the presence of Howell-Jolly and Pappenheimer bodies in RBCs on the peripheral blood film. In the lungs, pulmonary infarction from sickling in the microvasculature causes acute chest syndrome.

Acute chest syndrome is characterized by fever, chest pain, and presence of pulmonary infiltrates on the chest radiograph and is the leading cause of death among adults with SCD. Over 10% of adults with acute chest syndrome die from complications linked to chronic lung disease and pulmonary hypertension.[38] In children, acute chest syndrome generally is precipitated by infection characterized by fever, cough, and tachypnea. Acute chest syndrome is also linked with sPLA2, discussed previously. The level of sPLA2 has been shown to be a predictor of acute chest syndrome in patients with SCD[39] in that sPLA2 rises 24 to 48 hours before symptoms of acute chest syndrome begin.[40] In addition, a high sPLA2 level correlates with the degree of lung damage.

Pulmonary hypertension (PHT) is a serious and potentially fatal sequela of SCD. Among patients with SCD, PHT has a prevalence of about 33%, with 10% of patients manifesting a more severe version.[41] The mortality rate for sickle cell patients who develop PHT is 40% at 40 months.[41] An association has been documented between the development of PHT and the nitrous oxide (NO) pathway. NO is produced from the action of endothelial NO synthase (eNOS) on arginine, which causes vasodilation. Patients with SCD have a decrease in NO, and this leads to vasoconstriction and hypertension.[4,41] In addition, low NO levels in the blood fail to inhibit endothelin-1, a potent vasoconstrictor, which results in additional vasoconstriction and hypertension.[38] The connection between NO and SCD involves the hemolytic crisis. Erythrocyte hemolysis releases high levels of arginase, which degrades arginine; the result is less NO production from eNOS.[42,43] In addition, the free hemoglobin released from hemolyzed RBCs scavenges NO, which further reduces the levels and exacerbates the vasoconstriction and hypertension.[41] Blood arginine and NO levels drop a few days before the onset of acute chest syndrome,[37] a finding suggesting that the NO pathway is a connection between SCD, PHT, and asthma.[38,44] Treatment with large doses of arginine reduces pulmonary artery pressure, but the effect is not sustainable and does not reduce mortality. An increased tricuspid regurgitation velocity (TRV) and blood NT-ProBNP levels above 160 ng/L were found to be good predictors of pulmonary hypertension and are associated with a higher mortality rate.[33] Bosentan is the treatment of choice for pulmonary hypertension, but liver enzymes should be monitored for liver toxicity.[33]

Bacterial infections pose a major problem for SCD patients. These patients have increased susceptibility to life-threatening infection from *Staphylococcus aureus*, *Streptococcus pneumoniae*, and *Haemophilus influenzae*. Acute infections are common causes of hospitalization and have been the most frequent cause of death, especially in the first 3 years of life.[1] Bacterial infections of the blood (septicemia) are exacerbated by the autosplenectomy effect as the spleen gradually loses its ability to function as a secondary lymphoid tissue to effectively clear organisms from the blood.

Chronic hemolytic anemia is characterized by shortened RBC survival of between 16 and 20 days,[45] with a corresponding decrease in hemoglobin and hematocrit, an elevated reticulocyte count, and jaundice. Continuous screening and removal of sickle cells by the spleen perpetuate the chronic hemolytic anemia and autosplenectomy effect. Because other conditions, such as hepatitis and gallstones, may cause jaundice, chronic hemolysis is difficult to diagnose in sickle cell

patients.[21] RBC hemolysis releases free hemoglobin, which disrupts the arginine–nitric oxide pathway, resulting in the sequestration and lowering of nitric oxide.[31,45] Decreased NO leads to endothelial cell activation, vasoconstriction, adherence of RBCs to the endothelium, and pulmonary hypertension previously discussed.[45] Another major sequelae of hemolysis is renal dysfunction, which can be detected early by an increased glomerular filtration rate of 140 mL/min per 1.73 m3 found in 71% of patients with SCD.[46] Progression of renal dysfunction can be identified by detecting microalbuminuria (>4.5 mg/mmol), followed by proteinuria and terminating in elevated BUN and creatinine levels. Angiotensin-converting enzyme inhibitors (ACEI) have been shown to lower proteinuria in SCD patients.[33]

Megaloblastic episodes result from the sudden arrest of erythropoiesis due to folate depletion. Folic acid deficiency as a cause of exaggerated anemia in SCD is extremely rare in the United States. It is common practice to prescribe prophylactic folic acid for patients with SCD, however.[8]

Aplastic episodes (bone marrow failure) are the most common life-threatening hematologic complications and are usually associated with infection, particularly parvovirus infection.[34] Aplastic episodes present clinical problems similar to those seen with other hemolytic disorders.[47] Sickle cell patients usually can compensate for the decrease in RBC survival by increasing bone marrow output. When the bone marrow is suppressed temporarily by bacterial or viral infections, however, the hematocrit decreases substantially with no reticulocyte compensation. The spontaneous recovery phase is characterized by the presence of nucleated RBCs and an increase in the number of reticulocytes in the peripheral blood. Most aplastic episodes are short-lived and require no therapy. If anemia is severe and the bone marrow remains aplastic, transfusions become necessary. If patients are not transfused in a timely fashion, death can occur.[47]

Patients also experience cardiac defects, including enlarged heart and heart murmurs. In patients with severe anemia, cardiomegaly can develop as the heart works harder to maintain adequate blood flow and tissue oxygenation. Increased cardiac workload along with increased bone marrow erythropoiesis increases calorie burning, contributing to a reduced growth rate.[48] When patients enter childbearing age, pregnancy becomes risky.[4]

Impaired blood supply to the head of the femur and humerus results in a condition called *avascular necrosis* (AVN). About 50% of patients with SCD develop AVN by 35 years of age.[49] Physical therapy and surgery to relieve intramedullary pressure within the head of the long bones are effective, but hip and/or shoulder implants become necessary in most patients experiencing AVN.[49] Similarly, leg ulcers are a common complication of SCD. Ulcers tend to heal slowly, develop unstable scars, and recur at the same site, becoming a chronic problem, with associated chronic pain.[47]

Microstrokes can lead to headaches, poor school performance, reduced intelligence quotient (IQ), and overt central nervous system dysfunction. A neurologic examination followed by magnetic resonance imaging and, if available, transcranial

Doppler ultrasonography or magnetic resonance angiography is recommended to detect microstrokes.[48]

Incidence with Malaria and Glucose-6-Phosphate Dehydrogenase Deficiency

The sickle gene occurs with greatest frequency in Central Africa, the Near East, the region around the Mediterranean, and parts of India. The frequency of the gene parallels the incidence of *P. falciparum* and seems to offer some protection against cerebral falciparum malaria in young patients. Malarial parasites are living organisms within the RBCs that use the oxygen within the cells. This reduced oxygen tension causes the cells to sickle, which results in injury to the cells. These injured cells tend to become trapped within the blood vessels of the spleen and other organs, where they are easily phagocytized by scavenger WBCs. Selective destruction of RBCs containing parasites decreases the number of malarial organisms and increases the time for immunity to develop. One explanation for this phenomenon is that the infected cell is uniquely sickled and destroyed, probably in an area of the spleen or liver, where phagocytic cells are plentiful, and the oxygen tension is significantly decreased.[50]

Because of the high incidence of glucose-6-phosphate dehydrogenase (G6PD) deficiency in patients with SCD, it has been suggested that G6PD deficiency has a protective effect in these patients,[51] although this correlation has not been confirmed through studies. It also has been postulated that hemolytic episodes are more common in these patients. In the first 42 months of life, patients with SCD and G6PD deficiency had lower steady-state hemoglobin levels, higher reticulocyte counts, three times more acute anemia events, and more frequent blood transfusions—vasoocclusive and infectious events than matched sickle cell patients without G6PD deficiency.[30] Because of the presence of young cells rich in G6PD, however, the increased hemolysis is more likely caused by the enzyme abnormality when the population is shifted to the oldest cells during an aplastic crisis.[52]

Laboratory Diagnosis

The anemia of SCD is a chronic hemolytic anemia, classified morphologically as normocytic, normochromic. The characteristic diagnostic cell observed on a Wright-stained peripheral blood film is a long, curved cell with a point at each end (Figure 27-5). Because of its appearance, the cell was named a *sickle cell*.[32] The peripheral blood film shows marked poikilocytosis and anisocytosis with normal RBCs, sickle cells, target cells, nucleated RBCs along with a few spherocytes, basophilic stippling, Pappenheimer bodies, and Howell-Jolly bodies. The presence of sickle cells and target cells is the hallmark of SCD. There is moderate to marked polychromasia with a reticulocyte count between 10% and 25%, corresponding with the hemolytic state and the resultant bone marrow response. The RBC distribution width (RDW) is increased owing to moderate anisocytosis. The mean cell volume (MCV) is not as elevated as one would expect, however, given the elevated reticulocyte count. An aplastic crisis can be heralded by a decreased reticulocyte count. Moderate leukocytosis is usually present (sometimes 40 to 50 × 10⁹ WBC/L) with neutrophilia and a mild shift toward immature granulocytes. The leukocyte alkaline phosphatase score is not elevated when neutrophilia is caused by sickle cell crisis alone when no underlying infection is present. Thrombocytosis is usually present. The bone marrow shows erythroid hyperplasia, reflecting an attempt to compensate for the anemia, which results in polychromasia and an increase in reticulocytes and nucleated RBCs in the peripheral blood. Levels of immunoglobulins, particularly immunoglobulin A, are elevated in all forms of SCD. Serum ferritin levels are normal in young patients but tend to be elevated later in life; however, hemochromatosis is rare. Chronic hemolysis is evidenced by elevated levels of indirect and total bilirubin with the accompanying jaundice.

The diagnosis of SCD is generally a two-step process by first demonstrating the insolubility of deoxygenated Hb S in solution followed by confirmation of its presence using hemoglobin electrophoresis, high-performance liquid chromatography (HPLC), or capillary electrophoresis. For more complicated

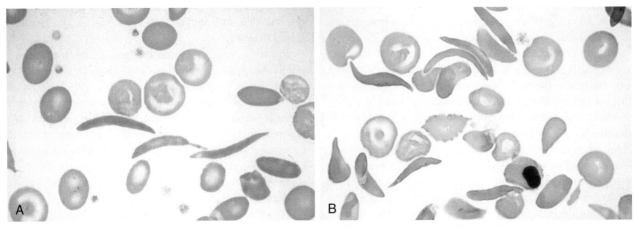

Figure 27-5 A, Peripheral blood film for a patient with sickle cell disease (SCD) showing anisocytosis, polychromasia, three sickle cells, target cells, and normal platelets (×1000). **B,** Peripheral blood film for an SCD patient showing anisocytosis, poikilocytosis, sickle cells, target cells, and one nucleated RBC (×1000). Platelets are not present in this field, but their numbers were adequate in this patient. (Courtesy Ann Bell, University of Tennessee, Memphis.)

cases, isoelectric focusing, tandem mass spectrometry, or DNA analysis may be needed. An older screening test detects Hb S insolubility by inducing sickle cell formation on a glass slide. A drop of blood is mixed with a drop of 2% sodium metabisulfite (a reducing agent) on a slide, and the mixture is sealed under a coverslip. The hemoglobin inside the RBCs is reduced to the deoxygenated form; this induces polymerization and the resultant sickle cell formation, which can be identified microscopically. This method is slow and cumbersome and is rarely used.

The most common screening test for Hb S, called the hemoglobin solubility test, capitalizes on the decreased solubility of deoxygenated Hb S in solution, producing turbidity. Blood is added to a buffered salt solution containing a reducing agent, such as sodium hydrosulfite (dithionite), and a detergent-based lysing agent (saponin). The saponin dissolves membrane lipids, causing the release of hemoglobin from the RBCs, and the dithionite reduces the iron from the ferrous to the ferric oxidation state. Ferric iron is unable to bind oxygen, converting the hemoglobin to the deoxygenated form. Deoxygenated Hb S polymerizes in solution, which renders it turbid, whereas solutions containing nonsickling hemoglobins remain clear (Figure 27-6). False-positive results for Hb S can occur with hyperlipidemia, a few rare hemoglobinopathies, and when too much blood is added to the test solution; false-negative results can occur in infants less than 6 months of age and with low hematocrits. Other hemoglobins that give a positive result on the solubility test include Hb C-Harlem (Georgetown), Hb C-Ziguinchor, Hb S-Memphis, Hb S-Travis, Hb S-Antilles, Hb S-Providence, Hb S-Oman, Hb Alexander, and Hb Porte-Alegre.[4,8] All of these hemoglobins have two amino acid substitutions: the Hb S substitution ($\beta^{6Glu \rightarrow Val}$) and another

unrelated substitution. Hb S-Antilles is particularly important because it can cause sickling in the heterozygous state.

Alkaline hemoglobin electrophoresis is a common first step in the confirmation of hemoglobinopathies, including SCD. Electrophoresis is based on the separation of hemoglobin molecules in an electric field due primarily to differences in total molecular charge. In alkaline electrophoresis, hemoglobin molecules assume a negative charge and migrate toward the anode (positive pole). Historically, alkaline hemoglobin electrophoresis was performed on cellulose acetate medium but is being replaced by electrophoresis on agarose medium. Nonetheless, because some hemoglobins have the same charge and, therefore, the same electrophoretic mobility patterns, hemoglobins that exhibit an abnormal electrophoretic pattern at an alkaline pH may be subjected to electrophoresis at an acid pH for definitive separation. In an acid pH some hemoglobins assume a negative charge and migrate toward the anode, while others are positively charged and migrate toward the cathode (negative pole). For example, Hb S migrates with Hb D and Hb G on alkaline electrophoresis but separates from Hb D and Hb G on acid electrophoresis. Similarly, Hb C migrates with Hb E and Hb O on alkaline electrophoresis but separates on acid electrophoresis. Figure 27-7 shows electrophoretic patterns for

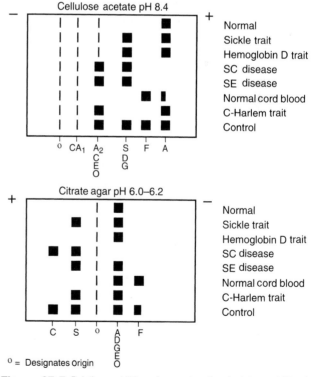

Figure 27-7 Relative mobilities of normal and variant hemoglobins in various conditions measured by electrophoresis on cellulose acetate at an alkaline pH and citrate agar at an acid pH. The relative amount of hemoglobin is not proportional to the size of the band; for example, in sickle cell trait (Hb AS), the bands may appear equal, but the amount of Hb A exceeds that of Hb S. (From Schmidt RM, Brosious EF: *Basic laboratory methods of hemoglobinopathy detection*, ed 6, HEW Pub No (CDC) 77-8266, Atlanta, 1976, Centers for Disease Control and Prevention.)

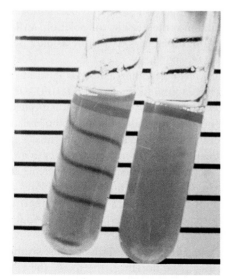

Figure 27-6 Tube solubility screening test for the presence of hemoglobin S. In a negative test result (*left*), the solution is clear and the lines behind the tube are visible. In a positive test result (*right*), the solution is turbid and the lines are not visible. (Courtesy Ann Bell, University of Tennessee, Memphis.)

normal and abnormal hemoglobins. Figure 27-8 shows the electrophoretic separation of a normal adult and a patient with sickle cell disease (Hb SS) at an alkaline pH. HPLC and capillary electrophoresis are gaining in popularity because these methods are more automated, the instruments are more user friendly, and they can be used to confirm hemoglobin variants observed with electrophoresis (Figure 27-9).

HPLC separates hemoglobin types in a cation exchange column and usually requires only one sample injection. Unlike electrophoresis, HPLC can identify and quantitate low levels of Hb A_2 and Hb F, but comigration of Hb A_2 and Hb E occurs. Therefore, HPLC is best used in the diagnosis of thalassemias rather than hemoglobinopathies because quantitation of low levels of normal and abnormal hemoglobin levels is necessary to distinguish thalassemias. HPLC is also commonly used to quantitate Hb A1c levels to monitor diabetic patients.

Capillary electrophoresis, like agarose electrophoresis, separates hemoglobin types based on charge in an alkaline buffer but does so using smaller volumes and produces better separation than traditional agarose electrophoresis. Semiautomated systems like the Capillarys® system (Sebia, Evry, France) allow for the testing of up to eight samples in parallel with computerized analysis of results. Capillary electrophoresis is also economical, since each capillary can accommodate at least 3000 runs.[1] In 2009 hemoglobin electrophoresis in agarose medium was still the most commonly used technique to identify hemoglobin variants, but capillary electrophoresis and HPLC are gaining in popularity.[53]

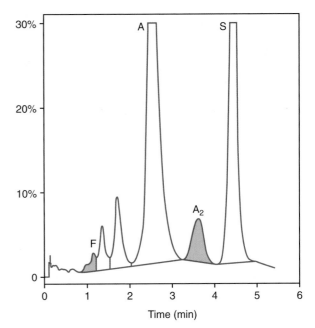

Figure 27-9 Ion-exchange high-performance liquid chromatography (HPLC) separation of hemoglobins (Hbs) in a patient with sickle cell trait demonstrating Hbs F, A, A_2, and an abnormal Hb in the S window (Bio-Rad Variant Classic Hb Testing System, BioRad Laboratories, Philadelphia). (Modified from Elghetany MT, Banki K: Erythrocytic disorders. In McPherson RA, Pincus MR: *Henry's Clinical Diagnosis and Management by Laboratory Methods*, ed 22, Philadelphia, 2011, Elsevier, p. 578.)

Isoelectric focusing (IEF) is a confirmatory technique that is expensive and complex, requiring well-trained and experienced laboratory personnel. The method uses an electric current to push the hemoglobin molecules across a pH gradient. The charge of the molecules change as they migrate through the pH gradient until the hemoglobin species reaches its isoelectric point (net charge of zero). With a net charge of zero, migration stops and the hemoglobin molecules accumulate at their isoelectric position. Molecules with isoelectric point differences of as little as 0.02 pH units can be effectively separated.[1]

Neonatal screening requires a more sophisticated approach, often using three techniques: adapted IEF, HPLC, and reversed-phase HPLC. This multisystem approach is needed to distinguish not only the multitude of hemoglobin variants but also the numerous thalassemias. The more progressive laboratories use a combination of two or more techniques to improve identification of hemoglobin variants. Some reference laboratories may use mass spectroscopy, matrix-assisted laser desorption-ionization time-of-flight (MALDI-TOF) mass spectrometry, or isoelectric focusing to separate hemoglobin types, or nucleic acid identification of the genetic mutation.[1,54]

Patients with Hb SS or Hb SC disease lack normal β-globin chains, so they have no Hb A. In Hb SS, the Hb S level is usually greater than 80%. The Hb F level is usually increased (1% to 20%), and when Hb F constitutes more than 20% of hemoglobin, it has a tendency to modulate the severity of the disease. This is especially true in newborns and in

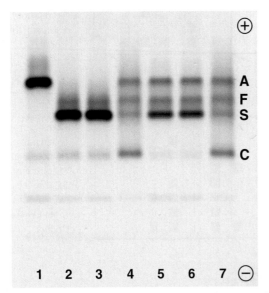

Figure 27-8 Electrophoretic separation of hemoglobins (Hb) at alkaline pH. **1,** Normal adult; **2** and **3,** 17-year-old patient with sickle cell anemia (Hb SS); **5** and **6,** patient with sickle cell anemia, recently transfused (note the presence of Hb A from the transfused red blood cells); **4** and **7,** Hbs A/F/S/C standard (Hydragel 7 Hemoglobin/Hydrasys System, Sebia Electrophoresis, Norcross, GA). (Modified from Elghetany MT, Banki K: Erythrocytic disorders. In McPherson RA, Pincus MR: *Henry's Clinical Diagnosis and Management by Laboratory Methods*, ed 22, Philadelphia, 2011, Elsevier, p. 578.)

patients with hereditary persistence of fetal hemoglobin.[31] The Hb A_2 level is normal or slightly increased (2% to 5%), and Hb A_2 quantitation is useful in differentiating Hb SS from Hb S–β^0-thalassemia, in which Hb A_2 is increased (Chapter 28). Hb G, Hb D, and Hb S all migrate in the same position on alkaline cellulose acetate and alkaline agarose electrophoresis, but Hb G and Hb D do not give a positive result on the tube solubility test.

The typical sequelae of SCD may be predicted, and the effectiveness of treatment monitored, if reliable biomarkers of inflammation can be identified. Among the common indicators of inflammation, WBC is a good predictor of sickle cell events and mortality, whereas the erythrocyte sedimentation rate and C-reactive protein (CRP) level exhibit variability too great to reliably predict events. However, CRP and sPLA$_2$ are both elevated during vasoocclusive crisis and acute chest syndrome. Other markers such as interleukin-6 (IL-6), IL-10, and protein S are showing promise as useful indicators in clinical practice.[55] Annexin A5, a protein bound to lipids in the plasma membrane of endothelial cells and platelets, has been shown to elevate before and during VOC.[56] Lipid damage from oxidative stress can be predicted by plasma elevations of malondialdehyde (MDA) and depleted α-tocopherol. In addition, α-tocopherol rises with CRP during bouts of inflammation. Of all the biomarkers evaluated, IL-6, IL-10, vascular cell adhesion molecule 1 (VCAM-1), and sPLA$_2$ are the most promising at predicting impending crisis.[57]

Treatment

Supportive care has been the mainstay of therapy for SCD. New therapies have evolved, however, that are actually modifying the genetic pathogenesis of the disease. Neonatal screening, childhood prophylactic penicillin therapy, bone marrow transplantation, and treatment with hydroxyurea (hydroxycarbamide) in adults may extend the life of the SCD patient further.

The main components of supportive therapy include adequate hydration, prophylactic vitamin therapy, avoidance of low-oxygen environments, analgesia for pain, and aggressive antibiotic therapy with the first signs of infection. Hydration maintains good blood flow and reduces vasoocclusive crises. Prophylactic oral penicillin V at a dose of 125 mg twice per day by the age of 3 months to 3 years of age is recommended to avoid infection and the associated morbidity and mortality. The penicillin dosage is increased to 250 mg twice per day from 3 to 5 years of age.[58] When infections occur, prompt antibiotic treatment reduces the associated morbidity and mortality.[9] Avoidance of strenuous exercise, high altitudes, and unpressurized air travel maintains high oxygen tensions and reduces the sickling phenomenon. Treatment for painful episodes includes ensuring optimal hydration, rapidly treating associated infection, oxygen therapy, and effectively relieving pain. Analgesics are the foundation of pain management, with nonsteroidal antiinflammatory drugs like paracetamol (acetaminophen) and nefopam administered to manage mild ischemic attacks. Opioids like meperidine (pethidine or demerol) or tramadol are recommended when pain becomes chronic.[59]

Acute VOC attacks are often treated with morphine in the emergency department or when in transit. Blood exchange transfusion (BET) is the treatment of choice for severe VOC attacks and acute chest syndrome (ACS).[33] Painful crises tend to increase with age, and physicians must be aware of opiate tolerance and rebound pain following opiate therapy, called central sensitization. Repeated painful crises can result in hypersensitivity to repeated pain by increasing peripheral inflammation, increased neurotransmitter release, increased calcium influx into postsynaptic junctions, and other pathways that increase pain signals to the brain.[45] This phenomenon can be misinterpreted as drug intolerance, causing inappropriate dose escalation, or as drug-seeking behavior, causing inappropriate termination of treatment. The most appropriate response to opioid tolerance and central sensitization is a gradual dose reduction to reset the pain receptors followed by switching to opioids such as methadone and buprenorphine that are less sensitive to this phenomenon.[45] The patient should be examined on a regular basis, and routine testing should be done to establish baseline values for the patient during nonsickling periods.

Children younger than 3 years often experience *hand-foot syndrome*, characterized by pain and swelling in the hands and feet.[33] Treatment usually consists of increasing intake of fluids and giving analgesics for pain.

Pneumococcal disease has been a leading cause of morbidity and mortality in children, especially children younger than 6 years. With immunization and prophylactic antibiotics, however, this is now a preventable complication.[7] Immunization with heptavalent conjugated pneumococcal vaccine is recommended at 2, 4, and 6 months of age. The 23-valent pneumococcal vaccine is recommended at 2 years, with a booster at the age of 5 years. Standard childhood vaccinations should be given as scheduled. In addition, annual administration of influenza vaccine is recommended beginning at 6 months of age.[42] The risk of bacterial infection probably increases in mature patients with Hb SC disease and homozygous SCD.[20]

Transfusions can be used to prevent the complications of SCD. More specifically, periodic transfusions, given at a frequency of eight or more per year, are effective at preventing stroke, symptomatic anemia, brain injury, priapism, leg ulcers, PHT, delayed pubescence, splenomegaly, and chronic pain and improving school attendance, IQ, energy, exercise tolerance, mood, and sense of well-being. In other circumstances, such as central nervous system infarction, hypoxia with infection, stroke, episodes of acute chest syndrome, and preparation for surgery, transfusions are used to decrease blood viscosity and the percentage of circulating sickle cells. Before all but simple surgeries, Hb SS patients are transfused with normal Hb AA blood to bring the volume of Hb S to less than 50% or to achieve a hemoglobin of 10 g/dL in an effort to prevent complications in surgery.[58,60] Maintenance transfusions should be given in pregnancy if the mother experiences vasoocclusive or anemia-related problems or if there are signs of fetal distress or poor growth.[20] Nonetheless, transfusion therapy has the potential to cause transfusion reactions, transfusion-related infections, and iron overload. Of the three, iron overload is the most frequent.

Iron overload has been associated with endocrine dysfunction[61] and cardiac disease.[62] Deferoxamine has been effective in treating iron overload by chelating and removing much of the excess iron from the body. Deferoxamine must be administered intravenously, however, and treatment requires at least 8 hours each day for a week. An oral iron chelator, deferasirox, was approved by the Food and Drug Administration in 2005.[63] Deferasirox is consumed in the morning as a slurry by dissolving several pills, but its effectiveness is yet to be determined.

Bone marrow or hematopoietic stem cell transplantation has proved successful for some individuals, but few patients qualify due to the lack of HLA-matched, related donors.[64] The event-free survival rates for patients receiving transplants from HLA-identical related donors are between 80% and 90% for SCD.[65-68] Patients chosen for transplantation are generally children younger than age 17 with severe complications of SCD (i.e., stroke, acute chest syndrome, and refractory pain). In addition, morbidity and mortality following transplantation increase with age, which places another restriction on transplantation therapy.[69] There is evidence that transplantation restores some splenic function, but its effect on established organ damage is unknown.[70] Transplantation of cord blood stem cells from HLA-identical related and unrelated donors is associated with a disease-free survival rate of 90%.[71] The primary benefit of using cord blood as a source of stem cells is that banking of cord blood increases the number of units available to achieve an HLA match.[71] Some researchers are now focusing on the use of in utero stem cell transplantation to produce engraftment while the immune system of the fetus is prone to HLA tolerance. Others are attempting to genetically alter fetal hematopoietic stems cells to overcome HLA mismatches.[72]

Hydroxycarbamide (hydroxyurea) therapy has offered some promise in relieving the sickling disorder by increasing the proportion of Hb F in the erythrocytes of individuals with SCD.[73] Hydroxyurea, given at 25 to 30 mg/kg, has been shown to reduce symptoms and prolong life, in part by increasing Hb F levels. Daily dosing produces a better HbF response compared to sequential weekly dosing.[74] Because Hb F does not copolymerize with Hb S, if the production of Hb F can be sufficiently augmented, the complications of SCD might be avoided. The severity of the disease expression and the number of irreversible sickle cells are inversely proportional to the extent to which Hb F synthesis persists. Individuals in whom Hb F levels stabilize at 12% to 20% of total hemoglobin may have little or no anemia and few, if any, vasoocclusive attacks. Levels of 4% to 5% Hb F may modulate the disease, and levels of 5% to 12% may suppress the severity of hemolysis and lessen the frequency of severe episodes.[34] Drug compliance is best monitored by an increasing MCV, while a decreasing LD might be an indicator of treatment response.[33] Response to hydroxycarbamide is variable among SCD patients, but high baseline Hb F level, neutrophil levels, and reticulocyte count are the best predictors of Hb F response.[75]

Prevention of intracellular RBC dehydration reduces intracellular HbS polymerization thus reducing VOC. The uses of senicapoc to inhibit Gardos channels and Mg^{++} to modulate K^+-Cl^- transport systems show increased hemoglobin levels and decreased numbers of dense RBCs, resulting in reduced hemolysis but no clear reduction in VOC.[76-80]

Course and Prognosis

Proper management of SCD has increased the life expectancy of patients from 14 years in 1973 to the current average life span of 50 years.[81] For men and women who are compound heterozygotes for Hb SC, the average life span is 60 and 68 years, respectively, with a few patients living into their seventies.[30,82] Individuals with Hb SS can pursue a wide range of vocations and professions. They are discouraged, however, from jobs that require strenuous physical exertion or exposure to high altitudes or extreme environmental temperature variations.

Newborn screening for hemoglobinopathies has significantly reduced mortality in children with SCD by enabling prompt and comprehensive medical care. The most common form of screening is HPLC followed by confirmation using hemoglobin electrophoresis and genotyping methods.[83]

Sickle Cell Trait

The term *sickle cell trait* refers to the heterozygous state (Hb AS) and describes a benign condition that generally does not affect mortality or morbidity except under conditions of extreme exertion. The trait occurs in approximately 8% of African Americans. It also can be found in Central Americans, Asians, and people from the region around the Mediterranean.[1]

Individuals with sickle cell trait are generally asymptomatic and present with no significant clinical or hematologic manifestations. Under extremely hypoxic conditions, however, systemic sickling and vascular occlusion with pooling of sickled cells in the spleen, focal necrosis in the brain, rhabdomyolysis, and even death can occur. In circumstances such as severe respiratory infection, unpressurized flight at high altitudes, and anesthesia in which pH and oxygen levels are sufficiently lowered to cause sickling, patients may develop splenic infarcts.[8] Failure to concentrate urine is the only consistent abnormality found in patients with sickle cell trait.[84] This abnormality is caused by diminished perfusion of the vasa recta of the kidney, which impairs concentration of urine by the renal tubules. Renal papillary necrosis with hematuria has been described in some patients.[8]

Although much controversy exists as to the potential connection between strenuous exercise and severe to fatal adverse events in patients with sickle cell trait, at least 46 cases have been documented in the literature (39 military recruits and 7 athletes).[85] The causes of these deaths were largely due to cardiac failures, renal failures, rhabdomyolysis, and heart illness. Opponents of the connection of sickle cell trait and fatal events argue that these events occur in sickle cell–negative people, many people with sickle cell trait do not develop adverse events, fatal sickle crisis cannot be adequately established in the patients encountering events, and similar events have not been clearly documented in patients with sickle cell disease. However, it has been shown that military recruits with sickle cell trait have a 21 times greater risk of exercise-related death than recruits with normal hemoglobin.[85] Similar data have not been established in athletes with sickle cell trait.[85]

The peripheral blood film of a patient with sickle cell trait shows normal RBC morphology, with the exception of a few target cells. No abnormalities in the leukocytes and thrombocytes are seen. The hemoglobin solubility screening test yields positive results, and sickle cell trait is diagnosed by detecting the presence of Hb S and Hb A on hemoglobin electrophoresis or HPLC. In individuals with sickle cell trait, electrophoresis reveals approximately 40% or less Hb S and approximately 60% or more Hb A, Hb A_2 level is normal or slightly increased, and Hb F level is within the reference interval. Levels of Hb S less than 40% can be seen in patients who also have α-thalassemia or iron or folate deficiency.[20] No treatment is required for this benign condition, and the patient's life span is not affected by sickle cell trait.

HEMOGLOBIN C

Hb C was the next hemoglobinopathy after Hb S to be described and in the United States is found almost exclusively in the African-American population. Spaet and Ranney reported this disease in the homozygous state (Hb CC) in 1953.[8]

Prevalence, Etiology, and Pathophysiology

Hb C is found in 17% to 28% of people of West African extraction and in 2% to 3% of African Americans.[4] It is the most common nonsickling variant encountered in the United States and the third most common in the world.[4] Hb C is defined by the structural formula $\alpha_2\beta_2^{6Glu\rightarrow Lys}$, in which lysine is substituted for glutamic acid in position 6 of the β chain. Lysine has a $+1$ charge and glutamic acid has a -1 charge, so the result of this substitution is a net change in charge of $+2$, which has a different structural effect on the hemoglobin molecule than the Hb S substitution.

Hb C is inherited in the same manner as Hb S but manifests as a milder disease. Similar to Hb S, Hb C polymerizes under low oxygen tension, but the structure of the polymers differs. Hb S polymers are long and thin, whereas the polymers in Hb C form a short, thick crystal within the RBCs. The shorter Hb C crystal does not alter RBC shape to the extent that Hb S does, so there is less splenic sequestration and hemolysis. In addition, vasoocclusive crisis does not occur.

Laboratory Diagnosis

A mild to moderate, normochromic, normocytic anemia occurs in homozygous Hb C disease. Occasionally, some microcytosis and mild hypochromia may be present. There is a marked increase in the number of target cells, a slight to moderate increase in the number of reticulocytes, and nucleated RBCs may be present in the peripheral blood.

Hexagonal crystals of Hb C form within the erythrocyte and may be seen on the peripheral blood film (Figure 27-10). Many

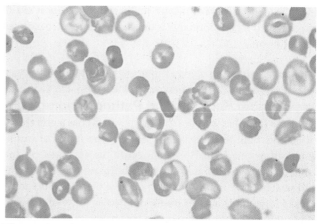

Figure 27-10 Peripheral blood film for a patient with hemoglobin C disease showing one Hb C crystal and target and folded cells ($\times$1000). (Courtesy Ann Bell, University of Tennessee, Memphis.)

crystals appear extracellularly with no evidence of a cell membrane.[86,87] In some cells, the hemoglobin is concentrated within the boundary of the crystal. The crystals are densely stained and vary in size and appear oblong with pyramid-shaped or pointed ends. These crystals may be seen on wet preparations by washing RBCs and resuspending them in a solution of sodium citrate.[11]

Hb C yields a negative result on the hemoglobin solubility test, and definitive diagnosis is made using electrophoresis or HPLC. No Hb A is present in Hb CC disease. In addition, Hb C is present at levels of greater than 90%, with Hb F at less than 7% and Hb A_2 at approximately 2%. In Hb AC trait, about 60% Hb A and 30% Hb C are present. On cellulose acetate electrophoresis at an alkaline pH, Hb C migrates in the same position as Hb A_2, Hb E, and Hb O-Arab (Figure 27-7). Hb C is separated from these other hemoglobins on citrate agar electrophoresis at an acid pH (Figure 27-7). No specific treatment is required. This disorder becomes problematic only if infection occurs or if mild chronic hemolysis leads to gallbladder disease.

HEMOGLOBIN C-HARLEM (HEMOGLOBIN C-GEORGETOWN)

Hb C-Harlem (Hb C-Georgetown) has a double substitution on the β chain.[5,20] The substitution of valine for glutamic acid at position 6 of the β chain is identical to the Hb S substitution, and the substitution at position 73 of aspartic acid for asparagine is the same as that in the Hb Korle Bu mutation. The double mutation is termed *Hb C-Harlem (Hb C-Georgetown)* because the abnormal hemoglobin migrates with Hb C on cellulose acetate electrophoresis at an alkaline pH. Patients heterozygous for this anomaly are asymptomatic, but patients with compound heterozygosity for Hb S and Hb C-Harlem have crises similar to those in Hb SS disease.[88]

A positive solubility test result may occur with Hb C-Harlem, and hemoglobin electrophoresis or HPLC is necessary to confirm the diagnosis. On cellulose acetate at pH 8.4, Hb C-Harlem migrates in the C position (Figure 27-7). Citrate agar electrophoresis at pH 6.2, however, shows migration of Hb C-Harlem in the S position (Figure 27-7). Because so few cases have been identified, the clinical outcome for homozygous individuals affected with this abnormality is uncertain,[88] but heterozygotes appear normal.

HEMOGLOBIN E

Prevalence, Etiology, and Pathophysiology

Hb E was first described in 1954.[89] The variant has a prevalence of 30% in Southeast Asia. As a result of the influx of immigrants from this area, Hb E prevalence has increased in the United States.[90] It occurs infrequently in African Americans and whites. Hb E is a β chain variant in which lysine is substituted for glutamic acid in position 26 ($\alpha_2\beta_2^{26Glu \rightarrow Lys}$). As with Hb C, this substitution results in a net change in charge of +2, but because of the position of the substitution, hemoglobin polymerization does not occur. However, the amino acid substitution at codon 26 inserts a cryptic splice site that causes abnormal alterative splicing and decreased transcription of functional mRNA for the Hb E globin chain.[91] Thus the Hb E mutation is both a qualitative defect (due to the amino acid substitution in the globin chain) and a quantitative defect with a β-thalassemia phenotype (due to the decreased production of the globin chain).[91]

Clinical Features

The homozygous state (Hb EE) manifests as a mild anemia with microcytes and target cells. The RBC survival time is shortened. The condition is not associated with clinically observable icterus, hemolysis, or splenomegaly. The main concern in identifying homozygous Hb E is differentiating it from iron deficiency, β-thalassemia trait, and Hb E–β-thal (Chapter 28).[91] The disease, Hb EE, resembles thalassemia trait. Because the highest incidence of the Hb E gene is in the areas of Thailand where malaria is most prevalent, it is thought that *P. falciparum* multiplies more slowly in Hb EE RBCs than in Hb AE or Hb AA RBCs and that the mutation may give some protection against malaria.[1] Hb E trait is asymptomatic. When Hb E is combined with β-thalassemia, however, the disease becomes more severe than Hb EE and more closely resembles β-thalassemia major, requiring regular blood transfusions.[1]

Laboratory Diagnosis

Hb E does not produce a positive hemoglobin solubility test result and must be confirmed using electrophoresis or HPLC. In the homozygous state there is greater than 90% Hb E, a very low MCV (55 to 65 fL), few to many target cells, and a normal reticulocyte count. The heterozygous state has a mean MCV of 65 fL, slight erythrocytosis, target cells[1] (Figure 27-11), and approximately 30% to 40% Hb E. On cellulose acetate electrophoresis at an alkaline pH, Hb E migrates with Hb C, Hb O, and Hb A_2 (Figure 27-7). On citrate agar electrophoresis at an acid pH, Hb E can be separated from Hb C, but it comigrates with Hb A and Hb O (Figure 27-7).

Treatment and Prognosis

No therapy is required with Hb E disease and trait. Some patients may experience splenomegaly and fatigue, however.

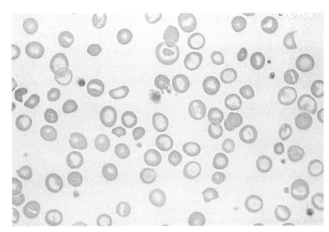

Figure 27-11 Microcytes and target cells in a patient with hemoglobin E trait. (From Hematology tech sample H-1, Chicago, 1991, American Society of Clinical Pathologists.)

Genetic counseling is recommended, and the Hb E gene mutation should be discussed in the same manner as a mild β-thalassemia allele.[91]

HEMOGLOBIN O-ARAB

Hb O-Arab is a β chain variant caused by the substitution of lysine for glutamic acid at amino acid position 121 ($\alpha_2\beta_2^{121Glu \rightarrow Lys}$).[5,20,32] It is a rare disorder found in Kenya, Israel, Egypt, and Bulgaria and in 0.4% of African Americans. No clinical symptoms are exhibited by individuals who carry this variant, except for a mild splenomegaly in homozygotes.[5] When Hb O-Arab is inherited with Hb S, however, severe clinical conditions similar to those in Hb SS result.[5]

Homozygous individuals have a mild hemolytic anemia, with many target cells on the peripheral blood film and a negative result on the hemoglobin solubility test. The presence of this hemoglobin variant must be confirmed using electrophoresis or HPLC. Because Hb O-Arab migrates with Hb A_2, Hb C, and Hb E on cellulose acetate at an alkaline pH, citrate agar electrophoresis at an acid pH is required to differentiate it from Hb C (Figure 27-7). Hb O-Arab is the only hemoglobin to move just slightly away from the point of application toward the cathode on citrate agar at an acid pH. No treatment is generally necessary for individuals with Hb O-Arab.

HEMOGLOBIN D AND HEMOGLOBIN G

Hb D and Hb G are a group of at least 16 β chain variants (Hb D) and 6 α chain variants (Hb G) that migrate in an alkaline pH at the same electrophoretic position as Hb S.[4,8,20,92] This is because their α and β subunits have one fewer negative charge at an alkaline pH than Hb A, as does Hb S. They do not sickle, however, when exposed to reduced oxygen tension.

Most variants are named for the place where they were discovered. Hb D-Punjab and Hb D-Los Angeles are identical hemoglobins in which glutamine is substituted for glutamic acid at position 121 in the β chain ($\alpha_2\beta_2^{121Glu \rightarrow Gln}$). Hb D-Punjab occurs in about 3% of the population in northwestern India, and Hb D-Los Angeles is seen in fewer than 2% of African Americans.

Hb G-Philadelphia is an α chain variant of the G hemoglobins, with a substitution of asparagine by lysine at position 68 ($\alpha_2^{68Asn \rightarrow Lys}\beta_2$).[5] The Hb G-Philadelphia variant is the most common G variant encountered in African Americans and is seen with greater frequency than the Hb D variants. The Hb G variant is also found in Ghana.[4,8,20,92]

Hb D and Hb G do not sickle and yield a negative hemoglobin solubility test result. On alkaline electrophoresis, Hb D and Hb G have the same mobility as Hb S (Figure 27-7). Hb D and Hb G can be separated from Hb S on citrate agar at pH 6.0 (Figure 27-7). These variants should be suspected whenever a hemoglobin is encountered that migrates in the S position on alkaline electrophoresis and has a negative result on the hemoglobin solubility test. In the homozygous state (Hb DD), there is greater than 95% Hb D, with normal amounts of Hb A_2 and Hb F.[30] Hb DD can be confused with the compound heterozygous state for Hb D and β⁰-thalassemia. The two disorders can be differentiated on the basis of the MCV, levels of Hb A_2, and family studies.[4,8,20,92]

Hb D and Hb G are asymptomatic in the heterozygous state. Hb D disease (Hb DD) is marked by mild hemolytic anemia and chronic nonprogressive splenomegaly. No treatment is required.[4,8,20,92]

COMPOUND HETEROZYGOSITY WITH HEMOGLOBIN S AND ANOTHER β-GLOBIN GENE MUTATION

Compound heterozygosity is the inheritance of two different mutant genes that share a common genetic locus—in this case the β-globin gene locus.[93-96] Because there are two β-globin genes, these compound heterozygotes have inherited Hb S from one parent and another β chain hemoglobinopathy or thalassemia from the other parent. Compound heterozygosity of Hb S with Hb C, Hb D, Hb O, or β-thalassemia may produce hemolytic anemia of variable severity. Inheritance of Hb S with

other hemoglobins, such as Hb E, Hb G-Philadelphia, and Hb Korle Bu, causes disorders of no clinical consequence.[93]

Hemoglobin SC

Hb SC is the most common compound heterozygous syndrome that results in a structural defect in the hemoglobin molecule in which different amino acid substitutions are found on each of two β-globin chains. At position 6, glutamic acid is replaced by valine (Hb S) on one β-globin chain and by lysine (Hb C) on the other β-globin chain. The frequency of Hb SC is 25% in West Africa. The incidence in the United States is approximately 1 in 833 births per year.[93,97]

Clinical Features

Hb SC disease resembles a mild SCD. Growth and development are delayed compared with normal children. Unlike Hb SS, Hb SC usually does not produce significant symptoms until the teenage years. Hb SC disease may cause all the vasoocclusive complications of sickle cell anemia, but the episodes are less frequent, and damage is less disabling. Hemolytic anemia is moderate, and many patients exhibit moderate splenomegaly. Proliferative retinopathy is more common and more severe than in sickle cell anemia.[98] Respiratory tract infections with *S. pneumoniae* are common.[8]

Patients with Hb SC disease live longer than patients with Hb SS and have fewer painful episodes, but this disorder is associated with considerable morbidity and mortality, especially after age 30.[99] In the United States, the median life span for men is 60 years and for women 68 years.[30]

Laboratory Diagnosis

The complete blood count shows a mild normocytic, normochromic anemia with many of the features associated with sickle cell anemia. The hemoglobin level is usually 11 to 13 g/dL, and the reticulocyte count is 3% to 5%. On the peripheral blood film, there are a few sickle cells, target cells, and intraerythrocytic crystalline structures. Crystalline aggregates of hemoglobin (SC crystals) form in some cells, where they protrude from the membrane (Figure 27-12).[93,96] Hb SC crystals often appear as a

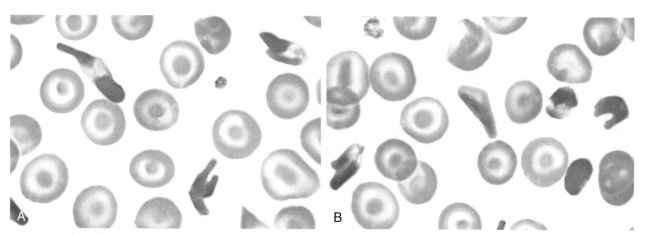

Figure 27-12 A and B, Peripheral blood film for a patient with hemoglobin SC. Note intraerythrocytic, blunt-ended SC crystals and target cells (×1000). (Courtesy Ann Bell, University of Tennessee, Memphis.)

hybrid of Hb S and Hb C crystals. They are longer than Hb C crystals but shorter and thicker than Hb S polymers and are often branched.

The result of the hemoglobin solubility screening test is positive because of the presence of Hb S. Electrophoretically, Hb C and Hb S migrate in almost equal amounts (45%) on cellulose acetate, and Hb F is normal. Hb C is confirmed on citrate agar at an acid pH, where it is separated from Hb E and Hb O. Hb A_2 migrates with Hb C, and its quantitation is of no consequence in Hb SC disease. Determination of Hb A_2 becomes vital, however, if a patient is suspected of having Hb C concurrent with β-thalassemia (Chapter 28).

Treatment and Prognosis

Therapy similar to that for SCD is given to individuals with Hb SC disease.[88]

Hemoglobin S–β-Thalassemia

Compound heterozygosity for Hb S and β-thalassemia is the most common cause of sickle cell syndrome in patients of Mediterranean descent and is second to Hb SC disease among all compound heterozygous sickle disorders. Hb S–β-thal usually causes a clinical syndrome resembling that of mild or moderate sickle cell anemia. The severity of this compound heterozygous condition depends on the β chain production of the affected β-thalassemia gene. If there is no β-globin chain production from the β-thalassemia gene (Hb S–β⁰-thal), the clinical course is similar to that of homozygous sickle cell anemia. If there is production of a normal β-globin chain (Hb S–β+-thal), patients tend to have a milder condition than patients with Hb SC. These patients can be distinguished from individuals with sickle cell trait because of the presence of greater amounts of Hb S than of Hb A, increased levels of Hb A_2 and Hb F, microcytosis from the thalassemia, hemolytic anemia, abnormal peripheral blood morphology, and splenomegaly (Chapter 28).[20,93]

Hemoglobin SD and Hemoglobin SG-Philadelphia

Hb SD is a compound heterozygous and Hb SG-Philadelphia a double heterozygous sickle cell syndrome.[20,92] Hb SG-Philadelphia is asymptomatic because Hb G is associated with an α gene mutation that still allows for sufficient Hb A to be produced. Hb SD syndrome may cause a mild to severe hemolytic anemia because both β chains are affected. Some patients with Hb SD may have severe vasoocclusive complications. The Hb D syndrome in African Americans is usually due to the interaction of Hb S with Hb D-Los Angeles (Hb D-Punjab).

The peripheral blood film findings for Hb SD disease are comparable to those seen in less severe forms of Hb SS disease. Because Hb D and Hb G comigrate with Hb S on cellulose acetate electrophoresis at an alkaline pH, citrate agar electrophoresis at an acid pH is necessary to separate Hb S from Hb D and Hb G. The clinical picture is valuable in differentiating Hb SD and Hb SG. The treatment for Hb SD disease is similar to that

for patients with SCD and is administered according to the severity of the clinical condition.

Hemoglobin S/O-Arab and HbS/D-Punjab

Hb S/O-Arab and Hb S/D-Punjab are rare compound heterozygous hemoglobinopathies that cause severe chronic hemolytic anemia with vasoocclusive episodes.[8,20,92] Both mutations replace glutamic acid at position 121; O-Arab substitutes lysine and D-Punjab substitutes glutamine. Glutamic acid at position 121 is located on the outer surface of the hemoglobin tetramer, which enhances the polymerization process involving Hb S. Hb S/O-Arab can be mistaken for Hb SC on cellulose acetate electrophoresis at an alkaline pH because Hb C and Hb O-Arab migrate at the same position; however, differentiation is easily made on citrate agar at an acid pH. Therapy for these patients is similar to that for patients with SCD. Similarly, Hb D-Punjab comigrates with Hb S on alkaline electrophoresis, making this mutation look like SCD. Hb O-Arab and Hb D-Punjab are not clinically significant in either the heterozygous or the homozygous form.[1]

Hemoglobin S-Korle Bu

Hb Korle Bu is a rare hemoglobin variant with substitution of aspartic acid for asparagine at position 73 of the β chain.[20] When inherited with Hb S, it interferes with lateral contact between Hb S fibers by disrupting the hydrophobic pocket for β₆ valine, which inhibits Hb S polymerization. The compound heterozygous condition Hb S-Korle Bu is asymptomatic.

CONCOMITANT CIS MUTATIONS WITH HEMOGLOBIN S

A concomitant cis mutation with Hb S involves a second mutation on the same gene along with Hb S. Three cis mutations will be described: Hb C-Harlem, Hb S-Antilles, and Hb S-Oman.

Hemoglobin C-Harlem

Hb C-Harlem has two substitutions on the β chain: the sickle mutation and the Korle Bu mutation. Patients heterozygous for only Hb C-Harlem are asymptomatic. The compound heterozygous Hb S–Hb C-Harlem state resembles Hb SS clinically. Hb C-Harlem yields a positive result on the hemoglobin solubility test and migrates to the Hb C position on cellulose acetate electrophoresis at an alkaline pH and to the Hb S position on citrate agar electrophoresis at an acid pH.

Hemoglobin S-Antilles and Hemoglobin S-Oman

Hb S-Antilles bears the Hb S mutation ($β^{6Glu→Val}$) along with a substitution of isoleucine for valine at position 23.[100] Hb S-Oman also has the Hb S mutation with a second substitution of lysine for glutamic acid at position 121.[101] In both of these hemoglobin variants, the second mutation enhances Hb S such that significant sickling can occur even in heterozygotes.[1]

Table 27-2 summarizes common clinically significant hemoglobinopathies, including general characteristics and treatment options.

TABLE 27-2 Common Clinically Significant Hemoglobinopathies

Hemoglobin Disorder	Abnormal Hemoglobin	Structural Defect	Groups Primarily Affected	Hemoglobin Solubility Test Results	Hemoglobins Present	Red Blood Cell Morphology	Symptoms/Organ Defects	Treatment
Sickle cell anemia (homozygous)	Hb S	$\alpha_2\beta_2^{6Glu\rightarrow Val}$	African, African American, Middle Eastern, Indian, Mediterranean	Positive	0% Hb A, >80% Hb S, 1%—20% Hb F, 2%—5% Hb A$_2$	Sickle cells, target cells, nucleated RBCs, polychromasia, Howell-Jolly bodies, basophilic stippling	Vasoocclusion, bacterial infections, hemolytic anemia, aplastic episodes; bones, lungs, liver, spleen, penis, eyes, central nervous system, urinary tract	Transfusions, antibiotics, analgesics, bone marrow transplant, hydroxyurea
Hb C disease (homozygous)	Hb C	$\alpha_2\beta_2^{6Glu\rightarrow Lys}$	African, African American	Negative	0% Hb A, >90% Hb C, <7% Hb F, 2% Hb A$_2$	Hb C crystals, target cells, nucleated RBCs, occasionally some microcytes	Mild splenomegaly, mild hemolysis	Usually none, antibiotics
Hb SC-Harlem* (Hb C-Georgetown)	Hb C-Harlem, Hb S	$\alpha_2\beta_2^{6Glu\rightarrow Val}$ and $\alpha_2\beta_2^{73Asp\rightarrow Asn}$ on same gene and $\alpha_2\beta_2^{6Glu\rightarrow Val}$	Rare, so uncertain; African, African American	Positive	Hb C-Harlem migrates with Hb C at alkaline pH; migrates with Hb S at acid pH	Target cells	Compound heterozygotes with Hb SC-Harlem have symptoms similar to Hb SS	Similar to Hb SS
Hb E disease (homozygous)	Hb E	$\alpha_2\beta_2^{26Glu\rightarrow Lys}$	Southeast Asian, African, African American	Negative	0% Hb A, 95% Hb E, 2%–4% Hb A$_2$; migrates with Hb A$_2$, Hb C, and Hb O at alkaline pH	Target cells, microcytes	Mild anemia, mild splenomegaly, no symptoms	Usually none
Hb O-Arab (homozygous)	Hb O-Arab	$\alpha_2\beta_2^{121Glu\rightarrow Lys}$	Kenyan, Israeli, Egyptian, Bulgarian, African American	Negative	0% Hb A, 95% Hb O, 2%–4% Hb A$_2$; migrates with Hb A$_2$, Hb C, and Hb E at alkaline pH	Target cells	Mild splenomegaly	Usually none
Hb D disease (rare homozygous)	Hb D-Punjab (Hb-D Los Angeles)	$\alpha_2\beta_2^{121Glu\rightarrow Gln}$	Middle Eastern, Indian	Negative	95% Hb D, normal Hb A$_2$ and Hb F; migrates with Hb S at alkaline pH	Target cells	Mild hemolytic anemia, mild splenomegaly	Usually none

Continued

TABLE 27-2 Common Clinically Significant Hemoglobinopathies—cont'd

Hemoglobin Disorder	Abnormal Hemoglobin	Structural Defect	Groups Primarily Affected	Hemoglobin Solubility Test Results	Hemoglobins Present	Red Blood Cell Morphology	Symptoms/Organ Defects	Treatment
Hb G disease (rare homozygous)	Hb G, Hb G-Philadelphia	$\alpha_2^{68Asn\rightarrow Lys}\beta_2$	African American, Ghanaian	Negative	95% Hb G, normal Hb A$_2$ and Hb F; migrates with S at alkaline pH	Target cells	Mild hemolytic anemia, mild splenomegaly	Usually none
Hb SC* disease	Hb S, Hb C	$\alpha_2\beta_2^{6Glu\rightarrow Val}$ and $\alpha_2\beta_2^{6Glu\rightarrow Lys}$	Same as Hb S	Positive	45% Hb S, 45% Hb C, 2%–4% Hb A$_2$, 1% Hb F	Sickle cells, Hb SC crystals, target cells	Same as those for Hb SS except milder	Similar to that for Hb SS but less intensive
Hb S–β-thalassemia*	Hb S + β-thalassemia mutation	$\alpha_2\beta_2^{6Glu\rightarrow Val}$ and β^0 or β^+	Same as Hb S	Positive	Hb S variable, some Hb A in β^+, increased Hb A$_2$ and Hb F	Sickle cells, target cells, microcytes	Hemolytic anemia, splenomegaly	Similar to that for Hb SS; varies depending on amount of Hb A present
Hb SD* disease	Hb S, Hb D	$\alpha_2\beta_2^{6Glu\rightarrow Val}$ and $\alpha_2\beta_2^{121Glu\rightarrow Gln}$	Same as Hb S	Positive	45% Hb S, 45% Hb D, 2%–4% Hb A$_2$, 1% Hb F; Hb S and D comigrate at alkaline pH	Sickle cells, target cells	Similar to those for Hb SS but milder	Similar to that for Hb SS but less intensive
Hb SG†	Hb S, Hb G	$\alpha_2\beta_2^{6Glu\rightarrow Val}$ and $\alpha_2^{68Asn\rightarrow Lys}\beta_2$	Same as Hb S	Positive	45% Hb S, 45% Hb G, 2%–4% Hb A$_2$, 1% Hb F; Hb S and G comigrate at alkaline pH	Target cells	No symptoms	Usually none
Hb SO-Arab*	Hb S, Hb O-Arab	$\alpha_2\beta_2^{6Glu\rightarrow Val}$ and $\alpha_2\beta_2^{121Glu\rightarrow Lys}$	Same as Hb S	Positive	45% Hb S, 45% Hb O, 2%–4% Hb A$_2$, 1% Hb F	Sickle cells, target cells	Similar to those for Hb SS	Similar to that for Hb SS

*Compound heterozygous.
†Double heterozygous.
Asn, Asparagine; *Asp,* aspartic acid; *Gln,* glutamine; *Glu,* glutamic acid; *Hb,* hemoglobin; *Lys,* lysine; *Val,* valine.

HEMOGLOBIN M

Hb M is caused by a variety of mutations in the α-, β-, and γ-globin genes, all of which result in the production of methemoglobin—hence the Hb M designation.[92,102] These genetic mutations result in a structural abnormality in the globin portion of the molecule. Most M hemoglobins involve a substitution of a tyrosine amino acid for either the proximal (F_8) or the distal (E_7) histidine amino acid in the α, β, or γ chains. These substitutions cause heme iron to auto-oxidize, which results in methemoglobinemia. Hb M has iron in the ferric state (Fe^{3+}) and is unable to carry oxygen, which produces cyanosis. Seven hemoglobin variants affecting the α or β chains have been classified as M hemoglobins: Hb M-Boston, Hb M-Iwate, and Hb Auckland (α chain variants); and Hb Chile, Hb M-Saskatoon, Hb M-Milwaukee-1, and Hb M-Milwaukee-2 (β chain variants), all named for the locations in which they were discovered.[5] Two variants affect the γ chain—Hb F-M-Osaka and Hb F-M-Fort Ripley[5]—but symptoms disappear when Hb A replaces Hb F at 3 to 6 months of age.

Hb M variants have altered oxygen affinity and are inherited as autosomal dominant disorders. Affected individuals have 30% to 50% methemoglobin (healthy individuals have less than 1%) and may appear cyanotic. Ingestion of oxidant drugs, such as sulfonamides, can increase methemoglobin to life-threatening levels. Methemoglobin causes the blood specimen to appear brown. Heinz bodies may be seen sometimes on wet preparations because methemoglobin causes globin chains to precipitate (see Figure 14-11). Diagnosis is made by spectral absorption of the hemolysate or by hemoglobin electrophoresis. The absorption spectrum peaks are determined at various wavelengths. The unique absorption range of each Hb M variant is identified when these are compared with the spectrum of normal blood.

Before electrophoresis, all hemoglobin types are converted to methemoglobin by adding potassium cyanide to the sample so that any migration differences observed are only due to an amino acid substitution, not differences in iron states. On cellulose acetate, Hb M migrates slightly more slowly than Hb A. The electrophoresis should be performed on agar gel at pH 7.1 for clear separation. Further confirmation may be obtained using HPLC or deoxyribonucleic acid (DNA)–based globin gene analysis. No treatment is necessary. Diagnosis is essential to prevent inappropriate treatment for other conditions, such as cyanotic heart disease.

UNSTABLE HEMOGLOBIN VARIANTS

Unstable hemoglobin variants result from genetic mutations to globin genes creating hemoglobin products that precipitate in vivo, producing Heinz bodies and causing a hemolytic anemia.[92,102] More than 140 variants of unstable hemoglobin exist.[5] The majority of these are β chain variants, and most others are α chain variants. Only a few are γ and δ chain variants. Most unstable hemoglobin variants have no clinical significance, although the majority has an increased oxygen affinity. About 25% of unstable hemoglobins are responsible for hemolytic anemia, which varies from compensated mild anemia to severe hemolytic episodes.

At one time, the anemia was referred to as *congenital nonspherocytic hemolytic anemia* or *congenital Heinz body anemia*. This disorder is more properly called *unstable hemoglobin disease*. The syndrome appears at or just after birth, depending on the globin chains involved. It is inherited in an autosomal dominant pattern. All patients are heterozygous; apparently the homozygous condition is incompatible with life. The instability of the hemoglobin molecule may be due to (1) substitution of a charged for an uncharged amino acid in the interior of the molecule, (2) substitution of a polar for a nonpolar amino acid in the hydrophobic heme pocket, (3) substitution of an amino acid in the α and β chains at the intersubunit contact points, (4) replacement of an amino acid with proline in the α helix section of a chain, and (5) deletion or elongation of the primary structure.

Clinical Features

The unstable hemoglobin disorder is usually detected in early childhood in patients with hemolytic anemia accompanied by jaundice and splenomegaly. Fever or ingestion of an oxidant exacerbates the hemolysis. The severity of the anemia depends on the degree of instability of the hemoglobin molecule. The unstable hemoglobin precipitates in vivo and in vitro in response to factors that do not affect normal hemoglobins, such as drug ingestion and exposure to heat or cold. The hemoglobin precipitates in the RBC as Heinz bodies. The precipitated hemoglobin attaches to the cell membrane, causing clustering of band 3, attachment of autologous immunoglobulin, and macrophage activation. In addition, Heinz bodies can be trapped mechanically in the splenic sieve, which shortens RBC survival. The oxygen affinity of these cells is also abnormal.

The most prevalent unstable hemoglobin is Hb Köln. Other unstable hemoglobins include Hb Hammersmith, Hb Zurich, Hb Gun Hill, and Hb Hammersmith.[5] Because of the large variability in the degree of instability in these hemoglobins, the extent of hemolysis varies greatly. For some of the variants, such as Hb Zurich, the presence of an oxidant is required for any significant hemolysis to occur.

Laboratory Diagnosis

The RBC morphology varies. It may be normal or show slight hypochromia and prominent basophilic stippling, which possibly is caused by excessive clumping of ribosomes. Before splenectomy, the hemoglobin level ranges from 7 to 12 g/dL, with a 4% to 20% reticulocyte count. After splenectomy, anemia is corrected, but reticulocytosis persists. Heinz bodies can be shown using a supravital stain (see Figure 14-11). After splenectomy, Heinz bodies are larger and more numerous. Many patients excrete dark urine that contains dipyrrole.

Many unstable hemoglobins migrate in the normal AA pattern and thus are not detected on electrophoresis. Other tests used to detect unstable hemoglobins include the isopropanol precipitation test, which is based on the principle that an isopropanol solution at 37° C weakens the bonding forces of the hemoglobin molecule. If unstable hemoglobins are present, rapid precipitation occurs in 5 minutes, and heavy flocculation occurs after 20 minutes. Normal hemoglobin does not begin to precipitate until after approximately 40 minutes. The heat denaturation test also can be used. When incubated at 50° C for 1 hour, heat-sensitive unstable hemoglobins show a flocculent precipitation, whereas normal hemoglobin shows little or no precipitation. Significant numbers of Heinz bodies appear after splenectomy, but even in individuals with intact spleens, with longer incubation and the addition of an oxidative substance such as acetylphenylhydrazine, unstable hemoglobins form more Heinz bodies than does the blood from individuals with normal hemoglobins. Other techniques, such as isoelectric focusing, can resolve many hemoglobin variants with only a slight alteration in their isoelectric point, and globin chain analysis can be performed by HPLC or DNA-based globin gene analysis.

Treatment and Prognosis

Patients are treated to prevent hemolytic crises. In severe cases, the spleen must be removed to reduce sequestration and rate of removal of RBCs. Because unstable hemoglobin disease is rare, prognosis in the affected individuals is unclear. Patients are cautioned against the use of sulfonamides and other oxidant drugs. They also should be informed of the potential for febrile illnesses to trigger a hemolytic episode.

HEMOGLOBINS WITH INCREASED AND DECREASED OXYGEN AFFINITY

More than 150 hemoglobin variants have been discovered to have abnormal oxygen affinity.[4,102-104] Most are high-affinity variants and have been associated with familial erythrocytosis. The remaining hemoglobin variants are characterized by low oxygen affinity. Many of these are associated with mild to moderate anemia.[2]

As described in Chapter 10, normal Hb A undergoes a series of allosteric conformational changes as it converts from a fully deoxygenated to a fully oxygenated form. These conformational changes affect hemoglobin function and its affinity for oxygen. When normal hemoglobin is fully deoxygenated (tense state), it has low affinity for oxygen and other heme ligands and high affinity for allosteric effectors, such as Bohr protons and 2,3-bisphosphoglycerate. In the oxygenated (relaxed) state, hemoglobin has a high affinity for heme ligands, such as oxygen, and a low affinity for Bohr protons and 2,3-bisphosphoglycerate. The transition from the tense to the relaxed state involves a series of structural changes that have a marked effect on hemoglobin function. If an amino acid substitution lowers the stability of the tense structure, the transition to the relaxed state occurs at an earlier stage in ligand binding, and the hemoglobin has increased oxygen affinity and decreased heme-heme interaction or cooperativity (Chapter 10). One example of a β chain variant is Hb Kempsey. This unstable hemoglobin variant has amino acid substitutions at sites crucial to hemoglobin function.

Hemoglobins with Increased Oxygen Affinity

The high-affinity variants, like other structurally abnormal hemoglobins, show an autosomal dominant pattern of inheritance. Affected individuals have equal volumes of Hb A and the abnormal variant. Exceptions to this are compound heterozygotes for Hb Abruzzo and β-thalassemia and for Hb Crete and β-thalassemia, in which the proportion of abnormal hemoglobin is greater than 85%.

More than 90 variant hemoglobins with high oxygen affinity have been discovered. Such hemoglobins fail to release oxygen on demand, and hypoxia results. The kidneys sense the hypoxia and respond by increasing the release of erythropoietin, which leads to a compensatory erythrocytosis. These variants differ from unstable hemoglobin, which also may have abnormal oxygen affinity, in that they do not precipitate in vivo to produce hemolysis and there is no abnormal RBC morphology.

Most individuals are asymptomatic and show no physical symptoms except a ruddy complexion. Erythrocytosis is usually detected during routine examination because the patient generally has a high RBC count, hemoglobin, and hematocrit. The WBC count, platelet count, and peripheral blood film findings are generally normal. In some cases, hemoglobin electrophoresis may establish a diagnosis. An abnormal band that separates from the A band is present on cellulose acetate in some variants; however, if a band is not found, the diagnosis of increased oxygen affinity cannot be ruled out. In some cases the abnormal hemoglobin can be separated by using citrate agar (pH 6.0) or by gel electrophoresis. Measurement of oxygen affinity is required for definitive diagnosis.

Patients with high-oxygen-affinity hemoglobins live normal lives and require no treatment. Diagnosis should be made to avoid unnecessary treatment of the erythrocytosis as a myeloproliferative neoplasm or a secondary erythrocytosis.

Hemoglobins with Decreased Oxygen Affinity

Hemoglobins with decreased oxygen affinity quickly release oxygen to the tissues, which results in normal to decreased hemoglobin concentration and slight anemia. The best known of these hemoglobins is Hb Kansas, which has an amino acid substitution of asparagine by threonine at position 102 of the β chain. These hemoglobins may be present when cyanosis and a normal arterial oxygen tension coexist, and most may be detected by starch gel electrophoresis, HPLC, or DNA-based globin gene analysis.

GLOBAL BURDEN OF HEMOGLOBINOPATHIES

The prevalence of hemoglobinopathies has already been presented in this chapter, and the bulk of these conditions occurs in underdeveloped countries. However, as developing countries work to decrease deaths from malnutrition, infectious diseases, and other conditions, more patients with hemoglobinopathies will survive and remain consumers of the health care system. For example, in 1944 thalassemia was first identified in Cypress. However, during the post–World War II recovery period, as the death rate decreased, the prevalence of thalassemias increased.[2] In 1970 it was estimated that in the absence of systems to control the disease, within 40 years 78,000 units of blood would be needed each year, requiring that 40% of the population serve as donors.[2] If left unchecked, the cost to maintain thalassemia therapy would exceed the country's total health care budget. In contrast, efforts to de-

velop prenatal screening and genetic counseling programs have reduced the birth rate of SCD.[2] It is clear that hemoglobinopathies are a worldwide problem requiring planning, investment, and interventions from around the globe to optimize the impact on patients with the disease without debilitating the health care systems of developing countries where the disease is prevalent.

SUMMARY

- Hemoglobinopathies are genetic disorders of globin genes that produce structurally abnormal hemoglobins with altered amino acid sequences, which affect hemoglobin function and stability.
- Hb S is the most common hemoglobinopathy, resulting from a substitution of valine for glutamic acid at position 6 of the β globin chain, and primarily affects people of African descent.
- Hb S polymerizes in the RBCs because of abnormal interaction with adjacent tetramers when it is in the deoxygenated form, producing sickle-shaped RBCs.
- In homozygous Hb SS, the polymerization of hemoglobin may result in severe episodic conditions; however, factors other than hemoglobin polymerization may account for vasoocclusive episodes in sickle cell patients.
- The most clinically significant hemoglobinopathies are Hb SS, Hb SC, and Hb S–β-thalassemia; Hb SS causes the most severe disease.
- Individuals with sickle cell trait (Hb AS) are clinically asymptomatic.
- Sickle cell anemia (Hb SS) is a normocytic, normochromic anemia, characterized by a single band in the S position on hemoglobin electrophoresis, a single Hb S peak on HPLC, and a positive hemoglobin solubility test.
- The median life expectancy of patients with SCD has been extended to approximately 50 years.
- Hb C and Hb E are the next most common hemoglobinopathies after Hb S and cause mild hemolysis in the homozygous state. In

the heterozygous states, these hemoglobinopathies are asymptomatic.
- Hb C is found primarily in people of African descent.
- On peripheral blood films from patients with Hb CC, hexagonal crystals may be seen with and without apparent RBC membrane surrounding them.
- Hb EE results in a microcytic anemia and is found primarily in people of Southeast Asian descent.
- Other variants, such as unstable hemoglobins and hemoglobins with altered oxygen affinity, can be identified, and many cause no clinical abnormality.
- Laboratory procedures employed for diagnosis of hemoglobinopathies are the CBC, peripheral blood film evaluation, reticulocyte count, hemoglobin solubility test, and methods to quantitate normal hemoglobins and variants including hemoglobin electrophoresis (acid and alkaline pH), high-performance liquid chromatography, and capillary electrophoresis.
- Advanced techniques available for hemoglobin identification include isoelectric focusing and DNA-based analysis of the globin genes.

Now that you have completed this chapter, go back and read again the case study at the beginning and respond to the questions presented.

REVIEW QUESTIONS

Answers can be found in the Appendix.

1. A qualitative abnormality in hemoglobin may involve all of the following *except:*
   a. Replacement of one or more amino acids in a globin chain
   b. Addition of one or more amino acids in a globin chain
   c. Deletion of one or more amino acids in a globin chain
   d. Decreased production of a globin chain

2. The substitution of valine for glutamic acid at position 6 of the β chain of hemoglobin results in hemoglobin that:
   a. Is unstable and precipitates as Heinz bodies
   b. Polymerizes to form tactoid crystals
   c. Crystallizes in a hexagonal shape
   d. Contains iron in the ferric (Fe^{3+}) state

3. Patients with SCD usually do not exhibit symptoms until 6 months of age because:
   a. The mother's blood has a protective effect
   b. Hemoglobin levels are higher in infants at birth
   c. Higher levels of Hb F are present
   d. The immune system is not fully developed

4. Megaloblastic episodes in SCD can be prevented by prophylactic administration of:
   a. Iron
   b. Folic acid
   c. Steroids
   d. Erythropoietin

5. Which of the following is the most definitive test for Hb S?
   a. Hemoglobin solubility test
   b. Hemoglobin electrophoresis at alkaline pH
   c. Osmotic fragility test
   d. Hemoglobin electrophoresis at acid pH

6. A patient presents with mild normochromic, normocytic anemia. On the peripheral blood film, there are a few target cells, rare nucleated RBCs, and hexagonal crystals within and lying outside of the RBCs. Which abnormality in the hemoglobin molecule is most likely?
   a. Decreased production of β chains
   b. Substitution of lysine for glutamic acid at position 6 of the β chain
   c. Substitution of tyrosine for the proximal histidine in the β chain
   d. Double amino acid substitution in the β chain

7. A well-mixed specimen obtained for a CBC has a brown color. The patient is being treated with a sulfonamide for a bladder infection. Which of the following could explain the brown color?
   a. The patient has Hb M.
   b. The patient is a compound heterozygote for Hb S and thalassemia.
   c. The incorrect anticoagulant was used.
   d. Levels of Hb F are high.

8. Through routine screening, prospective parents discover that they are both heterozygous for Hb S. What percentage of their children potentially could have sickle cell anemia (Hb SS)?
   a. 0%
   b. 25%
   c. 50%
   d. 100%

9. Painful crises in patients with SCD occur as a result of:
   a. Splenic sequestration
   b. Aplasia
   c. Vasoocclusion
   d. Anemia

10. The screening test for Hb S that uses a reducing agent, such as sodium dithionite, is based on the fact that hemoglobins that sickle:
    a. Are insoluble in reduced, deoxygenated form
    b. Form methemoglobin more readily and cause a color change
    c. Are unstable and precipitate as Heinz bodies
    d. Oxidize quickly and cause turbidity

11. DNA analysis documents a patient has inherited the sickle mutation in both β-globin genes. The two terms that best describe this genotype are:
    a. Homozygous/trait
    b. Homozygous/disease
    c. Heterozygous/trait
    d. Heterozygous/disease

12. In which of the following geographic areas is Hb S most prevalent?
    a. India
    b. South Africa
    c. United States
    d. Sub-Saharan Africa

13. Which hemoglobinopathy is more common in Southeast Asian patients?
    a. Hb S
    b. Hb C
    c. Hb O
    d. Hb E

14. Which of the following Hb S compound heterozygote exhibits the mildest symptoms?
    a. Hb S-β-Thal
    b. Hb SG
    c. Hb S-C-Harlem
    d. Hb SC

15. A 1-year-old Indian patient presents with anemia, and both parents claim to have an "inherited anemia" but can't remember the type. The peripheral blood shows target cells, and the hemoglobin solubility is negative. Alkaline hemoglobin electrophoresis shows a single band at the "Hb C" position and a small band at the "Hb F" position. Acid hemoglobin electrophoresis shows two bands. The most likely diagnosis is:
    a. Hb CC
    b. Hb AC
    c. Hb CO
    d. Hb SC

16. Unstable hemoglobins show all of the following findings EXCEPT:
    a. Globin chains precipitate intracellularly
    b. Heinz body formation
    c. Elevated reticulocyte count
    d. Only homozygotes are symptomatic

REFERENCES

1. Wajeman, H., & Moradkhani, K. (2011). Abnormal hemoglobins: detection and characterization. *Indian J Med Res, 134,* 538–546.
2. Weatherall, D. J. (2010). The inherited diseases of hemoglobin are an emerging global health burden. *Blood, 115*(22), 4331–4336.
3. Bauer, D. E., & Orkin, S. H. (2011). Update on fetal hemoglobin gene regulation in hemoglobinopathies. *Curr Opin Pediatr, 23,* 1–8.
4. Wang, W. C. (2009). Sickle cell anemia and other sickling syndromes. In Greer, J. P., Foerster, J., Rodgers, G. M., et al., (Eds.), *Wintrobe's Clinical Hematology.* (Vol. 1, 12th ed., pp. 1038–1082). Philadelphia: Wolters Kluwer Health/Lippincott Williams & Wilkins.
5. Patrinos, G. P., Giardine, B., Riemer, C., et al. (2004). Improvements in the HbVar database of human hemoglobin variants and thalassemia mutations for population and sequence variation studies. *Nucl Acids Res, 32*(database issue), D537–541. Retrieved from http://globin.cse.psu.edu/hbvar/menu.html. Accessed 29.11.13.
6. Fishleder, A. J., & Hoffman, G. C. (1987). A practical approach to the detection of hemoglobinopathies. Part II: the sickle cell disorders. *Lab Med, 18,* 441–443.
7. Konotey-Ahulu, F. I. (1974). The sickle cell diseases. Clinical manifestations including the "sickle crisis." *Arch Intern Med, 133,* 611–619.
8. Beutler, E. (2010). Disorders of hemoglobin structure: sickle cell anemia and related abnormalities. In Kaushansky, K., Lichtman, M. A., Beutler, E., Kipps, T. J., Seligsohn, U., Pechal, J. T., (Eds.), *Williams Hematology.* (8th ed., pp. 709–742). New York: McGraw-Hill.
9. Serjeant, G. R. (2001). Historical review: the emerging understanding of sickle cell disease. *Br J Haematol, 112,* 3–18.
10. Park, K. W. (2004). Sickle cell disease and other hemoglobinopathies. *Int Anesth Clin, 42,* 77–93.
11. Rees, D. C., Williams, T. N., & Gladwn, M. T. (2010). Sickle-cell disease. *Lancet, 376,* 2018–2031.
12. Piel, F. B., Patil, A. B., Howes, R. E., et al. (2013). Global epidemiology of sickle haemoglobin in neonates: a contemporary geostatistical model-based map and population estimates. *Lancet, 381,* 142–151.
13. Smith, J. A., Kinney, T. R., & Sickle Cell Disease Guideline Panel. (1994). Sickle cell disease: guideline and overview. *Am J Hematol, 47,* 152–154.
14. Shah, A. (2004). Hemoglobinopathies and other congenital hemolytic anemia. *Ind J Med Sci, 58,* 490–493.
15. Wishner, B. C., Ward, K. B., Lattman, E. E., et al. (1975). Crystal structure of sickle-cell deoxyhemoglobin at 5 A resolution. *J Mol Biol, 98,* 179–194.
16. Dykes, G., Crepeau, R. H., & Edeltein, S. J. (1978). Three-dimensional reconstruction of the fibers of sickle cell haemoglobin. *Nature, 272,* 506–510.
17. Dykes, G. W., Crepeau, R. H., & Edelstein, S. J. (1979). Three-dimensional reconstruction of the 14-filament fiber of hemoglobin S. *J Mol Biol, 130,* 451–472.
18. Crepeau, R. H., Edelstein, S. J., Szalay, M., et al. (1981). Sickle cell hemoglobin fiber structure altered by alpha-chain mutation. *Proc Natl Acad Sci U S A, 78,* 1406–1410.
19. Gibbs, N. M., & Larach, D. R. (2013). Anesthetic management during cardiopulmonary bypass. In Hensley, F. A., Gravlee, G. P., & Martin, D. E., (Eds.), *A Practical Approach to Cardiac Anesthesia.* (5th ed., pp. 214–237). Philadelphia: Lippincott, Williams & Wilkins.
20. Kawthalkar, S. M. (2013). Anemias due to excessive red cell destruction. In Kawthalkar, S. M. *Essentials of Hematology.* (2nd ed., pp. 171–184). New Delhi: Jaypee Brothers Medical Publishers.
21. de Jong, K., Larkin, S. K., Styles, L. A., et al. (2001). Characterization of the phosphatidylserine-exposing subpopulation of sickle cells. *Blood, 98,* 860–867.
22. Yasin, Z., Witting, S., & Palascak, M. B. (2003). Phosphatidylserine externalization in sickle red blood cell: associations with cell age, density, and hemoglobin F. *Blood, 102,* 365–370.
23. de Jong, K., Rettig, M. P., Low, P. S., et al. (2002). Protein kinase C activation induces phosphatidylserine exposure on red blood cells. *Biochemistry, 41,* 12562–12567.
24. de Jong, K., & Kuypers, F. A. (2006). Sulfhydral modifications alter scamblase activity in murine sickle cell disease. *Br J Haematol, 133,* 427–432.
25. Manodori, A. B., Barabino, G. A., Lubin, B. H., et al. (2000). Adherence of phosphatidylserine-exposing erythrocytes to endothelial matrix thrombomodulin. *Blood, 95,* 1293–1300.
26. Stuart, M. L., & Setty, B. N. (2001). Hemostatic alterations in sickle cell disease: relationships to disease pathophysiology. *Pediatr Pathol Mol Med, 20,* 27–46.
27. Setty, B. N., Kulkarni, S., & Stuart, M. J. (2002). Role of erythrocyte phosphatidylserine in sickle red cell-endothelial adhesion. *Blood, 99,* 1564–1571.
28. Kuypers, F. A., & Styles, L. A. (2004). The role of secretory phospholipase A2 in acute chest syndrome. *Cell Mol Biol, 50,* 87–94.
29. Neidlinger, N. A., Larkin, S. K., Bhagat, A., et al. (2006). Hydrolysis of phosphatidylserine-exposing red blood cells by secretory phospholipase A2 generates lysophosphatidic acid and results in vascular dysfunction. *J Biol Chem, 281,* 775–781.
30. Benkerrou, M., Alberti, C., Couque, N., et al. (2013). Impact of glucose-6-phosphate dehydrogenase deficiency on sickle cell expression in infancy and early childhood: a prospective study. *Br J Haematol, 163,* 646–654.
31. Noguchi, C. T., Rodgers, G. P., Sergeant, G., et al. (1988). Level of fetal hemoglobin necessary for treatment of sickle cell disease. *N Engl J Med, 318,* 96–99.
32. Diggs, L. W. (1965). Sickle cell crises. *J Clin Pathol, 44,* 1–19.
33. Bartolucci, P., & Galacteros, F. (2012). Clinical management of adult sickle cell disease. *Curr Opin Hematol, 19,* 149–155.
34. Embury, S. H., Hebbel, R. P., Steinberg, M. H., et al. (1994). Pathogenesis of vasoocclusion. In Embury, S. H., Hebbel, R. P., Mohandas, N., et al., (Eds.), *Sickle Cell Disease: Basic Principles and Clinical Practice.* (pp. 311–323). Philadelphia: Lippincott Williams & Wilkins.
35. Jandl, J. H. (1996). *Blood: Textbook of Hematology.* (2nd ed., pp. 531–577). Boston: Little, Brown.
36. Hebbel, R. P., Yamada, O., Moldow, C. F., et al. (1980). Abnormal adherence of sickle erythrocytes to cultured vascular endothelium: possible mechanism to microvascular occlusion in sickle cell disease. *J Clin Invest, 65,* 154–160.
37. Bunn, H. F. (1997). Pathogenesis and treatment of sickle cell disease. *N Engl J Med, 337,* 762–769.
38. Hagar, W., & Vichinsky, E. (2008). Advances in clinical research in sickle cell disease. *Br J Haematol, 141,* 346–356.
39. Styles, L. A., Schalkwijk, C. G., Aarsman, A. J., et al. (1996). Phospholipase A2 levels in acute chest syndrome of sickle cell disease. *Blood, 87,* 2573–2578.
40. Styles, L. A., Aareman, A. J., Vichinski, E. P., et al. (2000). Secretory phospholipase A2 predicts impending acute chest syndrome in sickle cell disease. *Blood, 96,* 3276–3278.
41. Morris, C. R., Kuypers, F. A., Larkin, S., et al. (2000). Patterns of arginine and nitrous oxide in patients with sickle cell disease with vaso-occlusive crisis and acute chest syndrome. *J Pediatr Haematol Oncol, 22,* 515–520.
42. Morris, C. R., Kato, G. J., Poljakovic, M., et al. (2005). Dysregulated arginine metabolism, hemolysis-associated pulmonary hypertension, and mortality in sickle cell disease. *JAMA, 294,* 81–90.

43. Hsu, L. L., Champion, H. C., Campbell-Lee, S. C., et al. (2007). Hemolysis in sickle cell mice causes pulmonary hypertension due to global impairment in nitric oxide bioavailability. *Blood, 109,* 3088–3098.

44. Onyekwere, O. C., Campbell, A., Teshome, M., et al. (2008). Pulmonary hypertension in children and adolescence with sickle cell disease. *Pediat Cardiol, 29*(2), 309–312.

45. Wright, J., & Ahmedzai, S. H. (2010). The management of painful crisis in sickle cell disease. *Curr Opin Support Palliat Care, 4,* 97–106.

46. Day, T. G., Drasar, E. R., Fulford, T., et al. (2011). Association between hemolysis and albuminuria in adults with sickle cell anemia. *Haematologica, 97,* 201–205.

47. Kelleher, J. F., Luban, N. L. C., Cohen, B. J., et al. (1984). Human serum parvovirus as a cause of aplastic crisis in sickle cell disease. *Am J Dis Child, 138,* 401–403.

48. Wethers, D. L. (2000). Sickle cell disease in childhood: Part I. Laboratory diagnosis, pathophysiology and health maintenance. *Am Fam Physician, 62,* 1013–1020.

49. Agular, C., Vichinsky, E., & Neumayr, L. (2005). Bone and joint disease in sickle cell disease. *Hematol Oncol Clin North Am, 19,* 929–941, viii.

50. Bunn, H. F. (2013). The triumph of good over evil: protection by the sickle gene against malaria. *Blood, 121,* 20–25.

51. Beutler, E., Johnson, C., Powars, D., et al. (1974). Prevalence of glucose-6-phosphate dehydrogenase deficiency in sickle cell disease. *N Engl J Med, 290,* 826–828.

52. Steinberg, M. H., West, M. S., Gallagher, D., et al. (1988). Effects of glucose-6 phosphate dehydrogenase deficiency upon sickle cell anemia. *Blood, 71,* 748–752.

53. Welsh, S. (2009). Hemoglobinopathies and thalassemias. The ABCs of Lab Evaluation. *Clin Lab News, 35*(10). Retrieved from http://www.aacc.org/publications/cln/2009/october/Pages/Series1009.aspx#. Accessed 05.05.10.

54. Clarke, G. M., & Higgins, T. N. (2000). Laboratory investigation of hemoglobinopathies and thalassemias: review and update. *Clin Chem, 46,* 1284–1290.

55. Bargoma, E. M., Mitsuyashi, J. K., Larkin, S. K., et al. (2005). Serum C-reactive protein parallels secretory phospholipase A2 in sickle cell disease patients with vaso-occlusive crisis or acute chest syndrome. *Blood, 105,* 3384–3385.

56. Célérier, E., González, J. R., Maldonado, R., et al. (2006). Opioid-induced hyperalgesia in a murine model of postoperative pain: role of nitric oxide generated from the inducible nitric oxide synthase. *Anesthesiology, 104,* 546–555.

57. Walters, P. B., Fung, E. B., Killilea, D. W., et al. (2006). Oxidative stress and inflammation in iron-overloaded patients with beta-thalassemia or sickle cell disease. *Br J Haematol, 135,* 254–263.

58. National Institutes of Health, National Heart, Lung, and Blood Institute Division of Blood Diseases and Resources. (2002, June). *The Management of Sickle Cell Disease.* (4th ed., p. 75). NIH Publication 02–2117. Retrieved from http://www.nhlbi.nih.gov/health/prof/blood/sickle/sc_mngt.pdf.

59. Preboth, M. (2000). Management of pain in sickle cell disease. *Am Fam Physician, 61,* 1–7.

60. Bunn, H. F., & Forget, B. G. (1986). Sickle cell disease—clinical and epidemiological aspects. In Bunn, H. F., & Forget, B. G., (Eds.), *Hemoglobin: Molecular, Genetic and Clinical Aspects* (pp. 503–510). Philadelphia: Saunders.

61. Fung, E. B., Harmatz, P. R., Lee, P. D., et al. (2006). Increased prevalence of iron-overload associated endocrinopathy in thalassemia verses sickle cell disease. *Br J Haematol, 135,* 574–582.

62. Fung, E. B., Harmatz, P. R., Milet, M., et al. (2007). Morbidity and mortality in chronically transfused subjects with thalassemia and sickle cell disease. *Am J Hematol, 82,* 255–265.

63. Vichinsky, E., Onyekwere, O., Porter, J., et al. (2007). A randomized comparison of deferasirox verses deferoxamine for the treatment of transfusional iron overload in sickle cell disease. *Br J Haematol, 136,* 501–508.

64. Walters, M. C., Patience, M., Leisenring, M., et al. (1996). Barriers to bone marrow transplant for sickle cell anemia. *Biol Bone Marrow Transplant, 2,* 100–104.

65. Bernaudin, F., Socie, G., Kuentz, M., et al. (2007). Long-term results of related, myeloablative stem cell transplantation to cure sickle cell disease. *Blood, 110,* 2749–2756.

66. Panepinto, J. A., Walters, M. C., Carreras, J., et al. (2007). Matched-related donor transplantation for sickle cell disease: report from the Center for International Blood and Transplant Research. *Br J Haematol, 137,* 479–485.

67. Vermylen, C., Cornu, G., Ferster, Y., et al. (1998). Haermatopoietic stem cell transplantation for sickle cell anaemia: the first 50 inpatients transplanted in Belgium. *Bone Marrow Transplant, 22,* 1–6.

68. Walters, M. C., Storb, R., Patience, M., et al. (2000). Impact of bone marrow transplantation for symptomatic sickle cell disease: an interim report. Multicenter investigation of bone marrow transplantation for sickle cell disease. *Blood, 95,* 1918–1924.

69. Walters, M. C., Patience, M., Leisenring, M., et al. (1997). Collaborative multicenter investigation of marrow transplantation for sickle cell disease: current results and future directions. *Biol Bone Marrow Transplant, 3,* 310–315.

70. Martin, H. S. (1996). Review: sickle cell disease: present and future treatment. *Am J Med Sci, 312,* 166–174.

71. Pinto, F. O., & Roberts, I. (2008). Cord blood stem cell transplantation for haemoglobinopathies. *Br J Haematol, 141,* 309–324.

72. Surbek, D., Schoeberlein, A., Wagner, A. (2008). Perinatal stem cell and gene therapy for hemoglobinopathies. *Semin Fetal Neonatal Med, 13,* 282–290.

73. Reid, C. D., Charache, S., Lubin, B., et al. (1995). *Management and Therapy of Sickle Cell Disease.* (3rd ed.). Pub No 95–2117. Bethesda, Md: National Heart, Lung and Blood Institute.

74. Paule, I., Sassi, H., Habibi, A., et al. (2011). Population pharmacokinetics and pharmacodynamics of hydroxyurea in sickle cell anemia patients, a basis for optimizing the dosing regimen. *Orphanet J Rare Dis, 6,* 30.

75. Steinberg, M. H., Lu, Z. H., Barton, F. B., et al. (1997). Fetal hemoglobin in sickle cell anemia: determinants of response to hydroxyurea. Multicenter study of hydroxyurea. *Blood, 89,* 1078–1088.

76. Lionnet, F., Arlet, J-B., Bartolucci, P., et al. (2009). Guidelines for management of adult sickle cell disease. *Rev Méd Interne, 30*(Suppl. 3), S162–S223.

77. Rees, D. C., Olujohungbe, A. D., Parker, N. E., et al. (2003). Guidelines for the management of the acute painful crisis in sickle cell disease. *Br J Haematol, 120,* 744–752.

78. Nagalla, S., & Ballas S. K. (2012) Drugs for preventing red blood cell dehydration in people with sickle cell disease. *Cochrane Database Syst Rev, 7,* CD003426. doi: 10.1002/14651858.CD003426.pub4.

79. Uzun, B., Kekec, Z., & Gurkan, E. (2010). Efficacy of tramadol vs meperidine in vasoocclusive sickle cell crisis. *Am J Emerg Med, 28,* 445–449.

80. Bartolucci, P., El Murr, T., Roudot-Thoraval, F., et al. (2009). A randomized, controlled clinical trial of ketoprofen for sickle-cell disease vaso-occlusive crises in adults. *Blood, 114,* 3742–3747.

81. Claster, S., & Vichinsky, E. (2003). Managing sickle cell disease. *BMJ, 327,* 1151–1155.

82. Steinberg, M. H., Ballas, S. K., Brunson, C. Y., et al. (1995). Sickle cell anemia in septuagenarians. *Blood, 86,* 3997–3998.

83. Michlitsch, J., Azimi, M., Hoppe, C., et al. (2009). Newborn screening for hemoglobinopathies in California. *Pediatr Blood Cancer, 52,* 486–490.

84. Schlitt, L. E., & Keital, H. G. (1960). Renal manifestations of sickle cell disease: a review. *Am J Med Sci, 239,* 773–778.

85. Kark, J. A. & Ward, F. T. (1994). Exercise and hemoglobin S. *Seminars in Hematology 31*(3), 181–225.

86. Diggs, L. W., & Bell, A. (1965). Intraerythrocytic hemoglobin crystals in sickle cell hemoglobin C disease. *Blood, 25,* 218–223.

87. Bell, A. (1974). *Homozygous C Disease, Hematology Tech Sample H-71.* Chicago: American Society of Clinical Pathologists.

88. Steinberg, M. H. (2009). Other sickle hemoglobinopathies. In Steinberg, M. H., Forget, B. G., Higgs, D. R., et al., (Eds.), *Disorders of Hemoglobin: Genetics, Pathophysiology and Clinical Management.* (2nd ed., pp. 564–588). Cambridge: Cambridge University Press.

89. Fairbanks, V. F., Gilchrist, G. S., Brimhall, B., et al. (1979). Hemoglobin E trait reexamined: a cause of microcytosis and erythrocytosis. *Blood, 53,* 109–115.

90. Anderson, H. M., & Ranney, H. M. (1990). Southeast Asian immigrants: the new thalassemias in America. *Semin Hematol, 27,* 239–246.

91. Vichinsky, E. (2007). Hemoglobin E syndromes. *Hematology Am Soc Hematol Educ Program, 2007,* 79–83.

92. Safko, R. (1990). Anemia of abnormal globin development—hemoglobinopathies. In Stiene-Martin, E. A., Lotspeich-Steininger, C., & Koepke, J. A., (Eds.), *Clinical Hematology: Principles, Procedures, Correlations.* (2nd ed., pp. 192–216). Philadelphia: Lippincott–Raven Publishers.

93. Randolph, T. R. (2008). Pathophysiology of compound heterozygotes involving hemoglobinopathies and thalassemias. *Clin Lab Sci, 21*(4), 240–248.

94. Hoffman, G. C. (1990). The sickling disorders. *Lab Med, 21,* 797–807.

95. Moewe, C. (1993). Hemoglobin SC: a brief review. *Clin Lab Sci, 6,* 158–159.

96. Nagel, R. L., & Lawrence, C. (1991). The distinct pathobiology of sickle cell-hemoglobin C disease: therapeutic implications. *Hematol Oncol Clin North Am, 5,* 433–451.

97. Lawrence, C., Fabry, M. E., & Nagel, R. L. (1991). The unique red cell heterogeneity of SC disease: crystal formation, dense reticulocytes and unusual morphology. *Blood, 78,* 2104–2112, 1991.

98. Platt, O. S., Thorington, B. D., Brambilla, D. J., et al. (1991). Pain in sickle cell disease: rates and risk factors. *N Engl J Med, 325,* 11–16.

99. Steinberg, M. H. (1996). Review: sickle cell disease: present and future treatment. *Am J Med Sci, 312,* 166–174.

100. Monplaisir, N., Merault, G., Poyart, C., et al. (1986). Hemoglobin S Antilles: a variant with lower solubility than hemoglobin S and producing sickle cell disease in heterozygotes. *Proc Natl Acad Sci U S A, 83,* 9363–9367.

101. Nagel, R. L., Daar, S., Romero, J. R., et al. (1998). HbS-Oman heterozygote: a new dominant sickle cell syndrome. *Blood, 92,* 4375–4782.

102. Steinberg, M. (2009). Hemoglobins with altered oxygen affinity, unstable hemoglobins, M-hemoglobins, and dyshemoglobinemias. In Greer, J. P., Foerster, J., Rodgers, G. M., et al., (Eds.), *Wintrobe's Clinical Hematology.* (12th ed., pp. 1132–1142). Philadelphia; Wolters Kluwer Health/Lippincott Williams & Wilkins.

103. Williamson, D. (1993). The unstable haemoglobins. *Blood Rev, 7,* 146–163.

104. Bunn, H. F. (1986). Hemoglobinopathy due to abnormal oxygen binding. In Bunn, H. F., Forget, B. G., (Eds.), *Hemoglobin: Molecular, Genetic and Clinical Aspects,* (pp. 595–616). Philadelphia: Saunders.

28

Thalassemias

*Elaine M. Keohane**

OBJECTIVES

After completion of this chapter, the reader will be able to:

1. Describe the hemoglobin defect found in thalassemias.
2. Discuss the geographic distribution of thalassemia and its association with malaria.
3. Name the chromosomes that contain the α-globin gene and the β-globin gene clusters and the globin chains produced by each.
4. Describe the type of genetic mutations that result in α- and β-thalassemias.
5. Explain the pathophysiologic effects caused by the imbalance of globin chain synthesis in α-and β-thalassemias.
6. Describe the four major clinical syndromes of β-thalassemia and the clinical expression of each heterozygous and homozygous form.
7. Recognize the pattern of laboratory findings in heterozygous and homozygous β-thalassemias, including hereditary persistence of fetal hemoglobin (HPFH).
8. Describe the treatment of homozygous β-thalassemias, the risks involved, and the reason it is necessary to monitor iron levels.
9. Correlate the clinical syndromes of α-thalassemia with the number of α genes present.
10. Recognize the laboratory findings associated with various α-thalassemia syndromes.
11. Describe the clinical syndromes of thalassemia associated with common structural hemoglobin variants.
12. Specify tests that are used for screening for β-thalassemia carriers.
13. Discuss the role of the complete blood count, peripheral blood film review, supravital stain, hemoglobin fraction quantification (using hemoglobin electrophoresis, high-performance liquid chromatography, and/or capillary zone electrophoresis), and molecular genetic testing in diagnosis of thalassemia syndromes.
14. Differentiate β-thalassemia minor from iron deficiency anemia.

CASE STUDY

After studying the material in this chapter, the reader should be able to respond to the following case study:

A 24-year-old male medical student in the United States was found to have a hemoglobin level of 10.2 g/dL in a hematology laboratory class. During discussion of the family history with this student, a hematologist at the university discovered that his mother had always been anemic, had periodically been given iron therapy, and had a history of several acute episodes of gallbladder disease (attacks). Both of the student's parents had been born in Sicily. A cousin on his mother's side had two children who died of thalassemia major at the ages of 4 and 5 years and had a third young daughter with thalassemia major who was being treated with regular blood transfusions. The student's laboratory test results were as follows:

Continued

* The author extends appreciation to Martha Payne, who provided the foundation of this chapter, and Rakesh P. Mehta, who authored this chapter in previous editions.

CASE STUDY—cont'd

	Patient Results	Reference Interval
RBC ($\times 10^{12}$/L)	5.74	4.60–6.00
HGB (g/dL)	10.2	14.0–18.0
HCT (%)	35	40–54
MCV (fL)	61.0	80–100
MCH (pg)	17.8	26–32
MCHC (g/dL)	29.1	32–36

Peripheral blood RBCs exhibited moderate microcytosis, slight hypochromia, and slight poikilocytosis with occasional target cells, and several RBCs had basophilic stippling. Hb A_2 was 4.9% of total hemoglobin by high-performance liquid chromatography (reference interval, 0% to 3.5%). Serum ferritin level was 320 ng/mL (reference interval, 15 to 400 ng/mL).

1. Why was the family history so important in this case, and what diagnosis did it suggest?

2. What laboratory values helped confirm the diagnosis?
3. From what other disorders should this anemia be differentiated? What laboratory tests would be helpful? Why is differentiation important?
4. If this individual was planning to have children, what genetic counseling should be done?

DEFINITIONS AND HISTORY

The thalassemias are a diverse group of inherited disorders caused by genetic mutations that reduce or prevent the synthesis of one or more of the globin chains of the hemoglobin (Hb) tetramer. In 1925, Cooley and Lee first described four children with anemia, splenomegaly, mild hepatomegaly, and mongoloid facies.[1] These characteristics would later become typical findings in young children with untreated β-thalassemia major, often referred to as *Cooley's anemia*. Seven years later, Whipple and Bradford published a paper outlining the detailed autopsy studies of children who died of this disorder.[2] Because of the high incidence of patients of Mediterranean descent with this disorder, Whipple called the disease *Thalassic* (Greek for "great sea") anemia, which was subsequently changed to *thalassemia*.[2] Several investigators in the 1940s demonstrated the genetic basis for this anemia and were able to show that in patients who were homozygous for this condition (thalassemia major), the disease had a severe course. The heterozygotes, however, not only were carriers but also had a milder anemia (thalassemia minor). In the 1950s, thalassemias resulting from defects in the α-globin chain were described.[2]

Thalassemia results from a reduced or absent synthesis of one or more of the globin chains of hemoglobin. A wide variety of mutations in hemoglobin genes lead to clinical outcomes that are extremely wide ranging, with certain mutations causing no anemia and others leading to death in utero, childhood, or early adulthood. Thalassemias are named according to the chain with reduced or absent synthesis. Mutations affecting the α- or β-globin gene are most clinically significant because Hb A ($\alpha_2\beta_2$) is the major adult hemoglobin. The decreased or absent synthesis of one of the

chains not only leads to a decreased production of hemoglobin but results in an imbalance in the α/β chain ratio.[3] The unaffected gene continues to produce globin chains at normal levels, and the accumulation of the unpaired normal chains damages the red blood cells (RBCs) or their precursors resulting in their premature destruction. This exacerbates the anemia and makes some forms of thalassemia particularly severe.

EPIDEMIOLOGY

The morbidity and mortality due to thalassemia significantly contributes to the global health burden. Approximately 5% of the world's population is a carrier of a clinically significant mutation for a hemoglobinopathy or thalassemia.[4] Annually an estimated 56,000 infants are born with a form of thalassemia major.[4,5] Although thalassemia occurs in all parts of the world, its distribution is concentrated in the "thalassemia belt" that extends from the Mediterranean east through the Middle East and India to Southeast Asia and south to Northern Africa (Figure 27-3).[6] The carrier frequency of β-thalassemia depends on the region, with Sardinia, Cyprus, and Greece having the highest frequency in Europe (6% to 19%) and India, Thailand, and Indonesia having the highest frequency in Asia and Southeast Asia (0.3% to 15%).[6] The carrier frequency of α-thalassemia varies considerably. In Europe, Cyprus has the highest carrier frequency at 14%.[6] The carrier frequency reaches 50% to 60% in Eastern Saudi Arabia and parts of Asia and Africa, and may be as high as 75% to 80% in certain groups in Nepal, India, Thailand, and Papua New Guinea.[6]

The geographic location of the thalassemia belt coincides with areas in which malaria is prevalent (Figure 27-3). Thalassemia minor (heterozygous thalassemia) appears to impart resistance to malaria. This allowed the selective advantage that established thalassemia in high frequency in areas in which malaria is endemic.[7,8] Several case-control studies evaluated the incidence of thalassemia in patients with severe malaria compared with a control population and consistently found a lower incidence of thalassemia in the population with malaria than in the population without malaria. One study demonstrated that the risk of death from malaria was 40% lower in patients with $\alpha\alpha/-\alpha$ thalassemia and more than 60% lower in those with $-\alpha/-\alpha$ thalassemia.[8] The mechanism of this resistance is still not fully elucidated; however, two major theories have been put forward: defective growth of the parasite in the affected cell and increased phagocytosis of the infected cell.[9,10] Although the exact mechanism is not known, the geographic distribution and the case-control studies corroborate the protective nature of the thalassemias in promoting resistance to malaria.

GENETICS OF GLOBIN SYNTHESIS

The normal hemoglobin molecule is a tetramer of two α-like chains (α or ζ) with two β-like chains (β, γ, δ, or ϵ). Combinations of these chains produce six normal hemoglobins. Three are embryonic hemoglobins: Hb Gower-1 ($\zeta_2\epsilon_2$), Hb Gower-2 ($\alpha_2\epsilon_2$), and Hb Portland ($\zeta_2\gamma_2$). The others are fetal hemoglobin (Hb F, $\alpha_2\gamma_2$) and two adult hemoglobins (Hb A, $\alpha_2\beta_2$, and Hb A$_2$, $\alpha_2\delta_2$). The α-like globin gene cluster is located on chromosome 16, whereas the β-like globin gene cluster is on chromosome 11. The α-like globin gene cluster contains three functional genes: *HBZ* (ζ-globin), *HBA1* (α_1-globin), and *HBA2* (α_2-globin).[11,12] The β-like globin gene cluster contains five functional genes: *HBE* (ϵ-globin), *HBG2* ($^G\gamma$-globin), *HBG1* ($^A\gamma$-globin), *HBD* (δ-globin), and *HBB* (β-globin).[3,11,12] These genes are positioned in the order that corresponds with their developmental stage of expression.[11] During the first 2 months of gestation, the genes for the embryonic ζ and ϵ chains are expressed, generating Hb Gower-1 ($\zeta_2\epsilon_2$). Expression of the genes for the α and γ chains begins in the second month of gestation, generating two additional embryonic hemoglobins: Hb Gower-2 ($\alpha_2\epsilon_2$) and Hb Portland ($\zeta_2\gamma_2$). By 10 weeks gestation, the genes for the embryonic ζ and ϵ chains are switched off and silenced, while the genes for α and γ chains are upregulated (called the ζ to α switch on chromosome 16, and the ϵ to γ switch on chromosome 11).[11] The γ chains combine with the α chains to make Hb F ($\alpha_2\gamma_2$), the predominant hemoglobin of fetal life. The gene for the β chain is initially activated during the second month of gestation, but β chain production occurs at low levels throughout most of fetal life.[13] Shortly before birth, however, the expression of the γ-globin gene is downregulated, while expression of the β-globin gene is upregulated (called the γ to β switch), so by 6 months of age and through adult life, Hb A ($\alpha_2\beta_2$) is the predominant hemoglobin. The gene for the δ chain is activated shortly before birth, but owing to its weak promoter, only produces a relatively small amount of δ chain, resulting in a low level of Hb A$_2$ ($\alpha_2\delta_2$) (Chapter 10 and Figure 10-6).[3,11] Table 28-1 contains the reference intervals for the normal hemoglobins in adults.

TABLE 28-1 Reference Intervals for Normal Hemoglobins in Adults

Hb A ($\alpha_2\beta_2$)	95%–100%
Hb A$_2$ ($\alpha_2\delta_2$)	0%–3.5%
Hb F ($\alpha_2\gamma_2$)	0%–2%

The γ-globin genes code for two globin chains ($^G\gamma$ and $^A\gamma$) that differ at position 136 by a single amino acid (glycine and alanine, respectively).[13] Both of these globin chains are found in Hb F, with no functional difference identified between them. Similarly, the α-globin gene loci are duplicated on each chromosome 16 and also code for two globin chains (α_1 and α_2). Either of these genes can contribute to the two α-globin chains in the hemoglobin tetramer, and no functional difference has been identified between the two. Interspersed between the functional genes on these chromosomes are four functionless gene-like loci or pseudogenes that are designated by the prefixed symbol ψ. The purpose of these pseudogenes is unknown.[13] The organization of these genes on chromosomes 16 and 11 is shown in Figure 28-1.

An individual inherits one cluster of the five functional genes on chromosome 11 from each parent. The genotype for normal β chain synthesis is designated β/β. Because two α-globin genes (α_1 and α_2) are inherited on each chromosome 16, a normal genotype is designated $\alpha\alpha/\alpha\alpha$.

CATEGORIES OF THALASSEMIA

The thalassemias are divided into β-thalassemias, which include all the disorders of reduced globin chain production arising from the β-globin gene cluster on chromosome 11, and α-thalassemias, which involve the genes for the α_1 and α_2 chains on chromosome 16. Various deletional and nondeletional mutations can cause each of these disorders, and individuals with similar clinical manifestations are often heterogeneous at the genetic level.[3,11,13]

The β-thalassemias affect mainly the β chain production but also may involve the δ, $^G\gamma$, $^A\gamma$, and ϵ chains. In the β-thalassemias, β^0 is the designation for the various mutations in the β-globin gene in which no β chains are produced. In the homozygous state (β^0/β^0), an individual does not produce Hb A ($\alpha_2\beta_2$). β^+ is the designation for the various mutations in the β-globin gene that result in a partial deficiency of β chains (5% to 30% of normal) and a decrease in production of Hb A.[3] Some mutations in the β-globin gene lead to minimal reductions in β chain production and are associated with mild or silent clinical states. The designation β^{silent} for silent carrier has been used for those mutations. The designation $\delta\beta^0$ is used for mutations in the δ- or β-globin genes in which no δ or β chains are produced. In the homozygous state ($\delta\beta^0/\delta\beta^0$), no Hb A ($\alpha_2\beta_2$) or Hb A$_2$ ($\alpha_2\delta_2$) are produced. The designation $\delta\beta^{Lepore}$ indicates a fusion of the δ- and β-globin genes that produces Hb Lepore.

The most common mutations in α-thalassemia are deletions involving the α_1- and/or α_2-globin genes.[11,12] The designation

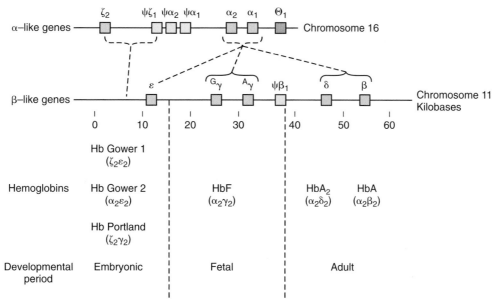

Figure 28-1 Chromosome organization of globin genes and their expression during development. The *light blue boxes* indicate functional globin genes; the *tan boxes* indicate pseudogenes. The scale of the depicted chromosomal segments is in kilobases of DNA. The switch from embryonic to fetal hemoglobin (Hb) occurs by 10 weeks of gestation, and the switch from fetal to adult hemoglobin occurs in the third trimester. (From Cunningham MJ, Sankaran VG, Nathan DG, et al: Chapter 20. The Thalassemias. In: Orkin SH, Nathan DG, Ginsberg D, et al (eds). Nathan and Oski 's hematology of infancy and childhood, ed 7, 2009, Saunders, an imprint of Elsevier, page 1017.)

α^+ is used to indicate a deletion of *either* the α_1- or the α_2-globin gene on chromosome 16 (also called the – α haplotype). This results in a decreased production of α chains from that chromosome. The designation α^0 is used to indicate a deletion of *both* the α_1- and α_2-globin genes on chromosome 16 (also called the – – *haplotype*). This results in no production of α chains from that chromosome.[3,11,13] Non-deletional mutations in the α-globin gene can also result in α-thalassemia, but these are less common.[12] The designation α^T is used for these mutations.[13] The major gene designations in thalassemia are summarized in Table 28-2.

GENETIC DEFECTS CAUSING THALASSEMIA

Types of genetic defects that cause a decrease or absent production of a particular globin chain include single nucleotide (or point) mutations, small insertions or deletions, or large deletions.[12,13] The mechanisms[3,11,13] by which these mutations interfere with globin chain production include:

- *Reduced or absent transcription of messenger ribonucleic acid (mRNA)* due to mutations in the promoter region or initiation codon of a globin gene, as well as mutations in polyadenylation sites that decrease mRNA stability
- *mRNA processing errors* due to mutations that add or remove splice sites resulting in no globin chain or altered globin chain production
- *Translation errors* due to mutations that change the codon reading frame (frameshift mutations), substitute an incorrect amino acid codon (missense mutations), add a stop codon causing premature chain termination (nonsense mutations), or remove a stop codon, which results in an elongated

and unstable mRNA that produces a dysfunctional globin chain
- *Deletion of one or more globin genes* resulting in the lack of production of the corresponding globin chains

All of these heterogeneous genetic mutations cause a reduction or lack of synthesis of one or more globin chains, resulting in the thalassemia syndromes (Figure 28-2).

PATHOPHYSIOLOGY

The clinical manifestations of thalassemia stem from:

1. A reduced or absent production of a particular globin chain, which diminishes hemoglobin synthesis and produces microcytic, hypochromic RBCs; and
2. An unequal production of the α- or β-globin chains causing an imbalance in the α/β chain ratio; this leads to a markedly decreased survival of RBCs and their precursors.[3,11,13]

The α/β chain imbalance is more significant and determines the clinical severity of the thalassemia.[11] The mechanism and the degree of shortened RBC survival are different for the β-thalassemias and α-thalassemias.

Mechanisms in β-Thalassemias

In the β-thalassemias, the unpaired, excess α chains precipitate in the developing RBCs, forming inclusion bodies; this causes oxidative stress and damage to cellular membranes.[14] Apoptosis is triggered, and the damaged and apoptotic RBC precursors are subsequently phagocytized and destroyed in the bone marrow by activated macrophages.[14] In addition, iron accumulation in the RBC precursors (discussed below) and inflammatory cytokines may also contribute to the

TABLE 28-2 Genetic Designations in Thalassemia

Designation	Definition
Designations for Normal β-Globin and α-Globin Genes	
β	Normal β-globin gene; normal amount of β chains produced; one gene located on each chromosome 11
αα	Normal α_1- and α_2-globin genes on one chromosome (haplotype αα); normal amount of α chains produced; two genes located on each chromosome 16
Designations for the Major Thalassemic Genes	
β^0	β-globin gene mutation in which no β chains are produced
β^+	β-globin gene mutation that results in 5% to 30% decrease in β chain production
β^{silent}	β-globin gene mutation that results in mildly decreased β chain production
$\delta\beta^0$	δβ-globin gene deletional or non-deletional mutation in which no δ or β chains are produced; accompanied by some increase in γ chain production
$\delta\beta^{Lepore}$	δβ-globin gene fusion that produces a small amount of fusion product, hemoglobin Lepore; no δ or β chains are produced; accompanied by some increase in γ chain production
HPFH	Hereditary persistence of fetal hemoglobin; δβ-globin gene deletional or non-deletional mutation in γ-globin gene promoter in which no δ or β chains are produced; accompanied by increase in γ chain production
α^0	Deletion of both α-globin genes on one chromosome (haplotype, − −) that results in no α chain production
α^+	Deletion of one α-globin gene on one chromosome (haplotype, − α) that results in decreased α chain production
α^T	Non-deletional mutation in one α-globin gene on one chromosome (haplotype $\alpha^T\alpha$) that results in decreased α chain production (T denotes thalassemia)

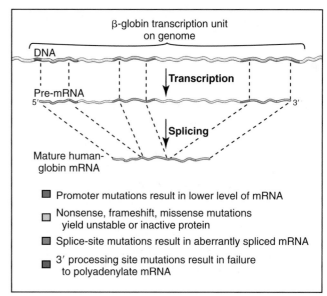

Figure 28-2 The transcription unit of the β-globin gene. The nucleotide sequence of the DNA template is transcribed into a complementary pre-mRNA. The pre-mRNA is processed by removing introns and splicing together the protein coding exons (orange). The DNA sequences required for expression of a functional β-globin chain are indicated in different colors. Mutations in any of these sequences can lead to decreased or absent β-globin chain production. (From Corden JL, Chapter 15. Gene Expression. In Pollard TD, Earnshaw WC. Cell Biology, ed 2. Philadelphia, 2008, Saunders, An imprint of Elsevier, Figure 15-2.)

apoptosis.[14] The premature death of RBC precursors in the bone marrow is called *ineffective erythropoiesis*.[11,14] In this situation, the bone marrow attempts to produce RBCs but is not able to release sufficient viable cells into the circulation. The cells that are released into the periphery are laden with inclusion bodies and are rapidly sequestered and destroyed by macrophages in the spleen (extravascular hemolysis).[11] Therefore, in β-thalassemia the anemia is multifactorial and results from ineffective production and increased destruction. Typically, individuals with severe β-thalassemia are asymptomatic during fetal life and through approximately 6 months of age because Hb F ($\alpha_2\gamma_2$) is the predominant circulating hemoglobin. Symptoms usually begin to appear between 6 and 24 months of age, after completion of the γ to β switch.[3,13,15] To compensate for the decreased expression of the β-globin gene, the γ- and/or δ-globin genes are usually upregulated, but in β-thalassemia major, this increase is insufficient to correct the α/β chain imbalance.[3]

In β-thalassemia major, the profound anemia stimulates an increase in erythropoietin production by the kidney and results in massive (but ineffective) erythroid hyperplasia.[11] In untreated or inadequately treated patients, marked bone changes and deformities occur due to the massive bone marrow expansion. A reduction in bone mineral density and a thinning of the cortex of the bone increases the risk of pathologic fractures.[3,11] In children, radiographs of the long bones may exhibit a lacy or lucent appearance.[3] Skull radiographs may demonstrate a typical "hair on end" appearance due to vertical striations of bony trabeculae (Figure 28-3).[3,11] A typical facies occurs, with prominence of the forehead (also known as frontal bossing), cheekbones, and upper jaw. Extramedullary erythropoiesis causes hepatosplenomegaly, and foci of hematopoietic tissue can appear in other body areas. Sequestration of blood cells in the enlarged spleen can worsen the anemia and can also cause neutropenia and thrombocytopenia.[11] The release of hemoglobin from the excessive destruction of RBCs and their precursors leads to an increase in the level of plasma indirect bilirubin. The bilirubin can diffuse into the tissues, causing jaundice (Chapter 23). Patients also have an increased risk of developing thrombosis.[3,11]

Iron accumulation in various organs is a serious complication in β-thalassemia major and is a significant cause of

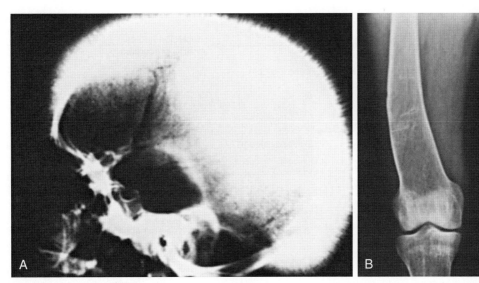

Figure 28-3 Radiologic abnormalities in a patient with homozygous β-thalassemia who receives blood transfusions infrequently (thalassemia intermedia). **A,** Skull radiograph illustrating the typical "hair on end" appearance. **B,** Severe osteoporosis, pseudofractures, thinning of the cortex, and bowing of the femur. (From Cunningham MJ, Sankaran VG, Nathan DG, et al. Chapter 20. The Thalassemias. In: Orkin SH, Nathan DG, Ginsberg D, et al. Nathan and Oski's hematology of infancy and childhood, ed 7, 2009, Saunders, an imprint of Elsevier.)

morbidity and mortality in adults.[3] In children, excess iron causes growth retardation and absence of sexual maturity; in adults, it causes cardiomyopathy, fibrosis and cirrhosis of the liver, and dysfunction of exocrine glands.[3,15] The risk of organ damage due to iron accumulation begins to increase after 10 to 11 years of age.[15] The iron overload is predominantly due to the regular RBC transfusions required in β-thalassemia major (discussed later). However, the extreme degree of erythropoiesis also suppresses hepcidin production by the liver, resulting in more iron absorption by the intestinal enterocytes (Chapter 11).[3,16] This increase in intestinal iron absorption further adds to the iron overload burden.[3,16] The pathophysiology of β-thalassemia major is summarized in Figure 28-4.

Mechanisms in α-Thalassemia

In α-thalassemia, the decreased production of α chains can manifest in utero because the α chain is a component of both fetal and adult hemoglobins. However, the accumulation of non–α chains has different consequences compared to β-thalassemia. In the fetus and newborn, a decrease in production of α chains results in an excess of γ chains. These γ chains accumulate in proportion to the number of deleted or defective α genes.[11,13] The γ chains are more stable and do not precipitate but instead form hemoglobin tetramers (γ_4) called *Hb Bart*.[13] After 6 months of age and through adulthood when the γ to β switch is completed, the decrease in α chain production results in excess β chains. The excess β chains are also relatively stable and form tetramers (β_4), called *Hb H*.

Because Hb H and Hb Bart do not precipitate to any significant degree in the developing RBCs in the bone marrow, patients with α-thalassemia do not have severe ineffective erythropoiesis.[11] As the mature RBCs age in the circulation, however, the β_4 tetramers in Hb H eventually precipitate and form inclusion bodies.[11] The macrophages in the spleen recognize and remove these abnormal RBCs from the circulation, and the patient manifests a moderate hemolytic anemia.

In addition to the decreased production and shortened RBC survival mechanisms, a third mechanism is involved in the anemia of α-thalassemia. Hb Bart and Hb H cannot deliver oxygen to tissues due to their very high affinity for oxygen.[13] A fetus cannot survive with only Hb Bart (found with a deletion of all four α-globin genes). The marked tissue hypoxia causes heart failure and massive edema (hydrops fetalis) and hepatomegaly, and the fetus usually dies in utero or shortly after birth.[3] This is discussed in the α-thalassemia section later in the chapter.

β-GLOBIN GENE CLUSTER THALASSEMIAS

There is great heterogeneity in the mutations in the β-globin gene cluster that leads to the clinical syndrome of β-thalassemia.[12] More than 300 genetic abnormalities have been discovered, including mutations affecting the β-, δ-, and γ-globin genes individually or in combination.[12,13] A small subset of mutations, however, accounts for the majority of the mutant alleles within a single ethnic group or geographic area in which β-thalassemia is found.[3,15] Because multiple mutations are present in each population, most individuals with severe β-thalassemia are compound heterozygotes for two different β-thalassemia mutations.[11] A comprehensive list of hemoglobin gene mutations is maintained in the HbVar mutation database, which is available online.[12]

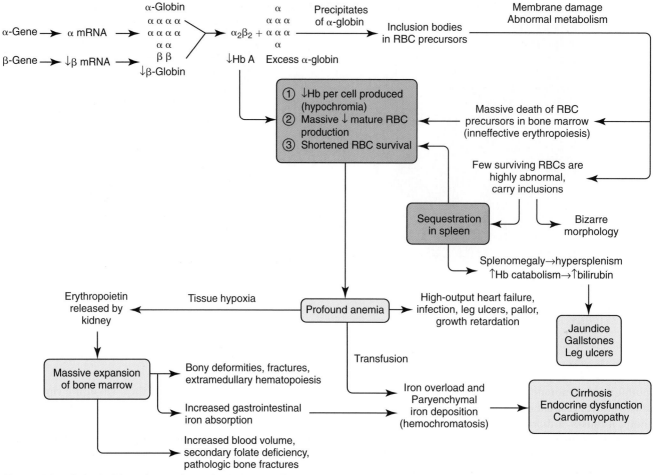

Figure 28-4 Pathophysiology of severe forms of β-thalassemia. The diagram outlines the pathogenesis of clinical abnormalities resulting from the primary defect in β-globin chain synthesis. *RBC*, Red blood cell. (From Giardina PJ, Rivella S: Thalassemia Syndromes. In: Hoffman R, Benz EJ, Jr, Silberstein LE, et al, editors: Hematology: basic principles and practice, ed 6, Philadelphia, 2013, Saunders, an imprint of Elsevier.)

Clinical Syndromes of β-Thalassemia

β-thalassemia is divided into four categories based on clinical manifestations (Table 28-3):[3,13]

- β-thalassemia silent carrier (heterozygous state) with *no* hematologic abnormalities or clinical symptoms
- β-thalassemia minor (heterozygous state) with mild hemolytic anemia, microcytic/ hypochromic RBCs, and no clinical symptoms
- β-thalassemia major (homozygous or compound heterozygous state) with severe hemolytic anemia, microcytic/hypochromic RBCs, severe clinical symptoms, and transfusion-dependence
- β-thalassemia intermedia with mild to moderate hemolytic anemia, microcytic/hypochromic RBCs, moderate clinical symptoms, and transfusion independence

The clinical manifestations of the various mutations depend on whether one or both of the β-globin genes are affected and the extent to which the affected gene or genes are expressed. Some mutations result in the complete absence of β chain production, and genes with these mutations are designated as β⁰. Other mutations lead to production of the β chains but at a significantly reduced rate, and these are designated as β⁺ mutations. The range of β chain production in these β⁺ mutations varies from 5% to 30% of normal β chain synthesis.[3] Still other mutations only minimally reduce β chain production, and genes with those mutations are designated as βˢⁱˡᵉⁿᵗ (Table 28-2).

β-thalassemia is inherited in an autosomal recessive pattern. If both parents are carriers of a β-thalassemia gene mutation, they have a 25% chance of having a child with two mutated β-globin genes (homozygote or compound heterozygote) and clinical manifestations of β-thalassemia major or intermedia.

Silent Carrier State of β-Thalassemia

The designation βˢⁱˡᵉⁿᵗ includes the various heterogeneous β-globin gene mutations that produce only a small decrease in production of the β chains. The silent carrier state (βˢⁱˡᵉⁿᵗ/β) results in nearly normal α-β chain ratios and no hematologic abnormalities.[3,11,13] It was first recognized through a study of families in which the affected children had a more severe β-thalassemia syndrome than a parent with typical β-thalassemia minor.[13] The parents had normal levels of Hb A₂ and a slight microcytosis. Some individuals who are homozygous for a

TABLE 28-3 Clinical Syndromes of β-Thalassemia with Examples of Genotypes

Genotype	Hb A	Hb A$_2$	Hb F	Hb Lepore
Normal (Normal Hematologic Parameters)				
β/β	N	N	N	0
Silent Carrier State (Asymptomatic; Normal Hematologic Parameters)				
β^{silent}/β	N	N	N	0
Thalassemia Minor (Asymptomatic; Mild Hemolytic Anemia; Microcytic, Hypochromic)				
β$^+$/β	↓	↑	N to Sl ↑	0
β^0/β	↓	↑	N to Sl ↑	0
δβ^0/β	↓	N to ↓	5%–20%	0
δβ^{Lepore}/β	↓	↓	↑	5%–15%
Thalassemia Major (Severe Hemolytic Anemia; Transfusion-Dependent; Microcytic, Hypochromic)				
β$^+$/β$^+$	↓↓	V	↑↑	0
β$^+$/β^0	↓↓↓	V	↑↑	0
β^0/β^0	0	V	↑↑	0
δβ^{Lepore}/δβ^{Lepore}	0	0	80%	20%
Thalassemia Intermedia (Mild to Moderate Hemolytic Anemia; Transfusion-Independent*; Microcytic, Hypochromic)*				
β^{silent}/β^{silent}	↓	↑	↑	0
β$^+$/β^{silent} or β^0/β^{silent}	↓	↑	↑	0
δβ^0/δβ^0	0	0	100%	0
β^0/δβ^0	0	N	↑↑	0

*Patients who are transfusion-independent do not require regular transfusions for survival, but may need transfusions occasionally, such as during pregnancy or infections.

**Other genotypes are included in this category such as dominantly inherited β-thalassemia (heterozygous for a very severe β-globin gene mutation) and coinheritance of a triplicated α-globin gene (ααα/αα) with thalassemia minor.

↑, Increased; ↓, decreased; 0, absent; *Hb*, hemoglobin; *N*, normal; *Sl*, slight; *V*, variable.

silent thalassemia gene mutation (β^{silent}/β^{silent}) have been described.[13,17] They present with a mild β-thalassemia intermedia phenotype with an increased level of Hb F and Hb A$_2$.[13,17]

β-Thalassemia Minor

β-thalassemia minor (also called β-thalassemia trait) results when one β-globin gene is affected by a mutation that decreases or abolishes its expression, whereas the other β-globin gene is normal (heterozygous state). It usually presents as a mild, asymptomatic anemia with hemoglobin ranging from 12.4 to 14.2 g/dL in affected men and 10.8 to 12.8 g/dL in affected women.[11] The RBC count is within the reference interval or slightly elevated.[3,13] The RBCs are microcytic and hypochromic, with a mean cell volume (MCV) less than 75 fL and a mean cell hemoglobin (MCH) less than 26 pg.[3] The reticulocyte count is within the reference interval or slightly increased.[3] Some degree of poikilocytosis (including target cells and elliptocytes) and basophilic stippling in the RBCs may be seen on a Wright-stained peripheral blood film (Figure 28-5). The bone marrow shows mild to moderate erythroid hyperplasia, with minimal ineffective erythropoiesis. Hepatomegaly and splenomegaly are seen in a few patients. In the most common β-thalassemia minor syndromes (β^0/β and β$^+$/β), the Hb A level is 92% to 95% and the Hb A$_2$ level is characteristically elevated and can vary from 3.5% to 7.0%.[3,13,15.] The Hb F level usually ranges from 1% to 5%.[3,13] Less common types of β-thalassemia minor exist, such as δβ^0/β and δβ^{Lepore}/β. Other rare types have atypical features, such as Dutch β^0-thalassemia minor that shows the expected elevation in Hb A$_2$ level but an Hb F level in the 5% to 20% range,[18] and another mutant found in a Sardinian family in which the Hb A$_2$ level is normal.[19]

β-Thalassemia Major

β-Thalassemia major is characterized by a severe anemia that requires regular transfusion therapy. It is usually diagnosed between 6 months and 2 years of age (after completion of the γ to β switch) when the child's Hb A level does not increase as expected.[3,13]

In untreated β-thalassemia major, the hemoglobin level can fall as low as 3 to 4 g/dL.[3,13] The MCV ranges from 50 to 70 fL.[11,15] The peripheral blood film shows marked microcytosis, hypochromia, anisocytosis, and poikilocytosis, including target cells, teardrop cells, and elliptocytes. Polychromasia and nucleated red blood cells may be observed (Figure 28-6). RBC inclusions are commonly found, including basophilic stippling, Howell-Jolly bodies, and Pappenheimer bodies, the latter as a result of the excess nonheme iron in the RBCs. The reticulocyte count is only mildly to moderately elevated and is inappropriately lower in relation to the amount of RBC hyperplasia and hemolysis present.[3] The inappropriate reticulocytosis results from the apoptosis of RBC precursors in the bone marrow (ineffective erythropoiesis).

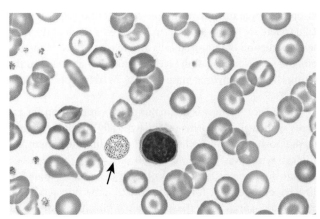

Figure 28-5 Red blood cells (RBCs) from a patient with β-thalassemia minor, showing microcytic, hypochromic RBCs with target cells, other poikilocytes, and basophilic stippling (*arrow*).

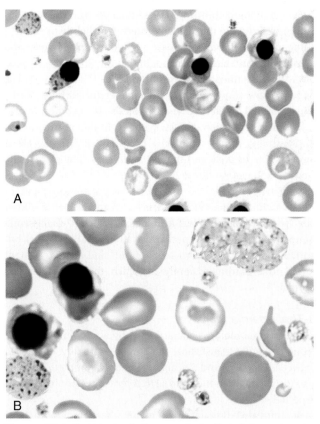

Figure 28-6 Red blood cells from a patient with β-thalassemia major. Note basophilic stippling, microcytosis, hypochromia, target cells, nucleated red blood cells, and red cell fragments. **A,** ×500. **B,** ×1000. (Adapted from Carr JH, Rodak BF: Clinical hematology atlas, ed 4, Philadelphia, 2013, Saunders.)

Hb A is absent or decreased, depending on the specific genotype, which determines whether none (β^0/β^0) or a decreased amount (β^+/β^+ or β^0/β^+) of β chains are produced. Hb A is produced only if a β^+ mutation is present, and usually ranges from 10 to 30%.[3,15] Hb F ranges from 70% to greater than 90%, depending on the genotype and amount of Hb A.[13,15] The level of Hb A_2 is variable and can be within or above the reference interval.[11] The bone marrow shows marked erythroid hyperplasia, with a myeloid-to-erythroid (M:E) ratio of 1:20 (reference interval is 1.5:1 to 3.3:1). As a result of the massive destruction of erythroid cells and release of free hemoglobin, the serum haptoglobin level is reduced or absent, and the serum lactate dehydrogenase activity is markedly elevated (Chapter 23).

Transfusion therapy is the major therapeutic option for patients with thalassemia major and typically is initiated when the hemoglobin drops to less than 7 g/dL and the patient has clinical symptoms.[3,20] Typically, 10 to 15 mL/kg of RBCs are transfused every 2 to 5 weeks.[3] RBCs that are less than 7 to 10 days old are used for transfusion to allow for maximum donor RBC survival in the patient.[3] Typing the patient for the major blood group antigens and transfusing antigen-negative donor RBCs are recommended to reduce the risk of alloimmunization.[11,15]

Administration of RBC transfusions at regular intervals began in the mid-1970s. The pretransfusion hemoglobin level is usually maintained between 9 and 10.5 g/dL.[3,21] Such transfusion regimens are termed *hypertransfusion* and are used not only to correct the anemia but to also suppress the marked erythropoiesis. With erythropoiesis suppressed, the marked marrow expansion does not occur, and therefore the bone changes do not take place. In addition, the reduction in erythropoiesis decreases the amount of iron absorbed in the intestinal enterocytes.[16] Children receiving this therapy do not develop hepatosplenomegaly and have much-improved growth and development.[3] The transfusion regimens, however, lead to an excess iron burden. Because there is no effective physiologic pathway for iron excretion in the body, the iron contained in the transfused RBCs accumulates in the body. This iron is stored in organs outside the bone marrow (e.g., liver, heart, pancreas), which results in organ damage. The accumulation of iron in the liver leads to cirrhosis, and the deposition of iron in the heart leads to cardiac dysfunction and arrhythmias. In the past, with transfusion therapy alone, thalassemic patients died in their teens, typically from cardiac failure. Now patients undergo iron chelation therapy with the transfusion therapy. Iron chelating agents bind excess iron so that it can be excreted in the urine and stool. The standard chelation therapy is a daily infusion of deferoxamine, usually administered subcutaneously with an infusion pump over 8 to 12 hours.[3,11] Owing to the cost, inconvenience, and side effects, patients may have poor compliance with the regimen.[3,11] Two oral iron chelators, deferasirox and deferiprone, have been approved by the U.S. Food and Drug Administration, which may improve compliance, but their long-term efficacy compared to deferoxamine is still being evaluated.[3,13,22] Additional oral iron chelating drugs are in development. Iron chelation treatment has been able to prevent iron accumulation and the subsequent complications of iron overload, helping to extend life expectancy of patients with β-thalassemia major into the fourth and fifth decade and beyond.[3,15,22]

Hematopoietic stem cell transplantation (HSCT) is the only curative therapy for thalassemia major.[3,23] In patients with a good risk profile (on a regular chelation therapy regimen, with no hepatomegaly or liver fibrosis), the average overall and thalassemia-free survival rates are greater than 90% and 80%, respectively.[15,23] The highest survival rates occur in young patients with an HLA identical sibling donor.[23] Because there is only a 25% chance that a sibling will have the identical HLA genotype, this option is not available to all patients. A well-matched unrelated donor can be used, but survival is not as high, and finding an immunologic match in an unrelated donor is less likely.

Hemoglobin F induction agents, such as hydroxyurea, 5-azacytidine, short chain fatty acids, erythropoietic-stimulating agents, and thalidomide derivatives have been evaluated for therapy in thalassemia major because of their ability to "switch on" the γ-globin gene to produce more γ chains.[24] The γ chains then combine with the excess α chains to form Hb F, thus partially correcting the α/β chain imbalance. Hydroxyurea therapy has benefited a few β-thalassemia major patients, allowing them to become transfusion-independent, but has not been beneficial in the majority of patients.[3,24] Studies with the other Hb F-inducing agents have shown initial promising results.[24] However, larger and better-designed studies are needed to determine the efficacy of these agents in thalassemia major.[24]

In 2010, a successful lentilviral β-globin gene transfer was reported in an adult with severe Hb E-β[0]-thalassemia who became transfusion-independent.[25] Based on this success, clinical trials have opened at multiple sites using lentalviral vectors for β- and γ-globin gene transfer.[26] In addition, research on the use of gene therapy to increase expression of the patient's own γ-globin genes has also intensified.[26] Ideally, in the future, gene therapy will be able to correct the genetic defect.

β-Thalassemia Intermedia

Thalassemia intermedia is a term used to describe anemia that is more severe than β-thalassemia minor but does not require regular transfusions to maintain hemoglobin level and quality of life (transfusion-independent).[3,11] Although patients with thalassemia intermedia typically maintain a hemoglobin level greater than 7 g/dL, it is the clinical features rather than the hemoglobin level that determine the diagnosis.[3,11] In these patients, the α/β chain imbalance falls between that observed in β-thalassemia minor and β-thalassemia major but without the need for regular transfusion therapy. The genotypes of thalassemia intermedia show great heterogeneity. Patients can be homozygous for mutations that cause a mild decrease in β-globin expression. Conversely, they may be compound heterozygous, with one gene causing a mild decrease in β chain production and the other causing a marked reduction in β chain production.[3,11] In rare instances, only one of the β-globin genes carries a mutation, but it is severe enough to cause a significant anemia. These cases are sometimes called *dominantly inherited* β-thalassemia.[13] Many of the thalassemia intermedia phenotypes are generated from the coinheritance of one or two abnormal β-globin genes with another hemoglobin defect, such as abnormal α-globin genes or unstable hemoglobins.[3,11] The coinheritance of α-thalassemia may permit homozygotes with more severe β-thalassemia mutations to remain transfusion independent because the α/β chain ratio is more balanced and fewer free α chains are available to precipitate and cause hemolysis.[3] Less severe clinical manifestations also occur when a β-thalassemia mutation is combined with a mutation that increases the expression of the γ-globin gene.[3] The increase in Hb F production ($\alpha_2\gamma_2$) helps to compensate for the reduction in Hb A, while helping to correct the α/β balance. Examples of these situations are the deletional forms of δβ[0]-thalassemia. Individuals homozygous for these mutations, or compound heterozygotes for δβ[0]-thalassemia and a β-thalassemia mutation, have thalassemia intermedia with increased γ chain and Hb F synthesis.[3,13] Conversely, coinheritance of a triplicated α-globin gene locus (ααα) (see section on α-thalassemia) is also a cause of thalassemia intermedia in some individuals heterozygous for β-thalassemia due to the production of more α chains and greater imbalance of the α/β chain ratio.[3,27]

Because of the genetic heterogeneity of β-thalassemia intermedia, the laboratory and clinical features vary. The degree of anemia and jaundice varies, depending on the extent to the α/β chain imbalance. Because of the presence of splenomegaly, the platelet and neutrophil counts may be low. The clinical course varies from minimal symptoms (despite moderately severe anemia) to severe exercise intolerance and pathologic fractures.[11] Patients with thalassemia intermedia also have iron overload even though they do not receive transfusions.[3] The markedly accelerated ineffective erythropoiesis suppresses hepcidin production by the liver, which results in more iron absorption by the intestinal enterocytes.[16] Cardiac, liver, and endocrine complications, however, present 10 to 20 years later in thalassemia intermedia patients than in patients who receive regular transfusions.[3]

Other Thalassemias Caused by Defects in the β-Globin Gene Cluster

Other thalassemias may be caused by deletion, inactivation, or fusion of a combination of genes of the β-globin gene cluster, such as hereditary persistence of fetal hemoglobin (HPFH), δβ[0]-thalassemia, and Hb Lepore thalassemia.[3,11,28]

Thalassemias with Increased Levels of Fetal Hemoglobin

HPFH and δβ[0]-thalassemia are closely related, heterogeneous conditions in which Hb F is expressed at increase levels beyond infancy into adulthood. These conditions have similarities but can be differentiated by the clinical presentation, hemoglobin level, MCV, and amount of Hb F produced.[13]

In HPFH, the β-globin gene cluster typically contains a deletion in the δβ region that leads to the increased production of Hb F. However, there are also HPFH conditions that have intact β-globin gene clusters with non-deletional mutations in the promoter region of the γ-globin genes that lead to the increased Hb F production.[11,13,29] Because individuals with these mutations are characteristically asymptomatic, this condition is of little significance except when it interacts with other forms of thalassemia or structural hemoglobin variants, such as Hb S. The additional γ chains produced are able to replace the missing β chains and help to restore the balance of α and non-α chains (γ or β). Significant variation is seen in heterozygotes for deletional-type HPFH, but these patients typically are asymptomatic with a normal MCV and Hb F levels of 10% to 35%, depending on the mutation.[3,11] Homozygotes for deletional-type HPFH are also asymptomatic. They have a normal to slightly increased hemoglobin level, 100% Hb F, with slightly hypochromic and microcytic RBCs.[13] The increase in hemoglobin observed in some patients is likely a response to the slight hypoxia induced by the higher oxygen affinity of Hb F compared with Hb A.[3] When assessed using the Kleihauer-Betke acid elution stain (discussed later), the distribution of Hb F in HPFH is usually pancellular (deletional-types), but it can be heterocellular (non-deletional-types). In contrast, the Hb F distribution in the other β-globin gene cluster thalassemias is always heterocellular.[3,30]

The $\delta\beta^0$-thalassemias are also characterized by deletions in the δ- and β-globin genes and an increase in Hb F in adult life. Non-deletional types have also been described.[11] In this condition, however, the increase in production of the γ chains is not sufficient to completely restore the balance between the α and non-α chains. Heterozygous $\delta\beta^0$-thalassemia individuals ($\delta\beta^0/\beta$) have a decreased level of Hb A, normal or decreased level of Hb A_2, and 5% to 20% Hb F.[11,13] They have a β-thalassemia minor phenotype, with a slight decrease in hemoglobin level and hypochromic, microcytic RBCs. Homozygous $\delta\beta^0$-thalassemia individuals ($\delta\beta^0/\delta\beta^0$) have hypochromic, microcytic RBCs, 100% Hb F, and a β-thalassemia intermedia phenotype[11,13] (Table 28-3).

Hemoglobin Lepore Thalassemia

Hemoglobin Lepore ($\delta\beta^{Lepore}$) is structural variant and rare type of $\delta\beta$-thalassemia caused by a fusion of the $\delta\beta$-globin genes.[12] This mutation occurs during meiosis due to nonhomologous crossover between the δ-globin locus on one chromosome and the β-globin locus on the other chromosome. The Lepore globin chain expressed by the $\delta\beta$ fusion gene contains the first 22 to 87 amino acids of the N-terminus of the δ chain and the last 31 to 97 amino acids of the C-terminus of the β chain, depending on the variant.[12] The $\delta\beta$ fusion gene produces a reduced level of the Lepore globin chain because its transcription is under the control of the δ-globin gene promoter, which is much less active than the β-globin gene promoter.[3] Conversely, in the reciprocal fusion on the other chromosome (called *anti-Lepore*), the β-globin gene locus is intact, so normal production of the β chain occurs.[3,13] In heterozygotes ($\delta\beta^{Lepore}/\beta$), there is a decreased level of Hb A and Hb A_2, an increase in Hb F, and approximately 5% to 15% Hb Lepore.[3,13] The clinical manifestations are similar to β-thalassemia minor. In homozygotes ($\delta\beta^{Lepore}/\delta\beta^{Lepore}$), there are no normal δ- or β-globin genes, no production of Hb A and Hb A_2, and approximately 80% Hb F and 20% Hb Lepore.[13] The clinical manifestations are similar to β-thalassemia major[3] (Table 28-3).

Screening for β-Thalassemia Minor

Because of the high carrier frequency of β-thalassemia mutations worldwide, screening has become an important global health issue.[5,6] Mass-screening programs in Italy and Greece combined with prenatal diagnosis have led to a significant reduction in the number of children born with β-thalassemia major.[13] Carrier parents have a 25% risk of having a child with thalassemia major or thalassemia intermedia, depending on the particular β globin gene mutations.[12] Potential carriers of these disorders can be initially identified by measuring the hemoglobin level, MCV, and the Hb A_2 and Hb F levels.[13,31] Other causes of microcytic anemias, such as iron deficiency, need to be ruled out. Molecular genetic testing of the *HBB* gene is performed for carrier detection in couples seeking preconception counseling and prenatal testing.[15]

α-THALASSEMIAS

In contrast to β-thalassemia, in which point mutations in the β-globin gene cluster are the most common type of mutation, in α-thalassemia large deletions involving the α_1- and/or α_2-globin genes are the predominant genetic defect.[11-13] Non-deletional mutations (mostly point mutations) also occur in α-thalassemia but are uncommon.[12,13,32] The extent of decreased production of the α chain depends on the specific mutation, the number of α-globin genes affected, and whether the affected α-globin gene is α_2 or α_1.[11] The α_2-globin gene produces approximately 75% of the α chains in normal RBCs, so mutations in the α_2-globin gene generally cause more severe anemia than mutations affecting the α_1-globin gene.[11,13,32] The notation for the normal α-globin gene complex or haplotype is $\alpha\alpha$, which signifies the two normal genes (α_2 and α_1) on one chromosome 16. A normal genotype is $\alpha\alpha/\alpha\alpha$.

The α-thalassemias are divided into two haplotypes: α^0-thalassemia and α^+-thalassemia. In the α^0-thalassemia haplotype (originally named α-thal-1), a deletion of both α-globin genes on chromosome 16 results in no α chain production from that chromosome. The designation, – –, is used for the α^0-thalassemia haplotype.[11,13] There are 21 known mutations that produce the α^0-thalassemia haplotype and involve deletion of both of the α-globin genes or the entire α-globin gene cluster (including the ζ-globin gene) on one chromosome.[12] The α^0 haplotype (– –) is found in approximately 4% of the population in Southeast Asia, is found less frequently in the Mediterranean region, and occurs infrequently in other parts of the world.[6]

In the α^+-thalassemia haplotype (originally named α-thal-2), a deletional or non-deletional mutation in one of the two α-globin genes on chromosome 16 results in decreased α chain production from that chromosome.[11] The designation, – α, is used for the deletional mutations, while the designation, $\alpha^T\alpha$, is used for the non-deletional mutations. The deletional α^+ haplotype (– α) is by far the most common of the α-thalassemia haplotypes. It is widely distributed throughout the thalassemia belt and central Africa (Figure 27-3), with a carrier frequency reaching 50% to 80% in some regions of Saudi Arabia, India, Southeast Asia, and Africa.[6] The deletional α^+ haplotype (– α) is also found in about 30% of African Americans.[32] The non-deletional α^+ haplotype ($\alpha^T\alpha$) is relatively uncommon.[13,32] More than 40 different mutations are known, the majority of which are point mutations that affect the predominant α_2 gene.[12] The $\alpha^T\alpha$ haplotype produces unstable α chains or fewer α chains than in the – α haplotype and generally results in a more severe anemia.[13,32]

One of the most common non-deletional α-globin gene mutations is Constant Spring ($\alpha_2^{142Stop\rightarrow Gln}$), also called α^{CS}, haplotype, $\alpha^{CS}\alpha$.[12,13] It is the result of a point mutation in the α_2-globin gene that changes the stop codon at 142 to a glutamine codon.[12,13,32] As a result, additional bases are added to the end of the mRNA during transcription until the next stop codon is reached. The elongated mRNA is very unstable and produces only a small amount of the α^{CS} chain.[3,33,34] The α^{CS} chains (with an additional 31 amino acids added to the C-terminal end) combine with β chains to form Hb Constant Spring, but the incorporation of a longer α chain makes the tetramer unstable.[34] Because of the instability of both the mRNA and the Hb tetramer, the circulating level of Hb Constant Spring is very low.[13,32,34] Consequently, hemoglobin

Constant Spring is difficult to detect by alkaline hemoglobin electrophoresis, and when present, is visualized as a faint, slow-moving band near the point of origin.[13]

Clinical Syndromes of α-Thalassemia

Four clinical syndromes are present in α-thalassemia, depending on the gene number, *cis* or *trans* pairing, and the amount of α chains produced.[11,13] The four syndromes are[11,13] (Table 28-4):

- Silent carrier state
- α-thalassemia minor
- Hb H disease
- Hb Bart hydrops fetalis syndrome

Silent Carrier State

The deletion of one α-globin gene, leaving three functional α-globin genes (– α/αα), is the major cause of the silent carrier

state. The α/β chain ratio is nearly normal, and no hematologic abnormalities are present.[11,13] Because one α-globin gene is absent, there is a slight decrease in α chain production. There is a slight excess of γ chains at birth that form tetramers of Hb Bart (γ_4) in the range of 1% to 2%.[11,13] There is no reliable way to diagnose silent carrier state other than genetic analysis. A non-deletional α^+ mutation in one α-globin gene ($\alpha^T\alpha/\alpha\alpha$) also results in the silent carrier state. In the heterozygous mutation, $\alpha^{CS}\alpha/\alpha\alpha$, Hb Constant Spring is less than 1% of the total hemoglobin.[13]

α-Thalassemia Minor

Deletion of two α-globin genes is the major cause of α-thalassemia minor. It exists in two forms: homozygous α^+ (– α/– α) or heterozygous α^0 (– –/αα).[11,13] This syndrome is asymptomatic and characterized by a mild anemia (typical hemoglobin concentration is 12 to 13 g/dL) with microcytic, hypochromic RBCs. At birth, the proportion of Hb Bart is in the range of 5% to 15%.[13] In adults, the production of α and β chains is balanced, so Hb H (β_4) is not usually present. Homozygosity for non-deletional mutations in both α_2-globin genes ($\alpha^T\alpha/\alpha^T\alpha$) produces a mild to moderate hemolytic anemia, often with jaundice and hepatosplenomegaly.[13,34] In the homozygous mutation, $\alpha^{CS}\alpha/\alpha^{CS}\alpha$, Hb Constant Spring is 5% to 6% of the total hemoglobin and the hemoglobin concentration is 9 to 11 gm/dL.[11,13,34]

Hemoglobin H Disease

Deletion of three α-globin genes is the major cause of Hb H disease in which only one α-globin gene remains to produce α chains (– –/– α).[11,13] This genetic abnormality is particularly common in Asians because of the prevalence of the α^0 gene haplotype (– –). It is characterized by the accumulation of excess unpaired β chains that form tetramers of Hb H in adults. In the newborn, Hb Bart comprises 10% to 40% of the hemoglobin, with the remainder being Hb F and Hb A. After the γ to β switch, Hb H replaces most of the Hb Bart, so Hb H is in the range of 1% to 40%, with a reduced amount of Hb A_2, traces of Hb Bart, and the remainder Hb A.[11,13,32,33] The non-deletional α^+ haplotype, when combined with the α^0 haplotype (– –/$\alpha^T\alpha$), generally produces a more severe Hb H disease with a higher level of Hb H than the α^0 interaction with the deletional α^+ haplotype (– –/– α).[13,32,34] Hb H-Hb Constant Spring (– –/$\alpha^{CS}\alpha$) is an example.[13,34-36]

Hb H disease is characterized by a mild to moderate, chronic hemolytic anemia with hemoglobin concentrations averaging 7 to 10 g/dL, and reticulocyte counts of 5% to 10%, although a wide variability in clinical and laboratory findings exists.[11,36] The bone marrow exhibits erythroid hyperplasia, and the spleen is usually enlarged. Patients with deletional Hb H disease are transfusion-independent, that is, they do not require regular transfusions. However, infection, pregnancy, or exposure to oxidative drugs may cause a hemolytic crisis requiring transfusions on a temporary basis.

Hemolytic crises often lead to the detection of the disease because individuals with Hb H disease may otherwise be asymptomatic. The RBCs are microcytic and hypochromic, with marked poikilocytosis, including target cells and bizarre

TABLE 28-4 Clinical Syndromes of α-Thalassemia

Genotype	Hb A	Hb Bart (in Newborn)	Hb H (in Adult)	Hb Constant Spring
Normal (Normal Hematologic Parameters)				
αα/αα	N	0	0	0
Silent Carrier State (Asymptomatic; Normal Hematologic Parameters)				
– α/αα	N	1%–2%	0	0
$\alpha^{CS}\alpha$/αα	N	1%–3%	0	<1%
α-Thalassemia Minor (Asymptomatic; Mild Hemolytic Anemia; Microcytic, Hypochromic)				
– –/αα	SI↓	5%–15%	0	0
– α/– α	SI↓	5%–15%	0	0
$\alpha^{CS}\alpha/\alpha^{CS}\alpha$*	SI↓	5%–15%	0	<6%
Hb H Disease (Mild to Moderate Hemolytic Anemia; Transfusion-Independent; Microcytic, Hypochromic)**				
– –/– α	↓	10%–40%	1%–40%	0
– –/$\alpha^{CS}\alpha$†	↓	↑↑	↑↑	<1%
Hb Bart Hydrops Fetalis Syndrome (Severe Anemia; Usually Infants are Stillborn or Die Shortly after Birth)				
– –/– –	0	80%–90% (remainder Hb Portland)	NA	0

*$\alpha^{CS}\alpha/\alpha^{CS}\alpha$ genotype results in mild to moderate hemolytic anemia with jaundice and hepatosplenomegaly.

**Patients who are transfusion-independent do not require regular transfusions for survival, but may need transfusions occasionally, such as during pregnancy or infections.

†– –/$\alpha^{CS}\alpha$ genotype and other non-deletional genotypes (– –/$\alpha^T\alpha$) result in Hb H disease that is moderate to severe and may require more frequent transfusions than the deletional – –/– α genotype.

↓, Decreased; ,↑↑ increased more than – –/– α; 0, absent; <, less than; *CS*, Constant Spring; *Hb*, hemoglobin; *N*, normal; *NA*, not applicable.

shapes. Hb H is vulnerable to oxidation and gradually precipitates in the circulating RBCs to form inclusion bodies of denatured hemoglobin.[11] These inclusions alter the shape and viscoelastic properties of the RBCs, contributing to the decreased RBC survival. Splenectomy is beneficial in patients with markedly enlarged spleens.[32] When incubated with brilliant cresyl blue or new methylene blue, RBCs with Hb H display fine, evenly distributed, granular inclusions. These inclusions are typically removed as the RBC passes through the spleen. Before splenectomy, only a portion of the cells have this characteristic, but after the spleen is removed, most of the RBCs are full of these inclusions. These cells are often described as "golf balls" or "raspberries" (Figure 28-7).

Two distinct conditions are associated with Hb H disease and congenital physical and intellectual abnormalities: alpha-thalassemia retardation-16 (ATR-16) syndrome and alpha-thalassemia X-linked intellectual disability (ATRX) syndrome. Patients with the ATR-16 syndrome inherit or acquire a large deletion in the short arm of chromosome 16, which removes the ζ- and α-globin genes as well as all the flanking genes to the terminus of the chromosome.[33] Patients have physical deformities, intellectual disabilities, and Hb H disease.[32,33,35] The ATRX syndrome is due to mutations of the *ATRX* gene located on the X chromosome.[37,38] The ATRX protein is a component of a large complex that regulates expression of various genes, including the α-globin genes.[33,38] The regulation is accomplished by DNA remodeling and/or methylation, thus affecting the transcription, replication, and repair of the target genes.[32,33,36,38] Therefore, when the *ATRX* gene is mutated, patients have decreased α chain production.[32,33,35,38] Affected males with ATRX syndrome have pronounced intellectual disability, physical deformities, developmental delay, and Hb H disease. An acquired Hb H disease with mutations in the *ATRX* gene has been found in myelodysplastic syndrome.[33,38,39]

Hb Bart Hydrops Fetalis Syndrome

Homozygous α[0]-thalassemia (– –/– –) results in the absence of all α chain production and usually results in death in utero or shortly after birth.[3,11] The fetus is severely anemic, which leads to cardiac failure and edema in the fetal subcutaneous tissues (hydrops fetalis). Hb Bart (γ_4) is the predominant hemoglobin, along with a small amount of Hb Portland ($\zeta_2\gamma_2$) and traces of Hb H.[3,11] Hb Bart has a very high oxygen affinity; it does not deliver oxygen to the tissues.[11,13] The fetus can survive until the third trimester because of Hb Portland, but this hemoglobin cannot support the later stages of fetal growth, and the affected fetus is severely anoxic.[11] The fetus is delivered prematurely and is usually stillborn or dies shortly after birth. In addition to anemia, edema, and ascites, the fetus has gross hepatosplenomegaly and cardiomegaly.[3,11] At delivery, there is a severe microcytic, hypochromic anemia (hemoglobin concentration of 3 to 8 gm/dL) with numerous nucleated RBCs in the peripheral blood.[33] The bone marrow cavity is expanded, and marked erythroid hyperplasia is present, along with foci of extramedullary erythropoiesis.

Hydropic pregnancies are hazardous to the mother, resulting in toxemia and severe postpartum hemorrhage.[11] Hydropic changes are detected in midgestation by means of ultrasound testing.[40] If both parents carry one α[0]-thalassemia haplotype (– –/αα), prenatal diagnosis of homozygosity can be made by molecular genetic testing of fetal cells from chorionic villus sampling or amniotic fluid.[33] Absence of the α-globin genes establishes the diagnosis. Early termination of the pregnancy prevents the serious maternal complications.[11]

THALASSEMIA ASSOCIATED WITH STRUCTURAL HEMOGLOBIN VARIANTS

Hemoglobin S-Thalassemia

Sickle cell anemia (Hb SS)- α-thalassemia is a genetic abnormality due to the coinheritance of two abnormal β-globin genes for Hb S and an α-thalassemia haplotype. Hb SS-α[+]-thalassemia is fairly common because the genes for Hb S and the α[+]-thalassemia haplotype, – α, are common in populations of African ancestry. Individuals with Hb SS–α[+]-thalassemia have a milder anemia with higher hemoglobin levels and lower reticulocyte counts than those with sickle cell anemia alone.[41] In one study, Hb SS individuals with the genotypes, αα/αα, – α/αα, and – α/– α, had average hemoglobin concentrations of 8.4, 9.0, and 9.5 g/dL, respectively, and reticulocyte counts of 10.8%, 8.8%, and 6.9%, respectively.[41]

Hb S-β-thalassemia is a compound heterozygous condition that results from the inheritance of a β-thalassemia gene from one parent and an Hb S gene from the other. This syndrome has been reported in the populations of Africa, the Mediterranean area, the Middle East, and India.[13] The clinical expression of Hb S-β-thalassemia depends on the type of β-thalassemia mutation inherited.[11,13] Individuals with Hb S-β[+]-thalassemia produce variable amounts of normal β chains. Patients have mostly Hb S with slightly elevated Hb A_2 and variable amounts of Hb F and Hb A, depending on the specific abnormal β[+] gene inherited. These patients can be distinguished from those with sickle cell anemia by the presence of microcytosis, splenomegaly, an elevated Hb A_2 level, and an Hb A level that is less than the Hb S level.

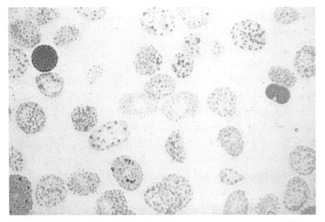

Figure 28-7 Red blood cells from a patient with hemoglobin H disease, incubated with brilliant cresyl blue, which have acquired fine, evenly dispersed granular inclusions and "golf ball" appearance. (From the American Society for Hematology slide bank.)

The interaction of β^{silent}-thalassemia (in which β chains are produced at mildly reduced levels) and Hb S results in a condition that may be slightly more severe than sickle cell trait. Typically, there is mild hemolytic anemia with splenomegaly. These patients can be distinguished from patients with sickle cell trait by the presence of microcytosis and splenomegaly. Hemoglobin electrophoresis or HPLC confirms this condition when the quantity of Hb S exceeds that of Hb A. In sickle cell trait, Hb A is the predominant hemoglobin.

The combination of β^0-thalassemia and Hb S produces a phenotype similar to sickle cell anemia with a similar incidence of stroke and a similar life expectancy.[42] Both conditions lack Hb A and produce severe painful crises as the predominant symptom. Typically, the microcytosis and elevated Hb A_2 level in Hb S-β^0-thalassemia distinguish it from sickle cell anemia.

Hemoglobin C-Thalassemia

Hb C-β-thalassemia produces moderately severe hemolysis, splenomegaly, hypochromia, microcytosis, and numerous target cells. The hemoglobin electrophoresis pattern varies, depending on the type of β-thalassemia gene defect, with higher Hb C concentrations in patients when there is minimal or no β chain production.[13]

Hemoglobin E-Thalassemia

Hb E-β-thalassemia is a significant concern in Southeast Asia and Eastern India owing to the high prevalence of both genetic mutations.[13] Hb E is due to a point mutation that inserts a splice site in the β-globin gene, and results in decreased production of Hb E.[3] In the homozygous state (Hb EE) the clinical symptoms are similar to a mild β-thalassemia. (Chapter 27) When the mutations are coinherited in the compound heterozygous state, there is a marked reduction of β chain production. The clinical symptoms are similar to β-thalassemia intermedia or β-thalassemia major, depending on the particular β-globin gene mutation.[13] Table 28-5 summarizes some compound heterozygous states of β-thalassemia combined with a structural β-globin defect.

DIAGNOSIS OF THALASSEMIA

History and Physical Examination

Individual and family histories are paramount in the diagnosis of thalassemia. The ethnic background of the individual should be investigated because of the increased prevalence of specific gene mutations in certain populations. In the clinical examination, findings that suggest thalassemia include pallor (due to the anemia); jaundice (due to the hemolysis); splenomegaly (caused by sequestration of the abnormal RBCs, excessive extravascular hemolysis, and some extramedullary erythropoiesis); and skeletal deformities (due to the massive expansion of the bone marrow cavities). These findings are particularly prominent in untreated or partially treated β-thalassemia major.[13] Table 28-6 contains a summary of tests for the diagnosis of thalassemia.

Laboratory Methods

Complete Blood Count with Peripheral Blood Film Review

Although most thalassemias result in a microcytic and hypochromic anemia, laboratory results can vary from borderline abnormal to markedly abnormal; this depends on the type and number of globin gene mutations. The hemoglobin and hematocrit are decreased, but the RBC count can be disproportionately high relative to the degree of anemia, which can generate a very low MCV and mean cell hemoglobin (MCH). The mean cell hemoglobin concentration (MCHC) is also decreased. The RBC distribution width (RDW) is elevated (reflecting anisocytosis) in untreated β-thalassemia major, but it is often normal in β-thalassemia minor. On a Wright-stained peripheral blood film, the RBCs are typically microcytic and hypochromic, except in the silent carrier

TABLE 28-5 β-Thalassemia Associated with Structural β-Globin Variants (Compound Heterozygotes)

Genotype	Hb A	Hb A_2	Hb F	Other Hb	RBC Morphology	Clinical Manifestations*	Treatment
Hb S-β^+-thalassemia	↓↓	↑	N to ↑	Hb S > Hb A	Microcytes, sickle cells, target cells	Ranges from mild to severe anemia with recurrent vasoocclusive crises	Ranges from no treatment to transfusion support and pain control
Hb S-β^0-thalassemia	0	↑	N to ↑	Hb S			
Hb C-β^+-thalassemia	↓↓	†	↑	Hb C > Hb A	Microcytes, Hb C crystals, target cells	Ranges from moderate to severe anemia	Usually no treatment needed
Hb C-β^0-thalassemia	0	†	↑	Hb C			
Hb E-β^+-thalassemia	↓↓	†	↑↑	Hb E > Hb A	Microcytes, target cells	Ranges from mild to severe anemia with transfusion dependency	Ranges from no treatment to transfusion support
Hb E-β^0-thalassemia	0	†	↑↑	Hb E			

↑, Increased; ↓, decreased; 0, absent; *Hb,* hemoglobin; *N,* normal; *RBC,* red blood cell.
*Clinical manifestations depend on the amount of Hb A produced; compound heterozygotes with the β^0 gene have more severe symptoms.
†Not all methods can quantitate Hb A_2 in the presence of the abnormal hemoglobin. High-performance liquid chromatography can separate Hb A_2 from Hb C; capillary zone electrophoresis can separate Hb A_2 from Hb E.

TABLE 28-6 Laboratory Diagnosis of Thalassemias[15,31,33,43]

Screening tests	Complete blood count	HGB, HCT, MCV, MCH, MCHC: ↓
	Peripheral blood film review	RETIC: sl to mod ↑
		Varying degrees of microcytosis, hypochromia, target cells, anisocytosis, poikiloctosis, RBC inclusions, NRBCs
	Iron studies (to rule out IDA)	Serum ferritin and serum iron: N or ↑; TIBC: N
Presumptive diagnosis	Supravital stain	α-thal: Hb H inclusions
	Hemoglobin fraction quantification by electrophoresis, HPLC, and/or CZE	β-thal: Hb A ↓ or 0; Hb A₂ ↑ (carriers); Hb F: usually ↑; Hb Lepore; other mutants
		α-thal: Hb A: ↓ or 0 (hydrops fetalis); Hb A₂ ↓; Hb Bart, Hb H, Hb Constant Spring, other mutants
Definitive* diagnosis	Molecular genetic tests: β-thal: >250 mutations** in *HBB* α-thal: >100 mutations** in *HBA1* and/or *HBA2*	Step 1: Targeted mutation analysis: β-thal: initial screen for four to six most common mutations if specific ethnic group known α-thal: initial screen for seven most common deletions If negative, Step 2: DNA sequence analysis If negative, Step 3: Deletion/duplication analysis (e.g., MLPA, aCGH)

*Required for prenatal diagnosis, preconception risk assessment/carrier detection in couples, diagnosis of rare or complex mutations, determining prognosis in young children,
**From reference 12 (HbVar database, accessed May 10, 2014).
aCGH, Array comparative genomic hybridization; *CZE,* capillary zone electrophoresis; *Hb,* hemoglobin; *HCT,* hematocrit; *HGB,* hemoglobin level (g/dL); *IDA,* iron deficiency anemia; *MCH,* mean cell hemoglobin; *MCHC,* mean cell hemoglobin concentration; *MCV,* mean cell volume; *MLPA,* multiplex ligation-dependent probe amplification; *mod,* moderate; *RETIC,* reticulocyte count; *RBCs,* red blood cells; *NRBCs,* nucleated red blood cells; *sl,* slight; *thal,* thalassemia.

phenotypes, in which the RBCs appear normal. In β-thalassemia minor, α-thalassemia minor, and Hb H disease, the cells are microcytic with target cells and slight to moderate poikilocytosis. In homozygous and compound heterozygous β-thalassemia, extreme poikilocytosis may be present, including target cells and elliptocytes, in addition to polychromasia, basophilic stippling, Howell-Jolly bodies, Pappenheimer bodies, and nucleated RBCs.

Reticulocyte Count

The reticulocyte count is elevated, which indicates that the bone marrow is responding to a hemolytic process. In Hb H disease, the typical reticulocyte count is 5% to 10%.[13] In homozygous β-thalassemia, it is typically 2% to 8%, disproportionately low relative to the degree of anemia.[13] An inadequate reticulocytosis reflects the ineffective erythropoiesis.

Supravital Staining

In α-thalassemia minor, Hb H disease, and silent carrier α-thalassemia, brilliant cresyl blue or new methylene blue stain may be used to induce precipitation of the intrinsically unstable Hb H.[35,43] Hb H inclusions (denatured β-globin chains) typically appear as small, multiple, irregularly shaped greenish-blue bodies that are uniformly distributed throughout the RBC. They produce a pitted pattern on the RBCs similar to the pattern of a golf ball or raspberry (Figure 28-7). In Hb H disease, almost all RBCs contain Hb H inclusions.[35] In α-thalassemia minor, only a few cells may contain these inclusions, and in silent carrier α-thalassemia, only a rare cell does. These inclusions appear different from Heinz bodies, which are larger and fewer in number and most often appear eccentrically along the inner membrane of the RBC. This test is very sensitive in detecting Hb H in the α-thalassemia conditions.[43]

Assessment of Normal and Variant Hemoglobins

The major clinical laboratory methods used to identify and quantify normal and variant hemoglobins include hemoglobin electrophoresis, cation-exchange high-performance liquid chromatography (HPLC), and capillary zone electrophoresis (CZE).[44] Each of these methods has advantages and limitations, and no one method is able to identify and quantify all hemoglobins. Therefore, a combination of at least two of the above methods is used for confirmation of a hemoglobin variant.[45] Molecular genetic testing is required to detect specific mutations in globin genes and definitively identify the type of thalassemia or hemoglobinopathy. Molecular genetic testing is not usually required in adults with typical findings on the CBC, electrophoresis, and/or HPLC, but it is required for prenatal diagnosis, preconception risk assessment/carrier detection in couples, diagnosis of rare or complex mutations, and determining prognosis in young children.[15,31,33,44]

Hemoglobin electrophoresis at alkaline pH has been the traditional tool for thalassemia and hemoglobinopathy diagnosis. In this method, patient RBC lysate is spotted on a solid support (such as agarose) and subjected to an electrical current in an alkaline buffer. Normal and variant hemoglobins will migrate and separate on the support according to their charge. The support is stained, and each hemoglobin band is quantified by scanning densitometry and reported as a percentage of the total hemoglobin.[45] This technique is able to distinguish the common hemoglobins, such as Hb A, Hb F, Hb S, Hb C, and the fast-moving hemoglobins, Hb H and Hb Bart.[44-46] Electrophoresis, however, has several limitations: it is labor-intensive and cannot accurately quantify Hb A₂ and Hb F. In addition, Hb S and Hb C must be confirmed by another method because Hb D and Hb G comigrate with Hb S, and Hb E and Hb O^Arab comigrate with Hb C.[45] Methods used for confirmation usually include agar electrophoresis at acid pH,

HPLC, or CZE, or in the case of Hb S, the solubility test (Figures 27-6, 27-7, 27-8, 27-9). Figure 28-8 shows the relative hemoglobin mobilities in alkaline electrophoresis for various thalassemias and hemoglobinopathies.

In HPLC, patient RBC lysate in buffer is injected into a cation-exchange column. Both normal and variant hemoglobins will bind to the column. An elution buffer is injected and forms a gradient of varying ionic strength.[45] The various hemoglobin types will be differentially eluted from the column, each having a specific column retention time. As each hemoglobin fraction passes near the end of the column, a detector measures the absorbance of the fraction at 415 nm, which is recorded as a peak on a chromatogram.[45] The area under the peak is used to quantify the hemoglobin fraction, which is reported as a percentage of total hemoglobin. With the availability of fully automated instruments, HPLC has replaced hemoglobin electrophoresis in many laboratories as the routine screening method for analysis of hemoglobins.[44] The method is ideal for thalassemia screening because it can accurately and quickly quantitate Hb A, Hb A_2, and Hb F with 100% sensitivity and 90% specificity if no hemoglobin variants are present (Figure 28-9).[46] The precise and accurate quantification of Hb A_2 is particularly important in screening individuals for β-thalassemia minor (trait). HPLC can also presumptively identify and quantify hemoglobin variants even in low concentration.[44,45] HPLC, however, requires specialized instrumentation and extensive experience and training to accurately interpret the complex chromatograms.[44,45,47] Additional limitations of HPLC include the following: Hb A_2 and Hb E have the same retention time and therefore cannot be accurately quantified by this method; Hb A_2 can be overestimated in the presence of Hb S due to overlapping peaks and underestimated in the presence of Hb D^{Punjab}; and it is not able to identify all variants.[44-47] A manual microcolumn method is also available for the measurement of Hb A_2.[45]

In capillary zone electrophoresis (CZE), patient RBC lysate is introduced into a thin silica glass capillary tube in an alkaline buffer. When a current is applied, the various hemoglobin fractions migrate to the cathode at different velocities due to electro-endoosmotic flow.[45] As each hemoglobin fraction passes near the end of the capillary, a detector measures the absorbance of the fraction at 415 nm, which is recorded as a peak on a electrophoretogram. The instrument calculates the percentage of each hemoglobin fraction using an integration of the area under the peak and the migration time.[45] Fully automated systems are available that provide rapid and accurate identification and quantification. The peaks are placed into zones in the electrophoretogram for easier identification, and it can presumptively identify hemoglobin variants, including those in low concentration (Figure 28-9).[45] An advantage of CZE over HPLC is that it can separate and quantify Hb A_2 in the presence of Hb E.[44] However, because there is overlap in the peaks for Hb A_2 and Hb C, it cannot quantify Hb A_2 in the presence of Hb C.[44] As with HPLC, it also cannot detect all variants.[44,45] Complementing electrophoresis, HPLC, and/or CZE results, however, have minimized the limitations of all these methods.[47] Other technologies such as isoelectric focusing and mass spectrometry are used in newborn screening programs for detection of common hemoglobin variants.[44-45]

Molecular Genetic Testing

For mutations in the *HBB* gene, targeted mutation analysis using polymerase chain reaction (PCR)-based methods can be initially performed for detection and quantification of the four to six most common mutations if an individual's ethnicity is known.[3,15] This strategy allows a mutation detection rate of 91% to 95% in Mediterranean, Middle East, Thai, and Chinese populations, and 75% to 80% in African and African-American populations.[15] In multiethnic individuals or if the ethnicity is unknown, DNA sequencing of the *HBB* gene is performed including exons, intervening sequences, splice sites, and 5′ and 3′ untranslated regulatory regions.[15,46] This strategy enables detection of approximately 95% of known mutants.[15,31] If sequencing is not successful, testing can reflex to deletion/duplication analysis (such as multiplex ligation-dependent probe amplification or array-based comparative genomic hybridization) (Chapter 31).[15,31,46]

For mutations in the *HBA1* or *HBA2* genes, PCR-based targeted mutation analysis can also be initially performed for the seven most common deletional mutations.[33] This strategy detects approximately 90% of all alleles, but the detection rate varies by method.[33,36] If the above screening is not successful, DNA sequencing of the *HBA1* and *HBA2* genes or deletion/duplication analysis can be performed as described above.[33]

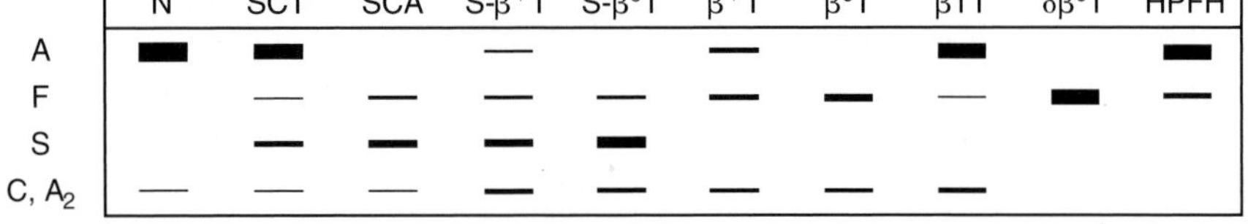

Figure 28-8 Relative electrophoretic mobilities on cellulose acetate (pH 8.4) of various hemoglobins (Hbs) important in the diagnosis of thalassemia syndromes and hemoglobinopathies. $\beta^0 T$, β⁰-thalassemia major, β⁰/β⁰ (no Hb A, increased Hb F, slight increase in Hb A_2); $\beta^+ T$, β⁺-thalassemia major, β⁺/β⁺ (decreased Hb A, increased Hb F, slight increase in Hb A_2); βTT, β-thalassemia minor (slight decrease in Hb A, increased Hb A_2, some Hb F); $\delta\beta^0 T$, δβ⁰-thalassemia, homozygous, δβ⁰/δβ⁰ (100% Hb F); *HPFH*, hereditary persistence of fetal hemoglobin, heterozygous (mostly Hb A, some Hb F, no Hb A_2); *N*, normal; *SCA*, sickle cell anemia (no Hb A, mostly Hb S, increased Hb F, normal Hb A_2); *SCT*, sickle cell trait (Hb A > Hb S, normal Hb A_2 and F); S-$\beta^0 T$, sickle cell-β⁰-thalassemia (no Hb A, increased Hb A_2 and F, mostly Hb S); S-$\beta^+ T$, sickle cell-β⁺-thalassemia (Hb A < Hb S, increased Hb A_2 and F).

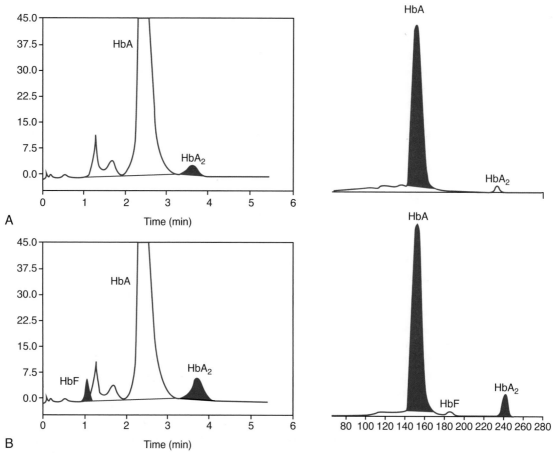

Figure 28-9 Separation and quantification of hemoglobin fractions by high performance liquid chromatography (Bio-Rad, left) and capillary electrophoresis (Sebia, right). **A,** Healthy adult with Hb F < 1% and Hb A$_2$ < 3.5%; **B,** Adult with β-thalassemia minor with increased Hb F and Hb A$_2$. (Modified from Giordano PC: Strategies for basic laboratory diagnostics of the hemoglobinopathies in multiethnic societies: interpretation of results and pitfalls. Int Jnl Lab Hem 35: 465-479, 2013, Figure 3, p. 472.)

When the parents' mutation is known, analysis for the specific mutation in fetal cells can be done on specimens from amniocentesis (at 15 to 18 weeks' gestation), chorionic villus sampling (at 10 to 12 weeks' gestation), or with preimplantation genetic diagnosis using a cell from a 3-day-old embryo after in vitro fertilization.[15,33]

Other Procedures

The classic *alkali denaturation* test is accurate and precise to quantify Hb F in the 0.2% to 50% range.[48] Most human hemoglobins are denatured on exposure to a strong alkali, but Hb F is not. The Hb F can be separated and its concentration compared with that of other hemoglobins. Consistent methodology is required to ensure accurate results.[48] However, automated HPLC is now often used to quantify Hb F.[45,46]

In the Kleihauer-Betke acid elution slide test, peripheral blood films are ethanol-fixed and immersed in a citrate-acid buffer (pH 3.3). Adult hemoglobins are eluted from the RBCs, whereas Hb F resists acid elution and remains in the cell. When the cells are subsequently stained, RBCs containing Hb F will take up the stain, whereas RBCs containing only adult hemoglobin will appear as "ghosts." This test determines if the Hb F distribution in RBCs is pancellular (found in all RBCs in deletional HPFH cases) or heterocellular (found in some but not all RBCs in β-globin gene cluster thalassemias and nondeletional HPFH cases).[35,45] The Kleihauer-Betke slide test is also used to estimate the volume of fetal-maternal hemorrhage to determine if an increased dose of Rh immune globulin is needed for an Rh-negative mother who delivers an Rh-positive baby. Because the Kleihauer-Betke slide test is cumbersome to perform and results are difficult to replicate, flow cytometry is becoming the standard test to measure fetal-maternal hemorrhage quickly and accurately.[49]

In underdeveloped countries with limited technology, a single-tube osmotic fragility test has been used to screen populations for thalassemia carriers.[11] This is based on the fact that carriers have hypochromic RBCs, resulting in decreased osmotic fragility.[46,50] An aliquot of anticoagulated blood is incubated in 0.375% saline for 5 minutes.[44] Because the solution is hypotonic, normal RBCs will lyse and the solution will clear. However, patients with thalassemia have hypochromic RBCs that will not lyse in 0.375% saline, and the solution will remain turbid. This test is not specific for thalassemia and will be positive for any condition causing hypochromia, including iron deficiency anemia.

Differential Diagnosis of Thalassemia Minor and Iron Deficiency Anemia

The RBCs in thalassemia minor are microcytic and hypochromic, and this disease must be differentiated from iron deficiency anemia and other microcytic, hypochromic anemias. The differential diagnosis for microcytic, hypochromic anemias is relatively limited (Table 20-1). Differentiating thalassemia minor from iron deficiency is important to avoid unnecessary tests or treatments. An incorrect presumption that a patient has iron deficiency may lead to inappropriate iron therapy or to unnecessary diagnostic procedures, such as a colonoscopy, to identify a source of blood loss.

Clinical history is crucial. A family history of thalassemia raises the suspicion for this diagnosis. A history of previously normal hemoglobin levels and RBC indices, significant bleeding, or pica leads to the diagnosis of iron deficiency.[51] *Pica* means cravings for nonfood items such as clay, dirt, or starch. The most common pica symptom in the United States is pagophagia, the craving to chew on ice.[51]

Iron deficiency and β-thalassemia minor are best differentiated using serum ferritin level, serum iron level, total iron-binding capacity, transferrin saturation, and Hb A_2 level, along with a complete blood count (CBC) and examination of a peripheral blood film.[51,52] Additional testing may also include soluble transferrin receptor and zinc protoporphyrin levels (Chapter 20).[51]

Before evaluating Hb A_2 levels for β-thalassemia minor, iron deficiency should be ruled out. Low iron levels in patients with β-thalassemia minor decrease the Hb A_2 levels.[52] The iron stores need to be replenished before the laboratory analysis for thalassemia is undertaken.

A mild erythrocytosis (high RBC count) and marked microcytosis (low MCV) are found more commonly in β-thalassemia minor. In iron deficiency anemia, the RBC count and MCV may be normal or decreased, depending on whether the deficiency is developing or long-standing.[53-55] The RDW can be normal or increased in both β-thalassemia minor and iron deficiency anemia, with a significant overlap of values; therefore, the RDW alone cannot distinguish these conditions.[52-54] Various discrimination indices have been proposed to distinguish β-thalassemia minor from iron deficiency anemia using a calculation based on the RBC count, hemoglobin level, MCV, MCH, and/or RDW (such as the Mentzer, Green and King, England and Fraser, Shine and Lal, and Srivastava indices).[52-54] Unfortunately, the sensitivity of these indices in discriminating β-thalassemia minor and iron deficiency anemia ranged from 60% to 96% in various studies, which leads to a high number of false-negative results. Thus their use for screening is not appropriate.[3,11,51-53] The peripheral blood film may demonstrate basophilic stippling in β-thalassemia minor, which can distinguish it from iron deficiency. Because target cells can be found in both conditions, however, their presence does not help discriminate between the two disorders.

SUMMARY

- Thalassemias are a group of heterogeneous disorders in which one or more globin chains are reduced or absent.
- Thalassemias result in a hypochromic, microcytic anemia due to decreased production of hemoglobin. The imbalance of globin chain synthesis causes an excess of the normally produced globin chain that damages the RBCs or their precursors and results in hemolysis.
- β-Thalassemia is caused by mutations that affect the β-globin gene complex. It is clinically manifested as silent carrier state, thalassemia minor, thalassemia intermedia, or thalassemia major.
- In the silent carrier state (β^{silent}/β), the blood picture is completely normal. β-thalassemia minor (β^0/β or β^+/β) is a mild, asymptomatic, microcytic, hypochromic anemia; it is usually characterized by an elevated Hb A_2 level, which aids in diagnosis. β-thalassemia major is a severe anemia leading to transfusion dependence. β-thalassemia intermedia manifests abnormalities with a severity between those of β-thalassemia major and β-thalassemia minor, and does not require regular transfusions.
- The α-thalassemias are usually caused by a deletion of one, two, three, or all four of the α-globin genes, resulting in reduced or absent production of α chains.
- In α-thalassemias, tetramers of γ chains form Hb Bart in the fetus and newborn, and tetramers of β chains form Hb H in the adult.
- The α-thalassemias are divided clinically into silent carrier state, α-thalassemia minor, Hb H disease, and Hb Bart hydrops fetalis syndrome.

- Silent carrier α-thalassemia is a result of the deletion, or rarely a non-deletional mutation, of one of four α-globin genes (– α/αα) or ($\alpha^T\alpha/\alpha\alpha$); it is associated with a normal RBC profile and is asymptomatic. α-Thalassemia minor is a result of the deletion of two α-globin genes (– α/– α or – –/αα) and is clinically similar to β-thalassemia minor except that Hb A_2 is not increased.
- Hb H disease is a result of the deletion of three of the four α-globin genes (– –/– α); Hb H inclusions (β_4) precipitate in older circulating RBCs, causing a hemolytic anemia. The RBCs are microcytic and hypochromic, and the disease is clinically similar to β-thalassemia intermedia. In Hb Bart hydrops fetalis syndrome, all four of the α-globin genes are deleted (– –/– –). There is severe anemia, and fetal death usually occurs in utero or shortly after birth. The predominant hemoglobin is Hb Bart (γ_4).
- The preliminary diagnosis of thalassemia is made from the complete blood count results and RBC morphology, hemoglobin electrophoresis, high-performance liquid chromatography, or capillary zone electrophoresis. Molecular genetic testing is required for definitive diagnosis.
- Thalassemia trait must be differentiated from other microcytic, hypochromic anemias, especially iron deficiency anemia. Iron studies are important for this differentiation.

Now that you have completed this chapter, go back and read again the case study at the beginning and respond to the questions presented.

REVIEW QUESTIONS

Answers can be found in the Appendix.

1. The thalassemias are caused by:
   a. Structurally abnormal hemoglobins
   b. Absent or defective synthesis of a polypeptide chain in hemoglobin
   c. Excessive absorption of iron
   d. Abnormal or defective protoporphyrin synthesis

2. Thalassemia is more prevalent in individuals from areas along the tropics because it confers:
   a. Heat resistance to those heterozygous for a thalassemia gene
   b. Selective advantage against tuberculosis
   c. Selective advantage against malaria
   d. Resistance to mosquito bites

3. The hemolytic anemia associated with the thalassemias is due to:
   a. Imbalance of globin chain synthesis
   b. Microcytic, hypochromic cells
   c. Ineffective erythropoiesis caused by immune factors
   d. Structurally abnormal hemoglobin

4. β-Thalassemia minor (heterozygous) usually exhibits:
   a. Increased Hb Constant Spring
   b. 50% Hb F
   c. No Hb A
   d. Increased Hb A_2

5. RBC morphologic features in β-thalassemia would most likely include:
   a. Microcytes, hypochromia, target cells, elliptocytes, stippled cells
   b. Macrocytes, acanthocytes, target cells, stippled cells
   c. Microcytes, sickle cells
   d. Macrocytes, hypochromia, target cells, stippled cells

6. The predominant hemoglobin present in β^0-thalassemia major is:
   a. Hb A
   b. Hb A_2
   c. Hb F
   d. Hb C

7. Heterozygous HPFH is characterized by:
   a. 10% to 35% Hb F with normal RBC morphology
   b. 100% Hb F with slightly hypochromic, microcytic cells
   c. A decreased amount of Hb F with normal RBC morphology
   d. 5% to 15% Hb F with hypochromic, macrocytic cells

8. Hb H is composed of:
   a. Two α and two β chains
   b. Two ε and two γ chains
   c. Four β chains
   d. Four γ chains

9. Hb Bart is composed of:
   a. Two α and two β chains
   b. Two ε and two γ chains
   c. Four β chains
   d. Four γ chains

10. When one α gene is deleted ($\alpha-/\alpha\alpha$), a patient has:
    a. Normal hemoglobin levels
    b. Mild anemia (hemoglobin range 9 to 11 g/dL)
    c. Moderate anemia (hemoglobin range 7 to 9 gm/dL)
    d. Marked anemia requiring regular transfusions

11. In which part of the world is the α gene mutation causing Hb Bart hydrops fetalis (– –/– –) most common?
    a. Northern Africa
    b. Mediterranean
    c. Middle East
    d. Southeast Asia

12. The condition Hb S-β^0-thalassemia has a clinical course that resembles:
    a. Sickle cell trait
    b. Sickle cell anemia
    c. β-Thalassemia minor
    d. β-Thalassemia major

13. Hb H inclusions in a supravital stain preparation appear as:
    a. A few large, blue, round bodies in the RBCs with aggregated reticulum
    b. Uniformly stained blue cytoplasm in the RBC
    c. Small, evenly distributed, greenish-blue granules that pit the surface of RBCs
    d. Uniform round bodies that adhere to the RBC membrane

14. Which of the following laboratory findings is *inconsistent* with β-thalassemia minor?
    a. A slightly elevated RBC count and marked microcytosis
    b. Target cells and basophilic stippling on the peripheral blood film
    c. Hemoglobin level of 10 to 13 g/dL
    d. Elevated MCHC and spherocytic RBCs

15. A 4-month-old infant of Asian heritage is seen for a well-baby check. Because of pallor, the physician suspects anemia and orders a CBC. The RBC count is 4.5×10^9/L, Hb concentration is 10 g/dL, and MCV is 77 fL, with microcytosis, hypochromia, poikilocytosis, and mild polychromasia noted on the peripheral blood film. These findings should lead the physician to suspect:
    a. β-Thalassemia major
    b. α-Thalassemia silent carrier state
    c. Iron deficiency anemia
    d. Homozygous α-thalassemia (– –/– –)

REFERENCES

1. Cooley, T. B., & Lee, P. (1925). A series of cases of spleno-megaly in children with anemia and peculiar bone changes. *Trans Am Pediatr Soc, 37*, 29–30.

2. Lichtman, M. A., Spivak, J. L., Boxer, L. A., et al. (2000). Hematology: landmark papers of the twentieth century, San Diego: Academic Press.

3. Giardina, P. J., & Rivella, S. (2013). Thalassemia syndromes. In Hoffman, R., Benz, E. J., Jr., Silberstein, L. E., et al., (Eds.), *Hematology: Basic Principles and Practice.* (6th ed.). Philadelphia: Saunders, an imprint of Elsevier.

4. Modell, B., & Darlison, M. (2008). Global epidemiology of haemoglobin disorders and derived service indicators. *Bull World Health Org, 86*, 480–487.

5. Weatherall, D. J. (2010). The inherited diseases of hemoglobin are an emerging global health burden. *Blood, 115*, 4331–4336.

6. Weatherall, D. J., & Clegg, J. B. (2001). Inherited haemoglobin disorders: an increasing global health problem. *Bull World Health Organ, 79*, 704–712.

7. Mockenhaupt, F. P., Ehrhardt, S., Gellert, S., et al. (2004). Alpha(+)-thalassemia protects African children from severe malaria. *Blood, 104*, 2003–2006.

8. Williams, T. N., Wambua, S., Uyoga, S., et al. (2005). Both heterozygous and homozygous α+ thalassemia protect against severe and fatal *Plasmodium falciparum* malaria on the coast of Kenya. *Blood, 106*, 368–371.

9. Pattanapanyasat, K., Yongvanitchit, K., Tongtawe, P., et al. (1999). Impairment of *Plasmodium falciparum* growth in thalassemic red blood cells: further evidence by using biotin labeling and flow cytometry. *Blood, 93*, 3116–3119.

10. Ayi, K., Turrini, F., Piga, A., et al. (2004). Enhanced phagocytosis of ring-parasitized mutant erythrocytes: a common mechanism that may explain protection against *falciparum* malaria in sickle trait and beta-thalassemia trait. *Blood, 104*, 3364–3371.

11. Borgna-Pignatti, C., & Galanello, R. (2009). Thalassemias and related disorders: quantitative disorders of hemoglobin synthesis. In Greer, J. P., Foerster, J., Rodgers, G. M., et al., (Eds.), *Wintrobe's Clinical Hematology.* (12th ed., pp. 1083–1131). Philadelphia: Wolters Kluwer Health/Lippincott Williams & Wilkins.

12. Patrinos, G. P., Giardine, B., Riemer, C., et al (2004). Improvements in the HbVar database of human hemoglobin variants and thalassemia mutations for population and sequence variation studies. *Nucl Acids Res, 32*, Database issue: D537–541. Retrieved from http://globin.cse.psu.edu/hbvar/menu.html. Accessed 10.05.14.

13. Weatherall, D. J. (2010). Chapter 47. The Thalassemias: Disorders of Globin Synthesis. In Lichtman, M. A., Kipps, T. J., Seligsohn, U., Kaushansky, K., Prchal, J. T., (Eds.), *Williams Hematology.* (8th ed.). New York, NY: McGraw-Hill. Retrieved from http://accessmedicine.mhmedical.com.libproxy2.umdnj.edu/content.aspx?bookid=358&Sectionid=39835865. Accessed 10.05.14.

14. Ribeil, J-A., Arlet, J-B., Dussiot, M., et al. (2013). Ineffective erythropoiesis in β-thalassemia. *Scientific World Journal, 394295.* doi:10.1155/2013/394295.

15. Cao, A., Galanello, R., & Origa, R. (1993-2014). Beta-thalassemia. 2000 Sep 28 [Updated 2013 Jan 24]. In Pagon, R. A., Adam, M. P., Ardinger, H. H., et al., (Eds.), *GeneReviews®* [Internet]. Seattle (WA): University of Washington, Seattle. Retrieved from http://www.ncbi.nlm.nih.gov/books/NBK1426/. Accessed 24.05.14.

16. Nemeth, E. (2010). Hepcidin in β-thalassemia. *Ann N Y Acad Sci, 1202*, 31–35.

17. Basran, R. K., Reiss, U. M., Luo, H-Y., et al. (2008). β-Thalassemia intermedia due to compound heterozygosity for two β-globin gene promoter mutations, including a novel TATA box deletion. *Pediatr Blood Cancer, 50*, 363–366.

18. Gilman, J. G., Huisman, T. H., & Abels, J. (1984). Dutch beta 0-thalassaemia: a 10 kilobase DNA deletion associated with significant gamma-chain production. *Br J Haematol, 56*, 339–348.

19. Oggiano, L., Pirastu, M., Moi, P., et al. (1987). Molecular characterization of a normal Hb A₂ beta-thalassaemia determinant in a Sardinian family. *Br J Haematol, 67*, 225–229.

20. Modell, B., Khan, M., & Darlison, M. (2000). Survival in beta-thalassaemia major in the UK: Data from the UK Thalassaemia Register. *Lancet, 355*, 2051–2052.

21. Borgna-Pignatti, C., Rugolotto, S., De Stefano, P., et al. (2004). Survival and complications in patients with thalassemia major treated with transfusion and deferoxamine. *Haemotologica, 89*, 1187–1193.

22. Angelucci, E., Barosi, G., Camaschella, C., et al. (2008). Italian Society of Hematology practice guidelines for the management of iron overload in thalassemia major and related disorders. *Haematologica, 93*, 741–752.

23. Angelucci, E., Matthes-Martin, S., Baronciani, D., et al. (2014). Hematopoietic stem cell transplantation in thalassemia major and sickle cell disease: indications and management recommendation from an international expert panel. *Haematologica, 99*, 811–820.

24. Musallam, K. M., Taher, A. T., Cappellini, M. D., et al. (2013). Clinical experience with fetal hemoglobin induction therapy in patients with β-thalassemia. *Blood, 121*, 2199–2212.

25. Cavazzana-Calvo, M., Payen, E., Negre, O., et al. (2010). Transfusion independence and *HMGA2* activation after gene therapy of human β-thalassaemia. *Nature, 467*, 318–322.

26. Chandrakasan, S., & Malik, P. (2014). Gene therapy for hemoglobinopathies: The state of the field and the future. *Hematol Oncol Clin N Am, 28*, 199–216.

27. Oron, V., Filon, D., Oppenheim, A., et al. (1994). Severe thalassaemia intermedia caused by interaction of homozygosity for alpha-globin gene triplication with heterozygosity for beta zero-thalassaemia. *Br J Haematol, 86*, 377–379.

28. Bollekens, J. A., & Forget, B. G. (1991). Delta beta thalassemia and hereditary persistence of fetal hemoglobin. *Hematol Oncol Clin North Am, 5*, 399–422.

29. Tuan, D., Feingold, E., Newman, M., et al. (1983). Different 3' end points of deletions causing delta beta-thalassemia and hereditary persistence of fetal hemoglobin: implications for the control of gamma-globin gene expression in man. *Proc Natl Acad Sci U S A, 80*, 6937–6941.

30. Stephens, A. D., Angastiniotis, M., Baysal, E., et al. (2012). ICSH recommendations for measurement of haemaglobin F. *Int J Lab Hem, 34*, 14–20.

31. Harteveld, C. L. (2014). State of the art and new developments in molecular diagnostics for hemoglobinopathies in multiethnic societies. *Int J Lab Hem, 36*, 1–12.

32. Chui, D. H., Fucharoen, S., Chan, V. (2003). Hemoglobin H disease: not necessarily a benign disorder. *Blood, 101*, 791–800.

33. Origa, R., Moi, P., Galanello, R., et al. (1993-2014). Alpha-Thalassemia. 2005 Nov 1 [Updated 2013 Nov 21]. In Pagon, R. A., Adam, M. P., Ardinger, H. H., et al., (Eds.), *GeneReviews®* [Internet]. Seattle (WA): University of Washington, Seattle. Retrieved from http://www.ncbi.nlm.nih.gov/books/NBK1435/. Accessed 25.05.14.

34. Singsanan, S., Fucharoen, G., Savongsy, O., et al. (2007). Molecular characterization and origins of Hb Constant Spring and Hb Pakse in Southeast Asian populations. *Ann Hematol, 86*, 665–669.

35. Fucharoen, S., & Viprakasit, V. (2009). Hb H disease: clinical course and disease modifiers. *Am Soc Hematol Educ Program, 26*–34.

36. Vinchinsky, E. (2012). Advances in treatment of alpha-thalassemia. *Blood Rev Apr, 26*(Suppl. 1), S31–S34.

37. Wilkie, A. O., Zeitlin, H. C., Lindenbaum, R. H., et al. (1990). Clinical features and molecular analysis of the alpha thalassemia/mental retardation syndromes. II. Cases without detectable abnormality of the alpha globin complex. *Am J Hum Genet, 46,* 1127–1140.

38. Higgs, D. R. (2004). Gene regulation in hematopoiesis: new lessons from thalassemia. *Hematology Am Soc Hematol Educ Program,* 1–13.

39. Nelson, M. E., Thurmes, P. J., Hoyer, J. D., et al. (2005). A novel 5′ ATRX mutation with splicing consequences in acquired α thalassemia-myelodysplastic syndrome. *Haematologica, 90,* 1463–1470.

40. Ko, T. M., Tseng, L. H., Hsu, P. M., et al. (1995). Ultrasonographic scanning of placental thickness and the prenatal diagnosis of homozygous alpha-thalassaemia 1 in the second trimester. *Prenat Diagn, 15,* 7–10.

41. Steinberg, M. H., Rosenstock, W., Coleman, M. B., et al. (1984). Effects of thalassemia and microcytosis on the hematologic and vasoocclusive severity of sickle cell anemia. *Blood, 63,* 1353–1360.

42. Quinn, C. T., Rogers, Z. R., & Buchanan, G. R. (2004). Survival of children with sickle cell disease. *Blood, 103,* 4023–4027.

43. Pan, L. L., Eng, H. L., Kuo, C. Y., et al. (2005). Usefulness of brilliant cresyl blue staining as an auxiliary method of screening for alpha-thalassemia. *J Lab Clin Med, 145*(2), 94–97.

44. Gallivan, M. V. E., & Giordano, P. C. (2012). Analysis of hemoglobinopathies, hemoglobin variants and thalassemias. In Kottke-Marchant, K., & Davis, B. H., (Eds.), *Laboratory Hematology Practice.* Oxford England (UK) United Kingdom.

45. Stephens, A. D., Angastiniotis, M., Baysal, E., et al. (2012). ICSH recommendations for the measurement of haemoglobin A₂. *Int J Lab Hem, 34,* 1–13.

46. Giordano, P. C. (2013). Strategies for basic laboratory diagnostics of the hemoglobinopathies in multi-ethnic societies: interpretation of results and pitfalls. *Int J Lab Hem, 35,* 465–479.

47. Keren, D. F. (2008). Comparison of Sebia Capillarys capillary electrophoresis with the Primus high-pressure liquid chromatography in the evaluation of hemoglobinopathies. *Am J Clin Pathol, 130,* 824–831.

48. Wild, B. J., & Bain, B. J. (2004). Detection and quantitation of normal and variant haemoglobins: an analytic review. *Ann Clin Biochem, 41,* 355–369.

49. Mundee, Y., Bigelow, N. C., Davis, B. H., et al. (2000). Simplified flow cytometric method for fetal hemoglobin containing red blood cells. *Cytometry, 42,* 389–393.

50. Singh, S. P., & Gupta, S. C. (2008). Effectiveness of red cell osmotic fragility test with varying degrees of saline content in detection of beta-thalassemia trait. *Singapore Med J, 49,* 823–826.

51. Cook, J. D. (2005). Diagnosis and management of iron-deficiency anaemia. *Best Pract Res Clin Haematol, 18,* 319–332.

52. Beyan, C., Kaptan, K., & Ifran, A. (2007). Predictive value of discrimination indices in differential diagnosis of iron deficiency anemia and beta-thalassemia trait. *Eur J Haematol, 78,* 524–526.

53. Ntaios, G., Chatzinikolaou, A., Saouli, Z., et al. (2007). Discrimination indices as screening tests for β-thalassemia trait. *Ann Hematol, 86,* 487–491.

54. Demir, A., Yarali, N., Fisgin, T., et al. (2002). Most reliable indices in differentiation between thalassemia trait and iron deficiency anemia. *Pediatr Int, 44,* 612–616.

55. Means, R. T., Jr., & Glader, B. (2009). Anemia: general considerations. In Greer, J. P., Foerster, J., Rodgers, G. M., et al., (Eds.), *Wintrobe's Clinical Hematology.* (12th ed., pp. 779–809). Philadelphia: Wolters Kluwer Health/Lippincott Williams & Wilkins.

Nonmalignant Leukocyte Disorders 29

Steven Marionneaux

OBJECTIVES

After the completion of this chapter, the reader will be able to:

1. Describe the basic genetic defect and the morphologic consequences in Pelger-Huët anomaly.
2. Discuss how Pelger-Huët cells might be confused with the presence of a neutrophilic left shift.
3. Compare and contrast two genetic causes of neutrophilic hypersegmentation.
4. Describe the basic genetic defect and the morphologic consequences in Alder-Reilly anomaly, Chédiak-Higashi syndrome, and May-Hegglin anomaly.
5. Indicate how inclusions in Alder-Reilly anomaly and May-Hegglin anomaly might be confused with morphologically similar conditions.
6. Discuss the defect and functional consequences of chronic granulomatous disease.
7. Describe the cellular deficiencies and functional consequences of leukocyte adhesion disorders.
8. Describe the characteristic macrophage morphology associated with the mucopolysaccharidoses, Gaucher disease, and Niemann-Pick disease.
9. Describe the basic defect in genetic disorders leading to decreased T lymphocyte production, decreased B lymphocyte production, and the combined decrease of T, B, and natural killer lymphocytes.
10. Define what is meant by *neutrophilia, neutropenia, lymphocytosis, lymphocytopenia, monocytosis, monocytopenia, eosinophilia, eosinopenia,* and *basophilia,* and give some examples of conditions in which each occurs.
11. Describe the nonmalignant alterations in granulocyte, monocyte, and lymphocyte morphology that are associated with infection, inflammation, or other causes.
12. Outline pathogenesis; and clinical/laboratory features of infectious mononucleosis.

CASE STUDIES

After studying the material in this chapter, the reader should be able to respond to the following case studies:

Case 1

A 5-year-old boy has a long history of recurring infections, including gastroenteritis, pneumonia, severe staphylococcal infections, and a liver abscess. He was treated with antibiotics in each case and responded well, albeit slowly. The CBC was essentially normal, and no morphologic abnormalities were detected. His neutrophils were tested and were shown to migrate normally and to respond to chemotactic agents. His neutrophils also phagocytized normally; however, they were not able to reduce nitroblue tetrazolium to its insoluble formazan.

1. What is the most likely cause of this child's recurring infections?
2. Genetically and biochemically speaking, what is the specific nature of the problem?
3. What is the prognosis as it relates to treatment?
4. How is this disorder transmitted genetically in the majority of cases?

Case 2

A 66-year-old retired male professor presents with malaise, weakness, a fever of 102° F, anorexia, and weight loss. Blood cultures ×8 were negative for pathogens. Ova and parasite examinations ×5 produced negative findings. Tuberculosis and fungal serologic testing were negative. The CBC revealed a mild normocytic, normochromic anemia; a WBC count of $4.0 \times 10^9/L$; and a platelet count of $130 \times 10^9/L$. The differential count showed a neutrophilic

Continued

CASE STUDIES—cont'd

After studying the material in this chapter, the reader should be able to respond to the following case studies:

left shift, 20% lymphocytes, 28% monocytes, and 1% basophils. Neutrophils contained toxic granulation and large vacuoles. Monocytes were large and highly vacuolated. The patient's erythrocyte sedimentation rate was 70 mm/hour.

1. Based on the differential results, what cells should the medical laboratory scientist look for on the patient's blood film?

2. Where on the blood film should the examination be made and why?

3. What is the significance if the suspected cells are found?

4. What preparation other than a blood film might be helpful in this situation?

This chapter concentrates on nonmalignant disorders of WBCs—etiologies underlying changes in number and morphology of neutrophils, lymphocytes, monocytes, eosinophils, and basophils. Both hereditary and acquired causes are presented. In recent years, the genetic origin of many of these disorders has come to light and the chapter has been updated to reflect these findings.

QUALITATIVE DISORDERS OF LEUKOCYTES

Morphologic Abnormalities with and without Functional Defects

Pelger-Huët Anomaly

Pelger-Huët anomaly (PHA), also known as true or congenital PHA, is an autosomal dominant disorder characterized by decreased nuclear segmentation (bilobed, unilobed) and a characteristic coarse chromatin clumping pattern potentially affecting all leukocytes, although morphologic changes are most obvious in mature neutrophils.[1] The prevalence of PHA is approximately 1 in 4785 in the United States.[1] The disorder is a result of a mutation in the *lamin β-receptor* gene.[2] The lamin β receptor is an inner nuclear membrane protein that combines β-type lamins and heterochromatin and plays a major role in leukocyte nuclear shape changes that occur during normal maturation.[1] Mutations in the *lamin β-receptor* gene result in the morphologic changes characteristic of PHA, although the exact pathological mechanisms are not known.[1] The nuclei may appear round, ovoid, or peanut shaped. Bilobed forms—the characteristic spectacle-like ("pince-nez") morphology with the nuclei attached by a thin filament—can also be seen (Figure 29-1).[3] In homozygous PHA, all neutrophils are affected and demonstrate round nuclei, whereas in the heterozygote, 55% to 93% of the neutrophil population are affected, and there is generally a mixture of all of the aforementioned nuclear shapes.[4] Neutrophils in Pelger-Huët anomaly appear to function normally.[5]

Pseudo- or Acquired Pelger-Huët Anomaly

Neutrophils with PHA morphology can be observed in patients with hematologic malignancies such as myelodysplastic syndromes (MDS), acute myeloid leukemia, and chronic myeloproliferative neoplasms. Pseudo-PHA neutrophils can also be seen in patients with HIV infection,

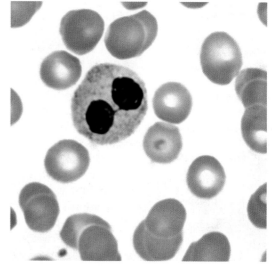

Figure 29-1 Pelger-Huët cell. Pince-nez form with two rounded segments connected by a filament. Notice the dense chromatin pattern.

tuberculosis, *Mycoplasma pneumoniae* and severe bacterial infections. Drugs known to induce pseudo-PHA include mycophenolate mofetil, valproate, sulfisoxazole, ganciclovir, ibuprofen, and chemotherapies such as paclitaxel and docetaxel.[6]

Laboratory Issues in Pelger-Huët Anomaly (True/Congenital and Pseudo/Acquired)

Differentiating between true PHA and pseudo-PHA can be challenging. (1) An important consideration is the number of cells present with PHA morphology. In true PHA, the number of affected cells is much higher than in pseudo-PHA (63% to 93% vs. <38%, respectively).[4,7] (2) Also in true PHA, all WBC lineages are potentially affected in terms of nuclear shape and chromatin structure. (3) In pseudo-PHA the phenomenon is usually seen only in neutrophils, except for some cases of MDS where monocytes, eosinophils, and basophils may exhibit PHA morphology. (4) Furthermore, if true PHA is suspected, a careful examination of peripheral blood smears of family members may reveal similar findings. (5) Hypogranular neutrophils are a common finding in MDS-related pseudo-PHA. In true PHA, neutrophils exhibit normal granulation.

In both true and pseudo-PHA there are potential challenges for the clinical lab related to cell identification. Because the nuclei of Pelger-Huët neutrophils may appear round, oval, or peanut shaped, the cells may be classified and counted as myelocytes, metamyelocytes, or band neutrophils, mimicking a neutrophilic left shift and triggering a clinical workup to uncover the cause. A careful examination of the chromatin structure can help to differentiate between Pelger-Huët cells, which are mature, and neutrophils, which are less mature.[2] Also, immature neutrophils such as metamyelocytes and myelocytes should show some degree of cytoplasmic basophilia. PHA cells are mature, so the cytoplasm is nearly colorless, except for the color imparted by normal cytoplasmic granulation.

Another laboratory challenge is determining the most appropriate label to use for reporting Pelger-Huët cells. PHA neutrophils may be unilobed or bilobed, so "segmented neutrophil" seems inappropriate. "Band neutrophil" is also not suitable for reasons stated above. It is suggested that one label should be applied to all morphologic variants of PHA neutrophils. Laboratories should address this concern and develop standardized labels to be used for all morphologic variants of PHA, the goal being to ensure that the clinician understands that PHA cells are present and that lineage maturity is not left shifted. One suggested approach would be to count Pelger-Huët neutrophils as "others" and then define "others" as Pelger-Huët neutrophils.

Neutrophil Hypersegmentation

Normal neutrophils contain three to five lobes that are separated by filaments. Hypersegmented neutrophils have more than five lobes and are most often associated with the megaloblastic anemias, where the neutrophil is also larger than normal (Figure 29-2). Hypersegmented neutrophils can also be seen in the myelodysplastic syndromes and represent a form of myeloid dysplasia. Much less frequently, hypersegmented neutrophils can be found in **hereditary neutrophil hypersegmentation**. In this disorder, patients are asymptomatic and have no signs of megaloblastic anemia.

Myelokathexis refers to a rare hereditary condition characterized by normal granulocyte production; however, there is impaired release into circulation that leads to neutropenia. Neutrophil morphology is also affected. Neutrophils appear hypermature. There may be hypersegmentation, hypercondensed chromatin, and pyknotic changes. Cytoplasmic vacuoles may also be observed.[8] Myelokathexis is a component of an extremely rare inherited disorder, **WHIM**, a syndrome in which warts, neutropenia, hypogammaglobulinemia, infections, and myelokathexis are common findings.[9,10] Mutations in *CXCR4* result in a hyperfunctional CXCR4 receptor and ligand binding, which impairs cellular homeostasis and trafficking, leading to neutropenia, lymphopenia, and hypogammaglobulinemia.[11,12]

Alder-Reilly Anomaly

Alder-Reilly anomaly is transmitted as a recessive trait and is characterized by granulocytes with large, darkly staining metachromatic cytoplasmic granules composed primarily of partially digested mucopolysaccharides. The granules are referred to as Alder-Reilly bodies or Reilly bodies. The morphology may resemble heavy toxic granulation, which is discussed later (Figure 29-3). Neutrophilia, Döhle bodies, and left shift, which are usually associated with toxic granulation, are not seen in Alder-Reilly anomaly. Also, in some patients with Alder-Reilly anomaly, the granules are found in lymphocytes and monocytes, ruling out toxic granulation, which is exclusive for neutrophils. The basic defect is the incomplete degradation of mucopolysaccharides. Reilly bodies are most commonly associated with Hurler syndrome, Hunter syndrome, and Maroteaux-Lamy polydystrophic dwarfism.[13] Leukocyte function is not affected in Alder-Reilly anomaly.

Chédiak-Higashi Syndrome

Chédiak-Higashi syndrome is a rare, fatal, autosomal recessive disease. In 2008, only 800 cases were reported worldwide.[14]

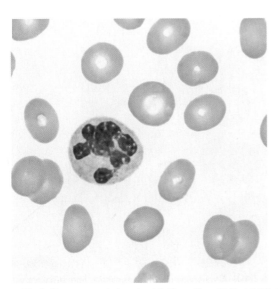

Figure 29-2 Hypersegmented neutrophil. (From Carr JH, Rodak BF: *Clinical hematology atlas*, ed 4, St. Louis, 2013, Saunders.)

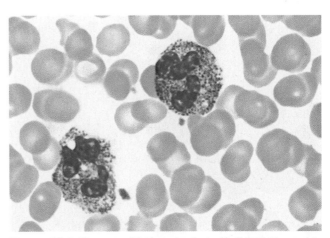

Figure 29-3 Two neutrophils from a patient with Alder-Reilly anomaly. Note the dark granules present in both cells. Such granules may also be seen in eosinophils and basophils. (Courtesy Dennis R. O'Malley, MD, US Labs, Irvine, CA.)

The disease is characterized by abnormal fusion of granules in most cells that contain granules throughout the body. The fused granules are large and mostly dysfunctional. Hematopoietic cells are affected, but disease manifestations can be found in hair, skin, adrenal and pituitary glands, and nerves. Hematologic findings in Chédiak-Higashi syndrome include giant lysosomal granules in granulocytes, monocytes, and lymphocytes (Figure 29-4). These fused granules result in leukocyte dysfunction and recurrent pyogenic infections. Patients often have bleeding issues due to abnormal dense granules in platelets.[15] Chédiak-Higashi syndrome is associated with a mutation in the *CHS1 LYST* gene on chromosome 1q42.1-2 that encodes for a protein involved in vesicle fusion or fission.[15]

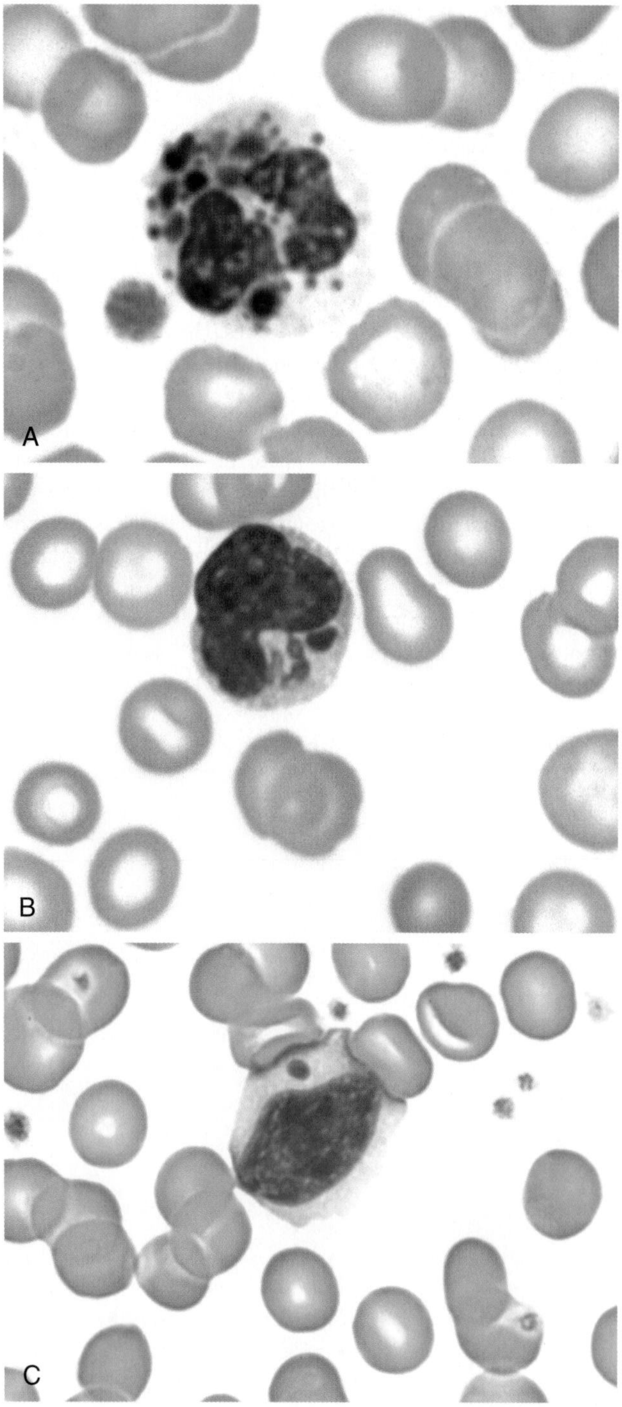

May-Hegglin Anomaly

May-Hegglin anomaly is a rare, autosomal dominant platelet disorder characterized by variable thrombocytopenia, giant platelets, and large Döhle body–like inclusions in neutrophils, eosinophils, basophils, and monocytes (Figure 29-5). May-Hegglin anomaly is caused by a mutation in the *MYH9* gene on chromosome 22q12-13.[16] There is disordered production of myosin heavy chain type IIA which affects megakaryocyte maturation and platelet fragmentation.[16] The basophilic Döhle body–like leukocyte inclusions in May-Hegglin anomaly are composed of precipitated myosin heavy chains. Döhle bodies are composed of lamellar rows of rough endoplasmic reticulum. Clinically, the majority of individuals with May-Hegglin anomaly are asymptomatic, but a few have mild bleeding tendencies that are related to the degree of thrombocytopenia.

A summary of morphologic changes and clinical findings associated with the above disorders is shown in Box 29-1.

Normal Morphology with Functional Abnormalities

The majority of genetic functional leukocyte disorders, with the exception of some of the storage disorders, are not characterized by specific morphologic alterations in leukocytes. Box 29-2 outlines the causes and clinical findings seen in these disorders.

Chronic Granulomatous Disease

Chronic granulomatous disease is a rare inherited disorder caused by the decreased ability of phagocytes to produce superoxide and reactive oxygen species. Following phagocytosis of

Figure 29-4 Three cells from a patient with Chédiak-Higashi syndrome. **A,** Neutrophil with large dark lysosomal granules. **B,** Monocyte with large azure granules. **C,** Lymphocyte with one large azure granule.

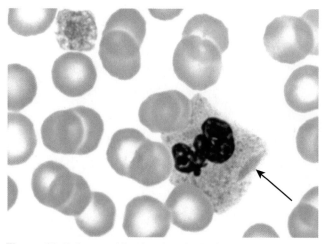

Figure 29-5 A neutrophil and a giant platelet from a patient with May-Hegglin anomaly. Note the large, elongated, bluish inclusion in the neutrophil cytoplasm.

BOX 29-1 Morphologic Abnormalities of Neutrophils with and without Functional Defects

Morphologic Abnormality	Morphologic Changes	Clinical Findings
Pelger-Huët anomaly	Decreased nuclear segmentation in neutrophils; sometimes also affects other WBCs	Asymptomatic
Pseudo-Pelger-Huët-anomaly	Decreased nuclear segmentation in neutrophils	Depends on underlying condition
Neutrophil hypersegmentation	>5 nuclear lobes in neutrophils	Depends on underlying cause
Alder-Reilly anomaly	Granulocytes contain large, darkly staining metachromatic cytoplasmic granules	Normal neutrophil function. Clinical findings, if present, are due to associated condition
Chédiak-Higashi disease	Giant lysosomal granules in granulocytes, monocytes, and lymphocytes	Leukocyte dysfunction and recurrent pyogenic infections; bleeding due to abnormal dense granules in platelets
May-Hegglin anomaly	Thrombocytopenia, giant platelets and large Döhle body–like inclusions in neutrophils, eosinophils, basophils, and monocytes	Usually asymptomatic; sometimes mild bleeding related to the degree of thrombocytopenia

---

Box 29-2 Normal Morphology of Neutrophils with Functional Abnormalities

Disorder	Cause(s)	Clinical Findings
Chronic granulomatous disease	Mutation(s) in *NADPH oxidase* genes leads to failure of neutrophil respiratory burst following phagocytosis of organism	Heterogeneous, however most experience recurrent bacterial and fungal infections; granulomas may obstruct organs (liver, spleen, others)
Leukocyte adhesion disorder – I	Mutation in gene(s) responsible for β_2 integrin subunits, leads to decreased or truncated β_2 integrin, needed for neutrophil adhesion to endothelial cells, recognition of bacteria, and outside-in signaling	Recurrent infections, neutrophilia, lymphadenopathy, splenomegaly, and skin lesions; variable severity and survival
Leukocyte adhesion disorder – II	Mutation in *SLC35C1* which codes for a fucose transporter involved in synthesis of selectin ligands. Results in decreased amount or function of selectin ligands and defective leukocyte recruitment	Physical growth retardation, coarse face, and/or other physical deformities; neurological defects, recurring infections, and absent blood group H antigen
Leukocyte adhesion disorder – III	Mutations in *Kindlin-3* and defective protein product Kindlin-3, needed for β integrin activation and leukocyte rolling. Failed response to external signals that would normally result in leukocyte activation.	Recurrent bacterial and fungal infections (less severe than LAD-I). Decreased platelet integrin GPIIbβ3, resulting in bleeding

---

microorganisms, there is no respiratory burst that normally results in the production of these antimicrobial agents. The basic defect is one or more mutations in genes responsible for proteins that make up a complex known as *NADPH oxidase* (NADPH is the reduced form of nicotinamide adenine dinucleotide phosphate). Under normal conditions, phagocytosis of foreign organism leads to phosphorylation and binding of cytosolic $p47_{phos}$ and $p67_{phos}$.[17] Primary granules containing antibacterial neutrophil elastase and cathepsin G and secondary granules containing the cytochrome complex $gp91_{phox}$ and $gp22_{phox}$ migrate to the phagolysosome. NADPH oxidase forms when $p47_{phos}$ and $p67_{phos}$ along with $p40_{phox}$ and RAC2 combine with the cytochrome complex. Superoxide is generated in the phagolysosome when an electron from NADPH is added to oxygen. NADPH has additional regulatory functions in the generation of other antimicrobial agents. Most cases of chronic granulomatous disease are due to mutations in gp91phox or p47. The majority of cases (approximately 60% to 65%)

are X-linked recessive, whereas 35% to 40% are autosomal recessive.[18]

The disease is heterogeneous, and survival is based on the type of mutation, which in turn determines the level of superoxide produced.[17] Most patients experience bacterial and fungal infections of the lung, skin, lymph nodes, and liver. Macrophage-rich granulomas can be found in the liver, spleen, and other organs. These granulomas sometimes obstruct the intestines, urinary tract, and lungs. Advancements in treatment, in particular antifungal agents have greatly increased survival rates, where 90% of patients survive well into adulthood.[19] In the nitroblue tetrazolium reduction test, normal neutrophils, when stimulated, reduce the yellow water-soluble nitroblue tetrazolium to a dark blue insoluble formazan. Neutrophils in chronic granulomatous disease cannot perform this reduction (Figure 29-6). The disease can also be diagnosed through flow cytometry, which uses a fluorescent probe, such as dihydrorhodamine-123,

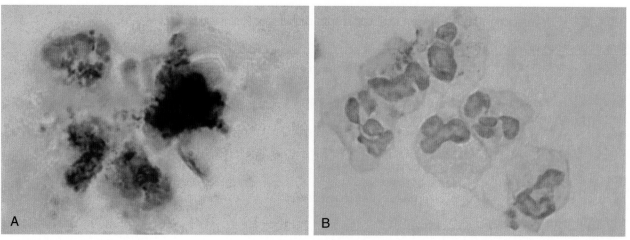

Figure 29-6 Two nitroblue tetrazolium preparations. **A,** Neutrophils from a normal control that have reduced the NBT to a dark formazan. **B,** Neutrophils from a patient with chronic granulomatous disease. (Courtesy Valerie Evans, University of Arizona Medical Center, Tucson, AZ.)

to measure intracellular production of reactive oxygen species.[18]

Leukocyte Adhesion Disorders

Recruitment of leukocytes to the site of inflammation involves capture of leukocytes from peripheral blood, followed by rolling along a vessel wall. This process is mediated through selectins, which interact with their ligands on the surface of leukocytes.[20] Ligand binding induces high-affinity binding of integrins with endothelial cell receptors. The cytoskeleton in leukocytes is reorganized, and cell spreading occurs, which ultimately leads to transmigration of the leukocyte out of the blood and into the tissues.

Leukocyte adhesion disorders (LADs) are rare autosomal recessive inherited disorders that result in the inability of neutrophils and monocytes to adhere to endothelial cells and to transmigrate from the blood to the tissues. The consequence is increased and potentially lethal bacterial infections. The basic defect is a mutation in the genes responsible for the formation of cell adhesion molecules (Chapter 12).

Leukocyte adhesion disorders have been subdivided into three subcategories. LAD I is caused by a mutation in exons 5 to 9 in the gene(s) responsible for β_2 integrin subunits, resulting in either a decreased or truncated form of the β_2 integrin,[21] which is necessary for adhesion to endothelial cells, recognition of bacteria, and outside-in signaling.[22] In addition to experiencing recurrent infections, patients with LAD I frequently have neutrophilia, lymphadenopathy, splenomegaly, and skin lesions. The clinical severity, including number of infections and survival, depends on the amount of the β_2 integrins produced.[23]

LAD II is considerably rarer than LAD I and presents in a similar manner (recurrent infection and neutrophilia), but the leukocytes have normal β_2 integrins. There are molecular defects in *SLC35C1*, which codes for a fucose transporter that moves fucose from the endoplasmic reticulum to the Golgi region.[24] Fucose is needed for posttranslational fucosylation of glycoconjugates, which is required for synthesis of selectin ligands.[25] Clinically, LAD II patients have growth retardation, a coarse face, and other physical deformities.[26] In LAD II the defective fucose transporter leads to an inability to produce functional selectin ligands and defective leukocyte recruitment, which leads to recurring infections. Other clinical findings related to defective fucose transport are absence of blood group H antigen, growth retardation, and neurological defects.[27]

LAD III is a very rare autosomal recessive disease. In LAD III, leukocytes and platelets have normal expression of integrins, but there is failure in response to external signals that would normally result in leukocyte activation.[23] Mutations in *Kindlin-3* have recently been identified as the culprit.[28] Kindlin-3 protein along with talin are required for activation of β integrin and leukocyte rolling. Clinically LAD III patients experience a mild LAD I–like immunodeficiency with recurrent bacterial and fungal infections. In addition, in LAD III, there is decreased platelet integrin GPIIbβ3, resulting in bleeding similar to what is seen in Glanzmann thrombasthenia (Chapter 41).

Miscellaneous Granulocyte Disorders

Myeloperoxidase (MPO) deficiency is characterized by a deficiency in myeloperoxidase in the primary granules of neutrophils and lysosomes of monocyte. Myeloperoxidase normally stimulates production of hypochlorite and hypochlorous acid, which are oxidant agents that attack phagocytized microbes. The disorder is inherited in an autosomal dominant manner with a prevalence of approximately 1 in 2000 individuals.[29] The defect originates through mutation in the *MPO* gene on chromosome 17. Most patients do not experience problematic recurring infections because compensatory pathways are utilized for microbe killing that do not involve myeloperoxidase.[29] Acquired myeloperoxidase deficiency can present in association with hematologic neoplasms and lead poisoning.[30] In the hematology laboratory, MPO deficiency can be easily detected by the Siemens Advia analyzer, which uses myeloperoxidase to identify cells in the automated differential.

Monocyte/Macrophage Lysosomal Storage Diseases

Monocyte/macrophage lysosomal storage diseases can be subdivided into mucopolysaccharide (or glycosaminoglycan [GAG]) storage diseases and lipid storage diseases (Table 29-1). As a group, they represent inherited enzyme deficiencies or defects that result in flawed degradation of phagocytized material and buildup of the partially digested material within the phagocyte. All cells containing lysosomes can be affected, including T lymphocytes.[31]

The *mucopolysaccharidoses* (MPSs) are a family of inherited disorders of GAG degradation. Each MPS is caused by deficient activity of an enzyme necessary for the degradation of dermatan sulfate, heparan sulfate, keratan sulfate, and/or chondroitin sulfate. The partially degraded GAG builds up in the lysosomes and eventually results in physical abnormality and sometimes mental retardation. The MPSs have been subdivided according to which enzyme is defective, which GAG is being stored, and whether the symptoms are severe or attenuated (Table 29-1).[32]

The peripheral blood of a patient with MPSs may appear relatively normal; however, metachromatic Reilly bodies may be seen in neutrophils, monocytes, and lymphocytes (Figure 29-7). Bone marrow may reveal macrophages with large amounts of metachromatic material. Diagnosis relies on assays for the specific enzymes involved. Treatment has consisted of enzyme replacement therapy or hematopoietic stem cell transplantation.[32]

Lipid storage diseases are inherited disorders in which lipid catabolism is defective (Figure 29-8). Two of these disorders are characterized by macrophages with distinctive morphology and are discussed here.

Gaucher disease is the most common of the lysosomal lipid storage diseases. It is an autosomal recessive disorder caused by a defect or deficiency in the catabolic enzyme β-glucocerebrosidase (gene located at *1q21*), which is necessary for glycolipid metabolism. At least 1 in 17 Ashkenazi Jews

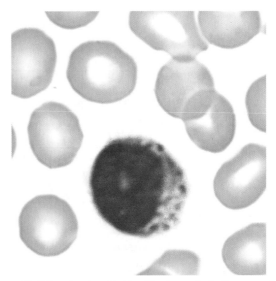

Figure 29-7 Lymphocyte on the blood film for a patient with a mucopolysaccharide storage disorder known as Hurler disease. Notice the dark cytoplasmic granules.

are carriers.[33] More than 300 genetic mutations have been reported,[34] and while some correlations have been found with specific mutations and disease severity and course, the majority of cases (phenotypes) cannot be predicted by genotype. In Gaucher disease there is an accumulation of unmetabolized substrate sphingolipid glucocerebroside in macrophages throughout the body, including osteoclasts in bone and microglia in the brain.

The clinical triad used in diagnosis is hepatomegaly, Gaucher cells in the bone marrow, and increase in serum phosphatase. Gaucher disease has been subdivided into three types based on clinical signs and symptoms (Table 29-2).[35] Neurologic symptoms play a key role in differentiating between the three subtypes. The phenotype is quite heterogeneous, with some patients being completely asymptomatic (seen in Type I),

TABLE 29-1 Variants of Monocyte/Macrophage Lysosomal Storage Disorders

Type	Name	Deficient Enzyme	Substance Stored
Mucopolysaccharidosis			
MPS I—severe	Hurler syndrome	α-l-iduronidase	Dermatan sulfate, heparan sulfate
MPS I—attenuated	Scheie syndrome	α-l-iduronidase	Dermatan sulfate, heparan sulfate
MPS II— severe	Hunter syndrome	Iduronate sulfatase	Dermatan sulfate, heparan sulfate
MPS III	Sanfilippo syndrome type A	Heparan *N*-sulfatase	Heparan sulfate
	Sanfilippo syndrome type B	α-*N*-acetylglucosaminidase	Heparan sulfate
	Sanfilippo syndrome type C	Acetyl–coenzyme A:α-glucosaminide *N*-acetyltransferase	Heparan sulfate
MPS IV	Morquio syndrome type A	Galactose-6-sulfatase	Keratan sulfate, chondroitin-6-sulfate
	Morquio syndrome type B	β-Galactosidase	Keratan sulfate
Lipid Storage Diseases			
Gaucher disease		β-Glucocerebrosidase	Glucocerebroside
Niemann-Pick disease		Sphingomyelinase	Sphingomyelin
Fabry disease		α-Galactosidase	Ceramide trihexoside
Tay-Sachs disease, Sandhoff disease		Hexosaminidase A	G_{M2} ganglioside

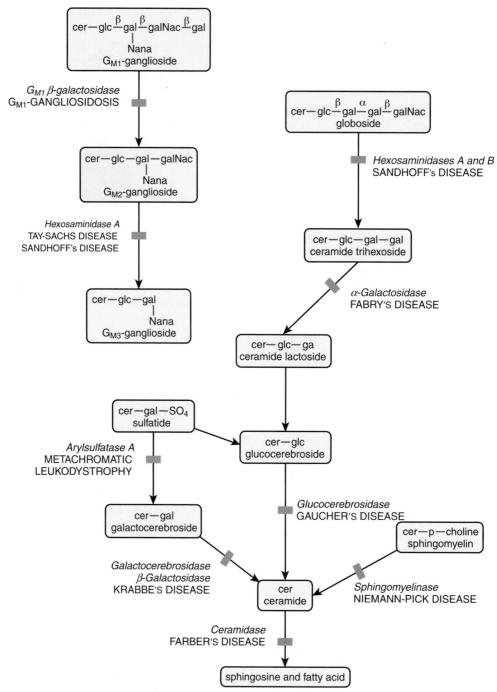

Figure 29-8 Pathways and diseases of sphingolipid metabolism. (From Orkin SH, Fisher DE, Look AT, et al: *Nathan and Oski's hematology of infancy and childhood,* ed 7, Philadelphia, 2009, Saunders.)

TABLE 29-2 Clinical Subtypes of Gaucher Disease

Clinical Features	Type I: Nonneuropathic	Type II: Acute Neuropathic	Type III: Subacute Neuropathic
Clinical onset	Childhood/adulthood	Infancy	Childhood
Hepatosplenomegaly	+	+	+
Skeletal abnormality	+	−	+
Neurodegeneration	−	+++	++
Death	Variable	By 2 years	Second to fourth decade
Ethnic predilection	Ashkenazi Jews	Panethnic	Swedes

NOTE: Absence and severity of features are indicated by − to +++.

while others experience a multitude of clinical problems. Clinical findings are mostly related to the patient's age and the degree of the enzyme deficiency.

Hematologic features include anemia and thrombocytopenia as a result of hypersplenism that is common in these patients. Bone marrow replacement by Gaucher cells may contribute to peripheral cytopenias. The bone marrow contains Gaucher cells, distinctive macrophages occurring individually or in clusters, that have an abundant fibrillar blue-gray cytoplasm with a striated or wrinkled appearance (sometimes described as onion skin–like) (Figure 29-9).[36] A useful test in terms of determining the level of glucocerebroside in storage is chitotriosidase.[37] This biomarker can be used in diagnosis and monitoring of the disease. The periodic acid-Schiff stain tests for mucopolysaccharides in Gaucher cells. Polymerase chain reaction is sometimes used in Ashkenazi Jews to screen for the most common mutations, but to confirm a diagnosis of Gaucher disease, gene sequencing is often needed. In all three forms of the disease, there is a fifteenfold increase for developing hematologic malignancies such as plasma cell neoplasm, chronic lymphocytic leukemia, lymphoma, and acute leukemia.[38]

Treatment of Gaucher disease includes the use of enzyme replacement therapy with recombinant glucocerebrosidase.[39,40] Agents are also available that reduce the amount of the substrate glucocerebroside. Stem cell transplantation offers the potential for cure, but safety is always a concern in allogeneic transplant, where the mortality rate associated with the procedure is high.[41] Another treatment approach is the use of pharmacologic chaperones that are active site-specific competitive glucocerebroside inhibitors.[42]

Pseudo-Gaucher cells can be found in the bone marrow in some patients with thalassemia,[43] chronic myelogenous leukemia,[44] and acute lymphoblastic leukemia.[45] In these diseases, pseudo-Gaucher cells form as a result of excessive cell turnover and overwhelming the glucocerebrosidase enzyme rather than a true decrease in the enzyme. Electron microscopy can distinguish between the two cells because pseudo-Gaucher cells do not contain the tubular inclusions described in Gaucher cells.

Niemann-Pick disease is an autosomal recessive lipid storage disease that has three subtypes: A, B, and C. Types A and B are characterized by recessive mutations in the *SMPD1* gene, which leads to a deficiency in the lysosomal hydrolase enzyme acid sphingomyelinase (ASM) and a subsequent buildup of the substrate sphingomyelin in the liver, kidney, and lungs. In type A, the brain is also affected. In types A and B, Niemann-Pick cells are usually found in the bone marrow. These are macrophages with a foamy cytoplasm packed with lipid-filled lysosomes that appear as vacuoles after staining (Figure 29-10). Type A presents in infancy and is associated with a failure to thrive, hepatosplenomegaly, and a rapid neurodegenerative decline that results in death, usually by age 3 years. In type A, there is less than 5% of normal sphingomyelinase activity. Type B patients have approximately 10% to 20% normal enzyme activity,[46] and the disease presents later in life with a variable clinical course. These patients have little or no neurological symptoms, but many experience severe and progressive hepatosplenomegaly, heart disease, and pulmonary insufficiency.[47]

In Niemann-Pick type C disease there is a decrease in cholesterol effluxing from the intracellular endosome/lysosome to the cytosol. In normal conditions this process is under control of two proteins: Niemann-Pick C I and Niemann-Pick C II. Mutations in these genes results in Niemann-Pick type C disease, where cholesterol, bisphosphate, and sphingolipids build up in lysosomal storage organelles of macrophages.[48] Patients with type C disease present with systemic, neurologic, and psychiatric symptoms.[49] The prognosis in type C is poor. Most patients die before the age of 25 years. The diagnosis can be confirmed through gene sequencing that identifies mutations

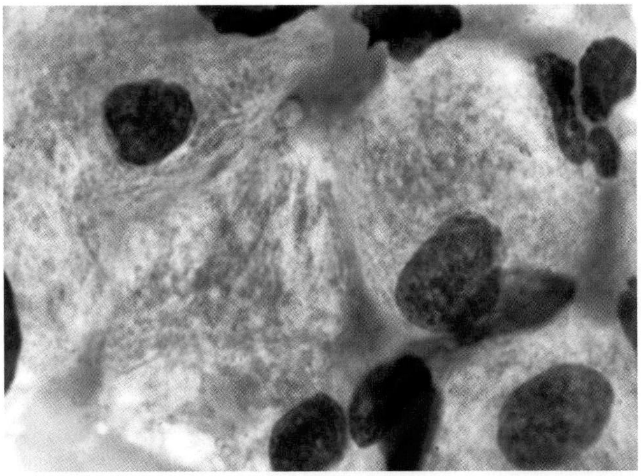

Figure 29-9 Characteristic macrophages with cytoplasmic striations found in the bone marrow of a patient with Gaucher disease. (From Carr JH, Rodak BF: *Clinical hematology atlas*, ed 4, St. Louis, 2013, Saunders.)

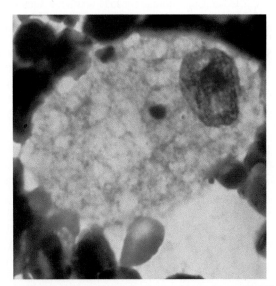

Figure 29-10 Niemann-Pick cell with eccentric nucleus and bubble-like pattern of storage deposit in the cytoplasm. (From Carr JH, Rodak BF: *Clinical hematology atlas*, ed 4, St. Louis, 2013, Saunders.)

in *NPC1* in 95% of cases. Five percent of patients will have mutations in *NPC2*.[50,51]

Morphology, disease characteristics and associated laboratory tests for Gaucher and Niemann-Pick disease are highlighted in Box 29-3.

Genetic B and T Lymphocyte Abnormalities

Functional B and T lymphocyte abnormalities are genetic disorders that generally result in the decreased production of B cells, T cells, or both. They are all associated with an increased risk of infection and secondary malignancy.

T lymphocyte abnormality is best represented by a condition known as *DiGeorge syndrome*. This syndrome is characterized by the absence or underdevelopment of the thymus and thus markedly decreased numbers of T lymphocytes. It is associated with a microdeletion in chromosome band 22q11.2, which is the most common chromosome deletion and occurs in approximately 1 in 3500 births. Individuals with this deletion have a broad range of abnormalities, including defective parathyroid glands, cardiac abnormalities, abnormal facial development, neurologic disorders, and hypocalcemia. Less than 1% of patients with this deletion are athymic, a condition sometimes referred to as *complete DiGeorge syndrome*.[52] Many of these patients are treated with thymus transplantation, with an approximately 75% survival rate.[53]

Sex-linked agammaglobulinemia (XLA) is a B cell disease that is caused most frequently by a mutation in the gene encoding Bruton tyrosine kinase (BTK). Such mutations result in decreased production of BTK, which is important for B cell development, differentiation, and signaling. Without BTK, B lymphocytes fail to reach maturity and will die prematurely.[54,55] Infants with XLA start to display symptoms after 1 to 2 months, once maternal antibodies have been cleared. Recurring bacterial infections ensue and can be life-threatening.

Combined B lymphocyte/T lymphocyte abnormalities include severe combined immunodeficiency (SCID) and Wiskott-Aldrich syndrome. SCID can be divided into two types: adenosine deaminase deficiency and X-linked SCID. Both result in depletions of T, B, and natural killer (NK) lymphocytes. Adenosine deaminase deficiency results in excess amounts of its natural substrates (adenosine and 2′-deoxyadenosine), which cause lymphocyte depletion through a variety of mechanisms.[56]

X-linked SCID is the more common of the two and is caused by a mutation in the gene encoding the IL-2 receptor γ chain, which is shared by several interleukins. The mutation results in T cell lymphopenia, B cells that are dysfunctional, and a lack of NK cells.[57]

Wiskott-Aldrich syndrome is also X-linked and is caused by a mutation in a gene that encodes a protein called *WASp*. The mutation results in low levels or absence of the protein, and affected individuals have immunodeficiency, eczema, and thrombocytopenia. Absence of WASp affects migration, adhesion, and activation of a variety of leukocytes, including T cells, B cells, and NK cells.[58]

QUANTITATIVE ABNORMALITIES OF LEUKOCYTES

Neutrophils

The age-specific reference range for leukocyte subsets is listed in the cover of this book. An increase in neutrophils above 7.0×10^9/L in adults and 8.5×10^9/L in children is referred to as *neutrophilia*. The normal relative neutrophil count is approximately 50% to 70%; however, neutrophilia should always be evaluated using absolute values. The absolute neutrophil count (ANC) is determined by adding the number of segmented and band neutrophils. Some laboratories calculate

---

Box 29-3   Lipid Storage Disease Characteristics and Associated Laboratory Tests

Disease	Morphologic Changes	Clinical Findings	Laboratory Test
Gaucher	Macrophages with blue-gray cytoplasm appear striated or wrinkled (onion skin–like)	Variable depending on subtype: includes neurologic symptoms, hypersplenism, anemia, thrombocytopenia	Chitotriosidase: determines level of storage glucocerebrosidase Periodic-acid-Schiff: stains glucocerebrosidase in macrophages, polymerase chain reaction and gene sequencing: screens for associated genetic mutations
Niemann-Pick type A	Macrophages contain foamy cytoplasm packed with lipid-filled lysosomes that appear as vacuoles after staining	Failure to thrive in infancy, hepatosplenomegaly, rapid neurodegenerative decline that results in death, usually by age 3 years	Acid sphingomyelinase activity level distinguishes type A vs. B
Niemann-Pick type B	Same as above	Presents in first decade to adulthood, hepatosplenomegaly, heart disease, and pulmonary insufficiency, no neurological symptoms	Acid sphingomyelinase activity level distinguishes type A vs. B
Niemann-Pick type C	Same as above	Systemic, neurologic, and psychiatric symptoms, poor prognosis, most patients die before the age of 25 years	Gene sequencing to screen for *NPC1* mutations (95% of cases) or *NPC2* (5% of cases)

the ANC differently and include metamyelocytes, or metamyelocytes and myelocytes in the count. An increase in neutrophils can be related to several factors, including catecholamine-induced demargination or a shift in neutrophils from the marginal pool (cells normally adhering to vessel walls) to the circulating pool. This can occur from strenuous exercise, emotional stress, shock, burns, trauma, labor, or an increase in epinephrine. Neutrophilia also occurs in conditions that result in an increase in bone marrow production or in the shift of neutrophils from the bone marrow storage pool to the peripheral blood. The latter is almost always accompanied by a shift to the left (presence of immature neutrophils). Table 29-3 lists the major causes of neutrophilia.

The term *leukemoid reaction* refers to a reactive leukocytosis above $50 \times 10^9/L$ with neutrophilia and a marked left shift (presence of immature neutrophilic forms). Leukemoid reactions are mostly a result of acute and chronic infection, metabolic disease, inflammation, or response to a malignancy. Leukemoid reaction most often refers to neutrophils, but the increased count may be due to an increase in other types of leukocytes. A neutrophilic leukemoid reaction may be confused with chronic myelogenous leukemia. There are several distinguishing features between the two that are listed in Box 29-4.

The term *leukoerythroblastic reaction* refers to the presence of immature neutrophils, nucleated red blood cells, and teardrop RBCs in the same sample. Leukoerythroblastic reactions are often accompanied by neutrophilia, but not always. Leukoerythroblastic reactions point to the possibility of a space-occupying lesion in the bone marrow. A space-occupying lesion can be a metastatic tumor, fibrosis, lymphoma, leukemia, or simply a marked increase in one of the normal marrow cells (e.g., erythroid hyperplasia seen in hemolytic anemia). A leukoerythroblastic reaction is also strongly associated with primary myelofibrosis.

Neutropenia refers to a decrease in the absolute neutrophil count (ANC) below $2.0 \times 10^9/L$ in white adults and $1.3 \times 10^9/L$ in black adults. The risk of infection increases as the ANC lowers, especially below $1.0 \times 10^9/L$. Severe neutropenia ($<0.5 \times 10^9/L$) further increases the risk. *Agranulocytosis* refers to neutrophil counts of less than $0.5 \times 10^9/L$. Some causes of neutropenia are an increased rate of

TABLE 29-3   Causes of Nonmalignant Neutrophilia and Neutropenia

Neutrophilia	Neutropenia	Neutrophilia	Neutropenia
• Emotional	• Drugs	• Uremia	• Sjögren syndrome
• Strenuous exercise	• **Analgesic/Antiinflammatory:** acetaminophen, ibuprofen, indomethacin	• Eclampsia	• Felty syndrome
• Trauma/injury		• Malignancy	• Overwhelming infections
• Pregnancy: labor and delivery	• **Antibiotics:** cephalosporins, chloramphenicol, clindamycin, gentamicin, penicillin, vancomycin, tetracycline	• Leukocyte adhesion deficiency	• Splenomegaly
• Postsurgery		• Familial cold urticaria	• Hemodialysis
• Acute hemorrhage	• **Anticonvulsants:** carbamazepine, mephenytoin, phenytoin	• Hereditary neutrophilia	• Decreased or ineffective hematopoiesis
• Infections: bacterial, some viral			• Copper deficiency
• Burns	• **Antidepressants:** amitriptyline, amoxapine, doxepin		• Alcoholism
• Surgery			• Babies born from hypertensive mothers
• Myocardial infarction	• **Antihistamines:** cimetidine, ranitidine		• Constitutional
• Pancreatitis	• **Antimalarials:** chloroquine, dapsone, quinine		• Shwachman-Diamond syndrome
• Vasculitis	• **Cardiovascular:** methyldopa, propranolol, captopril		• Severe congenital neutropenia
• Colitis			• Cyclic neutropenia
• Autoimmune disease	• **Diuretics:** chlorothiazide, hydrochlorothiazide		• Fanconi anemia
• Acute hemorrhage/ hemolysis	• **Antianxiety/hypnotics:** benzodiazepines, meprobamate		• Dyskeratosis congenita
• Steroids	• **Hypoglycemics:** chlorpropamide, tolbutamide		• Common variable immunodeficiency syndrome
• Lithium	• **Phenothiazides:** chlorpromazine, phenothiazines		• Hyper-IgM syndrome
• Colony-stimulating factors (G-CSF)	• **Others:** allopurinol, clozapine, levamisole		• X-linked agammaglobulinemia
• Smoking	• Radiation		• Reticular dysgenesis
• Chronic blood loss	• Toxins		• Glycogen storage disease, type Ib
• Metabolic ketoacidosis	• Immune mediated		• Chediak-Higashi syndrome
	• Alloimmune neonatal neutropenia		• Griscelli syndrome, type 2
	• Autoimmune neutropenia		• Hermansky-Pudlak syndrome, type 2
	• Lupus erythematosus		• Myelokathexis/WHIM syndrome
	• Rheumatoid arthritis		• Barth syndrome
			• Cohen syndrome

Adapted from Kaushansky K: *Williams hematology,* ed 8, New York, 2010, McGraw-Hill, pp 951-950; and Foucar K: *Bone marrow pathology,* ed 3, Chicago, 2010, ASCP Press, p 209.

BOX 29-4 Distinguishing between Chronic Myelogenous Leukemia and Leukemoid Reaction

Chronic Myelogenous Leukemia (Malignant)

Increases in all granulocytes, including eosinophils and basophils. Occasional blast may be seen.

Dyspoietic morphology such as mixed eosinophil/basophil granulation and pseudo-Pelger-Huët cells may be encountered.

Involvement of platelets (may be increased), including giant, hypogranular, and/or bizarre forms.

Leukocyte alkaline phosphatase score is markedly decreased.

Leukemoid Reaction (Reactive)

Increase in neutrophils, including immature forms. Blasts are only rarely seen.

Reactive morphologic changes, including toxic granulation, Döhle bodies, and, less commonly, cytoplasmic vacuolization, are present.

Normal platelet morphology and number.

Increased leukocyte alkaline phosphatase score.

---

removal/destruction of neutrophils from the blood; fewer neutrophils being released from the bone marrow to the blood as a result of decreased production or ineffective hematopoiesis, where neutrophils are present in the bone marrow but are not released into the blood because they are defective; changes in ratio of circulating versus marginal pool of neutrophils; or a combination of the above.

Neutropenia can also be classified as inherited or acquired. Table 29-3 lists the causes of neutropenia. Acquired causes of neutropenia are much more common than inherited causes. Immune-mediated neutropenia is caused by antibody binding to neutrophil antigens. In **alloimmune neonatal neutropenia**, maternal IgG crosses the placenta and binds to neutrophil-specific antigens inherited from the father, such as FcγRIIIb, NB1, or HLA.[59,60] Alloimmune neonatal neutropenia occurs in approximately 1 in 2000 births. The severity of the neutropenia varies. Neutrophil counts rise after a few months, consistent with the half-life of the maternal antibody. **Autoimmune neutropenia in children** is a primary illness, with moderate to severe neutropenia developing as a result of antibodies to HNA-1. The disease tends to be self-limiting, with resolution of neutrophil counts after 7 to 24 months.[61] **Secondary autoimmune neutropenia** is associated with autoimmune disorders such as rheumatoid arthritis and associated Felty syndrome, systemic lupus erythematosis, and Sjogren syndrome. In addition to antineutrophil antibodies, other factors may also induce neutropenia in secondary autoimmune neutropenia, including immune complex deposition, granulopoiesis-inhibiting cytokines, and splenomegaly. Over 100 drugs in use today are associated with neutropenia. Table 29-3 contains a partial listing. The annual rate of occurrence is 3 to 12 cases per million.[62,63] The mechanism of drug-induced neutropenia may be related to a dose-dependent toxicity on cell replication in hematopoiesis. Another cause may be immunologic and occurs when a particular drug is given subsequent to the initial exposure that resulted in antibody formation.[64]

Neutropenia may also result from infection, such as viral infection of hematopoietic progenitor cells, suppression of hematopoiesis by inflammatory cytokines, and increased usage of neutrophils due to overwhelming infection.

Intrinsic (constitutional/congenital) neutropenias are a relatively rare group of inherited disorders that usually present at birth. They are due to either decreased production from marrow hypoplasia or proliferation defect. Clinical presentation can be quite heterogeneous, but bacterial infections are the biggest risk. These infections can be life-threatening and/or diminish quality of life. However, antibiotic prophylaxis and therapy and the use of colony-stimulating factors such as G-CSF have lowered this risk and improved the quality of life for the majority of these patients.[65] All of the congenital neutropenias have an increased risk for developing secondary hematologic neoplasms, and G-CSF has been linked with an increased risk for secondary leukemia.[66,67] The intrinsic causes of neutropenia are listed in Table 29-3.

Shwachman-Diamond syndrome, or **Shwachman-Bodian-Diamond syndrome**, is an autosomal recessive disorder characterized by marrow failure, pancreatic insufficiency, and skeletal abnormalities. Intermittent neutropenia that fluctuates from severely low to near normal is the most common hematologic finding, affecting 88% to 100% of patients.[68] Mild normocytic to macrocytic normochromic anemia and reticulocytopenia is seen in approximately 80% of patients.[69,70] Thrombocytopenia occurs in 24% to 88% of patients.[71,72] Dysplastic changes involving all three granulocyte lineages are not uncommon. There is an increased risk for transformation to myelodysplasia and acute myeloid leukemia, which for many patients is a terminal event.

Congenital severe neutropenia consists of Kostmann syndrome and related diseases. Kostmann syndrome, or infantile genetic agranulocytosis, is an autosomal recessive disease characterized by severe neutropenia (often $< 0.2 \times 10^9$/L) that presents shortly after birth and bone marrow granulocyte hypoplasia with maturation arrest at the promyelocyte stage. In cyclic neutropenia, approximately 50% of patients have mutations in *ELANE/ELA2*, the gene that codes for neutrophil elastase.[73] Patients with cyclic neutropenia have periods of severe neutropenia every 21 days, during which time there is increased risk for fevers, bacterial infections, mouth ulcers, and sometimes gangrene, bacteremia, and septic shock. Administration of G-CSF has greatly reduced these neutropenia-associated events.[74]

Chronic idiopathic neutropenia in adults predominantly affects women 18 to 35 years of age. The bone marrow is quite variable between patients but generally shows more immature neutrophils than mature neutrophils, suggesting that cells are lost during maturation. Clinical severity is related to the degree of neutropenia. G-CSF has been shown to be a very useful treatment in these patients.

Fanconi anemia is a rare autosomal recessive or X-linked inherited disease characterized by variable degrees of bone marrow failure, peripheral cytopenias, and an increased risk for hematologic malignancies and other cancers.[75] Chapter 22 contains more information about Fanconi anemia.

Dyskeratosis congenita is a sex-linked recessive, autosomal dominant or autosomal recessively inherited disorder with a heterogeneous presentation.[76] In the classic form of the disease, patients have mucocutaneous abnormalities, abnormal skin pigmentation, nail dystrophy, and leukoplakia. Most patients also have bone marrow failure and increased risk for malignancy. Chapter 22 has more information about dyskeratosis congenita.

Eosinophils

Several factors influence the number of eosinophils in circulation: bone marrow proliferation rate and release into the bloodstream, movement from the blood into the extravascular tissues, and cell survival/destruction once the eosinophils have moved into the tissues. *Eosinophilia* is defined as an absolute eosinophil count above 0.4×10^9/L. Nonmalignant causes of eosinophilia are generally a result of cytokine stimulation, especially from interleukin-3 and interleukin-5 (IL3 and IL5).[77,78] Most causes of eosinophilia can be divided into two broad categories, depending on geography. In underdeveloped areas of the world, increased peripheral blood eosinophils are seen in patients with parasite infestation, especially helminthes and protozoa. A major function of eosinophils is degranulation, where substances are released that damage an offending organism (i.e., parasites) or target cell.[79] In developed countries eosinophilia is most often associated with allergic conditions, including asthma, hay fever, urticarial, and atopic dermatitis.[80,81] Eosinophilia is also seen in scarlet fever, HIV, fungal infections, autoimmune disorders, and hypersensitivity to antibiotics and antiseizure medications. In addition, abnormalities in cytokine regulation and expression in some neoplasms result in a reactive eosinophilia. For example, reactive eosinophilia is seen in acute lymphoblastic leukemia, subtype t(5;14).[82] In some cancers, eosinophils are able to penetrate solid tumors, allowing tumoricidal cytokines to bring about tumor necrosis.[83] If an individual is found to have eosinophilia ($>1.5 \times 10^9$/L) lasting more than 6 months without an identifiable cause, the diagnosis is most likely *hypereosinophilic syndrome,* or HES.[84] HES is considered to be a myeloproliferative neoplasm and will therefore not be discussed further in this chapter.

Eosinopenia is defined as an absolute eosinophil count of less than 0.09×10^9/L and can be difficult to detect because the normal eosinophil reference range is very low. Eosinopenia is most often associated with conditions that result in marrow hypoplasia, specifically involving leukocytes. Another common cause of decreased eosinophils is infection or inflammation that is accompanied by neutrophilia. Eosinophils move into the tissues under these circumstances, and marrow release of eosinophils may be inhibited. Absolute eosinopenia has also been reported in autoimmune

disorders, steroid therapy, stress, sepsis, and acute inflammatory states.[85,86]

Basophils

Basophilia is defined as an absolute basophil count greater than 0.15×10^9/L. The most common cause of basophilia is the presence of a malignant myeloproliferative neoplasm such as chronic myelogenous leukemia, which is covered in Chapter 33. Nonmalignant causes of basophilia are rare and include allergic rhinitis, hypersensitivity to drugs or food, chronic infections, hypothyroidism, chronic inflammatory conditions, radiation therapy, and bee stings.[87,88]

Monocytes

Monocytosis is defined as an absolute monocyte count greater than 1.0×10^9/L in adults and greater than 3.5×10^9/L in neonates. Monocytosis is associated with a wide range of nonmalignant conditions because of their participation in acute and chronic inflammation and infections, immunologic conditions, hypersensitivity reactions, and tissue repair. Monocytosis is frequently the first sign of recovery from acute overwhelming infection or severe neutropenia (most commonly after cancer chemotherapy). Monocytosis in these conditions is considered a positive sign of recovery. Monocytosis when due to administration of G-CSF or GM-CSF may be accompanied by reactive changes in monocyte morphology. Monocytosis is associated with a number of neutropenic disorders. In cyclic neutropenia, monocytosis occurs inversely with neutropenia in the 21-day cycle. A listing of the conditions associated with nonmalignant monocytosis is provided in Table 29-4.[89-97]

Monocytopenia, defined as an absolute monocyte count of less than 0.2×10^9/L, is very rare in conditions that do not also involve cytopenias of other lineage(s), such as aplastic anemia or chemotherapy-induced cytopenias. However, absolute monocytopenia has been found in patients receiving steroid therapy[98] or hemodialysis, or in sepsis.[99] Viral infections, especially those due to the Epstein-Barr virus (EBV), can cause monocytopenia (Table 29-4).[100]

Lymphocytes

The definition of *lymphocytosis* varies with the age of the individual. Children older than 2 weeks and younger than 8 to 10 years normally have higher absolute lymphocyte counts than adults. Lymphocytosis in young children is defined as an absolute lymphocyte count greater than 10.0×10^9/L, whereas in adults it is defined as a count greater than 4.5×10^9/L. As can be seen from the tables inside the front cover of this book, newborn infants have lymphocyte counts very similar to those of adults. The reference range for relative lymphocytes is approximately 20% to 40%. This number, however, should not be used to define lymphocytosis. Blood smear review criteria should be based on the absolute numbers rather than the relative percentage of lymphocytes present.

Lymphocytoses can be subdivided into those with and those without reactive morphologic alterations. See Table 29-5 for a listing of disorders that result in benign lymphocytosis.

TABLE 29-4 Reactive Causes of Monocytosis

Monocytosis

Infection
- Tuberculosis
- Viral
- Malaria
- Brucellosis
- Leishmaniasis
- Fungal
- Subacute bacterial endocarditis
- Syphilis
- Protozoal

Recovery from acute infection

Recovery from neutropenia

Immunologic/Autoimmune
- Systemic lupus erythematosus
- Rheumatoid arthritis
- Autoimmune neutropenia
- Inflammatory bowel disease
- Myositis
- Sarcoidosis

Hematologic
- Acute/chronic neutropenia
- Cyclic neutropenia
- Wiskott-Aldrich syndrome
- Drug-induced neutropenia
- Hemolysis
- Immune thrombocytopenia

Drugs
- Colony-stimulating factors
- Olanzapine
- Carbamazepine
- Phenytoin
- Phenobarbital
- Valproic acid

Cancer
- Carcinoma
- Sarcoma
- Plasma cell dyscrasias
- Lymphoma

Stress
- Trauma
- Myocardial infarction
- Intense exercise

Splenectomy

Gastointestinal disease
- Alcoholic liver disease
- Sprue

Adapted from Foucar K: *Bone marrow pathology,* ed 3, Chicago, 2010, ASCP Press, p 199.

The definition of *lymphocytopenia* is age-dependent. Lymphocytopenia in young children is defined as an absolute lymphocyte count below $2.0 \times 10^9/L$, whereas in adults it is defined as a count below $1.0 \times 10^9/L$. Nonmalignant causes of lymphocytopenia can be subdivided into inherited and acquired and are listed in Table 29-5.

TABLE 29-5 Causes of Nonmalignant Lymphocytosis and Lymphocytopenia

Lymphocytosis	Lymphocytopenia
Reactive Morphology	**Inherited**

Lymphocytosis — **Reactive Morphology**

Infection
- Infectious mononucleosis
- Cytomegalovirus Infection
- Hepatitis
- Acute HIV infection
- Adenovirus
- Chickenpox
- Herpes
- Influenza
- Paramyxovirus (mumps)
- Rubella (measles)
- Roseola
- Mumps
- ß-Hemolytic streptococci
- Brucellosis
- Paratyphoid fever
- Toxoplasmosis
- Typhoid fever
- Listeria
- Mycoplasma
- Syphilis

Miscellaneous
- Idiosyncratic drug reactions
- Postvaccination
- Sudden onset of stress from myocardial infarction
- Allergic reaction
- Hyperthyroidism
- Malnutrition

Nonreactive Morphology
- Bordetella pertussis (whooping cough)
- Acute infectious lymphocytosis
- Polyclonal B-lymphocytosis

Lymphocytopenia — **Inherited**

Congenital immunodeficiency diseases
- Severe combined immunodeficiency disease
- Common variable immune deficiency
- Ataxia-telangiectasia
- Wiskott-Aldrich syndrome
- Others

Acquired

Aplastic anemia

Infections
- Acquired immunodeficiency syndrome
- Severe acute respiratory syndrome
- West Nile
- Hepatitis
- Influenza
- Herpes
- Measles
- Tuberculosis
- Typhoid fever
- Pneumonia
- Rickettsiosis
- Ehrichiosis
- Sepsis
- Malaria

Iatrogenic
- Immunosuppressive agents
- Stevens-Johnson syndrome
- Chemotherapy
- Radiation
- Platelet or stem cell apheresis collection
- Major surgery

Systemic disease
- Autoimmune diseases
- Hodgkin lymphoma
- Carcinoma
- Primary myelofibrosis
- Protein-losing enteropathy
- Renal failure

Nutritional/dietary
- Ethanol abuse
- Zinc deficiency

Adapted from Kaushansky K: *Williams hematology,* ed 8, New York, 2010, McGraw-Hill, pp. 1141-1151; and Foucar K: *Bone marrow pathology,* ed 3, Chicago, 2010, p 450.

QUALITATIVE (MORPHOLOGIC) CHANGES

Neutrophils

Neutrophil reaction to infection, inflammation, stress, or administration of recombinant colony-stimulating factor (CSF) therapy may affect the number and types of circulating neutrophils (left shift), induce morphologic change, or both. While these changes may be considered "abnormal," they usually reflect a normal, reactive response. Depending on the severity of the infection, inflammation, or dose/reaction to CSF, the left shift can range from mild (an increase in band neutrophils and metamyelocytes) to moderate (metamyelocytes, myelocytes, and an occasional promyelocyte) to marked (myelocytes, promyelocytes, and an occasional blast form).

Reactive morphologic changes in neutrophils include toxic granulation, Döhle bodies, cytoplasmic vacuoles, hypersegmentation, and pyknosis. *Toxic granulation* of neutrophils appears as dark, blue-black granules in the cytoplasm of neutrophils: segmented, bands, and metamyelocytes. Toxic granules are peroxidase positive and reflect an increase in acid mucosubstance within primary, azurophilic granules of neutrophils.[101] The result is a lowered pH in phagolysosomes that enhances microbial killing.[101] There is a positive correlation between levels of C-reactive protein (acute phase protein) and the percentage of neutrophils with toxic granulation;[102] therefore, the intensity of toxic granulation is a general measure of the degree of inflammation.[103] In addition, toxic granulation can be seen in various infections as well as in patients who have received CSF. Toxic granulation, especially when intense, can mimic the granulation found in the mucopolysaccharidoses and Alder-Reilly anomaly. One helpful defining characteristic of toxic granulation is that in most patients not all neutrophils are equally affected (Figure 29-11). Box 29-5A highlights reactive neutrophil morphologic changes and associated conditions.

Döhle bodies are cytoplasmic inclusions consisting of remnants of ribosomal ribonucleic acid (RNA) arranged in parallel rows.[104] Döhle bodies are typically found in band and segmented neutrophils (Figure 29-12) and often in cells containing toxic granulation. They appear as intracytoplasmic, pale blue round or elongated bodies between 1 and 5 μm in diameter. They are usually located in close apposition to cellular membranes. A delay in preparing the blood after collection in EDTA tube may affect Döhle body appearance in that they are more gray than blue and in some cases may not be visible. Döhle bodies are relatively nonspecific. Their presence has been associated with a wide range of conditions, including bacterial infections, sepsis, and normal pregnancy.[104,105]

Cytoplasmic vacuolation of neutrophils is seen less often than toxic granules and Döhle bodies. Vacuoles generally reflect phagocytosis, either of self (autophagocytosis) or of extracellular material. Autophagocytic vacuoles tend to be small (approximately 2 μm) and distributed throughout the cytoplasm. In addition, autophagocytosis can be induced by drugs such as sulfonamides and chloroquine,[100] storage in EDTA (artefactual) for more than 2 hours, autoantibodies,[106] acute alcoholism,[107] and exposure to high doses of radiation.[108] Phagocytic vacuoles caused by either bacteria or fungi are often seen in septic patients. Phagocytic vacuoles are large (up to 6 μm) and are frequently accompanied by toxic granulation (Figure 29-13). When vacuoles are seen, especially when not accompanied by toxic granulation, Döhle bodies, or both, artefactual causes should be suspected. The blood collection time should be compared with when the smear was made. As stated above, this time should not exceed 2 hours.

When phagocytic vacuoles are seen, a careful examination should be made for bacteria or yeast within the vacuoles. Cases of ehrlichiosis and anaplasmosis have been increasing in the United States over the past decade.[109] *Ehrlichia* and *Anaplasma* are small, obligate, intracellular bacteria transmitted by ticks to humans and other vertebrate hosts. These organisms grow as a cluster (morula) in neutrophils (*A. phagocytophilum* and *E. ewingii*) (Figure 29-14, *A*) and in monocytes (*E. chaffeensis*) (Figure 29-14, *B*). Leukopenia, thrombocytopenia, and elevated liver enzymes are common laboratory findings, and anemia may develop in about half the cases of human monocytic ehrlichiosis.[110] Intracellular aggregates in neutrophils or monocytes may occasionally be detected in the first week of infection on a Wright-Giemsa–stained peripheral blood film or a buffy coat preparation. Immunofluorescent antibody titers or polymerase chain reaction testing may help to confirm the diagnosis.[110] Early diagnosis is essential because antibiotic treatment with doxycycline is very effective and can prevent serious complications.

Pyknotic nuclei in neutrophils generally indicate imminent cell death. In a pyknotic nucleus, nuclear water has been lost and the chromatin becomes very dense and dark; however, filaments can still be seen between segments.[111,112] Pyknotic nuclei should not be confused with necrotic nuclei found in dead cells. Necrotic nuclei are rounded fragments of nucleus with no filaments and no chromatin pattern (Figure 29-15).

Degranulation is a common finding in activated neutrophils and eosinophils (Figure 29-16). Both primary and secondary granules are emptied into phagosomes, and secondary granules are also secreted into the extracellular space.[113] In vitro degranulation in eosinophils often occurs when cellular membranes are

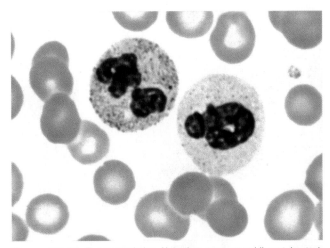

Figure 29-11 Toxic granulation. Note that one neutrophil contains toxic granulation and the other does not. Also note that the toxic granules are clustered in some areas of the cytoplasm. Both of these findings help in distinguishing toxic granulation from poor staining or from the dark granules seen in Alder-Reilly anomaly.

Box 29-5A Reactive Morphologic Changes in Neutrophils

Reactive Change	Morphology	Associated with
Toxic granulation	Dark, blue-black cytoplasmic granules	Inflammation, infection, administration of granulocyte colony stimulation factor (G-CSF)
Dohle bodies	Intracytoplasmic pale blue round or elongated bodies between 1 and 5 μm in diameter, usually adjacent to cellular membranes.	Nonspecific finding, or associated with bacterial infections, sepsis, and pregnancy
Cytoplasmic vacuolization of neutrophils	Small to large circular clear areas in cytoplasm, rarely may contain organism	Septicemia or other infection; autophagocytosis secondary to drug ingestion, acute alcoholism, or storage artifact; vacuoles are sometimes seen in conjunction with toxic granulation.

---

disrupted during the process of making the blood film. Eosinophils are fragile.

Cytoplasmic swelling may be caused by actual osmotic swelling of the cytoplasm or by increased adhesion to the glass slide by stimulated neutrophils. Regardless of the cause, the result is a variation in neutrophil size or neutrophil anisocytosis (Figure 29-17).

Monocytes

Occasional immature monocytes may be seen in the peripheral blood in response to infection or inflammation, but this is not as common as a neutrophilic left shift (Figure 29-18). Reactive changes may be seen in monocytes in infections, during recovery from bone marrow aplasia, and after GM-CSF administration. The nucleus can become thin and band-like in areas and may appear to be segmenting (Figure 29-19). Reactive changes also include increased cytoplasmic volume, increased numbers of cytoplasmic granules, and evidence of phagocytic activity

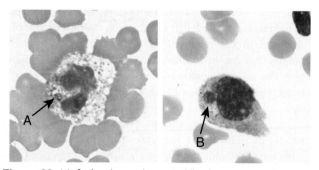

Figure 29-14 A, *Anaplasma phagocytophilum* in a neutrophil. **B,** *Ehrlichia chaffeensis* in a monocytic cell. (Courtesy J. Stephen Dumler, MD, Division of Medical Microbiology, The Johns Hopkins Medical Institution, Baltimore, MD.)

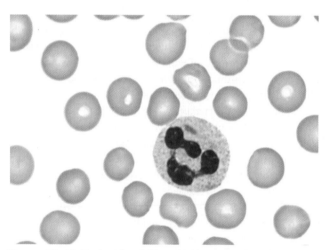

Figure 29-12 Neutrophil containing a bluish cytoplasmic inclusion known as a Döhle body.

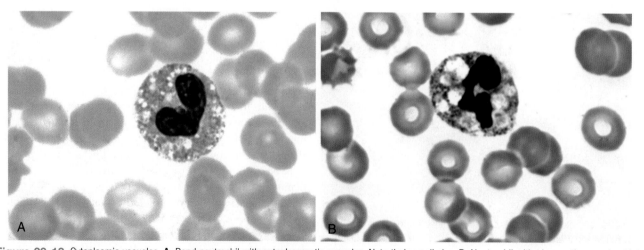

Figure 29-13 Cytoplasmic vacuoles. **A,** Band neutrophil with autophagocytic vacuoles. Note their small size. **B,** Neutrophil with phagocytic vacuoles. Note their larger size. Other evidence of toxicity in this cell is the pyknotic nucleus.

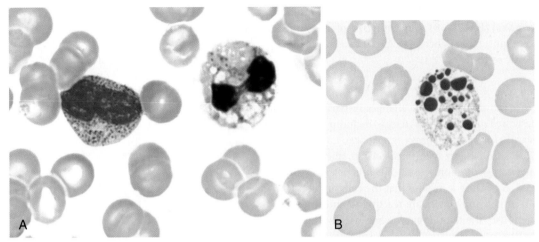

Figure 29-15 A, Upper cell is a neutrophil whose nucleus is dehydrated, which makes it very dark and dense. Note that there is still a filament between the segments. This is referred to as a pyknotic cell. The cell is also highly vacuolated. **B,** Neutrophil that has died. Note that the nucleus has disintegrated into numerous rounded spheres of DNA with no filaments. This is referred to as a necrotic or necrobiotic cell. (**B** from Carr JH, Rodak BF: *Clinical hematology atlas,* ed 3, St. Louis, 2009, Saunders.)

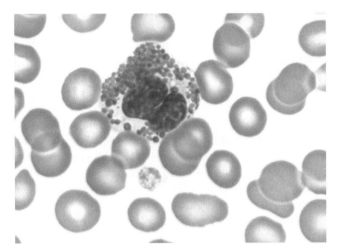

Figure 29-16 Partially degranulated eosinophil. This cell was found on the blood film for a patient with trichinosis.

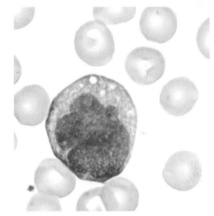

Figure 29-18 Immature monocyte. (From Carr JH, Rodak BF: *Clinical hematology atlas,* ed 4, St. Louis, 2013, Saunders.)

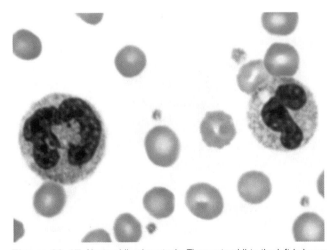

Figure 29-17 Neutrophil anisocytosis. The neutrophil to the left is larger than the other neutrophil. This is often caused by cytoplasmic swelling.

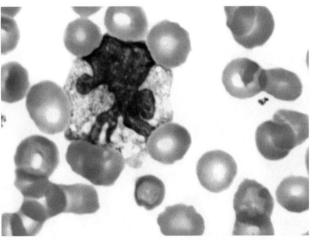

Figure 29-19 Reactive monocyte with contorted nucleus. Other evidence of toxicity is the several vacuoles in the cytoplasm.

(cytoplasmic vacuolation, intracellular debris, and irregular cytoplasmic borders) (Box 29-5B). Large numbers of immature monocytes occur most often in hematologic neoplasms involving the monocytic series.

Lymphocytes

Over the years, reactive morphologic changes in lymphocytes have been described using various terms, including *variant lymphocytes, reactive lymphocytes, effector lymphocytes, transformed lymphocytes, Turk cells, Downey cells, immunoblasts,* and *atypical lymphocytes. Atypical* is commonly used, but it is probably the least suitable of all because it implies that the cells are abnormal when in fact the lymphocytes are reacting to antigen in a normal manner. Also, the term *atypical,* when used by the cytology lab in a Pap smear result, suggests a suspicious, possibly precancerous lesion. Regardless of the labels that are applied, it is very important that the clinical staff understand the meaning behind the terms the lab uses to describe the reactive and malignant-appearing lymphocytes reported in the WBC differential.

Reactive lymphocytes are the result of complex morphologic and biochemical events that occur as lymphocytes are stimulated when interacting with antigens in peripheral lymphoid organs (Figures 29-20 and 29-21). B and T lymphocyte activation results in the transformation of small, resting lym-

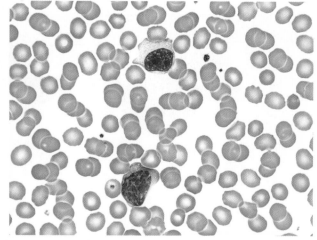

Figure 29-21 Reactive (variant) lymphocytes from a patient with infectious mononucleosis.

phocytes into proliferating larger cells. These lymphocytes spill into peripheral circulation, which is what is encountered upon smear review. Reactive lymphocytes often present as a heterogeneous population of various shapes and sizes. There is variation in the nuclear/cytoplasmic ratio, nuclear shape, and the chromatin pattern, which is generally clumped, but some cells may demonstrate chromatin patterns that are less mature (less clumped). Nucleoli may be visible. Most obvious in reactive lymphocytes is an increase in basophilic cytoplasm that may vary in intensity within and between cells. The cytoplasm may be indented by surrounding RBCs, but it is important to realize that other cells, including blasts, may also show similar indentation. A *plasmacytoid lymphocyte* is a type of reactive lymphocyte that has some of the morphologic features of plasmacytes (Figure 29-22). However, because reactive lymphocytes may be activated T or B cells, it is important to understand that *plasmacytoid* is a morphologic term and does not imply lineage. Features of reactive lymphocytes are summarized in Box 29-5C.

Box 29-5B Reactive Morphologic Changes in Monocytes

Morphology	Associated with
Thin and band-like, or segmentation of nucleus; increased cytoplasmic volume and granulation, and/or evidence of phagocytic activity (cytoplasmic vacuolation, intracellular debris, and irregular cytoplasmic borders)	Infection, recovery from bone marrow aplasia, and granulocyte monocyte colony stimulating factor (GM-CSF) administration

---

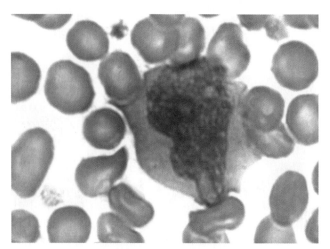

Figure 29-20 Reactive (variant) lymphocyte.

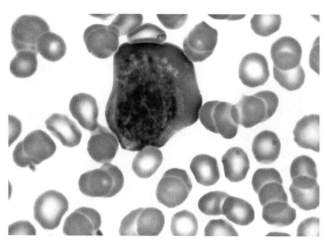

Figure 29-22 Reactive (variant) lymphocyte (plasmacytoid).

Box 29-5C Morphologic Changes in Reactive Lymphocytes

- Heterogeneous population of various shapes and sizes.
- Cells exhibit increased amount of variably basophilic cytoplasm.
- Lymphocyte population exhibits variation in nuclear/cytoplasmic ratio and/or nuclear shape.
- Chromatin is usually clumped however some cells may demonstrate less mature (less clumped) pattern.
- Nucleoli may be visible.
- The cytoplasm may be indented by surrounding RBCs

Box 29-6 Infectious Mononucleosis: Clinical and Lab Findings

Clinical Manifestations	Laboratory Test Results

• Common
  • Sore throat
  • Dysphagia
  • Fever
  • Chills
  • Cervical lymphadenopathy
  • Fatigue
  • Headache
• Less common
  • Hepatomegaly
  • Elevated transaminases
  • Splenomegaly
  • Hemolytic anemia
  • Thrombocytopenia
	• WBC: 10–30 x 10^9/L due to an absolute lymphocytosis
	• Reactive lymphocyte morphology
	• Positive heterophile antibody test
	• Positive EBV specific antigen & antibody tests

Epstein-Barr Virus (EBV)–Related Infections

Most humans are subclinically infected with EBV, which has been associated with several benign and malignant diseases but has only been proven to be the causative agent in a few, including infectious mononucleosis.

INFECTIOUS MONONUCLEOSIS (IM)

When primary infection with Epstein-Barr virus occurs in childhood, it often goes unnoticed. Infectious mononucleosis is the symptomatic illness that ensues whenever adolescents and adults are infected. The incubation period of infectious mononucleosis is about 3 to 7 weeks, and during this time the virus preferentially infects B lymphocytes through attachment of viral envelope glycoprotein 350/220 to CD21 (C3d complement receptors).[114] The oropharynx epithelial cells are also infected, but the mechanism is unclear because these cells do not express CD21. The cellular response in IM is important in the control of the infection and is characterized by proliferation and activation of natural killer (NK) lymphocytes, CD4$^+$ T cells, and CD8$^+$ memory cytotoxic T cells (EBV-CTLs) in response to B cell infection. Most of the circulating reactive lymphocytes seen in circulation represent activated T cells.

Common clinical manifestations include sore throat, dysphagia, fever, chills, cervical lymphadenopathy, fatigue, and headache. Hematologic findings resemble those seen in many viral disorders. The WBC count is usually elevated to a range of 10—30 × 10^9/L or more with an absolute lymphocytosis. There is a wide variation in lymphocyte morphology, with up to 50% or higher exhibiting reactive features. Complications that may occur are generally mild and include hepatosplenomegaly (and elevated transaminases), hemolytic anemia, and moderate thrombocytopenia. In rare cases patients may develop aplastic anemia, disseminated intravascular coagulation, thrombotic thrombocytopenic purpura, hemolytic uremic syndrome, Guillain-Barré syndrome, or other neurologic complications.[115] The incidence of IM in the United States is 500 cases per 100,000 annually. It has its highest frequency in young adults, aged 15 to 24 years,[116] although infections have been reported in patients 3 months to 70 years of age.

Testing for infectious mononucleosis includes rapid screening tests for the detection of heterophile antibodies, antibodies stimulated by the EBV that cross-react with antigens found on sheep and horse red cells. However, not everyone with infectious mononucleosis will produce heterophile antibodies, especially children. Definitive testing for EBV infection includes a panel of antigen and antibody tests for VCA, EBNA, and IgG/IgM antibodies against VCA and EBNA. Cytomegalovirus is capable of causing a mononucleosis syndrome with similar clinical features.

Clinical and laboratory findings associated with infectious mononucleosis are summarized in Box 29-6.

SUMMARY

- Pelger-Huët anomaly is a genetic disorder resulting in hypolobulated mature leukocytes. These cells can be confused with immature neutrophils. An acquired form of hyposegmentation called *pseudo-PHA* can be seen in some malignant myeloproliferative neoplasms.
- Alder-Reilly anomaly is a manifestation of the mucopolysaccharidosis characterized by metachromatic granules in leukocytes, which can be confused with toxic granulation.

- Chediak-Higashi syndrome is an inherited lethal disorder characterized by giant lysosomes in granular cells and dysfunctional leukocytes.
- May-Hegglin anomaly is characterized by thrombocytopenia, giant platelets, and Döhle body–like inclusions in leukocytes. Most affected individuals are asymptomatic.
- Chronic granulomatous disease is an inherited disorder of the NADPH oxidase system resulting in neutrophils that are incapable

of killing many microorganisms due to a failure in the respiratory burst, which is necessary to produce antibacterial agents.

- Leukocyte adhesion disorders are a group of disorders caused by mutations in the genes for adhesive molecules required for cells to migrate from the blood into the tissues.

- The mucopolysaccharidoses are a group of disorders, each of which is associated with a specific defect in an enzyme necessary for the degradation of GAGs such as heparan sulfate, keratan sulfate, dermatan sulfate, and chondroitin sulfate. The result is the buildup of partially digested GAGs within macrophages and leukocytes and clinical symptoms.

- The lipid storage diseases are a group of disorders, each of which is associated with a specific defect in an enzyme necessary for the degradation of lipids. The two lipid storage diseases with characteristic macrophage morphology are Gaucher disease and Niemann-Pick disease.

- Inherited lymphocyte disorders include DiGeorge syndrome, in which the lack or underdevelopment of the thymus results in decreased T cells; sex-linked agammaglobulinemia, in which the lack of a kinase results in blocked B cell development; and two types of severe combined immunodeficiency. Wiskott-Aldrich syndrome is a third inherited disorder affecting both T and B cells.

- Reactive changes in granulocytes include a left shift, Döhle bodies, toxic granulation, vacuoles, degranulation, and cytoplasmic swelling.

- Reactive changes in monocytes include occasional immature forms, contorted nuclei, and the presence of more immature forms.

- Reactive changes in lymphocytes include cell enlargement, increased basophilic cytoplasm, and morphologic heterogeneity.

Now that you have completed this chapter, go back and read again the case studies at the beginning and respond to the questions presented.

REVIEW QUESTIONS

Answers can be found in the Appendix.

1. Which of the following inherited leukocyte disorders is caused by a mutation in the lamin B receptor?
   a. Pelger-Huët anomaly
   b. Chédiak-Higashi disease
   c. Alder-Reilly anomaly
   d. May-Hegglin anomaly

2. Which of the following inherited leukocyte disorders is one of a group of disorders with mutations in nonmuscle myosin heavy-chain IIA?
   a. Pelger-Huët anomaly
   b. Chédiak-Higashi disease
   c. Alder-Reilly anomaly
   d. May-Hegglin anomaly

3. Which of the following inherited leukocyte disorders might be seen in Hurler syndrome?
   a. Pelger-Huët anomaly
   b. Chédiak-Higashi disease
   c. Alder-Reilly anomaly
   d. May-Hegglin anomaly

4. Which of the following lysosomal storage diseases is characterized by macrophages with striated cytoplasm and storage of glucocerebroside?
   a. Sanfilippo syndrome
   b. Gaucher disease
   c. Fabry disease
   d. Niemann-Pick disease

5. The neutrophils in chronic granulomatous disease are incapable of producing:
   a. Hydrogen peroxide
   b. Hypochlorite
   c. Superoxide
   d. All of the above

6. Individuals with X-linked SCID have a mutation that affects their ability to synthesize:
   a. Deaminase
   b. Oxidase
   c. IL-2 receptor
   d. IL-8 receptor

7. An absolute lymphocytosis with reactive lymphocytes suggests which of the following conditions?
   a. DiGeorge syndrome
   b. Bacterial infection
   c. Parasitic infection
   d. Viral infection

8. What leukocyte cytoplasmic inclusion is composed of ribosomal RNA?
   a. Primary granules
   b. Toxic granules
   c. Döhle bodies
   d. Howell-Jolly bodies

9. The expected complete blood count (CBC) results for women in active labor would include:
   a. High total white blood cell (WBC) count with increased lymphocytes
   b. High total WBC count with a slight shift to the left in neutrophils
   c. Normal WBC count with increased eosinophils
   d. Low WBC count with increased monocytes

10. Which of the following is true of an absolute increase in lymphocytes with reactive morphology?
    a. The population of lymphocytes appears morphologically homogeneous.
    b. They are usually effector B cells.
    c. The reactive lymphocytes have increased cytoplasm with variable basophilia.
    d. They are most commonly seen in bacterial infections.

REFERENCES

1. Colella, R., & Hollensead, S. C. (2012, Mar). Understanding and recognizing the Pelger-Huët anomaly. *Am J Clin Pathol, 137*(3), 358–366.
2. Speeckaert, M. M., Verhelst, C., Koch, A., Speeckaert, R., & Lacquet, F. (2009). Pelger-Huët anomaly: a critical review of the literature. *Acta Haematologica, 121*(4), 202–206.
3. Klein, A., Hussar, A. E., & Bornstein, S. (1955, Dec 15). Pelger-Huët anomaly of the leukocytes. *N Engl J Med, 253*(24), 1057–1062.
4. Skendzel, L. P., & Hoffman, G. C. (1962, Mar). The Pelger anomaly of leukocytes: forty-one cases in seven families. *Am J Clin Pathol, 37,* 294–301.
5. Johnson, C. A., Bass, D. A., Trillo, A. A., Snyder, M. S., & DeChatelet, L. R. (1980, Mar). Functional and metabolic studies of polymorphonuclear leukocytes in the congenital Pelger-Huët anomaly. *Blood, 55*(3), 466–469.
6. Cunningham, J. M., Patnaik, M. M., Hammerschmidt, D. E., & Vercellotti, G. M. (2009, Feb). Historical perspective and clinical implications of the Pelger-Huët cell. *Am J Hematol, 84*(2), 116–119.
7. Shetty, V. T., Mundle, S. D., & Raza, A. (2001, Aug 15). Pseudo Pelger-Huët anomaly in myelodysplastic syndrome: hyposegmented apoptotic neutrophil? *Blood, 98*(4), 1273–1275.
8. Gorlin, R. J., Gelb, B., Diaz, G. A., Lofsness, K. G., Pittelkow, M. R., & Fenyk, J. R., Jr. (2000, Apr 24). WHIM syndrome, an autosomal dominant disorder: clinical, hematological, and molecular studies. *Am J Med Genet, 91*(5), 368–376.
9. Zuelzer, W. W. (1964, Apr 2). "Myelokathexis"—a new form of chronic granulocytopenia. Report of a case. *N Engl J Med, 270,* 699–704.
10. Diaz, G. A., & Gulino, A. V. (2005, Sep). WHIM syndrome: a defect in CXCR4 signaling. *Current allergy and asthma reports, 5*(5), 350–355.
11. Dotta, L., Tassone, L., & Badolato, R. (2011, Jun). Clinical and genetic features of Warts, Hypogammaglobulinemia, Infections and Myelokathexis (WHIM) syndrome. *Curr Mol Med, 11*(4), 317–325.
12. Sokolic, R. (2013, Jan). Neutropenia in primary immunodeficiency. *Curr Opin Hematol, 20*(1), 55–65.
13. Groover, R. V., Burke, E. C., Gordon, H., & Berdon, W. E. (1972, Oct). The genetic mucopolysaccharidoses. *Semin Hematol, 9*(4), 371–402.
14. Introne, W., Boissy, R. E., & Gahl, W. A. (1999, Oct). Clinical, molecular, and cell biological aspects of Chediak-Higashi syndrome. *Mol Genet Metab, 68*(2), 283–303.
15. Kaplan, J., De Domenico, I., & Ward, D. M. (2008, Jan). Chediak-Higashi syndrome. *Curr Opin Hematol, 15*(1), 22–29.
16. Kunishima, S., Kojima, T., Tanaka, T., Kamiya, T., Ozawa, K., Nakamura, Y., et al. (1999, Nov). Mapping of a gene for May-Hegglin anomaly to chromosome 22q. *Hum Genets, 105*(5), 379–383.
17. Holland, S. M. (2013, Feb). Chronic granulomatous disease. *Hematol Oncol Clin North Am, 27*(1), 89–99.
18. Stasia, M. J., & Li, X. J. (2008, Jul). Genetics and immunopathology of chronic granulomatous disease. *Semin Immunopathol, 30*(3), 209–235.
19. Martire, B., Rondelli, R., Soresina, A., Pignata, C., Broccoletti, T., Finocchi, A., et al. (2008, Feb). Clinical features, long-term follow-up and outcome of a large cohort of patients with Chronic Granulomatous Disease: an Italian multicenter study. *Clin Immunol, 126*(2), 155–164.
20. Lawrence, M. B., Kansas, G. S., Kunkel, E. J., & Ley, K. (1997, Feb 10). Threshold levels of fluid shear promote leukocyte adhesion through selectins (CD62L,P,E). *J Cell Biol, 136*(3), 717–727.
21. Roos, D., & Law, S. K. (2001, Nov-Dec). Hematologically important mutations: leukocyte adhesion deficiency. *Blood Cells Mol Dis, 27*(6), 1000–1004.
22. Harris, E. S., McIntyre, T. M., Prescott, S. M., & Zimmerman, G. A. (2000, Aug 4). The leukocyte integrins. *J Biol Chem, 275*(31), 23409–23412.
23. Schmidt, S., Moser, M., & Sperandio, M. (2013, Aug). The molecular basis of leukocyte recruitment and its deficiencies. *Mol Immunol, 55*(1), 49–58.
24. Luhn, K., Wild, M. K., Eckhardt, M., Gerardy-Schahn, R., & Vestweber, D. (2001, May). The gene defective in leukocyte adhesion deficiency II encodes a putative GDP-fucose transporter. *Nat Genet, 28*(1), 69–72.
25. Sperandio, M., Gleissner, C. A., & Ley, K. (2009, Jul). Glycosylation in immune cell trafficking. *Immunol Rev, 230*(1), 97–113.
26. Marquardt, T., Brune, T., Luhn, K., Zimmer, K. P., Korner, C., Fabritz, L., et al. (1999, Jun). Leukocyte adhesion deficiency II syndrome, a generalized defect in fucose metabolism. *J Pediatr, 134*(6), 681–688.
27. Gazit, Y., Mory, A., Etzioni, A., Frydman, M., Scheuerman, O., Gershoni-Baruch, R., et al. (2010, Mar). Leukocyte adhesion deficiency type II: long-term follow-up and review of the literature. *J Clin Immunol, 30*(2), 308–313.
28. Moser, M., Nieswandt, B., Ussar, S., Pozgajova, M., & Fassler, R. (2008, Mar). Kindlin-3 is essential for integrin activation and platelet aggregation. *Nat Med, 14*(3), 325–330.
29. Hansson, M., Olsson, I., & Nauseef, W. M. (2006, Jan 15). Biosynthesis, processing, and sorting of human myeloperoxidase. *Arch Biochem Biophys, 445*(2), 214–224.
30. Nauseef, W. M. (1990). Myeloperoxidase deficiency. *Hematol Pathol, 4*(4), 165–178.
31. Bruck, W., Goebel, H. H., & Dienes, P. (1991, Jun). B and T lymphocytes are affected in lysosomal disorders—an immunoelectron microscopic study. *Neuropathol Appl Neurobiol, 17*(3), 219–222.
32. Muenzer, J. (2004 May). The mucopolysaccharidoses: a heterogeneous group of disorders with variable pediatric presentations. *J Pediatr, 144*(5 Suppl), S27–34.
33. Beutler, E., Nguyen, N. J., Henneberger, M. W., Smolec, J. M., McPherson, R. A., West, C., et al. (1993, Jan). Gaucher disease: gene frequencies in the Ashkenazi Jewish population. *Am J Hum Genet, 52*(1), 85–88.
34. Hruska, K. S., LaMarca, M. E., Scott, C. R., & Sidransky, E. (2008, May). Gaucher disease: mutation and polymorphism spectrum in the glucocerebrosidase gene (GBA). *Hum Mutat, 29*(5), 567–583.
35. Ron, I., & Horowitz, M. (2005, Aug 15). ER retention and degradation as the molecular basis underlying Gaucher disease heterogeneity. *Hum Mol Genet, 14*(16), 2387–2398.

36. Naito, M., Takahashi, K., & Hojo, H. (1988, May). An ultrastructural and experimental study on the development of tubular structures in the lysosomes of Gaucher cells. *Lab Invest, 58*(5), 590–598.

37. Hollak, C. E., van Weely, S., van Oers, M. H., & Aerts, J. M. (1994, Mar). Marked elevation of plasma chitotriosidase activity. A novel hallmark of Gaucher disease. *J Clin Invest, 93*(3), 1288–1292.

38. Rosenbloom, B. E., Weinreb, N. J., Zimran, A., Kacena, K. A., Charrow, J., & Ward, E. (2005, Jun 15). Gaucher disease and cancer incidence: a study from the Gaucher Registry. *Blood, 105*(12), 4569–4572.

39. Brady, R. O. (2006). Enzyme replacement for lysosomal diseases. *Annu Rev Med, 57*, 283–296.

40. Valayannopoulos, V. (2013). Enzyme replacement therapy and substrate reduction therapy in lysosomal storage disorders with neurological expression. *Handb Clin Neurol, 113*, 1851–1857.

41. Somaraju, U. R., & Tadepalli, K. (2012). Hematopoietic stem cell transplantation for Gaucher disease. *Cochrane Database Syst Rev, 7*, 1–8. CD006974.

42. Li, Z., Li, T., Dai, S., Xie, X., Ma, X., Zhao, W., et al. (2013, Jul 8). New insights into the pharmacological chaperone activity of c2-substituted glucoimidazoles for the treatment of Gaucher disease. *Chembiochem, 14*(10), 1239–1247.

43. Sharma, P., Khurana, N., & Singh, T. (2007, Oct). Pseudo-Gaucher cells in Hb E disease and thalassemia intermedia. *Hematology, 12*(5), 457–459.

44. Lee, R. E., & Ellis, L. D. (1971, Apr). The storage cells of chronic myelogenous leukemia. *Lab Invest, 24*(4), 261–264.

45. Carrington, P. A., Stevens, R. F., & Lendon, M. (1992, Apr). Pseudo-Gaucher cells. *J Clin Pathol, 45*(4), 360.

46. Schuchman, E. H. (2009). The pathogenesis and treatment of acid sphingomyelinase-deficient Niemann-Pick disease. *Int J Clin Pharmacol Ther, 47* Suppl 1:S48–57.

47. Schuchman, E. H. (2010, May 3). Acid sphingomyelinase, cell membranes and human disease: lessons from Niemann-Pick disease. *FEBS Lett, 584*(9), 1895–900.

48. Choudhury, A., Sharma, D. K., Marks, D. L., & Pagano, R. E. (2004, Oct). Elevated endosomal cholesterol levels in Niemann-Pick cells inhibit rab4 and perturb membrane recycling. *Mol Biol Cell, 15*(10), 4500–4511.

49. Patterson, M. C., Hendriksz, C. J., Walterfang, M., Sedel, F., Vanier, M. T., Wijburg, F., et al. (2012, Jul). Recommendations for the diagnosis and management of Niemann-Pick disease type C: an update. *Mol Genet Metab, 106*(3), 330–344.

50. Dvorakova, L., Sikora, J., Hrebicek, M., Hulkova, H., Bouckova, M., Stolnaja, L., et al. (2006, Aug). Subclinical course of adult visceral Niemann-Pick type C1 disease. A rare or underdiagnosed disorder? *J Inherit Metab Dis, 29*(4), 591.

51. Fensom, A. H., Grant, A. R., Steinberg, S. J., Ward, C. P., Lake, B. D., Logan, E. C., et al. (1999, Feb). An adult with a non-neuronopathic form of Niemann-Pick C disease. *J Inherit Metab Dis, 22*(1), 84–86.

52. McLean-Tooke, A., Spickett, G. P., & Gennery, A. R. (2007, Jul). Immunodeficiency and autoimmunity in 22q11.2 deletion syndrome. *Scand J Immunol, 66*(1), 1–7.

53. Markert, M. L., Devlin, B. H., Alexieff, M. J., Li, J., McCarthy, E. A., Gupton, S. E., et al. (2007, May 15). Review of 54 patients with complete DiGeorge anomaly enrolled in protocols for thymus transplantation: outcome of 44 consecutive transplants. *Blood, 109*(10), 4539–4547.

54. Vetrie, D., Vorechovsky, I., Sideras, P., Holland, J., Davies, A., Flinter, F., et al. (2012 Apr, 1). The gene involved in X-linked agammaglobulinaemia is a member of the Src family of protein-tyrosine kinases. 1993. *J Immunol, 188*(7), 2948–2955.

55. Tsukada, S., Saffran, D. C., Rawlings, D. J., Parolini, O., Allen, R. C., Klisak, I., et al. (2012, Apr 1). Deficient expression of a B cell cytoplasmic tyrosine kinase in human X-linked agammaglobulinemia. 1993. *J Immunol, 188*(7), 2936–2947.

56. Perez-Aguilar, M. C., Goncalves, L., & Bonfante-Cabarcas, R. (2012, Sep). [Adenosine deaminase in severe combined immunodeficiency syndrome]. *Invest Clin, 53*(3), 315–324.

57. Uribe, L., & Weinberg, K. I. (1998, Oct). X-linked SCID and other defects of cytokine pathways. *Semin Hematol, 35*(4), 299–309.

58. Notarangelo, L. D., Miao, C. H., & Ochs, H. D. (2008, Jan). Wiskott-Aldrich syndrome. *Curr Opin Hematol, 15*(1), 30–36.

59. Puig, N., de Haas, M., Kleijer, M., Montoro, J. A., Perez, A., Villalba, J. V., et al. (1995, Aug). Isoimmune neonatal neutropenia caused by Fc gamma RIIIb antibodies in a Spanish child. *Transfusion, 35*(8), 683–687.

60. Bux, J. (2008, May). Human neutrophil alloantigens. *Vox Sang, 94*(4), 277–285.

61. Bux, J., Behrens, G., Jaeger, G., & Welte, K. (1998, Jan 1). Diagnosis and clinical course of autoimmune neutropenia in infancy: analysis of 240 cases. *Blood, 91*(1), 181–186.

62. van Staa, T. P., Boulton, F., Cooper, C., Hagenbeek, A., Inskip, H., & Leufkens, H. G. (2003, Apr). Neutropenia and agranulocytosis in England and Wales: incidence and risk factors. *Am J Hematol, 72*(4), 248–254.

63. Andres, E., & Maloisel, F. (2008, Jan). Idiosyncratic drug-induced agranulocytosis or acute neutropenia. *Curr Opin Hematol, 15*(1), 15–21.

64. Claas, F. H. (1996). Immune mechanisms leading to drug-induced blood dyscrasias. *Eur J Haematol Suppl, 60*, 64–68.

65. Dale, D. C. (1998). The discovery, development and clinical applications of granulocyte colony-stimulating factor. *Trans Am Clin Climatol Assoc, 109*, 27–36.

66. Barkaoui, M., Fenneteau, O., Bertrand, Y., et al. (2005, Jan). Analysis of risk factors for myelodysplasias, leukemias and death from infection among patients with congenital neutropenia. Experience of the French Severe Chronic Neutropenia Study Group. *Haematologica, 90*(1), 45–53.

67. Rosenberg, P. S., Alter, B. P., Bolyard, A. A., Bonilla, M. A., Boxer, L. A., Cham, B., et al. (2006, Jun 15). The incidence of leukemia and mortality from sepsis in patients with severe congenital neutropenia receiving long-term G-CSF therapy. *Blood, 107*(12), 4628–4635.

68. Dokal, I., Rule, S., Chen, F., Potter, M., & Goldman, J. (1997, Oct). Adult onset of acute myeloid leukaemia (M6) in patients with Shwachman-Diamond syndrome. *Br J Haematol, 99*(1), 171–173.

69. Thornley, I., Dror, Y., Sung, L., Wynn, R. F., & Freedman, M. H. (2002, Apr). Abnormal telomere shortening in leucocytes of children with Shwachman-Diamond syndrome. *Br J Haematol, 117*(1), 189–192.

70. Woods, W. G., Krivit, W., Lubin, B. H., & Ramsay, N. K. (1981). Aplastic anemia associated with the Shwachman syndrome. In vivo and in vitro observations. *The American journal of pediatric hematology/oncology. Winter, 3*(4):347–351.

71. Kuijpers, T. W., Nannenberg, E., Alders, M., Bredius, R., & Hennekam, R. C. (2004, Sep). Congenital aplastic anemia caused by mutations in the SBDS gene: a rare presentation of Shwachman-Diamond syndrome. *Pediatrics, 114*(3):e387–e391.

72. Fleitz, J., Rumelhart, S., Goldman, F., Ambruso, D., Sokol, R. J., Pacini, D., et al. (2002, Jan). Successful allogeneic hematopoietic stem cell transplantation (HSCT) for Shwachman-Diamond syndrome. *Bone Marrow Transplant, 29*(1), 75–79.

73. Klein, C. (2009). Congenital neutropenia. *Hematology Am Soc Hematol Educ Program.* Vol 2009, no 1, 344–350.

74. Dale, D. C., & Welte, K. (2011). Cyclic and chronic neutropenia. *Cancer Treat Res, 157*, 97–108.

75. Bakker, S. T., de Winter, J. P., & te Riele, H. (2013, Jan). Learning from a paradox: recent insights into Fanconi anaemia through studying mouse models. *Dis Model Mech, 6*(1), 40–47.

76. Dokal, I. (2011). Dyskeratosis congenita. *Hematology Am Soc Hematol Educ Program, 2011:* 480–486.

77. Korenaga, M., Hitoshi, Y., Yamaguchi, N., Sato, Y., Takatsu, K., & Tada, I. (1991, Apr). The role of interleukin-5 in protective immunity to *Strongyloides venezuelensis* infection in mice. *Immunology, 72*(4), 502–507.

78. Simon, D., & Simon, H. U. (2007, Jun). Eosinophilic disorders. *The Journal of allergy and clinical immunology, 119*(6), 1291–1300.

79. Shurin, S. B. (1988, Mar). Pathologic states associated with activation of eosinophils and with eosinophilia. *Hematol Oncol Clin North Am, 2*(1):171–179.

80. Simon, D., Braathen, L. R., & Simon, H. U. (2004, Jun). Eosinophils and atopic dermatitis. *Allergy, 59*(6), 561–570.

81. Filley, W. V., Holley, K. E., Kephart, G. M., & Gleich, G. J. (1982, Jul 3). Identification by immunofluorescence of eosinophil granule major basic protein in lung tissues of patients with bronchial asthma. *Lancet, 2*(8288), 11–16.

82. Roufosse, F., Garaud, S., & de Leval, L. (2012, Apr). Lymphoproliferative disorders associated with hypereosinophilia. *Semin Hematol, 49*(2), 138–148.

83. Mingomataj, E. C. (2008). Eosinophil-induced prognosis improvement of solid tumors could be enabled by their vesicle-mediated barrier permeability induction. *Med Hypotheses, 70*(3), 582–584.

84. Leiferman, K. M., & Gleich, G. J. (2004, Jan). Hypereosinophilic syndrome: case presentation and update. *J Allergy Clin Immunol, 113*(1), 50–58.

85. Abidi, K., Khoudri, I., Belayachi, J., Madani, N., Zekraoui, A., Zeggwagh, A. A., et al. (2008). Eosinopenia is a reliable marker of sepsis on admission to medical intensive care units. *Crit Care, 12*(2), R59.

86. Abidi, K., Belayachi, J., Derras, Y., Khayari, M. E., Dendane, T., Madani, N., et al. (2011, Jul). Eosinopenia, an early marker of increased mortality in critically ill medical patients. *Intensive Care Med, 37*(7), 1136–1142.

87. Jimenez, C., Gasalla, R., et al. (1987). Incidence and clinical significance of peripheral and bone marrow basophilia. *J Med, 18*(5–6), 293–303.

88. May, M. E., & Waddell, C. C. (1984, Mar). Basophils in peripheral blood and bone marrow. A retrospective review. *Am J Med, 76*(3), 509–511.

89. Cooke, M. E., Potena, L., Luikart, H., & Valantine, H. A. (2006, Dec 15). Peripheral blood leukocyte counts in cytomegalovirus infected heart transplant patients: impact of acute disease versus subclinical infection. *Transplantation, 82*(11), 1419–1424.

90. Gulen, H., Basarir, F., Hakan, N., Ciftdogan, D. Y., Tansug, N., & Onag, A. (2005, Nov). Premature labor and leukoerythroblastosis in a newborn with parvovirus B19 infection. *Haematologica, 90* Suppl:ECR38.

91. Hong, Y. J., Jeong, M. H., Ahn, Y., Yoon, N. S., Lee, S. R., Hong, S. N., et al. (2007, Aug). Relationship between peripheral monocytosis and nonrecovery of left ventricular function in patients with left ventricular dysfunction complicated with acute myocardial infarction. *Circ J, 71*(8), 1219–1224.

92. Jubinsky, P. T., Shanske, A. L., Pixley, F. J., Montagna, C., & Short, M. K. (2006, Dec 15). A syndrome of holoprosencephaly, recurrent infections, and monocytosis. *Am J Med Genet A, 140*(24), 2742–2748.

93. Kratz, A., Lewandrowski, K. B., Siegel, A. J., Chun, K. Y., Flood, J. G., Van Cott, E. M., et al. (2002, Dec). Effect of marathon running on hematologic and biochemical laboratory parameters, including cardiac markers. *Am J Clin Pathol, 118*(6), 856–863.

94. Robinson, R. L., Burk, M. S., & Raman, S. (2003, Jan-Mar). Fever, delirium, autonomic instability, and monocytosis associated with olanzapine. *J Postgrad Med, 49*(1), 96.

95. Tsolia, M., Drakonaki, S., Messaritaki, A., Farmakakis, T., Kostaki, M., Tsapra, H., et al. (2002, May). Clinical features, complications and treatment outcome of childhood brucellosis in central Greece. *J Infect, 44*(4), 257–262.

96. Walsh, D. S., Thavichaigarn, P., Pattanapanyasat, K., Siritongtaworn, P., Kongcharoen, P., Tongtawe, P., et al. (2005, Dec). Characterization of circulating monocytes expressing HLA-DR or CD71 and related soluble factors for 2 weeks after severe, non-thermal injury. *J Surg Res, 129*(2), 221–230.

97. William, B. M., & Corazza, G. R. (2007 Feb). Hyposplenism: a comprehensive review. Part I: basic concepts and causes. *Hematology, 12*(1), 1–13.

98. Chakraborty, A., Blum, R. A., Cutler, D. L., & Jusko, W. J. (1999, Mar). Pharmacoimmunodynamic interactions of interleukin-10 and prednisone in healthy volunteers. *Clin Pharmacol Ther, 65*(3), 304–318.

99. Nockher, W. A., Wiemer, J., & Scherberich, J. E. (2001, Jan). Haemodialysis monocytopenia: differential sequestration kinetics of CD14+CD16+ and CD14++ blood monocyte subsets. *Clin Exp Immunol, 123*(1), 49–55.

100. Savard, M., & Gosselin, J. (2006, Aug). Epstein-Barr virus immunossuppression of innate immunity mediated by phagocytes. *Virus Res, 119*(2), 134–145.

101. van de Vyver, A., Delport, E. F., Esterhuizen, M., & Pool, R. (2010, Jul). The correlation between C-reactive protein and toxic granulation of neutrophils in the peripheral blood. *S Afr Med J, 100*(7), 442–444.

102. Kabutomori, O., Iwatani, Y., & Kanakura, Y. (2000, Nov 27). Toxic granulation neutrophils and C-reactive protein. *Arch Intern Med, 160*(21), 3326–3327.

103. Al-Gwaiz, L. A., & Babay, H. H. (2007). The diagnostic value of absolute neutrophil count, band count and morphologic changes of neutrophils in predicting bacterial infections. *Med Princ Pract, 16*(5), 344–347.

104. Prokocimer, M., & Potasman, I. (2008, Nov). The added value of peripheral blood cell morphology in the diagnosis and management of infectious diseases—part 1: basic concepts. *Postgrad Med J, 84*(997), 579–585.

105. Abernathy, M. R. (1966, Mar). Döhle bodies associated with uncomplicated pregnancy. *Blood, 27*(3), 380–385.

106. Boxer, L. A., & Stossel, T. P. (1974, Jun). Effects of anti-human neutrophil antibodies in vitro. Quantitative studies. *J Clin Invest, 53*(6), 1534–1545.

107. Davidson, R. J., & McPhie, J. L. (1980, Dec). Cytoplasmic vacuolation of peripheral blood cells in acute alcoholism. *J Clin Pathol, 33*(12), 1193–1196.

108. Holley, T. R., Van Epps, D. E., Harvey, R. L., Anderson, R. E., & Williams, R. C., Jr. (1974, Apr). Effect of high doses of radiation on human neutrophil chemotaxis, phagocytosis and morphology. *Am J Pathol, 75*(1), 61–72.

109. Dahlgren, F. S., Mandel, E. J., Krebs, J. W., Massung, R. F., & McQuiston, J. H. (2011, Jul). Increasing incidence of Ehrlichia chaffeensis and *Anaplasma phagocytophilum* in the United States, 2000-2007. *Am J Trop Med Hyg, 85*(1), 124–131.

110. Ismail, N., Bloch, K. C., & McBride, J. W. (2010, Mar). Human ehrlichiosis and anaplasmosis. *Clin Lab Med, 30*(1), 261–292.

111. Taneja, R., Parodo, J., Jia, S. H., Kapus, A., Rotstein, O. D., & Marshall, J. C. (2004, Jul). Delayed neutrophil apoptosis in sepsis is associated with maintenance of mitochondrial transmembrane potential and reduced caspase-9 activity. *Crit Care Med, 32*(7), 1460–1469.

112. Son, Y. O., Jang, Y. S., Heo, J. S., Chung, W. T., Choi, K. C., & Lee, J. C. (2009, Jun). Apoptosis-inducing factor plays a critical role in caspase-independent, pyknotic cell death in hydrogen peroxide-exposed cells. *Apoptosis: an international journal on programmed cell death, 14*(6), 796–808.

113. Gallin, J. I. (1984, Sep). Neutrophil specific granules: a fuse that ignites the inflammatory response. *Clin Res, 32*(3), 320–328.

114. Fingeroth, J. D., Weis, J. J., Tedder, T. F., Strominger, J. L., Biro, P. A., & Fearon, D. T. (1984, Jul). Epstein-Barr virus receptor of human B lymphocytes is the C3d receptor CR2. *Proc Natl Acad Sci U S A, 81*(14), 4510–4514.

115. Luzuriaga, K., & Sullivan, J. L. (2010, May 27). Infectious mononucleosis. *N Engl J Med, 362*(21), 1993–2000.

116. Crawford, D. H., Macsween, K. F., Higgins, C. D., Thomas, R., McAulay, K., Williams, H., et al. (2006, Aug 1). A cohort study among university students: identification of risk factors for Epstein-Barr virus seroconversion and infectious mononucleosis. *Clinical Infectious Diseases, 43*(3), 276–282.

30

Cytogenetics

Gail H. Vance

OBJECTIVES

After completion of this chapter, the reader will be able to:

1. Describe chromosome structure and the methods used in G-banded chromosome identification.
2. Explain the basic laboratory techniques for preparing chromosomes for analysis.
3. Differentiate between numeric and structural chromosome abnormalities.
4. Discuss the importance of karyotype in the diagnosis of hematologic cancer.
5. Explain the basic technique of fluorescence in situ hybridization (FISH).
6. Discuss the advantage of using FISH analysis in conjunction with G-banded analysis of cells.
7. Describe the types of chromosomal abnormalities that are detectable with cytogenetic methods.
8. Given a diagram of a G-banded chromosome, name the structures identifiable by light microscopy.
9. Given the designation of a chromosome mutation, be able to determine whether the abnormality is numeric or structural, which chromosomes are affected, what type of abnormality it is, and what portion of the chromosome is affected.
10. Define chromosomal microarray analysis.

CASE STUDY

After studying the material in this chapter, the reader should be able to respond to the following case study:

A 54-year-old man came to his physician with a history of fatigue, weight loss, and increased bruising over a 6-month period. His WBC count was elevated at 200×10^9/L. A bone marrow aspirate was sent for cytogenetic analysis. G-banded chromosome analysis of 20 cells from bone marrow cultures showed all cells to be positive for the Philadelphia chromosome, t(9;22)(q34;q11.2), as seen in chronic myelogenous leukemia (Figure 30-1). FISH studies using

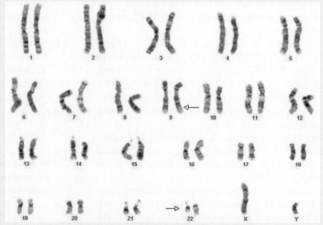

Figure 30-1 Karyogram for the patient in the case study showing a translocation between chromosomes 9 and 22, which is characteristic of chronic myelogenous leukemia. (Courtesy the Cytogenetics Laboratory, Indiana University School of Medicine, Indianapolis, IN.)

After studying the material in this chapter, the reader should be able to respond to the following case study:

the *BCR* and *ABL1* gene probes (Abbott Molecular, Des Plaines, IL) produced dual fusion signals, one located on the derivative chromosome 9 and one on the derivative chromosome 22, characteristic of the translocation between chromosomes 9 and 22 leading to the rearrangement of *BCR* and *ABL1* oncogenes (Figure 30-2). The patient was treated with imatinib mesylate for the next 2 months. Another cytogenetic study was performed on a second bone marrow aspirate. This analysis showed that 12 of 20 cells analyzed were normal, 46,XY[12]; however, there were still 8 cells positive for the Philadelphia chromosome, 46,XY,t(9;22)(q34; q11.2)[8].

1. What is G-banded chromosome analysis?
2. Is the described mutation an example of a numeric or a structural abnormality? What type? Which chromosomes are involved? Explain.
3. What is FISH, and how does it complement standard chromosome analysis?

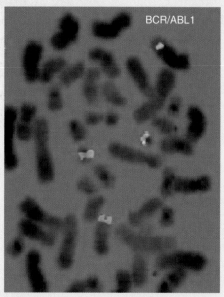

Figure 30-2 Bone marrow metaphase cell from the patient in the case study hybridized with probes for BCR (green) and ABL1 (red) (Abbott Molecular, Des Plaines, IL). The fusion signals (yellow) represent the translocated chromosomes 9 and 22 (der(9) and der(22)). (Courtesy the Cytogenetics Laboratory, Indiana University School of Medicine, Indianapolis, IN.)

Human cytogenetics is the study of chromosomes, their structure, and their inheritance. There are approximately 25,000 genes in the human genome, most of which reside on the 46 chromosomes normally found in each somatic cell.[1]

Chromosome disorders are classified as structural or numerical and involve the loss, gain, or rearrangement of either a piece of a chromosome or the entire chromosome. Because each chromosome contains thousands of genes, a chromosomal abnormality that is observable by light microscopy involves, on average, 3 to 5 megabases (Mb) of DNA and represents the disruption or loss of hundreds of genes. Such disruptions often have a profound clinical effect. Chromosomal abnormalities are observed in approximately 0.65% of all live births.[2] The gain or loss of an entire chromosome, other than a sex chromosome, is usually incompatible with life and accounts for approximately 50% of first-trimester spontaneous abortions.[3] In leukemia, cytogenetic abnormalities are observed in more than 50% of bone marrow specimens.[4] These recurring abnormalities often define the leukemia and frequently indicate clinical prognosis.

REASONS FOR CHROMOSOME ANALYSIS

Chromosome analysis is an important diagnostic procedure in clinical medicine. Not only are chromosomal anomalies major causes of reproductive loss and birth defects, but also nonrandom chromosome abnormalities are recognized in many forms of cancer.

Physicians who care for patients of all ages may order chromosome analysis or karyotyping for patients with mental retardation, infertility, ambiguous genitalia, short stature, fetal loss, risk of genetic or chromosomal disease, and cancer (Table 30-1). In the following discussion, basic cytogenetic concepts are presented. Supplementation of this chapter with the material in Chapter 31 is recommended.

CHROMOSOME STRUCTURE

Cell Cycle

The cell cycle is divided into four stages: G_1, the growth period before synthesis of deoxyribonucleic acid (DNA); S phase, the period during which DNA synthesis takes place; G_2, the period after DNA synthesis; and M, the period of mitosis or cell division, the shortest phase of the cell cycle (Figure 6-5). During mitosis, chromosomes are maximally condensed. While in mitosis, cells can be chemically treated to arrest cell progression through the cycle so that the chromosomes may be isolated and analyzed.

Chromosome Architecture

A chromosome is formed from a double-stranded DNA molecule that contains a series of genes. The complementary

TABLE 30-1 Common Translocations in Hematopoietic and Lymphoid Neoplasia and Sarcoma*

Tumor Type	Karyotype	Genes
Myeloid Leukemias		
CML (and pre-B-ALL)	t(9;22)(q34;q11.2)	BCR/ABL1
Also see Box 31-1		
B Cell Leukemias/Lymphomas		
B lymphoblastic leukemia	t(12;21)(p13;q22)	ETV6/RUNX1
	t(1;19)(q23.3;p13.3)	PBX1/TCF3
	t(4;11)(q21;q23)	AFF1/MLL(KMT2A)
Burkitt lymphoma	t(8;14)(q24;q32.3)	MYC/IGH
	t(2;8)(p12;q24)	IGK/MYC
	t(8;22)(q24;q11.2)	MYC/IGL
Mantle cell lymphoma	t(11;14)(q13;q32.3)	CCND1/IGH
Follicular lymphoma	t(14;18)(q32.3;q21.3)	IGH/BCL2
Diffuse large B cell lymphoma	t(3;14)(q27;q32.3)	BCL6/IGH
Lymphoplasmacytic lymphoma	t(9;14)(p13.2;q32.3)	PAX5/IGH
MALT lymphoma	t(14;18)(q32.3;q21)	IGH/MALT1
	t(11;18)(q22;q21)	BIRC3/MALT1
	t(1;14)(p22;q32.3)	BCL10/IGH
T Cell Leukemias/Lymphomas		
T lymphoblastic leukemia	del(1)(p32p32)	STIL/TAL1
	t(7;11)(q34;p13)	TRB/LMO2
ALCL	t(2;5)(p23;q35.1)	ALK/NPM1
Sarcomas and Tumors of Bone and Soft Tissue		
Alveolar rhabdomyo-sarcoma	t(2;13)(q36.1;q14.1)	PAX3/FOXO1A
	t(1;13)(p36.13;q14.1)	PAX7/FOXO1A
Ewing sarcoma/PNET	t(11;22)(q24;q12.2)	FLI1/EWSR1
	t(21;22)(q22.3;q12.2)	ERG/EWSR1
	t(7;22)(p22;q12.2)	ETV1/EWSR1
Clear cell sarcoma	t(12;22)(q13;q12.2)	ATF1/EWSR1
Myxoid liposarcoma	t(12;16)(q13;p11.2)	DDIT3/FUS
	t(12;22)(q13;q12.2)	DDIT3/EWSR1
Synovial sarcoma	t(X;18)(p11.2;q11.2)	SSX1 or SSX2/SS18
Alveolar soft part sarcoma	t(X;17)(p11.2;q25)	TFE3/ASPSCR1

ALCL, Anaplastic large cell leukemia; *ALL,* acute lymphoblastic leukemia; *AML,* acute myeloid leukemia; *CML,* chronic myelogenous leukemia; *CMML,* chronic myelomonocytic leukemia; *MALT,* mucosa-associated lymphoid tissue; *PNET,* primitive neuroectodermal tumor.
*Modified per the Hugo Nomenclature Database, May 2013

double-helix structure of DNA was established in 1953 by Watson and Crick.[5] The backbone is a sugar-phosphate-sugar polymer. The sugar is deoxyribose. Attached to the backbone and filling the center of the helix are four nitrogen-containing bases. Two of these, adenine (A) and guanine (G), are purines; the other two, cytosine (C) and thymine (T), are pyrimidines (Figure 31-6).

The chromosomal DNA of the cell resides in the cell's nucleus. This DNA and its associated proteins are referred to as *chromatin.* During the cell cycle, at mitosis, the nuclear chromatin condenses approximately 10,000-fold to form

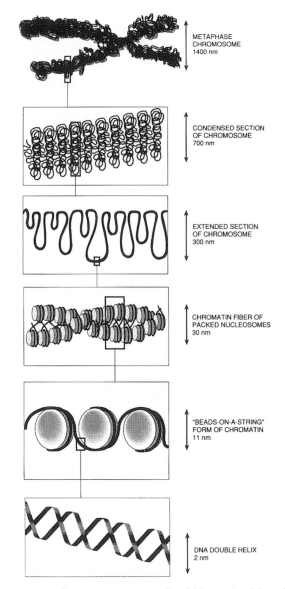

Figure 30-3 Chromosome structure. The folding and twisting of the DNA double helix. (From Gelehrter TD, Collins FS, Ginsberg D: *Principles of medical genetics,* ed 2, Philadelphia, 1998, Lippincott Williams & Wilkins.)

chromosomes.[6] Each chromosome results from progressive folding, compression, and compaction of the entire nuclear chromatin. This condensation is achieved through multiple levels of helical coiling and supercoiling (Figure 30-3).

Metaphase Chromosomes

Metaphase is the stage of mitosis where the chromosomes align on the equatorial plate. Electron micrographs of metaphase chromosomes have provided models of chromosome structure. In the "beads-on-a-string" model of chromatin folding, the DNA helix is looped around a core of histone proteins.[7] This packaging unit is known as a *nucleosome* and measures approximately 11 nm in diameter.[8] Nucleosomes are coiled into twisted forms to create an approximately 30-nm chromatin fiber. This fiber, called a *solenoid,* is condensed further and bent into a loop configuration. These loops extend at an angle from the main chromosome axis.[9]

CHROMOSOME IDENTIFICATION

Chromosome Number

In 1956, Tijo and Levan[10] identified the correct number of human chromosomes as 46. This is the *diploid* chromosome number and is determined by counting the chromosomes in dividing somatic cells. The designation for the diploid number is *2n.* Gametes (ova and sperm) have half the diploid number (23). This is called the *haploid* number of chromosomes and is designated as *n.* Different species have different numbers of chromosomes. The reindeer has a relatively high chromosome number for a mammal (2n = 76), whereas the Indian muntjac, or barking deer, has a very low chromosome number (2n = 7 in the male and 2n = 6 in the female).[11]

Chromosome Size and Type

In the 1960s, before the discovery of banding, chromosomes were categorized by overall size and the location of the centromere (primary constriction) and were assigned to one of seven groups: A through G. Group A includes chromosome pairs 1, 2, and 3. These are the largest chromosomes, and their centromeres are located in the middle of the chromosome; that is, they are metacentric. Group B chromosomes, pairs 4 and 5, are the next largest chromosomes; their centromeres are off center, or submetacentric. Group G consists of the smallest chromosomes, pairs 21 and 22, whose centromeres are located at one end of the chromosomes and are designated as acrocentric (Figure 30-4).

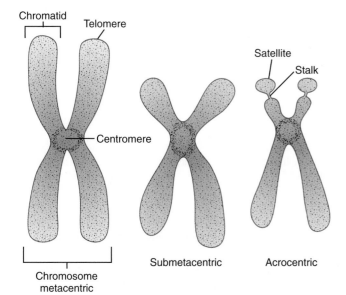

Figure 30-4 Chromosome morphology. The three shapes of chromosomes are metacentric, submetacentric, and acrocentric. This figure also shows the position of the centromere and telomere as well as the two sister chromatids that comprise a metaphase chromosome.

TECHNIQUES FOR CHROMOSOME PREPARATION AND ANALYSIS

Chromosome Preparation

Tissues used for chromosome analysis contain cells with an inherently high mitotic rate (bone marrow cells) or cells that can be stimulated to divide in culture (peripheral blood lymphocytes). Special harvesting procedures are established for each tissue type. Mitogens such as phytohemagglutinin or pokeweed mitogen are added to peripheral blood cultures. Phytohemagglutinin primarily stimulates T cells to divide,[12] whereas pokeweed preferentially stimulates B lymphocytes.[13]

Chromosomes may be obtained from replicating cells by arresting the cell in metaphase. Cells from the peripheral blood or bone marrow are cultured in media for 24 to 72 hours. In standard peripheral blood cultures, since the cells are terminally differentiated, a mitogen is added to stimulate cellular division. Neoplastic cells are spontaneously dividing and generally do not require stimulation with a mitogen. After the cell cultures have grown for the appropriate period, Colcemid, an analogue of colchicine, is added to disrupt the mitotic spindle fiber attachment to the chromosome. Following culture and treatment with Colcemid, cells are exposed to a hypotonic (potassium chloride) solution that lyses red cells and causes the chromosomes to spread apart from one another. A fixative of 3:1 methanol and acetic acid is added that "hardens" cells and removes proteinaceous material. Cells are dropped onto cold, wet glass slides to achieve optimal dispersal of the chromosomes. The slides are then aged, typically by exposure to heat, before banding.

Chromosome Banding

Analysis of each chromosome is made possible by staining with a dye. The name *chromosome* is derived from the Greek words *chroma,* meaning "color," and *soma,* meaning "body." Hence *chromosome* means "colored body." In 1969, Caspersson and colleagues[14] were the first investigators to stain chromosomes successfully with a fluorochrome dye. Using quinacrine mustard, which binds to adenine-thymine–rich areas of the chromosome, they were able to distinguish a banding pattern unique to each chromosome. This banding pattern, called *Q-banding,* differentiates the chromosome into bands of differing widths and relative brightnesses (Figure 30-5). The most brightly fluorescent bands of the 46 human chromosomes include the distal end of the Y chromosome, the centromeric regions of chromosomes 3 and 4, and the short arms of the acrocentric chromosomes (13, 14, 15, 21, and 22).

Other stains are used to identify chromosomes, but in contrast to Q-banding, these methods normally necessitate some pretreatment of the slide to be analyzed. Giemsa (G) bands are obtained by pretreating the chromosomes with the proteolytic enzyme trypsin. *GTG banding* means "G banding by Giemsa with the use of trypsin." Giemsa, like quinacrine mustard, stains AT-rich areas of the chromosome. The dark bands are called *G-positive* (+) bands. Guanine-cytosine–rich areas of the chromosome have little affinity for the dye and are referred to

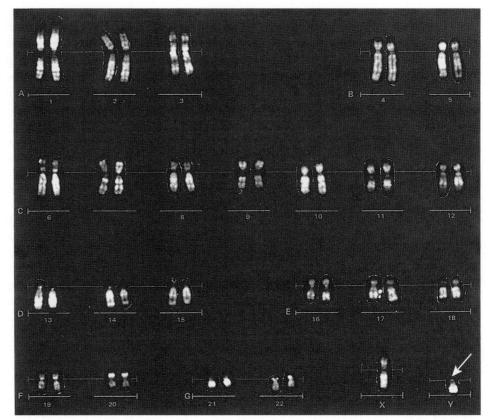

Figure 30-5 Q-banded preparation. Note the intense brilliance of Yq. (Courtesy the Cytogenetics Laboratory, Indiana University School of Medicine, Indianapolis, IN.)

as *G-negative* (−) bands. G+ bands correspond with the brightly fluorescing bands of Q-banding (Figures 30-6 and 30-7). G-banding is the most common method used for staining chromosomes.

C-banding stains the centromere (primary constriction) of the chromosome and the surrounding condensed heterochromatin. Constitutive heterochromatin is a special type of late-replicating repetitive DNA that is located primarily at the centromere of the chromosome. In C-banding, the chromosomes are treated first with an acid and then with an alkali (barium hydroxide) before Giemsa staining. C-banding is most intense in human chromosomes 1, 9, and 16 and the Y chromosome.

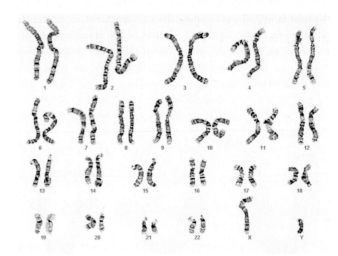

Figure 30-7 Normal male karyogram, GTG-banded preparations. (Courtesy the Cytogenetics Laboratory, Indiana University School of Medicine, Indianapolis, IN.)

Polymorphisms from different individuals are also observed in the C-bands. These polymorphisms have no clinical significance (Figure 30-8).

Specific chromosomal regions that are associated with the nucleoli in interphase cells are called *nucleolar organizer regions* (NORs). NORs contain tandemly repeated ribosomal nucleic acid (RNA) genes. NORs can be differentially stained in chromosomes by a silver stain in a method called *AG-NOR–banding*.

Chromosome banding is visible after chromosome condensation, which occurs during mitosis. The banding pattern

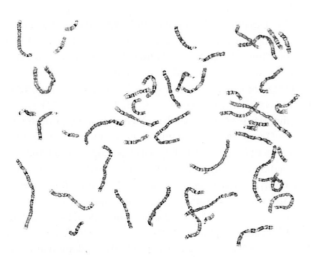

Figure 30-6 Normal male metaphase chromosomes.

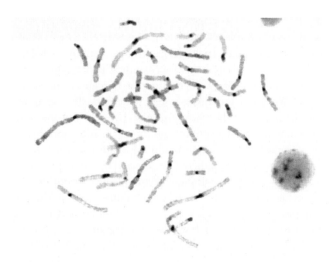

Figure 30-8 C-banded male metaphase chromosomes. Note the stain at the centromere and heterochromatic regions of the chromosomes. (Courtesy the Cytogenetics Laboratory, Indiana University School of Medicine, Indianapolis, IN.)

observed depends on the degree of condensation. By examination of human chromosomes early in mitosis, it has been possible to estimate a total haploid genome (23 chromosomes) with approximately 2000 AT-rich (G+) bands.[15] The later the stage of mitosis, the more condensed the chromosome and the fewer total G+ bands observed.

Metaphase Analysis

After banding, prepared slides with dividing cells are scanned under a light microscope with a low-power objective lens (10×). When a metaphase cell has been selected for analysis, a 63× or 100× oil immersion objective lens is used. Each metaphase cell is analyzed first for a chromosome number. Then each chromosome pair is analyzed for its banding pattern. A normal somatic cell contains 46 chromosomes, which

includes two sex chromosomes and 22 pairs of autosomes (chromosomes 1 through 22). The technologist records his or her summary of the analysis using chromosome nomenclature. This summary is called a *karyotype*. Any variation in number and banding pattern is recorded by the technologist. At least 20 metaphase cells are analyzed from leukocyte cultures. If abnormalities are noted, the technologist may need to analyze additional cells. Computer imaging or photography is used to confirm and record the microscopic analysis. A picture of all the chromosomes aligned from 1 to 22 including the sex chromosomes is called a *karyogram*.

Fluorescence In Situ Hybridization

The use of molecular methods coupled with standard karyotype analysis has improved chromosomal mutation detection beyond that of the light microscope. DNA or RNA probes labeled with either fluorescent or enzymatic detection systems are hybridized directly to metaphase or interphase cells on a glass microscope slide. These probes usually belong to one of three classes: probes for repetitive DNA sequences, primarily generated from centromeric DNA; whole-chromosome probes that include segments of an entire chromosome; and specific loci or single-copy probes.

Fluorescence in situ hybridization (FISH) is a molecular technique commonly used in cytogenetic laboratories. FISH studies are a valuable adjunct to the diagnostic workup. In FISH, the DNA or RNA probe is labeled with a fluorophore. Target DNA is treated with heat and formamide to denature the double-stranded DNA, which renders it single-stranded. The target DNA anneals to a similarly denatured, single-stranded, fluorescently labeled DNA or RNA probe with a complementary sequence. After hybridization, the unbound probe is removed through a series of stringent washes, and the cells are counterstained for visualization (Figure 30-9).

In situ hybridization with centromere or whole-chromosome painting probes can be used to identify individual chromosomes

General FISH Protocol

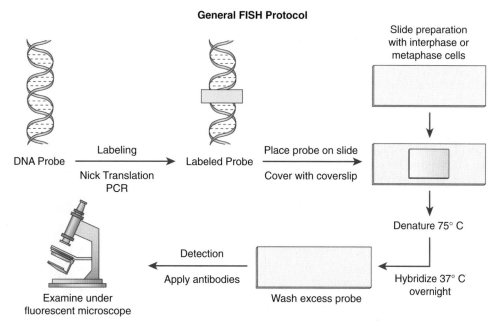

Figure 30-9 General protocol for fluorescence in situ hybridization. *PCR,* Polymerase chain reaction.

(Figure 30-10). Marker chromosomes represent chromatin material that has been structurally altered and cannot be identified by a G-band pattern. FISH using a centromere or paint probe, or both, is often helpful in identifying the chromosome of origin (Figure 30-11).[16] Specific loci probes can be used to detect both structural and numerical abnormalities but are especially helpful in identifying chromosomal translocations or inversions.

The FISH procedure has many advantages and has advanced the detection of chromosomal abnormalities beyond that of G-banded analysis. Both dividing (metaphase) and nondividing (interphase) cells can be analyzed with FISH. Performance of FISH on uncultured cells, such as bone marrow smears, provides a quick test result that can be reported in 24 hours. Also, in cultured bone marrow samples submitted for G-band analysis, the number of dividing cells may be insufficient for cytogenetic diagnosis. In such cases, FISH performed on interphase (nondividing) cells with probes for a specific translocation or structural abnormality may provide the diagnosis. FISH also can be performed on paraffin-embedded tissue sections, specimens obtained by fine needle aspiration, and touch preparations from lymph nodes or solid tumors.

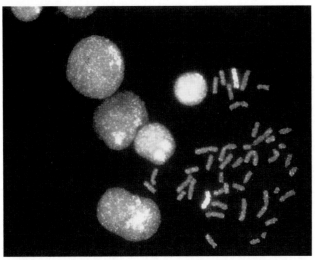

Figure 30-10 Metaphase preparation is "painted" with multiple probes for chromosome 7, producing a fluorescent signal. (Courtesy the Cytogenetics Laboratory, Indiana University School of Medicine, Indianapolis, IN.)

Locus-specific probes Chromosome paint probes Centromere probes	
Detection of numerical chromosome abnormalities	**Detection of structural chromosome abnormalities**
Trisomy Monosomy Polyploidy	Deletions Duplications Inversions Translocations Ring chromosomes Marker chromosomes Dicentric chromosomes

Figure 30-11 Fluorescence in situ hybridization in the clinical laboratory.

CYTOGENETIC NOMENCLATURE

Banding techniques enabled scientists to identify each chromosome pair by a characteristic banding pattern. In 1971, a Paris conference for nomenclature of human chromosomes was convened to designate a system to describe the regions and specific bands of the chromosomes. The chromosome arms were designated *p* (petite) for the short arm and *q* for the long arm. The regions in each arm and the bands contained within each region were numbered consecutively, from the centromere outward to the telomere or end of the chromosome. To designate a specific region of the chromosome, the chromosome number is written first, followed by the designation of either the short or long arm, then the region of the arm, and finally the specific band. *Xq21* designates the long arm of the X chromosome, region 2, band 1. To designate a subband, a decimal point is placed after the band designation, followed by the number assigned to the subband, as in Xq21.1 (Figure 30-12).

Cytogenetic (and FISH) nomenclature represents a uniform code used by cytogeneticists around the world to communicate chromosome abnormalities. In this nomenclature each string begins with the modal number of chromosomes, followed by the sex chromosome designation. A normal male karyotype is designated 46,XY, and a normal female karyotype is designated 46,XX. If abnormalities are observed in the cell, the designation is written to include abnormalities of modal chromosome number, sex chromosomes, and then the autosomes. A cell from a bone marrow specimen with trisomy of chromosome 8 (three copies of chromosome 8) in a male is written as 47,XY,+8 (no intervening spaces). The number of cells with this abnormality is indicated in brackets. If 20 cells were examined, trisomy 8 was found in 10 cells, and the remainder were normal, the findings would be written as 47,XY,+8[10]/46,XY[10]. Translocations

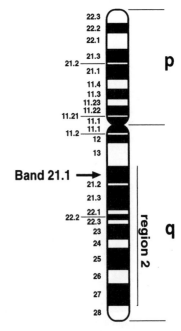

Figure 30-12 Banding pattern of the human X chromosome at the 550 average band level. Arrow indicates the location of Xq21.1.

(exchange of material between two chromosomes) are designated *t*, with the lowest chromosome number listed first. Thus a translocation between the short arm of chromosome 12 at band p13 and the long arm of chromosome 21 at band q22 is written as t(12;21)(p13;q22). A semicolon is used to separate the chromosomes and the band designations. A translocated chromosome is called a *derivative chromosome*. Using the previous example, chromosomes 12 and 21 are referred to as der(12) and der(21). Deletions are written with the abbreviation *del* preceding the chromosome. A deletion of the long arm of chromosome 5 at band 31 is written as del(5)(q31). No spaces are entered in these designations except between abbreviations.[17]

CHROMOSOME ABNORMALITIES

There are many types of chromosome abnormalities, such as deletions, inversions, ring formations, trisomies, and polyploidy. All these defects can be grouped into two major categories: defects involving an abnormality in the *number* of chromosomes and defects involving *structural* changes in one or more chromosomes.

Numeric Abnormalities

Numeric abnormalities often are subclassified as aneuploidy or polyploidy. *Aneuploidy* refers to any abnormal number of chromosomes that is not a multiple of the haploid number (23 chromosomes). The common forms of aneuploidy in humans are trisomy (the presence of an extra chromosome) and monosomy (the absence of a single chromosome). Aneuploidy is the result of nondisjunction, the failure of chromosomes to separate normally during cell division. Nondisjunction can occur during either of the two types of cell division: mitosis or meiosis. During normal mitosis, a cell divides once to produce two cells that are identical to the parent cell. In mitosis, each daughter cell contains 46 chromosomes. Meiosis is a special type of cell division that generates male and female gametes (sperm and ova). In contrast to mitosis, meiosis entails two cell divisions: meiosis I and meiosis II. The end result is a cell with 23 chromosomes, which is the haploid number (n).

In polyploidy, the chromosome number is higher than 46 but is always an exact multiple of the haploid chromosome number of 23. A karyotype with 69 chromosomes is called *triploidy (3n)* (Figure 30-13). A karyotype with 92 chromosomes is called *tetraploidy (4n)*.

In cancer, numerical abnormalities in the karyotype may be classified further based on the modal number of chromosomes in a neoplastic clone. *Hypodiploid* refers to a cell with fewer than 46 chromosomes; *near-haploid* cells have from 23 up to approximately 34 chromosomes (Figure 30-14); *hyperdiploid* cells have more than 46 chromosomes. *High hyperdiploidy* refers to a chromosome number of more than 50.[18] Finally the term *pseudodiploid* is used to describe a cell with 46 chromosomes and structural abnormalities.

Structural Abnormalities

Structural rearrangements result from breakage of a chromosome region with loss or subsequent rejoining in an abnormal

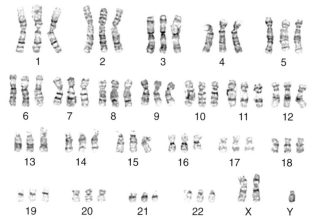

Figure 30-13 Triploid karyotype, 69,XXY. (Courtesy the Cytogenetics Laboratory, Indiana University School of Medicine, Indianapolis, IN.)

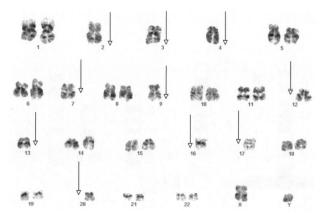

Figure 30-14 Hypodiploid karyotype with 36 chromosomes (arrows indicate missing chromosomes).

combination. Structural rearrangements are defined as *balanced* (no loss or gain of genetic chromatin) or *unbalanced* (gain or loss of genetic material). Structural rearrangements of single chromosomes include inversions, deletions, isochromosomes, ring formations, insertions, translocations, and duplications. Inversions (inv) involve one or two breaks in a single chromosome, followed by a 180-degree rotation of the segment between the breaks with no loss or gain of material. If the chromosomal material involves the centromere, the inversion is called *pericentric*. If the material that is inverted does not include the centromere, the inversion is called *paracentric* (Figure 30-15).

Interstitial *deletions* arise after two breaks in the same chromosome arm and loss of the segment between the breaks. Terminal deletions (loss of chromosomal material from the end of a chromosome) and interstitial deletions involve the loss of genetic material. The clinical consequence to the individual with a deletion depends on the extent and location of the deleted chromosomal material (Figure 30-16).

Isochromosomes arise from either abnormal division of the centromeres in which division is perpendicular to the long axis of the chromosome rather than parallel to it or from breakage and reunion in chromatin adjacent to the centromere. Each resulting daughter cell has a chromosome in which the short arm or the long arm is duplicated.

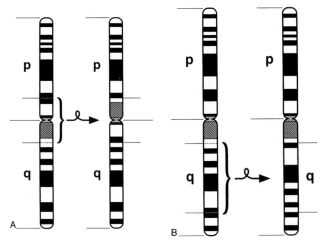

Figure 30-15 **A,** Pericentric inversion involves the centromere. **B,** Paracentric inversion occurs in either the short or long arm of the chromosome.

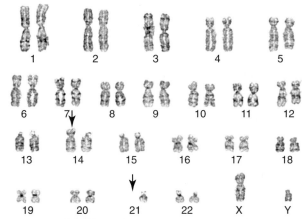

Figure 30-17 Balanced Robertsonian translocation between chromosomes 14 and 21. The nomenclature for this karyogram is written 45,XY,der(14;21)(q10;q10). (Courtesy the Cytogenetics Laboratory, Indiana University School of Medicine, Indianapolis, IN.)

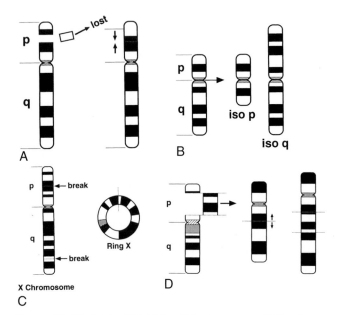

Figure 30-16 **A,** Interstitial deletion. **B,** Isochromosome. **C,** Ring chromosome. **D,** Insertion.

Ring chromosomes can result from breakage and reunion of a single chromosome with loss of chromosomal material outside the break points. Alternatively, one or both telomeres (chromosome ends) may join to form a ring chromosome without significant loss of chromosomal material.

Insertions involve movement of a segment of a chromosome from one location of the chromosome to another location of the same chromosome or to another chromosome. The segment is released as a result of two breaks, and the insertion occurs at the site of another break.

Duplication means partial trisomy for part of a chromosome. This can result from an unbalanced insertion or unequal crossing over in meiosis or mitosis.

Translocations occur when there is breakage in two chromosomes and each of the broken pieces reunites with another chromosome. If chromatin is neither lost nor gained, the

exchange is called a *balanced reciprocal translocation*. A reciprocal translocation is balanced if all chromatin material is present. The loss or gain of chromatin material results in partial monosomy or trisomy for a segment of the chromosome, which is designated an *unbalanced rearrangement*.

Another type of translocation involving breakage and reunion near the centromeric regions of two acrocentric chromosomes is known as a *Robertsonian translocation*. Effectively this is a fusion between two whole chromosomes rather than exchange of material, as in a reciprocal translocation. These translocations are among the most common balanced structural rearrangements seen in the general population with a frequency of 0.09% to 0.1%.[19] All five human acrocentric autosomes (13, 14, 15, 21, and 22) are capable of forming a Robertsonian translocation. In this case, the resulting balanced karyotype has only 45 chromosomes, which include the translocated chromosomes (Figure 30-17).

CANCER CYTOGENETICS

Cancer cytogenetics is a field that has been built upon discovery of nonrandom chromosome abnormalities in many types of cancer. In hematologic neoplasias, specific structural rearrangements are associated with distinct subtypes of leukemia that have characteristic morphologic and clinical features. Cytogenetic analysis of malignant cells can help determine the diagnosis and often the prognosis of a hematologic malignancy, assist the oncologist in the selection of appropriate therapy, and aid in monitoring the effects of therapy. Bone marrow is the tissue most frequently used to study the cytogenetics of a hematologic malignancy. Unstimulated peripheral blood and bone marrow trephine biopsy samples also may be analyzed. Cytogenetic analysis of cancers involving other organ systems can be performed using solid tissue obtained during surgery or by needle biopsy. Chromosomal defects in cancer include a wide range of numeric abnormalities and structural rearrangements, as discussed earlier (Table 30-1).

Cancer results from multiple and sequential genetic mutations occurring in a somatic cell. At some juncture, a critical mutation occurs, and the cell becomes self-perpetuating or clonal. A *clone* is a cell population derived from a single progenitor.[17] A cytogenetica clone exists if two or more cells contain the same structural abnormality or supernumerary marker chromosome or if three or more cells are missing the same chromosome. The primary aberration or stemline of a clone is a cytogenetic abnormality that is frequently observed as the sole abnormality associated with the cancer. The secondary aberration or sideline includes abnormalities additional to the primary aberration.[17] In chronic myelogenous leukemia, the primary aberration is the Philadelphia chromosome resulting from a translocation between the long arms of chromosomes 9 and 22, t(9;22)(q34;q11.2). A sideline of this clone would include secondary abnormalities, such as trisomy for chromosome 8, written as +8,t(9;22)(q34;q11.2).

Leukemia

Leukemias are clonal proliferations of malignant leukocytes that arise initially in the bone marrow before disseminating to the peripheral blood, lymph nodes, and other organs. They are broadly classified by the type of blood cell giving rise to the clonal proliferation (lymphoid or myeloid) and by the clinical course of the disease (acute or chronic). The four main leukemia categories are acute lymphoblastic leukemia (ALL), acute myeloid leukemia (AML), chronic lymphocytic leukemia (CLL), and chronic myelogenous leukemia (CML). The World Health Organization (WHO) classification for myeloid malignancies has categorized AML into seven subtypes: AML with recurrent genetic abnormalities; AML with myelodysplasia-related changes; therapy-related myeloid neoplasms; AML not otherwise specified; myeloid sarcoma; myeloid proliferations related to Down syndrome; and blastic plasmacytoid dendritic cell neoplasm (Chapter 35).[20] "AML with recurrent genetic abnormalities" is a classification based on the cytogenetic abnormalities observed (Box 30-1). Some of the divisions of the French-American-British (FAB) classification[21] are included in the "not otherwise classified" category. The WHO has classified lymphoid leukemias by precursor cell type, B or T (Chapter 35).

BOX 30-1 Acute Myeloid Leukemia (AML) with Recurrent Genetic Abnormalities*

AML with t(8;21)(q22;q22);*RUNX1T1/RUNX1*

AML with inv(16)(p13.1q22) or t(16;16)(p13.1;q22); */MYH11/CBFB*

Acute promyelocytic leukemia with t(15;17)(q24.1;q21.1);*PML/RARA*

AML with t(9;11)(p22;q23);*MLLT3/MLL(KMT2A)*

AML with t(6;9)(p23;q34);*DEK/NUP214*

AML with inv(3)(q21q26.2) or t(3;3)(q21.3;q26.2);*RPN1/MECOM*

AML (megakaryoblastic) with t(1;22)(p13;q13);*RBM15/MKL1*

AML with normal chromosomes and mutated *NPM1*(5q35.1)

AML with normal chromosomes and mutated *CEBPA*(19q13.1)

Modified from Swerdlow SH, Campo E, Harris NL, et al, editors: *WHO classification of tumours of haematopoietic and lymphoid tissues*, ed 4, Lyon, France, 2008, IARC Press.
*Updated per Hugo Nomenclature Database, May 2013

Chronic Myelogenous Leukemia

The first malignancy to be associated with a specific chromosome defect was CML, in which approximately 95% of patients were found to have the Philadelphia chromosome translocation, t(9;22)(q34;q11.2) by G-banded analysis.[22,23] The Philadelphia chromosome (derivative chromosome 22) is characterized by a balanced translocation between the long arms of chromosomes 9 and 22. At the molecular level, the gene for *ABL1*, an oncogene on chromosome 9, joins a gene on chromosome 22 named *BCR*. The result of the fusion of these two genes is a new fusion protein of about 210 kD with growth-promoting capabilities that override normal cell regulatory mechanisms (Figures 30-18 and 30-19) (Chapter 33).[24]

BCR/ABL1

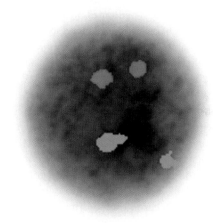

Figure 30-18 Normal bone marrow interphase cell hybridized with the *BCR* (green) and *ABL1* (red) genes (Abbott Molecular, Des Plaines, IL). The two red and two green signals represent the genes on the normal chromosomes 9 and 22. (Courtesy the Cytogenetics Laboratory, Indiana University School of Medicine, Indianapolis, IN.)

BCR/ABL1

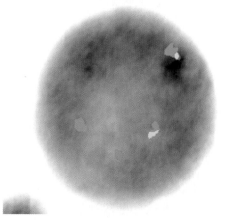

Figure 30-19 Abnormal bone marrow interphase cell with one *BCR* (green) and one *ABL1* (red) signal (Abbott Molecular, Des Plaines, IL.) representing the normal chromosomes and two fusion signals from the derivative chromosomes 9 and 22. (Courtesy the Cytogenetics Laboratory, Indiana University School of Medicine, Indianapolis, IN.)

The fusion protein activates tyrosine kinase signaling to drive proliferation of the cell. This signaling can be blocked by imatinib mesylate (Gleevec; Novartis Pharmaceuticals, East Hanover, NJ) or another tyrosine kinase inhibitor.[25] Patient response to imatinib is monitored by cytogenetic analysis and FISH. At diagnosis, the characteristic karyotype is the presence of the Philadelphia chromosome in all cells analyzed. After treatment with imatinib for several months, the karyotype typically has a mixture of abnormal and normal cells indicating patient response to therapy. *Complete response* is defined as a bone marrow karyotype with only normal cells. Therapeutic response is often monitored using peripheral blood instead of a bone marrow aspirate. In contrast to the bone marrow, the peripheral blood does not contain spontaneously dividing cells. As a result, chromosomal analysis of a specimen of unstimulated peripheral blood may be unsuccessful because of the absence of dividing cells. In these cases, FISH with probes for the specific abnormality is performed on 200 or more interphase (nondividing) cells of the peripheral blood specimen to search for chromosomally abnormal cells. The detection of cytogenetic abnormalities in interphase (nondividing) cells is an important advantage of FISH technology.

Acute Leukemia

The Philadelphia chromosome is also observed in acute leukemia. It is seen in about 20% of adults with ALL, 2% to 5% of children with ALL, and 1% of patients with AML.[26-28] In childhood ALL, chromosome number is critical for predicting the severity of the leukemia. Children whose leukemic cells contain more than 50 chromosomes (hyperdiploid karyotype) have the best prognosis for complete recovery with therapy. Recurring translocations observed in ALL include t(4;11) (q21;q23), t(12;21)(p13;q22), and t(1;19)(q23;p13.3). Each translocation is associated with a prognostic outcome and assists oncologists in determining patient therapy. The t(4;11) translocation is the one most commonly found in infants with acute lymphoblastic leukemia. Rearrangements of the *AFF1* gene on chromosome 4 and the *MLL* gene on chromosome 11 occur in this translocation.[29,30] Disruption of the *MLL* gene is seen in both ALL and AML (Figures 30-20 and 30-21).

The AMLs are subdivided into several morphologic classifications ranging from M0 to M7 according to the FAB classification (Chapter 35).[31,32] Characteristic chromosome translocations are associated with some subgroups and were incorporated into the WHO classification. Among them is a translocation between the long arms of chromosomes 8 and 21, t(8;21) (q22;q22), which is representative of AML with maturation. Acute promyelocytic leukemia is associated with a translocation between the long arms of chromosomes 15 and 17, t(15;17) (q24;q21) (Figure 30-22). A pericentric inversion of chromosome 16, inv(16)(p13.2q22), is seen in AML with increased eosinophils. The inversion juxtaposes the core the binding factor beta (*CBFB*) gene on 16q with the myosin heavy chain gene (*MYH11*) on 16p to form a new fusion protein (Figure 30-23).[33] These recurring translocations have enabled researchers to localize genes important for cell growth and regulation. As with acute lymphoblastic leukemia, the specific translocation

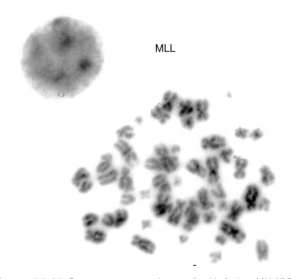

Figure 30-20 Bone marrow metaphase cell with fusion *MLL(KMT2A)* signal on the normal chromosome 11 and split red and green signals on the translocated chromosomes, representing a disruption of the *MLL(KMT2A)* gene. (Courtesy the Cytogenetics Laboratory, Indiana University School of Medicine, Indianapolis, IN.)

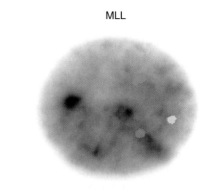

Figure 30-21 Bone marrow interphase cell with a fusion signal (normal chromosome 11) and split red and green signals from the *MLL(KMT2A)* gene representing a rearrangement. (Courtesy the Cytogenetics Laboratory, Indiana University School of Medicine, Indianapolis, IN.)

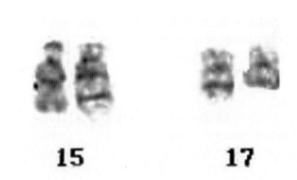

Figure 30-22 Bone marrow metaphase chromosomes 15 and 17 homologues showing a translocation between the long arms of chromosomes 15 and 17, t(15;17)(q24.1;q21.1), diagnostic of acute promyelocytic leukemia. The abnormal chromosomes are on the right. (Courtesy the Cytogenetics Laboratory, Indiana University School of Medicine, Indianapolis, IN.)

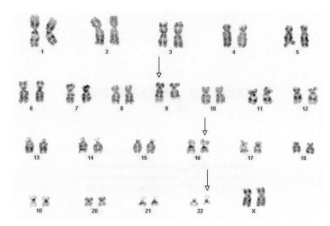

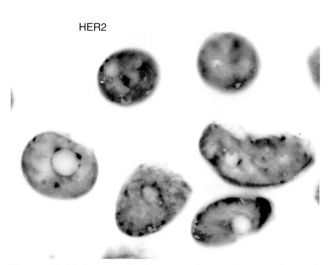

Figure 30-23 Bone marrow karyogram for a patient with acute myeloid leukemia (AML) showing a translocation, t(9;22)(q34;q11.2), and an inverted chromosome 16, inv(16)(p13.1q22). (Courtesy the Cytogenetics Laboratory, Indiana University School of Medicine, Indianapolis, IN.)

Figure 30-25 Tissue section from a breast cancer demonstrating amplification of *HER2*. The tissue was hybridized with fluorescence in situ hybridization probes for *HER2* (red) and the chromosome 17 centromere probe (green) (Abbott Molecular, Des Plaines, IL). The number of *HER2* signals exceeds the number of centromere signals, which indicates selective amplification of *HER2*.

in AML often predicts patient prognosis and response to therapy. Understanding the molecular consequences of the cytogenetic mutations, such as the *BCR/ABL1* translocation, provides the fundamental information for the development of targeted therapies.

Solid Tumors

Just as recurring structural and numeric chromosome defects have been observed in the hematologic malignancies, a wide range of nonrandom abnormalities have also been found in solid tumors. Most of these abnormalities confer a proliferative advantage on the malignant cell and serve as useful prognostic indicators. Amplification (increased copy number) of the gene *HER2* (also called *ERBB2*) on chromosome 17, a transmembrane growth factor receptor, is associated with an aggressive form of invasive breast cancer.[34,35] FISH with probes for the *HER2* gene and an internal control (17 centromere) can determine if there is gene amplification in the tumor (Figure 30-24).[36] If FISH testing

shows amplification to be present, the patient is eligible for targeted therapy with a monoclonal antibody, trastuzumab (Figure 30-25).[37] FISH for *HER2* typically is performed on tissue sections from the paraffin-embedded tumor block.

CHROMOSOMAL MICROARRAY ANALYSIS

Chromosomal microarray (CMA) is a fluorescence-based molecular technique for submicroscopic analysis of genomic DNA. CMA testing increases the detection of clinically significant imbalances over a karyotype.[38] CMA is performed utilizing a glass slide or chip platform. Chromosomal microarrays, like standard cytogenetic analysis, look at the entire genome but with higher levels of resolution (base pair or kilobase level) determined by the number and composition of targets on the array. Using a SNP-based array, patient DNA is hybridized to a chip composed of greater than 2 million markers that detect copy number variation (gains and losses) and SNP polymorphisms. Single nucleotide polymorphism (SNP) probes detect position-specific markers that have different forms (polymorphic). Analysis of the SNP data from a specimen allows for detection of copy neutral loss of heterozygosity or uniparental disomy, as well as gains and losses of genomic DNA. Regions of imbalance (copy gain or copy loss) in the patient specimen are assessed relative to a reference control. The yield of detection of abnormalities is increased from an average of 3% to 11% due to the high resolution of the array (Figures 30-26 and 30-27).[38-40] This technique is presently used primarily for diagnosis of constitutional (inherited) disorders, but emerging applications for cancer are in development.

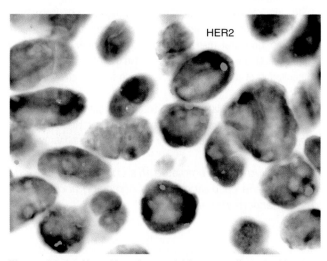

Figure 30-24 Normal interphase nuclei from a paraffin-embedded tissue section hybridized with probes for *HER2* (red) and the chromosome 17 centromere (green) (Abbott Molecular, Des Plaines, IL). Two green and two red signals are seen per cell.

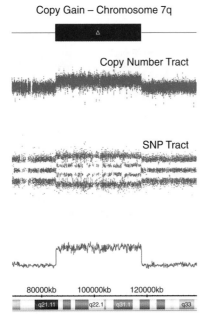

Figure 30-26 Chromosomal microarray diagram demonstrating approximately a 32.4-Mb gain of genetic material between bands 7q21 and 7q31. (Courtesy of the Cytogenetics Laboratory, Indiana University School of Medicine, Indianapolis, IN.)

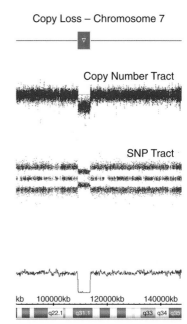

Figure 30-27 Chromosomal microarray diagram demonstrating approximately a 4.6 Mb loss at band 7q31.1. (Courtesy of the Cytogenetics Laboratory, Indiana University School of Medicine, Indianapolis, IN.)

SUMMARY

- Cytogenetics is the study of chromosome structure and inheritance.
- Chromosome disorders are secondary to structural or numeric chromosomal abnormalities involving the rearrangement or the loss or gain of a piece of a chromosome or the entire chromosome.
- Nonrandom chromosome abnormalities are associated with cancer.
- A chromosome is composed of a double helix strand of DNA. Attached to the backbone of deoxyribose are adenine (A), guanine (G), cytosine (C), and thymine (T).
- During mitosis, cells can be chemically treated to arrest cell progression in metaphase so that chromosomes can be analyzed.
- Q-banding differentiates chromosomes into bands of different widths and relative brightness, revealing a banding pattern unique to each individual chromosome.
- Other stains used to identify chromosomes may require pretreatment of the slide for analysis. These include G-banding, C-banding, and AG-NOR–banding.
- FISH, a molecular cytogenetic technique, uses DNA or RNA probes and fluorescence microscopy to identify individual chromosomes and targeted chromosomal loci. Metaphase and interphase cells can be analyzed by FISH.

- Tissues used for chromosome analysis typically include bone marrow cells and peripheral blood lymphocytes, amniotic fluid, nonneoplastic tissue, and tumors.
- A normal cell contains 46 chromosomes, which includes 2 sex chromosomes (XX or XY).
- Defects in chromosomes can be categorized as numeric or structural. Numeric abnormalities can be subclassified as aneuploidy and polyploidy.
- Structural rearrangements include inversions, deletions, isochromosomes, ring formations, insertions, translocations, and duplications.
- Specific structural rearrangements are associated with distinct subtypes of leukemias and may assist in diagnosis, prognosis, and monitoring of therapy. Solid tumors also may be analyzed using cytogenetics.
- Chromosomal microarray testing utilizes a microarray platform to detect abnormalities at a submicroscopic level of resolution. The higher resolution increases the detection of chromosomal abnormalities.

Now that you have completed this chapter, go back and read again the case study at the beginning and respond to the questions presented.

REVIEW QUESTIONS

Answers can be found in the Appendix.

1. *G-banding* refers to the technique of staining chromosomes:
   a. To isolate those in the G group (i.e., chromosomes 21 and 22)
   b. In the G_0 or resting stage
   c. Using Giemsa stain
   d. To emphasize areas high in guanine residues

2. Which of the following compounds is used to halt mitosis in metaphase for chromosome analyses?
   a. Imatinib
   b. Fluorescein
   c. Trypsin
   d. Colchicine

3. One arm of a chromosome has 30 bands. Which band would be nearest the centromere?
   a. Band 1
   b. Band 15
   c. Band 30

4. Which of the following is *not* an advantage of the use of FISH?
   a. It can be used on nondividing cells.
   b. It can be used on paraffin-embedded tissue.
   c. It can detect mutations that do not result in abnormal banding patterns.
   d. It must be performed on dividing cells.

5. Which of the following types of mutations would likely *not* be detectable with cytogenetic banding techniques?
   a. Point mutation resulting in a single amino acid substitution
   b. Transfer of genetic material from one chromosome to another
   c. Loss of genetic material from a chromosome that does not appear on any other chromosome
   d. Duplication of a chromosome resulting in 3n of that genetic material

6. Which of the following describes a chromosomal deletion?
   a. Point mutation resulting in a single amino acid substitution
   b. Transfer of genetic material from one chromosome to another
   c. Loss of genetic material from a chromosome that does not appear on any other chromosome
   d. Duplication of a chromosome resulting in 3n of that genetic material

The chromosome analysis performed on a patient's leukemic cells is reported as 47, XY,+4,del(5)(q31)[20]. Answer questions 7 to 9 based on this description.

7. This patient's cells have which of the following mutations?
   a. Loss of the entire number 31 chromosome
   b. Loss of the entire number 5 chromosome
   c. Loss of a portion of the short arm of chromosome 4
   d. Loss of a portion of the long arm of chromosome 5

8. What other mutation is present in this patient's cells?
   a. Polyploidy
   b. Tetraploidy
   c. An extra chromosome 4
   d. Four copies of chromosome 5

9. This patient's leukemic cells demonstrate:
   a. Structural chromosomal defects only
   b. Numeric chromosomal defects only
   c. Both structural and numeric chromosomal defects

10. *Aneuploidy* describes the total chromosome number:
    a. That is a multiple of the haploid number
    b. That reflects a loss or gain of a single chromosome
    c. That is diploid but has a balanced deletion and duplication of whole chromosomes
    d. In gametes; *diploid* is the number in somatic cells

REFERENCES

1. International Human Genome Sequencing Consortium. (2004). Finishing the euchromatic sequence of the human genome. *Nature, 431,* 931–945.
2. Benn, P. (2010). Prenatal diagnosis of chromosomal abnormalities through amniocentesis. In Milunsky, A., & Milunsky, J. M., (Eds.), *Genetic disorders and the fetus.* (6th ed., pp. 194–195). Baltimore: Wiley-Blackwell.
3. Boué, J., Boué, A., & Lazar, P. (1975). Retrospective and prospective epidemiological studies of 1500 karyotyped spontaneous human abortions. *Teratology, 12,* 11–26.
4. Rowley, J. D. (2008). Chromosomal translocations: revisited yet again. *Blood, 112,* 2183–2189.
5. Watson, J. D., & Crick, F. H. C. (1983). Molecular structure of nucleic acids: a structure for deoxyribose nucleic acid. *Nature, 171,* 737–738.
6. Earnshaw, W. C. (1988). Mitotic chromosome structure. *Bioessays, 9,* 147–150.
7. Olins, A. L., & Olins, D. E. (1974). Spheroid chromatin units. *Science, 183,* 330–332.
8. Oudet, P., Gross-Bellard, M., & Chambon, P. (1975). Electron microscopic and biochemical evidence that chromatin structure is a repeating unit. *Cell, 4,* 281–300.
9. Rattner, J. B. (1988). Chromatin hierarchies and metaphase chromatin structure. In Adolph, K. W., (Ed.), *Chromosomes and chromatin,* vol 3. (pp. 30). Boca Raton, Fla: CRC Press.
10. Tijo, J. H., & Levan, A. (1956). The chromosome number of man. *Hereditas, 42,* 1–6.
11. Hsu, T. C. (1979). *Human and mammalian cytogenetics* (pp. 6–7). New York: Springer-Verlag.

12. Nowell, P. C. (1960). Phytohemagglutinin: an initiator of mitosis in culture of normal human leukocytes. *Cancer Res, 20,* 462–466.

13. Farnes, P., Barker, B. E., Brownhill, L. E., et al. (1964). Mitogenic activity of *Phytolacca americana* (pokeweed). *Lancet, 2,* 1100–1101.

14. Caspersson, T., Zech, L., Modest, E. J., et al. (1969). Chemical differentiation with fluorescent alkylating agents in *Vicia faba* metaphase chromosomes. *Exp Cell Res, 58,* 128–140.

15. Yunis, J. J. (1979). Cytogenetics. In Henry, J. B., (Ed.). *Clinical diagnosis and management by laboratory methods.* (16th ed., p. 825). Philadelphia: Saunders.

16. Plattner, R., Heerema, N. A., Yurov, Y. B., et al. (1993). Efficient identification of marker chromosomes in 27 patients by stepwise hybridization with alpha satellite DNA probes. *Hum Genet, 91,* 131–140.

17. Shaffer, L. G., McGowan-Jordan, J., & Schmid, J. M., (Eds.). (2013). ISCN 2013. *An international system for human cytogenetic nomenclature.* Basel, Switzerland: S. Karger.

18. Moorman, A. V., Richards, S. M., Martineau, M., et al. (2003). Outcome heterogeneity in childhood high-hyperdiploid acute lymphoblastic leukemia. *Blood, 102,* 2756–2762.

19. Turleau, C., Chavin-Colin, F., & de Grouchy, J. (1979). Cytogenetic investigation in 413 couples with spontaneous abortions. *Eur J Obstet Gynecol Reprod Biol, 9,* 65–74.

20. Swerdlow, S. H., Campo, E., Harris, N. L., et al., (Eds.). (2008). *WHO classification of tumours of haematopoietic and lymphoid tissues.* (4th ed.). Lyon, France: IARC Press.

21. Bennett, J. M., Catovsky, D., Daniel, M. T., et al. (1976). Proposals for classification of the acute leukaemias. French-American-British (FAB) Co-operative Group. *Br J Haematol, 33,* 451–458.

22. Nowell, P. C., & Hungerford, D. A. (1960). A minute chromosome in human chronic granulocytic leukemia. *Science, 132,* 1497 (abstract).

23. Rowley, J. D. (1973). A new consistent chromosomal abnormality in chronic myelogenous leukemia identified by quinacrine fluorescence and Giemsa staining. *Nature, 243,* 290–293.

24. Ben-Neriah, Y., Daley, G. Q., Mes-Masson, A., et al. (1986). The chronic myelogenous leukemia–specific P210 protein is the product of the *BCR/ABL* hybrid gene. *Science, 233,* 212–214.

25. Druker, B. J., Tamura, S., Buchdunger, E., et al. (1996). Effects of a selective inhibitor of the Abl tyrosine kinase on the growth of BCR-ABL positive cells. *Nat Med, 2,* 561–566.

26. Third International Workshop on Chromosomes in Leukemia. (1981). Chromosomal abnormalities in acute lymphoblastic leukemia: structural and numerical changes in 234 cases. *Cancer Genet Cytogenet, 4,* 101–110.

27. Ribeiro, R. C., Abromowitch, M., Raimondi, S. C., et al. (1987). Clinical and biologic hallmarks of the Philadelphia chromosome in childhood acute lymphoblastic leukemia. *Blood, 70,* 948–953.

28. Crist, W., Carroll, A., Shuster, J., et al. (1990). Philadelphia chromosome positive acute lymphoblastic leukemia: clinical and cytogenetic characteristics and treatment outcome. A Pediatric Oncology Group study. *Blood, 76,* 489–494.

29. Morrissey, J., Tkachuk, D. C., Milatovich, A., et al. (1993). A serine/proline-rich protein is fused to HRX in t(4;11) acute leukemias. *Blood, 81,* 1124–1131.

30. Hayne, C. C., Winer, E., Williams, T., et al. (2006). Acute lymphoblastic leukemia with a 4;11 translocation analyzed by multi-modal strategy of conventional cytogenetics, FISH, morphology, flow cytometry, molecular genetics and review of the literature. *Exp Mol Pathol, 81,* 62–71.

31. Bennett, J. M., Catovsky, D., Daniel, M. T., et al. Proposed revised criteria for the classification of acute myeloid leukemia: a report of the French-American-British Cooperative Group. *Ann Intern Med, 103,* 620–625.

32. Bennett, J. M., Catovsky, D., Daniel, M. T., et al. (1985). Criteria for the diagnosis of acute leukemia of megakaryocytic lineage (M7): a report of the French-American-British Cooperative Group. *Ann Intern Med, 103,* 460–462.

33. Claxton, D. F., Liu, P., Hsu, H. B., et al. (1994). Detection of fusion transcripts generated by the inversion 16 chromosome in acute myelogenous leukemia. *Blood, 83,* 1750–1756.

34. Slamon, D. J., Godolphin, W., Jones, L. A., et al. (1989). Studies of the HER-2 proto-oncogene in human breast and ovarian cancer. *Science, 244,* 707–712.

35. Perez, E. A., Roche, P. C., Jenkins, R. B., et al. (2002). HER2 testing in patients with breast cancer: poor correlation between weak positivity by immunohistochemistry and gene amplification by fluorescence in situ hybridization. *Mayo Clin Proc, 77,* 148–154.

36. Wolff, A. C., Hammond, E., Schwartz, J. N., et al. (2007). American Society of Clinical Oncology/College of American Pathologists guideline recommendations for human epidermal growth factor receptor 2 testing in breast cancer. *J Clin Oncol, 25*(1), 118–145.

37. Slamon, D. J., Leyland-Jones, B., Shak, S., et al. (2001). Use of chemotherapy plus a monoclonal antibody against HER2 for metastatic breast cancer that overexpresses HER2. *N Engl J Med, 344,* 783–792.

38. Miller, D. T., Adam, M. P., Aradhya, S., Biesecker, L. G., Brothman, A. R., et al. (2010). Consensus statement: chromosomal microarray is the first-tier clinical diagnostic test for individuals with developmental disabilities or congenital anomalies. *Am J Hum Genet, 86,* 749–764.

39. Kearney, H. M., Thorland, E. C., Brown, K. K., et al. (2011). American College of Medical Genetics standards and guidelines for interpretation and reporting of postnatal constitutional copy number variants. *Genet Med, 13,* 680–685.

40. Kearney, H. M., South, S. T., Wolff, D. J., Lamb, A., et al. (2011). American College of Medical Genetics recommendations for the design and performance expectations for clinical genomic copy number microarrays intended for use in the postnatal setting for detection of constitutional abnormalities. *Genet Med, 13,* 676–679.

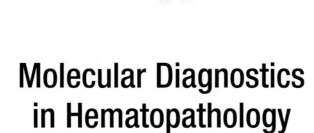

Molecular Diagnostics in Hematopathology

31

Cynthia L. Jackson and Shashi Mehta*

OUTLINE

OBJECTIVES

After completion of this chapter, the reader will be able to:

1. Describe the structure of DNA, including the composition of a nucleotide, the double helix, and the antiparallel complementary strand orientation.
2. Predict the nucleotide sequence of a complementary strand of DNA or RNA given the nucleotide sequence of a DNA template.
3. Explain the relationship between DNA structure and protein structure.
4. Discuss the process of DNA replication, including replication origin, replication fork, primase, primer, DNA polymerase, Okazaki fragments, leading strand, and lagging strand.
5. Determine the appropriate patient specimen required for DNA isolation to identify an inherited or somatic mutation.
6. Discuss common methods of DNA and RNA isolation.
7. Explain the principle of polymerase chain reaction (PCR), reverse transcriptase PCR, and nucleic acid hybridization.
8. Compare and contrast the methods for detecting target DNA including: gel electrophoresis using intercalating dyes or capillary gel electrophoresis; cleavage-based signal amplification; restriction fragment length polymorphism; and probe hybridization techniques such as Southern blotting.
9. Describe the principle of qualitative real-time PCR and contrast it with endpoint PCR.
10. Discuss the use of quantitative real-time PCR for monitoring minimal residual disease.
11. Explain traditional Sanger DNA sequencing and contrast it with pyrosequencing, and next-generation sequencing (massively parallel sequencing).
12. Describe the use of microarray-based comparative genomic hybridization (aCGH) and single nucleotide polymorphism array (SNP-A) karyotyping for the detection of chromosome copy number alterations.

CASE STUDY**

After studying the material in this chapter, the reader should be able to respond to the following case study:

A 42-year-old man came to the emergency room complaining of pain behind his right knee. He had observed swelling below the knee for the previous 2 days. The patient was in no apparent distress and was experiencing no chest pain, shortness of breath, dyspnea, or hemoptysis. The patient reported no history of trauma except for a right femur break 20 years before. He reported that he was taking no medications and was in good general health. Five years previously, he experienced an episode of deep vein thrombosis (DVT) in his right lower leg and was treated with intravenous heparin followed by oral warfarin (Coumadin) for 3 months. Subsequent to treatment, he experienced occasional pain behind both knees, which he treated with aspirin. He noted that his mother had been diagnosed with carpal tunnel syndrome and had developed DVT, for which she has been taking oral warfarin for 15 years. The patient's job requires frequent long airplane flights. He flies first class and walks around occasionally during the long flights. His leg pain began 1 week after a flight to Europe.

Continued

---

*The authors acknowledge Dr. Mark E. Lasbury, whose work in prior editions formed the foundation for this chapter.

CASE STUDY**—cont'd

On physical examination, the patient had no evidence of rash or oral ulcers. No petechiae or purpura were noted. He had mild pretibial pitting edema. His right leg measured 36.5 cm at 25 cm distal to the superior aspect of the patella, whereas his left leg measured 33.5 cm in the same location. CBC findings were unremarkable, and both the prothrombin time and activated partial prothrombin time were within the reference intervals. Doppler ultrasonography revealed complete occlusion of the distal superficial femoral vein, anterior tibial vein, and popliteal vein. The diagnosis was DVT without pulmonary emboli. The patient was hospitalized, and a heparin drip was started. The hematologist ordered a factor V (*F5*) Leiden mutation analysis on blood drawn in an EDTA tube. Figure 31-1 illustrates the results of the mutation analysis.

1. What type of specimen is appropriate when analyzing DNA for a hereditary mutation?
2. Examine the gel electrophoresis result (Figure 31-1). Are the correct controls present?
3. What band sizes (in base pairs or bp) appear in the patient's sample?
4. What band sizes are expected for an individual who is homozygous for the factor V (*F5*) Leiden mutation, heterozygous for the mutation, and free of the mutation?
5. Does this patient have the factor V (*F5*) Leiden gene mutation?

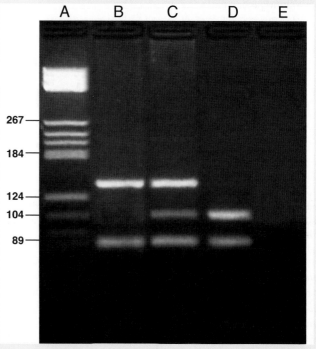

Figure 31-1 Results of the factor V (*F5*) Leiden mutation test on the patient in the case study. Lane **A,** molecular size marker; **B,** positive control (homozygous for factor V Leiden mutation); **C,** patient's sample; **D,** negative control (no mutation); **E,** no-DNA control. The expected banding pattern on an agarose gel for the factor V (*F5*) Leiden mutation test is as follows: homozygous for the mutation, 141 and 82 bp bands; heterozygous for the mutation, 141, 104, and 82 bp bands; no mutation (normal or wild-type), 104 and 82 bp bands. A band at 37 bp is barely visible and is difficult to detect on an agarose gel. However, this band is not essential for interpreting the results.

**This case was provided by George A. Fritsma, MS, MLS, manager, The Fritsma Factor: Your Interactive Hemostasis Resource, http://www.fritsmafactor.com, sponsored by Precision BioLogic, Inc., Cambridge, Nova Scotia.

M olecular biology techniques enhance the diagnostic team's ability to predict or identify an increasing number of diseases in the clinical laboratory. Molecular techniques also enable clinicians to monitor disease progression during treatment, make accurate prognoses, and predict the response to therapeutics. The short interval required to perform molecular diagnostic tests and analyze their results is an additional positive aspect of this type of testing, resulting in more efficient patient management, especially in cases of infection. The five main areas of hematopathologic molecular testing include detection of mutations, gene rearrangements, and chromosomal abnormalities for diagnosis and prognosis of hematologic malignancies (Box 31-1); detection and quantification of minimal residual disease to monitor treatment of hematologic malignancies; detection of mutations in inherited hematologic disorders (Box 31-2); pharmacogenetic testing to detect

genetic variation affecting certain drug therapies (Box 31-3); and identification of hematologically important infectious diseases (Box 31-4).

STRUCTURE AND FUNCTION OF DNA

The Central Dogma: DNA to RNA to Protein

Much of the stored information needed to carry out cell processes resides in deoxyribonucleic acid (DNA); therefore, proper cellular storage, maintenance, and replication of DNA are necessary to ensure homeostasis. Because molecular testing takes advantage of DNA structure and replication, a review of molecular biology is helpful.

The *central dogma* in genetics is that information stored in the DNA is *replicated* to daughter DNA, *transcribed* to messenger ribonucleic acid (mRNA), and *translated* into a functional protein (Figure 31-2). This process is essential to carry out cellular

---

BOX 31-1 Major Hematologic Malignancies in Which Molecular Methods Are Performed for Diagnosis and Monitoring Minimal Residual Disease

For Diagnosis:

Acute leukemias
  Myeloid
  Lymphoblastic
Myeloproliferative neoplasms
  Chronic myelogenous leukemia
  Polycythemia vera
  Essential thrombocythemia
  Primary myelofibrosis
Myelodysplastic syndromes
Mature lymphoid neoplasms
  Chronic lymphocytic leukemia
  Lymphomas

For Monitoring Minimal Residual Disease:

Acute leukemias
  Quantification of fusion mRNA transcripts due to translocations
  Quantification of specific B and T cell receptor rearrangements
Chronic myelogenous leukemia
  Quantification of fusion mRNA transcripts due to translocation

---

BOX 31-2 Inherited Hematologic Disorders Detected by Molecular Methods

Erythrocyte disorders
  Hemoglobinopathies/thalassemias
  Membrane abnormalities
  Enzyme deficiencies
  Erythropoietic porphyrias
Leukocyte disorders
  Quantitative disorders
  Functional disorders
  Storage disorders
Platelet disorders
  Quantitative disorders
  Functional disorders
Bone marrow failure syndromes
Coagulopathies
Thrombophilia

BOX 31-3 Pharmacogenetic Testing for Genetic Variation Affecting Therapy

Warfarin sensitivity
  Cytochrome P450 2C9 variants, CYP2C9*2, CYP2C9*3
  VKORC1 variants
Clopidogrel sensitivity
  Cytochrome P450 2C19 variants, CYP2C19*17, others
Thiopurine sensitivity
  Thiopurine S-methyltransferase, TPMT*2, TPMT*3C, TPMT*3A
Imatinib resistance
  ABL1 mutation analysis

BOX 31-4 Hematologically Important Pathogens Detected by Molecular Methods

Parasitic pathogens
  Plasmodium
  Filaria
  Babesia
  Leishmania
  Trypanosoma
Fungal pathogens
Bacterial pathogens
Viral pathogens
  Parvovirus B19
  Cytomegalovirus
  Epstein-Barr virus
  Human immunodeficiency virus types 1 and 2
  Human T-cell lymphotropic virus type 1

Modified from Paessler M, Bagg A: Use of molecular techniques in the analysis of hematologic diseases. In Hoffman R, Benz EJ Jr, Shattil SJ, et al, editors: *Hematology: basic principles and practice,* ed 4, Philadelphia, 2005, Churchill Livingstone, pp. 2713-2726.

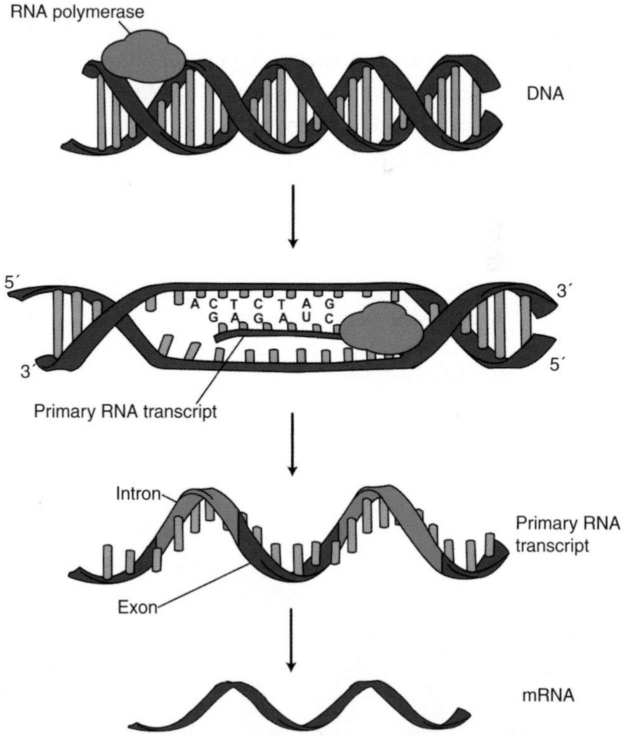

Figure 31-2 RNA polymerase binds to a sequence of DNA called the *promoter region,* which causes the DNA strands to separate. Using one of the DNA strands as a template, RNA polymerase moves along and simultaneously reads the DNA strand, forming the primary messenger RNA (mRNA) transcript by joining the complementary ribonucleotides. The primary mRNA transcript consists of sequences called exons that provide coding information and introns that are excised from the mature mRNA. The spliced mRNA then leaves the nucleus and enters the cytoplasm of the cell where the ribosomes translate the mRNA into protein.

functions while preserving a record of the stored information. In eukaryotes, the initial DNA sequence is composed of *translated* exons separated by *untranslated* introns. The introns are enzymatically excised following transcription from DNA to RNA, and the mature mRNA sequence is then translated. Translation is an enzymatic process wherein mRNA three-nucleotide base sequences called *codons* drive the addition of individual amino acids to the growing peptide. The mature protein then carries out its cellular function, which may be structural or may involve recognition, regulation, or enzymatic activity.

The structural units that carry DNA's message are called *genes*. The human β-globin gene, part of the hemoglobin molecule, provides a good example of replication and transcription, because it was one of the first sequenced and demonstrates the result of aberrant sequence maintenance. A normal (or *wild-type*) β-globin gene contains a sequence of bases that code for a β-globin peptide of 146 amino acids (Chapter 10). One inherited mutation changes a single DNA base. This is called a *point mutation*. The mutation occurs in the portion of the sequence that codes for the sixth amino acid of β-globin. The mutation substitutes the amino acid *valine* for *glutamic acid* in the growing peptide. Valine modifies the overall charge, producing a protein that polymerizes in a low-oxygen environment. This leads to sickled erythrocytes, circulatory ischemia, and poor oxygen exchange between blood and tissues.[1,2] A mutation in one of the two copies (*alleles*) of this gene inherited from the parents results in a heterozygous condition, or sickle cell trait. In a *heterozygote,* the symptoms of the disease are often unseen or are present only during times of physical stress. If both alleles are mutated, there is overt *homozygous* sickle cell disease, and the symptoms are severe.

Every active gene is translated. Human somatic cells contain 20,000 to 25,000 genes in 2 meters of DNA.[3,4] Significant packing (Figure 30-3) takes place to reduce the volume of the nucleic acid to the size of chromosomes.

DNA at the Molecular Level

DNA is a duplex molecule composed of two complementary hydrogen-bonded *nucleotide* strands (Figure 31-3). Deoxyribo-

nucleotides and ribonucleotides are the building blocks of DNA and RNA, respectively. Each nucleotide is composed of a 5-carbon sugar (pentose), a nitrogenous base, and a phosphate group. The numbers one prime (1′) to five prime (5′) designate the pentose's carbons. In DNA, the pentose is a ribose in which the hydroxyl group on the 2′ carbon is replaced by a hydrogen molecule, hence 2′-deoxyribose (Figure 31-4, *A*). In RNA, the 2′ ribose retains the 2′ hydroxyl group. The hydroxyl group present on the 3′ carbon of the sugar is crucial for polymerization of the nucleotide monomers to form the nucleic acid strand.

The nitrogenous base is linked to the sugar by a glycosidic bond at the 1′ carbon. Four different bases form DNA, but the linkage to the sugar is the same for each. The phosphate group is linked to the sugar at the 5′ carbon by a phosphodiester bond (Figure 31-4, *B, C*). The phosphate group is also crucial

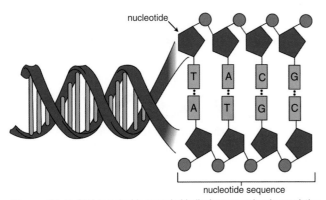

Figure 31-3 DNA is a double-stranded helical macromolecule consisting of nucleotide subunits joined in sequence by deoxyribose molecules (pentagons) and phosphate radicals (circles). The bases thymine (T), adenine (A), cytosine (C), and guanine (G) are illustrated in their standard pairs: thymine to adenine, cytosine to guanine.

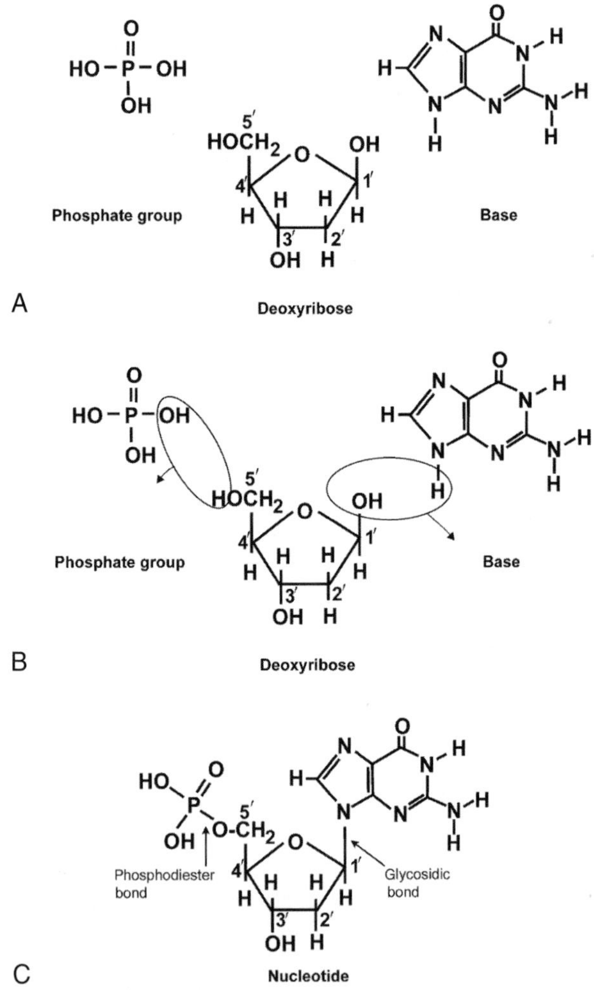

Figure 31-4 A, The pentose sugar, deoxyribose, a phosphate group, and a nitrogenous base compose a DNA nucleotide. The carbons of the deoxyribose molecule are numbered 1′ through 5′. The hydroxyl group on the 2′ carbon of ribose is replaced by a hydrogen molecule, making the structure a deoxyribose. **B,** A nucleotide results from the formation of a glycosidic bond between the nitrogenous base and the hydroxyl group on the 1′ carbon of deoxyribose and a phosphodiester bond between the phosphate group and the hydroxyl group on the 5′ carbon of deoxyribose. **C,** A nucleotide illustrating the glycosidic and phosphodiester bonds.

for addition of nucleotides to the growing polymer. A sugar, whether ribose or deoxyribose, linked to a nitrogenous base but without a phosphate group, is called a *nucleoside*. A nucleoside cannot be incorporated into DNA, and neither can a nucleotide consisting of only one phosphate group (deoxynucleotide monophosphate, or dNMP). To be incorporated into a growing strand of DNA, the nucleotide must have three phosphate groups linked to one another, referred to as the α-, β-, and γ-phosphates with the α-phosphate linked to the sugar (Figure 31-5).

Creation of a phosphodiester bond between the 3′ hydroxyl group of the existing strand and the 5′ α-phosphate of the nucleotide monomer requires the enzyme *DNA polymerase*. This enzyme recognizes the hydroxyl group on the 3′ carbon of the sugar and bonds the 3′ hydroxyl group of one nucleotide with the α-phosphate group of another (Figure 31-5). Polymerization of subsequent nucleotides forms a DNA strand.

DNA consists of two strands that are *antiparallel* and *complementary* (Figure 31-6). One strand begins with a phosphate group attached to the 5′ carbon of the first nucleotide and ends with the hydroxyl group on the 3′ carbon of the last nucleotide. This strand is in the 5′-to-3′ direction. The other strand runs in the 3′-to-5′ direction, or antiparallel. The nucleotide sequences composing these strands provide the encoded messages of our genes. Therefore, the addition of nucleotides is highly regulated.

One regulation mechanism arises from the complementary characteristic of the nucleotides. A nucleotide's identity depends on the type of nitrogenous base present on the template. There are two categories of nitrogenous bases in nucleic acids: *purines* and *pyrimidines* (Figure 31-7). The bases *adenine* (A) and *guanine* (G) are double-ringed purines, whereas *thymine* (T) and *cytosine* (C) are single-ringed pyrimidines. Adenine forms hydrogen bonds at two points with thymine (A:T), whereas guanine forms hydrogen bonds at three points with cytosine (G:C). If a strand has a 5′-CTAG-3′ sequence, the complementary nucleotides on the 3′-to-5′ strand are 3′-GATC-5′. In RNA, the pyrimidine *uracil* (U) takes the place of thymine and forms

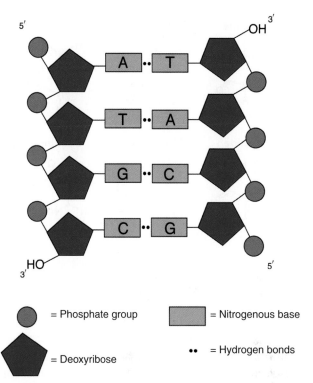

= Phosphate group   = Nitrogenous base

= Deoxyribose   ·· = Hydrogen bonds

Figure 31-6 DNA consists of two antiparallel and complementary strands. One strand begins with a 5′ phosphate group and ends with a 3′ hydroxyl group. This strand is read in the 5′-to-3′ direction. The other strand begins with a 3′ hydroxyl group and ends with a 5′ phosphate group. This strand is shown in the 3′-to-5′ orientation.

hydrogen bonds with adenine. Hydrogen bonds between A:T and G:C hold the strands together (Figure 31-8). RNA is most often single-stranded but can have significant secondary structure.

In addition to conferring identity to the nucleotide, the nitrogenous bases assist in maintaining a constant width between the strands of a DNA molecule. DNA resembles a ladder, with the repeating sugar and phosphate groups forming the

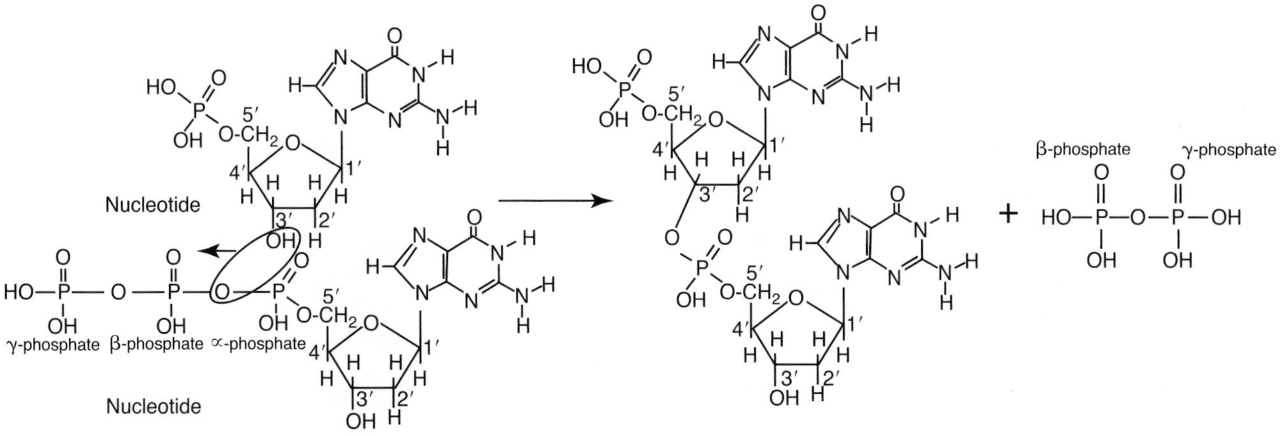

Figure 31-5 The enzyme DNA polymerase catalyzes the reaction between the hydroxyl group on the 3′ carbon of one nucleotide with the phosphate group bound to the 5′ carbon of the downstream nucleotide. The α-phosphate group is split by the 3′-OH, with release of the β- and γ-phosphates.

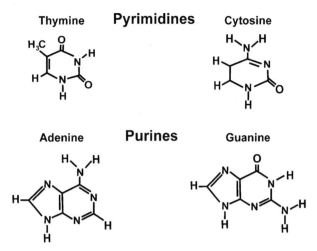

Figure 31-7 The single-ringed pyrimidines (thymine and cytosine) and the double-ringed purines (adenine and guanine) are the code-carrying nitrogenous bases of DNA.

sides of the ladder and the bases forming the rungs. The pairing of a double-ringed purine on one strand with a single-ringed pyrimidine on the other maintains a consistent distance between the DNA strands. This makes DNA flexible, which allows the molecule to twist into a helix. Twisting stabilizes the molecule and protects the bases from their environment.

Transcription and Translation

DNA provides a permanent set of instructions. The cellular enzyme *RNA polymerase* transcribes the code. RNA polymerase recognizes starter sequences called *promoters*. Promoters lie upstream of coding sequences and bind RNA polymerase which separates the DNA strands. The enzyme then slides along the 3′ to 5′ template DNA strand, "reading" the code and polymerizing (assembling) the complementary ribonucleotides. As the complementary ribonucleotides form hydrogen bonds with the bases of the exposed DNA strand, the RNA polymerase creates phosphodiester bonds to extend the single-stranded primary RNA transcript (Figure 31-2). If the nucleo-

tide sequence of the template DNA strand is 3′-CTAG-5′, the primary RNA transcript is 5′-GAUC-3′, where uracil is substituted for thymine.

Primary mRNA transcripts are composed of *introns* and *exons*. Introns are untranslated intervening sequences located between the coding portions of genes. Their functions remain unclear, although they may play a role in regulation of gene expression.[5] Exons are the sequences that encode the gene product. Before mRNA can serve as a translation template, the introns must be excised from the primary transcript and the exons adjoined. The mature mRNA is completed by the addition of a 5′ cap and a tail of many repeated adenine nucleotides (polyA tail).[6] The mature mRNA leaves the nucleus and enters cytoplasm to be translated by the ribosomes.

Ribosomes translate the mRNA code into a peptide sequence. Complexes of proteins and structural ribosomal RNAs (rRNAs) form both large and small ribosome subunits. Mature cytoplasmic mRNA is bound by the small ribosomal subunit at the translation start site. At this point, another series of elements is introduced, *transfer RNAs* (tRNAs), each bound to its specific amino acid. Because there are 20 natural amino acids, there are 20 tRNAs. Each tRNA has a specific nucleic acid sequence located at the point of interaction with the mRNA, complementary to the nucleotide sequence of the mRNA. Each tRNA interacting sequence (anticodon) complements a specific three-nucleotide sequence (codon) of the mRNA.

The mRNA codon AUG is the most common translation start site and codes for the amino acid methionine. The first step in translation is hydrogen bonding of the appropriately charged tRNA (with a bound methionine) to the start codon of the mRNA. The appropriate tRNA is then bonded to the adjacent codon, and a peptide bond is catalyzed between the two amino acids. The peptide bond forms between the carboxyl terminus of the methionine in the existing peptide chain and the amino terminus of the amino acid to be added. Hydrogen bonding of tRNAs to the codons and the formation of the peptide bonds are mediated by the ribosome. With addition of more amino acids, translation proceeds until a termination codon is reached. Three termination codons exist that do not

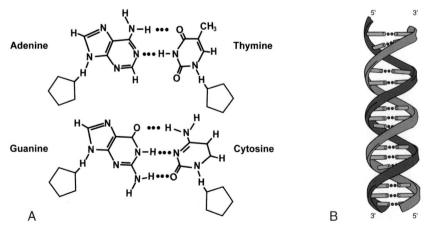

Figure 31-8 A, The purine adenine forms two hydrogen bonds with the pyrimidine thymine. The purine guanine forms three hydrogen bonds with the pyrimidine cytosine. **B,** The two strands maintain a consistent distance from each other, which allows DNA to twist into a helix.

code for any amino acid and terminate translation: UAA, UAG, and UGA. The ribosome then dissociates, and the peptide folds to its functional shape.

DNA Replication and the Cell Cycle

After cells carry out their functions, they either divide via mitosis or die via *apoptosis,* also called *programmed cell death* (Chapter 6). The cell cycle progresses through a defined sequence (Figure 31-9). *Interphase* is made up of the G_1, S, and G_2 phases. During the G_1 phase, the cell grows rapidly and performs its cellular functions. S phase is the synthesis stage, in which DNA is replicated. The G_2 phase is the period when the cell produces materials essential for cell division. The *M phase* refers to mitosis, during which two identical daughter cells are produced, each of which receives one entire set of the DNA that was replicated during S phase. Checkpoints occur at the end of G_1 before DNA replication in the S phase, and at the end of G_2 before mitosis in the M phase. The checkpoints have complex mechanisms to stop the progression of the cell cycle if a problem is detected, at which point the cell will undergo apoptosis. Some cells exit the cell cycle during the G_1 phase and enter a phase called G_0. Cells in G_0 normally do not reenter the cell cycle and remain alive performing their function until apoptosis occurs.

DNA replication during the S phase requires a complex orchestration of events; this discussion focuses on those events that are exploited for molecular diagnostic testing. Contained within the double-stranded DNA helix are multiple *origins of replication*. At each origin, the enzyme *helicase* disrupts the hydrogen bonds, and untwists and separates the DNA strands producing two *replication forks*. Here a deoxyribonucleotide (deoxynucleotide triphosphate, or dNTP) polymerizes to form new complementary strands (Figure 31-10). DNA replication occurs bidirectionally from the two replication origin sites. Each DNA strand in the replication fork serves as a template for the formation of a daughter or complementary strand through the activity of DNA polymerase.[7] The DNA polymerase substrate is the *free hydroxyl group* located on the 3' carbon of a deoxyribonucleotide. DNA polymerase recognizes this group

and catalyzes the joining of the complementary deoxyribonucleotide. DNA polymerase reads the DNA template in the 3'-to-5' direction, and the complementary strand is synthesized in the 5'-to-3' direction.

A *primer* is required to provide the free 3' hydroxyl group that is necessary for DNA polymerase activity. The enzyme *primase* synthesizes short RNA polymers complementary to the template that serve as primers to initiate DNA synthesis. At the replication origin, the primer hybridizes to the 3' end of the 5'-to-3' (top) template strand (Figure 31-10). Then DNA polymerase recognizes the free hydroxyl group on the 3' carbon of the last nucleotide in the primer and catalyzes the formation of phosphodiester bonds between the correct complementary nucleotide triphosphate and the primer, releasing the β- and γ-phosphate groups. DNA polymerase continues adding deoxyribonucleotides along the replication fork, going to the left of the replication origin, producing the complementary strand called the *leading strand.*

The second template strand, called the *lagging strand,* is also read in the 3'-to-5' direction. To form a complementary strand, a primer hybridizes to the exposed 3' end of the replication fork. To proceed in the 5'-to-3' direction, nucleotides are added in fragments toward the origin of replication. As the left replication fork extends to open more of the template strands for replication, additional primers are hybridized, and DNA polymerase uses the primers to initiate the formation of the complementary strand, continuing until it meets a previously hybridized primer.

DNA polymerase not only joins nucleotides, but it also degrades the RNA primers and fills in the correct complementary deoxyribonucleotides. Because the replication of the lagging strand produces many small fragments, it is called *discontinuous* replication, and the fragments are called *Okazaki fragments.* Finally, the enzyme *ligase* joins the discontinuous fragments. The replication fork to the right (downstream) is replicated in the same fashion, although the lagging strand is now formed complementary to the top (5'-to-3') strand, and the leading strand is formed from the 3'-to-5' strand; the opposite of the situation described occurs for the left replication fork (Figure 31-10).

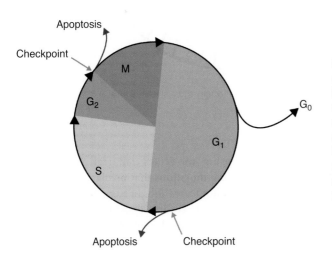

Figure 31-9 The cell cycle consists of interphase and mitosis. Interphase is divided into G_1, S, and G_2 phases. Cell growth occurs during G_1. During the S phase, DNA synthesis or replication occurs. The cell prepares for mitosis during the G_2 phase. During mitosis the cell divides, producing two identical daughter cells. The cells may also enter a quiescent phase called G_0, where the cell functions but does not divide. There are two critical times in the cell cycle that are checkpoints where the cell will either continue through the cell cycle or undergo apoptosis. The first checkpoint is before S phase and DNA replication, and the second checkpoint is at the end of G_2, where the cell will either enter mitosis or undergo apoptosis.

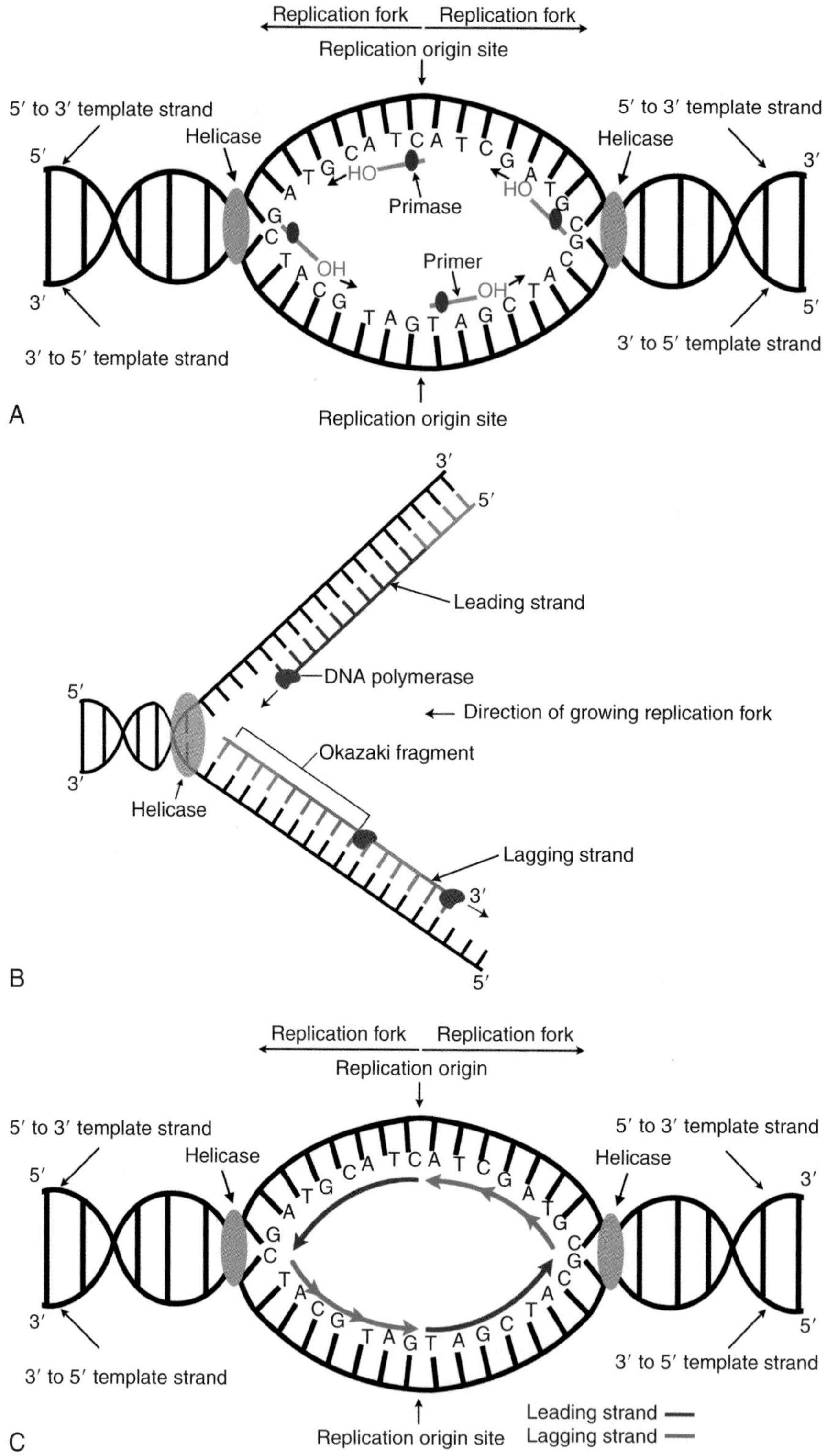

Figure 31-10 DNA Replication. **A,** Primases synthesize RNA primers that anneal to the single-stranded template strands. The primers must be oriented in such a way that the hydroxyl group on the 3′ end of the primers is available for deoxyribonucleotide addition by DNA polymerase. **B,** DNA polymerase extends the primer located on the 5′-to-3′ coding strand, producing the complementary leading strand (*blue*). On the 3′-to-5′ template strand, DNA polymerase extends the primers, producing Okazaki fragments. The primer ribonucleotides (*red*) are replaced with deoxynucleotides by DNA polymerase to produce the complementary lagging strand (*green*). **C,** Bidirectional DNA replication shown in which the 5′-to-3′ parent strand serves as the template for producing the continuous leading strands on a replication fork to the left of an origin. The 3′-to-5′ parent strand is the template for the lagging strands, which are produced in a discontinuous manner. The continuous and discontinuous strands are reversed on the replication fork to the right.

The cell cycle is highly regulated. At certain critical points within the cycle, decisions are made to continue or begin cell death via apoptosis. This decision may depend on the state of the DNA replicated. Normally, the cell detects errors made during replication and either corrects them or begins apoptosis. This prevents the persistence of daughter cells with genetic errors. If the sensing molecules fail, cell division may continue. Debilitating mutations that mediate cell cycle control may result in tumor formation. In summary, DNA synthesis and accurate cell cycle control demand that the integrity of the nucleotide sequence be maintained during DNA replication.

MOLECULAR DIAGNOSTIC TESTING OVERVIEW

DNA or RNA sequences are used to diagnose and monitor solid tumors, acute leukemia, myeloproliferative disorders, myelodysplastic neoplasms, inherited thrombosis risk factors, and viral, parasitic, and bacterial infections. Molecular diagnostic testing exploits the enzymes and processes of DNA *replication*. Most molecular testing methods use replication—for example, polymerase chain reaction (PCR)—to make millions of *amplicons* (copies) of a DNA sequence of interest. Further, creation of synthetic DNA requires the use of short sequences used as either *primers* or *probes* to locate specific DNA or RNA sequences within vast populations of nucleic acids.

Specific mutations are associated with hematologic disease. These are detected by allele-specific amplification methods, DNA sequencing, or restriction fragment length polymorphism analysis of amplified material. Messenger and ribosomal RNA also may be amplified through a process called *reverse transcriptase PCR* (RT-PCR). Using mRNA, the existence of mutations that are being actively translated can be detected. Assessment of mRNA shows whether a mutation is expressed in a certain cell type or tissue and can be used to quantitatively determine the level of transcription of a gene. It can also be used to detect and monitor chromosome translocations that produce novel chimeric mRNA transcripts in conditions where the breakpoints are too widely separated to be detected by PCR amplification of DNA.

Most molecular tests use DNA amplification such as PCR, generating multiple amplicons of the target sequence. Amplification is meant to be specific to the sequence of interest in the sample being tested; however, it will amplify any DNA that is present in the reaction. Consequently, it is critical to eliminate contamination of newly isolated target DNA with amplicons from previously amplified samples. Contamination can be avoided by designating separate laboratory locations for each step, having a unidirectional work flow, and employing appropriate controls. Operators routinely employ ultraviolet (UV) light and bleach to induce strand breaks in contaminating DNA on work surfaces and a *uracil-N-glycosylase* system that destroys previously amplified DNA can also be incorporated into the PCR reactions.

In genetically based hematologic disease, mutations and polymorphisms can occur that do not affect function. Individuals vary in genetic sequences coding for identical proteins. Such single nucleotide polymorphisms are commonly detected but might not be associated with disease. With these caveats in mind, several techniques are presented and an example from hematopathology is given for each. Box 31-5 is a summary of molecular methods with hematopathology applications.

NUCLEIC ACID ISOLATION

Isolating DNA from Clinical Specimens

Most molecular diagnostic tests begin with the isolation of DNA or RNA from a patient specimen. To test for a mutation

---

> **BOX 31-5** Molecular Methods with Hematopathology Applications
>
> Nucleic acid isolation
>   DNA
>   RNA
> Amplification of nucleic acid
>   Polymerase chain reaction (PCR)
>   Reverse transcriptase PCR
> Detection of amplified DNA
>   Electrophoresis
>   Restriction endonuclease methods
>   Nucleic acid hybridization and Southern blotting
>   Cleavage-based signal amplification
>   DNA sequencing
> Real-time PCR
>   Qualitative
>   Quantitative
>   Minimal residual disease in leukemia
>   Mutation enrichment strategies
> Chromosomal microarrays
> Pathogen detection and infectious disease load
> Current developments
>   Mass spectrometry
>   Digital PCR
>   Next-generation sequencing

---

in patient DNA, the patient's DNA is isolated. To test for microorganism DNA, as in an infection, DNA is also isolated from the patient specimen because it will include the organism DNA. The preferred nucleic acid for clinical diagnosis is DNA because it is inherently more stable than RNA and is less labor intensive to isolate.

The molecular laboratory isolates nucleic acid from a wide variety of clinical specimen types. Patient specimens for human DNA isolation may include peripheral blood, bone marrow, tissue biopsy specimens (both fresh and formalin fixed paraffin-embedded), needle aspirates, body fluids, saliva, and cheek swabs. Blood, saliva, or cheek swab specimens are all appropriate for identifying an inherited defect, although blood is the most common specimen type. Every nucleated cell contains a full complement of DNA. If individuals inherit a mutation, it is present in the DNA of all their nucleated cells, both gamete and non-gamete (*somatic*) cells. Thus the DNA in the nucleus of white blood cells can reveal inherited mutations. In solid tumors, *somatic* (acquired) *mutations* are detected by analyzing DNA from the suspect tissue. For identification of infectious disease organisms by molecular techniques, DNA must also be isolated from the affected tissues. Peripheral blood is adequate for infections with viruses such as human immunodeficiency virus (HIV) and cytomegalovirus (CMV) that infect blood cells, whereas cerebrospinal fluid is required for meningeal infections.

Whole blood is preferentially collected in an ethylenediaminetetraacetic acid (EDTA) tube to prevent clotting and to inhibit enzymes that may digest DNA, although other tubes may also be acceptable. The red blood cells (RBCs) are removed by taking advantage of the differential lysis in hypotonic buffer due to differing osmotic fragility between white and red blood cells. Incubation in hypotonic buffer will result in the red blood cells lysing before the white blood cells, thus allowing the WBCs to be removed from the hemoglobin and lysed RBCs by centrifugation. Hemoglobin is a potent inhibitor of PCR and other downstream procedures.[8]

DNA from tissue suspected of being cancerous can be isolated from formalin-fixed, paraffin-embedded tissue sections mounted on glass microscope slides or whole sections cut directly into a microfuge tube. Tissue is obtained from the entire section or from a portion of the section by microdissection, either by scraping or by laser. The tissue is degraded by an enzyme called *proteinase K* to break open the cells and release the DNA. The sample is then purified using an automated or manual extraction kit as described below.[9] In addition to paraffin-embedded samples, fresh or frozen tissue samples are also appropriate for DNA isolation. Quickly thawing and mincing the frozen tissue prepares the sample for DNA isolation. The minced tissue is mixed with an extraction buffer to release the DNA from the cells, and it is then purified.

There are a number of automated extraction systems as well as manual extraction kits available for DNA extraction. Most of these systems use a solid phase extraction system that takes advantage of the binding of DNA to silica under high salt conditions. Manual kits use columns that can be spun in a microcentrifuge with the eluent collected in microfuge tubes. Cells that have been lysed and protease treated are applied to a column in a high salt buffer. The column is washed to remove impurities and the DNA eluted in a low-ionic-strength buffer and collected in a microfuge tube.[10] Automated extractors have reagents packaged in sets and can be programmed to extract and purify the DNA automatically. There are a variety of models to choose from, depending on the number and type of samples. Isolated DNA can be stored at −20°C. If a delay in the molecular testing is necessary, the isolated DNA sample can be stored at −80°C indefinitely.

Isolating RNA from Clinical Specimens

RNA isolation poses greater technical challenges than DNA isolation. Ubiquitous *ribonucleases* (RNases) degrade RNA. These enzymes are the body's primary defense against pathogens and are found on mammalian epidermal surfaces; therefore, they contaminate all laboratory surfaces.[11] Clinical laboratories that isolate RNA must be RNase free, which necessitates costly precautions and decontamination steps.[12]

The isolated total RNA includes mRNA, rRNA, and tRNA, all of which participate in protein synthesis. Depending on cell type, mRNA may comprise only 3% to 5% of the total cellular RNA; therefore, a large specimen may be needed to obtain adequate mRNA. The mRNA does not represent all the information stored in the DNA, only those genes being expressed. Consequently, mRNA provides quantitative information on the genes being expressed in a cell at the time the specimen is collected.

RNA may be purified using either liquid or solid phase procedures. The steps of RNA isolation using a liquid phase method are (1) RNA release by cell lysis combined with RNase inhibition by homogenization or incubation in a strongly denaturing solution containing chemical agents such as urea or guanidine isothiocyanate, (2) protein and DNA removal, and (3) RNA precipitation using alcohols. In step 2, extraction is performed using acidic phenol chloroform and guanidine isothiocyanate.

These separate the DNA and protein into the organic phase, while the RNA remains in the aqueous phase. RNA resists acidic pH, whereas DNA is readily depurinated because acid cleaves the bond between the purine base and the deoxyribose sugar. Therefore, acidic phenol preferentially isolates and preserves RNA, while the genomic DNA (all the DNA) is partitioned along with contaminating proteins, lipids, and carbohydrates. Precipitating the RNA from the aqueous phase requires the addition of salt to neutralize the charge of the phosphodiester backbone and ethanol to make the nucleic acid insoluble.[13,14] Purification of RNA using column-based methods is similar to DNA except that the RNA is suspended in a high-salt buffer that preferentially binds RNA greater than 200 nucleotides to the column to remove smaller RNAs such as tRNA and 5S RNA.

AMPLIFICATION OF NUCLEIC ACIDS BY POLYMERASE CHAIN REACTION

Polymerase Chain Reaction for Amplifying DNA

Polymerase chain reaction (PCR) is the principal technique in the clinical molecular laboratory. PCR is an enzyme-based method for amplifying a specific target sequence to allow its detection from a small amount of highly complex material.[15] Sickle cell anemia results from a single β-globin nucleotide substitution (point mutation) in which an adenine replaces a thymine. Detecting this mutation from among 6 billion nucleotides in the human genome would be like finding a needle in a haystack if only a few cells were assessed. When millions of β-globin copies are produced, however, the mutation is easily detected.[16] There are two categories of PCR reactions: endpoint PCR and real-time PCR. The amplification for both categories is basically the same. The major difference is in the method of detection of the PCR product. With endpoint or standard PCR, the amplification products must be detected using another technique such as gel electrophoresis, which is described later in the chapter. In real-time PCR, the amplicons are detected during the PCR cycles by using fluorescence detection. This is also described in further detail later in the chapter.

As with natural DNA replication, PCR amplification requires primers that anneal (bind) to complementary nucleotide sequences on either side of the target region. In testing for the sickle cell mutation, for example, selected primers flank (i.e., bind on either side of) the β-globin gene sequence containing the mutation. The total base pair (bp) length of the primer sequences plus the target sequence can vary, but in this example, it is 110 bp for the β-globin gene, a typical sequence length for many mutation sites (Figure 31-11).[16] Besides

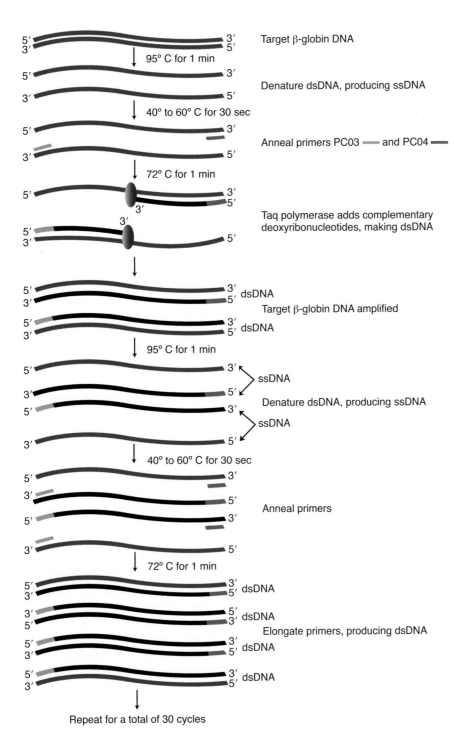

Target β-globin DNA

95° C for 1 min

Denature dsDNA, producing ssDNA

40° to 60° C for 30 sec

Anneal primers PC03 ━━ and PC04 ━━

72° C for 1 min

Taq polymerase adds complementary deoxyribonucleotides, making dsDNA

dsDNA
Target β-globin DNA amplified
dsDNA

95° C for 1 min

ssDNA
Denature dsDNA, producing ssDNA
ssDNA

40° to 60° C for 30 sec

Anneal primers

72° C for 1 min

dsDNA
dsDNA
Elongate primers, producing dsDNA
dsDNA
dsDNA

Repeat for a total of 30 cycles

Figure 31-11 Application of PCR to target ß-globin DNA. PCR amplifies the target DNA, making millions of copies of the target DNA after 30 cycles. Flanking forward and reverse primers (PCO3 and PCO4) are used to amplify the target ß-globin DNA. One primer (PCO3, *orange*) anneals to the 3′ end of the 3′-to-5′ DNA strand. The other primer (PCO4, *green*) anneals to the 3′ end of the 5′-to-3′ DNA strand. These primers provide the 3′-OH end for extension in the 5′ to 3′ direction during the PCR reaction and set the boundaries for the size of the amplicon. *dsDNA,* double-stranded DNA; *ssDNA,* single-stranded DNA.

primers, the PCR *master mix* reagents include a heat-insensitive DNA polymerase—for example, *Taq polymerase*—isolated from the thermophilic bacterium *Thermus aquaticus* and a mixture of the four deoxyribonucleotides—deoxyadenosine triphosphate (dATP), deoxythymidine triphosphate (dTTP), deoxyguanosine triphosphate (dGTP), and deoxycytidine triphosphate (dCTP)—in a magnesium buffer.

The DNA is first *denatured* at 95° C, which separates the strands; then cooled to the primer *annealing (binding) temperature* of 40° to 60° C; and then warmed to 72° C to promote specific chain *extension*, in which nucleotides are added to the

primers by DNA polymerase. The annealing temperature is optimized for each set of primers. A *thermocycler* is used to accurately produce and monitor the rapid temperature changes.

Once the double-stranded DNA is denatured, one primer anneals to the 3′ end of the 5′-to-3′ strand and the other primer to the 3′ end of the complementary 3′-to-5′ strand. Both primers possess a free 3′ hydroxyl group. The *DNA poly-merase* recognizes this hydroxyl group, reads the template, and catalyzes formation of the phosphodiester bond joining the first complementary deoxyribonucleotide to the primer. The polymerase rapidly continues down the template strand at

1000 nucleotides per second, extending the complementary strand in the 5′-to-3′ direction to eventually produce a complete daughter strand that continues to the 5′ end of the template.[17] This completes one PCR cycle. In the second cycle, the temperature changes are repeated, and the first-cycle product becomes the template for a daughter strand. After the second cycle, daughter strands are produced that are bounded by the primer sequences at the 5′ and 3′ ends, resulting in a fragment of DNA of the desired length. In 25 to 40 subsequent cycles, this DNA of specific length and sequence, called an *amplicon*, is reproduced millions of times.[18,19]

Primer annealing accounts for PCR specificity, and primer design is crucial for achieving confidence in the test results regardless of the application. Wherever primers anneal, specifically or nonspecifically, they become starting points for extension.

Commercial kits contain primer sets that have been tested for annealing specificity, but care must be taken to use the optimal annealing temperature. Even if the primer is properly designed, it can anneal to noncomplementary regions if the annealing temperature is too low. Several online primer design programs are available from genome centers and company websites. One such program that can help determine the uniqueness and therefore specificity of the primers is the Basic Local Alignment Sequence Tool (BLAST).[20] These programs will also analyze pairs of primers to avoid complementarity between the primers themselves to prevent hybridization to one another, which forms undesirable *primer dimers.*

Controls are essential for the accurate interpretation of a PCR result. The three controls required for PCR are the negative, positive, and "no-DNA" or no template (NTC) controls. All three are included in each run. In addition, in most applications, a sensitivity control will be included that consists of a low positive sample at the lowest concentration detected. The negative control consists of DNA known to lack the sequence of interest; the positive control contains the target sequence. Comparison of the amplification in the patient sample to results in the negative and positive controls determines whether the target DNA sequence is present in the patient's DNA. The no-DNA control detects master mix contamination. Amplification in the no template control indicates DNA contamination, which renders the entire test result unreliable.[21]

Reverse Transcription Polymerase Chain Reaction for Amplifying RNA

Some hematology molecular tests such as those for translocations, require mRNA as the starting material. Genetically altered mRNA sequences often translate to an altered protein. The classic example is the Philadelphia chromosome (Ph′), carrying the chromosome translocation t(9;22)(q34;q11.2) (Chapter 33). This translocation is present in 95% of chronic myelogenous leukemia (CML) cases, as well as 20% of adult acute lymphoblastic leukemia (ALL) and 5% of pediatric ALL cases, and in rare instances in acute myeloid leukemia.[22,23] Ph′ results from a reciprocal translocation of the *ABL1* (Ableson) gene on chromosome 9 to the breakpoint cluster region (*BCR*) of chromosome 22, producing a *BCR-ABL1* hybrid or chimeric gene (Figure 31-12A).[24-26] Transcription of *BCR-ABL1* produces a chimeric mRNA made up of exons from both the *BCR* and *ABL1* genes. Translation generates a fusion protein, *tyrosine kinase,* that alters normal cell cycle control, which results in unrestrained cell proliferation.[27] RT-PCR of the chimeric mRNA is the standard method to detect this mutation. Although the mutation is present at the DNA level, the nucleotide position at which the two chromosome sections join is variable, whereas the chimeric mRNA is always the same. The DNA also includes untranslated introns, which make the chimera too long to replicate. The physiologic excision and splicing of mRNA yields a much shorter target that is more easily amplified.

In RT-PCR, the *reverse transcriptase* enzyme produces *complementary* DNA (cDNA) from mRNA present in a total RNA sample extracted from patient specimens such as blood or bone marrow (Figure 31-12). PCR subsequently amplifies the cDNA.

The first step is to transcribe the RNA into DNA using reverse transcriptase and a primer to produce an RNA-cDNA hybrid. The primer can be *oligo(dT),* a series of thymine nucleotides complementary to the string of adenine nucleotides on the 3′ end of most mRNAs, called the *polyA tail;* a set of short random primers that prime the cDNA synthesis more evenly; or a specific primer for the gene of interest. The primer anneals to the complementary sequence of the mRNA. Reverse transcriptase recognizes the hydroxyl group on the last nucleotide of the primer and reads the mRNA template strand, then adds the correct complementary deoxyribonucleotide. Reverse transcriptase continues along the mRNA template strand, joining the complementary deoxyribonucleotides to the growing cDNA strand to form the mRNA-cDNA hybrid. Subsequently, heat denaturation breaks the hydrogen bonds between the mRNA-cDNA hybrid, separating the two strands. The cDNA strand then acts as a template for replication by DNA polymerase. The cDNA synthesis can be done separately from the PCR amplification step in a two-step procedure or combined with the PCR in a single reaction. For example, with the *BCR-ABL1* translocation, the single-stranded cDNA is amplified as in DNA-based PCR using one primer specific for a target sequence in the *BCR* gene and a second primer specific for the *ABL1* gene. DNA polymerase extends the primers, forming a double-stranded cDNA of the target chimeric gene. Only the cDNA containing the translocation, and therefore both primer binding sites, will be amplified, resulting in millions of copies of the *BCR-ABL1* sequence.[28,29]

DETECTION OF AMPLIFIED DNA

Although many molecular tests are now performed using real-time PCR, there are still circumstances where amplicons are produced using endpoint PCR and the product must be detected using downstream techniques. Amplified target DNA may be detected by gel electrophoresis using fluorescent dyes. PCR can also be combined with restriction enzyme digestion of the amplicons followed by gel electrophoresis or cleavage-based signal amplification (Invader) technology for detection (discussed later in the chapter).

Gel Electrophoresis

Nucleic acid phosphate groups confer a net negative charge to DNA fragments. Consequently, in electrophoresis, the rate at

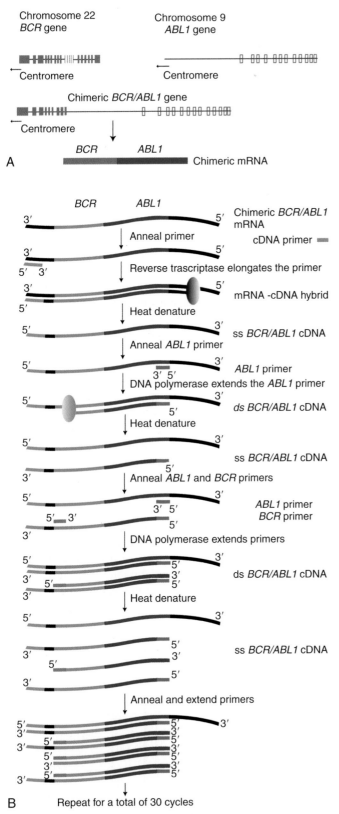

A, The *BCR* gene is present on chromosome 22, and the *ABL1* gene is located on chromosome 9. The Ph' chromosome results from the translocation of the *ABL1* gene to chromosome 22, which places the *ABL1* gene next to the *BCR* gene and produces a chimeric *BCR/ABL1* gene. The transcription of the *BCR/ABL1* gene produces a chimeric messenger RNA (mRNA) consisting of a portion of the *BCR* gene and a portion of the *ABL1* gene. **B,** Reverse transcriptase polymerase chain reaction (RT-PCR) produces complementary DNA (cDNA) from messenger RNA (mRNA). This diagram shows the RT-PCR steps used to produce amplified *BCR/ABL1* cDNA. Initially, a gene-specific primer or short random primers anneal to the chimeric *BCR/ABL1* mRNA. Reverse transcriptase elongates the primer, producing an mRNA-cDNA hybrid. Heat denaturation breaks the hydrogen bonds, holding the hybrid molecule together, releasing the single-stranded (ss) *BCR/ABL1* cDNA. Next, a primer specific for the *ABL1* gene is annealed to the cDNA. DNA polymerase elongates the primer, producing the double-stranded (ds) *BCR/ABL1* cDNA. The cDNA becomes single stranded by heat denaturation. Then the *ABL1* primer as well as a primer specific for the *BCR* gene anneal to the ss cDNA. DNA polymerase elongates the primers, producing ds *BCR/ABL1* cDNA. The cycle is repeated 20 to 40 times, producing millions of copies of the ds *BCR/ABL1* cDNA.

which DNA fragments (amplicons) migrate through gels is proportional to their mass only and, unlike proteins, not their relative charge. DNA fragment mass is a function of the length in base pairs (bp) or kilobase pairs (kb, 1000 × bp). Fragments are sieved through an *agarose* or *polyacrylamide* gel matrix by passing a current through the gel as it is bathed in a buffered conducting salt solution. Electrophoresis gel *pore diameter* is a function of gel concentration. The pores of an agarose gel are larger than the pores of a polyacrylamide gel. When larger fragments (500 bp to 50 kb) are to be separated, an agarose gel is most effective. For smaller DNA fragments (5 to 1000 bp), a polyacrylamide gel is used.[30]

In slab gel electrophoresis, PCR products (amplicons) of patients and controls, and a mass marker or *ladder* are pipetted into the sample wells in the gel slab near the negative electrode (cathode). An electrical current moves the negatively charged fragments toward the positive electrode (anode). Smaller fragments move faster and migrate farther than larger fragments. The ladder, composed of fragments of known masses (sizes), measured in base pairs or kilobase pairs, runs alongside the patient and control lanes and is used to determine the mass (size) of any DNA fragments in the patient and control samples (Figure 31-13). Fluorescent dyes such as ethidium bromide and Gel Red® (which intercalate between the base pairs of the DNA helix) or SYBR green® (which binds to the minor groove of the DNA helix) are employed to visualize the DNA fragments of the patient, controls, and size markers in the gel. The newer dyes (e.g., Gel Red and SYBR green) have largely replaced ethidium bromide because they are much less toxic. Gels are soaked in a solution of diluted dye and then exposed to UV light, which causes the nucleic acid to appear as fluorescent bands. The mass of the bands in the patient and control lanes is determined by comparing the distance they migrated in the gel with the distance migrated by the bands of the size markers. Gel electrophoresis is appropriate

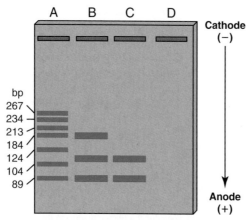

Figure 31-13 Electrophoresis pattern of a DNA sample on a slab gel. **A,** Molecular size marker (ladder); **B,** positive control; **C,** negative control; **D,** no-DNA control. DNA samples are placed in wells at the cathode (negative pole) and migrate to the anode (positive pole) due to the negative charge of the DNA molecules. By comparing the bands present in the gel with the molecular size markers, the mass of each band, measured in base pairs, is determined. For example, in the positive control sample, the three bands are 184, 110, and 89 bp. Positive, negative, and no-DNA controls must be used when performing gel electrophoresis. The positive control contains the target DNA sequence, and the negative control lacks this sequence. The no-DNA control sample lacks DNA. No banding should be present in the no-DNA control. If bands are present, contamination of samples occurred during the testing process.

when the goal is qualitative—that is, to determine the presence or absence of the target DNA.

Another method of fractionating DNA fragments by mass (size) is capillary gel electrophoresis. In this type of electrophoresis, long fused silica capillaries filled with derivatized acrylamide polymer are used for separation of single-stranded negatively charged DNA fragments on the basis of size or number of base pairs. The sample is applied to the capillary using electrokinetic injection, and the DNA fragments are separated using a high voltage as they migrate through the capillary from the negative electrode to the positive electrode. Smaller DNA fragments

move faster through the polymer in the capillary compared to larger fragments. Detection of the separated fragments occurs by incorporating a fluorescent label into the PCR-amplified DNA. Before reaching the positive electrode the fluorescently labeled DNA fragments cross the path of a laser beam and detector. When the laser beam hits a fluorescent DNA fragment, light is emitted at a specific wavelength. The light emission is read by the detector, and the signal produces a peak on an electropherogram (Figure 31-14).

Capillary electrophoresis offers a number of advantages over traditional gel electrophoresis. The injection, separation, and detection of the fragments are automated. The separation can be quite rapid with excellent resolution. The time of fragment elution and the peak height information are stored for easy retrieval. Size ladders can be labeled with different fluorescent dyes and run in the same capillary as the sample providing more accurate sizing.[31] This method of separation is used in a number of applications including B and T cell clonality testing, bone marrow engraftment analysis, and screening for the internal tandem duplication mutation in the *FLT3* gene in acute myeloid leukemia (AML) (Chapter 35).[32]

Restriction Endonuclease Methods

One method to determine whether an amplified target DNA fragment contains a mutation of interest uses enzymes called *restriction endonucleases* (also known as *restriction enzymes*). These enzymes are produced naturally in bacteria and are so named because they restrict foreign (phage) DNA from entering and destroying the bacterium. Each restriction enzyme recognizes a specific nucleotide sequence and cuts both strands of the target DNA at the sequence, producing *restriction fragments*. *Recognition sequences* can be 4 to 15 nucleotides long. There are hundreds of commercially available restriction endonucleases, which allow recognition of many sequences. The number of restriction fragments produced depends on the number of restriction sites present in the amplified target.[33,34] Enzyme action at one restriction site produces two restriction

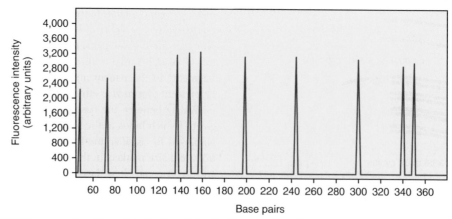

Figure 31-14 An electropherogram of capillary gel electrophoresis showing the separation of fluorescently labeled DNA fragments by size (number of base pairs). Fragments migrate through the matrix in the capillary from the negative to the positive pole and emerge from the capillary in size order (smaller fragments first). Before reaching the positive electrode, the fluorescently labeled DNA fragments are detected by passing one at a time between a laser beam and the detector. Each fragment is represented by a peak on the electropherogram.

fragments, action at two restriction sites produce three restriction fragments, and so on.

A restriction enzyme detects even a single base substitution if the mutation alters the recognition sequence and prevents digestion at the site or creates a new site resulting in an additional fragment. A *restriction fragment length polymorphism* (RFLP) is a mutation or polymorphism-induced change in the recognition site of the restriction enzyme that alters the length (number of base pairs) of the restriction fragment. A mutation in the coagulation factor V gene (*F5* Leiden mutation) is an excellent example of RFLP. Individuals possessing this mutation have an increased risk of venous thrombosis. This mutation results from the replacement of guanine with adenine at nucleotide position 1691 (G1691A) of the *F5* gene.[35,36] The mutation alters a restriction site normally detected and cut by the restriction enzyme *Mnl* I. The wild-type (normal) *F5* amplicon is 223 bp long with two *Mnl* I-specific sites. After PCR amplification and incubation with *Mnl* I, the

wild-type amplicon is cut into three restriction fragments, separable using slab gel or capillary electrophoresis. The fragments are 37, 82, and 104 bp long. The mutant gene generates only two fragments with lengths of 82 and 141 bp. A sample from an individual homozygous for the wild-type gene generates the three expected fragments 37, 82, and 104 bp. A sample from an individual homozygous for the *F5* Leiden mutation possesses two copies of the mutated *F5* gene and generates only two bands: 82 and 141 bp. A sample from a heterozygous individual possesses one normal and one mutated *F5* gene and produces four bands of lengths 37, 82, 104, and 141 bp (Figure 31-15 and Figure 31-1).

Nucleic Acid Hybridization and Southern Blotting

Once used in a number of molecular tests, including B and T cell clonality assays, as well as the detection of chromosome translocations, Southern blots are now largely used for samples

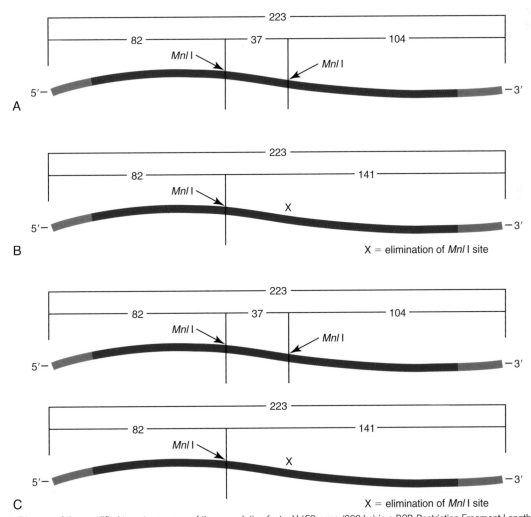

Figure 31-15 Diagram of the amplified target sequence of the coagulation factor V (*F5*) gene (223 bp) in a PCR-Restriction Fragment Length Polymorphism (RFLP) method to detect the *F5* Leiden mutation. **A,** The amplified target sequence for the normal (wild-type) *F5* gene contains two restriction sites for *Mnl* I, so three restriction fragments of 37, 82, and 104 bp are produced. **B,** In the *F5* Leiden mutation, the substitution of an A for a G in position 1691 of the *F5* gene eliminates one of the restriction sites for *Mnl* I. Thus the mutated *F5* Leiden gene possesses only one restriction site for *Mnl* I. In individuals homozygous for the mutation, only two restriction fragments of 82 and 141 bp are produced. **C,** An individual who is heterozygous for the *F5* Leiden mutation has a normal and a mutated *F5* gene. *Mnl* I produces four restriction fragments of 37, 82, 104, and 141 bp.

that do not provide a result using standard PCR methods or for research applications. Southern blots can only be performed on high-quality genomic DNA or PCR amplicons. Briefly, DNA is digested with a restriction enzyme, size fractionated using agarose gel electrophoresis, denatured to become single stranded, and then finally transferred to a solid support—typically a nylon or nitrocellulose membrane and then detected with a labeled probe.

In the classic Southern blot procedure, detection of the band containing the sequence of interest requires a radioactive or enzyme (horseradish peroxidase or alkaline phosphatase)–conjugated, single-stranded probe complementary to the target sequence. The probe hybridizes to the target DNA, unhybridized probe is washed off, and the hybridized bands are visualized, depending on the labeling system chosen. Most probes today are detected using a chemiluminescence detection by autoradiography (Figure 31-16).[37-41]

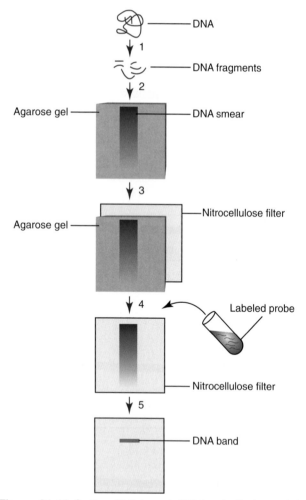

Figure 31-16 Southern blot steps. *1*, DNA is cut with the restriction endonuclease *Eco*RI, which produces many restriction fragments. *2*, DNA fragments are separated on an agarose gel. *3*, DNA fragments are transferred to a nitrocellulose filter. *4*, A labeled probe is hybridized to the DNA fragments on the filter. *5*, Autoradiography is used to visualize the hybridized DNA probe, the detection of which indicates the presence of the given DNA sequence in the sample.

Cleavage-Based Signal Amplification

Cleavage-based amplification is an isothermal signal amplification method marketed as Invader® (Hologic, Inc., Bedford, MA). In the primary reaction, the 3' end of a test probe and an Invader oligo probe anneal to complementary sequences on the target DNA template forming a specific substrate site recognized by a Cleavase enzyme (Figure 31-17). The 5' end of the test probe (5' flap) does not anneal to the target. The Cleavase enzyme cuts and releases the 5' flap of the test probe. In a coupled secondary reaction, the 5' flap of the test probe anneals to a complementary signal probe that has a FRET (fluorescence resonance energy transfer) reporter. The signal probe and reporter (called a *FRET cassette*) is specific for the 5' flap of the test probe. The FRET reporter is a fluorescent dye bound to the signal probe in close proximity to a quencher; the quencher prevents the reporter dye from emitting a fluorescent signal. The combination of the 5' flap of the test probe and the FRET cassette forms another specific substrate site for the Cleavage enzyme. Cleavage of the 5' end of the FRET cassette results in separation of the fluorescent reporter from the quencher and production of a fluorescent signal. Repeated binding and cleavage result in the signal amplification. Two reactions are done simultaneously using different fluorescent molecules for detection of either the wild-type or mutant sequence. Because the mutant sequence is different from the wild-type sequence, the wild type test probe will not anneal to the mutant target, and no fluorescent signal will occur. This technique can be used to detect single base pair changes, small insertions, and deletions. It is also FDA-approved for the detection of mutations associated with thrombophilia, including the factor V (*F5*) Leiden mutation, the prothrombin G20210A mutation in the *F2* gene, and methylenetetrahydrofolate reductase (*MTHFR*) gene mutations.[42]

DNA Sequencing

The ability to read the sequence of the nucleic acid has been just as important as PCR in the development of molecular biology. A combination of these two important techniques (cycle sequencing) has made DNA sequencing an integral part of molecular diagnostics. In cycle sequencing, the order of the nucleotide bases is determined after amplification.[43] Cycle sequencing is applied in molecular testing to assess amplified sequences for insertions, deletions, or point mutations, such as the *FLT3* internal tandem duplication (ITD) or point mutations in the *KIT* gene that occur in AML (Chapter 35).[44-46]

Cycle sequencing is based on *dideoxynucleotide terminator* sequencing.[47] The addition of nucleotides to a growing DNA polymer requires a 3' hydroxyl group on the last added nucleotide and a triphosphate group on the 5' end of the next nucleotide to be added (Figure 31-5). If a nucleotide lacks the 3' hydroxyl group, it can be incorporated into the newly synthesized strand of the DNA but cannot be extended, so the fragment terminates at the "defective" base. If low concentrations of the terminators, dideoxyadenosine triphosphate, dideoxycytosine triphosphate, dideoxyguanine triphosphate, and dideoxythymine triphosphate, are included in the single primer PCR master mix used for sequencing, over a number of cycles

Mutant target DNA plus mutant (MUT) test probe

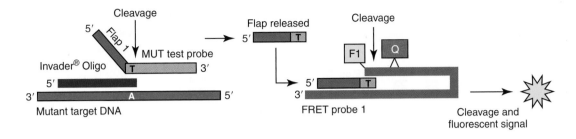

Mutant target DNA plus wild-type (WT) test probe

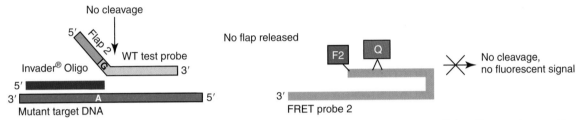

Figure 31-17 Cleavage-based signal amplification. The Cleavage-based DNA Signal Amplification Assays use a Cleavase® enzyme to recognize and cleave specific structures formed by the addition of two oligonucleotide probes to a nucleic acid target. Two oligonucleotide probes (a test probe and an Invader® oligo probe) hybridize in tandem to the target DNA to form an overlapping structure. The 5′ end of the test probe includes a 5′ flap that does not hybridize to the target DNA. The 3′ nucleotide of the bound Invader® oligo overlaps the test probe. The Cleavase® enzyme recognizes this overlapping structure and cleaves off the unpaired 5′ flap of the test probe, releasing it as a target-specific product. In the secondary reaction, each released 5′ flap anneals to a fluorescence resonance energy transfer (FRET™) probe to create another overlapping structure that is recognized and cleaved by the Cleavase® enzyme. When the FRET™ probe is cleaved, the fluorophore (F) and quencher (Q) on the FRET™ probe are separated, generating detectable fluorescence signal. The initial and secondary reactions run concurrently in the same well. Two different fluorescent labels are used, one to identify the presence of the wild-type allele and one to identify the presence of the mutant allele.

a series of DNA fragments is produced that terminate at each successive base with each fragment differing in length by one nucleotide. This is called a *ladder* or *nested series* of fragments.

In the dye terminator method each of the four dideoxynucleotides in the PCR reaction is labeled with a different fluorescent dye so that each DNA fragment terminates in a labeled dideoxynucleotide corresponding to the sequence of the target DNA (Figure 31-18, *A*). The specific fluorescent color of the DNA fragment identifies the terminal nucleotide. Alternatively, in the dye primer method, the primers are labeled with four different fluorescent dyes (corresponding to each nucleotide), and in separate tubes, each labeled primer is subjected to PCR with unlabeled dideoxynucleotides (Figure 31-18, *B*). As in the dye terminator method, the specific fluorescent color of the DNA fragments corresponds to the terminal nucleotide.

The fluorescently labeled fragments are subjected to capillary electrophoresis (described earlier in the chapter). The DNA fragments migrate through the capillary and separate based on their size. Near the end of the capillary, the fragments pass one by one through the beam of a laser in an order based on their length (with the shortest fragments emerging first). A detector reads the specific fluorescent color of each fragment and displays the signal as a peak on an electropherogram; this allows the sequence to be read (Figure 31-18, *C*).

In order to unambiguously read the nucleotide at each position, the PCR reaction for cycle sequencing contains only a single primer that produces *single-sided* PCR. Two separate reactions are typically carried out, one using the forward primer and a second using the reverse primer. This produces complementary sequences from both strands. After the cycle sequencing reactions, the nested products are purified and denatured before loading on the capillary sequencer. The injection, separation, and detection are automated, but the operator can set the parameters such as amount of sample injected, length of capillaries, and the type of polymer. Capillary DNA sequencing instruments are equipped with base calling software that will read the base sequence of the DNA fragment sequenced. Software packages will also identify alterations in the sequence such as single nucleotide polymorphisms (SNPs), point mutations, and insertions or deletions based on comparison to a specific reference sequence.

Pyrosequencing is another sequencing method that is useful for the determination of point mutations and short sequence analysis. This method uses a "sequencing by synthesis" principle and the detection of pyrophosphate release upon nucleotide incorporation. Nucleotides are added sequentially to a single-stranded template, and when the complementary base is added, it is incorporated, resulting in pyrophosphate release. The pyrophosphate

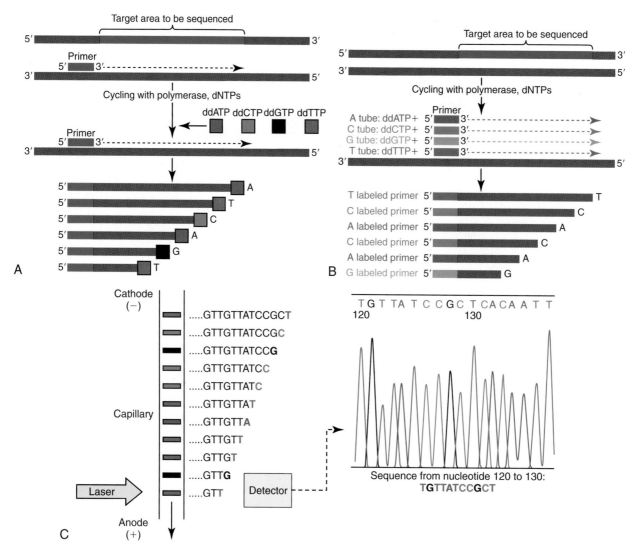

Figure 31-18 Dideoxy Chain Termination (Sanger) DNA Sequencing. Cycle sequencing of a DNA template produces a nested series of fragments that differ by one nucleotide each. The template is amplified by polymerase chain reaction (PCR) using a single primer sequence (single-sided PCR). The PCR master mix includes small amounts of dideoxynucleotides. When a dideoxynucleotide is incorporated into the growing DNA polymer, chain extension terminates. **A,** Dye terminator method in which each of the four dideoxynucleotides are labeled with a different fluorescent dye. The identity of the terminal nucleotide corresponds to its specific fluorescent color. **B,** Dye primer method in which the primer is labeled with four different fluorescent dyes, corresponding to each nucleotide. Again, the identity of the terminal nucleotide corresponds to the specific color of the primer. **C,** Capillary gel electrophoresis in which fluorescently labeled fragments pass between a laser and detector in size order (smallest fragments first). The fluorescent color of the fragment identifies the terminal nucleotide. The signals appear as peaks on an electropherogram, with each peak representing a specific terminal nucleotide in sequence order.

released is then converted to ATP by sulfurylase in the presence of adenosine 5′ phosphosulfate. This reaction is coupled to the luminescent conversion of luciferin to oxyluciferin by the enzyme luciferase, resulting in the release of light. Luminescent reactions resulting from the incorporation of nucleotides are represented as peaks on a pyrogram. The intensity of the light determines if there are multiple nucleotides that are identical because the peak height in the pyrogram will be proportional to the number of nucleotides.[48]

Sanger DNA sequencing is considered the gold standard for the detection of point mutations and single nucleotide polymorphisms. With a point mutation, for example, sequencing of either strand will show whether the mutation (for example, adenine to thymine) is present by comparison of the sequence to the reference sequence. Each cell has two copies (alleles) of

somatic genes; therefore, sequencing will produce a nested series of fragments from each allele. If the patient is a homozygote, the two nested series of fragments will be identical, whether wild-type or mutant. If the patient is a heterozygote, both wild-type and mutant fragments will be produced in the single-sided PCR, generating two nested series of fragments. In analysis of this sequence, both signals will be present at the position of the mutation, but half the templates will contain each sequence.

Next-generation sequencing (NGS), also known as massively parallel sequencing (MPS), is a new technique that is being increasingly applied in all areas of molecular diagnostics, including hematology. The technology is still rapidly changing, but most of the currently available methods sequence short fragments multiple times and use bioinformatics to reassemble the sequence. The process of NGS can be divided into several steps, including template preparation, sequencing and detection, and finally data analysis and assembly. Currently available commercial systems use a variety of methods. One commonly used method involves the immobilization of molecules on a solid phase followed by amplification to produce clonally amplified clusters. Sequencing by synthesis reactions are carried out using cyclic reversible terminators in four colors and fluorescent detection by lasers following each base addition. A second commonly used method also amplifies the sequencing template but uses emulsion PCR to accomplish it. The sequencing technology takes advantage of the hydrogen ion released when a base is added and uses semiconductor technology to translate that into a nucleotide sequence by the sequential addition of bases and the measurement of the voltage produced when the correct nucleotide base is added. Both methods use proprietary software and alignment to a reference sequence to produce the final template sequence. There are also numerous programs available as open source or from commercial vendors for analysis. Current applications for NGS have been mainly limited to the sequencing of panels of genes associated with a particular disease. This makes the bioinformatics analysis more manageable and limits the number of variants of unknown significance (VUS) that are identified.[49-51]

REAL-TIME POLYMERASE CHAIN REACTION

In contrast to *end-point* PCR, *real-time* PCR measures the change in nucleic acid amplification as replication progresses using fluorescent marker dyes. There are several commercially available instruments that vary in their capacity, sample volume, and optics.[52] There are a variety of choices in the optics for fluorescent detection. A tungsten lamp is commonly used for excitation, and different filters are used to select the excitation and emission wavelength. Light emitting diodes (LEDs) or lasers for excitation can also be coupled with emission detection, depending on the instrument. Real-time PCR can be used in quantitative or qualitative assays. The time interval, expressed as the number of replication cycles, required to reach a selected fluorescence threshold is proportional to the *copy number* of target molecules in the original sample.[53] The PCR cycle at which amplification crosses the threshold is denoted as the *Ct* for *threshold value* or the *Cp* for *crossing point value*. Importantly these values are calculated from the exponential portion of the amplification curve. The Ct value is inversely related to the amount of target so that the more starting DNA or cDNA that is present in the reaction, the lower the number of PCR cycles that are required to reach the threshold and exponential phase of the reaction (Figure 31-19).

Real-time PCR requires the use of fluorescent detection, and there are several different options available. The simplest and the most straightforward option is to add a fluorescent dye, such as SYBR® green, to the PCR reaction. These dyes bind to double-stranded DNA so that the fluorescence increases in proportion to the number of copies of the PCR product. The disadvantage of this approach is that these dyes do not differentiate between

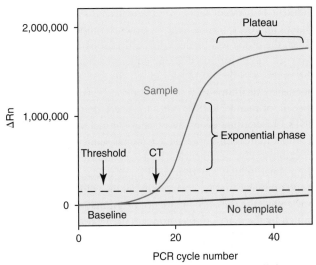

Figure 31-19 Real-time PCR amplification curve illustrating the important features of the curve, including the threshold CT value and the exponential phase of the curve.

specific and nonspecific PCR amplicons, so the PCR reaction must be free of mispriming and primer dimers (primers that partially anneal to one another and are extended by the polymerase, forming very short amplicons). A more specific method of detection adds a probe in addition to the forward and reverse PCR primers, which also binds to the amplicon, providing additional specificity. There are several methods commonly employed, including hybridization probes, Taqman probes, and molecular beacon and Scorpion probes. Hybridization probes utilize two oligonucleotide probes that bind to the amplicon adjacent (within one to five bases) to one another. One of the oligos has a 3' donor fluorophore and the other a 5' acceptor. The 3' fluorophore is excited, and the energy is transferred to the acceptor, which then fluorescences at a detectable wavelength. This is called fluorescence resonance energy transfer, or FRET.[54] Hybridization probe technology in combination with melting curve analysis is used in some commercial thrombophilia assays.

Taqman probes consist of a single oligonucleotide that anneals between the forward and reverse primers. This probe contains a fluorophore on the 5' end and a quencher on the 3' end. This method takes advantage of the 5'-to-3' exonuclease activity of DNA polymerase. As the amplicon is synthesized by DNA polymerase, the probe is degraded. This separates the fluorophore from the quencher and results in fluorescence. As the number of amplicons increases, there is more target to anneal to the probe and greater fluorescence as the probes are degraded.[55] Molecular beacons and Scorpion probes use a hairpin structure to juxtapose the reporter and quencher. When the probe binds to the target, the hairpin unfolds and separates the fluorophore from the quencher, and fluorescence is detected.[56]

Qualitative Real-Time Polymerase Chain Reaction

Taqman assays are used to detect point mutations such as the common point mutations in hereditary hemochromatosis (Chapter 20). Two Taqman probes are synthesized with a different fluorescent label, complementary to either the wild-type or mutant sequence. If the sequence is complementary to the target, the probe will be degraded as described above, and fluorescence will be produced. If the sequence contains a mismatch, the probe will be displaced and the fluorescence will remain quenched. Real-time PCR can also be combined with sequence-specific primer PCR (SSP-PCR) to detect point mutations or SNPs. This method takes advantage of the fact that the 3′ end of a primer in PCR must match the template sequence exactly to be extended by the polymerase. This is in contrast to the 5′ end of the primer, which can have additional nucleotides added. By using primers complementary to either the wild-type or mutant nucleotide, the presence or absence of a mutation can be determined by the reaction that produces the PCR product.[57] There are several modifications of this technique. One widely used technique, called SNaPshot®, uses dideoxynucleotides, each labeled with a different fluorophore and primers of different size in a multiplex reaction to detect several different nucleotide changes simultaneously. The different-sized PCR products are then identified by size fractionation using capillary gel electrophoresis (Figure 31-20).[58] There are other variations on this technique as well that are not discussed here. It is clear, however, that there are an increasing number of applications of real-time PCR in hematology, and multiple different techniques can be used to detect the same mutation. Applications of these techniques include the detection of resistance mutations in viruses or bacteria, as well as somatic mutations in cancer cells and germline mutations in genetic diseases.[59]

Quantitative Real-Time Polymerase Chain Reaction

Real-time quantitative PCR can be done in two ways: relative quantitation, which normalizes to a reference gene used when measuring gene expression, or absolute quantitation, where a standard curve of known copy number of diluted standards is run along with the patient samples. Once the relationship between the copy number of the standards and the Ct value is determined using the standard curve, the copy number of the patient sample can be determined from the crossing point value. This is used to monitor residual disease in chronic myelogenous leukemia by quantifying the amount of the BCR-ABL1 transcript (Chapter 33) as well as viral loads in infectious disease (Figure 31-21).[60-66]

High Resolution Melting Curve (HRM) analysis is a real-time PCR method that uses the quantitative analysis of the melting curve to detect sequence differences in PCR amplicons. Melting curves are often run in conjunction with real-time PCRs to confirm specificity of the product by heating the amplicon in increasing intervals from 65° C to 95° C and measuring the fluorescence. When the double-stranded DNA melts, the fluorescence will sharply decrease. High-resolution melt curves use narrower temperature increments and a saturating fluorescent dye to determine the melting curve. This allows the determination of sequence differences in PCR amplicons. This method requires a thermocycler with good temperature stability and a software package for HRM analysis. The advantage of HRM is that it will detect any sequence difference in an amplicon and the exact mutation does not have to be known in advance.[67]

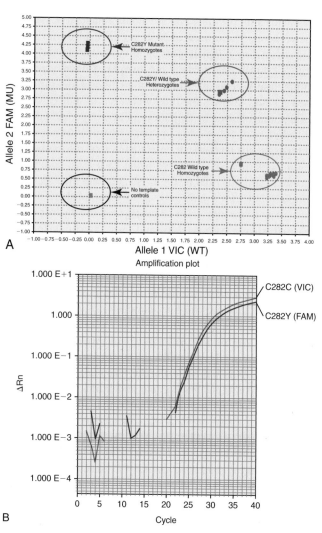

Figure 31-20 Qualitative real-time PCR for hereditary hemochromatosis, *HFE* C282 gene mutation detection. The mutation replaces the amino acid cysteine (C) with tyrosine (Y) in position 282 of the HFE protein. The method uses two Taqman amplification probes, one for the wild-type (normal) and one for the mutant allele, each labeled with a different fluorescent reporter. **A,** Taqman allelic discrimination plot demonstrating the three genotypic populations for the *HFE* gene and no template controls. The scatter plots are derived from the total fluorescence of the amplification curve for both fluorescent probes. The genotype can be determined from the position on the scatter plot. **B,** Real-time PCR amplification curves of a heterozygous C282C/Y mutant patient showing fluorescence with the two Taqman probes: VIC for the wild-type and FAM for the mutant allele.

Minimal Residual Disease in Leukemia

Real-time quantitative PCR provides the opportunity to follow disease burden and to measure *minimal residual disease* (MRD) in leukemia, a key indicator of treatment efficacy, clinical remission, and prognosis.[61,62] Currently, chemotherapy, radiation therapy, and hematopoietic stem cell transplantation reduce leukemic cells to levels undetectable first by visual examination of a bone marrow smear or peripheral blood film and later by flow cytometry assay.[68] The persistence of disease after treatment that is only detected by molecular assays is called *minimal residual disease*. Real-time quantitative PCR identifies the specific nucleic acid sequence in residual leukemic cells and helps guide the types and

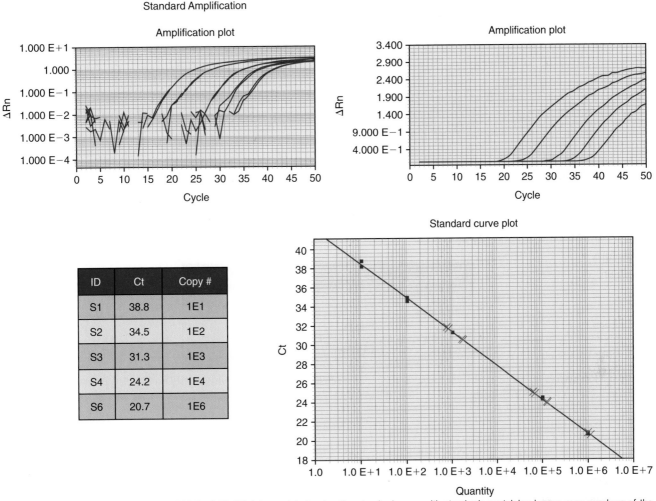

Figure 31-21 Quantitative real-time PCR for BCR-ABL1 transcript showing the standard curve with standards containing known copy numbers of the *BCR-ABL1* cDNA. Plotting the crossing point threshold value (CT) on the *y*-axis versus the log of the copy number on the *x*-axis generates a standard curve.

intensity of therapy with the goal of "molecular" remission. Real-time reverse transcriptase quantitative PCR to assess the fusion transcript levels for CML is regarded as the "gold standard" for the detection and quantification of minimal residual disease. Subsequent to remission, periodic real-time quantitative PCR assays are used to detect early relapse and drug resistance, enabling the hematologist to initiate appropriate follow-up therapy.[69]

Real-time quantitative PCR may detect a few malignant cells within a population of a million cells, providing unparalleled sensitivity. Current assays to assess MRD can detect one leukemic cell among 10^5 to 10^6 normal cells. Current applications include detection of BCR-ABL1 transcripts in CML and some acute leukemias (Figure 31-22); *JAK2* ("just another kinase" or Janus kinase) mutations in the myeloproliferative neoplasms, polycythemia vera, and essential thrombocythemia (Chapter 33); the t(15;17) (q22;q21) or PML-RARA fusion transcript in *acute promyelocytic leukemia* (Chapter 35); and *gene rearrangements* in mature lymphoid neoplasms (Chapter 36).[70]

A major issue with quantitative assays has been the lack of reproducibility between different laboratories due to the specimen type and quality, the choice of housekeeping gene for normalization, and the specific assay used. Recently an international standard for BCR-ABL1 has been developed and made available by the World Health Organization (WHO). This standard will serve as a universal standard and allow for interlaboratory comparison.[71]

Mutation Enrichment Strategies

In order to detect low levels of disease or emerging resistance, it is helpful to be able to enrich for the presence of the mutation. There are currently several methods to accomplish this, all of which seek to selectively amplify the mutant sequence in the presence of an excess of wild-type sequence. Peptide-nucleic acid (PNA) and locked nucleic acid (LNA) both contain normal nucleotide bases for hybridization but different backbones from the phosphodiester backbone of DNA and RNA.[72] This gives these probes the ability to hybridize more tightly when used as probes in PCR reactions. When the probes span and match the wild-type sequence, they can inhibit the amplification of the wild-type allele, thus enriching for the mutant allele.[73]

COLD-PCR (**co**-amplification at **l**ower **d**enaturation temperature–PCR) is another mutation enrichment technique based on PCR amplification. COLD-PCR is based on the principle that DNA containing a mismatch will melt at a

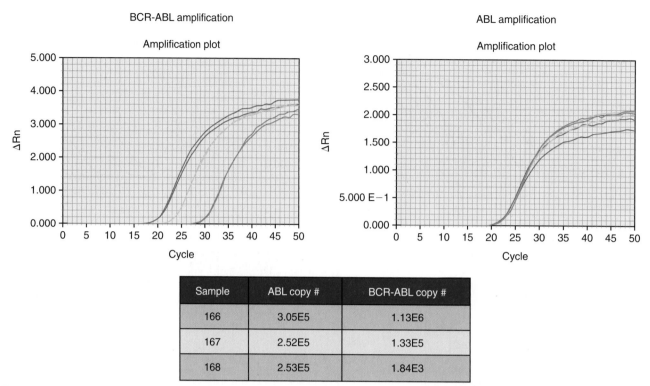

BCR-ABL amplification

Amplification plot

ABL amplification

Amplification plot

Sample	ABL copy #	BCR-ABL copy #
166	3.05E5	1.13E6
167	2.52E5	1.33E5
168	2.53E5	1.84E3

Figure 31-22 Quantitative real-time PCR for BCR-ABL1 transcript. Using the standard curve, the copy number of BCR-ABL1 transcripts in unknown samples can be determined. Two amplification graphs are shown. The graph on the left shows the amplification of the BCR-ABL1 transcript, and the graph on the right shows the amplification of the ABL1 transcript as a control for sample quality.

slightly lower temperature than completely matched sequences. Designing the PCR cycle temperatures to maximize that difference results in a preferential amplification of the mutant sequence in a mixed sample of mutant and wild-type DNA, even when the mutant is in very low concentrations. This is accomplished by carrying out the denaturation step at the temperature that will have mutant-wild-type heteroduplexes in a single-stranded state, while wild-type homoduplexes will not yet have denatured.[74] All of these methods, although useful to enrich for mutant alleles, are technically demanding and therefore are not yet in widespread usage in molecular laboratories.

CHROMOSOME MICROARRAYS

Chromosomal microarray analysis is a methodology used to measure gains and losses of genomic DNA. The advantage of microarrays compared to karyotyping is that it is a higher-resolution method and will detect genetic changes that cannot be observed by karyotyping (Chapter 30). In addition, chromosome microarrays have the advantage of also detecting aneuploidy and large chromosomal duplications and insertions.

There are two different types of chromosome microarrays: comparative genomic hybridization (aCGH) and single nucleotide polymorphism array (SNP-A) karyotyping. Both types of arrays can identify variation in copy number. Due to differences in methodology, however, they detect different types of variants (Figure 31-23).

In an array-based assay, the specimen DNA is isolated, denatured, and hybridized to a chip or array containing thousands of probes with known sequences. For comparative genome hybridization, the patient and a control DNA are labeled with different fluorescent dyes, and after hybridization, the relative intensity of the two fluorescent signals is used to determine if there are any genomic gains or losses. Duplications result in a higher-intensity fluorescence relative to control, and deletions result in a lower-intensity fluorescence. CGH is most useful in the detection of relatively large duplications or deletions.[75]

In SNP arrays only the patient DNA is labeled, denatured, and hybridized to an array containing probes with known SNPs. Again, the signal intensity is used to determine the copy number. SNP arrays are able to detect runs of homozygosity that can indicate uniparental disomy or consanguinity.[76] Because each of these methods has both advantages and disadvantages, array platforms have been developed that contain both types of sequences: SNPs and larger clones used in CGH. This provides a more uniform coverage over the entire genome. In certain situations, arrays are replacing or used as an adjunct to conventional karyotyping and fluorescence in situ hybridization (FISH) (Chapter 30). Arrays are useful to detect copy number variants but do not detect balanced translocations.[77-78]

PATHOGEN DETECTION AND INFECTIOUS DISEASE LOAD

Box 31-4 contains a listing of hematologically important pathogens detected by molecular methods. Real-time quantitative PCR can detect and quantitate a number of blood-borne viruses: hepatitis B and C viruses, human papillomavirus,

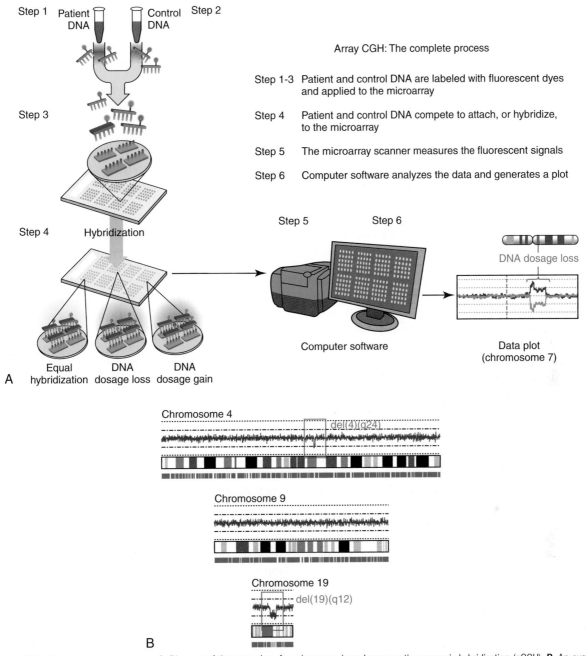

Figure 31-23 Chromosomal microarrays. **A,** Diagram of the procedure for microarray-based comparative genomic hybridization (aCGH). **B,** An example of a single nucleotide polymorphism array (SNP-A) karyogram from a patient with a secondary acute myeloid leukemia with microdeletions on chromosomes 4 and 19 and normal chromosome 9. (© 2008 SLACK, Inc. Modified from Shaffer L. G. & Bejjani B. A. Using microarray-based molecular cytogenetic methods to identify chromosome abnormalities. Pediatric Annals 38, 440-447 (2009) doi: 10.3928/00904481-20090723-08.)

CMV, Epstein-Barr virus, and HIV.[79] Human bacterial pathogens such as β-hemolytic streptococcus from throat swabs, anaerobes from wound swabs, and bacteria from urine or other body fluids can be detected within hours of collection. Antibacterial therapy can be initiated based upon the rapid results of molecular susceptibility testing. Real-time quantitative PCR is the reference method for detection and quantification of methicillin-resistant *Staphylococcus aureus* (MRSA), vancomycin-resistant enterococcus, and opportunistic *Clostridium difficile*. Molecular diagnostic techniques are effective in identifying

and monitoring malarial and other blood-borne parasites. The challenge to primer and probe developers is to select sequences that are specific enough to avoid false positives caused by non-pathogenic strains, sensitive enough to positively identify infectious strains, and flexible enough to remain effective as pathogenic microorganisms mutate and evolve. There are currently multiple FDA approved assays for the detection of viral and bacterial pathogens. A current listing of these tests can be found in the test directory on the Association for Molecular Pathology web site (amp.org).

Clinical relevance is important when assessing infectious disease using molecular techniques. These methods allow millions of copies to be generated from a single DNA or RNA sequence from a microorganism or virus. Theoretically, the presence of a single organism can lead to a positive test result, but a single organism may not be clinically relevant. Standard curves of template number are crucial to data interpretation. Also, because DNA survives the organism, a positive result on a test for a given sequence does not guarantee that the organism was viable at the time of sampling.

CURRENT DEVELOPMENTS

Molecular diagnostics is a rapidly growing area of the clinical laboratory, and the technology continues to develop. It promises to revolutionize laboratory techniques in all disciplines, and the technologies of genomics are being extended to proteomics (the molecular analysis of proteins) and metabolomics (the molecular analysis of metabolism). Methods continue to be automated and miniaturized, providing ever greater sensitivity and reliability coupled with short turnaround time and technical simplification. In many situations, assays are moving from single analyte assays to multiplex assays detecting panels of analytes. In the case of leukemias such as AML, mutations in multiple genes are incorporated into the WHO guidelines.[80] Methods such as the SNaPshot technique described previously are being applied to detect multiple mutations simultaneously.

Another technique being applied to the detection of mutation panels is Matrix-assisted laser desorption/ionization—time of flight (MALDI-TOF) mass spectrometry. This methodology uses PCR coupled to a single-base extension reaction that adds labeled nucleotides so that the extension products containing different mutations have different masses. These reactions are also multiplexed to increase throughput, detecting hundreds of mutations in a single panel assay.[81]

Digital PCR (ddPCR) is a technique with very high sensitivity that can be used to detect resistance mutations to tyrosine kinase inhibitors used to treat CML (such as the T315I resistance mutation in the *BCR-ABL1* gene)[82] (Chapter 33) or to quantify virus copy number.[83] This technique uses various methods—for example, a droplet generator to create nanoliter droplets that partition template molecules, which are then amplified by PCR. The amplicons are detected by fluorescence and either read by a droplet reader or other detection mechanism. For translocation detection, wells containing an amplified housekeeping gene, translocation product, or both are then quantitated. This method is extremely sensitive, detecting a few molecules per sample, and can be applied to both DNA and RNA applications.

NGS will continue to play an increasingly important role in molecular diagnostics. In addition to sequencing panels of genes, this technology has been used to sequence whole genomes, exomes (the coding exons), as well as RNA sequencing (RNAseq)[84,85] (Figure 31-24). This technology is also being applied to the determination of the epigenome[86]—modifications such as methylation that affect gene regulation and expression.

Small microRNAs (miR; ~20 nucleotides long) that were once thought to be insignificant are evolving as biomarkers for the progression of hematologic malignancies. The dysregulation of miRs affects normal hematopoiesis, and their atypical expression is beginning to be established in T and B cell leukemias and lymphomas.[87] These miRs target genes in the 3' UTR (3' untranslated region) and are hypothesized to inhibit the translation of mRNA to proteins.[88] These miRs can be detected by many molecular-based techniques such as PCR, NGS, and microarray technology. Their clinical role in hematologic cancer therapy as a prognostic marker is now starting to be recognized. A link between p53 expression and possible therapeutic efficacy is shown with miR-181a/b dysregulation in chronic lymphocytic leukemia (CLL) patients in a recent study.[89] Another example is a report by Seca and colleagues[90] that lists many functions of miR-21, including the upregulation of the BCR-ABL1 protein and induction of chemoresistance. An overexpression of miR-21 has been demonstrated in patients who are fludarabine nonresponders.[91] The overexpression of plasma miR-155 is correlated to the identification of B-CLL in patients,[92] and association of miR-21 is established with drug resistance in plasma cell myeloma.[93] The listed studies demonstrate that the ability to measure the expression of miR has expanded the repertoire of diagnostic, prognostic, and therapeutic efficacy markers in hematologic malignancies.

The future molecular technologies will increase the efficiency and sensitivity for detection of all types of genome alterations, including point mutations, insertion and deletion mutations, copy number variants, and chromosome rearrangements. It will facilitate the discovery of new chromosome rearrangements as well as the diagnosis of microbial infections. It will result in refined classification and improved treatment of hematological diseases.

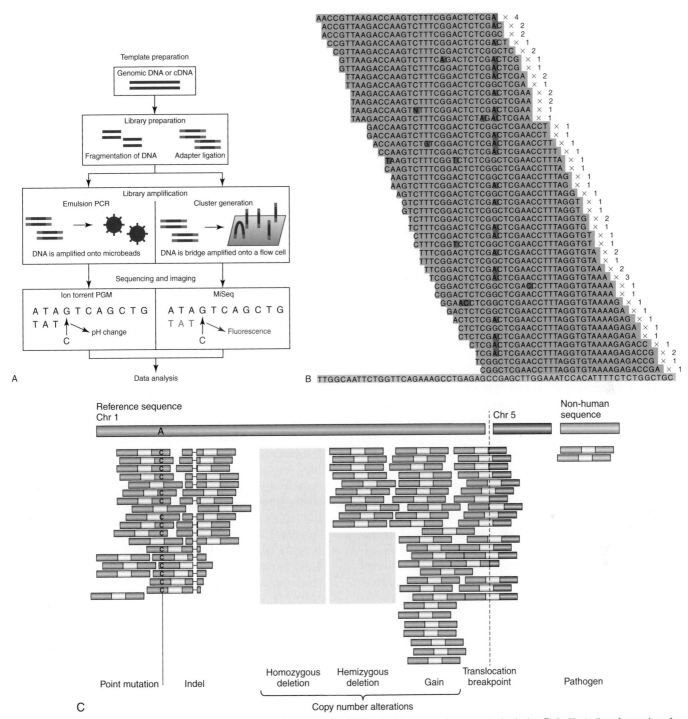

Figure 31-24 A, Diagram of the procedure for next-generation sequencing (NGS) using the two most common technologies. **B,** An illustration of a number of NGS reads for a 32-nucleotide sequence aligned with the genomic reference sequence in blue on the bottom (sequence mismatches are in red). The center of the alignment shows a variant present in the heterozygous state. **C,** Sequenced fragments are depicted as bars with colored tips representing the sequenced ends and the unsequenced portion of the fragment in gray. Reads are aligned to the reference genome (for example, mostly chromosome 1 in this example). The colors of the sequenced ends show where they align. Different types of genomic alterations can be detected. From left to right, point mutations (in this example, A to C) and small insertions and deletions (indels) (in this example, a deletion shown by a dashed line) are detected by identifying multiple reads that show non-reference sequence; changes in sequencing depth (relative to a normal control) are used to identify copy number changes (shaded boxes represent absent or decreased reads in a tumor sample); paired-ends that map to different genomic loci (in this case, chromosome 5) are evidence of rearrangements; and sequences that map to nonhuman sequences are evidence for the potential presence of genomic material from pathogens. (**A** from Grada A, Weinbrecht K: Next-generation sequencing: methodology and application. *Journal of Investigative Dermatology* 133, 248-251, 2013; **B** from Almomani R, van der Heijden J, Ariyurek Y, et al: Experiences with array-based sequence capture; toward clinical applications. *European Journal of Human Genetics* 19:50-55, 2011; **C** from Meyerson M, Gabriel S, Getz G: Advances in understanding cancer genomes through second generation sequencing, *Nature Reviews Genetics* 11: 685-696, 2010.)

SUMMARY

- DNA directs cell function as described by the *central dogma*. DNA retains the genetic code and reproduces itself through *replication*.
- The genetic code is *transcribed* from DNA to mRNA. mRNA consists of coding exons and noncoding introns that are excised after transcription. The processed mRNA then transports the code from the nucleus to the cytoplasm, where it is *translated* by the cytoplasmic ribosomes. Translation depends on tRNA, small RNA molecules designed to transport and add amino acid to growing peptide chains in cytoplasmic ribosomes.
- DNA consists of a five-carbon sugar (deoxyribose), a phosphate group, and a nitrogenous base. The bases are either purines or pyrimidines. The purines in DNA are adenine (A) and guanine (G). The pyrimidines in DNA are thymine (T) and cytosine (C).
- DNA is a double-stranded molecule held together by hydrogen bonding between the bases, A to T and G to C. Heat denatures double-stranded DNA by breaking the hydrogen bonds to produce single-stranded DNA. DNA strands are antiparallel.
- RNA is a single-stranded molecule that contains the sugar ribose instead of the deoxyribose found in DNA and the pyrimidine uracil in place of thymine.
- RNA polymerase recognizes a sequence of deoxyribonucleotides called the *promoter* within DNA. RNA polymerase separates the DNA strands and begins adding ribonucleotides, forming an initial RNA transcript consisting of introns and exons.
- Proteins function as structural components of the cell, as enzymes involved in metabolism or regulation, as receptors to regulate cellular functions, or as antibodies for the immune system. Mutation within a gene ultimately alters the protein produced, which often affects the function of the protein.
- Five areas of hematopathologic molecular testing include detection of mutations, gene rearrangements, and chromosomal abnormalities for diagnosis and prognosis of hematologic malignancies; detection and quantification of minimal residual disease to monitor treatment of hematologic malignancies; detection of mutations in inherited hematologic disorders; pharmacogenetic testing to detect genetic variation affecting certain drug therapies; and identification of hematologically important infectious diseases.
- Peripheral blood, bone marrow, tissue biopsy samples (both fresh and formalin fixed paraffin-embedded), fine-needle aspirates, body fluids, saliva, and cheek swabs are specimens used for DNA and RNA isolation.
- DNA is amplified by in vitro endpoint polymerase chain reaction (PCR) and real-time PCR. RNA targets can be amplified by PCR by first converting the RNA target to complementary DNA or cDNA.
- In endpoint PCR, amplified DNA is detected by electrophoresis (slab gel or automated capillary gel electrophoresis) or cleavage-based signal amplification (Invader) technology. Endpoint PCR can also be combined with restriction enzyme digestion of the amplicons, followed by detection of the restriction fragments by one of the methods mentioned above. In real-time PCR, the amplicons are detected during the PCR cycles by fluorescence detection.
- Real-time PCR can be used qualitatively to determine the presence or absence of a target or can quantify the copy number of a target DNA or RNA. PCR can be used to amplify RNA targets by first converting them to cDNA with reverse transcriptase activity.
- The dideoxy chain termination (Sanger) method for DNA sequencing is based on the principle that synthesis of a DNA polymer is terminated upon incorporation of a dideoxynucleotide. The target DNA template is amplified over a number of cycles, which produces a series of DNA fragments that terminate at each successive base with each fragment differing in length by one nucleotide. DNA fragments are detected by labeling either the dideoxynucleotide or the primer with a fluorescent dye. Other methods for DNA sequencing include pyrosequencing and next-generation sequencing (NGS).
- Chromosomal microarrays measure gains and losses of genomic DNA. They provide much greater sensitivity in detecting small genomic changes compared to conventional karyotyping. There are two types: microarray-based comparative genomic hybridization (aCGH) and single nucleotide polymorphism array (SNP-A) karyotyping. CGH requires the use of a control DNA.
- Molecular testing permits clinicians to make more accurate diagnostic, therapeutic, and prognostic decisions. It also allows a more sensitive assessment of minimal residual disease and therapeutic efficacy, resulting in better patient management.

Now that you have completed this chapter, go back and read again the case study at the beginning and respond to the questions presented.

Review Questions

Answers can be found in the Appendix.

1. If the DNA nucleotide sequence is 5′-ATTAGC-3′, then the mRNA sequence transcribed from this template is:
   a. 5′-GCUAAU-3′
   b. 5′-AUUAGC-3′
   c. 5′-TAATCG-3′
   d. 5′-UAAUCG-3′

2. Cells with damaged DNA and mutated or nonfunctioning cell cycle regulatory proteins:
   a. Are arrested in G_1 and the DNA is repaired
   b. Continue to divide, which leads to tumor progression
   c. Divide normally, producing identical daughter cells
   d. Go through apoptosis

3. To start DNA replication, DNA polymerase requires an available 3′ hydroxyl group found on the:
   a. Leading strand
   b. mRNA
   c. Parent strand
   d. Primer

4. Ligase joins Okazaki fragments of the:
   a. 5′-to-3′ template strand
   b. Lagging strand
   c. Leading strand
   d. Primer fragments

5. A 40-year-old patient enters the hospital with a rare form of cancer caused by faulty cell division regulation. This cancer localized in the patient's spleen. An ambitious laboratory developed a molecular test to verify the type of cancer present. This molecular test would require patient samples taken from which two tissues?
   a. Abnormal growths found on the skin and in the bone marrow
   b. Normal splenic tissue and cancerous tissue
   c. Cancerous tissue in spleen and bone marrow
   d. Peripheral blood and cancerous tissue in the spleen

6. One main difference between PCR and reverse transcriptase PCR is that:
   a. PCR requires primers
   b. PCR uses reverse transcriptase to elongate the primers
   c. Reverse transcriptase PCR forms millions of cDNA fragments
   d. Reverse transcriptase PCR requires ligase to amplify the target DNA

7. Which one of the following statements about gel electrophoresis is *false*?
   a. The gel is oriented in the chamber with the wells at the positive terminal.
   b. A buffer solution is required to maintain the electrical current.
   c. The matrix of a polyacrylamide gel is tighter than that of an agarose gel.
   d. The larger DNA fragments will be closest to the wells of the gel.

8. Autoradiography of DNA is the:
   a. Detection of radioactive or chemoluminescent oligonucleotides
   b. Exposure of the gel to UV light
   c. Transfer of DNA to a nitrocellulose filter
   d. Use of ethidium bromide to visualize the DNA banding pattern

9. One major difference between endpoint PCR and real-time PCR is that:
   a. Endpoint PCR requires thermostable DNA polymerase, deoxynucleotides, and primers
   b. Endpoint PCR requires a separate step to detect the amplicons formed in the reaction
   c. Real-time PCR uses capillary gel electrophoresis to detect amplicons during PCR cycling
   d. Real-time PCR detects and quantifies amplicons using cleavage-based signal amplification

10. Which of the following statements about minimal residual disease is *true*?
    a. Clinical remission of hematologic cancers is determined by molecular techniques such as PCR and flow cytometry.
    b. Real-time quantitative PCR–determined copy number of *BCR/ABL1* transcripts will always be lower in molecular remission than in clinical remission.
    c. Qualitative PCR that uses a known copy number of a target sequence is of use in determining minimal residual disease levels.
    d. Minimal residual disease assessment can aid physicians in making treatment decisions but does not yet offer insights into prognosis.

REFERENCES

1. Kaufman, R. E. (1999). Synthesis of sickle and normal hemoglobins: laboratory and clinical implications. *Lab Med, 30,* 129–133.
2. Mayo, M. M., & Samuel, S. M. (1999). Clinical pathology rounds: diagnosing hemoglobin SC. *Lab Med, 30,* 98–101.
3. International Human Genome Sequencing Consortium. (2004). Finishing the euchromatic sequence of the human genome. *Nature, 431,* 931–945.
4. Calladine, C. R., Drew, H. R., & Luisi, B. F. (2004). *Understanding DNA: The Molecule and How it Works.* (3rd ed., pp. 1–17). San Diego: Academic Press.
5. Mattick, J. S., & Makunin, I. V. (2006). Non-coding RNA. *Hum Mol Genet, 15,* R17–R29.
6. Lewin, B. (2008). Messenger RNA. In *Genes IX.* (3rd ed., pp. 127–150). Sudbury, Mass: Jones & Bartlett.
7. Basic molecular genetic mechanisms. (2012). In Lodish, H., Berk, A., Kaiser, C. A., et al., (Eds.), *Molecular Cell Biology.* (7th ed., pp. 115–169). New York: WH Freeman.
8. Bartlett, J. M. S., & White, A. (2003). Extraction of DNA from whole blood. In Bartlett, J. M. S., & Stirling, D., (Eds.), *PCR Protocols.* (2nd ed., pp. 29–31). Totowa, NJ: Humana Press.

9. Shimizu, H., & Burns, J. C. (1995). Extraction nucleic acids: sample preparation from paraffin-embedded tissues. In Innis, M. A., Gelfand, D. H., & Sninsky, J. J., (Eds.), *PCR Strategies* (pp. 32–38). San Diego: Academic Press.

10. Cao, W., Hashibe, M., Rao, J. Y., et al. (2003). Comparison of methods for DNA extraction from paraffin-embedded tissues and buccal cells. *Cancer Detect Prevent, 27*, 397–404.

11. Harder, J., & Schroder, J. M. (2002). RNase 7, a novel innate immune defense antimicrobial protein of healthy human skin. *J Biol Chem, 277*, 46779–46784.

12. Bogner, P. N., & Killeen, A. A. (2006). Extraction of nucleic acids. In Coleman, W. B., & Tsongalis, G. J., (Eds.), *Molecular Diagnostics for the Clinical Laboratorian* (pp. 25–30). Totowa, NJ: Humana Press.

13. Miller, W. H., Kakizuka, A., Frankel, S. R., et al. (1992). Reverse transcription polymerase chain reaction for the rearranged retinoic acid receptor α clarifies diagnosis and detects minimal residual disease in acute promyelocytic leukemia. *Proc Natl Acad Sci U S A, 89*, 2694–2698.

14. Schwartz, R. C., Sonenshein, G. E., Bothwell, A., et al. (1981). Multiple expression of Ig δ-chain encoding RNA species in murine plasmacytoma cells. *J Immunol, 126*, 2104–2108.

15. Mullis, K. B., & Faloona, F. A. (1987). Specific synthesis of DNA in vitro via a polymerase-catalyzed chain reaction. *Methods Enzymol, 155*, 335–350.

16. Saiki, R. K., Scharf, S., Faloona, F., et al. (1985). Enzymatic amplification of β-globin genomic sequences and restriction site analysis for diagnosis of sickle cell anemia. *Science, 230*, 1350–1354.

17. Studwell, P. S., & O'Donnell, M. (1990). Processive replication is contingent on the exonuclease subunit of DNA polymerase III holoenzyme. *J Biol Chem, 265*, 1171–1178.

18. Saiki, R. K., Gelfand, D. H., Stoffel, S., et al. (1988). Primer-directed enzymatic amplification of DNA with a thermostable DNA polymerase. *Science, 239*, 487–491.

19. Cha, R. S., & Thilly, W. G. (1995). Specificity, fidelity and efficiency of PCR. In Dieffenbach, C. W., & Dveksler, G. S., (Eds.), *PCR Primer: a Laboratory Manual.* (pp. 37–52). Cold Spring Harbor, NY: Cold Spring Harbor Press.

20. Altschul, S. F., Gish, W., Miller, W., et al. (1990). Basic local alignment search tool. *J Mol Biol, 215*, 403–410.

21. Mifflin, T. E. (2003). Setting up a PCR laboratory. In Dieffenbach, C. W., & Dveksler, G. S., (Eds.), *PCR Primer: A Laboratory Manual.* (2nd ed., pp. 5–14). Cold Spring Harbor, NY: Cold Spring Harbor Laboratory Press.

22. Najfeld, V. (2013). Conventional and molecular cytogenetic basis of hematologic malignancies. In Hoffman, R., Benz, E. J. Jr, Silberstein, L. E., et al., (Eds.), *Hematology: Basic Principles and Practice.* (6th ed., pp. 728–780). Philadelphia: Saunders, an imprint of Elsevier.

23. Bhatt, V. R., Akhtari, M., Bociek, R, G., et al. (2014). Allogeneic stem cell transplantation for Philadelphia chromosome-positive acute myeloid leukemia. *J Natl Compr Canc Netw, 12*, 963–968.

24. Keung, Y. K., Beaty, M., Powell, B. L., et al. (2004). Philadelphia chromosome positive myelodysplastic syndrome and acute myeloid leukemia—retrospective study and review of literature. *Leuk Res, 28*, 579–586.

25. Bartram, C. R., de Klein, A., Hagemeijer, A., et al. (1983). Translocation of the *c-abl* oncogene correlates with the presence of a Philadelphia chromosome in chronic myelocytic leukemia. *Nature, 306*, 277–280.

26. Heisterkamp, N., Stephenson, J. R., Groffen, J., et al. (1983). Localization of the *c-abl* oncogene adjacent to a translocation break point in chronic myelocytic leukemia. *Nature, 306*, 239–242.

27. Clark, S. S., McLaughlin, J., Crist, W. M., et al. (1987). Unique forms of the abl tyrosine kinase distinguish Ph1-positive CML from Ph1-positive ALL. *Science, 235*, 85–88.

28. Preudhomme, C., Revillion, F., Merlat, A., et al. (1999). Detection of BCR-ABL transcripts in chronic myeloid leukemia (CML) using a "real-time" quantitative RT-PCR assay. *Leukemia, 13*, 957–964.

29. Luu, M. H., & Press, R. D. (2013). BCR-ABL PCR testing in chronic myelogenous leukemia: molecular diagnosis for targeted cancer therapy and monitoring. *Expert Rev Mol Diagn, 13*, 749–762.

30. Sambrook, J., & Russell, D. W. (2001). Gel electrophoresis of DNA and pulsed-field agarose gel electrophoresis. In Sambrook, J., & Russell, D. W., (Eds.), *Molecular Cloning: A Laboratory Manual.* (3rd ed., pp. 5.4–5.86). Cold Spring Harbor, NY: Cold Spring Harbor Laboratory Press.

31. Dubrow, R. S. (1992). Capillary gel electrophoresis. In Grossman, P. D., & Colburn, J. C., (Eds.), *Capillary Gel Electrophoresis Theory and Practice.* (pp. 146–154). San Diego: Academic Press.

32. Van Dongen, J., Langerak, A. W., Bruggemann, M., et al. (2003). Design and standardization of PCR primers and protocols for the detection of immunoglobulin and T cell receptor gene rearrangements in suspect lymphoproliferations. Report of the BIOMED-2 Concerted Action BMH4-CT98-3936. *Leukemia, 12*, 2257–2317.

33. Nathans, D., & Smith, H. O. (1975). Restriction endonucleases in the analysis and restructuring of DNA molecules. *Annu Rev Biochem, 44*, 273–293.

34. Ross, D. W. (1990). Restriction enzymes. *Arch Pathol Lab Med, 114*, 906.

35. De Stefano, V., Finazzi, G., & Mannucci, P. M. (1996). Inherited thrombophilia: pathogenesis, clinical syndromes, and management. *Blood, 87*, 3531–3544.

36. Liu, X. Y., Nelson, D., Grant, C., et al. (1995). Molecular detection of a common mutation in coagulation F5 causing thrombosis via hereditary resistance to activated protein C. *Diagn Mol Pathol, 4*, 191–197.

37. Southern, E. M. (1975). Detection of specific sequences among DNA fragments separated by gel electrophoresis. *J Mol Biol, 98*, 503–517.

38. Chen, C. Y., Shiesh, S. C., & Wu, S. J. (2004). Rapid detection of K-ras mutations in bile by peptide nucleic acid-mediated PCR clamping and melting curve analysis: comparison with restriction fragment length polymorphism analysis. *Clin Chem, 50*, 481–489.

39. Saiki, R. K., Walsh, P. S., Levenson, C. H., et al. (1989). Genetic analysis of amplified DNA with immobilized sequence-specific oligonucleotide probes. *Proc Natl Acad Sci U S A, 86*, 6230–6234.

40. Yuen, E., & Brown, R. D. (2005). Southern blotting of IgH rearrangements in B-cell disorders. In Brown, R. D., & Ho, P., (Eds.), *Multiple Myeloma.* (pp. 85–103). Totowa, NJ: Humana Press.

41. Thorpe, G. H., & Kricka, L. J. (1986). Enhanced chemiluminescent reactions catalyzed by horseradish peroxidase. *Methods Enzymol, 133*, 331–353.

42. Kwiatkowski, R. W., Lyamichev, V., de Arruda, M., et al. (1999). Clinical, genetic and pharmacogenetic applications of the Invader assay. *Mol Diagn, 4*, 353–364.

43. Buckingham, L. (2012). DNA sequencing. In Buckingham, L., (Ed.), *Molecular Diagnostics: Fundamentals, Methods, and Clinical Applications.* (2nd ed., pp. 222–240). Philadelphia: FA Davis.

44. Schnittger, S., Schoch, C., Dugas, M., et al. (2002). Analysis of FLT3 length mutations in 1003 patients with acute myeloid leukemia: correlation to cytogenetics, FAB subtype and prognosis in the AMLCG study and usefulness as a marker for the detection of minimal residual disease. *Blood, 100*, 59–66.

45. Furtado, L. V., Weiglin, H. C., Elenitoba-Johnson, K. S. J., et al. (2013). A multiplexed fragment analysis-based assay for the detection of JAK2 exon 12 mutations. *J Mol Diagn, 15*, 592–599.

46. Nybakken, G. E., & Bagg, A. (2014). The genetic basis and expanding role of molecular analysis in the diagnosis, prognosis and therapeutic design for myelodysplastic syndrome. *J Mol Diagn, 16*, 145–158.

47. Sanger, F., Nicklen, S., & Coulson, A. R. (1977). DNA sequencing with chain-terminating inhibitors. *Proc Natl Acad Sci U S A, 74*, 5463–5467.

48. Fakhrai-Rad, H., Pourmand, N., & Ronaghi, M. (2002). Pyrosequencing: an accurate detection platform for single nucleotide polymorphisms. *Hum Mutat, 19*, 479–485.

49. Myerson, M., Gabriel, S., & Getz, G. (2010). Advances in understanding cancer genomes through second-generation sequencing. *Nat Rev Genet, 11*, 685–696.

50. Mullighan, C. G. (2013). Genome sequencing of lymphoid malignancies. *Blood, 122*, 3899–3907.

51. White, B. S., & DiPersio, J. F. (2014). Genomic tools in acute myeloid leukemia: From the bench to the bedside. *Cancer, 120*, 1134–1144.

52. Templeton, K. E., & Claas, E. C. J. (2003). Comparison of four real-time PCR detection systems. In Dieffenbach, C. W., & Dveksler, G. S., (Eds.), *PCR Primer: A Laboratory Manual*. (2nd ed., pp. 187–198). Cold Spring Harbor, NY: Cold Spring Harbor Laboratory Press.

53. van der Velden, V. H. J., Hochhaus, A., Cazzaniga, G., et al. (2003). Detection of minimal residual disease in hematologic malignancies by real-time quantitative PCR: principles, approaches, and laboratory aspects. *Leukemia, 17*, 1013–1034.

54. Ahmad, A. I., & Ghasemi, J. B. (2007). New FRET primers for quantitative real-time PCR. *Anal Bioanal Chem, 387*, 2737–2743.

55. Luthra, R., & Medeiros, L. J. (2006). TaqMan reverse transcriptase-polymerase chain reaction coupled with capillary electrophoresis for quantification and identification of bcr-abl transcript type. *Methods Mol Biol, 335*, 135–145.

56. Tan, W., Wang, K., & Drake, T. J. (2004). Molecular beacons. *Curr Opin Chem Biol, 8*, 547–553.

57. Rudert, W. A., Braun, E. R., & Faas, S. J. (1997). Double labeled fluorescent probes for 5′ nuclease assays: purification and performance evaluation. *BioTechniques, 22*, 1140–1145.

58. Fanis, P., Kousiappa, I., Phylactides, M., et al. (2014). Genotyping of BCL11A and HBSIL-MYB SNPs associated with fetal haemoglobin levels: a SNaPshot minisequencing approach. *BMC Genomics, 15*, 108. doi:10.1186/1471-2164-15-108.

59. Latini, F. R., Gazito, D., Amoni, C. P., et al. (2014). A new strategy to identify rare blood donors: single polymerase chain reaction multiplex SNaPshot reaction for detection of 16 blood group alleles. *Blood Transfus, 12*(Suppl. 1), s256–263.

60. Le Guillou-Guillemette, H., Lunel-Fabiani, F. (2009). Detection and quantification of serum or plasma HCV RNA: mini review of commercially available assays. *Methods Mol Biol, 510*, 3–14.

61. Kern, W., Voskova, D., Schoch, C., et al. (2004). Determination of relapse risk based on assessment of minimal residual disease during complete remission by multiparameter flow cytometry in unselected patients with acute myeloid leukemia. *Blood, 104*, 3078–3085.

62. Fenk, R., Ak, M., Kobbe, G., et al. (2004). Levels of minimal residual disease detected by quantitative molecular monitoring herald relapse in patients with multiple myeloma. *Haematologica, 89*, 557–566.

63. Brüggemann, M., Schrauder, A., Raff, T., et al; European Working Group for Adult Acute Lymphoblastic Leukemia (EWALL); International Berlin-Frankfurt-Münster Study Group (I-BFM-SG). (2010). Standardized MRD quantification in European ALL trials: proceedings of the Second International Symposium on MRD assessment in Kiel, Germany, 18-20 September 2008. *Leukemia, 24*, 521–535.

64. Stentoft, J., Pallisgaard, N., Kjeldsen, E., et al. (2001). Kinetics of BCR-ABL fusion transcript levels in chronic myeloid leukemia patients treated with ST1571 measured by quantitative real-time polymerase chain reaction. *Eur J Haematol, 67*, 302–308.

65. Gabert, J., Beillard, E., van der Velden, V. H., et al. (2003). Standardization and quality control studies of "real-time" quantitative reverse transcriptase polymerase chain reaction of fusion transcripts for residual disease detection in leukemia—a Europe Against Cancer program. *Leukemia, 17*, 2318–2357.

66. Wittek, M., Stürmer, M., Doerr, H. W., et al. (2007). Molecular assays for monitoring HIV infection and antiretroviral therapy. *Expert Rev Mol Diagn, 7*, 237–746.

67. Wittwer, C., Gudrun, H. R., Gundry, C. N., et al. (2003). High-resolution genotyping by amplicon melting analysis using LC Green. *Clin Chem, 49*, 853–860.

68. Kantarjian, H., Schiffer, C., Jones, D., et al. (2008). Monitoring the response and course of chronic myeloid leukemia in the modern era of BCR-ABL tyrosine kinase inhibitors: practical advice on the use and interpretation of monitoring methods. *Blood, 111*, 1774–1780.

69. Parker, W. T., Lawrence, R. M., Ho, M., et al. (2011). Sensitive detection of BCR-ABL1 mutations with chronic myeloid leukemia after imatinib resistance is predictive of outcome during subsequent therapy. *J Clin Oncol, 29*, 4250–4259.

70. Lobetti-Bodoni, C., Mantoan, B., Monitillo, L., et al. (2013). Clinical implications and prognostic role of minimal residual disease detection in follicular lymphoma. *Ther Adv Hematol, 4*, 189–198.

71. White, H. E., Matejtschuk, P., Rigsby, P., et al. (2010). Establishment of the first World Health Organization International Genetic Reference Panel for quantitation of BCR-ABL mRNA. *Blood, 116*, e111–e117.

72. Porcheddu, A., & Giacomelli, G. (2005). Peptide nucleic acids (PNAs), a chemical overview. *Curr Med Chem, 12*, 2561–2599.

73. Oh, J. E., Lim, H. S., An, C. H., et al. (2010). Detection of low-level KRAS mutations using PNA-mediated asymmetric PCR clamping and melting curve analysis with unlabeled probes. *J Mol Diagn, 12*, 418–424.

74. Milbury, C. A., Li, J., Liu, P., et al. (2011). COLD-PCR: Improving the sensitivity of molecular diagnostics assays. *Expert Rev Mol Diagn, 11*, 159–169.

75. Shao, L., Kang, S-H., Li, J., et al. (2010). Array comparative genomic hybridization detects chromosomal abnormalities in hematological cancers that are not detected by conventional cytogenetics. *J Mol Diagn, 12*, 670–679.

76. Hagenkord, J., & Chang, C. C. (2009). The reward and challenges of array-based karyotyping for clinical oncology applications. *Leukemia, 23*, 829–833.

77. Schweighofer, C. D., Coombes, K. R., Majewski, T., et al. (2013). Genomic variation by whole genome SNP mapping assays predicts time to event outcome in patients with chronic lymphocytic leukemia. *J Mol Diagn, 15*, 196–209.

78. Kwong, Y. L., Pang, A. W., Leung, A. Y., et al. (2014). Quantification of circulating Epstein-Barr virus DNA in NK/T-cell lymphoma treated with the SMILE protocol: diagnostic and prognostic significance. *Leukemia, 28*, 865–870.

79. Chevaliez, S., Bouvier-Alias, M., Rodriguez, C., et al. (2013). The COBAS Ampliprep/COBAS TaqMan HCV test v2.0, real-time PCR assay accurately quantifies hepatitis C virus genotype 4 RNA. *J Clin Microbiol, 51*, 1078–1082.

80. Arber, D. A., Brunning, R. D., Le Beau, M. M. et al. (2008). Acute myeloid leukemia with recurrent genetic abnormalities: In Swerdlow, S. H., Campo, E., Harris, N. L., et al., (Eds.), *Who Classification of Tumours of Haematopoietic and Lymphoid Tissues*. (4th ed.). Lyon: International Agency for Research on Cancer.

81. Dunlap, J., Beadling, C., Warrick, A., et al. (2012). Multiplex high-throughput gene mutation analysis in acute myeloid leukemia. *Hum Pathol, 43*, 2167–2176.

82. Jennings, L. J., George, D., Czech, J., et al. (2014). Detection and quantification of BCR-ABL1 fusion transcripts by droplet digital PCR. *J Mol Diagn, 16*, 174–179.

83. Hall Sedlak, R., & Jerome, K. R. (2014). The potential advantages of digital PCR for clinical virology diagnostics. *Expert Rev Mol Diagn, 14*, 501–507.

84. Ferreira, P. G., Jares, P., Rico, D., et al. (2014). Transcriptome characterization by RNA sequencing identifies a major molecular and clinical subdivision in chronic lymphocytic leukemia. *Genome Res, 24*, 212–226.

85. Koboldt, D. C., Steinberg, K. M., Larson, D. E., et al. (2013). The next-generation sequencing revolution and its impact on genomics. *Cell, 155*, 27–38.

86. Rivera, C. M., & Ren, B. (2013). Mapping human epigenomes. *Cell, 155*, 39–55.

87. Zhao, H., Wang, D., Du, W., et al. (2010). MicroRNA and leukemia: tiny molecule, great function. *Crit Rev Oncol Hematol, 74*, 149–155.

88. Undi, R. B., Kandi, R., & Gutti, R. K. (2013). MicroRNA as haematopoiesis regulators. *Adv Hematol, 2013*, 1–20.

89. Zhu, D. X., Zhu, W., Fang, C., et al. (2012). miR-181a/b significantly enhances drug sensitivity in chronic lymphocytic leukemia cells via targeting multiple anti-apoptosis genes. *Carcinogenesis, 33*, 1294–1301.

90. Seca, H., Lima, R. T., Lopes-Rodrigues, V., et al. (2013). Targeting miR-21 induces autophagy and chemosensitivity of leukemia cells. *Curr Drug Targets, 14*, 1135–1143.

91. Ferracin, M., Zagatti, B., Rizzotto, L., et al. (2010). MicroRNAs involvement in fludarabine refractory chronic lymphocytic leukemia. *Mol Cancer, 9*, 123.

92. Ferraioli, A., Shanafelt, T. D., Shimizu, M., et al. (2013). Prognostic value of miR-155 in individuals with monoclonal B-cell lymphocytosis and patients with B chronic lymphocytic leukemia. *Blood, 122*, 1891–1899.

93. Ma, J., Liu, S., & Wang, Y. (2014). MicroRNA-21 and multiple myeloma: small molecule and big function. *Med Oncol, 31*, 94.

Flow Cytometric Analysis in Hematologic Disorders

Magdalena Czader

OBJECTIVES

After completion of this chapter, the reader will be able to:

1. Describe the technique of flow cytometry, including specimen selection and preparation, instrumentation, data collection, and a design of an antibody panel.
2. Discuss the pattern recognition approach to analysis of flow cytometric data for diagnosis and follow-up of hematologic malignancies.
3. Identify basic cell populations defined by flow cytometric parameters.
4. Recognize the key immunophenotypic features of normal bone marrow, peripheral blood, and lymph node tissue, and specimens from patients with acute leukemia or lymphoma.
5. Discuss novel applications of flow cytometry beyond the immunophenotyping of hematologic malignancies.

CASE STUDIES

After studying the material in this chapter, the reader should be able to respond to the following case studies:

Case 1

A 58-year-old man had a 5-month history of extensive right cervical lymphadenopathy and night sweats. His complete blood count (CBC) results were within normal limits. Physical examination showed additional bilateral axillary lymphadenopathy. The cervical lymph node was excised. Histologic examination revealed nodular architecture with predominantly medium-sized lymphoid cells with irregular nuclear outlines. Flow cytometric data are presented in Figure 32-1.

1. What cell subpopulation predominates on the forward scatter (FS)/side scatter (SS) scattergram?
2. List antigens positive in this population.
3. Does the pattern of light chain expression support the diagnosis of lymphoma?

Case 2

A 3-year-old girl was brought to the physician because of fatigue and fevers. The CBC revealed a WBC count of 3×10^9/L, HGB level of 8.3 g/dL, and platelet count of 32×10^9/L. Review of the peripheral blood film showed rare undifferentiated blasts with occasional cytoplasmic blebs. No granules or Auer rods were identified. Bone marrow examination showed a marked increase in blasts (79%) and decreased trilineage hematopoiesis. Flow cytometric analysis was performed. In addition to the markers shown in Figure 32-2, the population of interest was positive for CD34, CD33, CD41, and HLA-DR.

1. What abnormal features are observed on the CD45/SS scattergram?
2. What is the most likely diagnosis considering the constellation of markers expressed by the predominant population?

Continued

After studying the material in this chapter, the reader should be able to respond to the following case studies:

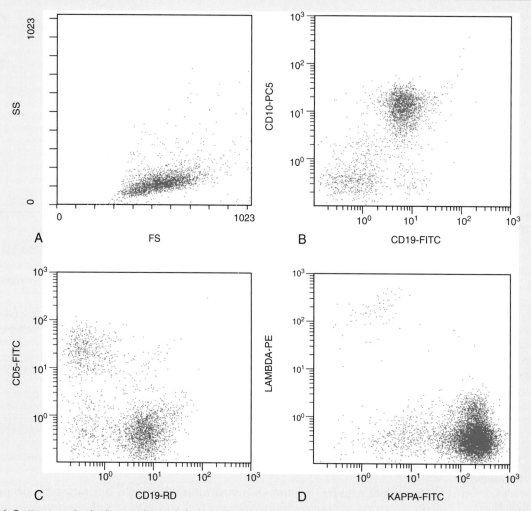

Figure 32-1 Scattergrams showing immunophenotypic features of lymphoid cells from the patient in Case 1. *FITC,* fluorescein isothiocyanate; *FS,* Forward scatter; *RD,* rhodamine; *SS,* side scatter.

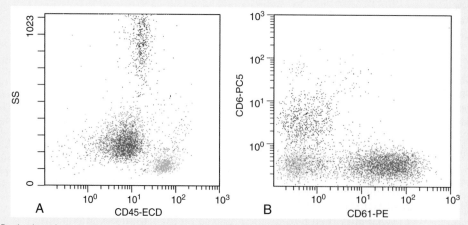

Figure 32-2 Predominant bone marrow population for the patient in Case 2. *ECD,* phycoerythrin-Texas Red; *PE,* phycoerythrin; *SS,* Side scatter.

low cytometry was originally designed to measure physical properties of cells based on their ability to deflect light. Over the years, it has evolved to include detection of fluorescent signals emitted by dyes bound directly to specific molecules or attached to proteins through monoclonal antibodies. The development of monoclonal antibodies is the most significant factor contributing to today's broad application of flow cytometry. Although the term *flow cytometry* implies the measurement of a cell, this technique is applied successfully to study other particles, including chromosomes, microorganisms, and proteins. The main advantage of flow cytometry over other techniques is its ability to rapidly and simultaneously analyze multiple parameters in a large number of cells. When one adds the capability of identifying and quantifying rare-event cells in a heterogeneous cell population, the value of flow cytometry to clinical hematology becomes obvious. Currently, this technique not only is applied to analysis of cell lineage in acute leukemia or a detection of clonality in lymphoid populations but also makes it possible to discern abnormal populations in chronic myeloid neoplasms, quantitate minimal residual disease, and monitor immunodeficiency states. Immunophenotypes that originally were used to supplement morphologic classification frequently correlate with specific cytogenetic or molecular abnormalities. According to the classification of hematopoietic neoplasms recommended by the World Health Organization,[1] one no longer can rely solely on morphology for a diagnosis of hematologic malignancies. Current diagnostic algorithms integrate morphologic, immunophenotypic, and genotypic information. This approach emphasizes the central role that flow cytometry plays in the hematopathology laboratory.

The focus of this chapter is on the use of flow cytometry in a routine hematopathology laboratory. The chapter follows a "life" of a flow cytometric specimen that starts with specimen processing and ends with a final diagnosis. The discussion is divided into preanalytical (specimen processing), analytical (flow cytometric instrumentation and analysis), and postanalytical (immunophenotypic features of hematopoietic disorders) sections.

SPECIMEN PROCESSING

Flow cytometric analysis is particularly useful in diagnosing hematologic malignancies. The specimens most commonly analyzed are bone marrow, peripheral blood, and lymphoid tissues. In addition, immunophenotyping is often performed on body cavity fluids and solid tissues when they are suspected to harbor a hematologic malignancy.[2]

Prolonged transport or transport under inappropriate conditions may render a specimen unsuitable for analysis. Peripheral blood and bone marrow specimens should be processed within 24 to 48 hours from the time of collection. Certain specimens, such as body cavity fluids or samples from neoplasms with a high proliferative activity, may require even more rapid processing.

When cells are suspended in a fluid, as in peripheral blood and bone marrow, minimal sample preparation is required. These specimens are collected into a tube or container with an anticoagulant, preferably heparin, and are transported to a flow cytometry laboratory at room temperature. Bone marrow biopsy specimens and solid tissue specimens, including core biopsy samples, are submitted in culture media to maintain viability or on saline-moistened gauze. Tissue fragments are mechanically dissociated to yield a cell suspension, usually by mincing with a scalpel.

To obtain a pure population of nucleated cells, red blood cells (RBCs) are lysed. The analytical process depends on cellularity and viability of a specimen; both are routinely assessed before a sample is stained. Cell count can be obtained using automated cell counters or flow cytometry. A specimen is stained with propidium iodide or 7-amino actinomycin to test viability. A cytocentrifuge slide (Chapter 18) is prepared for a morphologic inspection of a cell suspension.

As soon as these steps are completed, a sample is stained with a cocktail of fluorochrome-conjugated monoclonal antibodies. The analysis of intracytoplasmic markers requires an additional fixation and permeabilization step to allow antibodies to pass through a cell membrane. A predetermined panel of antibodies may be used to detect membrane-bound and intracellular markers. Simultaneous analysis of multiple markers, known as *multicolor* or *multiparameter flow cytometry,* has numerous advantages. It facilitates visualization of antigen expression and maturation patterns, which are often disturbed in hematopoietic malignancies. In addition, regardless of a complexity of a specimen, analysis can be accomplished using few tubes and with a lower total number of cells, which saves reagents, time, and data storage. There is no consensus on the standardized panel of antibodies to be used in routine flow cytometric evaluation. The U.S.-Canadian Consensus Project in Leukemia/Lymphoma Immunophenotyping recommends the comprehensive approach with multiple markers for myeloid and lymphoid lineage.[3] Selected markers commonly analyzed by flow cytometry are presented in Table 32-1.

FLOW CYTOMETRY: PRINCIPLE AND INSTRUMENTATION

The most significant discovery that led to the advancement of flow cytometry and its subsequent widespread application in clinical practice was the development of monoclonal antibodies.[4] In the original *hybridoma* experiments, lymphocytes with predetermined antibody specificity were co-cultured with a myeloma cell line to form immortalized hybrid cells producing specific monoclonal antibodies. For this discovery, which not only fueled the development of flow cytometry but also had innumerable research and, more recently, clinical applications, Köhler and Milstein received a Nobel Prize in 1984. Over the years, numerous antibodies were produced and tested for their lineage specificity. Categorization of these antibodies and associated antigens is accomplished through workshops on human leukocyte differentiation antigens that have been held regularly since 1982. These workshops provide a forum for reporting new antigens and antibodies and define a cluster of antibodies recognizing the same antigen, called *cluster of differentiation* (CD) (Table 32-2; see also Table 32-1). Consecutive numbers are assigned to each new reported antigen. The Ninth International Conference on Human Leukocyte Differentiation Antigens brought to over 350 the total number of antigens characterized.[5]

TABLE 32-1 Lineage-Associated Markers Commonly Analyzed in Routine Flow Cytometry

Lineage	Markers
Immature	CD34
	CD117
	Terminal deoxynucleotidyl transferase
Granulocytic/monocytic	CD33
	CD13
	CD15
	CD14
Erythroid	CD71
	Glycophorin A
Megakaryocytic	CD41
	CD42
	CD61
B lymphocytes	CD19
	CD20
	CD22
	κ Light chain
	λ Light chain
T lymphocytes	CD2
	CD3
	CD4
	CD5
	CD7
	CD8

Monoclonal antibodies have various applications, including immunohistochemistry, immunofluorescence, and Western blot. These methods study cellular proteins in fixed tissues or in cellular extracts; however, they do not provide the ability to examine antigens in their native state and cannot decipher composite cell populations with a complex antigen makeup. In contrast, flow cytometry can define antigen expression on numerous viable cells. Currently, 17 antigens can be detected simultaneously on an individual cell.[6] This is accomplished by the conjugation of monoclonal antibodies to a variety of fluorochromes that can be detected directly by a flow cytometer. In a flow cytometer, particles are suspended in fluid and pass one by one in front of a light source. As particles are illuminated, they emit fluorescent signals registered by detectors. These results are later converted to digital output and analyzed using flow cytometry software. The flow cytometer consists of fluidics, a light source (laser), a detection system, and a computer. A brief discussion of these basic components is presented.

To be analyzed individually, cells must pass separately, one by one, through the illumination and detection system of a flow cytometer. This passage is accomplished by injecting a cell suspension into a stream of sheath fluid. This technique, called *hydrodynamic focusing*, creates a central core of individually aligned cells surrounded by a sheath fluid (Figure 32-3). The central alignment is essential for consistent illumination of cells as they pass before a laser light source.

A laser is composed of a tube filled with gas, most commonly argon or helium-neon, and a power supply. Current is

TABLE 32-2 Hematolymphoid Antigens Commonly Used in Clinical Flow Cytometry

Cluster of Differentiation	Function	Cellular Expression
CD1a	T cell development	Precursor T cells
CD2	T cell activation	Precursor and mature T cells, NK cells
CD3	Antigen recognition	Precursor and mature T cells
CD4	Co-receptor for HLA class II	Precursor T cells, helper T cells, monocytes
CD5	T cell signaling	Precursor and mature T cells, subset of B cells
CD7	T cell activation	Precursor and mature T cells, NK cells
CD8	Coreceptor for HLA class I	Precursor T cells, suppressor/cytotoxic T cells, subset of NK cells
CD10	B cell regulation	Precursor B cells, germinal center B cells, granulocytes
CD11b	Cell adhesion	Granulocytic and monocytic lineage, NK cells
CD13	Unknown	Granulocytic and monocytic lineage
CD14	Monocyte activation	Mature monocytes
CD15	Ligand for selectins	Granulocytic and monocytic lineage
CD16	Low-affinity IgG Fc receptor	Granulocytic and monocytic lineage, NK cells
CD18	Cell adhesion and signaling	Granulocytic and monocytic lineage
CD19	B cell activation	Precursor and mature B cells
CD20	B cell activation	Precursor and mature B cells
CD22	B cell activation and adhesion	Precursor and mature B cells
CD31	Cell adhesion	Megakaryocytes, platelets, leukocytes
CD33	Cell proliferation and survival	Granulocytic and monocytic lineage
CD34	Cell adhesion	Hematopoietic stem cells
CD36	Cell adhesion	Megakaryocytes, platelets, erythroid precursors, monocytes
CD38	Cell activation and proliferation	Hematopoietic cells, including activated lymphocytes and plasma cells
CD41	Cell adhesion	Megakaryocytes, platelets
CD42b	Receptor for von Willebrand factor	Megakaryocytes, platelets
CD45	T and B cell receptor activation	Hematopoietic cells
CD56	Cell adhesion	NK cells, subset of T cells

TABLE 32-2 Hematolymphoid Antigens Commonly Used in Clinical Flow Cytometry—cont'd

Cluster of Differentiation	Function	Cellular Expression
CD61	Cell adhesion	Megakaryocytes, platelets
CD62P	Homing	Platelets
CD63	Cell development, activation, growth, and motility	Platelets
CD64	High-affinity IgG Fc receptor	Granulocytic and monocytic lineage
CD71	Iron uptake	High density on erythroid precursors, low to intermediate density on other proliferating cells
CD79a	B cell receptor signal transduction	Precursor and mature B cells
CD117	Stem cell factor receptor	Hematopoietic stem cells, mast cells

Ig, Immunoglobulin; *NK,* natural killer.

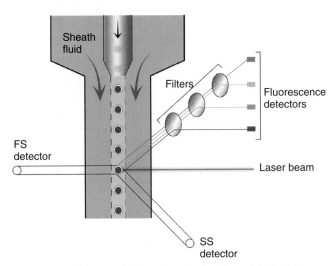

Figure 32-3 Diagram of a flow cytometer. As cells are injected into pressurized sheath fluid, they are positioned in the center of the stream and one by one exposed to the laser light. Forward scatter (FS) and side scatter (SS) are collected by separate detectors.

applied to the gas to raise electrons of a gas to an excited state. When electrons return to a ground state, they emit photons of light. Through an amplification system, a strong beam of light with light waves of identical direction, polarization plane, and wavelength is produced. This narrow coherent beam of light is used to illuminate individual cells, each stained with antibodies conjugated to specific fluorochromes.

After absorption of laser light, the electrons of fluorochromes are raised from a ground state to a higher energy state (Figure 32-4). The return to the original ground level is accompanied by a loss of energy, emitted as light of a specific wavelength. Flow cytometers are equipped with several photodetectors, each specific for light of a unique color (wavelength). The fluorescence from an individual cell is partitioned into its different wavelengths through a series of filters (dichroic mirrors) and directed to the corresponding photodetector. Fluorescent signals derived from different fluorochromes attached to particular antibodies are registered separately.

In addition to fluorescence, scatter signals are recorded. The detector situated directly in line with the illuminating laser beam measures forward scatter (FS or FSC), which is proportional to particle volume or size. A photodetector located to the side measures side scatter (SS or SSC), which reflects surface complexity and internal structures such as granules and

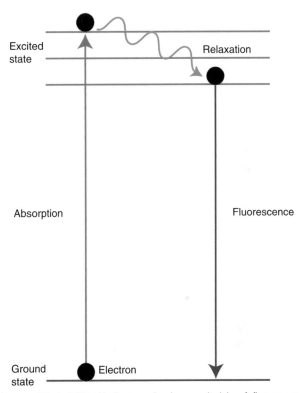

Figure 32-4 Jablonski diagram showing a principle of fluorescence. When electrons absorb energy, they are raised to the excited state. Subsequently, on their return to ground state, the absorbed energy is emitted in a form of fluorescence.

vacuoles. FS, SS, and fluorescence are displayed simultaneously on the instrument screen and registered by the computer system.

PATTERN RECOGNITION APPROACH TO ANALYSIS OF FLOW CYTOMETRIC DATA

Concept of Gating

Cell populations with similar physical properties such as size, cytoplasmic complexity, and expression of a specific antigen form *clusters* on data displays generated by flow cytometers. A *gate* is an electronic boundary an operator uses to delineate cell clusters. Thus, gating is a process of selecting, with a cursor or computer mouse, a population of interest as defined by one or more flow cytometric parameters.

Gating can be applied at the time of data acquisition (live gate) or at the time of analysis. For diagnostic purposes, data are collected ungated; that is, all events detected by the flow cytometer are recorded. This allows comprehensive testing and retention of positive and negative internal controls. In addition, unexpected abnormal populations are detected. Gating is most commonly applied after a specimen is run through a flow cytometer, when a target population is already known. In contrast, live gating focuses on the acquisition of data for a specific cell population as defined by flow cytometric parameters. For example, one can collect data only on CD19+ B cells to facilitate detection of a small population of monoclonal B cells.

Analysis of Flow Cytometric Data

As with microscopic examination, an evaluation of flow cytometric data is based on the inspection of visual patterns. First, the data are scanned to detect abnormal populations. Subsequent analysis focuses on the antigenic properties of these abnormal cells.

Analysis begins with inspection of dot plots presenting cell size, cytoplasmic complexity, and expression of pan-hematopoietic antigen CD45. As in microscopic examination at low magnification, an operator detects specific cell populations based on their physical properties (Figure 32-5). The identification of particular populations can be confirmed and further resolved on the scattergram of CD45 antigen density and SS (Figure 32-6). This display also provides information on the relative proportion of specific cell populations in the flow cytometric sample. Lymphocytes show the highest density of CD45, with approximately 10% of the cell membrane occupied by this antigen. Granulocytic series show intermediate CD45 density; late erythroid precursors and megakaryocytes are negative for CD45. The CD45/SS display is particularly useful for detection of blasts, which overlap with lymphocytes, monocytes, or both on the FS/SS display.[7,8]

The FS/SS and CD45/SS displays allow the initial identification of the target population. Further analysis focuses on patterns of antigen expression, including qualitative data (antigen presence or absence) and fluorescence intensity as a relative measure of an antigen density.

CELL POPULATIONS IDENTIFIED BY FLOW CYTOMETRY

The surface and cytoplasmic markers expressed in hematologic malignancies resemble those of normal hematopoietic cell differentiation. Frequently, neoplastic cells are arrested at a particular stage of development and display aberrant antigenic patterns. Diagnosis and classification of hematologic neoplasms is based on the knowledge of normal hematopoietic maturation pathways.

In the past, the differentiation of hematopoietic cells was defined by morphologic criteria. Over time, it became clear that specific morphologic stages of development are accompanied by distinct changes in immunophenotype. Approximate morphologic-immunophenotypic correlates exist; however, because hematopoiesis is a continuous process, transitions between various developmental phases are not discrete.

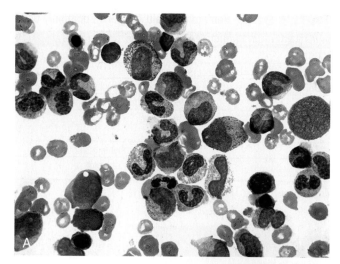

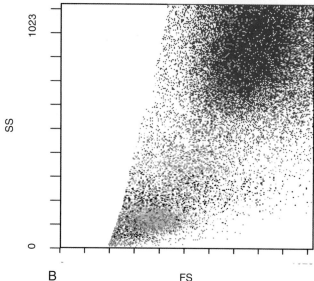

Figure 32-5 Main cell subpopulations of normal bone marrow. **A,** Bone marrow is composed of a heterogeneous population of cells of different sizes and variable complexity of cytoplasm (Wright-Giemsa stain, ×1000). **B,** Dot plot of forward scatter (FS, cell size) versus side scatter (SS, internal complexity) reflects the heterogeneity of bone marrow subpopulations. Lymphocytes are smallest with negligible amount of agranular cytoplasm and are located closest to the origins of the axes (*aqua*). Monocytes are slightly larger with occasional granules and vacuoles (*green*). Granulocytic series shows prominent granularity (*navy*).

All hematopoietic progeny are derived from pluripotent stem cells. These cells are morphologically unrecognizable and are defined by their functional and antigenic characteristics. They usually express a combination of CD34, CD117 (*c-kit*), CD38, and HLA-DR antigens.[9] As hematopoietic cells mature, they lose stem cell markers and acquire lineage-specific antigens. A brief discussion of the maturation sequence of major hematopoietic cell lineages is presented in the following sections.

Granulocytic Lineage

The stages of granulocytic lineage development, as defined by the expression of specific antigens, correspond closely to the morphologic sequence.[10] The first morphologically recognizable cell committed to the granulocytic lineage is a

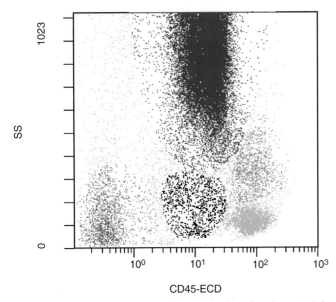

Figure 32-6 Scattergram showing differential densities of pan-hematopoietic marker CD45 on marrow leukocytes. Lymphocytes (*aqua*) and monocytes (*green*) show highest density of CD45 antigen. Intermediate expression of CD45 is seen in the granulocytic population (*navy*) and blasts (*black*). Erythroid precursors (*red*) are CD45−. *ECD*, phycoerythrin-Texas Red; *SS*, Side scatter.

myeloblast (Chapter 12). A myeloblast is characterized by an expression of immature cell markers CD34, CD38, HLA-DR, and stem cell factor receptor CD117. Pan-myeloid markers CD13 and CD33, present on all myeloid progeny, are first expressed at this stage. As a myeloblast matures to a promyelocyte, it loses CD34 and HLA-DR and acquires the CD15 antigen. Further maturation to a myelocyte stage leads to an expression of CD11b, a temporary loss of CD13, and a gradual decrease in the density of CD33. Finally, as granulocytic cells near a band stage, CD16 is acquired, and the density of CD13 increases.

Monocytic Lineage

The earliest immunophenotype stage of monocytic development is defined by a gradual increase in the density of CD13, CD33, and CD11b antigens. Subsequent acquisition of CD15 and CD14 marks the transition to a promonocyte and mature monocyte. In contrast to the granulocytic series, strong expression of CD64 and HLA-DR antigens persists throughout monocytic maturation.

Erythroid Lineage

The majority of erythroid precursors do not express pan-hematopoietic marker CD45. The earliest marker of erythroid differentiation is the transferrin receptor, CD71. The density of this antigen increases starting in the pronormoblast stage and is rapidly downregulated in reticulocytes.[11] In contrast, glycophorin A, although present on reticulocytes and erythrocytes, first appears at the basophilic normoblast stage.

Megakaryocytic Lineage

The maturation sequence of megakaryocytes is less well defined. CD41 and CD61, referred to as *glycoprotein IIb/IIIa complex*,

appear as the first markers of megakaryocytic differentiation. These antigens are present on a small subset of CD34+ cells believed to represent early megakaryoblasts.[9] CD31 and CD36, although not entirely specific for megakaryocytic lineage, also are present on megakaryoblasts. Subsequent maturation to megakaryocytes and platelets is characterized by the appearance of additional glycoproteins, CD42, CD62P, and CD63.

Lymphoid Lineage

The B and T lymphocytes are derived from lymphoid progenitors that express CD34, terminal deoxynucleotidyl transferase (TdT), and HLA-DR. Lymphoid differentiation is characterized by a continuum of changes in the expression of surface and intracellular antigens. The earliest B cell markers include CD19, cytoplasmic CD22, and cytoplasmic CD79.[12] As B cell precursors mature, they acquire the CD10 antigen. The appearance of the mature B cell marker CD20 coincides with the decrease in CD10 antigen expression. Another specific immature B cell marker is the cytoplasmic μ chain that eventually is transported to the surface and forms the B cell receptor. At this stage, the immunoglobulin chains in so-called naive B cells have become rearranged. The normal mature B cell population shows a mix of κ and λ light chain–expressing cells. The exclusive expression of only κ or λ molecules is a marker of monoclonality, seen frequently in mature B cell neoplasms. The differentiation of mature naive B cells, often recapitulated by B cell malignancies, is discussed in detail in Chapter 36.

Similar to B cell precursors, immature T cells express CD34 and TdT.[13] The first markers associated with T cell lineage include CD2, CD7, and cytoplasmic CD3. CD2 and CD7 are also present in natural killer (NK) cells and, along with the CD56 molecule, are used to detect NK cell–derived neoplasms. In T cells, the expression of CD2, CD7, and cytoplasmic CD3 is followed by the appearance of CD1a and CD5 and coexpression of CD4 and CD8 antigens. Finally, the CD3 antigen appears on the cell surface, and CD4 or CD8 is lost. The sequential transition from double-negative (CD4−CD8−) through double-positive (CD4+CD8+) stages generates a population of mature helper (CD4+) and suppressor (CD8+) T cells. T cell differentiation occurs in the thymus.

FLOW CYTOMETRIC ANALYSIS OF MYELOID NEOPLASMS (ACUTE MYELOID LEUKEMIAS AND CHRONIC MYELOID NEOPLASMS)

In myeloid malignancies, flow cytometry is used for initial diagnosis, follow-up, and prognostication. Specific immunophenotypes are associated with select cytogenetic abnormalities. Because most myeloid malignancies are stem cell disorders, the evaluation of blast population and maturing myeloid component is considered mandatory. Almost invariably, blasts are characterized by a low-density expression of CD45 antigen. In normal bone marrow, a blast gate includes a relatively low number of cells showing the immature myeloid immunophenotype (Figure 32-6). In acute myeloid and lymphoblastic leukemias, this region becomes densely populated by immature cells, which reflects the increased number of blasts seen in the bone marrow (Figure 32-7). The exact position of the immature population on the CD45/SS

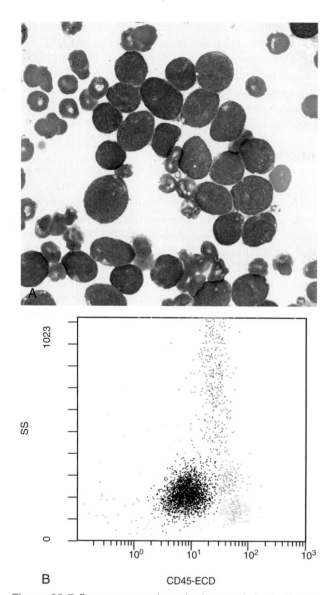

Figure 32-7 Bone marrow specimen showing acute leukemia. Note uniform cytologic and flow cytometric characteristics. **A,** Bone marrow aspirate from a patient with acute lymphoblastic anemia (Wright-Giemsa stain, ×500). **B,** CD45 versus side scatter (SS) plot shows a homogeneous population of blasts with a marked decrease in normal hematopoietic elements. Compare with the heterogeneous pattern of normal bone marrow in Figure 33-6. *ECD,* Phycoerythrin-Texas Red.

displays depends on the subtype of acute myeloid leukemia (AML). In this chapter, the immunophenotypic features of AML and chronic myeloid neoplasms are discussed in the context of the World Health Organization classification, which introduced categories defined by recurrent cytogenetic abnormalities.[1] These leukemias often show specific immunophenotypes and are discussed separately in the following sections.

Acute Myeloid Leukemias with Recurrent Cytogenetic Abnormalities

In most cases, AML with t(8;21)(q22;q22);*RUNX1/RUNX1T1* shows an immature myeloid immunophenotype with high-density CD34 and coexpression of CD19 (Figure 32-8).[14] In

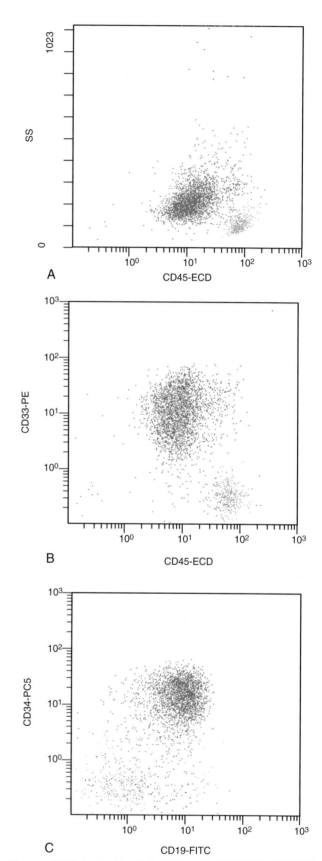

Figure 32-8 Acute myeloid leukemia with t(8;21)(q22;q22);*RUNX1-RUNX1T1.* **A,** CD45 versus side scatter (SS) showing increase in blasts (*red*) with residual lymphocytes (*aqua*). **B** and **C,** Blasts are positive for CD33 and CD34 with characteristic coexpression of CD19 antigen. *ECD,* Phycoerythrin-Texas Red; *FITC,* fluorescein isothiocyanate.

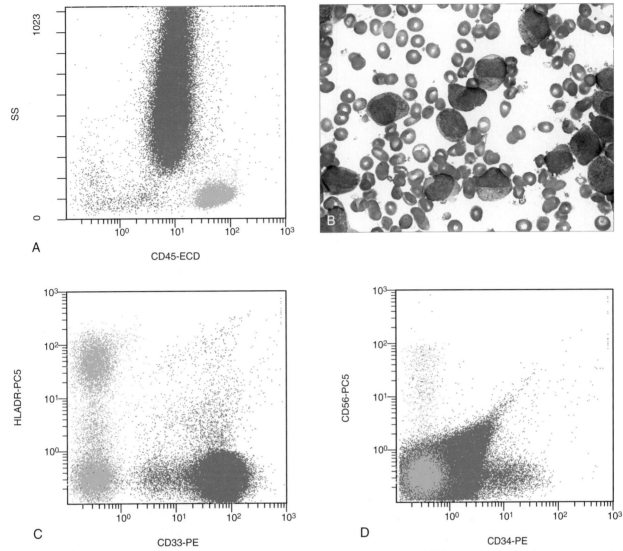

Figure 32-9 Acute promyelocytic leukemia. **A,** Typical side scatter (SS) pattern in acute promyelocytic leukemia corresponding to prominent granularity of leukemic cells (*red*). Residual lymphocytes are shown in aqua. **B,** Numerous leukemic promyelocytes with distinct granules and occasional Auer rods (Wright-Giemsa stain, ×1000). **C,** Leukemic cells show high-density expression of CD33 antigen and lack HLA-DR. **D,** Similarly, CD34 antigen is absent or present in only a few leukemic cells. *ECD,* phycoerythrin-Texas Red; *PC5,* phycoerythrin-cyanine 5; *PE,* phycoerythrin; *SS,* Side scatter.

addition, numerous myeloid antigens, including CD33, CD13 and myeloperoxidase, are expressed. Frequently, there is asynchronous coexpression of CD34 and CD15. TdT is commonly present.

AML with inv(16)(p13.1q22) or t(16;16)(p13.1;q22);*CBFB/ MYH11* is characterized by the presence of immature cells with expression of CD34, CD117, and TdT and a subpopulation of maturing cells showing monocytic (CD14, CD11b, CD4) and granulocytic (CD15) markers.[15] The aberrant coexpression of CD2 on the monocytic population is common.

Acute promyelocytic leukemia, AML with t(15;17)(q22;q12); *PML/RARA,* shows a specific immunophenotype. In contrast to most less-differentiated myeloid leukemias, acute promyelocytic leukemia manifests with high SS, which reflects the granular cytoplasm of leukemic cells (Figure 32-9). The constellation of immunophenotypic features used to diagnose acute promyelocytic leukemia includes lack of CD34 and HLA-DR antigens, presence of homogeneous strong CD33 along with myeloperoxidase, and variable CD13 and CD15.[16]

AMLs with t(9;11)(p22;q23);*MLLT3/MLL* in adults most commonly present with monocytic differentiation. The immunophenotypic features are nonspecific and can be seen in any acute myelomonocytic or monocytic leukemia (negative for CD34 and positive for CD33, CD13, CD14, CD4, CD11b, and CD64).

Acute Myeloid Leukemias Not Otherwise Specified

In the least-differentiated AMLs—AML with minimal differentiation and AML without maturation—blasts are present in the region of low-density CD45 antigen and display low SS reflecting their relatively agranular cytoplasm. Even the least differentiated AML with minimal differentiation is usually positive for myeloid markers. The expression of CD13, CD33, and CD117 is common. Primitive hematopoietic antigens such as CD34 and HLA-DR are often seen. Myeloperoxidase is absent or is expressed in only a few cells. The immunophenotypic profile of AML with maturation is similar, but more

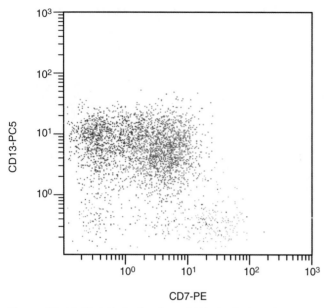

Figure 32-10 Myeloblasts of acute myeloid leukemia show aberrant co-expression of CD7 antigen. *PE*, Phycoerythrin; *PC5*, phycoerythrin-cyanine 5.

mature myeloid markers such as CD15 and myeloperoxidase are often expressed.

Occasionally, there is aberrant coexpression of antigens. Simultaneous expression of early and late markers of myeloid differentiation on the leukemic blasts is not uncommon (asynchronous antigen expression). Similarly, markers specific for other lineages, such as lymphoid lineage may be seen on myeloid blasts. The most common example is CD7 antigen, which is usually present in the T/NK cell population (Figure 32-10).

Acute myelomonocytic leukemia and acute monoblastic leukemia usually show higher expression of CD45, similar to normal monocytic precursors. In addition, in acute myelo-monocytic leukemia, a population of primitive myeloid blasts is often seen (Figure 32-11). The expression of myeloid markers and antigens associated with monocytic lineage, such as CD14, CD4, CD11b, and CD64, is commonly seen. Although CD14 is present on all mature monocytes, it may be absent in monocytic leukemias.[17] More immature monocytic markers, such as CD64, are more consistently expressed.

Acute erythroid leukemias are categorized into two subtypes: pure erythroid leukemia and erythroleukemia (erythroid/myeloid

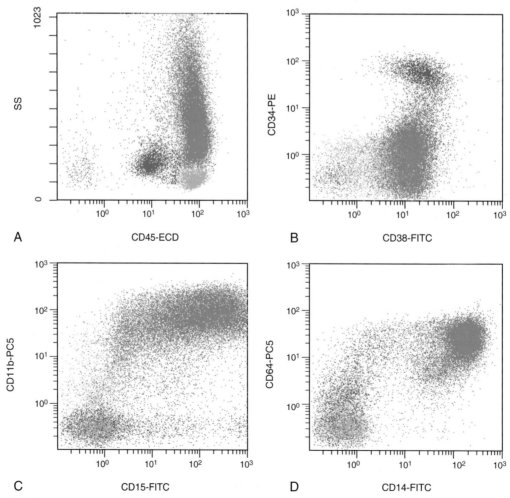

Figure 32-11 Peripheral blood immunophenotyping in acute myelomonocytic leukemia. **A,** CD45 versus side scatter (SS) display shows myeloid blasts (*red*) and a monocytic population (*green*). **B** through **D,** Primitive leukemic blasts are positive for CD34 and negative for CD14. In contrast, monocytic population does not express CD34 and shows positivity for mature monocyte marker CD14 and characteristic monocytic pattern of CD11b and CD15 expression. *ECD*, Phyco-erythrin-Texas Red; *FITC*, fluorescein isothiocyanate; *PC5*, phycoerythrin-cyanine 5.

leukemia). In the latter, primitive myeloid blasts and erythroid precursors are present. Leukemic cells are positive for erythroid markers such as CD71, glycophorin A, and hemoglobin (HGB). In more immature erythroid leukemias, glycophorin A and hemoglobin may be absent. In these cases, the diagnosis is based on the absence of myeloid markers, high expression of CD71, and scatter characteristics.

Acute megakaryoblastic leukemia usually shows low SS and low to absent CD45. Early megakaryocytic markers, CD41 and CD61, are frequently expressed.[18] Occasionally, the late megakaryocytic marker CD42 is present. The expression of stem cell markers CD34 and HLA-DR on the population of leukemic megakaryoblasts varies.

Myeloproliferative Neoplasms and Myelodysplastic Syndromes

The knowledge of antigen expression in the normal differentiation of myeloid lineages allows us to define the aberrant expression patterns frequently seen in chronic myeloid disorders. The abnormalities detected by flow cytometry reflect morphologic features (e.g., hypogranulation of neutrophils in myelodysplastic syndrome detected by low SS) and show changes in antigen expression. Qualitative (presence or absence of a particular antigen) and quantitative abnormalities (differences in the number of antigen molecules) can be used for diagnostic purposes. The interested reader is referred to review articles discussing the details of immunophenotyping in myelodysplastic syndromes and myeloproliferative neoplasms.[19-21] A few examples are highlighted to illustrate the role of flow cytometry in diagnosing these diseases.

SS abnormalities related to hypogranulated neutrophils are seen in approximately 70% of myelodysplastic syndromes (Figure 32-12). In high-grade myelodysplastic syndrome and myeloproliferative neoplasms undergoing transformation, the increase in immature cells is detected easily. Blasts have a variety of aberrant immunophenotypic features, most commonly coexpression of CD7 and CD56 antigens. Blasts and maturing granulocytic precursors may show asynchronous expression of myeloid markers, including retention of CD34 and HLA-DR in late stages of maturation or late myeloid markers presenting early in differentiation, such as CD15 on myeloblasts. Asynchronous coexpression of markers can also be seen in monocytic and erythroid lineages. Aberrant immunophenotypes are seen in 98% of cases of myelodysplastic syndrome. More importantly, immunophenotypic abnormalities can be seen in cases with minimal or no morphologic dysplasia.[19] Other studies underscore the significance of immunophenotypic abnormalities in predicting the outcome after stem cell transplantation.[22,23]

The utility of flow cytometry in myeloproliferative neoplasms is less well established. Specifically, the application of flow cytometry as a diagnostic tool in chronic myelogenous leukemia is limited to the accelerated or blast phase, in which a lineage of an expanding blast population needs to be determined. In the chronic phase, the presence of *BCR/ABL1* rearrangement (Philadelphia chromosome) demonstrated by conventional karyotyping or molecular studies remains the defining feature of the disease. Other myeloproliferative neoplasms are not well studied. In general, flow cytometric

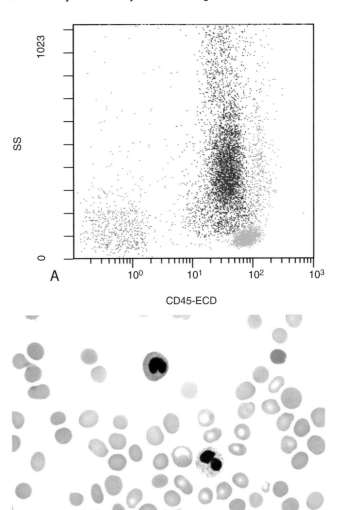

Figure 32-12 A, Low side scatter (SS) of hypogranular neutrophils seen in most cases of myelodysplastic syndrome (*navy*). **B,** Corresponding photomicrograph of markedly dysplastic, hypogranulated neutrophils in myelodysplastic syndrome (Wright-Giemsa stain, ×1000). *ECD,* Phycoerythrin-Texas Red.

abnormalities are seen in most cases with abnormal karyotype.[20] No consistent set of immunophenotypic features that can be routinely used in the workup of myeloproliferative states has been described.

FLOW CYTOMETRIC ANALYSIS OF LYMPHOID NEOPLASMS (LYMPHOBLASTIC LEUKEMIA/LYMPHOMA AND MATURE LYMPHOID NEOPLASMS)

Similar to myeloid neoplasms, a diagnosis of lymphoid malignancies relies on the expression of lineage-associated markers corresponding to specific stages of lymphoid development. No single marker can be used for lineage assignment, and a diagnosis is typically based on the presence of several B cell or T cell antigens. The sentinel feature of mature B and T cells is the presence of surface receptor complexes. The immune system responds to a wide array of antigens; in healthy individuals, B and T cells express a great diversity of surface immunoglobulin and T cell receptor complexes (polyclonal populations). A neoplastic lymphoid population is characterized by the monoclonal expression of a single B or T cell receptor. In most cases, clonality confirms the malignant nature of lymphoid proliferation. In contrast, lymphoid precursors are generally negative for surface immunoglobulin and T cell receptors and instead carry immature markers. In lymphoblastic (precursor-derived) neoplasms, an expansion of a population with homogeneous marker expression, rather than clonality, is diagnostic of malignancy. The following section presents the key immunophenotypic features of lymphoblastic leukemias and lymphomas. Selected examples of the association between the immunophenotype and the genotype are discussed.

B Lymphoblastic Leukemia/Lymphoma

B lymphoblastic leukemia/lymphoma (B-LL) is also referred to as B acute lymphoblastic leukemia or B lymphoblastic lymphoma. B lymphoblasts are positive for CD19, CD22, CD79a, HLA-DR, and TdT (Figure 32-13). The expression of CD34 and CD10 is frequently seen. Surface immunoglobulin light chains are not present. Cytoplasmic μ chain or surface immunoglobulin M may be detected, however. Because B-LL can arise at any stage of B cell differentiation, the presence of several specific markers usually defines early precursor, intermediate, and pre-B stages. Frequently, immunophenotypes correlate with specific cytogenetic and clinical features. In routine practice, confirmation of cytogenetic abnormality using conventional karyotyping or molecular techniques is necessary.

B Lymphoblastic Leukemia/Lymphoma with t(v;11q23);MLL Rearranged

MLL gene rearrangements occur most frequently in infant B-LL. Unlike in most B-LLs, blasts in this leukemia are negative for CD10 antigen.[24] CD19, CD34, TdT, and occasional myeloid markers are present. The more mature B cell marker CD20 is absent.

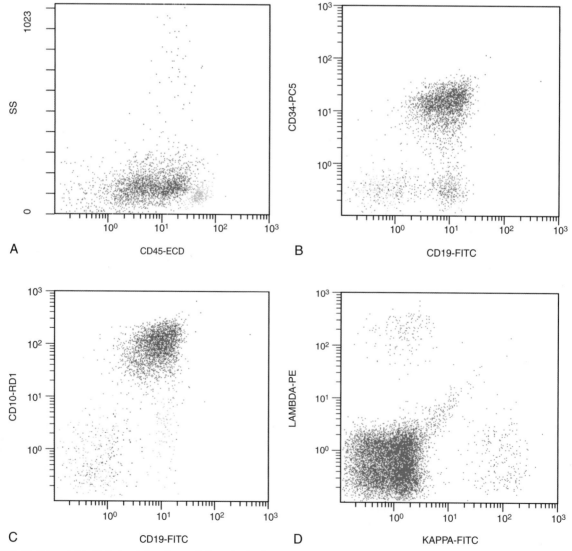

Figure 32-13 B lymphoblastic leukemia/lymphoma. **A,** Low-density CD45 antigen characteristic of the blast population. **B,** Uniform expression of CD34 and CD19 on leukemic blasts. **C,** High-density CD10 on CD19+ blasts. **D,** Lack of surface κ and λ light chains signifies immature B cell population. *ECD,* phycoerythrin-Texas Red; *FITC,* fluorescein isothiocyanate; *PC5,* phycoerythrin-cyanine 5; *PE,* phycoerythrin; *SS,* Side scatter.

B Lymphoblastic Leukemia/Lymphoma with t(9;22) (q34;q11.2);BCR/ABL1

Philadelphia chromosome, t(9;22);*BCR/ABL1*, is a hallmark of chronic myelogenous leukemia but also can occur in pediatric and adult B-LL. These cases benefit from an addition of tyrosine kinase inhibitor to the chemotherapy regimen, so it is important to identify them promptly. Most *BCR/ABL1*–positive cases have a classic intermediate or common B-LL immunophenotype with the expression of CD19, CD10, CD34, and TdT. The expression of myeloid markers CD13 and CD33 and the lack or decreased expression of CD38 antigen on leukemic blasts are common. The density of antigens and their homogeneous or heterogeneous expression within leukemic populations correlates closely with the presence of *BCR-ABL1*.[25]

T Lymphoblastic Leukemia/Lymphoma

T lymphoblastic leukemia/lymphoma (T-LL) is derived from immature cells committed to T cell lineage. Designation of leukemia or lymphoma depends on the primary site of involvement:

bone marrow or lymph node. T-LL expresses a combination of markers reflecting the stage of T cell differentiation. CD3 is the most specific T cell marker. As with normal T cells, this antigen is seen initially in the cytoplasm before appearing on the cell surface. Other T cell antigens include CD2, CD7, CD5, CD1a, CD4, and CD8. Usually a series of these antigens is detected, recapitulating the T cell differentiation (Figure 32-14). CD34 and CD10 may be present. As in other lymphoid neoplasms, the panel of markers determines the lineage.

Mature Lymphoid Neoplasms

B and T cell lymphomas display immunophenotypes resembling their normal counterparts. The immunophenotypic features of lymphomas are discussed in detail in Chapter 36 and are summarized in Table 36-2. The flow cytometric workup of lymphomas is facilitated by the *clonal* origin of mature lymphoid neoplasms, which implies that the malignant population is derived from a single cell. Therefore, all neoplastic cells typically show similar genetic and immunophenotypic features. This stands in strong

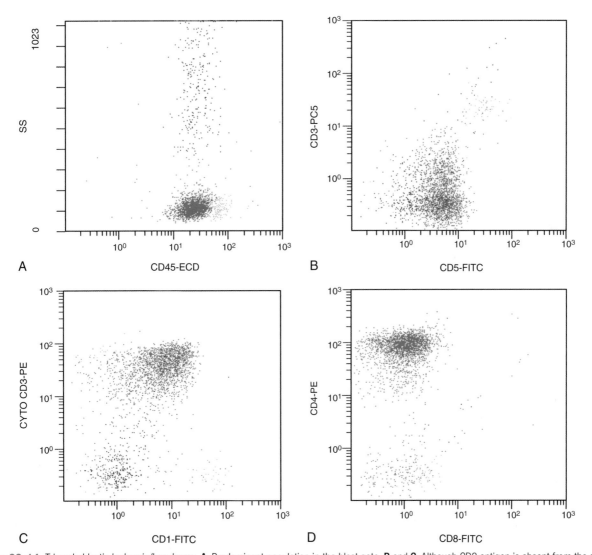

Figure 32-14 T lymphoblastic leukemia/lymphoma. **A,** Predominant population in the blast gate. **B** and **C,** Although CD3 antigen is absent from the surface of leukemic cells, it is present in blast cytoplasm, confirming the precursor T cell origin of the leukemia **(C)**. Note residual normal T cells (*aqua*) positive for surface CD3 and CD5 antigens. **D,** Simultaneous expression of CD4 and CD8 antigens. *ECD,* phycoerythrin-Texas Red; *FITC,* fluorescein isothiocyanate; *PC5,* phycoerythrin-cyanine 5; *PE,* phycoerythrin; *SS,* Side scatter.

contrast to variable immunophenotypes of normal lymphoid populations, reflecting a process of antigen-driven selection.

Mature B Cell Neoplasms

Normal precursor B cells randomly rearrange immunoglobulin heavy and light chain genes. As a result, a mature B cell population expresses a mix of heavy and light chains (Figure 32-15, *A*). In contrast, a monoclonal surface light chain expression, exclusively κ or λ, is seen in most B cell lymphomas (Figure 32-15, *B*). Light chain monoclonality along with the expression of pan–B cell markers is diagnostic of B cell lymphoma. Rarely, lymphomas may lose the expression of surface light chains, a feature not seen in normal mature B cells.[26] In most cases of plasma cell myeloma, neoplastic plasma cells lack surface immunoglobulin light chains and express only cytoplasmic κ or λ.

Mature T Cell Neoplasms

In T cells, similar to B cells, clonality in most cases indicates malignancy. In the past, the clonality of T cells could only be confirmed by using a molecular analysis of T cell receptor genes. Recently, a flow cytometric assay has been shown to detect clonality in most cases of T cell lymphoma.[27] This technique uses a broad array of antibodies against variable regions of T cell receptors. Because this methodology is not widely available, often a diagnosis of T cell lymphoma is based on aberrant immunophenotype. In most cases, a loss or atypical expression of a lymphoid marker can be shown using flow cytometry. For example, mycosis fungoides/Sézary syndrome is characterized by a mature T cell immunophenotype with expression of CD2, surface CD3, CD5, and CD4 and with a loss of the CD7 antigen (Figure 32-16). Over the

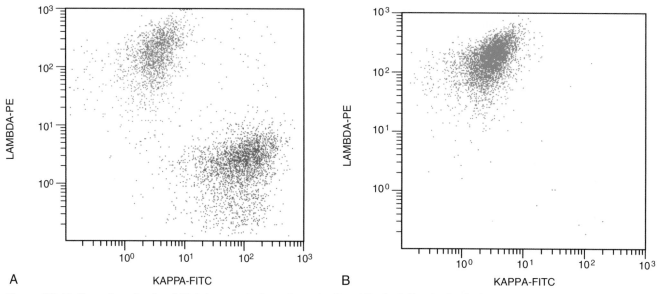

Figure 32-15 Comparison of surface light chain expression in reactive and malignant B cells. **A,** Reactive B cells show heterogeneous expression of κ and λ. **B,** B cell lymphomas are monoclonal, with the entire lymphoma population expressing only one type of light chain. *FITC,* Fluorescein isothiocyanate; *PE,* phycoerythrin.

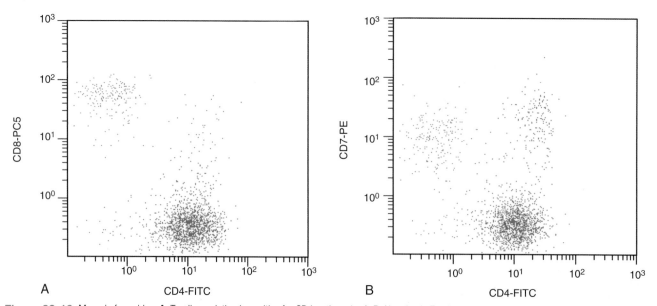

Figure 32-16 Mycosis fungoides. **A,** T cell population is positive for CD4 antigen (*red*). **B,** Neoplastic T cells show loss of CD7. Red represents CD4 and the expression of CD7 (*green*) is very low. *FITC,* Fluorescein isothiocyanate; *PE,* phycoerythrin; *PC5,* phycoerythrin-cyanine 5.

years it has been shown that the aberrant immunophenotype is a reliable diagnostic feature when the neoplastic population is sizeable. However, small numbers of T cells with unusual antigen makeup can appear in inflammatory conditions;[28] thus the aberrant immunophenotype alone cannot be considered pathognomonic of T cell malignancy.

OTHER APPLICATIONS OF FLOW CYTOMETRY BEYOND IMMUNOPHENOTYPING OF HEMATOLOGIC MALIGNANCIES

The immunophenotyping of hematolymphoid neoplasms is one of many applications of flow cytometry. Other common applications include a diagnosis and monitoring of immunodeficiency states, diagnosis of paroxysmal nocturnal hemoglobinuria (PNH), stem cell enumeration, cell cycle analysis, detection of fetal hemoglobin, and monitoring of sepsis.

Select primary (inherited) and secondary (acquired) immunodeficiencies can be diagnosed using flow cytometry. Both a loss of specific antigens (e.g., CD11/CD18 in leukocyte adhesion deficiency) and functional defects (e.g., oxidative burst evaluation in chronic granulomatous disease) can be assayed by flow cytometry.

Human immunodeficiency virus infection causes a progressive decrease in the number of CD4+ helper T cells. The absolute number of helper T cells in peripheral blood correlates with the stage of the disease and with patient prognosis. The enumeration of T cells and their subsets is easily accomplished by flow cytometry using antibodies against CD4 and CD8 antigens. The absolute numbers are derived by performing a routine white blood cell (WBC) count on the concurrent peripheral blood specimen or by running calibrating beads simultaneously with the patient sample. The CD4:CD8 ratio in healthy individuals is typically greater than 1. There is a significant decrease in numbers of CD4 positive T cells in HIV-positive patients resulting in a reversed CD4:CD8 ratio. Since the CD4 lymphocyte depletion is associated with various infections, the absolute number of CD4 positive lymphocytes serves also as a guide for antibiotic prophylaxis in HIV positive patients.

The diagnostic approach to PNH is a prime example of how an application of flow cytometry increases understanding of hematologic disorders and directly contributes to clinical decision making (Chapter 24).[29] Before the development of the flow cytometric assay, PNH diagnosis was based on detection of increased susceptibility of RBCs to lysis by the Ham or sucrose hemolysis tests, both of which showed inconsistent sensitivity. Flow cytometry significantly improved the sensitivity and specificity of PNH testing. The absence or decreased expression of glycosylphosphatidylinositol-anchored proteins on RBCs, granulocytes, and monocytes as measured by flow cytometry is diagnostic of PNH. In addition, the levels of CD59 expression correlate with clinical symptoms (Figure 32-17).

Another important application of flow cytometry is cell sorting. During sorting, a heterogeneous cell population is physically divided into subsets according to their physical or

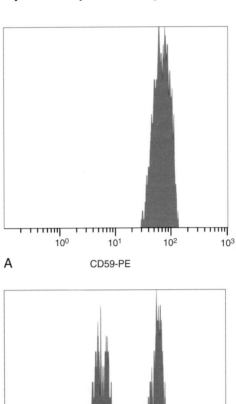

A   CD59-PE

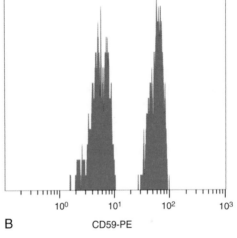

B   CD59-PE

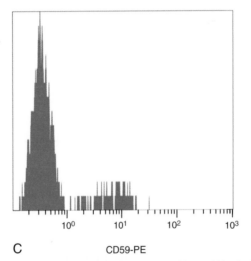

C   CD59-PE

Figure 32-17 Diagnosis of paroxysmal nocturnal hemoglobinuria (PNH) is based on the decreased expression of glycosylphosphatidylinositol (GPI)–linked molecules. Different levels of GPI-anchored proteins are best visualized in red blood cells (RBCs) using an antibody against CD59 antigen. **A,** RBCs from a healthy volunteer show a high number of CD59 molecules and correspond with type I cells. **B,** Varying percentages of type I cells (normal level of CD59 antigen) and a population with slight decrease in CD59 expression (type II cells) can be seen in PNH patients. **C,** Granulocytes with a complete loss of CD59 (type III cells) in a patient with PNH. This patient received numerous red blood cell transfusions; the loss of CD59 is best shown in granulocytic and monocytic populations. *PE,* Phycoerythrin.

immunophenotypic properties. High-speed sorting is achieved by charging droplets containing individual cells of interest. As the charged droplet passes through the electrostatic field, it is isolated from the remainder of the sample and collected into a separate container. The primary clinical application of cell sorting is in stem cell transplantation.

For years, flow cytometry remained confined to the hematopathology and research laboratories. Currently, this methodology is used in bone marrow transplantation, transfusion medicine, coagulation, microbiology, molecular pathology, and drug development. Specific examples of novel applications include tissue typing, molecular testing for neoplasia-associated translocations, and follow-up of drug response, such as by monitoring platelet activation after antiplatelet therapy.

Flow cytometry is a mature field that in recent years experienced a revival with a focus on high-throughput testing for simultaneous analysis of multiple biologic constituents. New approaches to a single-cell analysis such as spectral flow cytometry and an integration of mass spectrometry with single-cell fluidics provide a superior resolution and expand the number of parameters that can be measured in any given cell. These methodologies are in development and open new avenues to diagnostic immunophenotyping in hematopathology.[30,31]

SUMMARY

- Flow cytometry measures physical, antigenic, and functional properties of particles suspended in a fluid.
- Multiparameter flow cytometry is a technique routinely used for a diagnosis and follow-up of hematologic disorders.
- The characterization of complex specimens is achieved through the analysis of individual cells for multiple parameters and the simultaneous display of data for thousands of cells. The cell size, cytoplasmic complexity, and immunophenotypic features detected by monoclonal antibodies directly conjugated to various fluorochromes are analyzed in clinical specimens.
- A key starting point in flow cytometric analysis is a high-quality fresh specimen.
- A flow cytometer consists of fluidics, a light source (laser), multiple detectors, and a computer.
- As with microscopic examination, an evaluation of flow cytometric data is based on the inspection of visual patterns. Initially, the entire sample is scanned for the presence of abnormal populations. Subsequently, detailed immunophenotypic features of cell subsets are studied.
- The immunophenotyping of hematologic specimens is based on knowledge of the maturation patterns of hematopoietic cells. In comparison, myeloid and lymphoid malignant cells and cell populations in nonneoplastic hematologic disorders show significant qualitative and quantitative differences in antigen expression.
- Flow cytometric analysis of acute leukemia determines a lineage of leukemic cells. In select entities, immunophenotype corresponds to the underlying genetic lesion.
- Immunophenotyping of myelodysplastic syndromes and chronic myeloproliferative neoplasms is an emerging application of clinical flow cytometry.
- The clonality of mature B cell and T cell neoplasms can be detected by flow cytometry.
- Flow cytometric analysis is used for diagnosis and monitoring of immunodeficiencies, stem cell enumeration, detection of fetal hemoglobin, tissue typing, molecular analysis, and drug testing.

Now that you have completed this chapter, go back and read again the case studies at the beginning and respond to the questions presented.

REVIEW QUESTIONS

Answers can be found in the Appendix.

1. What is the most common clinical application of flow cytometry?
   a. Diagnosis of platelet disorders
   b. Detection of fetomaternal hemorrhage
   c. Diagnosis of leukemias and lymphomas
   d. Differentiation of anemias

2. Which of the following is true of CD45 antigen?
   a. It is present on every cell subpopulation in the bone marrow.
   b. It is expressed on all hematopoietic cells, with the exception of megakaryocytes and late erythroid precursors.
   c. It is not measured routinely in flow cytometry.
   d. It may be present on nonhematopoietic cells.

3. Erythroid precursors are characterized by the expression of:
   a. CD71
   b. CD20
   c. CD61
   d. CD3

4. In Figure 32-2A, the cell population colored in aqua represents:
   a. Monocytes
   b. Nonhematopoietic cells
   c. Granulocytes
   d. Lymphocytes

5. Antigens expressed by B-LL include:
   a. CD3, CD4, and CD8
   b. CD19, CD34, and CD10
   c. There are no antigens specific for B-LL.
   d. Myeloperoxidase

6. Which of the following is true of flow cytometric gating?
   a. It is best defined as selection of a target population for flow cytometric analysis.
   b. It can be done only at the time of data acquisition.
   c. It can be done only at the time of final analysis and interpretation of flow cytometric data.
   d. It is accomplished by adjusting flow rate.

7. Collection of ungated events:
   a. Facilitates comprehensive analysis of all cells
   b. Does not help in detection of unexpected abnormal populations
   c. Allows the collection of data on a large number of rare cells
   d. Is used for leukemia diagnosis only

8. Mycosis fungoides is characterized by:
   a. Loss of certain antigens compared with the normal T cell population
   b. Polyclonal T cell receptor
   c. Immunophenotype indistinguishable from that of normal T cells
   d. Expression of CD3 and CD8 antigens

9. Mature granulocytes show the expression of:
   a. CD15, CD33, and CD34
   b. CD15, CD33, and CD41
   c. CD15, CD33, and CD13
   d. CD15, CD33, and CD7

10. During the initial evaluation of flow cytometric data, cell size, cytoplasmic complexity, and expression of CD45 antigen are used to define cell subpopulations. Which of the following parameters defines cytoplasmic complexity/granularity?
    a. SS
    b. FS
    c. CD45
    d. HLA-DR

11. The most important feature of the mature neoplastic B cell population is:
    a. The presence of a specific immunophenotype with expression of CD19 antigen
    b. A clonal light chain expression (i.e., exclusively κ- or λ-positive population)
    c. A clonal T cell receptor expression
    d. Aberrant expression of CD5 antigen on CD19$^+$ cells

REFERENCES

1. Swerdlow, S. H., Campo, E., Harris, N. L., et al., (Eds.). (2008). *WHO Classification of Tumours of Haematopoietic and Lymphoid Tissues.* (4th ed.). Lyon, France: IARC Press.
2. Czader, M., Ali, S. Z. (2003). Flow cytometry as an adjunct to cytomorphologic analysis of serous effusions. *Diagn Cytopathol, 29,* 74–78, 2003.
3. Wood, B. L., Arroz, M., Barnett, D., et al. (2007). 2006 Bethesda International Consensus recommendations on the immunophenotypic analysis of hematolymphoid neoplasia by flow cytometry: optimal reagents and reporting for the flow cytometric diagnosis of hematopoietic neoplasia. *Cytometry B Clin Cytom, 72,* S14–S22.
4. Köhler, G., & Milstein, C. (1975). Continuous cultures of fused cells secreting antibody of predefined specificity. *Nature, 256,* 495–497.
5. Human Cell Differentiation Molecules. Retrieved from http://hcdm.org. Accessed 06.11.14.
6. Perfetto, S. P., Chattopadhyay, P. K., & Roederer, M. (2004). Seventeen-colour flow cytometry: unravelling the immune system. *Nat Rev Immunol, 4,* 648–655.
7. Stelzer, G. T., Shults, K. E., & Loken, M. R. (1993). CD45 gating for routine flow cytometric analysis of human bone marrow specimens. *Ann N Y Acad Sci, 677,* 265–281.
8. Borowitz, M. J., Guenther, K. L., Shults, K. E., et al. (1993). Immunophenotyping of acute leukemia by flow cytometric analysis: use of CD45 and right-angle light scattered to gate on leukemic blasts in three-color analysis. *Am J Clin Pathol, 100,* 534–540.
9. Macedo, A., Orfao, A., Ciudad, J., et al. (1995). Phenotypic analysis of CD34 subpopulations in normal human bone marrow and its application for the detection of minimal residual disease. *Leukemia, 9,* 1896–1901.
10. Terstappen, L. W., Safford, M., & Loken, M. R. (1990). Flow cytometric analysis of human bone marrow: III. Neutrophil maturation. *Leukemia, 4,* 657–663.
11. Loken, M. R., Shah, V. O., Dattilio, K. L., et al. (1987). Flow cytometric analysis of human bone marrow: I. Normal erythroid development. *Blood, 69,* 255–263.
12. Ciudad, J., Orfao, A., Vidriales, B., et al. (1998). Immunophenotypic analysis of CD19+ precursors in normal human adult bone marrow: implications for minimal residual disease detection. *Haematologica, 83,* 1069–1075.
13. Terstappen, L. W., Huang, S., & Picker, L. J. (1992). Flow cytometric assessment of human T-cell differentiation in thymus and bone marrow. *Blood, 79,* 666–677.
14. Andrieu, V., Radford-Weiss, I., Troussard, X., et al. (1996). Molecular detection of t(8;21)/AML1-ETO in AML M1/M2: correlation with cytogenetics, morphology and immunophenotype. *Br J Haematol, 92,* 855–865.
15. Adriaansen, H., Boekhorst, P. A. W., Hagemeijer, A. M., et al. (1993). Acute myeloid leukemia M4 with bone marrow eosinophilia (M4Eo) and inv(16)(p13q22) exhibits a specific immunophenotype with CD2 expression. *Blood, 81,* 3043–3051.
16. Lo Coco, F., Avvisati, G., Diverio, D., et al. (1991). Rearrangements of the RAR-alpha gene in acute promyelocytic leukaemia: correlations with morphology and immunophenotype. *Br J Haematol, 78,* 494–499.
17. Krasinskas AM, Wasik MA, Kamoun M, et al: The usefulness of CD64, other monocyte-associated antigens, and CD45 gating in the subclassification of acute myeloid leukemias with monocytic differentiation. *Am J Clin Pathol 110,* 797–805, 1998.
18. Helleberg, C., Knudsen, H., Hansen, P. B., et al. (1994). CD34$^+$ megakaryoblastic leukaemic cells are CD38$^−$, but

CD61$^+$ and glycophorin A$^+$: improved criteria for diagnosis of AML-M7? *Leukemia, 11*, 830–834.

19. Stetler-Stevenson, M., Arthur, D. C., Jabbour, N., et al. (2001). Diagnostic utility of flow cytometric immunophenotyping in myelodysplastic syndrome. *Blood, 98*, 979–987.

20. Kussick, S. J., Wood, B. L. (2003). Four-color flow cytometry identifies virtually all cytogenetically abnormal bone marrow samples in the workup of non-CML myeloproliferative disorders. *Am J Clin Pathol, 120*, 854–865.

21. Zhang, S., Zhou, J., Nassiri, M., Czader, M. (2013). Diagnostic approach to myelodysplastic syndrome. In Sayar, H., (Ed.), *Myelodysplastic Syndrome*. Nova Science Publishers, Hauppauge NY chapter 2, pages 25–60.

22. Ogata, K., Nakamura, K., Yokose, N., et al. (2002). Clinical significance of phenotypic features of blasts in patients with myelodysplastic syndrome. *Blood, 100*, 3887–3896.

23. Wells, D. A., Benesch, M., Loken, M. R., et al. Myeloid and monocytic dyspoiesis as determined by flow cytometric scoring in myelodysplastic syndrome correlates with the IPSS and with outcome after hematopoietic stem cell transplantation. *Blood, 102*, 394–403.

24. Harbott, J., Mancini, M., Verellen-Dumoulin, C., et al. (1998). Hematological malignances with a deletion of 11q23: cytogenetic and clinical aspects. *Leukemia, 12*, 823–827.

25. Tabernero, M. D., Bortoluci, A. M., Alaejos, I., et al. (2001). Adult precursor B-ALL with *BCR/ABL* gene rearrangements displays a unique immunophenotype based on the pattern of CD10, CD34, CD13 and CD38 expression. *Leukemia, 15*, 406–414.

26. Li, S., Eshleman, J. R., Borowitz, M. J. (2002). Lack of surface immunoglobulin light chain expression by flow cytometric immunophenotyping can help diagnose peripheral B-cell lymphoma. *Am J Clin Pathol, 118*, 229–234.

27. Beck, R. C., Stahl, S., O'Keefe, C. L., et al. (2003). Detection of mature T-cell leukemias by flow cytometry using anti T-cell receptor V beta antibodies. *Am J Clin Pathol, 120*, 785–794.

28. Alaibac, M., Pigozzi, B., Belloni-Fortina, A., et al. (2003). CD7 expression in reactive and malignant human skin T-lymphocytes. *Anticancer Res, 23*, 2707–2710.

29. Richards, S. J., Rawstron, A. C., & Hillmen, P. (2004). Application of flow cytometry to the diagnosis of paroxysmal nocturnal hemoglobinuria. *Cytometry, 42*, 223–233.

30. Sander, C. K., & Mourant, J. R. (2013). Advantages of full spectrum flow cytometry. *J Biomed Opt, 18*, 037004, 1–8.

31. Bendall, S. C., Simonds, E. F., Qiu, P., Amir, el-A. D., et al. (2011). Single-cell mass cytometry of differential immune and drug responses across a human hematopoietic continuum. *Science, 332*, 687–696.

Myeloproliferative Neoplasms

33

Tim R Randolph

OBJECTIVES

After completion of this chapter, the reader will be able to:

1. Define myeloproliferative neoplasms (MPNs), list the most common diseases included in the World Health Organization (WHO) classification of MPNs, and recognize their abbreviations.
2. Define chronic myelogenous leukemia (CML), and describe the cell lines involved, the clinical phases, and the expected clinical manifestations, key peripheral blood and bone marrow findings, and diagnostic criteria applicable to each stage.
3. Discuss the cytogenetics, molecular genetics, and molecular pathophysiology of CML and relate it to treatment approaches, monitoring minimal residual disease, mechanisms of drug resistance.
4. Define polycythemia vera (PV), and describe the cell lines involved, clinical manifestations, key peripheral blood and bone marrow findings, and the diagnostic criteria.
5. Discuss the *JAK2* mutation and the proposed pathogenic mechanism in PV.
6. Discuss the progression of PV and treatment modalities to include JAK inhibitors.
7. Define essential thrombocythemia (ET), and describe the cell lines involved, clinical manifestations, key peripheral blood and bone marrow findings, and the diagnostic criteria.
8. Discuss common mutations, pathophysiology, and two complications that may occur in patients with ET.
9. Define primary myelofibrosis (PMF), and describe the cell lines involved, clinical manifestations, key patho-logic features in peripheral blood, bone marrow, and tissues, and the diagnostic criteria.
10. Describe the mutations that occur in PMF and relate them to disease progression and current therapy.
11. Briefly discuss the potential interrelationships between the mutations and hypotheses for disease development and progression among between ET, PV, and PMF.
12. Briefly describe the other myeloproliferative disorders outlined in this chapter.
13. Given complete blood count and cytogenetic, molecu-lar, and other laboratory results, recognize the findings consistent with each major MPN.
14. Recommend follow-up testing for suspected MPN and interpret the results of testing.

CASE STUDY

After studying the material in this chapter, the reader should be able to respond to the following case study:

A 34-year-old woman came to the physician with a 2-month history of increasing weakness, persis-tent nonproductive cough, fever and chills accompanied by night sweats, and a 13-pound weight loss over a 6-month period. Results of chest radiographs and purified protein derivative test (for tuberculosis) were negative. The patient was treated with ciprofloxacin and her cough improved, but she continued to grow weaker and was able to consume only small quantities of food. The patient appeared pale and cachectic. Tenderness and fullness were present in the left upper quadrant, and the spleen was palpable below the umbilicus. No hepatomegaly or peripheral adenopathy was noted. Her laboratory results were as follows:

WBCs—248 × 10^9/L
HGB—9.5 g/dL

Continued

CASE STUDY—cont'd

After studying the material in this chapter, the reader should be able to respond to the following case study:

HCT—26.3%

Platelets—449 × 10⁹/L

Segmented neutrophils—44%

Band neutrophils—4%

Lymphocytes—10%

Eosinophils—3%

Basophils—7%

Myelocytes—30%

Promyelocytes—1%

Myeloblasts—1%

Nucleated RBCs—2 per 100 WBCs

Reticulocytes—3%

Leukocyte alkaline phosphatase (LAP) score—20 (reference range, 40 to 130)

Lactate dehydrogenase—692 IU (reference range, 140 to 280 IU)

Uric acid—8.1 mg/dL (reference range, 4 to 6 mg/dL)

1. What is the significance of the elevated WBC count and abnormal WBC differential?
2. How does the LAP score aid in the diagnosis?
3. Justify the use of cytogenetic studies in a patient with test results similar to those in this case study.
4. Predict the results of the cytogenetic studies.
5. Describe the molecular mutation resulting from the cytogenetic abnormality.
6. What is the usual treatment for this disorder?
7. Briefly discuss mechanisms of drug resistance.

The myeloproliferative neoplasms (MPNs) are clonal hematopoietic disorders caused by genetic mutations in the hematopoietic stem cells that result in expansion, excessive production, and accumulation of erythrocytes, granulocytes, and platelets. Myeloproliferation is due to hypersensitivity or independence of normal cytokine regulation that reduces cytokine levels through negative feedback systems normally induced by mature cells.[1,2] Expansion occurs in varying combinations in the bone marrow, peripheral blood, and tissues.[3-6] The MPNs have pathogenetic similarities, as well as common clinical and laboratory features.[7]

MPNs are predominantly chronic with accelerated, subacute, or acute phases. In certain patients it is difficult to make a clear delineation between subacute and chronic phases using clinical and morphologic findings.

The World Health Organization (WHO) has classified the MPNs into four predominant disorders: chronic myelogenous leukemia (CML); polycythemia vera (PV), also known as *polycythemia rubra vera*; essential (primary) thrombocythemia (ET); and primary myelofibrosis (PMF), also known as *agnogenic myelofibrosis with myeloid metaplasia* and *chronic idiopathic myelofibrosis*. Several other less common MPN conditions have been described and are classified as chronic neutrophilic leukemia (CNL); chronic eosinophilic leukemia (CEL), not otherwise specified; mastocytosis; and myeloproliferative disorder, unclassified.[8] CML and PV are defined by their overproduction of granulocytes and erythrocytes, respectively.[4,9,10] PMF is a combination of overproduction of hematopoietic cells and stimulation of fibroblast production leading to ineffective hematopoiesis with resultant peripheral blood cytopenias.[11] ET is characterized by increased megakaryocytopoiesis and peripheral blood thrombocytosis.[12]

MPNs present as stable chronic disorders that may transform first to a subacute, then to an aggressive cellular growth phase, such as acute myeloid leukemia (AML) or acute lymphoblastic leukemia (ALL). They may manifest a depleted cellular phase, such as bone marrow hypoplasia, or exhibit clinical symptoms and morphologic patterns characteristic of a subacute followed by a more aggressive cellular expression. Familial MPNs have been described in families in which two or more members are affected.[13]

CHRONIC MYELOGENOUS LEUKEMIA

Chronic myelogenous leukemia (CML) is an MPN arising from a single genetic translocation in a pluripotential hematopoietic stem cell producing a clonal overproduction of the myeloid cell line, resulting in a preponderance of immature cells in the neutrophilic line. CML begins with a chronic clinical phase and, if untreated, progresses to an accelerated phase in 3 to 4 years and often terminates as an acute leukemia. The clinical features are frequent infection, anemia, bleeding, and splenomegaly, all secondary to massive pathologic accumulation of myeloid progenitor cells in bone marrow, peripheral blood, and extramedullary tissues. Neutrophilia with all maturational stages present, basophilia, eosinophilia, and often thrombocytosis are noted in peripheral blood. The clonal origin of hematopoietic cells in CML has been verified in studies of females heterozygous for glucose-6-phosphate dehydrogenase. Only one isoenzyme is active in affected cells, whereas two isoenzymes are active in nonaffected cells.[14]

Incidence

CML occurs at all ages but is seen predominantly in those aged 46 to 53 years. It represents about 20% of all cases of leukemia, is slightly more common in males than in females, and carried a mortality rate of 1.5 per 100,000 per year in the era prior the development of imatinib mesylate (Gleevec). Imatinib is a tyrosine kinase inhibitor that has changed the prognosis and treatment for CML and is described in detail later.

Symptoms associated with clinical onset are usually of minimal intensity and include fatigue, decreased tolerance of exertion, anorexia, abdominal discomfort, weight loss, and symptomatic effects from splenic enlargement.

Cytogenetics of the Philadelphia Chromosome

A unique chromosome, the Philadelphia chromosome, is present in proliferating hematopoietic stem cells and their progeny in CML and must be identified to confirm the diagnosis. Although the cause of Philadelphia chromosome formation is unknown, it appears more frequently in populations exposed to ionizing radiation.[15,16] In most patients, a cause cannot be identified. Appearance of the Philadelphia chromosome in donor cells after allogeneic bone marrow transplantation indicates the possibility of a transmissible agent.[17] The Philadelphia chromosome was first identified as a short chromosome 22 in 1960 by Nowell and Hungerford in Philadelphia.[18] In 1973 Rowley, of the University of Illinois at Chicago, discovered that the Philadelphia chromosome is a reciprocal translocation between the long arms of chromosomes 9 and 22 (Chapter 30).[19] This acquired somatic mutation specifically reflects the translocation of an *ABL* proto-oncogene from band q34 of chromosome 9 to the breakpoint cluster region (BCR) of band q11 of chromosome 22, resulting in a unique chimeric gene, *BCR-ABL1*.[20] This new gene produces a 210-kD BCR/ABL fusion protein (p210BCR/ABL) that expresses enhanced tyrosine kinase activity from the ABL moiety compared with its natural enzymatic counterpart.

Molecular Genetics

The t(9;22) translocation that produces the *BCR/ABL1* chimeric gene has been observed in four primary molecular forms that produce three versions of the BCR/ABL chimeric protein: p190, p210, and p230 (Figure 33-1). The four genetic variations are based on the area of the *BCR* gene that houses the breakpoint on chromosome 22, because the breakpoint on chromosome 9 occurs in the same location. The wild-type (normal) *ABL1* gene on chromosome 9 is a relatively large gene of approximately

230 kilobases (kb) containing 11 exons. The breakpoint consistently occurs 5′ of the second exon such that exons 2 to 11 are contributed to the *BCR/ABL1* fusion gene.[20]

There are four *BCR* genes in the human genome: *BCR1, BCR2, BCR3,* and *BCR4.* It is the *BCR1* gene that is involved in the Philadelphia translocation. The wild-type (normal) *BCR1* gene is approximately 100 kb with 20 exons. In 1984 Groffen and colleagues identified the BCR on chromosome 22 as a 5-exon region involving exons 12 to 16 that was the area of breakage in the traditional t(9;22) translocation.[21] This area was later termed the *major BCR.* Two other areas of breakage were identified on chromosome 22, one near the 5′ (head) of the *BCR1* gene, called the *minor BCR,* and one in the 3′ end (tail) of the *BCR1* gene, termed the *micro BCR.* Therefore, two areas of breakage in the major BCR, one breakpoint area in the minor BCR, and one breakpoint region in the micro BCR produce four versions of the *BCR* gene that combine with the *ABL1* gene to form four versions of the *BCR/ABL1* chimeric gene.

Within the major BCR two specific breakpoints account for the t(9;22) translocation involved in the development of CML. Breakage in the *BCR1* gene in the major BCR contributes exons 1 to 13 or 1 to 14, whereas the *ABL1* gene contributes exons 2 to 11. Because the two breakpoints in the major BCR differ by only one exon, the chimeric protein product is essentially the same size and is designated as the p210 protein. Breakage in the minor BCR contributes only exon one from *BCR1,* which joins with the same exons 2 to 11 of *ABL1* to produce a p190 protein. The micro BCR breakpoint contributes exons 2 to 19 from *BCR1,* which fuse with *ABL1* exons 2 to 11, producing the p230 protein. Therefore, the four possible *BCR1* breakpoints produce four different chimeric genes, resulting in a total of three different protein products.[22]

Pathogenetic Mechanism

To understand the aberrant function of the BCR/ABL fusion protein, it is first helpful to understand both the normal BCR and ABL proteins. The wild-type ABL protein, when in its usual location on chromosome 9, codes for p125, which exhibits normal tyrosine kinase activity. The *BCR1* gene produces p160, expresses serine and threonine kinase activity, and is thought to function in the regulation of cell growth. Protein kinases are enzymes that catalyze the transfer of phosphate groups from adenosine triphosphate (ATP), guanosine triphosphate, and other phosphate donors to receiver proteins. A tyrosine kinase transfers the phosphate group to a tyrosine amino acid on the receiver protein. For the kinase activity of the ABL protein to occur, the ABL protein must first be phosphorylated. This is often accomplished through autophosphorylation. The ABL protein has three primary domains called *SH1, SH2,* and *SH3* that together express and regulate the kinase activity. SH1 is the binding site for ATP; SH2 is the docking point for phosphate receiver proteins; and SH3 is the domain that controls the phosphorylation activity. When ATP binds to the ATP binding site, the phosphate is transferred to the SH2 region of the ABL protein, which initiates a conformational change that alters the tertiary structure of the protein and exposes the active site of the kinase enzyme. When a second ATP binds the ATP binding

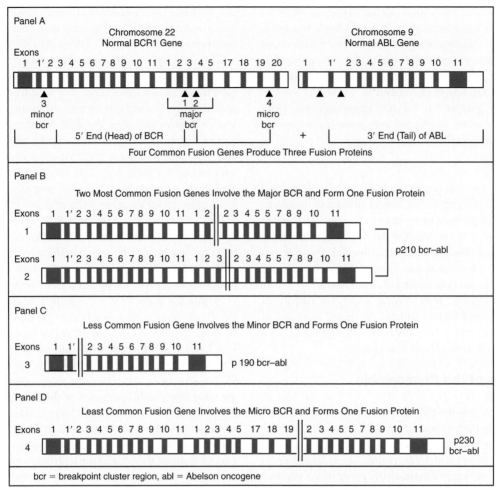

Figure 33-1 Molecular biology of the *BCR/ABL* fusion gene. **A,** Normal *BCR1* gene on chromosome 22 and *ABL* gene on chromosome 9. **B,** Two BCR fusion gene products from the major *BCR*. **C,** Fusion gene product from the minor *BCR*. **D,** Fusion gene product from the micro *BCR*.

site and a receiver protein docks in the SH2 domain, the phosphate group is transferred to the receiver protein. In most physiologically normal intracellular pathways, protein phosphorylation activates the receiver proteins (Figure 33-2). This phosphorylation initiates a cascade of phosphorylation events, each activating the next protein until a transcription factor becomes activated. These activation cascades, called *signal transduction pathways,* are designed to activate genes necessary to control cell proliferation, differentiation, and natural cell death, called *apoptosis.* There are several signal transduction pathways activated by the ABL tyrosine kinase that function in concert to activate these genes in a precise order and at the required level of activation to control these cellular events.[22,23]

In the case of CML, the *BCR/ABL1* translocation occurs next to the SH3 domain of the *ABL1* moiety, which is designed to control the rate and timing of phosphorylation. Therefore, the BCR/ABL tyrosine kinase loses the ability to shut off kinase activity and is said to have constitutive tyrosine kinase activity. The BCR/ABL enzyme continuously adds phosphate groups to tyrosine residues on cytoplasmic proteins, activating several signal transduction pathways. These pathways stimulate gene expression, keeping the myeloid cells proliferating, reducing differentiation, reducing adhesion of cells to bone marrow

stroma, and virtually eliminating apoptosis. The result is increased clonal proliferation of myeloid cells secondary to a reduction in or loss of sensitivity to protein regulators.[24] There is an increase in growth factor–independent cellular proliferation from activation of the *RAS* gene and a decrease in or resistance to apoptosis. New clones of stem cells vulnerable to additional genetic changes lead to the accelerated and blast phases of CML. In addition, the BCR/ABL protein localizes in the cytoplasm rather than in the nucleus, as does the normal ABL protein. The mutation affects maturation and differentiation of hematopoietic and lymphopoietic cells, whose progeny eventually dominates in the affected individual. Progeny cells that exhibit this chromosome include neutrophils, eosinophils, basophils, monocytes, nucleated erythrocytes, megakaryocytes, and B lymphocytes.[9,25]

In addition, the loss of genetic segments in the 5′ end of the *ABL1* gene results in an altered protein-binding affinity for F-actin, which leads to a reduction in contact binding of hematopoietic CML cells to stromal cells, causing premature release of cells into the circulation.[23] Abnormal adhesion between stem cells and stroma may dysregulate hematopoiesis. One action of interferon-α therapy is to reverse the loss of adhesion of CML progenitor cells, which reduces the premature release of these cells into the circulation.[26]

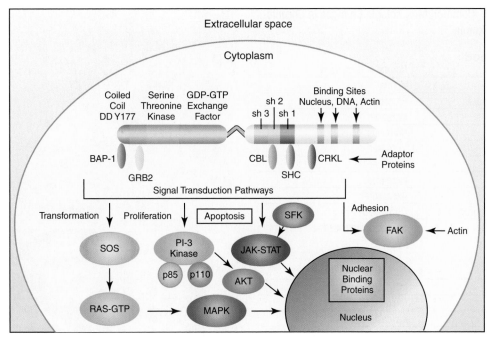

Figure 33-2 Signal transduction pathways influenced by the BCR/ABL fusion protein.

Apoptotic functions are lost because the BCR/ABL fusion protein has a propensity to be sequestered in the cytoplasm, which has antiapoptotic functions. The p210 is necessary for CML transformation of the hematopoietic stem cell.

The *BCR/ABL1* fusion gene is also identified with Philadelphia chromosome–positive ALL. The chromosome appears in 20% of adults and 2% to 5% of children with this disease. The minor chimeric *BCL/ABL1* gene that transcribes and translates to a p185/p190 protein is present in 50% of Philadelphia chromosome–positive ALL cases in adults and 75% of Philadelphia chromosome–positive ALL cases in children. The micro *BCR*, when fused with the *ABL1* gene, produces a large p230 protein that is associated with chronic neutrophilic leukemia and is the least common version found.

Peripheral Blood and Bone Marrow

There are dramatic morphologic changes in the peripheral blood and bone marrow that reflect the expansion of the granulocyte pool, particularly in the later maturational stages. Table 33-1 lists the qualitative changes in the peripheral blood, bone marrow, and extramedullary tissues that are commonly observed at the time of diagnosis. A dramatic left shift is noted that extends down to the promyelocyte stage and occasionally even produces a few blasts in the peripheral blood. The platelet count is often elevated, reflecting the myeloproliferative nature of the disease. Extramedullary granulopoiesis may involve sinusoids and medullary cords in the spleen and sinusoids, portal tract zones, and solid areas of the liver.

Figure 33-3 illustrates a common pattern in the peripheral blood film of chronic phase CML at the time of diagnosis. Leukocytosis is readily apparent at scanning microscopic powers. Segmented neutrophils, bands, metamyelocytes, and myelocytes predominate, and immature and mature eosinophils

and basophils are increased. Myeloblasts and promyelocytes are present at a rate of approximately 1% and 5%, respectively. Lymphocytes and monocytes are present and often show an absolute increase in number but a relative decrease in percentage. Nucleated red blood cells (NRBCs) are rare. Platelets are normal or increased, and some may exhibit abnormal morphology.

Bone marrow changes are illustrated in Figure 33-4. An intense hypercellularity is present due to granulopoiesis, marked by broad zones of immature granulocytes, usually perivascular or periosteal, differentiating into more centrally placed mature granulocytes. Normoblasts appear reduced in number. Megakaryocytes are normal or increased in number and, when increased, may appear in clusters and exhibit dyspoietic cytologic changes. They often appear small with reduced nuclear size (by approximately 20%) and reduced nuclear lobulations. Reticulin fibers are increased in approximately 20% of patients. Increased megakaryocyte density is associated with an increase in myelofibrosis.[27] The presence of pseudo-Gaucher cells (Chapter 29) usually occurs.

Other Laboratory Findings

Hyperuricemia and uricosuria from increased cell turnover may be associated with secondary gout, urinary uric acid stones, and uric acid nephropathy.[28] Approximately 15% of patients exhibit total white blood cell (WBC) counts greater than 300×10^9/L.[29] Symptoms in these patients are secondary to vascular stasis and possible intravascular consumption of oxygen by the leukocytes. Symptoms are reversible with the lowering of the total WBC count.[30]

In patients with the typical peripheral blood findings discussed above, the diagnosis of CML is confirmed by demonstrating the presence of the t(9;22) translocation by cytogenetic

TABLE 33-1 Common Morphologic Changes in Chronic Myelogenous Leukemia

Peripheral Blood

Erythrocytes	Normal or decreased
Reticulocytes	Normal
Nucleated red blood cells	Present
Total white blood cells	Increased
Lymphocytes	Normal or increased
Neutrophils	Increased
Basophils	Increased
Eosinophils	Increased
Myelocytes	Increased
Leukocyte alkaline phosphatase	Decreased
Platelets	Normal or increased

Bone Marrow

Cellularity	Increased
Granulopoiesis	Increased
Erythropoiesis	Decreased
Megakaryopoiesis	Increased or normal
Reticulin	Increased

Macrophages

Gaucherlike	Sea blue
Green-gray crystals	Increased

Megakaryocytes

Small	Increased

Extramedullary Tissue

Splenomegaly	Present
Sinusoidal	Present
Medullary	Present
Hepatomegaly	Present
Sinusoidal	Present
Portal tract	Present
Local infiltrates	Present

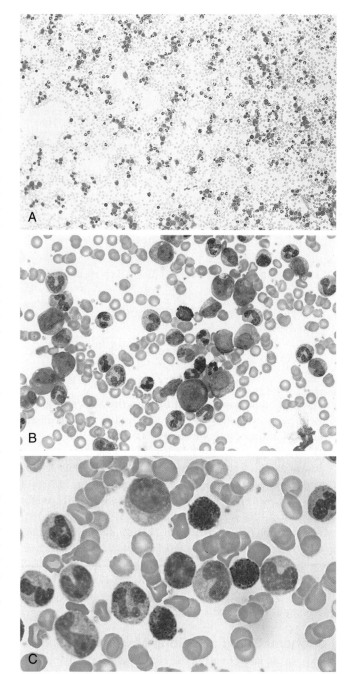

Figure 33-3 Peripheral blood films in the chronic phase of chronic myelogenous leukemia. **A,** Leukocytosis is evident at scanning power (×100). **B,** Bimodal population of segmented neutrophils and myelocytes (×500). **C,** Increased basophils and immature neutrophils (×1000).

analysis (Figure 30-1), detection of the *BCR/ABL1* fusion gene using fluorescence in situ hybridization (Figures 30-2 and 30-21), and/or detecting the *BCR/ABL1* fusion transcript by qualitative reverse transcriptase polymerase chain reaction (Figure 31-12).

Although molecular techniques are more commonly used to diagnose CML, initial testing of the cells for leukocyte alkaline phosphatase (LAP) enzyme activity may be useful in some setting for preliminary differentiation of CML from a leukemoid reaction due to severe infections (Chapter 29).

LAP is an enzyme found in the membranes of secondary granules of neutrophils. In the procedure a blood film is incubated with a naphthol-phosphate substrate and diazo dye at an alkaline pH. The LAP enzyme hydrolyzes the substrate, and the liberated naphthol reacts with the dye producing a colored precipitate on the granules. The slide is examined microscopically and 100 segmented neutrophils and bands are counted and rated from 0 to 4+ based on the intensity of the staining. The LAP score is calculated by multiplying each score by the number of cells, and adding the products. For example, 5 cells with 4+ staining, 5 cells with 3+, 25 cells with 2+, 45 cells with 1+, and 20 cells with 0 staining calculates to a LAP score of 130. Because scoring is subjective, the mean score of two examiners is reported, and they should agree within 10%.

A sample reference interval for the LAP score is 15 to 170, but every laboratory establishes its own. The LAP score is decreased in untreated CML, and normal or increased in

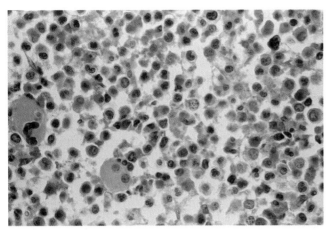

Figure 33-4 Bone marrow biopsy specimen in the chronic phase of chronic myelogenous leukemia, showing hypercellularity with increased granulocytes and megakaryocytes (hematoxylin and eosin stain, ×400).

leukemoid reactions. Individuals with polycythemia vera or those in the third trimester of pregnancy also have higher LAP scores.

Progression

In the pre-imatinib era, most cases of this disease would eventually transform into acute leukemia.[31] Before blastic transformation, some patients proceed through an intermediate *metamorphosis* or *accelerated* phase. Disease progression is accompanied by an increase in the frequency and number of clinical symptoms, adverse changes in laboratory values, and poorer response to therapy than in the chronic phase. Additional chromosome abnormalities reflect evolution of the malignant clone and may appear, associated with enhanced dyshematopoietic cell maturation patterns and increases in morphologic and functional abnormalities in blood cells. There is often an increasing degree of anemia and, in the peripheral blood, fewer mature leukocytes, more basophils, and fewer platelets, with a greater proportion of abnormal platelets, micromegakaryocytes, and megakaryocytic fragments. The circulating blast count increases to 10% to 19%. This total blast percentage, or a combination of 20% blasts and promyelocytes, has been proposed as a diagnostic criterion for the accelerated phase.[32]

Blast crisis involves the peripheral blood, bone marrow, and extramedullary tissues. Based on acute leukemia definitions, blasts constitute more than 20% of total bone marrow cellularity, and the peripheral blood exhibits increased blasts.[31] Blast crisis leukemia usually is AML or ALL, but origins from other hematopoietic clonal cells are possible. Extramedullary growth may occur as lymphocytic or myelogenous cell proliferations; the latter are often referred to as *granulocytic sarcoma*. Extramedullary sarcoma is observed at many sites or locations in the body and may precede a marrow blast crisis. The clinical symptoms of blast crisis mimic those of acute leukemia, including severe anemia, leukopenia of all WBCs except blasts, and thrombocytopenia. Chromosome abnormalities such as additional Philadelphia chromosome(s), isochromosome 17, trisomy 8, loss of Y chromosome, and trisomy 19 accumulate with disease progression.[33,34] These

generally occurred in approximately 75% of patients in the pre-imatinib era.

Related Diseases

Several diseases exist that are clinically similar to CML but do not exhibit the Philadelphia chromosome and express only a few pseudo-Gaucher cells. Chronic neutrophilic leukemia is another MPN that manifests with peripheral blood, bone marrow, and extramedullary infiltrative patterns similar to those of CML, except that only neutrophilic granulocytes are present and fewer than 10% of peripheral blood neutrophils are immature.[35] Similarly, chronic monocytic leukemia involves a comparable expansion of monocytes, including functional monocytes.[36]

Juvenile myelomonocytic leukemia and adult chronic myelomonocytic leukemia are classified by the WHO as myelodysplastic/myeloproliferative diseases because of the overlap in clinical, laboratory, or morphologic findings. Juvenile myelomonocytic leukemia is observed in children younger than 4 years of age and is accompanied by an expansion in the number of monocytes and granulocytes, including immature granulocytes, and manifestations of dyserythropoiesis.[37]

The peripheral blood of adults with chronic myelomonocytic leukemia may have characteristics similar to those seen in the refractory anemias, such as oval macrocytes and reticulocytopenia. The peripheral WBC concentration may reach 100×10^9/L. According to WHO criteria, absolute monocytosis (more than 1×10^9 monocytes/L) must be present to make the diagnosis. Clinical features include prominent splenomegaly, symptoms of anemia, fever, bleeding, and infection. Before the presence of the Philadelphia chromosome was established as a requirement for the diagnosis of CML, some cases that were classified as Philadelphia chromosome–negative CML likely represented misdiagnoses of chronic myelomonocytic leukemia.[38] Chronic myelomonocytic leukemia is discussed further with myelodysplastic syndromes in Chapter 34.

A puzzling group of patients exhibit Philadelphia chromosome–positive acute leukemia. Studies reveal that 2% of patients with AML exhibit Philadelphia chromosome in a significant proportion of blasts. Further, 5% of patients with childhood-onset ALL and 20% of those with adult-onset ALL test positive for Philadelphia chromosome.[39-42] The proper alignment of these cases within the spectrum of CML is speculative. It is understood that some of these cases likely represent undiagnosed CML that rapidly progressed to an acute leukemia prior to diagnosis. However, because rapidly dividing malignant cells are more prone to genetic mutation, the presence of the Philadelphia chromosome in acute leukemias may reflect a late-stage mutation that contributed little to acute leukemia leukemogenesis.

Treatment

Early treatment approaches for CML were unable to produce remission, so the goal of therapy became the reduction of tumor burden. The first forms of therapy for CML included alkylating agents such as nitrogen mustard,[43] introduced in the late 1940s, and busulfan,[44] which came into use in the early 1950s. Later, busulfan in combination with 6-thioguanine was used to achieve the goal of tumor burden reduction. Other drugs like hydroxyurea and 6-mercaptopurine were introduced later and found to improve patient survival. The discovery of interferon-α in 1983 dramatically improved outcomes of patients with CML by inducing the suppression of the Philadelphia chromosome, reducing the rate of cellular progression to blast cells, and increasing the frequency of long-term patient survival.[45]

Interferon-α stimulates a cell-mediated antitumor host response that reduces myeloid cell numbers, induces cytogenetic remissions, and increases survival.[46] It improves the frequency and duration of hematologic remission and reduces the frequency of detection of the Philadelphia chromosome. In some patients, a complete cytogenetic remission is achieved for a time.

In 1997 it was discovered that cytarabine given with interferon-α improved the frequency of hematologic remissions but did not eliminate the *BCR/ABL1* gene, which was still detected by molecular and fluorescent methods.[47] Also, in some patients the side effects of therapy became severe, drug resistance appeared, and relapse rates were not improved compared with other chemotherapies.

Bone marrow and stem cell transplantation with either autologous or allogeneic hematopoietic stem cells have been reported as curative, especially in patients younger than age 55. Relapses occur, but long-term, disease-free survival is possible. Optimal survival occurs when the patient is treated during the chronic phase within 1 year of diagnosis and is younger than age 50. Treatment requires ablative chemotherapy followed by transplantation of mobilized normal progenitor cells that exhibit CD34+ surface markers. Allogeneic bone marrow transplants are more successful in patients up to age 55 when donors are matched for HLA antigens A, B, and

DR. Donor-matched lymphocyte infusions after allogeneic transplantation of marrow from a sibling donor may assist in producing complete remissions.[48]

Modern therapies involve the use of synthetic proteins that bind the abnormal BCR/ABL protein, blocking the constitutive tyrosine kinase activity and reducing signal transduction activation. Imatinib mesylate is a synthetic tyrosine kinase inhibitor designed to selectively bind the ATP binding site and thus inhibit the tyrosine kinase activity of the BCR/ABL fusion protein. When imatinib binds the ATP binding site, ATP is unable to bind to provide the phosphate group necessary for kinase activity. Imatinib binds the BCR/ABL protein in the inactive conformation, which precedes the autophosphorylation necessary to generate the kinase active site (Figure 33-5).[49]

Goals of therapy include complete hematologic, cytogenetic, and molecular remission indicated by a normalized CBC and differential, absence of Ph1 by karyotype analysis, and absence of measurable BCR/ABL transcripts, respectively. Complete remission from imatinib therapy is induced in part by the reactivation of apoptotic pathways.[50] The effectiveness of imatinib therapy and stem cell transplantation is best monitored by measuring BCR/ABL transcripts using quantitative real-time reverse transcriptase polymerase chain reaction (RT-PCR). These monitoring tools are used to determine the extent of molecular remission. The most sensitive measure of the effectiveness of imatinib therapy is the number of log reductions of *BCR/ABL* transcripts using real-time RT-PCR.[51] Remission milestones indicating effective imatinib therapy are complete hematologic remission in 3 to 6 months, complete cytogenetic response in 6 months to 1 year, and a 2- to 3-log reduction in

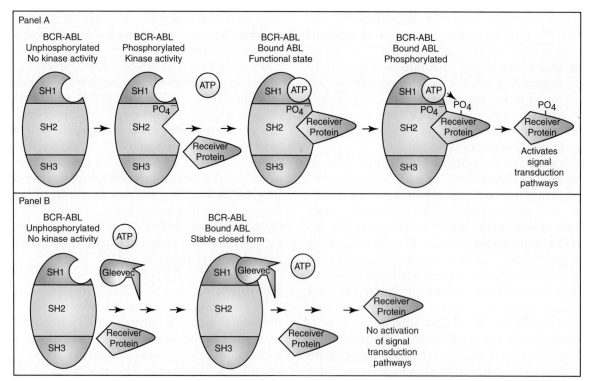

Figure 33-5 Mechanism of imatinib mesylate inhibition of BCR/ABL tyrosine kinase activity. **A,** Mechanism of tyrosine kinase activity of the BCR/ABL fusion protein. **B,** Mechanism of tyrosine kinase inhibition by imatinib mesylate.

BCR/ABL transcripts. When real-time RT-PCR is used, the greatest log reduction possible is a more than 4 log reduction, which represents the maximum sensitivity of the assay. However, discontinuation of imatinib therapy in patients who achieve a more than 4-log reduction usually results in relapse.

Although imatinib has proven to be a successful form of therapy, a major limitation is the development of imatinib resistance resulting in relapse. Approximately 25% to 30% of patients with newly diagnosed CML will discontinue imatinib therapy within 5 years due to lack of remission, resistance, or toxicity.[52] The two major categories of imatinib resistance are primary and secondary. Primary resistance is defined as the inability to reach the remission milestones. This form of resistance accounts for most treatment failures and probably results from the presence of mutations other than the *BCR/ABL1* mutation at the time of diagnosis. Secondary resistance involves the loss of a previous response and occurs at a rate of 16% at 42 months. The majority of cases of imatinib resistance result from two primary causes: acquisition of additional *BCR/ABL1* mutations and expression of point mutations in the ATP binding site. Additional *BCR/ABL1* mutations can occur through the usual translocation of the remaining unaffected chromosomes 9 and 22, which converts the hematopoietic stem cell from heterozygous to homozygous for the *BCR/ABL1* mutation. A double dose of *BCR/ABL1* can also be acquired from gene duplication during mitosis and accounts for 10% of secondary mutations. An additional *BCR/ABL1* mutation will double the tyrosine kinase activity, making the imatinib dosage inadequate. In these cases higher doses of imatinib will restore remission in most patients (Figure 33-6). The majority of patients who do not respond to higher doses of imatinib express point mutations in the ATP binding site. Over 60 mutations have been identified in the ATP binding site, and these account for the remaining 50% to 90% of secondary mutations. Mutations in the ATP binding site reduce the binding affinity of imatinib, producing some level of resistance (Figure 33-7). Three second-generation tyrosine kinase inhibitors—dasatinib (Sprycel), nilotinib (Dasigna), and bosutinib (Bosulib)—overcome the ATP binding site mutations because they have a much higher binding affinity than imatinib. All three are FDA approved for first-line therapy and are effective at rescuing patients resistant to imatinib, except patients who have developed the T315I mutation. The T315I mutation places a large, bulky isoleucine residue in the center of the ATP binding site, and all four FDA-approved tyrosine kinase inhibitors are resistant to this mutation. However, a third-generation tyrosine kinase inhibitor, ponatinib (Iclusig), inhibits the *T315I* mutation as well as drugs designed to bind the A loop (receiver protein binding site) will also inhibit tyrosine kinase activity and

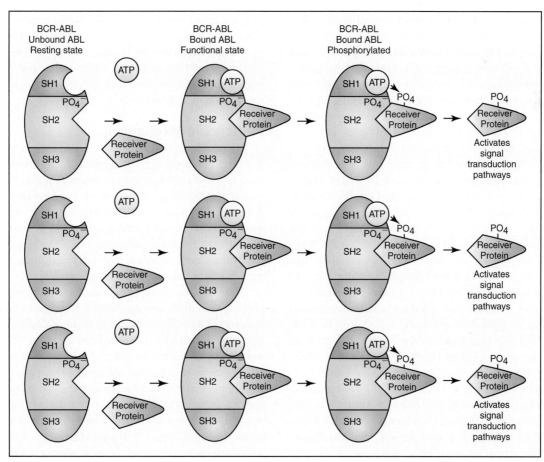

Figure 33-6 Mechanism of imatinib mesylate resistance due to an increased copy number of *BCR/ABL* genes. The increased copies produce more BCR/ABL fusion proteins, which results in an increased tyrosine kinase activity requiring a higher dosage of imatinib to restore remission.

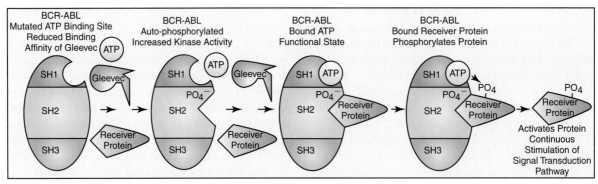

Figure 33-7 Mechanism of imatinib mesylate resistance due to point mutations in the adenosine triphosphate (ATP) binding site. The mutations reduce the binding affinity of imatinib, allowing ATP to bind; this restores the increased tyrosine kinase activity that drives the phenotype and pathogenesis of the disease.

overcome the T315I mutation.[53-55] Currently, studies are under way to evaluate modification of the dosage of imatinib used, to identify and develop other tyrosine kinase inhibitors, and to discover new classes of inhibitors that may be more effective than currently known tyrosine kinase inhibitors.

The development of a care plan for treating a patient with newly diagnosed CML is an ongoing commitment requiring not only the formulation of alternative approaches to achieve and maintain complete cellular remission but also the establishment of laboratory monitoring parameters to follow that confirm long-term success of therapy. Historically, chemotherapy has provided cellular remission but usually has not prevented clinical progression to accelerated or blast phases. Bone marrow transplantation for patients who qualify is likely the preferred choice, but the long-term success (cure) rate remains at 50% to 70%, and most patients will not qualify. For a patient to qualify for transplantation, the patient must be younger than 50 years of age, in the first year of the disease, and have CML that is still in the chronic phase, and a histocompatible donor must be available. For the past 15 years, imatinib has been considered first-line therapy for all patients with newly diagnosed CML. For the small subset of patients who qualify for hematopoietic stem cell transplantation, imatinib is used to induce hematologic remission prior to transplantation. For all other CML patients, imatinib has been used as first-line therapy unless remission is not achieved (primary resistance) or until relapse occurs following remission (secondary resistance). Once the cause of relapse has been determined by cytogenetic and molecular testing, either a higher dosage of imatinib can be given (for an additional *BCR/ABL1* mutation) or a second- or third-generation tyrosine kinase inhibitor (dasatinib, nilotinib, bosutinib) can be prescribed, unless the mutation is the T315I mutation in the ATP binding site. If the T315I mutation is detected, the patient can be given Ponatinib or an A-loop inhibitor (ONO12380) or other drugs like Omacetaxine, MK 0457, or BIRB-796 that inhibit the T315I mutation.[54] Physicians are beginning to prescribe dasatinib, nilotinib and bosutinib as first-line therapy to replace imatinib in hopes that tyrosine kinase inhibitors with higher binding affinities will extend remissions by reducing the rate of mutation-induced relapses. Among the second-generation TKIs, bosutinib shows the most promise because it demonstrates high potency, has the ability to overcome

most P-loop mutations (except T315I), and shows fewer side effects like neutropenia, thrombocytopenia, cardiotoxicity, and pancreatitis compared to nilotinib and dasatinib. Ponatinib and A-loop inhibitors can be used to rescue patients treated with second-generation tyrosine kinase inhibitors, particularly those who develop the T315I mutation.[52]

POLYCYTHEMIA VERA

Polycythemia vera (PV) is a neoplastic clonal myeloproliferative disorder that commonly manifests with panmyelosis in the bone marrow and increases in erythrocytes, granulocytes, and platelets in the peripheral blood.[2] Splenomegaly is common. The disease arises in a hematopoietic stem cell. The hypothesis of a clonal origin for PV is supported by studies of X-linked restriction fragment-length deoxyribonucleic acid (DNA) polymorphisms that demonstrate monoclonal X chromosome inactivation in all blood cells.[56]

Pathogenic Mechanism

In PV, neoplastic clonal stem cells are hypersensitive to, or function independently of, erythropoietin for cell growth. Trace levels of erythropoietin in serum stimulate the growth of erythroid progenitor cells in in vitro colony-forming growth systems. There is preservation of hypersensitive and normosensitive erythroid colony-forming units, however, which indicates some level of normal hematopoiesis.[57] Adverse clinical progression seems to correlate with the propagation of the erythropoietin-sensitive colony-forming units.[58]

Understanding of the pathologic mechanism explaining this phenomenon in PV was significantly advanced in 2005 with the discovery of a consistent mutation in the *JAK2* gene. The specific *JAK2* mutation, *JAK2* V617F, is detected in 90% to 97% of patients with PV. Shortly after the *JAK2* V617F mutation was reported, several groups corroborated the finding using other approaches and showed that the mutation is acquired, clonal, present in the hematopoietic stem cell, constitutively active, and capable of activating the erythropoietic signal transduction pathway in the absence of erythropoietin.[59,60] The point mutation replaces guanine with thymine at exon 14 of the gene, which changes the amino acid at position 617 from valine to phenylalanine. This one amino acid change prevents the inhibition conformation of the tyrosine kinase, causing it to remain in the active conformation. More specifically, the phenylalanine mutation in the kinase domain is unable to bind the corresponding amino acid in the pseudokinase domain, as can the valine in the wild-type counterpart, which prevents the protein from folding into the inactive conformation (Figure 33-8).[61,62]

Normally, erythropoietin is released from the kidney into the blood in response to hypoxia and binds to erythropoietin receptors on the surface of erythroid precursor cells. The resulting conformational change in the erythropoietin receptor causes two erythropoietin receptors to dimerize. This produces a docking point for the head of the inactive *JAK2* protein at a domain known as FERM (Band-4.1, ezrin, radixin, and moesin). Docking of *JAK2* stimulates a phosphorylation event, causing a conformational change, and the valine releases from the pseudokinase domain, converting it to an active tyrosine kinase. *JAK2* can also bind to several other receptors to include MPL (myeloproliferative leukemia, aka TPO-R [thrombopoietin receptor]), GCSF-R (granulocyte colony stimulating factor receptor), prolactin receptor, growth hormone receptor, GM-CSF-R (granulocyte/monocyte colony stimulating factor receptor), IL-3-R (interleukin-3 receptor), IL-5-R (interleukin-5 receptor), and INF-γ2-R (interferon gamma 2 receptor).[62] The diversity in ligand receptor binding explains the range of myeloid proliferation observed in PV (erythroid), ET (thrombopoietic), and neutrophilic (PMF). Once activated, *JAK2* phosphorylates several cytoplasmic proteins, but the STAT (signal transducer and activator of transcription) proteins are the main targets. A cascade of phosphorylation reactions through the STAT proteins produce activated transcription factors that activate a host of genes designed to drive and control cell proliferation and differentiation while also initiating apoptosis (Figure 33-9). Constitutive tyrosine kinase activity of the *JAK2* protein causes continuous activation of several signal transduction pathways that are normally activated following erythropoietin stimulation via the erythropoietic receptor. Active *JAK2* will phosphorylate STAT proteins in the absence of erythropoietin or will overphosphorylate in its presence (Figure 33-10).

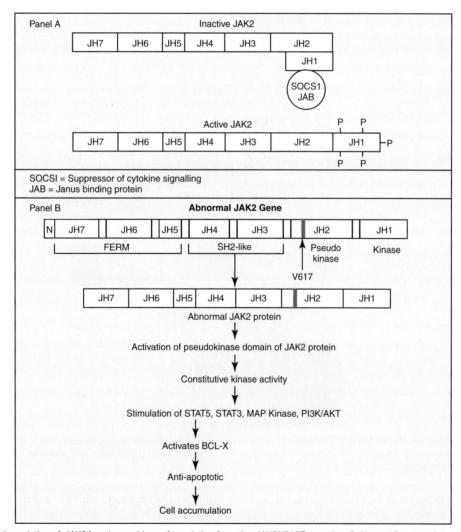

Figure 33-8 Normal regulation of *JAK2* function and loss of regulation from the *JAK2* V617F mutation. **A,** Normal function of the *JAK2* protein and regulation of phosphorylation by *JAK2* intrachain folding and the binding of *JAK2* inhibitors SOCS1 and JAB proteins. **B,** The *JAK2* V617F mutation and the loss of normal *JAK2* folding and inhibitor binding resulting in phosphorylation, activation, and the stimulation of STAT, MAP kinase, and PI3K/AKT signal transduction pathways.

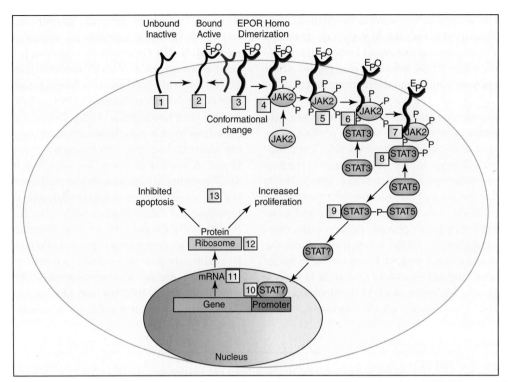

Figure 33-9 Normal erythropoiesis involving erythropoietin binding to erythropoietin receptors and stimulation of the JAK/STAT pathway via the normal *JAK2* protein.

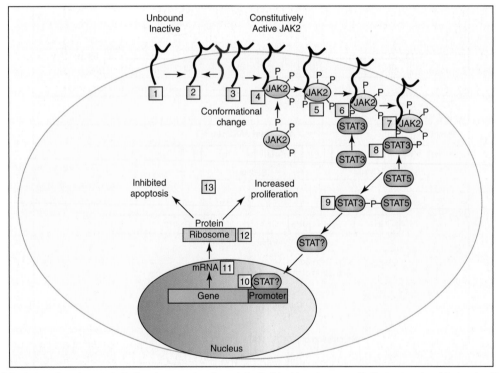

Figure 33-10 Stimulation of erythropoiesis in the absence of erythropoietin that is driven by a constitutively phosphorylated and activated *JAK2* protein resulting from the *JAK2* V617F mutation.

Hematopoietic stem cells that bear the *JAK2* mutation are resistant to erythropoietin-deprivation apoptosis by upregulation of BCL-X, an antiapoptotic protein. PV progenitor cells do not divide more rapidly but accumulate because they do not die normally.[63-65] In addition to the role of mutated *JAK2* in the abrogation of STAT signaling, it has also been shown to influence chromatin structure[66,67] and to decrease methyltransferase activity.[68] Lastly, homozygosity of *JAK2* V617F occurs more commonly in PV, whereas *JAK2* heterozygosity occurs more commonly in ET. Therefore, disease progression from ET to PV may partially be explained by the dosage effect of *JAK2* mutations.[62]

Because approximately 5% of PV patients do not possess the *JAK2* V617F mutation and because PV has a familial predisposition, it is thought that other mutations must be involved in the pathogenesis of PV and some must precede and possibly predispose the *JAK2* V617F mutation. Since the original discovery of a mutation in the thrombopoietic receptor gene *MPL* in 2006,[69] several gain-of-function mutations have been identified. Most *MPL* mutations occur in exon 10 where tryptophan 515 is substituted for a leucine, lysine, asparagine, or alanine.[69-72] Tryptophan 515 is located on the cytosolic side of the membrane and is key in transducing the signal that thrombopoietin (TPO) has bound to the receptor. These mutations cause the MPL receptor to be hypersensitive to TPO and in some cases to assume the active conformation in the absence of TPO. A similar mutation, *MPL* S505N, was initially described in familial PV but has since been found in sporadic MPN.[69,72] These types of *MPL* mutations have since been identified in up to 15% of *JAK2* V617F–negative ET and PMF patients.[73]

In 2007 a second type of *JAK2* mutation was identified in exon 12, usually between amino acid residues 536 and 547, that also resulted in a gain of function similar to the *JAK2* V617F.[74] Exon 12 is not located in the pseudokinase domain, but it is hypothesized that the mutation can modify the structure of the JH2 domain, rendering the protein incapable of forming the inactive conformation.[62] *JAK2* exon 12 mutations have been found in 3% of patients with PV and are not associated with ET or PMF but can be found in patients who progress to secondary myelofibrosis.[74,75]

Experts hypothesize that mutations in signaling molecules alone are insufficient to initiate MPNs, suggesting that other mutations are necessary prior to *JK2* V617F to induce disease and later to drive progression. Four lines of evidence support this hypothesis: familial MPN expresses a classic PV or ET phenotype in the absence of *JAK2* V617F or *MPL* W515L mutations and transmits in an autosomal dominant fashion; in some ET and PV clones that were erythropoietin independent, *JAK2* V617F was identified in a minority of cells, indicating that a pre–*JAK2* mutation drove the disease; approximately 50% of patients who developed acute leukemia from a *JAK2* V617F form of MPN expressed wild-type *JAK2*, suggesting a line of clonal evolution independent of *JAK2*; and in patients with PV and ET at diagnosis, the *JAK2* V617F allele burden in HSCs was low compared to the allele burden in later stages of hematopoiesis, suggesting that *JAK2* V617F confers a weak proliferative advantage to HSCs.[62]

Three reports in 2010 identified a germline haplotype block that predisposes patients to *JAK2* mutations.[76-78] This haplotype block was identified as a single nucleotide polymorphism (rs10974944) located in intron 12 of the *JAK2* gene, increasing the development of MPN by three- to fourfold.[61]

Also in 2010, mutations were discovered in the adapter protein LNK (aka Src homology 2 B3–SH2B3), which downregulates JAK-STAT signaling pathways by regulating *JAK2* activation. Approximately 3% to 6% of patients with MPN bear an *LNK* mutation,[79,80] with approximately 13% of mutations appearing in the blast phase versus the chronic phase of the disease.[81] Following the binding of the corresponding ligand to its receptor, LNK binds to erythropoietin receptor (EPO-R), thrombopoietin receptor (MPL), and *JAK2* to downregulate the JAK-STAT pathway as a negative modulator. Mutations in *LNK* produce a loss of function that removes a level of inhibitory control, increasing the proliferation of erythrocytes and thrombocytes. This loss of function mutation is accentuated in the presence of *JAK2* V617F and *MPL* W515L mutations, resulting in the PV and ET phenotypes, respectively.[61] More recently, somatic mutations have been identified in genes that control DNA methylation in patients with PV and other MPNs. The most notable are *TET2*, *IDH1*, and *IDH2*. *TET2* (Ten Eleven Translocation 2) is one of three members of the *TET* family of genes (*TET1* and *TET3*) and the only one identified with sequence alterations. *TET2* appears to be highly mutagenic for three reasons: mutations have been identified in all types of myeloid disorders to include MPNs, MDSs, and AMLs; mutations have been found in all coding regions of the gene; and mutations are often biallelic (homozygous).[82] *TET2* catalyzes the reaction that oxidizes the 5-methyl group of cytosine (5-mC) to 5-hydroxymethycytosine (5-hmC).[83] It is hypothesized that 5-hmC serves as an intermediate base in the demethylation of DNA. Methylation of histones serves to silence genes. Therefore, *TET2* mutations produce a loss of function effect, resulting in hypermethylation and a loss of gene activation (inactivation of tumor suppressor genes).[61] In addition, it appears that *TET2* mutations precede *JAK2* mutations based on three observations: *TET2* mutations are expressed in CD34+ hematopoietic stem cells (HSC); *TET2* mutations have been identified in all forms of myeloid disorders; and all patients with both *TET2* and *JAK2* mutations produced clones with both mutations and clones that were *TET2* positive and *JAK2* negative but none that were *JAK2* positive and *TET2* negative. Therefore, *TET2* mutations may create abnormal clones that predispose to *JAK2* mutations.[82] *TET2* mutations have been identified in 9.8% to 16% of PV, 4.4% to 5% of ET, and 7.7% to 17% of PMF patients.[61]

Mutations in the genes that code for the citric acid cycle enzymes isocitrate dehydrogenase 1 (IDH1) and isocitrate dehydrogenase 2 (IDH2) have been associated with hypermethylation of DNA in patients with MPN and AML.[84] Normally these enzymes function to convert isocitrate to α-ketoglutarate, requiring the reduction of NAD(P)+ to NADPH as the energy source. In patients with MPNs, mutations in *IDH1/2* occur most frequently at the IDH2 R140 residue, the *IDH1* R132 residue, and the IDA2 R172 residue.[85] These mutations are thought to alter enzyme function, causing the conversion of α-ketoglutarate to 2-hydroxyglutarate (2-HG).[86] It is hypothesized that because *TET2* is dependent on α-ketoglutarate, the *IDH1/2* mutations would result in less α-ketoglutarate, thus impairing the function of *TET2* and exacerbating the hypermethylation function of mutated *TET2* protein products.[84] *IDH1/2* mutations occur most frequently (21.6% of patients) in late-stage PV and ET patients during blast transformation compared to an incidence of 1% to 5% in patients with early PV (1.9%), ET (0.8%), and PMF (4.2%).[61] As expected, *IDH1/2* mutations are associated with adverse overall survival, raising the potential of using *IDH1/2* mutational analysis and/or 2-HG detection as poor prognostic indicators.

Mutations in two additional genes involved in epigenetic modification, *EZH2* and *ASXL1*, have been implicated in MPN, MDS, and MDS/MPN and, along with *TET2*, may precede *JAK2* V617F mutations. *EZH2* and *EZH1* function as two of several proteins that form the polychrome repressive complex 2 (PRC2) that regulates chromatin structure. More specifically, *EZH1* and *EZH2* provide the functional domain for the PRC2 complex to methylate histone H3 at lysine 27.[87] The array of mutations noted in *EZH2* to date function to either eliminate protein production or abrogate methyltransferase activity. Mutations in *EZH2* have been identified in 3% of PV patients, 13% of PMF patients, 12.3% of MDS/MPN patients, and 5.8% to 23% of MDS patients.[88,89] *ASXL1* (Additional Sex Combs–like 1) mutations have been identified in most myeloid malignancies and at a frequency similar to *TET2*.[62] *ASXL1* normally functions in conjunction with *ASXL2* and *ASXL3* to deubiquinate histone H2 to balance the activity of PRC1 to monoubiquinate target genes to modify chromatin structure.[90,91] Ubiquination tags proteins for natural removal, thus regulating their function. The function of *ASXL1* in hematopoiesis is poorly understood, but the loss of function mutations have been identified in less than 7% of PV and ET and from 19% to 40% in PMF.[92,93]

Disease progression to blast crisis occurs in less than 10% of PV and ET patients, but several genetic mutation are implicated in this transformation.[94-96] In addition to those that modulate epigenetic changes previously discussed (*IDH1/2* and *TET2*), mutations in *TP53* and *RUNX1* are involved in blast transformation. *TP53* produces the P53 protein that is known to be a tumor suppressor gene. P53 controls cell cycle checkpoints and apoptosis, and loss-of-function mutations are implicated in a host of cancers to include disease progression in the classic MPNs. *TP53* mutations have not been identified in MPNs in the chronic phase but have been found in 20% of patients with MPNs who have progressed to AML.[97-99] The protein product of the *RUNX1/AML1* gene is a transcription factor that is important in hematopoiesis. *RUNX1* mutations were observed in 30% of post–MPN-AML patients, making it a candidate for the most frequent mutation involved in MPN transformation to AML.[62]

Diagnosis

Based on the WHO standards, the diagnosis of PV requires that two major criteria and one minor criterion be met or that the first major criterion listed and two minor criteria be met. The two major criteria are an elevated hemoglobin (Hb) level (>18.5 g/dL in men and >16.5 g/dL in women) and the identification of the *JAK2* V617F mutation, the *JAK2* exon 12 mutation, or a similar *JAK2* mutation. The three minor criteria are panmyelosis in the bone marrow; low serum erythropoietin levels; and autonomous, in vitro erythroid colony formation.[8] Additional diagnostic features of PV include an increased RBC mass of 36 mL/kg or greater in males and 32 mL/kg or greater in females, an arterial oxygen saturation of 92% (normal) or greater, and splenomegaly. Other features of PV are thrombocytosis of greater than 400×10^9 platelets/L; leukocytosis of greater than 12×10^9 cells/L without fever or infection; and increases in leukocyte alkaline phosphatase (LAP), serum vitamin B_{12}, or unbound vitamin B_{12} binding capacity.[100,101] Recent research indicates that the *JAK2* V617F mutation can be expected in more than 90% to 95% of cases.[8] The WHO criteria for the diagnosis of PV are summarized in Box 33-1.

It is not always easy to assign an early diagnosis of PV. Erythrocytosis secondary to hypoxia or erythropoietin-producing neoplasms are the most difficult to diagnose correctly. In individuals with these conditions, the bone marrow exhibits erythroid hyperplasia without granulocytic or megakaryocytic hyperplasia. Patients with stress or spurious erythrocytosis exhibit increased hemoglobin and hematocrit (HCT) without increased erythrocyte mass or splenomegaly.

Peripheral Blood and Bone Marrow

Common peripheral blood, bone marrow, and tissue findings in the early or proliferative phase of PV are listed in Table 33-2. Figures 33-11 and 33-12 show common morphologic patterns in peripheral blood and bone marrow morphologic and cellular changes. Not only are quantitative changes seen, but bone marrow normoblasts may collect in large clusters, megakaryocytes are enlarged and exhibit lobulated nuclei, and bone marrow sinuses are enlarged without fibrosis. Pseudo-Gaucher cells are rare.[28] Approximately 80% of patients manifest bone marrow panmyelosis, and 100% of bone marrow volume may exhibit hematopoietic cellularity. Although the bone marrow pattern may mimic that of other MPNs, the peripheral blood cells appear normal, with normocytic, normochromic erythrocytes; mature granulocytes; and normal-sized, granulated

---

BOX 33-1 World Health Organization Criteria for the Diagnosis of Polycythemia Vera

Diagnosis requires the presence of both major criteria and one minor criterion or the presence of the first major criterion together with two minor criteria.

Major Criteria
1. Hemoglobin >18.5 g/dL in men, >16.5 g/dL in women or other evidence of increased red blood cell volume*
2. Presence of *JAK2* V617F or other functionally similar mutation such as *JAK2* exon 12 mutation

Minor Criteria
1. Bone marrow biopsy specimen showing hypercellularity for age with trilineage growth (panmyelosis) with prominent erythroid, granulocytic, and megakaryocytic proliferation
2. Serum erythropoietin level below the reference range for normal
3. Endogenous erythroid colony formation in vitro

*Hemoglobin or hematocrit >99th percentile of method-specific reference range for age, sex, altitude, or residence, or hemoglobin >17 g/dL in men, >15 g/dL in women if associated with a documented and sustained increase of at least 2 g/dL from an individual's baseline value that cannot be attributed to correction of iron deficiency, or elevated red cell mass >25% above mean normal predicted value.

From Vardiman JW, Thiele J, Arber DA, et al: The 2008 revision of the World Health Organization (WHO) classification of myeloid neoplasms and acute leukemia: rationale and important changes. *Blood* 114:937-951, 2009.

TABLE 33-2 Common Morphologic Changes in Polycythemia Vera

Peripheral Blood

Hemoglobin	Increased
Hematocrit	Increased
Red blood cell volume	Increased
Erythrocyte morphology	Normocytic/Normochromic
Total white blood cells	Increased
Granulocytes	Increased
Platelets	Increased
Leukocyte alkaline phosphatase	Normal or increased

Bone Marrow

Normoblasts	Increased
Granulocytes	Increased
Megakaryocytes	Increased
Reticulin	Increased

Extramedullary Tissue

Splenomegaly	Present
Sinusoidal	Present
Medullary	Present
Hepatomegaly	Present
Sinusoidal	Present

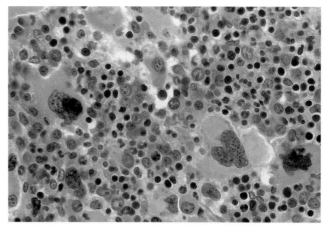

Figure 33-12 Bone marrow biopsy specimen in stable phase polycythemia vera showing panmyelosis (hematoxylin and eosin stain, ×400).

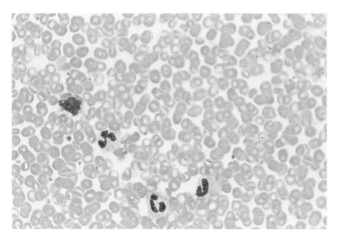

Figure 33-11 Peripheral blood film in stable phase polycythemia vera with essentially normocytic, normochromic erythrocytes (×500).

platelets. The other 20% of patients exhibit lesser degrees of cellularity in the bone marrow and peripheral blood. Splenomegaly, hepatomegaly, generalized vascular engorgement, and circulatory disturbances increase the risk of hemorrhage, tissue infarction, and thrombosis.

Clinical Presentation

PV initially manifests in a proliferative phase independent of normal regulatory mechanisms. PV is always associated with increased RBC mass. This is the stable phase of PV, which progresses to a spent phase in a few patients. In the spent phase, patients experience progressive splenomegaly (palpable

spleen) or hypersplenism (large spleen with bone marrow hyperplasia and peripheral blood cytopenias) and pancytopenia. They may also exhibit the triad of bone marrow fibrosis, splenomegaly, and anemia with teardrop-shaped poikilocytes. The latter pattern is called *postpolycythemic myeloid metaplasia*, and its morphologic features are similar to those of PMF. Peripheral WBC and RBC counts vary, and nucleated erythrocytes, immature granulocytes, and large platelets are present. Usually, splenomegaly is secondary to extramedullary hematopoiesis.[102] Myelofibrosis occurs within the bone marrow and may come to occupy a significant proportion of bone marrow volume, with subsequent ineffective hematopoiesis.[103]

Treatment and Prognosis

The treatment of choice for PV is therapeutic phlebotomy at a frequency necessary to maintain the hematocrit at less than 45%. Low-dose aspirin has been shown efficacious to minimize thrombosis in all risk categories.[104] The alkylating agent hydroxyuria is recommended in high-risk patients with PV and can be substituted for INF-γ in younger patients[105, 106] and busulfan in older patients who develop intolerance or resistance to hydroxyuria.[107] Prognosis for patients with PV is good, with a median survival exceeding 15 to 20 years.[108] However, the disease progresses to acute leukemia in 15% of patients. The use of myelosuppressive therapy such as phosphorus P 32 (^{32}P) or alkylating agents seems to increase the risk.[101] Only 1% to 2% of patients treated with phlebotomy alone experience leukemic transformation. However, the risk of thrombosis and bleeding is increased in patients treated with phlebotomy alone, so the use of alkylating myelosuppressive agents may be required to control these complications. Some patients may manifest a temporary disease pattern similar to myelodysplasia, and the cell morphology in transformation to acute leukemia may be difficult to classify. Patients with both early and advanced PV may show clinical, peripheral blood, bone marrow, and extramedullary features that mimic those of other MPNs.

Treatment with modern JAK inhibitors has provided important benefits to patients with PV. A total of 34 patients intolerant or refractive to hydroxyuria were enrolled in the phase II study and treated with INCB018424 (ruxolitinib) at a dose of

10 mg b.i.d. Of the 34 patients, 15 (45%) had a complete remission.[109] In addition, 97% (32 patients) achieved phlebotomy independence, and 80% (27 patients) achieved a 50% decrease in spleen size, as well as a reduction in pruritus, bone pain, and night sweats.[110] CEP-701 (Lestaurtinib) was studied on 27 PV and 12 ET patients refractory or intolerant to hydroxyuria, and the outcomes were less promising. In 15 of the 39 patients who completed 18 weeks of treatment, 83% (15/18) achieved some degree of spleen size reduction, 60% (3/5) had a reduction in phlebotomy requirements, 20% (3/15) had a 15% decrease in *JAK2* allele burden, and 15% developed thrombosis; gastrointestinal events were frequent.[111]

ESSENTIAL THROMBOCYTHEMIA

Essential thrombocythemia (ET) is a clonal MPN with increased megakaryopoiesis and thrombocytosis, usually with a count greater than 600×10^9/L and sometimes with a count greater than 1000×10^9/L.[112] However, WHO criteria require a sustained thrombocytosis with a platelet count of 450×10^9/L or greater. Over the years, ET has been known as *primary thrombocytosis, idiopathic thrombocytosis,* and *hemorrhagic thrombocythaemia.*[3,113]

Incidence

In the absence of a well-defined diagnostic algorithm, determining the true incidence of ET has been difficult. When the diagnostic system developed by the Polycythemia Vera Study Group (PVSG) is applied, however, the incidence is estimated to be between 0.6 and 2.5 cases per 100,000 persons per year. The majority of cases occur in individuals between the ages of 50 and 60 years, but a second peak occurs primarily in women in the childbearing years, approximately 30 years of age.[113]

Pathogenic Mechanism

Most of the mutations described in PV also occur in ET but usually at a lower frequency. The *JAK2* V617F occurs in approximately 55% of patients with ET.[114] *MPL* exon 10 mutations (*MPL* W515L/K) are observed in 3% of ET patients, as well as several other mutations previously discussed to include *TET2* (4.4% to 5%), *ASXL1* (5.6%), *LNK* (3% to 6%), and *IDH1/2* (0.8%).[61] The manner in which these mutations alter normal cellular functions is similar to PV, as previously described.

Clinical Presentation

In more than one half of the patients diagnosed with ET, the disorder is discovered in the laboratory by virtue of an unexpectedly elevated platelet count on a routine complete blood count; the remaining patients see a physician due to vascular occlusion or hemorrhage. Vascular occlusions are often the result of microvascular thromboses in the digits or thromboses in major arteries and veins that occur in a variety of organ systems, including splenic or hepatic veins, as in Budd-Chiari syndrome. Bleeding occurs most frequently from mucous membranes in the gastrointestinal and upper respiratory tracts. Splenomegaly is observed at presentation in 50% of patients when the PVSG

diagnostic criteria are used but at a much lower frequency when the WHO standards are applied. This difference is largely due to the elimination of the diagnosis of ET in patients who meet the criteria for PMF in the prefibrotic stage.[113]

Diagnosis

ET must be differentiated from secondary or reactive thrombocytoses and from other MPNs. Thrombocytosis may be secondary to chronic active blood loss, hemolytic anemia, chronic inflammation or infection, or nonhematogenous neoplasia. The diagnostic criteria for ET first proposed by the PVSG were intended to distinguish ET from other MPNs. These features included a platelet count of greater than 600×10^9/L, a hemoglobin of less than 13 g/dL or a normal erythrocyte mass, and stainable iron in the bone marrow or a failure of iron therapy. Philadelphia chromosome negativity, absence of marrow collagen fibrosis (less than one third of a biopsy specimen is fibrous), no splenomegaly, absence of leukoerythroblastic reaction, and no known cause of reactive thrombocytosis all support the diagnosis.[115]

The newest WHO group now requires the documentation of four major criteria to establish a diagnosis of ET. First, the WHO group lowered the platelet count threshold to 450×10^9/L or greater to capture patients who would eventually meet diagnostic criteria but who were experiencing hemorrhage or thrombosis with platelet counts of between 450×10^9/L and 600×10^9/L.[113] Because a lower platelet threshold could lead to false-positive ET diagnoses, all the WHO criteria must be met to eliminate such patients. Second, the bone marrow must show significant megakaryopoiesis characterized by large, mature-looking megakaryocytes with no substantial increase in erythropoiesis or granulopoiesis or left shift in the neutrophil line. Third, the condition cannot meet the criteria of any other MPN, myelodysplasia, or other myeloid neoplasm. Fourth, patients must demonstrate either the *JAK2* V617F or other clonal mutation or, in the absence of a clonal marker, the absence of reactive thrombocytosis. Careful analysis of the bone marrow biopsy specimen is useful in distinguishing ET from myelodysplastic syndromes (MDSs) associated with the del(5q) mutation, refractory anemia with ringed sideroblasts with thrombocytosis, and the prefibrotic phase of PMF. Likewise, the identification of the *JAK2* V617F mutation excludes cases of reactive thrombocytosis.[113]

The *JAK2* V617F mutation is found in 50% to 60% of ET patients and supports the diagnosis of ET.[116,117] WHO diagnostic criteria were modified to include a minimum platelet count of 450×10^9/L when the *JAK2* mutation is present.[118] *JAK2* mutations have not been identified in the germline of any patient with MPN disorder, which supports the view that the mutation is acquired. *MPL* W515K/L, a mutation in the thrombopoietin receptor (*MPL*), has been reported in 3% of ET cases and is also used to exclude a diagnosis of reactive thrombocytosis.[114] Other genetic mutations are uncommon but have been reported to be found in 5% to 10% of cases when the diagnostic criteria proposed by the PVSG are applied. The most commonly reported additional mutations are +8, 9q, and (del)20q.[113]

Peripheral Blood and Bone Marrow

Figure 33-13 shows a peripheral blood film that exhibits early-phase thrombocytosis with variation in platelet diameter and shape, including giantism, agranularity, and pseudopods. Commonly, platelets are present in clusters and tend to accumulate near the thin edge of the blood film. Segmented neutrophils may be increased; basophils are not. Erythrocytes are normocytic and normochromic, unless iron deficiency is present secondary to excessive bleeding.

Early-phase bone marrow shows marked megakaryocytic hypercellularity, clustering of megakaryocytes, and increased megakaryocyte diameter with nuclear hyperlobulation and density (Figure 33-14). Special studies reveal increased numbers of smaller and less mature megakaryocytes.[119] Increased granulopoiesis and erythropoiesis may contribute to bone marrow hypercellularity, and, in a few patients, reticulin fibers may be increased. The major peripheral blood, bone marrow, and extramedullary findings are listed in Table 33-3.

A diagnosis of ET is questionable in patients with a platelet count of more than $450 \times 10^9/L$ if certain features are observed

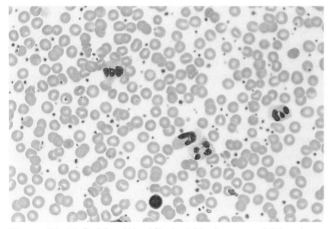

Figure 33-13 Peripheral blood film in stable phase essential thrombocythemia showing increased numbers of platelets and mature neutrophils (×500).

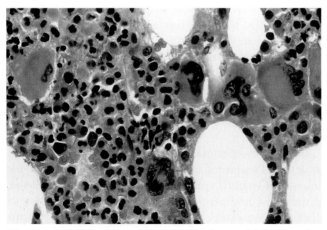

Figure 33-14 Bone marrow biopsy specimen in essential thrombocythemia showing marked megakaryocytic hypercellularity (hematoxylin and eosin stain, ×400).

TABLE 33-3 Common Morphologic Changes in Essential Thrombocythemia

Peripheral Blood

Hemoglobin	Slightly decreased
Hematocrit	Slightly decreased
Red blood cell volume	Normal
Total white blood cells	Normal or slightly increased
Neutrophils	Normal or slightly increased
Platelets	Increased
Platelet function	Decreased

Bone Marrow

Normoblasts	Normal or increased
Granulocytes	Normal or slightly increased
Megakaryocytes	
Clusters	Present
Large	Present
Hyperlobulated	Present
Dense nuclei	Present
Variability in size	Increased
Reticulin	Normal or slightly increased

Extramedullary Tissue

Splenomegaly	Present
Sinusoidal	Present
Medullary	Present
Megakaryocytic proliferation	Present

on the bone marrow biopsy specimen. For example, increased erythropoiesis or granulopoiesis in the bone marrow is a questionable finding for ET and suggests an alternative diagnosis of PV or PMF, respectively, especially if bizarre or significantly atypical megakaryocytes are also observed. Dyserythropoiesis and/or dysgranulopoiesis suggests a myelodysplastic disorder and should prompt an investigation for (del)5q, (inv)3, and/or t(3;3).[113]

Treatment and Prognosis

Treatment involves prevention or early alleviation of hemorrhagic or vasoocclusive complications that occur as the platelet count increases. The production of platelets must be reduced by suppressing marrow megakaryocyte production with an alkylating agent like hydroxyuria. As observed in PV, ET patients so treated may incur an increased risk for disease transformation to acute leukemia or myelofibrosis. However, malignant transformation occurs at a frequency of less than 5%.[114] Hydroxyurea therapy may achieve a desired reduction of peripheral platelets without the risk of complications experienced with myelosuppressive agents. This may relate to the youth of ET patients, in whom the risk of leukemic transformation seems relatively low. For patients who develop intolerance or resistance to hydroxyuria, cytoreduction can be achieved with interferon-α in younger patients[105] and busulfan in older patients.[120] Low-dose aspirin is also recommended to prevent thrombosis.[114]

JAK2 inhibitors are being investigated in ET patients who are refractory or intolerant to hydroxyuria or are otherwise high risk. INCB018424 (ruxolitinib) was studied in 39 patients with ET at a dose of 25 mg b.i.d. In all 39 patients, the median platelet count reduced from 884 to 558 $\times$ 10^9/L, and the 11 patients who had leukocytosis achieved a normal WBC count after 6 months of treatment. Four patients who demonstrated splenomegaly showed spleen size reduction; 40% to 75% of patients had a 50% or greater improvement in one or more of the following: pruritus, bone pain, night sweats, and peripheral tingling/numbness. Only 13% (5 patients), achieved complete remission. However, a follow-up report at 10.4 months of treatment showed that 92% were still participating in the study, no grade 3 or 4 hematologic complications were noted, and although cytopenias were observed in 10% to 20%, they were grade 2 (mild).[110] CEP701 (Lestaurtinib) was studied in 27 patients with PV and 12 patients with ET who were refractory or intolerant to hydroxyuria. In 15 of the 39 patients who completed 18 weeks of treatment, 83% (15/18) achieved some degree of spleen size reduction, 20% (3/15) had a 15% decrease in *JAK2* allele burden, and 15% developed thrombosis and had frequent gastrointestinal events.[111]

Patients with ET experience relatively long survival provided they remain free of serious thromboembolic or hemorrhagic complications. Clinical symptoms associated with thromboembolic vasoocclusive events include the syndrome of erythromelalgia (throbbing and burning pain in the hands and feet, accompanied by mottled redness of areas), transient ischemic attacks, seizures, and cerebral or myocardial infarction. Other symptoms include headache, dizziness, visual disturbances, and dysesthesias (decreased sensations). Hemorrhagic complications include bleeding from oral and nasal mucous membranes or gastrointestinal mucosa and the appearance of cutaneous ecchymoses (Chapter 40).

The median survival for patients with ET is 20 years, including cases in which the process arises in younger patients.[121] However, some patients may develop post-ET myelofibrosis, which reduces survival. Patients whose cells manifest chromosome abnormalities may have a poorer prognosis.[39]

PRIMARY MYELOFIBROSIS

Primary myelofibrosis (PMF), previously known as *chronic idiopathic myelofibrosis, agnogenic myelofibrosis,* and *myelofibrosis with myeloid metaplasia,* is a clonal MPN[6] in which there is splenomegaly and ineffective hematopoiesis associated with areas of marrow hypercellularity, fibrosis, and increased megakaryocytes. Megakaryocytes are enlarged with pleomorphic nuclei, coarse segmentation, and areas of hypochromia. The peripheral blood film exhibits immature granulocytes and normoblasts, dacryocytes (teardrop-shaped RBCs), and other bizarre RBC shapes.

PMF clonality was manifest in studies in which cytogenetic abnormalities were detected in normoblasts, neutrophils, macrophages, basophils, and megakaryocytes. Female patients heterozygous for glucose-6-phosphate dehydrogenase isoenzymes have PMF cells of a single enzyme isotype, whereas tissue cells, including marrow fibroblasts, contain both enzyme isotypes.[6]

Myelofibrosis

The myelofibrosis in this disease consists of three of the five types of collagen: I, III, and IV. Increases in type III collagen are detected by silver impregnation techniques, increases in type I by staining with trichrome, and increases in type IV by the presence of osteosclerosis, which may be diagnosed from increased radiographic bone density.[122] In approximately 30% of patients, biopsy specimens show no fibrosis.[39] Increases in these collagens are not a part of the clonal proliferative process but are considered secondary to an increased release of fibroblastic growth factors, such as platelet-derived growth factor, transforming growth factor α from megakaryocyte α-granules, tumor necrosis factor-α, and interleukin-1α and interleukin-1β. Marrow fibrosis causes expansion of marrow sinuses and vascular volume, with an increased rate of blood flow. Bone marrow fibrosis is not the sole criterion for the diagnosis of PMF because increases in marrow fibrosis may reflect a reparative response to injury from benzene or ionizing radiation, may be a consequence of immunologically mediated injury, or may represent a reactive response to other hematologic conditions.

Type IV collagen and laminin normally are discontinuous in sinusoidal membranes but appear as stromal sheets in association with neovascularization and endothelial cell proliferation in regions of fibrosis. In addition, deposition of type VII collagen is observed, and this may form a linkage between type I fibers, type III fibers, and type I plus type III fibers.[123]

Hematopoiesis and Extramedullary Hematopoiesis

Extramedullary hematopoiesis, clinically recognized as hepatomegaly or splenomegaly, seems to originate from release of clonal stem cells into the circulation.[124] The cells accumulate in the spleen, liver, or other organs, including adrenals, kidneys, lymph nodes, bowel, breasts, lungs, mediastinum, mesentery, skin, synovium, thymus, and lower urinary tract. The cause of extramedullary hematopoiesis is unknown. In experimental animal models, chemicals, hormones, viruses, radiation, and immunologic factors have been implicated. The disease is associated with an increase in circulating hematopoietic cells, but fibroblasts are a secondary abnormality and not clonal.[125] B and T cells may be involved.[126] There is an increase in circulating unilineage and multilineage hematopoietic progenitor cells,[127] and the number of CD34$^+$ cells may be 300 times normal.[128] The increase in circulating CD34$^+$ cells separates PMF from other MPNs and predicts the degree of splenic involvement and risk of conversion to acute leukemia.

Body cavity effusions containing hematopoietic cells may arise from extramedullary hematopoiesis in the cranium, the intraspinal epidural space, or the serosal surfaces of pleura, pericardium, and peritoneum. Portal hypertension, with its attendant consequences of ascites, esophageal and gastric varices, gastrointestinal hemorrhage, and hepatic encephalopathy, arises from the combination of a massive increase in splenoportal blood flow and a decrease in hepatic vascular compliance secondary to fibrosis around the sinusoids and hematopoietic cells within the sinusoids.[129]

Pathogenetic Mechanism

As with PV and ET, the *JAK2* V617F mutation is involved in the pathogenesis and is found in 65% of PMF patients.[114] The *MPL* W515L/K occurs in an additional 10% of patients, along with most of the other mutations previously discussed, to include *CBL* (6%),[130] *TET2* (7.7% to 17%), *ASXL1* (13% to 23%), *LNK* (3% to 6%), *EZH2* (13%), and *IDH1/2* (4.2%).[61]

Incidence and Clinical Presentation

The disease occurs in patients older than age 60 and may be asymptomatic. PMF generally presents with fatigue, weakness, shortness of breath, palpitations, weight loss, and discomfort or pain in the left upper quadrant associated with splenomegaly.

Peripheral Blood and Bone Marrow

PMF presents with a broad range of changes in laboratory test values and peripheral blood film results, but examination of the bone marrow biopsy specimen provides most of the information for diagnosis. Changes commonly observed in peripheral blood and bone marrow examinations are summarized in Table 33-4.

Abnormalities in erythrocytes noted on peripheral blood films include the presence of dacryocytes, other bizarre shapes, nucleated RBCs, and polychromatophilia. Granulocytes are increased, normal, or decreased in number and may include immature granulocytes, blasts, and cells with nuclear or cytoplasmic anomalies. Platelets may be normal, increased, or decreased in number, with a mixture of normal and abnormal morphologic features (Figure 33-15). Micromegakaryocytes may be observed (Figure 33-16).

Bone marrow biopsy specimens exhibit intense fibrosis, granulocytic and megakaryocytic hypercellularity, dysmegakaryopoiesis, dysgranulopoiesis, and numerous dilated sinuses containing luminal hematopoiesis. Neutrophils may exhibit impairment of physiologic functions such as phagocytosis, oxygen consumption, and hydrogen peroxide generation, and decreased myeloperoxidase and glutathione reductase activities. Platelets show impaired aggregation in response to epinephrine, decreased adenosine diphosphate concentration in dense granules, and decreased activity of platelet lipoxygenase.

Immune Response

Humoral immune responses are altered in approximately 50% of patients and include the appearance of autoantibodies to erythrocyte antigens, nuclear proteins, gamma globulins, phospholipids, and organ-specific antigens.[131] Circulating immune complexes, increased proportions of marrow-reactive lymphocytes, and the development of amyloidosis are evidence for active immune processes. Collagen disorders coexist with PMF, which suggests that immunologic processes may stimulate marrow fibroblast activity.

Treatment and Prognosis

A diverse spectrum of therapies has been implemented to alleviate symptoms or modify clinical problems in patients with

TABLE 33-4 Common Morphologic Changes in Primary Myelofibrosis

Peripheral Blood

Hemoglobin	Normal or decreased
Anisocytosis	Present
Poikilocytosis	Present
Teardrop-shaped erythrocytes	Present
Nucleated red blood cells	Present
Polychromasia	Normal or increased
Total white blood cells	Normal, decreased, or increased
Immature granulocytes	Increased
Blasts	Present
Basophils	Present
Leukocyte anomaly	Present
Leukocyte alkaline phosphatase	Increased, normal, or decreased
Platelets	Increased, normal, or decreased
Abnormal platelets	Present
Megakaryocytes	Present

Bone Marrow

Cellularity	Increased
Granulopoiesis	Increased
Megakaryocytes	Increased
Erythropoiesis	Normal or increased
Myelofibrosis	Increased
Sinuses	Increased
Dysmegakaryopoiesis	Present
Dysgranulopoiesis	Present

Extramedullary Tissue

Splenomegaly	Present
Sinusoidal	Present
Medullary	Present
Hepatomegaly	Present
Sinusoidal	Present
Portal tract	Present
Local infiltrates	Present
Other tissues	Present

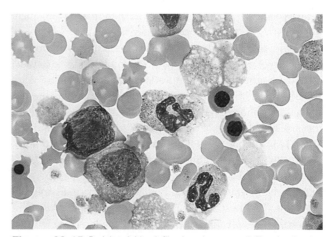

Figure 33-15 Peripheral blood film in primary myelofibrosis showing nucleated red blood cells, giant platelets, and immature myeloid cells (×1000).

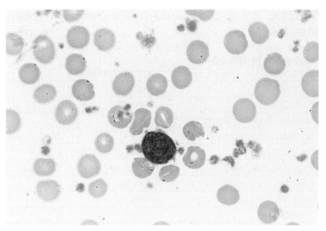

Figure 33-16 Peripheral blood film in primary myelofibrosis exhibiting increased platelets and a micromegakaryocyte (×1000).

PMF, but none has been disease-modifying, so treatment approaches have been largely palliative. Treatment has been targeted at the amelioration of anemia, hepatosplenomegaly, and constitutional symptoms. Between 34% and 54% of PMF patients present with a hemoglobin of less than 10 g/dL.[132,133] Severe anemia has been treated with androgen therapy, prednisone, danazol,[134] thalidomide,[135,136] or lenalidomide,[137] and hemolytic anemia with glucocorticosteroids. Approximately 20% of patients respond with an average duration of 1 to 2 years. Thalidomide and lenalidomide must be used with caution due to the occurrence of neuropathies and myelosuppression, particularly if the patient has been identified with del(5q31).[138]

Splenomegaly is present in 90% of patients with PMF, and 50% show hepatomegaly.[132,133] The most common first-line therapy for splenomegaly is hydroxyuria, but caution must be exercised so as not to exacerbate preexisting cytopenias.[139,140] Splenectomy and local radiation to the spleen and liver have been used in patients refractory to hydroxyuria, but patients must be carefully monitored for postoperative thrombosis, bleeding, infections, and cytopenias.[141]

The most common constitutional symptoms encountered by patients with PMF include fatigue (84%), bone pain (47%), night sweats (56%), pruritus (50%), and fever (18%).[142,143] However, treatment to alleviate these symptoms are minimally effective.

The development and testing of JAK inhibitors were directed at PMF because the symptoms and outcomes are worse compared to those of PV and ET. Among the JAK2 inhibitors tested, the four that showed the most promise were two JAK1/2 inhibitors, INCB018424 (ruxolitinib) and CYT387; one JAK2 inhibitor, TG101348; and one non-JAK inhibitor, CEP-701 (Lestaurtinib).

INCB018424 (ruxolitinib) was evaluated in a phase I/II trial at a dose of 25 mg b.i.d. and 100 mg q.d. on 153 patients with high- and moderate-risk PMF, both with primary disease and those who progressed from PV and ET. Clinical improvement associated with splenomegaly reduction (smaller spleen without progressive disease or increase in severity of anemia, thrombocytopenia, or neutropenia) was reported in 44% (16/140), and 14% (4/28) who were transfusion dependent showed anemia

improvement, while 25% (38/153) withdrew from the study due largely to grade 3 thrombocytopenia and anemia (27%) that reduced to 16% following dose reduction to 10 mg b.i.d.[144] A majority of patients reported a 50% improvement in symptoms, probably due to a measurable reduction in proinflammatory cytokines. However, there was no appreciable reduction in JAK2 V617F allele burden.[114,143] A phase III trial (COMFORT-1) of INCB018424 (ruxolitinib) is under way.

A phase I trial of TG101348 was conducted on 59 patients with high- and moderate-risk PMF at a maximum tolerated dose (MTD) of 680 mg q.d. Low-grade, transient nausea; vomiting; and diarrhea occurred in up to 69% of subjects, and along with adverse events, 45% withdrew from the study. Increases in serum lipase, transaminases, and creatinine occurred in approximately 25% of patients without any associated symptoms. Over 50% of subjects reported improvement in early satiety, night sweats, fatigue, pruritus, and cough along with a greater than 50% reduction in spleen size among 68% of the subjects. Thrombocytosis was normalized in 90% of patients and leukocytosis was normalized in 57%. In addition, 78% of patients had a 50% reduction in JAK2 V617F burden, while 13% increased and 9% remained unchanged.[145]

CYT387 is in phase I trials using 36 patients with high- and moderate-risk PMF, including 28% who were previously treated with INCB018424 or TG101348. At an MTD of 300 mg/day, all subjects continued after 15 weeks of treatment. Drug-related thrombocytopenia was observed in 22% (grade 3 or 4), anemia in 3% (grade 3), first-dose effect of lightheadedness and hypotension in 36% (grade 1), and several incidences of grade 3 adverse events, including elevations in liver and pancreatic enzymes, headaches, and QTc prolongations on ECG tracings. Reduction in splenomegaly was observed in 97% of subjects, with 37% achieving a greater than 50% response. The majority of patients reported a reduction in fatigue, pruritus, night sweats, cough, bone pain, and fever, and 41% of patients with pretreatment anemia showed clinical improvement.[146]

CEP-701 (lestaurtinib) was evaluated in phase II clinical trials at a dose of 80 mg b.i.d. using 20 patients who were JAK2 V617F positive. Twenty patients (91%) withdrew from the study for a variety of reasons, including diarrhea (73%), nausea (50%), vomiting (27%), headache (32%), mucositis (14%), peripheral neuropathy (14%), elevated transaminases (27%), anemia (27%), and thrombocytopenia (23%). Neither JAK2 V617F allele burden nor serum levels of proinflammatory cytokines were affected by therapy. However, 27% of subjects reported clinical improvement in anemia splenomegaly reduction.[147] A new phase I/II trial is under way with a new formulation of CEP-701 at higher doses.[148]

Reduction of myelofibrosis and of marrow and tissue hypercellularity has been accomplished with busulfan hydroxyurea and, in a few patients, interferon-α and interferon-γ. Radiotherapy is considered for patients with severe splenic pain, patients with massive splenomegaly who are not clinical candidates for splenectomy, patients with ascites secondary to serosal implants (metastatic nodules), and patients with localized bone pain and localized extramedullary fibrohematopoietic masses in other areas, especially in the epidural space. Splenectomy is performed to end severe pain, excessive transfusion requirements, or severe thrombocytopenia and to correct severe portal hypertension.

Chemotherapy is partially successful in reducing the number of CD34$^+$ cells and immature hematopoietic cells, marrow fibrosis, and splenomegaly.[149] Single-agent chemotherapy is most helpful in the early clinical phases of the disease, and agents such as busulfan, 6-thioguanine, and chlorambucil, alone or in combination with other chemotherapy, are useful. Other therapies include interferon-α, hydroxyurea, and combinations of the previously mentioned drugs.[150] The most successful treatment to date for patients younger than age 60 is allogeneic stem cell transplantation. Five-year survival approaches 50% in patients undergoing transplantation, but 1-year mortality is 27%, and graft-versus-host disease occurs in 33%.[151]

Average survival from the time of diagnosis is about 5 years, but patients have lived as long as 15 years. During this time, increasing numbers and pleomorphy of megakaryocytes lead to progressive marrow failure. Marrow blasts may increase.[39] Adverse prognostic indicators include more severe anemia and thrombocytopenia, greater hepatomegaly, unexplained fever, and hemolysis. Mortality is associated with infection, hemorrhage, postsplenectomy complications, and transformation to acute leukemia.

SUMMARY OF CURRENT THERAPY OF NON-*BCR/ABL1*, PRIMARY MPNs

JAK2 inhibitors are most effective in patients with PMF due in part to the more severe symptoms in PMF compared to PV and ET. INCB018424, TG101348, and CYT387 appear to have a significant effect on decreasing splenomegaly—one of the more serious symptoms in PMF patients—within the first cycle of therapy, which peaks in 3 months. Splenic responses are dose dependent, durable through 12 treatment cycles, and limited by concomitant myelosuppression. Splenomegaly quickly returns with cessation of *JAK2* inhibitors either within days for INCB018424 or within weeks for TG101348, due largely to their respective half-lives and possibly mode of action. The same three *JAK2* inhibitors improve constitutional symptoms and appear to be durable. Treatment-related anemia is associated more with some JAK1/2 inhibitors (INCB018424) than others (CYT387) and is also associated with some *JAK2* inhibitors (TG101348).[114]

In contrast, adverse events are dissimilar across the JAK inhibitors. For example, gastrointestinal events occur more frequently with the *JAK2* inhibitor (TG101348) and with the non–*JAK2* inhibitor (CEP-701), which might be due to the off-target FLT3 inhibition. Acute relapse of symptoms with drug discontinuation is seen in only one particular JAK1/2 inhibitor (INCB018424), which may be due to a "cytokine flare." Lastly, only one of the JAK1/2 inhibitors (CYT387) produces first-dose symptoms of transient hypotension, flushing, and lightheadedness. Future JAK inhibitor treatment may start with an induction dose to maximize response, followed by a maintenance dose with the addition and removal of other therapies tailored to the unique symptoms of each patient. For example, treatment-related myelosuppression could be ameliorated with

pomalidomide, androgens, erythropoietin, and transfusions, and constitutional symptoms can also be managed through a host of traditional therapies. Outcomes in PV and ET are not as impressive, and the need to modulate symptoms is not as critical. Nonetheless, the JAK2 inhibitor TG101348 is most useful due its ability to normalize leukocytosis and thrombocytosis.[114,145]

INTERCONNECTION AMONG ESSENTIAL THROMBOCYTHEMIA, POLYCYTHEMIA VERA, AND PRIMARY MYELOFIBROSIS

The discovery of the *JAK2* V617F mutation has advanced our understanding of the MPNs but has also raised questions about the interconnection of three of the primary myeloproliferative conditions: ET, PV, and PMF. Why is the *JAK2* mutation found in more than 90% to 95% of patients with PV but in only 50% to 60% of patients with ET and PMF, and how can the same mutation produce three distinct phenotypes?

Currently four hypotheses exist to account for this apparent discordance. One prevailing thought suggests that the resulting phenotype is dependent on the stage of differentiation of the hematopoietic stem cell. For example, if the hematopoietic stem cell has developed a predilection toward platelet development at the time of the *JAK2* mutation, ET will develop. Reports have described differences in differentiation programs[152,153] and in *JAK2* mutations among ET, PV, and PMF.[154] A second hypothesis proposes that the genetic background of the patient predisposes the patient to a particular phenotype. Mutations in the erythropoietin receptor, thrombopoietin receptor (MPL), and granulocyte colony-stimulating factor receptor have all been implicated.[155] The third hypothesis suggests that the phenotype depends on the level of *JAK2* tyrosine kinase activity, called the *dosage effect*. Patients diagnosed with PV showed greater tyrosine kinase activity than patients presenting with an ET phenotype. Experiments in which erythroid progenitors were collected from these patients and tested in colony-forming assays showed that nearly all the cell cultures developing a PV phenotype were homozygous for the *JAK2* mutation, whereas the ET phenotype was observed in the vast majority of cell cultures expressing a heterozygous genotype.[156,157] This phenomenon was corroborated in experiments with transgenic mice.[158,159] The last hypothesis proposes that a pre-*JAK2* mutation produces a premalignant clone,[160-162] predisposing the hematopoietic stem cell to a particular phenotype, and that the *JAK2* mutation drives the malignant transformation. Groups have reported mutations coexisting with the *JAK2* V617F mutation, like *BCR/ABL*,[163,164] MPL mutations,[165] and another version of the *JAK2* mutation.[166,167] Familial MPN provides the strongest support for a pre–*JAK2* mutation.[168,169]

The most appealing model includes all of the hypotheses previously presented and suggests that ET, PV, and PMF may represent a continuum of diseases. It seems reasonable to assume that a pre–*JAK2* mutation occurs in the hematopoietic stem cell most if not all of the time to create a hyperproliferative clone that predisposes to additional mutations like the *JAK2* mutation. The pre–*JAK2* mutation can be familial, congenital, or somatic. Because MPL is expressed in high levels on megakaryocyte precursors, one *JAK2* V617F mutation (heterozygous) is sufficient to induce MPL signaling and thus stimulate megakaryocyte production. This could lead to the ET phenotype. In contrast, the erythropoietin receptor is expressed in low density on the surface of erythroid precursors, which requires the higher amount of *JAK2* V617F tyrosine kinase that is produced by two *JAK2* mutations (homozygous). This could lead to the PV phenotype. Because MPL stimulation begins with the first *JAK2* mutation and continues with the second *JAK2* mutation, the MPL receptor undergoes continuous stimulation. It has been shown that excessive thrombopoietin stimulation leads to myelofibrosis, which may result in a progression to PMF.[170] The identification of additional mutations in the *BCR/ABL1* negative MPNs to include negative regulators of signaling pathways (*LNK, c-CBL, SOCs*), tumor suppressor genes (*IZF1, TP53*), and epigenetic regulators (*TET2, IDH1/2, ASXL1, EZH2*) combines to set the disease on a particular course. *JAK2* and MPL mutations serve as the drivers for the disease, but mutations in the negative regulators of signaling pathways may synergize with the driver mutations. Mutations in the epigenetic regulator genes may be early events that precede *JAK2* but can also appear late to promote progression. Tumor suppressor gene mutations tend to occur during phases of disease progression.[62] More than likely, most, if not all, of the hypotheses previously described function together to drive the *BCR/ABL1* negative MPNs down a particular phenotype and through the phases of clonal expansion and disease progression.

OTHER MYELOPROLIFERATIVE NEOPLASMS

Chronic Neutrophilic Leukemia

Chronic neutrophilic leukemia (CNL) is a clonal disorder in which a hyperproliferation of neutrophilic cells in the bone marrow produces sustained neutrophilia in the peripheral blood and hepatosplenomegaly. CNL must be differentiated from CML, based on the absence of the Philadelphia chromosome and the *BCR/ABL* fusion gene, as well as from both a reactive neutrophilic process and other MPNs.[171]

Incidence

The incidence of CNL is not known, but it is a rare disorder of which about 150 cases have been reported. However, if the WHO criteria had been applied in these cases, many might have been reclassified as reactive rather than neoplastic conditions.[171]

Clinical Presentation

Hepatosplenomegaly is the most common finding, but 25% to 30% of patients report bleeding from mucocutaneous sites like the gastrointestinal tract. Other symptoms include gout from WBC turnover and pruritus that may be associated with neutrophil infiltration of tissues and organs.[171]

Peripheral Blood and Bone Marrow

Patients have a WBC count of more than 25×10^9/L with a slight left shift. Neutrophils dominate, but the increase in bands, metamyelocytes, myelocytes, and promyelocytes in combination usually comprise fewer than 5% of WBCs but can

be as many as 10%. Neutrophils do not appear dysplastic, but they often contain toxic granules. RBC and platelet morphology are normal in the peripheral blood.[171]

The bone marrow reflects the peripheral blood in that it is hypercellular with predominantly a proliferation of neutrophils, including myelocytes, metamyelocytes, bands, and segmented neutrophils. The myeloid-to-erythroid ratio is at least 20:1. RBCs and platelets are normal in number, and no cell line exhibits significant dysplastic morphology.[171]

Diagnosis

The WBC count must be greater than 25×10^9/L, with greater than 90% mature neutrophils, fewer than 10% immature neutrophilic cells, and fewer than 1% blasts in the peripheral blood. The bone marrow shows an increase in normal-appearing neutrophilic cells with fewer than 5% myeloblasts. Megakaryocytes are normal or slightly left-shifted. Splenomegaly must be present and is often accompanied by hepatomegaly. Reactive neutrophilia must be excluded by eliminating infection, inflammation, and tumors as a cause of the neutrophilia. A diagnosis of CNL can still be made in the presence of a reactive process if clonality of the myeloid line can be documented by karyotyping or molecular analysis. There must be no evidence of the Philadelphia chromosome, *BCR/ABL* mutation, or rearrangements of the *PDGFRA, PDGFRB,* or *FGRF1* genes. Lastly, there can be no evidence of PV, PMF, ET, MDS, or MDS/MPN disorders.[171]

Genetics

Approximately 90% of CNL patients have a normal karyotype, but chromosomal abnormalities are observed, particularly as the disease progresses, including +8, +9, +21, del(20q), del(11q), and del(12p). The Philadelphia chromosome or a *BCR/ABL* mutation cannot be expressed in CNL; otherwise, a diagnosis of CML is required. *JAK2* mutations have been observed, but rarely.[171]

Prognosis

CNL is a slow, smoldering condition, and patient survival ranges from as short as 6 months to longer than 20 years. The neutrophilia does progress, and some patients develop myelodysplasia and can experience transformation into AML.[171]

Chronic Eosinophilic Leukemia, Not Otherwise Specified

Chronic eosinophilic leukemia (CEL) is a clonal proliferation of eosinophils from eosinophil precursors that dominate in the bone marrow and peripheral blood. Eosinophils are found in other peripheral tissues, including heart, lungs, central nervous system, gastrointestinal tract, and skin. Hepatosplenomegaly is observed in approximately 30% to 50% of patients. Infiltrating eosinophils degranulate to release cytokines, enzymes, and other granular proteins that damage the surrounding tissue, which results in organ dysfunction.[172]

Clinical Presentation

Although some patients may be asymptomatic when found to have eosinophilia, most have signs and symptoms of fever, fatigue, cough, angioedema, muscle pain, and pruritus. A more severe sequela of CEL involves the heart. Fibrosis can form in the heart (endomyocardial fibrosis), which can evolve into cardiomegaly. Within the heart, scar tissue may form in the mitral and tricuspid valves, affecting valve function and predisposing to thrombi formation. Other serious complications include peripheral neuropathy, central nervous system dysfunction, pulmonary symptoms from eosinophilic infiltrates, and rheumatologic problems.[172]

Peripheral Blood and Bone Marrow

Peripheral eosinophilia must be observed, with the majority of eosinophils appearing normal. Some evidence of eosinophil abnormality is found, however, and includes the presence of eosinophilic myelocytes and metamyelocytes, hypogranulation, and vacuolization. Neutrophilia is a common finding; other features such as mild monocytosis, basophilia, and the presence of blasts are less common. The bone marrow is hypercellular owing to eosinophilic proliferation and can demonstrate Charcot-Leyden crystals. Myeloblast numbers are elevated but below the 20% threshold necessary to classify the disorder as an acute leukemia. Erythrocytes and megakaryocytes are normal in number but sometimes demonstrate dysplastic morphologic features. Bone marrow fibrosis occurs due to the release of eosinophilic basic protein and eosinophilic cationic proteins from the eosinophil granules. Bone marrow fibrosis contributes to the premature release of eosinophils into the circulation, and they deposit in a variety of tissues.[172]

Diagnosis

The diagnosis of CEL requires eosinophilia with a count of more than 1.5×10^9 cells/L and the presence of malignant features, and the elimination of reactive eosinophilia and other malignancies that have concomitant eosinophilia. Reactive conditions like parasitic infections, allergies, Loeffler syndrome (pulmonary disease), cyclical eosinophilia, angiolymphoid hyperplasia of the skin, collagen vascular disorders, and Kimura disease must be excluded in the differential diagnosis. Likewise, other malignancies that can produce a concomitant eosinophilia include T cell lymphoma, Hodgkin lymphoma, systemic mastocytosis, chronic myelomonocytic leukemia, atypical CML, and ALL. These disorders lead to the release of a variety of interleukins that can drive a secondary eosinophil reaction. No single genetic abnormality is specific for CEL, but CEL can be ruled out by the presence of several karyotypic abnormalities, such as *PDGFRA*, *PDGFRB*, *FGFR1*, and *BCR/ABL*. Common myeloid mutations like +8, i(17q), and *JAK2* can support a diagnosis of CEL.[172]

Prognosis

Survival is variable, but approximately 80% of patients will live 5 years after diagnosis. Features of dysplasia, an increase in karyotype abnormalities, or an increase in blasts indicates an unfavorable prognosis.[172]

Mastocytosis

Mastocytosis is a broad term referring to a clonal neoplastic proliferation of mast cells, which accumulate in one or more organ systems, but it can present differently and manifest in a range of severities. The WHO group has classified mastocytosis into seven subcategories: cutaneous mastocytosis, indolent systemic mastocytosis, systemic mastocytosis with associated clonal hematologic non–mast-cell-lineage disease, aggressive systemic mastocytosis, mast cell leukemia, mast cell sarcoma, and extracutaneous mastocytoma.[173]

Incidence

Mastocytosis can occur at any age, with cutaneous mastocytosis seen most often in children. Babies can be born with cutaneous mastocytosis, and half of affected children develop the disease before 6 months of age. In contrast, systemic mastocytosis generally occurs after the second decade of life. Approximately 80% of patients with mastocytosis show skin involvement regardless of the type of mastocytosis diagnosed. Cutaneous mastocytosis occurs in the skin; systemic mastocytosis usually involves the bone marrow and other organ systems like the spleen, lymph nodes, liver, and gastrointestinal tract; and mast cell leukemia is characterized by mast cells in the peripheral blood.[173]

Clinical Presentation

Patients present with urticarial lesions (wheel and flare) that may become activated when stroked upon physical examination. Skin lesions also tend to have melanin pigmentation. Four categories of symptom severity have been described in mastocytosis: constitutional systems like fatigue and weight loss; skin manifestations; mediator-related systemic events such as abdominal pain, gastrointestinal distress, headache, and respiratory symptoms; and musculoskeletal complaints like bone pain, arthralgias, and myalgias. Hematologic findings include anemia, leukocytosis, eosinophilia, neutropenia, and thrombocytopenia. In patients with systemic mastocytosis with associated clonal hematologic non–mast-cell-lineage disease the most common associated hematologic finding is chronic myelomonocytic leukemia, but any myeloid or lymphoid malignancy can occur, although myeloid versions predominate.[173]

Diagnosis

The typical skin lesion is the first diagnostic clue to mastocytosis. Cutaneous mastocytosis occurs in three forms: urticaria pigmentosa, diffuse cutaneous mastocytosis, and mastocytosis of the skin, all of which occur predominantly in children. In urticaria pigmentosa, mast cells are confined to the skin and form aggregates in the dermis, whereas in diffuse cutaneous mastocytosis, mast cells are found in more than one cutaneous location. In systemic mastocytosis, mast cells are observed in one area of the bone marrow with fibrosis, other areas of the bone marrow are hypercellular with panmyelosis, and/or mast cells are identified in other extracutaneous sites. In addition to the major criteria just described, at least one of four minor criteria must be met. These include (1) more than 25% of mast cells must be immature or have atypical morphology, like a spindle shape; (2) mast cells must express a *KIT* mutation at codon 816; (3) mast cells must express normal markers and CD2 and/or CD25; and (4) total serum tryptase must be above

20 mg/mL. Key diagnostic features distinguish the six types of systemic mastocytosis. Indolent systemic mastocytosis is characterized by a low–mast cell burden. Systemic mastocytosis with associated clonal hematologic non–mast-cell-lineage disease presents with myelodysplastic syndrome, myeloproliferative neoplasm, AML, lymphoma, or another hematopoietic neoplasm. Aggressive systemic mastocytosis usually does not manifest with skin lesions or mast cells in circulation but does have mast cells in bone marrow, dysplastic hematopoietic changes, and/or hepatosplenomegaly. Mast cell leukemia is characterized by more than 20% atypical mast cells in the bone marrow and more than 10% in the peripheral blood. Mast cell sarcoma presents as a single unifocal mast cell tumor with a high-grade pathology. Extracutaneous mastocytoma also exhibits a unifocal mast cell tumor, but it is of low-grade pathology.[173]

Genetics

The most common genetic mutation in patients with mastocytosis involves codon 816 in the *KIT* gene and occurs in about 95% of adults and 33% of children with systemic mastocytosis. This mutation replaces aspartic acid with valine, which alters the tyrosine kinase receptor activity so as to cause constitutive kinase activity in the absence of ligand. Usually the mutation is somatic, but a few cases of familial *KIT* mutations have been reported. Additional mutations can push proliferation of hematopoietic clones, causing systemic mastocytosis with associated clonal hematologic non–mast-cell-lineage disease. These include mutations of *RUNX1/RUNX1T* in AML, *JAK1* in MPN, and *FIP1L1/PDGFRA* in myeloid neoplasms with eosinophilia.[173]

Prognosis

Cutaneous mastocytosis in children has a favorable prognosis and may regress spontaneously around puberty. Milder versions like cutaneous mastocytosis and indolent cutaneous mastocytosis follow a benign course and are associated with a normal life span. Hematologic involvement usually evolves into the corresponding hematologic disease. Patients with aggressive systemic mastocytosis, mast cell leukemia, and mast cell sarcoma are often treated with cytoreductive chemotherapy but may survive only a few months after diagnosis. Signs and symptoms that predict a poorer prognosis include elevated lactate dehydrogenase and alkaline phosphatase, anemia, thrombocythemia, abnormal peripheral blood morphology, bone marrow hypercellularity, and hepatosplenomegaly.[173]

Myeloproliferative Neoplasm, Unclassifiable

The category *myeloproliferative neoplasm, unclassifiable* (MPN-U) is designed to capture disorders that clearly express myeloproliferative features but either fail to meet the criteria of a specific condition or have features that overlap two or more specific conditions. Most patients with MPN-U fall into one of three groups: patients with an early stage of PV, ET, or PMF in which the criteria that define the disorders are not yet fully developed; patients presenting with features indicative of advanced disease resulting from clonal evolution that masks the potential underlying condition; and patients who have clear evidence of an MPN but who have a concomitant condition like a second neoplasm or an inflammatory condition that alters the MPN features. MPN-U may account for as many as 10% to 15% of MPN disorders, but caution should be exercised so that morphologic changes caused by the patient's cytotoxic drug therapy or growth factor therapy or poor collection of samples are not confused with the features of MPN-U. In patients with MPN-U in the early stages of development or with a concomitant disorder like inflammation, the MPN-U may be reclassified to a specific category of MPN once the disease begins to express typical features or the secondary condition subsides. Likewise, in patients with an advanced MPN, the disorder may be reclassified as an acute leukemia once the blast criterion of more than 20% blasts in the bone marrow is met.[174]

SUMMARY

- MPNs are clonal hematopoietic stem cell disorders that result in excessive production and overaccumulation of erythrocytes, granulocytes, and platelets in some combination in bone marrow, peripheral blood, and body tissues.
- Within the classification of MPN, the four major conditions are CML, PV, ET, and PMF.
- In CML, there are large numbers of myeloid precursors in the bone marrow, peripheral blood, and extramedullary tissues.
- The peripheral blood exhibits leukocytosis with increased myeloid series, particularly the later maturation stages, often with increases in eosinophils and basophils.
- The LAP score is dramatically decreased in CML.
- The Philadelphia chromosome, t(9;22), either at the chromosomal or molecular level, must be present in all cases of CML.
- In CML, the bone marrow exhibits intense hypercellularity with a predominance of myeloid precursors. Megakaryocyte numbers are normal to increased.

- Patients with CML progress from a chronic stable phase through an accelerated phase into transformation to acute leukemia.
- Bone marrow transplantation has been successful in CML, and imatinib mesylate, a tyrosine kinase inhibitor, produces remission in most cases.
- Approximately 4% of CML patients given imatinib as first-line therapy develop imatinib resistance.
- Dosage escalation or administration of second-generation tyrosine kinase inhibitors restores remission in most patients with imatinib resistance.
- PV manifests with panmyelosis in the bone marrow with increases in erythrocytes, granulocytes, and platelets.
- The clinical diagnosis of PV requires a hemoglobin of greater than 18.5 g/dL in men and greater than 16.5 g/dL in women or other evidence of increased RBC volume and the presence of *JAK2* V617F or another mutation in the *JAK2* gene. If only one of these major criteria is met, two of the minor criteria must be satisfied.

- The *JAK2* V617F mutation is found in 90% to 95% of PV patients and contributes to the pathogenesis of the disease.
- PV is currently treated with phlebotomy, hydroxyuria, and low-dose aspirin, and then with *JAK2* inhibitors in the future.
- ET involves an increase in megakaryocytes with a sustained platelet count greater than 450×10^9/L.
- Other diagnostic criteria include normal RBC mass, stainable iron in the bone marrow, absence of the Philadelphia chromosome, lack of marrow collagen fibrosis, absence of splenomegaly or leukoerythroblastic reaction, and absence of any known cause of reactive thrombocytosis.
- In the early phases of ET, peripheral blood shows increased numbers of platelets with abnormalities in size and shape. Bone marrow megakaryocytes are increased in number and in size.
- Complications of ET include thromboembolism and hemorrhage.
- The *JAK2* V617F mutation is observed in 50% to 60% of patients with ET and PMF and contributes to the pathogenesis of the disorders.
- PMF manifests with ineffective hematopoiesis, sparse areas of marrow hypercellularity (especially with increased megakaryocytes), bone marrow fibrosis, splenomegaly, and hepatomegaly.
- The peripheral blood in PMF exhibits immature granulocytes and nucleated RBCs; teardrop-shaped cells are a common finding.
- Platelets may be normal, increased, or decreased in number with abnormal morphology. Micromegakaryocytes may be present.
- Immune responses are altered in about 50% of patients.
- Treatment of PMF includes a variety of approaches to include transfusions, hydroxyuria, INF-γ, busulfan, androgens, erythropoietin, and others.
- JAK inhibitors improve splenomegaly and constitutional symptoms in patients with PMF to a greater degree than in ET or PV.
- Other MPNs include CNL, CEL not otherwise specified, mastocytosis, and unclassifiable MPN.

Now that you have completed this chapter, go back and read again the case study at the beginning and respond to the questions presented.

REVIEW QUESTIONS

Answers can be found in the Appendix.

1. A peripheral blood film that shows increased neutrophils, basophils, eosinophils, and platelets is highly suggestive of:
   a. AML
   b. CML
   c. MDS
   d. Multiple myeloma

2. Which of the following chromosome abnormalities is associated with CML?
   a. t(15;17)
   b. t(8;14)
   c. t(9;22)
   d. Monosomy 7

3. A patient has a WBC count of 30×10^9/L and the following WBC differential:
   Segmented neutrophils—38%
   Bands—17%
   Metamyelocytes—7%
   Myelocytes—20%
   Promyelocytes—10%
   Eosinophils—3%
   Basophils—5%
   Which of the following test results would be helpful in determining whether the patient has CML?
   a. Nitroblue tetrazolium reduction product increased
   b. Myeloperoxidase increased
   c. Periodic acid–Schiff staining decreased
   d. FISH positive for *BCR/ABL1* fusion

4. A patient in whom CML has previously been diagnosed has circulating blasts and promyelocytes that total 30% of leukocytes. The disease is considered to be in what phase?
   a. Chronic stable phase
   b. Accelerated phase
   c. Transformation to acute leukemia
   d. Temporary remission

5. The most common mutation found in patients with primary PV is:
   a. *BCR/ABL*
   b. Philadelphia chromosome
   c. *JAK2* V617F
   d. t(15;17)

6. The peripheral blood in PV typically manifests:
   a. Erythrocytosis only
   b. Erythrocytosis and thrombocytosis
   c. Erythrocytosis, thrombocytosis, and granulocytosis
   d. Anemia and thrombocytopenia

7. A patient has a platelet count of 700×10^9/L with abnormalities in the size, shape, and granularity of platelets; a WBC count of 12×10^9/L; and hemoglobin of 11 g/dL. The Philadelphia chromosome is not present. The most likely diagnosis is:
   a. PV
   b. ET
   c. CML
   d. Leukemoid reaction

8. Complications of ET include all of the following *except:*
   a. Thrombosis
   b. Hemorrhage
   c. Seizures
   d. Infections

9. Which of the following patterns is characteristic of the peripheral blood in patients with PMF?
   a. Teardrop-shaped erythrocytes, nucleated RBCs, immature granulocytes
   b. Abnormal platelets only
   c. Hypochromic erythrocytes, immature granulocytes, and normal platelets
   d. Spherocytes, immature granulocytes, and increased numbers of platelets

10. The myelofibrosis associated with PMF is a result of:
    a. Apoptosis resistance in the fibroblasts of the bone marrow
    b. Impaired production of normal collagenase by the mutated cells
    c. Enhanced activity of fibroblasts owing to increased stimulatory cytokines
    d. Increased numbers of fibroblasts owing to cytokine stimulation of the pluripotential stem cells

REFERENCES

1. Delhommeau, F., Pisani, D. F., James, C., et al. (2006). Oncogenic mechanisms in myeloproliferative disorders. *Cell Mol Life Sci, 63*(24), 2939–2953.
2. Campbell, P. J., & Green, A. R. (2006). The myeloproliferative disorders. *N Engl J Med, 7,* 355(23), 2452–2466.
3. Fialkow, P. J., Jacobson, R. J., & Papayannopoulou, T. (1977). Chronic myelocytic leukemia: clonal origin in a stem cell common to the granulocytic, erythrocytic, platelet and monocyte/macrophage. *Am J Med, 63,* 125–130.
4. Adamson, J. W., Fialkow, P. J., Murphy, S., et al. (1976). Polycythemia vera: stem-cell and probable clonal origin of the disease. *N Engl J Med, 295,* 913–916.
5. Fialkow, P. J., Faguet, G. B., Jacobson, R. J., et al. (1981). Evidence that essential thrombocythemia is a clonal disorder with origin in a multipotent stem cell. *Blood, 58,* 916–919.
6. Jacobson, R. J., Salo, A., & Fialkow, P. J. (1978). Agnogenic myeloid metaplasia: a clonal proliferation of hematopoietic stem cells with secondary myelofibrosis. *Blood, 51,* 189–194.
7. Dameshek, W. (1951). Some speculations on the myeloproliferative syndromes. *Blood, 6,* 372 (editorial).
8. Vardiman, J. W., Thiele, J., Arber, D. A., et al. (2009). The 2008 revision of the World Health Organization (WHO) classification of myeloid neoplasms and acute leukemia: rationale and important changes. *Blood, 114,* 937–951.
9. Whang, J., Frei, E. III., Tijo, J. H., et al. (1963). The distribution of the Philadelphia chromosome in patients with chronic myelogenous leukemia. *Blood, 22,* 664–673.
10. Spiers, A. S., Bain, B. J., & Turner, J. E. (1977). The peripheral blood in chronic granulocytic leukemia: study of 50 untreated Philadelphia-positive cases. *Scand J Hematol, 18,* 25–28.
11. Ward, H. P., & Block, M. H. (1971). The natural history of agnogenic myeloid metaplasia (AMM) and a critical evaluation of its relationship with the myeloproliferative syndrome. *Medicine (Baltimore), 150,* 357–420.
12. Mitus, A. J., & Schafer, A. I. (1990). Thrombocytosis and thrombocythemia. *Hematol Oncol Clin North Am, 4,* 157–178.
13. Gilbert, H. S. (1998). Familial myeloproliferative disease. *Ballieres Clin Haematol, 11,* 849–858.
14. Barr, R. D., & Fialkow, P. J. (1973). Clonal origin of chronic myelocytic leukemia. *N Engl J Med, 289,* 307–309.
15. Bizzozzero, O. J., Johnson, K. G., & Ciocco, A. (1966). Radiation-related leukemia in Hiroshima and Nagasaki, 1946-1964: I. Distribution, incidence, and appearance time. *N Engl J Med, 274,* 1095–1101.
16. Brown, W. M., & Doll, R. (1965). Mortality from cancer and other causes after radiotherapy for ankylosing spondylitis. *BMJ, 5474,* 1327–1332.
17. Marmont, A., Frassoni, F., Bacigalupo, A., et al. (1984). Recurrence of Ph¹-positive leukemia in donor cells after marrow transplantation for chronic granulocytic leukemia. *N Engl J Med, 310,* 903–906.
18. Nowell, P., & Hungerford, D. A. (1960). A minute chromosome in human granulocytic leukemia. *Science, 132,* 1497–1499.
19. Rowley, J. D. (1973). A new consistent chromosome abnormality in chronic myelogenous leukemia identified by quinacrine fluorescence and Giemsa banding. *Nature, 243,* 290–293.
20. Stam, K., Heisterkamp, N., Grosveld, G., et al. (1985). Evidence of a new chimeric bcr/c-abl mRNA in patients with chronic myelocytic leukemia and the Philadelphia chromosome. *N Engl J Med, 313,* 1429–1433.
21. Groffen, J., Stephenson, J. R., Heisterkamp, N., et al. (1984). Philadelphia chromosomal breakpoints are clustered within a limited region, bcr, on chromosome 22. *Cell, 36*(1), 93–99.
22. Randolph, T. R. (2005). Chronic myelocytic leukemia part I: history, clinical presentation, and molecular biology. *Clin Lab Sci, 18*(1), 38–48.
23. Faderl, S., Talpaz, M., Estrov, Z., et al. (1999). Mechanisms of disease: the biology of chronic myeloid leukemia. *N Engl J Med, 341*(3), 164–172.
24. Epner, D. E., & Koeffler, H. P. (1990). Molecular genetic advances in chronic myelogenous leukemia. *Ann Intern Med, 113,* 3–6.
25. Douer, D., Levine, A. M., Sparkes, R. S., et al. (1981). Chronic myelocytic leukemia: a pluripotent haemopoietic cell is involved in the malignant clone. *Br J Haematol, 49,* 615–619.
26. Bhatia, R., & Verfaillie, C. M. (1998). The effects of interferon-alpha on beta-1 integrin mediated adhesion and growth regulation in chronic myelogenous leukemia. *Leuk Lymphoma, 28,* 241–254.
27. Georgii, A., Buesche, G., & Krept, A. (1998). The histopathology of chronic myeloproliferative disorders: review. *Ballieres Clin Haematol, 11,* 721–749.
28. Klineberg, J. R., Bluestone, R., Schlosstein, L., et al. (1973). Urate deposition disease: how it is regulated and how can it be modified? *Ann Intern Med, 78,* 99–111.
29. Lichtman, M. A., & Rowe, J. M. (1982). Hyperleukocytic leukemias: rheological, clinical and therapeutic considerations. *Blood, 60,* 279–283.
30. Lichtman, M. A., Heal, J., & Rowe, J. M. (1987). Hyperleukocytic leukemia. *Ballieres Clin Haematol, 1,* 725–746.
31. Muehleck, S. D., McKenna, R. D., Arthur, D. C., et al. (1984). Transformation of chronic myelogenous leukemia: clinical, morphologic and cytogenetic features. *Am J Clin Pathol, 82,* 1–14.
32. Vardiman, J. W., Melo, J. V., Baccarani, M., et al. (2008). Chronic myelogenous leukemia. BCR-ABL1 positive. In Swerdlow, S. H.,

Campo, E., Harris, N. L., et al., (Eds.), *WHO classification of tumours of haematopoietic and lymphoid tissues.* (4th ed., pp. 32–37). Lyon, France: IARC Press.

33. Bernstein, R. (1988). Cytogenetics of chronic myelogenous leukemia. *Semin Hematol, 25,* 20–34.

34. Sandberg, A. A. (1978). Chromosomes in the chronic phase of CML. *Virchows Arch B Cell Pathol, 29,* 51–55.

35. Bareford, D., & Jacobs, P. (1980). Chronic neutrophilic leukemia. *Am J Clin Pathol, 73,* 837.

36. Bearman, R. M., Kjeldsburg, C. R., Pangalis, G. A., et al. (1981). Chronic monocytic leukemia in adults. *Cancer, 48,* 2239–2255.

37. Thomas, W. J., North, R. B., Poplack, D. G., et al. (1981). Chronic myelomonocytic leukemia in childhood. *Am J Hematol, 10,* 181–194.

38. Mijovic, A., & Mufti, G. J. (1998). The myelodysplastic syndromes: towards a functional classification. *Blood Rev, 12,* 73–83.

39. Kurzrock, R., Gutterman, J. U., & Talpaz, M. (1988). The molecular genetics of Philadelphia chromosome positive leukemias. *N Engl J Med, 319,* 990–998.

40. Specchia, G., Mininni, D., Guerrasio, A., et al. (1995). Ph positive acute lymphoblastic leukemia in adults: molecular and clinical studies. *Leuk Lymphoma, 18*(Suppl.), 37–42.

41. Faderl, S., Talpaz, M., Estrov, A., et al. (1999). Chronic myelogenous leukemia: biology and therapy. *Ann Intern Med, 131,* 207–219.

42. Catovsky, D. (1979). Ph[1]-positive acute leukemia and chronic granulocytic leukemia: one or two diseases? *Br J Haematol, 42,* 493–498.

43. Wintrobe, M. M., Huguley, C. M., McLennan, M. T., et al. (1947). Nitrogen mustard as a therapeutic agent for Hodgkin's disease, lymphosarcoma and leukemia. *Ann Intern Med, 27,* 529–539.

44. Galton, D. A. (1953). The use of myleran in chronic myeloid leukemia: results of treatment. *Lancet, 264,* 208–213.

45. Lion, T., Gaiger, A., Henn, T., et al. (1995). Use of quantitative polymerase chain reaction to monitor residual disease in chronic myelogenous leukemia during treatment with interferon. *Leukemia, 9,* 1353–1360.

46. Sawyers, C. L. (1999). Chronic myeloid leukemia. *N Engl J Med, 340,* 1330–1340.

47. Guilhot, F., Chastang, C., Michallet, M., et al. (1997). Interferon alpha 2b combined with cytarabine versus interferon alone in chronic myelogenous leukemia. *N Engl J Med, 337,* 223–229.

48. O'Brien, S. G. (1997). Autografting for chronic myeloid leukemia. *Baillieres Clin Haematol, 10,* 369–388.

49. Atwell, S., Adams, J. M., Badger, J., et al. (2004). A novel mode of Gleevec binding is revealed by the structure of spleen tyrosine kinase. *J Biol Chem, 279*(53), 55827–55832.

50. Druker, B. J., Talpaz, M., Resta, D. J., et al. (2001). Efficacy and safety of a specific inhibitor of the BCR-ABL tyrosine kinase in chronic myeloid leukemia. *N Engl J Med, 344,* 1031–1037.

51. Lin, F., Drummond, M., O'Brien, S., et al. (2003). Molecular monitoring in chronic myeloid leukemia patients who achieve complete remission on imatinib. *Blood, 102,* 1143 (letter).

52. Bhamidipati, P. K., Kantarjian, H., Cortex, J., et al. (2013). Management of imatinib-resistant patients with chronic myeloid leukemia. *Ther Adv Hem, 4*(2), 103–117.

53. Nardi, A., Azam, M., & Daley, G. O. (2004). Mechanisms and implications of imatinib resistance mutations in BCR-ABL. *Curr Opin Hematol, 11,* 35–43.

54. Kantarjian, H. M., Talpaz, M., Giles, F., et al. (2006). New insights into the pathophysiology of chronic myeloid leukemia and imatinib resistance. *Ann Intern Med, 145,* 913–923.

55. Narayanan, V., Pollyea, D. A., Gutman, J. A., et al. (2013). Ponatinib for the treatment of chronic myeloid leukemia and Philadelphia chromosome-positive acute lymphoblastic leukemia. *Drugs Today, 49*(4), 261–269.

56. Gilliland, D. G., Blanchard, K. L., Levy, J., et al. (1991). Clonality in myeloproliferative disorders: analysis by means of the polymerase chain reaction. *Proc Natl Acad Sci U S A, 88,* 6848–6852.

57. Prchal, J. F., Adamson, J. W., Murphy, S., et al. (1978). Polycythemia vera: the in vitro response of normal and abnormal stem cell lines to erythropoietin. *J Clin Invest, 61,* 1044–1047.

58. Adamson, J. W., Singer, J. W., Catalano, P., et al. (1980). Polycythemia vera: further in vitro studies of hematopoietic regulation. *J Clin Invest, 66,* 1363–1368.

59. Tefferi, A., Thiele, J., & Vardiman, J. W. (2009). The World Health Organization classification system for myeloproliferative neoplasms: order out of chaos. *Cancer, 115*(17), 3842–3847.

60. Kralovicics, R., Guan, Y., & Prchal, J. T. (2002). Acquired uniparental disomy of chromosome 9p is a frequent stem cell defect in polycythemia vera. *Exp Hematol, 30*(3), 229–236.

61. Wahab-Abdel, O. (2011). Genetics of the myeloproliferative neoplasms. *Curr Opin Hematol, 18,* 117–123.

62. Vainchenker, W., Delhommeau, F., Constantinescu, S. N., et al. (2011). New mutations and pathogenesis of myeloproliferative neoplasms. *Blood, 118*(7), 1723–1735.

63. James, C., Ugo, V., Le Couedic, J. P., et al. (2005). A unique clonal JAK2 mutation leading to constitutive signalling causes polycythemia vera. *Nature, 434,* 1144–1148.

64. Baxter, E. J., Scott, L. M., Campbell, P. J., et al. (2005). Acquired mutation of the tyrosine kinase JAK2 in human myeloproliferative disorders. *Lancet, 365,* 1054–1061.

65. Levine, R. L., Wadleigh, M., Cools, J., et al. (2005). Activating mutation in the tyrosine kinase JAK2 in polycythemia vera, essential thrombocythemia, and myeloid metaplasia with myelofibrosis. *Cancer Cell, 7,* 387–397.

66. Shi, S., Calhgoun, H. C., Xai, F., et al. (2006). JAK signaling globally counteracts heterochromatic gene silencing. *Nat Genet, 38*(9), 1071–1076.

67. Shi, S., Larson, K., Guo, D., et al. (2008). Drosophila STAT is required for directly maintaining HP1localization and heterochromatin stability. *Nat Cell Biol, 10*(4), 489–496.

68. Liu, F., Zhao, X., Pema, F., et al. (2011). JAK2V617F-mediated phosphorylation of PRMT5 downregulates its methyltransferase activity and promotes myeloproliferation. *Cancer Cell, 19*(2), 283–294.

69. Pikman, Y., Lee, B. H., Mercher, T., et al. (2006). MPLW515L is a novel somatic activating mutation in myelofibrosis with myeloid metaplasia. *PLoS Med, 3,* e270.

70. Beer, P. A., Campbell, P. J., Scott, L. M., et al. (2008). MPL mutations in myeloproliferative disorders; analysis of the PT-1 cohort. *Blood, 112*(1), 141–149.

71. Boyd, E. M., Bench, A. J., Goday-Fernandez, A., et al. (2010). Clinical utility of routing MPL exon 10 analysis in the diagnosis of essential thrombocythaemia and primary myelofibrosis. *Br J Haematol, 149*(2), 250–257.

72. Chaligne, R., Tonetti, C., Besancenot, R., et al. (2008). New mutations in MPL in primitive myelofibrosis: only the MPL W515L mutations promote a G1/S-phase transition. *Leukemia, 22*(8), 1557–1566.

73. Pietra, D., Brisci, A., Rumi, E., et al. (2011). Deep sequencing reveals double mutations in cis of MPL exon 10 in myeloproliferative neoplasms. *Haematologica, 96*(4), 607–611.

74. Scott, L. M., Tong, W., Levine, R. L., et al. (2007). JAK2 exon 12 mutations in polycythemia vera and idiopathic erythrocytosis. *N Engl J Med, 356,* 459–468.

75. Passamonti, F., Elena, C., Schnittger, S., et al. (2011). Molecular and clinical features of the myeloproliferative neoplasm associated with JAK2 exon 12 mutations [published online ahead of print January 11, 2011]. *Blood,* doi:10.1182/blood-2010-11-316810.

76. Jones, A. V., Chase, A., Silver, R. T., et al. (2009). JAK2 haplotype is a major risk factor for the development of myeloproliferative neoplasms. *Nat Genet, 41,* 446–449.

77. Kilpivaara, O., Mukherjee, S., Schram, A. M., et al. (2009). A germline JAK2 SNP is associated predisposition to the development of JAK2(V617F)-positive myeloproliferative neoplasms. *Nat Genet, 41,* 455–459.

78. Olcaydu, D., Harutyunyan, A., Jager, R., et al. (2009). A common JAK2 haplotype confers susceptibility to myeloproliferative neoplasms. *Nat Genet, 41,* 450–454.

79. Lasho, T. L., Pardanani, A., Tefferi, A. (2010). LNK mutations in JAK2 mutation-negative erythropoiesis. *N Engl J Med, 363,* 1189–1190.

80. Oh, S. T., Simonds, E. F., Jones, C., et al. (2010). Novel mutations in the inhibitory adaptor protein LNK drive JAK-STAT signaling in patients with myeloproliferative neoplasms. *Blood, 116,* 988–992.

81. Pardanani, A., Lasho, T., Finke, C., et al. (2010). LNK mutation studies in blast-phase myeloproliferative neoplasms, and in chronic–phase disease with TET2, IDH, JAK2 or MPL mutations. *Leukemia, 24*(10), 1713–1718.

82. Delhommeau, F., Dupont, S., Della Valle, V., et al. (2009). Mutations in TET2 in myeloid cancers. *N Engl J Med, 360,* 2289–2301.

83. Tahiliani, M., Koh, K. P., Shen, Y., et al. (2009). Conversion of 5-methylcytosine to 5-hydroxymethylcytosine in mammalian DNA by MLL partner TET1. *Science, 324,* 930–935.

84. Figueroa, M., Abdel-Wahab, O., Lu, C., et al. (2010). Leukemic IDH1 and IDH2 mutations result in a hypermethylation phenotype, disrupt TET2 function, and impair hematopoietic differentiation. *Cancer Cell, 18,* 553–567.

85. Tefferi, A., Lasho, T. L., Abdel-Wahab, O., et al. (2010). IDH1 and IDH2 mutation studies in 1473 patients with chronic-, fibrotic-, or blast-phase essential thrombocythemia, polycythemia vera or myelofibrosis. *Leukemia, 24,* 1302–1309.

86. Dang, L., White, D. W., Gross, S., et al. (2009). Cancer-associated IDH1 mutations produce 2-hydroxyglutarate. *Nature, 462,* 739–744.

87. Cao, R. & Zhang, Y. (2004). The functions of E(Z)/EZH2-mediated methylation of lysine 27 in histone H3. *Curr Opin Genet Dev, 14*(2), 155–164.

88. Ernest, T., Chase, A. J., Score, J., et al. (2010). Inactivating mutations of the histone methyltransferase gene EZH2 in myeloid disorders. *Nat Genet, 42,* 722–776.

89. Nikoloski, G., Langemeijer, S. M., Kuiper, R. P., et al. (2010). Somatic mutations of the histone methyltransferase gene EZH2 in myelodysplastic syndromes. *Nat Genet, 42,* 665–667.

90. Sauvageau, M., & Sauvaheau, G. (2010). Polycomb group proteins: multi-faceted regulators of somatic stem cells and cancer. *Cell Stem Cell, 7*(3), 299–313.

91. Scheuermann, J. C., de Ayala Alonso, A. G., Oktaba, K., et al. (2010). Histone H2A deubiquitinas activity of the Polycomb repressor complex PR-DUB. *Nature, 465*(7295), 243–247.

92. Carbuccia, N., Murati, A., Trouplin, V., et al. (2009). Mutations of ASXL1 gene in myeloproliferative neoplasms. *Leukemia, 23*(11), 2183–2186.

93. Tefferi, A. (2010). Novel mutations and their functional clinical relevance in myeloproliferative neoplasms: JAK2, MPL, TET2, ASXL1, CBL, IDH and IKZF1. *Leukemia, 24*(6), 1128–1138.

94. Najean, Y., & Rain, J. D. (1997). The very long-term evolution of polycythemia vera: an analysis of 318 patients initially treated by phlebotomy or 32P between 1969 and 1981. *Semin Hematol, 34*(1), 6–16.

95. Campbell, P. J., Baxter, E. J., Beer, P. A., et al. (2006). Mutation of JAK2 in the myeloproliferative disorders: timing, clonality studies, cytogenetic associations, and role in leukemic transformation. *Blood, 108*(10), 3548–3555.

96. Mesa, R. A., Li, C. Y., Ketterling, R. P., et al. (2005). Leukemic transformation in myelofibrosis with myeloid metaplasia: a single-institution experience with 91 cases. *Blood, 105*(3), 973–977.

97. Beer, P. A., Delhommeau, F., LeCouedic, J. P., et al. (2010). Two routes to leukemic transformation after a JAK2 mutation-positive myeloproliferative neoplasm. *Blood, 115*(14), 2891–2900.

98. Harutyunyan, A., Klampfl, T., Cazzola, M., et al. (2011). p53 lesions in leukemic transformation. *N Engl J Med, 364*(5), 488–490.

99. Beer, P. A., Ortmann, C. A., Campbell, P. J., et al. (2010). Independently acquired biallelic JAK2 mutations are present in a minority of patients with essential thrombocythemia. *Blood, 116*(6), 1013–1014.

100. Berlin, N. (1975). Diagnosis and classification of the polycythemias. *Semin Hematol, 12,* 339–351.

101. Berk, P. D., Goldberg, J. N., Donovan, P. B., et al. (1986). Therapeutic recommendations in polycythemia vera based on Polycythemia Vera Study Group protocols. *Semin Hematol, 23,* 132–143.

102. Wolf, B. C., Bank, P. M., Mann, R. B., et al. (1988). Splenic hematopoiesis in polycythemia vera: a morphologic and immunohistologic study. *Am J Clin Pathol, 89,* 69–75.

103. Ellis, J. T., Peterson, P., Geller, S. A., et al. (1986). Studies of the bone marrow in polycythemia vera and the evolution of myelofibrosis and second hematologic malignancies. *Semin Hematol, 23,* 144–155.

104. Landolfi, R., Marchioli, R., Kutti, J., et al. (2004). Efficacy and safety of low-dose aspirin in polycythemia vera. *N Engl J Med, 350,* 114–124.

105. Quintas-Cardama, A., Kantarjian, H., Manshouri, T., et al. (2009). Pegylated interferon alfa-2a yields high rates of hematologic and molecular response in patients with advanced essential thrombocythemia and polycythemia vera. *J Clin Oncol, 27,* 5418–5424.

106. Kiladjian, J. J., Cassinat, B., Chevret, S., et al. (2008). Pegylated interferon-alfa-2a induces complete hematologic and molecular responses with low toxicity in polycythemia vera. *Blood, 112,* 3065–3072.

107. "Leukemia and Hematosarcoma" Cooperative Group, European Organization for research on Treatment of Cancer (E.O.R.T.C.). (1981). Treatment of polycythaemia vera by radiophosphorus or busulphan: a randomized trial. *Br J Cancer, 44,* 75–80.

108. Angat, N., Strand, J., Li, C. Y., et al. (2007). Leucocytosis in polycythemia vera predicts both inferior survival and leukaemic transformation. *Br J Haematol, 138,* 354–358.

109. Barosi, G., Birgegard, G., Finazzi, G., et al. (2009). Response criteria for essential thrombocythemia and polycythemia vera: results of a European LeukemiaNet consensus conference. *Blood, 113,* 4829–4833.

110. Verstovsek, S., Passamonti, F., Rambaldi, A., et al. (2009). A phase 2 study of INCB018424, an oral, selective JAK1/JAK2 inhibitor, in patients with advanced polycythemia vera (PV) and essential thrombocythemia (ET) refractory to hydroxyurea. *Blood, 113,* 4829–4833.

111. Moliterno, A. R., Hexner, E., Roboz, G. J., et al. (2009). An open-label study of CEP-701 in patients with JAK2 V617F-positive PV and ET: update of 39 enrolled patients. *Blood, 114,* abstract 753.

112. Mitus, A. J., & Schafer, A. (1990). Thrombocytosis and thrombocythemia. *Hematol Oncol Clin North Am, 4,* 157–178.

113. Thiele, J., Kvasnicka, H. M., Orazi, A., et al. (2008). Essential thrombocythemia. In Swerdlow, S. H., Campo, E., Harris, N. L., et al., (Eds.), *WHO classification of tumours of haematopoietic and lymphoid tissues.* (4th ed., pp. 48–53). Lyon, France: IARC Press.

114. Pardanani, A., & Tefferi, A. (2011). Targeting myeloproliferative neoplasms with JAK inhibitors. *Curr Opin Hematol, 18,* 105–110.

115. Murphy, S., Iland, H., Rosenthal, D., et al. (1986). Essential thrombocythemia: an interim report from the Polycythemia Vera Study Group. *Semin Hematol, 23,* 177–182.

116. Eu, P. J., Scott, L. M., Buck, G., et al. (2005). Definitions of subtypes of essential thrombocythemia and relation to polycythemia vera based on JAK2 V617F mutation status: a prospective study. *Lancet, 366*, 1945–1953.

117. Vannucchi, A. M., Antonioli, E., Guglielmelli, P., et al. (2008). Characteristics and clinical correlates of MPL 515W.L/K mutation in essential thrombocythemia. *Blood, 112*, 844–847.

118. Tefferi, A., & Vardiman, J. W. (2008). Classification and diagnosis of myeloproliferative neoplasms: the 2008 World Health Organization criteria and point-of-care diagnostic algorithms. *Leukemia, 22*, 14–22.

119. Kuecht, H., & Streuli, R. A. (1985). Megakaryopoiesis in different forms of thrombocytosis and thrombocytopenia: identification of megakaryocyte precursors by immunostaining of intracytoplasmic factor VIII-related antigen. *Acta Haematol, 74*, 208–212.

120. Shvidel, L., Sigler, E., Haran, M., et al. (2007). Busulphan is safe and effective treatment in elderly patients with essential thrombocythemia. *Leukemia, 21*, 2071–2072.

121. Passamonti, F., Rumi, E., Arcaini, L., et al. (2008). Prognostic factors for thrombosis, myelofibrosis, and leukemia in essential thrombocythemia: a study of 605 patients. *Haematologica, 93*, 1645–1651.

122. McCarthy, D. M. (1985). Fibrosis of the bone marrow, content and causes. *Br J Haematol, 59*, 1–7 (annotation).

123. Reilly, I. F. (1994). Pathogenesis of idiopathic myelofibrosis: present status and future directions. *Br J Haematol, 88*, 1–8.

124. Wang, J. C., Cheung, C. P., Fakhiuddin, A., et al. (1983). Circulating granulocyte and macrophage progenitor cells in primary and secondary myelofibrosis. *Br J Haematol, 54*, 301–307.

125. Jacobson, R. J., Salo, A., & Fialkow, P. J. (1978). Agnogenic myeloid metaplasia: a clonal proliferation of hematopoietic stem cells with secondary myelofibrosis. *Blood, 51*, 189–194.

126. Buschle, M., Janssen, J. Y., Drexler, H., et al. (1988). Evidence for pluripotent stem cell origin of idiopathic myelofibrosis: clonal analysis of a case characterized by a N-ras gene mutation. *Leukemia, 2*, 658–660.

127. Juvonen, E. (1988). Megakaryocyte colony formation in chronic myeloid leukemia and myelofibrosis. *Leuk Res, 12*, 751–756.

128. Barosi, G., Viarengo, G., Pecci, A., et al. (2001). Diagnostic and clinical relevance of the number of circulating CD34(+) cells in myelofibrosis with myeloid metaplasia. *Blood, 98*, 3249–3255.

129. Jacobs, P., Maze, S., Tayob, F., et al. (1985). Myelofibrosis, splenomegaly, and portal hypertension. *Acta Haematol, 74*, 45–48.

130. Grand, F. H., Hidalgo-Curtis, C. E., Ernst, T., et al. (2009). Frequent CBL mutations associated with 11q acquired uniparental disomy in myeloproliferative neoplasms. *Blood, 113*, 6182–6192.

131. Vellenga, E., Mulder, N., The, T., et al. (1982). A study of the cellular and humoral immune response in patients with myelofibrosis. *Clin Lab Haematol, 4*, 239–246.

132. Cervantes, F., Dupriez, B., Pereira, A., et al. (2009). New prognostic scoring system for primary myelofibrosis based on a study of the International Working Group for Myelofibrosis Research and Treatment. *Blood, 113*, 2895–2901.

133. Gangat, N., Caramazza, D., Vaidya, R., et al. (2010). DIPSS-Plus: a refined dynamic international prognostic scoring system (DIPSS) for primary myelofibrosis that incorporates prognostic information from karyotype, platelet count and transfusion status. *J Clin Oncol* (Epub ahead of print).

134. Cervantes, S., Mesa, R., & Barosi, G. (2007). New and old treatment modalities in primary myelofibrosis. *Cancer J, 13*, 377–383.

135. Elliott, M. A., Mesa, R., & Barosi, G. (2002). Thalidomide treatment in myelofibrosis with myeloid metaplasia. *Br J Haematol, 117*, 288–296.

136. Thomas, D. A., Giles, F. J., Albitar, M., et al. (2006). Thalidomide therapy for myelofibrosis with myelometaplasia. *Cancer, 106*, 1974–1984.

137. Tefferi, A., Cortez, J., Verstovsek, S., et al. (2006). Lenalidomide therapy in myelofibrosis with myeloid metaplasia. *Blood, 108*, 1158–1164.

138. Tefferi, A., Lasho, T. L., Mesa, R. A., et al. (2007). Lenalidomide therapy in del(5)(q31)-associated myelofibrosis: cytogenetic and JAK2V617F molecular remissions. *Leukemia, 21*, 1827–1828.

139. Martinez-Trillos, A., Gaya, A., Maffioli, M., et al. (2010). Efficacy and tolerability of hydroxyuria in the treatment of the myeloproliferative manifestations of myelofibrosis: results of 40 patients. *Ann Hematol, 89*, 1233–1237.

140. Siragusa, S., Vaidya, R., & Tefferi, A. (2009). Hydroxyurea effect on marked splenomegaly associated with primary myelofibrosis: response rates and correlation with JAK2V617F allele burden. *Blood, 114*, abstract 4971.

141. Mishchenko, E., & Tefferi, A. (2010). Treatment options for hydroxyuria-refractory disease complications in myeloproliferative neoplasms: JAK2 inhibitors, radiotherapy, splenectomy and transjugular intrahepatic portosystemic shunt. *Eur J Haematol, 85*, 192–199.

142. Mesa, R. A., Schwager, S., Radia, D., et al. (2009). The Myelofibrosis Symptom Assessment Form (MFSAF): an evidence-based brief inventory to measure quality of life and symptomatic response to treatment in myelofibrosis. *Leuk Res, 33*, 1199–1203.

143. Mesa, R. A., Niblack, J., Wadleigh, M., et al. (2007). The burden of fatigue and quality of life in myeloproliferative disorders (MPDs): an international Internet-based survey of 1179 MPD patients. *Cancer, 109*, 68–76.

144. Tefferi, A., Barosa, G., Mesa, R. A., et al. (2006). International Working Group (IWG) consensus criteria for treatment response in myelofibrosis with myeloid metaplasia for the IWG for Myelofibrosis Research and Treatment (IWG-MRT). *Blood, 108*, 1497–1503.

145. Pardanani, A., Gotlib, J. R., Jamieson, C., et al. (2010). Longer-term follow up with TG101348 therapy in myelofibrosis confirms sustained improvement in splenomegaly, disease-related symptoms, and JAK2V617F allele burden. *Blood, 116*, abstract 459.

146. Pardanani, A., George, G., Lasho, T. L., et al. (2010). A Phase I/II study of CYT387, an oral JAK-1/2 Inhibitor, in myelofibrosis: significant response rates in anemia, splenomegaly, and constitutional symptoms. *Blood, 116*, abstract 460.

147. Santos, F. P., Kantarjian, H. M., Jain, N., et al. (2010). Phase 2 study of CEP-701, an orally available JAK2 inhibitor, in patients with primary or postpolycythemia vera/essential thrombocythemia myelofibrosis. *Blood, 115*, 1131–1136.

148. Hexner, E., Goldberg, J. D., Prchal, J. T., et al. (2009). A multicenter, open label phase I/II study of CEP701 (Lestaurtinib) in adults with myelofibrosis: a report on phase I: a study of the Myeloproliferative Disorders Research Consortium (MPD-RC). *Blood, 114*, abstract 754.

149. Pegrum, G. D., Foadi, M., Boots, M., et al. (1981). How should we manage myelofibrosis? *J R Coll Physicians Lond, 15*, 17–18.

150. Tefferi, A., & Silverstein, M. N. (1996). Current perspective in agnogenic myeloid metaplasia. *Leuk Lymphoma, 22*(Suppl. 1), 169–171.

151. Guardiola, P., Anderson, J. E., Bandini, G., et al. (1999). Allogeneic stem cell transplantation for agnogenic myeloid metaplasia: a European Group for Blood and Marrow Transplantation, Société Française de Greffe de Moelle, Gruppo Italiano per il Trapianto del Midollo Osseo, and Fred Hutchinson Cancer Research Center Collaborative Study. *Blood, 93*, 2831–2838.

152. Xu, M., Bruno, E., Chao, J., et al. (2005). The constitutive mobilization of bone marrow–repopulating cells into the peripheral blood in idiopathic myelofibrosis. *Blood, 105,* 1699–1705.

153. Ishii, T., Zhao, Y., Sozer, S., et al. (2007). Behavior of CD34+ cells isolated from patients with polycythemia vera in NOD/SCID mice. *Exp Hematol, 35,* 1633–1640.

154. James, C., Mazurier, F., Dupont, S., et al. (2008). The hematopoietic stem cell compartment of JAK2V617F-positive myeloproliferative disorders is a reflection of disease heterogeneity. *Blood, 112,* 2429–2438.

155. Pardanani, A., Fridley, B. L., Lash, T. L., et al. (2008). Host genetic variation contributes to phenotypic diversity in myeloproliferative disorders. *Blood, 111,* 2785–2789.

156. Dupont, S., Masse, A., James, C., et al. The JAK2 617 V>F mutation triggers erythrocyte hypersensitivity and terminal erythroid amplification in primary erythroid cells from patients with polycythemia vera. *Blood, 110,* 1013–1021.

157. Scott, L. M., Scott, M. A., Campbell, P. J., et al. (2006). Progenitors homozygous for the V617F mutation occur in most patients with polycythemia vera but not essential thrombocythemia. *Blood, 108,* 2435–2437.

158. Xing, S., Wanting, T. H., Zhao, W., et al. (2008). Transgenic expression of JAK2V617F causes myeloproliferative disorders in mice. *Blood, 111,* 5109–5117.

159. Tiedt, R., Hao-Shin, S., Sobas, M. A., et al. (2008). Ratio of mutant JAK2-V617F to wild-type JAK2 determines the MPD phenotype in transgenic mice. *Blood, 111,* 3931–3940.

160. Kiladjian, J. J., Elkassar, N., Cassinat, B., et al. (2006). Essential thrombocythemias without V617F JAK2 mutation are clonal hematopoietic stem cell disorders. *Leukemia, 20,* 1181–1183.

161. Levine, R. L., Belisle, C., Wadleigh, M., et al. (2006). X-inactivation-based clonality analysis and quantitative JAK2V617F assessment reveal a strong association between clonality and JAK2V617F in PV but not ET/MMM, and identifies a subset of JAK2V617F-negative ET and MMM patients with clonal hematopoiesis. *Blood, 107,* 4139–4141.

162. Kralovics, R., Teo, S. S., Li, S. S., et al. (2006). Acquisition of the V617F mutation of JAK2 is a late genetic event in a subset of patients with myeloproliferative disorders. *Blood, 108,* 1377–1380.

163. Hussein, K., Bock, O., Seegers, A., et al. (2007). Myelofibrosis evolving during imatinib treatment of chronic myeloproliferative disease with coexisting *BCR/ABL* translocation and JAK2V617F mutation. *Blood, 109,* 4106–4107.

164. Kramer, A., Reiter, A., Kruth, J., et al. (2007). JAK2-V617F mutation in a patient with Philadelphia-chromosome positive chronic myeloid leukemia. *Lancet Oncol, 8,* 658–660.

165. Pardanani, A. D., Levine, R. L., Lasho, T., et al. (2006). MPL515 mutations in myeloproliferative and other myeloid disorders: a study of 1182 patients. *Blood, 108,* 3472–3476.

166. Li, S., Kralovics, R., De Libero, G., et al. (2008). Clonal heterogeneity in polycythemia vera patients with JAK2 exon 21 and JAK2-V617F mutations. *Blood, 111,* 3863–3866.

167. Petra, D., Li, S., Brisci, A., et al. (2008). Somatic mutations of JAK2 exon 12 in patients with JAK2 (V617F)–negative myeloproliferative disorders. *Blood, 111,* 1686–1689.

168. Kralovics, R., Stockton, D., Prchal, J., et al. (2003). Clonal hematopiesis in familial polycythemia vera suggests the involvement of multiple mutational events in the early pathogenesis of the disease. *Blood, 102,* 3793–3796.

169. Bellanne-Chantelot, C., Chaumarel, I., Labopin, M., et al. (2006). Genetic and clinical implications of the Val617Phe JAK2 mutation in 72 families with myeloproliferative disorders. *Blood, 108,* 346–352.

170. Villeval, J. L., Cohen-Solal, K., Tulliez, M., et al. (1997). High thrombopoietin production by hematopoietic cells induces a fatal myeloproliferative syndrome in mice. *Blood, 90,* 4369–4383.

171. Bain, B. J., Brunning, R. D., Vardiman, J. W., et al. (2008). Chronic neutrophilic leukemia. In Swerdlow, S. H., Campo, E., Harris, N. L., et al., (Eds.), *WHO classification of tumours of haematopoietic and lymphoid tissues.* (4th ed., pp. 38–39). Lyon, France: IARC Press.

172. Bain, B. J., Gilliland, D. G., Vardiman, J. W., et al. (2008). Chronic eosinophilic leukaemia, not otherwise specified. In Swerdlow, S. H., Campo, E., Harris, N. L., et al., (Eds.), *WHO classification of tumours of haematopoietic and lymphoid tissues.* (4th ed., pp. 51–53). Lyon, France: IARC Press.

173. Horny, H. P., Metcalfe, D. D., Bennett, J. M., et al. (2008). Mastocytosis. In Swerdlow, S. H., Campo, E., Harris, N. L., et al., (Eds.), *WHO classification of tumours of haematopoietic and lymphoid tissues.* (4th ed., pp. 54–63). Lyon, France: IARC Press.

174. Kvasnicka, H. M., Bain, B. J., Thiele, J., et al. (2008). Myeloproliferative neoplasm, unclassifiable. In Swerdlow, S. H., Campo, E., Harris, N. L., et al., (Eds.), *WHO classification of tumours of haematopoietic and lymphoid tissues.* (4th ed., pp. 64–65). Lyon, France: IARC Press.

Myelodysplastic Syndromes

34

Bernadette F. Rodak

OBJECTIVES

After completion of this chapter, the reader will be able to:

1. Define myelodysplastic syndromes (MDSs).
2. Explain the etiology of MDS.
3. Recognize morphologic features of dyspoiesis in bone marrow and peripheral blood.
4. Discuss abnormal functions of granulocytes, erythrocytes, and thrombocytes in MDS.
5. Correlate peripheral blood, bone marrow, and cytogenetic and molecular findings in MDS with classification systems.
6. Compare and contrast the French-American-British and the 2008 World Health Organization classifications of MDS.
7. Discuss prognostic indicators in MDS.
8. Indicate modes of management for MDS.
9. Review the epidemiology of MDS and apply it as a contributor in differential diagnosis.
10. Suggest laboratory tests and their results that would rule out MDS in the differential diagnosis.
11. Explain the rationale for the category of myelodysplastic/myeloproliferative neoplasms (MDS/MPN).
12. Correlate peripheral blood, bone marrow, and cytogenetic findings in MDS/MPN with disease classification.
13. Review prognostic indicators in MDS.
14. Discuss treatment in MDS, including novel therapies.

CASE STUDY

After studying the material in this chapter, the reader should be able to respond to the following case study:

A 43-year-old man experienced fatigue and malaise. He presented with pancytopenia (WBC count of 2.2×10^9/L, hemoglobin of 6.1 g/dL, platelet count of 51×10^9/L). The WBC differential was essentially normal. Mean cell volume was 132 fL (reference range, 80 to 100 fL), and vitamin B_{12} and folate levels were normal. The bone marrow was normocellular with a myeloid-to-erythroid ratio of 1:1 and adequate megakaryocytes. The erythroid component was dysplastic with megaloblastic features. No abnormal localization of immature precursors was noted. Chromosome analysis indicated direct duplication of chromosome 1q. The patient was maintained with transfusions over the next 6 years. At that time, his bone marrow revealed increased erythropoiesis, decreased granulopoiesis, and megakaryopoiesis, all with dysplastic changes. There were 50% to 60% ring sideroblasts.

1. What should be included in the differential diagnosis of patients with pancytopenia and elevated mean cell volume?
2. Given the normal vitamin B_{12} and folate levels, what is the patient's probable diagnosis?
3. In which WHO 2008 classification does this disorder belong?

For decades, laboratory professionals have observed a group of morphologic abnormalities in peripheral blood films and bone marrow smears of elderly patients. The findings were heterogeneous and affected all cell lines, and the condition either remained stable for years or progressed rapidly to death.

Historically, this pattern of abnormalities was referred to as *refractory anemia, smoldering leukemia, oligoblastic leukemia,* or *preleukemia.*[1-3] In 1982 the French-American-British (FAB) Cooperative Leukemia Study Group proposed terminology and a specific set of morphologic criteria to describe what are now known as *myelodysplastic syndromes* (MDSs).[4] In 1997 a group from the World Health Organization (WHO) proposed a new classification that included molecular, cytogenetic, and immunologic criteria in addition to morphologic features.[5,6] The WHO classification was revised in 2008. Both the FAB and WHO classifications are discussed in this chapter.

MDSs are a group of acquired clonal hematologic disorders characterized by progressive cytopenias in the peripheral blood, reflecting defects in erythroid, myeloid, and/or megakaryocytic maturation.[7,8] The median age at diagnosis is 70. MDSs rarely affect individuals younger than age 50 unless preceded by chemotherapy or radiation for another malignancy.[1,9] Cases in young adults and children have been reported, however.[10,11] The incidence of these disorders seems to be increasing, but this apparent increase may be attributable in part to improved techniques for identifying these diseases and to improved classification.[12-14] At this time, the fastest-growing segment of the population is the group older than 60 years of age. MDSs are becoming a more common finding in the hematology laboratory, and familiarity with these disorders is an essential part of the body of knowledge of all medical laboratory professionals.

ETIOLOGY

MDS may arise de novo (primary MDS) or as a result of therapy (therapy-related MDS). Although MDSs are a group of heterogeneous diseases, all are the result of proliferation of abnormal stem cells.[7,8,15] The initiating defect in most cases is at the level of the myeloid stem cell, because primarily the erythroid, myeloid, and megakaryocytic cells are affected. It may be that the affected hematopoietic stem cell has lost its lymphopoietic potential, because only rarely does MDS transform to acute lymphoblastic leukemia.[16,17] The abnormal stem cell may be the result of the cumulative effects of environmental exposure in susceptible individuals. Mutations may be caused by chemical insult, radiation, or viral infection. There also may be an association with smoking.[18] An association with inherited hematologic disorders has also been found.[19] The mutated stem cell produces a pathologic clone of cells that expands in size at the expense of normal cell production.[20] Because each mutation produces a unique clone with a specific cellular defect, MDSs have a multitude of expressions. Two morphologic findings are common to all types of MDSs, however; the presence of progressive cytopenias despite cellular bone marrows and dyspoiesis in one or more cell lines.

Disruption of apoptosis may be responsible for the ineffective hematopoiesis in MDS.[21-26] Apoptosis (programmed cell death) regulates cell population by decreasing cell survival. In MDS, apoptosis is increased in early disease, when peripheral blood cytopenias are evident. Later in MDS, when progression toward leukemia is apparent, apoptosis has been shown to be decreased, which allows increased neoplastic cell survival and expansion of the abnormal clone.[27-30] Other important factors include the levels of antiangiogenic cytokines, tumor necrosis factor, and cellular components of the immune system, as well as the interaction between MDS clonal cells and the hematopoietic inductive microenvironment. Patients with MDS have increased levels of angiogenic growth factors, including vascular endothelial growth factor.[31,32]

Therapy-related MDS (t-MDS) occurs in patients who have been treated previously with chemotherapy or radiotherapy or both. Median onset of therapy-related MDS varies with the agents used and is usually 4 to 7 years after therapy was initiated.[20,33] Patients who have received cytokines, such as G-CSF or GM-CSF, for bone marrow stimulation are also at an increased risk for developing t-MDS.[34] Therapy-related MDS often is more aggressive and may evolve quickly into acute myeloblastic leukemia (AML).[20,33,35] The 2008 WHO classification places therapy-related MDSs into the AML category of therapy-related myeloid neoplasms (Chapter 35).

MORPHOLOGIC ABNORMALITIES IN PERIPHERAL BLOOD AND BONE MARROW

In MDS each of the three major myeloid cell lines has dyspoietic morphologic features. The following sections provide descriptions of common abnormal morphologic findings.[4,9,19] These descriptions are not all-inclusive because of the large number of possible cellular mutations and combinations of mutations.

Dyserythropoiesis

In the peripheral blood, the most common morphologic finding in dyserythropoiesis is the presence of oval macrocytes (Figure 34-1). When these cells are seen in the presence of normal vitamin B_{12} and folate values, MDS should be included in the differential diagnosis. Hypochromic microcytes in the presence of adequate iron stores also are seen in MDS. A dimorphic red blood cell (RBC) population (Figure 34-2) is another indication of the clonality of this disease. Poikilocytosis, basophilic stippling, Howell-Jolly bodies, and siderocytes also are indications that the erythrocyte has undergone abnormal development.[36]

Dyserythropoiesis in the bone marrow is evidenced by RBC precursors with more than one nucleus or abnormal nuclear shapes. The normally round nucleus may have lobes or buds. Nuclear fragments may be present in the cytoplasm

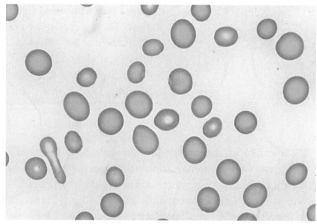

Figure 34-1 Oval macrocytes in peripheral blood (×1000).

(Figure 34-3). Internuclear bridging is occasionally present (Figure 34-4).[37] Abnormal cytoplasmic features may include basophilic stippling or heterogeneous staining (Figure 34-5). Ring sideroblasts are a common finding. Megaloblastoid cellular development in the presence of normal vitamin B_{12} and folate values is another indication of MDS. The bone marrows in these cases may have erythrocytic hyperplasia or hypoplasia (Box 34-1).

Dysmyelopoiesis

Dysmyelopoiesis in the peripheral blood is suspected when there is a persistence of basophilia in the cytoplasm of otherwise mature white blood cells (WBCs), indicating nuclear-cytoplasmic asynchrony (Figure 34-6). Abnormal granulation of the cytoplasm of neutrophils, in the form of larger than normal granules, hypogranulation, or the absence of granules, is a common finding. Agranular bands can be easily misclassified

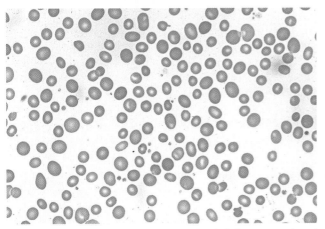

Figure 34-2 Dimorphic erythrocyte population, including macrocytic and microcytic cells (in peripheral blood, ×500).

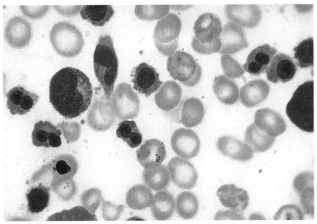

Figure 34-3 Bone marrow specimen showing erythroid hyperplasia and nuclear budding in erythroid precursors (×1000).

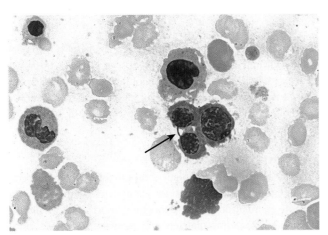

Figure 34-4 Erythroid precursors showing nuclear bridging (*arrow*) (bone marrow, ×1000).

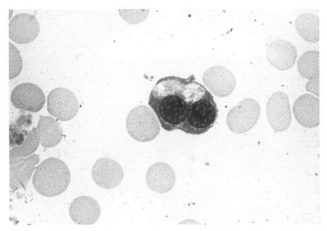

Figure 34-5 Bone marrow specimen showing heterogeneous staining in a bilobed erythroid precursor (×1000).

BOX 34-1 **Morphologic Evidence of Dyserythropoiesis**

Oval macrocytes
Hypochromic microcytes
Dimorphic red blood cell (RBC) population
RBC precursors with more than one nucleus
RBC precursors with abnormal nuclear shapes
RBC precursors with uneven cytoplasmic staining
Ring sideroblasts

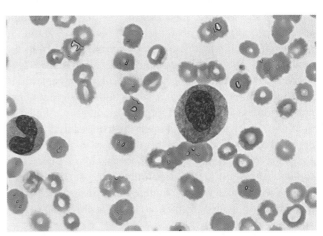

Figure 34-6 This myelocyte (*right*) in peripheral blood has a nucleus with clumped chromatin and a basophilic immature cytoplasm showing asynchrony. Note also the agranular myeloid cell (*left*) (×1000).

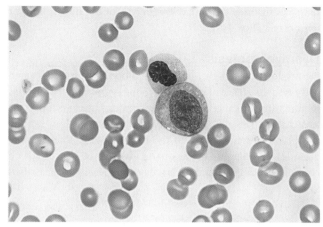

Figure 34-7 Agranular myeloid cells (peripheral blood, ×1000).

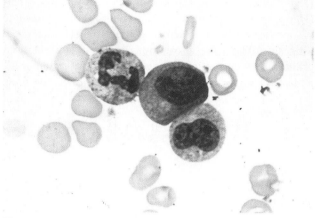

Figure 34-9 Uneven staining of white blood cell cytoplasm (bone marrow, ×1000).

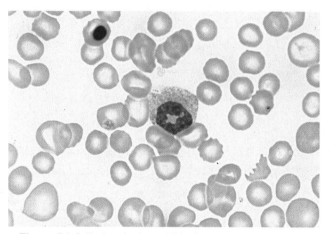

Figure 34-8 Nuclear ring in myeloid cell (peripheral blood, ×1000).

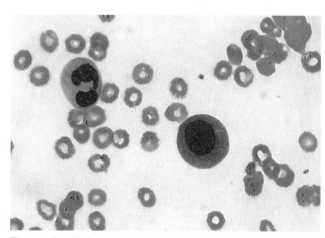

Figure 34-10 Promyelocyte or myelocyte devoid of granules and an agranular neutrophil (bone marrow, ×1000).

as monocytes (Figure 34-7). Abnormal nuclear features may include hyposegmentation, hypersegmentation, or nuclear rings (Figure 34-8).[38]

In the bone marrow, dysmyelopoiesis may be represented by nuclear-cytoplasmic asynchrony. Cytoplasmic changes include uneven staining, such as a dense ring of basophilia around the periphery with a clear unstained area around the nucleus or whole sections of cytoplasm unstained, with the remainder of the cytoplasm stained normally (Figure 34-9). There may be abnormal granulation of the cytoplasm in which promyelocytes or myelocytes or both are devoid of primary granules (Figure 34-10), primary granules may be larger than normal, or secondary granules may be reduced in number or absent, and there may be an occasional Auer rod.[39,40] Agranular promyelocytes may be mistaken for blasts; this could lead to misclassification of the disease in the AML scheme. Abnormal nuclear findings may include hypersegmentation or hyposegmentation and possibly ring-shaped nuclei (Box 34-2).

The bone marrow may exhibit granulocytic hypoplasia or hyperplasia. Monocytic hyperplasia is a common finding in dysplastic marrows.

BOX 34-2 Morphologic Evidence of Dysmyelopoiesis

Persistent basophilic cytoplasm
Abnormal granulation
Abnormal nuclear shapes
Uneven cytoplasmic staining

Abnormal localization of immature precursors is a characteristic finding in bone marrow biopsy specimens from patients with MDS.[41] Normally, myeloblasts and promyelocytes reside along the endosteal surface of the bone marrow. In some cases of MDS, these cells tend to cluster centrally in marrow sections.

Dysmegakaryopoiesis

Platelets also exhibit dyspoietic morphology in the peripheral blood. Common changes include giant platelets and abnormal platelet granulation, either hypogranulation or agranulation (Figure 34-11). Some platelets may possess large fused granules. Circulating micromegakaryocytes may be present in peripheral blood from patients with MDS (Figure 34-12).[9]

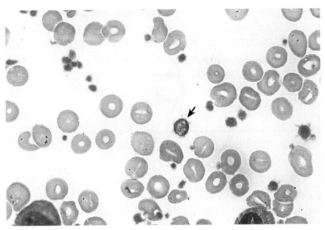

Figure 34-11 Abnormal platelet granulation (*arrow*) (peripheral blood, ×1000).

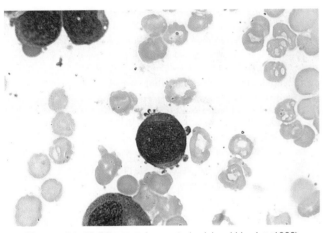

Figure 34-12 Micromegakaryocyte (peripheral blood, ×1000).

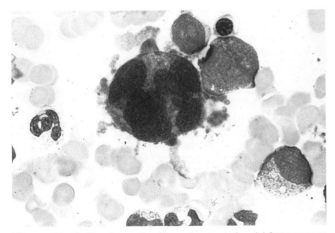

Figure 34-13 Megakaryocyte with small separated nuclei (bone marrow, ×1000).

The megakaryocytic component of the bone marrow may exhibit abnormal morphology: large mononuclear megakaryocytes, micromegakaryocytes, or micromegakaryoblasts. The nuclei in these cells may be bilobed or have multiple small, separated nuclei (Figure 34-13; Box 34-3).[9]

BOX 34-3 Morphologic Evidence of Dysmegakaryopoiesis

Giant platelets
Platelets with abnormal granulation
Circulating micromegakaryocytes
Large mononuclear megakaryocytes
Micromegakaryocytes or micromegakaryoblasts or both
Abnormal nuclear shapes in the megakaryocytes/blasts

DIFFERENTIAL DIAGNOSIS

Dysplasia by itself is not sufficient evidence for MDS, because several other conditions can cause similar morphologic features. Some examples are vitamin B_{12} or folate deficiency, which can cause pancytopenia and dysplasia, and exposure to heavy metals. Copper deficiency may cause reversible myelodysplasia.[9] Some congenital hematologic disorders, such as Fanconi anemia and congenital dyserythropoietic anemia, may also present with dysplasia. Parvovirus B19 and some chemotherapeutic agents may give rise to dysplasia similar to that in MDS. Paroxysmal nocturnal hemoglobinuria has similar features, as does human immunodeficiency virus (HIV).[42] Therefore, a thorough history and physical examination, including questions about exposure to drugs and chemicals, are essential.[9]

ABNORMAL CELLULAR FUNCTION

The cells produced by abnormal maturation not only have an abnormal appearance but also have abnormal function.[9,43] The granulocytes may have decreased adhesion,[44,45] deficient phagocytosis,[45] decreased chemotaxis,[44,45] or impaired microbicidal capacity.[46] Decreased levels of myeloperoxidase and alkaline phosphatase may be found.[47] The RBCs may exhibit shortened survival,[48] and erythroid precursors may have a decreased response to erythropoietin that may contribute to anemia.[49] Patients may experience increased bleeding despite adequate platelet numbers.[9,50,51] The type and degree of dysfunction depend on the mutation present in the hematopoietic stem cell.

CLASSIFICATION OF MYELODYSPLASTIC SYNDROMES

French-American-British Classification

In an effort to standardize the diagnosis of MDSs, the FAB created five classes of MDS, each with a specific set of morphologic criteria. The categories were defined by the amount of dysplasia and the number of blasts in the bone marrow. The diagnosis of acute leukemia required at least 30% blasts in the bone marrow.[4] The FAB classification included the following:

1. Refractory anemia
2. Refractory anemia with ring sideroblasts (RARS)
3. Refractory anemia with excess blasts (RAEB)
4. Chronic myelomonocytic leukemia (CMML)
5. Refractory anemia with excess blasts in transformation (RAEB-t)

The FAB classification provided a framework for discussion of a seemingly heterogeneous group of disorders; however, its reliance on morphology alone limited its usefulness as a prognostic indicator. In addition, the FAB classification did not view MDSs in their totality because it did not address therapy-related or hereditary forms, and childhood MDS was not considered. Advances in medical knowledge, including molecular analysis, have allowed integration of clinical, immunologic, genetic, and molecular data with morphologic features. The WHO classification retains many of the FAB features, while recognizing molecular, cytogenetic, and immunologic characteristics of these disorders. The WHO classification also removed the problematic categories of CMML and RAEB-t and placed them in MDS/MPD and acute leukemia, respectively.[19,52]

World Health Organization Classification

The original modifications from the FAB classification of MDS included a reduction in the percentage of blasts required for diagnosis of AML from 30% to 20% and the recognition of two new classifications: refractory cytopenia with multilineage dysplasia (RCMD) and del(5q) syndrome. The 2008 revision of the WHO criteria added the category of refractory cytopenia with unilineage dysplasia (RCUD), refined some categories, and added the provisional category of childhood MDS, also called *refractory cytopenia of childhood.* The 2008 WHO classification is outlined in Box 34-4 and detailed in Table 34-1. The classification is extensive, and only the highlights are presented in this chapter.[19]

BOX 34-4 World Health Organization Classification of Myelodysplastic Syndromes (2008)

Refractory cytopenia with unilineage dysplasia
Refractory anemia with ring sideroblasts
Refractory cytopenia with multilineage dysplasia
Refractory anemia with excess blasts
Myelodysplastic syndrome with isolated del(5q)
Myelodysplastic syndrome, unclassifiable
Childhood myelodysplastic syndrome (provisional)

From Swerdlow SH, Campo E, Harris NL, et al, editors: *WHO classification of tumours of haematopoietic and lymphoid tissues,* ed 4, Lyon, France, 2008, IARC Press.

TABLE 34-1 Peripheral Blood and Bone Marrow Findings in Myelodysplastic Syndromes (MDSs)

Disease	Blood Findings	Bone Marrow Findings
Refractory cytopenia with unilineage dysplasia (RCUD); refractory anemia (RA); refractory neutropenia (RN); refractory thrombocytopenia (RT)	Unicytopenia* No or rare blasts (<1%)†	Unilineage dysplasia: ≥10% of cells in one myeloid lineage <5% blasts <15% of erythroid precursors are ring sideroblasts
Refractory anemia with ring sideroblasts (RARS)	Anemia No blasts	≥15% of erythroid precursors are ring sideroblasts Erythroid dysplasia only <5% blasts
Refractory cytopenia with multilineage dysplasia (RCMD)	Cytopenia(s) No or rare blasts (<1%)† No Auer rods <1 × 10⁹/L monocytes	Dysplasia in ≥10% of cells in two or more myeloid lineages (neutrophil and/or erythroid precursors and/or megakaryocytes) <5% blasts in marrow No Auer rods ±15% ring sideroblasts
Refractory anemia with excess blasts 1 (RAEB-1)	Cytopenia(s) <5% blasts No Auer rods <1 × 10⁹/L monocytes	Unilineage or multilineage dysplasia 5%–9% blasts† No Auer rods
Refractory anemia with excess blasts 2 (RAEB-2)	Cytopenia(s) 5%–19% blasts ± Auer rods‡ <1 × 10⁹/L monocytes	Unilineage or multilineage dysplasia 10%–19% blasts† ± Auer rods‡
Myelodysplastic syndrome, unclassified (MDS-U)	Cytopenia(s) ≤1% blasts†	Unequivocal dysplasia in <10% of cells in one or more myeloid cell lines when accompanied by a cytogenetic abnormality considered as presumptive evidence for a diagnosis of MDS <5% blasts
MDS associated with isolated del(5q)	Anemia Usually normal or increased platelet count No or rare blasts (<1%)	Normal to increased megakaryocytes with hypolobulated nuclei <5% blasts Isolated del(5q) cytogenetic abnormality No Auer rods

From Swerdlow SH, Campo E, Harris NL, et al, editors: *WHO classification of tumours of haematopoietic and lymphoid tissues,* ed 4, Lyon, France, 2008, IARC Press.
*Bicytopenia may occasionally be observed. Cases with pancytopenia should be classified as MDS-U.
†If the marrow myeloblast percentage is less than 5%, but there are 2% to 4% myeloblasts in the blood, the diagnostic classification is RAEB-1. Cases of RCUD and RCMD with 1% myeloblasts in the blood should be classified as MDS-U.
‡Cases with Auer rods and less than 5% myeloblasts in the blood and less than 10% myeloblasts in the marrow should be classified as RAEB-2.

Refractory Cytopenia with Unilineage Dysplasia

Presenting symptoms of RCUD are related to the cytopenia—namely, fatigue or shortness of breath if anemia is present; increased infections from neutropenia; and petechiae, bruising, or bleeding if thrombocytopenia is present. This category includes MDS cases with less than 1% blasts in the peripheral blood and less than 5% blasts in the bone marrow. Dysplasia must be present in more than 10% of a single myeloid lineage. Included in RCUD is refractory anemia with only dyserythropoiesis (but less than 15% ring sideroblasts), refractory neutropenia, and refractory thrombocytopenia.[52] Although cytogenetic abnormalities may be seen in up to 50% of cases of refractory anemia, none is specific to the diagnosis. Median survival is generally 2 to 5 years, with only a 2% risk of transformation to acute leukemia.[52,53]

Refractory Anemia with Ring Sideroblasts

In RARS, anemia and dyserythropoiesis are present, and more than 15% of the bone marrow erythroid precursors are ring sideroblasts. To be considered a ring sideroblast, an erythroid precursor must contain at least five iron granules per cell, and these iron-containing mitochondria must circle at least one third of the nucleus (Figure 34-14).[54] In the peripheral blood there may be a dimorphic picture, with a population of hypochromic cells along with a majority of normochromic cells. RARS occurs primarily in the older population. Mean survival is 69 to 108 months.[55] Refractory anemia with ring sideroblasts and marked thrombocytosis and *JAK2* V617F mutation are discussed with the myelodysplastic/myeloproliferative neoplasms.[56] Acquired sideroblastic anemia, which is not considered MDS, is discussed in Chapter 20.

Refractory Cytopenia with Multilineage Dysplasia

RCMD is categorized by one or more cytopenias, dysplasia in two or more myeloid cell lines, less than 1% blasts in peripheral blood, and less than 5% blasts in the bone marrow. In RCMD, the myeloblasts do not contain Auer rods; if Auer rods are noted, the disorder is classified as RAEB-2.[57] Some cases of RCMD have more than 15% ring sideroblasts, but the dyspoiesis in more than the erythroid line places them in the RCMD

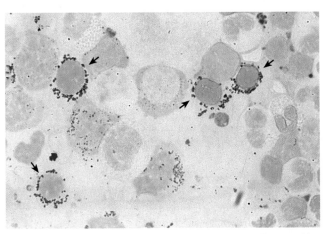

Figure 34-14 Ring sideroblast (*arrows*) (bone marrow, Prussian blue stain, ×1000).

rather than the RARS category.[53] This distinction is important, because RCMD has a more aggressive course than RARS.[33]

Refractory Anemia with Excess Blasts

Trilineage cytopenias, as well as significant dysmyelopoiesis, dysmegakaryopoiesis, or both, are common in RAEB. According to the WHO classification, the peripheral blood must contain 2% to 19% blasts. In the bone marrow, blasts number 5% to 19%. RAEB is distinguished from RCMD by myeloblast percentage. Because there are significant differences in survival and because evolution to AML may occur, the WHO classification divided RAEB into two types, depending on the percentage of blasts in blood and bone marrow:

RAEB-1—5% to 9% blasts in the bone marrow or 2% to 4% blasts in the peripheral blood

RAEB-2—10% to 19% blasts in the bone marrow and 5% to 19% blasts in the peripheral blood

The presence of Auer rods, regardless of blast count, qualifies a case as RAEB-2. RAEB with greater than 10% myeloblasts has a more aggressive course, with a greater percentage of cases transforming to AML.[53,57]

Myelodysplastic Syndrome with Isolated del(5q) (5q– Syndrome)

In patients who have only the deletion of 5q (5q–), MDS represents a fairly well-defined syndrome, affecting predominantly women and occurring at a median age of 67. These patients typically have refractory anemia without other cytopenias and/or thrombocytosis, hypolobulated megakaryocytes, and erythroid hypoplasia.[58-60] There are less than 1% blasts in the peripheral blood, and Auer rods are not seen.[61] Patients with MDS with isolated del(5q) have long-term stable disease (median survival, 145 months). The thalidomide analogue lenalidomide (Revlimid) has proven to be effective in patients with isolated del(5q), as well as in those with del(5q) and additional cytogenetic abnormalities.[58-60]

Myelodysplastic Syndrome, Unclassifiable

The category of *myelodysplastic syndrome, unclassifiable* refers to subtypes of MDS that initially lack the specific changes necessary for classification into other MDS categories. If characteristics of a specific subtype develop later, the case should be reclassified into the appropriate group.[62]

Childhood Myelodysplastic Syndromes

De novo MDS in children is very rare, and although some of the characteristics of adult MDS are present, there are also some distinct differences. The 2008 WHO classification introduced a provisional category of *refractory cytopenia of childhood*. Several authors have addressed this provisional category in detail.[10,52]

MYELODYSPLASTIC/MYELOPROLIFERATIVE NEOPLASMS

The MDS/MPN category includes myeloid neoplasms with clinical, laboratory, and morphologic features that are characteristic of both MDS and MPN. Included in this classification are chronic myelomonocytic leukemia; atypical chronic myeloid leukemia; juvenile myelomonocytic leukemia; and MDS/MPN, unclassifiable, with a provisional subtype of refractory anemia with ring sideroblasts and thrombocytosis (Box 34-5).[52]

Chronic Myelomonocytic Leukemia

CMML is characterized by a persistent monocytosis of more than 1.0 monocyte $\times$ 10^9/L, absence of the *BCR/ABL1* fusion gene, less than 20% blasts and promonocytes in the peripheral blood and bone marrow, and dysplasia in one or more myeloid cell line. Patients usually have an increased leukocyte count with absolute monocytosis. Dysgranulopoiesis is evident, but neutrophil precursors make up less than 10% of the total leukocytes.[63] Splenomegaly may be present due to infiltration of leukemic cells. Although cytogenetic abnormalities are found in up to 40% of patients, there is none specific for CMML. Prognosis varies, depending on the number of blasts plus promonocytes. If there are less than 5% blasts and promonocytes in the peripheral blood and less than 10% in the bone marrow, the disease is classified as CMML-1 and the prognosis is better than in those cases in which there are 5% to 19% blasts and promonocytes in the peripheral blood or 10% to 19% in the bone marrow (classified as CMML-2).[52,63]

Atypical Chronic Myeloid Leukemia, *BCR/ABL1* Negative

Atypical CML, *BCR/ABL1* negative (aCML), is characterized by leukocytosis with morphologically dysplastic neutrophils and their precursors. Basophilia may be present, but it is not a prominent feature. Multilineage dysplasia is common. The *BCR/ABL1* fusion gene is not present, but a variety of other karyotypic abnormalities may be seen. Dyspoiesis may be seen in all cell lines, but it is most remarkable in the neutrophils, which may exhibit Pelger-Huët–like cells, hypogranularity, and bizarre segmentation.[64,65] The prognosis is poor for patients with aCML, who either progress to AML or succumb to bone marrow failure.[66]

Juvenile Myelomonocytic Leukemia

Juvenile myelomonocytic leukemia is a clonal disorder characterized by proliferation of the granulocytic and monocytic cell lines and affects children from 1 month to 14 years of age. There is a strong association with neurofibromatosis type 1.[67]

Allogeneic stem cell transplantation is effective in about 50% of patients.[68]

Myelodysplastic/Myeloproliferative Neoplasm, Unclassifiable

The designation *MDS/MPN, unclassifiable* is used for cases that meet the criteria for MDS/MPN but do not fit into one of the specified subcategories.[69] Within this group there is a provisional entity that has features of refractory anemia with ring sideroblasts and thrombocytosis (RARS-T) and also carries the *JAK2* V617F mutation.[56]

CYTOGENETICS, MOLECULAR GENETICS, AND EPIGENETICS

Cytogenetics

Chromosome abnormalities are found in about 50% of cases of de novo MDS and 90% to 95% of t-MDS.[70] Karyotype has a major effect on prognosis in MDS patients, and specific karyotypes can be used cautiously to predict response to certain treatments.[70] Balanced translocations, which are common among patients with AML, are found only rarely in cases of de novo MDS.[19,70] Except for del(5q), no cytogenetic abnormality is specific to subtype. The most common abnormalities involve chromosomes 5, 7, 8, 11, 13, and 20.[9,19] The most common single abnormalities are trisomy 8 and monosomy 7.[71,72] Less common abnormalities in MDS are 12p–, iso 17, –22, and loss of the Y chromosome.[73]

Molecular Alterations

Advances in molecular genetic testing have made testing more available for routine use, and such information could be used to strengthen other prognostic indicator schemes.[74] Likewise, identification of genetic defects may allow development of targeted therapies.[75] Although not specific to MDS, the most common mutations include those in the *TP53* gene,[74] *RUNX1*,[76,77] and *TET2*.[78] *NRAS* has been detected in a small percentage of MDS patients.[79,80] It appears that a multistep process is required for transformation of MDS to AML. Some gene mutations, such as *TET2*, confer a more favorable prognosis,[78] while others such as *TP53* confer a higher risk of transformation.[79]

Epigenetics

The term *epigenetics* describes changes in gene expression that occur without altering the DNA sequence. Gene function is affected through selective activation or inactivation, rather than a change in the primary nucleotide sequence itself.[81,82] In oncogenesis, regions of a gene with specific regulatory functions, such as apoptosis, may be hypermethylated.[83] Incorporation of demethylating agents into the DNA appears to slow the progression of MDS, although the mechanism is not clearly understood.[82-84]

PROGNOSIS

In 1997 the International Prognostic Scoring System (IPSS) was developed to predict prognosis of patients with primary

TABLE 34-2 Revised International Prognostic Scoring System for MDS

	SCORE VALUE						
	0	0.5	1	1.5	2	3	4
Cytogenetics	Very Good	—	Good	—	Intermediate	Poor	Very Poor
BM Blasts (%)	≤2%	—	>2% to <5%	—	5% to 10%	>10%	—
Hemoglobin (g/dL)	≥10	—	8 to <10	<8	—	—	—
Platelets (×10⁹/L)	≥100	50 to <100	<50	—	—	—	—
ANC (×10⁹/L)	≥0.8	<0.8	—	—	—	—	—

Risk Score and Median Survival (All Ages)		Karotype	
Very Low	≤1.5 (8.8 years)	Very Good	−Y, del(11q)
Low	>1.5 to 3 (5.3 years)	Good	Normal, del(5q), del(12p), del(20q), double incl del 5(q)
Intermediate	>3 to 4.5 (3.0 years)	Intermediate	Del(7q), +8, +19, i(17q), any other single or double abnormality
High	>4.5 to 6 (1.6 years)	Poor	−7, inv(3)/t/del(3q), double incl −7/del(7q), complex 3 abnormalities
Very High	>6 (0.8 years)	Very Poor	Complex >3 abnormalities

Median survival is also adjusted for age and decreases with age

Adapted from Greenberg et al. Revised international prognostic scoring system for myelodysplastic syndromes. Blood 2012;120(12):2454-2465.

untreated MDS.[85] In 2012 a refinement of the IPSS scoring system integrated newer cytogenetic groupings and depth of cytopenias into the equation, defining five major prognostic categories. The basis of the revised system retained three of the original parameters—cytogenetics, bone marrow blast percentage, and cytopenias—but divided the cytogenetic groups into five rather than the original three, split the blast percentage into more groups, and addressed the depth of cytopenias. Other features that affected survival but not transformation into AML included patient age, serum ferritin, patient performance status, and lactate dehydrogenase levels.[86] Recently, levels of specific cytokines have been shown to affect disease progression in MDS.[87] Table 34-2 summarizes the revised IPSS.

TREATMENT

Treatment of MDS patients is challenging because many are older and have coexisting illnesses, and the heterogeneity of the disease makes the use of one standard treatment impossible. The overall goal of treatment is to provide improved quality of life and to prolong survival.

Supportive care has been the predominant mode of treatment for most MDS patients, except those who qualify for stem cell transplantation. Supportive care includes administration of blood products (RBCs and platelets as necessary) and prevention or treatment of infections with antibiotics.

Recently, however, three drugs (lenalidomide, azacitidine, and decitabine) have been approved by the U.S. Food and Drug Administration (FDA) that show promise when used either alone or in combination with other therapies.[84,88] Azacitidine and decitabine belong to a group of drugs that deplete intracellular methyltransferases (DMNTs) and are effective in low dose, with minimal side effects, and have improved the quality of life for patients with high-grade MDS.[84] Therapies are usually stratified into those used in low-risk disease and those in higher-risk MDS cases.

Treatment for patients with low-risk MDS is aimed at maintaining residual function of the bone marrow through the use of hematopoietic growth factors such as erythropoietin, thrombopoietin, and granulocyte colony-stimulating factor. Although levels of these growth factors are often normal in MDS patients, there is a subset of patients who respond to their use.[88-90]

In patients with low-risk MDS, immunosuppressive therapy with drugs such as antithymocyte globulin and cyclosporine has resulted in decreased risk of leukemic transformation.[90-92]

Lenalidomide (Revlimid; Celgene, Summit, NJ), a thalidomide analogue that is less toxic than thalidomide, was approved by the FDA in 2005 for use in patients with low- or intermediate-risk MDS.[93-95] It has shown remarkable promise, especially in patients with the 5q chromosome arm deletion. Transfusion independence was achieved in 64% of patients, and a median increase of 3.9 g/dL of hemoglobin was achieved in patients taking the drug. Complete cytogenetic remission was seen in 55% of MDS patients taking lenalidomide, whereas in MDS patients taking erythropoietin, cytogenetic remission is rare.[93] Lenalidomide has immunomodulatory and antiangiogenic effects.[88-90] The apparent efficacy of lenalidomide must be weighed against its ability to cause significant myelosuppression.[88,93]

NRAS is mutated in about 20% of MDS patients. Farnesyltransferase inhibitors interfere with this process.[90,96] Patients with high-risk MDS benefit from treatment with hypomethylating agents such as azacitidine and, to a lesser extent, decitabine.[81,82,84,88,97-99]

The only cure is hematopoietic stem cell transplantation. Patients with an IPSS score of intermediate 2 or higher and patients with more than 10% blasts should be considered for allogeneic stem cell transplantation.[100,101] Stem cell transplantation is most successful in patients younger than age 70 with no comorbidity.[9]

Future Directions

As research addressing the role of apoptosis in MDS continues, future therapies may be aimed at controlling apoptosis, with or without the use of chemotherapeutic agents. Because effective treatment for MDS remains limited, it has been suggested that patients be provided with information on the prognosis for their type of MDS, available therapies, and success rates and should take part in making decisions regarding their treatment.[102,103] As more is learned about the molecular biology of MDS, it may be possible to develop customized treatment plans for individual patients.[104]

SUMMARY

- MDSs are a group of clonal disorders characterized by progressive cytopenias and dyspoiesis of the myeloid, erythroid, and megakaryocytic cell lines.
- The dyspoiesis is evidenced by abnormal morphologic appearance and abnormal function of the cell lines affected.
- The WHO classification of MDSs is based on morphologic, molecular, cytogenetic, and immunologic characteristics of blood cell lines.
- Prognosis in MDS depends on several factors, including percentage of bone marrow blasts, depth of cytopenias, and karyotypic abnormalities.
- Treatment of MDS depends on the prognosis. If the prognosis is favorable, patients may receive only supportive therapy.

- Other treatments that have met with limited success include chemotherapeutic agents and epigenetic modifiers.
- Currently, the only cure for MDS is bone marrow or hematopoietic stem cell transplantation.
- Future treatment possibilities include the use of apoptosis-controlling drugs.

Now that you have completed this chapter, go back and read again the case study at the beginning and respond to the questions presented.

REVIEW QUESTIONS

Answers can be found in the Appendix.

1. MDSs are most common in which age group?
   a. 2 to 10 years
   b. 15 to 20 years
   c. 25 to 40 years
   d. Older than 50 years

2. What is a major indication of MDS in the peripheral blood and bone marrow?
   a. Dyspoiesis
   b. Leukocytosis with left shift
   c. Normal bone marrow with abnormal peripheral blood features
   d. Thrombocytosis

3. An alert hematologist should recognize all of the following peripheral blood abnormalities as diagnostic clues in MDS *except:*
   a. Oval macrocytes
   b. Target cells
   c. Agranular neutrophils
   d. Circulating micromegakaryocytes

4. For an erythroid precursor to be considered a ring sideroblast, the iron-laden mitochondria must encircle how much of the nucleus?
   a. One quarter
   b. One third
   c. Two thirds
   d. Entire nucleus

5. According to the WHO classification of MDS, what percentage of blasts would constitute transformation to an acute leukemia?
   a. 5%
   b. 10%
   c. 20%
   d. 30%

6. A patient has anemia, oval macrocytes, and hypersegmented neutrophils. Which of the following tests would be most efficient in differential diagnosis of this disorder?
   a. Serum iron and ferritin levels
   b. Erythropoietin level
   c. Vitamin B_{12} and folate levels
   d. Chromosome analysis

7. A 60-year-old woman comes to the physician with fatigue and malaise. Her hemoglobin is 8 g/dL, hematocrit is 25%, RBC count is 2.00×10^{12}/L, platelet count is 550×10^9/L, and WBC count is 3.8×10^9/L. Her WBC differential is unremarkable. Bone marrow shows erythroid hypoplasia and hypolobulated megakaryocytes; granulopoiesis appears normal. Ring sideroblasts are rare. Chromosome analysis reveals the deletion of 5q only. Based on the classification of this disorder, what therapy would be most appropriate?
   a. Supportive therapy; lenalidomide if the disease progresses
   b. Aggressive chemotherapy
   c. Bone marrow transplantation
   d. Low-dose cytosine arabinoside, accompanied by *cis*-retinoic acid

8. Which of the following is *least* likely to contribute to the death of patients with MDS?
   a. Neutropenia
   b. Thrombocytopenia
   c. Organ failure
   d. Neuropathy

9. Into what other hematologic disease does MDS often convert?
   a. Megaloblastic anemia
   b. Aplastic anemia
   c. AML
   d. Myeloproliferative disease

10. Chronic myelomonocytic leukemia is classified in the WHO system as:
    a. A myeloproliferative neoplasm
    b. Myelodysplastic syndrome, unclassified
    c. MDS/MPN
    d. Acute leukemia

REFERENCES

1. Layton, D. M., Mufti, G. J. (1986). Myelodysplastic syndromes: their history, evolution and relation to acute myeloid leukemia. *Blood, 53,* 423–436, 1986.
2. Mufti, G. J., Galton, D. A. G. (1986). Myelodysplastic syndromes: natural history and features of prognostic significance. *Clin Haematol, 15,* 953–971.
3. Cheson, B. D., Bennett, J. M., Kantarjian, H., et al. (2000). Report of an international working group to standardize response criteria for myelodysplastic syndromes. *Blood, 96,* 3671–3674.
4. Bennett, J. M., Catovsky, D., Daniel, M. T., et al. (1982). Proposals for the classification of the myelodysplastic syndromes. *Br J Haematol, 51,* 189–199.
5. Harris, N. L., Jaffe, E. S., Diebold, J., et al. (2000). The World Health Organization classification of hematological malignancies report of the Clinical Advisory Committee Meeting, Airlie House, Virginia, November 1997. *Mod Pathol, 13,* 193–207.
6. Vardiman, J. W., Harris, N. L., & Brunning, R. D. (2002). The World Health Organization (WHO) classification of the myeloid neoplasms. *Blood, 100,* 2292–2302.
7. Janssen, J. W. G., Buschle, M., Layton, M., et al. (1989). Clonal analysis of myelodysplastic syndromes: evidence of multipotential stem cell origin. *Blood, 73,* 248–254.
8. Greenberg, P. L. (1987). Biologic nature of the myelodysplastic syndromes. *Acta Haematol, 78*(suppl 1),94–99.
9. DeAngelo, D. J., & Stone, R. M. (2012). Myelodysplastic syndromes: biology and treatment. In Hoffman, R., Benz, E. J. Jr., Silberstein, L. E., et al., (Eds.), *Hematology: Basic Principles and Practice.* (6th ed.). Philadelphia: Saunders Elsevier, Chapter 59.
10. Hasle, H., Niemeyer, C. M., Chessells, J. M., et al. (2003). A pediatric approach to the WHO classification of myelodysplastic and myeloproliferative diseases. *Leukemia, 17,* 277–282.
11. Niemeyer, C. M., & Baumann, I. (2008). Myelodysplastic syndrome in children and adolescents. *Semin Hematol, 45*(1), 60–70.
12. National Cancer Institute. (2000-2009). Surveillance, Epidemiology, and End Results (SEER) program. Age-adjusted SEER incidence rates and 95% confidence intervals by cancer sites. *All Ages, All Races, Both Sexes.* Myelodysplastic Syndromes. Retrieved from http://seer.cancer.gov/faststats/selections.php? Accessed 23.04.13.
13. Ma, X., Does, M., Raza, A., et al. (2007). Myelodysplastic syndromes: incidence and survival in the United States. *Cancer, 109,* 1536–1542.
14. Werner, C. A. (2011, Nov). *The Older Population: 2010. 2010 Census Briefs.* United States Census Bureau. Retrieved from http://www.census.gov/prod/cen2010/briefs/c2010br-09.pdf. Accessed 23.04.13.
15. Tsukamoto, N., Morita, K., Maehara, T., et al. (1993). Clonality in myelodysplastic syndromes: demonstration of pluripotent stem cell origin using X-linked restriction fragment length polymorphisms. *Br J Haematol, 83,* 589–594.
16. Kroef, M. J., Fibbe, W. E., Mout, R., et al. (1993). Myeloid, but not lymphoid cells carry the 5q deletion: polymerase chain reaction analysis of loss of heterozygosity using mini-repeat sequences on highly purified cell fractions. *Blood, 81,* 1849–1854.
17. van Kamp, H., Fibbe, W. E., Jansen, R. P. M., et al. (1992). Clonal involvement of granulocytes and monocytes, but not of T and B lymphocytes and natural killer cells in patients with myelodysplasia: analysis by X-linked restriction fragment length polymorphism and polymerase chain reaction of phosphoglycerate kinase gene. *Blood, 80,* 1774–1980.
18. Du, Y., Fryzek, J., Sekeres, M. A., et al. (2010). Smoking and alcohol intake as risk factors for myelodysplastic syndromes (MDS). *Leuk Res, 34,* 1–5.
19. Brunning, R. D., Orazi, A., Germing, U., et al. (2008). Myelodysplastic syndromes/neoplasms, overview. In Swerdlow, S. H., Campo, E., Harris, N. L., et al., (Eds.), *WHO Classification of Tumours of Haematopoietic and Lymphoid Tissues.* (4th ed., pp. 88–93). Lyon, France: IARC Press.
20. Mufti, G. J. (2004). Pathobiology, classification, and diagnosis of myelodysplastic syndrome. *Best Pract Res Clin Haematol, 17*(4), 543–557.
21. Yoshida, Y., & Mufti, G. J. (1999). Apoptosis and its significance in MDS: controversies revisited. *Leuk Res, 23,* 777–785.
22. Yoshida, Y. (1993). Hypothesis: apoptosis may be the mechanism responsible for the premature intramedullary cell death in the myelodysplastic syndrome. *Leukemia, 7,* 144–146.
23. Yoshida, Y., Stephenson, J., & Mufti, G. J. (1993). Myelodysplastic syndromes: from morphology to molecular biology: Part I. Classification, natural history and cell biology of myelodysplasia. *Int J Hematol, 57,* 87–97.
24. Yoshida, Y., Anzai, N., & Kawabata, H. (1995). Apoptosis in myelodysplasia: a paradox or paradigm. *Leuk Res, 19,* 887–891.
25. DiGiuseppe, J. A., & Kastan, M. B. (1997). Apoptosis in haematological malignancies. *J Clin Pathol, 50,* 361–364.
26. Lepelley, P., Campergue, L., Grardel, N., et al. (1996). Is apoptosis a massive process in myelodysplastic syndromes? *Br J Haematol, 95,* 368–371.
27. Greenberg, P. L. (1998). Apoptosis and its role in the myelodysplastic syndromes: implication for disease natural history and treatment. *Leuk Res, 22,* 1123–1126.
28. Raza, A., Gezer, S., Mundle, S., et al. (1995). Apoptosis in bone marrow biopsy samples involving stromal and hematopoietic cells in 50 patients with myelodysplastic syndromes. *Blood, 86,* 268–276.
29. Rajapaksa, R., Ginzton, N., Rott, L. S., et al. (1996). Altered oncoprotein expression and apoptosis in myelodysplastic syndrome marrow cells. *Blood, 88,* 4275–4287.

30. Parker, J. E., & Mufti, G. J. (2001). The role of apoptosis in the pathogenesis of the myelodysplastic syndromes. *Int J Hematol, 73,* 416–428.

31. Wimazal, F., Krauth, M-T., Vales, A., et al. (2006). Immunohistochemical detection of vascular endothelial growth factor (VEGF) in the bone marrow in patients with myelodysplastic syndromes: correlation between VEGF expression and the FAB category. *Leuk Lymphoma, 47,* 451–460.

32. Brunner, B., Gunsilius, E., Schumacher, P., et al. (2002). Blood levels of angiogenin and vascular endothelial growth factor are elevated in myelodysplastic syndromes and in some acute myeloid leukemia. *J Hematother Stem Cell Res, 11,* 119–125.

33. Perkins, S. L., & McKenna, R. W. (2010). Myelodysplastic syndromes. In Kjeldsberg, C. R., Perkins, S. L., (Eds.), *Practical Diagnosis of Hematologic Disorders.* (5th ed., pp. 547–582). Chicago: ASCP Press, chap 45.

34. Hershman, D., Neugut, A. I., Jacobson, J. S., et al. (2007). Acute myeloid leukemia or myelodysplastic syndrome following use of granulocyte colony-stimulating factors during breast cancer adjuvant therapy. *J Natl Cancer Inst, 99,* 196–205.

35. Tsurusawa, M., Manabe, A., Hayashi, Y., et al. (2005). Therapy-related myelodysplastic syndrome in childhood: a retrospective study of 36 patients in Japan. *Leuk Res, 29,* 625–632.

36. Rodak, B. F., & Leclair, S. J. (2002). The new WHO nomenclature: introduction and myeloid neoplasms. *Clin Lab Sci, 15,* 44–54.

37. Head, D. R., Kopecky, K., Bennett, J. M., et al. (1989). Pathologic implications of internuclear bridging in myelodysplastic syndrome. An Eastern Cooperative Oncology Group/Southwest Oncology Group Cooperative Study. *Cancer, 64,* 2199–2202.

38. Langenhuijsen, M. M. (1984). Neutrophils with ring-shaped nuclei in myeloproliferative disease. *Br J Haematol, 58,* 227–230.

39. Doll, D. C., & List, A. F. (1989). Myelodysplastic syndromes. *West J Med, 151,* 161–167.

40. Seymour, J. F., & Estey, E. H. (1993). The prognostic significance of Auer rods in myelodysplasia. *Br J Haematol, 85,* 67–76.

41. Tricot, G., De Wolf-Peeters, R., Vlietinck, R., et al. (1984). Bone marrow histology in myelodysplastic syndromes. *Br J Haematol, 58,* 217–225.

42. Leguit, R. J., & van den Tweel, J. G. (2010). The pathology of bone marrow failure. *Histopathology, 57,* 655–670. Review.

43. Barbui, T., Cortelazzo, S., Viero, P., et al. (1993). Infection and hemorrhage in elderly acute myeloblastic leukemia and primary myelodysplasia. *Hematol Oncol, 11*(suppl 1), 15–18.

44. Mazzone, A., Ricevuti, G., Pasotti, D., et al. (1993). The CD11/CD18 granulocyte adhesion molecules in myelodysplastic syndromes. *Br J Haematol, 83,* 245–252.

45. Mittelman, M., Karcher, D., Kammerman, L., et al. (1993). High Ia (HLA-DR) and low CD11b (Mo1) expression may predict early conversion to leukemia in myelodysplastic syndromes. *Am J Hematol, 43,* 165–171.

46. Pomeroy, C., Oken, M. M., Rydell, R. E., et al. (1991). Infection in the myelodysplastic syndromes. *Am J Med, 90,* 338–344.

47. Boogaerts, M. A., Nelissen, V., Roelant, C., et al. (1983). Blood neutrophil function in primary myelodysplastic syndromes. *Br J Haematol, 55,* 217–227.

48. Verhoef, G. E., Zachee, P., Ferrant, A., et al. (1992). Recombinant human erythropoietin for the treatment of anemia in the myelodysplastic syndromes: a clinical and erythrokinetic assessment. *Ann Hematol, 64,* 16–21.

49. Merchav, S., Nielsen, O. J., Rosenbaum, H., et al. (1990). In vitro studies of erythropoietin-dependent regulation of erythropoiesis in myelodysplastic syndromes. *Leukemia, 4,* 771–774.

50. Lintula, R., Rasi, V., Ikkala, E., et al. (1981). Platelet function in preleukemia. *Scand J Haematol, 26,* 65–71.

51. Raman, B. K., Van Slyck, E. J., Riddle, J., et al. (1989). Platelet function and structure in myeloproliferative disease, myelodysplastic syndrome and secondary thrombocytosis. *Am J Clin Pathol, 91,* 647–655.

52. Vardiman, J. W., Thiele, J., Arber, D. A., et al. (2009). The 2008 revision of the World Health Organization (WHO) classification of myeloid neoplasms and acute leukemia: rationale and important changes. *Blood, 114,* 937–951.

53. Germing, U., Strupp, C., Kuemdgen, A., et al. (2006). Prospective validation of the WHO proposals for the classification of myelodysplastic syndromes. *Haematologica, 91*(12), 1596–1604.

54. Mufti, G. J., Bennett, J. M., Goasguen, J., et al. (2008). Diagnosis and classification of myelodysplastic syndrome: International Working Group on Morphology of myelodysplastic syndrome (IWGM-MDS) consensus proposals for the definition and enumeration of myeloblasts and ring sideroblasts. *Haematologica, 93,* 1712–1717.

55. Hasserjian, R. P., Gattermann, N., Bennett, J. M., et al. (2008). Refractory anemia with ring sideroblasts. In Swerdlow, S. H., Campo, E., Harris, N. L., et al., (Eds.), *WHO Classification of Tumours of Haematopoietic and Lymphoid Tissues.* (4th ed., pp. 96–97). Lyon, France: IARC Press.

56. Szpurka, H., Tiu, R., Murugesan, G., et al. (2006). Refractory anemia with ringed sideroblasts assoiciated with marked thrombocytosis (RARS-T), another myeloproliferative condition characterized by JAK2 V617F mutation. *Blood, 108,* 2173–2181.

57. Brunning, R. D., Bennett, J. M., Matutes, E., et al. (2008). Refractory cytopenia with multilineage dysplasia. In Swerdlow, S. H., Campo, E., Harris, N. L., et al., (Eds.), *WHO Classification of Tumours of Haematopoietic and Lymphoid Tissues.* (4th ed., pp. 98–99). Lyon, France: IARC Press.

58. Giagounidis, A. A., Germing, U., Wainscoat, J. S., et al. (2004). The 5q– syndrome. *Hematology, 9,* 271–277.

59. Giagounidis, A. A., Germing, U., Haase, S., et al. (2004). Clinical, morphological, cytogenetic, and prognostic features of patients with myelodysplastic syndromes and del(5q) including band q31. *Leukemia, 18,* 113–119.

60. Giagounidis, A. A., Haase, S., Heinsch, M., et al. (2007). Lenalidomide in the context of complex karyotype or interrupted treatment: case reviews of del(5q) MDS patients with unexpected responses. *Ann Hematol, 86,* 133–137.

61. Hasserjian, R. P., LeBeau, M. M., List, A. F., et al. (2008). Myelodysplastic syndrome with isolated del(5q). In Swerdlow, S. H., Campo, E., Harris, N. L., et al., (Eds.), *WHO Classification of Tumours of Haematopoietic and Lymphoid Tissues.* (4th ed., p. 102). Lyon, France: IARC Press.

62. Orazi, A., Brunning, R. D., & Baumann, I. (2008). Myelodysplastic syndrome, unclassifiable. In Swerdlow, S. H., Campo, E., Harris, N. L., et al., (Eds.), *WHO Classification of Tumours of Haematopoietic and Lymphoid Tissues.* (4th ed., p. 103). Lyon, France: IARC Press.

63. Orazi, A., Bennett, J. M., Germing, U., et al. (2008). Chronic myelomonocytic leukemia. In Swerdlow, S. H., Campo, E., Harris, N. L., et al., (Eds.), *WHO Classification of Tumours of Haematopoietic and Lymphoid Tissues,* (4th ed., p. 76). Lyon, France: IARC Press.

64. Vardiman, J. W., Bennett, J. M., Bain, B. J., et al. (2008). Atypical chronic myeloid leukemia, *BCR-ABL1* negative. In Swerdlow, S. H., Campo, E., Harris, N. L., et al., (Eds.), *WHO Classification of Tumours of Haematopoietic and Lymphoid Tissues.* (4th ed., pp. 80–81). Lyon, France: IARC Press.

65. Xubo, G., Xingguo, L., Xiaanguo, W., et al. (2009). The role of peripheral blood, bone marrow aspirate and especially bone marrow trephine biopsy in distinguishing atypical chronic myeloid leukemia from chronic granulocytic leukemia and chronic myelomonocytic leukemia. *Eur J Haematol, 83,* 1292–1301.

66. Breccia, M., Biondo, F., Latagliata, R., et al. (2006). Identification of risk factors in atypical chronic myeloid leukemia. *Haematologica, 91,* 1566–1568.

67. Niemeyer, C. M., Aricó, M., Basso, G., et al. (1997). Chronic myelomonocytic leukemia in childhood: a retrospective analysis of 110 cases. *Blood, 89,* 3534–3543.

68. Locatelli, F., Nöllke, P., Zecca, M., et al. (2005). Hematopoietic stem cell transplantation (HSCT) in children with juvenile myelomonocytic leukemia (JMML): results of the EWOG-MDS/EBMT trial. *Blood, 105*, 410–419.

69. Vardiman, J. W., Bennett, J. M., Bain, B. J., et al. (2008). Myelodysplastic/myeloproliferative neoplasm, unclassifiable. In Swerdlow, S. H., Campo, E., Harris, N. L., et al., (Eds.), *WHO Classification of Tumours of Haematopoietic and Lymphoid Tissues.* (4th ed., pp. 85–86). Lyon, France: IARC Press.

70. Pedersen-Bjergaard, J., Andersen, M. T., Andersen, M. K. (2007). Genetic pathways in the pathogenesis of therapy-related myelodysplasia and acute myeloid leukemia. *Hematology Am Soc Hematol Educ Program*, 391–397.

71. Bernasconi, P., Klersy, C., Boni, M., et al. (2005). Incidence and prognostic significance of karyotype abnormalities in de novo primary myelodysplastic syndromes: a study on 331 patients from a single institution. *Leukemia, 19*, 1424–1431.

72. Paulsson, K., Johansson, B. (2007). Trisomy 8 as the sole chromosomal aberration in acute myeloid leukemia and myelodysplastic syndromes. *Pathol Biol (Paris), 55*, 37–48.

73. Geddes, A. D., Bowen, D. T., Jacobs, A. (1990). Clonal karyotype abnormalities and clinical progress in the myelodysplastic syndrome. *Br J Haematol, 76*, 194–202.

74. Horiike, S., Kita-Sasai, Y., Nakao, M., et al. (2003). Configuration of the TP53 gene as an independent prognostic parameter of myelodysplastic syndrome. *Leuk Lymphoma, 44*, 915–922.

75. Cilloni, D., Messa, E., Messa, F., et al. (2006). Genetic abnormalities as targets for molecular therapies in myelodysplastic syndromes. *Ann N Y Acad Sci, 1089*, 411–423.

76. Chen, C. Y., Lin, L. I., Tang, J. L., et al. (2007). RUNX1 gene mutation in primary myelodysplastic syndrome—the mutation can be detected early at diagnosis or acquired during disease progression and is associated with poor outcome. *Br J Haematol, 139*, 405–414.

77. Harada, H., Harada, Y., Niimi, H., et al. (2004). High incidence of somatic mutations in the *AML1/RUNX* gene in myelodysplastic syndrome and low blast percentage myeloid leukemia with myelodysplasia. *Blood, 103*, 2316–2324.

78. Kosmider, O., Gelsi-Boyer, V., Cheok, M., et al. (2009). TET2 mutation is an independent favorable prognostic factor in myelodysplastic syndromes (MDSs). *Blood, 114*, 3285–3291.

79. Greenberg, P. L. (2011). Molecular and genetic features of myelodysplastic syndromes. *Int J Lab Hematol, 34*, 215–22.

80. Epling-Burnette, P. K., & List, A. F. (2009). Advancements in the molecular pathogenesis of myelodysplastic syndrome. *Curr Opin Hematol, 16*, 70–76.

81. Nakao, M. (2001). Epigenetics: interaction of DNA methylation and chromatin. *Gene, 278*, 25–31.

82. Musolino, C., Sant'Antonio, E., Penna, G., et al. (2010). Epigenetic therapy in myelodysplastic syndromes. *Eur J Haematol, 84*, 463–473.

83. Quesnel, B. (2006). Methylation and myelodysplastic syndromes: when and where? *Leuk Res, 30*, 1327–1329 (editorial).

84. Griffiths, E. A., & Gore, S. D. (2013). Epigenetic therapies in MDS and AML. *Adv Exp Med Biol, 754*, 253–283.

85. Greenberg, P., Cox, C., & LeBeau, M. M. (1997). International scoring system for evaluating prognosis in myelodysplastic syndromes. *Blood, 89*, 2079–2088.

86. Greenberg, P. L., Tuechler, H., Schanz, J., et al. (2012). Revised international scoring system for myelodysplastic syndromes. *Blood, 120*, 2454–2465.

87. Pardanani, A., Finke, C., Lasho, T. L., et al. (2012). IPSS-independent prognostic value of plasma CXCL 10, IL-7 and IL-6 levels in myelodysplastic syndromes. *Leukemia, 26*, 693–699.

88. Sekeres, M. A. (2009). Treatment of MDS; something old, something new, something borrowed. *Hematology Am Soc Hematol Educ Program*, 656–663.

89. Hellström-Lindberg, E., & Malcovati, L. (2008). Supportive care, growth factors, and new therapies in myelodysplastic syndromes. *Blood Rev, 22*, 75–91.

90. Loaiza-Bonilla, A., Gore, S., & Carraway, H. E. (2010). Novel approaches for myelodysplastic syndromes: beyond hypomethylating agents. *Curr Opin Hematol, 17*, 104–109.

91. Sloand, E. M., Wu, C. O., Greenberg, P., et al. (2008). Factors affecting response and survival in patients with myelodysplasia treated with immunosuppressive therapy. *J Clin Oncol, 26*, 2505–2511.

92. Jonásová, A., Neuwirtová, R., Cermák, J., et al. (1998). Cyclosporin A therapy in hypoplastic MDS patients and certain refractory anaemias without hypoplastic bone marrow. *Br J Haematol, 100*, 304–309.

93. List, A., Kurtin, S., Roe, D., et al. (2005). Efficacy of lenalidomide in myelodysplastic syndromes. *N Engl J Med, 352*, 549–557.

94. Chustecka, Z. (2013, Mar 07). *Dramatic Changes in the Treatment Landscape of MDS.* Retrieved from http://www.medscape.com/viewarticle/780319. Accessed 29.04.13.

95. University of Texas MD Anderson Cancer Center. *Patient Education.* Myelodysplastic syndrome. Retrieved from http://www2.mdanderson.org/app/pe/index.cfm?pageName=opendoc&docid=304. Updated 4/23/09. Accessed 29.04.13.

96. Lancet, J. E., & Karp, J. E. (2003). Farnesyltransferase inhibitors in hematologic malignancies: new horizons in therapy. *Blood, 102*, 3880–3889.

97. Cheson, B. D., Bennett, J. M., Kantarijian, H., et al. (2000). Report of an international working group to standardize response criteria for myelodysplastic syndromes. *Blood, 96*, 3671–3674.

98. Silverman, L. R., Demakos, E. P., Peterson, B. L., et al. (2002). Randomized controlled trial of azacytidine in patients with the myelodysplastic syndrome: a study of the Cancer and Leukemia Group B. *J Clin Oncol, 20*, 2429–2440.

99. Kornblith, A. B., Herndon, J. E. 2nd, Silverman, L. R., et al. (2002). Impact of azacytidine on the quality of life of patients with myelodysplastic syndrome treated in a randomized phase trial III, a Cancer and Leukemia Group study B. *J Clin Oncol, 20*, 2441–2452.

100. Appelbaum, F. R. (2011). The role of hematopoietic cell transplantation as therapy for myelodysplasia. *Best Pract Res Clin Haematol, 24*, 541–547.

101. Gerds, A. T., & Deeg, H. J. (2012). Transplantation for myelodysplastic syndrome in the era of hypomethylating agents. *Curr Opin Hematol, 19*, 71–75.

102. Sekeres, M. A., Stowell, S. A., Berry, C. A., et al. (2013). Improving the diagnosis and treatment of patients with myelodysplastic syndromes through a performance improvement initiative. *Leuk Res, 37*, 422–426.

103. Besson, D., Rannou, S., Elmaaroufi, H., et al. (2012). Disclosure of myelodysplastic syndrome diagnosis: improving patients' understanding and experience. *Eur J Haematol, 90*, 151–156.

104. Scott, B. L., & Deeg, H. J. (2010). Myelodysplastic syndromes. *Annu Rev Med, 61*, 345–358.

35

Acute Leukemias

Woodlyne Roquiz, Pranav Gandhi, and Ameet R. Kini

OBJECTIVES

After completion of this chapter, the reader will be able to:

1. Discuss the causes and development of acute leukemia.
2. Characterize the diagnostic criteria used for acute myeloid and acute lymphoblastic leukemias.
3. Compare and contrast acute lymphoblastic and myeloid leukemias by morphology, presenting signs and symptoms, laboratory findings, and prognosis.
4. Interpret the results of diagnostic tests for acute leukemias.
5. Discuss tumor lysis syndrome, including risk, cause, and laboratory findings.
6. Discuss the cell staining patterns for the following tests: myeloperoxidase, Sudan black B, and esterases.

CASE STUDY

After studying the material in this chapter, the reader should be able to respond to the following case study:

A 5-year-old child was seen by her family physician because of weakness and headaches. She had been in good health except for the usual communicable diseases of childhood. Physical examination revealed a pale, listless child with multiple bruises. The WBC count was 15×10^9/L, the hemoglobin was 8 g/dL, and the platelet count was 90×10^9/L. She had "abnormal cells" in her peripheral blood (Figure 35-1). Cytogenetic studies revealed hyperdiploidy.

1. What is the most likely diagnosis?
2. What characteristics of this disease indicate a positive prognosis?
3. What prognosis is associated with the hyperdiploidy?

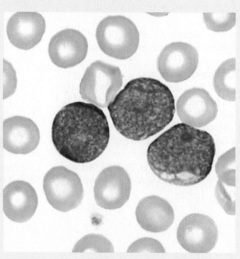

Figure 35-1 Peripheral blood film for the patient in the case study (×1000). (From Carr JH, Rodak BF: *Clinical hematology atlas*, ed 4, St. Louis, 2013, Saunders.)

INTRODUCTION

The broad term *leukemia* is derived from the ancient Greek words *leukos* (λευκός), meaning "white," and *haima* (αἷμα), meaning "blood."[1] As defined today, acute leukemia refers to the rapid, clonal proliferation in the bone marrow of lymphoid or myeloid progenitor cells known as lymphoblasts and myeloblasts, respectively. When proliferation of blasts overwhelms the bone marrow, blasts are seen in the peripheral blood and the patient's symptoms reflect suppression of normal hematopoiesis.

For most cases of acute leukemia, the causes directly related to the development of the malignancy are unknown. The exceptions that exist are certain toxins that can induce genetic changes leading to a malignant phenotype. Environmental exposures known to lead to hematopoietic malignancies include radiation and exposure to organic solvents, such as benzene. Rarely, leukemias can be seen in patients with known familial cancer predisposition syndromes. Alkylating agents and other forms of chemotherapy used to treat various forms of cancer can induce deoxyribonucleic acid (DNA) damage in hematopoietic cells, leading to therapy-related leukemias.

Regardless of the mechanism of initial genetic damage, the development of leukemia is currently believed to be a stepwise progression of mutations or "multiple hits" involving mutations in genes that give cells a proliferative advantage, as well as mutations that hinder differentiation.[2,3] These mutations result in transformation of normal hematopoietic stem cells or precursors into leukemic stem cells (LSCs). The LSCs then initiate, proliferate, and sustain the leukemia.[4]

CLASSIFICATION SCHEMES FOR ACUTE LEUKEMIAS

The French-American-British (FAB) classification of the acute leukemias was devised in the 1970s and was based on morphologic examination along with cytochemical stains to distinguish lymphoblasts from myeloblasts (Figure 35-2). The use of cytochemical stains continues to be a useful adjunct for differentiation of hematopoietic diseases, especially acute leukemias. The details of the cytochemical stains are addressed at the end of this chapter. In addition to morphologic and cytochemical stains, techniques commonly used to diagnose hematopoietic malignancies include flow cytometry and genetic/molecular studies. Findings of these techniques are discussed throughout the chapter in relation to specific leukemias.

Hematologists and pathologists are now moving toward more precise classification of many of the leukocyte neoplasms based on recurring chromosomal and genetic lesions found in many patients. These lesions are related to disruptions of oncogenes, tumor suppressor genes, and other regulatory elements that control proliferation, maturation, apoptosis, and other vital cell functions. In 2001 the World Health Organization (WHO) published new classification schemes for nearly all of the tumors of hematopoietic and lymphoid tissues,[5] and in some cases WHO melded the older morphologic schemes with the newer schemes. For instance, in the WHO classification scheme for acute myeloid leukemias (AMLs), there are some remnants of the old FAB classification, but new classifications were introduced for leukemias associated with consistently recurring chromosomal translocations. According to the WHO classification, a finding of at least 20% blasts in the bone marrow is required for diagnosis of the majority of acute leukemias, and testing must be performed to detect the presence or absence of genetic anomalies. In 2008 the WHO classification of hematologic malignancies was revised to reflect advances in the field.[6] In-depth discussion of each of the subclassifications is beyond the scope of this book, so only the most common subtypes of acute lymphoblastic leukemia and acute myeloid leukemia are detailed here.

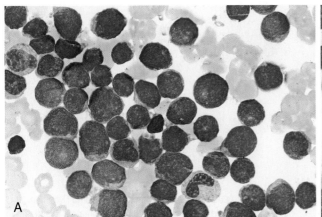
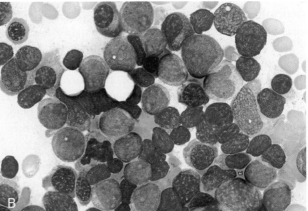

Figure 35-2 A, Lymphoblasts (bone marrow, Wright stain, ×500). Cells have a diameter two to three times the normal lymphocyte diameter, scant blue cytoplasm, coarse chromatin, deeper staining than myeloblasts, and inconspicuous nucleoli. **B,** Myeloblasts (bone marrow, Wright stain, ×500). Cells have a diameter three to five times the lymphocyte diameter, moderate gray cytoplasm, uniform fine chromatin, two or more prominent nucleoli, and possibly Auer rods.

ACUTE LYMPHOBLASTIC LEUKEMIA

Acute lymphoblastic leukemia (ALL) is primarily a disease of childhood and adolescence, accounting for 25% of childhood cancers and up to 75% of childhood leukemia.[7] The peak incidence of ALL in children is between 2 and 5 years of age.[8] Although ALL is rare in adults, risk increases with age; most adult patients are older than 50 years of age. The subtype of ALL is an important prognostic indicator for survival.[6] Adults have a poorer outlook: 80% to 90% experience complete remission, but the cure rate is less than 40%.[9,10]

Patients with B cell ALL typically present with fatigue (caused by anemia), fever (caused by neutropenia and infection), and mucocutaneous bleeding (caused by thrombocytopenia). Lymphadenopathy, including enlargement, is often a symptom.[11] Enlargement of the spleen (splenomegaly) and of the liver (hepatomegaly) may be seen. Bone pain often results from intramedullary growth of leukemic cells.[11] Eventual infiltration of malignant cells into the meninges, testes, or ovaries occurs frequently, and lymphoblasts can be found in the cerebrospinal fluid.[12]

In T cell ALL, there may be a large mass in the mediastinum leading to compromise of regional anatomic structures. Similar to B-ALL, T-ALL may present with anemia, thrombocytopenia, organomegaly, and bone pain, although the degree of leukopenia is often less severe.[13]

World Health Organization Classification

B lymphoblastic leukemia/lymphoma (B-ALL) is subdivided into seven subtypes that are associated with recurrent cytogenetic abnormalities.[14] These entities are linked with unique clinical, phenotypic, or prognostic features (Box 35-1). Cases of B cell ALL that do not exhibit the specific genetic abnormalities are classified as B lymphoblastic leukemia/lymphoma, not otherwise specified. Although 50% to 70% of patients with T lymphoblastic leukemia/lymphoma have abnormal gene rearrangements, none of the abnormalities is clearly associated with specific biologic features, and thus T-ALL is not further subdivided clinically.[14]

Morphology

Lymphoblasts vary in size but fall into two morphologic types. The most common type seen is a small lymphoblast (1.0 to 2.5 times the size of a normal lymphocyte) with scant blue cytoplasm and indistinct nucleoli (Figure 35-2); the second type of lymphoblast is larger (two to three times the size of a lymphocyte) with prominent nucleoli and nuclear membrane irregularities (Figure 35-3).[13] These cells may be confused with the blasts of acute myeloid leukemia (AML).

Prognosis

Prognosis in ALL has improved dramatically over the past decades as a result of improvement in algorithms for treatment.[13] The prognosis for ALL depends on age at the time of diagnosis, lymphoblast load (tumor burden), immunophenotype, and

---

> **BOX 35-1** B Lymphoblastic Leukemia/Lymphoma with Recurrent Genetic Abnormalities (2008 World Health Organization Classification)
>
> B lymphoblastic leukemia/lymphoma with t(9;22)(q34;q11.2);*BCR-ABL1*
> B lymphoblastic leukemia/lymphoma with t(v;11q23);*MLL* rearranged
> B lymphoblastic leukemia/lymphoma with t(12;21)(p13;q22);*TEL-AML1 (ETV6-RUNX1)*
> B lymphoblastic leukemia/lymphoma with hyperdiploidy
> B lymphoblastic leukemia/lymphoma with hypodiploidy
> B lymphoblastic leukemia/lymphoma with t(5;14)(q31;q32);*IL3-IGH*
> B lymphoblastic leukemia/lymphoma with t(1;19)(q23;p13.3);*E2A-PBX1(TCF3-PBX1)*

From Swerdlow SH, Campo E, Harris NL, et al, editors: *WHO classification of tumours of haematopoietic and lymphoid tissues,* ed 4, Lyon, France, 2008, IARC Press.

genetic abnormalities. Children rather than infants or teens do the best. Chromosomal translocations are the strongest predictor of adverse treatment outcomes for children and adults. Peripheral blood lymphoblast counts greater than 20 to 30×10^9/L, hepatosplenomegaly, and lymphadenopathy all are associated with worse outcome. The effects of other variables previously associated with a poorer prognosis, such as sex and ethnic group, have been eliminated when patients have been given equal access to treatment in trials carried out at a single institution.[15]

Immunophenotyping

Although morphology is the first tool used to distinguish ALL from AML, immunophenotyping and genetic analysis are the most reliable indicators of a cell's origin. Because both B and T cells are derived from lymphoid progenitors, both usually express CD34, terminal deoxynucleotidyl transferase (TdT),

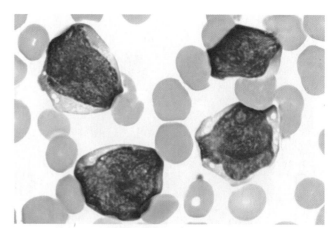

Figure 35-3 Acute lymphoblastic leukemia. Large lymphoblast with prominent nucleoli and membrane irregularities (peripheral blood, ×1000). (From Carr JH, Rodak BF: *Clinical hematology atlas,* ed 4, St. Louis, 2013, Saunders.)

and HLA-DR. Four types of ALL have been identified by immunologic methods: early B-ALL (pro-B, or pre-pre-B), intermediate (common) B-ALL, pre-B-ALL, and T-ALL (Table 35-1). B-ALL is characterized by specific B cell antigens that are expressed at different stages of B cell development. In general, B cells express CD19, CD20, CD22, CD24, C79a, CD10, cytoplasmic μ, and PAX-5 (B cell specific activator protein). The degree of differentiation of B-lineage lymphoblasts often correlates with genetics and plays an important role in treatment decisions.[6,13,16] In the earliest stage of differentiation (pre-pre B or pro-B), blasts express CD34, CD19, cytoplasmic CD22, and TdT. The incidence of pro-B ALL is about 5% in children and 11% in adults. In intermediate or *common* B-ALL, CD10 is expressed. The most mature B-ALL is called *pre-B-ALL*, in which CD34 is typically negative, but there is characteristic expression of cytoplasmic μ heavy chain. Pre-B-ALL accounts for 15% of childhood cases and 10% of adult B-ALL.[17]

T-ALL is seen most often in teenaged males with a mediastinal mass, elevated peripheral blast counts, meningeal involvement, and infiltration of extra marrow sites.[18,19] The common T cell markers CD2, CD3, CD4, CD5, CD7, and CD8 are usually present. Most cases express TdT. A distinct subtype of T-ALL, ETP-ALL (early T cell precursor ALL), contains a characteristic immunophenotype (CD8-, CD5dim) and has a poor response to chemotherapy, low rates of remission, and overall poor survival.[20,21]

Genetic and Molecular Findings

Cytogenetic abnormalities are seen in the majority of B and T cell ALL, which produce changes that affect normal B and T cell development and underlie the pathogenesis of these neoplasms. A majority of T-ALL have been shown to have gain-of-function mutations involving the *NOTCH1* gene, which alters the Notch receptor signaling pathway responsible for normal T cell development.[22]

In T-ALL, however, the cytogenetic alterations show less specificity and less correlation with prognosis and treatment outcome than in B-ALL. B lymphoblastic leukemia/lymphoma with the t(9;22)(q34;q11.2);*BCR-ABL1* mutation (Philadelphia chromosome–positive ALL) has the worst prognosis among ALLs. It is more common in adults than in children. Imatinib, which has shown success in treating chronic myelogenous leukemia, has improved survival (Chapter 33).

TABLE 35-1 Immunophenotypic Characteristics of Acute Lymphoblastic Leukemia

ALL Subtype	Immunophenotype
Early (pro/pre-pre) B-ALL	CD34, CD19, cytoplasmic CD22, TdT
Intermediate (common) B-ALL	CD34, CD19, CD10, cytoplasmic CD22, TdT
Pre-B-ALL	CD34, CD19, cytoplasmic CD22, cytoplasmic μ, TdT (variable)
T-ALL	CD2, CD3, CD4, CD5, CD7, CD8, TdT

B lymphoblastic leukemia/lymphoma with t(v;11q23);*MLL* rearranged is more common in very young infants, and the translocation may even occur in utero.[23] This leukemia has a very poor prognosis. About 25% of childhood ALL cases show a t(12;21)(p13;q22);*ETV6-RUNX1* translocation and appear to derive from a B cell progenitor rather than the hematopoietic stem cell.[24] This translocation is rare in adults. In children, it carries an excellent prognosis, with a cure rate of over 90%. Hyperdiploidy in B lymphoblastic leukemia/lymphoma is common in childhood B-ALL, accounting for 25% of cases, but it is much less common in adults. This genotype is associated with a very favorable prognosis in children. Conversely, hypodiploidy (less than 46 chromosomes) conveys a poor prognosis in both children and adults.

ACUTE MYELOID LEUKEMIA

AML is the most common type of leukemia in adults, and the incidence increases with age. AML is less common in children. The French-American-British (FAB) classification of AML was based on morphology and cytochemistry; the WHO classification relies heavily on cytogenetics and molecular characterization (Chapters 30 and 31).[6,14]

Clinical Presentation

The clinical presentation of AML is nonspecific but reflects decreased production of normal bone marrow elements. Most patients with AML have a total WBC count between 5 and 30 × 10⁹/L, although the WBC count may range from 1 to 200 × 10⁹/L. Myeloblasts are present in the peripheral blood in 90% of patients. Anemia, thrombocytopenia, and neutropenia give rise to the clinical findings of pallor, fatigue, fever, bruising, and bleeding. In addition, disseminated intravascular coagulation and other bleeding abnormalities can be significant.[25] Infiltration of malignant cells into the gums and other mucosal sites and skin also can be seen.

Splenomegaly is seen in half of AML patients, but lymph node enlargement is rare. Cerebrospinal fluid involvement in AML is rare and does not seem to be as ominous a sign as in ALL. Patients with AML tend to have few symptoms related to the central nervous system, even when it is infiltrated by blasts.

Common abnormalities in laboratory test results include hyperuricemia (caused by increased cellular turnover), hyperphosphatemia (due to cell lysis), and hypocalcemia (the latter two are also involved in progressive bone destruction). Hypokalemia is also common at presentation. During induction chemotherapy, especially when the WBC is quite elevated, tumor lysis syndrome may occur. Tumor lysis syndrome is a group of metabolic complications that can occur in patients with malignancy, most notably lymphomas and leukemias, with and without treatment of the malignancy. These complications are caused by the breakdown products of dying cancer cells, which in turn cause acute uric acid nephropathy and renal failure. Tumor lysis syndrome is characterized by hyperkalemia, hyperphosphatemia, hyperuricemia and hyperuricosuria, and hypocalcemia.[26] The hyperkalemia alone can be life-threatening. Aggressive prophylactic measures to prevent or reduce the clinical manifestations of tumor lysis syndrome are critical.[27]

Subtypes of Acute Myeloid Leukemia and Related Precursor Neoplasms

Laboratory diagnosis of AML begins with a complete blood count, peripheral blood film examination, and bone marrow aspirate and biopsy specimen examination. The total WBC count may be normal, increased, or decreased; anemia is usually present, along with significant thrombocytopenia. The bone marrow is usually hypercellular, and greater than 20% of cells typically are marrow blasts, although if certain genetic abnormalities are present, the 20% blast threshold is not necessary for the diagnosis of AML.[6] Each category is discussed, and a summary of the classification is presented in Box 35-2.

The 2008 WHO classification for myeloid malignancies has categorized AMLs with recurrent cytogenetic abnormalities into subgroups based on the primary cytogenetic aberrations (Box 35-3).[6,14]

BOX 35-2 Acute Myeloid Leukemia and Related Precursor Neoplasms (2008 World Health Organization Classification)

Acute myeloid leukemia with recurrent genetic abnormalities
Acute myeloid leukemia with myelodysplasia-related changes
Therapy-related myeloid neoplasms
Acute myeloid leukemia, not otherwise specified
Myeloid sarcoma
Myeloid proliferations related to Down syndrome
Blastic plasmacytoid dendritic cell neoplasm

From Swerdlow SH, Campo E, Harris NL, et al, editors: *WHO classification of tumours of haematopoietic and lymphoid tissues*, ed 4, Lyon, France, 2008, IARC Press.

BOX 35-3 Acute Myeloid Leukemia with Recurrent Genetic Abnormalities (2008 World Health Organization Classification)

AML with t(8;21)(q22;q22); *RUNX1-RUNX1T1*
AML with inv(16)(p13.1q22) or t(16;16)(p13.1;q22); *CBFB-MYH11*
APL with t(15;17)(q22;q12); *PML-RARA*
AML with t(9;11)(p22;q23); *MLLT3-MLL*
AML with t(6;9)(p23;q34); *DEK-NUP214*
AML with inv(3)(q21q26.2) or t(3;3)(q21;q26.2); *RPN1-EVI1*
AML with t(1;22)(p13;q13) *RBM15-MKL1*
Provisional entity: AML with mutated *NPM1*
Provisional entity: AML with mutated *CEBPA*

From Swerdlow SH, Campo E, Harris NL, et al, editors: *WHO classification of tumours of haematopoietic and lymphoid tissues*, ed 4, Lyon, France, 2008, IARC Press.

AML with Recurrent Genetic Abnormalities

Acute Myeloid Leukemia with t(8;21)(q22;q22);RUNX1/RUNX1T1. The t(8;21)(q22;q22);*RUNX1/RUNX1T1* mutation is found in about 5% of AML cases. Seen predominantly in children and young adults, AML with this translocation has myeloblasts with dysplastic granular cytoplasm, Auer rods, and some maturation (Figure 35-4), similar to the FAB M2 classification (see later in chapter). Various anomalies, such as pseudo–Pelger-Huët cells and hypogranulation, can be seen. Eosinophilia is possible. Prognosis is generally favorable but may be negatively impacted if unfavorable additional abnormalities, such as monosomy 7, occur.[28] The diagnosis of this subtype is based on the genetic abnormality, regardless of blast count.[6]

Acute Myeloid Leukemia with inv(16)(p13.1q22) or t(16;16)(p13.1;q22);CBFB-MYH11. Accounting for approximately 5% to 8% of all AML cases, core-binding factor (CBF) AML occurs at all ages, but it is found predominantly in younger patients.[6] The genetic aberration is sufficient for diagnosis regardless of blast count.[6,29] Myeloblasts, monoblasts, and promyelocytes are seen in the peripheral blood and bone marrow. In the bone marrow there may be eosinophilia with dysplastic changes (Figure 35-5). The incidence of extramedullary disease is higher than in most types of AML, and the central nervous system is a common site for relapse.[6,29] The remission rate is good, but only one half of patients are cured.[29]

Acute Myeloid Leukemia with t(15;17)(q22;q12); PML-RARA. Also known as *acute promyelocytic leukemia* (APL), AML with the t(15;17)(q22;q12);*PML-RARA* mutation comprises 5% to 10% of AML cases. It occurs in all age groups but is seen most commonly in young adults. This disorder is characterized by a differentiation block at the promyelocytic stage. The abnormal promyelocytes are considered to be comparable to blasts for the purpose of diagnosis. Detection of the 15;17 translocation is sufficient for diagnosis regardless of blast count.[6,28] Characteristic of this presentation are the

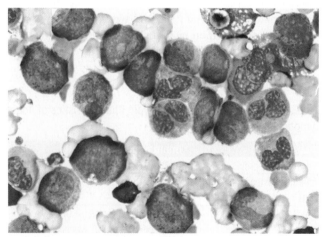

Figure 35-4 Acute myeloid leukemia with t(8;21). Myeloblasts with granular cytoplasm and some maturation (bone marrow, ×500). (From Carr JH, Rodak BF: *Clinical hematology atlas*, ed 4, St. Louis, 2013, Saunders.)

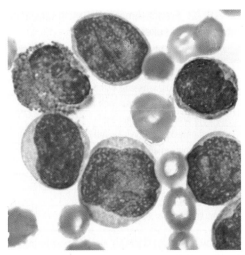

Figure 35-5 Acute myeloid leukemia with inv(16). There is an increase in myeloid and monocytic lines. Eosinophilia may also be present (peripheral blood, ×1000). (From Carr JH, Rodak BF: *Clinical hematology atlas*, ed 4, St. Louis, 2013, Saunders.)

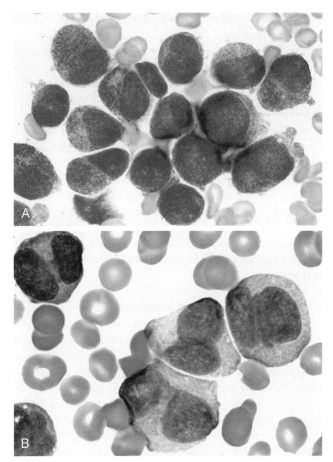

Figure 35-6 Acute myeloid leukemia with t(15;17), or promyelocytic leukemia. **A,** Low-power view of the more common hypergranular variant (peripheral blood, ×500). **B,** Oil immersion view of the microgranular variant showing bilobed nuclear features (peripheral blood, ×1000). (**B** from Carr JH, Rodak BF: *Clinical hematology atlas*, ed 4, St. Louis, 2013, Saunders.)

abnormal hypergranular promyelocytes, some with Auer rods (Figure 35-6). When promyelocytes release primary granule contents, their procoagulant activity initiates disseminated intravascular coagulation; however, thromboembolic events may occur at presentation and during treatment.[30] In one variant of APL, the granules are so small that because of the limits of light microscopy, the cells give the appearance of having no granules. This microgranular variant, accounting for 30% to 40% of APL cases, may be confused with other presentations of AML, but the presence of occasional Auer rods, the "butterfly" or "coin-on-coin" nucleus, and the clinical presentation are clues. The treatment of APL is significantly different from all other types of acute myeloid leukemia, and it is therefore important to arrive at an accurate diagnosis. Treatment includes all-*trans*-retinoic acid (ATRA) and arsenic trioxide.[31] ATRA is a vitamin A analogue and induces differentiation of the malignant promyelocytes. In adults who achieve a complete remission, the prognosis is better than for any other type of AML.[28] There are a few variants in *RARA* translocations that confer a poor diagnosis because the cells do not respond to ATRA therapy.[6,14]

Acute Myeloid Leukemia with t(9;11)(p22;q23);MLLT3-MLL. AML with t(9;11)(p22;q23);*MLLT3-MLL* represents a specific subgroup of the previous classification of AML with 11q23 abnormalities, and AMLs with other *MLL* abnormalities should not be placed in this group.[14] AML with t(9;11) is a rare leukemia (6% of AML cases) that presents with an increase in monoblasts and immature monocytes (Figure 35-7). The blasts are large with abundant cytoplasm and fine nuclear chromatin. The cells may have motility, with pseudopodia seen frequently. Granules and vacuoles can be observed in the blasts. Typically this disease occurs in children and may be associated with gingival and skin involvement and/or disseminated intravascular coagulation. The prognosis is intermediate to poor.[28]

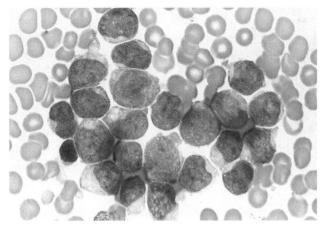

Figure 35-7 Acute myeloid leukemia with t(9;11) abnormalities. Both monoblasts and immature monocytes are increased (bone marrow, ×500).

Acute Myeloid Leukemia with t(6;9)(p23;q34);DEK-NUP214, Acute Myeloid Leukemia with inv(3)(q21q26.2) or t(3;3)(q21;q26.2);RPN1-EVI1, and Acute Myeloid Leukemia (Megakaryoblastic) with t(1;22)(p13;q13);RBM15-MKL1. These are rare leukemias included in the 2008 WHO classification. Detailed description of these entities is beyond the scope of this chapter.

Acute Myeloid Leukemia with Myelodysplasia-Related Changes

AML with myelodysplasia affects primarily older adults and has a poor prognosis. This subcategory of AML with myelodysplasia-related changes incorporates leukemias with at least 20% blasts, multilineage dysplasia, a history of MDS or MDS/myeloproliferative neoplasm (MPN), or a specific MDS-associated cytogenetic abnormality and the absence of AML with recurrent genetic abnormalities.[28,32] Significant dysplastic morphology includes pancytopenia with neutrophil hypogranulation or hypergranulation, pseudo–Pelger-Huët cells, and unusually segmented nuclei. Erythrocyte precursors have vacuoles, karyorrhexis, megaloblastoid features, and ringed sideroblasts. There may be dysplastic micromegakaryocytes and dysplastic megakaryocytes. Genetic findings are similar to those found in MDS, with complex karyotypes and −7/del(7q) and −5/del(5q) being the most common.[6,33]

Therapy-Related Myeloid Neoplasms

Treatment with alkylating agents, radiation, or topoisomerase II inhibitors has been associated with the development of a secondary AML, MDS, or MDS/MPN.[6,28,34,35] These therapy-related neoplasms account for 10% to 20% of AMLs, MDSs, and MDSs/MPNs. Generally these disorders occur following treatment for a prior malignancy, but they have also been associated with intensive treatment of patients with nonmalignant disorders requiring cytotoxic therapy.[6,34,36] Therapy-related myeloid neoplasms are similar in morphology to AML with myelodysplasia, monocytic/monoblastic leukemia, or AML with maturation, and the prognosis is generally poor, although therapy-related neoplasms with the t(15;17) and inv(16) mutations behave more like the de novo counterparts.[6,28]

Acute Myeloid Leukemia, Not Otherwise Specified

Because the leukemias in the "not otherwise specified" category do not fit easily into the WHO subtypes described earlier, they are grouped according to morphology, flow cytometric phenotyping (Chapter 32), and limited cytochemical reactions, as in the FAB classification. The FAB classification was based on the cell of origin, degree of maturity, cytochemical reactions, and limited cytogenetic features (Table 35-2).[37,38] A blast percentage of at least 20% in the peripheral blood or bone marrow is required for diagnosis. This category accounts for about 25% of all AML, but as more genetic subgroups are recognized, the number in this group will diminish.[14]

Acute Myeloid Leukemia with Minimal Differentiation.

The blasts in AML with minimal differentiation are CD13[+], CD33[+], CD34[+], and CD117[+] (Figure 35-8).[6,39] Auer rods typically are absent, and there is no clear evidence of cellular maturation. The cells yield negative results with the cytochemical stains myeloperoxidase and Sudan black B. These cases account for less than 5% of AML, and patients are generally either infants or older adults.

Acute Myeloid Leukemia without Maturation.   Closely aligned with the blasts in minimally differentiated AML, the

TABLE 35-2 French-American-British Classification of the Acute Myeloid Leukemias

Subtype	Description
M0	Acute myeloid leukemia, minimally differentiated
M1	Acute myeloid leukemia without maturation
M2	Acute myeloid leukemia with maturation
M3	Acute promyelocytic leukemia
M4	Acute myelomonocytic leukemia
M4eo	Acute myelomonocytic leukemia with eosinophilia
M5a	Acute monocytic leukemia, poorly differentiated
M5b	Acute monocytic leukemia, well differentiated
M6	Acute erythroleukemia
M7	Acute megakaryocytic leukemia

Data from Bennett JM, Catovsky D, Daniel MT, et al: Proposals for the classification of the acute leukemias. French-American-British (FAB) co-operative group, *Br J Haematol* 33:451-458, 1976; and Bennett JM, Catovsky D, Daniel MT, et al: Proposed revised criteria for the classification of acute myeloid leukemia. A report of the French-American-British Cooperative Group, *Ann Intern Med* 103:620-625, 1985.

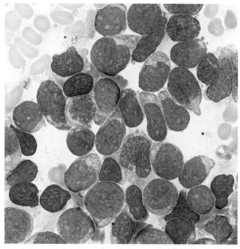

Figure 35-8 Acute myeloid leukemia, minimally differentiated (French-American-British classification M0). Blasts lack myeloid morphologic features and yield negative results with myeloperoxidase and Sudan black B staining. Auer rods are not seen. CD34 is frequently present (bone marrow, ×500). (From Carr JH, Rodak BF: *Clinical hematology atlas*, ed 4, St. Louis, 2013, Saunders.)

blasts in AML without maturation are also CD13[+], CD33[+], and CD117[+], and CD34 is present in about 70% of cases (Figure 35-9).[6] Blasts may comprise 90% of nonerythroid cells in the bone marrow, and fewer than 10% of the leukocytes show maturation to the promyelocyte stage or beyond. Blasts have Auer rods and usually give positive results with myeloperoxidase or Sudan black B stains.[6,28]

Acute Myeloid Leukemia with Maturation.   AML with maturation is a common variant that presents with greater than 20% blasts, at least 10% maturing cells of neutrophil lineage (Figure 35-10), and fewer than 20% precursors with monocytic lineage. Auer rods and other aspects of dysplasia are present.[6]

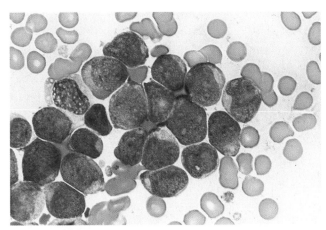

Figure 35-9 Acute myeloid leukemia without maturation (French-American-British classification M1). Blasts constitute 90% of the nonerythroid cells; there is less than 10% maturation of the granulocytic series beyond the promyelocyte stage (bone marrow, ×500).

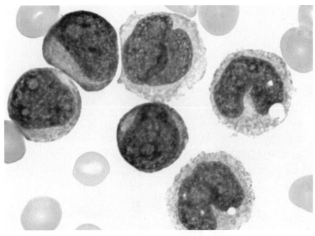

Figure 35-11 Acute myelomonocytic leukemia. Both myeloid and monocytic cells are present. Monocytic cells comprise at least 20% of all marrow cells, with monoblasts and promonocytes present (peripheral blood, ×1000). (From Carr JH, Rodak BF: *Clinical hematology atlas,* ed 4, St. Louis, 2013, Saunders.)

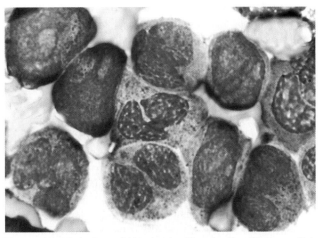

Figure 35-10 Acute myeloid leukemia with maturation. Blasts constitute 20% or more of the nucleated cells of the bone marrow, and there is maturation beyond the promyelocyte stage in more than 10% of the nonerythroid cells (bone marrow, ×1000).

Acute Myelomonocytic Leukemia.

Acute myelomonocytic leukemia is characterized by a significantly elevated WBC count and the presence of myeloid and monocytoid cells in the peripheral blood and bone marrow (Figure 35-11). Monocytic cells (monoblasts and promonocytes) constitute at least 20% of all marrow cells. The monoblasts are large with abundant cytoplasm containing small granules and pseudopodia. The nucleus is large and immature and may contain multiple nucleoli. Promonocytes also are present and may have contorted nuclei. The cells are positive for the myeloid antigens CD13 and CD33 and the monocytic antigens CD14, CD4, CD11b, CD11c, CD64, and CD36. Nonspecific cytogenetic changes are found in most cases.[6]

Acute Monoblastic and Monocytic Leukemias.

In these leukemias, which are divided into monoblastic and monocytic based on the degree of maturity of the monocytic cells present in the marrow and peripheral blood, more than

80% of the marrow cells are of monocytic origin. These cells are CD14+, CD4+, CD11b+, CD11c+, CD36+, CD64+, and CD68+. Blasts are large with abundant, often agranular cytoplasm and large prominent nucleoli (Figure 35-12, *A*). When some evidence of maturation is present, the cells are called *promonocytes.* Promonocytes in monocytic leukemias with differentiation are considered to be blast equivalents (Figure 35-12, *B*). Nonspecific esterase testing usually yields positive results. Acute monoblastic/monocytic leukemia comprises fewer than 5% of cases of AML and is most common in younger individuals. Extramedullary involvement, including cutaneous and gingival infiltration, and bleeding disorders are common. Nonspecific cytogenetic abnormalities are seen in most cases.[6,40]

Acute Erythroid Leukemia.

According to the WHO classification, there are two subtypes of acute erythroid leukemia, based on the presence of a significant component of myeloblasts. The first is *acute erythroleukemia* (erythroid/myeloid), in which 50% or more of nucleated bone marrow cells are normoblasts and greater than 20% are myeloblasts. In the FAB classification, this subtype was known as *M6.*

The second type is *pure erythroid leukemia.* In this type, 50% or more nucleated cells are pronormoblasts and 30% or more are basophilic normoblasts. Together, these two erythroid components comprise more than 80% of the bone marrow. The myeloblast component is not significant. Complex rearrangements and hypodiploid chromosome number are common. Chromosomes 5 and 7 are frequently affected.[6]

The red blood cell (RBC) precursors have significant dysplastic features, such as multinucleation, megaloblastoid asynchrony, and vacuolization. The nucleated RBCs in the peripheral blood may account for more than 50% of the total number of nucleated cells. Ringed sideroblasts, Howell-Jolly bodies, and other inclusions may be present (Figure 35-13). Abnormal megakaryocytes may be seen. Both types of erythroid leukemia have an aggressive and rapid clinical course.[6]

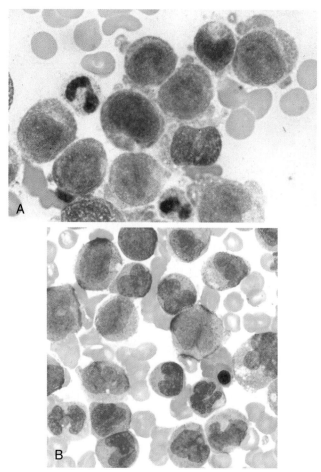

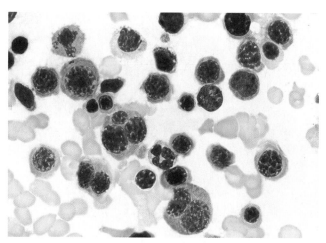

Figure 35-13 Acute erythroid leukemia. Erythroid precursors showing dysplastic features, including multinucleation and megaloblastic asynchrony (bone marrow, ×500). (From Carr JH, Rodak BF: *Clinical hematology atlas,* ed 4, St. Louis, 2013, Saunders.)

Acute Megakaryoblastic Leukemia.   Patients with acute megakaryoblastic leukemia usually have cytopenias, although some may have thrombocytosis. Dysplastic features are often present in all cell lines. Diagnosis requires the presence of at least 20% blasts, of which at least 50% must be of megakaryocyte origin. This category excludes AML with MDS-related changes and Down syndrome–related cases, as well as those with recurrent genetic abnormalities, as discussed previously.

Megakaryoblast diameters vary from that of a small lymphocyte to three times their size. Chromatin is delicate with prominent nucleoli. Immature megakaryocytes may have light blue cytoplasmic blebs (Figure 35-14, *A*). Megakaryoblasts are identified by immunostaining, employing antibodies specific for cytoplasmic von Willebrand factor or platelet membrane antigens CD41 (glycoprotein IIb), CD42b (glycoprotein Ib) (Figure 35-14, *B*), or CD61 (glycoprotein IIIa).[6]

Figure 35-12 A, Acute monoblastic leukemia. More than 80% of the bone marrow cells are of monocytic origin (bone marrow, ×500). **B,** Acute monocytic leukemia with promonocytes. Promonocytes are considered blast equivalents. (**B** from Carr JH, Rodak BF: *Clinical hematology atlas,* ed 4, St. Louis, 2013, Saunders.)

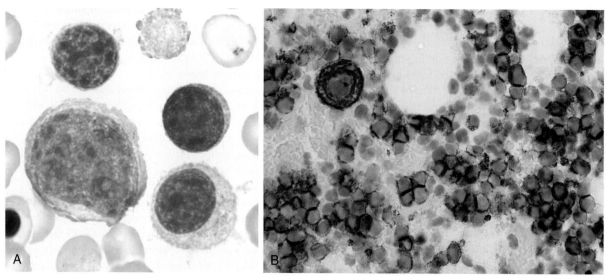

Figure 35-14 Acute megakaryocytic leukemia. **A,** Note heterogeneity of blasts, one small with scant cytoplasm, two with cytoplasmic blebbing, and one quite large (peripheral blood ×1000). **B,** Positive reaction for CD42b (bone marrow, ×1000). (**A** from Carr JH, Rodak BF: *Clinical hematology atlas,* ed 4, St. Louis, 2013, Saunders.)

Myeloid Sarcoma

Myeloid sarcoma refers to extramedullary proliferation of blasts of one or more myeloid lineages that disrupts tissue architecture. Tissue architecture must be effaced for the neoplasm to qualify for this diagnosis.[6,28]

Myeloid Proliferations Related to Down Syndrome

Unique patterns of malignancy occur in persons with trisomy 21 resulting in Down syndrome. Somatic mutations of the *GATA1* gene have also been detected and are linked to both leukemogenesis and high cure rates.[41] Approximately 10% of newborns with Down syndrome present with transient abnormal myelopoiesis, which is morphologically indistinguishable from AML. Spontaneous remission generally occurs within a few months. Among individuals with Down syndrome, there is a fiftyfold increased incidence of AML during the first 5 years of life compared with individuals without Down syndrome. The leukemia is of megakaryocytic lineage, and young children respond well to chemotherapy, although older children do not fare as well.[6,41]

Blastic Plasmacytoid Dendritic Cell Neoplasm

Blastic plasmacytoid cell neoplasm is a rare clinically aggressive tumor derived from precursors of plasmacytoid dendritic cells. It presents with skin lesions and may ultimately progress to involve peripheral blood and bone marrow.[6,14]

ACUTE LEUKEMIAS OF AMBIGUOUS LINEAGE

Acute leukemias of ambiguous lineage (ALALs) include leukemia in which there is no clear evidence of differentiation along a single cell line and are commonly referred to as *acute undifferentiated leukemias* (AULs). Other cases of ALAL that demonstrate a multiplicity of antigens where it is not possible to determine a specific lineage are called *mixed phenotype acute leukemias* (MPALs). The 2008 WHO classification significantly revised the criteria for this designation and is shown in Box 35-4.[6]

BOX 35-4 Classification of Acute Leukemia of Ambiguous Lineage (ALAL) (2008 World Health Organization Classification)

Acute undifferentiated leukemia (AUL)—synonyms: ALAL without differentiation, primitive acute leukemia, stem cell leukemia
Mixed phenotype acute leukemia (MPAL)—synonyms: biphenotypic acute leukemia, bilineal leukemia, mixed lineage acute leukemia, dual lineage acute leukemia, hybrid acute leukemia:
  MPAL with t(9;22)(q34;q11.2);*BCR-ABL1*
  MPAL with t(v;11q23);*MLL* rearranged
  MPAL B/myeloid, not otherwise specified
  MPAL T/myeloid, not otherwise specified

From Swerdlow SH, Campo E, Harris NL, et al, editors: *WHO classification of tumours of haematopoietic and lymphoid tissues*, ed 4, Lyon, France, 2008, IARC Press.

FUTURE DIRECTONS IN THE CLASSIFICATION OF ACUTE LEUKEMIAS

A number of recent studies have shown the importance of gene mutations in the pathogenesis of acute leukemias.[42,43] These mutations also have prognostic importance and are likely to be incorporated into future classifications. Important mutated genes include *KIT, FLT3, ASXL1, TP53, CEBPA,* and *NPM1.* AML with mutated *NPM1* and AML with mutated *CEBPA* are provisional entities in the 2008 WHO classification.[6]

CYTOCHEMICAL STAINS AND INTERPRETATIONS

Techniques such as flow cytometry, cytogenetic analysis, and molecular testing are now commonly used in the diagnosis of acute leukemias. However, older techniques such as cytochemical stains still retain their importance. An advantage of cytochemical stains is that they are relatively cheap and can be performed by laboratories throughout the world, including in areas where resources and access to advanced techniques are limited. The cytochemical stains are summarized in Table 35-3.

Myeloperoxidase

Myeloperoxidase (MPO) (Figures 35-15 and 35-16) is an enzyme found in the primary granules of granulocytic cells (neutrophils, eosinophils, and, to a certain extent, monocytes). Lymphocytes do not exhibit MPO activity. This stain is useful for differentiating the blasts of acute myeloid leukemia (AML) from those of acute lymphoblastic leukemia (ALL).

Interpretation

MPO is present in the primary granules of most granulocytic cells, beginning at the promyelocyte stage and continuing throughout maturation. Leukemic myeloblasts are usually positive for MPO. In many cases of the AMLs (without maturation, with maturation, and promyelocytic leukemia), it has been found that more than 80% of the blasts show MPO activity. Auer rods found in leukemic blasts and promyelocytes test strongly MPO positive.

TABLE 35-3 Acute Leukemia Cytochemical Reaction Chart

Condition	MPO	SBB	NASDA	ANBE	ANAE
ALL	−	−	−	−/+ (focal)	−/+ (focal)
AML	+	+	+	−	−
AMML	+	+	+	+ (diffuse)	+ (diffuse)
AMoL	−	−/+	−	+ (diffuse)	+ (diffuse)
Megakaryocytic leukemia	−	−	−	−	+ (localized)

+, Positive reaction; −, negative reaction; −/+, negative or positive reaction; *ALL,* acute lymphoblastic leukemia; *AML,* acute myeloid leukemia; *AMML,* acute myelomonocytic leukemia; *AMoL,* acute monocytic leukemia; *ANAE,* α-naphthyl acetate esterase; *ANBE,* α-naphthyl butyrate esterase; *MPO,* myeloperoxidase; *NASDA,* naphthol AS-D chloroacetate esterase; *SBB,* Sudan black B.

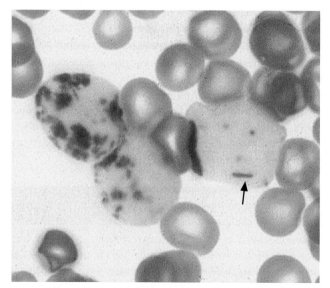

Figure 35-15 Positive reaction to myeloperoxidase stain in early myeloid cells. Note Auer rod at arrow (bone marrow, ×1000).

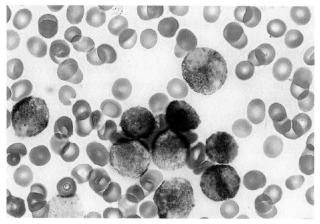

Figure 35-16 Strong positive reaction to myeloperoxidase stain in leukemic promyelocytes from a patient with acute promyelocytic leukemia (bone marrow, ×1000).

In contrast, lymphoblasts in ALL and lymphoid cells are MPO negative. It is important that the reaction only in the blast cells be used as the determining factor for the differentiation of acute leukemias. This is true for MPO and for the other cytochemical stains used in determining cell lineage that are mentioned in this chapter. The fact that maturing granulocytes are MPO positive is normal and has little or no diagnostic significance.

Sudan Black B

SBB staining (Figure 35-17) is another useful technique for the differentiation of AML from ALL. SBB stains cellular lipids. The staining pattern is quite similar to that of MPO; SBB staining is possibly a little more sensitive for the early myeloid cells.

Interpretation

Granulocytes (neutrophils) show a positive reaction to SBB from the myeloblast through the maturation series. The staining becomes more intense as the cell matures as a result of the increase in the numbers of primary and secondary granules.

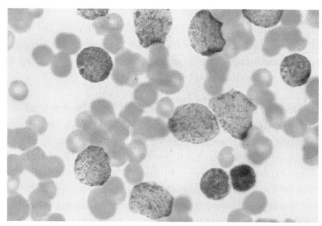

Figure 35-17 Sudan black B reaction. The positivity increases with the maturity of the granulocytic cell (bone marrow, ×1000).

Monocytic cells can demonstrate negative to weakly positive staining due to various changes that occur during differentiation. Lymphoid cells generally do not stain. In ALL, fewer than 3% of the blast cells show a positive reaction.[44-46]

Esterases

Esterase reactions are used to differentiate myeloblasts and neutrophilic granulocytes from cells of monocytic origin. Nine isoenzymes of esterases are present in leukocytes. Two substrate esters commonly used are α-naphthyl acetate and α-naphthyl butyrate (both nonspecific). Naphthol AS-D chloroacetate (specific) also may be used. "Specific" refers to the fact that only granulocytic cells show staining, whereas nonspecific stains may produce positive results in other cells as well.

Interpretation

Esterase stains can be used to distinguish acute leukemias that are granulocytic from leukemias that are primarily of monocytic origin. When naphthol AS-D chloroacetate is used as a substrate, the reaction is positive in the granulocytic cells and negative to weak in the monocytic cells (Figure 35-18). Chloroacetate esterase is present in the primary granules of neutrophils. Leukemic

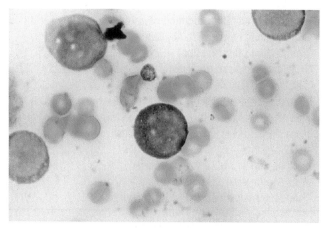

Figure 35-18 Positive reaction to AS-D chloroacetate esterase stain in two granulocytic cells (bone marrow, ×1000).

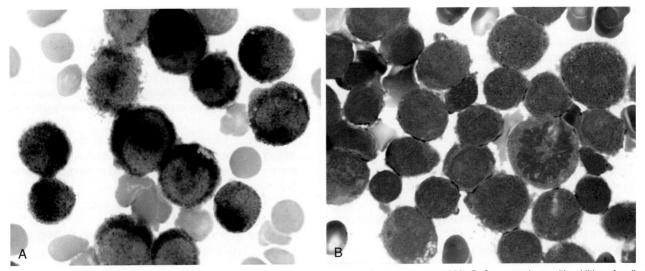

Figure 35-19 A, Positive reaction to α-naphthyl acetate esterase stain in monocytes (bone marrow, ×1000). **B,** Same specimen with addition of sodium fluoride. The esterase reaction in the monocytes is inhibited (bone marrow, ×1000).

myeloblasts generally show a positive reaction. Auer rods show positivity as well.

α-Naphthyl acetate, in contrast to naphthol AS-D chloroacetate, reveals strong esterase activity in monocytes that can be inhibited with the addition of sodium fluoride.[44,46] Granulocytes and lymphoid cells generally show a negative result on nonspecific esterase staining (Figure 35-19).

A diffuse positive α-naphthyl butyrate esterase reaction is seen in monocytes. α-Naphthyl butyrate is less sensitive than α-naphthyl acetate, but it is more specific. Granulocytes and lymphoid cells generally show a negative reaction (Figure 35-20), although a small positive dot may be seen in lymphocytes. In myelomonocytic leukemia, positive AS-D chloroacetate activity and positive α-naphthyl butyrate or α-naphthyl acetate activity should be seen because myeloid and monocytic cells are present. In myelomonocytic leukemia, at least 20% of the cells must show monocytic differentiation that is nonspecific esterase positive and is inhibited by sodium fluoride. In the pure monocytic leukemias, 80% or more of the blasts are nonspecific esterase positive and specific esterase negative.

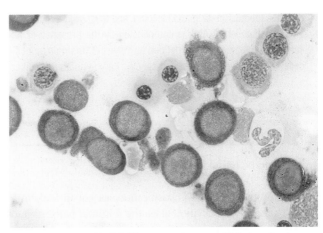

Figure 35-20 α-Naphthyl butyrate esterase positivity in cells of monocytic origin from a patient with acute monoblastic/monocytic leukemia. Note the negativity of myeloid and erythroid precursors (bone marrow, ×1000).

SUMMARY

- The development of leukemia is currently believed to be a step-wise progression of mutations, or "multiple-hits," involving mutations that give leukemic stem cells a proliferative advantage and also hinder differentiation.
- For most acute leukemias, causes directly related to the development of the malignancy are unknown, but a few exceptions exist. Some known causes include environmental toxins, certain viruses, previous chemotherapy, and familial predisposition.
- There are several classification schemes for leukocyte neoplasia, including the FAB system, based primarily on morphology and cytochemical staining, and the WHO system, which retains some

elements of the FAB scheme but emphasizes molecular and cytogenetic changes.
- Only half of patients with ALL have leukocytosis, and many do not have circulating lymphoblasts, but neutropenia, thrombocytopenia, and anemia are usually present.
- In children ALL is a disease in which the "good prognosis" subtypes are associated with a 95% rate of complete remission, but adults with ALL have a poorer outlook.
- Infiltration of malignant cells into the meninges can occur, with lymphoblasts found in the cerebrospinal fluid, testes, and ovaries.

- Prognosis in ALL depends primarily on age at the time of diagnosis, lymphoblast load (tumor burden), and immunophenotype. Chromosomal translocations seem to be the strongest predictor of adverse treatment outcomes for children and adults.
- The t(12;21) marker is found in a significant number of patients with childhood ALL.
- There are two main subtypes of ALL according to the WHO classification system: B lymphoblastic leukemia/lymphoma and T lymphoblastic leukemia/lymphoma.
- Tumor lysis syndrome is an increasingly common complication of treatment, especially in patients with a high tumor burden.
- Although morphology is the first tool in distinguishing ALL from AML, immunophenotyping is often the only reliable indicator of a cell's origin.
- The incidence of AML in adults increases with age.
- The clinical presentation of a patient with AML is nonspecific and reflects the decreased production of normal bone marrow elements, an elevated WBC count, and the presence of myeloblasts. Anemia, thrombocytopenia, and neutropenia give rise to the clinical findings of pallor, fatigue, bruising and bleeding, and fever with infections.
- The classification of AML is complicated by the presence or absence of multiple cell lines defined as "myeloid" in origin, specific cells within these cell lines, and specific karyotype abnormalities.

- Leukemias with ambiguous lineage include leukemias in which there is no clear evidence of differentiation along a single cell line.
- Cytochemical techniques are often used in conjunction with morphologic analysis, immunohistochemical methods, flow cytometry, cytogenetic analysis, and molecular biologic techniques in establishing a diagnosis.
- Cytochemical reactions may be enzymatic or nonenzymatic. Fresh smears must be used to detect enzymatic activity, whereas nonenzymatic procedures may be performed on specimens that have been stored at room temperature.
- MPO stains primary granules and is useful in differentiating granulocytic from lymphoid cells.
- SBB stains lipids and results parallel those with the MPO stain.
- Esterases help differentiate granulocytes and their precursors from cells of monocytic origin. Butyrate esterase testing gives positive results in monocytes but not in granulocyte precursors, whereas naphthol AS-D chloroacetate esterase stains granulocyte precursors.

Now that you have completed this chapter, go back and read again the case study at the beginning and respond to the questions presented.

REVIEW QUESTIONS

Answers can be found in the Appendix.

1. According to the WHO classification, except in leukemias with specific genetic anomalies, the minimal percentage of blasts necessary for a diagnosis of acute leukemia is:
   a. 10%
   b. 20%
   c. 30%
   d. 50%

2. A 20-year-old patient has an elevated WBC count with 70% blasts, 4% neutrophils, 5% lymphocytes, and 21% monocytes in the peripheral blood. Eosinophils with dysplastic changes are seen in the bone marrow. AML with which of the following karyotypes would be most likely to be seen?
   a. AML with t(8;21)(q22;q22)
   b. AML with t(16;16)(p13;q22)
   c. AML with t(15;17)(q22;q12)
   d. AML with t(9;11)(p22;q23)

3. Which of the following would be considered a sign of potentially favorable prognosis in children with ALL?
   a. Hyperdiploidy
   b. Presence of CD 19 and 20
   c. Absence of trisomy 8
   d. Presence of *BCR/ABL* gene

4. Signs and symptoms of cerebral infiltration with blasts are more commonly seen in:
   a. AML with recurrent cytogenetic abnormalities
   b. Therapy-related myeloid neoplasms
   c. AML with myelodysplasia-related changes
   d. ALL

5. An oncology patient exhibiting signs of renal failure with seizures after initial chemotherapy may potentially develop:
   a. Hyperleukocytosis
   b. Tumor lysis syndrome
   c. Acute leukemia secondary to chemotherapy
   d. Myelodysplasia

6. Disseminated intravascular coagulation is more often seen in association with leukemia characterized by which of the following mutations?
   a. t(12;21)(p13;q22)
   b. t(9;22)(q34;q11.2)
   c. inv(16)(p13;q22)
   d. t(15;17)(q22;q12)

7. Which of the following leukemias affects primarily children, is characterized by an increase in monoblasts and monocytes, and often is associated with gingival and skin involvement?
   a. Pre-B lymphoblastic leukemia
   b. Pure erythroid leukemia
   c. AML with t(9;11)(p22;q23)
   d. AML with t(15;17)(q22;q12)

8. A 20-year-old patient presents with fatigue, pallor, easy bruising, and swollen gums. Bone marrow examination reveals 82% cells with delicate chromatin and prominent nucleoli that are CD14$^+$, CD4$^+$, CD11b$^+$, and CD36$^+$. Which of the following acute leukemias is likely?
   a. Minimally differentiated leukemia
   b. Leukemia of ambiguous lineage
   c. Acute monoblastic/monocytic leukemia
   d. Acute megakaryoblastic leukemia

9. Pure erythroid leukemia is a disorder involving:
   a. Pronormoblasts only
   b. Pronormoblasts and basophilic normoblasts
   c. All forms of developing RBC precursors
   d. Equal numbers of pronormoblasts and myeloblasts

10. A patient with normal chromosomes has a WBC count of 3.0 × 10^9/L and dysplasia in all cell lines. There are 60% blasts of varying sizes. The blasts stain positive for CD61. The most likely type of leukemia is:
    a. Acute lymphoblastic
    b. Acute megakaryoblastic
    c. Acute monoblastic
    d. AML with t(15;17)

11. SBB stains which of the following component of cells?
    a. Glycogen
    b. Lipids
    c. Structural proteins
    d. Enzymes

12. The cytochemical stain α-naphthyl butyrate is a nonspecific esterase stain that shows diffuse positivity in cells of which lineage?
    a. Erythroid
    b. Monocytic
    c. Granulocytic
    d. Lymphoid

REFERENCES

1. Anderson, D. M., Novak, P. D., Elliot, M. A., et al. (1994). Leukemia. *Mosby's Medical, Nursing & Allied Health Dictionary.* (4th ed.). Mosby-YearBook. St. Louis.
2. Reilly, J. T. (2005, Jan) Pathogenesis of acute myeloid leukaemia and inv(16)(p13;q22): a paradigm for understanding leukaemogenesis? *Br J Haematol, 128*(1), 18–34.
3. Bachas, C., Schuurhuis, G. J., Hollink, I. H., et al. (2010, Oct 14). High-frequency type I/II mutational shifts between diagnosis and relapse are associated with outcome in pediatric AML: implications for personalized medicine. *Blood, 116*(15), 2752–2758.
4. Lane, S. W., & Gilliland, D. G. (2010). Leukemia stem cells. *Semin Cancer Biol, 20*(2), 71–76.
5. World Health Organization. (2001). *WHO Classification of Tumours: Pathology and Genetics of Tumours of Haematopoietic and Lymphoid Tissues.* Lyon, France: IARC Press.
6. World Health Organization. (2008). *WHO Classification of Tumours of Haematopoietic and Lymphoid Tissues.* (4th ed.). Lyon, France: IARC Press.
7. Stanulla, M., & Schrauder, A. (2009, Jun). Bridging the gap between the north and south of the world: the case of treatment response in childhood acute lymphoblastic leukemia. *Haematologica, Jun, 94*(6), 748–752.
8. Inaba, H., Greaves, M., & Mullighan, C. G. (2013, Mar 21). Acute lymphoblastic leukaemia. *Lancet. 9881*, 1943–55.
9. Advani, A., Jin, T., Bolwell, B., et al. (2009, Jul). A prognostic scoring system for adult patients less than 60 years of age with acute lymphoblastic leukemia in first relapse. *Leuk Lymphoma, 50*(7), 1126–1131.
10. Pui, C. H., & Evans, W. E. (2006, Jan 12). Treatment of acute lymphoblastic leukemia. *N Engl J Med, 354*(2), 166–178.
11. Redaelli, A., Laskin, B. L., Stephens, J. M., Botteman, M. F., & Pashos, C. L. (2005, Mar). A systematic literature review of the clinical and epidemiological burden of acute lymphoblastic leukaemia (ALL). *Eur J Cancer Care (Engl), 14*(1), 53–62.
12. Hutter, J. (2010). Childhood Leukemia. *Pediatr Rev 31*, 234–241. Retrieved from http://pedsinreview.aappublications.org/cgi/content/full/31/6/234. Accessed 10.10.13.
13. Onciu, M. (2009, Aug). Acute lymphoblastic leukemia. *Hematol Oncol Clin North Am, 23*(4), 655–674.
14. Vardiman, J. W., Thiele, J., Arber, D. A., et al. (2009, Jul 30). The 2008 revision of the World Health Organization (WHO) classification of myeloid neoplasms and acute leukemia: rationale and important changes. *Blood, 114*(5), 937–951.
15. Pilozzi, E., Pulford, K., Jones, M., et al. (1998, Oct). Co-expression of CD79a (JCB117) and CD3 by lymphoblastic lymphoma. *J Pathol, 186*(2), 140–143.
16. Thomas, D. A., O'Brien, S., & Kantarjian, H. M. (2009, Oct). Monoclonal antibody therapy with rituximab for acute lymphoblastic leukemia. *Hematol Oncol Clin North Am, 23*(5), 949–971, v.
17. Hoelzer, D. G. N. (2009). *Acute Lymphoblastic Leukemias in Adults,* Chapter 66. (5th ed.). Philadelphia: Churchill Livingstone.
18. Attarbaschi, A., Mann, G., Dworzak, M., Wiesbauer, P., Schrappe, M., & Gadner, H. (2002, Dec). Mediastinal mass in childhood T-cell acute lymphoblastic leukemia: significance and therapy response. *Med Pediatr Oncol, 39*(6), 558–565.
19. Goldberg, J. M., Silverman, L. B., Levy, D. E., et al. (2003, Oct 1). Childhood T-cell acute lymphoblastic leukemia: the Dana-Farber Cancer Institute acute lymphoblastic leukemia consortium experience. *J Clin Oncol, 21*(19), 3616–3622.
20. Coustan-Smith, E., Mulligan, C. G., Onciu, M., et al. (2009, Feb). Early T-cell precursor leukaemia: a subtype of very high-risk acute lymphoblastic leukaemia. *Lancet Oncol, 10*(2), 147–156.
21. Inukai, T., Kiyokawa, N., Campana, D., et al. (2012, Feb). Clinical significance of early T-cell precursor acute lymphoblastic leukaemia: results of the Tokyo Children's Cancer Study Group Study L99-15. *Br J Haematol, 156*(3), 358–365.
22. Van Vlierberghe, P., & Ferrando, A. (2012, Oct 1). The molecular basis of T cell acute lymphoblastic leukemia. *J Clin Invest, 122*(10), 3398–3406.
23. Gale, K. B., Ford, A. M., Repp, R., et al. (1997, Dec 9). Backtracking leukemia to birth: identification of clonotypic gene fusion sequences in neonatal blood spots. *Proc Natl Acad Sci U S A, 94*(25), 13950–13954.

24. Castor, A., Nilsson, L., Astrand-Grundstrom, I., et al. (2005, Jun). Distinct patterns of hematopoietic stem cell involvement in acute lymphoblastic leukemia. *Nat Med, 11*(6), 630–637.

25. Uchiumi, H., Matsushima, T., Yamane, A., et al. (2007, Aug). Prevalence and clinical characteristics of acute myeloid leukemia associated with disseminated intravascular coagulation. *Int J Hematol, 86*(2), 137–142.

26. Montesinos, P., Lorenzo, I., Martin, G., et al. (2008, Jan). Tumor lysis syndrome in patients with acute myeloid leukemia: identification of risk factors and development of a predictive model. *Haematologica, 93*(1), 67–74.

27. Cairo, M. S., & Bishop, M. (2004, Oct). Tumour lysis syndrome: new therapeutic strategies and classification. *Br J Haematol, 127*(1), 3–11.

28. Heerema-McKenney, A., & Arber, D. A. (2009, Aug). Acute myeloid leukemia. *Hematol Oncol Clin North Am, 23*(4), 633–654.

29. Mrozek, K., Marcucci, G., Paschka, P., & Bloomfield, C. D. (2008, Nov). Advances in molecular genetics and treatment of core-binding factor acute myeloid leukemia. *Curr Opin Oncol, 20*(6), 711–718.

30. Stein, E., McMahon, B., Kwaan, H., Altman, J. K., Frankfurt, O., & Tallman, M. S. (2009, Mar). The coagulopathy of acute promyelocytic leukaemia revisited. *Best Pract Res Clin Haematol, 22*(1), 153–163.

31. Nasr, R., Lallemand-Breitenbach, V., Zhu, J., Guillemin, M. C., & de The, H. (2009, Oct 15). Therapy-induced PML/RARA proteolysis and acute promyelocytic leukemia cure. *Clin Cancer Res, 15*(20), 6321–6326.

32. Weinberg, O. K., Seetharam, M., Ren, L., et al. (2009, Feb 26). Clinical characterization of acute myeloid leukemia with myelodysplasia-related changes as defined by the 2008 WHO classification system. *Blood, 113*(9), 1906–1908.

33. Ngo, N., Lampert, I. A., & Naresh, K. N. (2008, Feb). Bone marrow trephine findings in acute myeloid leukaemia with multilineage dysplasia. *Br J Haematol, 140*(3), 279–286.

34. Czader, M., & Orazi, A. (2009, Sep). Therapy-related myeloid neoplasms. *Am J Clin Pathol, 132*(3), 410–425.

35. Vardiman, J. W. (2010, Mar 19). The World Health Organization (WHO) classification of tumors of the hematopoietic and lymphoid tissues: an overview with emphasis on the myeloid neoplasms. *Chem Biol Interact, 184*(1–2), 16–20.

36. Anderson, L. A., Pfeiffer, R. M., Landgren, O., Gadalla, S., Berndt, S. I., & Engels, E. A. (2009, Mar 10). Risks of myeloid malignancies in patients with autoimmune conditions. *Br J Cancer, 100*(5), 822–828.

37. Bennett, J. M., Catovsky, D., Daniel, M. T., et al. (1976, Aug). Proposals for the classification of the acute leukaemias. French-American-British (FAB) co-operative group. *Br J Haematol, 33*(4), 451–458.

38. Bennett, J. M., Catovsky, D., Daniel, M. T., et al. (1985, Oct). Proposed revised criteria for the classification of acute myeloid leukemia. A report of the French-American-British Cooperative Group. *Ann Intern Med, 103*(4), 620–625.

39. Kaleem, Z., Crawford, E., Pathan, M. H., et al. (2003, Jan). Flow cytometric analysis of acute leukemias. Diagnostic utility and critical analysis of data. *Arch Pathol Lab Med, 127*(1), 42–48.

40. Villeneuve, P., Kim, D. T., Xu, W., Brandwein, J., & Chang, H. (2008, Feb). The morphological subcategories of acute monocytic leukemia (M5a and M5b) share similar immunophenotypic and cytogenetic features and clinical outcomes. *Leuk Res, 32*(2), 269–273.

41. Xavier, A. C., Ge, Y., & Taub, J. W. (2009, Sep). Down syndrome and malignancies: a unique clinical relationship: a paper from the 2008 William Beaumont Hospital symposium on molecular pathology. *J Mol Diagn, 11*(5), 371–380.

42. Grossmann, V., Schnittger, S., Kohlmann, A., et al. (2012, Oct 11). A novel hierarchical prognostic model of AML solely based on molecular mutations. *Blood, 120*(15), 2963–2972.

43. Ley, T. J., Miller, C., King, L. (2013, May 30). Genomic and epigenomic landscapes of adult de novo acute myeloid leukemia. *N Engl J Med, 368*(22), 2059–2074.

44. Scott, C. S., Den Ottolander, G. J., Swirsky, D., et al. (1993, Sep). Recommended procedures for the classification of acute leukaemias. International Council for Standardization in Haematology (ICSH). *Leuk Lymphoma, 11*(1–2):37–50.

45. Cheson, B. D., Cassileth, P. A., Head, D. R., et al. (1990, May). Report of the National Cancer Institute-sponsored workshop on definitions of diagnosis and response in acute myeloid leukemia. *J Clin Oncol, 8*(5), 813–819.

46. Head, D. R. (1996, Nov). Revised classification of acute myeloid leukemia. *Leukemia, 10*(11), 1826–1831.

Mature Lymphoid Neoplasms

36

Magdalena Czader

OBJECTIVES

After completion of this chapter, the reader will be able to:

1. Describe normal lymph node morphology and discuss the function of various compartments and constituent cells.
2. Outline the most common histologic patterns of reactive lymphadenopathies.
3. Describe the peripheral blood findings in chronic lymphocytic leukemia and hairy cell leukemia.
4. Describe the approach to the diagnosis of lymphomas as outlined by the World Health Organization classification.
5. Discuss the most commonly occurring mature B and T cell neoplasms, including epidemiology, clinical presentation, pathophysiology, lymph node histologic features, peripheral blood or bone marrow findings, and diagnostic test results.
6. Interpret diagnostic test results to identify lymphoproliferative disorders.

CASE STUDY

After studying the material in this chapter, the reader should be able to respond to the following case study:

A 46-year-old previously healthy man came for evaluation of an enlarged left cervical lymph node. The patient had discovered this isolated lymphadenopathy 2 weeks previously and did not complain of any other symptoms. The lymph node measured approximately 2 cm. The findings of his physical examination were otherwise unremarkable. The lymph node was excised, and microscopic examination showed the histologic features presented in Figure 36-1, *A.* Immunohistochemical stains showed CD20 (Figure 36-1, *B*), CD10, and BCL-6 positivity and focal CD30 antigen expression.

1. What is your diagnosis based on the histologic and immunophenotypic features?

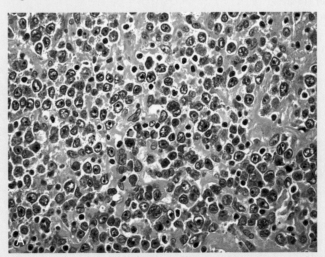

Figure 36-1 Histologic lymph node findings for the patient in the case study. **A,** Lymph node (hematoxylin and eosin stain, ×500).

Continued

After studying the material in this chapter, the reader should be able to respond to the following case study:

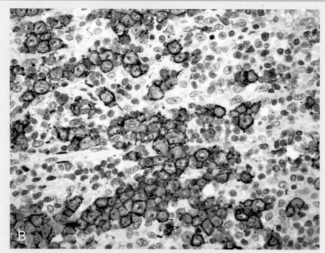

Figure 36-1,cont'd   **B,** CD20 antigen expression in the lymphoid population (immunoperoxidase stain, ×500).

2. What additional immunophenotypic features that confirm the diagnosis could be seen using flow cytometry?

3. Is it likely that this patient would show disseminated disease, including bone marrow involvement?

Lymphomas are neoplasms of the lymphoid system. Original microscopic observations and immunophenotypic and molecular studies confirmed that these malignancies recapitulate specific stages of normal lymphoid differentiation. The diagnosis is based on a combination of biologic features such as morphology, immunophenotype and molecular genetic characteristics, and clinical information.[1] Therefore, during initial sample processing, the appropriate steps must be taken to ensure tissue preservation and availability for microscopic examination and immunophenotypic and molecular studies.

Knowledge of normal lymphoid differentiation is a prerequisite for understanding the lymphoid neoplasms. This chapter describes the morphologic and immunophenotypic features of normal lymph nodes and selected common lymphomas and lymphoproliferative disorders. Reactive lymphoid hyperplasias, which can resemble lymphoid neoplasms, also are discussed.

MORPHOLOGIC AND IMMUNOPHENOTYPIC FEATURES OF NORMAL LYMPH NODES

Lymphoid organs serve as sites of antigen recognition, antigen processing, and lymphopoiesis. Most of the lymphoid tissue is concentrated in lymph nodes, which are round to oval encapsulated organs serving as primary sites of immunologic response. They are particularly prominent at sites with an environmental interface. Large groups of lymph nodes are found draining specific peripheral areas (e.g., cervical, axillary, or inguinal). Similarly, internal organs are served by regional lymph nodes (e.g., mediastinal, hilar, and mesenteric). Respiratory and digestive tracts have additional aggregates of lymphoid tissue located directly in the mucosa called *mucosa-associated lymphoid tissue* (MALT). These aggregates are the primary sites of antigenic contact and drain directly into regional lymph nodes.

Histologic components of a lymph node include cortex, paracortex, medullary cords, and sinuses (Figure 36-2). They are both structural and functional compartments serving as sites of immunologic reactions for specific antigenic stimuli.

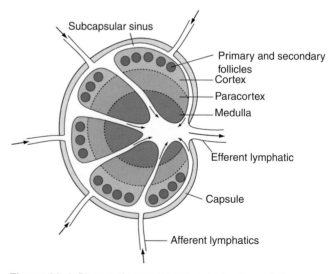

Figure 36-2 Diagram of a normal lymph node showing cortical, paracortical, and medullary compartments.

Cortex

The lymph node is surrounded by a capsule of fibrous tissue. Immediately below the capsule is the cortex, the most superficial portion of the lymph node consisting of primary and secondary follicles. Primary follicles are microscopic aggregates of small naive B lymphocytes. These lymphocytes express pan-B cell markers, including CD19 and CD20 and are frequently CD5[+] (Figure 36-3). The formation of secondary follicles with germinal centers and their functions are assisted by follicular dendritic cell meshworks, best visualized by immunohistochemical stains such as CD21.[2,3] On antigen encounter, naive B lymphocytes undergo transformation, proliferation, and differentiation into precursors of antibody-producing plasma cells and memory B cells (Figure 36-3). The remaining naive B cells are displaced into the periphery of the germinal center and form the mantle zone.

Germinal center B cells have a specific immunophenotype. In addition to pan-B cell markers, they express germinal center cell antigens CD10 and BCL6, and, in contrast to circulating B cells, they lack anti-apoptotic BCL2 protein. Functional compartments of the germinal center include the dark zone occupied by centroblasts, large B cells with round vesicular nuclei, small nucleoli adjacent to nuclear membrane, and basophilic cytoplasm (Figure 36-4). The dark zone is a site of high proliferative activity and somatic mutations of B cell immunoglobulin variable regions. The latter process allows for the production of immunoglobulins with the best affinity for a particular antigen.

After completing somatic mutations, centroblasts differentiate into centrocytes, smaller cells with dense chromatin and irregular nuclear outlines, which form the light zone (Figure 36-4). Subsequently, centrocytes with low-affinity ("unfit") surface immunoglobulins undergo apoptosis and are phagocytized by germinal center macrophages (tingible-body macrophages). The presence of numerous macrophages with apoptotic debris contributes to

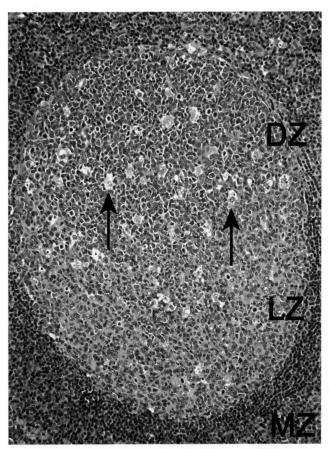

Figure 36-4 Secondary follicle with well-developed polarization in germinal center showing dark zone (DZ) and light zone (LZ). Note the presence of numerous tingible body macrophages (*arrows*). A distinct mantle zone (MZ) also is present at the periphery of the germinal center (hematoxylin and eosin stain, ×100).

the characteristic "starry sky" pattern of the germinal center. Centrocytes with immunoglobulins with high affinity for a particular antigen lose their germinal center antigens (CD10 and BCL6) and differentiate into memory B cells that form a marginal zone at the periphery of the mantle zone. Marginal zone lymphocytes are medium sized with abundant clear cytoplasm and indented nuclei.

In the final step of B cell differentiation are plasma cells that reside in medullary cords of lymph nodes and that also migrate to bone marrow. Plasma cells are negative for pan-B cell antigens and surface immunoglobulins; however, they express CD138, CD38, and cytoplasmic immunoglobulins.

Paracortex

The paracortex occupies the area separating the follicles and extends toward medullary cords. This compartment generates immunocompetent T cells and is occupied predominantly by T cells, interdigitating dendritic cells (antigen-presenting cells), and high-endothelial venules. The last are specialized vessels serving as a gate of entry for lymphocytes from peripheral blood into lymph nodes. T cells express pan-T cell antigens such as CD3, CD5, CD2, and CD7. Both CD4[+] and CD8[+] T lymphocytes are seen in paracortex. Similar to B cells, T cells

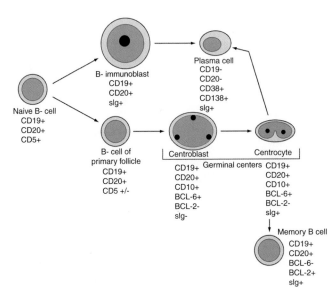

Figure 36-3 Differentiation stages of mature B cells. Note changes in immunophenotype at specific stages of differentiation. *BCL*, B cell lymphoma; *sIg*, surface immunoglobin.

transform in response to antigen stimulation. In this process, small lymphocytes become immunoblasts: large lymphoid cells with vesicular nuclei; prominent, often single, nucleoli; and abundant basophilic cytoplasm. The paracortex also contains numerous B immunoblasts.

Medulla

The medulla represents the innermost portion of the lymph node surrounding the hilum. This area is composed of medullary cords with plasma cells and medullary sinuses.

Sinuses

The filtration of lymphatic fluid through lymph nodes is accomplished via afferent lymphatics communicating with a subcapsular sinus, which is situated immediately beneath the capsule (Figure 36-2). The subcapsular sinus drains into cortical sinuses, which run through the cortex and empty to medullary sinuses. The latter converge into the efferent lymphatic vessel at the hilum. The sinuses are filled with macrophages or sinus histiocytes. These cells play an important role in antigen capture and processing.

LYMPH NODE PROCESSING

Current approach to diagnosis of lymphomas incorporates routine light microscopic examination and ancillary techniques. During processing of excised lymph nodes, appropriate steps should be taken to ensure adequate preservation of the tissue and its availability for all necessary studies. The appropriate transport conditions need to be maintained to preserve tissue integrity and prevent drying. Immediately after excision, the lymph node should be transported to the pathology laboratory in a sealed sterile jar on gauze pads moistened with sterile saline or in tissue culture media. The fresh lymph node is cut into 3-mm-thick sections for the evaluation of nodal architecture. If areas of granulomas or suppuration are present, a portion of the tissue should be sent for cultures.

Touch imprints can be prepared to ensure the adequacy of the specimen and to perform special studies. To obtain an adequate imprint, a freshly cut tissue surface is gently touched to the glass slide and pulled away. Touch imprints can be fixed in formalin or alcohol solution or air-dried for subsequent Wright-Giemsa staining. Storing of fixed touch imprints for immunocytochemical studies is optional because currently immunophenotyping is most commonly performed on paraffin-embedded tissue or using flow cytometry. The latter is particularly helpful in confirming monoclonal light chain expression.

Several thin lymph node sections are placed in 10% buffered formalin for paraffin embedding. Some pathology laboratories fix additional tissue samples in a variety of fixatives with protein-precipitating properties (B5 fixative, zinc chloride formalin) for better preservation of cytologic detail.[4] Regardless of fixative used, thin sectioning of a fresh lymph node is crucial for proper tissue permeation and fixation. A portion of lymph node is placed in culture medium (Roswell Park Memorial Institute medium) and transported to a flow cytometry laboratory for immunophenotyping. The remaining fresh tissue can be stored at −70° C for further studies.

REACTIVE LYMPHADENOPATHIES

Lymphadenopathy, lymph node enlargement, can occur in benign/reactive and malignant conditions. Reactive lymphadenopathies can affect any compartment of a lymph node and present as expansion of normal nodal structures. Reactive hyperplasias are classified into several patterns, as follows:
1. Follicular
2. Paracortical
3. Sinusoidal
4. Mixed

Follicular Pattern

Follicular hyperplasia is the most common form of reactive lymphadenopathies. It is frequently seen in lymph nodes and tonsils of children and adolescents as a reaction to infections. In adults, it occurs in association with infections, autoimmune disorders (rheumatoid arthritis, systemic lupus erythematosus), syphilis, and early human immunodeficiency virus (HIV) infection. Microscopically, an expansion of reactive follicles can be prominent and extend beyond the cortex into the medulla (Figure 36-5). Secondary follicles retain all the hallmarks of reactive germinal centers, including distinct polarization, presence of tingible-body macrophages, abundant mitotic figures, and preserved mantle zones (Figure 36-4).

Paracortical Pattern

Paracortical expansion is associated with viral infections (e.g., infectious mononucleosis) and drug reactions and is also seen in patients with chronic skin diseases (dermatopathic lymphadenopathy). In addition to small lymphocytes, the paracortex shows numerous immunoblasts, increased mitotic activity, and vascular proliferation (Figure 36-6). Focal areas of necrosis may also be seen. In dermatopathic lymphadenopathy, the paracortex has a characteristic mottled appearance as a result of an increased number of large cells with abundant clear cytoplasm scattered among small lymphoid cells (Figure 36-7).

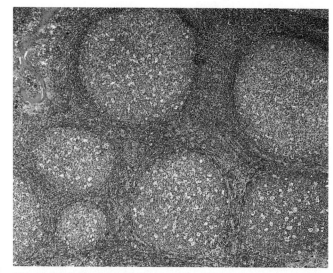

Figure 36-5 Reactive follicular hyperplasia with numerous secondary follicles scattered throughout the lymph node (hematoxylin and eosin stain, ×40).

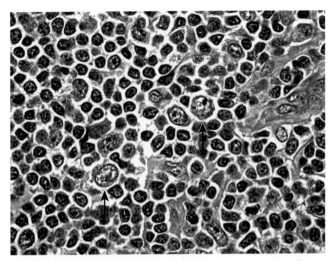

Figure 36-6 Immunoblasts (*arrows*) scattered in the paracortex (hematoxylin and eosin stain, ×1000).

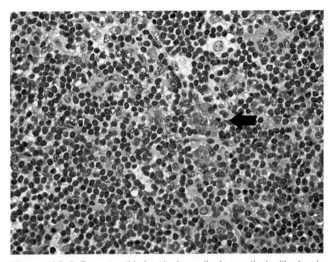

Figure 36-8 Dermatopathic lymphadenopathy in a patient with chronic skin rash. Scattered pigment-laden macrophages (*arrow*) are present in the paracortical area (hematoxylin and eosin stain, ×400).

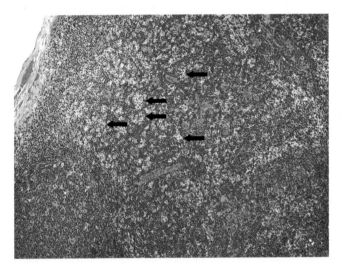

Figure 36-7 Paracortical hyperplasia. Note mottled appearance of the paracortex resulting from multiple scattered histiocytes with abundant cytoplasm (*arrows*) (hematoxylin and eosin stain, ×40).

These cells include histiocytes, often carrying melanin pigment, and Langerhans cells (Figure 36-8). Scattered immunoblasts, plasma cells, eosinophils, and vascular proliferation are also encountered.

Sinusoidal Pattern

Expanded subcapsular, cortical, and medullary sinuses are often seen in lymph nodes draining limbs, abdominal organs, various inflammatory lesions, and malignancies. In select cases, the prominent sinuses compress the nodal parenchyma. They may be completely filled with histiocytes showing abundant cytoplasm, a small oval nucleus with inconspicuous nucleolus, and delicate chromatin. Monocytoid B cells with abundant cytoplasm and oval indented nuclei that may mimic histiocytes are seen in HIV-associated lymphadenopathy and *Toxoplasma* lymphadenitis (Figure 36-9, *A*). Numerous malignant lesions show predilection for sinuses, such as Langerhans cell histiocytosis, B and T cell lymphomas, and carcinomas;

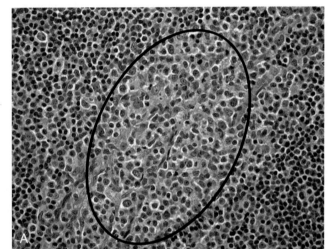

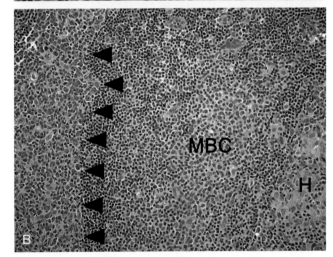

Figure 36-9 *Toxoplasma* lymphadenitis. **A,** Monocytoid B cells are medium sized with irregular nuclear outlines and abundant cytoplasm (shown in *center circle*) (hematoxylin and eosin stain, ×400). **B,** Classic triad of reactive changes seen in *Toxoplasma* lymphadenitis includes follicular hyperplasia with focal aggregates of histiocytes (H) and monocytoid B cells (MBC). An irregular outline of a secondary follicle is seen on the left (*arrowheads*) (hematoxylin and eosin stain, ×100).

therefore, a thorough evaluation of expanded sinuses under high magnification is always necessary.

Mixed Pattern

A classic example of mixed-pattern hyperplasia is seen in *Toxoplasma gondii* infection, a common protozoal infection typically seen after ingestion of raw meat or contamination by cat feces. The expansion of all lymph node compartments is seen (Figure 36-9). Florid follicular hyperplasia is accompanied by paracortical expansion, aggregates of histiocytes encroaching on germinal centers, and expanded sinuses. Sinuses are focally filled with a specific subset of B cells, so-called monocytoid B cells.

LYMPHOMAS

Approximately 86,000 new cases of lymphoma are diagnosed annually in the United States.[5] Most lymphomas develop in previously healthy individuals. The strongest risk factor for development of lymphoproliferative disorder is altered immune function as seen in immunocompromised patients or individuals with autoimmune diseases.[6,7] Similarly, certain viral and bacterial infections are associated with a higher risk for the development of lymphoma.[8] Accumulating evidence indicates that exposure to chemicals and herbicides may predispose to lymphoid neoplasms. Most lymphomas present in lymph nodes. Certain types show a predilection for extranodal sites. The frequency of bone marrow and peripheral blood (leukemic phase) involvement varies, depending on the lymphoma subtype.

Over the years, numerous classification systems have been proposed based mainly on the morphology and clinical characteristics (e.g., Rappaport classification, Kiel classification, Working Formulation). With increased understanding of the development and function of the immune system, however, it became clear that lymphomas, like myeloid neoplasms, recapitulate normal stages of lymphoid differentiation. In addition, the elucidation of specific molecular events occurring in lymphomagenesis helped in devising clinically relevant classification, especially for morphologically heterogeneous entities. Currently, numerous types of lymphoma are distinguished based on morphology, immunophenotype, molecular genetics, and clinical and laboratory characteristics. The integration of these features is mandatory for comprehensive lymphoma diagnosis. On the basis of cellular origin, lymphomas can be categorized into lesions of lymphoid precursors and neoplasms of mature lymphoid cells (Table 36-1).

TABLE 36-1 2008 World Health Organization Classification of Mature Lymphoid Neoplasms

Type of Lymphoma	Examples
Mature B cell lymphomas	Chronic lymphocytic leukemia/small lymphocytic lymphoma
	B cell prolymphocytic leukemia
	Splenic B cell marginal zone lymphoma
	Hairy cell leukemia
	Splenic B cell lymphoma/leukemia, unclassifiable
	Splenic diffuse red pulp small B cell lymphoma
	Hairy cell leukemia-variant
	Lymphoplasmacytic lymphoma
	Heavy chain diseases
	Gamma heavy chain disease
	Mu heavy chain disease
	Alpha heavy chain disease
	Plasma cell neoplasms
	Monoclonal gammopathy of undetermined significance (MGUS)
	Plasma cell myeloma
	Solitary plasmacytoma of bone
	Extraosseous plasmacytoma
	Monoclonal immunoglobulin deposition diseases
	Extranodal marginal zone lymphoma of mucosa-associated lymphoid tissue (MALT lymphoma)
	Nodal marginal zone lymphoma
	Follicular lymphoma
	Primary cutaneous follicle center lymphoma
	Mantle cell lymphoma
	Diffuse large B cell lymphoma (DLBCL), not otherwise specified
	T cell/histiocyte-rich large B cell lymphoma
	Primary DLBCL of the central nervous system
	Primary cutaneous DLBCL, leg type
	Epstein-Barr virus (EBV)–positive DLBCL of the elderly
	DLBCL associated with chronic inflammation
	Lymphomatoid granulomatosis
	Primary mediastinal (thymic) large B cell lymphoma

TABLE 36-1 2008 World Health Organization Classification of Mature Lymphoid Neoplasms—cont'd

Type of Lymphoma	Examples
	Intravascular large B cell lymphoma
	ALK-positive large B cell lymphoma
	Plasmablastic lymphoma
	Large B cell lymphoma arising in human herpesvirus 8–associated multicentric Castleman disease
	Primary effusion lymphoma
	Burkitt lymphoma
	B cell lymphoma, unclassifiable, with features intermediate between those of DLBCL and Burkitt lymphoma
	B cell lymphoma, unclassifiable, with features intermediate between those of DLBCL and classical Hodgkin lymphoma
Mature T cell lymphomas	T cell prolymphocytic leukemia
	T cell large granular lymphocytic leukemia
	Chronic lymphoproliferative disorder of natural killer (NK) cells
	Aggressive NK cell leukemia
	EBV-positive T cell lymphoproliferative diseases of childhood
	Systemic EBV-positive T cell lymphoproliferative diseases of childhood
	Hydroa vacciniforme–like lymphoma
	Adult T cell leukemia/lymphoma
	Extranodal NK/T cell lymphoma, nasal type
	Enteropathy-associated T cell lymphoma
	Hepatosplenic T cell lymphoma
	Subcutaneous panniculitis-like T cell lymphoma
	Mycosis fungoides
	Sézary syndrome
	Primary cutaneous CD30+ T cell lymphoproliferative disorders
	Primary cutaneous peripheral T cell lymphomas, rare subtypes
	Primary cutaneous gamma-delta T cell lymphoma
	Primary cutaneous CD8+ aggressive epidermotropic cytotoxic T cell lymphoma
	Primary cutaneous CD4+ small/medium T cell lymphoma
	Peripheral T cell lymphoma, not otherwise specified
	Angioimmunoblastic T cell lymphoma
	Anaplastic large cell lymphoma, ALK positive
	Anaplastic large cell lymphoma, ALK negative

In this chapter, only mature B cell and T cell neoplasms are discussed; the precursor malignancies are covered in Chapter 35.

Mature B Cell Lymphomas

Mature B cell lymphomas are derived from various stages of B cell differentiation. Although they show significant morphologic and immunophenotypic heterogeneity, all B cell lymphomas produce monoclonal light chain immunoglobulins, clonal immunoglobulin gene rearrangements, or both. Follicular lymphoma and diffuse large B cell lymphoma (DLBCL) are the most common subtypes of B cell lymphoma.[9] Most cases are lymph node based and occur in elderly individuals. However, leukemic involvement (peripheral blood and bone marrow) can occur with any lymphoma type. The most common mature B cell neoplasms are discussed in the following paragraphs and are summarized in Table 36-2.

Chronic Lymphocytic Leukemia/Small Lymphocytic Lymphoma

Definition.   Chronic lymphocytic leukemia (CLL) and small lymphocytic lymphoma (SLL) are characterized by accumulation of small lymphoid cells in peripheral blood, bone marrow, and lymphoid organs. The exact cell of origin in CLL/SLL is not known, however gene expression profiling has shown that antigen-experienced B cells, both memory B cells and marginal zone B cells, are likely candidates.[10] The World Health Organization (WHO) classification scheme considers CLL and SLL as one entity with different clinical presentations.[1] The diagnosis of CLL/SLL is based on the predominant site of involvement. CLL presents mostly in peripheral blood and bone marrow. SLL primarily involves lymph nodes and other lymphoid organs.

Morphology.   In CLL, bone marrow and peripheral blood films show small lymphoid cells with a characteristically coarse chromatin ("soccer-ball" pattern), absent or inconspicuous nucleoli, and scant cytoplasm[1,11] (Figure 36-10). According to the 2008 International Workshop on Chronic Lymphocytic Leukemia, up to 55% of the cells in CLL may include prolymphocytes (larger lymphoid cells with pale blue cytoplasm, less condensed chromatin, and a distinct nucleolus), lymphoid cells with cleaved nuclei, or large lymphoid cells with an

TABLE 36-2 Morphologic and Immunophenotypic Features of Mature B-Cell Lymphomas

Subtype	Architectural Features	Cytologic Characteristics	Immunophenotype/ Cytogenetics	Cell of Origin
Chronic lymphocytic leukemia/small lymphocytic lymphoma	Diffuse lymphocytic proliferation with growth centers	Small lymphoid cells	CD20$^+$, CD19$^+$, CD5$^+$, CD23$^+$, LEF1	Memory and marginal zone B cells
B cell prolymphocytic leukemia	Diffuse proliferation	Medium-sized lymphoid cells with distinct "punched-out" nucleoli and abundant cytoplasm	CD20$^+$, CD19$^+$, FMC7$^+$, CD5$^{+/-}$	Unknown mature B cell
Mantle cell lymphoma	Diffuse, nodular, or mantle zone pattern	Medium-sized lymphocytes with irregular nuclei	CD20$^+$, CD19$^+$, CD5$^+$, FMC7$^+$, SOX11, cyclin D1$^+$, t(11;14)	Mantle zone cell
Follicular lymphoma	Follicular pattern	Medium-sized lymphocytes with indented nuclei and variable numbers of large lymphoid cells	CD20$^+$, CD19$^+$, CD10$^+$, BCL6$^+$, BCL2$^+$, t(14;18)	Germinal center cell
Extranodal marginal zone lymphoma of mucosa-associated lymphoid tissue	Diffuse lymphoid proliferation, occasionally marginal zone or nodular pattern	Medium-sized lymphocytes with irregular nuclei and clear abundant cytoplasm	CD20$^+$, CD19$^+$, CD43$^{+/-}$	Marginal zone cell
Plasma cell myeloma, plasmacytoma	Sheets or large aggregates of plasma cells	Plasma cells, frequently with cytologic atypia	CD20$^-$, CD19$^{+/-}$, CD38$^+$, CD138$^+$, cytoplasmic light chain$^+$	Plasma cell
Diffuse large B cell lymphoma	Diffuse proliferation	Large lymphoid cells	CD20$^+$, CD19$^+$, CD10$^{+/-}$, BCL6$^{+/-}$, BCL2$^{+/-}$, CD5$^{+/-}$	Different stages of mature B cells
Burkitt lymphoma	Diffuse lymphoid proliferation with "starry sky" pattern	Medium-sized lymphocytes with evenly distributed chromatin, inconspicuous nucleoli	CD20$^+$, CD19$^+$, CD10$^+$, BCL6$^+$, BCL2$^-$, high proliferative activity, t(8;14)	Germinal center cell

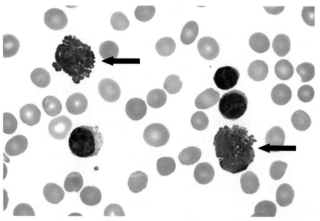

Figure 36-10 Chronic lymphocytic leukemia/small lymphocytic lymphoma. Peripheral blood film showing small lymphocytes and smudge cells (*arrows*) (Wright-Giemsa stain, ×1000).

atypical appearance.[12] The French-American-British (FAB) Cooperative Group has proposed, and other groups have supported, a morphologic classification of CLL consisting of two major types: typical CLL (>90% small mature lymphocytes and <10% prolymphocytes) and an atypical CLL category.[13,14,15,16] The 2008 WHO classification of lymphoid malignancies does not divide CLL into typical and atypical types.[1]

Smudge cells, representing disintegrated lymphoid cells, are typically seen on peripheral blood films of CLL patients. Smudge cells are helpful in the diagnosis because they are not often seen in other subtypes of malignant lymphoma. The bone marrow biopsy specimen shows nodular, diffuse, or interstitial infiltrates of small lymphoid cells (Figure 36-11).

Lymph nodes involved by SLL show an effacement of normal nodal architecture by a diffuse proliferation of small, round lymphoid cells with coarse chromatin, indistinct nucleoli, and scant cytoplasm (Figure 36-12, *A*). In addition, scattered nodules (so-called pseudofollicles, growth centers, or proliferation centers) composed of medium-sized and large lymphoid cells with dispersed chromatin and distinct nucleoli are observed (Figure 36-12, *B*). The diffuse proliferation of small lymphoid cells with pseudofollicles is pathognomonic for SLL.

Diagnosis and Immunophenotype. CLL is diagnosed based on a sustained increase in the monoclonal B lymphocytes with CLL immunophenotype which is equal or greater than 5000/uL. The CLL immunophenotype includes an expression of CD19, CD20, and CD23, with aberrant expression of CD5.[1] Expression of CD20 and CD79b is weaker than in normal B cells.[1] Immunophenotyping also demonstrates

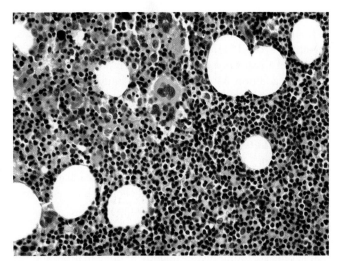

Figure 36-11 Chronic lymphocytic leukemia/small lymphocytic lymphoma. Bone marrow biopsy specimen with nodular (*right*) and interstitial lymphoid infiltrate composed of small lymphocytes (hematoxylin and eosin stain, ×400).

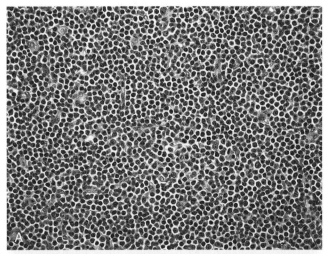

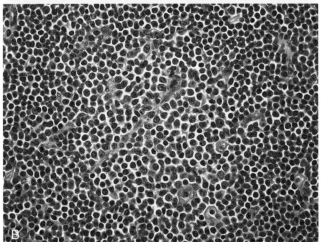

Figure 36-12 Chronic lymphocytic leukemia/small lymphocytic lymphoma in a lymph node. **A,** Diffuse proliferation of small lymphoid cells (hematoxylin and eosin stain, ×100). **B,** Proliferation center with large and medium-sized lymphoid cells in a background of small lymphocytes (hematoxylin and eosin stain, ×400).

expression of kappa *or* lambda light chains (clonal light chain restriction).[1,12]

CD23 and LEF1 (lymphoid-enhancer-binding factor 1) expression and the absence of FMC7, cyclin D1, and SOX11 distinguish CLL/SLL from mantle cell lymphoma. The presence of less than 5000/μL of circulating monoclonal B cells with a CLL/SLL immunophenotype can be found in a small proportion of healthy individuals and has been designated a monoclonal B-cell lymphocytosis.[1,17] Therefore, the demonstration of these cells by flow cytometry must always be interpreted in the context of other clinical and laboratory features.[17]

Clinical Features and Prognosis. CLL/SLL generally affects older adults, however approximately 24% of patients are less than 55 years old.[18] In CLL most patients are asymptomatic at diagnosis. The first indication of disease is often an incidental finding of lymphocytosis on a routine CBC in a blood count ordered for a different reason.

CLL is a heterogeneous disease in terms of clinical behavior. A variety of features have been used over the years to predict patient outcomes, including staging systems based on the extent of lymphoid organ involvement and degree of cytopenias. More recently, a growing number of biologic and molecular markers are being used which have enabled a more accurate assessment of disease status and prognosis.

The somatic mutation status of the variable region of the immunoglobulin heavy chain (*IGVH*) locus has divided the disease into two groups with considerably different outcomes.[11] Approximately 55% of CLL patients have mutated *IGVH*, indolent disease, and a median survival time of 24 years.[19,20] On the other hand, patients with unmutated *IGVH* have aggressive disease and a median survival of approximately 8 years.[19,20] At diagnosis, patients can be routinely screened using techniques such as fluorescent in situ hybridization (FISH) for the presence of chromosomal abnormalities, del13q14.3, del11q22-23, trisomy 12, and del17p13, which provide information regarding predicted survival (good, poor, intermediate, and very poor, respectively).[20] Next generation sequencing has recently identified additional significant genetic mutations such as EZH2, *NOTCH1*, *SF3B1*, and *BIRC3*, which can be used for an assessment of prognosis.[21] The timing as well as selection of the most appropriate treatment approach has also been the subject of intense research. Independent of the course of the original disease, approximately 5% of patients with CLL/SLL develop a high-grade diffuse large B cell lymphoma (called *Richter syndrome*) with a survival of less than 1 year.[16]

Prolymphocytic Leukemia

Definition. Prolymphocytic leukemia (PLL) is a rare mature lymphoid leukemia that can be derived from B or T cells. Both B cell and T cell types involve peripheral blood, bone marrow, and spleen. Lymph node involvement is more commonly seen in T cell PLL. This lymphoproliferative disease is distinct from CLL, and its diagnosis requires that more than 55% of circulating lymphoid cells have the morphology of a prolymphocyte.

Morphology and Immunophenotype. The pathogno-monic cell of B cell PLL is a prolymphocyte of medium size with round nucleus, moderately abundant cytoplasm, and distinct "punched-out" nucleolus (Figure 36-13). The cell size (twice that of a normal lymphocyte) and prominent central nucleolus allow PLL to be distinguished from CLL/SLL. The peripheral blood involvement in PLL is prominent, with a white blood cell count frequently in excess of 100×10^9/L. Bone marrow shows interstitial and/or nodular proliferation of prolymphocytes. Both white and red splenic pulp are infiltrated by PLL. B cell PLL is positive for pan–B cell markers CD20, CD19, CD22, and FMC7. The density of CD20 and surface light chain is higher than in typical cases of CLL/SLL. A proportion of cases are positive for CD5 antigen. In such cases, distinguishing the PLL from mantle cell lymphoma presenting with a leukemic involvement might be challenging and requires cytogenetic or molecular studies to exclude the presence of t(11;14) (refer to the section on mantle cell lymphoma).

Morphologic features of T cell PLL are not as distinct as those of the B cell type. Neoplastic cells seen in peripheral blood films are small to medium size, with round or irregular nuclei, the latter resembling Sézary cells. Prominent nucleoli are seen only in a proportion of cases. Cytoplasmic blebbing is common. Bone marrow, spleen, lymph node, and occasionally skin involvement is diffuse, with accentuation in nodal paracortical areas and around the vessels in dermis. The diagnosis of T cell PLL is challenging when attempted using morphologic features alone. A combination of morphologic, clinical, and immunophenotypic features is most helpful in making the diagnosis. T prolymphocytes are positive for T cell markers such as CD3, CD2, and CD5. In contrast to many T cell lymphomas, T cell PLL is positive for CD7 antigen. Most commonly CD4 antigen is expressed. A minority of cases can be double positive for CD4 and CD8, or positive for CD8.

Clinical Features and Prognosis. Like CLL/SLL, PLL is a disease of the elderly (mean age of presentation is 70 years). Overall prognosis is poor (median survival is 3 years for B cell

PLL), partly due to the high incidence of mutation in the tumor suppressor gene *TP53* and the unavailability of targeted therapy.[22] T cell PLL is an aggressive disease with a median survival of 1 year when conventional chemotherapies are used. Recently, addition of monoclonal antibody therapy against CD52 (alemtuzumab) has significantly improved treatment response and survival of patients with T cell PLL.

Hairy Cell Leukemia
Definition. Hairy cell leukemia is characterized by small B lymphocytes with abundant cytoplasm and fine ("hairy") cytoplasmic projections. The postulated cell of origin is the peripheral B cell of post–germinal center stage (memory B cell).

Morphology and Immunophenotype. Hairy cell leukemia cells are found predominantly in bone marrow and the red pulp of the spleen. A low number of neoplastic B cells are seen in peripheral blood. Lymph node involvement is rare. The bone marrow infiltrates are interstitial and are composed of small to medium-sized lymphoid cells with abundant cytoplasm (Figure 36-14, *A*). The bone marrow involvement may be subtle with preservation of normal hematopoiesis. As a result of the production of fibrogenic cytokines by leukemic cells, a bone marrow biopsy specimen shows an increase in reticulin fibers. The characteristic cytologic features of neoplastic cells are best appreciated in bone marrow aspirate and peripheral blood films. Neoplastic cells display an oval or indented nucleus, abundant cytoplasm, and fine, hairlike cytoplasmic projections (Figure 36-14, *B*).

Typical cases of hairy cell leukemia show strong positivity for B cell markers (CD19, CD20, CD22) coupled with bright expression of CD11c, CD25, CD103, tartrate-resistant acid phosphatase (TRAP, demonstrated by immunohistochemical analysis or cytochemical stain), DBA-44, CD123, and annexin A1. CD123 and annexin A1 are the most specific markers for classic hairy cell leukemia and can help in differentiating hairy cell leukemia from splenic marginal zone lymphoma. These antibodies, available for both flow cytometry and paraffin-embedded tissues, replaced the TRAP cytochemical stain previously commonly used to establish the diagnosis of hairy cell leukemia.

Clinical Features and Prognosis. Hairy cell leukemia is a rare lymphoproliferative disorder occurring in middle-aged individuals (median age, 55 years). The presenting signs include splenomegaly and pancytopenia. Durable remissions can be achieved using purine analogues. Conventional lymphoma therapy is not effective.

Mantle Cell Lymphoma
Definition. Mantle cell lymphoma is a lymphoproliferative disorder characterized by medium-sized lymphoid cells with irregular nuclear outlines derived from the follicular mantle zone.[23]

Morphology and Immunophenotype. The main sites of presentation are lymph nodes. Bone marrow, peripheral blood, spleen, and gastrointestinal tract also are frequently involved. Most commonly, lymph nodes show a replacement of

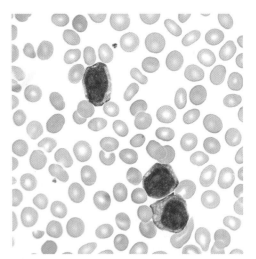

Figure 36-13 Peripheral blood film showing a characteristic morphology of prolymphocytes (medium size, abundant cytoplasm, distinct nucleoli) (×1000).

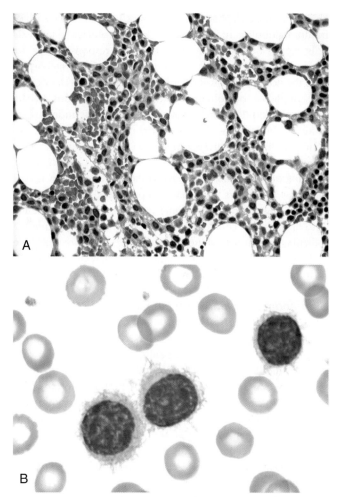

Figure 36-14 Hairy cell leukemia. **A,** Interstitial bone marrow infiltrate composed of widely spaced lymphoid cells with abundant cytoplasm and irregular nuclei (hematoxylin and eosin stain, ×1000). **B,** Lymphoid cells of hairy cell leukemia show characteristic cytoplasmic projections, which are supported by the peripheral cytoplasmic network of polymerized actin (peripheral blood, Wright-Giemsa stain, ×1000).

normal nodal architecture with a diffuse proliferation of monotonous, medium-sized lymphoid cells with irregular nuclear outlines (Figure 36-15, *A*). Occasionally, lymph nodes demonstrate a vaguely nodular pattern or partial preservation of nodal architecture with a prominent thickening of mantle zones (Figure 36-15, *B*). Peripheral blood involvement by mantle cell lymphoma can mimic PLL (Figure 36-15, *C*).

Like other B cell lymphoproliferative disorders, mantle cell lymphoma shows expression of pan–B cell markers (CD19, CD20) and high-density clonal surface light chains. There is coexpression of CD5 antigen; however, CD23 antigen is absent. In contrast to CLL/SLL, the expression of CD20 and light chains is strong, and there is immunoreactivity for cyclin D1 and SOX11. *Cyclin D1* (*BCL1*) is a proto-oncogene involved in the regulation of G₁ to S phase transition. In mantle cell lymphoma, this gene is constitutively expressed through its translocation to the immunoglobulin heavy chain gene, t(11;14). This cytogenetic abnormality is present in the majority of mantle cell lymphomas. Cyclin D1–negative cases are positive for SOX11, a recently described diagnostic

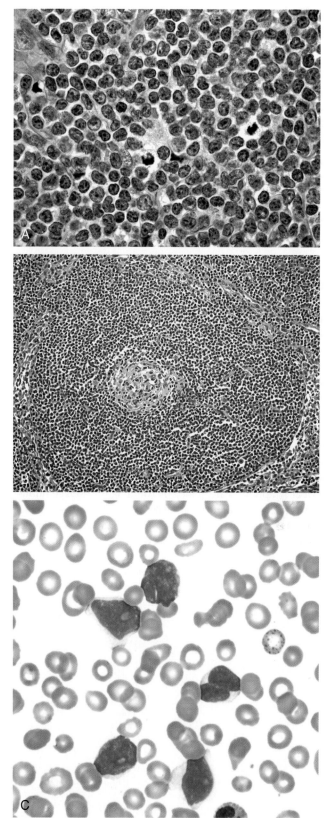

Figure 36-15 Mantle cell lymphoma. **A,** Diffuse proliferation of medium-sized lymphoid cells with irregular nuclei (hematoxylin and eosin stain, ×1000). **B,** Mantle zone pattern. Regressed germinal center is seen in the center (hematoxylin and eosin stain, ×100). **C,** Circulating mantle cell lymphoma cells with a few showing indented nuclei reminiscent of the cleaved nuclei seen in histologic sections (peripheral blood film, Wright-Giemsa stain, ×1000).

and prognostic marker present in the majority of cases of mantle cell lymphoma.

Clinical Features and Prognosis. Mantle cell lymphoma is an aggressive lymphoproliferative disorder with a median survival time of 3 to 5 years. Most patients present with disseminated disease, including bone marrow involvement. This lymphoma is incurable with currently available chemotherapy, but stem cell transplantation is successful in a proportion of patients.

Follicular Lymphoma

Definition. Follicular lymphoma originates from germinal center B cells and in most cases recapitulates follicular architecture.

Morphology and Immunophenotype. Numerous closely spaced follicles replace the normal nodal architecture (Figure 36-16). The neoplastic proliferation may extend into perinodal adipose tissue. In contrast to the reactive secondary follicles, in follicular lymphoma the mantle zone and polarization are absent. The neoplastic follicles are composed of medium-sized lymphoid cells with angular or indented nuclei, cytologically similar to centrocytes, with a variable admixture of large lymphoid cells. The latter resemble centroblasts and show oval nuclei with vesicular chromatin and several nucleoli located close to nuclear membrane. The relative proportion of medium-sized and large lymphoid cells is of prognostic significance. Cases with high numbers of large cells show a more aggressive clinical course, similar to that of DLBCL. Therefore, follicular lymphomas are graded by counting the average number of large cells per high-power field.[1] Two grades are recognized: grade 1-2 shows rare scattered large lymphocytes, and grade 3 follicular lymphomas are composed of numerous centroblasts.

The immunophenotype reflects the follicle center cell origin of this disease. Pan–B cell markers (CD19, CD20) are present, along with the coexpression of CD10, BCL6, and clonal surface immunoglobulin. In contrast to reactive follicles, neoplastic cells express BCL2 protein. This protein is responsible for the decreased sensitivity of lymphoma cells to apoptosis and allows the accumulation of neoplastic lymphocytes. The expression of BCL-2 by follicular lymphoma cells is due to the t(14;18)(q32;q21), which places the *BCL2* gene under a promoter of the immunoglobulin heavy chain gene. This cytogenetic abnormality is present in 95% of cases.[24]

Clinical Features and Prognosis. The median age at diagnosis is 59 years. Most patients present with disseminated disease. Bone marrow involvement is present in approximately 50% of cases. The course of the disease is indolent in grade 1-2 follicular lymphoma, whereas grade 3 cases are more aggressive and are treated in a manner similar to DLBCL with doxorubicin (Adriamycin)–based regimens.

Extranodal Marginal Zone Lymphoma of Mucosa-Associated Lymphoid Tissue

Definition. Three subtypes of marginal zone lymphomas are recognized: nodal, extranodal (MALT lymphoma), and splenic. In this chapter, we focus on the extranodal variant derived from marginal zone cells of MALT. In this lymphoma, the neoplastic proliferation is usually heterogeneous, encompassing small and medium-sized lymphocytes, plasma cells, and scattered large lymphoid cells. MALT lymphoma is frequently associated with autoimmune conditions (e.g., Sjögren syndrome, Hashimoto thyroiditis) or infections (*Helicobacter pylori* gastritis or hepatitis C).[25] Persistent immune stimulation leads to the accumulation of reactive lymphoid tissue and subsequently to the development of marginal zone lymphoma. The importance of continuous antigenic stimulation in the early stages of these lymphomas is shown by the remission of the disease, when associated infection is eradicated with antibiotic therapy.[26]

Morphology and Immunophenotype. In most cases, the neoplastic population is composed of a mixture of medium-sized lymphocytes, plasma cells, and occasional large lymphoid cells. There is a predominance of medium-sized marginal zone cells with irregular nuclei (Figure 36-17, *A*). Residual reactive germinal centers may be present, which are colonized to variable degrees by neoplastic cells. A characteristic feature of MALT lymphoma is the presence of so-called lympho-epithelial lesions, representing the invasion of the neoplastic lymphocytes into the glandular epithelium (Figure 36-17, *B*). This feature is usually absent from reactive lymphoid proliferations associated with autoimmune processes or infections.

The neoplastic cells of marginal zone lymphoma express CD20, CD19, and monoclonal immunoglobulin chains. CD5 and CD10 are absent. CD43 antigen is coexpressed in 30% of cases and can be a helpful feature in diagnosing marginal zone lymphoma when there is a significant residual reactive component. In select cases, the demonstration of clonality by flow cytometry or by polymerase chain reaction (PCR) analysis of immunoglobulin heavy chain (IgH) gene rearrangements may be necessary to confirm the diagnosis.

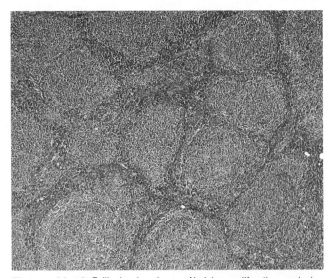

Figure 36-16 Follicular lymphoma. Nodular proliferation replacing normal elements of lymph node architecture (hematoxylin and eosin stain, ×40).

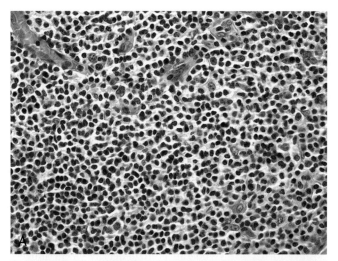

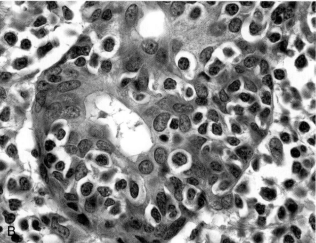

Figure 36-17 Mucosa-associated lymphoid tissue lymphoma. **A,** Heterogeneous population of medium-sized lymphoid cells with abundant clear cytoplasm and occasional large cells (hematoxylin and eosin stain, ×500). **B,** Lymphoepithelial lesion. Malignant lymphocytes invading glandular epithelium (hematoxylin and eosin stain, ×1000).

Antigenic stimulation and interference with the apoptotic pathway play an important role in the pathogenesis of MALT lymphoma. Approximately 30% of cases show a translocation involving apoptosis-inhibitor gene *API2* and the *MLT* gene, the t(11;18)(q21;q21).[27]

Clinical Features and Prognosis. The gastrointestinal tract is the most common site for extranodal marginal zone lymphoma. The lung, thyroid, ocular adnexa, and breast are other primary sites of involvement. In most cases, the disease is localized to a primary site and regional lymph nodes. Bone marrow is less frequently involved than in other types of indolent lymphoma.[28] In cases of gastric MALT lymphoma positive for *H. pylori*, the antibiotic treatment of the infection may induce a remission of the associated lymphoma. Other cases may benefit from local therapy.

Plasma Cell Neoplasms

Definition. Plasma cell neoplasms are characterized by a monoclonal proliferation of terminally differentiated B cells

(i.e., plasma cells). These disorders can present as a localized or disseminated process most commonly involving bone marrow and bone. The clinical features and the primary site of involvement define distinct clinicopathologic entities (Table 36-3).

Plasma cell myeloma is a multifocal accumulation of malignant plasma cells in bone marrow presenting as lytic bone lesions. In most cases, monoclonal immunoglobulin produced by neoplastic plasma cells is detected in serum, urine, or both (monoclonal gammopathy). The overt disease may be preceded by an asymptomatic period of monoclonal gammopathy with only mild bone marrow plasmacytosis (fewer than 10% plasma cells). Approximately 25% of asymptomatic patients with clonal serum immunoglobulin progress to symptomatic plasma cell myeloma.[29] The term *monoclonal gammopathy of undetermined significance* (MGUS) is used to encompass the entire patient population with clonal serum immunoglobulin and only mild marrow plasmacytosis. Plasmacytoma, a localized form of plasma cell neoplasm, may present as a solitary bone lesion or involve an extraosseous or extramedullary site, most commonly the nasopharynx, oropharynx, or sinuses.

Morphology and Immunophenotype. Plasma cell myeloma is characterized by marked bone marrow plasmacytosis. Large aggregates and sheets of plasma cells, frequently with cytologic atypia, are present and often constitute more than 30% of marrow cellularity (Figure 36-18, *A*). Atypical cytologic features seen in plasma cell myeloma include a high nuclear-to-cytoplasmic ratio, dispersed chromatin pattern, and distinct nucleoli (Figure 36-18, *B*). These changes are rarely seen in reactive conditions and MGUS. Similarly, in reactive plasmacytosis associated with infections and autoimmune disorders,

TABLE 36-3 Clinicopathologic Features of Selected Plasma Cell Neoplasms

Plasma Cell Disorder	Defining Features
Plasma cell myeloma	Monoclonal protein in serum or urine
	Clonal plasma cells in bone marrow or presence of plasmacytoma
	Organ or tissue impairment (CRAB: hyper*c*alcemia, *r*enal insufficiency, *a*nemia, *b*one lesions)
Plasma cell leukemia	Clonal plasma cell population in bone marrow and other features of plasma cell myeloma in conjunction with peripheral blood involvement: >2 × 10⁹/L or >20% circulating plasma cells
	May present with involvement of spleen, liver, and body cavity fluid including cerebrospinal fluid
Monoclonal gammopathy of undetermined significance	Bone marrow plasmacytosis (<10% plasma cells)
	Monoclonal gammopathy (<30 g/L)
	No lytic bone lesions or organ/tissue impairment
Solitary plasmacytoma of bone	Localized bone mass composed of plasma cells
Extraosseous plasmacytoma	Localized extraosseous mass composed of plasma cells

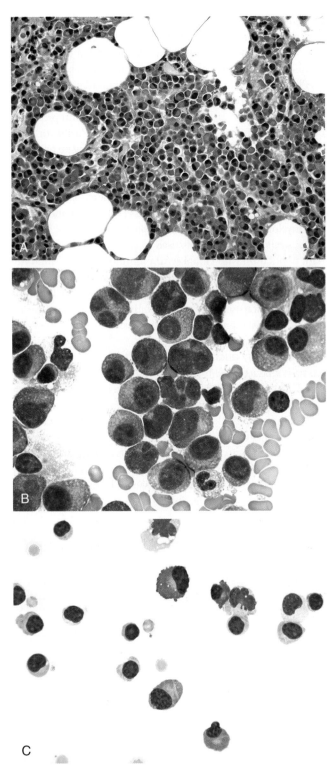

Figure 36-18 Plasma cell myeloma. **A,** Bone marrow biopsy specimen showing large aggregates of plasma cells (hematoxylin and eosin stain, ×400). **B,** Neoplastic plasma cells with cytologic atypia (bone marrow, Wright-Giemsa stain, ×1000). **C,** Plasma cells in the pleural fluid of a patient with plasma cell myeloma (Wright-Giemsa stain, ×1000).

plasma cells appear scattered throughout the marrow and form small clusters around the vessels. Large aggregates and sheets of plasma cells, which are commonly seen in plasma cell myeloma, are not present in reactive conditions. Rarely, patients with plasma cell myeloma show a marked increase in circulating plasma cells. The term *plasma cell leukemia* is reserved for cases with more than 20% circulating plasma cells or plasma cell counts exceeding 2×10^9/L. Neoplastic plasma cells can also infiltrate spleen, liver, or lymph nodes and involve body cavity fluids (Figure 36-18, *C*). Plasmacytoma represents a localized, mass-forming, monoclonal plasma cell proliferation.

Neoplastic plasma cells show an immunophenotype similar to that of their normal counterparts. At this terminal stage of differentiation, pan–B cell markers CD19 and CD20 and surface immunoglobulin chains are usually absent. Plasma cells are positive for CD138 (syndecan-1), high-density CD38 antigen, and monoclonal cytoplasmic immunoglobulins. These monoclonal proteins, in the form of complete immunoglobulin— most commonly IgG or IgA or isolated clonal light chains—are secreted by the neoplastic plasma cells and are seen in serum and urine as monoclonal spikes. In addition, neoplastic plasma cells can show an expression of other antigens typically not expressed by normal plasma cells, such as CD56 and myeloid markers.

Clinical Features and Prognosis. Plasma cell myeloma is a disease of older individuals (median age, 70 years).[30] Bone pain and pathologic fractures are directly related to the proliferation of neoplastic plasma cells. These cells produce factors that cause localized bone destruction (lytic lesions on radiographic examination) and hypercalcemia. Renal insufficiency is triggered by the obstruction or direct damage of renal tubules by monoclonal protein. Cytopenias are related to the replacement of normal trilineage hematopoiesis by massive plasma cell infiltrates. Depressed normal immunoglobulin levels result in a susceptibility to infections, which commonly occur in patients with plasma cell myeloma. High levels of serum immunoglobulins also may interfere with the coagulation cascade and impair circulation through an increase in serum viscosity. Tissue deposits of clonal immunoglobulins, called *amyloidosis,* may compromise kidney, heart, and liver function and cause peripheral neuropathies.

Most of the cases show a rapidly progressive course, and the median survival is 3 years. The prognosis is closely related to the number of plasma cells in the bone marrow and to clinical features reflecting overall tumor burden. Patients with more than 50% bone marrow plasma cells, associated renal failure, and severe anemia have a shorter survival than patients with fewer than 20% plasma cells and preserved renal function.

Typically, patients with bone and extraosseous plasmacytomas are younger and respond favorably to local radiation therapy. Approximately 15% progress to plasma cell myeloma.

Asymptomatic monoclonal gammopathy (MGUS) occurs in fewer than 5% of individuals older than 70 years.[29] As discussed earlier, 25% of patients with MGUS develop overt myeloma. That is why all individuals with MGUS should be monitored closely with repeat measurements of serum immunoglobulin levels and bone marrow examinations.

Diffuse Large B Cell Lymphoma

Definition. The defining feature of DLBCL is the large cell size. In contrast to the neoplastic cells in the lymphoproliferative disorders discussed so far, DLBCL cells are significantly larger than normal lymphocytes. Most show a diffuse histologic growth pattern and can differ significantly in cytologic appearance and immunophenotype. DLBCL is one of the most common lymphomas, accounting for 30% to 40% of all non-Hodgkin lymphoma cases.[9]

Morphology and Immunophenotype. The most common type, DLBCL not otherwise specified, shows a diffuse proliferation of large lymphoid cells replacing normal nodal architecture. Cells are at least twice the size of normal small lymphocytes and show single or multiple nucleoli and ample cytoplasm (Figure 36-19). In rare cases, in addition to neoplastic large lymphoid cells, there is a considerable admixture of background histiocytes and small lymphocytes.

As in other B cell lymphomas, pan–B cell antigens are expressed. DLBCL can originate from a variety of stages in B cell development—hence the coexpression of other markers is heterogeneous. CD5, CD10, BCL6, CD30, and CD138 can be present (Table 36-2).

Clinical Features and Prognosis. Although, as with most lymphomas, the median age at diagnosis is in the sixties, DLBCL can be seen in children and young adults. Most commonly, it presents as a localized disease involving a group of lymph nodes. Bone marrow involvement is rare at presentation but can occur later in the course of the disease. DLBCL can also be seen in extranodal sites, including the gastrointestinal tract, central nervous system, bone, and serous effusions. DLBCL is an aggressive neoplasm with a proliferation rate frequently exceeding 40%, which makes it more sensitive to multiagent chemotherapy. The prognosis depends on a variety of clinical parameters, such as patient age, the extent of disease, and the site of involvement. The original morphologic subclassification of DLBCL was flawed by poor intraobserver and interobserver reproducibility.[31] However, recent results of gene microarray studies have shown that patients with DLBCL of follicle center origin have better survival than patients with other subtypes.[32]

Burkitt Lymphoma

Definition. Burkitt lymphoma is characterized by medium-sized, highly proliferating lymphoid cells with basophilic vacuolated cytoplasm. The WHO classification lists three variants of this lymphoma: endemic (occurring predominantly in Africa), sporadic, and immunodeficiency associated.

Morphology and Immunophenotype. The lymphoid proliferation is diffuse and at low magnification shows a prominent "starry sky" pattern imparted by numerous tingible-body macrophages (Figure 36-20, *A*). The macrophages are responsible for phagocytosing apoptotic debris, a by-product of the extremely high proliferative activity. Lymphoma cells are medium size with round nuclei, finely distributed chromatin, and small nucleoli. The cytoplasm is deeply basophilic and highly vacuolated, a feature best displayed on touch imprints or other cytologic preparations (Figure 36-20, *B*).

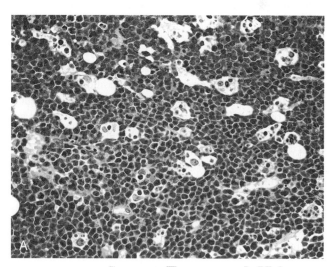

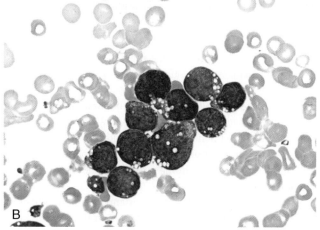

Figure 36-20 Burkitt lymphoma. **A,** "Starry sky" pattern imparted by numerous macrophages with apoptotic debris (hematoxylin and eosin stain, ×400). **B,** Touch preparation showing characteristic cells of Burkitt lymphoma. Note the deeply basophilic cytoplasm with numerous vacuoles (Wright-Giemsa stain, ×1000).

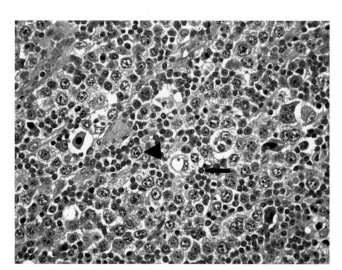

Figure 36-19 Diffuse large B cell lymphoma with proliferation of large lymphoid cells. Note the size difference between small lymphocytes (*arrow*) and neoplastic B cells (*arrowhead*) (hematoxylin and eosin stain, ×500).

The immunophenotype of Burkitt lymphoma reflects germinal center origin. CD19, CD20, CD10, and BCL6 antigens are present. There is surface expression of monoclonal immunoglobulin light chains. BCL2 is absent. The hallmark of Burkitt lymphoma is a high proliferation rate. Nearly 100% of Burkitt lymphoma cells are actively proliferating. This feature is linked to the constitutive expression of *MYC* gene (cell cycle gatekeeping gene) secondary to its translocation under the promoter of immunoglobulin heavy or light chain genes [t(8;14), t(2;8), or t(8;22)]. This translocation is pathognomonic for Burkitt lymphoma, and its demonstration is required for a definitive diagnosis.

Clinical Features and Prognosis. The clinical presentation of Burkitt lymphoma is dependent on the variant (endemic, sporadic, or immunodeficiency associated). The endemic form presents in young children (4 to 7 years of age), most commonly as a jawbone mass. The sporadic variant, seen in the United States and Europe, occurs in children and young adults most commonly as an abdominal mass. Gastrointestinal tract and abdominal lymph nodes are often involved. Other extranodal sites, such as gonads and breasts, can be a site of primary disease. Immunodeficiency-associated Burkitt lymphoma presents most often as nodal disease. Independent of the presentation, Burkitt lymphoma commonly involves the central nervous system, bone marrow, and peripheral blood (Burkitt leukemia). Epstein-Barr virus (EBV) is present in a proportion of patients.

A diagnosis of Burkitt lymphoma is a medical emergency. Because of its high proliferation rate, the doubling time is extremely short. The chemotherapy is significantly different from that used for other types of high-grade lymphoma. These highly aggressive treatment regimens take into account the high proliferative activity and contribute to high cure rates for childhood and adult Burkitt lymphoma: 60% to 90%, depending on the stage of the disease.[33,34] Immunodeficiency-associated Burkitt lymphoma occurs predominantly in HIV-positive patients. Its prognosis is not as favorable as for other variants.

Mature T Cell and Natural Killer Cell Lymphomas

Lymphomas derived from mature T cells and natural killer cells are much less common than the previously discussed mature B cell neoplasms and account for approximately 10% of all lymphomas. The incidence of the specific subtypes of T cell lymphoma shows geographic and ethnic variability. In certain geographic regions, T cell malignancies may be more prevalent than in the United States. Compared with B cell lymphomas, T cell neoplasms occur more frequently in extranodal sites. The most common skin lymphoma, mycosis fungoides, is of T cell phenotype.

Although morphology is an important criterion in the diagnosis of T cell lymphomas, a significant morphologic and cytologic variability is seen within specific subtypes. Similarly, the immunophenotypic features are not as specific as those seen in B cell malignancies. Due to the significant morphologic and immunophenotypic variability, an integration of morphologic, immunophenotypic, cytogenetic, molecular, and clinical information, as recommended by the WHO classification, is crucial in diagnosing T cell and natural killer cell malignancies. Until recently, the demonstration of clonality in T cell proliferations was limited to molecular methods showing T cell receptor gene rearrangements. The development of multiple antibodies directed against the variable region of the T cell receptor enables the determination of T cell clonality by flow cytometry.[35]

Mycosis Fungoides and Sézary Syndrome

Definition. Mycosis fungoides is the most common cutaneous lymphoma. It is composed of small to medium-sized lymphoid cells with irregular nuclear outlines (cerebriform nuclei). These cells show a predilection for the epidermis (epidermotropism) and dermis and may spread to regional lymph nodes. Sézary syndrome presents as a disseminated disease with widespread skin involvement (erythroderma), lymphadenopathy, and circulating lymphoma cells (Sézary cells with characteristic cerebriform nuclei) (Figure 36-21, *A*).

Morphology and Immunophenotype. In mycosis fungoides, the extent of cutaneous infiltrate is related to the stage of the disease. Early lesions show patchy or lichenoid infiltrate of the dermis by small to medium-sized lymphoid cells with irregular nuclear outlines (Figure 36-21, *B*). The aggregates of neoplastic lymphocytes in epidermis, called Pautrier microabscesses, are frequently seen in mycosis fungoides (Figure 36-21, *C*). Later in the course of the disease, cutaneous infiltrates may become more dense and form tumor-like lesions. The involvement of regional lymph nodes and peripheral blood may be present, especially in advanced stages of the disease.

The immunophenotype is similar to that of T lymphocytes normally present in the skin. The expression of pan–T cell markers CD3, CD5, and CD2 is seen along with CD4 antigen. An important feature, rarely seen in benign lymphoid infiltrates, is the absence of CD7 antigen. The T cell receptor gene is clonally rearranged.

Sézary syndrome is by definition a disseminated disease with leukemic presentation and skin and lymph node involvement.[36,37] The malignant cells are medium size with cerebriform nuclei. Skin and lymph node involvement is more pronounced than in early stages of mycosis fungoides and shows diffuse, monotonous lymphoid infiltrates. Due to low interobserver reproducibility, the determination of peripheral blood involvement based purely on morphology is not recommended. Currently, both morphologic and immunophenotypic evaluations are performed in order to demonstrate at least 1000 Sézary cells/µL, a CD4-to-CD8 ratio of more than 10 (due to significant numbers of circulating CD4+ Sézary cells), and an aberrant immunophenotype.[1] The latter is defined as a significant loss of CD7, CD26, or T cell marker(s) on CD4+ T cells.

Clinical Features and Prognosis. The incidence of mycosis fungoides increases with age, and the average age at presentation is 55 to 60 years. The survival of patients with early-stage disease is excellent, because progression and development of disseminated lymphoma are very slow.[36] In this patient group, 10-year disease-specific survival was reported as 97% to 98%. In most cases, only local treatment is necessary. In contrast, Sézary syndrome is an aggressive lymphoma with a low (10% to 20%) 5-year survival rate.[37]

Peripheral T Cell Lymphoma, Unspecified

Definition.   Peripheral T cell lymphoma, unspecified, comprises a morphologically heterogeneous group of lymphomas with mature T cell phenotype.

Morphology and Immunophenotype.   Lymph node involvement is usually diffuse with a prominent vascular proliferation. The cytologic features are variable with medium-sized to large cells with atypical and occasionally pleomorphic nuclei (Figure 36-22). Certain variants show a considerable admixture of reactive small lymphocytes, immunoblasts, histiocytes, and eosinophils. Bone marrow is frequently involved, but a significant circulating lymphoma component is rarely seen at presentation. Most cases are derived from CD4$^+$ T cells and retain this immunophenotype. Variable loss of pan–T cell antigens, including CD7, is seen.

Clinical Features and Prognosis.   Peripheral T cell lymphoma is an aggressive disease occurring predominantly in older adults (average age of 60 years). Generalized lymphadenopathy and a variety of constitutional symptoms, such as fever, night sweats, weight loss, and pancytopenia, are present at diagnosis. The 3-year survival rate is reported to be approximately 40%.[38] Biologic features and advanced stage at presentation contribute to the dismal prognosis. In addition, few treatment regimens have been developed specifically for T cell lymphomas; aggressive B cell lymphoma protocols are commonly used to treat these disorders.

Anaplastic Large Cell Lymphoma

Definition.   Although considerable morphologic variability can be seen, a typical case of anaplastic large cell lymphoma

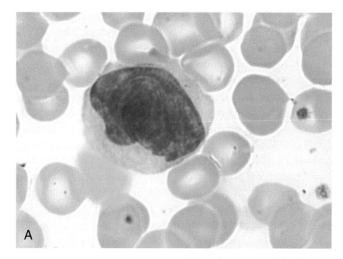
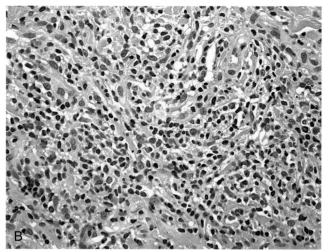
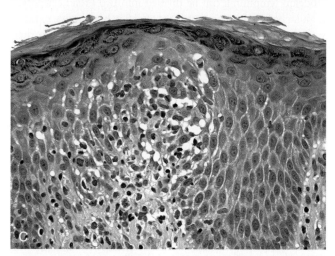

Figure 36-21 Mycosis fungoides. **A,** Sezary cell (Wright-Giemsa stain, × 1000) **B,** Dermal infiltrate of medium-sized lymphoid cells with angulated nuclei (hematoxylin and eosin stain, ×400). **C,** Neoplastic lymphocytes invading the epidermis (hematoxylin and eosin stain, ×400).

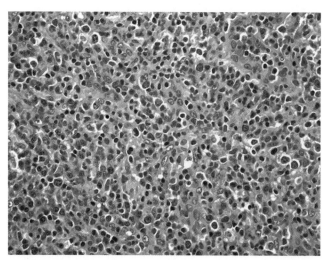

Figure 36-22 Peripheral T cell lymphoma showing heterogeneous population of small, medium-sized, and large lymphoid cells (hematoxylin and eosin stain, ×500).

is characterized by large atypical cells with pleomorphic nuclei and abundant cytoplasm. The expression of CD30 antigen and ALK-1 protein is seen in the majority of cases.

Morphology and Immunophenotype. Numerous morphologic variants have been described, depending on the predominant architectural and cytologic features. The lymph node architecture is most often diffusely effaced by malignant lymphoid cells (Figure 36-23, *A*). Occasionally, lymph node involvement may be partial with characteristic infiltrates of nodal sinuses. When significant fibrosis is present, anaplastic large cell lymphoma may resemble classical Hodgkin lymphoma. Regardless of the histologic variant, in almost every case, at least a proportion of cells are large with abundant cytoplasm and pleomorphic, eccentric, kidney-shaped nuclei, so-called hallmark cells. Leukemic involvement is not frequent, but it may be seen in the small cell variant. In such cases, the peripheral blood film shows atypical lymphoid cells with indented nuclei reminiscent of Sézary cells (Figure 36-23, *B*). Immunophenotyping is instrumental for prompt diagnosis.

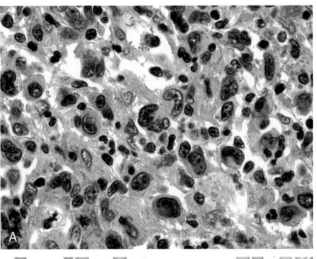

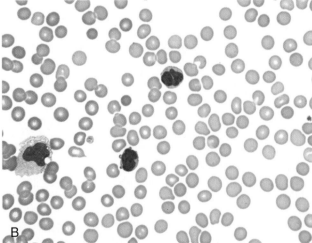

Figure 36-23 A, Anaplastic large cell lymphoma with large pleomorphic cells (hematoxylin and eosin stain, ×1000). **B,** Peripheral blood involvement by small cell variant of anaplastic large cell lymphoma (Wright-Giemsa stain, ×1000).

CD30 antigen and, in most cases, ALK-1 protein are defining immunophenotypic features of this lymphoma. The overexpression of ALK-1 is most often due to t(2;5)(p23;35) between the *ALK-1* and nucleophosmin genes. Alternative partner genes for *ALK-1* translocation have also been identified. The cytotoxic T cell origin of this lymphoma can be demonstrated by immunohistochemistry showing expression of cytotoxic antigens such as TIA-1, granzyme, and perforin.[39] Pan–T cell markers (CD3, CD7, CD5) are often absent. The most commonly expressed T cell lineage–associated antigens are CD4 and CD2. Pan-hematopoietic antigen CD45 is expressed only in a proportion of cases (Table 36-4). By flow cytometry, the coexpression of myeloid markers such as CD13, CD33, and CD15 is seen in approximately 50% of cases. In cases negative for the T cell–associated antigens and ALK-1 protein, the demonstration of clonal T cell receptor gene rearrangement can help to render a definitive diagnosis.

Clinical Features and Prognosis. Anaplastic large cell lymphoma is less frequent in adults. However, it is one of the most common lymphomas in the pediatric population, representing 10% to 15% of childhood lymphomas. Anaplastic large cell lymphoma presents as disseminated nodal disease with constitutional symptoms. Extranodal sites, including skin, can also be involved. The most important prognostic feature is the expression of ALK-1 protein. ALK-1$^+$ disease has a favorable prognosis, whereas ALK-1$^-$ disease shows survival rates more comparable to those of peripheral T cell lymphoma, unspecified.

Hodgkin Lymphoma

Hodgkin lymphoma can be divided into two broad categories: nodular lymphocyte-predominant Hodgkin lymphoma and classical Hodgkin lymphoma.[1] Although both disorders occur preferentially in young individuals and share certain morphologic characteristics, more recent studies have shown that they are biologically distinct entities, and they are discussed separately.

Nodular Lymphocyte-Predominant Hodgkin Lymphoma

Definition. Nodular lymphocyte-predominant Hodgkin lymphoma is a B cell neoplasm composed of relatively rare

TABLE 36-4 Immunophenotypic Features of Lymphomas Composed of Large Lymphoid Cells

Antigen	NLPHL	Classical HL	DLBCL	ALCL
CD30	−	+	+/−	+
CD15	−	+	−	−
CD45	+	−	+	+/−
CD20	+	+/−*	+	−
CD3	−	−	−	+/−†

ALCL, Anaplastic large cell lymphoma; *DLBCL,* diffuse large B cell lymphoma; *HL,* Hodgkin lymphoma; *NLPHL,* nodular lymphocyte-predominant Hodgkin lymphoma.
*If positive, the immunoreactivity is weak and present only in a proportion of neoplastic cells.
†Other T cell markers, such as CD2 and CD4, are more often present.

neoplastic cells (lymphocytic/histiocytic or "popcorn" cells) scattered within nodules of reactive lymphocytes.

Morphology and Immunophenotype. The normal architecture of a lymph node is replaced by a nodular proliferation of small lymphocytes and scattered lymphocytic/histiocytic or popcorn cells, the latter being the neoplastic cells of nodular lymphocyte-predominant Hodgkin lymphoma (Figure 36-24). These are large lymphoid cells with abundant cytoplasm and vesicular multilobated nuclei (popcorn nuclei). The nucleoli are inconspicuous.

The lymphocytic/histiocytic cells are of follicle center cell origin and are positive for B cell markers, including CD20 antigen, BCL6, and immunoglobulin chains (Table 36-4).[40] The neoplastic cells do not show evidence of EBV infection. In addition to neoplastic cells, the nodules are composed of CD20+ small B cells, T lymphocytes, and CD21 positive follicular dendritic cell meshworks.

Clinical Features and Prognosis.
Most patients are males in their thirties and present with localized peripheral lymphadenopathy. Mediastinal lymph node involvement is rare. As for classical Hodgkin lymphoma, the prognosis is excellent, with survival rates of 80% to 90% when the disease is diagnosed in the early stages.[41]

Classical Hodgkin Lymphoma

Definition. Classical Hodgkin lymphoma comprises a heterogeneous group of lymphoid neoplasms derived from the germinal center.[42] It is characterized by the presence of relatively few diagnostic neoplastic cells, Reed-Sternberg cells, in a rich reactive background. The incidence of this disease varies in different geographic regions. In the United States and Europe, it is a common form of lymphoma occurring in young adults. In the United States, approximately 7400 new cases are diagnosed annually.[5] A bimodal age distribution is observed, with incidence peaks between 15 and 34 years and older than 54 years.

Morphology and Immunophenotype. On the basis of architectural features, the composition of the reactive background, and relative proportion of neoplastic cells, classical Hodgkin lymphoma can be divided into four subtypes (Table 36-5):
1. Nodular sclerosis
2. Mixed cellularity
3. Lymphocyte rich
4. Lymphocyte depleted

Reed-Sternberg cells are present in all subtypes of classical Hodgkin lymphoma. The typical Reed-Sternberg cell is large with a bilobed nucleus or two nuclei with prominent eosinophilic nucleoli and abundant cytoplasm (Figure 36-25, *A*). When encountered in an appropriate background, Reed-Sternberg cells are pathognomonic for the diagnosis. However, not all neoplastic cells of classical Hodgkin lymphoma show the typical morphology of Reed-Sternberg cells. Variants of neoplastic cells, including Hodgkin cells, mummified cells, and lacunar cells, are often encountered in a single lymph node. Hodgkin cells are large mononuclear lymphoid cells with an oval nucleus, thick nuclear membrane, distinct eosinophilic nucleolus, and abundant cytoplasm. Mummified cells are degenerated or apoptotic cells with a pyknotic nucleus and condensed cytoplasm. Lacunar cells occur predominantly in the nodular sclerosis variant of classical Hodgkin lymphoma and are characterized by a lobated nucleus and artifactual retraction of cytoplasm secondary to formalin fixation. Because of this artifact, the cells appear to be situated in a clear space (i.e., lacuna).

In all subtypes of classical Hodgkin lymphoma, Reed-Sternberg cells and their variants have a similar immunophenotype (Table 36-5). They are CD30+ in all cases (Figure 36-25, *B*) and CD15+ in approximately 80% of cases. The CD15

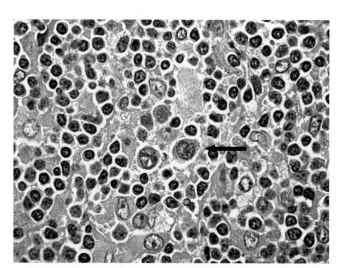

Figure 36-24 Characteristic popcorn (lymphocytic/histiocytic) cells of nodular lymphocyte-predominant Hodgkin lymphoma (*arrow*) (hematoxylin and eosin stain, ×1000).

TABLE 36-5 Morphologic Subtypes of Classical Hodgkin Lymphoma

Subtype	Neoplastic Cells	Additional Morphologic Features
Nodular sclerosis	RS cells; Hodgkin cells; lacunar cells	Fibrotic bands; background of small lymphocytes, histiocytes, and eosinophils
Mixed cellularity	RS cells; Hodgkin cells	Background of small lymphocytes, eosinophils, neutrophils, histiocytes, plasma cells; no fibrotic bands
Lymphocyte rich	RS cells; Hodgkin cells	Diffuse nodular background of small lymphocytes; no or few eosinophils and neutrophils
Lymphocyte depleted	RS cells; Hodgkin cells	Numerous RS cells and Hodgkin lymphoma cells; few background lymphocytes

RS, Reed-Sternberg.

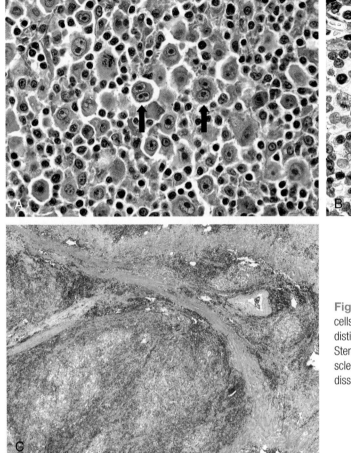

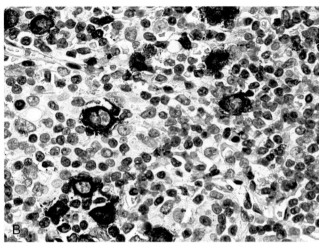

Figure 36-25 Classical Hodgkin lymphoma. **A,** Typical Reed-Sternberg cells (*arrows*) of classical Hodgkin lymphoma with two nuclear lobes and distinct nucleoli (hematoxylin and eosin stain, ×500). **B,** CD30⁺ Reed-Sternberg cells and their variants (immunoperoxidase, ×500). **C,** Nodular sclerosis type of classical Hodgkin lymphoma showing broad fibrotic bands dissecting the lymph node (hematoxylin and eosin stain, ×40).

immunoreactivity may be weak and seen in only a few malignant cells. The expression of B cell marker CD20 is weak to absent. Similarly, CD45 antigen is absent. The frequency of EBV infection depends on the subtype of classical Hodgkin lymphoma. The background small lymphocytes are predominantly CD4⁺ T cells.

Nodular Sclerosis Classical Hodgkin Lymphoma. The defining feature of the nodular sclerosis subtype is the presence of broad collagen bands transecting the lymph node and thickening of nodal capsule (Figure 36-25, *C*). The background cellularity includes small lymphocytes, eosinophils, and histiocytes. This is the most common subtype of classical Hodgkin lymphoma, accounting for 70% of cases. The frequency of immunohistochemically demonstrable EBV infection is lowest in this variant.

Mixed Cellularity Classical Hodgkin Lymphoma. In the mixed cellularity subtype, Reed-Sternberg cells and their variants are scattered among the diffuse background composed of small lymphocytes, histiocytes, eosinophils, neutrophils, and plasma cells. Typical Reed-Sternberg cells, mononuclear Hodgkin cells, and mummified cells are seen; however, lacunar cells are absent. Similarly, fibrotic bands and capsular thickening are not present. Approximately 20% of classical Hodgkin

lymphomas show this morphology. An association with EBV infection is seen in 75% of cases.

Lymphocyte-Rich Classical Hodgkin Lymphoma. In the lymphocyte-rich subtype, scattered mononuclear Hodgkin and Reed-Sternberg cells are seen together with a vaguely nodular background of small lymphocytes. Nodules represent remnants of mantle zones and germinal centers. Compared with other subtypes of classical Hodgkin lymphoma, the background cellularity is less heterogeneous.

Lymphocyte-Depleted Classical Hodgkin Lymphoma. The lymphocyte-depleted subtype is an uncommon variant of classical Hodgkin lymphoma occurring predominantly in immunodeficient patients. There is a paucity of reactive background, and neoplastic Reed-Sternberg cells and their variants are much more frequent. In most cases, neoplastic cells show evidence of EBV infection.

Clinical Features and Prognosis. With the exception of the lymphocyte-rich variant, which occurs in a slightly older population, classical Hodgkin lymphoma is a disease of young adults with a peak incidence at 15 to 35 years. Mostly peripheral lymph nodes are involved, except in the nodular sclerosis variant, which often shows mediastinal lymphadenopathy.

With the contemporary treatment protocols combining chemotherapy and radiotherapy, the cure rates are 80% to 90%, depending on the stage of the disease, patient age, and clinical symptoms. The best prognosis is seen in the nodular sclerosis subtype. Lymphocyte-depleted Hodgkin lymphoma is the most aggressive variant of classical Hodgkin lymphoma, especially in

HIV-positive patients. In this patient group, Hodgkin lymphoma also may manifest in unusual extranodal sites, including bone marrow. Patients with classical Hodgkin lymphoma treated with a combination of chemotherapy and radiotherapy are at high risk of developing secondary malignancies, including lung and breast carcinomas and acute leukemia.

SUMMARY

- Histologic components of normal lymph nodes include the cortex, paracortex, medullary cords, and sinuses. These are structural and functional compartments from which reactive hyperplasias and neoplasms originate.
- Lymphomas are neoplasms of the lymphoid system arising at specific stages of lymphoid differentiation.
- Modern lymphoma classification incorporates morphologic, immunophenotypic, molecular, laboratory data, and clinical characteristics.
- Lymphomas are broadly divided into neoplasms derived from precursor (immature) and mature lymphoid cells, and B cell and T cell malignancies.
- The most common mature B cell neoplasms are follicular lymphoma and DLBCL.
- The T cell neoplasms most common in the United States and Europe are peripheral T cell lymphoma, unspecified, and anaplastic large cell lymphoma.
- In CLL, the peripheral blood and bone marrow display smudge cells and small lymphoid cells with coarse chromatin, inconspicuous nucleoli, and scant cytoplasm.

- In HCL, small B lymphocytes have abundant cytoplasm and fine cytoplasmic projections.
- Hodgkin lymphoma has been shown to be of B cell origin.
- Hodgkin lymphoma is subclassified based on morphologic and immunophenotypic features.
- B cell and T cell lymphomas and Hodgkin lymphoma involve mainly lymph nodes; the involvement of extranodal sites and bone marrow or peripheral blood occurs with varying frequency.
- In general, lymphomas occur in elderly individuals; however, specific subtypes such as Hodgkin lymphoma show a predilection for younger age groups.
- The prognosis depends on lymphoma subtype. Indolent lymphomas show a protracted course but are largely incurable with current chemotherapeutic regimens. In contrast, aggressive lymphomas have a more rapidly progressive course, and the cure rates are higher.

Now that you have completed this chapter, go back and read again the case study at the beginning and respond to the questions presented.

REVIEW QUESTIONS

Answers can be found in the Appendix.

1. In most cases, the diagnosis of lymphoma relies on all of the following *except:*
   a. Microscopic examination of affected lymph nodes
   b. Immunophenotyping using immunohistochemistry or flow cytometry
   c. Molecular or cytogenetic analysis
   d. Peripheral blood examination and a complete blood count

2. The most common lymphoma occurring in young adults is:
   a. Follicular lymphoma
   b. DLBCL
   c. Hodgkin lymphoma
   d. Mycosis fungoides

3. In a normal lymph node, the medulla includes predominantly:
   a. T cells
   b. B cells
   c. Tingible-body macrophages
   d. Plasma cells

4. The t(11;14) is the defining feature of:
   a. Follicular lymphoma
   b. Hodgkin lymphoma
   c. CLL
   d. Mantle cell lymphoma

5. The immunophenotype of mycosis fungoides is:
   a. The normal T cell immunophenotype
   b. An abnormal T cell immunophenotype with expression of CD4 and loss of CD7 antigen
   c. A mix of CD4$^+$ and CD8$^+$ T cells
   d. An abnormal T cell immunophenotype with expression of CD8 and loss of CD7 antigen

6. What is the major morphologic difference between Hodgkin lymphoma and other B cell lymphomas?
   a. The extent of the lymph node involvement
   b. The presence of numerous reactive lymphocytes and only a few malignant cells in Hodgkin lymphoma
   c. The presence of numerous tingible-body macrophages in Hodgkin lymphoma
   d. The preservation of normal lymph node architecture in Hodgkin lymphoma

7. Which morphologic diagnosis has to be confirmed with molecular studies demonstrating the presence of t(8;14)?
   a. Mantle cell lymphoma
   b. Burkitt lymphoma
   c. Follicular lymphoma
   d. Sézary syndrome

8. What is the function of the germinal center?
   a. Generation of B cells producing immunoglobulins with the highest affinity for a particular antigen through the process of somatic mutation
   b. Production of plasma cells that secrete specific immunoglobulins following antigenic stimulation
   c. T cell maturation following T cell education in the thymus
   d. Generation of dendritic cells with unique antigen-processing capabilities

9. Marked paracortical expansion is most commonly seen in:
   a. Rheumatoid arthritis
   b. Syphilis
   c. Dermatopathic lymphadenopathy
   d. Follicular lymphoma

10. MGUS is best described as:
   a. The presence of monoclonal immunoglobulin in serum with only mild bone marrow plasmacytosis
   b. The presence of monoclonal serum or urine immunoglobulin with significant bone marrow plasmacytosis
   c. The presence of significant bone marrow plasmacytosis in a patient with only a few clinical symptoms of plasma cell myeloma
   d. The presence of monoclonal immunoglobulin in a patient with a solitary mass composed of plasma cells

REFERENCES

1. Swerdlow, S. H., Campo, E., Harris, N. L., et al., (Eds.). (2008). *WHO Classification of Tumours of Haematopoietic and Lymphoid Tissues.* (4th ed.). Lyon, France: IARC Press.
2. MacLennan, I. C. (2008). B cells: The follicular dimension of the marginal zone. *Immunol Cell Biol, 86,* 219–220.
3. Manser, T. (2004). Textbook germinal centers? *J Immunol, 172,* 3369–3375.
4. Herman, G. E., Chlipala, E., Bochenski, G., et al. (1988). Zinc formalin fixative for automated tissue processing. *J Histotechnol, 11,* 85–89.
5. American Cancer Society. (2014). *Cancer Facts & Figures 2014.* Atlanta: American Cancer Society. Retrieved from http://www.cancer.org/acs/groups/content/
6. Parvaneh, N., Filipovich, A. H., & Borkhardt, A. (2013). Primary immunodeficiencies predisposed to Epstein-Barr virus-driven haematological diseases. *Br J Haematol, 162*(5), 573–586.
7. Mueller, N. (1999). Overview of the epidemiology of malignancy in immune deficiency. *J Acquir Immune Defic Syndr, 21*(Suppl. 1), S5–S10.
8. Fisher, S. F., & Fisher, R. I. (2004). The epidemiology of non-Hodgkin's lymphoma. *Oncogene, 23,* 6524–6534.
9. The Non-Hodgkin's Lymphoma Classification Project: A clinical evaluation of the International Lymphoma Study Group Classification of non-Hodgkin's lymphoma. *Blood, 89,* 3909–3918.
10. Gaidano, G., Foà, R., Dalla-Favera, R. (2012). Molecular pathogenesis of chronic lymphocytic leukemia. *J Clin Invest, 122,* 3432–3438.
11. Stilgenbauer, S., Bullinger, L., Lichter, P., et al. (2002). Review: genetics of chronic lymphocytic leukemia: genomic aberrations and VH gene mutation status in pathogenesis and clinical course. *Leukemia, 16,* 993–1007.
12. Hallek, M., Cheson, B. D., Catovsky, D., et al. (2008). Guidelines for the diagnosis and treatment of chronic lymphocytic leukemia: a report from the International Workshop on Chronic Lymphocytic Leukemia updating the National Cancer Institute-Working Group 1996 guidelines. *Blood, 111,* 5446–5456.
13. Bennett, J. M., Catovsky, D., Daniel, M. T., et al. (1989). Proposals for the classification of chronic (mature) B and T lymphoid leukaemias. French-American-British (FAB) Cooperative Group. *J Clin Pathol, 42,* 567–584.
14. Matutes, E., & Polliack, A. (2000). Morphological and immunophenotypic features of chronic lymphocytic leukemia. *Rev Clin Exp Hematol, 4,* 22–47.
15. Matutes, E., Attygalle, A., Wotherspoon, A., et al. (2010). Diagnostic issues in chronic lymphocytic leukaemia (CLL). *Best Pract Res Clin Haematol, 23,* 3–20.
16. Johnston, J. B., Selftel, M., & Gibson, S. B. (2014). Chronic lymphocytic leukemia. In Greer, J. P., Arber, D. A., Glader, B., et al., (Eds.), *Wintrobe's Clinical Hematology.* Philadelphia: Lippincott Williams & Wilkins.
17. Shanafelt, T. D., Ghia, P., Lanasa, M. C., et al. (2010). Monoclonal B-cell lymphocytosis (MBL): biology, natural history and clinical management. *Leukemia, 24,* 512–520.
18. Shanafelt, T. D., Rabe, K. G., Kay, N. E., et al. (2010). Age at diagnosis and the utility of prognostic testing in patients with chronic lymphocytic leukemia. *Cancer, 116,* 4777–4787.
19. Hamblin, T. J., Davis, Z., Gardiner, A., et al. (1999). Unmutated IgV(H) genes are associated with a more aggressive form of chronic lymphocytic leukemia. *Blood, 94,* 1848–1854.
20. Chiorazzi, N. (2012). Implications of new prognostic markers in chronic lymphocytic leukemia. *Hematology Am Soc Hematol Educ Program,* 76–87.
21. Rossi, D., Rasi, S., Spina, V., et al. (2013). Integrated mutational and cytogenetic analysis identifies new prognostic subgroups in chronic lymphocytic leukemia. *Blood, 121,* 1403–1412.
22. Dohner, H., Fischer, K., Bentz, M., et al. (1995). p53 gene deletion predicts for poor survival and non-response to therapy with purine analogs in chronic B-cell leukemias. *Blood, 85,* 1580–1589.
23. Swerdlow, S. H., & Williams, M. E. (2002). From centrocytic to mantle cell lymphoma: a clinicopathologic and molecular review of three decades. *Hum Pathol, 33,* 7–20.
24. Horsman, D. E., Gascoyne, R. D., Coupland, R. W., et al. (1995). Comparison of cytogenetic analysis, southern analysis, and polymerase chain reaction for the detection of t(14;18) in follicular lymphoma. *Am J Clin Pathol, 103,* 472–478.
25. Thieblemont, C., Berger, F., & Coiffier, B. (1995). Mucosa-associated lymphoid tissue lymphomas. *Curr Opin Oncol, 7,* 415–420.
26. Parsonnet, J., & Isaacson, P. (2004). Bacterial infection and MALT lymphoma. *N Engl J Med, 350,* 213–215.
27. Streubel, B., Lamprecht, A., Dierlamm, J., et al. (2003). T(14;18)(q32;21) involving IGH and MALT1 is a frequent chromosomal aberration in MALT lymphoma. *Blood, 101*(6), 2335–2339.
28. Thieblemont, C., Berger, F., Dumontet, C., et al. (2000). Mucosa-associated lymphoid tissue lymphoma is a disseminated

disease in one third of 158 patients analyzed. *Blood, 95,* 802–806.

29. Kyle, R. A., Therneau, T. M., Rajkumar, S. V., et al. (2004). Long-term follow-up of 241 patients with monoclonal gammopathy of undetermined significance: the original Mayo Clinic series 25 years later. *Mayo Clin Proc, 79,* 859–866.

30. Kyle, R. A., & Rajkumar, S. V. (2004). Multiple myeloma. *N Engl J Med, 351,* 1860–1873.

31. Harris, N. L., Jaffe, E. S., Stein, H., et al. (1994). A revised European-American classification of lymphoid neoplasms: a proposal from the International Lymphoma Study Group. *Blood, 84,* 1361–1392.

32. Alizadeh, A. A., Eisen, M. B., Davis, R. E., et al. (2000). Distinct types of diffuse large B-cell lymphoma identified by gene expression profiling. *Nature, 403,* 503–511.

33. Blum, K. A., Lozanski, G., & Byrd, J. C. (2004). Adult Burkitt leukemia and lymphoma. *Blood, 104,* 3009–3020.

34. Cairo, M. S., Sposto, R., Perkins, S. L., et al. (2003). Burkitt's and Burkitt-like lymphoma in children and adolescents: a review of the Children's Cancer Group experience. *Br J Haematol, 120,* 660–670.

35. Clark, D. M., Boylston, A. W., Hall, P. A., et al. (1986). Antibodies to T cell antigen receptor beta chain families detect monoclonal T cell proliferation. *Lancet, 2,* 835–837.

36. Fink-Puches, R., Zenahlik, P., Bäck, B., et al. (2002). Primary cutaneous lymphomas: applicability of current classification schemes (European Organization for Research and Treatment of Cancer, World Health Organization) based on clinicopathologic features observed in a large group of patients. *Blood, 99,* 800–805.

37. Hristov, A. C., Vonderheid, E. C., & Borowitz, M. J. (2011). Simplified flow cytometric assessment in mycosis fungoides and Sezary syndrome. *Am J Clin Pathol, 136*(6), 944–953.

38. Escalon, M. P., Liu, N. S., Yang, Y., et al. (2005). Prognostic factors and treatment of patients with T-cell non-Hodgkin lymphoma. *Cancer, 103,* 2091–2098.

39. Foss, H. D., Anagnostopoulos, I., Araujo, I., et al. (1996). Anaplastic large-cell lymphomas of T-cell and null-cell phenotype express cytotoxic molecules. *Blood, 88,* 4005–4011.

40. Braeuninger, A., Kuppers, R., Strickler, J. G., et al. (1997). Hodgkin and Reed-Sternberg cells in lymphocyte predominant Hodgkin disease represent clonal populations of germinal center–derived tumor B cells. *Proc Natl Acad Sci U S A, 94,* 9337–9342.

41. Diehl, V., Sextro, M., Franklin, J., et al. (1999). Clinical presentation, course, and prognostic factors in lymphocyte-predominant Hodgkin's disease and lymphocyte-rich classical Hodgkin's disease: report from the European Task Force on Lymphoma Project on Lymphocyte-Predominant Hodgkin's Disease. *J Clin Oncol, 17,* 776–783.

42. Thomas, R. K., Re, D., Wolf, J., et al. (2004). Part I: Hodgkin's lymphoma—molecular biology of Hodgkin and Reed-Sternberg cells. *Lancet Oncol, 5,* 11–18.

Normal Hemostasis and Coagulation 37

Margaret G. Fritsma and George A. Fritsma

OUTLINE

Overview of Hemostasis
Vascular Intima in Hemostasis
Anticoagulant Properties of Intact Vascular Intima
Procoagulant Properties of Damaged Vascular Intima
Fibrinolytic Properties of Vascular Intima
Platelets
Coagulation System
Nomenclature of Procoagulants
Classification and Function of Procoagulants
Plasma-Based (In Vitro) Coagulation: Extrinsic, Intrinsic, and Common Pathways
Cell-Based (In Vivo, Physiologic) Coagulation
Coagulation Regulatory Mechanisms
Tissue Factor Pathway Inhibitor
Protein C Regulatory System
Antithrombin and Other Serine Protease Inhibitors (Serpins)
Fibrinolysis
Plasminogen and Plasmin
Plasminogen Activation
Control of Fibrinolysis
Fibrin Degradation Products and D-Dimer

OBJECTIVES

After completion of this chapter, the reader will be able to:

1. List the systems that interact to provide hemostasis.
2. Describe the properties of the vascular intima in the initiation and regulation of hemostasis and fibrinolysis.
3. List the hemostatic functions of tissue factor-bearing cells and blood cells, especially platelets, in hemostasis.
4. Describe the relationships among platelet function, von Willebrand factor, and fibrinogen, and their impact on hemostasis.
5. Describe the nature, origin, and function of each of the tissue and plasma factors necessary for normal coagulation.
6. Explain the role of vitamin K in the production and function of the prothrombin group of plasma clotting factors.
7. Distinguish between coagulation pathway serine proteases and cofactors.
8. Describe six roles of thrombin in hemostasis.

9. Diagram fibrinogen structure, fibrin formation, fibrin polymerization, and fibrin cross-linking.
10. For each coagulation complex—extrinsic tenase, intrinsic tenase, and prothrombinase—identify the serine protease and the cofactor forming the complex, the type of cell involved, and the substrate(s) activated.
11. List the factors in order of reaction in the plasma-based extrinsic, intrinsic, and common pathways.
12. Describe the cell-based in vivo coagulation process and the role of tissue factor–bearing cells and platelets.
13. Show how tissue factor pathway inhibitor, the protein C pathway, and the serine protease inhibitor antithrombin function to regulate coagulation and prevent thrombosis.
14. Describe the fibrinolytic pathway, its regulators, and its products.

CASE STUDY

After studying the material in this chapter, the reader should be able to respond to the following case study:

A pregnant woman developed a blood clot in her left leg (deep vein thrombosis, or DVT). Her mother reportedly had a history of thrombophlebitis. She had a brother who was diagnosed with a DVT following a flight from Los Angeles to Sydney, Australia.
1. Is this hemostatic disorder typical of an acquired or an inherited condition?
2. Are these symptoms most likely caused by a deficiency of a procoagulant or an inhibitor?

Hemostasis is a complex physiologic process that keeps circulating blood in a fluid state and then, when an injury occurs, produces a clot to stop the bleeding, confines the clot to the site of injury, and finally dissolves the clot as the wound heals. When hemostasis systems are out of balance, hemorrhage (bleeding) or thrombosis (pathological clotting) can be life-threatening. The absence of a single plasma procoagulant may destine the individual to lifelong *anatomic hemorrhage*, chronic inflammation, and transfusion dependence. Conversely, absence of a control protein allows coagulation to proceed unchecked and results in thrombosis, stroke, pulmonary embolism, deep vein thrombosis, and cardiovascular events.

Understanding the major systems of hemostasis—blood vessels, platelets, and plasma proteins—is essential to interpreting laboratory test results and to prevent, predict, diagnose, and manage hemostatic disease.

OVERVIEW OF HEMOSTASIS

Hemostasis involves the interaction of vasoconstriction, platelet adhesion and aggregation, and coagulation enzyme activation to stop bleeding. The coagulation system, similar to other humoral amplification mechanisms, is complex because it translates a diminutive physical or chemical stimulus into a profound lifesaving event.[1] The key cellular elements of hemostasis are the cells of the vascular intima, extravascular tissue factor (TF)–bearing cells, and platelets. The plasma components are the coagulation and fibrinolytic proteins and their inhibitors.

Primary hemostasis (Table 37-1) refers to the role of blood vessels and platelets in response to a vascular injury, or to the commonplace *desquamation* of dying or damaged endothelial cells. Blood vessels contract to seal the wound or reduce the blood flow (vasoconstriction). Platelets become activated, adhere to the site of injury, secrete the contents of their granules, and aggregate with other platelets to form a platelet plug. Vasoconstriction and platelet plug formation comprise the initial, rapid, short-lived response to vessel damage, but to control major bleeding in the long term, the plug must be reinforced by fibrin. Defects in primary hemostasis such as collagen abnormalities, thrombocytopenia, qualitative platelet disorders, or von Willebrand disease can cause debilitating, sometimes fatal, chronic hemorrhage.

Secondary hemostasis (Table 37-1) describes the activation of a series of coagulation proteins in the plasma, mostly serine proteases, to form a fibrin clot. These proteins circulate as inactive zymogens (proenzymes) that become activated during the process of coagulation and, in turn, form complexes that activate other zymogens to ultimately generate thrombin, an enzyme that converts fibrinogen to a localized fibrin clot. The final event of hemostasis is fibrinolysis, the gradual digestion and removal of the fibrin clot as healing occurs.[2]

Although the vascular intima and platelets are associated with primary hemostasis, and coagulation and fibrinolysis are associated with secondary hemostasis, all systems interact in early- and late-hemostatic events. For example, platelets, although a key component of primary hemostasis, also secrete coagulation factors stored in their granules and provide an essential cell membrane phospholipid on which coagulation complexes form. The remainder of this chapter examines vascular intima, platelets, normal coagulation, coagulation control, and fibrinolysis in detail.

VASCULAR INTIMA IN HEMOSTASIS

The vascular intima provides the interface between circulating blood and the body tissues. The innermost lining of blood vessels is a monolayer of metabolically active *endothelial cells* (*EC*) (Box 37-1; Figure 37-1).[3] Endothelial cells are complex and heterogeneous and are distributed throughout the body. They display unique structural and functional characteristics, depending on their environment and physiologic requirements, not only in subsets of blood vessels such as arteries *versus* veins but also in the various tissues and organs of the body.[4,5] ECs play essential roles in immune response, vascular permeability, proliferation, and, of course, hemostasis.

ECs form a smooth, unbroken surface that eases the fluid passage of blood. An elastin-rich internal elastic lamina (basement membrane) and its surrounding layer of connective tissues support the ECs. In all blood vessels, fibroblasts occupy the connective tissue layer and produce collagen. Smooth muscle cells in arteries and arterioles, but not in the walls of veins, venules, or capillaries, contract during primary hemostasis.

Anticoagulant Properties of Intact Vascular Intima

Normally, the intact vascular endothelium prevents thrombosis by inhibiting platelet aggregation, preventing coagulation activation and propagation, and enhancing fibrinolysis. Several specific anticoagulant mechanisms prevent intravascular thrombosis (Box 37-2; Figure 37-2). First, ECs are rhomboid and contiguous, providing a smooth inner surface of the blood vessel that prevents harmful turbulence that otherwise may activate platelets and coagulation enzymes. ECs form a physical barrier separating procoagulant proteins and platelets in blood from *collagen* in the internal elastic lamina that promotes platelet adhesion, and *tissue factor* in fibroblasts and smooth muscle cells that activates coagulation.

TABLE 37-1 Primary and Secondary Hemostasis

Primary Hemostasis	Secondary Hemostasis
Activated by desquamation and small injuries to blood vessels	Activated by large injuries to blood vessels and surrounding tissues
Involves vascular intima and platelets	Involves platelets and coagulation system
Rapid, short-lived response	Delayed, long-term response
Procoagulant substances exposed or released by damaged or activated endothelial cells	The activator, tissue factor, is exposed on cell membranes

---

BOX 37-1 Vascular Intima of the Blood Vessel

Innermost Vascular Lining
Endothelial cells (endothelium)

Supporting the Endothelial Cells
Internal elastic lamina composed of elastin and collagen

Subendothelial Connective Tissue
Collagen and fibroblasts in veins
Collagen, fibroblasts, and smooth muscle cells in arteries

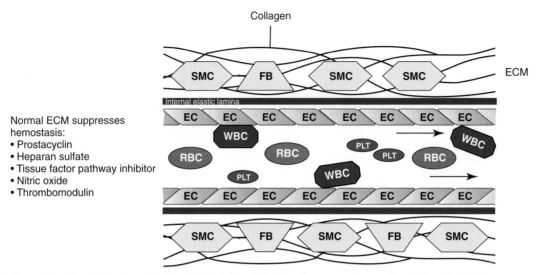

Figure 37-1 Normal blood flow in intact vessels. Smooth, rhomboid endothelial surfaces promote even flow. RBCs and platelets are concentrated toward the center, WBCs roll along the endothelium. The endothelium contains or secretes several hemostasis-suppressing materials. *EC,* Endothelial cell; *ECM,* extracellular matrix; *FB,* fibroblast; *PLT,* platelet; *RBC,* red blood cell; *SMC,* smooth muscle cell; *WBC,* white blood cell; *lines* indicate collagen.

BOX 37-2 Anticoagulant Properties of Intact Endothelium

Composed of rhomboid cells presenting a smooth, contiguous surface

Secretes the eicosanoid platelet inhibitor *prostacyclin*

Secretes vascular "relaxing" factor *nitric oxide*

Secretes the anticoagulant glycosaminoglycan *heparan sulfate*

Secretes coagulation extrinsic pathway regulator *tissue factor pathway inhibitor*

Expresses endothelial protein C receptor

Expresses cell membrane *thrombomodulin,* a protein C coagulation control system activator

Secretes TPA, thereby activating *fibrinolysis*

ECs synthesize and secrete a variety of substances that maintain normal blood flow. Prostacyclin, a platelet inhibitor and a vasodilator, is synthesized through the eicosanoid pathway (Chapter 13) and prevents unnecessary or undesirable platelet activation in intact vessels.[6] Nitric oxide is synthesized in ECs, vascular smooth muscle cells, neutrophils, and macrophages. Nitric oxide induces smooth muscle relaxation and subsequent vasodilation, inhibits platelet activation, and promotes angiogenesis and healthy arterioles.[7,8] An important EC-produced anticoagulant is *tissue factor pathway inhibitor* (TFPI), which controls activation of the tissue factor pathway, also called the extrinsic coagulation pathway.

Figure 37-2 Anticoagulant functions of normal intact endothelial cells and procoagulant properties of endothelial cells when damaged. *EC,* Endothelial cells; *PGI₂,* prostacyclin or prostaglandin I₂; *TFPI,* tissue factor pathway inhibitor; *EPCR,* endothelial cell protein C receptor; *TPA,* tissue plasminogen activator; *VWF,* von Willebrand factor; *ADAMTS-13,* a disintegrin and metalloproteinase with a thrombospondin type 1 motif, member 13; *TF,* tissue factor; *PAI-1,* plasminogen activator inhibitor-1; *TAFI,* thrombin-activatable fibrinolysis inhibitor.

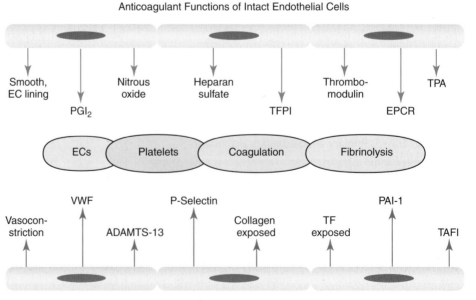

Finally, ECs synthesize and express on their surfaces inhibitors of thrombin formation, *thrombomodulin,* facilitated by *endothelial protein C receptor (EPCR),* and *heparan sulfate.* EPCR binds protein C, and thrombomodulin catalyzes the activation of the protein C pathway. The protein C pathway downregulates coagulation by digesting activated factors V and VIII, thereby inhibiting thrombin formation. Heparan sulfate is a glycosaminoglycan that enhances the activity of antithrombin, a serine protease inhibitor.[9] The pharmaceutical anticoagulant *heparin,* manufactured from porcine gut tissues, resembles EC heparan sulfate in its antithrombin activity. Heparin is used extensively as a therapeutic agent to prevent propagation of the thrombi that cause coronary thrombosis, strokes, deep vein thromboses, and pulmonary emboli.

Procoagulant Properties of Damaged Vascular Intima

Although the intact endothelium has anticoagulant properties, when damaged, the vascular intima promotes coagulation. First, any harmful local stimulus, whether mechanical or chemical, induces vasoconstriction in arteries and arterioles (Table 37-2; Figure 37-2). Smooth muscle cells contract, the vascular lumen narrows or closes, and blood flow to the injured site is minimized. Although veins and capillaries do not have smooth muscle cells, bleeding into surrounding tissues creates extravascular pressure on the blood vessel, effectively minimizing the escape of blood.

Second, the subendothelial connective tissues of arteries and veins are rich in collagen, a flexible, elastic structural protein that binds and activates platelets. Some connective tissue degeneration occurs naturally in aging, which leads to an increased bruising tendency.

Third, ECs secrete von Willebrand factor (VWF) from storage sites called *Weibel-Palade* bodies when activated by vasoactive agents such as thrombin. VWF is a large multimeric glycoprotein that is necessary for platelets to adhere to exposed subendothelial collagen in arterioles.[10]

Fourth, on activation, ECs secrete and coat themselves with *P-selectin,* an adhesion molecule that promotes platelet and leukocyte binding.[11] ECs also secrete immunoglobulin-like adhesion molecules called *intercellular adhesion molecules* (ICAMs) and *platelet endothelial cell adhesion molecules* (PECAMs) that further promote platelet and leukocyte binding.[12]

Finally, subendothelial smooth muscle cells and fibroblasts support the constitutive membrane protein tissue factor.[13] Physiologically, EC disruption exposes tissue factor in subendothelial cells and activates the coagulation system through contact with plasma factor VII. In pathological conditions, tissue factor may also be expressed on bloodborne monocytes during inflammation and sepsis and by tissue factor–positive microparticles derived from membrane fragments of activated or apoptotic vascular cells and possibly on the surface of some ECs.[14] Activation of the TF:VIIa:Xa complex within the circulation is limited by TFPI.

Fibrinolytic Properties of Vascular Intima

ECs support fibrinolysis (Figure 37-2), the removal of fibrin to restore vessel patency, with the secretion of tissue plasminogen activator (TPA). During thrombus formation, both TPA and plasminogen bind to polymerized fibrin. TPA activates fibrinolysis by converting plasminogen to plasmin, which gradually digests fibrin and restores blood flow. ECs also regulate fibrinolysis by providing inhibitors to prevent excessive plasmin generation. ECs, as well as other cells, secrete *plasminogen activator inhibitor 1* (PAI-1), a TPA control protein that inhibits plasmin generation and fibrinolysis.[15] Another inhibitor of plasmin generation, *thrombin-activatable fibrinolysis inhibitor* (TAFI), is activated by thrombin bound to EC membrane thrombomodulin.[16] Elevations in PAI-1 or TAFI can slow fibrinolysis and increase the tendency for thrombosis.

Although the significance of the vascular intima in hemostasis is well recognized, there are few valid laboratory methods to assess the integrity of ECs, smooth muscle cells, fibroblasts, and their collagen matrix.[17] The diagnosis of blood vessel disorders is often based on clinical symptoms, family history, and laboratory tests that rule out platelet or coagulation disorders.

PLATELETS

Platelets are produced from the cytoplasm of bone marrow megakaryocytes (Chapter 13).[18] Although platelets are only 2 to 3 μm in diameter on a fixed, stained peripheral blood film, they are complex, metabolically active cells that interact with their environment and initiate and control hemostasis.[19]

At the time of an injury, platelets adhere, aggregate, and secrete the contents of their granules (Table 37-3).[20,21] *Adhesion* is the property by which platelets bind nonplatelet surfaces such as subendothelial collagen (Figures 37-3 and 37-4). Further, VWF links platelets to collagen in areas of high shear stress such as arteries and arterioles, whereas platelets may bind directly to collagen in damaged veins and capillaries. VWF binds platelets through their glycoprotein GP Ib/IX/V membrane receptor.[22] The importance of platelet adhesion is underscored by bleeding disorders such as Bernard-Soulier syndrome, in which the platelet GP Ib/IX/V receptor is absent,

TABLE 37-2 Procoagulant Properties of the Damaged Vascular Intima

Structure	Procoagulant Property
Smooth muscle cells in arterioles and arteries	Induce vasoconstriction
Exposed subendothelial collagen	Binds VWF and platelets
Damaged or activated ECs	Secrete VWF
	Secrete adhesion molecules: P-selectin, ICAMs, PECAMs
Exposed smooth muscle cells and fibroblasts	Tissue factor exposed on cell membranes
ECs in inflammation	Tissue factor is induced by inflammation

ECs, endothelial cells; *ICAMs,* Intercellular adhesion molecules; *PECAMs,* platelet endothelial cell adhesion molecules; *VWF,* von Willebrand factor.

TABLE 37-3 Platelet Function

Function	Characteristics
Adhesion: platelets roll and cling to nonplatelet surfaces	Reversible; seals endothelial gaps, some secretion of growth factors, in arterioles VWF is necessary for adhesion
Aggregation: platelets adhere to each other	Irreversible; platelet plugs form, platelet contents are secreted, requires fibrinogen
Secretion: platelets discharge the contents of their granules	Irreversible; occurs during aggregation, platelet contents are secreted, essential to coagulation

and von Willebrand disease, in which VWF is missing or defective.

Aggregation is the property by which platelets bind to one another (Figure 37-5). When platelets are activated, a change in the GP IIb/IIIa receptor allows binding of fibrinogen, as well as VWF and fibronectin.[23] Fibrinogen binds to GP IIb/IIIa receptors on adjacent platelets and joins them together in the presence of ionized calcium (Ca^{2+}). Fibrinogen binding is essential for platelet aggregation, as evidenced by bleeding and compromised aggregation in patients with afibrinogenemia or in patients who lack the GP IIb/IIIa receptor (Glanzmann thrombasthenia). In in vitro platelet aggregation

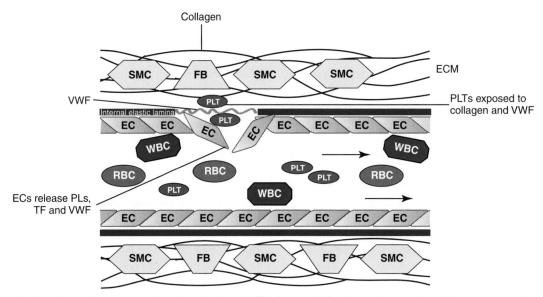

Figure 37-3 Platelet adhesion. Upon desquamation of endothelial cells (*EC*), platelets (*PLT*) adhere to the internal elastic lamina or extracellular matrix (ECM) and fill in until new ECs grow. *FB,* Fibroblast; *PL,* phospholipid; *RBC,* red blood cell; *SMC,* smooth muscle cell; *TF,* tissue factor; *VWF,* von Willebrand factor; *WBC,* white blood cell; *lines* indicate collagen.

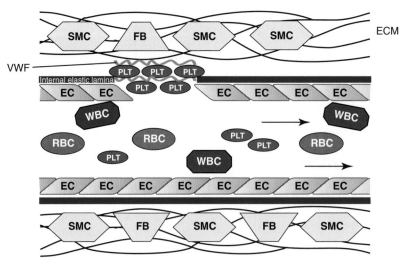

Figure 37-4 Interaction of platelets (*PLT*), von Willebrand factor (*VWF*), and collagen. In arterioles and arteries, where blood flows rapidly, platelets adhere by binding VWF. The larger VWF multimers form a fibrillar carpet on which the platelets assemble. Though a protective mechanism, a white clot consisting of PLTs and VWF may occlude the vessel, causing acute myocardial infarction, stroke, or peripheral artery disease. *EC,* Endothelial cell; *ECM,* extracellular matrix; *SMC,* smooth muscle cell; *FB,* fibroblast; *RBC,* red blood cell; *WBC,* white blood cell; *lines* indicate collagen.

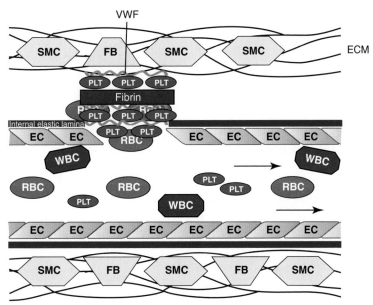

Figure 37-5 Platelet aggregation. In veins and venules, the bulky "red clot" consists of platelets *(PLT)*, von Willebrand factor *(VWF)*, fibrin, and red blood cells *(RBC)*. Though a protective mechanism, the red clot may occlude the vessel, causing venous thromboembolic disease. *EC,* Endothelial cell; *ECM,* extracellular matrix; *FB,* fibroblast; *WBC,* white blood cell; *SMC,* smooth muscle cell; *lines* indicate collagen.

studies, the most commonly used agonists to induce aggregation are thrombin (or thrombin receptor activation peptide, TRAP), arachidonic acid, adenosine diphosphate (ADP), collagen, and epinephrine, which bind to their respective platelet membrane receptors.[24]

Platelets secrete the contents of their granules during adhesion and aggregation, with most secretion occurring late in the platelet activation process. Platelets secrete procoagulants, such as factor V, VWF, factor VIII, and fibrinogen, as well as control proteins, Ca^{2+}, ADP, and other hemostatic molecules. See Table 37-4 for a summary of the contents of platelet α-granules and dense bodies (dense granules).

During activation, ADP and Ca^{2+} activate phospholipase A_2, which converts membrane phospholipid to arachidonic acid. *Cyclooxygenase* converts arachidonic acid into prostaglandin endoperoxides. In the platelet, thromboxane synthetase converts

prostaglandins into thromboxane A_2, which causes Ca^{2+} to be released and promotes platelet aggregation and vasoconstriction (Figure 37-6). Aspirin acetylation permanently inactivates cyclooxygenase, blocking thromboxane A_2 production and causing impairment of platelet function (aspirin effect).[25]

Chapter 13 provides an in-depth description of platelet structure and function. Platelet disorders are considered in detail in Chapters 40 and 41.

The platelet membrane is the key surface for coagulation enzyme-cofactor-substrate complex formation.[26] Platelets supply Ca^{2+}, the membrane phospholipid phosphatidylserine, procoagulant factors, and receptors. Coagulation is initiated on tissue factor–bearing cells (such as fibroblasts) with the formation of the extrinsic tenase complex TF:VIIa:Ca^{2+}, which activates factors IX and X and produces enough thrombin to activate platelets and factors V, VIII, and XI in a feedback loop. Coagulation is then propagated on the surface of the platelet with the formation of the intrinsic tenase complex (IXa:VIIIa:phospholipid:Ca^{2+}) and the prothrombinase complex (Xa:Va:phospholipid:Ca^{2+}), ultimately generating a burst of thrombin at the site of injury. See subsequent text for more details.

Erythrocytes, monocytes, and lymphocytes also participate in hemostasis. Erythrocytes add bulk and structural integrity to the fibrin clot; there is a tendency to bleed in anemia. In inflammatory conditions, monocytes and lymphocytes, and possibly ECs, provide surface-borne tissue factor that may trigger coagulation. Leukocytes also have a series of membrane integrins and selectins that bind adhesion molecules and help stimulate the production of inflammatory cytokines that promote the wound-healing process.[27]

TABLE 37-4   Platelet Granule Contents

Platelet α-Granules	Platelet Dense Granules (Dense Bodies)
Large Molecules	**Small Molecules**
β-Thromboglobulin	Adenosine diphosphate (activates neighboring platelets)
Factor V	Adenosine triphosphate
Factor XI	Calcium
Protein S	Serotonin (vasoconstrictor)
Fibrinogen	
VWF	
Platelet factor 4 (heparin inhibitor)	
Platelet-derived growth factor	

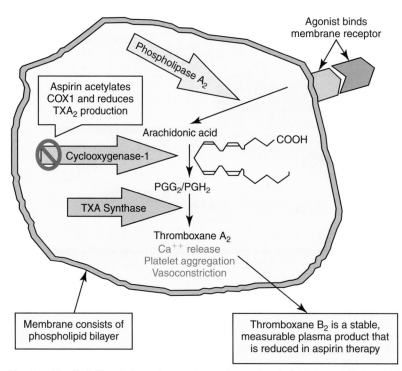

Figure 37-6 Arachidonic acid and aspirin effect. Phospholipase A$_2$ converts membrane phospholipids to arachidonic acid during platelet activation. Arachidonic acid is converted to prostaglandin endoperoxides (PGG$_2$/PGH$_2$) by cyclooxygenase, then to thromboxane A$_2$ (TXA$_2$). TXA$_2$ causes release of Ca^{2+}, which promotes platelet aggregation and vasoconstriction. Aspirin permanently blocks the action of cyclooxygenase-1 and TXA$_2$ synthesis, impairing platelet function.

COAGULATION SYSTEM

Nomenclature of Procoagulants

Plasma transports at least 16 procoagulants, also called *coagulation factors.* Nearly all are glycoproteins synthesized in the liver, although monocytes, ECs, and megakaryocytes produce a few (Table 37-5; Figure 37-7). Eight are enzymes that circulate in an inactive form called *zymogens.* Others are *cofactors* that bind, stabilize, and enhance the activity of their respective enzymes. The sequence of activation is shown in Figure 37-8. During clotting, the procoagulants become activated and produce a localized thrombus. In addition, there are plasma glycoproteins that act as controls to regulate the coagulation process. See subsequent text for more details.

In 1958 the International Committee for the Standardization of the Nomenclature of the Blood Clotting Factors officially named the plasma procoagulants using Roman numerals in the order of their initial description or discovery.[28] When a procoagulant becomes activated, a lowercase *a* appears behind the numeral; for instance, activated factor VII is VIIa. Both zymogens and cofactors become activated in the coagulation process.

We customarily call factor I *fibrinogen* and factor II *prothrombin,* although occasionally they are identified by their numerals. The numeral III was given to *tissue thromboplastin,* a crude mixture of tissue factor and phospholipid. Now that the precise structure of tissue factor has been described, the numeral designation is seldom used. The numeral IV identified the plasma cation calcium (Ca^{2+}); however, calcium is referred to by its name or chemical symbol, not by its numeral. The numeral VI was assigned to a procoagulant that later was determined to be activated factor V; VI was withdrawn from the naming system and never reassigned. Factor VIII, antihemophilic factor, is a cofactor that circulates linked to a large carrier protein, VWF. Prekallikrein (pre-K), also called *Fletcher factor,* and high-molecular-weight kininogen (HMWK), also called *Fitzgerald factor,* have never received Roman numerals because they belong to the kallikrein and kinin systems, respectively, and their primary functions lie within these systems. Platelet phospholipids, particularly phosphatidylserine, are required for the coagulation process but were given no Roman numeral; instead they were once called collectively *platelet factor 3.*

Classification and Function of Procoagulants

The plasma procoagulants may be serine proteases or cofactors, except for factor XIII, which is a transglutaminase (Table 37-6).[29] Serine proteases are proteolytic enzymes of the trypsin family and include the procoagulants thrombin (factor IIa); factors VIIa, IXa, Xa, XIa, and XIIa; and pre-K.[30] Each member has a reactive seryl amino acid residue in its active site and acts on its substrate by hydrolyzing peptide bonds, digesting the primary backbone, and producing smaller polypeptide fragments. Serine proteases are synthesized as inactive zymogens consisting of a single peptide chain. Activation occurs when the zymogen is cleaved at one or more specific sites by the action of another protease during the coagulation process.

The procoagulant cofactors that participate in complex formation are tissue factor, located on membranes of fibroblasts and smooth muscle cells, and soluble plasma factors V, VIII, and HMWK. The remaining components of the coagulation pathway are fibrinogen, factor XIII, phospholipids, calcium, and VWF (Box 37-3). Fibrinogen is the ultimate substrate of the coagulation pathway. When hydrolyzed by thrombin,

TABLE 37-5 Plasma Procoagulants: Function, Molecular Weight, Plasma Half-Life, and Plasma Concentration

Factor	Name	Function	Molecular Weight (Daltons)	Half-Life (Hours)	Mean Plasma Concentration
I*	Fibrinogen	Thrombin substrate, polymerizes to form fibrin	340,000	100–150	200–400 mg/dL
II*	Prothrombin	Serine protease	71,600	60	10 mg/dL
III*	Tissue factor	Cofactor	44,000	Insoluble	None
IV*	Ionic calcium	Mineral	40	NA	8–10 mg/dL
V	Labile factor	Cofactor	330,000	24	1 mg/dL
VII	Stable factor	Serine protease	50,000	6	0.05 mg/dL
VIII	Antihemophilic factor	Cofactor	260,000	12	0.01 mg/dL
VWF	von Willebrand factor	Factor VIII carrier and platelet adhesion	600,000–20,000,000	24	1 mg/dL
IX	Christmas factor	Serine protease	57,000	24	0.3 mg/dL
X	Stuart-Prower factor	Serine protease	58,800	48–52	1 mg/dL
XI	Plasma thromboplastin antecedent (PTA)	Serine protease	143,000	48–84	0.5 mg/dL
XII	Hageman factor	Serine protease	84,000	48–70	3 mg/dL
Prekallikrein	Fletcher factor, pre-K	Serine protease	85,000	35	35–50 µg/mL
High-molecular-weight kininogen	Fitzgerald factor, HMWK	Cofactor	120,000	156	5 mg/dL
XIII	Fibrin-stabilizing factor (FSF)	Transglutaminase, transamidase	320,000	150	2 mg/dL
Platelet factor 3	Phospholipids, phosphatidyl-serine, PF3	Assembly molecule	—	Released by platelets	—

*These factors are customarily identified by name rather than Roman numeral.
From Greenberg DL, Davie EW: The blood coagulation factors: their complementary DNAs, genes, and expression. In Colman RW, Marder VJ, Clowes, AM, et al, editors: *Hemostasis and thrombosis: basic principles and clinical practice,* ed 5, Philadelphia, 2006, Lippincott Williams & Wilkins, pp. 21-58.

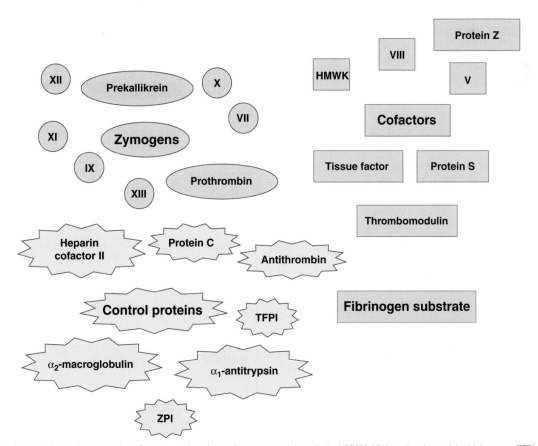

Figure 37-7 Procoagulants (zymogens), cofactors, and anticoagulants (control proteins). *HMWK,* High-molecular-weight kininogen; *TFPI,* tissue factor pathway inhibitor; *ZPI,* protein Z-dependent protease inhibitor.

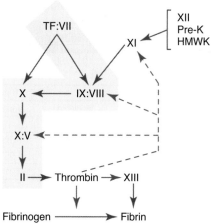

Figure 37-8 Simplified coagulation pathway. Exposed tissue factor (*TF*) activates factor VII, which activates factors IX and X. Factor IXa:VIIIa complex also activates X, and the factor Xa:Va complex activates prothrombin (factor II). The resulting thrombin cleaves fibrinogen to form fibrin and activates factor XIII to stabilize the clot. Thrombin also activates factors V, VIII, XI, and platelets. In vitro exposure to negatively charged surfaces activates the contact factors XII, pre-kallikrein (*pre-K*) and high-molecular-weight kininogen (*HMWK*), which activate factor XI.

TABLE 37-6   Plasma Procoagulant Serine Proteases

Inactive Zymogen	Active Protease	Cofactor	Substrate
Prothrombin (II)	Thrombin (IIa)	—	Fibrinogen, V, VIII, XI, XIII
VII	VIIa	Tissue factor	IX, X
IX	IXa	VIIIa	X
X	Xa	Va	Prothrombin
XI	XIa	—	IX
XII	XIIa	High-molecular-weight kininogen	XI
Prekallikrein	Kallikrein	High-molecular-weight kininogen	XI

BOX 37-3 Other Plasma Procoagulants

Fibrinogen
Factor XIII
Phospholipids
Calcium
VWF

---

fibrinogen forms the primary structural protein of the fibrin clot, which is further stabilized by factor XIII.[31]

Calcium is required for the assembly of coagulation complexes on platelet or cell membrane phospholipids. Serine proteases bind to negatively charged phospholipid surfaces, predominantly phosphatidylserine, through positively charged calcium ions. Activation is a localized cell-surface process, limited to the site of injury and controlled by regulatory mechanisms. If zymogen activation is uncontrolled and generalized, the condition is called *disseminated intravascular coagulation (DIC)*, a serious, often life-threatening condition (Chapter 39).

The molecular weights, plasma concentrations, and plasma half-lives of the procoagulants are given in Table 37-5. These essential pieces of clinical information assist in the interpretation of laboratory tests, monitoring of anticoagulant therapy, and design of effective replacement therapies in deficiency-related hemorrhagic diseases. For example, factor VIII has a short half-life of 12 hours, so replacement therapy for hemophilic individuals who are deficient in factor VIII is administered every 12 hours. For most factors, the level that achieves hemostatic effectiveness is 25% to 30%. This is the minimum level that must be maintained to prevent bleeding in factor-deficient patients. Therapy for a hemophilic patient is designed to maintain the factor level above 30%. A higher level may be desirable, such as in a patient preparing for surgery. The half-life is also important in monitoring anticoagulant therapy, especially warfarin (Coumadin), because even though factor VII becomes reduced in 6 hours, the reduction of prothrombin takes 4 to 5 days. Therefore, the full effect of warfarin is not realized until approximately 5 days after therapy has begun.

Vitamin K–Dependent Prothrombin Group

Prothrombin (factor II), factors VII, IX, and X and the regulatory proteins protein C, protein S, and protein Z are vitamin K–dependent (Table 37-7). These are named the *prothrombin group* because of their structural resemblance to prothrombin. All seven proteins have 10 to 12 glutamic acid units near their amino termini. All except proteins S and Z are serine proteases when activated; S and Z are cofactors.

Vitamin K is a quinone found in green leafy vegetables (Box 37-4) and is produced by the intestinal organisms *Bacteroides*

TABLE 37-7   Vitamin K–Dependent Coagulation Factors

Procoagulants	Regulatory Proteins
Prothrombin (II)	Protein C
VII	Protein S
IX	Protein Z
X	

BOX 37-4 Food Sources High in Vitamin K

Kale
Spinach
Turnip greens
Collards
Mustard greens
Swiss chard
Brussels sprouts
Broccoli
Asparagus
Cabbage
Green onions
Lettuce: Boston, romaine, or Bibb
Avocado
Cauliflower
Parsley, fresh

fragilis and *Escherichia coli*. Vitamin K catalyzes an essential posttranslational modification of the prothrombin group proteins: γ-carboxylation of amino-terminal glutamic acids (Figure 37-9). Glutamic acid is modified to γ-carboxyglutamic acid when a second carboxyl group is added to the γ carbon. With two ionized carboxyl groups, the γ-carboxyglutamic acids gain a net negative charge, which enables them to bind ionic calcium (Ca^{2+}). The bound calcium enables the vitamin K–dependent proteins to bind to negatively charged phospholipids to form coagulation complexes.

In vitamin K deficiency or in the presence of warfarin, a vitamin K antagonist, the vitamin K–dependent procoagulants are released from the liver without the second carboxyl group added to the γ carbon. These are called *des-γ-carboxyl proteins* or *proteins in vitamin K antagonism* (PIVKAs). Because they lack the second carboxyl group, they cannot bind to Ca^{2+} and phospholipid, so they cannot participate in the coagulation reaction. Vitamin K antagonism is the basis for oral anticoagulant (warfarin, Coumadin) therapy (Chapter 43).

Vitamin K–dependent procoagulants are essential for the assembly of three membrane complexes leading to the generation of thrombin (Figure 37-10). Each complex is composed of a vitamin K–dependent serine protease, its non-enzyme cofactor, and Ca^{2+}, bound to the negatively charged phospholipid membranes of activated platelets or tissue factor–bearing cells. The initial complex, extrinsic tenase, is composed of factor

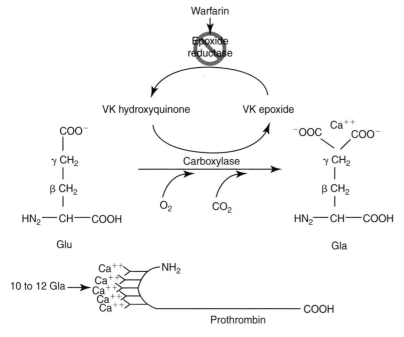

Figure 37-9 Vitamin K (*K*) posttranslational γ-carboxylation of coagulation factors II (prothrombin), VII, IX, and X, and control proteins C, S, and Z. Vitamin K hydroxyquinone transfers a carboxyl (COO^-) group to the γ carbon of glutamic acid (*Glu*), creating γ-carboxyglutamic acid (*Gla*). The negatively charged pocket formed by the two carboxyl groups attracts ionic calcium, which enables the molecule to bind to phosphatidylserine. Vitamin K hydroxyquinone is oxidized to vitamin K epoxide by *carboxylase* in the process of transferring the carboxyl group but is subsequently reduced to the hydroxyquinone form by *epoxide reductase*. Warfarin suppresses *epoxide reductase*, which slows the reaction and prevents γ-carboxylation. "Des-carboxy" proteins are unable to participate in coagulation. There are typically 10 to 12 γ-carboxyglutamic acid molecules near the amino terminus of the vitamin K–dependent factors.

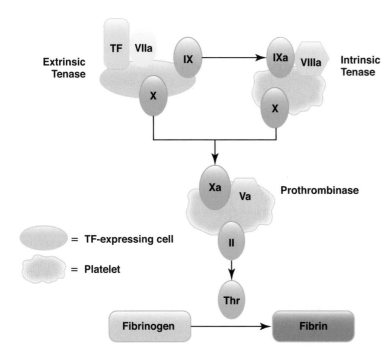

Figure 37-10 Coagulation complexes. Coagulation complexes form on TF-bearing cells (TF:VIIa) and on platelet phospholipid membranes (IXa:VIIIa and Xa:Va). Each complex consists of a vitamin K–dependent serine protease, a cofactor, and Ca^{2+}, bound to the cell membrane. *Extrinsic tenase complex* is factor VIIa and tissue factor (TF) on the membrane of a TF-bearing cell. This complex activates both factors IX and X. *Intrinsic tenase complex*, which is factor IXa and its cofactor VIIIa on platelet membranes, activates factor X also. *Prothrombinase complex* is factor Xa and its cofactor Va, bound to the surface of platelets. Prothrombinase cleaves prothrombin to the active enzyme, thrombin.

TABLE 37-8 Coagulation Complexes

Complex	Components	Activates
Extrinsic tenase	VIIa, tissue factor, phospholipid, and Ca²⁺	IX and X
Intrinsic tenase	IXa, VIIIa, phospholipid, and Ca²⁺	X
Prothrombinase	Xa, Va, phospholipid, and Ca²⁺	Prothrombin

VIIa and tissue factor, and it activates factors IX and X, which are components of the next two complexes, intrinsic tenase and prothrombinase, respectively (Table 37-8). Intrinsic tenase is composed of factor IXa and its cofactor VIIIa; it also activates factor X much more efficiently than the TF:VIIa complex. Prothrombinase is composed of factor Xa and its cofactor Va; this converts prothrombin to thrombin in a multistep hydrolytic process that releases thrombin and a peptide fragment called prothrombin fragment 1.2 (F 1.2). Prothrombin fragment 1.2 in plasma is thus a marker for thrombin generation.

Cofactors in Hemostasis

Procoagulant cofactors are tissue factor, factor V, factor VIII, and HMWK. Coagulation control cofactors are thrombomodulin, protein S, and protein Z (Table 37-9).[32] Thrombomodulin is also a cofactor in control of fibrinolysis. Each cofactor binds its particular serine protease. When bound to their cofactors, serine proteases gain stability and increased reactivity.

Tissue factor is a transmembrane receptor for factor VIIa and is found on extravascular cells such as fibroblasts and smooth muscle cells, but under normal conditions, it is not found on blood vessel ECs.[33] Vessel injury exposes blood to the subendothelial tissue factor–bearing cells and leads to activation of coagulation through VIIa. Tissue factor is expressed in high levels in cells of the brain, lung, placenta, heart, kidney, and testes. In inflammatory conditions and sepsis, leukocytes and other cells can also express tissue factor and initiate coagulation.[34]

Factors V and VIII are soluble plasma proteins. Both are activated by thrombin and inactivated by protein C. Factor V is a glycoprotein circulating in plasma and also present in platelet α-granules. During platelet activation and secretion, platelets release partially activated factor V at the site of injury. Factor Va is a cofactor to Xa in the prothrombinase complex in

TABLE 37-9 Hemostasis Cofactors

Cofactor	Function	Binds
Tissue factor	Procoagulant	VIIa
V	Procoagulant	Xa
VIII	Procoagulant	IXa
High-molecular-weight kininogen	Procoagulant	XIIa, prekallikrein
Thrombomodulin	Control (Protein C)	Thrombin
	Antifibrinolytic (TAFI)	Thrombin
Protein S	Control	Protein C, TFPI
Protein Z	Control	ZPI

coagulation. The prothrombinase complex accelerates thrombin generation more than 300,000-fold compared to Xa alone.[35] As described below, thrombomodulin-bound thrombin activates protein C, which inactivates Va to Vi. Therefore, factor V is both activated and then ultimately inactivated by the generation of thrombin, as is factor VIII. Factor VIII is a cofactor to factor IX, which together form the intrinsic tenase complex, discussed in the next section. High-molecular-weight kininogen is a cofactor to factor XIIa and prekallikrein in the intrinsic contact factor complex, a mechanism for activating coagulation in conditions where foreign objects such as mechanical heart valves or bacterial membranes and/or high levels of inflammation are present.

Thrombomodulin, a transmembrane protein constitutively expressed by vascular ECs, is a thrombin cofactor. Together, thrombomodulin and thrombin activate protein C, a coagulation regulatory protein, and thrombin activatable fibrinolysis inhibitor (TAFI), a fibrinolysis inhibitor. In one of many examples of negative feedback regulation in coagulation, once thrombin is bound to thrombomodulin, it loses its procoagulant ability to activate factors V and VIII, and, through activation of protein C, leads to destruction of factors V and VIII, thus suppressing further generation of thrombin.

Both protein S and protein C are cofactors in the regulation and control of coagulation, discussed later in this chapter. Protein S is a cofactor to protein C, as well as TFPI. Protein Z is a cofactor to Z-dependent protease inhibitor (ZPI).

Factor VIII and Von Willebrand Factor

Factor VIII has a molecular mass of 260,000 Daltons and is produced primarily by hepatocytes, but also by microvascular ECs in lung and other tissues.[36] Free factor VIII is unstable in plasma; it circulates bound to VWF. During coagulation, thrombin cleaves factor VIII from VWF and activates it. Factor VIIIa binds to activated platelets and forms the intrinsic tenase complex with factor IXa and Ca²⁺. Like factor Va, factor VIIIa is also inactivated by protein C.

Factor VIII and factor IX are the two plasma procoagulants whose production is governed by genes carried on the X chromosome. Hemophilia A (factor VIII deficiency) and hemophilia B (factor IX deficiency) are therefore sex-linked disorders occurring almost exclusively in males. Males with hemophilia A have diminished factor VIII activity but normal VWF levels.[37] Factor VIII is a cofactor, but its importance in hemostasis cannot be overstated, as evidenced by the severe bleeding and symptoms associated with hemophilia A.

Factor VIII deteriorates more rapidly than the other coagulation factors in stored blood. In thawed component plasma, the factor VIII level drops to approximately 50% after 5 days.[38] Treatment for hemophilia bleeding episodes consists of replacement therapy transfused according to the 12-hour half-life of factor VIII.

VWF is a large multimeric glycoprotein that participates in platelet adhesion and transports the procoagulant factor VIII. VWF is composed of multiple subunits of 240,000 Daltons each.[39] The subunits are produced by ECs and megakaryocytes, where they combine to form multimers that range from 600,000 to 20,000,000 Daltons.[40] VWF molecules are stored in α-granules in platelets and in Weibel-Palade bodies in ECs. The molecules are released from storage into the plasma, and they circulate at a concentration of 7 to 10 µg/mL. ECs release ultralarge multimers of VWF into plasma, where they are normally degraded into smaller multimers by a VWF-cleaving protease, ADAMTS-13 (*a d*isintegrin *a*nd *m*etalloproteinase with a *t*hrombo*s*pondin type 1 motif, member *13*), in blood vessels with high shear stress. In thrombotic thrombocytopenic purpura (TTP), inherited or acquired defective ADAMTS-13 enzyme activity is associated with the presence of ultralarge VWF multimers in plasma, resulting in platelet aggregation and microvascular thrombosis.[41]

VWF has receptor sites for both platelets and collagen (Figure 37-11) and helps to bind platelets to exposed subendothelial collagen during platelet adhesion, especially in arteries and arterioles where the flow of blood is faster. The primary platelet surface receptor for VWF is GP Ib/IX/V. Arginineglycine-aspartic acid (RGD) sequences in VWF also bind a second platelet integrin, GP IIb/IIIa, during platelet aggregation.

A third site on the VWF molecule binds collagen, and a fourth site binds the plasma procoagulant cofactor, factor VIII. VWF is decreased in von Willebrand disease (VWD), a relatively common disorder that occurs in 1% to 2% of the general population. Because factor VIII depends on VWF for stability, individuals with VWD who have diminished VWF also have diminished factor VIII activity levels. Typically, factor VIII levels decrease to hemorrhagic levels (less than 30%) only in severe VWD. The level of VWF also varies in people according to their ABO blood type. Group O individuals have lower levels of VWF than other ABO types.[42] VWF is an acute phase protein, as is factor VIII, and levels increase in pregnancy, trauma, infections, and stress.

Factor XI and the Contact Factors

The "contact factors," also called intrinsic accessory pathway proteins, are factor XII, high-molecular-weight kininogen (HMWK, Fitzgerald factor), and prekallikrein (pre-K, Fletcher factor). They are so named because they are activated by contact with negatively charged foreign surfaces. Factor XIIa transforms pre-K, a glycoprotein that circulates bound to HMWK, into its active form kallikrein, which cleaves HMWK to form bradykinin.

Factor XII and pre-K are zymogens that are activated to become serine proteases; HMWK is a nonenzymatic cofactor.

The contact factor complex (HMWK:pre-K:FXII) activates factor XI; factor XIa is an activator of factor IX (Figure 37-8). Deficiencies of factor XII, HMWK, or pre-K do not cause clinical bleeding disorders. However, deficiencies do prolong laboratory tests and necessitate investigation. Factor XII is activated in vitro by negatively charged surfaces such as nonsiliconized glass, kaolin, or ellagic acid in partial thromboplastin time (PTT) reagents. In vivo, foreign materials such as stents or valve prostheses may activate contact factors to cause thrombosis.

Factor XI is activated by the contact factor complex and, more significantly, by thrombin during coagulation generated from tissue factor activation. Factor XIa activates factor IX, and the reaction proceeds as described previously. Deficiencies of factor XI (Rosenthal syndrome) usually result in mild and variable bleeding.[43] Factor XI supplements or boosts factor IX activation, so deficiencies of factor XI are less severe clinically than deficiencies of the other factors such as IX or VIII.

Thrombin

The primary function of thrombin is to cleave fibrinopeptides A and B from the α and β chains of the fibrinogen molecule, triggering spontaneous fibrin polymerization (Figure 37-12). In addition, thrombin amplifies the coagulation mechanism by activating cofactors V and VIII and factor XI by a positive feedback mechanism (Figure 37-8). Thrombin also activates factor XIII, which forms covalent bonds between the D domains of the fibrin polymer to cross-link and stabilize the fibrin clot. Thrombin also initiates aggregation of platelets. Thrombin bound to thrombomodulin activates the protein C pathway to suppress coagulation, and it activates TAFI to suppress fibrinolysis. Thrombin, therefore, plays a role in coagulation (fibrin), in platelet activation, in coagulation control (protein C), and in controlling fibrinolysis (TAFI). Because of its multiple autocatalytic functions, thrombin is considered the key protease of the coagulation pathway.

Fibrinogen Structure and Fibrin Formation, Factor XIII

Fibrinogen is the primary substrate of thrombin, which converts soluble fibrinogen to insoluble fibrin to produce a clot. Fibrinogen is also essential for platelet aggregation because it links activated platelets through their GP IIb/IIIa platelet fibrinogen receptor. Fibrinogen is a 340,000 Dalton glycoprotein synthesized in the liver. The normal plasma concentration of fibrinogen ranges from 200 to 400 mg/dL, the most concentrated of all the plasma procoagulants. Fibrinogen is an acute phase reactant protein, whose level increases in inflammation, infection, and other stress conditions. Platelet α-granules absorb, transport, and release abundant fibrinogen.[44]

The fibrinogen molecule is a mirror-image "trinodular" dimer, each half consisting of three nonidentical polypeptides, designated Aα, Bβ, and γ, united by disulfide bonds (Figure 37-13). The six N-terminals assemble to form a bulky central region called the E domain. The carboxyl terminals assemble at the outer ends of the molecule to form two D domains.[45]

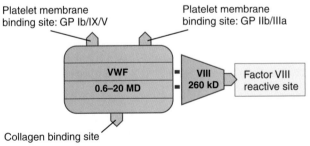

Figure 37-11 Von Willebrand factor (*VWF*)–factor VIII complex. Factor VIII circulates covalently bound to VWF. VWF provides three other active receptor sites: VWF binds to collagen and binds to glycoprotein Ib/IX/V to support platelet adhesion and binds to glycoprotein IIb/IIIa to facilitate platelet aggregation.

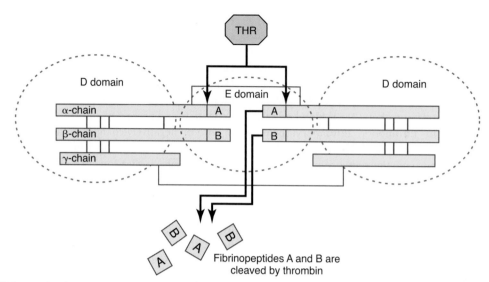

Figure 37-12 Fibrinogen domains and cleavage by thrombin. Each molecule of fibrinogen or fibrin has three "domains": two D domains (the carboxyl ends of the molecule) and one E domain (the central portion of the molecule), as shown in this diagram. Thrombin (*THR*) cleaves fibrinopeptides A and B from the alpha and beta chains in the E domain.

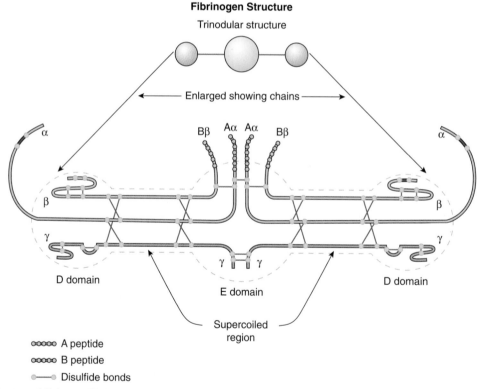

Figure 37-13 Structure of fibrinogen. Fibrinogen is a trinodular structure composed of three pairs (Aα, Bβ, and γ) of disulfide-bonded polypeptide chains. The central node is known as the *E domain*. Thrombin cleaves small peptides, A and B, from the α and β chains in this region to form fibrin. The central nodule is joined by supercoiled α-helices to the terminal nodules known as the *D domains*. (From McKenzie SB, Williams JL: *Clinical laboratory hematology*, ed 2, Upper Saddle River, NJ, 2009, Pearson, p 653.)

Thrombin cleaves fibrinopeptides A and B from the protruding N-termini of each of the two α and β chains of fibrinogen, reducing the overall molecular weight by 10,000 Daltons. The cleaved fibrinogen is called *fibrin monomer*. The exposed fibrin monomer α and β chain ends (E domain) have an immediate affinity for portions of the D domain of neighboring

monomers, spontaneously polymerizing to form *fibrin polymer* (Figure 37-14).

Thrombin also activates factor XIII, a heterodimer whose α subunit is produced mostly by megakaryocytes and monocytes, and whose β subunit is produced in the liver.[46] Factor XIIIa covalently crosslinks fibrin polymers to form a stable

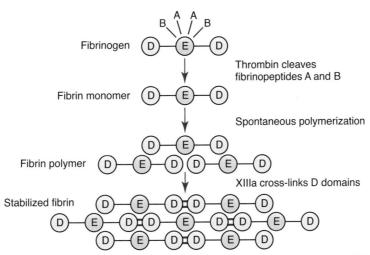

Figure 37-14 Formation of a stabilized fibrin clot. Thrombin cleaves fibrinopeptides A and B to form fibrin monomer. Fibrin monomers polymerize due to the affinity of thrombin-cleaved positively charged E domains for negatively charged D domains of other monomers. Factor XIIIa catalyzes the covalent cross-linking of γ chains of adjacent D domains to form an insoluble stable fibrin clot.

insoluble fibrin clot. Factor XIIIa is a transglutaminase that catalyzes the formation of covalent bonds between the carboxyl terminals of γ chains from adjacent D domains in the fibrin polymer. These bonds link the ε-amino acid of lysine moieties and the γ-amide group of glutamine units. Multiple cross-links form to provide an insoluble meshwork of fibrin polymers linked by their D domains, providing physical strength to the fibrin clot. Factor XIIIa reacts with other plasma and cellular structural proteins and is essential to wound healing and tissue integrity. Cross-linking of fibrin polymers by factor XIIIa covalently incorporates fibronectin, a plasma protein involved in cell adhesion, and α$_2$-antiplasmin, rendering the fibrin mesh resistant to fibrinolysis. Plasminogen, the primary serine protease of the fibrinolytic system, also becomes covalently bound via lysine moieties, as does TPA, a serine protease that ultimately hydrolyzes and activates bound plasminogen to initiate fibrinolysis.

Plasma-Based (In Vitro) Coagulation: Extrinsic, Intrinsic, and Common Pathways

In the past, two coagulation pathways were described, both of which activated factor X at the start of a common pathway leading to thrombin generation (Figure 37-15). The pathways were characterized as cascades in that as one enzyme became activated, it in turn activated the next enzyme in sequence. Most coagulation experts identified the activation of factor XII as the primary step in coagulation because this factor could be found in blood, whereas tissue factor could not. Consequently, the reaction system that begins with factor XII and culminates in fibrin polymerization has been called the *intrinsic pathway*. The coagulation factors of the intrinsic pathway, in order of reaction, are XII, pre-K, HMWK, XI, IX, VIII, X, V, prothrombin (II), and fibrinogen. The laboratory test that detects the absence of one or more of these factors is the activated partial thromboplastin time (APTT or PTT; Chapter 42). We now know that the contact factors XII, pre-K, and HMWK do not play a significant role in in vivo coagulation with trauma-type

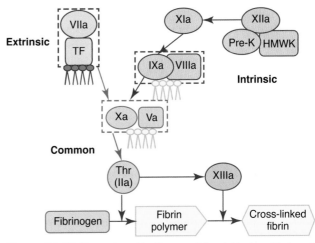

Figure 37-15 Plasma-based in vitro coagulation: intrinsic, extrinsic, and common pathways. In the intrinsic pathway, the contact factors XII, prekallikrein (*pre-K*), and high-molecular-weight kininogen (*HMWK*) are activated and proceed to activate factors XI, IX, VIII, X, and V and prothrombin, which converts fibrinogen to fibrin. In the extrinsic pathway, exposed tissue factor (*TF*) on subendothelial cells activates factor VII, which activates factors X, V, and prothrombin, cleaving fibrinogen to fibrin. Both the intrinsic and extrinsic pathways converge with the activation of factor X, so factors X, V, prothrombin, and fibrinogen are called the common pathway.

injuries, although their deficiencies prolong the in vitro laboratory tests of the intrinsic pathway, in particular, the PTT.

Formation of TF:VIIa has since proven to be the primary in vivo initiation mechanism for coagulation. Because tissue factor is not present in blood, the tissue factor pathway has been called the *extrinsic pathway*. This pathway includes the factors VII, X, V, prothrombin, and fibrinogen. The test used to measure the integrity of the extrinsic pathway is the prothrombin time test (PT; Chapter 42).

The PT and PTT are assays often used in tandem to screen for coagulation factor deficiencies. Factor VIII and factor IX are not considered to be part of the extrinsic pathway, because the PT fails to identify their absence or deficiency. But clearly, the IXa:VIIIa complex in the intrinsic pathway is crucial to the activation of factor X. Deficiencies of either one of these components—factor VIII in hemophilia A, or factor IX in hemophilia B—can result in severe and life-threatening hemorrhage.

The two pathways have in common factor X, factor V, prothrombin, and fibrinogen; this portion of the coagulation pathway is often called the *common pathway*. These designations—intrinsic, extrinsic, and common—are used extensively to interpret in vitro laboratory testing and to identify factor deficiencies; however, they do not adequately describe the complex interdependent reactions that occur in vivo.

Cell-Based (In Vivo, Physiologic) Coagulation

An intricate combination of cellular and biochemical events function in harmony to keep blood liquid within the veins and arteries, to prevent blood loss from injuries by the formation of thrombi, and to reestablish blood flow during the healing process.[47] As noted above, the series of cascading proteolytic reactions traditionally known as the *extrinsic* and *intrinsic coagulation pathways* do not fully describe how coagulation occurs in vivo. These pathways are not distinct, independent, alternative mechanisms for generating thrombin but are actually interdependent. For example, a deficiency of factor VII in the extrinsic pathway can cause significant bleeding, even when the intrinsic pathway is intact. Similarly, deficiencies of factors VIII and IX may cause severe bleeding, regardless of the presence of a normal extrinsic pathway.[48]

In addition to procoagulant and anticoagulant plasma proteins, normal physiologic coagulation requires the presence of two cell types for formation of coagulation complexes: cells that express tissue factor (usually extravascular) and platelets (intravascular) (Figure 37-16).[49] Operationally, coagulation can be described as occurring in two phases: initiation, which occurs on tissue factor–expressing cells and produces 3% to 5% of the total thrombin generated, and propagation,

occurring on platelets, which produces 95% or more of the total thrombin.[50]

Initiation

In vivo, the principle mechanism for generating thrombin is begun by formation of the extrinsic tenase complex, rather than the intrinsic pathway. The initiation phase refers to extrinsic tenase complex formation and generation of small amounts of factor Xa, factor IXa, and thrombin (Figure 37-16).

Damage to the endothelium spills blood and platelets into the extravascular tissue and triggers a localized response. The magnitude of the response depends largely on the extent of the injury: how large the bleed is, how much tissue is damaged, and how many platelets are available.

About 1% to 2% of factor VIIa is present normally in blood in the activated form, but it is inert until bound to tissue factor[51] and is unaffected by TFPI and other inhibitors. Fibroblasts and other subendothelial cells provide tissue factor, a cofactor to factor VIIa. Factor VIIa binds to tissue factor on the membrane of subendothelial cells, and the extrinsic tenase complex TF:VIIa is formed.

TF:VIIa activates low levels of both factor IX and factor X. Minute amounts of thrombin are generated by membrane-bound Xa and Xa:Va prothrombinase complexes. Factor Va comes from the activation of plasma factor V by thrombin, by platelets if there has been an injury, or by noncoagulation proteases.[52]

Coagulation complexes bound to cell membranes are relatively protected from inactivation by most inhibitors. However, if Xa:Va dissociates from the cell, it is rapidly inactivated by the protease inhibitors TFPI, antithrombin, and protein Z–dependent protease inhibitor (ZPI) until a threshold of Xa:Va activity is reached.

Even though the amount of thrombin generated in this phase is minute, platelets, cofactors, and procoagulants become activated; fibrin formation begins; and the initial platelet

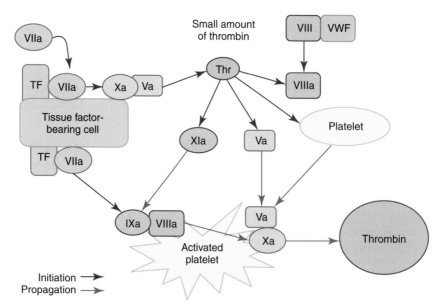

Figure 37-16 Cell-based in vivo physiologic coagulation. VIIa binds to tissue factor (*TF*) and activates both factors X and IX. Cell-bound factor Xa combines with Va and generates a small amount of thrombin (Thr), which activates platelets, V, VIII, and XI and begins fibrin formation. Factor IXa, activated by both TF:VIIa and XIa, combines with factor VIIIa on the platelet surface to activate X, which forms prothrombinase (Xa:Va) and produces a burst of thrombin.

plug is formed. The low level of thrombin generated in the initiation phase (1) activates platelets through cleavage of protease activated receptors PAR-1 and PAR-4; (2) activates factor V released from platelet α-granules; (3) activates factor VIII and dissociates it from VWF; (4) activates factor XI, the intrinsic accessory procoagulant that activates more factor IX; and (5) splits fibrinogen peptides A and B from fibrinogen and forms a preliminary fibrin network.

Cleavage of fibrinopeptides occurs at the end of the initiation phase and beginning of the propagation phase. In most clot-based coagulation assays, this is the visual endpoint of the assay.[45] It occurs with only 10 to 30 nmol/L of thrombin, or approximately 3% of the total thrombin generated.

Propagation

More than 95% of thrombin generation occurs during propagation. In this phase the reactions occur on the surface of the activated platelet, which now has all the components needed for coagulation. Large numbers of platelets adhere to the site of injury, localizing the coagulation response. Platelets are activated at the site of injury by both the low-level thrombin generated in the initiation phase and by adhering to exposed collagen (Figure 37-16). They are sometimes referred to as COAT-platelets: platelets partially activated by *co*llagen *a*nd *t*hrombin.[53]

These partially activated COAT-platelets have a higher level of procoagulant activity than platelets exposed to collagen alone. They also provide a surface for formation and amplification of intrinsic tenase and prothrombinase complexes.

The cofactors Va and VIIIa activated by thrombin in the initiation phase bind to platelet membranes and become receptors for Xa and IXa. IXa generated in the initiation phase binds to VIIIa on the platelet membrane to form the intrinsic tenase complex IXa:VIIIa. More factor IXa is also generated by platelet-bound factor XIa. This intrinsic tenase complex activates factor X at a 50- to 100-fold higher rate than the extrinsic tenase complex.[49] Factor Xa binds to Va to form the prothrombinase complex, which activates prothrombin and generates a burst of thrombin. Thrombin cleaves fibrinogen into a fibrin clot, activates factor XIII to stabilize the clot, binds to thrombomodulin to activate the protein C control pathway, and activates TAFI to inhibit fibrinolysis.

Since coagulation depends on the presence of both tissue factor–bearing cells and activated platelets, clotting is localized to the site of injury. Protease inhibitors and intact endothelium prevent clotting from spreading to other parts of the body.

It may be helpful operationally to think of the extrinsic or tissue factor pathway as occurring on the tissue factor–bearing cell and the intrinsic pathway (minus factors XII, HMWK, and pre-K) as occurring on the platelet surface. However, these are not separate and redundant pathways; they are interdependent and occur in parallel until blood flow has ceased and termination by control mechanisms takes place.

Both platelets and tissue factor–bearing cells are essential for physiologic coagulation. Deficiencies of any of the key proteins of coagulation complex formation and activity (VII, IX, VIII, X, V, or prothrombin) compromise thrombin generation and manifest as significant bleeding disorders.

COAGULATION REGULATORY MECHANISMS

Inhibitors and their cofactors regulate serine proteases and cofactors in the coagulation system. They also provide feedback loops to maintain a complex and delicate balance between thrombosis and abnormal bleeding. These inhibitors, or natural anticoagulants, function to slow the activation of procoagulants and suppress thrombin production. They ensure that coagulation is localized and is not a systemic response, and they prevent excessive clotting or thrombosis. The principal regulators are TFPI, antithrombin (AT), and activated protein C, the endpoint of the protein C pathway. Acquired or inherited deficiencies of these proteins may be associated with increased incidence of venous thromboembolic disease, as the hemostatic balance is shifted more toward coagulation than termination of the activated pathway. Figure 37-17 illustrates coagulation mechanism regulatory points. Characteristics of these and other coagulation regulatory proteins are summarized in Table 37-10.

Tissue Factor Pathway Inhibitor

TFPI is a Kunitz-type serine protease inhibitor and is the principal regulator of the tissue factor pathway. The Kunitz-2 domain binds to and inhibits factor Xa, and Kunitz-1 binds to and inhibits VIIa:TF.[54] TFPI is synthesized primarily by ECs and is also expressed on platelets. In the initiation of coagulation, factor VIIa and tissue factor combine to activate factors IX and X. TFPI inhibits coagulation in a two-step process by first binding and inactivating Xa. The TFPI:Xa complex then binds to TF:VIIa, forming a quaternary complex and preventing further activation of X and IX (Figure 37-18).[55,56] Alternatively, TFPI may bind to Xa in the TF:VIIa:Xa complex and inactivate Xa and TF:VIIa. TFPI provides feedback inhibition, because it is not actively engaged until coagulation is initiated and factor X is activated. Protein S, the cofactor of activated protein C

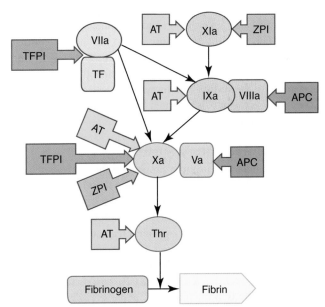

Figure 37-17 Coagulation pathway showing regulatory points. *TFPI*, Tissue factor pathway inhibitor; *AT*, antithrombin; *APC*, activated protein C; *ZPI*, protein Z–dependent protease inhibitor.

TABLE 37-10 Coagulation Regulatory Proteins

Name	Function	Molecular Mass (Daltons)	Half-Life (Hours)	Mean Plasma Concentration
Tissue factor pathway inhibitor	With Xa, binds TF:VIIa	33,000	Unknown	60–80 ng/mL
Thrombomodulin	EC surface receptor for thrombin	450,000	Does not circulate	None
Protein C	Serine protease	62,000	7–9	2–6 μg/mL
Protein S	Cofactor	75,000	Unknown	20–25 μg/mL
Antithrombin	Serpin	58,000	68	24–40 mg/dL
Heparin cofactor II	Serpin	65,000	60	30–70 μg/mL
Z-dependent protease inhibitor	Serpin	72,000	Unknown	1.5 μg/mL
α_1-Protease inhibitor (α_1-antitrypsin)	Serpin	60,000	Unknown	250 mg/dL
α_2-Macroglobulin	Serpin	725,000	60	150–400 mg/dL

Serpin, Serine protease inhibitor; *EC,* endothelial cell.

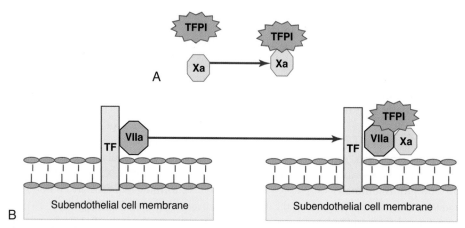

Figure 37-18 Tissue factor pathway inhibitor. *TFPI* binds the complex of tissue factor (*TF*) and factors VIIa and Xa in a Xa-dependent feedback mechanism. **A,** TFPI first binds to factor Xa and inactivates it. **B,** The TFPI:Xa complex then binds and inactivates TF:VIIa, preventing more activation of Xa. Alternatively, TFPI may bind directly to Xa and VIIa in the TF:VIIa:Xa complex.

(APC), is also a cofactor of TFPI and enhances factor Xa inhibition by TFPI tenfold.[57-59] Because of the inhibitory action of TFPI, the TF:VIIa:Xa reaction is short-lived. Once TFPI shuts down extrinsic tenase and Xa, additional Xa and IXa production shifts to the intrinsic pathway.[60] Propagation of coagulation occurs as factor X is activated by IXa:VIII and more factor IX is activated by factor XIa.

Protein C Regulatory System

During coagulation, thrombin propagates the clot as it cleaves fibrinogen and activates factors V, VIII, XI, and XIII. In intact normal vessels, where coagulation would be inappropriate, thrombin avidly binds the EC membrane protein *thrombomodulin* and triggers an essential coagulation regulatory system called the *protein C anticoagulant system.*[61] The protein C system revises thrombin's function from a procoagulant enzyme to an anticoagulant. EC protein C receptor (EPCR) is a transmembrane protein that binds both protein C and APC adjacent to the thrombomodulin-thrombin complex and augments the action of thrombin-thrombomodulin at least fivefold in activating protein C to a serine protease (Figure 37-19).[62,63] APC dissociates

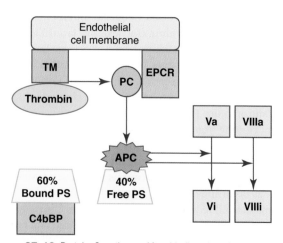

Figure 37-19 Protein C pathway. After binding thrombomodulin (*TM*), thrombin activates protein C (*PC*), bound by endothelial cell protein C receptor (*EPCR*). Free protein S (*PS*) [not bound to C4b binding protein (*C4bBP*)] binds and stabilizes activated protein C (*APC*). The APC/protein S complex digests and inactivates factors Va (Vi, inhibited factor V) and VIIIa (VIIIi, inhibited factor VIII).

from EPCR and binds its cofactor, free plasma protein S. The stabilized APC-protein S complex hydrolyzes and inactivates factors Va and VIIIa, slowing or blocking thrombin generation/coagulation.

Protein S, the cofactor that binds and stabilizes APC, is synthesized in the liver and circulates in the plasma in two forms. About 40% of protein S is free, but 60% is covalently bound to the complement control protein C4b-binding protein (C4bBP).[64] Bound protein S cannot participate in the protein C anticoagulant pathway; only free plasma protein S can serve as the APC cofactor. Protein S-C4bBP binding is of particular interest in inflammatory conditions because C4bBP is an acute phase reactant. When the plasma C4bBP level increases, additional protein S is bound, and free protein S levels become proportionally decreased, which may increase the risk of thrombosis. Chronic acquired or inherited protein C or protein S deficiency or mutations of protein C, protein S, or factor V compromise the normal downregulation of factors Va and VIIIa and may be associated with recurrent venous thromboembolic disease (Chapter 39). Underscoring the importance of the protein C regulatory system, neonates who completely lack protein C have a massive thrombotic condition called *purpura fulminans* and die in infancy unless treated with protein C replacement and anticoagulation.[65,66]

Antithrombin and Other Serine Protease Inhibitors (Serpins)

Antithrombin (AT) was the first of the coagulation regulatory proteins to be identified and the first to be assayed routinely in the clinical hemostasis laboratory.[67] Other members of the serpin family include heparin cofactor II, protein Z-dependent protease inhibitor (ZPI), protein C inhibitor, α_1-protease inhibitor (α_1-antitrypsin), α_2-macroglobulin, α_2-antiplasmin, and PAI-1.[68]

AT is a serine protease inhibitor (serpin) that binds and neutralizes serine proteases, including thrombin (factor IIa) and factors IXa, Xa, XIa, XIIa, prekallikrein, and plasmin.[69] Heparin cofactor II is a serpin that primarily inactivates thrombin. AT and heparin cofactor II both require heparin for effective anticoagulant activity. In vivo, heparin is available from endothelium-associated mast cell granules or as EC heparan sulfate, a natural glycosaminoglycan that activates AT, although not to the same intensity as therapeutic unfractionated heparin. AT's activity is accelerated 2000-fold by binding to heparin and is the basis for the anticoagulant activity of pharmaceutical heparin. Therapeutically, heparin is administered as unfractionated heparin, low-molecular-weight heparin, or heparin pentasaccharide. Unfractionated heparin consists of chains of greater than 18 sugar units and accelerates inactivation of thrombin through heparin-dependent conformational changes and bridging mechanisms (Figure 37-20). With low-molecular-weight and pentasaccharide heparins lacking long polysaccharide chains for thrombin inactivation, AT preferentially inactivates factor Xa (Chapter 43).

In vivo, antithrombin covalently binds thrombin, forming an inactive thrombin-antithrombin complex (TAT), which is then released from the heparin molecule. Laboratory measurement of TAT is used as an indicator for thrombosis, since it measures both the generation of thrombin and its inhibition.

ZPI, in the presence of its cofactor, protein Z, is a potent inhibitor of factor Xa.[70,71] ZPI covalently binds protein Z and factor Xa in a complex with Ca^{2+} and phospholipid. Protein Z is a vitamin K–dependent plasma glycoprotein that is synthesized in the liver. Although protein Z has a structure similar to that of the other vitamin K–dependent proteins (factors II, VII, IX, and X and protein C), it lacks an activation site and, like protein S, is nonproteolytic. Protein Z increases the ability of

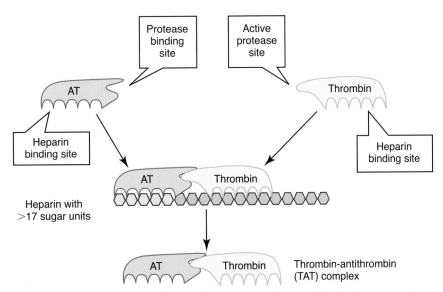

Figure 37-20 Unfractionated heparin potentiates antithrombin-thrombin reaction. Antithrombin (*AT*) attaches to a specific pentasaccharide sequence in unfractionated heparin. The thrombin binding site for heparin is adjacent to the AT site. The AT is sterically modified to covalently bind and inactivate the thrombin active protease site. Thrombin and AT, covalently bound, release from heparin and form measurable plasma thrombin-antithrombin (*TAT*) complexes, useful as a marker of coagulation activation.

ZPI to inhibit factor Xa 2000-fold.[72] ZPI also inhibits factor XIa, in a separate reaction that does not require protein Z, phospholipid, and Ca^{2+}. The inhibition of factor XIa is accelerated twofold by the presence of heparin.

Protein C inhibitor is a nonspecific, heparin-binding serpin that inhibits a variety of proteases, including APC, thrombin, factor Xa, factor XIa, and urokinase. It is found not only in plasma but also in many other body fluids and organs. Depending on its target, it can function as an anticoagulant (inhibits thrombin), as a procoagulant (inhibits thrombin-thrombomodulin and APC), or as a fibrinolytic inhibitor.

The serpins α_1-protease inhibitor and α_2-macroglobulin are able to inhibit serine proteases reversibly. See Table 37-11 and the section on fibrinolysis for further information on α_2-antiplasmin and PAI-1.

FIBRINOLYSIS

Fibrinolysis, the final stage of coagulation (Figure 37-21), begins a few hours after fibrin polymerization and cross-linking. Two activators of fibrinolysis, TPA and UPA, are released in response to inflammation and coagulation. Fibrinolytic proteins assemble on fibrin during clotting. Plasminogen, plasmin, TPA, UPA, and PAI-1 become incorporated into the fibrin clot as they bind to lysine through their "kringle" loops, thereby concentrating and localizing them to the fibrin clot. Fibrinolysis is the systematic, accelerating hydrolysis of fibrin by bound plasmin. TPA and UPA activate fibrin-bound plasminogen several hours after thrombus formation, degrading fibrin and restoring normal blood flow during vascular repair. Again, there is a delicate balance between activators and inhibitors. Excessive fibrinolysis can cause bleeding due to

TABLE 37-11   Proteins of the Fibrinolysis Pathway

Name	Function	Molecular Mass (Daltons)	Half-Life	Mean Plasma Concentration
Plasminogen	Plasma serine protease, plasmin digests fibrin/fibrinogen	92,000	24–26 hr	15–21 mg/dL
Tissue plasminogen activator	Serine protease secreted by activated endothelium, activates plasminogen	68,000	Unknown	4–7 μg/dL
Urokinase	Serine protease secreted by kidney, activates plasminogen	54,000	Unknown	—
Plasminogen activator inhibitor-1	Secreted by endothelium, inhibits tissue plasminogen activator	52,000	1 hr	14–28 mg/dL
α_2-Antiplasmin	Inhibits plasmin	51,000	Unknown	7 mg/dL
Thrombin-activatable fibrinolysis inhibitor	Suppresses fibrinolysis by removing fibrin C-terminal lysine binding sites	55,000	8–10 min	5 μg/mL

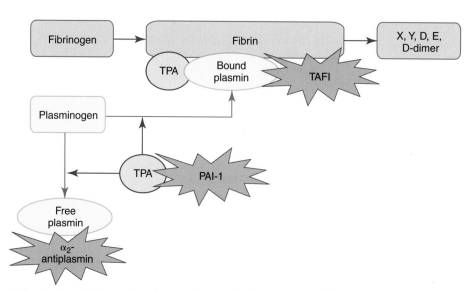

Figure 37-21 Fibrinolysis pathway and inhibitors. Plasminogen and tissue plasminogen activator (*TPA*) are bound to fibrin during coagulation. TPA converts bound plasminogen to plasmin, which slowly digests fibrin to form fibrin degradation products (FDPs) X, Y, D, E, and D-D (D-dimer). D-dimer is produced from cross-linked fibrin. Free plasmin is neutralized by α_2-antiplasmin. TPA is neutralized by plasminogen activator inhibitor-1 (*PAI-1*). Thrombin-activatable fibrinolysis inhibitor (*TAFI*) inhibits fibrinolysis by cleaving lysine residues on fibrin, preventing the binding of plasminogen, plasmin, and TPA.

premature clot lysis before wound healing is established, whereas inadequate fibrinolysis can lead to clot extension and thrombosis.

Plasminogen and Plasmin

Plasminogen is a 92,000 Dalton plasma zymogen produced by the liver (Table 37-11).[73,74] It is a single-chain protein possessing five glycosylated loops termed *kringles*. Kringles enable plasminogen, along with activators TPA and UPA, to bind fibrin lysine molecules during polymerization (Figure 37-22). This fibrin-binding step is essential to fibrinolysis. Fibrin-bound plasminogen becomes converted into a two-chain active plasmin molecule when cleaved between arginine at position 561 and valine at position 562 by neighboring fibrin-bound TPA or UPA. Plasmin is a serine protease that systematically digests fibrin polymer by the hydrolysis of arginine-related and lysine-related peptide bonds.[75] Bound plasmin digests clots and restores blood vessel patency. Its localization to fibrin through lysine binding prevents systemic activity. As fibrin becomes digested, the exposed carboxy-terminal lysine residues bind additional plasminogen and TPA, which further accelerates clot digestion.[76,77] Free plasmin is capable of digesting plasma fibrinogen, factor V, factor VIII, and fibronectin, causing a potentially fatal primary fibrinolysis. However, plasma α_2-antiplasmin rapidly binds and inactivates any free plasmin in the circulation.

Plasminogen Activation

Tissue Plasminogen Activator (TPA)

ECs secrete TPA, which hydrolyzes fibrin-bound plasminogen and initiates fibrinolysis. TPA, with two glycosylated kringle regions, forms covalent lysine bonds with fibrin during polymerization and localizes at the surface of the thrombus with plasminogen, where it begins the digestion process by converting plasminogen to plasmin. Circulating TPA is bound to inhibitors such as PAI-1 and is cleared from plasma. Synthetic recombinant TPAs mimic intrinsic TPA and are a family of drugs used to dissolve pathologic clots that form in venous and arterial thrombotic disease.

Urokinase Plasminogen Activator (UPA)

Urinary tract epithelial cells, monocytes, and macrophages secrete another intrinsic plasminogen activator called *urokinase plasminogen activator*. UPA circulates in plasma at a concentration of 2 to 4 ng/mL and becomes incorporated into the mix of fibrin-bound plasminogen and TPA at the time of thrombus formation. UPA has only one kringle region, does not bind firmly to fibrin, and has a relatively minor physiologic effect. Like TPA, purified UPA preparations are used to dissolve thrombi in myocardial infarction, stroke, and deep vein thrombosis.

Control of Fibrinolysis

Plasminogen Activator Inhibitor 1 (PAI-1)

PAI-1 is the principal inhibitor of plasminogen activation, inactivating both TPA and UPA and thus preventing them from converting plasminogen to the fibrinolytic enzyme plasmin.

PAI-1 is a single-chain glycoprotein serine protease inhibitor and is produced by ECs, megakaryocytes, smooth muscle cells, fibroblasts, monocytes, adipocytes, hepatocytes, and other cell types.[78,79] Platelets store a pool of PAI-1, accounting for more than half of its availability and for its delivery to the fibrin clot. PAI-1 is present in excess of the TPA concentration in plasma, and circulating TPA normally becomes bound to PAI-1. Only at times of EC activation, such as after trauma, does the level of TPA secretion exceed that of PAI-1 to initiate fibrinolysis. Binding of TPA to fibrin protects TPA from PAI-1 inhibition.[80] Plasma PAI-1 levels vary widely. PAI-1 deficiency has been associated with chronic mild bleeding due to increased fibrinolysis. PAI-1 is an acute phase reactant and is increased in many conditions, including metabolic syndrome, obesity, atherosclerosis, sepsis, and stroke.[79] Increased PAI-1 levels correlate with reduced fibrinolytic activity and increased risk of thrombosis.

α_2-Antiplasmin

α_2-Antiplasmin (AP) is synthesized in the liver and is the primary inhibitor of free plasmin. AP is a serine protease inhibitor with the unique characteristic of both N- and C-terminal extensions.[81] During thrombus formation, the N-terminus of AP is covalently linked to fibrin by factor XIIIa (Figure 37-22).[82] The C-terminal contains lysine, which is capable of reacting with the lysine-binding kringles of plasmin. Free plasmin produced by activation of plasminogen can bind either to fibrin, where it is protected from AP because its lysine-binding site is occupied, or to the C-terminus of AP, which rapidly and irreversibly inactivates it. Thus AP with its C-terminal lysine slows fibrinolysis by competing with lysine residues in fibrin for plasminogen binding and by binding directly to plasmin and inactivating it.

The therapeutic lysine analogues, tranexamic acid and ϵ-aminocaproic acid, are similarly antifibrinolytic through their affinity for kringles in plasminogen and TPA. Both inhibit the proteolytic activity of plasmin.

Thrombin-Activatable Fibrinolysis Inhibitor

TAFI is a plasma procarboxypeptidase synthesized in the liver that becomes activated by the thrombin-thrombomodulin complex. This is the same complex that activates the protein C pathway; however, the two functions are independent. Activated TAFI functions as an antifibrinolytic enzyme. It inhibits fibrinolysis by cleaving exposed carboxy-terminal lysine residues from partially degraded fibrin, thereby preventing the binding of TPA and plasminogen to fibrin and blocking the formation of plasmin (Figure 37-22).[83] In coagulation factor–deficient states, such as hemophilia, decreased thrombin production may reduce the activation of TAFI, resulting in increased fibrinolysis that contributes to more bleeding. Conversely, in thrombotic disorders, increased thrombin generation may increase the activation of TAFI. The resulting decreased fibrinolysis may contribute further to thrombosis. TAFI also may play a role in regulating inflammation and wound healing.[84]

Fibrin Degradation Products and D-Dimer

Plasmin cleaves fibrin and produces a series of identifiable fibrin fragments: X, Y, D, E, and D-D (Figure 37-23).[85] Several

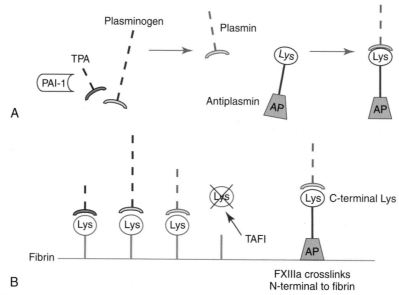

Figure 37-22 Schematic diagram of the action of fibrinolytic proteins. **A,** Tissue plasminogen activator (*TPA*) activates plasminogen to the serine protease, plasmin. TPA is inhibited by plasminogen activator inhibitor-1 (*PAI-1*). α_2-Antiplasmin (*AP*) rapidly inactivates free plasmin. **B,** Fibrinolytic proteins TPA, plasminogen, and plasmin bind to fibrin C-terminal lysine (*Lys*) during clotting. Thrombin activatable fibrinolysis inhibitor (*TAFI*) inhibits fibrinolysis by removing the C-terminal Lys from fibrin, thereby reducing binding of fibrinolytic proteins. AP N-terminus is bound to fibrin by FXIIIa. The AP C-terminus Lys competes with fibrin C-terminus Lys to bind plasmin and inactivates it.

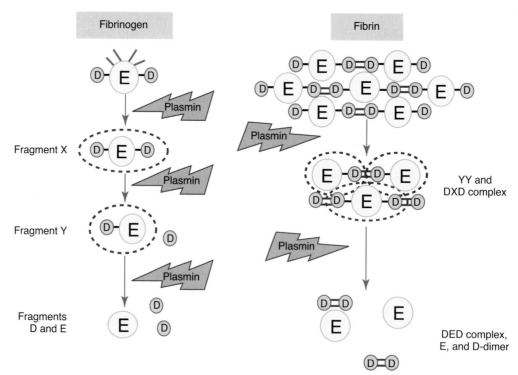

Figure 37-23 Degradation of fibrinogen and fibrin by plasmin. Plasmin systematically degrades fibrinogen and fibrin by digestion of small peptides and cleavage of D-E domains. From fibrinogen, fragment X consists of a central E domain with two D domains (D-E-D); further cleavage produces fragment Y (D-E), with eventual degradation to D and E domains. From cross-linked fibrin, plasmin digestion produces fragment complexes from one or more monomers. D-dimer consists of two D domains from adjacent monomers that have been cross-linked by factor XIIIa in the process of fibrin formation (thrombosis).

of these fragments inhibit hemostasis and contribute to hemorrhage by preventing platelet activation and by hindering fibrin polymerization. Fragment X is described as the central E domain with the two D domains (D-E-D), minus some peptides cleaved by plasmin. Fragment Y is the E domain after cleavage of one D domain (D-E). Eventually these fragments are further digested to individual D and E domains.

The D-D fragment, called *D-dimer,* is composed of two D domains from separate fibrin molecules cross-linked by the action of factor XIIIa. Fragments X, Y, D, and E are produced by digestion of either fibrin or fibrinogen by plasmin, but D-dimer is a specific product of digestion of cross-linked fibrin only and is therefore a marker of thrombosis and fibrinolysis—that is, thrombin, factor XIIIa, and plasmin activation.

The various fragments may be detected by quantitative or semiquantitative immunoassay to reveal fibrinolytic activity. D-dimer is separately detectable by monoclonal antibody for D-dimer antigen, using a wide variety of automated quantitative laboratory immunoassays and other formats including point-of-care tests performed on whole blood.[86,87] The D-dimer immunoassay is used to identify chronic and acute DIC and to rule out venous thromboembolism in suspected cases of deep venous thrombosis or pulmonary embolism.

SUMMARY

- The vascular intima, platelets, tissue factor–bearing cells, and coagulation and fibrinolytic proteins interact to maintain hemostasis.
- Intact vascular intima prevents coagulation through synthesis of prostacyclin, nitric oxide, TFPI, thrombomodulin, and heparan sulfate.
- Damaged intima promotes coagulation by vasoconstriction, exposure of tissue factor and collagen, and secretion of VWF and other adhesion molecules.
- Platelets function in primary and secondary hemostasis through adhesion, aggregation, and secretion of granular contents.
- Platelets adhere to collagen through VWF and use fibrinogen to aggregate.
- Most coagulation factors are produced in the liver.
- The plasma factors of the prothrombin group (prothrombin; factors VII, IX, and X; protein C; protein S; and protein Z) require vitamin K in their production.
- Plasma coagulation factors include trypsin-like enzymes called serine proteases and cofactors that stabilize the proteases. Factor XIIIa is a transamidase.
- The extrinsic pathway of coagulation consists of the membrane receptor tissue factor and coagulation factors VII, X, V, II, and I. The PT is a screening test for these factors.
- The intrinsic pathway factors are XII, pre-K, HMWK, XI, IX, VIII, X, V, II, and I. The PTT is a screening test for these factors.

- Activation of coagulation pathways produces thrombin, which converts fibrinogen to a fibrin polymer. Thrombin also activates platelets and factors V, VIII, XI, and XIII, and binds to thrombomodulin to activate protein C and TAFI.
- Fibrinogen is cleaved by thrombin to form first fibrin monomer, then fibrin polymer, and finally, when acted on by factor XIIIa, cross-linked fibrin.
- In vivo, coagulation is initiated on tissue factor–bearing cells. TF:VIIa activates factors IX and X, generating enough thrombin to activate platelets and factors V, VIII, and XI. Coagulation proceeds on activated platelet phospholipid membranes with the formation of IXa:VIIIa and Xa:Va complexes, which produces a burst of thrombin that cleaves fibrinogen to fibrin.
- The coagulation pathway is regulated by TFPI, APC, and the serpins, including antithrombin and ZPI. These control proteins prevent thrombosis and confine clotting to the site of injury.
- The fibrinolytic pathway digests the thrombus. Plasminogen is converted to plasmin by TPA. Plasmin degrades fibrin to fragments X, Y, D, and E, and D-dimer. Control proteins are PAI-1, α_2-antiplasmin, and TAFI.

Now that you have completed this chapter, go back and read again the case study at the beginning and respond to the questions presented.

REVIEW QUESTIONS

Answers can be found in the Appendix.

1. What intimal cell synthesizes and stores VWF?
   a. Smooth muscle cell
   b. Endothelial cell
   c. Fibroblast
   d. Platelet

2. What subendothelial structural protein triggers coagulation through activation of factor VII?
   a. Thrombomodulin
   b. Nitric oxide
   c. Tissue factor
   d. Thrombin

3. What coagulation plasma protein should be assayed when platelets fail to aggregate properly?
   a. Factor VIII
   b. Fibrinogen
   c. Thrombin
   d. Factor X

4. What role does vitamin K play for the prothrombin group factors?
   a. Provides a surface on which the proteolytic reactions of the factors occur
   b. Protects them from inappropriate activation by compounds such as thrombin
   c. Accelerates the binding of the serine proteases and their cofactors
   d. Carboxylates the factors to allow calcium binding

5. What is the source of fibrinopeptides A and B?
   a. Plasmin proteolysis of fibrin polymer
   b. Thrombin proteolysis of fibrinogen
   c. Proteolysis of prothrombin by factor Xa
   d. Plasmin proteolysis of cross-linked fibrin

6. What serine protease forms a complex with factor VIIIa, and what is the substrate of this complex?
   a. Factor VIIa, factor X
   b. Factor Va, prothrombin
   c. Factor Xa, prothrombin
   d. Factor IXa, factor X

7. What protein secreted by endothelial cells activates fibrinolysis?
   a. Plasminogen
   b. TPA
   c. PAI-1
   d. TAFI

8. What two regulatory proteins form a complex that digests activated factors V and VIII?
   a. TFPI and Xa
   b. Antithrombin and protein C
   c. APC and protein S
   d. Thrombomodulin and plasmin

9. Coagulation factor VIII circulates bound to:
   a. VWF
   b. Factor IX
   c. Platelets
   d. Factor V

10. Most coagulation factors are synthesized in:
    a. The liver
    b. Monocytes
    c. Endothelial cells
    d. Megakaryocytes

REFERENCES

1. Aird, W. C. (2003). Hemostasis and irreducible complexity. *J Thromb Haemost, 1*, 227–230.
2. Collen, D., & Lijnen, H. R. (2004). Tissue-type plasminogen activator: a historical perspective and personal account. *J Thromb Haemost, 2*, 541–546.
3. Ruggeri, Z. M. (2003). Von Willebrand factor, platelets and endothelial cell interactions. *J Thromb Haemost, 1*, 1335–1342.
4. Aird, W. C. (2007). Phenotypic heterogeneity of the endothelium: structure, function, and mechanisms. *Circ Res, 100*, 158–173.
5. Aird, W. C. (2007). Phenotypic heterogeneity of the endothelium: representative vascular beds. *Circ Res, 100*, 174–190.
6. Mitchell, J. A., Ferhana, A., Bailey, L., Moreno, L., & Harrington, L. S. (2008). Role of nitric oxide and prostacyclin as vasoactive hormones released by the endothelium. *Experimental Physiology, 93*, 141–147.
7. Looft-Wilson, R. C., Billaud, M., Johnstone, S. R., Straub, A. C., & Isakson, B. E. (2012). Interaction between nitric oxide signaling and gap junctions: effects on vascular function. *Biochim Biophys Acta, 1818*(8), 1895–1902.
8. Moncada, S. P., Palmer, R. M. J., & Higgs, A. J. (1991). Nitric oxide: physiology, pathophysiology and pharmacology. *Pharmacol Rev, 43*, 109–142.
9. Huntington, J. A. (2003). Mechanisms of glycosaminoglycan activation of the serpins in hemostasis. *J Thromb Haemost, 1*, 1535–1549.
10. Furlan, M. (1996). Von Willebrand factor: molecular size and functional activity. *Ann Hematol, 72* (6),341–348.
11. Bevilacqua, M. P., & Nelson, R. M. (1993). Selectins. *J Clin Invest, 91*, 379–387.
12. Kansas, G. S. (1996). Selectins and their ligands: current concepts and controversies. *Blood, 88*, 3259–3287.
13. Mackman, N., Tilley, R. A., & Key, N. S. (2007). Role of the extrinsic pathway of blood coagulation in hemostasis and thrombosis. *Arterioscler Thromb Vasc Biol, 27*, 1687–1693.
14. Kretz, C. A., Vaezzadeh, N., & Gross, P. L. (2010). Tissue factor and thrombosis models. *Arterioscler Thromb Vasc Biol, 30*, 900–908.
15. Dellas, C., & Loskutoff, D. J. (2005). Historical analysis of PAI-1 from its discovery to its potential role in cell motility and disease. *Thromb Haemost, 93*, 631–640.
16. Foley, J. H., Kim, P. Y., Mutch, N. J., & Gils, A. (2013). Insights into thrombin activatable fibrinolysis inhibitor function and regulation. *J Thromb Haemost, 11*(Suppl. 1), 306–315.
17. Polgar, J., Matuskova, J., & Wagner, D. D. (2005). The P-selectin, tissue factor, coagulation triad. *J Thromb Haemost, 3*, 1590–1596.
18. Bordé, E. C., & Vainchenker, W. (2012). Platelet production: cellular and molecular regulation. In Marder, V. J., Aird, W. C., Bennett, J. S., Schulman, S., & White G. C., II, (Eds.), *Hemostasis and Thrombosis: Basic Principles and Clinical Practice*. (6th ed., pp. 349–364). Philadelphia: Lippincott Williams & Wilkins.
19. Fritsma, G. A. (1988). Platelet production and structure. In Corriveau, D. M., & Fritsma, G. A., (Eds.), *Hemostasis and Thrombosis in the Clinical Laboratory* (pp. 206–228). Philadelphia: JB Lippincott.
20. Bennett, J. S. (2012). Overview of megakaryocyte and platelet biology. In Marder, V. J., Aird, W. C., Bennett, J. S., Schulman, S., & White G. C., II, (Eds.), *Hemostasis and Thrombosis: Basic Principles and Clinical Practice*. (6th ed., pp. 341–348). Philadelphia: Lippincott Williams & Wilkins.

21. Abrams, C. S., & Brass, L. F. (2012). Platelet signal transduction. In Marder, V. J., Aird, W. C., Bennett, J. S., Schulman, S., & White G. C., II, (Eds.), *Hemostasis and Thrombosis: Basic Principles and Clinical Practice.* (6th ed., pp. 449–461). Philadelphia: Lippincott Williams & Wilkins.

22. Berndt, M. C., & Andrews, R. K. (2012). Major platelet glycoproteins. GP Ib/IX/V. In Marder, V. J., Aird, W. C., Bennett, J. S., Schulman, S., & White G. C., II, (Eds.), *Hemostasis and Thrombosis: Basic Principles and Clinical Practice.* (6th ed., pp. 382–385). Philadelphia: Lippincott Williams & Wilkins.

23. Ye, F., & Ginsberg, M. H. (2012). Major platelet glycoproteins. Integrin α2bβ3 (GP IIb/IIIa). In Marder, V. J., Aird, W. C., Bennett, J. S., Schulman, S., & White G. C., II, (Eds.), *Hemostasis and Thrombosis: Basic Principles and Clinical Practice.* (6th ed., pp. 386–392). Philadelphia: Lippincott Williams & Wilkins.

24. McGlasson, D. L., & Fritsma, G. A. (2009). Whole blood platelet aggregometry and platelet function testing. *Semin Thromb Hemost, 35,* 168–180.

25. Rao, A. K. (2013). Inherited platelet function disorders: overview and disorders of granules, secretion, and signal transduction. *Hematol Oncol Clin North Am, 27,* 585–611.

26. Walsh, P. N. (2012). Role of platelets in blood coagulation. In Marder, V. J., Aird, W. C., Bennett, J. S., Schulman, S., & White G. C., II, (Eds.), *Hemostasis and Thrombosis: Basic Principles and Clinical Practice.* (6th ed., pp. 468–474). Philadelphia: Lippincott Williams & Wilkins.

27. Zarbock, A., Polanowska-Grabowska, R. K., & Ley, K. (2007). Platelet-neutrophil-interactions: linking hemostasis and inflammation. *Blood Rev, 21,* 99–111.

28. Sherry, S. (1990). The founding of the International Society on Thrombosis and Haemostasis: how it came about. *Thromb Haemost, 64,* 188–191.

29. Saito, H. (1996). Normal hemostatic mechanisms. In Ratnoff, O. D., & Forbes, C. D., (Eds.), *Disorders of Hemostasis.* (3rd ed., pp. 23–52). Philadelphia: WB Saunders.

30. Coughlin, S. R. (2005). Protease-activated receptors in hemostasis, thrombosis and vascular biology. *J Thromb Haemost, 3,* 1800–1814.

31. Mosesson, M. W. (2005). Fibrinogen and fibrin structure and functions. *J Thromb Haemost, 3,* 1894–1904.

32. Lane, D. A., Philippou, H., & Huntington, J. A. (2005). Directing thrombin. *Blood, 106,* 2605–2612.

33. Mackman, N., Tilley, R. E., & Key, N. S. (2007). Role of the extrinsic pathway of blood coagulation in hemostasis and thrombosis. *Arterioscler Thromb Vasc Biol, 27,* 1687–1693.

34. Broze, G. J. (1995). Tissue factor pathway inhibitor and the revised theory of coagulation. *Ann Rev Med, 46,* 103–112.

35. Mann, K. G., Saulius, B., & Brummel, K. (2003). The dynamics of thrombin formation. *Arterioscler Thromb Vasc Biol, 23,* 17–25.

36. Shahani, T., Lavend'homme, R., Luttun, A., Saint-Remy, J. M., Peerlinck, K., & Jacquemin, M. (2010, Jun 10). Activation of human endothelial cells from specific vascular beds induces the release of a FVIII storage pool. *Blood, 115,* 4902–4909.

37. Jacquemin, M., De Maeyer, M., D'Oiron, R., et al. (2003). Molecular mechanisms of mild and moderate hemophilia A. *J Thromb Haemost, 1,* 456–463.

38. Scott, E., Puca, K., Heraly, J., Gottschall, J., & Friedman, K. (2009). Evaluation and comparison of coagulation factor activity in fresh-frozen plasma and 24-hour plasma at thaw and after 120 hours of 1-6 C storage. *Transfusion, 49* (8), 1584–1591.

39. Sadler, J. E. (1991). Von Willebrand factor. *J Biol Chem, 266,* 22777–22780.

40. Blann, A. D. (2006). Plasma von Willebrand factor, thrombosis, and the endothelium: the first 30 years. *Thromb Haemost, 95,* 49–55.

41. Tsai, H. M. (2006). ADAMTS13 and microvascular thrombosis. *Expert Rev Cardiovasc Ther, 4,* 813–825.

42. Gill, J. C., Endres-Brooks, J., Bauer, P. J., Marks, W. J. Jr., & Montgomery, R. R. (1987). The effect of ABO group on the diagnosis of von Willebrand disease. *Blood, 69,* 1691–1695.

43. Roberts, H. R., & Escobar, M. A. (2013). Less common congenital disorders of hemostasis. In Craig, S., Kitchens, M. D., Barbara, A., Konkle, M. D., Craig, M., & Kessler, M. D., (Eds.), *Consultative Hemostasis and Thrombosis.* (2nd ed., pp. 60–78) Philadelphia: Saunders Elsevier.

44. Harrison, P., Wilborn, B., Devilli, N., et al. (1989). Uptake of plasma fibrinogen into the alpha granules of human megakaryocytes and platelets. *J Clin Invest, 84,* 1320–1324.

45. Mosesson, M. W. (2005). Fibrinogen and fibrin structure and functions. *J Thromb Haemost, 3,* 1894–1904.

46. Lorand, L. (2005). Factor XIII and the clotting of fibrinogen: from basic research to medicine. *J Thromb Haemost, 3,* 1337–1348.

47. Corriveau, D. M. (1988). Major elements of hemostasis. In Corriveau, D. M., & Fritsma, G. A., (Eds.), *Hemostasis and thrombosis in the clinical laboratory* (pp. 1–33). Philadelphia: JB Lippincott.

48. Monroe, D. M., & Hoffman, M. (2006). What does it take to make the perfect clot? *Arterioscler Thromb Vasc Biol, 26,* 41–48.

49. Hoffman, M. (2003). Remodeling the blood coagulation cascade. *J Thromb Thrombolysis, 16,* 17–20.

50. Mann, K. G., Brummel, K., & Butenas, S. (2003). What is all that thrombin for? *J Thromb Haemost, 1,* 1504–1514.

51. Morrissey, J. H., Macik, B. G., Neuenschwander, P. F., & Comp, P. C. (1993). Quantitation of activated factor VII levels in plasma using a tissue factor mutant selectively deficient in promoting factor VII activation. *Blood, 81,* 734–744.

52. Hoffman, M., & Monroe, D. M. (2007). Coagulation 2006: a modern view of hemostasis. *Hematol Oncol Clin North Am, 21,* 1–11.

53. Hoffman, M., & Cichon, L. J. H. (2013). Practical coagulation for the blood banker. *Transfusion, 53,* 1594–1602.

54. Broze, G. J. Jr., & Girard, T. J. (2013). Tissue factor pathway inhibitor: structure-function. *Front Biosci, 17,* 262–280.

55. Lwaleed, B. A., & Bass, P. S. (2006). Tissue factor pathway inhibitor: structure, biology, and involvement in disease. *J Pathol, 208,* 327–339.

56. Monroe, D. M., & Key, N. S. (2007). The tissue factor–factor VIIa complex: procoagulant activity, regulation, and multitasking. *J Thromb Haemost, 5,* 1097–1105.

57. Hakeng, T. M., Maurissen, L. F. A., Castoldi, E., et al. (2009). Regulation of TFPI function by protein S. *J Thromb Haemost, 7*(Suppl. 1), 165–168.

58. Hakeng, T. M., & Rosing, J. (2009). Protein S as cofactor for TFPI. *Arterioscler Thromb Vasc Biol, 29,* 2015–2020.

59. Hakeng, T. M., Sere, K. M., Tans, G., et al. (2006). Protein S stimulates inhibition of the tissue factor pathway by tissue factor pathway inhibitor. *Proc Natl Acad Sci U S A, 103,* 3106–3111.

60. Golino, P. (2002). The inhibitors of the tissue factor: factor VII pathway. *Thromb Res, 106,* V257–V265.

61. Dahlback, B. (1995). The protein C anticoagulant system: inherited defects as basis for venous thrombosis. *Thromb Res, 77,* 1–43.

62. Taylor, F. B., Jr., Peer, G. T., Lockhart, M. S., Ferrell, G., & Esmon, C. T. (2001). Endothelial cell protein C receptor plays an important role in protein C activation in vivo. *Blood, 97,* 1685–1688.

63. Van Hinsbergh, V. W. M. (2012). Endothelium-role in regulation of coagulation and inflammation. *Semin Immunopathol, 34,* 93–106.

64. Griffin, J. H., Gruber, A., & Fernandez, J. A. (1992). Reevaluation of total free, free, and bound protein S and C4b-binding protein levels in plasma anticoagulated with citrate or hirudin. *Blood, 79,* 3203.

65. Dreyfus, M., Magny, J. F., Bridey, F., Schwartz, H. P., Planche, C., Dehan, M., & Tchernia, G. (1991). Treatment of homozygous protein C deficiency and neonatal purpura fulminans with a purified protein C concentrate. *N Engl J Med, 325,* 1565–1568.

66. Price, V. E., Ledingham, D. L., Krumpel, A., & Chan, A. K. (2011). Diagnosis and management of neonatal purpura fulminans. *Semin Fetal Neonatal Med, 16,* 318–322.

67. de Moerloose, P., Bounameaux, H. R., & Mannucci, P. M. (1998). Screening test for thrombophilic patients: which tests, for which patient, by whom, when, and why? *Semin Thromb Hemost, 24,* 321–327.

68. Rau, J. C., Beaulieu, L. M., Huntington, J. A., et al. (2007). Serpins in thrombosis, hemostasis and fibrinolysis. *J Thromb Haemost, 5*(Suppl. 1), 102–115.

69. Bock, S. (2013). Antithrombin and the serpin family. In Marder, V. J., Aird, W. C., Bennett, J. S., Schulman, S., & White G. C., II, (Eds.), *Hemostasis and Thrombosis: Basic Principles and Clinical Practice.* (6th ed., pp. 286–299). Philadelphia: Lippincott Williams & Wilkins.

70. Corral, J., Gonzalez-Conejero, R., Hernandez-Espinosa, D., et al. (2007). Protein Z/Z-dependent protease inhibitor (PZ/ZPI) anticoagulant system and thrombosis. *Br J Haematol, 137*(2), 99–108.

71. Broze, G. J., Jr. (2001). Protein Z-dependent regulation of coagulation. *Thromb Haemost, 86,* 8–13.

72. Chung, D. W., Xu, W., & Davie, E. W. (2013). The blood coagulation factors and inhibitors: their primary structure, complementary DNAs, genes, and expression. In Marder, V. J., Aird, W. C., Bennett, J. S., Schulman, S., & White G. C., II, (Eds.), *Hemostasis and Thrombosis: Basic Principles and Clinical Practice.* (6th ed., pp. 110–145). Philadelphia: Lippincott Williams & Wilkins.

73. Mutch, N. J., & Booth, N. A. (2013). Plasminogen activation and regulation of fibrinolysis. In Marder, V. J., Aird, W. C., Bennett, J. S., Schulman, S., & White G. C., II, (Eds.), *Hemostasis and Thrombosis: Basic Principles and Clinical Practice.* (6th ed., pp. 314–333). Philadelphia: Lippincott Williams & Wilkins.

74. Bennett, B., & Ogston, D. (1996). Fibrinolytic bleeding syndromes. In Ratnoff, O. D., & Forbes, C. D., (Eds.), *Disorders of hemostasis.* (3rd ed., pp. 296–322). Philadelphia: WB Saunders.

75. Kolev, K., & Machovich, R. (2003). Molecular and cellular modulation of fibrinolysis. *Thromb Haemost, 89,* 610–621.

76. Fay, W. P., Garg, N., & Sunkar, M. (2007). Vascular functions of the plasminogen activation system. *Arterioscler Thromb Vasc Biol, 27,* 1237.

77. Esmon, C. T., & Esmon, N. L. (2013). Regulatory mechanisms in hemostasis. In Hoffman, R., Benz, E. J., Jr., Silberstein, L. E., Heslop, H. E., Weitz, J. I., & Anastasi, J., (Eds.), *Hematology: Basic Principles and Practice.* (6th ed., pp. 1842–1846). Philadelphia: Elsevier.

78. Dellas, C., & Loskutoff, D. J. (2005). Historical analysis of PAI-1 from its discovery to its potential role in cell motility and disease. *Thromb Haemost, 93,* 631–640.

79. Cesari, M., Pahor, M., & Incalzi, R. A. (2010). Plasminogen activator inhibitor-1 (PAI-1): a key factor linking fibrinolysis and age-related subclinical and clinical conditions. *Cardiovasc Ther, 28,* 72–91.

80. Weisel, J. W., & Dempfle, C. (2013). Fibrinogen structure and function. In Marder, V. J., Aird, W. C., Bennett, J. S., Schulman, S., & White G. C., II, (Eds.), *Hemostasis and Thrombosis: Basic Principles and Clinical Practice.* (6th ed., pp. 254–271). Philadelphia: Lippincott Williams & Wilkins.

81. Coughlin, P. B. (2005). Antiplasmin: The forgotten serpin? *FEBS Journal, 272,* 4852–4857.

82. Rau, J. C., Beaulieu, L. M., Huntington, J. A., & Church, F. C. (2007). Serpins in thrombosis, hemostasis and fibrinolysis. *J Thromb Haemost, 5* (Suppl. 1), 102–115.

83. Bouma, B. N., & Meijers, J. C. M. (2003). Thrombin-activatable fibrinolysis inhibitor (TAFI, plasma procarboxypeptidase B, procarboxypeptidase R, procarboxypeptidase U). *J Thromb Haemost, 1,* 1566–1574.

84. Bouma, B. N., & Mosnier, L. O. (2003/2004). Thrombin activatable fibrinolysis inhibitor (TAFI) at the interface between coagulation and fibrinolysis. *Pathophysiol Haemost Thromb, 33,* 375–381.

85. Lowe, G. D. (2005). Circulating inflammatory markers and risks of cardiovascular and non-cardiovascular disease. *J Thromb Haemost, 3,* 1618–1627.

86. Adam, S. S., Key, N. S., & Greenberg, C. S. (2009). D-dimer antigen: current concepts and future prospects. *Blood, 113,* 2878–2887.

87. Geersing, G. J., Janssen, K. J. M., & Oudega, R., et al. (2009). Excluding venous thromboembolism using point of care D-dimer tests in outpatients: a diagnostic meta-analysis. *BMJ, 339,* b2990.

Hemorrhagic Disorders and Laboratory Assessment

38

George A. Fritsma*

OUTLINE

OBJECTIVES

After completion of this chapter, the reader will be able to:

1. Distinguish among the causes of localized versus generalized, soft tissue versus mucocutaneous, and acquired versus congenital bleeding.
2. List and interpret laboratory tests that differentiate among acquired hemorrhagic disorders of trauma, liver disease, vitamin K deficiency, and kidney failure.
3. Discuss the laboratory monitoring of therapy for acquired hemorrhagic disorders.
4. Interpret laboratory assay results that diagnose, subtype, and monitor the treatment of von Willebrand disease.
5. Use the results of laboratory tests to identify and monitor the treatment of congenital single coagulation factor deficiencies such as deficiencies of factors VIII, IX, and XI.
6. Explain the principle and rationale for the use of each laboratory test for the detection and monitoring of hemorrhagic disorders.

CASE STUDY

After studying this chapter, the reader will be able to respond to the following case study:

A 55-year-old man comes to the emergency department with epistaxis (uncontrolled nosebleed). He reports that he has "bleeder's disease" and has had multiple episodes of inflammatory hemarthroses (joint bleeding). Physical examination reveals swollen, immobilized knees; mild jaundice; and an enlarged liver and spleen. CBC results indicate that the patient is anemic and has thrombocytopenia with a platelet count of 74,400/μL (reference interval, 150,000 to 450,000/μL). The PT is 18 seconds (reference interval, 12 to 14 seconds), and the PTT is 43 seconds (reference interval, 25 to 35 seconds).

1. What is the most likely diagnosis?
2. What treatment does the patient need?

BLEEDING SYMPTOMS

Hemorrhage is severe bleeding that requires physical intervention. Hemorrhage may be *localized* or *general, acquired* or *congenital*. To establish the cause of a patient's tendency to bleed or a bleeding event, the physician obtains a complete patient and family history and performs a physical examination before ordering diagnostic laboratory tests.[1]

Localized Versus Generalized Hemorrhage

Bleeding from a single location commonly indicates injury, infection, tumor, or an isolated blood vessel defect and is

---

*The author acknowledges the substantial contributions of Marisa B. Marques, MD, to Chapter 41 of the third edition of this textbook, many of which remain in this edition.

called *localized bleeding* or *localized hemorrhage.* An example of localized bleeding is an inadequately cauterized or ineffectively sutured surgical site. Localized bleeding seldom implies a blood vessel defect, a qualitative platelet defect, a reduced platelet count (thrombocytopenia), or a coagulation factor deficiency.

Bleeding from multiple sites, spontaneous and recurring bleeds, or a hemorrhage that requires physical intervention and transfusions is called *generalized bleeding.* Generalized bleeding is potential evidence for a disorder of *primary hemostasis* such as blood vessel defects, platelet defects, or thrombocytopenia, or *secondary hemostasis* characterized by single or multiple coagulation factor deficiencies.

Mucocutaneous Versus Anatomic Hemorrhage

Generalized bleeding may exhibit a *mucocutaneous* (*systemic*) or a soft tissue (*anatomic*) pattern. Mucocutaneous hemorrhage may appear as *petechiae,* pinpoint hemorrhages into the skin (Figure 40-1, *A*); *purpura,* purple lesions of the skin greater than 3 mm caused by extravasated (seeping) red blood cells (RBCs) (Figure 40-1, *B*); or *ecchymoses* (bruises) greater than 1 cm typically seen after trauma (Fig. 40-1, *C*).[2] The unprovoked presence of more than one such lesion may indicate a disorder of primary hemostasis. Other symptoms of a primary hemostasis defect include bleeding from the gums, epistaxis (uncontrolled nosebleed), hematemesis (vomiting of blood), and menorrhagia (profuse menstrual flow). Although nosebleeds are common and mostly innocent, especially in children, they suggest a primary hemostatic defect when they occur repeatedly, last longer than 10 minutes, involve both nostrils, or require physical intervention or transfusions.

Mucocutaneous hemorrhage tends to be associated with thrombocytopenia (platelet count lower than 150,000/μL; Chapter 40), qualitative platelet disorders (Chapter 41), von Willebrand disease (VWD), or vascular disorders such as scurvy or telangiectasia (Chapters 13 and 37). A careful history and physical examination distinguish between mucocutaneous and anatomic bleeding; this distinction helps direct investigative laboratory testing and subsequent treatment.

Anatomic (soft tissue) hemorrhage is seen in acquired or congenital defects in secondary hemostasis, or *plasma coagulation factor* deficiencies (coagulopathies).[3] Examples of anatomic bleeding include recurrent or excessive bleeding after minor trauma, dental extraction, or a surgical procedure. In such cases, hemorrhage may immediately follow a primary event, but it is often delayed or recurs minutes or hours after the event. Anatomic bleeding episodes may even be spontaneous. Most anatomic bleeds are internal, such as bleeds into joints, body cavities, muscles, or the central nervous system, and may initially have few visible signs. Because joint bleeds (*hemarthroses*) cause swelling and acute pain, they may not be immediately recognized as hemorrhages, although experienced hemophilia patients usually recognize the symptoms at their outset. Repeated hemarthroses cause painful swelling and

inflammation, and they may culminate in permanent cartilage damage that immobilizes the joint. Bleeds into soft tissues such as muscle or fat may cause nerve compression and subsequent temporary or permanent loss of function.[4] When bleeding involves body cavities, it causes symptoms related to the organ that is affected. Bleeding into the central nervous system, for instance, may cause headaches, confusion, seizures, and coma and is managed as a medical emergency. Bleeds into the kidney may present as *hematuria* and may be associated with acute kidney failure.

Hemostasis laboratory testing is essential whenever a mucocutaneous or soft tissue disorder is suspected. Box 38-1 lists symptoms that suggest generalized hemorrhagic disorders. Besides a complete blood count that includes a platelet count, most laboratory directors offer the prothrombin time (PT), partial thromboplastin time (PTT), and fibrinogen assay (Table 38-1).[5] In 2000, laboratory practitioners began to add *thromboelastography* performed using the Thromboelastograph® (TEG, Haemoscope Corporation, Niles, IL) or subsequently *thromboelastometry* (TEM) using the rotational thromboelastometer (ROTEM®, Pentapharm GmbH, Munich, Germany; FDA-cleared 2011) (Chapter 44). TEG and TEM are coagulometers that measure

---

BOX 38-1 Generalized Bleeding Signs Heralding a Possible Hemostatic Defect

- Purpura—recurrent, chronic bruising in multiple locations; called *petechiae* when less than 3 mm in diameter, *ecchymoses* when greater than 1 cm in diameter
- Epistaxis—nosebleeds that are recurrent, last longer than 10 minutes, or require physical intervention
- Recurrent or excessive bleeding from trauma, surgery, or dental extraction
- Bleeding into multiple body cavities, joints, or soft tissue
- Simultaneous hemorrhage from several sites
- Menorrhagia (menstrual hemorrhage)
- Bleeding that is delayed or recurrent
- Bleeding that is inappropriately brisk
- Bleeding for no apparent reason
- Hematemesis (vomiting of blood)

TABLE 38-1 Screening Tests for a Generalized Hemostatic Disorder

Test	Assesses
Hemoglobin, hematocrit; reticulocyte count	Anemia associated with chronic bleeding; bone marrow response
Platelet count	Thrombocytopenia
Prothrombin time (PT)	Deficiencies of factors II (prothrombin), V, VII, or X (clotting time prolonged)
Partial thromboplastin time (PTT)	Deficiencies of all factors except VII and XIII (clotting time prolonged)
Thrombin time or fibrinogen assay	Hypofibrinogenemia and dysfibrinogenemia

whole blood clotting.[6] Both report clot onset, clot strength, and fibrinolysis within 15 minutes of blood collection. Experienced laboratory practitioners must interpret TEG or TEM results.

Acquired Versus Congenital Bleeding Disorders

Liver disease, kidney failure, chronic infections, autoimmune disorders, obstetric complications, dietary deficiencies such as vitamin C or vitamin K deficiency, blunt or penetrating trauma, and inflammatory disorders may all associate with bleeding. If a patient's bleeding episodes begin after childhood, are associated with some disease or physical trauma, and are not duplicated in relatives, they are probably acquired, not congenital. When an adult patient comes for treatment of generalized hemorrhage, the physician first looks for an underlying disease or event and records a personal and family history (Box 38-2). The important elements of patient history are age, sex, current or past pregnancy, any systemic disorders such as diabetes or cancer, trauma, and exposure to drugs, including prescription drugs, over-the-counter drugs, alcohol abuse, or drug abuse. The physician determines the trigger, location, and volume of bleeding, and then orders laboratory assays (Table 38-1). These tests take on clinical significance when the history and physical examination already have established the existence of abnormal bleeding. Owing to their propensity for false positives, they are not effective when employed indiscriminately as screens for healthy individuals (Chapter 5).[7]

Congenital hemorrhagic disorders are uncommon, occurring in fewer than 1 per 100 people, and are usually diagnosed in infancy or during the first years of life.[8] There may be relatives with similar symptoms. Congenital bleeding disorders lead to repeat hemorrhages that may be spontaneous or may occur following minor injury or in unexpected locations, such as joints, body cavities, retinal veins and arteries, or the central nervous system. Patients with mild congenital hemorrhagic disorders may have no symptoms until they reach adulthood or experience some physical challenge, such as trauma, dental extraction, or a surgical procedure. The most common congenital deficiencies are VWD, factor VIII and IX deficiencies (hemophilia A and B), and platelet function disorders. Inherited deficiencies of fibrinogen, prothrombin, and factors V, VII, X, XI, and XIII are rare.

BOX 38-2 Indications of Congenital Hemorrhagic Disorders

- Relatives with similar bleeding symptoms
- Onset of bleeding in infancy or childhood
- Bleeding from umbilical cord or circumcision wound
- Repeated hemorrhages in childhood, adulthood
- Hemorrhage into joints, central nervous system, soft tissues, peritoneum

---

ACQUIRED COAGULOPATHIES

Far more patients experience acquired bleeding disorders secondary to trauma, drug exposure, or chronic disease than possess inherited coagulopathies. Chronic disorders commonly associated with bleeding are *liver disease, vitamin K deficiency,* and *renal failure.* In all cases, laboratory test results are necessary to confirm the diagnosis and guide the management of acquired hemorrhagic events.[1,9]

Acute Coagulopathy of Trauma-Shock

In North America, unintentional injury is the leading cause of death among those aged 1 to 45 years. The total rises when statisticians include self-inflicted, felonious, and combat injuries. In the United States alone, trauma causes 93,000 deaths per year.[10] Severe neurologic displacement accounts for 50% of trauma deaths, with most occurring before the patient arrives at the hospital; however, of initial survivors, 20,000 die of hemorrhage within 48 hours.[11] *Acute coagulopathy of trauma-shock* (ACOTS) accounts for most fatal hemorrhage, and 3000 to 4000 of these deaths are preventable. Coagulopathy is defined as any hemostasis deficiency, and ACOTS is triggered by the combination of injury-related *acute inflammation, platelet activation, tissue factor release, hypothermia, acidosis,* and *hypoperfusion* (poor distribution of blood to tissues caused by low blood pressure), all of which are elements of systemic shock. For in-transit fluid resuscitation, colloid plasma expanders such as 5% dextrose are used by most emergency medical technicians to counter hypoperfusion, though in 2013 some trauma specialists advocate for plasma instead of colloids as a means to control coagulopathy.[12] Colloids dilute plasma procoagulants, which become further diluted by emergency department transfusion of RBCs. Although colloids and RBCs are essential, they intensify the coagulopathy, as does subsequent surgical intervention.

Massive transfusion, defined as administration of more than 3 RBC units within 1 hour or 8 to 10 units within 24 hours, is essential in otherwise healthy trauma victims when the systolic blood pressure is below 110 mm Hg, pulse is greater than 105 beats/min, pH is less than 7.25, hematocrit is below 32%, hemoglobin is below 10 g/dL, and PT is prolonged to more than 1.5 times the mean of the reference interval or generates an international normalized ratio (INR) of 1.5.[13]

Acute Coagulopathy of Trauma-Shock Management: RBCs

According to the American Society of Anesthesiologists surgical practice guidelines, RBC transfusions are required when the hemoglobin is less than 6.0 g/dL and are contraindicated when the hemoglobin is greater than 10.0 g/dL.[14] For hemoglobin concentrations between 6.0 and 10.0 g/dL, the decision to transfuse is based upon the acuity of the patient's condition as determined by *physical evidence of blood loss; current blood loss rate; blood pressure; arterial blood gas values, especially pH and oxygen saturation; urine output;* and *laboratory evidence for coagulopathy* provided there is time for specimens to be collected and laboratory assays completed.

Acute Coagulopathy of Trauma-Shock Management: Plasma

Plasma remains a key component of ACOTS management. Before 2005, donor services centrifuged donor blood units and separated and froze the supernatant plasma within 8 hours of collection, yielding fresh-frozen plasma (FFP). Most donor services now separate plasma within 24 hours of donor collection, officially naming the product FP-24 instead of FFP; however, laboratory practitioners, nurses, and physicians still say and write "FFP" from habit.[15] FP-24 or FFP may also be thawed and stored at 1° C to 6° C for up to 5 days, a product called "thawed plasma."[16] Von Willebrand factor (VWF) and coagulation factor V and VIII activities decline to approximately 60% after 5 days of refrigerator storage, so thawed plasma may be ineffective in von Willebrand disease or hemophilia. High-volume trauma centers and mobile emergency services may maintain a small inventory of thawed plasma ready for emergency administration.

Frozen plasma is thawed, warmed to 37° C, and transfused when there is microvascular bleeding and the PT is prolonged to greater than 1.5 times the mean of the PT reference interval or if the PTT is prolonged to greater than 2 times the mean of the PTT reference interval. Plasma is also transfused when the patient is known to have a preexisting single coagulation factor deficiency such as factor VIII deficiency and no factor concentrate is available, when there has been significant volume replacement with colloid plasma expanders and RBCs, and when hemorrhage is complicated by or caused by *Coumadin overdose* (Chapter 43).

Most transfusion service directors recommend that 1 plasma unit be administered per 4 RBC units to retain coagulation stability; however, evidence from retrospective studies on battlefield casualties in Iraq and Afghanistan have led to consideration of a ratio of 1 plasma unit to each RBC unit. The 1:1 ratio appears to provide better coagulation stability, and many transfusion services have modified their massive transfusion protocols to approximate the new ratios.[17,18]

The standard adult plasma dosage is 10 to 15 mL/kg in continuous infusion. Theoretically, plasma should be transfused until 30% coagulation factor activity has been reached for all factors; however, the actual volume that may be administered is limited by the risk of *transfusion-associated circulatory overload* (TACO).[19]

TACO and *transfusion-related acute lung injury* (TRALI) are potential adverse effects of plasma administration.[20] TACO and TRALI can lead to potentially fatal acute *adult respiratory distress syndrome* (ARDS). Plasma therapy may also cause *thrombosis*, *anaphylaxis*, and *multiple organ failure*.

Acute Coagulopathy of Trauma-Shock Management: Platelet Concentrate

During surgery, coagulopathy is assessed based on *microvascular bleeding*, which is evaluated by estimating the volume of blood that fills suction canisters, surgical sponges, and surgical drains. *Platelet concentrate* is ordered when the platelet count is less than 50,000/μL or higher when the surgeon anticipates blood loss.[21] Platelet concentrate therapy is generally ineffective when the patient is known to have *immune thrombocytopenic purpura, thrombotic thrombocytopenic purpura,* or *heparin-induced thrombocytopenia*. In patients with these conditions, therapeutic platelets are rapidly consumed, and their administration may therefore be contraindicated, although they may provide temporary rescue. Platelet concentrate is never ordered when the platelet count is greater than 100,000/μL. Platelet administration may be necessary when the platelet count is between 50,000 and 100,000/μL and there is bleeding into a confined space such as the brain or eye; if the patient is taking antiplatelet agents, aspirin, clopidogrel, prasugrel, or ticagrelor; if there is a known platelet disorder such as a release defect, Glanzmann thrombasthenia, or Bernard-Soulier syndrome (Chapters 40 and 41); or if the surgery involves cardiopulmonary bypass, which suppresses platelet activity.[14]

Acute Coagulopathy of Trauma-Shock Management: Components and Concentrates

In an effort to reduce the risk of TACO and TRALI, improve patient outcomes, and conserve resources, transfusion service directors employ components and concentrates to augment or even replace plasma administration. Activated prothrombin complex concentrate (PCC, FEIBA® [factor eight inhibitor bypassing activity], Baxter Healthcare Corp., Deerfield, IL, or Autoplex T®, Nabi Biopharmaceuticals, Inc., Boca Raton, FL) may be used at a dosage of 50 units/kg every 12 hours, not to exceed 200 units/kg in 24 hours.[22,23] The dose-response relationship of FEIBA or Autoplex T varies among recipients, and because both contain activated coagulation factors, their use raises the risk of disseminated intravascular coagulation (DIC). Nonactivated PCCs such as four-factor concentrate Kcentra® (CLS Behring, King of Prussia, PA) are safer and may also be employed. Kcentra was FDA-cleared in 2013 to treat hemorrhage in Coumadin overdose, but its use in ACOTS is off-label (not FDA cleared).[24,25]

PCCs, either activated or nonactivated, may be used in conjunction with the antifibrinolytic lysine analogue *tranexamic acid* (TXA, Cyklokapron®, Pharmacia & Upjohn Co., Division of Pfizer Inc., New York, NY).[26] TXA may be infused at a loading dose of 1 g administered over 10 minutes followed by infusion of 1 g over 8 hours.[27] First FDA-cleared in 1986 to prevent bleeding in hemophilic patients who are about to undergo invasive procedures, TXA is effective for ACOTS, but this is an off-label use.

Administration of *cryoprecipitate* or *fibrinogen concentrate* (RiaSTAP®, CLS Behring, King of Prussia, PA) is indicated when there is microvascular bleeding and the fibrinogen concentration is less than 100 mg/dL.[28] A 15 to 20 mL unit of cryoprecipitate provides 150 to 250 mg of fibrinogen, and the risk of TACO is lower than that with colloids or plasma. The fibrinogen concentrate dose is 70 mg/kg of body weight infused at less than 5 mL/minute, and a target fibrinogen level of 100 mg/dL should be maintained. Von Willebrand factor and factor VIII concentrates may also be used when the patient is deficient. Plasma and PCCs may all provide reduced factor VIII levels.[29,30]

Recombinant activated coagulation factor VII (rVIIa, Novo-Seven, Novo Nordisk Inc., Princeton, NJ) was FDA-cleared in 1999 for treating hemophilia A or B when factor VIII or factor IX inhibitors are present, respectively; its application in the treatment of ACOTS is off-label. A NovoSeven dosage of 30 µg/kg is rapidly effective in halting microvascular hemorrhage in nonhemophilic trauma victims, and NovoSeven does not cause DIC.[9,31-33] However, one study found a possible link between off-label NovoSeven use and arterial and venous thrombosis in patients with existing thrombotic risk factors.[34]

Acute Coagulopathy of Trauma-Shock: Monitoring Therapy

A skilled operator employing TEG or TEM technology may monitor plasma, PCCs, activated PCC, four-factor PCC, TXA, and rFVIIa. Fibrinogen concentrate or cryoprecipitate efficacy may be measured using the fibrinogen assay. Also, laboratory directors characteristically advise surgeons and emergency department physicians to monitor the effectiveness of all ACOTS therapy indirectly by checking for the correction of platelet count, PT, and PTT to within their respective reference intervals. Platelet aggregometry may be used to measure post-therapy platelet function, and coagulation factor assays are valuable as follow-ups to PT and PTT to determine if the target activity of 30% has been met. While PT, PTT, platelet count, and platelet function assays are accepted approaches, TEG and TEM provide immediate feedback and may be more sensitive to small physiologic improvements.[35] Once ACOTS has been stabilized, additional hemostasis-related therapy is seldom required.

Liver Disease Coagulopathy

The bleeding associated with liver disease may be localized or generalized, mucocutaneous or anatomic. Enlarged and collateral esophageal vessels called *esophageal varices* are a complication of chronic alcoholic cirrhosis; hemorrhaging from varices is localized bleeding, not a coagulopathy, though often fatal. Mucocutaneous bleeding occurs in liver disease–associated thrombocytopenia, often accompanied by decreased platelet function. Soft tissue bleeding is the consequence of procoagulant dysfunction and deficiency.

Procoagulant Deficiency in Liver Disease

The liver produces nearly all of the plasma coagulation factors and regulatory proteins. Hepatitis, cirrhosis, obstructive jaundice, cancer, poisoning, and congenital disorders of bilirubin metabolism may suppress the synthetic function of hepatocytes, reducing either the concentrations or activities of the plasma coagulation factors to below hemostatic levels (less than 30% of normal).

Liver disease predominantly alters the production of the vitamin K–dependent factors II (prothrombin), VII, IX, and X and control proteins C, S, and Z. In liver disease, these seven factors are produced in their *des-γ-carboxyl* forms, which cannot participate in coagulation (Chapter 37). At the onset of liver disease, factor VII, which has the shortest plasma half-life at 6 hours, is the first coagulation factor to exhibit decreased activity. Because the PT is particularly sensitive to factor VII activity, it is characteristically prolonged in mild liver disease, serving as a sensitive early marker.[36] Vitamin K deficiency caused by dietary insufficiency independent of liver disease produces a similar effect on the PT (see the case study in this chapter).

Declining coagulation factor V activity is a more specific marker of liver disease than deficient factor II, VII, IX, or X because factor V is non–vitamin K dependent and is not affected by dietary vitamin K deficiency. The factor V activity assay, performed in conjunction with the factor VII assay, may be used to distinguish liver disease from vitamin K deficiency.[37]

Fibrinogen is an acute phase reactant that is frequently elevated in early or mild liver disease. Moderately and severely diseased liver produces fibrinogen that is coated with excessive sialic acid, a condition called *dysfibrinogenemia*, in which the fibrinogen functions poorly. Dysfibrinogenemia causes generalized soft tissue bleeding associated with a prolonged thrombin time and an exceptionally prolonged reptilase clotting time.[38] In end-stage liver disease, the fibrinogen level may fall to less than 100 mg/dL, which is a mark of liver failure.[39]

VWF and factors VIII and XIII are acute phase reactants that may be unaffected or elevated in mild to moderate liver disease.[40,41] In contrast to the other coagulation factors, VWF is produced from endothelial cells and megakaryocytes and is stored in endothelial cells and platelets.

Platelet Abnormalities in Liver Disease

Moderate *thrombocytopenia* occurs in a third of patients with liver disease. Platelet counts of less than 150,000/µL may result from sequestration and shortened platelet survival associated with portal hypertension and resultant hepatosplenomegaly.[42] In alcoholism-related hepatic cirrhosis, acute alcohol toxicity also suppresses platelet production. Platelet aggregation and secretion properties are often suppressed; this is reflected in reduced platelet aggregometry and lumiaggregometry results (Chapter 42). Occasionally platelets are hyperreactive. Aggregometry may be used to predict bleeding and thrombosis risk.[43]

Disseminated Intravascular Coagulation in Liver Disease

Chronic or compensated DIC (Chapter 39) is a significant complication of liver disease that is caused by decreased liver production of regulatory antithrombin, protein C, or protein S and by the release of activated procoagulants from degenerating liver cells. The failing liver cannot clear activated coagulation factors. In primary or metastatic liver cancer, hepatocytes may also produce procoagulant substances that trigger chronic DIC, leading to ischemic complications.

In acute, uncompensated DIC, the PT, PTT, and thrombin time are prolonged; the fibrinogen level is reduced to less than 100 mg/dL; and fibrin degradation products, including D-dimers, are significantly increased.[44] If the DIC is chronic and compensated, the only elevated test result may be the

D-dimer assay value, a hallmark of unregulated coagulation and fibrinolysis. Although DIC can be resolved only by removing its underlying cause, its hemostatic deficiencies may be corrected temporarily by administering RBCs, plasma, activated or nonactivated PCC, TXA, platelet concentrates, or antithrombin concentrates.[45]

Hemostasis Laboratory Tests in Liver Disease

The PT, PTT, thrombin time, fibrinogen concentration, platelet count, and D-dimer concentration are used to characterize the hemostatic abnormalities in liver disease (Table 38-2). Factor V and VII assays may be used in combination to differentiate liver disease from vitamin K deficiency. Both factors are decreased in liver disease, but factor V is not decreased in vitamin K deficiency.

Plasminogen deficiency and an elevated D-dimer confirm systemic fibrinolysis. The *reptilase time* test occasionally may be useful to confirm dysfibrinogenemia. This test duplicates the thrombin time test except that venom of the reptile *Bothrops atrox* (common lancehead viper) is substituted for thrombin reagent. The *Bothrops* venom triggers fibrin

TABLE 38-2   Hemostasis Laboratory Tests in Liver Disease

Assay	Interpretation
Fibrinogen	>400 mg/dL in early, mild liver disease; <200 mg/dL in moderate to severe liver disease, causing hypofibrinogenemia or dysfibrinogenemia
Thrombin time	Prolonged in dysfibrinogenemia, hypofibrinogenemia, elevation of fibrin degradation products, and therapy with unfractionated heparin
Reptilase time	Prolonged in hypofibrinogenemia, significantly prolonged in dysfibrinogenemia; not affected by heparin; assay rarely used
Prothrombin time (PT)	Prolonged even in mild liver disease due to des-γ-carboxyl factors replacing normal factors II (prothrombin), VII, IX, and X. Report PT in seconds, not international normalized ratio (INR), when testing for liver disease.
Partial thromboplastin time (PTT)	Mildly prolonged in severe liver disease due to disseminated intravascular coagulation (DIC) or des-γ-carboxyl factors II (prothrombin), IX, and X
Factor V assay	Factor V level becomes reduced in liver disease, but is unaffected by vitamin K deficiency so the factor V level helps distinguish the conditions
Platelet count	Mild thrombocytopenia, platelet count <150,000/μL
Platelet aggregometry	Mild suppression of platelet aggregation and secretion in response to most agonists
D-dimer	>240 ng/mL by quantitative assay

polymerization by cleaving fibrinopeptide A but not fibrinopeptide B from the fibrinogen molecule. The subsequent polymerization is slowed by structural defects, which prolong the time interval to clot formation. The reptilase time test is unaffected by standard unfractionated heparin therapy and can be used to assess fibrinogen function even when there is heparin in the sample.[46]

Hemostatic Treatment to Resolve Liver Disease–Related Hemorrhage

Oral or intravenous vitamin K therapy may correct the bleeding associated with nonfunctional des-γ-carboxyl factors II (prothrombin), VII, IX, and X; however, the therapeutic effect of vitamin K is short-lived compared to its effect in dietary vitamin K deficiency because of the liver's impaired synthetic ability. In severe liver disease, plasma transfusion provides all of the coagulation factors in hemostatic concentrations, although VWF and factors V and VIII may be reduced. Owing to its small concentration and short half-life of factor VII, plasma is unlikely to return the PT to within the reference interval.

A unit of plasma has a volume of 200 to 280 mL. The typical adult plasma dose for liver disease is 2 units, but the dose varies widely, depending on the indication and the ability of the patient's cardiac and renal system to rapidly excrete excess fluid. TACO is likely to occur when 30 mL/kg has been administered, but it may occur with even smaller volumes in patients with compromised cardiac or kidney function.

If the fibrinogen level is less than 50 mg/dL, spontaneous bleeding is imminent, and cryoprecipitate or fibrinogen concentrate may be selected for therapy. Plasma and cryoprecipitate present a theoretical risk of virus transmission, as do other untreated single-donor biologic blood products, and allergic transfusion reactions are more common with plasma-containing products. Other therapeutic options for patients with liver disease–related bleeding are platelet concentrates, PCC, antithrombin concentrate (Thrombate III, Telacris® Biotherapeutics, Inc., Research Triangle Park, NC), rFVIIa, and TXA.

Chronic Renal Failure and Hemorrhage

Chronic renal failure of any cause is often associated with *platelet dysfunction* and *mild to moderate mucocutaneous bleeding*.[47] Platelet adhesion to blood vessels and platelet aggregation are suppressed, perhaps because the platelets become coated by *guanidinosuccinic acid* or dialyzable *phenolic compounds*.[48] Decreased RBC mass (anemia) and thrombocytopenia contribute to the bleeding and may be corrected with dialysis, *erythropoietin* or RBC transfusions, and interleukin-11 therapy.[49-52]

Hemostasis activation syndromes that deposit fibrin in the renal microvasculature reduce glomerular function. Examples of such disorders are DIC, *hemolytic uremic syndrome*, and thrombotic thrombocytopenic purpura. Although these are by definition thrombotic disorders, they invariably cause thrombocytopenia, which may lead to mucocutaneous bleeding. Fibrin also may be deposited in renal transplant rejection and in the glomerulonephritis syndrome of systemic lupus erythematosus. This may be associated with a rise in quantitative plasma D-dimer, thrombin-antithrombin complexes, or prothrombin fragments 1 + 2, which are markers of coagulation activation (Chapter 42).[53]

Laboratory tests for bleeding in renal disease provide only modest information with little predictive or management value. The bleeding time test may be prolonged, but it is too unreliable to provide an accurate diagnosis or to assist in monitoring treatment.[54] Platelet aggregometry test results may predict bleeding.[55] The PT and PTT are expected to be normal.

Management of renal failure–related bleeding typically focuses on the severity of the hemorrhage without reliance on laboratory test results. Renal dialysis temporarily activates platelets and may ultimately improve platelet function, particularly when anemia is well controlled.[56,57] Desmopressin acetate may be administered intravenously (DDAVP) or intranasally (Stimate®, CSL Behring, King of Prussia, PA) to increase the plasma concentration of high-molecular-weight multimers of VWF, which also aids platelet adhesion and aggregation.[58] Patients with renal failure should not take aspirin, clopidogrel, prasugrel, ticagrelor, or other platelet inhibitors, because these drugs increase the risk of hemorrhage.

Nephrotic Syndrome and Hemorrhage

Nephrotic syndrome is a state of increased glomerular permeability associated with a variety of conditions, such as chronic glomerulonephritis, diabetic glomerulosclerosis, systemic lupus erythematosus, amyloidosis, and renal vein thrombosis.[59] In nephrotic syndrome, low-molecular-weight proteins are lost through the glomerulus into the glomerular filtrate and the urine. Coagulation factors II (prothrombin), VII, IX, X, and XII have been detected in the urine, as have the coagulation regulatory proteins antithrombin and protein C. In 25% of cases, loss of regulatory proteins takes precedence over loss of procoagulants and leads to a tendency toward venous thrombosis.

Vitamin K Deficiency and Hemorrhage

Vitamin K is ubiquitous in foods, especially green leafy vegetables, and the daily requirement is small, so pure dietary deficiency is rare. Body stores are limited, however, and become exhausted when the usual diet is interrupted, as when patients are fed only with parenteral (intravenous) nutrition for an extended period or when people embark upon fad diets. Also, because vitamin K is fat soluble and requires bile salts for absorption, biliary duct obstruction (*atresia*), fat malabsorption, and chronic diarrhea may cause vitamin K deficiency. Broad-spectrum antibiotics that disrupt normal gut flora may cause a slight reduction because they destroy bacteria that produce vitamin K. The degree of reduction is insignificant when the diet is otherwise normal but may become an important issue when the patient is receiving only parenteral nutrition.[60]

Hemorrhagic Disease of the Newborn Caused by Vitamin K Deficiency

Because of their sterile intestines and the minimal concentration of vitamin K in human milk, newborns are constitutionally vitamin K deficient.[61] Hemorrhagic disease of the newborn was common in the United States before routine administration of vitamin K to infants was legislated in the 1960s, and it

still occurs in developing countries. The activity levels of factors II (prothrombin), VII, IX, and X are lower in normal newborns than in adults, and premature infants have even lower concentrations of these factors. Breastfeeding prolongs the deficiency because passively acquired maternal antibodies delay the establishment of gut flora.

Vitamin K Antagonists: Coumadin

The γ-carboxylation cycle of coagulation factors is interrupted by coumarin-type oral anticoagulants such as Coumadin (warfarin) that disrupt the vitamin K epoxide reductase and vitamin K quinone reductase reactions (Figure 38-1).[62] In this situation, the liver releases dysfunctional des-γ-carboxyl factors II (prothrombin), VII, IX, and X, and proteins C, S, and Z; these inactive forms are called *proteins in vitamin K antagonism* (*PIVKA*). Therapeutic overdose or the accidental or felonious administration of warfarin-containing rat poisons may result in moderate to severe hemorrhage because of the lack of functional factors. The effect of *brodifacoum* or "superwarfarin," often used as a rodenticide, lasts for weeks to months, and treatment of poisoning with this substance requires repeated administration of vitamin K with follow-up PT monitoring.[63] Coumadin overdose is the single most common reason for hemorrhage-associated emergency department visits.

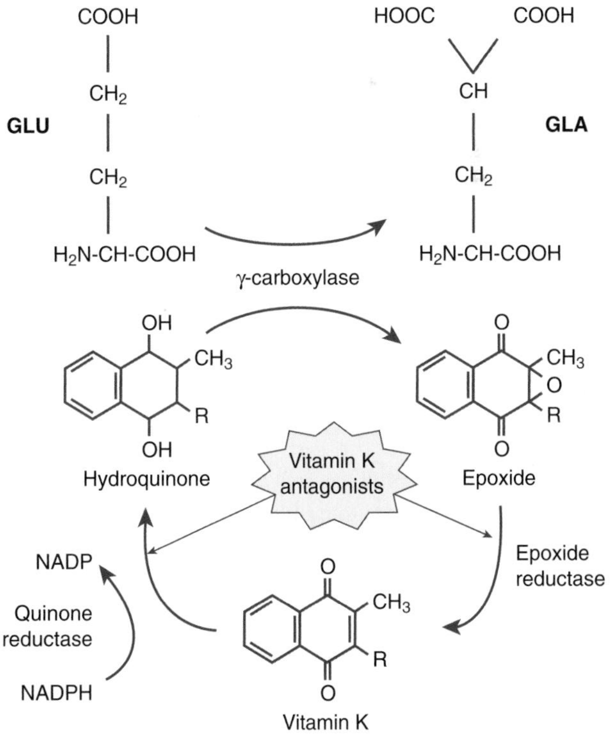

Figure 38-1 Glutamic acid (GLU) gains a carboxyl group to become γ-carboxyglutamic acid (GLA) when catalyzed by γ-carboxylase. This posttranslational modification enables the vitamin K-dependent coagulation factors II (prothrombin), VII, IX, and X and proteins C, S, and Z to bind ionic calcium necessary for normal coagulation. Vitamin K donates the carboxyl group through the quinone reductase pathway. Warfarin inactivates quinone reductase and epoxide reductase to prevent carboxylation. *NADP,* Nicotinamide adenine dinucleotide phosphate; *NADPH,* reduced form of nicotinamide adenine dinucleotide phosphate; *R,* any side chain.

Detection of Vitamin K Deficiency or Proteins in Vitamin K Antagonism

Clinical suspicion of vitamin K deficiency is supported by a prolonged PT with or without a prolonged PTT. In PT and PTT mixing studies, if pooled platelet-free normal plasma (NP; Cryocheck, Precision BioLogic, Inc., Dartmouth, Nova Scotia) is combined with patient plasma, the mixture yields normal (corrected) PT and PTT results, which indicates that factor deficiencies were the cause of the prolonged screening test times. Specific single-factor assays always detect low factor VII because of its short half-life, followed in turn by decreases in factors IX, X, and II (prothrombin).

The standard therapy for vitamin K deficiency is oral—or, in an emergency, intravenous—vitamin K. Because synthesis of functional vitamin K–dependent coagulation factors requires at least 3 hours, in the case of severe bleeding, plasma, activated or nonactivated PCC, four-factor PCC, or rFVIIa may be administered. The only assays for plasma, PCC, or rFVIIa efficacy are TEG or TEM, which are not available everywhere, but the patient's recovery may be monitored indirectly using the PT/INR.

Autoanti-VIII Inhibitor and Acquired Hemophilia

Acquired autoantibodies that specifically inhibit factors II (prothrombin), V, VIII, IX, and XIII and VWF have been described in nonhemophilic patients.[64] Autoanti-VIII is the most common. Patients who develop an autoantibody to factor VIII, which is diagnostic of acquired hemophilia, are frequently older than age 60 and have no apparent underlying disease. Acquired hemophilia is occasionally associated with rheumatoid arthritis, inflammatory bowel disease, systemic lupus erythematosus, or lymphoproliferative disease. Pregnancy appears to trigger acquired hemophilia 2 to 5 months after delivery. Patients with inhibitor autoantibodies are prescribed immunosuppressive therapy, although autoantibodies that develop after pregnancy typically disappear spontaneously. Acquired hemophilia has an overall incidence of 1 per million people per year. Patients experience sudden and severe bleeding in soft tissues or bleeding in the gastrointestinal or genitourinary tract. Acquired hemophilia, even when treated, remains fatal in at least 20% of cases. Autoantibodies to other procoagulants are less frequent but create similar symptoms.[65]

Clot-Based Assays in Acquired Hemophilia

Laboratory directors recommend the PT, PTT, and thrombin time for any patient with sudden onset of anatomic hemorrhage that resembles acquired hemophilia. In the presence of a factor VIII inhibitor, which is the most common inhibitor, the PTT is likely to be prolonged, whereas the lab practitioner expects the PT and thrombin time to be normal. A factor assay should reveal factor VIII activity to be less than 30% and often undetectable.

The laboratory professional confirms the presence of the inhibitor with clot-based mixing studies. The PTT prolongation may be corrected initially by the addition of normal plasma (NP) to the test specimen in a 1:1 ratio, but PTT again becomes prolonged after incubation of the 1:1 NP–patient plasma mixture at 37° C for 1 to 2 hours. The return of prolongation after incubation occurs because factor VIII autoantibodies are frequently of the immunoglobulin G4 isotype, which are time and temperature dependent. Consequently, the inhibitor effect may be evident only after the patient's inhibitor is allowed to interact with the factor VIII in the NP for 1 to 2 hours at 37° C before testing. A few high-avidity inhibitors may cause immediate prolongation of the PTT; in this case an incubated mixing study is unnecessary.

The in vitro kinetics of factor VIII neutralization by an autoantibody are nonlinear. Although there is early rapid loss of factor VIII activity, residual activity remains, which indicates that the reaction has reached equilibrium. This is called *type II kinetics* (Figure 38-2). In contrast, alloantibodies to factor VIII, which develop in 20% to 25% of patients with severe hemophilia in response to factor VIII therapy, exhibit type I kinetics. In the latter, there is linear in vitro neutralization of factor VIII activity over 1 to 2 hours, which results in complete inactivation. In type I kinetics, in vitro measurement is relatively accurate, whereas in type II kinetics, the titration of inhibitor activity is semiquantitative.[66]

Quantitation of autoanti-VIII inhibitor is accomplished using the *Bethesda assay*, which is ordinarily employed to measure inhibitors in hemophilic patients with alloantibodies to factor VIII (see Hemophilia A and Factor VIII Inhibitors). Titer results help the clinician choose the proper therapy to control bleeding. Repeat titers are used to follow the response to immunosuppressive drugs but are not needed for management of the bleeding symptoms.

Factor Inhibitors Other Than Autoanti-Factor VIII

Anticoagulation factor II (anti-prothrombin) antibodies, detectable by immunoassay, develop in approximately 30% of patients with lupus anticoagulant.[67] Although lupus anticoagulant is associated with thrombosis, some patients with antiprothrombin antibodies experience bleeding and have a prolonged PT. A finding of reduced activity on prothrombin assay and a positive test result for lupus anticoagulant confirm the diagnosis. Antiprothrombin antibodies not associated with lupus anticoagulant are rare.

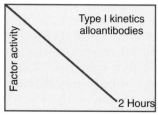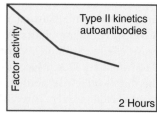

Figure 38-2 In type I linear kinetics, the inhibitor fully inactivates the factor in vitro. This is typical of alloantibodies such as factor VIII inhibitors in patients with severe hemophilia A. In type II kinetics, the inhibitor and factor reach equilibrium. This is typical of autoantibodies such as the factor VIII inhibitor in acquired hemophilia A. Because of the type II kinetics, the Bethesda titer is considered a semiquantitative measure in acquired hemophilia, although the results are commonly used to distinguish low-titer from high-titer antibodies.

Factor V and XIII inhibitors have been documented in patients receiving isoniazid treatment for tuberculosis.[68,69] Antibodies to factor IIa (thrombin) and factor V may arise after exposure to topical bovine thrombin or fibrin glue.[70] Fibrin glue–generated autoantibodies have become less prevalent since 2008 when fibrin glue preparations began to use recombinant human thrombin instead of bovine thrombin. Autoanti-X antibodies are rare; however, factor X deficiency in amyloidosis may be caused by what seems to be an absorptive mechanism.[71] In many cases of acquired inhibitors, mixing studies show uncorrected prolongation without incubation (immediate mixing study), and inhibitor titers may be determined by the Bethesda procedure.

Acquired Hemophilia Management

Activated PCC or rFVIIa may bypass the coagulation factor VIII inhibitor in acquired hemophilia and thereby control acute bleeding. Patients who have low titers of inhibitor (less than 5 Bethesda units) may respond to administration of desmopressin acetate (DDAVP) or factor VIII concentrates, but close monitoring of their response to therapy with serial coagulation factor VIII activity assays is warranted. Once bleeding is controlled, immunosuppressive therapy may reduce the inhibitor titer.[72] Plasma exchange may also be used in severe cases, but the response is less reliable than the response to immunosuppression.

Acquired von Willebrand Disease

Acquired VWF deficiency, with symptoms similar to those of congenital VWD, has been described in association with hypothyroidism; autoimmune, lymphoproliferative, and myeloproliferative disorders; benign monoclonal gammopathies; Wilms tumor; intestinal angiodysplasia; congenital heart disease; pesticide exposure; and hemolytic uremic syndrome.[73] The pathogenesis of acquired VWD varies and may involve decreased production of VWF, presence of an autoantibody, or adsorption of VWF to abnormal cell surfaces, as seen in association with lymphoproliferative disorders and Wilms tumor.[74]

Acquired VWD manifests with moderate to severe mucocutaneous bleeding and may be suspected in any patient with recent onset of bleeding who has no significant medical history. Although the PT is not affected, the PTT may be moderately prolonged if the VWF reduction is severe enough to cause a deficiency of coagulation factor VIII, for which VWF serves as a carrier molecule. As in congenital VWD, the diagnosis is based on a finding of diminished VWF activity (ristocetin cofactor [VWF:RCo] assay) and diminished VWF antigen (VWF:Ag) by immunoassay. It may be difficult to differentiate between mild, previously asymptomatic congenital VWD and acquired VWD.

If the patient requires treatment for bleeding, DDAVP or a plasma-derived factor VIII/VWF concentrate such as Humate-P® (CSL Behring, King of Prussia, PA), Wilate® (Octapharma, Hoboken, NJ), or Alphanate® (Grifols, Los Angeles, CA) is effective at controlling the symptoms. Cryoprecipitate is no longer recommended for treatment of VWD because it does not undergo viral inactivation.

Disseminated Intravascular Coagulation

DIC, although characteristically identified through its hemorrhagic symptoms, is classified as a thrombotic disorder and is described in Chapter 39.

CONGENITAL COAGULOPATHIES

Von Willebrand Disease

VWD is a common mucocutaneous bleeding disorder first described by Finnish professor Erik von Willebrand in 1926. VWD is caused by any one of dozens of germline mutations that result in quantitative or structural abnormalities of VWF. Both quantitative and structural abnormalities lead to decreased adhesion by platelets to injured vessel walls, causing impaired primary hemostasis. VWD is the most prevalent of the congenital bleeding disorders and is found in approximately 1% of the population. It affects both sexes because of its autosomal dominant inheritance pattern. The parameters of and laboratory testing guidelines for VWD are established and defined in the National Heart, Lung, and Blood Institute (NHLBI) publication *The Diagnosis, Evaluation, and Management of von Willebrand Disease*.[75]

Molecular Biology and Functions of von Willebrand Factor

VWF is a glycoprotein whose molecular mass ranges from 800,000 to 20,000,000 Daltons, the largest molecule in human plasma. Its plasma concentration is 0.5 to 1.0 mg/dL, but a great deal more is readily available on demand from storage organelles. VWF is synthesized in the endoplasmic reticulum of endothelial cells and stored in cytoplasmic *Weibel-Palade bodies* of endothelial cells. It is also synthesized in megakaryocytes and stored in the α-granules of platelets (Chapter 13). Weibel-Palade bodies and α-granules release VWF in response to a variety of hemostatic stimuli.[76]

The VWF gene consists of 52 exons spanning 178 kilobase pairs (kb) on chromosome 12.[77] The translated protein is a monomer of 2813 amino acids that, after glycosylation, forms dimers that are transferred to the aforementioned storage organelles, where the dimers polymerize to form enormous multimers. At the time of storage, a signal sequence and a propeptide, known as *VWF antigen II*, are cleaved so that the mature monomers, already polymerized, consist of 2050 amino acids.[78]

As described in Chapter 37, VWF-cleaving protease (ADAMTS-13) cleaves the ultra-large VWF multimers of the Weibel-Palade bodies at their moment of release into monomers of various size. ADAMTS-13 deficiency allows for release of the ultra-large multimers, the basis for the devastating disorder, thrombotic thrombocytopenic purpura (Chapter 40)

Each VWF monomer has four functional domains that bind factor VIII, platelet glycoprotein Ib/IX/V, platelet glycoprotein IIb/IIIa, and collagen (Chapter 13). Upon release from intracellular stores, VWF forms a complex with coagulation factor VIII. This complex is named *VIII/VWF* (Figure 38-3). VWF protects factor VIII from proteolysis, prolonging its plasma half-life from a few minutes without VWF to 8 to 12 hours with

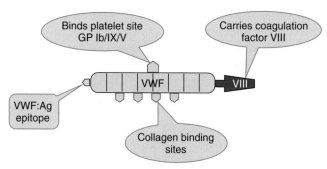

Figure 38-3 Large von Willebrand factor (VWF) multimers bind intimal collagen upon desquamation of endothelial cells or more extensive injury and expand under shear force to form a "carpet" to which platelets adhere through platelet glycoprotein (GP) Ib/IX/V binding sites. VWF binds and stabilizes factor VIII, serving as a carrier protein. The VWF antigen (VWF:Ag) is the target of quantitative immunoassays.

VWF. Table 38-3 lists the nomenclature entries for the structural and functional components of the factor VIII/VWF molecule.

Although VWF is the factor VIII carrier molecule, its primary function is to mediate platelet adhesion to subendothelial collagen in areas of high flow rate and high shear force, as in capillaries and arterioles. VWF first binds fibrillar intimal collagen exposed during the desquamation of endothelial cells. Subsequently, platelets adhere through their glycoprotein Ib/IX/V receptor to the VWF "carpet." The largest VWF multimers are

TABLE 38-3 Nomenclature Relating to the Factor VIII/ von Willebrand Factor Complex

Term	Meaning
VIII/VWF	Customary term for the plasma combination of factor VIII and VWF.
VIII	Procoagulant factor VIII, the protein transported on VWF. Factor VIII binds activated factor IX to form the complex of VIIIa-IXa, which digests and activates factor X. Factor VIII deficiency is called *hemophilia A*.
VWF:Ag	Epitope that is the antigenic target for the VWF immunoassay.
VWF:RCo	Ristocetin cofactor activity, also called *VWF activity*. VWF activity is measured by the ability of ristocetin to cause agglutination of reagent platelets by the patient's VWF.
VWF:CBA	Collagen binding assay, a second method for assaying VWF activity. Large VWF multimers bind immobilized target collagen, predominantly collagen III.
VWF:Immunoactivity	Automated nephelometric activity assay that employs latex microparticles and monoclonal anti-glycoprotein I-VWF receptor, a third method for assaying VWF activity.
VIII:C	Factor VIII coagulant activity as measured in factor-specific clot-based assays.

best equipped to serve the adhesion function. When VWF binds glycoprotein Ib/IX/V, platelets become activated and express a second VWF binding site, glycoprotein IIb/IIIa. This receptor binds VWF and fibrinogen to mediate irreversible platelet-to-platelet aggregation. The adhesion and aggregation sequences are essential to normal hemostasis.

Pathophysiology of von Willebrand Disease

Structural (qualitative) or quantitative VWF abnormalities reduce platelet adhesion, which leads to mucocutaneous hemorrhage of varying severity: epistaxis, ecchymosis, menorrhagia, gastrointestinal tract bleeding, hematemesis, and surgical bleeding. Symptoms vary over time and within kindreds because VWF production and release are susceptible to a variety of physiologic influences. Severe quantitative VWF deficiency creates in addition factor VIII deficiency owing to the inability to protect nonbound factor VIII from proteolysis. Many people have VWF levels in the intermediate range of 30% to 50% of normal and maintain a factor VIII level sufficient for competent coagulation.[79] When factor VIII levels decrease to less than 30% of normal, anatomic soft tissue bleeding accompanies the typical mucocutaneous bleeding pattern of VWD.

Von Willebrand Disease Types and Subtypes

Type 1 von Willebrand Disease. Type 1 VWD is a quantitative VWF deficiency caused by one of several autosomal dominant frameshifts, nonsense mutations, or deletions.[80,81] Type 1 is seen in approximately 75% of VWD patients. The plasma concentrations of all VWF multimers and factor VIII are variably, although proportionally, reduced (Figure 38-4).[82] There is mild to moderate bleeding, usually following a hemostatic challenge such as dental extraction or surgery. In women, menorrhagia is a common complaint that leads to the diagnosis of VWD.

Type 2 von Willebrand Disease. Type 2 VWD comprises a variety of qualitative VWF abnormalities. VWF levels

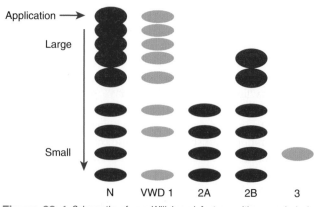

Figure 38-4 Schematic of von Willebrand factor multimer analysis by polyacrylamide gel electrophoresis shows diminished concentration but normal ratios in von Willebrand disease (VWD) type 1, absence of large and intermediate multimers in subtype 2A, absence of large forms in subtype 2B, and absence of all multimers in type 3.

may be normal or moderately decreased, but VWF function is consistently reduced.

Subtype 2A von Willebrand Disease.

Ten percent to 20% of VWD patients have subtype 2A, which arises from well-characterized autosomal dominant point mutations in the A2 structural domain of the VWF molecule. These mutations render VWF more susceptible to proteolysis by ADAMTS-13, which leads to a predominance of small-molecular-weight multimers in the plasma (Figure 38-4). The smaller multimers support less platelet adhesion activity than the normal high- or intermediate-molecular-weight multimers. Patients with subtype 2A VWD have normal or slightly reduced VWF:Ag levels, with markedly reduced VWF activity as a result of the loss of the high-molecular-weight and intermediate-molecular-weight multimers essential for platelet adhesion.[83]

Subtype 2B von Willebrand Disease.

In subtype 2B VWD, rare mutations within the A1 domain raise the affinity of VWF for platelet glycoprotein Ib/IX/V, its customary binding site; these are thus "gain-of-function" mutations. Large VWF multimers spontaneously bind resting platelets and are unavailable for normal platelet adhesion. Consequently, the electrophoretic multimer pattern is characterized by lack of high-molecular-weight multimers but presence of intermediate-molecular-weight multimers (Figure 38-4). There also may be moderate thrombocytopenia caused by chronic platelet activation because multimer-coated platelets indiscriminately bind the endothelium.

A platelet mutation that increases glycoprotein Ib/IX/V affinity for normal VWF multimers creates a clinically similar disorder called *platelet-type VWD* or *pseudo-VWD*. In this instance, the large multimers also are lost from the plasma, and platelets become adhesive. Both clinically and in the laboratory, the two entities are indistinguishable.

Subtype 2M von Willebrand Disease.

Subtype 2M VWD describes a qualitative variant of VWF that has decreased platelet receptor binding but a normal multimeric pattern in electrophoresis. The distinguishing feature of subtype 2M that separates it from type 1 is a discrepancy between the concentration of VWF:Ag and its activity as measured using the VWF:RCo assay.

Subtype 2N von Willebrand Disease (Normandy Variant; Autosomal Hemophilia).

A rare autosomal VWF missense mutation impairs its factor VIII binding site. This condition results in factor VIII deficiency despite normal VWF:Ag concentration and activity and a normal multimeric pattern. The disorder is also known as *autosomal hemophilia* because its clinical symptoms are indistinguishable from the symptoms of hemophilia except that it affects both males and females. Subtype 2N is suspected when a girl or woman is diagnosed with hemophilia after soft tissue bleeding symptoms. In boys or men, subtype 2N is suspected when a patient misdiagnosed with hemophilia A fails to respond to factor VIII concentrate therapy. The poor response occurs because the factor has a plasma

half-life of mere minutes when it cannot be bound by VWF. The diagnosis of VWD subtype 2N is confirmed using a molecular assay that detects the specific mutation responsible for the abnormal factor VIII binding to VWF.

Type 3 von Willebrand Disease.

Autosomal recessive VWF gene translation or deletion mutations produce severe mucocutaneous and anatomic hemorrhage in compound heterozygotes or, in consanguinity, homozygotes. In this rare disorder, VWF is absent or nearly absent from plasma (Figure 38-4). Factor VIII is also proportionally diminished or absent, and primary and secondary hemostasis is impaired.

Laboratory Detection and Classification of von Willebrand Disease

Definitive diagnosis of VWD depends on the combination of a personal and family history of mucocutaneous bleeding and the laboratory demonstration of decreased VWF activity. A CBC is necessary to rule out thrombocytopenia as the cause of mucocutaneous bleeding, and PT and PTT, which assess the coagulation system, are part of the initial VWD workup. No longer recommended, according to the 2009 NHLBI VWD guidelines, are the *bleeding time* test and the PFA-100 or other automated functional platelet assays (Chapters 42 and 44). These traditional screening tests generate "conflicting" sensitivity and specificity data.[84]

The standard VWD test panel includes three assays: a *quantitative VWF* test (VWF:Ag assay) employing enzyme immunoassay or automated latex immunoassay methodology, such as the Liatest (Diagnostica Stago, Asnières-sur-Seine, France); the *VWF activity* test, which determines the factor's ability to bind to platelets, also known as the *VWF:RCo assay;* and a factor VIII activity assay. The VWF:RCo assay employs preserved reagent platelets. The agonist ristocetin supports platelet agglutination in the presence of VWF.

When the ratio of the VWF:RCo assay value to the VWF:Ag concentration is less than 0.5, 0.6, or 0.7 (ratio cutoff is generated from reference interval studies by local laboratories), the laboratory professional infers qualitative or type 2 VWD. Additional tests are needed to confirm type 2 VWD and to differentiate subtype 2A from subtype 2B. *Low-dose ristocetin-induced platelet aggregometry* (RIPA), also called the *ristocetin response curve*, identifies subtype 2B. The low-dose RIPA test is performed on platelet-rich plasma. In subtype 2B the patient's platelets, because they are coated with abnormal VWF multimers, agglutinate in response to less than 0.5 mg/mL ristocetin; sometimes they even agglutinate in response to 0.1 mg/mL ristocetin. In comparison, normal platelets or platelets from a patient with subtype 2A agglutinate only at ristocetin concentrations greater than 0.5 mg/mL.

VWF *multimer analysis* by *sodium dodecyl sulfate–polyacrylamide gel electrophoresis* further differentiates between VWD subtypes 2A and 2B. Although both 2A and 2B lack high-molecular-weight multimers, intermediate multimers are present in the electrophoretic pattern of subtype 2B VWD samples but are absent from the pattern of a patient with subtype 2A VWD. Multimer analysis is technically demanding and is performed mainly in reference laboratories for differentiation of VWD subtypes. Table 38-4 lists the expected test results for all VWD types and subtypes.

Because acquired VWD may mimic any one of the VWD types and subtypes, results of the laboratory workup do not help to differentiate it from the inherited condition. Review of the clinical history with emphasis on age at onset of bleeding, comorbid conditions, and family history may signal acquired disease rather than the congenital form.

Pitfalls in von Willebrand Disease Diagnosis

Varying genetic penetrance, ABO blood group, inflammation, hormones, age, and physical stress influence VWF activity.[85] Increased estrogen levels during the second and third trimesters of pregnancy nearly normalize plasma VWF activity even in women with moderate VWF deficiency. However, VWF function and concentration decrease rapidly after delivery, which may lead to acute postpartum hemorrhage, for which the obstetrician is watchful. Oral contraceptive use and hormone replacement therapy also raise VWF activity, and activity waxes and wanes with the menstrual cycle.

VWF activity rises substantially in acute inflammation such as occurs postoperatively, subsequent to trauma, or during an infection. Physical stress such as cold, exertion, or children's crying or struggling during venipuncture causes VWF activity to rise. VWF activity rises when the phlebotomist allows the tourniquet to remain tied for more than 1 minute prior to venipuncture and drops if the specimen is stored in the refrigerator prior to testing. VWD patients experience fluctuation in disease severity over time, and the clinical manifestations of the disease vary from person to person within kindred, despite the assumption that everyone in the family possesses the same mutation. When the clinical presentation suggests VWD, the VWD laboratory assay panel should be repeated until the results are conclusive.[86]

Adding to VWD diagnostic confusion is concern over the variability in the results of the VWF:RCo assay, which is based on platelet aggregometry but is performed using a variety of instruments and methods, including at least one automated

device, the BCS XP System® with von Willebrand reagent (Siemens Healthcare Diagnostics, Inc., Deerfield, IL). Ristocetin avidity varies from lot to lot. In the United States, proficiency surveys consistently reveal VWF:RCo assays to have an unimpressive interlaboratory coefficient of variation of 30% and a least detectable activity range of 6% to 12%.[87]

Concern over the poor reproducibility of results of the VWF activity assay has led to attempts at developing alternative assays, the most promising of which is the *VWF collagen binding (VWF:CB) assay*. VWF:CB employs type III collagen as its solid-phase target antigen. Developed in 1990, the VWF:CB assay produces results that more closely match those of the VWF:RCo assay than of VWF:Ag assays, because collagen type III binds predominantly large VWF multimers; however, the target collagen composition requires standardization before this assay achieves standard assay status.[88] The VWF:CB assay has better precision than the VWF:RCo assay.[89]

Many reference laboratories add the VWF:CB assay to their initial VWD screening profile. They argue that the VWF:CB assay detects abnormalities of VWF collagen binding, whereas the VWF:RCo assay detects abnormalities of VWF platelet binding and cite instances in which the VWF:CB value was abnormal when the VWF:RCo value was normal, and vice versa.[90]

A second alternative to VWF:RCo is the automated HemosIL von Willebrand Factor Activity assay (Instrumentation Laboratory Company [IL], Bedford, MA). This nephelometric immunoassay employs latex microparticles coated with monoclonal antibodies directed to the VWF glycoprotein I binding site. Results compare well with the cofactor assay when the immunoassay is performed on IL instrumentation.[91]

In an effort to more closely reflect clinical reality and reduce false-positive type 1 VWD diagnoses, the 2009 NHLBI VWD guidelines have coined the nondisease description *"low VWF"* for the condition in which VWF activity and antigen concentrations are between 30% and 50% of normal, the ratio of VWF:RCo to VWF:Ag is greater than 0.5, and factor VIII activity is greater than 50% of normal. This suggested category reflects the difficulty in distinguishing mucocutaneous bleeding from self-reported "easy bruising" and recognizes that low VWF

TABLE 38-4 Laboratory Detection and Classification of von Willebrand Disease: Typical Results*

Laboratory Test	Type 1	Type 2A	Type 2B	Type 3
VWF activity via ristocetin cofactor, collagen binding, or immunoactivity assay	Low	Low	Low	Very low or absent
VWF antigen	Low	Normal to slightly decreased	Normal to slightly decreased	Very low or absent
VWF activity to VWF antigen ratio	>0.5	<0.5	<0.5	N/A
Platelet count	Normal	Normal	Decreased	Normal
Partial thromboplastin time (PTT)	Normal to slightly prolonged	Normal	Normal	Prolonged
RIPA	Decreased	Decreased	Increased	Absent
Factor VIII activity	Mildly low	Normal	Normal	<5%
VWF multimers	Normal pattern	Large and intermediate forms absent	Large forms absent	All forms absent

*Expected results are given, but results vary over time and within affected kindred.
N/A, Not applicable; *RIPA*, ristocetin-induced platelet aggregometry with 1 mg/mL ristocetin; *VWF*, von Willebrand factor.

activity and bleeding often associate coincidentally. To make a definite type 1 VWD diagnosis, 30% of normal VWF activity is used as the cutoff. Molecular confirmation of type 1 VWD, currently but a dream because of the plethora of contributing mutations, may soon become routine as molecular microchip technology meets the challenge.

VWF activity varies by ABO blood group, and expert panels have in the past recommended that laboratory directors maintain separate reference intervals for each group, as provided in Table 38-5. The 2009 NHLBI VWD guidelines have recommended against this practice, noting that "despite the ABO blood grouping and associated reference ranges, the major determinant of bleeding risk is low VWF." Therefore, VWF test result reference intervals are now population based rather than ABO stratified. The internationally generalized cutoff of 50% for low VWF and 30% for VWD is clinically reasonable, although laboratory directors may choose to validate and adjust this cutoff in internal reference interval studies.

In a well-managed tertiary care facility, laboratory professionals and physicians communicate regularly with medical staff who are challenged with VWD management—for example, nurses, pharmacists, emergency department and primary care physicians, internists, surgeons, gynecologists, and hematologists. Laboratory professionals ensure that those who manage VWD patients are aware of the effects of ABO group, estrogen levels, inflammation, and physical stress on VWF activity and that they understand the strengths and limitations of VWF laboratory assay panels, the proper interpretation of assay results, and the availability of follow-up and confirmatory assays.

Treatment of von Willebrand Disease

Mild bleeding may resolve with the use of localized measures, such as limb elevation, pressure, and application of ice packs (the athlete's acronym is *RICE* for rest, ice, compression, and elevation).[92] Moderate bleeding may respond to *estrogen* and *desmopressin acetate*, which trigger the release of VWF from storage organelles. Therapeutic dosages are monitored when necessary using serial VWF:Ag concentration assays. Desmopressin acetate (1-desamino-8-D arginine vasopressin) is an antidiuretic hormone analogue used to control incontinence in diabetes mellitus and bed-wetting; release of VWF from storage organelles is a side effect. Desmopressin acetate in its oral form, DDAVP, or nasal spray form, Stimate (both from

CSL Behring, King of Prussia, PA), is consistently effective for type 1 VWD and generally useful for subtype 2A. It is contraindicated for subtype 2B, however, because it causes the release of abnormal VWF with increased affinity for platelet receptors, which may intensify thrombocytopenia and lead to increased platelet activation and consumption. Because of its antidiuretic property, repeated doses may lead to hyponatremia (low serum sodium). For this reason, it is necessary to monitor and regulate electrolytes during desmopressin acetate therapy.

The lysine analogues ε-aminocaproic acid (EACA; Amicar) and TXA (Cyklokapron) inhibit fibrinolysis and may help control bleeding when used alone or in conjunction with desmopressin acetate. Therapy using nonbiological preparations is preferred over human plasma-derived biologic therapy because nonbiologicals eliminate the risk of viral disease transmission and circumvent religious objections to receipt of human blood products.

For treatment of severe VWD (type 3) and subtype 2B, three commercially prepared human plasma-derived high-purity preparations are available that provide a mixture of VWF and coagulation factor VIII: Humate-P, Alphanate, and Wilate (Wilate was FDA-cleared in December 2009).[92] The calculation of the proper dosage follows principles identical to those used for treatment of hemophilia A provided in the next section. Laboratory monitoring by the VWF:Ag assay is essential to determine if the given amount produced the target level of VWF and to follow its degradation between doses.

Recombinant and affinity-purified factor VIII preparations contain no VWF and cannot be used to treat VWD. Cryoprecipitate and plasma are less desirable alternatives because of the risk of virus transmission, and the necessary plasma volume per dose may cause TACO. Therapy for bleeding secondary to acquired VWD follows the same principles as delineated previously, plus treatment of the primary disease, if applicable.[93] Therapeutic recommendations for VWD are summarized in Table 38-6.

Hemophilia A (Factor VIII Deficiency)

The hemophilias are congenital single-factor deficiencies marked by anatomic soft tissue bleeding. Second to VWD in prevalence among congenital bleeding disorders, hemophilias occur in 1 in 10,000 individuals. Of those affected, 85% are deficient in factor VIII, 14% are deficient in factor IX, and 1%

TABLE 38-5 Von Willebrand Factor (VWF) Reference Intervals by Blood Group

Blood Group	Reference Interval
O	36%–157%
A	48%–234%
B	57%–241%
AB	64%–238%
Population based: "Low VWF"	<50%
Population based: von Willebrand disease	<30%

TABLE 38-6 Therapeutic Strategies in von Willebrand Disease

Type	Primary Approach	Other Options
1	Estrogen, DDAVP, EACA or TXA	Factor VIII/VWF concentrate
2A	Estrogen, DDAVP, EACA or TXA	Factor VIII/VWF concentrate
2B	Factor VIII/VWF concentrate	EACA
2N	Factor VIII/VWF concentrate	EACA
3	Factor VIII/VWF concentrate	Platelet transfusions

DDAVP, Desmopressin acetate; *EACA,* ε-aminocaproic acid; *TXA,* tranexamic acid; *VWF,* von Willebrand factor.

are deficient in factor XI or one of the other coagulation factors, such as factor II (prothrombin), V, VII, X, or XIII. Congenital deficiency of factor VIII is called *classic hemophilia* or *hemophilia A*.[94]

Factor VIII Structure and Function

Factor VIII is a two-chain, 285,000 Dalton protein translated from the X chromosome.[95] When the coagulation cascade is activated, thrombin cleaves plasma factor VIII and releases a large polypeptide called the *B domain* that dissociates from the molecule. This leaves behind a calcium-dependent heterodimer that detaches from its VWF carrier molecule to bind phospholipid and factor IXa. The VIIIa/IXa complex, sometimes called *tenase complex*, cleaves and activates coagulation factor X at a rate 10,000 times faster than free IXa can cleave factor X. Consequently, factor VIII deficiency significantly slows the coagulation pathway's production of thrombin and leads to hemorrhage. In vitro, factor VIII (like factor V) is labile and deteriorates at about 5% an hour at room temperature.

Hemophilia A Genetics

The gene for factor VIII spans 186 kb of the X chromosome and is the site of various deletions, stop codons, and nonsense and missense mutations. Most of these mutations result in quantitative disorders in which the factor VIII coagulant activity and antigen concentration match, but in rare cases low activity is seen despite normal antigen concentration.[96] The latter cases are due to qualitative or structural factor VIII abnormalities traditionally known as *cross-reacting material positive* disorders.[97]

Male hemizygotes, whose sole X chromosome contains a factor VIII gene mutation, experience anatomic bleeding, but female heterozygotes, who are carriers, do not.[98] When a female carrier has children with an unaffected man, the chances of hemophilia A inheritance are 25% chance of a normal daughter, 25% chance of a carrier daughter, 25% chance of a normal son, and 25% chance of a hemophilic son. All sons of men with hemophilia A and noncarrier women are normal, whereas all daughters are obligate carriers of the disease.[99] In addition, approximately 30% of newly diagnosed cases arise as a result of spontaneous germline mutations in individuals who have no family history of hemophilia A.[100] Rarely, the symptoms of hemophilia A may be seen in females. This phenomenon could be due to true homozygosity or double heterozygosity, such as in the female offspring of a hemophilic father and a carrier mother. Other possibilities include a spontaneous germline mutation in the otherwise normal allele of a heterozygous female or a disproportional inactivation of the X chromosome with the normal gene, termed *extreme lyonization*. Finally, VWD of the Normandy subtype may present as mild hemophilia A in males and females.

Hemophilia A Clinical Manifestations

Hemophilia A causes anatomic bleeds with deep muscle and joint hemorrhages; hematomas; wound oozing after trauma or surgery; and bleeding into the central nervous system, peritoneum, gastrointestinal tract, and kidneys. Acute joint bleeds (hemarthroses) are exquisitely painful and cause temporary immobilization. Chronic joint bleeds cause inflammation and eventual permanent loss of mobility, whereas bleeding into muscles may cause nerve compression injury, with first temporary and then lasting disability. Cranial bleeds lead to severe, debilitating, and durable neurologic symptoms, such as loss of memory, paralysis, seizures, and coma, and may be rapidly fatal. Bleeding may begin immediately after a triggering event or may become manifest after a delay of several hours. Some bleeding seems to be spontaneous.

The diagnosis of hemophilia A begins with laboratory testing after the birth of an infant to a mother who has a family history of hemophilia. In the absence of a family history, abnormal bleeding in the neonatal period, which may appear as easy bruising, bleeding from the umbilical stump, postcircumcision bleeding, hematuria, or intracranial bleeding, is considered suspicious for hemophilia. Severe hemophilia usually is diagnosed in the first year of life, whereas mild hemophilia may not become apparent until a triggering event such as trauma, surgery, or dental extraction occurs in late childhood, adolescence, or adulthood.

The laboratory diagnosis of coagulopathies in the newborn or older infant is complicated by the requirement for an unhemolyzed specimen of at least 2 mL in volume from tiny veins and by the typically low newborn levels of some coagulation factors. Medical laboratory practitioners expect the PT and PTT to be prolonged because of physiologically low levels of factors II (prothrombin), VII, IX, and X, even in full-term infants. Factor VIII levels are similar to the levels in adults, even in infants who are born prematurely; this allows skillful laboratory staff to provide the correct diagnosis of hemophilia A using a factor VIII activity assay.

The severity of hemophilia A symptoms is inversely proportional to factor VIII activity. Laboratory professionals classify an activity level of less than 1% as severe, associated with spontaneous or exaggerated bleeding in the neonatal period. Activity levels of 1% to 5% are seen in moderate hemophilia, which is usually diagnosed in early childhood after symptoms become apparent. In mild hemophilia, with activity levels of 5% to 30%, hemorrhage follows significant trauma and becomes a risk factor mainly in surgery or dental extractions, and patients may go for long periods without symptoms.

Hemophilia A Complications

As a result of frequent bleeds, hemophilia patients often have debilitating and progressive musculoskeletal lesions and deformities and neurologic deficiencies after intracranial hemorrhage. In addition, other effects of chronic diseases, such as limited productivity, low self-esteem, poverty, drug dependency, and depression, are common problems. Before the advent of sterilized and recombinant factor concentrates, chronic hepatitis often resulted from repeated exposure to blood products. Tragically, 70% of hemophiliacs treated before 1984 are human immunodeficiency virus (HIV) positive or have died from acquired immunodeficiency syndrome.[101]

Hemophilia A Laboratory Diagnosis

The laboratory workup for a suspected congenital single coagulation factor deficiency starts with the PT, PTT, and thrombin time and continues with factor assays based on the results of the screening tests. Before the physician initiates laboratory testing, however, he or she records a history of the patient's hemorrhagic symptoms. In hemophilia A, the PT and thrombin time are likely to be normal, and the PTT is prolonged, provided that the PTT reagent is sensitive to factor VIII deficiencies at or less than the 30% plasma level. Table 38-7 lists the expected results for each clot-based screening assay for any single-factor deficiency associated with bleeding, including deficiencies of fibrinogen and factors II (prothrombin), V, VII, VIII, IX, X, and XI. Deficiencies of contact factors (factor XII, high-molecular-weight kininogen, and prekallikrein) have no relationship to bleeding, and these factors do not appear in Table 38-7.

Hemophilia A Carrier Detection

Approximately 90% of female carriers of hemophilia A are detected by measuring the ratio of factor VIII activity to VWF:Ag value (VIII:VWF). This ratio is effective because VWF production is unaffected by factor VIII deficiency. Using a ratio, rather than a factor VIII assay value alone, normalizes for some of the physiologic variables that affect factor VIII activity and VWF:Ag assays, such as estrogen levels, inflammation, stress, and exercise.

The laboratory professional establishes a reference interval for the VIII:VWF ratio using plasmas from at least 30 women who do not have factor VIII deficiency. If the ratio of the individual being tested is below the lower limit of the interval, she is likely to be a carrier. These results may be influenced by excessive lyonization, variation in VWF production, and analytical variables; consequently, if carrier status is suspected and the VIII:VWF ratio is greater than the lower limit of the reference range, genetic testing may be necessary to detect one of the many polymorphisms associated with factor VIII deficiency.

Hemophilia A Treatment

The goal of on-demand hemophilia A treatment is to raise the patient's factor VIII activity to hemostatic levels whenever he or she experiences or suspects a bleeding episode or anticipates a hemostatic challenge such as a surgical procedure. The target activity level depends on the nature of the bleeding and the procedure, but it is seldom necessary to reach activity greater than 75%. Target activity should be maintained until the threat is resolved. In the case of a bleed into soft tissue or a body cavity, the sooner the target factor level is reached, the less painful the episode, and the less likely the patient is to experience inflammation or nerve damage. Because factor VIII has a half-life of 8 to 12 hours, twice-a-day infusions are required.

With the availability of abundant recombinant factor VIII concentrate, many hemophilic patients maintain themselves on a steady prophylactic dosage designed to constantly keep their factor VIII activity at hemostatic levels.[102] Although it is initially more expensive, the prophylactic approach conserves downstream resources by ameliorating the adverse effects of repeated hemorrhages and their long-term consequences.[103]

Many hemophilic patients' factor VIII activity rises upon administration of desmopressin acetate in the form of DDAVP or Stimate (nasal formulation), alone or in combination with an antifibrinolytic such as EACA or TXA. When desmopressin acetate treatment proves ineffective, intravenous factor VIII concentrates are the next option. High-purity factor VIII concentrates are produced from mammalian cells using recombinant DNA technology or are derived from human plasma using factor VIII–specific monoclonal antibodies and column separation.[104,105] The human plasma-derived concentrates Alphanate, Humate-P, and Wilate are prepared by chemical fractionation of human plasma and contain VWF, fibrinogen, and noncoagulant proteins, in addition to factor VIII. All plasma-derived concentrates undergo viral inactivation steps, and since 1985, none has transmitted lipid-envelope viruses such as HIV, hepatitis B virus, or hepatitis C virus. Plasma-derived factor VIII concentrates, however, may transmit nonlipid viruses such as parvovirus B19 and hepatitis A virus.[106] Recombinant products may use human albumin in the manufacturing process, which introduces the theoretical risk of Creutzfeldt-Jakob disease transmission; however, manufacturers now provide products free of all human protein, such as Bioclate (Pfizer, New York, NY).[107]

TABLE 38-7 Results of Clot-Based Screening Assays in Congenital Single-Factor Deficiencies*

Deficient Factor	PT	PTT	TCT	Reflex Test
Fibrinogen	Prolonged	Prolonged	Prolonged	Fibrinogen assay
Prothrombin	Prolonged	Prolonged	Normal	Prothrombin, V, VII, and X assays
V	Prolonged	Prolonged	Normal	Prothrombin, V, VII, and X assays
VII	Prolonged	Normal	Normal	VII assay
VIII	Normal	Prolonged	Normal	VIII, IX, and XI assays
IX	Normal	Prolonged	Normal	VIII, IX, and XI assays
X	Prolonged	Prolonged	Normal	Prothrombin, V, VII, and X assays
XI	Normal	Prolonged	Normal	VIII, IX, and XI assays
XIII	Normal	Normal	Normal	Factor XIII quantitative assay

PT, Prothrombin time; *PTT*, partial thromboplastin time; *TCT*, thrombin clotting time.
*Results are valid when no anticoagulants are in use. Results may vary in response to reagent sensitivities.

When hematologists treat a hemophilic patient, they base their factor VIII concentrate dosage calculations on the definition of a unit of factor VIII activity, which is the mean amount present in 1 mL of normal plasma and is synonymous with 100% activity. They further calculate the desired increase after factor VIII concentrate infusion by subtracting the patient's preinfusion factor activity from the target activity level. The desired increase is multiplied by the patient's plasma volume to compute the dosage. The patient's plasma volume may be estimated from blood volume and hematocrit.[108] The blood volume is approximately 65 mL/kg of body weight, and the plasma volume is the plasmacrit (100% − hematocrit %) × blood volume, as in the following formulas:

$$\text{Plasma volume} = \text{weight in kilograms} \times 65 \text{ mL/kg} \times (1 - \text{hematocrit})$$
$$\text{Factor VIII concentrate dose} = \text{plasma volume} \times (\text{target factor VIII level} - \text{initial factor VIII level})$$

This formula is also used in the treatment of VWD. Overdosing seems to confer no thrombotic risk, but it wastes resources. Regardless of the dose administered, laboratory monitoring and close clinical observation are essential to prevent or halt bleeding and its complications. Repeat dosing is done on an 8- to 12-hour schedule reflecting the half-life of factor VIII. The second administration of factor VIII uses half the concentration of the first dose.

Hemophilia A and Factor VIII Inhibitors

Alloantibody inhibitors of factor VIII arise in response to treatment in 30% of patients with severe hemophilia and 3% of those with moderate hemophilia. The laboratory practitioner suspects the presence of an inhibitor when bleeding persists or when the plasma factor VIII activity fails to rise to the target level after appropriate concentrate administration. Most factor VIII inhibitors are immunoglobulin G4, non-complement-fixing, warm-reacting antibodies. It is impossible to predict which patients are likely to develop inhibitors based on genetics, demographics, or the type of concentrate used.[109]

The first step in inhibitor detection is a factor VIII assay. If the factor VIII activity exceeds 30%, no inhibitor is present. If the level is less than 30%, the laboratory practitioner proceeds to mixing studies. When the test plasma from the bleeding patient has a prolonged PTT, it is mixed 1:1 with normal plasma (NP), it is incubated 1 to 2 hours at 37° C, and the PTT of the mixture is measured. If no inhibitor is present, the incubated mixture should produce a PTT result within 10% of the incubated NP PTT. If an inhibitor is present, however, the factor VIII from the normal plasma is partially neutralized, and the mixture's PTT remains prolonged or "uncorrected," presumptive evidence of the inhibitor.

If mixing studies and the therapeutic results suggest the presence of a factor VIII inhibitor, a *Bethesda assay* is used to quantitate the inhibitor. NP with 100% factor activity is mixed at increasing dilutions in a series of tubes with the full-strength patient plasma. Factor VIII assays are performed on each mixture. The operator then compares the results of the various dilutions and expresses the titer as Bethesda units. One Bethesda unit is the reciprocal of the dilution that caused neutralization of 50% of the factor VIII from the NP. The same assay is employed to measure factor VIII inhibitors in acquired hemophilia. Although the complex kinetics of acquired autoantibodies diminishes the accuracy of the results in acquired hemophilia, this method is adequate to monitor therapy.

Hemophilia patients with inhibitors are classified as *low* or *high responders*. Low responders generate inhibitor titers of 5 Bethesda units or lower and their inhibitor titers do not increase significantly following factor VIII administration. High responders generate inhibitor titers that exceed 5 Bethesda units and their antibody titers further rise in response to therapy. Low responders may be managed with raised factor VIII doses alone, whereas high responders may require activated prothrombin complex concentrate such as FEIBA (factor eight inhibitor bypassing activity) to control bleeding plus steroid or immunomodulation therapy to reduce the inhibitor antibody titer. Each laboratory director may choose to maintain a database of hemophilia patients who have inhibitors because previous titers often predict future inhibitor behavior.

Hemophilia A Treatment in Patients with Inhibitors

Every hemophilic patient with an inhibitor needs an individualized treatment plan to control bleeding episodes. Low responders often experience cessation of bleeding upon administration of large doses of factor VIII concentrate and may be so maintained. High responders may gain no benefit from factor VIII concentrates and instead are treated with activated PCC, Autoplex T or FEIBA, which generates thrombin in the presence of factor VIII inhibitors. The activated PCC dosage should not exceed 200 units/kg per day, distributed in two to four injections, because the activated factors may trigger DIC. NovoSeven also bypasses the physiologic factor VIII requirement, because it promotes thrombin formation through the tissue factor pathway.[110] The discussions in this chapter of ACOTS and acquired hemophilia provide additional detail on activated PCC dosages.

Hemophilia B (Factor IX Deficiency)

Hemophilia B, also called *Christmas disease*, totals approximately 14% of hemophilia cases in the United States, although its incidence in India nearly equals that of hemophilia A.[94] Hemophilia B is caused by deficiency of factor IX, one of the vitamin K–dependent serine proteases. Factor IX is a substrate for both factors XIa and VIIa because it is cleaved by either to form dimeric factor IXa (Figure 38-5). Subsequently, factor IXa complexes with factor VIIIa to cleave and activate its substrate, factor X. Factor IX deficiency reduces thrombin production and causes soft tissue bleeding that is indistinguishable from that in hemophilia A. It also is a sex-linked, markedly heterogeneous disorder involving numerous separate mutations resulting in a range of mild to severe bleeding manifestations. Determination of female carrier status is less successful in

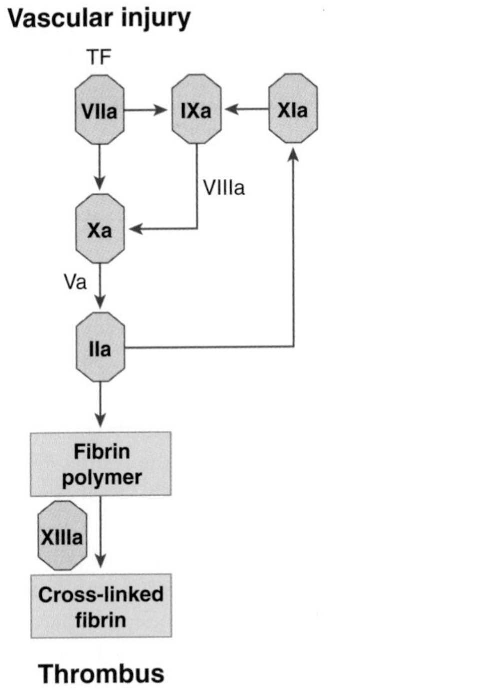

Vascular injury

Figure 38-5 Simplified coagulation cascade mechanism showing positions of all factors whose absence may cause hemorrhage. *TF*, Tissue factor.

hemophilia B than in hemophilia A because of the large number of factor IX mutations and the lack of a linked molecule such as VWF that can be used as a normalization index. DNA analysis occasionally may be used to establish carrier status when hemophilia B has been diagnosed and its specific mutation identified in a relative.

The laboratory is essential to the diagnosis of hemophilia B. The PTT typically is prolonged, whereas the PT is normal. If the clinical symptoms suggest hemophilia B, the factor IX assay should be performed even if PTT is within the reference range, because the PTT reagent may be insensitive to mild factor IX deficiency.

Recombinant or column-purified plasma-derived factor IX concentrates are used to treat hemophilia B. Dosing is calculated the same way as for factor VIII concentrates in hemophilia A and VWD, with the exception that the calculated initial dose is doubled to compensate for factor IX distribution into the extravascular space. Repeat doses of factor IX are given every 24 hours, reflecting the half-life of the factor. The second and subsequent doses, if needed, are half the initial dose, provided that factor assays determine that the target level of factor IX was achieved.

Inhibitors to factor IX arise in only 3% of hemophilia B patients. Anti-factor IX alloantibodies react avidly with factor IX and may be detected using the Bethesda assay. Bleeding in patients with inhibitors is treated as in patients with factor VIII inhibitors using activated PCC or rFVIIa.

Hemophilia C (Rosenthal Syndrome, Factor XI Deficiency)

Factor XI deficiency is an autosomal dominant hemophilia with mild to moderate bleeding symptoms. More than half of the cases have been described in Ashkenazi Jews, but individuals of any ethnic group may be affected. The frequency and severity of bleeding episodes do not correlate with factor XI levels, and laboratory monitoring of treatment serves little purpose after the diagnosis is established. The physician treats hemophilia C with frequent plasma infusions during times of hemostatic challenge.[111] In the laboratory, the PTT is prolonged and the PT is normal.

Other Congenital Single-Factor Deficiencies

The remaining congenital single-factor deficiencies listed in Table 38-8 are rare, are caused by autosomal recessive mutations, and are often associated with consanguinity. The PT, PTT, and thrombin time may be employed to distinguish among these disorders, as shown in Table 38-7. In addition, immunoassays may be performed to distinguish among the more prevalent quantitative and the less prevalent qualitative abnormalities. In qualitative disorders, often called *dysproteinemias*,

TABLE 38-8 Rare Congenital Single-Factor Deficiencies

Deficiency	Factor Levels	Symptoms	Therapy
Afibrinogenemia	No measurable fibrinogen	Severe anatomic bleeding	CRYO or fibrinogen concentrate to raise to >100 mg/dL
Hypofibrinogenemia	Fibrinogen activity assay <100 mg/dL	Moderate systemic bleeding	
Dysfibrinogenemia	Fibrinogen activity assay <100 mg/dL	Mild systemic bleeding	
Prothrombin deficiency	Factor II <30%	Mild systemic bleeding	PCC or plasma to raise to 75%
Factor V deficiency	Factor V <30%	Mild systemic bleeding	Plasma to raise to 75%
Factor VII deficiency	Factor VII <30%	Moderate to severe anatomic bleeding	NovoSeven, PCC, four-factor PCC, plasma
Factor X deficiency	Factor X <30%	Severe anatomic bleeding	PCC or plasma to raise to 75%
Factor XI deficiency	Factor XI <50%	Anatomic bleeding	Plasma to raise to 75%
Factor XIII deficiency	Factor XIII <1%	Moderate to severe systemic bleeding, poor wound healing	Plasma or CRYO every 3 weeks

CRYO, Cryoprecipitate; *PCC*, prothrombin complex concentrate.

the ratio of factor activity to antigen is less than 0.7. The bleeding symptoms in the dysproteinemias may be more severe than in quantitative deficiencies, but the risk of inhibitor formation is theoretically lower. The clot-based measurement of factors II (prothrombin) and X may be supplemented or replaced by more reproducible chromogenic substrate assays. Fibrinogen is usually measured using the Clauss clot-based assay, a modification of the thrombin time, but it also may be measured by turbidimetry or immunoassay.

Because platelets transport about 20% of circulating factor V, the platelet function in *factor V deficiency* may be diminished, which is reflected in a prolonged bleeding time but normal platelet aggregation.[112] The PT and PTT are prolonged. Because of the concentration of factor V in platelet α-granules, normal platelet concentrate is an effective form of therapy for factor V deficiency. A combined factor V and VIII deficiency may be caused by a genetic defect traced to chromosome 18 that affects transport of both factors by a common protein in the Golgi apparatus.[113]

Factor VII deficiency causes moderate to severe anatomic hemorrhage. The bleeding does not necessarily reflect the factor VII activity level. The half-life of factor VII is approximately 6 hours, which affects the frequency of therapy. NovoSeven at 30 µg/mL and nonactivated four-factor PCC preparations are effective and may provide a target factor VII level of 10% to 30%. Many factor VII deficiencies are dysproteinemias.[114] The PT, but not the PTT, is prolonged in factor VII deficiency.

Factor X deficiency causes moderate to severe anatomic hemorrhage that may be treated with plasma or nonactivated PCC to produce therapeutic levels of 10% to 40%.[115] The half-life of factor X is 24 to 40 hours. Acquired factor X deficiency has been described in amyloidosis, in paraproteinemia, and in association with antifungal drug therapy. The hemorrhagic symptoms may be life-threatening. The PT and PTT are both prolonged in factor X deficiency. In the *Russell viper venom time* test, which activates the coagulation mechanism at the level of

factor X, clotting time is prolonged in deficiencies of factors X and V, prothrombin, and fibrinogen. The venom used is harvested from the Russell viper, the most dangerous snake in Asia. This test may be useful in distinguishing a factor VII deficiency, which does not affect the results, from deficiencies in the common pathway, although specific factor assays are the standard approach.

Plasma factor XIII is a tetramer of paired α and β monomers. The intracellular form is a homodimer (two α chains) and is stored in platelets, monocytes, placenta, prostate, and uterus. The α chain contains the active enzyme site, and the β chain is a binding and stabilizing portion. Factor XIII deficiency occurs in three forms related to the affected chain, as shown in Table 38-9. Patients with factor XIII deficiency have a normal PT, PTT, and thrombin time despite anatomic bleeds and poor wound healing. They form weak (non-cross-linked) clots that dissolve within 2 hours when suspended in a 5-M urea solution, a traditional factor XIII screening assay.[116] To confirm factor XIII deficiency, factor activity may be measured accurately using a chromogenic substrate assay such as the Behring Behrichrom FXIII assay (Behring Diagnostics, King of Prussia, PA).

Finally, autosomally inherited deficiencies of the fibrinolytic regulatory proteins α₂-antiplasmin and plasminogen activator inhibitor-1 (PAI-1) have been reported to cause moderate to severe bleeding. Both are rare and may be diagnosed using chromogenic substrate assays.

TABLE 38-9   Factor XIII Deficiency

Type of Deficiency	Incidence	Factor XIII Activity	β-Protein	α-Protein
Type I	Rare	Absent	Absent	Absent
Type II	Frequent	Absent	Normal	Low
Type III	Rare	Low	Absent	Low

SUMMARY

- Hemorrhage is classified as localized versus generalized, acquired versus congenital, and anatomic soft tissue hemorrhage versus systemic mucocutaneous hemorrhage.
- Acquired hemorrhagic disorders that are diagnosed in the hemostasis laboratory include thrombocytopenia of various etiologies (Chapter 40), the acute coagulopathy of trauma-shock, liver and renal disease, vitamin K deficiency, acquired hemophilia or VWD, and DIC.
- VWD is the most common congenital bleeding disorder, and the diagnosis and classification of the type and subtypes require a series of clinical laboratory assays.

- The hemophilias are congenital single-factor deficiencies that cause moderate to severe anatomic hemorrhage. The clinical laboratory plays a key role in diagnosis, classification, and treatment monitoring in hemophilia.

Now that you have completed this chapter, go back and read again the case study at the beginning and respond to the questions presented.

REVIEW QUESTIONS

Answers can be found in the Appendix.

1. What is the most common acquired bleeding disorder?
   a. Vitamin K deficiency
   b. Liver disease
   c. ACOTS
   d. VWD

2. Which is a typical form of anatomic bleeding?
   a. Epistaxis
   b. Menorrhagia
   c. Hematemesis
   d. Soft tissue bleed

3. What factor deficiency has the speediest effect on the prothrombin time?
   a. Prothrombin deficiency
   b. Factor VII deficiency
   c. Factor VIII deficiency
   d. Factor IX deficiency

4. Which of the following conditions causes a prolonged thrombin time?
   a. Antithrombin deficiency
   b. Prothrombin deficiency
   c. Hypofibrinogenemia
   d. Warfarin therapy

5. In what subtype of VWD is the RIPA test result positive when ristocetin is used at a concentration of less than 0.5 mg/mL?
   a. Subtype 2A
   b. Subtype 2B
   c. Subtype 2N
   d. Type 3

6. What is the typical treatment for vitamin K deficiency when the patient is bleeding?
   a. Vitamin K and PCC
   b. Vitamin K and plasma
   c. Vitamin K and platelet concentrate
   d. Vitamin K and factor VIII concentrate

7. If a patient has anatomic soft tissue bleeding and poor wound healing, but the PT, PTT, thrombin time, platelet count, and platelet functional assay results are normal, what factor deficiency is indicated?
   a. Fibrinogen
   b. Prothrombin
   c. Factor XII
   d. Factor XIII

8. What therapy may be used for a hemophilic boy who is bleeding and who has a high titer of factor VIII inhibitor?
   a. rFVIIa
   b. Plasma
   c. Cryoprecipitate
   d. Factor VIII concentrate

9. What is the most prevalent form of VWD?
   a. Type 1
   b. Type 2A
   c. Type 2B
   d. Type 3

10. Which of the following assays is used to distinguish vitamin K deficiency from liver disease?
    a. PT
    b. Protein C assay
    c. Factor V assay
    d. Factor VII assay

11. Mucocutaneous hemorrhage is typical of:
    a. Acquired hemorrhagic disorders
    b. Localized hemorrhagic disorders
    c. Defects in primary hemostasis
    d. Defects in fibrinolysis

REFERENCES

1. Kessler, C. M. (2013). A systematic approach to the bleeding patient: correlation of clinical symptoms and signs with laboratory testing. In Kitchens, C. S., Kessler, C. M., Konkle, B. A., (Eds.), *Consultative Hemostasis and Thrombosis.* (3rd ed., pp. 16–32). St Louis: Elsevier-Saunders.
2. Kitchens, C. S. (2013). Purpura and other hematovascular disorders. In Kitchens, C. S., Kessler, C. M., & Konkle, B. A., (Eds.), *Consultative Hemostasis and Thrombosis.* (3rd ed., pp. 150–173). St Louis: Elsevier-Saunders.
3. Weiss, A. E. (1988). Acquired coagulation disorders. In Corriveau, D. M., & Fritsma, G. A., (Eds.), *Hemostasis and Thrombosis in the Clinical Laboratory* (pp. 169–205). Philadelphia: Lippincott.
4. Vanderhave, K. L., Caird, M. S., Hake, M., et al. (2012). Musculoskeletal care of the hemophiliac patient. *J Am Acad Orthop Surg, 20,* 553–563.
5. Funk, D. M. (2012). Coagulation assays and anticoagulant monitoring. *Hematology Am Soc Hematol Educ Program, 2012,* 460–465.

6. Shore-Lesserson, L., Manspeizer, H. E., DePerio, M., et al. (1999). Thromboelastography-guided transfusion algorithm reduces transfusions in complex cardiac surgery. *Anesth Analg, 88,* 312–319.

7. Chee, Y. L., Crawford, J. C., Watson, H. G., & Greaves, M. (2008). Guidelines on the assessment of bleeding risk prior to surgery or invasive procedures. British Committee for Standards in Haematology. *Br J Haematol, 140,* 496–504.

8. Fogarty, P. F., & Kessler, C. M. (2013). Hemophilia A and B. In Kitchens, C. S., Kessler, C. M., & Konkle, B. A., (Eds.), *Consultative Hemostasis and Thrombosis.* (3rd ed., pp. 45–59). St Louis: Elsevier-Saunders.

9. Boffard, K. D., Choog, P. I. T., Kloger, Y., et al. (2009). The treatment of bleeding is to stop the bleeding! Treatment of trauma-related hemorrhage. On behalf of the NovoSeven Trauma Study Group. *Transfusion, 49,* 240S–247S.

10. Go, A. S., Mozaffarian, D., Roger, V. L. et al. (2014). Heart disease and stroke statistics—2014 update: a report from the American Heart Association. *Circulation, 129,* e28–e292.

11. Duchesne, J. C., & Holcomb, J. B. (2009). Damage control resuscitation: addressing trauma-induced coagulopathy. *Br J Hosp Med (Lond), 70,* 22–25.

12. Holcomb, J. B., & Pati, S. (2013). Optimal trauma resuscitation with plasma as the primary resuscitative fluid: the surgeon's perspective. *Am Soc Hematol Educ Program, 2013,* 656–659.

13. Shakur, H., Roberts, I., Bautista, R., et al. (2010). CRASH-2 Trial Collaborators: Effects of tranexamic acid on death, vascular occlusive events, and blood transfusion in trauma patients with significant haemorrhage (CRASH-2): a randomised, placebo-controlled trial. *Lancet, 376* (9734). 23–32.

14. American Society of Anesthesiologists Task Force. (2006). Practice guidelines for perioperative blood transfusion and adjuvant therapies: an updated report by the American Society of Anesthesiologists Task Force on Perioperative Blood Transfusion and Adjuvant Therapies. *Anesthesiology, 105,* 198–208.

15. Lu, F. Q., Kang, W., Peng, Y., & Wang, W. M. (2011). Characterization of blood components separated from donated whole blood after an overnight holding at room temperature with the buffy coat method. *Transfusion, 51,* 2199–2207.

16. Benjamin, R. J., & McLaughlin, L. S. (2012). Plasma components: properties, differences, and uses. *Transfusion, 52*(Suppl. 1), 9S–19S.

17. Borgman, M. A., Spinella, P. C., Perkins, J. G., et al. (2007). The ratio of blood products transfused affect mortality in patients receiving massive transfusions in a combat support hospital. *J Trauma, 63,* 805–813.

18. McLaughlin, D. F., Niles, S. E., Salinas, J., et al. (2008). A predictive model for massive transfusion in combat casualty patients. *J Trauma, 64,* S57–S63.

19. Narick, C., Triulzi, D. J., & Yazer, M. H. (2012). Transfusion-associated circulatory overload after plasma transfusion. *Transfusion, 52,* 160–165.

20. Middelburg, R. A., van Stein, D., Briët, E., & van der Bom, J. G. (2008). The role of donor antibodies in the pathogenesis of transfusion-related acute lung injury: a systematic review. *Transfusion, 48,* 2167–2176.

21. Vostal, J. G. (2006). Efficacy evaluation of current and future platelet transfusion products. *J Trauma, 60*(Suppl. 6), S78–S82.

22. Duchesne, J. C., & Holcomb, J. B. (2009). Damage control resuscitation: addressing trauma-induced coagulopathy. *Br J Hosp Med (Lond), 70,* 22-25.

23. Wójcik, C., Schymik, M. L., & Cure, E. G. (2009). Activated prothrombin complex concentrate factor VIII inhibitor bypassing activity (FEIBA) for the reversal of warfarin-induced coagulopathy. *Int J Emerg Med, 2,* 217–225.

24. Ferreira, J., & DeLosSantos, M. (2013). The clinical use of prothrombin complex concentrate. *J Emerg Med, 44,* 1201–1210.

25. Quinlan, D. J., Eikelboom, J. W., & Weitz, J. I. (2013). Four-factor prothrombin complex concentrate for urgent reversal of vitamin K antagonists in patients with major bleeding. *Circulation, 128,* 1179–1181.

26. CRASH-2 trial collaborators. (2010). Effects of tranexamic acid on death, vascular occlusive events, and blood transfusion in trauma patients with significant haemorrhage (CRASH-2): a randomised, placebo-controlled trial. *The Lancet, 376,* 23–32.

27. Napolitano, L. M., Cohen, M. J., Cotton, B. A., Schreiber, M. A., & Moore, E. E. (2013). Tranexamic acid in trauma: how should we use it? *J Trauma Acute Care Surg, 74,* 1575–1586.

28. Wikkelsø, A., Lunde, J., Johansen, M., et al. (2013). Fibrinogen concentrate in bleeding patients. *Cochrane Database Syst Rev, 8.* doi:10.1002/14651858.CD008864.pub2.

29. Kakaiya, R., Aronson, C. A., & Julleis, J. (2008). Whole blood collection and component procession. In Roback, J. D., Combs, M. R., Grossma, B. J., et al., (Eds.), *Technical Manual.* (16th ed.). Bethesda MD: AABB.

30. Downes, K. A., Wilson, E., Yomtovian, R., et al. (2001). Serial measurement of clotting factors in thawed plasma stored for five days. *Transfusion, 41,* 570 (letter).

31. Hedner, U., Lee, C. A. (2011). First 20 years with recombinant FVIIa (NovoSeven). *Haemophilia, 17,* e172–e182.

32. Levi, M., Peters, M., & Buller, H. R. (2005). Efficacy and safety of recombinant factor VIIa for treatment of severe bleeding: a systematic review. *Crit Care Med, 33,* 883–890.

33. Tatoulis, J., Theodore, S., Meswani, M., et al. (2009). Safe use of recombinant activated factor VIIa for recalcitrant postoperative haemorrhage in cardiac surgery. *Interact Cardiovasc Thorac Surg, 9,* 459–462.

34. O'Connell, K. A., Wood, J. J., Wise, R. P., et al. (2006). Thromboembolic adverse events after use of recombinant human coagulation factor VIIa. *JAMA, 295,* 293–298.

35. da Luz, L. T., Nascimento, B., & Rizoli, S. (2013). Thrombelastography (TEG®): practical considerations on its clinical use in trauma resuscitation. *Scand J Trauma Resusc Emerg Med, 21,* 29. doi:10.1186/1757-7241-21-29.

36. Robert, A., & Chazouilleres, O. (1996). Prothrombin time in liver failure: time, ratio, activity percentage, or international normalized ratio? *Hepatology, 24,* 1392–1394.

37. Lisman, T., & Porte, R. J. (2013). Understanding and managing the coagulopathy of liver disease. In Kitchens, C. S., Kessler, C. M., & Konkle, B. A., (Eds.), *Consultative Hemostasis and Thrombosis.* (3rd ed., pp. 688–697). St Louis: Elsevier-Saunders.

38. Ratnoff, O. D. (1996). Hemostatic defects in liver and biliary tract disease and disorders of vitamin K metabolism. In Ratnoff, O. D., & Forbes, C. D., (Eds.), *Disorders of Hemostasis.* (3rd ed., pp. 422–442). Philadelphia: Saunders.

39. Lisman, T., Leebeek, F. W., & de Groot, P. G. (2002). Haemostatic abnormalities in patients with liver disease. *J Hepatol, 37,* 280–287.

40. Ferro, D., Quintarelli, C., Lattuada, A., et al. (1996). High plasma levels of von Willebrand factor as a marker of endothelial perturbation in cirrhosis: relationship to endotoxemia. *Hepatology 23,* 1377–1383.

41. Hollestelle, M. J., Geertzen, H. G., Straatsburg, J. H., et al. (2004). Factor VIII expression in liver disease. *Thromb Haemost, 91,* 267–275.

42. Fouad, Y. M. (2013). Chronic hepatitis C-associated thrombocytopenia: aetiology and management. *Trop Gastroenterol, 34,* 58–67.

43. Younger, H. M., Hadoke, P. W., Dillon, J. F., et al. (1997). Platelet function in cirrhosis and the role of humoral factors. *Eur J Gastroenterol Hepatol, 9,* 982–992.

44. Bates, S. M. (2012). D-dimer assays in diagnosis and management of thrombotic and bleeding disorders. *Semin Thromb Hemost, 38,* 673–682.

45. Wiedermann, C. J., & Kaneider, N. C. (2006). A systematic review of antithrombin concentrate use in patients with

disseminated intravascular coagulation of severe sepsis. *Blood Coagul Fibrinolysis, 17,* 521–526.

46. Cunningham, M. T., Brandt, J. T., Laposata, M., & Olson, J. D. (2002). Laboratory diagnosis of dysfibrinogenemia. *Arch Pathol Lab Med, 126,* 499–505.

47. Saito, H. (1996). Alterations of hemostasis in renal disease. In Ratnoff, O. D., & Forbes, C. D., (Eds.), *Disorders of Hemostasis.* (3rd ed., pp. 443–456). Philadelphia: Saunders.

48. Cohen, B. D. (2003). Methyl group deficiency and guanidino production in uremia. *Mol Cell Biochem, 244,* 31–36.

49. Galbusera, M., Remuzzi, G., & Boccardo, P. (2009). Treatment of bleeding in dialysis patients. *Semin Dial, 22,* 279–286.

50. Kahan, B. D. (2008). Fifteen years of clinical studies and clinical practice in renal transplantation: reviewing outcomes with de novo use of sirolimus in combination with cyclosporine. *Transplant Proc, 40,* S17–S20.

51. Leng, S. X., & Elias, J. A. (1997). Interleukin-11. *Int J Biochem Cell Biol, 29,* 1059–1062.

52. Wadhwa, M., & Thorpe, R. (2008). Haematopoietic growth factors and their therapeutic use. *Thromb Haemost, 99,* 863–873.

53. Ambuhl, P. M., Wuthrich, R. P., Korte, W., et al. (1997). Plasma hypercoagulability in haemodialysis patients: impact of dialysis and anticoagulation. *Nephrol Dial Transplant, 12,* 2355–2364.

54. Lind, S. E. (1991). The bleeding time does not predict surgical bleeding. *Blood, 77,* 2547–2552.

55. Brunzel, N. A. (2002). Renal and metabolic disease. In *Fundamentals of Urine and Body Fluid Analysis.* (2nd ed., pp. 271–310). Philadelphia: Saunders.

56. Knehtl, M., Ponikvar, R., & Buturovic-Ponikvar, J. (2013). Platelet-related hemostasis before and after hemodialysis with five different anticoagulation methods. *Int J Artif Organs, 36,* 717–724.

57. Daugirdas, J. T., & Bernardo, A. A. (2012). Hemodialysis effect on platelet count and function and hemodialysis-associated thrombocytopenia. *Kidney Int, 82,* 147–157.

58. Torres, V. E. (2008). Vasopressin antagonists in polycystic kidney disease. *Semin Nephrol, 28,* 306–317.

59. Khanna, R. (2011). Clinical presentation and management of glomerular diseases: hematuria, nephritic and nephrotic syndrome. *Mo Med, 108,* 33–36.

60. Bolan, C. D., & Klein, H. G. (2013). Blood component and pharmacologic therapy for hemostatic disorders. In Kitchens, C. S., Kessler, C. M., & Konkle, B. A., (Eds.), *Consultative Hemostasis and Thrombosis.* (3rd ed., pp. 496–525). St Louis: Elsevier-Saunders.

61. Burke, C. W. (2013). Vitamin K deficiency bleeding: overview and considerations. *J Pediatr Health Care, 27,* 215–221.

62. Patriquin, C., & Crowther, M. (2013). Antithrombotic agents. In Kitchens, C. S., Kessler, C. M., & Konkle, B. A., (Eds.), *Consultative Hemostasis and Thrombosis.* (3rd ed., pp. 477–495). St Louis: Elsevier-Saunders.

63. Misra, D., Bednar, M., Cromwell, C., et al. (2010). Manifestations of superwarfarin ingestion: a plea to increase awareness. *Am J Hematol, 85,* 391–392.

64. Kershaw, G., Jayakodi, D., & Dunkley, S. (2009). Laboratory identification of factor inhibitors: the perspective of a large tertiary hemophilia center. *Semin Thromb Hemost, 35,* 760–768.

65. Franchini, M., & Mannucci, P. M. (2013). Acquired haemophilia A: a 2013 update. *Thromb Haemost, 110,* 111–120.

66. Biggs, R., Austen, D. E. G., Denson, D. W. E., et al. (1972). The mode of action of antibodies which destroy factor VIII: II. Antibodies which give complex concentration graphs. *Br J Haematol, 23,* 137–155.

67. Miesbach, W., Matthias, T., & Scharrer, I. (2005). Identification of thrombin antibodies in patients with antiphospholipid syndrome. *Ann NY Acad Sci, 1050,* 250–256.

68. Krumdieck, R., Shaw, D. R., Huang, S. T., et al. (1991). Hemorrhagic disorder due to an isoniazid-associated acquired factor XIII inhibitor in a patient with Waldenström's macroglobulinemia. *Am J Med, 90,* 639–645.

69. Shapiro, S. S., & Hultin, M. (1975). Acquired inhibitors to the blood coagulation factors. *Semin Thromb Hemost, 1,* 336–385.

70. Bowman, L. J., Anderson, C. D., & Chapman, W. C. (2010). Topical recombinant human thrombin in surgical hemostasis. *Semin Thromb Hemost, 36,* 477–484.

71. Barker, B., Altuntas, F., Paranjape, G., et al. (2004). Presurgical plasma exchange is ineffective in correcting amyloid associated factor X deficiency. *J Clin Apheresis, 19,* 208–210.

72. von Depka, M. (2004). Immune tolerance therapy in patients with acquired hemophilia. *Hematology, 9,* 245–257.

73. Federici, A. B. (2011). Acquired von Willebrand syndrome associated with hypothyroidism: a mild bleeding disorder to be further investigated. *Semin Thromb Hemost, 37,* 35–40.

74. Franchini, M., & Lippi, G. (2007). Acquired von Willebrand syndrome: an update. *Am J Hematol, 82,* 368–375.

75. National Heart, Lung, and Blood Institute. (2009). *The Diagnosis, Evaluation, and Management of Von Willebrand Disease.* NIH Publication No. 08-5832, Bethesda, MD: US Department of Health and Human Services, National Institutes of Health.

76. James, A. H., Manco-Johnson, M. J., Yawn, B. P., et al. (2009). Von Willebrand disease: key points from the 2008 National Heart, Lung, and Blood Institute guidelines. *Obstet Gynecol, 114,* 674–678.

77. Lenting, P. J., Casari, C., Christophe, O. D., Denis, C. V. (2012). Von Willebrand factor: the old, the new and the unknown. *J Thromb Haemost, 10,* 2428–2437.

78. Schneppenheim, R., & Budde, U. (2011). Von Willebrand factor: the complex molecular genetics of a multidomain and multifunctional protein. *J Thromb Haemost, 9*(Suppl. 1), 209–215.

79. Lee, C. A., Abdul-Kadir, R. (2005). Von Willebrand disease and women's health. *Semin Hematol, 42,* 42–48.

80. Rick, M. E., & Konkle, B. A. (2013). Von Willebrand disease. In Kitchens, C. S., Kessler, C. M., & Konkle, B. A., (Eds.), *Consultative Hemostasis and Thrombosis.* (3rd ed., pp. 90–102). St Louis: Elsevier-Saunders.

81. Sadler, J. E., Rodeghiero, F., on behalf of the ISTH SSC Subcommittee on von Willebrand Factor. (2005). Provisional criteria for the diagnosis of VWD type 1. *J Thromb Haemost, 3,* 775–777.

82. Schneppenheim, R., & Budde, U. (2005). Phenotypic and genotypic diagnosis of von Willebrand disease: a 2004 update. *Semin Hematol, 42,* 15–28.

83. Gill, J. C., Endres-Brooks, J., Bauer, P. J., et al. (1987). The effect of ABO blood group on the diagnosis of von Willebrand disease. *Blood, 69,* 1691–1695.

84. Favaloro, E. J. (2008). Clinical utility of the PFA-100. *Semin Thromb Hemost, 34,* 709–733.

85. Favaloro, E. J., Bonar, R., Kershaw, G., et al. (2005). Royal College of Pathologists of Australasia Quality Assurance Program in Haematology: Laboratory diagnosis of von Willebrand disorder: use of multiple functional assays reduces diagnostic error rates. *Lab Hematol, 11,* 91–97.

86. Hayes, T. E., Brandt, J. T., Chandler, W. L., et al. (2006). External peer review quality assurance testing in von Willebrand disease: the recent experience of the United States College of American Pathologists proficiency testing program. *Semin Thromb Hemost, 32,* 499–504.

87. Favaloro, E. J., Kershaw, G., McLachlan, A. J., et al. (2007). Time to think outside the box? Proposals for a new approach to future pharmacokinetic studies of von Willebrand factor concentrates in people with von Willebrand disease. *Semin Thromb Hemost, 33,* 745–758.

88. Favaloro, E. J., Bonar, R., Kershaw, G., et al. (2006). Reducing errors in identification of von Willebrand disease: the experience of the Royal College of Pathologists of Australasia quality assurance program. *Semin Thromb Hemost, 32,* 505–513.

89. Rodeghiero, F., & Castaman, G. (2005). Treatment of von Willebrand disease. *Semin Hematol, 42,* 29–35.

90. Favaloro, E. J. (2007). An update on the von Willebrand factor collagen binding assay: 21 years of age and beyond adolescence but not yet a mature adult. *Semin Thromb Hemost, 33,* 727–744.

91. Chandler, W. L., Peerschke, E. I. B., Castellone, D. D., Meijer, P., on behalf of the NASCOLA Proficiency Testing Committee. (2011). Von Willebrand factor assay proficiency testing. The North American Specialized Coagulation Laboratory Association Experience. *Am J Clin Pathol, 135,* 862–869.

92. Berntorp, E., & Windyga, J. (2009). European Wilate Study Group: Treatment and prevention of acute bleedings in von Willebrand disease—efficacy and safety of Wilate, a new generation von Willebrand factor/factor VIII concentrate. *Haemophilia, 15,* 122–130.

93. Batlle, J., López-Fernández, M. F., Fraga, E. L., Trillo, A. R., Pérez-Rodríguez, M. A. (2009). Von Willebrand factor/factor VIII concentrates in the treatment of von Willebrand disease. *Blood Coagul Fibrinolysis, 20,* 89–100.

94. Fogarty, P. F., & Kessler, C. M. (2013). Hemophilia A and B. In Kitchens, C. S., Kessler, C. M., Konkle, B. A., (Eds.), *Consultative Hemostasis and Thrombosis.* (3rd ed., pp. 45–59). St Louis: Elsevier-Saunders.

95. Thompson, A. R. (2003). Structure and function of the factor VIII gene and protein. *Semin Thromb Hemost, 29,* 11–22.

96. Rossetti, L. C., Radic, C. P., Larripa, I. B., et al. (2005). Genotyping the hemophilia inversion hotspot by use of inverse PCR. *Clin Chem, 51,* 1154–1158.

97. Weiss, A. E. (1988). The hemophilias. In Corriveau, D. M., Fritsma, G. A., (Eds.), *Hemostasis and Thrombosis in the Clinical Laboratory* (pp. 128–168) Philadelphia: JB Lippincott.

98. Peake, I. R., Lillicrap, D. P., Boulyjenkov, V., et al. (1993). Hemophilia: strategies for carrier detection and prenatal diagnosis. *Bull World Health Org, 71,* 429–458.

99. Lusher, J. M., & Warrier, I. (1992). Hemophilia A. *Hematol Oncol Clin North Am, 6,* 1021–1033.

100. Evatt, B. L. (2005). Demographics of hemophilia in developing countries. *Semin Thromb Hemost, 31,* 489–494.

101. Evatt, B. L. (2006). The tragic history of AIDS in the hemophilia population, 1982-1984. *J Thromb Haemost, 4,* 2295–2301.

102. Gringeri, A., Lundin, V., von Mackensen, S., et al. (2009). Primary and secondary prophylaxis in children with haemophilia A reduces bleeding frequency and arthropathy development compared to on demand treatment; a 10-year, randomized clinical trial. *J Thromb Haemost, 7,* 780–786.

103. Schobess, R., Kurnik, K., Friedrichs, F., et al. (2008). Effects of primary and secondary prophylaxis on the clinical expression of joint damage in children with severe haemophilia A. Results of a multicenter non-concurrent cohort study. *Thromb Haemost, 99,* 71–76.

104. Bray, G. L., Gomperts, E. D., Courter, S., et al. (1994). A multicenter study of recombinant factor VIII (Recombinate): safety, efficacy, and inhibitor risk in previously untreated patients with hemophilia A. *Blood, 83,* 2428–2437.

105. Lusher, J. M., Arkin, S., Abildgaard, C. F., et al. (1993). Recombinant factor VIII for the treatment of previously untreated patients with hemophilia A. *N Engl J Med, 328,* 453–457.

106. Gröner, A. (2008). Pathogen safety of plasma-derived products—Haemate P/Humate-P. *Haemophilia, 14*(Suppl. 5), 54–71.

107. Kessler, C. M., Gill, J. C., White, G. C., et al. (2005). B-domain deleted recombinant factor VIII preparations are bioequivalent to a monoclonal antibody purified plasma-derived factor VIII concentrate: a randomized, three-way crossover study. *Haemophilia, 11,* 84–91.

108. Marques, M. B., & Fritsma, G. A. (2009). *Quick Guide to Coagulation Testing.* (2nd ed., p. 57). Washington, DC: American Association for Clinical Chemistry Press.

109. Franchini, M., Lippi, G., & Favaloro, E. J. (2012). Acquired inhibitors of coagulation factors: part II. *Semin Thromb Hemost, 38,* 447–453.

110. Franchini, M., Zaffanello, M., & Veneri, D. (2005). Recombinant factor VIIa: an update on its clinical use. *Thromb Haemost, 93,* 1027–1035.

111. Duga, S., & Salomon, O. (2013). Congenital factor XI deficiency: an update. *Semin Thromb Hemost, 39,* 621–631.

112. Miletich, J. P., Majerus, D. W., & Majerus, P. W. (1978). Patients with congenital factor V deficiency have decreased factor Xa binding sites on their platelets. *J Clin Invest, 62,* 824–831.

113. Nichols, W. C., Seligsohn, U., Zivelin, A., et al. (1997). Linkage of combined factors V and VIII deficiency to chromosome 18q by homozygosity mapping. *J Clin Invest, 99,* 596–601.

114. Mariani, G., & Bernardi, F. (2009). Factor VII deficiency. *Semin Thromb Hemost, 35,* 400–406.

115. Menegatti, M., & Peyvandi, F. (2009). Factor X deficiency. *Semin Thromb Hemost, 35,* 407–415.

116. Jenning, I., Kitchen, S., Woods, T. A. L., et al. (2003). Problems relating to the laboratory diagnosis of factor XIII deficiency: a UKNEQAS study. *J Thromb Haemost, 1,* 2603–2608.

Thrombotic Disorders and Laboratory Assessment

39

George A. Fritsma*

OBJECTIVES

After completion of this chapter, the reader will be able to:

1. Describe the prevalence of thrombotic disease in developed countries.
2. Define thrombophilia.
3. Distinguish between venous and arterial thrombosis.
4. Differentiate among acquired thrombosis risk factors related to lifestyle and disease, and congenital risk factors, listing which factors can be assessed in the hemostasis laboratory.
5. Discuss the frequency with which the heritable risk factors occur in various ethnic groups.
6. Offer a sequence of lupus anticoagulant antibody tests that provides the greatest diagnostic validity and interpret the results of the tests.
7. Describe the relevance of antithrombin assays, proteins C and S assays, activated protein C resistance, the factor V Leiden assay, and the prothrombin G20210A assay to assess venous thrombotic risk.
8. Describe the relevance of the tests for high-sensitivity C-reactive protein, homocysteine, fibrinogen, and lipoprotein (a) to assess arterial thrombotic risk.
9. Describe the causes and pathophysiology of disseminated intravascular coagulation (DIC).
10. Describe the assays comprising a primary test profile for diagnosis and management of DIC in an acute care facility.
11. Discuss the value of quantitative D-dimer assays.
12. Describe the cause and clinical significance of heparin-induced thrombocytopenia.
13. Describe the clinical diagnosis, laboratory diagnosis, and management of heparin-induced thrombocytopenia.

CASE STUDY

After studying the material in this chapter, the reader should be able to respond to the following case study:

A 42-year-old woman with no significant medical history developed sudden onset of shortness of breath and chest pain. She was taken to an emergency department, where a pulmonary embolism was diagnosed. After admission, she was treated with intravenous heparin and given a hypercoagulability workup.
1. For what conditions can the woman be tested while she is in the hospital?
2. List possible acquired risk factors for thrombosis that need to be excluded in this patient.
3. What would be the implications of diagnosing a congenital risk factor for thrombosis in this patient?

---

*The author acknowledges the substantial contributions of Marisa B. Marques, MD, to Chapter 42 of the third edition of this textbook, many of which continue in this edition.

DEVELOPMENTS IN THROMBOSIS RISK TESTING

Before 1992, medical laboratory professionals performed assays to detect only three inherited venous thrombosis risk factors: deficiencies of the coagulation control factors *antithrombin, protein C,* and *protein S*.[1] Taken together, these three deficiencies accounted for no more than 7% of cases of recurrent venous thromboembolic disease and bore no relationship to arterial thrombosis. Since the report by Dahlback and colleagues[2] of *activated protein C (APC) resistance* in 1993 and the characterization by Bertina and colleagues[3] of the *factor V. Leiden* (FVL) mutation as its cause in 1994, efforts devoted to thrombosis prediction and evaluation have redefined the hemostasis laboratory and increased its workload exponentially. The list of current assays includes *antithrombin, protein C, protein S, APC resistance, FVL mutation, prothrombin G20210A mutation, lupus anticoagulant (LA),* and several additional markers of both venous and arterial thrombotic disease described in this chapter. Technical improvements have enhanced the diagnostic efficacy of integrated LA detection kits, the quantitative D-dimer assay, and tests for localized coagulation activation markers such as *prothrombin fragment 1+2* (PF 1+2, PF 1.2) and *thrombin-antithrombin* (TAT) complex.[4]

ETIOLOGY AND PREVALENCE OF THROMBOSIS

Thrombosis Etiology

Thrombosis is a multifaceted disorder resulting from abnormalities in blood flow, such as stasis, and abnormalities in the coagulation system, platelet function, leukocyte activation molecules, and the blood vessel wall. Thrombosis is the inappropriate formation of platelet or fibrin clots that obstruct blood vessels. These obstructions cause *ischemia* (loss of blood supply) and *necrosis* (tissue death).[5]

Thrombophilia (once called *hypercoagulability*) is defined as the predisposition to thrombosis secondary to a congenital or acquired disorder. The theoretical causes of thrombophilia are the following:

- Physical, chemical, or biologic events such as chronic or acute inflammation that release prothrombotic mediators from damaged blood vessels or suppress blood vessel production of normal antithrombotic substances
- Inappropriate and uncontrolled platelet activation
- Uncontrolled blood coagulation system activation
- Uncontrolled fibrinolysis suppression

Prevalence of Thrombosis

From 2000 to 2010, the U.S. death rate attributable to venous and arterial thrombotic disease declined 31%, and the number of thrombosis-related deaths declined by 17% per year. Yet, in 2010 thrombosis accounted for one of every three deaths in the United States. Of these, 25% of initial thrombotic events were fatal, and many fatal thromboses went undiagnosed before autopsy.[6]

Prevalence of Venous Thromboembolic Disease

The annual incidence of venous thromboembolic disease (or *venous thromboembolic events,* VTE) in the unselected U.S. population has remained constant for at least 25 years at 1 in 1000 and is more prevalent in African Americans and in women of childbearing age.[7,8] The most prevalent VTE is *deep vein thrombosis,* caused by clots that form in the iliac, popliteal, and femoral veins of the calves and upper legs.[9] Large occlusive thrombi also may form, although less often, in the veins of the upper extremities, liver, spleen, intestines, brain, and kidneys. Thrombosis symptoms include localized pain, the sensation of heat, redness, and swelling. In deep vein thrombosis, the entire leg swells.

Fragments of thrombi, called *emboli,* may separate from the proximal end of a venous thrombus, move swiftly through the right chambers of the heart, and lodge in the arterial pulmonary vasculature, causing ischemia and necrosis of lung tissue.[10] Nearly 95% of these pulmonary emboli arise from thrombi in the deep leg and calf veins. Of the 250,000 U.S. residents per year who suffer pulmonary emboli, 10% to 15% die within 3 months. Many pulmonary emboli go undiagnosed because of the ambiguity of the symptoms, which may resemble those of heart disease or pneumonia. Predilection for deep venous thrombosis versus pulmonary embolism shows a familial distribution. Coagulation system imbalances, such as inappropriate activation, gain of coagulation factor function, inadequate control of thrombin generation, or suppressed fibrinolysis, are the mechanisms that cause VTE; components of cancer, or chronic heart, lung, or renal disease are often implicated in VTE.[11]

Prevalence of Arterial Thrombosis

Cardiovascular disease caused 380,000 premature U.S. deaths in 2010, and 790,000 strokes accounted for 1 in 19 premature deaths (deaths before 78 years of age). Approximately 80% of acute myocardial infarctions and 85% of strokes are caused by thrombi that block coronary arteries or carotid end arteries of the vertebrobasilar system, respectively.[12] Transient ischemic attacks and peripheral arterial occlusions are more frequent than strokes and coronary artery disease and, although not fatal, cause substantial morbidity.

One important mechanism for arterial thrombosis is the well-described vessel wall *unstable atherosclerotic plaque.* Activated platelets, monocytes, and macrophages embed the fatty plaque within the endothelial lining, suppressing the normal release of antithrombotic molecules such as nitric oxide and exposing prothrombotic substances such as *tissue factor* (Chapter 37). Small plaques rupture, occluding arteries and releasing mediators that trigger thrombotic events. The mediators activate platelets, which combine with von Willebrand factor to form arterial platelet plugs—the "white thrombi" that cause ischemia and necrosis of surrounding tissue (Chapter 13).

The hemostasis-related lesions we associate with arterial thrombosis are blood vessel wall destruction and platelet activation. Often these are inseparable. Researchers continue to examine new thrombosis markers that capture pathological events in platelets and endothelial cells before a thrombotic event occurs.

THROMBOSIS RISK FACTORS

Acquired Thrombosis Risk Factors

In life, we acquire a legion of habits and circumstances that either help maintain or damage our hemostasis systems. Their variety and interplay make it difficult to pinpoint the factors that contribute to thrombosis or to determine which have the greatest influence. These factors seem to contribute to venous and arterial thrombosis in varying degrees. Table 39-1 lists the nondisease risk factors implicated in thrombosis.[13]

Thrombosis Risk Factors Associated with Systemic Diseases

In addition to life events, several conditions and diseases threaten us with thrombosis. Some are listed in Table 39-2, with an indication of the laboratory's diagnostic contribution.[14]

TABLE 39-1 Nondisease Risk Factors That Contribute to Thrombotic Disease

Risk Factor	Comment	Contribution to Thrombosis	Laboratory Diagnosis
Age	Thrombosis after age 50	Risk doubles each decade after 50	
Immobilization	Distance driving, air travel, restriction to wheelchair or bed, obesity	Slowed blood flow raises thrombosis risk	
Diet	Fatty foods; inadequate folate, vitamin B_6, and vitamin B_{12}	Homocysteinemia associated with $2\times$ to $7\times$ increased risk for arterial or venous thrombosis	Plasma homocysteine, vitamin levels, and lipid profile
Lipid metabolism imbalance	Hyperlipidemia, hypercholesterolemia, dyslipidemia, elevated lipoprotein (a), decreased HDL-C, elevated LDL-C	Moderate arterial thrombosis association with LDL-C elevation and hypercholesterolemia, may be congenital	Lipid profile: total cholesterol, HDL-C, LDL-C, triglycerides, and lipoprotein (a)
Oral contraceptive use	30 μg, formulation with progesterone	$4\times$ to $6\times$ increased risk	
Pregnancy		$3\times$ to $5\times$ increased risk	
Hormone replacement therapy		$2\times$ to $4\times$ increased risk	
Femoral or tibial fracture		80% incidence of thrombosis if not treated with antithrombotic	
Hip, knee, gynecologic, prostate surgery		50% incidence of thrombosis if not treated with antithrombotic	
Smoking		Depends on degree	HSCRP
Inflammation	Chronic	Arterial thrombosis	HSCRP
Central venous catheter	Endothelial injury and activation	33% of children with central venous lines develop venous thrombosis	

HDL-C, High-density lipoprotein cholesterol; *HSCRP,* high-sensitivity C-reactive protein; *LDL-C,* low-density lipoprotein cholesterol.

TABLE 39-2 Diseases with Thrombotic Risk Components

Disease	Examples or Effects	Contribution to Thrombosis	Laboratory Diagnosis
Antiphospholipid syndrome	Chronic antiphospholipid antibody often secondary to autoimmune disorders	When chronic, $1.6\times$ to $3.2\times$ increased risk of stroke, myocardial infarction, recurrent spontaneous abortion, venous thrombosis	PTT mixing studies, lupus anticoagulant profile, anticardiolipin antibody and anti–β_2-glycoprotein I immunoassays
Myeloproliferative neoplasms	Essential thrombocythemia, polycythemia vera, chronic myelogenous leukemia	Increased risk due to plasma viscosity, platelet activation	Platelet counts and platelet aggregometry
Hepatic disease	Diminished production of most coagulation control proteins	Increased risk due to deranged coagulation pathways, excess thrombin production	Prothrombin time, proteins C and S, and antithrombin assays, factor assays
Cancer: adenocarcinoma	Trousseau syndrome, low-grade chronic DIC	$20\times$ increased risk of thrombosis; 10% to 20% of people with idiopathic venous thrombosis have cancer	DIC profile: platelet count, D-dimer, PTT, PT, fibrinogen, blood film examination
Leukemia	Acute promyelocytic leukemia (M3), acute monocytic leukemia, (M4-M5)	Increased risk for chronic DIC	DIC profile: platelet count, D-dimer, PTT, PT, fibrinogen, blood film examination
Paroxysmal nocturnal hemoglobinuria	Platelet-related thrombosis	Increased risk for deep vein thrombosis, pulmonary embolism, DIC	Flow cytometry phenotyping for CD55 and CD59; DIC profile: platelet count, D-dimer, PTT, PT, fibrinogen, blood film examination
Chronic inflammation	Diabetes, cancer, infection, autoimmune disorder, obesity, smoking		Fibrinogen, HSCRP

DIC, Disseminated intravascular coagulation; *PT,* prothrombin time; *PTT,* partial thromboplastin time, *HSCRP,* high-sensitivity C-reactive protein.

Together, transient and chronic antiphospholipid (APL) antibodies such as the *lupus anticoagulant* (LA), anticardiolipin (ACL) antibodies, and *anti–β2-glycoprotein* I (anti–β_2-GPI) antibodies may be detected in 1% to 2% of the unselected population.[15] Chronic APL antibodies confer a risk of venous or arterial thrombosis—a condition called the *antiphospholipid syndrome* (APS). Chronic APL antibodies often accompany autoimmune connective tissue disorders, such as lupus erythematosus. Some appear in patients without any apparent underlying disease.

Malignancies often are implicated in venous thrombosis. One mechanism is tumor production of tissue factor analogues that trigger chronic low-grade disseminated intravascular coagulation (DIC). In addition, venous and arterial stasis and inflammatory effects increase the risk of thrombosis. Migratory thrombophlebitis, or *Trousseau syndrome*, is a sign of occult adenocarcinoma such as cancer of the pancreas or colon.[16]

Myeloproliferative neoplasms such as *essential thrombocythemia* and *polycythemia vera* (Chapter 33) may trigger thrombosis, probably through platelet hyperactivity. A cardinal sign of *acute promyelocytic leukemia* (Chapter 35) is DIC secondary to the release of procoagulant granules from malignant promyelocytes. DIC can intensify during therapy at the time of vigorous cell lysis.[17] *Paroxysmal nocturnal hemoglobinuria* (PNH) (Chapter 24) is caused by a stem cell mutation that modifies membrane-anchored platelet activation suppressors. Venous or arterial thromboses occur in at least 40% of PNH cases.[18]

Chronic inflammatory diseases cause thrombosis through a variety of mechanisms, such as elevation of fibrinogen and factor VIII, suppressed fibrinolysis, promotion of atherosclerotic plaque formation, and reduced free protein S activity secondary to raised C4b-binding protein (C4bBP) levels. Diabetes mellitus is a particularly dangerous chronic inflammatory condition, raising the risk of cardiovascular disease sixfold.[19] Conditions associated with venous stasis, such as congestive heart failure, also are risk factors for venous thrombosis. Untreated atrial fibrillation increases the risk of ischemic strokes caused by clot formation in the right atrium and embolization to the brain.[20] Nephrotic syndrome creates protein imbalances that lead to thrombosis through loss of plasma proteins such as antithrombin. Nephrotic syndrome may also cause hemorrhage (Chapter 38).[21]

Congenital Thrombosis Risk Factors

Clinicians suspect congenital thrombophilia when a thrombotic event occurs in young adults; occurs in unusual sites such as the mesenteric, renal, or axillary veins; is recurrent; or occurs in a patient who has a family history of thrombosis (Table 39-3).[22] Because thrombosis is multifactorial, however, even patients with congenital thrombophilia are most likely to experience thrombotic events because of a combination of constitutional and acquired conditions.[23]

The *antithrombin* activity assay (previously called the antithrombin III or AT III assay) has been available since 1972, and *protein C* and *protein S* activity assays became available in the mid-1980s. The 1990s brought the *activated protein C (APC) resistance* assay and its confirmatory *factor V Leiden (FVL) mutation* molecular assay; the *prothrombin G20210A mutation* molecular assay; and tests for *dysfibrinogenemia, plasminogen deficiency, plasma TPA,* and *plasma PAI-1.*

APC resistance is found in 3% to 8% of Caucasians worldwide. APC resistance extends to Arabs and Hispanics, but the mutation is nearly absent from African and East Asian populations (Table 39-4).[24] APC resistance may exist in the absence of the FVL mutation and is occasionally acquired in pregnancy or in association with oral contraceptive therapy.[25]

TABLE 39-3 Predisposing Congenital Factors and Thrombosis Risk

Risk Factor	Comment	Risk of Thrombosis	Laboratory Tests
AT (previously AT III) deficiency	AT, enhanced by heparin, inhibits the serine proteases IIa (thrombin), IXa, Xa, and XIa	Heterozygous: increased 10× to 20× Homozygous: 100%, rarely reported	Clot-based and chromogenic AT activity assays, immunoassays for AT concentration (antigen)
PC deficiency	Activated PC is a serine protease that hydrolyzes factors Va and VIIIa, requires protein S as a stabilizing cofactor	Heterozygous: increased 2× to 5× Homozygous: 100%; causes neonatal purpura fulminans	Clot-based and chromogenic PC activity assays, immunoassay for PC concentration (antigen)
Free PS deficiency	PS is a stabilizing cofactor for activated protein C, 40% is free, 60% circulates bound to C4bBP	Heterozygous: increased 1.6× to 11.5× Homozygous: 100% but rarely reported; causes neonatal purpura fulminans	Clot-based free PS activity assays, free and total PS immunoassays for PS concentration (antigen)
APC resistance	Factor V Leiden (R506Q) mutation gain of function renders factor V resistant to APC	Heterozygous: increased 3× Homozygous: increased 18×	PTT-based APC resistance test and confirmatory molecular assay
Prothrombin G20210A	Mutation in prothrombin gene untranslated 3′ promoter region creates moderate elevation in prothrombin activity	Heterozygous: increased 1.6× to 11.5×	Molecular assay only; phenotypic assay provides no specificity
Hyperfibrinogenemia	Associated with arterial thrombosis	Under investigation: acute phase reactant	Clauss fibrinogen clotting assay, immunoassay, nephelometric assay

APC, Activated protein C; *AT,* antithrombin; *C4bBP,* complement component C4b binding protein; *PC,* protein C; *PS,* protein S; *PTT,* partial thromboplastin time.

TABLE 39-4 Prevalence of Congenital Thrombosis Risk Factors in the General Population and in Individuals with Recurrent Thrombotic Disease

Factor	Unselected Population	People with at Least One Thrombotic Event
Activated protein C resistance, factor V Leiden mutation	3% to 8% of Caucasians, rare in Asians or Africans	20%–25%
Prothrombin G20210A	2% to 3% of Caucasians, rare in Asians or Africans	4%–8%
Antithrombin deficiency	1 in 2000 to 1 in 5000	1%–1.8%
Protein C deficiency	1 in 300	2.5%–5.0%
Protein S deficiency	Unknown	2.8%–5.0%
Hyperhomocysteinemia associated with methylenetetrahydrofolate reductase gene mutations	11%	13.1%–26.7%

The FVL gene mutation is the most common inherited thrombophilia, and the prothrombin G20210A gene mutation is the second most common inherited thrombophilia tendency in patients with a personal and family history of deep vein thrombosis.[26] Altogether, protein C, protein S, and antithrombin deficiencies are found in only 0.2% to 1.0% of the world population. The incidences of dysfibrinogenemia and the various forms of abnormal fibrinolysis (plasminogen deficiency, TPA deficiency, and PAI-1 excess) are under investigation.

Double Hit

Thrombosis often is associated with a combination of genetic defect, disease, and lifestyle influences. Just because someone possesses protein C, protein S, or antithrombin deficiency does not mean that thrombosis is inevitable. Many heterozygotes experience no thrombotic event during their lifetimes, whereas others experience clotting only when two or more risk factors converge. A young woman who is heterozygous for the FVL mutation has a thirty-fivefold increase in thrombosis risk upon starting oral contraceptive therapy. In the Physicians' Health Study, homocysteinemia tripled the risk of idiopathic venous thrombosis, and the FVL mutation doubled it. When both were present, the risk of venous thrombosis was increased tenfold.[27]

LABORATORY EVALUATION OF THROMBOPHILIA

When thrombophilia is suspected, it is important to assess all known risk factors because it is the combination of positive results that determines the patient's cumulative risk of thrombosis.[28] Table 39-5 summarizes the commonly used thrombosis risk assays and indicates those that can be relied on while the patient is on antithrombotic therapy or while the patient is recovering from an acute thrombotic event.

TABLE 39-5 Thrombophilia Laboratory Test Profile

Assay	Reference Value/Interval	Comments
APC resistance	Ratio ≥1.8	Clot-based screen that employs PTT with factor V-depleted plasma.
Factor V Leiden mutation	Wild-type	Molecular assay performed as follow-up to APC resistance ratio that is <1.8.
Prothrombin G20210A	Wild-type	Molecular assay. There is no phenotypic assay for prothrombin G20210A.
LA profile*	Negative for LA	Minimum of two clot-based assays. Primary assays are based on PTT and DRVVT, secondary assays based on KCT, or dilute PT. All four include phospholipid neutralization follow-up test.
ACL antibody	IgG: <12 GPL IgM: <10 MPL	Immunoassay for immunoglobulins of APL family. ACL depends on β_2-GPI in reaction mix.
Anti–β_2-GPI antibody	<20 G units	Immunoassay for an immunoglobulin of APL family. β_2-GPI is key phospholipid-binding protein in family.
AT activity*	78%–126%	Serine protease inhibitor suppresses IIa (thrombin), IXa, Xa, XIa. When consistently below reference limit, follow up with AT antigen assay.
PC activity*	70%–140%	Digests VIIIa and Va. When consistently below reference limit, follow up with PC antigen assay.
PS activity*	65%–140%	PC cofactor. When consistently below reference limit, follow up with total and free PS antigen assay, C4b-binding protein assay.
Fibrinogen	220–498 mg/dL	Clot-based assay. Elevation may be associated with arterial thrombosis.

ACL, anticardiolipin; *APC*, activated protein C; *APL*, antiphospholipid antibody; *AT*, antithrombin; β_2-*GPI*, β_2-glycoprotein I; *DRVVT*, dilute Russell viper venom time; *GPL*, IgG antiphospholipid antibody unit; *Ig*, immunoglobulin; *KCT*, kaolin clotting time; *LA*, lupus anticoagulant; *MPL*, IgM antiphospholipid antibody unit; *PC*, protein C; *PS*, protein S; *PT*, prothrombin time; *PTT*, partial thromboplastin time.
*Inaccurate during active thrombosis or anticoagulant therapy. Perform 14 days after anticoagulant therapy is discontinued.

The presence or absence of laboratory-detected risk factors does not affect anticoagulant treatment when thrombosis is in progress.[29] However, it is important to realize that current anticoagulant therapy and ongoing or recent thrombotic events interfere with the interpretation of antithrombin, protein C, protein S, factor VIII, and LA testing. These assays should be performed at least 14 days after anticoagulant therapy is discontinued.

Antiphospholipid Antibodies

APL antibodies comprise a family of immunoglobulins that bind protein-phospholipid complexes.[30] APL antibodies include LAs, detected by clot-based profiles, and ACL and anti–β_2-GPI antibodies, detected by immunoassay. Chronic autoimmune APL antibodies are associated with APS, which is characterized by transient ischemic attacks, strokes, coronary and peripheral artery disease, venous thromboembolism, and recurrent pregnancy complications, including spontaneous abortions.[31,32]

APL antibodies arise as immunoglobulin M (IgM), IgG, or IgA isotypes. Because they may bind a variety of protein-phospholipid complexes, they are called *nonspecific inhibitors.* Their name implies that they were once thought to directly bind phospholipids; however, their target antigens are actually the proteins that assemble on anionic phospholipid surfaces.[33] The plasma protein most often bound by APL antibodies is β_2-GPI, although *annexin V* and *prothrombin* are sometimes implicated as APL targets. APL antibodies probably develop in response to newly formed protein-phospholipid complexes, and laboratory scientists continue to investigate how they cause thrombosis.[34,35]

Clinical Consequences of Antiphospholipid Antibodies

Between 1% and 2% of unselected individuals of both sexes and all races, and 5% to 15% of individuals with recurrent venous or arterial thrombotic disease have APL antibodies.[36] Most APL antibodies arise in response to a bacterial, viral, fungal, or parasitic infection or to treatment with numerous drugs (Box 39-1) and disappear within 12 weeks. These are mostly transient *alloimmune* APL antibodies and have no clinical consequences.[37] Nevertheless, the laboratory professional must follow up any positive results on APL antibody assays to determine their persistence.

BOX 39-1 Agents Known to Induce Antiphospholipid Antibodies

Various antibiotics
Phenothiazine
Hydralazine
Quinine and quinidine
Calcium channel blockers
Procainamide
Phenytoin
Cocaine
Elevated estrogens

Autoimmune APL antibodies are part of the family of autoantibodies that arise in collagen vascular diseases; 50% of patients with systemic lupus erythematosus have autoimmune APL antibodies. Autoimmune APL antibodies are also detected in patients with rheumatoid arthritis, scleroderma, and Sjögren syndrome but may arise spontaneously, a disorder called *primary APS.* Autoimmune APL antibodies may persist, and fully 30% are associated with arterial and venous thrombosis. Chronic presence of an autoimmune APL antibody not associated with a known underlying autoimmune disorder confers a 1.8-fold to 3.2-fold increased risk of thrombosis.

Detection and Confirmation of Antiphospholipid Antibodies

Clinicians suspect APS in unexplained venous or arterial thrombosis, thrombocytopenia, or recurrent fetal loss.[38] Specialized clinical hemostasis laboratories offer APL detection profiles that include clot-based assays for LA and immunoassays for ACL and anti–β_2-GPI antibodies. Occasionally, an LA is suspected because of an unexplained prolonged partial thromboplastin time (PTT) that does not correct in mixing studies (Figure 39-1; Chapter 42).[39,40]

Lupus Anticoagulant Test Profile

Clot-based assays with reduced reagent phospholipid concentrations are sensitive to LA. There are two commonly used test systems, and both are required for an LA profile. The need for two parallel assay systems arises from the multiplicity of LA reaction characteristics: a confirmed positive result in one system is conclusive despite a negative result in the other. The two most commonly recommended test systems are the dilute Russell viper venom time (DRVVT) and the silica-based partial thromboplastin time (PTT), both formulated with low-phospholipid concentrations designed to be LA sensitive.[41] Two older systems, still used in many institutions and available from specialty laboratories and coagulation reagent distributors, are the kaolin clotting time (KCT) and the dilute thromboplastin time (DTT, also named tissue thromboplastin inhibitor test, TTI).[42] As illustrated in Figure 39-2, the KCT and PTT initiate coagulation at the level of factor XII; DRVVT at factor X; and DTT at factor VII.

The 2009 International Society on Thrombosis and Haemostasis (ISTH) update of guidelines for LA detection provides the following sequence of assays:[43]

1. Prolonged phospholipid-dependent clot formation using an initial screen assay such as a low phospholipid PTT or DRVVT.
2. Failure to correct the prolonged clot time when mixing with normal platelet-poor control plasma and repeating the test (see mixing study below).
3. Shortening or complete correction of the prolonged screen assay result by addition of a reagent formulated with excess phospholipids.
4. Exclusion of other coagulopathies.

Performing the Clot-Based Lupus Anticoagulant Mixing Study. Laboratory practitioners perform the LA profile upon clinician request, often based on adverse thrombotic or obstetric

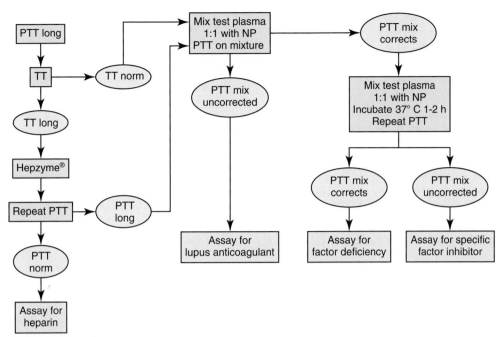

Figure 39-1 Mixing study employing a partial thromboplastin time (PTT) reagent with intermediate lupus anticoagulant sensitivity. Beginning at the top left, when the PTT result exceeds the upper limit of the PTT reference interval, perform a thrombin clotting time (TT) to detect unfractionated heparin. If the TT exceeds the TT reference interval, presume that heparin is present. Treat an aliquot of the specimen with Hepzyme and repeat the PTT. If the new PTT is normal, assay the original sample for heparin. If the PTT remains prolonged, or if the TT was normal, proceed by mixing the patient plasma with control normal plasma (NP) and perform a PTT on the mixture. If the PTT is still prolonged (uncorrected) in comparison to the NP, proceed to assay for the lupus anticoagulant. If the PTT mixture corrects, prepare a new 1:1 mix and incubate at 37° C for 1 to 2 hours and repeat the PTT, comparing the result to incubated NP. If the incubated PTT shows a correction, assay for a factor deficiency. If prolonged, assay for a lupus anticoagulant (Figs. 39-2 and 39-3) (a specific factor inhibitor such as anti-factor VIII associated with bleeding will also be detected in this manner).

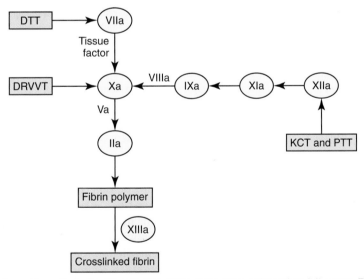

Figure 39-2 Simplified coagulation pathway illustrating the activation points of the lupus anticoagulant (LA) assays. The dilute Russell viper venom time (DRVVT) assay, regarded as the primary LA detection method, activates factor X (ten). DRVVT is typically accompanied by a low-phospholipid LA-sensitive partial thromboplastin time assay (PTT) that activates factor XII. The historic kaolin clotting time (KCT) also activates factor XII, and the dilute thromboplastin time test (DTT), still available, activates factor VII.

events, or when a prolonged PTT raises the presumption of an LA. Most laboratory protocols begin with a mixing study where the PTT is performed on patient plasma combined with control normal plasma (NP) (Figure 39-1; Chapter 42). The mixing study includes a 37° C incubation step, as many LAs and specific inhibitors require an incubation to enhance their avidity. Practitioners typically perform the mixing study using a PTT reagent with intermediate LA sensitivity but may substitute the prothrombin time (PT) reagent, DRVVT, or an LA-sensitive low-phospholipid PTT reagent. The mixing study includes a means for detecting unfractionated heparin, most often the thrombin clotting time or the chromogenic anti-Xa heparin assay. The practitioner may add heparinase (Hepzyme®, Siemens Healthcare USA, Inc., Malvern, PA) to the sample to neutralize heparin, although this may be unnecessary because many LA detection reagents provide heparin-neutralizing polybrene. Mixing studies that use a PT, a DRVVT, or an LA-sensitive PTT reagent seldom include the 37° C incubation step.

The NP that is mixed 1:1 with patient plasma will shorten a prolonged PTT. Each laboratory director decides what degree of PTT "shortening" constitutes "correction." Many use the Rosner index, which defines correction as a mixture result within 10% of the NP result.[44] Others define correction as return to a value within 5 seconds of the NP result or return to a value within the PTT reference interval.

In performing mixing studies, the laboratory professional employs only platelet-poor plasma—plasma centrifuged so that it has a platelet count of less than 10,000/μL (Chapter 42). The use of platelet-poor plasma avoids neutralization of LA by the platelet membrane phospholipids. Platelet membrane fragments that form during freezing and thawing can likewise neutralize LA and lead to a false-negative LA result.

Performing Clot-Based Lupus Anticoagulant Tests.

Following a mixing study that suggests the presence of an LA, specific testing for the LA is performed. Most LA protocols begin with the DRVVT, considered the most specific of the LA assays (Figure 39-3). If the DRVVT screening reagent-patient plasma result exceeds the NP result by a predetermined ratio, frequently near 1.2, LA is presumed. The practitioner then confirms LA by mixing an aliquot of the patient sample with the DRVVT high-phospholipid confirmatory reagent, comparing the result in seconds to the original DRVVT screening reagent patient plasma result. The reagent phospholipid neutralizes LA and shortens the DRVVT. If the original screening reagent result exceeds the DRVVT confirm reagent result by a predetermined ratio, again near 1.2, LA is confirmed.

If the original DRVVT screen ratio was less than 1.2, the practitioner turns to the silica-based low-phospholipid LA-sensitive PTT and repeats the steps used for the DRVVT, again basing results on a predetermined ratio, often 1.2.[45,46]

There exist numerous modifications to this algorithm. Many laboratory directors prefer to begin with the silica-based low-phospholipid PTT assay, and others include an intermediate NP mixing study step. Some incorporate the KCT or DTT. Some assay systems use an absolute difference, in seconds, instead of a ratio, often 8 seconds. The 1.2 ratio and the 8-second difference are examples; each institution establishes its own reference interval and threshold ratio or difference.

Some laboratory directors choose to normalize ratios using the mean of the reference interval (MRI) or the NP value. The formula for normalization using the MRI is:

$$\text{Normalized ratio} = \frac{\begin{array}{c}\text{Patient screen result in}\\\text{seconds/screen MRI}\end{array}}{\begin{array}{c}\text{Patient confirm result in}\\\text{seconds/confirm MRI}\end{array}} = \frac{\text{Screen ratio}}{\text{Confirm ratio}}$$

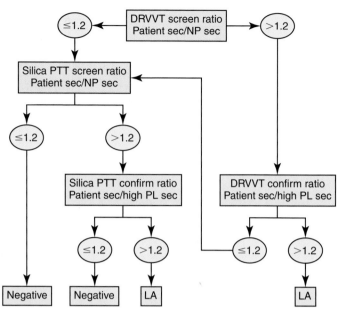

Figure 39-3 Lupus anticoagulant (LA) algorithm. When LA is suspected, perform a dilute Russell viper venom (DRVVT) screen, comparing the patient DRVVT screen result to the control normal plasma (NP) DRVVT screen result. If the ratio of patient to NP DRVVT in seconds is greater than 1.2, mix patient plasma 1:1 with high-phospholipid DRVVT confirm reagent and perform a new DRVVT. If the patient DRVVT screen result exceeds the DRVVT confirm/patient plasma result by greater than 1.2, LA is confirmed. If the ratio is 1.2 or less or if the original DRVVT screen ratio was 1.2 or less, proceed to a silica-based partial thromboplastin (PTT) screen and confirm. Compare the patient silica-based PTT screen to the NP screen result. If the ratio is 1.2 or less, no LA is present. If the ratio is greater than 1.2, mix the patient plasma with high-phospholipid silica-based PTT confirm reagent and perform a new PTT. If the patient PTT screen exceeds the patient PTT confirm by more than 1.2, LA is confirmed. If the ratio is 1.2 or less, LA is not present.

Anticardiolipin Antibody Immunoassay

LA and ACL antibodies coexist in 60% of cases, and both may be found in APS. The ACL test is an immunoassay that may be normalized among laboratories and is not affected by heparin therapy, oral anticoagulant therapy, current thrombosis, or factor deficiencies.

The manufacturer coats microplate wells with bovine heart cardiolipin and blocks (fills open receptor sites) with a bovine serum solution containing β_2-GPI. The laboratory practitioner pipettes test sera or plasmas to the wells alongside calibrators and controls (Figure 39-4). ACL binds the solid-phase cardiolipin–β_2-GPI target complex and cannot be washed from the wells. The practitioner adds enzyme-labeled anti–human IgG, IgM, or IgA conjugates subsequent to washing, followed by a color-producing substrate. A color change indicates the presence of ACL and color intensities of the patient, and control sample wells are compared with the calibrator curve wells. Results are expressed using GPL, MPL, or APL units, where 1 unit is equivalent to 1 μg/mL of an affinity-purified standard IgG, IgM, or IgA specimen.[47] Reference limits are established in each laboratory.[48]

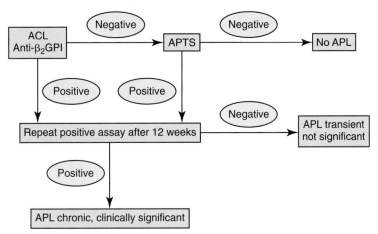

Figure 39-4 Antiphospholipid antibody (APL) immunoassay algorithm. If an APL is suspected, perform an anticardiolipin (ACL) or anti–β₂-glycoprotein I (anti–β₂-GPI) immunoassay. If either is positive, confirm chronicity using a new specimen collected at least 12 weeks later. If negative, perform immunoassay to detect an antiphosphatidyl serine (APTS) antibody. If positive, repeat after 12 weeks.

Anti–β₂-Glycoprotein I Immunoassay

The practitioner performs IgM and IgG anti–β₂-GPI immunoassays as a part of the profile that includes ACL assays. An anti–β₂-GPI result of greater than 20 IgG or IgM anti–β₂-GPI units correlates with thrombosis more closely than the presence of ACL antibodies. Any ACL or anti–β₂-GPI assay yielding positive results is repeated on a new specimen collected after 12 weeks to distinguish a transient alloantibody from a chronic autoantibody.

Antiphosphatidylserine Immunoassay

For cases in which an APL antibody is suspected but the routine LA, ACL, and β₂-GPI assay results are negative, the clinician may wish to order the antiphosphatidylserine immunoassay to detect APL antibodies specific for phosphatidylserine.[49] A result greater than or equal to 16 IgG or 22 IgM antiphosphatidylserine units is considered positive. The antiphosphatidylserine assay is available from specialty reference laboratories.

Activated Protein C Resistance and Factor V Leiden Mutation

Clinical Importance of Activated Protein C Resistance

The *activated protein C (APC)–protein S complex* normally hydrolyzes activated factors V and VIII (factors Va and VIIIa). A mutation in the factor V gene substitutes glutamine for arginine at position 506 of the factor V molecule (FV R506Q). The arginine molecule is a normal cleavage site for APC, so the substitution slows or resists APC hydrolysis (Figure 39-5). The resistant factor Va remains active and raises the production of thrombin, leading to thrombosis. The factor V R506Q mutation is named for the city in The Netherlands in which it was first described: Leiden [*factor V Leiden (FVL) mutation,* also referred to as *APC resistance*]. Between 3% and 8% of Northern European Caucasians possess the FVL mutation (Table 39-4).[50] Owing to its prevalence and the associated threefold higher

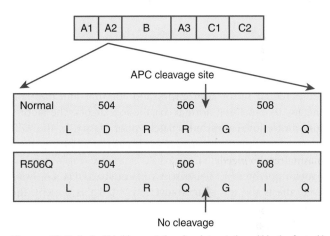

Figure 39-5 Factor V Leiden mutation. A point mutation within the factor V gene results in the substitution of amino acid glutamine for arginine at position 506 (R506Q) of the factor V molecule. The normal arginine at position 506 is a cleavage site for activated protein C (APC), so glutamine substitution slows or prevents cleavage of the factor V molecule. *D,* Aspartic acid; *G,* glycine; *I,* isoleucine; *L,* leucine; *R,* arginine, *Q,* glutamine.

thrombosis risk (eighteenfold higher for homozygotes), most acute care hemostasis laboratory directors provide APC resistance detection to screen for FVL.[51,52]

Activated Protein C Resistance Clot-Based Assay

In the APC resistance clot-based assay, patient plasma is mixed 1:4 with factor V–depleted plasma.[53] PTT reagent is added to two aliquots of the mixture and incubated for 3 minutes (Figure 39-6). A solution of calcium chloride is pipetted into one mixture, and the clot formation is timed. A solution of *calcium chloride with APC* is added to the second mixture, and clotting is timed. The time to clot formation of the second aliquot is at least 1.8 times the time to clot formation of the first (prolonged time to clot due to the increased amount of APC), so the normal ratio of PTT results between the two assays is 1.8 or greater. In APC resistance, the ratio is less than 1.8.[54]

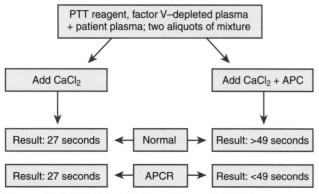

Figure 39-6 Activated protein C resistance ratio (APCR) measurement. Patient plasma is mixed 1:4 with factor V–depleted plasma and partial thromboplastin time (PTT) reagent. Two aliquots of this mixture are then tested: one aliquot is mixed with calcium chloride ($CaCl_2$) alone, and the other aliquot is mixed with $CaCl_2$ plus activated protein C (APC). The reaction in the mixture with the APC should be prolonged to a clotting time at least 1.8 times longer than the mixture without APC. A ratio of 1.8 or less implies APC resistance.

Performance Characteristics of the Activated Protein C Resistance Test.

Factor V–depleted plasma compensates for potential factor deficiencies and for oral anticoagulant therapy by providing normal coagulation factors. The laboratory professional uses only platelet-poor plasma in the APC resistance test to prevent loss of sensitivity caused by the abundant release of platelet factor 4. APC resistance reagent test kits contain polybrene or heparinase to neutralize UFH. LA, however, affects the test system adversely.[55] If LA is present, the molecular test for FVL is indicated.[56]

Factor V Leiden Mutation Assay

Most laboratories confirm the APC resistance diagnosis using the molecular FVL mutation test. The determination of zygosity is important to predict the risk for thrombosis and establish a treatment regimen.

Prothrombin G20210A

A guanine-to-adenine mutation at base 20210 of the 3′ untranslated region of the *prothrombin* (factor II) gene has been associated with mildly elevated plasma prothrombin levels, averaging 130%.[52] The increased risk of thrombosis in those with the mutation seems to be related to the elevated prothrombin activity.[53] The prevalence of this mutation among individuals with familial thrombosis is 5% to 18%, whereas prevalence worldwide is 0.3% to 2.4%, depending on race.[57] The risk of venous thrombosis in heterozygotes is only two to three times the baseline risk. Although the mutation may cause a slight prothrombin elevation, a phenotypic prothrombin activity assay is of little diagnostic value because there is considerable overlap between normal prothrombin levels and prothrombin levels in people with the mutation.[58,59]

Antithrombin

Antithrombin (previously named antithrombin III or ATIII) is a serine protease inhibitor (SERPIN) that neutralizes factors IIa

(thrombin), IXa, Xa, XIa, and XIIa, all the serine proteases except factor VIIa. Antithrombin activity is enhanced by unfractionated heparin (UFH), low-molecular-weight heparin (LMWH), and synthetic pentasaccharide (fondaparinux) (Figures 39-7 and 39-8). Antithrombin was the first of the plasma coagulation control proteins to be identified and the first to be assayed

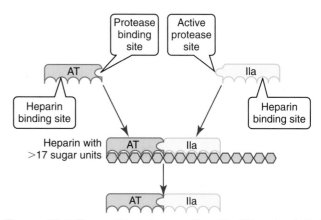

Figure 39-7 The reaction between antithrombin (AT) and activated coagulation factor II (IIa; thrombin) is supported by heparin. Standard unfractionated heparin, with a molecular weight of 5000 to 40,000 Daltons, provides polysaccharide chains of at least 17 sugar subunits. Heparin molecules of this length support the reaction between AT and IIa, as AT and IIa assemble on the heparin molecule. The AT molecule attaches to a specific pentasaccharide sequence. The IIa possesses a heparin-binding site that enables it to assemble on the heparin surface adjacent to the AT, a property called *approximation*. The AT becomes sterically modified (allostery), supporting a covalent reaction between the AT protease binding site and the IIa active protease site. Thrombin (IIa) and antithrombin, covalently bound, release from heparin and form measurable plasma thrombin-antithrombin (TAT) complexes, useful as a marker of coagulation activation.

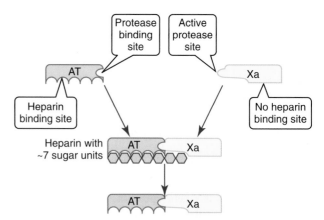

Figure 39-8 The reaction between antithrombin (AT) and activated coagulation factor X (Xa) is supported by low-molecular-weight heparin. Low-molecular-weight heparin, with a molecular weight of less than 8000 Daltons, provides polysaccharide chains of six or seven sugar subunits. Heparin molecules of this length support the reaction between AT and Xa. The AT molecule attaches to a specific pentasaccharide sequence. The Xa does not possess a heparin-binding site and does not need to assemble on the heparin surface adjacent to the AT. The AT becomes sterically modified (allostery), supporting a covalent reaction between the AT protease binding site and the Xa active protease site.

routinely in the clinical hemostasis laboratory.[55] Other members of the serpin family are heparin cofactor II, α_2-macroglobulin, α_2-antiplasmin, and α_1-antitrypsin. Typically, hemostasis specialty laboratories or reference laboratories are the only places that assay serpins other than the more commonly ordered antithrombin activity, which has found its way into laboratories at most acute care facilities.

Antithrombin Deficiency

Acquired antithrombin deficiency occurs in liver disease, in nephrotic syndrome, with prolonged heparin therapy, with asparaginase therapy, with the use of oral contraceptives, and in DIC, where antithrombin is rapidly consumed. Congenital deficiency is present in 1 in 2000 to 1 in 5000 of the general population and accounts for 1.0% to 1.8% of recurrent venous thromboembolic disease cases.[60] About 90% of cases of antithrombin deficiency are quantitative (reduced production), or type I; the remainder are caused by mutations creating structural abnormalities in the antithrombin *protease binding* site or the *heparin binding* site. Type II mutations do not reduce antithrombin production, but the molecules are nonfunctional.[61]

Antithrombin Reference Intervals

Adult plasma antithrombin activity ranges from 78% to 126%, whether measured by clot-based or chromogenic assay. Antithrombin antigen levels range from 22 to 39 mg/dL (68% to 128%) by latex microparticle immunoassay, and the plasma biologic half-life is 72 hours. Adult levels are reached by 3 months of age, and levels remain steady throughout adult life, except during periods of physiologic challenge, such as pregnancy. Antithrombin activity decreases with age.[62]

Antithrombin Activity Assay

Laboratory practitioners screen for antithrombin deficiency using a clot-based or chromogenic functional assay. The clot-based assay has been available since 1972, but most laboratory directors choose the chromogenic assay because of its stability and reproducibility. The operator mixes test plasma with a solution of heparin and factor Xa (Figure 39-9) and incubates the mixture at 37° C for several minutes. During incubation, the heparin-activated plasma antithrombin irreversibly binds a proportion of the reagent factor Xa. Residual factor Xa hydrolyzes a chromogenic substrate, added as a second reagent. The degree of hydrolysis, measurable by colored end product intensity, is inversely proportional to the activity of antithrombin in the test plasma.[63] The chromogenic substrate test for plasma antithrombin activity detects quantitative and qualitative antithrombin deficiencies and detects mutations affecting the proteolytic site but not the heparin binding site. Clot-based antithrombin assays are affected by, and therefore detect, mutations in both the proteolytic and heparin binding sites.

Antithrombin Antigen Assay

Antithrombin concentration is measured in a turbidometric microparticle immunoassay using a suspension of latex microbeads coated with antibody to antithrombin. In the absence of antithrombin, the wavelength of incident monochromatic

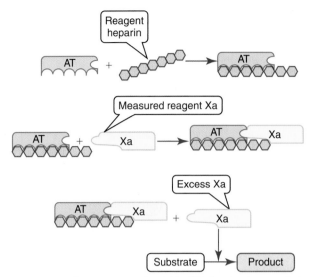

Figure 39-9 Chromogenic antithrombin (AT) functional assay. Patient plasma is pipetted into a reagent consisting of heparin, a measured concentration of activated coagulation factor X (Xa), and a chromogenic substrate. AT is activated by heparin and binds Xa. Excess Xa hydrolyzes the substrate and produces a yellow product, para-nitroaniline (pNA). The intensity of pNA color is inversely proportional to AT activity.

light exceeds the latex microparticle diameter, so the light passes through unabsorbed.[64] In the presence of antithrombin, the particles form larger aggregates. The antithrombin concentration is directly proportional to the rate of light absorption change. Antithrombin antigen levels are diminished in quantitative (type I) but not qualitative (type II) antithrombin deficiency. Oral anticoagulant Coumadin therapy may raise the antithrombin level and mask a mild deficiency. Antithrombin activity remains decreased for 10 to 14 days after surgery or a thrombotic event, so the assay should not be used to establish a congenital deficiency during this period.[65]

Heparin Resistance and the Antithrombin Assay

Antithrombin may become decreased during prolonged or intense heparin therapy and may be largely consumed if the patient has a congenital antithrombin deficiency. In this instance, heparin may be administered in therapeutic or higher dosages, but it neither exerts an anticoagulant effect nor is detected by the PTT. This is known as *heparin resistance*. In such cases, an antithrombin assay is necessary to confirm antithrombin deficiency. Antithrombin deficiency may be treated with antithrombin concentrate (Thrombate III; Grifols, Inc., Los Angeles, CA).[66]

Protein C Control Pathway

Thrombin is an important coagulation factor because it cleaves fibrinogen, activates platelets, and activates factors V, VIII, XI, and XIII. In the intact vessel where clotting would be pathological, thrombin binds endothelial cell membrane *thrombomodulin* and becomes an anticoagulant.[67] How does this paradox happen? The thrombin–thrombomodulin complex activates plasma protein C, and the APC binds free plasma protein S (Figure 39-10).[68] The stabilized APC–protein S complex, simultaneously bound to

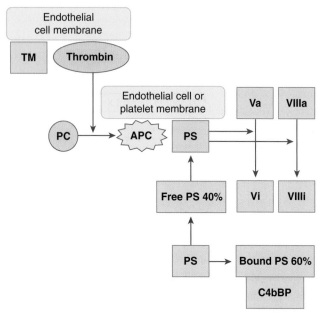

Figure 39-10 Protein C pathway. Thrombin (activated coagulation factor II or IIa) binds constitutive thrombomodulin (TM) on the endothelial cell membrane. The TM-thrombin complex activates protein C (PC). Activated protein C (APC) binds protein S (PS) on endothelial cell or platelet membrane phospholipids. The bound active complex hydrolyzes (inactivates) activated coagulation factors V and VIII (Va and VIIIa). PS can be in either a free (able to interact as described above) or bound state. *C4bBP*, C4b-binding protein; *Vi*, inactivated coagulation factor V; *VIIIi*, inactivated coagulation factor VIII.

the endothelial protein C receptor, hydrolyzes factors Va and VIIIa to slow coagulation. Recurrent venous thrombosis is the potential consequence of protein C or protein S deficiency.[69]

Protein S, the cofactor that binds and stabilizes APC, circulates in the plasma either free or covalently bound to the complement binding protein *C4bBP*. Bound protein S cannot participate in the protein C anticoagulant pathway; only free plasma protein S is available to serve as the APC cofactor. Protein S–C4bBP binding is of particular interest in inflammatory conditions, where acute phase reactant C4bBP level rises, binding additional protein S. Free protein S levels are proportionally decreased.

Protein C and Protein S Reference Ranges

Heterozygous protein C or protein S deficiency leads to a 1.6-fold to 11.5-fold increased risk of recurrent deep vein thrombosis and pulmonary embolism. Protein S deficiency also has been implicated in transient ischemic attacks and strokes, particularly in the young. The reference interval for both protein C and protein S activity and antigen levels is 65% to 140%, and levels ordinarily remain between 30% and 65% for heterozygotes.

Control proteins C and S (and Z) and factors II (prothrombin), VII, IX, and X are vitamin K-dependent. Because the half-life of protein C is 6 hours, its level decreases as rapidly as that of factor VII at the onset of Coumadin (warfarin, vitamin K antagonist) therapy. In heterozygous protein C deficiency, protein C activity may drop to less than 65% (a thrombotic level) more rapidly than the coagulation factor activities reach low

therapeutic levels (less than 30%). Consequently, in early Coumadin therapy a patient may experience *Coumadin-induced skin necrosis,* a paradoxical situation in which the anticoagulant therapy brings on thrombosis of the dermal vessels. This complication is suspected when the patient develops painful necrotic lesions that are preceded by severe itching, called pruritus. The necrosis may require surgical débridement. To avoid this risk, hematologists recommend coadministration of LMWH or synthetic pentasaccharide (fondaparinux) with Coumadin for any patient suspected of protein C deficiency or known to have previously suffered skin necrosis until a satisfactory and stable international normalized ratio (INR) is reached (Chapter 43).

Activity levels of protein C and protein S remain below normal for 10 to 14 days after cessation of Coumadin therapy. Similarly, for several days after surgery or a thrombotic event, these proteins are diminished even if Coumadin has not been used.[70] Their activities are depressed in pregnancy, liver or renal disease, vitamin K deficiency, DIC, and with oral contraceptive use. Protein C and protein S assays therefore cannot be used to identify a congenital deficiency when they are employed within 14 days after thrombosis or after the cessation of Coumadin therapy, during pregnancy, or in the presence of DIC, liver disease, renal disease, vitamin K deficiency, or oral contraceptive use.[71]

Homozygous protein C or protein S deficiency results in *neonatal purpura fulminans,* a condition that is rapidly fatal when untreated. Treatment includes administration of factor concentrates and lifelong Coumadin therapy.

Protein C Assays

Functional assays detect both quantitative and qualitative protein C deficiencies.[72] Either chromogenic or clot-based protein C activity assays are available. In the former, the laboratory professional first mixes the patient's plasma with Protac (Pentapharm, Inc., Basel, Switzerland), derived from the venom of the southern copperhead serpent *Agkistrodon contortrix,* which activates protein C. Subsequently, a chromogenic substrate is added, and its hydrolysis by the recently generated APC is measured by assessing the intensity of colored product, which is proportional to the activity of protein C (Figure 39-11). The assay detects abnormalities that affect the molecule's *proteolytic*

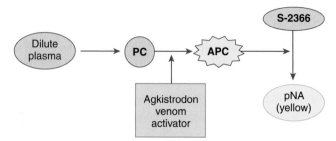

Figure 39-11 Chromogenic protein C (PC) assay. Patient plasma is pipetted into a reagent composed of *Agkistrodon contortrix* venom activator and chromogenic substrate (S-2366) specific to activated protein C (APC). The APC hydrolyzes the substrate to produce para-nitroaniline (pNA), a yellow product. The intensity of color is proportional to APC activity.

properties (active serine protease site) but misses those that affect protein C's phospholipid binding site or protein S binding site. In cases in which protein C chromogenic assays and immunoassays generate normal results but the clinical condition continues to indicate possible protein C deficiency, a clot-based protein C assay may detect abnormalities at these additional sites on the molecule.

The clot-based protein C assay is based on the ability of APC to prolong the PTT. The laboratory professional mixes plasma with protein C–depleted normal plasma to ensure normal levels of all factors except protein C. PTT reagent mixed with Protac and a heparin neutralizer is added, followed by calcium chloride, and the interval to clot formation is measured. Prolongation is proportional to plasma protein C activity. The clot-based protein C activity assay may be performed using an automated coagulation analyzer. Therapeutic heparin concentrations greater than 1 IU/mL consume the heparin neutralizer, prolong the PTT, and lead to overestimation of protein C. APC resistance, LA, and the presence of therapeutic *direct thrombin inhibitors* such as *argatroban* or *dabigatran* may prolong the PTT and falsely raise the protein C activity level in clot-based assays.

Enzyme immunoassay is used to measure protein C antigen when the functional activity is low and acquired causes have been ruled out. Microtiter plates coated with rabbit anti–human protein C antibody are used to capture test plasma protein C, and the concentration of antigen is measured by color development after the sequential addition of peroxidase-conjugated anti–human protein C and orthophenylenediamine substrate. The protein C antigen concentration assay detects most acquired deficiencies and quantitative congenital deficiencies, but it does not detect qualitative congenital abnormalities, which is why it is used only in response to an abnormally reduced protein C functional assay result.

Protein S Assays

As with testing for antithrombin and protein C deficiencies, protein S deficiency screening requires a functional assay. No chromogenic assay is available. The laboratory practitioner performs a clot-based assay by mixing the patient's plasma with protein S–depleted normal plasma to ensure normal levels of all factors other than protein S. APC and Russell viper venom are added in a buffer that contains a heparin neutralizer, followed by calcium chloride. The practitioner records the interval to clot formation. The more prolonged the test result, the higher the protein S activity (Figure 39-12). The clot-based protein S assay can be automated.

Therapeutic heparin levels greater than 1 IU/mL consume the heparin neutralizer and lead to overestimation of protein S activity. APC resistance, LA, and the presence of the therapeutic direct thrombin inhibitors argatroban or dabigatran may prolong the PTT and falsely raise the activity levels in clot-based protein S assays.[73] Coagulation factor VII activation may occur during prolonged refrigeration of plasma at 4° C to 10° C; this may cause underestimation of protein S activity and may affect prothrombin time-based coagulation factor assays such as factor V or factor X assays.[74]

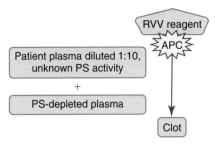

Figure 39-12 Clot-based protein S (PS) assay. Patient plasma is diluted and pipetted into a reagent composed of PS-depleted plasma. A second reagent is composed of Russell viper venom (RVV), which activates clotting at the level of factor X, and activated protein C (APC). The patient PS binds the reagent APC to prolong the clotting time. Clotting time is proportional to PS activity.

TABLE 39-6 Anticipated Protein S (PS) Test Results in Qualitative and Quantitative Deficiencies

	Type of PS Deficiency	PS Activity	PS Free Antigen	PS Total Antigen	C4bBP
I	Quantitative	<65%	<65%	<65%	Normal
II	Qualitative	<65%	>65%	>65%	Normal
III	Inflammation	<65%	<65%	>65%	Elevated

C4bBP, C4b-binding protein.

When there is clinical suspicion of primary protein S deficiency based on a low activity level, enzyme immunoassays are employed to measure both total and free protein S antigen. These assays detect most quantitative congenital deficiencies and aid in the diagnosis of qualitative type II congenital deficiencies characterized by normal antigen but decreased activity of protein S. In type III deficiency, the concentration of free antigen protein S and its activity, but not the total antigen, are reduced (Table 39-6). The concentration of plasma C4bBP, measured with an immunoassay available for research use only, aids in the classification of the type of protein S deficiency.

ARTERIAL THROMBOSIS PREDICTORS

Arterial thrombotic disease, including peripheral vascular occlusion, myocardial infarction (heart attack), and cerebrovascular ischemia (stroke), arises from atherosclerotic plaque. The traditional predictors of arterial thrombosis risk are elevated *total cholesterol* (TC) and *low-density lipoprotein cholesterol* (LDL-C), or an *elevated ratio of total cholesterol to high-density lipoprotein cholesterol* (TC:HDL-C) secondary to HDL-C deficiency. One third of primary cardiovascular and cerebrovascular events occur in patients whose lipid profiles are normal, however, and half of people with proven lipid risk factors never experience an arterial thrombotic event.[75]

Researchers have sought additional arterial thrombosis predictors by performing prospective randomized studies of lipoprotein subtypes, fibrinolytic pathway components, and markers of inflammation. The results of these studies have led to the identification of potential markers of arterial thrombosis risk (Table 39-7), of which *homocysteine* and *high-sensitivity CRP*

TABLE 39-7 Markers of Arterial Thrombosis Risk

Marker	Reference Interval	Comments
High-sensitivity C-reactive protein	0.3–1.7 mg/L	Marker of inflammation; stable, reproducible
Fibrinogen	220–498 mg/dL	Chronic level >300 mg/dL increases thrombotic risk; inadequate reproducibility with numerous test platforms
Homocysteine	4.6–12.1 μmol/L	Reference interval and predictive values vary with population; may be reduced with vitamin B_6, B_{12}, and folate supplementation
Total cholesterol (TC)	<200 mg/dL	Reproducible; some relationship with diet, exercise; risk prediction is partially dependent on inflammation
Ratio of total cholesterol to high-density lipoprotein cholesterol (TC : HDL-C)	<10	Reproducible; elevated ratio relates to diet, exercise; risk prediction is partially dependent on inflammation
Low-density lipoprotein cholesterol (LDL-C)	<130 mg/dL	Reproducible; may be significantly lowered with statin therapy
Lipoprotein (a)	2.2–49.4 mg/dL	Varies with race and age; lowered with statin therapy; inadequate reproducibility

have become a part of many institution's arterial thrombosis risk profiles. The role of platelets in arterial thrombosis is also under investigation.

C-Reactive Protein

CRP is a calcium-dependent pentameric ligand-binding member of the *pentraxin* family produced in the liver that circulates in plasma at a concentration below 0.55 mg/L. First described in 1930, CRP is an acute-phase reactant whose plasma concentration rises 1000-fold 6 to 8 hours after the onset of an inflammatory event such as an infection, trauma, or surgery. This rise remains stable over several days in vivo, and the protein is resistant to in vitro degradation.[76] Extremely high CRP levels are identified using one of several time-honored manual semiquantitative laboratory assays, all of which employ polyclonal anti-CRP antibodies that coats a suspension of visible latex particles. The test takes place on a slide or card. Laboratory professionals continue to use this simple and inexpensive assay to confirm inflammation and monitor the effectiveness of anti-inflammatory therapy.

A second CRP assay, high-sensitivity CRP (HSCRP), was developed in the late 1990s and is used to document modest but chronic CRP elevation. Both the manual HSCRP enzyme immunoassay and an automated latex microparticle immunoassay employ sensitive monoclonal antibodies that detect CRP at normal or slightly elevated concentrations. Chronic plasma HSCRP concentrations that remain at 1.5 mg/L or above indicate atherosclerosis secondary to low-grade inflammation that correlates to increased risk of myocardial infarction and stroke.[77] Consequently, HSCRP is a clinical measure, independent from the lipid profile, employed to predict cardiovascular or cerebrovascular disease (Table 39-8).[78] HSCRP may also be used in relationship with total cholesterol (Table 39-9) and the TC:HDL-C ratio (Table 39-10) to predict the risk of myocardial infarction. Laboratory professionals may also use HSCRP to monitor the anti-inflammatory effects of statins.[79-82]

Plasma Homocysteine

Homocysteine is a naturally occurring sulfur-containing amino acid formed in the metabolism of dietary *methionine*.[83,84] The

TABLE 39-8 Relative Risk for Myocardial Infarction or Stroke at Four Levels of High-Sensitivity C-Reactive Protein (HSCRP) Independent of Lipid Levels

Quartile	HSCRP	Men	Women
1	≤0.55 mg/L	1.0	1.0
2	0.56–1.14 mg/L	1.8	2.9
3	1.15–2.10 mg/L	2.5	3.5
4	≥2.11 mg/L	2.9	5.5

TABLE 39-9 Relative Risk for Myocardial Infarction at Three Levels of High-Sensitivity C-Reactive Protein (HSCRP) Related to Total Cholesterol

HSCRP	TOTAL CHOLESTEROL		
	Low: ≤191 mg/dL	Medium: 192–223 mg/dL	High: ≥224 mg/dL
Low: ≤0.72 mg/L	1.0	1.4	2.3
Medium: 0.73–1.69 mg/L	1.2	1.5	4.3
High: ≥1.70 mg/L	1.1	2.3	5.3

TABLE 39-10 Relative Risk for Myocardial Infarction at Three Levels of High-Sensitivity C-Reactive Protein (HSCRP) Related to Ratio of Total Cholesterol to High-Density Lipoprotein Cholesterol (TC : HDL-C Ratio)

HSCRP	TC : HDL-C RATIO		
	Low: ≤3.78	Medium: 3.79–5.01	High: ≥5.02
Low: ≤0.72 mg/L	1.0	1.2	2.8
Medium: 0.73–1.69 mg/L	1.1	2.5	3.4
High: ≥1.70 mg/L	1.3	2.8	4.4

homocysteine concentration in plasma depends on adequate protein intake and adequate levels of vitamin B_6, vitamin B_{12}, and folate. Its concentration is regulated by three enzymes: cystathionine β-synthase, which converts homocysteine to *cystathionine* in the presence of vitamin B_6; 5,10-*methylenetetrahydrofolate reductase* (MTHFR), required for the remethylation of homocysteine to methionine in the folic acid cycle; and methionine synthase, which requires vitamin B_{12}. Folate, B_6, or B_{12} deficiencies; common functional polymorphisms of the MTHFR gene; or an inherited deficiency of either cystathionine β-synthase or methionine synthase yields increased plasma homocysteine, *homocysteinemia*.[85]

Clinical Significance of Homocysteinemia

Fasting homocysteinemia is an independent risk factor for arterial thrombosis, with relative risk ratios of 1.7 for coronary artery disease, 2.5 for cerebrovascular disease, and 6.8 for peripheral artery disease.[86,87] Homozygosity for the MTHFR C677T mutation is associated with homocysteinemia but is not an independent thrombosis risk factor. Several theories link homocysteinemia with coronary artery disease, most citing damage to the endothelial cell.[88]

Homocysteine Reference Range and Therapy

The reference ranges for homocysteine differ for men and women, and they rise with age, as shown in Table 39-11. No clinical outcomes studies have correlated homocysteine reduction with reductions in adverse arterial thrombosis events.

Fibrinogen Activity

Laboratory professionals measure fibrinogen using immunoassay, nephelometry, or the Clauss clot-based method to detect dysfibrinogenemia, hypofibrinogenemia, or afibrinogenemia (Chapter 42). The same assays may be used to detect chronic hyperfibrinogenemia. Fibrinogen concentration correlates with relative risk of myocardial infarction in asymptomatic persons or patients with angina pectoris, as shown in Table 39-12.[89] The relative risk triples from the first to the fifth quintiles, and even chronic high-normal levels predict increased risk. There also exists a direct correlation between fibrinogen and total cholesterol (Figure 39-13). High fibrinogen concentrations can be used to predict hypercholesterolemia and identify patients who are at high risk for new coronary events. In contrast, low normal fibrinogen levels are associated with low risk of cardiovascular events, even in people with high total cholesterol levels.

TABLE 39-11 Homocysteine Enzyme Immunoassay Reference Intervals

Population	Reference Interval (μmol/L)
Females ≤60 yr	4.6–12.1
Females >60 yr	6.6–14.1
Males ≤60 yr	5.0–15.6
Males >60 yr	7.0–17.6

TABLE 39-12 Relative Risk of Coronary Events According to Concentration of Fibrinogen*

Fibrinogen Concentration Quintile	Relative Risk of Coronary Event
1	1.0
2	1.89
3	2.33
4	2.56
5	2.89

*The relative risks are shown for each of five quintiles of subjects defined according to the concentrations of each fibrinogen from 1, the group with the lowest concentration, to 5, the group with the highest concentration. Relative risks have been adjusted for all confounding factors. The group with the lowest values serves as the reference group.

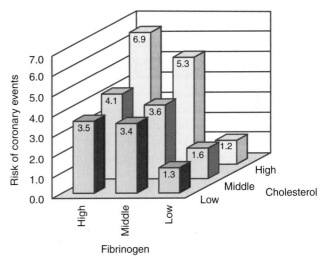

Figure 39-13 Coronary risk prediction by fibrinogen and cholesterol concentrations. Fibrinogen and total cholesterol synergistically predict coronary risk. Tertiles of fibrinogen concentration are shown in relation to tertiles of total cholesterol concentration with the relative risk of coronary events indicated for each combination.

Elevated fibrinogen supports coagulation and activates platelets by binding to their glycoprotein IIb/IIIa membrane receptors. Fibrinogen becomes integrated into atherothrombotic lesions and contributes to their thrombotic potential.

Although hyperfibrinogenemia predicts arterial thrombosis, the use of the fibrinogen assay for this purpose is limited. There are no independent therapeutic regimens that specifically lower fibrinogen, and no clinical trials suggest that fibrinogen reduction reverses the odds of thrombosis. Further, the various fibrinogen assay methods are not normalized. Nevertheless, statin therapy, smoking cessation, and exercise lower fibrinogen levels alongside LDL-C and total cholesterol levels, and the assay results parallel those for the other members of the risk prediction profile.

Lipoprotein (a)

Lipoprotein (a) is low-density lipoprotein that may be used to predict arterial thrombosis. The plasma level is measured by enzyme immunoassay, and its reference ranges are shown in Table 39-13. Although lipoprotein (a) concentrations are

TABLE 39-13 Normal Ranges for Lipoprotein (a) by Race and Sex

Race	Males	Females
African American	4.7–71.8 mg/dL	4.4–75.0 mg/dL
European American	2.2–49.4 mg/dL	2.1–57.3 mg/dL

higher in African Americans than in European Americans, the level is a stronger predictor of thrombosis in Caucasians.[90]

Lipoprotein (a) may contribute to thrombosis by its antifibrinolytic property. The molecule competes with plasminogen for binding sites on newly formed fibrin polymer, decreasing the plasmin activity available for clot degradation. It also may contribute to the overall concentration of LDL-C. Levels can be lowered with statin drugs, as can LDL-C levels.

DISSEMINATED INTRAVASCULAR COAGULATION

DIC, also named *defibrination syndrome* or *consumption coagulopathy*, is the generalized activation of hemostasis secondary to a systemic disease. DIC involves all hemostatic systems: vascular intima, platelets, leukocytes, coagulation, coagulation control pathways, and fibrinolysis.[91] In DIC, fibrin microthrombi partially occlude small vessels and consume platelets, coagulation factors, coagulation control proteins, and fibrinolytic enzymes. Fibrin/fibrinogen degradation products (FDPs, traditionally called *fibrin split products,* FSPs), including D-dimer, become elevated and interfere with normal fibrin formation.[92] This combination of events sets loose a series of toxic and inflammatory processes.[93]

DIC may be *acute and uncompensated*, with deficiencies of multiple hemostasis components, or *chronic*, with normal or even elevated clotting factor levels. In chronic DIC, liver coagulation factor production and bone marrow platelet production compensate for increased consumption.

Although DIC is a thrombotic process, the thrombi that form are small and ineffective, so systemic hemorrhage is often the first or most apparent sign. Acute DIC is often fatal and requires immediate medical intervention. The diagnosis relies heavily on the hemostasis laboratory, and medical laboratory professionals often perform a DIC profile under emergent circumstances.

Causes

Any disorder that contributes hemostatic molecules or promotes their endogenous secretion may cause DIC. Classifying and listing all the causes of DIC are impossible, but the major triggering mechanisms and examples of each are listed in Table 39-14.

The more acutely ill the patient, the more dangerous the symptoms. Chronic DIC may be associated with vascular tumors, tissue necrosis, liver disease, renal disease, chronic inflammation, use of prosthetic devices, and adenocarcinoma. The malignancies most associated with DIC are pancreatic, prostatic, ovarian, and lung cancers; multiple myeloma; and

TABLE 39-14 Conditions Associated with Disseminated Intravascular Coagulation Grouped by Mechanism

Mechanism	Examples of Conditions
Tissue factor is released into circulation through endothelial cell damage or monocyte activation	Physical trauma: crush or brain injuries, surgery Degradation of muscle; rhabdomyolysis Tissue ischemia; myocardial infarction Thermal injuries: burns or cold Adenocarcinoma
Exposure of subendothelial tissue factor during vasodilatation	Hypovolemic and hemorrhagic shock Malignant hypertension Asphyxia and hypoxia Heat stroke Vasculitis
Endotoxins that activate cytokines	Bacterial, protozoal, fungal, and viral infections, septicemia Toxic shock syndrome
Circulating immune complexes	Heparin-induced thrombocytopenia with thrombosis Drugs that trigger an immune response Acute hemolytic transfusion reactions Allergic reactions and anaphylaxis Bacterial and viral infections Graft rejection
Particulate matter from tissue injury	Eclampsia, preeclampsia, HELLP syndrome Retained dead fetus or missed abortion Amniotic fluid embolism Abruptio placentae Rupture of uterus Tubal pregnancy Fat embolism Heatstroke
Infusion of activated clotting factors	Activated prothrombin complex concentrate therapy
Secretion of proteolytic enzymes	Acute promyelocytic or myelomonocytic leukemia Bacterial, protozoal, fungal, and viral infections Pancreatitis
Toxins that trigger coagulation	Snake or spider envenomation Pancreatitis
Thrombotic disease or thrombogenic conditions	Thrombotic thrombocytopenic purpura, hemolytic uremic syndrome Pregnancy, postpartum period, estrogen therapy Deep vein thrombosis, pulmonary embolus Coagulation control system deficiencies Purpura fulminans, skin necrosis
Severe hypoxia or acidosis	Acute coagulopathy of trauma-shock Chronic inflammation Diabetes mellitus
Platelet activation	Vascular surgery, coronary artery bypass surgery Thrombocytosis, thrombocythemia, polycythemia Vascular tumors Vascular prostheses Aortic aneurysm

HELLP, Hemolysis, elevated liver enzymes, and low platelet count.

myeloproliferative diseases. Acute DIC is seen in association with obstetric emergencies, intravascular hemolysis, septicemia, viremia, burns, acute inflammation, crush injuries, dissecting aortic aneurysms, and cardiac disorders.

Pathophysiology

Triggering events may activate coagulation at any point in the pathway. When triggered, however, DIC proceeds in a predictable sequence of events. Circulating thrombin is the primary culprit because it activates platelets, activates coagulation proteins (positive feedback loops within the coagulation cascade), and catalyzes fibrin formation, of which the ensuing clots consume control proteins. The fibrinolytic system may become activated at the level of plasminogen or TPA subsequent to fibrin formation, and endothelial cells may become damaged, releasing coagulation-active substances. Finally, leukocytes—particularly monocytes—may be induced to secrete tissue factor by the cytokines released during inflammation.

Thrombin cleaves fibrinogen, creating fibrin monomers. In normal hemostasis, fibrin monomers spontaneously polymerize to form an insoluble gel. The polymer becomes strengthened through cross-linking, binding plasminogen as it forms. In DIC, a percentage of fibrin monomers fail to polymerize and circulate in plasma as *soluble fibrin monomers*. The monomers coat platelets and coagulation proteins, creating an anticoagulant effect (Figures 37-12 and 37-14).

Soluble fibrin monomers, fibrin polymer, and cross-linked fibrin all activate plasminogen. Normally, the active form of plasminogen—plasmin—acts locally to digest only the solid fibrin clot to which it is bound (Chapter 37). In DIC, plasmin circulates in the plasma and digests all forms of fibrinogen and fibrin.[94] Consequently, fibrin degradation products labeled X, Y, D, E, and D-dimer are detectable in the plasma in concentrations exceeding 20,000 ng/mL. D-dimer arises from cross-linked fibrin polymer, whereas the other fibrin degradation products may be produced from fibrinogen or fibrin monomers or polymers.[95]

Platelets become enmeshed in the fibrin polymer or are exposed to thrombin; both events trigger platelet activation, which further drives the coagulation system and produces thrombocytopenia. At the same time, coagulation pathway control is lost as protein C, protein S, and antithrombin are consumed. The combination of thrombin activation, circulating plasmin, loss of control, and thrombocytopenia contributes to the overall hemorrhagic outcome of DIC.

Free plasmin digests factors V, VIII, IX, and XI, as well as other plasma proteins. Plasmin also may trigger complement, which leads to hemolysis, and the kinin system, which results in inflammation, hypotension, and shock. During fibrinolytic therapy, in amyloidosis, and sometimes in liver disease, plasminogen becomes activated independently of the coagulation pathway. This condition, called *systemic fibrinolysis* or *primary fibrinolysis*, produces laboratory-measurable fibrinogen and fibrin degradation products, including D-dimer, and prolonged prothrombin time (PT) and PTT with a normal platelet count.[96]

Symptoms

The symptoms signaling DIC frequently are masked by the symptoms of the underlying disorder and may be chronic, acute, or even fulminant. Thrombosis in the microvasculature of major organs may produce symptoms of organ failure, such as renal function impairment, adult respiratory distress syndrome, and central nervous system manifestations. Skin, bone, and bone marrow necrosis may be seen. *Purpura fulminans* is seen in meningococcemia, chickenpox, and spirochete infections.

Laboratory Diagnosis

DIC is a clinical diagnosis that requires laboratory confirmation (Chapter 42). The initial laboratory profile includes a platelet count, blood film examination, PT, PTT, D-dimer, and fibrinogen assay. Table 39-15 lists anticipated DIC results. Prolonged PT and PTT reflect coagulation factor consumption. Fibrinogen concentrations may decrease in DIC, but because fibrinogen is an acute phase reactant that rises in inflammation, the fibrinogen concentration alone provides little reliable information and may exceed 400 mg/dL. The peripheral blood film platelet estimate confirms thrombocytopenia in nearly all cases, and the presence of *schistocytes* helps establish the diagnosis of DIC in about 50% of cases.[97,98] An elevated D-dimer level is essential to the diagnosis. D-dimer also may be elevated in inflammatory conditions, localized thrombosis, or renal disease in the absence of DIC; the PT, PTT, platelet count, blood film examination, and other laboratory assays must be performed alongside the D-dimer to rule out these disorders.

The D-dimer reference limit is typically 240 ng/mL, although the interval varies with location and technology. In 85% of DIC cases, D-dimer levels reach 10,000 to 20,000 ng/mL. A normal D-dimer assay result rules out DIC and rules out localized venous thromboembolic disease such as deep vein thrombosis or pulmonary emboli, in which levels rise to greater than 500 ng/mL but not to DIC levels.[99] D-dimer concentrations are typically elevated in inflammation, sickle cell crisis, pregnancy, and renal disease, so an abnormal result alone cannot be used to definitively diagnose venous thromboembolism.[100] The judicious use of the D-dimer assay reduces the requirement for

TABLE 39-15 Anticipated Results of Disseminated Intravascular Coagulation (DIC) Primary Laboratory Profile

Test	Reference Interval	Value in DIC
Platelet count	150,000–450,000/μL	<150,000/μL
Prothrombin time	11–14 sec	>14 sec
Partial thromboplastin time	25–35 sec	>35 sec
D-dimer	0–240 ng/mL	>240 ng/mL, often 10,000 to 20,000 ng/mL
Fibrinogen	220–498 mg/dL	<220 mg/dL, often higher, because fibrinogen is an acute phase reactant

invasive diagnostic tests such as pulmonary angiography when pulmonary embolism is suspected.[101]

Specialized Laboratory Tests That May Aid in Diagnosis

Table 39-16 lists specialized laboratory tests that may be used to diagnose and classify DIC in special circumstances. Results consistent with DIC and clinical comments are included. Many of these tests are available in acute care facilities, but they are not routinely applied to the diagnosis of DIC. Others are available only in tertiary care facilities and hemostasis reference laboratories.[102-104]

Protein C, protein S, and antithrombin typically are consumed in DIC, and their assay may contribute to the diagnosis. When thawed frozen plasma or antithrombin concentrate (Thrombate III) is used to treat DIC, these assays are useful in establishing the necessity for therapy and monitoring its effect.[105] Factor assays may clarify PT and PTT results. The thrombin time and the reptilase time also are sensitive DIC screens.

Tests of the fibrinolytic pathway include serum fibrin degradation products, now obsolete; chromogenic plasminogen activity assay; and TPA and PAI-1 immunoassays.[106] These tests are seldom offered in the acute care hemostasis laboratory because they require careful specimen management, but they may help in the diagnosis of primary fibrinolysis, which may occur after fibrinolytic therapy.

Treatment

To arrest DIC, the physician must diagnose and treat the underlying disorder. Surgery, anti-inflammatory agents, antibiotics, or obstetric procedures as appropriate may normalize hemostasis, particularly in chronic DIC. Supportive therapy, such as maintenance of fluid and electrolyte balance, always accompanies medical and surgical management.

In acute DIC, in which multiorgan failure from microthrombosis and bleeding threatens the life of the patient, heroic measures are necessary. Treatment falls into two categories: therapies that slow the clotting process and therapies that replace missing platelets and coagulation factors.

UFH may be used for its antithrombotic properties to stop the uncontrolled activation of the coagulation cascade. Because UFH may aggravate bleeding, careful observation and support are required. Repeated chromogenic anti-factor Xa heparin assays may be necessary to control heparin dosage because in DIC the PTT is ineffective for monitoring heparin therapy.

Thawed frozen plasma provides all the necessary coagulation factors and replaces blood volume lost during acute DIC hemorrhage. Prothrombin complex concentrate (Proplex T complex, Baxter Healthcare Corporation, Deerfield, IL; or Kcentra, CSL Behring, King of Prussia, PA), fibrinogen concentrate (RiaSTAP, CSL Behring, King of Prussia, PA), and factor VIII concentrate (ADVATE, Baxter, Deerfield, IL) may be used in place of plasma, particularly if there is concern for transfusion-associated circulatory overload. Repeated measurements of fibrinogen, PT, and PTT are necessary to confirm the effectiveness of these therapeutics. Platelet transfusions are necessary if thrombocytopenia is severe. The effectiveness of platelet concentrate and platelet consumption are monitored with platelet counts (Chapters 15 and 16). Red blood cells are administered as necessary to treat the resulting anemia. Antifibrinolytic therapy is contraindicated, except in proven systemic fibrinolysis.[107,108]

LOCALIZED THROMBOSIS MONITORS

In addition to D-dimer, several peptides and coagulation factor complexes are released into the plasma during coagulation. One complex, *thrombin-antithrombin complex* (TAT), and one peptide, *prothrombin fragment F 1+2* (PF 1+2 or PF 1.2), may be assayed as a means to detect and monitor localized venous or arterial thromboses. TAT and PF 1+2 immunoassays are sensitive and specific for thrombosis, which occurs in DIC, septicemia, eclampsia, pancreatitis, leukemia, liver disease, and

TABLE 39-16 Specialized Hemostasis Laboratory Assays Used to Diagnose and Classify Disseminated Intravascular Coagulation (DIC)

Assay	Value in DIC	Comments
Serum fibrin degradation products (FDP)	>10 μg/mL	Obsolete, replaced by quantitative D-dimer.
Soluble fibrin monomer	Positive	Hemagglutination assay provides valid measure of fibrin monomer. Avoid obsolete tests such as protamine sulfate solubility or ethanol gelation.
Thrombus precursor protein	>3.5 μg/mL	Immunoassay with no interference from fibrinogen or FDPs.
Protein C, protein S, and AT activity assays	<50%	Use to monitor therapy: plasma, AT concentrate, recombinant thrombomodulin.
Plasminogen, tissue plasminogen activator	Decreased	May be useful for analyzing systemic fibrinolysis. Specimen management protocol must be strictly observed.
Peripheral blood film exam	Anemia with schistocytes	Schistocytes (microangiopathic hemolytic anemia) are present in 50% of DIC cases; leukocytosis is common.
Localized thrombosis markers: prothrombin fragment 1+2, thrombin-antithrombin	Elevated	Most useful in diagnosis of localized thrombotic events, but may be used to monitor DIC therapy. Used in clinical trials.
Factor assays: II (prothrombin), V, VIII, X	<30%	Factors V and VIII rise in inflammation; assays may give misleading results.
Thrombin time, reptilase time	Prolonged	Fibrinogen levels <80 mg/dL, elevated FDPs, and soluble fibrin monomer all prolong thrombin time and reptilase time.

AT, Antithrombin; *FDP,* fibrin degradation product.

trauma.[108] These assays are of particular value in clinical trials of anticoagulants.

PF 1+2 is released from prothrombin at the time of its conversion to thrombin by the prothrombinase complex. It has a plasma half-life of 90 minutes and a reference range of 0.3 to 1.5 nmol/L. Elevated PF 1+2 may be seen in venous thromboembolism. Heparin or oral anticoagulant therapy reduces its plasma concentration.

The TAT covalent complex is formed when antithrombin neutralizes thrombin. This reaction is enhanced by the presence of heparin. TAT has a half-life of 3 minutes and a normal range of 0.5 to 5 ng/mL.

To avoid in vitro release or activation of PF 1+2 or TAT, plasma specimens are collected in 3.2% sodium citrate and are centrifuged and separated within minutes of collection; then the plasma is frozen until ready for assay.

HEPARIN-INDUCED THROMBOCYTOPENIA

Heparin-induced thrombocytopenia (HIT), also called *heparin-induced thrombocytopenia with thrombosis,* is an adverse effect of heparin treatment.

Cause and Clinical Significance

Between 1% and 5% of patients receiving unfractionated heparin (UFH) for more than 5 days develop an IgG antibody specific for heparin–platelet factor 4 complexes. In 30% to 50% of these cases, the immune complexes that are formed bind platelet Fc receptors, which leads to platelet activation, thrombocytopenia, and formation of microvascular thrombi.[109] HIT occurs with UFH administration at both prophylactic and therapeutic dosages, although it is more frequent with therapeutic doses.[110] Venous thrombosis predominates 5:1, but arterial thrombosis accounts for the most disturbing symptoms. Patients may develop pulmonary emboli, limb gangrene requiring amputation, stroke, and myocardial infarction. HIT is often a medical emergency, and the mortality rate is 20%.[111] LMWH also causes HIT. In most cases, HIT during LMWH therapy turns out to be a cross-reaction in a patient recently exposed to UFH; however, LMWH has been implicated as a primary cause at a rate of 1% of UFH-caused HIT. Likewise, protamine sulfate, a salmon sperm derivative that cardiac surgeons use to rapidly reduce UFH's anticoagulant may itself generate antibodies similar to anti–heparin-PF4 antibodies and cause thrombocytopenia and thrombosis symptoms indistinguishable from UFH-caused HIT.

Platelet Count

Patients receiving heparin must have platelet counts performed every other day. A platelet count decrease during heparin administration indicates HIT, but interpretation of the thrombocytopenia is confounded because 30% of patients receiving heparin develop an immediate, benign, and limited thrombocytopenia, sometimes called *HIT type I.*[112] This benign form of thrombocytopenia usually develops in 1 to 3 days, whereas thrombotic HIT, sometimes called *HIT type II*, develops after 5 days. However, thrombotic HIT may develop in 1 to 3 days in patients recently exposed to heparin. In HIT (HIT type II), the decrease in platelet count may exceed 40%, whereas in benign thrombocytopenia the decrease is relatively small; however, in both cases, the platelet count may remain within the normal range. The HIT diagnosis is made using the "4Ts" approach, provided in Table 39-17.

TABLE 39-17 The "4Ts" Scoring System: Laboratory and Clinical Pretest Probability of Heparin-Induced Thrombocytopenia (HIT)

Indicator	SCORE		
	2	1	0
Acute thrombocytopenia	>50% decrease in platelet count to nadir of ≥20,000/μL	30%–50% decrease in platelet count, >50% if directly resulting from surgery, or to nadir of 10,000–19,000/μL	<30% decrease in platelet count, or to nadir of <10,000/μL
Timing of platelet count decrease, thrombosis, or other sequelae of HIT (first day of heparin therapy is day 0)	Onset of decrease on days 5–10, or onset of decrease on day 1 if previous heparin exposure within past 5–30 days	Apparent decrease on days 5–10, but unclear due to missing platelet counts; or decrease after day 10; or decrease on day 1 if previous heparin exposure within past 31–100 days	Decrease at ≤4 days without recent heparin exposure
Thrombosis, skin lesions, acute system reaction	Proven new thrombosis or skin necrosis; acute systemic reaction after heparin exposure	Progressive, recurrent, or suspected thrombosis; erythematous skin lesions	None
Other causes for thrombocytopenia	No explanation for platelet count decrease is evident	Possible other cause is evident	Probable other cause is evident

From Crowther MA, Cook DJ, Albert M, et al: Canadian Critical Care Trials Group: the 4Ts scoring system for heparin-induced thrombocytopenia in medical-surgical intensive care unit patients, *J Crit Care* 25:287-293, 2010.
Maximum pretest probability score is 8; a score of 6 to 8 indicates high probability of HIT; 4 to 5, intermediate probability; 0 to 3, low probability.
The most immunizing heparin exposure is considered first; unfractionated heparin (UFH) received during cardiac surgery is more immunogenic than UFH or low-molecular-weight heparin received for acute coronary syndrome. The day the platelet count begins to fall is considered the day of onset of thrombocytopenia. It generally takes 1 to 3 days before an arbitrary threshold that defines thrombocytopenia, such as 150,000 platelets/μL, is passed.

Laboratory Tests for HIT

Because at least 10% of hospitalized patients receive heparin, the acute care laboratory must provide a procedure to confirm HIT and differentiate it from benign thrombocytopenia. Most acute care laboratories provide a heparin-induced antibody immunoassay but seldom as a stat assay (Chapter 40).[113] Owing to its sensitivity, the immunoassay result may be positive before clinical signs of HIT become evident. Further, the immunoassay result may be negative in a few HIT patients, possibly because peptides such as protamine sulfate may also form complexes with PF4. Microbial contamination, lipemia, and hemolysis may also invalidate immunoassay results. Conversely, patient specimen immune complexes or immunoglobulin aggregates may cause nonspecific binding and produce false-positive results.

Many laboratories provide aggregometry or lumiaggregometry methods to confirm HIT (Chapter 40).[114] Aggregometry is technically demanding and is only 50% sensitive for HIT. Also technically demanding, but perhaps more sensitive, is washed platelet suspension lumiaggregometry. The reference method is the washed platelet ^{14}C-serotonin release assay (serotonin release assay, SRA), provided by reference laboratories that possess radionuclide licenses.

Treatment

When heparin-induced antibodies are detected, the administration of UFH or LMWH is immediately discontinued, and the physician chooses an alternate form of anticoagulation. Complete cessation of anticoagulant therapy is risky because additional thrombotic events are likely to occur. Although LMWH causes HIT in only 1% of cases in which it is the sole anticoagulant, its use as a substitute for UFH is contraindicated owing to its tendency to react with the existing antibody. Likewise, Coumadin is discouraged; it may precipitate a potentially severe skin necrosis if given in high bolus dosages, but more importantly its onset is too slow to be practical in this setting. Synthetic pentasaccharide (fondaparinux), which mimics heparin's antithrombin-binding sequence, has been shown in several small case series to be useful for the management of patients with suspected HIT.[115]

Recombinant bivalirudin (Angiomax, The Medicines Company, Parsippany, NJ) is a direct thrombin inhibitor modeled after leech saliva. Argatroban (Mitsubishi Pharma Corporation, Tokyo, Japan) is an amino acid analogue direct thrombin inhibitor. Both bind the active thrombin protease site, and, in HIT, physicians administer either argatroban or bivalirudin as a continuous infusion. Laboratory practitioners may monitor either using the PTT. The activated clotting time (ACT); the ecarin clotting time, which uses a reagent derived from *Echis carinatus* snake venom (Diagnostica Stago, Inc., Parsippany, NJ); or the plasma-diluted thrombin time (HEMOCLOT Thrombin, Aniara, Hyphen Biomed, West Chester, OH) may also be employed to monitor these direct thrombin inhibitors (Chapter 43).

CONCLUSION

The importance of laboratory diagnosis has become evident in all forms of thrombotic disease: chronic and acute, arterial and venous, primary and secondary, and acquired and congenital. The future may give us markers of endothelial cell disease, measures of leukocyte adhesion, and specific markers of inflammation and platelet activity that will further enable us to predict and prevent thrombosis.

SUMMARY

- Thrombosis is the most prevalent condition in developed countries and accounts for most illnesses and premature death.
- Thrombosis may be arterial, causing peripheral artery disease, heart disease, and stroke, or venous, causing deep vein thrombosis and pulmonary emboli.
- Most thrombosis occurs as a result of lifestyle habits and aging, but many thrombotic disorders are related to congenital risk factors.
- Thrombosis risk profiles may be offered to clinicians for screening purposes in high-risk populations.
- The main hemostasis predictors of arterial thrombotic disease are elevated levels of CRP (measured by high-sensitivity assay), homocysteine, fibrinogen, lipoprotein (a), and coagulation factors.
- The main hemostasis predictors of venous thromboembolic disease are APL antibodies, antithrombin, PC, and PS deficiency, FVL mutation, and prothrombin G20210A.
- APL antibody testing requires a series of essential hemostasis laboratory assays—clot-based tests and immunoassays.
- Antithrombin may be assayed using chromogenic substrate and enzyme immunoassay analyses.
- The tests for evaluating the protein C pathway include protein C and protein S activity and concentration, APC resistance, FVL assay, and C4bBP assay.
- The molecular test for the prothrombin G20210A mutation predicts the risk of venous thrombosis.
- DIC is a clinical diagnosis confirmed by a series of assays in the acute care facility.
- Chronic thrombosis may be identified using the PF 1+2, TAT complex, and quantitative D-dimer assays.
- The laboratory provides confirmatory tests for HIT with thrombosis.

Now that you have completed this chapter, go back and read again the case study at the beginning and respond to the questions presented.

REVIEW QUESTIONS

Answers can be found in the Appendix.

1. What is the prevalence of venous thrombosis in the United States?
   a. 0.01
   b. 1 in 1000
   c. 10% to 15%
   d. 500,000 cases per year

2. What is thrombophilia?
   a. Predisposition to thrombosis secondary to a congenital or acquired disorder
   b. Inappropriate triggering of the plasma coagulation system
   c. A condition in which clots form uncontrollably
   d. Inadequate fibrinolysis

3. What acquired thrombosis risk factor is assessed in the hemostasis laboratory?
   a. Smoking
   b. Immobilization
   c. Body mass index
   d. Lupus anticoagulant

4. Trousseau syndrome, a low-grade chronic DIC, is often associated with what type of disorder?
   a. Renal disease
   b. Hepatic disease
   c. Adenocarcinoma
   d. Chronic inflammation

5. What is the most common heritable thrombosis risk factor in Caucasians?
   a. APC resistance (factor V Leiden mutation)
   b. Prothrombin G20210A mutation
   c. Antithrombin deficiency
   d. Protein S deficiency

6. In most LA profiles, what screening test is primary because it detects LA with the fewest interferences?
   a. Low-phospholipid PTT
   b. DRVVT
   c. KCT
   d. PT

7. A patient with venous thrombosis is tested for protein S deficiency. The protein S activity, antigen, and free antigen all are less than 65%, and the C4bBP level is normal. What type of deficiency is likely?
   a. Type I
   b. Type II
   c. Type III
   d. No deficiency is indicated, because the reference range includes 65%.

8. An elevated level of what fibrinolytic system assay is associated with arterial thrombotic risk?
   a. PAI-1
   b. TPA
   c. Factor VIIa
   d. Factor XII

9. How does lipoprotein (a) cause thrombosis?
   a. It causes elevated factor VIII levels.
   b. It coats the endothelial lining of arteries.
   c. It substitutes for plasminogen or TPA in the forming clot.
   d. It contributes additional phospholipid in vivo for formation of the Xase complex.

10. What test may be used to *confirm* the presence of LA?
    a. PT
    b. Bethesda titer
    c. Antinuclear antibody
    d. PTT using high-phospholipid reagent

11. What molecular test may be used to *confirm* APC resistance?
    a. Prothrombin G20210A
    b. MTHFR 1298
    c. MTHFR 677
    d. FVL

12. What therapeutic agent may occasionally cause DIC?
    a. Factor VIII
    b. Factor VIIa
    c. Antithrombin concentrate
    d. Activated prothrombin complex concentrate

13. Which is *not* a fibrinolysis control protein?
    a. Thrombin-activatable fibrinolysis inhibitor
    b. Plasminogen activator inhibitor-1
    c. α2-antiplasmin
    d. D-dimer

14. What is the most important application of the quantitative D-dimer test?
    a. Diagnose primary fibrinolysis
    b. Diagnose liver and renal disease
    c. Rule out deep venous thrombosis
    d. Diagnose acute myocardial infarction

REFERENCES

1. Francis, J. L. (1998). Laboratory investigation of hypercoagulability. *Semin Thromb Hemost, 24*, 111–126.

2. Dahlback, B., Carlsson, M., & Svensson, P. J. (1993). Familial thrombophilia due to a previously unrecognized mechanism characterized by poor anticoagulant response to activated protein C: prediction of a cofactor to activated protein C. *Proc Natl Acad Sci U S A, 90*, 1004–1008.

3. Bertina, R. M., Koeleman, B. P. C., Koster, T., et al. (1994). Mutation in blood coagulation factor V associated with resistance to activated protein C. *Nature, 369*, 64–67.

4. Nieuwdorp, M., Stroes, E. S., Meijers, J. C., et al. (2005). Hypercoagulability in the metabolic syndrome. *Curr Opin Pharmacol, 5*, 155–159.

5. Heit, J. A. (2013). Thrombophilia: clinical and laboratory assessment and management. In Kitchens, C. S., Kessler, C. M., & Konkle, B. A., (Eds.), *Consultative Hemostasis and Thrombosis.* (3rd ed., pp. 205–239). Philadelphia: Saunders.

6. Go, A. S., Mozaffarian, D., Roger, V. L., et al; on behalf of the American Heart Association Statistics Committee and Stroke Statistics Subcommittee. (2014). Heart disease and stroke statistics—2014 update: a report from the American Heart Association. *Circulation*, Published online December 18, 2013, doi:10.1161/01.cir0000441139.02102.80.

7. Heit, J. A. (2008). The epidemiology of venous thromboembolism in the community. *Arterioscler Thromb Vasc Biol, 28*, 370–372.

8. Zöller, B., Li, X., Sundquist, J., & Sundquist, K. (2012). Shared familial aggregation of susceptibility to different manifestations of venous thromboembolism: a nationwide family study in Sweden. *Br J Haematol, 157*, 146–148.

9. Jensen, R. (1997). The interface of the physician and the laboratory in the detection of venous thrombotic risk—part I. *Clin Hemost Rev, 11*, 1–4.

10. Stein, P. D., Matta, F., Musani, M. H., et al. (2010). Silent pulmonary embolism in patients with deep venous thrombosis: a systematic review. *Am J Med, 123*, 426–431.

11. Rosendaal, F. R., & Reitsma, P. H. (2009). Genetics of venous thrombosis. *J Thromb Haemost, 7*(Suppl. 1), 301–304.

12. Vemulapalli, S., & Becker, R. C. (2013). Hemostatic aspects of cardiovascular medicine. In Kitchens, C. S., Kessler, C. M., & Konkle, B. A., (Eds.), *Consultative Hemostasis and Thrombosis.* (3rd ed., pp. 342–394). Philadelphia: Saunders.

13. The Surgeon General's Call to Action to prevent deep vein thrombosis and pulmonary embolism. (2008). US Department of Health and Human Services. Office of the Surgeon General, US. http://www.ncbi.nlm.nih.gov/books/NBK44178/. Accessed 21.11.14.

14. Piazza, G., & Goldhaber, S. Z. (2010). Venous thromboembolism and atherothrombosis: an integrated approach. *Circulation, 121*, 2146–2150.

15. Rand, J. H., Wolgast, L. R. (2013). Antiphospholipid syndrome: pathogenesis, clinical presentation, diagnosis, and patient management. In Kitchens, C. S., Kessler, C. M., Konkle, B. A., (Eds.), *Consultative Hemostasis and Thrombosis.* (3rd ed., pp. 321–341). Philadelphia: Saunders.

16. Rak, J., Milsom, C., May, L., et al. (2006). Tissue factor in cancer and angiogenesis: the molecular link between genetic tumor progression, tumor neovascularization, and cancer coagulopathy. *Semin Thromb Hemost, 32*, 54–70.

17. Sanz, M. A., Grimwade, D., & Tallman, M. S. (2009). Management of acute promyelocytic leukemia: recommendations from an expert panel on behalf of the European Leukemia Net. *Blood, 13*, 1875–1891.

18. Rosse, W. F., & Ware, R. E. (1995). The molecular basis of paroxysmal nocturnal hemoglobinuria. *Blood, 86*, 3277–3286.

19. Gröntved, A., & Hu, F. B. (2011). Television viewing and risk of type 2 diabetes, cardiovascular disease, and all-cause mortality: a meta-analysis. *JAMA, 305*, 2448–2455.

20. Garg, N., Kumar, A., & Flaker, G. C. (2010). Antiplatelet therapy for stroke prevention in atrial fibrillation. *Mo Med, 107*, 44–47.

21. Bramham, K., Hunt, B. J., & Goldsmith, D. (2009). Thrombophilia of nephrotic syndrome in adults. *Clin Adv Hematol Oncol, 7*, 368–372.

22. Lane, D. A., Mannuci, P. M., Bauer, K. A., et al. (1996). Inherited thrombophilia: part 2. *Thromb Haemost, 76*, 824–834.

23. Johnson, C. M., Mureebe, L., & Silver, D. (2005). Hypercoagulable states: a review. *Vasc Endovasc Surg, 39*, 123–133.

24. Itakkura, H. (2005). Racial disparities in risk factors for thrombosis. *Curr Opin Hematol, 12*, 364–369.

25. Sedano-Balbás, S., Lyons, M., Cleary, B., et al. (2011). Acquired activated protein C resistance, thrombophilia and adverse pregnancy outcomes: a study performed in an Irish cohort of pregnant women. *J Pregnancy, 2011*, 1–9.

26. Berg, A. O., Botkin, J., Calonge, N., et al., Evaluation of Genomic Applications in Practice and Prevention (EGAPP) Working Group. (2011). Recommendations from the EGAPP Working Group: routine testing for Factor V Leiden (R506Q) and prothrombin (G20210A) mutations in adults with a history of idiopathic venous thromboembolism and their adult family members. *Genet Med, 13*, 67–76.

27. Ridker, P. M., Hennekens, C. H., Selhub, J., et al. (1997). Interrelation of hyperhomocysteinemia, factor V Leiden, and risk of future venous thromboembolism. *Circulation, 95*, 1777–1782.

28. Heit, J. A., O'Fallon, W. M., Petterson, T. M., et al. (2002). Relative impact of risk factors for deep vein thrombosis and pulmonary embolism: a population-based study. *Arch Intern Med, 162*, 1245–1248.

29. Reitsma, P. H., Versteeg, H. H., & Middeldorp, S. (2012). Mechanistic view of risk factors for venous thromboembolism. *Arterioscler Thromb Vasc Biol, 32*, 563–568.

30. Alarcon-Segovia, D., & Cabral, A. R. (2006). The concept and classification of antiphospholipid/cofactor syndromes. *Lupus, 5*, 364–367.

31. Lim, W., Crowther, M. A., & Eikelboom, J. W. (2006). Management of antiphospholipid antibody syndrome: a systematic review. *JAMA, 295*, 1050–1057.

32. Pengo, V., Tripodi, A., Reber, G., et al. (2009). Update of the guidelines for lupus anticoagulant detection. Subcommittee on Lupus Anticoagulant/Antiphospholipid Antibody of the Scientific and Standardisation Committee of the International Society on Thrombosis and Haemostasis. *J Thromb Haemost, 7*, 1737–1740.

33. Kandiah, D. A., Sheng, Y. H., & Krilis, S. A. (1996). Beta-2 glycoprotein I: target antigen for autoantibodies in the "antiphospholipid syndrome." *Lupus, 5*, 381–386.

34. Lie, J. T. (1966). Vasculopathy of the antiphospholipid syndromes revisited: thrombosis is the culprit and vasculitis the consort. *Lupus, 5*, 368–371.

35. Lopez-Pedrera, C., Buendia, P., Barbarroja, N., et al. (2006). Antiphospholipid-mediated thrombosis: interplay between anticardiolipin antibodies and vascular cells. *Clin Appl Thromb Hemost, 12*, 41–45.

36. Hughes, G. R. V. (1996). The antiphospholipid syndrome. *Lupus, 5*, 345–346.

37. Cohen, D., Berger, S. P., Steup-Beekman, G. M., et al. (2010). Diagnosis and management of the antiphospholipid syndrome. *BMJ, 340*, c2541.

38. Devreese, K., & Hoylaerts, M. F. (2010). Challenges in the diagnosis of the antiphospholipid syndrome. *Clin Chem, 56*, 930–940.

39. Marques, M. B., & Fritsma, G. A. (2009). *Quick guide to coagulation testing.* (2nd ed.). Washington, DC: AACC Press.

40. Fritsma, G. A., Dembitzer, F. R., Randhawa, A., Marques, M. B., Van Cott, E. M., Adcock-Funk, D., & Peerschke, E. I. (2012). Recommendations for appropriate activated partial thromboplastin time reagent selection and utilization. *Am J Clin Pathol, 137,* 904–908.

41. Sato, K., Kagami, K., Asai, M., et al. (1995). Detection of lupus anticoagulant using a modified diluted Russell's viper venom test. *Rinsho Byori, 43,* 263–268.

42. Brandt, J. T., Triplett, D. A., Alving, B., et al. (1995). Criteria for the diagnosis of lupus anticoagulants: an update. *Thromb Haemost, 74,* 1185–1190.

43. Pengo, V., Tripodi, A., Reber, G., et al. (2009). Update of the guidelines for lupus anticoagulant detection. Subcommittee on Lupus Anticoagulant/Antiphospholipid Antibody of the Scientific and Standardisation Committee of the International Society on Thrombosis and Haemostasis. *J Thromb Haemost, 7,* 1737–1740.

44. Devreese, K. M. (2007). Interpretation of normal plasma mixing studies in the laboratory diagnosis of lupus anticoagulants. *Thromb Res, 119,* 369–376.

45. Rauch, J., Tannenbaum, M., Neville, C., & Fortin, P. R. (1998). Inhibition of lupus anticoagulant activity by hexagonal phase phosphatidylethanolamine in the presence of prothrombin. *Thromb Haemost, 80,* 936-941.

46. Schouwers, S. M. E., & Devreese, K. M. J. (2010). Lupus anticoagulant testing in patients with inflammatory status: does C-reactive protein interfere with LAC test results? *Thrombosis Research, 125,* 102–104.

47. Tebo, A. E., Jaskowski, T. D., Phansalkar, A. R., et al. (2008). Diagnostic performance of phospholipid-specific assays for the evaluation of antiphospholipid syndrome. *Am J Clin Pathol, 129,* 870–875.

48. Forastiero, R., Martinuzzo, M., Pombo, G., et al. (2005). A prospective study of antibodies to beta$_2$-glycoprotein I and prothrombin, and risk of thrombosis. *J Thromb Haemost, 3,* 1231–1238.

49. Blank, M., & Shoenfeld, Y. (2004). Antiphosphatidylserine antibodies and reproductive failure. *Lupus, 13,* 661–665.

50. Bouaziz-Borgi, L., Nguyen, P., Hazard, N., et al. (2007). A case control study of deep venous thrombosis in relation to factor V G1691A (Leiden) and A4070G (HR2 Haplotype) polymorphisms. *Exp Mol Pathol, 83,* 480–483.

51. Favaloro, E. J., McDonald, D., & Lippi, G. (2009). Laboratory investigation of thrombophilia: the good, the bad, and the ugly. *Semin Thromb Hemost, 35,* 695–710.

52. Dahlback, B., & Hildebrand, B. (1994). Inherited resistance to activated protein C is corrected by anticoagulant cofactor activity found to be a property of factor V. *Proc Natl Acad Sci U S A, 91,* 1396–1400.

53. De Ronde, H., & Bertina, R. M. (1994). Laboratory diagnosis of APC-resistance: a critical evaluation of the test and the development of diagnostic criteria. *Thromb Haemost, 72,* 880–886.

54. Johnson, N. V., Khor, B., & Van Cott, E. M. (2012). Advances in laboratory testing for thrombophilia. *Am J Hematol, 87* (Suppl. 1), S108–S112.

55. Ragland, B. D., Reed, C. E., Eiland, B. M., et al. (2003). The effect of lupus anticoagulant in the second-generation assay for activated protein C resistance. *Am J Clin Pathol, 119,* 66–71.

56. Emadi, A., Crim, M. T., Brotman, D. J., et al. (2010). Analytic validity of genetic tests to identify factor V Leiden and prothrombin G20210A. *Am J Hematol, 85,* 264–270.

57. Poort, S. R., Rosendaal, F. R., Reitsma, P. Y., et al. (1996). A common genetic variation in the 3′ untranslated region of the prothrombin gene is associated with elevated plasma prothrombin levels and an increase in venous thrombosis. *Blood, 88,* 3698–3703.

58. Danckwardt, S., Hartmann, K., Gehring, N. H., et al. (2006). 3′ end processing of the prothrombin mRNA in thrombophilia. *Acta Haematol, 115,* 192–197.

59. Naeem, M. A., Anwar, M., Ali, W., et al. (2006). Prevalence of prothrombin gene mutation (G-A 20210 A) in general population: a pilot study. *Clin Appl Thromb Hemost, 12,* 223–226.

60. Thaler, E., & Lechner, K. (1981). Antithrombin III deficiency and thromboembolism. *Clin Haematol, 10,* 369–390.

61. De Stefano, V., & Rossi, E. (2013, Oct). Testing for inherited thrombophilia and consequences for antithrombotic prophylaxis in patients with venous thromboembolism and their relatives. A review of the Guidelines from Scientific Societies and Working Groups. *Thromb Haemost, 110,* 697–705.

62. Cooper, P. C., Coath, F., Daly, M. E., & Makris, M. (2011). The phenotypic and genetic assessment of antithrombin deficiency. *Int J Lab Hematol, 33,* 227–237.

63. Rosen, S. (2005). Chromogenic methods in coagulation diagnostics. *Hamostaseologie, 25,* 259–266.

64. Antovic, J., Söderström, J., Karlman, B., et al. (2001). Evaluation of a new immunoturbidimetric test (Liatest antithrombin III) for determination of antithrombin antigen. *Clin Lab Haematol, 23,* 313–316.

65. Wu, O., Robertson, L., Twaddle, S., et al. (2006). Screening for thrombophilia in high-risk situations: systematic review and cost-effectiveness analysis. The Thrombosis Risk and Economic Assessment of Thrombophilia Screening (TREATS) study. *Health Technol Assess, 10,* 1–110.

66. Spiess, B. D. (2008). Treating heparin resistance with antithrombin or fresh frozen plasma. *Ann Thorac Surg, 85,* 2153–2160.

67. Dahlback, B. (1995). The protein C anticoagulant system: inherited defects as basis for venous thrombosis. *Thromb Res, 77,* 1–43.

68. Heit, J. A. (2013). Epidemiology and risk factors for venous thromboembolism. In Marder, V. J., Aird, W. C., Bennett, J. S., Schulman, S., & White, G. C., (Eds.), *Hemostasis and Thrombosis: Basic Principles and Clinical Practice.* (6th ed., pp. 973–976). Philadelphia, PA: Lippincott, Williams, and Wilkins.

69. Mann, H. J., Short, M. A., & Schlichting, D. E. (2009). Protein C in critical illness. *Am J Health Syst Pharm, 15,* 1089–1096.

70. Desancho, M. T., Dorff, T., & Rand, J. H. (2010). Thrombophilia and the risk of thromboembolic events in women on oral contraceptives and hormone replacement therapy. *Blood Coagul Fibrinolysis, 21,* 534–538.

71. Khor, B., & Van Cott, E. M. (2010). Laboratory tests for protein C deficiency. *Am J Hematol, 85,* 440–442.

72. Van Cott, E. M., Ledford-Kraemer, M., Meijer, P., et al. (2005). NASCOLA Proficiency Testing Committee. Protein S assays: an analysis of North American Specialized Coagulation Laboratory Association proficiency testing. *Am J Clin Pathol, 123,* 778–785.

73. Clinical Laboratory and Standards Institute. (2008). *Collection, Transport, and Processing of Blood Specimens for Testing Plasma-Base Coagulation Assays, Approved Guideline.* (5th ed.). Document H21–A5, Wayne, Pa: Clinical Laboratory and Standards Institute.

74. Ens, G. E., & Newlin, F. (1995). Spurious protein S deficiency as a result of elevated factor VII levels. *Clin Hemost Rev, 9,* 18.

75. Ridker, P. M. (1999). Evaluating novel cardiovascular risk factors: can we better predict heart attacks? *Ann Intern Med, 130,* 933–937.

76. Yousuf, O., Mohanty, B. D., Martin, S. S., et al. (2013). High-sensitivity C-reactive protein and cardiovascular disease: a resolute belief or an elusive link? *J Am Coll Cardiol, 62,* 397–408.

77. Lelubre, C., Anselin, S., Buodjeltia, K. Z., et al. (2013). Interpretation of C-reactive protein concentrations in critically ill patients. *BioMed Research International, 2013,* 1–9.

78. Pepys, M. B., & Baltz, M. L. (1983). Acute phase proteins with special reference to C-reactive protein and related proteins (pentaxins) and serum amyloid A proteins. *Adv Immunol, 34,* 141–212.

79. Wilkins, J., Gallimore, R., Moore, E., et al. (1998). Rapid automated high sensitivity enzyme immunoassay of C-reactive protein. *Clin Chem, 44,* 1358–1361.

80. Ridker, P. M., Cushman, M., Stampfer, M. J., et al. (1997). Inflammation, aspirin, and the risk of cardiovascular disease in apparently healthy men. *N Engl J Med, 336*, 97–99.

81. Genest, J. (2010). C-reactive protein: risk factor, biomarker and/or therapeutic target? *Can J Cardiol, 26*(Suppl. A), 41A–44A.

82. Glynn, R. J., Koenig, W., Nordestgaard, B. G., et al. (2010). Rosuvastatin for primary prevention in older persons with elevated C-reactive protein and low to average low-density lipoprotein cholesterol levels: exploratory analysis of a randomized trial. *Ann Intern Med, 152*, 488–496.

83. Williams, R. H., & Maggiore, J. A. (1999). Hyperhomocysteinemia pathogenesis, clinical significance, laboratory assessment, and treatment. *Lab Med, 30*, 468–474.

84. Cacciapuoti, F. (2011). Hyper-homocysteinemia: a novel risk factor or a powerful marker for cardiovascular diseases? Pathogenetic and therapeutical uncertainties. *J Thromb Thrombolysis, 32*, 82–88.

85. Vizzardi, E., Bonadei, I., Zanini, G., et al. (2009). Homocysteine and heart failure: an overview. *Recent Pat Cardiovasc Drug Discov, 4*, 15–21.

86. Guba, S. C., Fonseca, V., & Fink, L. M. (1999). Hyperhomocysteinemia and thrombosis. *Semin Thromb Hemost, 25*, 291–309.

87. Ciaccio, M., & Bellia, C. (2010). Hyperhomocysteinemia and cardiovascular risk: effect of vitamin supplementation in risk reduction. *Curr Clin Pharmacol, 5*, 30–36.

88. Sainani, G. S., & Sainani, R. (2002). Homocysteine and its role in the pathogenesis of atherosclerotic vascular disease. *J Assoc Physicians India, 50*(Suppl. 1),16–23.

89. Franchini, M., & Veneri, D. (2005). Inherited thrombophilia: an update. *Clin Lab, 51*, 357–365.

90. Deb, A., & Caplice, N. M. (2004). Lipoprotein(a): new insights into mechanisms of atherogenesis and thrombosis. *Clin Cardiol, 27*, 258–264.

91. Mandernach, M. W., & Kitchens, C. S. (2013). Disseminated intravascular coagulation. In Kitchens, C. S., Kessler, C. M., & Konkle, B. A., (Eds.), *Consultative Hemostasis and Thrombosis.* (3rd ed., pp. 174–189). Philadelphia: Elsevier Saunders.

92. Giles, A. R. (1994). Disseminated intravascular coagulation. In Bloom, A. L., Forbes, C. D., Thomas, D. P., et al., (Eds.), *Haemostasis and Thrombosis.* (pp. 969–986). New York: Churchill Livingstone.

93. Levi, M., Feinstein, D. I., Colman, R. W., & Marder, V. J. (2013). Consumptive thrombohemorrhagic disorders. In Marder, V. J., Aird, W. C., Bennett, J. S., Schulman, S., Gilbert, C., White, G. C., (Eds.), *Hemostasis and Thrombosis: Basic Principles and Clinical Practice.* (pp. 1178–1196). Philadelphia: Lippincott Williams & Wilkins.

94. Vaughan, D. E., & Declerck, P. J. (2003). Regulation of fibrinolysis. In Loscalzo, J., & Schafer, A. I., (Eds.), *Thrombosis and hemorrhage.* (pp. 105–120). Philadelphia: Lippincott Williams & Wilkins.

95. Jensen, R. (1998). The diagnostic use of fibrin breakdown products. *Clin Hemost Rev, 12*, 1–2.

96. Wada, H., Kobayashi, T., Abe, Y., et al. (2006). Elevated levels of soluble fibrin or D-dimer indicate high risk of thrombosis. *J Thromb Haemost, 4*, 1253–1258.

97. Labelle, C. A., & Kitchens, C. S. (2005). Disseminated intravascular coagulation: treat the cause, not the lab values. *Cleve Clin J Med, 72*, 377–378, 383–385, 390.

98. Mos, I. C., Klok, F. A., Kroft, L. J., et al. (2009). Safety of ruling out acute pulmonary embolism by normal computed tomography pulmonary angiography in patients with an indication for computed tomography: systematic review and meta-analysis. *J Thromb Haemost, 7*, 1491–1498.

99. Khoury, J. D., Adcock, D. M., Chan, F., et al. (2010). Increases in quantitative D-dimer levels correlate with progressive disease better than circulating tumor cell counts in patients with refractory prostate cancer. *Am J Clin Pathol, 134*, 964–969.

100. Wada, H., Wakita, Y., Nakase, T., et al. (1999). Hemostatic molecular markers before the onset of disseminated intravascular coagulation. *Am J Hematol, 60*, 273–278.

101. Huisman, M. V., & Klok, F. A. (2013). Diagnostic management of acute deep vein thrombosis and pulmonary embolism. *J Thromb Haemost, 11*, 412–422.

102. Sawamura, A., Hayakawa, M., Gando, S., et al. (2009). Disseminated intravascular coagulation with a fibrinolytic phenotype at an early phase of trauma predicts mortality. *Thromb Res, 124*, 608–613.

103. Moresco, R. N., Vargas, L. C., Voegeli, C. F., et al. (2003). D-dimer and its relationship to fibrinogen/fibrin degradation products (FDPs) in disorders associated with activation of coagulation or fibrinolytic systems. *J Clin Lab Anal, 17*, 77–79.

104. Boisclair, M. D., Lane, D. A., Wilde, J. T., et al. (1990). A comparative evaluation of assays for markers of activated coagulation and/or fibrinolysis: thrombin-antithrombin complex, D-dimer and fibrinogen/fibrin fragment E antigen. *Br J Haematol, 74*, 471–479.

105. Gando, S., Saitoh, D., Ishikura, H., et al. (2013). A randomized, controlled, multicenter trial of the effects of antithrombin on disseminated intravascular coagulation in patients with sepsis. *Crit Care, 17*, R297.

106. Favaloro, E. J. (2010). Laboratory testing in disseminated intravascular coagulation. *Semin Thromb Hemost, 36*, 458–467.

107. Levi, M., de Jonge, E., van der Poll, T. (2006). Plasma and plasma components in the management of disseminated intravascular coagulation. *Best Pract Res Clin Haematol, 19*, 127–142.

108. Gorog, D. A. (2010). Prognostic value of plasma fibrinolysis activation markers in cardiovascular disease. *J Am Coll Cardiol, 15*, 2701–2709.

109. Brace, L. D. (1992). Testing for heparin-induced thrombocytopenia by platelet aggregometry. *Clin Lab Sci, 5*, 80–81.

110. Vermylen, J., Hoylaerts, M. F., & Arnout, J. (1997). Antibody-mediated thrombosis. *Thromb Haemost, 78*, 420–426.

111. Crowther, M. A., Cook, D. J., Albert, M., et al. (2010). Canadian Critical Care Trials Group. The 4Ts scoring system for heparin-induced thrombocytopenia in medical-surgical intensive care unit patients. *J Crit Care, 25*, 287–293.

112. Warkentin, T. E., & Greinacher, A. (2013). Heparin-induced thrombocytopenia. In Marder, V. J., Aird, W. C., Bennett, J. S., Schulman, S., & White, G. C., (Eds.), *Basic Principles and Clinical Practice.* (6th ed., pp. 1293–1307). Philadelphia: Lippincott Williams & Wilkins.

113. Warkentin, T. E., & Sheppard, J. A. (2006). Testing for heparin-induced thrombocytopenia antibodies. *Transfus Med Rev, 20*, 259–272.

114. Tan, C. W., Ward, C. M., & Morel-Kopp, M. C. (2012). Evaluating heparin-induced thrombocytopenia: the old and the new. *Semin Thromb Hemost, 38*, 135–143.

115. Warkentin, T. E., Pai, M., Sheppard, J. I., Schulman, S., Spyropoulos, A. C., Eikelboom, J. W. (2011). Fondaparinux treatment of acute heparin-induced thrombocytopenia confirmed by the serotonin-release assay: a 30-month, 16-patient case series. *J Thromb Haemost, 9*, 2389–2396.

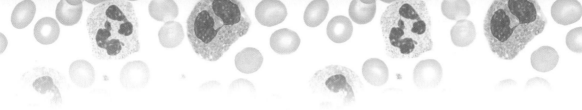

Thrombocytopenia and Thrombocytosis

40

Larry D. Brace

OBJECTIVES

After completion of this chapter, the reader will be able to:

1. Define thrombocytopenia and thrombocytosis, and state their associated platelet counts.
2. Compare and contrast the clinical symptoms of platelet disorders and clotting factor deficiencies.
3. Explain the primary pathophysiologic processes of thrombocytopenia.
4. Name and list the unique diagnostic features of at least four disorders included in congenital hypoplasia of the bone marrow and describe their inheritance patterns.
5. Differentiate between acute and chronic immune thrombocytopenia.
6. Describe the immunologic and nonimmunologic mechanisms by which drugs may induce thrombocytopenia.
7. Differentiate between neonatal isoimmune thrombocytopenia and neonatal autoimmune thrombocytopenia.
8. Explain the laboratory findings and pathophysiology associated with thrombotic thrombocytopenic purpura and hemolytic uremic syndrome.
9. Summarize the pathophysiology of thrombotic complications in heparin-induced thrombocytopenia and describe the sequence of treatment options.
10. Given clinical history and laboratory test results for patients with thrombocytopenia or thrombocytosis, suggest a diagnosis that is consistent with the information provided.

CASE STUDY

After studying the material in this chapter, the reader should be able to respond to the following case study:

An 18-month-old African-American girl sustained severe burns over 40% to 50% of her body, including both lower extremities. Within 1 month, she underwent a below-knee amputation of the left lower extremity. Over the next several years, she underwent skin-grafting surgeries, central venous line placement, and other burn-related surgeries. During these procedures, the patient was exposed to heparinized saline irrigation. Four years after the burn injury, thrombosis was noted in the right femoral artery during a grafting surgery. Unfractionated heparin was used during the surgery. Surgeons were unable to save the leg, and an above-knee amputation was necessary. At this time, hypercoagulability studies were ordered. Results were as follows:

	Patient Results	Reference Range
Protein C antigen	78%	70% to 137%
Protein S antigen	120%	63% to 156%
Antithrombin activity	111%	76% to 136%

The patient's results were normal on tests for the factor V Leiden and prothrombin G20210A mutations, and she was found not to have antiphospholipid antibody syndrome. Her platelet count had been decreasing steadily for 7 days before surgery but was still within the reference range.

1. Is the heparin used during the grafting surgeries significant in this patient's case?
2. What test should be ordered next?

Bleeding disorders resulting from platelet abnormalities, whether quantitative or qualitative, usually are manifested by bleeding into the skin or mucous membranes or both (mucocutaneous bleeding). Common presenting symptoms include petechiae, purpura, ecchymoses, epistaxis, and gingival bleeding. Similar findings also are seen in vascular disorders, but vascular disorders (e.g., Ehlers-Danlos syndrome, hereditary hemorrhagic telangiectasia) are relatively rare. In contrast, deep tissue bleeding, such as hematoma and hemarthrosis, is associated with clotting factor deficiencies.

THROMBOCYTOPENIA: DECREASE IN CIRCULATING PLATELETS

Although the reference range for the platelet count varies among laboratories, it is generally considered to be approximately 150,000 to 450,000/μL (150,000 to 450,000/mm^3 or 150 to 450 $\times$ 10^9/L). Thrombocytopenia (platelet count of fewer than 100,000/μL) is the most common cause of clinically important bleeding. True thrombocytopenia has to be differentiated from the thrombocytopenia artifact that can result from poorly prepared blood smears or automated cell counts when platelet clumping or platelet satellitosis are present (Chapters 15 and 16). The primary pathophysiologic processes that result in thrombocytopenia are decreased platelet production, accelerated platelet destruction, and abnormal platelet distribution (sequestration) (Box 40-1).

Small-vessel bleeding in the skin attributed to thrombocytopenia is manifested by hemorrhages of different sizes (Figure 40-1). *Petechiae* are small pinpoint hemorrhages about 1 mm in diameter, *purpura* are about 3 mm in diameter and generally round, and *ecchymoses* are 1 cm or larger and usually irregular in shape. Ecchymosis corresponds with the lay term *bruise*. Other conditions such as defective platelet function, vascular fragility, and trauma contribute to the hemorrhagic state.

Clinical bleeding varies and often is not closely correlated with the platelet count. It is unusual for clinical bleeding to occur when the platelet count is greater than 50,000/μL, but the risk of clinical bleeding increases progressively as the platelet count decreases from 50,000/μL. Patients with platelet counts of 20,000/μL or sometimes lower may have little or no bleeding symptoms. In general, patients with platelet counts of fewer than 10,000/μL are considered to be at high risk for a serious hemorrhagic episode.

Impaired or Decreased Platelet Production

Abnormalities in platelet production may be divided into two categories: One type is associated with megakaryocyte hypoplasia in the bone marrow, and the other type is associated with ineffective thrombopoiesis, as may be seen in disordered proliferation of megakaryocytes.

Inherited Thrombocytopenia/Congenital Hypoplasia

It is increasingly apparent that most inherited thrombocytopenias can be linked to fairly specific chromosomal abnormalities

---

BOX 40-1   Classification of Thrombocytopenia

Impaired or Decreased Production of Platelets
Congenital
    May-Hegglin anomaly
    Bernard-Soulier syndrome
    Fechtner syndrome
    Sebastian syndrome
    Epstein syndrome
    Montreal platelet syndrome
    Fanconi anemia
    Wiskott-Aldrich syndrome
    Thrombocytopenia with absent radii (TAR) syndrome
    Congenital amegakaryocytic thrombocytopenia
    Autosomal dominant and X-linked thrombocytopenia
Neonatal
Acquired
    Viral
    Drug induced

Increased Platelet Destruction
Immune
    Acute and chronic immune thrombocytopenic purpura

    Drug induced: immunologic
    Heparin-induced thrombocytopenia
    Neonatal alloimmune (isoimmune neonatal) thrombocytopenia
    Neonatal autoimmune thrombocytopenia
    Posttransfusion isoimmune thrombocytopenia
    Secondary autoimmune thrombocytopenia
Nonimmune
    Thrombocytopenia in pregnancy and preeclampsia
    Human immunodeficiency virus infection
    Hemolytic disease of the newborn
    Thrombotic thrombocytopenia purpura
    Disseminated intravascular coagulation
    Hemolytic uremic syndrome
    Drug induced

Abnormalities of Distribution or Dilution
Splenic sequestration
Kasabach-Merritt syndrome
Hypothermia
Loss of platelets: massive blood transfusions, extracorporeal circulation

From Colvin BT: Thrombocytopenia, *Clin Haematol* 14:661-681, 1985; and Thompson AR, Harker LA: *Manual of hemostasis and thrombosis*, ed 3, Philadelphia, 1983, FA Davis.

or specific genetic defects. Table 40-1 provides a list of inherited thrombocytopenias associated with specific gene and chromosomal abnormalities, mode of inheritance, and associated features.

Lack of adequate bone marrow megakaryocytes (megakaryocytic hypoplasia) is seen in a wide variety of congenital disorders, including Fanconi anemia (pancytopenia), thrombocytopenia with absent radius (TAR) syndrome, Wiskott-Aldrich syndrome, Bernard-Soulier syndrome, May-Hegglin anomaly, and several other less common disorders. Although thrombocytopenia is a feature of Bernard-Soulier syndrome and Wiskott-Aldrich syndrome, the primary abnormality in these disorders is a qualitative defect, and these disorders are discussed in Chapter 41.

May-Hegglin Anomaly. May-Hegglin anomaly is a rare autosomal dominant disorder; the exact frequency is unknown. Large platelets (20 μm in diameter) are present on the peripheral blood film, and Döhle-like bodies are present in neutrophils (Figure 40-2) and occasionally in monocytes. Other than the increase in size, platelet morphology is normal. Thrombocytopenia is present in about one third to one half of affected patients. Platelet function in response to platelet-activating agents is usually normal. In some patients, megakaryocytes are increased in number and have abnormal ultrastructure. Mutations in the *MYH9* gene that encodes for nonmuscle myosin heavy chain (a cytoskeletal protein in platelets) have been reported.[1] This mutation may be responsible for the abnormal size of platelets in this disorder. Most patients are asymptomatic unless severe thrombocytopenia is present, but bleeding times may be prolonged in some patients in the absence of bleeding complications (Table 40-1).

Three other disorders involving mutations of the *MYH9* gene have been reported: Sebastian syndrome, Fechtner syndrome, and Epstein syndrome.[2] Sebastian syndrome is inherited as an autosomal dominant disorder characterized by large platelets, thrombocytopenia, and granulocytic inclusions. Similar abnormalities are observed in Fechtner syndrome and are accompanied by deafness, cataracts, and nephritis. In Epstein syndrome, large platelets are associated with deafness, ocular problems, and glomerular nephritis.[3] These disorders are discussed in more detail in Chapter 41.

TAR Syndrome. TAR syndrome is a rare autosomal recessive disorder characterized by severe neonatal thrombocytopenia and congenital absence or extreme hypoplasia of the radial bones of the forearms with absent, short, or malformed ulnae and other orthopedic abnormalities. TAR syndrome is associated with a mutation in the *RBM8A* gene located on the long arm of chromosome 1 or a 200 Kb deletion involving the *RBM8A* gene (1q21.1). TAR can result from two deletions of the *RBM8A* gene, two mutations of the *RBM8A* gene, or, most commonly, a combination of the two (Table 40-1). In addition to bony abnormalities, patients tend to have cardiac lesions and a high incidence of transient leukemoid reactions with elevated white blood cell (WBC) counts (sometimes with counts above 100,000/μL) in 90% of patients.[4] Platelet counts

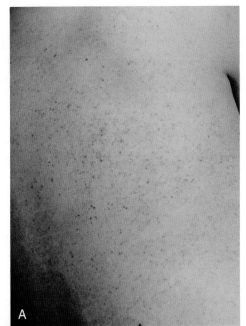

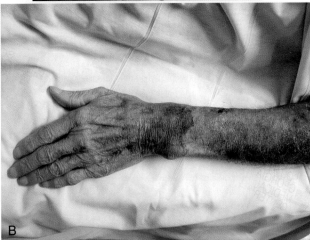

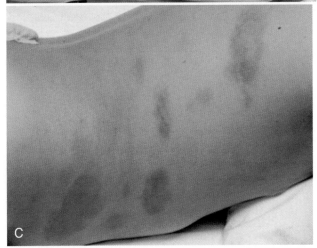

Figure 40-1 **A,** Petechiae, **B,** purpura, and **C,** ecchymoses indicate the various patterns of systemic (mucocutaneous) hemorrhage. (Fig. 40-1A and 40-1C from Gary P. Williams, MD, University of Wisconsin Clinical Science Center, Madison, WI.) (Fig. 40-1B from Kitchens CS, Alving BM, Kessler CM: *Consultative hemostasis and thrombosis*, Philadelphia, 2002, Saunders.)

TABLE 40-1 List of Inherited Thrombocytopenias

Disease (abbreviation, OMIM entry)	Frequency*/ Spontaneous Bleeding	Inheritance	Gene (chromosome localization)	Other Features
SYNDROMIC FORMS				
Wiskott-Aldrich syndrome (WAS, 301000)	++++/yes	XL	*WAS* (Xp11)	Severe immunodeficiency leading to death in infancy; small platelets
X-linked thrombocytopenia (XLT, 313900)				Mild immunodeficiency; small platelets
MYH9-related disease (*MYH9*-RD, nd)	++++/no	AD	*MYH9* (22q12-13)	Cataracts, nephropathy and/or deafness; giant platelets; also non-syndromic
Paris-Trousseau thrombocytopenia (TCPT, 188025/600588), Jacobsen syndrome (JBS, 147791)	++++/yes	AD	Large deletion (11q23-ter)	Cardiac and facial defects, developmental delay and/or other defects; large platelets
Thrombocytopenia with absent radii (TAR, 274000)	++++/yes	AR	*RBM8A* (1q21.1)	Platelet count tends to rise and often normalizes in adulthood; reduced megakaryocytes; normal-sized platelets. Bilateral radial aplasia and/or other malformations
GATA1-related disease (GATA1-RD) (Dyserythropoietic anemia with thrombocytopenia-nd, 300367- X-linked thrombocytopenia with thalassemia-XLTT, 314050)	++yes	XL	*GATA1* (Xp11)	Hemolytic anemia, possible unbalanced globin chain synthesis, possible congenital erythro-poietic porphyria; large platelets
Congenital thrombocytopenia with radio-ulnar synostosis (CTRUS, 605432)	+/yes	AD	*HOXA11* (7p15-14)	Radio-ulnar synostosis and/or other defects; possible evolution into aplastic anemia; normal sized platelets
Thrombocytopenia associated with sitosterolemia (STSL, 210250)	+/no	AR	*ABCG5*, ABCG8 (2p21)	Anemia, tendon xanthomas, atherosclerosis; large platelets; also non-syndromic
FLNA-related thrombocytopenia (FLNA-RT, nd)	+/yes	XL	*FLNA* (Xq28)	Periventricular nodular heterotopia (MIM 300049); large platelets; also non-syndromic
NON-SYNDROMIC FORMS				
Bernard-Soulier syndrome (BSS, 231200)				
Biallelic	++++/yes	AR	*GP1BA* (17p13),	Giant platelets
Monoallelic	+++/no	AD	*GP1BB* (22q11), *GP9* (3q21)	Large platelets
Congenital amegakaryocytic thrombo-cytopenia (CAMT, 604498)	+++/yes	AR	*MPL* (1p34)	Always evolves into bone marrow aplasia in infancy; normal-sized platelets
Familial platelet disorder and predis-position to acute myelogenous leukemia (FPD/AML, 601399)	++/no	AD	*RUNX1* (21q22)	High risk of developing leukemia or MDS; normal-sized platelets
Gray platelet syndrome (GPS, 139090)	++/yes	AR	*NBEAL2* (3p21.1)	High risk of developing evolutive myelofibrosis and splenomegaly; giant platelets
ANKRD26-related thrombocytopenia (THC2, 313900)	++/no	AD	*ANKRD26* (10p11-12)	May be at risk of leukemia; normal-sized platelets
ITGA2B/ITGB3-related thrombocyto-penia (*ITGA2B/ITGB3*-RT, nd)	+/no	AD	*ITGA2B* (17q21.31), *ITGB3* (17q21.32)	Large platelets
TUBB1-related thrombocytopenia (TUBB1-RT, nd)	+/no	AD	*TUBB1* (6p21.3)	Giant platelets
CYCS-related thrombocytopenia (THC4, 612004)	+/no	AD	*CYCS* (7p15.3)	Normal-sized platelets

AD, Autosomal dominant; *AR*, autosomal recessive; *MDS*, myelodysplastic syndrome; *nd*, not defined; *OMIM*, Online Mendelian Inheritance in Man; *XL*, X-linked. Some forms are categorized as both syndromic and non-syndromic. *++++, >100 families; +++, >50 families; ++ >10 families; +, <10 families.
From: Balduini CL, Savoia A, Seri M. Inherited thrombocytopenias frequently diagnosed in adults. *J Thromb Haemost* 2013;11:1006-1019.

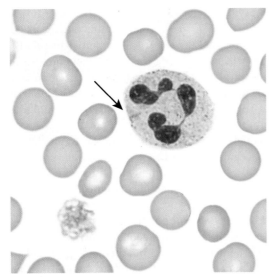

Figure 40-2 Döhle body in segmented neutrophil and giant platelets associated with May-Hegglin anomaly (peripheral blood, ×1000). (From Carr JH, Rodak BF: *Clinical hematology atlas*, ed 4, Philadelphia, 2013, Saunders.)

are usually 10,000 to 30,000/μL in infancy. Interestingly, platelet counts usually increase over time, with normal levels often achieved within 1 year of birth.

Fanconi Anemia.   Fanconi anemia is also associated with thrombocytopenia, although other abnormalities are extensive, including bony abnormalities, abnormalities of visceral organs, and pancytopenia. Chapter 22 contains a more detailed description.

Congenital Amegakaryocytic Thrombocytopenia

Congenital amegakaryocytic thrombocytopenia is an autosomal recessive disorder reflecting bone marrow failure.[5] Affected infants usually have platelet counts of fewer than 20,000/μL at birth, petechiae and evidence of bleeding at or shortly after birth, and frequent physical anomalies. About half of the infants develop aplastic anemia in the first year of life, and there are reports of myelodysplasia and leukemia later in childhood. Allogeneic stem cell transplantation is considered curative for infants with clinically severe disease or aplasia.[6] This disorder is caused by mutations in the *MPL* gene on chromosome 1 (1p34), resulting in complete loss of thrombopoietin receptor function (Table 40-1). This loss of function results in reduced megakaryocyte progenitors and high thrombopoietin levels.[7]

Autosomal Dominant Thrombocytopenia

Autosomal dominant thrombocytopenia has been mapped to a mutation(s) in the *ANKRD26* gene on the short arm of chromosome 10 (10p11-12). Mutations in this gene appear to lead to incomplete megakaryocyte differentiation and the resultant thrombocytopenia. Platelet morphology and size are usually normal. Until recently, autosomal dominant thrombocytopenia was considered a very rare disorder. However, *ANKRD26* mutations have recently been found in 21 of 210 thrombocytopenic pedigrees. This indicates that *ANKRD26* mutations may be responsible for approximately 10% of inherited

thrombocytopenias and is a relatively frequent form of autosomal dominant thrombocytopenia.[8] Bleeding in these patients is usually absent or mild, and platelet function is usually normal (Table 40-1).[9,10]

X-Linked Thrombocytopenia

X-linked thrombocytopenia can result from mutations in the *WAS* (Wiskott-Aldrich syndrome) gene on the X chromosome (Xp11) or mutations in the *GATA1* gene, also on the X chromosome at Xp11.[11-13] X-linked thrombocytopenias range from mild thrombocytopenia and small platelets and absent or mild bleeding to macrothrombocytopenia with severe bleeding (Table 40-1).

Other Inherited Thrombocytopenias

In addition to the inherited thrombocytopenias discussed above, there are several others that are due to gene mutations, including *HOXA11*, *ABCG5* and *ABCG8*, *FLNA*, *RUNX1*, *ITGA2B*, *ITGB3*, *TUBB1*, and *CYCS* (Table 40-1).

Neonatal Thrombocytopenia

Neonatal thrombocytopenia (platelet count <150,000/μL) is present in 1% to 5% of infants at birth. The causes of neonatal thrombocytopenia are numerous as illustrated in Table 40-2. In 75% of cases, the thrombocytopenia is present at or within 72 hours of birth. Only a minority of these patients have immunologic disorders or coagulopathy causing thrombocytopenia.

Causes of neonatal thrombocytopenia include infection with *Toxoplasma*, rubella, cytomegalovirus (CMV), herpes (TORCH), and human immunodeficiency virus (HIV), and in utero exposure to certain drugs, particularly chlorothiazide diuretics and the oral hypoglycemic tolbutamide and other agents. TORCH infections cause thrombocytopenia with characteristically small platelets. CMV is the most common infectious agent causing congenital thrombocytopenia, with an overall incidence of 0.5% to 1% of all births,[14] but only 10% to 15% of infected infants have symptomatic disease,[15] which suggests that the incidence of significant neonatal thrombocytopenia caused by CMV is about 1 in 1000 infants. Although the mechanism of thrombocytopenia is not well understood, reports suggest that CMV inhibits megakaryocytes and their precursors, which results in impaired platelet production.[16] About 1 in 1000 to 1 in 3000 infants are affected by congenital toxoplasmosis. About 40% of such infants develop thrombocytopenia.[17] While persistent thrombocytopenia is a prominent feature in infants with congenital rubella syndrome, it is now rare in countries with organized immunization programs.[18,19] Thrombocytopenia also is a feature of maternal transmission of HIV to the neonate and is a sign of intermediate to severe disease.[20]

Maternal ingestion of chlorothiazide diuretics or tolbutamide can have a direct cytotoxic effect on the fetal marrow megakaryocytes. Thrombocytopenia may be severe, with platelet counts of 70,000/μL and sometimes lower. Bone marrow examination reveals a marked decrease or absence of megakaryocytes. The thrombocytopenia develops gradually and is slow to regress when the drug is stopped. Recovery usually occurs within a few weeks after birth.[10,21,22]

TABLE 40-2 Classification of Fetal and Neonatal Thrombocytopenias

Fetal	Alloimmune
	Congenital infection (e.g., CMV, toxoplasma, rubella, HIV)
	Aneuploidy (e.g., trisomies 18, 13, 21, or triploidy)
	Autoimmune (e.g., ITP, SLE)
	Severe Rh hemolytic disease
	Congenital/inherited (e.g., Wiskott-Aldrich syndrome)
Early onset neonatal (<72 hours)	Placental insufficiency (e.g., preeclampsia, IUGR, diabetes)
	Perinatal asphyxia
	Perinatal infection (e.g., *E. coli*, group B streptococcus, *Haemophilus influenzae*)
	DIC
	Alloimmune
	Autoimmune (e.g., ITP, SLE)
	Congenital infection (e.g., CMV, toxoplasma, rubella, HIV)
	Thrombosis (e.g., aortic, renal vein)
	Bone marrow replacement (e.g., congenital leukemia)
	Kasabach-Merritt syndrome
	Metabolic disease (e.g., propionic and methylmalonic acidemia)
	Congenital/inherited (e.g., TAR, CAMT)
Late onset neonatal (>72 hours)	Late onset sepsis
	NEC
	Congenital infection (e.g., CMV, toxoplasma, rubella, HIV)
	Autoimmune
	Kasabach-Merritt syndrome
	Metabolic disease (e.g., propionic and methylmalonic acidemia)
	Congenital/inherited (e.g., TAR, CAMT)

CAMT, Congenital amegakaryocytic thrombocytopenia; *CMV*, cytomegalovirus; *DIC*, disseminated intravascular coagulation; *ITP*, immune thrombocytopenic purpura; *IUGR*, intrauterine growth restriction; *NEC*, necrotizing enterocolitis; *SLE*, systemic lupus erythematosus; *TAR*, thrombocytopenia with absent radii.
From: Roberts I, Murray NA. Neonatal thrombocytopenia: causes and management. *Arch Dis Child Fetal Neonatal Ed* 2003;88:F359-F364.

While infectious agents and certain drugs are well-known causes of neonatal thrombocytopenia, the overwhelming cause is impaired production. Most patients are preterm neonates born after pregnancies complicated by placental insufficiency and/or fetal hypoxia (preeclampsia and intrauterine growth restriction). These neonates have early-onset thrombocytopenia and impaired megakaryopoiesis in spite of increased levels of thrombopoietin (Table 40-2).

Increased platelet consumption/sequestration is another mechanism of neonatal thrombocytopenia accounting for approximately 2% to 25% of neonatal thrombocytopenia. Of these, 15% to 20% result from transplacental passage of maternal alloantibodies and autoantibodies (see neonatal alloimmune thrombocytopenia and neonatal autoimmune thrombocytopenia later in this chapter). Another 10% to 15% of cases are due to disseminated intravascular coagulation (DIC), almost always in very ill infants, particularly those with perinatal asphyxia or infections. Other examples include thrombosis, platelet activation, or immobilization at sites of inflammation (e.g., necrotizing enterocolitis). In very sick infants, splenic sequestration may be a contributing factor to thrombocytopenia.

Inherited thrombocytopenic syndromes are increasingly being recognized as causes of neonatal thrombocytopenia (Tables 40-1 and 40-2). Although considered to be rare, they may be more common than once believed.

Acquired (Drug-Induced) Hypoplasia

A wide array of chemotherapeutic agents used for the treatment of hematologic and nonhematologic malignancies suppress bone marrow megakaryocyte production and the production of other hematopoietic cells. Examples include the commonly used agents methotrexate, busulfan, cytosine arabinoside, cyclophosphamide, and cisplatin. The resulting thrombocytopenia may lead to hemorrhage, and the platelet count should be monitored closely. Drug-induced thrombocytopenia is often the dose-limiting factor for many chemotherapeutic agents. Recombinant interleukin-11 has been approved for treatment of chemotherapy-induced thrombocytopenia, and thrombopoietin may prove to be useful for this purpose.[23-25] Zidovudine (used for the treatment of HIV infection) is also known to cause myelotoxicity and severe thrombocytopenia.[26]

Several drugs specifically affect megakaryocytopoiesis without significantly affecting other marrow elements. Anagrelide is one such agent, although its mechanism of action is unknown. This characteristic has made anagrelide useful for treating the thrombocytosis of patients with essential thrombocythemia and other myeloproliferative disorders.[27]

Ingestion of ethanol for long periods (months to years) may result in persistent severe thrombocytopenia. Although the mechanism is unknown, studies indicate that alcohol can inhibit megakaryocytopoiesis in some individuals. Mild thrombocytopenia is a common finding in alcoholic patients, but other causes unrelated to ethanol use, such as portal hypertension, splenomegaly, and folic acid deficiency, should be excluded. The platelet count usually returns to normal within a few weeks of alcohol withdrawal, but thrombocytopenia may persist for longer periods. A transient rebound thrombocytosis may develop when alcohol ingestion is stopped.[10]

Interferon therapy commonly causes mild to moderate thrombocytopenia, although under certain circumstances, the thrombocytopenia can be severe and life-threatening. Interferon-α and interferon-γ inhibit stem cell differentiation and proliferation in the bone marrow, but the mechanism of action is unclear.[28]

Thrombocytopenia presumably caused by megakaryocyte suppression also has been reported to follow the administration of large doses of estrogen or estrogenic drugs such as diethylstilbestrol. Other drugs, such as certain antibacterial agents (e.g., chloramphenicol), tranquilizers, and anticonvulsants, also have been associated with thrombocytopenia caused by bone marrow suppression.[29-31]

Ineffective Thrombopoiesis

Thrombocytopenia is a usual feature of the megaloblastic anemias (pernicious anemia, folic acid deficiency, and vitamin B_{12} deficiency). Quantitative studies indicate that, as with erythrocyte production in these disorders, platelet production is ineffective. Although the bone marrow generally contains an increase in the number of megakaryocytes, the total number of platelets released into the circulation is decreased. Thrombocytopenia is caused by impaired DNA synthesis, and the bone marrow may contain grossly abnormal megakaryocytes with deformed, dumbbell-shaped nuclei, sometimes in large numbers. Stained peripheral blood films reveal large platelets that may have a decreased survival time and may have abnormal function. Thrombocytopenia is usually mild, and there is evidence of increased platelet destruction. Patients typically respond within 1 to 2 weeks to vitamin replacement.[22,32-34]

Miscellaneous Conditions

Viruses are known to cause thrombocytopenia by acting on megakaryocytes or circulating platelets, either directly or in the form of viral antigen-antibody complexes. Live measles vaccine can cause degenerative vacuolization of megakaryocytes 6 to 8 days after vaccination. Some viruses interact readily with platelets by means of specific platelet receptors. Other viruses associated with thrombocytopenia include CMV, varicella-zoster virus, rubella virus, Epstein-Barr virus (which causes infectious mononucleosis), and the virus that causes Thai hemorrhagic fever.[10]

Certain bacterial infections commonly are associated with the development of thrombocytopenia. This may be the result of toxins of bacterial origin, direct interactions between bacteria and platelets in the circulation, or extensive damage to the endothelium, as in meningococcemia. Many cases of thrombocytopenia in childhood result from infection. Purpura may occur in many infectious diseases in the absence of thrombocytopenia, presumably because of vascular damage (Chapter 41).[10,35]

A common cause of unexplained thrombocytopenia is infiltration of the bone marrow by malignant cells with a progressive decrease in marrow megakaryocytes as the abnormal cells replace normal marrow elements. Inhibitors of thrombopoiesis may be produced by these abnormal cells and may help to account for the thrombocytopenia associated with conditions such as myeloma, lymphoma, metastatic cancer, and myelofibrosis.[22,32,36]

Increased Platelet Destruction

Thrombocytopenia as a result of increased platelet destruction can be separated into two categories: increased platelet destruction caused by immunologic responses and increased destruction caused by mechanical damage or consumption or both. Regardless of the process, increased production is required to maintain a normal platelet count, and the patient becomes thrombocytopenic only when production capacity is no longer adequate to compensate for the increased rate of destruction.

Immune Mechanisms of Platelet Destruction

Immune (Idiopathic) Thrombocytopenic Purpura: Acute and Chronic. The term *idiopathic thrombocytopenic purpura (ITP)* was used previously to describe cases of thrombocytopenia arising without apparent cause or underlying disease state. Although the acronym for the disorder remains the same, the word *idiopathic* has been replaced by *immune* because of the realization that acute and chronic ITP are immunologically mediated.

Acute ITP. This is primarily a disorder of children, although a similar condition is seen occasionally in adults. The disorder is characterized by the abrupt onset of bruising, petechiae, and sometimes mucosal bleeding (e.g., epistaxis) in a previously healthy child. The primary hematologic feature is thrombocytopenia, which frequently occurs 1 to 3 weeks after an infection.

The infection is most often a nonspecific upper respiratory tract or gastrointestinal tract viral infection, but acute ITP also may occur after rubella, rubeola, chickenpox, or other viral illnesses and may follow live virus vaccination.[37] The incidence of acute ITP is estimated to be 4 in 100,000 children, with a peak frequency in children between 2 and 5 years of age. There is no sex predilection. In about 10% to 15% of the children initially thought to have acute ITP, the thrombocytopenia persists for 6 months or longer, and these children are reclassified as having chronic ITP.[38] The observation that acute ITP often follows a viral illness suggests that some children produce antibodies and immune complexes against viral antigens and that platelet destruction may result from the binding of these antibodies or immune complexes to the platelet surface.

The diagnosis of acute ITP in a child with severe thrombocytopenia almost always can be made without a bone marrow examination. If the child has recent onset of bleeding signs and symptoms, otherwise normal results on complete blood count (for all red and white blood cell parameters and cell morphology), and normal findings on physical examination (except for signs of bleeding), there is a high likelihood that the child has ITP. In addition, if the bleeding symptoms develop suddenly and there is no family history of hemorrhagic abnormalities or thrombocytopenia, the diagnosis of ITP is almost certain. There is, at present, no specific test that is diagnostic of acute or chronic ITP.

In mild cases of acute ITP, patients may have only scattered petechiae. In most cases of acute ITP, however, patients develop fairly extensive petechiae and some ecchymoses and may have hematuria or epistaxis or both. About 3% to 4% of acute ITP cases are considered severe, and typically generalized purpura is present, often accompanied by gastrointestinal bleeding, hematuria, mucous membrane bleeding, and retinal hemorrhage. Of patients with severe disease, 25% to 50% are considered to be at risk for intracranial hemorrhage, which is the primary complication that contributes to the overall 1% to 2% mortality rate for patients with acute ITP.[38] Most patients with life-threatening hemorrhage have a platelet count of less than

4000/µL.[39] Hemorrhage is rarely experienced by patients whose platelet count exceeds 10,000/µL.

Most patients with acute ITP recover with or without treatment in about 3 weeks, although for some, recovery may take 6 months. In a few children, recurrent episodes of acute ITP are occasionally seen after complete recovery from the first episode.[40] Most patients with acute ITP have relatively mild symptoms, and no treatment is needed. The most severe cases may need to be treated, however, and intravenous immunoglobulin (IVIG), platelet transfusions, and splenectomy (or some combination of these) seem to offer the most immediate benefit.[37,38]

Chronic ITP. This disorder can be found in patients of any age, although most cases occur in patients between the ages of 20 and 50 years. Females with this disorder outnumber males 2:1 to 3:1, with the highest incidence in women between 20 and 40 years of age. The incidence of chronic ITP ranges from 3.2 to 6.6 cases per 100,000 per year.[41] Chronic ITP usually begins insidiously, with platelet counts that are variably decreased and sometimes normal for periods of time. Presenting symptoms are those of mucocutaneous bleeding, with menorrhagia, recurrent epistaxis, and easy bruising (ecchymoses) being most common.

Platelet destruction in chronic ITP is the result of an immunologic process. The offending antibodies attach to platelets, and as a result, the antibody-labeled platelets are removed from the circulation by reticuloendothelial cells, primarily in the spleen. Autoantibodies that recognize platelet surface glycoproteins such as glycoprotein IIb (GP IIb) and GP IIIa (αIIb/β_3), GP Ia/IIa, and others can be demonstrated in 50% to 60% of ITP patients.[42,43] Because megakaryocytes also express GP IIb/IIIa and GP Ib/IX on their membranes, these cells are obvious targets of the antibodies. Platelet turnover studies have shown impaired platelet production in ITP. Overall, the life span of the platelet is shortened from the normal 7 to 10 days to a few hours, and the rapidity with which platelets are removed from the circulation correlates with the degree of thrombocytopenia. If plasma from a patient with ITP is infused into the circulation of a normal recipient, the recipient develops thrombocytopenia. The thrombocytopenia-producing factor in the plasma of the ITP patient is an immunoglobulin G (IgG) antibody that can be removed from serum by adsorption with normal human platelets. In addition, cytotoxic T cell-mediated lysis of platelets has been shown in vitro using CD3[+]CD8[+] lymphocytes from patients with active chronic ITP, although the in vivo significance of this mechanism is not known.[44]

The only abnormalities in the peripheral blood of patients with ITP are related to platelets. In most cases, platelets number between 30,000/µL and 80,000/µL. Patients with ITP undergo periods of remission and exacerbation, however, and their platelet counts may range from near normal to fewer than 20,000/µL during these periods (Figure 40-3). Morphologically, platelets appear normal, although larger in diameter than usual. This is reflected in an increased mean platelet volume as measured by electronic cell counters. The marrow typically is characterized by megakaryocytic hyperplasia. Megakaryocytes are increased in size, and young forms with a single nucleus,

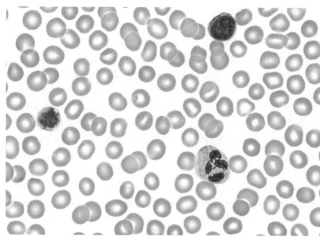

Figure 40-3 Typical peripheral blood cell morphology in immune thrombocytopenic purpura. Note scarce platelets and increased platelet size but normal red blood cell and leukocyte morphology (peripheral blood, ×500).

smooth contour, and diminished cytoplasm are commonly seen. In the absence of bleeding, infection, or other underlying disorder, erythrocyte and leukocyte precursors are normal in number and morphology. Coagulation tests showing abnormal results include tests dependent on platelet function. Although platelet-associated IgG levels are increased in most patients,[10,21,45] it has not been shown conclusively that any method of testing for platelet antibodies is sensitive or specific for ITP.

The initial treatment of chronic ITP depends on the urgency for increasing the platelet count. In ITP patients with platelet counts greater than 30,000/µL who receive no treatment, the expected mortality rate is equal to that of the general population. Unless there are additional risk factors, ITP patients with platelet counts greater than 30,000/µL should not be treated. If additional risk factors are present, such as old age, coagulation defects, recent surgery, trauma, or uncontrolled hypertension, the platelet count should be kept at 50,000/µL or higher, depending on the clinical situation. In patients in whom the need is considered urgent, IVIG remains the treatment of choice. For most patients, however, the initial treatment of chronic ITP consists principally of prednisone. About 70% to 90% of patients respond to this therapy, with an increase in platelet count and a decrease in hemorrhagic episodes. Although reported response rates vary widely, about 50% of patients have a long-term beneficial effect from corticosteroid treatment.[46] If the response to corticosteroids is inadequate or no response is seen, steroid therapy can be supplemented with IVIG or, in some cases, anti-D immunoglobulin.[47] For patients in whom prednisone is ineffective, intravenous rituximab should be tried. Responses to rituximab are usually seen within 3 to 4 weeks. In some patients splenectomy may become necessary. Splenectomy eliminates the primary site of platelet removal and destruction, but it also removes an organ containing autoantibody-producing lymphocytes. Splenectomy is an effective treatment for adult chronic ITP, with 88% of patients showing improvement and 66% having a complete and lasting response.[48] Vaccination with pneumococcal, meningococcal, and *Haemophilus influenzae* vaccines should be performed at least 2 weeks prior to surgery. The use of laparoscopic surgery speeds recovery and shortens hospitalization and is generally preferred to open splenectomy. In the most severe refractory cases, immunosuppressive (chemotherapeutic) agents such as azathioprine given alone or with steroids may be necessary. In such patients, platelet transfusions may be of transient benefit in treating severe hemorrhagic episodes but should not be given routinely.[45] IVIG given alone or just before platelet transfusion also may be beneficial.[37,45]

Chronic ITP occurring in association with HIV infection, with hemophilia, or with pregnancy presents special problems in diagnosis and therapy. Unexplained thrombocytopenia in otherwise healthy members of high-risk populations may be an early manifestation of acquired immune deficiency syndrome (AIDS).[36,45]

Differentiation of Acute Versus Chronic Immune Thrombocytopenic Purpura. The differences between acute and chronic ITP are summarized in Table 40-3. Acute ITP occurs most frequently in children 2 to 9 years of age and in young adults, whereas chronic ITP occurs in patients of all ages, although most frequently in adults aged 20 to 50 years, and more commonly in women. Of patients with acute ITP, 60% to 80% have a history of infection, usually viral (rubella, rubeola, chickenpox, and nonspecific respiratory tract infection), occurring 2 to 21 days before ITP onset. Acute ITP also may occur after immunization with live vaccine for measles, chickenpox, mumps, and smallpox.

TABLE 40-3 Clinical Picture of Acute and Chronic Immune Thrombocytopenic Purpura

Characteristic	Acute	Chronic
Age at onset	2–6 yr	20–50 yr
Sex predilection	None	Female over male, 3:1
Prior infection	Common	Unusual
Onset of bleeding	Sudden	Gradual
Platelet count	<20,000/µL	30,000–80,000/µL
Duration	2–6 wk	Months to years
Spontaneous remission	90% of patients	Uncommon
Seasonal pattern	Higher incidence in winter and spring	None
Therapy		
Steroids	70% response rate	30% response rate
Splenectomy	Rarely required	<45 yr, 90% response rate >45 yr, 40% response rate

From Triplett DA, editor: *Platelet function: laboratory evaluation and clinical application,* Chicago, 1978, American Society of Clinical Pathologists; Quick AJ: *Hemorrhagic diseases and thrombosis,* ed 2, Philadelphia, 1966, Lea & Febiger; and Bussel J, Cines D: Immune thrombocytopenia, neonatal alloimmune thrombocytopenia, and post-transfusion purpura. In Hoffman R, Benz EJ Jr, Shattil SJ, et al, editors: *Hematology: basic principles and practice,* ed 3, New York, 2000, Churchill Livingstone, pp 2096-2114.

Acute ITP usually is self-limited, and spontaneous remissions occur in 80% to 90% of patients, although the duration of the illness may range from days to months. In chronic ITP, there is typically a fluctuating clinical course, with episodes of bleeding that last a few days or weeks, but spontaneous remissions are uncommon and usually incomplete.[45]

Symptoms of acute ITP vary, but petechial hemorrhages, purpura, and often bleeding from the gums and gastrointestinal or urinary tract typically begin suddenly, sometimes over a few hours. Hemorrhagic bullae in the oral mucosa are often prominent in patients with severe thrombocytopenia of acute onset. Usually the severity of bleeding is correlated with the degree of thrombocytopenia.[45] In contrast, presenting symptoms of chronic ITP begin with a few scattered petechiae or other minor bleeding manifestations. Occasionally, a bruising tendency, menorrhagia, or recurrent epistaxis is present for months or years before diagnosis. Platelet counts range from 5000/µL to 75,000/µL and are generally higher than those in acute ITP. Giant platelets are commonly seen. Platelet-associated immunoglobulin levels are elevated in most patients, but the test lacks sensitivity and specificity.[45]

Treatment also varies for acute and chronic ITP. In chronic ITP, initial therapy often consists of glucocorticoids (corticosteroids), which interfere with splenic and hepatic macrophages to increase platelet survival time. If the ITP does not respond to corticosteroids or the patient cannot tolerate them because of the resultant immunosuppression and toxicity, splenectomy may be necessary. In acute ITP, treatment for all but the most severely thrombocytopenic and hemorrhagic patients is contraindicated. When treatment is necessary, a good response to IVIG or corticosteroids or both usually can be obtained, and splenectomy is rarely required.[37,38]

Immunologic Drug-Induced Thrombocytopenia. As can be seen from Box 40-2, many drugs can induce acute thrombocytopenia. Drug-induced immune-mediated thrombocytopenia can be divided into several types based on the interaction of the antibody with the drug and platelets. Mechanisms of drug-antibody binding are shown in Figure 40-4.

Drug-dependent antibodies. One mechanism of drug-dependent antibodies is typified by quinidine- and quinine-induced thrombocytopenia and has been recognized for more than 100 years. The antibody induced by drugs of this type interacts with platelets only in the presence of the drug. Drug-dependent antibodies typically occur after 1 to 2 weeks of exposure to a new drug. Many drugs can induce such antibodies, but quinine, quinidine, and sulfonamide derivatives do so more often than other drugs. When antibody production has begun, the platelet count falls rapidly and often may be fewer than 10,000/µL. Patients may have abrupt onset of bleeding symptoms. If this type of drug-induced thrombocytopenia develops in a pregnant woman, both she and her fetus may be affected. Quinine previously was used to facilitate labor but is no longer used for this purpose.

The initial studies of quinidine-induced thrombocytopenia suggested that the drug first combines with the antibody and that the antigen-antibody (immune) complex then attaches to

BOX 40-2 Common Drugs Causing Immune Thrombocytopenia

Analgesics
Salicylates
Acetaminophen
Phenylbutazone

Antibiotics
Cephalothin
Penicillin
Streptomycin
Aminosalicylic acid
Rifampin
Novobiocin
Various sulfa drugs (chlorthalidone, furosemide)

Alkaloids
Quinidine
Quinine

Sedatives, Anticonvulsants
Methoin
Troxidone
Chlorpromazine
Diphenylhydantoin
Meprobamate
Phenobarbital
Carbamazepine

Oral Hypoglycemics
Chlorpropamide
Tolbutamide

Heavy Metals
Gold
Mercury
Bismuth
Organic arsenicals

Miscellaneous
Chloroquine
Chlorothiazide
Insecticides

From Triplett DA, editor: *Platelet function: laboratory evaluation and clinical application,* Chicago, 1978, American Society of Clinical Pathologists; and Quick AJ: *Hemorrhagic diseases and thrombosis,* ed 2, Philadelphia, 1966, Lea & Febiger.

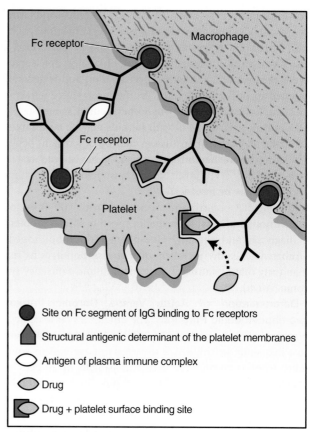

- ● Site on Fc segment of IgG binding to Fc receptors
- ◤ Structural antigenic determinant of the platelet membranes
- ◯ Antigen of plasma immune complex
- ⬭ Drug
- ◖ Drug + platelet surface binding site

Figure 40-4 Immunoglobulin binds a platelet membrane antigen or antigen and drug combination. Macrophage Fc receptors bind the Fc portion of the immunoglobulin. This may result in platelet removal and thrombocytopenia. *IgG,* immunoglobulin G. (From Rapaport SI: *Introduction to hematology,* ed 2, Philadelphia, 1987, JB Lippincott, p. 489.)

the platelet in an essentially nonspecific manner (the "innocent bystander" hypothesis). It now seems clear, however, that the antibodies responsible for drug-induced thrombocytopenia bind to the platelets by their Fab regions, rather than by attaching nonspecifically as immune complexes. The innocent bystander/immune complex explanation for this type of drug-induced thrombocytopenia should be abandoned. The Fab portion of the antibody binds to a platelet membrane constituent, usually the GP Ib/IX/V complex or the GP IIb/IIIa complex, only in the presence of drug.[49,50] The mechanism by which the drug promotes binding of a drug-dependent antibody to a specific target on the platelet membrane without covalently linking to the target or the antibody remains to be determined, however. Because the Fc portion of the immunoglobulin is not involved in binding to platelets, it is still available to the Fc receptors on phagocytic cells. This situation may contribute to the rapid onset and relatively severe nature of the thrombocytopenia. Most drug-induced platelet antibodies are of the IgG class, but in rare instances, IgM antibodies are involved.[45]

A similar pattern is seen with the antiplatelet/antithrombotic agents abciximab, tirofiban, and eptifibatide, although with these drugs thrombocytopenia tends to occur within several hours of exposure. Such immediate reactions are due to naturally occurring antibodies to the murine structural elements of abciximab (a mouse/human monoclonal antibody fragment) or to structural changes induced by binding of eptifibatide or tirofiban to platelet GP IIb/IIIa.

Hapten-induced antibodies. A second mechanism of drug-induced thrombocytopenia is induction of hapten-dependent antibodies. Some drug molecules are too small by themselves to trigger an immune response, but they may act as a hapten and combine with a larger carrier molecule (usually a plasma protein or protein constituent of the platelet membrane) to form a complex that can act as a complete antigen.[45] Penicillin and penicillin derivatives are the primary offending agents causing drug-induced thrombocytopenia by this mechanism. Drug-induced thrombocytopenia of this type is often severe. The initial platelet count may be fewer than 10,000/μL and sometimes fewer than 1000/μL. The number of bone marrow megakaryocytes is usually normal to elevated.[45] Bleeding is often severe and rapid in onset, and hemorrhagic bullae in the mouth may be prominent.

Drug-induced autoantibodies. Drug-induced autoantibodies represent a third mechanism of drug-induced thrombocytopenia. In this case, the drugs stimulate the formation of an autoantibody that binds to a specific platelet membrane glycoprotein with no requirement for the presence of free drug. Gold salts and procainamide are two examples of such drugs. Levodopa also may cause thrombocytopenia in the same way. The precise mechanism by which these drugs induce autoantibodies against platelets is not known with certainty.

Treatment for any drug-induced thrombocytopenia is first to identify the offending drug, immediately discontinue its use, and substitute another suitable therapeutic agent. This is often difficult to accomplish. Many patients are taking multiple drugs, and it is not always easy to determine which of the drugs is at fault for causing thrombocytopenia. Under these conditions, identifying the causative agent may be a trial-and-error procedure in which the most likely drugs are eliminated one at a time. In addition, even if the patient is taking only one agent, there may not be a suitable replacement, or a prolonged period may be required for the alternative drug to become effective. Drugs usually are cleared from the circulation rapidly, but dissociation of drug-antibody complexes may require longer periods, perhaps 1 to 2 weeks.[10] In some cases, such as those caused by gold salts, thrombocytopenia may persist for months. Platelet transfusions may be necessary for patients with life-threatening bleeds. Although it is true that the transfused platelets are destroyed rapidly, they may function to halt bleeding effectively before they are destroyed. In addition, high-dose IVIG may be used and is generally an effective treatment for most drug-induced immune thrombocytopenias. Laboratory testing to identify the specific drug involved is usually beyond the capabilities of most laboratories. This type of testing is performed by many reference laboratories, however.

Immune complex–induced thrombocytopenia. *Heparin-induced thrombocytopenia* (HIT) is a good example of another type of drug-induced thrombocytopenia. Heparin binds to platelet factor 4 (PF4), a heparin-neutralizing protein made and released by platelets (Figure 40-5). Binding of heparin by plasma PF4 or platelet membrane–expressed PF4 causes a conformational change in PF4, resulting in the exposure of neoepitopes. Exposure of these neoepitopes ("new antigens") stimulates the immune system of some individuals, which leads to the production of an antibody to one of the neoepitopes. In HIT, heparin and PF4 form a complex on the platelet surface or circulating free complexes to which the antibody binds. The Fab portion of the immunoglobulin molecule binds to an exposed neoepitope in the PF4 molecule; this leaves the Fc portion of the IgG free to bind with the platelet FcγIIa receptor, which causes platelet activation.[51,52] Because the Fc portions of the IgG molecules bind to platelet FcγIIa receptor, they are not available to the Fc receptors of the cells of the reticuloendothelial system. This may explain the less severe decline in platelet count in this thrombocytopenia. That does not mean, however, that the consequences are less serious. The opposite may be true. Because platelets are activated by occupancy of their FcγIIa receptor, in vivo platelet aggregation with thrombosis is possible. HIT sometimes is referred to as *heparin-induced thrombocytopenia and thrombosis* (Chapter 39). Heparin binding to PF4 is required to expose the neoepitope to which the antibody binds. The treatment for HIT is to discontinue heparin administration and replace it with another suitable anticoagulant. Low-molecular-weight heparin should not be used as a heparin replacement for this purpose, because the antibody cross-reacts with low-molecular-weight heparin and PF4 to result in platelet activation and aggregation.[53]

Heparin-induced thrombocytopenia. HIT is a relatively common side effect of unfractionated heparin administration,

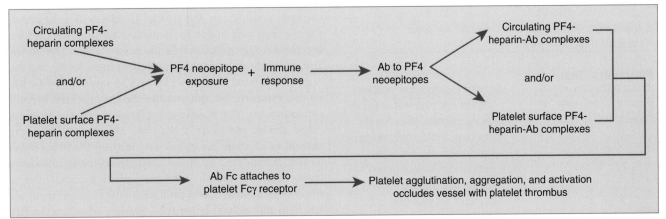

Figure 40-5 Heparin-induced thrombocytopenia with thrombosis. An antibody (Ab) binds the heparin–platelet factor 4 (PF4) complex in plasma or on the platelet surface. The Fc portion binds platelet Fc receptors and activates the platelet. The activated platelets aggregate to form platelet thrombi in the arterial circulation. Thrombi can also occur in the venous system.

with about 1% to 5% of patients developing this complication. Despite the thrombocytopenia, patients with HIT usually are not at significant risk of bleeding, because the platelet count typically does not fall below 40,000/μL. Ten percent to 30% of patients with HIT develop thrombotic complications, however. In patients who develop HIT, heparin therapy should be stopped as soon as the diagnosis is made, because continued heparin therapy can lead to significant morbidity and mortality, including gangrene of the extremities, amputation, and death. After discontinuation of heparin, the platelet count begins to increase and should return to normal within a few days.[54]

Because the immune system is involved in the development of HIT, the clinical signs of HIT typically are not seen until 7 to 14 days after the initiation of heparin therapy (the time necessary to mount an immune response on first exposure to an antigen). If the patient has been exposed to heparin previously, however, symptoms of HIT may be seen in 1 to 3 days. Because the platelet count may fall sharply in 1 day, it is recommended that platelet counts be measured daily in patients receiving unfractionated heparin therapy (Table 40-4).

One other sign of impending HIT in some patients is the development of *heparin resistance*. This is the clinical situation in which a patient who had experienced adequate anticoagulation at a certain heparin dosage suddenly requires increasing amounts of heparin to maintain the same level of anticoagulation. This situation can result from in vivo activation of platelets and release of PF4 and β-thromboglobulin from platelet α-granules. Both of these substances neutralize heparin, which leads to a normalization of results on the partial thromboplastin time test that is used to monitor heparin therapy. Heparin resistance often is seen before the development of thrombocytopenia.[55]

A common benign form of HIT that occurs on heparin administration is type I (non–immune mediated) HIT. It is important to distinguish benign type I from type II HIT. *Type I HIT* is associated with a rapid decrease in the platelet count after administration of heparin, but the thrombocytopenia is mild (the platelet count rarely decreases to fewer than 100,000/μL) and transient, and the platelet count returns rapidly to the preheparin level even if heparin therapy is continued. Careful attention should be paid to the platelet count and other signs of HIT so that this form of thrombocytopenia is not confused with the clinically significant *type II HIT*. Although the mechanism of type I HIT has not been completely described, it may be related to the well-documented proaggregatory effects of heparin.[53,56] Because activated or aggregated platelets are cleared from the circulation, these effects may explain the mild decrease in the platelet count that occurs during the first few days of heparin administration. This has not been clearly documented, however.

The binding of heparin and related compounds depends on polysaccharide chain length, composition, and degree of sulfation. Short-chain heparin polysaccharides (low-molecular-weight heparin) have lower affinity to PF4 and are less prone to cause type II HIT. Pentasaccharide and its synthetic derivatives (e.g., fondaparinux) do not seem to bind PF4 and are unlikely to cause type II HIT.

The detection of clinically significant HIT occurs by laboratory testing using immunoassays and platelet function tests (Table 40-4 and Chapter 42). Laboratory testing, however, is problematic because all tests lack sensitivity. Three methods are commonly used, but all depend on the presence of free heparin–induced antiplatelet antibodies in the patient's serum or plasma in sufficient quantity to cause a positive test result. HIT can be detected by a *platelet aggregation technique*.[57] In this method, serum from the patient is added to platelet-rich plasma from normal donors, heparin is added to the mixture, and platelet aggregation is typically monitored for 20 minutes. The specificity of the method is excellent (near 100%), but the sensitivity is quite low (about 50%). The sensitivity of the test can be improved, but this requires the use of several heparin concentrations and platelet-rich plasma from two or more blood donors, preferably of the same ABO blood type as the patient. In addition, the individuals donating blood for platelet-rich plasma must not have taken aspirin for 10 to 14 days before platelet donation because platelets from donors who have ingested aspirin produce a false-negative result for HIT.[53] In the author's experience, patients who develop HIT while receiving aspirin therapy rarely develop thrombotic complications, and the drop in their platelet counts is less precipitous, gradually decreasing over the course of several days

TABLE 40-4 Laboratory Tests for Heparin-Induced Thrombocytopenia

Laboratory Test	Comment
Platelet count	A >30% decrease from baseline may signal HIT, even if still within the reference interval.
Antigen Tests ELISAs: GTI PVS:PF4* Stago H:PF4* Hyphen BioMed Rapid tests (point-of-care): Akers PIFA* DiaMed Pa-GIA Coagulation instrument based tests: Milenia Biotec LFI-HIT HemosIL HIT-Ab	Use with a clinical scoring system (Table 39-17). Can be used as a first lab test to screen for the presence of HIT antibodies; due to high frequency of false positive results, functional tests should be performed to confirm a positive antigen test. False negative results can also occur.
Functional Tests Platelet Aggregation HIPA Lumi-Aggregation HIPA Serotonin Release Assay	Important to perform functional testing that detects platelet activation by HIT antibodies to confirm a diagnosis of HIT; sensitivities and specificities differ among tests with the SRA (washed platelet assay) being the most sensitive. Require skill and experience of the operator to obtain quality results.

HIPA, Heparin-induced platelet aggregation.
*FDA-cleared.

(unpublished observations). Given the efficacy of aspirin therapy in primary and secondary prevention of myocardial infarction and thrombotic stroke, it is increasingly difficult to find a sufficient pool of suitable (and willing) blood donors. Although the platelet aggregation procedure is time consuming, reasonable sensitivity can be obtained with sufficient attention to the details of the technique.[27]

Dense granules of platelets contain serotonin, and platelets have an active mechanism for rapid uptake and storage of serotonin in dense granules. This property of platelets is used in another test for HIT, the *serotonin release assay* (SRA), in which washed normal platelets from a donor are incubated with radioactive serotonin (Figure 40-6).[58] Radioactive serotonin is taken up rapidly and stored in the dense granules of the donor platelets, which are washed and resuspended. In the presence of heparin-dependent antiplatelet antibody and heparin, the donor platelets become activated and release the contents of their dense granules when the concentration of heparin in the test suspension is near the therapeutic range. The reappearance of radioactive serotonin in the plasma indicates the presence of a heparin-dependent antiplatelet antibody (i.e., HIT). Under these same conditions, supratherapeutic concentrations of heparin do not activate platelets, however, and if platelets release the contents of dense granules at both therapeutic and supratherapeutic concentrations of heparin, the test result is not positive for HIT. A similar phenomenon is observed in the test that uses platelet aggregometry.[53,59] The SRA is considered the gold standard for detection of HIT. Its major drawback is the requirement for radiolabeled serotonin. Most clinical laboratories no longer use isotopic techniques. As a result, this test is performed only in a few specialized centers. In addition, it has some of the same methodologic drawbacks as the platelet aggregation technique, in particular the need for platelets from drug-free donors. Nonetheless, when properly performed, this technique has similar specificity and superior sensitivity compared with the platelet aggregation method.

More recently, *enzyme-linked immunosorbent assays* (ELISAs) have been developed based on the knowledge that the antigenic target of the heparin-dependent antiplatelet antibody is a PF4-heparin complex (Figure 40-7). In this assay, PF4 and

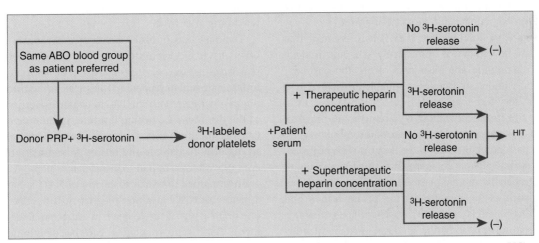

Figure 40-6 The serotonin release assay (SRA) for heparin-induced thrombocytopenia (HIT). Donor platelets in platelet-rich plasma (PRP) are labeled with tritiated (^{3}H) serotonin, washed, and suspended in a buffer to which patient plasma is added. Heparin in therapeutic and saturating doses is added to two aliquots. Release of radioactive serotonin in the therapeutic aliquot in combination with no release in the supratherapeutic system indicates HIT.

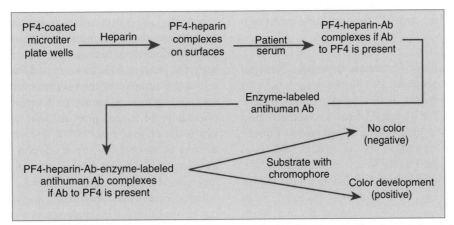

Figure 40-7 Enzyme immunoassay for heparin-induced thrombocytopenia (HIT). The solid-phase target antigen is a complex of platelet factor 4 (PF4) and heparin or a heparin surrogate. Anti–heparin-PF4 antibody in patient serum binds the antigen and is bound by enzyme-labeled anti–human antibody (Ab), a "sandwich" assay. The enzyme catalyzes the release of a chromophore from its substrate.

heparin (or a related compound) are coated to the surfaces of microplate wells. The serum or plasma from the patient suspected to have HIT is added to wells of the microtiter plate. If the antibody is present, it adheres to the PF4-heparin (or heparin-like compound) complex. The plate wells are washed, and enzyme-labeled monoclonal antibodies against human IgG and IgM are added. After an appropriate incubation period, the plate is washed, and a chromogenic substrate for the enzyme is added. Color development in the assay well indicates the presence of the heparin-dependent antiplatelet antibody in the patient specimen.[60] This assay has greater sensitivity than the platelet aggregation method and similar sensitivity to the SRA, but it has lower specificity than the serotonin release assay or the platelet aggregation method. Unlike the functional HIT assays (SRA and platelet aggregation), the ELISA can detect anti–PF4-heparin antibodies that are not pathologic; that is, the test result is positive, but the patient does not have clinical HIT. Some ELISA assays can detect both IgG and IgM antibodies to heparin-PF4 complexes. More recently, ELISA kits that detect only IgG antibodies have been developed and have a better correlation with the SRA. The ELISA method is considerably less labor intensive, does not require blood from healthy drug-free donors, and can be performed in most laboratories.

For patients who develop type II HIT, it is essential that heparin therapy be withdrawn immediately. It is not prudent, however, to discontinue administration of an anticoagulant/antithrombotic without substituting a suitable alternative. It is clear from the literature that under these circumstances, withdrawal of heparin treatment without replacement anticoagulant therapy results in an unacceptably high rate of thrombotic events. In the recent past, good alternatives for heparin were not available. Today, several alternative agents are suitable substitutes (although considerably more expensive), including *direct thrombin inhibitors* such as the intravenous use of argatroban and bivalirudin (Angiomax) (Chapter 43). Fondaparinux (Arixtra) is a synthetic heparin pentasaccharide, identical in chemical structure to the antithrombin binding sequence in heparin and heparin-derived agents such as low-molecular-weight heparins. Fondaparinux is given subcutaneously, and while its use in patients with HIT is "off-label" (not FDA approved), it is gaining favor in the clinical community as a second-line agent for the management of suspected HIT to avoid progression into acute HIT.

Neonatal Alloimmune Thrombocytopenia.

Neonatal alloimmune thrombocytopenia (NAIT) develops when the mother lacks a platelet-specific antigen (usually human platelet antigen 1a, or HPA-1a [P1^{A1}]) that the fetus has inherited from the father. HPA-1a is the most often involved (80% of cases), and HPA-5b accounts for another 10% to 15% of cases. Fetal platelet antigens may pass from the fetal to the maternal circulation as early as the fourteenth week of gestation.[61] If the mother is exposed to a fetal antigen she lacks, she may make antibodies to that fetal antigen. These antibodies cross the placenta, attach to the antigen-bearing fetal platelets, and result in thrombocytopenia in the fetus. In this regard, the pathophysiology of NAIT is the same as that of hemolytic disease of the newborn.

The most frequent cause of NAIT in whites is the HPA-1a antigen expressed on GP IIIa of the surface membrane GP IIb/IIIa complex, followed by HPA-5b (Br^a). The antigen HPA-3a (Bak^a) is present on GP IIb and is an important cause of neonatal thrombocytopenia in Asians. Platelet antigen HPA-4 (Penn and Yuk) accounts for the disorder in a few affected neonates.

Clinically significant thrombocytopenia develops in an estimated 1 in 1000 to 2000 newborns.[62] With the first pregnancy, about 50% of neonates born to mothers lacking a specific platelet antigen are affected, whereas with subsequent pregnancies the risk is 75% to 97%.[62] The incidence of intracranial hemorrhage or death or both in affected offspring is about 25%, and about half of the intracranial hemorrhages occur in utero in the second trimester.

Affected infants may appear normal at birth but soon manifest scattered petechiae and purpuric hemorrhages. In many infants with NAIT, serious hemorrhage does not develop, however, and the infants recover over a 1- to 2-week period as the level of passively transferred antibody decreases.[10,38] In symptomatic cases, platelet levels are usually below 30,000/μL and may diminish even further in the first few hours after birth.

The diagnosis of NAIT is one of exclusion of other causes of neonatal thrombocytopenia, including maternal ITP and maternal ingestion of drugs known to be associated with drug-induced thrombocytopenia. The presence of thrombocytopenia in a neonate with a HPA-1a–negative mother or a history of the disorder in a sibling is strong presumptive evidence in favor of the diagnosis. Confirmation should include platelet typing of both parents and testing for evidence of a maternal antibody directed at paternal platelets.[37]

In situations in which suspicion of NAIT is high or there is a history of NAIT in a first pregnancy, it may be necessary to test or treat the fetus to prevent intracranial hemorrhage in utero. Fetal genotypes now can be determined at 10 to 18 weeks of gestation using polymerase chain reaction methods on cells obtained by chorionic villus sampling or amniocentesis.[63] Periumbilical sampling to determine the fetal platelet count can be performed at about 20 weeks of gestation. When the fetus is thrombocytopenic, weekly maternal infusions of IVIG have been shown to be effective in increasing the fetal platelet count in most cases.[64] In cases in which the fetal platelet count does not increase with IVIG therapy, washed maternal platelets have been infused into the fetus with good results.[65] Treatment of the mother with high-dose corticosteroids (to decrease maternal antibody production) is not recommended because of potential fetal toxicity. In situations in which the diagnosis of NAIT is known or highly suspected, delivery should be by cesarean section to avoid fetal trauma associated with vaginal delivery. After delivery, the affected infant may be treated with transfusion of the appropriate antigen-negative platelets (usually maternal). In addition, IVIG can be used alone or in combination with platelet transfusion. IVIG should not be used as the sole treatment in a bleeding infant, because response to this therapy usually takes 1 to 3 days.[62]

Neonatal Autoimmune Thrombocytopenia. The diagnosis of ITP or systemic lupus erythematosus in the mother is a prerequisite for the diagnosis of neonatal autoimmune thrombocytopenia. Neonatal autoimmune thrombocytopenia is due to passive transplacental transfer of antibodies from a mother with ITP or, occasionally, systemic lupus erythematosus. The neonate does not have an ongoing autoimmune process per se, but rather is an incidental target of the mother's autoimmune process. During pregnancy, relapse is relatively common for women with ITP in complete or partial remission; this has been attributed to the facilitation of reticuloendothelial phagocytosis by the high estrogen levels in pregnant women. Women commonly develop chronic ITP during pregnancy. ITP in the mother tends to remit after delivery. Corticosteroids are the primary treatment for pregnant women with ITP, and at the dosages used, there is a relatively low incidence of adverse fetal side effects.[66] Neonatal autoimmune thrombocytopenia develops in only about 10% of the infants of pregnant women with autoimmune thrombocytopenia, and intracranial hemorrhage occurs in 1% or less. It is no longer recommended that high-risk infants be delivered by cesarean section to avoid the trauma of vaginal delivery and accompanying risk of hemorrhage in the infant, regardless of maternal platelet count.[67]

Affected newborns may have normal to decreased platelet numbers at birth and have a progressive decrease in the platelet count for about 1 week before the platelet count begins to increase. It has been speculated that the falling platelet count is associated with maturation of the infant's reticuloendothelial system and accelerated removal of antibody-labeled platelets by cells of the reticuloendothelial system. Neonatal thrombocytopenia typically persists for about 1 to 2 weeks but sometimes lasts for several months. It usually does not require treatment. Severely thrombocytopenic infants generally respond quickly to IVIG treatment. If an infant develops hemorrhagic symptoms, platelet transfusion, IVIG treatment, or corticosteroid therapy should be started immediately.[37]

Posttransfusion Purpura. Posttransfusion purpura (PTP) is a relatively rare disorder that typically develops about 1 week after transfusion of platelet-containing blood products, including fresh or frozen plasma, whole blood, and packed or washed RBCs. PTP is manifested by the rapid onset of severe thrombocytopenia and moderate to severe hemorrhage that may be life-threatening. The recipient's plasma is found to contain alloantibodies to antigens on the platelets or platelet membranes of the transfused blood product, directed against an antigen the recipient does not have. In more than 90% of cases, the antibody is directed against the HPA-1a antigen; in most of the remaining cases, the antibodies are directed against Pl^A2 or other epitopes on GP IIb/IIIa.[37] Involvement of other alloantigens, such as HPA-3a (Bak), HPA-4 (Penn), and HPA-5b (Br), has been reported. The mechanism by which the recipient's own platelets are destroyed is unknown. Most patients with this type of thrombocytopenia are multiparous middle-aged women. Almost all the other patients have a history of blood transfusion. PTP seems to be exceedingly rare in men who have never been transfused and in women who have never been pregnant or never been transfused.[68] PTP seems to require prior exposure to foreign platelet antigens and behaves in many respects like an anamnestic immune response.

No clinical trials have been conducted on the treatment of PTP, primarily because of the small number of cases. If PTP is untreated or treatment is ineffective, mortality rates may approach 10%.[69] In addition, untreated or unresponsive patients have a protracted clinical course, with thrombocytopenia typically lasting 3 weeks but in some cases up to 4 months. Plasmapheresis and exchange transfusion have been used with some success in the past, but the treatment of choice is now IVIG. Many patients with PTP respond to a 2-day course of IVIG, generally within the first 2 to 3 days, although a second course occasionally is necessary.[69] IVIG also is much easier to administer, and the response rates are higher than for plasmapheresis or exchange transfusion. Corticosteroid therapy is not particularly efficacious when used alone but may be beneficial in combination with other, more effective treatments.[37]

Secondary Thrombocytopenia, Presumed to Be Immune Mediated. Severe thrombocytopenia has been observed in patients receiving biologic response modifiers such as interferons, colony-stimulating factors, and interleukin-2.[70-72] The thrombocytopenia associated with use of these substances is reversible and, at least for interferon, may be immune mediated, because increased levels of platelet-associated IgG have been measured. Immune thrombocytopenia develops in about 5% to 10% of patients with chronic lymphocytic leukemia and in a smaller percentage of patients with other lymphoproliferative disorders.[73,74] Thrombocytopenia also is noted in 14% to 26% of patients with systemic lupus erythematosus.[75] The clinical picture is similar to that of ITP: the bone marrow has a larger than normal number of megakaryocytes, and increased levels of platelet-associated IgG frequently are found.[36] Parasitic infections also are known to cause thrombocytopenia. Malaria is the most studied in this group and is regularly accompanied by thrombocytopenia, the onset of which corresponds to the first appearance of antimalarial antibodies, a decrease in serum complement, and control of parasitemia. There is evidence for the adsorption of microbial antigens to the platelet surface and subsequent antibody binding via the Fab terminus.[76] Immune destruction of platelets seems to be the most likely mechanism for the thrombocytopenia.

Nonimmune Mechanisms of Platelet Destruction

Nonimmune platelet destruction may result from exposure of platelets to nonendothelial surfaces, from activation of the coagulation process, or from platelet consumption by endovascular injury without measurable depletion of coagulation factors.[36]

Thrombocytopenia in Pregnancy and Preeclampsia
Incidental Thrombocytopenia of Pregnancy. Incidental thrombocytopenia of pregnancy also is known as pregnancy-associated thrombocytopenia and gestational thrombocytopenia. This disorder is the most common cause of thrombocytopenia in pregnancy. Random platelet counts in pregnant and postpartum

women are slightly higher than normal, but about 5% of pregnant women develop a mild thrombocytopenia (100,000 to 150,000/μL), with 98% of such women having platelet counts greater than 70,000/μL. These women are healthy and have no prior history of thrombocytopenia. They do not seem to be at increased risk for bleeding or for delivery of infants with neonatal thrombocytopenia. The cause of this type of thrombocytopenia is unknown. Maternal platelet counts return to normal within several weeks of delivery. These women commonly experience recurrence in subsequent pregnancies.

Preeclampsia and other hypertensive disorders of pregnancy.   Approximately 20% of cases of thrombocytopenia of pregnancy are associated with hypertensive disorders. These disorders include the classifications preeclampsia, preeclampsia-eclampsia, preeclampsia with chronic hypertension, chronic hypertension, and gestational hypertension. Preeclampsia complicates about 5% of all pregnancies and typically occurs at about 20 weeks of gestation. The disorder is characterized by the onset of hypertension and proteinuria and may include abdominal pain, headache, blurred vision, or mental function disturbances.[77] Thrombocytopenia occurs in 15% to 20% of patients with preeclampsia, and about 40% to 50% of these patients progress to eclampsia (hypertension, proteinuria, and seizures).[78,79]

Some patients with preeclampsia have microangiopathic hemolysis, elevated liver enzymes, and a low platelet count, termed *HELLP syndrome*. HELLP syndrome affects an estimated 4% to 12% of women with severe preeclampsia[45,80,81] and seems to be associated with higher rates of maternal and fetal complications. This disorder may be difficult to differentiate from thrombotic thrombocytopenic purpura (TTP), hemolytic uremic syndrome (HUS), and disseminated intravascular coagulation (DIC).

The development of thrombocytopenia in these patients is thought to be due to increased platelet destruction. The mechanism of platelet destruction is unclear, however. Some evidence (elevated D-dimer) suggests that these patients have an underlying low-grade DIC.[82] Elevated platelet-associated immunoglobulin is commonly found in these patients, however, which indicates immune involvement.[83] Early reports suggested that there may be a component of in vivo platelet activation because low-dose aspirin therapy has been shown to prevent preeclampsia in high-risk patients.[84,85] When aspirin is used to prevent preeclampsia, however, reduction in risk is only 15%.

The treatment of preeclampsia is delivery of the infant whenever possible. After delivery, the thrombocytopenia usually resolves in a few days. In cases in which delivery is not possible (e.g., the infant would be too premature), bed rest and aggressive treatment of the hypertension may help to increase the platelet count in some patients. Such treatments include magnesium sulfate and other antiepileptic therapies to inhibit eclamptic seizures.

Other causes of thrombocytopenia during pregnancy. As has been discussed previously, ITP is a relatively common disorder in women of childbearing age, and pregnancy does nothing to ameliorate the symptoms of this disorder. ITP should be a part of the differential diagnosis of thrombocytopenia in a pregnant woman. There is little or no correlation between the level of maternal autoantibodies and the fetal platelet count. Other causes of thrombocytopenia during pregnancy include HIV infection, systemic lupus erythematosus, antiphospholipid syndromes, TTP, and HUS. Of all women who develop TTP, 10% to 25% manifest the disease during pregnancy or in the postpartum period, and TTP tends to recur in subsequent pregnancies.[86,87] Plasmapheresis is the treatment of choice, and the maternal mortality is 90% or greater without such treatment.

Hemolytic Disease of the Newborn.   Thrombocytopenia, usually moderate in degree, occurs frequently in infants with hemolytic disease of the newborn. Although the RBC destruction characteristic of this disorder is antibody induced, the antigens against which the antibodies are directed are not expressed on platelets. Platelets may be destroyed as a result of their interaction with products of RBC breakdown, rather than their direct participation in an immunologic reaction.[36]

Thrombotic Thrombocytopenic Purpura.   TTP, sometimes referred to as Moschcowitz syndrome, is characterized by the triad of microangiopathic hemolytic anemia, thrombocytopenia, and neurologic abnormalities.[88] In addition, fever and renal dysfunction (forming a pentad) are often present. Additional symptoms are present in most patients at the time of diagnosis and include diarrhea, anorexia, nausea, weakness, and fatigue. TTP is uncommon but not rare, and its incidence may be increasing. About twice as many women as men are affected, and it is most common in women 30 to 40 years of age.[34,89] About half of the patients who develop TTP have a history of a viral-like illness several days before the onset of TTP.

There seem to be at least four types of TTP. In most patients, TTP occurs as a single acute episode, although a small fraction of these patients may have recurrence at seemingly random intervals. Recurrent TTP occurs in 11% to 28% of TTP patients.[90,91] A third type of TTP is drug induced. The primary agents involved are the purinoreceptor (adenosine diphosphate) blocking agents ticlopidine (Ticlid) and clopidogrel (Plavix) used for inhibition of platelet function. Ticlopidine seems to cause TTP in about 0.025% of patients, whereas the incidence of clopidogrel-induced TTP is approximately four times less frequent.[89] The fourth type is chronic relapsing TTP, a rare form of TTP, in which episodes occur at intervals of approximately 3 months starting in infancy.[92,93]

Although it is unclear what triggers their deposition, hyaline thrombi are found in the end arterioles and capillaries. These hyaline thrombi are composed of platelets and von Willebrand factor (VWF) but contain very little fibrin or fibrinogen. As these platelet-VWF thrombi are deposited, thrombocytopenia develops. The degree of thrombocytopenia is directly related to the extent of microvascular platelet aggregation. RBCs flowing under arterial pressure are prone to fragmentation and hemolysis when they encounter the strands of these thrombi.

Hemolysis is usually quite severe, and most patients have less than 10 g/dL hemoglobin at the time of diagnosis. Examination of the peripheral blood film reveals a marked decrease in platelets, RBC polychromasia, and RBC fragmentation (microspherocytes, schistocytes, keratocytes), a triad of features characteristic of microangiopathic hemolytic anemias (Figure 40-8). Nucleated RBC precursors also may be present, depending on the degree of hemolysis. Other laboratory evidence of intravascular hemolysis includes reduction of haptoglobin, hemoglobinuria, hemosiderinuria, increased serum unconjugated bilirubin, and

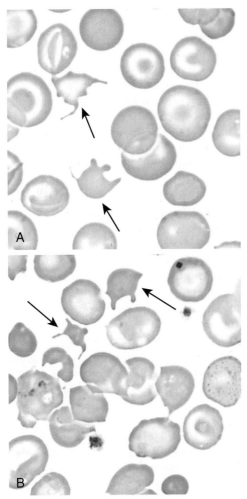

Figure 40-8 Microangiopathic hemolytic anemia. **A,** Thrombotic thrombocytopenic purpura (TTP); **B,** Hemolytic uremic syndrome (HUS). Abundant schistocytes (arrows) reflect the platelet rich clots in the microvasculature that occur with TTP and HUS. TTP and HUS have similar blood morphologies. (From Carr JH, Rodak BF: *Clinical hematology atlas,* ed 4, Philadelphia, 2013, Saunders.)

increased lactate dehydrogenase activity. Bone marrow examination reveals erythroid hyperplasia and a normal to increased number of megakaryocytes. The partial thromboplastin time, prothrombin time, fibrinogen, fibrin degradation products, and D-dimer test results are usually normal and may be useful in differentiating this disorder from DIC.

The thrombotic lesions also give rise to the other characteristic manifestations of TTP, because they are deposited in the vasculature of all organs. The thrombi occlude blood flow and lead to organ ischemia. Symptoms depend on the severity of ischemia in each organ. Neurologic manifestations range from headache to paresthesia and coma. Visual disturbances may be of neurologic origin or may be due to thrombi in the choroid capillaries of the retina or hemorrhage into the vitreous. Renal dysfunction is common and present in more than half of patients.[90,91] Symptoms of renal dysfunction include proteinuria and hematuria. Overwhelming renal damage with anuria and fulminant uremia usually does not occur, however, which helps to distinguish TTP from HUS.[10] Gastrointestinal bleeding occurs frequently in severely thrombocytopenic patients, and abdominal pain is occasionally present due to occlusion of the mesenteric microcirculation.

ADAMTS-13 and thrombotic thrombocytopenic purpura. The development of TTP seems to be directly related to the accumulation of ultra-large von Willebrand factor (ULVWF) multimers in the plasma of patients with TTP. VWF multimers are made by megakaryocytes and endothelial cells. The primary source of plasma VWF seems to be endothelial cells. Endothelial cells secrete VWF into the subendothelium and plasma and store it in Weibel-Palade bodies (storage granules). Endothelial cells and megakaryocytes make even larger VWF multimers (ULVWF multimers) than those found in plasma, and these are even more effective than the normal plasma VWF multimers at binding platelet GP Ib/IX or GP IIb/IIIa complexes under fluid shear stresses (Figure 40-9).[92] In the plasma, the ULVWF multimers are rapidly cleaved into the smaller VWF multimers normally found in the plasma by a VWF-cleaving protease, called *a disintegrin and metalloprotease with a thrombospondin type 1 motif, member 13* (ADAMTS-13). This metalloprotease seems to be more effective when VWF multimers are partially unfolded by high shear stress.[94,95]

Familial chronic relapsing TTP is a form characterized by recurrent episodes of thrombocytopenia with or without ischemic organ damage. In this type of TTP, the VWF-cleaving metalloprotease is completely deficient. The more common

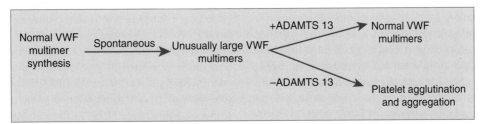

Figure 40-9 Mechanism for thrombotic thrombocytopenic purpura (TTP). Unusually large von Willebrand factor (ULVWF) multimers are normally digested by the VWF–cleaving protease ADAMTS-13 (a disintegrin and metalloprotease with a thrombospondin type 1 motif, member 13). In TTP, the absence of ADAMTS-13 allows the release of ULVWF, triggering platelet activation.

form of TTP (usually not familial) does not tend to recur, but patients also are deficient in the metalloprotease. In this more common form of TTP, the metalloprotease deficiency occurs through removal of the enzyme (or blockade of its function) by a specific autoantibody that is present during TTP but disappears during remission.[96,97] An assay to measure the VWF-cleaving enzyme has been introduced.[98] However, the test may take several days, and treatment decisions must usually be made before test results are available. In addition, the assay lacks sensitivity and specificity for TTP. Additional tests for ADAMTS-13 (and TTP) are in development and hold the promise for rapid diagnosis of TTP.

In patients with TTP, ULVWF multimers tend to be present in the plasma at the beginning of the episode. These ULVWF multimers, and usually the normal-sized plasma multimers, disappear as the TTP episode progresses and the thrombocytopenia worsens. Platelets and VWF are consumed during deposition of the microvascular hyaline thrombi characteristic of this disorder.[99] If the patient survives an episode of TTP and does not experience relapse, the plasma VWF multimers are usually normal after recovery. If ULVWF multimers are found in the plasma after recovery, however, it is likely that the patient will have recurrent episodes of TTP. The episodes may be infrequent and at irregular intervals (intermittent TTP) or frequent and at regular intervals, as is often the case when TTP episodes occur in early childhood or infancy.

The most effective treatment for TTP is plasma exchange using fresh-frozen plasma or cryoprecipitate-poor plasma (plasma lacking most of the fibrinogen, fibronectin, and VWF).[100] Either of these approaches may produce dramatic effects within a few hours. Because plasmapheresis is not available in all centers, the patient should be given corticosteroids and infusions of fresh-frozen plasma immediately. Plasma exchange should be arranged as quickly as possible. Plasmapheresis and replacement/infusion of plasma is effective on two fronts. First, some of the ULVWF multimers will be removed by apheresis, and plasma (fresh-frozen plasma or cryoprecipitate-poor plasma) supplies the deficient protease, which is able to degrade the ULVWF multimers in the blood of the patient. Because some patients with TTP have recovered while receiving immunosuppressive treatment (corticosteroids) alone, it is recommended that all patients with TTP be given high-dose corticosteroids in addition to undergoing plasma exchange. Plasma exchange typically is continued over a 5-day period. If a response is not seen within 5 days, or if the condition of the patient worsens during the first few days of plasma exchange, additional treatment is instituted. Such therapies include administering vincristine or azathioprine (or other immunosuppressive agents), performing splenectomy, or passing the patient's plasma over a staphylococcal A column to remove immune complexes. The use of antiplatelet agents, prostacyclin, heparin, or fibrinolytic agents is controversial and has not clearly been shown to be helpful. Platelet transfusions should be avoided unless intracranial bleeding or other serious hemorrhagic problems arise.[45]

Before 1990, TTP was fatal in more than 80% of patients. With the means for rapid diagnosis and the advent of exchange plasmapheresis, now 80% of patients who are treated early can be expected to survive. Because patients are known to experience relapse, however, platelet counts should be monitored on a regular basis until patients are in remission. The detection of ULVWF multimers in patient samples after complete remission has predicted relapse accurately in 90% of the patients tested[101]; this may prove to be useful in the long-term management of TTP.

Hemolytic Uremic Syndrome.   Clinically, HUS resembles TTP except that it is found predominantly in children 6 months to 4 years of age and is self-limiting. Approximately 90% of cases are caused by *Shigella dysenteriae* serotypes or enterohemorrhagic *Escherichia coli* OH serotypes, particularly O157:H7.[102] These organisms sometimes can be cultured from stool samples. The bloody diarrhea typical of childhood HUS is caused by colonization of the large intestine with the offending organism, which causes erosive damage to the colon. *S. dysenteriae* produces Shiga toxin, and enterohemorrhagic *E. coli* produces either Shiga-like toxin-1 (SLT-1) or SLT-2, which can be detected in fecal samples from patients with HUS. The toxins enter the bloodstream and attach to renal glomerular capillary endothelial cells, which become damaged and swollen and release ULVWF multimers.[102,103] This process leads to formation of hyaline thrombi in the renal vasculature and the development of renal failure, thrombocytopenia, and microangiopathic hemolytic anemia, although the RBC fragmentation is usually not as severe as that seen in TTP (this is, however, not a differentiating feature). The extent of renal involvement correlates with the rate of recovery. In more severely affected children, renal dialysis may be needed. The mortality rate associated with HUS in children is much lower than that for TTP, but there is often residual renal dysfunction that may lead to renal hypertension and severe renal failure. Because HUS in children is essentially an infectious disorder, it affects boys and girls equally and is often found in geographic clusters of cases rather than in random distribution.

The adult form of HUS is associated most often with exposure to immunosuppressive agents or chemotherapeutic agents or both, but it also may occur during the postpartum period. Usually the symptoms of HUS do not appear until weeks or months after exposure to the offending agent.[104] This disorder most likely results from direct renal arterial endothelial damage caused by the drug or one of its metabolic products. The damage to endothelial cells results in release of VWF (including ULVWF multimers), turbulent flow in the arterial system with increased shear stresses on platelets, and VWF-mediated platelet aggregation in the renal arterial system. The renal impairment in adults seems to be more severe than that in childhood HUS, and dialysis is usually required. The cause of HUS associated with pregnancy or oral contraceptive use is unclear, but it may be related to development of an autoantibody to endothelial cells. In outbreaks of HUS associated with consumption of *E. coli*–contaminated water, both children and adults have developed HUS.

The cardinal signs of HUS are hemolytic anemia, renal failure, and thrombocytopenia. The thrombocytopenia is usually mild to moderate in severity. Renal failure is reflected in elevated blood urea nitrogen and creatinine levels. The urine nearly always contains RBCs, protein, and casts. The hemolytic process is shown by a hemoglobin level of less than 10 g/dL, elevated reticulocyte count, and presence of schistocytes in the peripheral blood.

Differentiating the adult form of HUS from TTP may be difficult. The lack of neurologic symptoms, the presence of renal dysfunction, and the absence of other organ involvement suggest HUS. Also, in HUS the thrombocytopenia tends to be mild to moderate (platelet consumption occurs primarily in the kidneys), whereas in TTP the thrombocytopenia is usually severe. Similarly, fragmentation of RBCs and the resultant anemia tend to be milder than that observed in TTP, because RBCs are being fragmented primarily in the kidneys. In some cases of HUS, other organs become involved, and the differentiation between HUS and TTP becomes less clear. In such cases, it is prudent to treat as though the patient has TTP.

Disseminated Intravascular Coagulation. A common cause of destructive thrombocytopenia is activation of the coagulation cascade (by a variety of agents or conditions), resulting in a consumptive coagulopathy that entraps platelets in intravascular fibrin clots. This disorder is described in more detail in Chapter 39 but is discussed here briefly for the sake of completeness. DIC has many similarities to TTP, including microangiopathic hemolytic anemia and deposition of thrombi in the arterial circulation of most organs. In DIC, however, the thrombi are composed primarily of platelets and fibrinogen, whereas in TTP the thrombi are composed primarily of platelets and VWF.

One form of DIC is acute with rapid platelet consumption and results in severe thrombocytopenia. In addition, levels of factor V, factor VIII, and fibrinogen are decreased as a result of in vivo thrombin generation. The test for D-dimer (a breakdown product of stabilized fibrin) almost always yields positive results. This form of DIC is life-threatening and must be treated immediately.

In chronic DIC, there is an ongoing, low-grade consumptive coagulopathy. Clotting factors may be slightly reduced or normal, and compensatory thrombocytopoiesis results in a moderately low to normal platelet count.[34] D-dimer may not be detectable or may be slightly to moderately increased. Chronic DIC is not generally life-threatening, and treatment usually is not urgent. Chronic DIC is almost always due to some underlying condition. If that condition can be corrected, the DIC usually resolves without further treatment. Chronic DIC should be followed closely, however, because it can convert into the life-threatening acute form.

Drug-Induced Thrombocytopenia. A few drugs directly interact with platelets to cause thrombocytopenia. Ristocetin, an antibiotic no longer in clinical use, facilitates the interaction of VWF with platelet membrane GP Ib and leads to in vivo platelet agglutination and thrombocytopenia. Hematin, used for the treatment of acute intermittent porphyria, may give rise to a transient thrombocytopenia that seems to be caused by stimulation of platelet secretion and aggregation. Protamine sulfate and bleomycin may induce thrombocytopenia by a similar mechanism.[45]

Abnormalities in Distribution or Dilution

An abnormal distribution of platelets also may cause thrombocytopenia. The normal spleen sequesters approximately one third of the total platelet mass. Mild thrombocytopenia may be present in any of the "big spleen" syndromes. The total body platelet mass is often normal in these disorders, but numerous platelets are sequestered in the enlarged spleen, and consequently the venous blood platelet count is low. Disorders such as Gaucher disease, Hodgkin disease, sarcoidosis, lymphoma, cirrhosis of the liver, and portal hypertension may result in splenomegaly and lead to thrombocytopenia.

Lowering the body temperature to less than 25° C, as is routinely done in cardiovascular surgery, results in a transient but mild thrombocytopenia secondary to platelet sequestration in the spleen and liver. An associated transient defect in function also occurs with hypothermia. Platelet count and function return to baseline values on return to normal body temperature.[32]

Thrombocytopenia often follows surgery involving extracorporeal circulatory devices, as a consequence of damage and partial activation of platelets in the pump. In a few cases, severe thrombocytopenia, marked impairment of platelet function, and activation of fibrinolysis and intravascular coagulation may develop.[45]

The administration of massive amounts of stored whole blood may produce a temporary thrombocytopenia. This phenomenon is explained by the fact that stored blood contains platelets whose viability is severely impaired by the effects of storage and temperature. Under these conditions, the dead or damaged platelets are rapidly sequestered by the reticuloendothelial system of the patient. If this problem is encountered, it may be minimized by administering platelet concentrates or units of fresh whole blood along with the stored blood. This situation is only rarely encountered, however, because the practice of transfusing whole blood has been replaced almost completely by the use of specific components. Finally, mild thrombocytopenia may be encountered in patients with chronic renal failure, severe iron deficiency, megaloblastic anemia, postcompression sickness, and chronic hypoxia.

THROMBOCYTOSIS: INCREASE IN CIRCULATING PLATELETS

Thrombocytosis is defined as an abnormally high platelet count, typically more than 450,000/μL. The term *reactive thrombocytosis* is used to describe an elevation in the platelet count secondary to inflammation, trauma, or other underlying and seemingly unrelated conditions. In reactive thrombocytosis, the platelet count is elevated for a limited period and usually does not exceed 800,000/μL, although platelet counts greater than 1 million/μL are occasionally seen (Figure 40-10). A marked and persistent elevation in the platelet count is a hallmark of myeloproliferative disorders such as polycythemia vera, chronic myelogenous leukemia, and myelofibrosis with myeloid metaplasia (or primary myelofibrosis). In these conditions, the platelet count often exceeds 1 million/μL. Although the terms *thrombocythemia* and *thrombocytosis* are often used

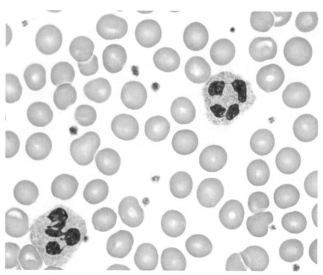

Figure 40-10 Peripheral blood film showing cell morphology in reactive thrombocytosis. Note the increased number of platelets but reasonably normal platelet morphology, characteristic of reactive thrombocytosis.

From Colvin BT: Thrombocytopenia, *Clin Haematol* 14:661-681, 1985; and Thompson AR, Harker LA: *Manual of hemostasis and thrombosis*, ed 3, Philadelphia, 1983, FA Davis.

BOX 40-3 Processes Resulting in Thrombocytosis

Conditions Associated with Reactive Thrombocytosis
Blood loss and surgery
Splenectomy
Iron deficiency anemia
Inflammation and disease
Stress or exercise

Myeloproliferative Disorders Associated with Thrombocytosis
Polycythemia vera
Chronic myelogenous leukemia
Myelofibrosis with myeloid metaplasia
Thrombocythemia: essential or primary

interchangeably, in this text the term *thrombocythemia* is used only as part of the description of the myeloproliferative disorder known as *essential thrombocythemia* (Figure 40-11). In essential thrombocythemia, platelet counts typically exceed 1 million/μL and may reach levels of several million.[34,105,106] Processes resulting in thrombocytosis are summarized in Box 40-3.

Reactive (Secondary) Thrombocytosis

Platelet counts between 450,000/μL and 800,000/μL with no change in platelet function can result from acute blood loss, splenectomy, childbirth, and tissue necrosis secondary to surgery, chronic inflammatory disease, infection, exercise, iron deficiency anemia, hemolytic anemia, renal disorders, and malignancy. Occasionally, patients manifest a platelet count of 1 to 2 million/μL (Figure 40-10). In reactive thrombocytosis, platelet production remains responsive to normal regulatory stimuli (e.g., thrombopoietin, a humoral factor that is produced in the kidney parenchyma), and morphologically normal platelets are produced at a moderately increased rate. This is in contrast to essential thrombocythemia, which is characterized by unregulated or autonomous platelet production and platelets of variable size.[105,106]

Examination of the bone marrow from patients with reactive thrombocytosis reveals a normal to increased number of megakaryocytes that are normal in morphology. Results of platelet function tests, including aggregation induced by various agents, and bleeding time are usually normal in reactive thrombocytosis but also may be normal in patients with elevated platelet counts accompanying myeloproliferative disorders.

Reactive thrombocytosis is not associated with thrombosis, hemorrhage, or abnormal thrombopoietin levels. It seldom produces symptoms per se and disappears when the underlying disorder is brought under control.[105,106]

Reactive Thrombocytosis Associated with Hemorrhage or Surgery

After acute hemorrhage, the platelet count may be low for 2 to 6 days (unless platelets have been transfused) but typically rebounds to elevated levels for several days before returning to the prehemorrhage level. A similar pattern of thrombocytopenia and thrombocytosis is seen after major surgical procedures in which there is significant blood loss. In both cases, the platelet count typically returns to normal 10 to 16 days after the episode of blood loss.

Postsplenectomy Thrombocytosis

Removal of the spleen typically results in platelet counts that can reach or exceed 1 million/μL regardless of the reason for splenectomy. The spleen normally sequesters about one third of the circulating platelet mass. After splenectomy, one would

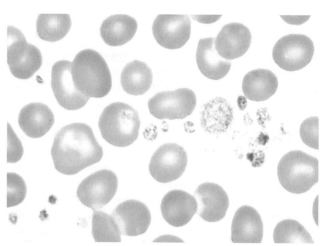

Figure 40-11 Peripheral blood film showing cell morphology in essential thrombocythemia. Note the increased number of platelets and wide variation in platelet size characteristic of essential thrombocythemia. Red and white blood cell morphology is characteristically normal. (From Carr JH, Rodak BF: *Clinical hematology atlas*, ed 4, Philadelphia, 2013, Saunders.)

expect an initial increase in the platelet count of approximately 30% to 50%. The platelet count, however, far exceeds levels that could result from rebalancing of the circulating platelet pool to incorporate the splenic platelet pool. The cause of the accelerated platelet production is unknown. Unlike after blood loss from hemorrhage or other types of surgery, the platelet count reaches a maximum 1 to 3 weeks after splenectomy and remains elevated for 1 to 3 months. In some patients who undergo splenectomy for treatment of chronic anemia, the count can remain elevated for several years.

Thrombocytosis Associated with Iron Deficiency Anemia

Mild iron deficiency anemia secondary to chronic blood loss is associated with thrombocytosis in about 50% of cases. Thrombocytosis can be seen in severe iron deficiency anemia, but thrombocytopenia also has been reported. In some cases of iron deficiency, the platelet count may be 2 million/µL. After iron therapy is started, the platelet count usually returns to normal within 7 to 10 days. It is believed that iron plays some role in regulating thrombopoiesis, because treatment of the iron deficiency with iron replacement has resulted in a normalization of the platelet count in thrombocytopenic patients and has been reported to induce thrombocytopenia in patients with normal platelet counts. Not enough research has been done, however, to elucidate the role of iron in thrombopoiesis.

Thrombocytosis Associated with Inflammation and Disease

Similar to elevations in C-reactive protein, fibrinogen, VWF, and other acute phase reactants, thrombocytosis may be an indication of inflammation. Thrombocytosis may be found in association with rheumatoid arthritis, rheumatic fever, osteomyelitis, ulcerative colitis, acute infections, and malignancy. In rheumatoid arthritis, the presence of thrombocytosis can be correlated with activation of the inflammatory process.

Kawasaki disease (Kawasaki syndrome) causes inflammation of the walls of small and medium-sized arteries throughout the body. It is also known as mucocutaneous lymph node syndrome because it affects lymph nodes, skin, and mucous membranes in the mouth, nose, and throat. It is an acute febrile illness of infants and young children. Boys are more likely than girls to develop the disease, and children of Japanese and Korean descent have higher rates of Kawasaki disease. It is a self-limited acute vasculitic syndrome of unknown origin, although an infectious etiology has been suspected. Although the disease is self-limiting, there can be lifelong sequelae, including coronary artery thrombosis and aneurysms. The acute febrile stage of the disease lasts 2 weeks or longer, with a fever of 40° C or higher, and is unresponsive to antibiotic therapy. The longer the fever continues, the higher the risk of cardiovascular complications. The subacute phase lasts an additional week to 10 days. During this phase, the platelet count usually is elevated, and counts of 2 million/µL have been reported. In addition, acute phase reactants such as C-reactive protein and sedimentation rate are elevated, consistent with an inflammatory component. The WBC count can be moderately to markedly elevated with a left shift, and many patients develop a mild normochromic, normocytic anemia. During this phase, cardiovascular complications and aneurysms develop. The higher the platelet count, the higher the risk of cardiovascular complication. After the subacute phase comes the convalescent phase, during which all signs of illness disappear and the acute phase reactants subside to normal. The highest incidence of Kawasaki disease is found in Japan and in individuals of Japanese descent, although the disease seems to occur in most, if not all, ethnic groups. There is no specific test for Kawasaki disease. Diagnosis is primarily by excluding other diseases that cause similar signs and symptoms (e.g., scarlet fever, juvenile rheumatoid arthritis, Stevens-Johnson syndrome, and toxic shock syndrome). The treatment for Kawasaki disease is administration of antiplatelet agents and immunoglobulin.

An elevated platelet count also may be early evidence of a tumor (e.g., Hodgkin disease) and various carcinomas. Finally, hemophilic patients often have platelet counts above normal limits, even in the absence of active bleeding.

Exercise-Induced Thrombocytosis

Strenuous exercise is a well-known cause of relative thrombocytosis and is likely due to the release of platelets from the splenic pool or hemoconcentration by transfer of plasma water to the extravascular compartment or both. Normally, the platelet count returns to its preexercise baseline level 30 minutes after completion of exercise.

Rebound Thrombocytosis

Thrombocytosis often follows the thrombocytopenia caused by marrow-suppressive therapy or other conditions. "Rebound" thrombocytosis usually reaches a peak 10 to 17 days after withdrawal of the offending drug (e.g., alcohol or methotrexate) or after institution of therapy for the underlying condition with which thrombocytopenia is associated (e.g., vitamin B_{12} deficiency).[45]

Thrombocytosis Associated with Myeloproliferative Disorders

Primary or autonomous thrombocytosis is a typical finding in four chronic myeloproliferative disorders: polycythemia vera, chronic myelogenous leukemia, myelofibrosis with myeloid metaplasia (primary myelofibrosis), and essential thrombocythemia. Depending on the duration and stage of the myeloproliferative disorder at the time of diagnosis, it may be difficult to differentiate among these diseases. Chapter 33 provides a more complete description of these disorders. In the other types of myeloproliferative disorders, the platelet count seldom reaches the extreme values characteristic of essential thrombocythemia. Diagnosis of essential thrombocythemia should not be based on the platelet count alone but should also take into account the physical examination findings, history, and other laboratory data.[34,106]

Essential (Primary) Thrombocythemia

Essential thrombocythemia is a clonal disorder related to other chronic myeloproliferative diseases and is the most common cause of primary thrombocytosis. It is characterized by peripheral blood platelet counts exceeding 1 million/µL and uncontrolled proliferation of marrow megakaryocytes. Although the platelet count may (or may not) be markedly elevated in other myeloproliferative disorders, persistent marked elevation of the platelet count is an absolute requirement for the diagnosis of essential thrombocythemia (Figure 40-11). There is evidence that essential thrombocythemia is caused by a clonal proliferation of a single abnormal pluripotential stem cell that eventually crowds out normal stem cells. As with most myeloproliferative disorders, essential thrombocythemia is neither congenital nor hereditary, is prevalent in middle-aged and older patients, and affects equal numbers of men and women. In contrast to other myeloproliferative disorders, however, the other marrow cell lines are not involved at the time of diagnosis.

The clinical manifestations of essential thrombocythemia are hemorrhage, platelet dysfunction, and thrombosis. Bleeding times are usually normal. There is no specific clinical sign, symptom, or laboratory test that establishes the diagnosis of essential thrombocythemia. The diagnosis must be made by ruling out the other myeloproliferative disorders and systemic illnesses that produce reactive thrombocytosis.

Thrombosis in the microvasculature is relatively common in essential thrombocythemia, and the incidence at the time of diagnosis is 10% to 20%. This thrombosis can lead to digital pain, digital gangrene, or erythromelalgia (throbbing, aching, and burning sensation in the extremities, particularly in the palms and soles).[106] The symptoms of erythromelalgia can be explained by arteriolar inflammation and occlusive thrombosis mediated by platelets and can be relieved for several days by a single dose of aspirin.[107] Thrombosis of large veins and arteries also may occur in essential thrombocythemia. The arteries most commonly involved are those in the legs, the coronary arteries, and the renal arteries, but involvement of the mesenteric, subclavian, and carotid arteries is not infrequent (in fact, neurologic complications are relatively common). Venous thrombosis may involve the large veins of the legs and pelvis, hepatic veins, or splenic veins.[108] The platelets of some patients who have experienced thrombotic episodes have been shown to have increased binding affinity for fibrinogen and to generate more than the usual quantities of thromboxane B_2, and these patients have elevated levels of thromboxane B_2 and β-thromboglobulin in the blood. These findings suggest enhanced in vivo platelet activation and perhaps an explanation for the thrombotic tendencies of patients with essential thrombocythemia. The primary cause of death of patients with essential thrombocythemia seems to be thrombosis. Hemorrhagic episodes occur less frequently than thrombotic episodes in patients with essential thrombocythemia.

As with bleeding secondary to platelet function disorders, the hemorrhagic manifestations of essential thrombocythemia are mucocutaneous in nature, with gastrointestinal tract bleeding occurring most frequently. Other sites of bleeding include the mucous membranes of the nose and mouth, the urinary tract, and the skin. Symptoms may be aggravated by aspirin use. In an occasional patient with essential thrombocythemia, there is a paradoxical combination of thromboembolic (clotting) and hemorrhagic episodes in association with this condition.

A patient with essential thrombocythemia who has had a thrombotic event may have a hemorrhagic event later.[109]

The bleeding manifestations may be related to a variety of qualitative abnormalities in the platelets, including deficiencies in epinephrine receptors and ultrastructural defects in granules, mitochondria, and microfilaments. Platelets may be agranular or hypogranular and have a clear, light blue appearance on a routine Wright-stained film of the peripheral blood. Although platelet size is heterogeneous, giant and bizarrely shaped platelets are characteristic of myeloproliferative diseases, and megakaryocyte fragments or nuclei are commonly encountered in the peripheral blood. Platelets may be notably clumped on blood films, exhibiting marked variation in size and shape. The number and volume of megakaryocytes are increased in the bone marrow, and they are predominantly large, show some cellular atypia, and tend to form clusters. Often the platelets are functionally defective when tested in vitro. Aggregation is usually absent in response to epinephrine and may be decreased with adenosine diphosphate but is usually normal with collagen. Lack of an epinephrine response may help to differentiate essential thrombocythemia from reactive thrombocytosis, because this response is usually normal in reactive thrombocytosis but absent in most cases of essential thrombocythemia. Platelet adhesion also may be decreased.[106]

The degree of thrombocytosis has not been found to predict hemorrhagic or thrombotic events reliably. The role of lowering platelet counts as a prophylactic treatment in this disease is not established. The risks from exposure to mutagenic alkylating agents used to decrease the platelet count may be greater than the risk of thrombosis or hemorrhage. When treatment is deemed necessary because of thrombotic tendencies or splenomegaly, a variety of myelosuppressive agents (e.g., melphalan, busulfan, hydroxyurea, or even radioactive phosphorus) can be used.[106] In patients with life-threatening hemorrhage or thrombosis and an extremely high platelet count, platelet apheresis may be used to reduce the platelet count rapidly. In these situations, a myelosuppressive agent is added for longer-term control of the platelet count.[110] Interferon-α has been used to treat essential thrombocythemia and is associated with an approximately 60% rate of complete remission, but 28% of patients given the drug cannot tolerate the dosages required.[111-113] A newer agent that has shown great promise in the treatment of essential thrombocythemia is anagrelide. The drug acts by inhibiting megakaryocyte maturation and platelet release.[114] In one large study, anagrelide decreased the platelet count in 93% of patients.[115] Many patients cannot tolerate anagrelide, however, and in these patients other, more traditional chemotherapeutic agents seem to be more effective. Despite the availability of newer treatments for essential thrombocythemia, whether a patient with essential thrombocythemia and an elevated platelet count who is asymptomatic should or should not be treated remains controversial.

In patients with essential thrombocythemia there is a low incidence of transformation to acute leukemia or fatal thrombotic or hemorrhagic complications. Therapy to prevent thrombotic complications seems to be effective in preventing morbidity but does not seem to improve survival, at least in high-risk patients.

SUMMARY

- Thrombocytopenia is the most common cause of clinically significant bleeding.
- Thrombocytopenia may be a result of decreased platelet production, increased destruction, or abnormal distribution of platelets and manifests with small-vessel bleeding in the skin.
- Decreased production of platelets can be attributed to megakaryocyte hypoplasia, ineffective thrombopoiesis, or replacement of marrow by abnormal cells.
- Patients experiencing increased platelet destruction become thrombocytopenic only when the rate of platelet production can no longer increase enough to compensate.
- Pathologic destruction of platelets can be caused by both immunologic and nonimmunologic mechanisms.
- Acute ITP commonly occurs in children after a viral illness, and there is usually spontaneous remission. Chronic ITP is more commonly seen in women and requires treatment if the platelet count decreases to fewer than 30,000/μL.

- Treatment of drug-induced thrombocytopenia must begin with identification of the causative drug and discontinuation of its use.
- TTP presents with a triad of symptoms that includes microangiopathic hemolytic anemia, thrombocytopenia, and neurologic abnormalities; these may be accompanied by fever and renal dysfunction.
- Abnormal distribution of platelets can be caused by splenic sequestration.
- Reactive thrombocytosis is secondary to inflammation, trauma, or a variety of underlying conditions. Platelet counts are increased for a limited time. The thrombocytosis seen in myeloproliferative disorders is marked and persistent.

Now that you have completed this chapter, go back and read again the case study at the beginning and respond to the questions presented.

REVIEW QUESTIONS

Answers can be found in the Appendix.

1. The autosomal dominant disorder associated with decreased platelet production is:
   a. Fanconi anemia
   b. TAR syndrome
   c. May-Hegglin anomaly
   d. Wiskott-Aldrich anomaly

2. Which of the following is *not* a hallmark of ITP?
   a. Petechiae
   b. Thrombocytopenia
   c. Large overactive platelets
   d. Megakaryocyte hypoplasia

3. The specific antigen most commonly responsible for the development of NAIT is:
   a. Bak
   b. HPA-1a
   c. GP Ib
   d. Lewis antigen a

4. A 2-year-old child with an unexpected platelet count of 15,000/μL and a recent history of a viral infection most likely has:
   a. HIT
   b. NAIT
   c. Acute ITP
   d. Chronic ITP

5. What is the first step in the treatment of HIT?
   a. Start low-molecular-weight heparin therapy
   b. Stop heparin infusion immediately
   c. Switch to warfarin (Coumadin) immediately
   d. Initiate a platelet transfusion

6. A defect in primary hemostasis (platelet response to an injury) often results in:
   a. Musculoskeletal bleeding
   b. Mucosal bleeding
   c. Hemarthroses
   d. None of the above

7. When a drug acts as a hapten to induce thrombocytopenia, an antibody forms against which of the following?
   a. Typically unexposed, new platelet antigens
   b. The combination of the drug and the platelet membrane protein to which it is bound
   c. The drug alone in the plasma, but the immune complex then binds to the platelet membrane
   d. The drug alone, but only when it is bound to the platelet membrane

8. *TAR* refers to:
   a. Abnormal platelet morphology in which the radial striations of the platelets are missing
   b. Abnormal appearance of the iris of the eye in which radial striations are absent
   c. Abnormal bone formation, including hypoplasia of the forearms
   d. Neurologic defects affecting the root (radix) of the spinal nerves

9. Neonatal autoimmune thrombocytopenia occurs when:
   a. The mother lacks a platelet antigen that the infant possesses, and she builds antibodies to that antigen, which cross the placenta
   b. The infant develops an autoimmune process such as ITP secondary to in utero infection
   c. The infant develops an autoimmune disease such as lupus erythematosus before birth
   d. The mother has an autoimmune antibody to her own platelets, which crosses the placenta and reacts with the infant's platelets

10. HUS in children is associated with:
   a. Diarrhea caused by *Shigella* species
   b. Meningitis caused by *Haemophilus* species
   c. Pneumonia caused by *Mycoplasma* species
   d. Pneumonia caused by respiratory viruses

REFERENCES

1. Kelley, M. J., Jawien, W., Ortel, T. L., et al. (2000). Mutations of MYH9, encoding for non-muscle myosin heavy chain A, in May Hegglin anomaly. *Nat Genet, 26,* 106–108.
2. The May Hegglin/Fechtner Syndrome Consortium. (2000). Mutations in MHY9 result in May-Hegglin anomaly, and Fechtner and Sebastian syndromes. *Nat Genet, 26,* 103–105.
3. Mhawech, P., & Saleem, A. (2000). Inherited giant platelet disorders: classification and literature review. *Am J Clin Pathol, 113,* 176–190.
4. Hall, J. G. (1987). Thrombocytopenia and absent radius (TAR) syndrome. *J Med Genet, 24,* 79–83.
5. Freedman, M. H., & Doyle, J. J. (1999). Inherited bone marrow failure syndromes. In Lilleyman, J. S., Hann, I. M., & Branchette, V. S., (Eds.), *Pediatric Hematology* (pp. 23–49). London: Churchill Livingstone.
6. Lackner, A., Basu, M., Bierings, M., et al. (2000). Haematopoietic stem cell transplantation for amegakaryocytic thrombocytopenia. *Br J Haematol, 109,* 773–775.
7. van den, Oudenrijn, S. M., Bruin, M., Folman, C. C., et al. (2000). Mutations in the thrombopoietin receptor, Mlp, in children with congenital amegakaryocytic thrombocytopenia. *Br J Haematol, 110,* 441–448.
8. Balduini, C. L., Savoia, A., & Seri, M. (2013). Inherited thrombocytopenias frequently diagnosed in adults. *J Thromb Haemost, 11,* 1006–1019.
9. Stormorken, H., Hellum, B., Egeland, T., et al. (1991). X-linked thrombocytopenia and thrombocytopathia: attenuated Wiscott-Aldrich syndrome: functional and morphological studies of platelets and lymphocytes. *Thromb Haemost, 65,* 300–305.
10. Thorup, O. A. (1987). *Leavell and Thorup's fundamentals of clinical hematology.* (5th ed.). Philadelphia: Saunders.
11. Villa, A. L., Notarangelo, P., Maachi, E., et al. (1999). X-linked thrombocytopenia and Wiskott-Aldrich syndrome are allelic diseases with mutations in the WASP gene. *Nat Genet, 9,* 414–417.
12. Mehaffey, M. G., Newton, A. L., Gandhi, M. J., et al. (2001). X-linked thrombocytopenia caused by a novel mutation of GATA-1. *Blood, 98,* 2681–2688.
13. Freson, K. K., Devriendt, G., Matthijs, G., et al. (2001). Platelet characteristics in patients with X-linked macrothrombocytopenia because of a novel GATA-1 mutation. *Blood, 98,* 85–92.
14. Casteels, A. A., Naessens, F., Cordts, L., et al. (1999). Neonatal screening for congenital cytomegalovirus infections. *J Perinat Med, 27,* 116–121.
15. Brown, H. L., Abernathy, M. P. (1998). Cytomegalovirus infection. *Semin Perinatol, 22,* 260–266.
16. Crapnell, K. E. D., Zanfani, A., Chaudhuri, J. L., et al. (2000). In vitro infection of megakaryocytes and their precursors by human cytomegalovirus. *Blood, 95,* 487–493.
17. McAuley, J., Boyer, D., Patel, D., et al. (1994). Early and longitudinal evaluations of treated infants and children and untreated historical patients with congenital toxoplasmosis: the Chicago Collaborative Treatment Trial. *Clin Infect Dis, 18,* 38–72.
18. Sullivan, E. M., Burgess, M. A., Forrest, J. M. (1999). The epidemiology of rubella and congenital rubella in Australia, 1992-1997. *Commun Dis Intell, 23,* 209–214.
19. Tookey, P. A., Peckham, C. S. (1999). Surveillance of congenital rubella in Great Britain, 1971-96. *BMJ, 318,* 769–770.
20. Tovo, P. A., de-Martino, M., Gabiano, C., et al. (1992). Prognostic factors and survival in children with perinatal HIV-1 infection. The Italian Register for HIV Infections in Children. *Lancet, 339,* 1249–1253.
21. Triplett, D. A., (Ed.). (1978). *Platelet function: laboratory evaluation and clinical application.* Chicago: American Society of Clinical Pathologists.
22. Brown, B. A. (1993). *Hematology: principles and procedures.* (6th ed.). Philadelphia: Lea & Febiger.
23. Aster, R. (2002). Drug-induced thrombocytopenia. In Michelson, A. D., (Ed.). *Platelets* (pp. 593–606). San Diego: Academic Press.
24. Vadhan-Raj, S. (2000). Clinical experience with recombinant human thrombopoietin in chemotherapy-induced thrombocytopenia. *Semin Hematol, 37,* 28–34.
25. Basser, R. L., Underhill, C., Davis, M. D., et al. (2000). Enhancement of platelet recovery after myelosuppressive chemotherapy by recombinant human megakaryocyte growth and development factor in patients with advanced cancer. *J Clin Oncol, 18,* 2852–2861.
26. Koch, M. A., Volberding, P. A., Lagakos, S. W., et al. (1992). Toxic effects of zidovudine in asymptomatic human immunodeficiency virus–infected individuals with CD4$^+$ cell counts of 0.5×10^9/L or less: detailed and updated results from Protocol 019 of the AIDS Clinical Trials Group. *Arch Intern Med, 152,* 2286–2292.
27. Silverstein, M. N., & Tefferi, A. (1999). Treatment of essential thrombocythemia with anagrelide. *Semin Hematol, 36,* 23–25.
28. Martin, T. G., & Shuman, M. A. (1998). Interferon-induced thrombocytopenia: is it time for thrombopoietin? *Hepatology, 28,* 1430–1432.
29. Colvin, B. T. (1985). Thrombocytopenia. *Clin Haematol, 14,* 661–681.
30. Sata, M., Yano, Y., Yoshiyama, et al. (1997). Mechanisms of thrombocytopenia induced by interferon therapy for chronic hepatitis B. *J Gastroenterol, 32,* 206–221.
31. Trannel, T. J., Ahmed, I., & Goebert, D. (2001). Occurrence of thrombocytopenia in psychiatric patients taking valproate. *Am J Psychiatry, 158,* 128–130.
32. Thompson, A. R., Harker, L. A. (1983). *Manual of hemostasis and thrombosis.* (3rd ed.). Philadelphia: FA Davis.
33. Taghizadeh, M. (1997). Megaloblastic anemias. In Harmening, D. M., (Ed.), *Clinical hematology and fundamentals of hemostasis.* (3rd ed., pp. 116–134). Philadelphia: FA Davis.

34. Corriveau, D. M., & Fritsma, G. A., (Eds.). (1988). *Hemostasis and thrombosis in the clinical laboratory.* Philadelphia: JB Lippincott.

35. Quick, A. J. (1966). *Hemorrhagic diseases and thrombosis.* (2nd ed.). Philadelphia: Lea & Febiger.

36. Davis, G. L. (1998). Quantitative and qualitative disorders of platelets. In Steine-Martin, E. A., Lotspeich-Steininger, C., & Koepke, J. A., (Eds.), *Clinical hematology: principle, procedures, correlations.* (2nd ed., pp. 717–734). Philadelphia: Lippincott Williams & Wilkins.

37. Bussel, J., & Cines, D. (2000). Immune thrombocytopenia, neonatal alloimmune thrombocytopenia, and post-transfusion purpura. In Hoffman, R., Benz, E. J., Shattil, S. J., et al., (Eds.), *Hematology: basic principles and practice.* (3rd ed., pp. 2096–2114). New York: Churchill Livingstone.

38. Kessler, C. M., Acs, P., & Mariani, G. (2006). Acquired disorders of coagulation: the immune coagulopathies. In Colman, R. W., Hirsh, J., & Marder, V. J., et al., (Eds.), *Hemostasis and thrombosis: basic principles and clinical practice.* (5th ed., pp. 1061–1085). Philadelphia: Lippincott Williams & Wilkins.

39. Woerner, S. J., Abildgaard, C. F., & French, B. N. (1981). Intracranial hemorrhage in children with idiopathic thrombocytopenic purpura. *Pediatrics, 67,* 453–460.

40. Dameshek, W., Ebbe, S., Greenberg, L., et al. (1963). Recurrent acute idiopathic thrombocytopenic purpura. *N Engl J Med, 269,* 646–653.

41. Stasi, R., & Provan, D. (2004). Management of immune thrombocytopenic purpura in adults. *Mayo Clin Proc, 79,* 504–522.

42. Kunicki, T. J., & Newman, P. J. (1992). The molecular immunology of human platelet proteins. *Blood, 80,* 1386–1404.

43. Beer, J. H., Rabaglio, M., Berchtold, P., et al. (1993). Autoantibodies against the platelet glycoproteins (GP) IIb/IIIa, Ia/IIa, and IV and partial deficiency in GPIV in a patient with a bleeding disorder and a defective platelet collagen interaction. *Blood, 82,* 820–829.

44. Olsson, B., Andersson, P., Jernas, M., et al. (2003). T-cell–mediated cytotoxicity toward platelets in chronic idiopathic thrombocytopenic purpura. *Nat Med, 9,* 1123–1124.

45. George, J. N., & Kojouri, K. (2006). Immune thrombocytopenic purpura. In Colman, R. W., Marder, V. J., Clowes, A. W., et al., (Eds.), *Hemostasis and thrombosis.* (5th ed., pp. 1085–1094). Philadelphia: Lippincott Williams & Wilkins.

46. Chong, B. H., & Ho, S-J. (2005). Autoimmune thrombocytopenia. *J Thromb Haemost, 3,* 1763–1772.

47. Jacobs, P., Wood, L., & Novitzky, N. (1994). Intravenous gammaglobulin has no advantages over oral corticosteroids as primary therapy for adults with immune thrombocytopenia: a prospective randomized clinical trial. *Am J Med, 1,* 55–59.

48. Kojouri, K., Vesely, S. K., Terrell, D. R., et al. (2004). Splenectomy for adult patients with idiopathic thrombocytopenic purpura. *Blood, 104,* 2623–2634.

49. Smith, M. E., Reid, D. M., Jones, C. E., et al. (1987). Binding of quinine- and quinidine-dependent drug antibodies to platelets is mediated by the Fab domain of the immunoglobulin G and is not Fc dependent. *J Clin Invest, 79,* 912–917.

50. Pfueller, S. L., Bilsont, R. A., Logan, D., et al. (1988). Heterogeneity of drug-dependent platelet antigens and their antibodies in quinine- and quinidine-induced thrombocytopenia: involvement of glycoproteins Ib, IIb, IIIa, and IX. *Blood, 11,* 190–198.

51. Chong, B. H., Fawaz, I., Chesterman, C. N., et al. (1989). Heparin-induced thrombocytopenia: mechanism of interaction of the heparin-dependent antibody with platelets. *Br J Haematol, 73,* 235–240.

52. Amiral, J., Bridley, F., Dreyfus, M., et al. (1992). Platelet factor 4 complexed to heparin is the target for antibodies generated in heparin-induced thrombocytopenia. *Thromb Haemost, 68,* 95 (letter).

53. Brace, L. D., Fareed, J., Tomeo, J., et al. (1986). Biochemical and pharmacological studies on the interaction of PK 10169 and its subfractions with human platelets. *Haemostasis, 16,* 93–105.

54. Warkentin, T. E. (2006). Heparin-induced thrombocytopenia. In Colman, R. W., Marder, V. J., Clowes, A. W., et al., (Eds.), *Hemostasis and thrombosis.* (5th ed., pp. 1649–1663). Philadelphia: Lippincott Williams & Wilkins.

55. Rhodes, G. R., Dixon, R. H., & Silver, D. (1977). Heparin-induced thrombocytopenia: eight cases with thrombotic-hemorrhagic complications. *Am Surg, 186,* 752–758.

56. Brace, L. D., & Fareed J. (1985). An objective assessment of the interaction of heparin and its subfractions with human platelets. *Semin Thromb Hemost, 11,* 190–198.

57. Fratantoni, J. C., Pollet, R., & Gralnick, H. R. (1975). Heparin-induced thrombocytopenia: confirmation by in vitro methods. *Blood, 45,* 395–401.

58. Sheridan, D., Carter, C., Kelton, J. G. (1986). A diagnostic test for heparin-induced thrombocytopenia. *Blood, 67,* 27–30.

59. Brace, L. D. (1992). Testing for heparin-induced thrombocytopenia by platelet aggregometry. *Clin Lab Sci, 5,* 80–81.

60. Collins, J. L., Aster, R. H., Moghaddam, M., et al. (1997). Diagnostic testing for heparin-induced thrombocytopenia (HIT): an enhanced platelet factor 4 complex enzyme linked immunosorbent assay (PF4 ELISA). *Blood, 90*(Suppl. 1), 461.

61. Gruel, Y., Boizard, B., Daffos, F., et al. (1986). Determination of platelet antigens and glycoproteins in the human fetus. *Blood, 68,* 488–492.

62. Mueller-Eckhardt, C., Kiefel, V., Grubert, A., et al. (1989). 348 cases of suspected neonatal alloimmune thrombocytopenia. *Lancet, 1,* 363–366.

63. McFarland, J. G., Aster, R. H., Bussel, J. B., et al. (1991). Prenatal diagnosis of neonatal alloimmune thrombocytopenia using allele-specific oligonucleotide probes. *Blood, 78,* 2276–2282.

64. Levin, A. B., & Berkowitz, R. L. (1991). Neonatal alloimmune thrombocytopenia. *Semin Perinatol, 15*(Suppl. 2), 35–40.

65. Kaplan, C., Daffos, F., Forestier, F., et al. (1988). Management of alloimmune thrombocytopenia: antenatal diagnosis and in utero transfusion of maternal platelets. *Blood, 72,* 340–343.

66. Rayburn, W. F. (1992). Glucocorticoid therapy for rheumatic diseases: maternal, fetal, and breast-feeding considerations. *Am J Reprod Immunol, 28,* 138–140.

67. Clerc, J. M. (1989). Neonatal thrombocytopenia. *Clin Lab Sci, 2,* 42–47.

68. Mueller-Eckhardt, C. (1986). Post-transfusion purpura. *Br J Haematol, 64,* 419–424.

69. Vogelsang, G., Kickler, T. S., & Bell, W. R. (1986). Post-transfusion purpura: a report of five patients and a review of the pathogenesis and management. *Am J Hematol, 21,* 259–267.

70. McLaughlin, P., Talpaz, M., Quesada, J. R., et al. (1985). Immune thrombocytopenia following α-interferon therapy in patients with cancer. *JAMA, 254,* 1353–1354.

71. Yoshida, Y., Hirashima, K., Asano, S., et al. (1991). A phase II trial of recombinant human granulocyte colony-stimulating factor in the myelodysplastic syndromes. *Br J Haematol, 78,* 378–384.

72. Paciucci, P. A., Mandeli, J., Oleksowicz, L., et al. (1990). Thrombocytopenia during immunotherapy with interleukin-2 by constant infusion. *Am J Med, 89,* 308–312.

73. Fink, K., & Al-Mondhiry, H. (1976). Idiopathic thrombocytopenic purpura in lymphoma. *Cancer, 37,* 1999–2004.

74. Carey, R. W., McGinnis, A., Jacobson, B. M., et al. Idiopathic thrombocytopenic purpura complicating chronic lymphocytic leukemia: management with sequential splenectomy and chemotherapy. *Arch Intern Med, 136,* 62–66.

75. Miller, M. H., Urowitz, M. B., & Gladman, D. D. (1983). The significance of thrombocytopenia in systemic lupus erythematosus. *Arthritis Rheum, 26,* 1181–1186.

76. Kelton, J. G., Keystone, J., Moore, J., et al. (1983). Immune-mediated thrombocytopenia of malaria. *J Clin Invest, 71,* 832–836.

77. Barron, W. M. (1992). The syndrome of preeclampsia. *Gastroenterol Clin North Am, 21,* 851–872.

78. Schindler, M., Gatt, S., Isert, P., et al. (1990). Thrombocytopenia and platelet function defects in pre-eclampsia: implications for regional anesthesia. *Anaesth Intensive Care, 18,* 169–174.

79. Gibson, W., Hunter, D., Neame, P. B., et al. (1982). Thrombocytopenia in preeclampsia and eclampsia. *Semin Thromb Hemost, 8,* 234–247.

80. Martin, J. N. Jr, Blake, P. G., Perry, K. G. Jr, et al. (1991). The natural history of HELLP syndrome: patterns of disease progression and regression. *Am J Obstet Gynecol, 164,* 1500–1509.

81. Green, D. (1988). Diagnosis and management of bleeding disorders. *Compr Ther, 14,* 31–36.

82. Trofatter, K. F. Jr, Howell, M. L., Greenberg, C. S., et al. (1989). Use of the fibrin D-dimer in screening for coagulation abnormalities in preeclampsia. *Obstet Gynecol, 73,* 435–440.

83. Burrows, R. F., Hunter, D. J. S., Andrew, M., et al. (1987). A prospective study investigating the mechanism of thrombocytopenia in preeclampsia. *Obstet Gynecol, 70,* 334–338.

84. Benigni, A., Gregorini, G., Frusca, T., et al. (1989). Effect of low-dose aspirin on fetal and maternal generation of thromboxane by platelets in women at risk for pregnancy-induced hypertension. *N Engl J Med, 321,* 357–362.

85. Schiff, E., Peleg, E., Goldenberg, M., et al. (1989). The use of aspirin to prevent pregnancy-induced hypertension and lower the ratio of thromboxane A_2 to prostacyclin in relatively high risk pregnancies. *N Engl J Med, 321,* 351–356.

86. Ezra, Y., Rose, M., & Eldor, A. (1996). Therapy and prevention of thrombotic thrombocytopenic purpura during pregnancy: a clinical study of 16 pregnancies. *Am J Hematol, 51,* 1–6.

87. Dashe, J. S., Ramin, S. M., & Cunningham, F. G. (1998). The long-term consequences of thrombotic microangiopathy (thrombotic thrombocytopenic purpura and hemolytic uremic syndrome) in pregnancy. *Obstet Gynecol, 91,* 662–668.

88. Moschcowitz, E. (1925). An acute febrile pleiochromic anemia with hyaline thrombosis of the terminal arterioles and capillaries: a hitherto undescribed disease. *Arch Intern Med, 36,* 89–93.

89. Moake, J. L. (2002). Thrombotic thrombocytopenic purpura and hemolytic uremic syndrome. In Michelson, A. D., (Ed.), *Platelets* (pp. 607–620). San Diego: Academic Press.

90. Bell, W. R., Braine, H. G., Ness, P. M., et al. (1991). Improved survival in thrombotic thrombocytopenic purpura–hemolytic uremic syndrome: clinical experience in 108 patients. *N Engl J Med, 325,* 398–403.

91. Rock, G. A., Shumak, K. H., Buskard, N. A., et al. (1991). Comparison of plasma exchange with plasma infusion in the treatment of thrombotic thrombocytopenic purpura. *N Engl J Med, 325,* 393–397.

92. Moake, J. L., Turner, N. A., Stathopoulos, N. A., et al. Involvement of large plasma von Willebrand factor (VWF) multimers and unusually large VWF forms derived from endothelial cells in shear-stress induced platelet aggregation. *J Clin Invest, 78,* 1456–1461, 1986.

93. Furlan, M., Robles, R., Solenthaler, M., et al. (1997). Deficient activity of von Willebrand factor-cleaving protease in chronic relapsing thrombotic thrombocytopenic purpura. *Blood, 89,* 3097–3103.

94. Furlan, M., Robles, R., & Lammle, B. (1996). Partial purification and characterization of a protease from human plasma cleaving von Willebrand factor to fragments produced by in vivo proteolysis. *Blood, 87,* 4223–4234.

95. Tsai, H. M. (1996). Physiologic cleaving of von Willebrand factor by a plasma protease is dependent on its conformation and requires calcium ion. *Blood, 87,* 4235–4244.

96. Tsai, H. M., & Lian, E. C. Y. (1998). Antibodies to von Willebrand factor–cleaving protease in acute thrombotic thrombocytopenic purpura. *N Engl J Med, 339,* 1585–1594.

97. Furlan, M., & Lammle, B. (1999). von Willebrand factor in thrombotic thrombocytopenic purpura. *Thromb Haemost, 82,* 592–600.

98. Gerritsen, H. E., Turecek, P. L., Schwarz, H. P., et al. (1999). Assay of von Willebrand factor (VWF)–cleaving protease based on decreased collagen binding affinity of degraded VWF: a tool for the diagnosis of thrombotic thrombocytopenic purpura (TTP). *Thromb Haemost, 82,* 1386–1389.

99. Moake, J. L., & McPherson, P. D. (1989). Abnormalities of von Willebrand factor multimers in thrombotic thrombocytopenic purpura and the hemolytic uremic syndrome. *Am J Med, 87,* 3–9.

100. Byrnes, J. J., Moake, J. L., Klug, P., et al. (1990). Effectiveness of the cryosupernatant fraction of plasma in the treatment of refractory thrombotic thrombocytopenic purpura. *Am J Hematol, 34,* 169–174.

101. Kwaan, H. C., & Soff, G. A. (1997). Management of thrombotic thrombocytopenic purpura and hemolytic uremic syndrome. *Semin Hematol, 34,* 159–166.

102. Karmali, M. A. (1992). The association of verotoxins and the classical hemolytic uremic syndrome. In Kaplan, B. S., Trompeter, R. S., & Moake, J. L., (Eds.), *Hemolytic-uremic syndrome and thrombotic thrombocytopenic purpura* (pp. 199–212). New York: Marcel Dekker.

103. Obrig, T. G. (1992). Pathogenesis of Shiga toxin (verotoxin)–induced endothelial cell injury. In Kaplan, B. S., Trompeter, R. S., & Moake, J. L., (Eds.), *Hemolytic-uremic syndrome and thrombotic thrombocytopenic purpura* (pp. 405–419). New York: Marcel Dekker.

104. Charba, D., Moake, J. L., Harris, M. A., et al. (1993). Abnormalities of von Willebrand factor multimers in drug-associated thrombotic microangiopathies. *Am J Hematol, 42,* 268–277.

105. Santhosh-Kumar, C. R., Yohannon, M. D., Higgy, K. E., et al. (1991). Thrombocytosis in adults: analysis of 777 patients. *J Intern Med, 229,* 493–495.

106. Mitus, A. J., & Schafer, A. I. (1990). Thrombocytosis and thrombocythemia. *Hematol Oncol Clin North Am, 4,* 157–178.

107. Michiels, J. J., & Ten Cate, F. J. (1992). Erythromelalgia in thrombocythemia of various myeloproliferative disorders. *Am J Hematol, 39,* 131–136.

108. Hoffman, R. (2000). Primary thrombocythemia. In Hoffman, R., Benz, E. J., Shattil, S. J., et al., (Eds.), *Hematology: basic principles and practice.* (3rd ed., pp 1188–1204). New York: Churchill Livingstone.

109. Schafer, A. I. (1984). Bleeding and thrombosis in the myeloproliferative disorders. *Blood, 64,* 1–12.

110. Panlilio, A. L., & Reiss, R. F. (1979). Therapeutic plateletpheresis in thrombocythemia. *Transfusion, 19,* 147–152.

111. Middelhoff, G., & Boll, I. (1992). A long term trial of interferon alpha-therapy in essential thrombocythemia. *Ann Hematol, 64,* 207–209.

112. Lazzarino, M., Vitale, A., Morra, E., et al. (1989). Interferon alpha-2b as treatment for Philadelphia-negative myeloproliferative disorders with excessive thrombocytosis. *Br J Haematol, 72,* 173–177.

113. Giles, F. J., Singer, C. R. J., Gray, A. G., et al. (1988). Alpha interferon for essential thrombocythemia. *Lancet, 2,* 70–72.

114. Petitt, R. M., Silverstein, M. N., Petrone, M. E. (1997). Anagrelide for control of thrombocythemia in polycythemia and other myeloproliferative disorders. *Semin Hematol, 34,* 51–54.

115. Tefferi, A., Silverstein, M. N., Petitt, R. M., et al. (1997). Anagrelide as a new platelet-lowering agent in essential thrombocythemia: mechanism of action, efficacy, toxicity, current indications. *Semin Thromb Hemost, 23,* 379–383.

Qualitative Disorders of Platelets and Vasculature

41

Larry D. Brace

OBJECTIVES

After completion of this chapter, the reader will be able to:

1. Describe the effect of aspirin on the cyclooxygenase pathway.
2. Describe the defect in each of the following hereditary disorders: storage pool disease, gray platelet syndrome, Glanzmann thrombasthenia, and Bernard-Soulier syndrome (BSS).
3. Discuss the mechanisms of action of antiplatelet drugs.
4. Explain the effects of paraproteins on platelet function.
5. Compare and contrast Glanzmann thrombasthenia and BSS.
6. Recognize the clinical presentation of patients with dysfunctional platelets.
7. Distinguish among the following types of inherited platelet disorders: membrane receptor abnormality, secretion disorder, and storage pool deficiency.
8. For each of the inherited platelet disorders listed, name useful laboratory tests and recognize diagnostic results.
9. Identify the most common type of hereditary platelet defect.
10. Discuss the mechanism of the platelet defects associated with myeloproliferative diseases, uremia, and liver disease.
11. Recognize conditions associated with acquired vascular disorders.

CASE STUDY

After studying the material in this chapter, the reader should be able to respond to the following case study:

A 19-year-old woman with a chief complaint of easy bruising, occasional mild nosebleeds, and heavy menstrual periods was examined by her physician. At the time of her examination, she had a few small bruises on her arms and legs, but no other problems. Initial laboratory data revealed a normal prothrombin time, and a normal partial thromboplastin time. A CBC, including platelet count and morphology, yielded normal results.

A detailed history revealed that the patient's bleeding problems occurred most frequently after aspirin ingestion. Her mother and one of her brothers also had some of the same symptoms. Blood was drawn for platelet function studies, and platelet aggregation tests were performed. Aggregation induced by ristocetin and adenosine diphosphate was near normal, arachidonic acid–induced aggregation was absent, epinephrine induced only primary aggregation,

and collagen-induced aggregation was decreased, although a near-normal aggregation response could be obtained with a high collagen concentration. Spontaneous aggregation was not observed.

1. What are three possible explanations for the test results so far?
2. Given the bleeding history in her family, which of the three explanations seems most likely?

A quantitative test for adenosine triphosphate (ATP) release was performed using the firefly luciferin-luciferase bioluminescence assay. The result of this test showed a marked decrease in the amount of ATP released when platelets were stimulated with thrombin.

3. Based on the ATP test results, what is the likely cause of the patient's bleeding symptoms?

Clinical manifestations of bleeding disorders can be divided into two broad, rather poorly defined groups: (1) superficial bleeding (e.g., petechiae, epistaxis, or gingival bleeding), usually associated with a platelet defect or vascular disorder; and (2) deep tissue bleeding (e.g., hematomas or hemarthrosis), usually associated with plasma clotting factor deficiencies.[1] This chapter describes platelet and vascular disorders. Bleeding problems resulting from defects in the coagulation mechanism are described in Chapter 38.

QUALITATIVE PLATELET DISORDERS

Excessive bruising, superficial (mucocutaneous) bleeding, and a prolonged bleeding time in a patient whose platelet count is normal suggest an acquired or a congenital disorder of platelet function. Congenital disorders have been described that result from abnormalities of each of the major phases of platelet function: adhesion, aggregation, and secretion. Rapid progress in this field began in the 1960s, mostly as a result of the development of instruments and test methods for measuring platelet function.[2]

Qualitative platelet disorders are summarized in Box 41-1.[3,4] This chapter discusses the individual qualitative platelet disorders grouped by the mechanism that causes the defect. A summary of the primary disorders is illustrated in Figure 41-1 for defects associated with surface components and Figure 41-2 for defects associated with intracellular components.[5]

Disorders of Platelet Aggregation Affecting GP IIb/IIIa Function

Glanzmann Thrombasthenia

Glanzmann thrombasthenia originally was described as a bleeding disorder associated with abnormal in vitro clot retraction and a normal platelet count. Clot retraction is the process of the compaction of a formed clot (reducing its volume), mediated by contraction of the intracellular actin-myosin cytoskeleton of the activated platelets incorporated in the clot. It is inherited as an autosomal recessive disorder and is seen most frequently in populations with a high degree of consanguinity. Heterozygotes are clinically normal, whereas homozygotes have serious bleeding problems. This rare disorder manifests itself clinically in the neonatal period or infancy, occasionally with bleeding after circumcision and frequently with epistaxis and gingival bleeding. Hemorrhagic manifestations include petechiae, purpura (Figure 40-1), menorrhagia, gastrointestinal bleeding, and hematuria. There are wide variations in the clinical symptoms. Some patients may have minimal symptoms, whereas others may have frequent and serious hemorrhagic complications. The severity of the bleeding episodes seems to decrease with age.[6,7]

The biochemical lesion responsible for the disorder is a deficiency or abnormality of the platelet membrane glycoprotein (GP) IIb/IIIa (integrin α_{IIb}/β_3) complex, a membrane receptor capable of binding fibrinogen, von Willebrand factor (VWF), fibronectin, and other adhesive ligands. Typically, the platelets of homozygous individuals lack surface-expressed GP IIb/IIIa, whereas the GP IIb/IIIa content of the platelets from

---

> **BOX 41-1**　Qualitative Abnormalities: Changes in Platelet Function (Thrombocytopathy)[3,4]
>
> **Disorders of Platelet Aggregation**
> Glanzmann thrombasthenia
> Hereditary afibrinogenemia
> Acquired defects of platelet aggregation:
> 　Acquired von Willebrand disease
> 　Acquired uremia
>
> **Disorders of Platelet Adhesion**
> Bernard-Soulier syndrome
> Von Willebrand disease
> Acquired defects of platelet adhesion:
> 　Myeloproliferative, lymphoproliferative disorders, dysproteinemias
> 　Antiplatelet antibodies
> 　Cardiopulmonary bypass surgery
> 　Chronic liver disease
> 　Drug-induced membrane modification
>
> **Disorders of Platelet Secretion (release reactions)**
> Storage pool diseases
> Thromboxane pathway disorders
> Hereditary aspirin-like defects:
> 　Cyclooxygenase or thromboxane synthetase deficiency
> Drug inhibition of the prostaglandin pathways
> Drug inhibition of platelet phosphodiesterase activity
>
> **Changes in Membrane Phospholipid Distribution**
> Scott syndrome
> Stormorken syndrome
>
> **Hyperactive Prothrombotic Platelets**

---

heterozygotes has been found to be 50% to 60% of normal.[8,9] Binding of fibrinogen to the GP IIb/IIIa complex mediates normal platelet aggregation responses. Failure of such binding results in a profound defect in hemostatic plug formation and the serious bleeding characteristic of thrombasthenia.[2,8,10-13]

More than 70 mutations are known to give rise to Glanzmann thrombasthenia.[14-16] GP IIb/IIIa is coded by the *ITGA2B* and *ITGB3* genes present on chromosome 17, and genetic defects are distributed widely over the two genes.[17] Rarely, thrombocytopenia and large platelets may be seen with some mutations in these genes (Table 40-1). α_{IIb} is synthesized in megakaryocytes as pro-α_{IIb}, which complexes β_3 in the endoplasmic reticulum. The complex is transported to the Golgi body, where α_{IIb} is cleaved to heavy and light chains to form the complete complex. Uncomplexed α_{IIb} and β_3 are not processed in the Golgi body. As with the GP Ib/IX/V complex, it is necessary for both proteins of the GP IIb/IIIa complex to be produced and assembled into a complex for the complex to be expressed on the platelet surface. Gene defects that lead to the absence of

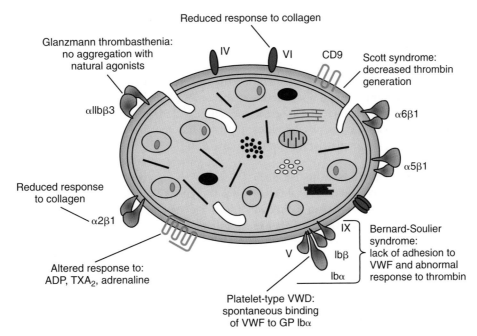

Figure 41-1 An illustration of the primary disorders associated with defects of the surface components of platelets. (From Nurden P and Nurder AT. Congenital disorders associated with platelet dysfunction. *Thromb Haemost* 2008;99:253-263.)

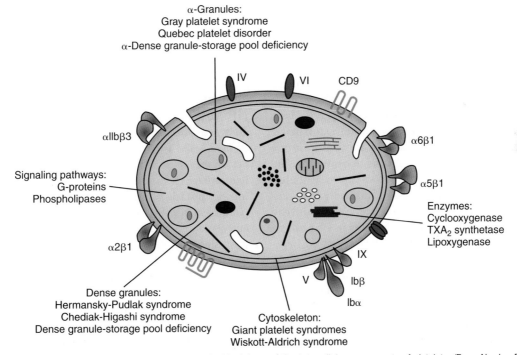

Figure 41-2 An illustration of the primary disorders associated with defects of the intracellular components of platelets. (From Nurden P and Nurder AT. Congenital disorders associated with platelet dysfunction. *Thromb Haemost* 2008;99:253-263.)

production of either protein lead to absence of the complex on the platelet surface. Defects that interfere with or prevent complex formation or affect complex stability have the same effect.

Numerous variants of Glanzmann thrombasthenia have been described in which the GP IIb/IIIa complex is qualitatively abnormal. α_{IIb} and β_3 are produced, form a complex, and are processed normally. One or more functions of the complex (e.g., fibrinogen binding or signal transduction) are abnormal, however. Bleeding in these patients ranges from mild to severe.

One component of the α_{IIb}/β_3 integrin, β_3, is a component of the vitronectin receptor, α_V/β_3, found on endothelial cells, osteoclasts, fibroblasts, monocytes, and activated B lymphocytes, where it acts as a receptor for a variety of adhesive protein ligands. Patients who have β_3 gene defects that result in the absence of α_{IIb}/β_3 integrin also lack the vitronectin receptor. These patients do not seem to have a more severe form of Glanzmann thrombasthenia.[18,19] The vitronectin receptor is thought to play a role in vascularization, but so far, no evidence for abnormal blood vessel development has been documented in individuals lacking the vitronectin receptor. It also is unclear whether platelet vitronectin receptors play any significant role in platelet functional processes.[14]

Rarely, a thrombasthenia-like state can be acquired. Such conditions include development of autoantibodies against GP IIb/IIIa, multiple myeloma in which the paraprotein is directed against GP IIIa, and afibrinogenemia. A thrombasthenia-like state also can be induced in individuals with otherwise normal platelet function by the therapeutic antiplatelet drugs ticlopidine and clopidogrel.[7,12]

Laboratory Features.   The typical laboratory features of Glanzmann thrombasthenia are a normal platelet count, normal platelet morphology, and a lack of platelet aggregation in response to all platelet activating agents (including ADP, collagen, thrombin, and epinephrine).[2,8,10,12] If the stimulating agent is strong enough (e.g., thrombin), the platelets undergo the release/secretion reaction, even in the absence of aggregation. Ristocetin-induced binding of VWF to platelets and the resulting platelet agglutination are normal. The results of the complete blood count (CBC) are usually normal, unless there is another underlying disorder or the patient has had a recent hemorrhagic episode. Tests for platelet procoagulant activity, previously called the platelet factor 3 test, usually show diminished activity.[2,9,20] There seem to be several reasons for this. When normal platelets are activated, procoagulant microvesicles are shed from the platelet surface, and coagulation factors assemble on the microvesicle surfaces during activation of the coagulation cascade. In Glanzmann thrombasthenia, markedly fewer microvesicles are produced. Second, prothrombin binds directly to GP IIb/IIIa. Because this complex is missing in Glanzmann thrombasthenia, significantly less thrombin is generated in response to tissue factor. Finally, Glanzmann thrombasthenia platelets are not as activated by thrombin as are normal platelets.[21-24]

A subdivision of Glanzmann thrombasthenia into type 1 and type 2 has been proposed. In general, individuals with type 2 disease have more residual GP IIb/IIIa complexes (10% to 20% of normal) than those with type 1 disease (0% to 5% of normal), although there is considerable variability within each subdivision.[25,26]

Treatment.   Thrombasthenia is one of the few forms of platelet dysfunction in which hemorrhage is severe and disabling. Bleeding of all types, including epistaxis, ecchymosis, hemarthrosis, subcutaneous hematoma, menorrhagia, and gastrointestinal and urinary tract hemorrhage, has been reported. Treatment of bleeding episodes in patients with Glanzmann thrombasthenia requires the transfusion of normal platelets. In Glanzmann thrombasthenia, the defective

platelets may interfere with the normal transfused platelets, and it may be necessary to infuse more donor platelets than expected to control bleeding. As in Bernard-Soulier syndrome or any situation in which repeated transfusions are required, patients with Glanzmann thrombasthenia may become alloimmunized. Strategies to reduce alloimmunization include use of single-donor platelet apheresis products, HLA-matched donor platelets, or ABO-matched donor platelets.[27]

A variety of treatments have been used successfully to control or prevent bleeding, alone or in combination with platelet transfusion. To a large extent, the site of hemorrhage determines the therapeutic approach used. Hormonal therapy (norethindrone acetate) has been used to control menorrhagia. If the patient is treated with oral contraceptives, excessive bleeding should be reduced. Menorrhagia at the onset of menses is uniformly severe and can be life-threatening, which has led some to suggest that birth control pills be started before menarche. Also, antifibrinolytic therapy (aminocaproic acid or tranexamic acid) can be used to control gingival hemorrhage or excessive bleeding after tooth extraction.[26] Recombinant factor VIIa has proved useful to treat severe bleeding in patients with isoantibodies to α_{IIb}/β_3 and in patients undergoing invasive procedures.[28] Recombinant factor VIIa (rVIIa, NovoSeven, Novo Nordisk Inc, Princeton, NJ) is thought to enhance thrombus formation at the site of a lesion by stimulating tissue factor-independent thrombus generation and fibrin formation.[29]

Disorders of Platelet Adhesion Affecting GP Ib/IX/V Complexes
Bernard-Soulier (Giant Platelet) Syndrome
Bernard-Soulier syndrome (BSS) is a rare disorder of platelet adhesion that is usually manifested in infancy or childhood with hemorrhage characteristic of defective platelet function: ecchymoses, epistaxis, and gingival bleeding. Hemarthroses and expanding hematomas are only rarely seen. BSS is inherited as an autosomal recessive disorder in which the GP Ib/IX/V complex is missing from the platelet surface or exhibits abnormal function. Heterozygotes who have about 50% of normal levels of GP Ib, GP V, and GP IX have normal or near-normal platelet function. Homozygotes have a moderate to severe bleeding disorder characterized by enlarged platelets, thrombocytopenia, and usually decreased platelet survival. Platelet counts generally range from 40,000/μL to near normal.[30] On peripheral blood films, platelets typically are 5 to 8 μm in diameter, but they can be 20 μm (Figure 41-3). Viewed by electron microscopy, BSS platelets contain a larger number of cytoplasmic vacuoles and membrane complexes, and these observations extend to megakaryocytes, in which the appearance of the demarcation membrane system is irregular.[2,3,8,10,31]

Four glycoproteins are required to form the GP Ib/IX/V complex: GP Ibα, GP Ibβ, GP IX, and GP V. In the complex, these proteins are present in the ratio of 2:2:2:1. The gene for GP Ibα is located on chromosome 17, the gene for GP Ibβ is located on chromosome 22, and the genes for GP IX and GP V

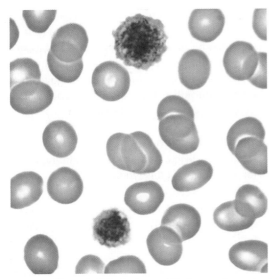

Figure 41-3 Giant platelets in Bernard-Soulier syndrome (peripheral blood, ×1000). (Modified from Carr JH, Rodak BF: *Clinical hematology atlas,* ed 3, Philadelphia, 2009, Saunders.)

are located on chromosome 3. For surface expression of the GP Ib/IX complex, it seems that synthesis of three proteins, GP Ibα, GP Ibβ, and GP IX, is required. Only GP V can be expressed alone in significant quantities on the surface of platelets, but the expression seems to be enhanced if the rest of the complex is present. The most frequent forms of BSS involve defects in GP Ibα synthesis or expression (Table 40-1). The presence of GP Ibα is essential to normal function because it contains binding sites for VWF and thrombin. Defects in the GP Ibβ and GP IX genes also are known to result in BSS.[32-34] Diseases causing mutations include missense, frameshift, and nonsense mutations.[35,36]

Variants. Several unusual variants of BSS have been described in which all or most of the GP Ib/IX/V complex is present, but mutations that affect binding domains affect interactions between elements of the complex, or result in truncation of a specific protein in the complex. In these cases, the complex fails to bind VWF or does so poorly.[33] In rare circumstances, an antibody to GP Ib/V can cause a Bernard-Soulier–like syndrome (*pseudo-BSS*), in which the GP Ib/IX/V complex is nonfunctional.

Mutations in the GP Ib/IX/V complex can also give rise to gain of function and result in *platelet-type VWD (pseudo-VWD)*. This gain of function results in spontaneous binding of plasma VWF to the mutated GP Ib/IX/V complex. As a consequence, platelets and large VWF multimers with their associated factor VIII are removed from the circulation, resulting in thrombocytopenia and reduced factor VIII clotting activity. GP Ibα mutations that give rise to platelet-type VWD are 233 Gly → Val or Ser and 239 Met → Val.[37,38] Loss of residues 421 to 429 in GP Ibα also has been reported to result in platelet-type VWD.[39]

Laboratory Features. BSS platelets have normal aggregation responses to adenosine diphosphate (ADP), epinephrine, collagen, and arachidonic acid but do not respond to

ristocetin and have diminished response to thrombin.[2,8,10] The lack of response to ristocetin is due to the lack of GP Ib/IX/V complexes and the inability of BSS platelets to bind VWF. Lack of binding to VWF also accounts for the inability of platelets to adhere to exposed subendothelium and the resultant bleeding characteristic of this disorder. This defect in adhesion shows the importance of initial platelet attachment in primary hemostasis. In many respects, this disorder resembles the defect seen in von Willebrand disease (VWD). In contrast to VWD, however, this abnormality cannot be corrected by the addition of normal plasma or cryoprecipitate, which is consistent with a defect that resides in the platelets.

Treatment. There is no specific treatment for BSS. Platelet transfusions are the therapy of choice, but patients invariably develop alloantibodies, so further platelet transfusion is not possible. BSS patients tend to do better if apheresis platelets are used for transfusion because this tends to limit the number of donors to which the patient is exposed, and the rate of alloimmunization tends to be lower.[8,10] Other treatments that have been used include desmopressin acetate (DDAVP) and, more recently, recombinant factor VIIa (rVIIa, NovoSeven, Novo Nordisk Inc, Princeton, NJ).

Inherited Giant Platelet Syndromes

In addition to BSS, there are several other inherited *giant platelet syndromes*. See Table 40-1 and Mhawech and Saleem[40] for a more complete discussion of these syndromes. Box 41-2 provides a listing of the inherited giant platelet syndromes.

Giant Platelets with Velocardiofacial Syndrome

This disorder is considered an autosomal recessive heterozygous variant of BSS. It is characterized by mild thrombocytopenia (with platelet counts ranging from 100 to 220 × 10⁹/L), giant platelets, and association with velocardiofacial syndrome (VCFS). The clinical picture of VCFS includes velopharyngeal insufficiency, conotruncal heart disease, and learning disabilities. VCFS is considered to be a milder form of DiGeorge syndrome (thymic hypoplasia, conotruncal cardiac defects, and cardiac abnormalities). No bleeding symptoms

---

BOX 41-2 Inherited Giant Platelet Disorders

Bernard-Soulier syndrome
Giant platelets with velocardiofacial syndrome
Giant platelets with abnormal surface glycoproteins and mitral valve insufficiency
Familial macrothrombocytopenia with GP IV abnormality
Montreal platelet syndrome
Gray platelet syndrome
May-Hegglin anomaly
Fechtner syndrome
Sebastian syndrome
Hereditary macrothrombocytopenia
Epstein syndrome
Mediterranean macrothrombocytopenia

have been reported. Other than increased platelet size, no ultrastructural abnormalities have been observed. GP Ibβ is mapped on chromosome 22q11.2,14, which is located in the same region that is deleted in most patients with VCFS. Therefore, patients with a 22q11 deletion are obligate heterozygous carriers for the GP Ibβ deletion and are heterozygotes for BSS.

Giant Platelets with Abnormal Surface Glycoproteins and Mitral Valve Insufficiency

This extremely rare autosomal recessive disorder is characterized by thrombocytopenia with platelet counts ranging from 50 to 60 × 10⁹/L, giant platelets, and mild bleeding symptoms in association with mitral valve insufficiency. Platelets generally are larger than 20 μm. Other than increased platelet size, ultrastructural characteristics are normal. These patients usually have a mild bleeding disorder expressed primarily as ecchymosis and epistaxis occurring early in childhood. This disorder is distinguished from other inherited giant platelet syndromes by mitral valve insufficiency. Platelet surface glycoproteins GP Ia, GP Ic, and GP IIa are absent, while GP Ib, GP IIb, and GP IIIa are normal. The surface glycoproteins absent in this disorder do not seem to have a clear role. However, the abnormal bleeding tendency clearly reflects a platelet dysfunction that could result from a defect in glycoprotein composition, the absence or defective function of an anchor protein necessary to attach the glycoproteins to the cytoskeleton, or both. The cause of large platelets is unclear.

Familial Macrothrombocytopenia with GP IV Abnormality

Familial macrothrombocytopenia with GP IV abnormality is an extremely rare, autosomal dominant disorder characterized by thrombocytopenia, giant platelets, and variable degrees of bleeding tendencies. The thrombocytopenia varies, and the platelet count ranges from 45 × 10⁹/L to normal. GP IV is present in normal concentration, but there seems to be a defect in its glycosylation. GP IV seems to be involved in the early stages of adhesion, and abnormal function may be related to the mild bleeding tendency. Peripheral blood smears show large platelets and neutrophils without inclusions. At this point, the cause of large platelets remains to be clarified.

Montreal Platelet Syndrome

Montreal platelet syndrome (MPS) is characterized by severe thrombocytopenia, giant platelets, spontaneous platelet aggregation, and bleeding symptoms, including significant bruising and episodes of hemorrhage. Of the inherited giant platelet syndromes, MPS patients have the most severe thrombocytopenia with platelet counts ranging from 5 to 40 × 10⁹/L. Ultrastructurally, the platelets are large with no other abnormalities. Glycoprotein analysis is normal. It has been suggested that calpain, which is known to be involved in the cleavage of cytoskeleton proteins—in particular, actin-binding protein and talin—may have a role in spontaneous platelet aggregation. Low calpain proteolytic activity in MPS platelets has been demonstrated and may result in defective regulation of binding sites of platelets for adhesive proteins. As a result, platelet binding sites may be abnormally exposed, leading to an abnormal binding of adhesive proteins to the exposed platelet surfaces and spontaneous aggregation. The pathogenesis of giant platelets, severe thrombocytopenia, spontaneous aggregation, and the role of calpain remain to be clarified.

Gray Platelet Syndrome

See α-Granule Deficiency: Gray Platelet Syndrome later in this chapter for a discussion of this syndrome.

May-Hegglin Anomaly

May-Hegglin anomaly (MHA) is characterized by the presence of giant platelets, thrombocytopenia with platelet counts 60 to 100 × 10⁹/L, Döhle body-like neutrophil inclusions, and mild bleeding symptoms (Figure 29-5). MHA is the most common of the inherited giant platelet disorders and is inherited as an autosomal dominant trait. There appear to be two populations of platelets in MHA. Normal-sized platelets have normal ultrastructure and function. The large platelets show clear evidence of abnormal distribution of the platelet microtubule system, and this may be responsible for the large size and defective platelet function that could lead to bleeding symptoms. The cause of the thrombocytopenia is unknown. Chapter 40 provides a detailed discussion of this disorder.

Fechtner Syndrome

Fechtner syndrome is characterized by thrombocytopenia with platelet counts ranging from 30 to 90 × 10⁹/L, giant platelets, and the development of deafness, cataracts, and nephritis. Its mode of inheritance appears to be autosomal dominant. Glaucoma and cataracts occur at an early age. Nephritis progresses to end-stage renal failure by the age of 20 to 40 years, necessitating hemodialysis and renal transplant. By the third decade of life, there is usually high-frequency hearing loss. Neutrophils and occasionally eosinophils contain one or more 1- to 2-μm irregularly shaped cytoplasmic inclusions that appear pale blue with Wright-Giemsa stain. They are smaller and less intensely stained than the inclusions found in May-Hegglin anomaly. The thrombocytopenia in this disorder may be due to ineffective megakaryocytopoiesis and thrombopoiesis as reflected by large numbers of megakaryocytes, abnormal morphology, and low platelet count.

Sebastian Syndrome

Sebastian syndrome is an extremely rare autosomal dominant thrombocytopenia characterized by giant platelets, neutrophil inclusions, a mild bleeding disorder, and no other clinical manifestations. The thrombocytopenia is mild with platelet counts ranging from 40 to 120 × 10⁹/L. Mild bleeding such as epistaxis may occur in early childhood, but severe postoperative hemorrhage has been observed. Peripheral blood smears show large platelets and faintly blue cytoplasmic inclusions in the neutrophils, similar in appearance to Döhle bodies. At the ultrastructural level, the platelets are enlarged but have normal structural elements. The pathogenesis of the thrombocytopenia and the neutrophil inclusions remains to be clarified.

Hereditary Macrothrombocytopenia

Hereditary macrothrombocytopenia is a rare disorder characterized by mild thrombocytopenia with platelet counts ranging from 50 to 123 $\times$ 10^9/L, giant platelets, bleeding tendency, and high-frequency hearing loss. It appears to be inherited in an autosomal dominant fashion. These patients have a mild bleeding tendency, the most frequent symptoms being gingival bleeding after brushing teeth, epistaxis, easy bruising, and menorrhagia. Bleeding symptoms appear early in childhood, but hearing loss appears later. Ultrastructurally, the platelets are large but have no additional abnormalities. Interestingly, flow cytometry studies have shown a distinct population of platelets in these patients that have glycophorin A on their surface. Glycophorin A is generally considered an erythroid-specific protein and is not expressed on normal platelets. However, the pathogenesis of thrombocytopenia and giant platelets remains unclear, as does the presence of glycophorin A on the surface of the giant platelets in this disorder.

Epstein Syndrome

Epstein syndrome is a very rare, autosomal dominant disorder characterized by thrombocytopenia, large platelets, and mild bleeding diathesis, in association with nephritis and high-frequency hearing loss. These patients also have persistent proteinuria, microscopic hematuria, and moderate hypertension. The mild bleeding tendency includes epistaxis, gastrointestinal bleeding, and female genital tract bleeding. Bleeding symptoms occur early in life but may disappear later. The thrombocytopenia is often severe, with platelet counts ranging from 30 to 60 $\times$ 10^9/L. The peripheral blood smear shows increased platelet size in approximately 50% of the platelets. Ultrastructurally, the giant platelets are spherical and have a prominent surface-connected open canalicular system leading to a sponge-like cytoplasm. The pathogenesis of the thrombocytopenia and large platelets has not been determined.

Mediterranean Macrothrombocytopenia

Mediterranean macrothrombocytopenia is characterized by thrombocytopenia and large platelets. There is no bleeding or others symptom. This disorder has a high prevalence among persons originating from Greece, Italy, and the Balkan Peninsula. The incidence is unknown. The thrombocytopenia is mild, with platelet counts ranging from 89 to 290 $\times$ 10^9/L. The peripheral blood smear shows large platelets, and electron microscopy reveals no other abnormalities. Of unknown significance, stomatocytes are also present on peripheral blood smears. The pathogenesis of this disorder remains to be elucidated.

Disorders of Platelet Secretion (Release Reactions)

Of the hereditary platelet function defects, disorders involving storage pool defects and the release reaction are the most common. The clinical features of this group of disorders are mucocutaneous hemorrhage and hematuria, epistaxis, and easy and spontaneous bruising. Petechiae are less common than in other qualitative platelet disorders. Hemorrhage is rarely severe but may be exacerbated by ingestion of aspirin or other antiplatelet agents. In most of these disorders, the platelet count is normal, and the bleeding time is usually, although not always, prolonged. Platelet aggregation abnormalities are usually seen but vary, depending on the disorder.[2,8,41,42]

Storage Pool Diseases

Platelet disorders of the storage pool type can be related to defects of the dense granules or defects of the α-granules. Box 41-3 lists these disorders.

Dense Granule Deficiencies. The inheritance of *dense granule deficiency* does not follow a single mode, and it is likely that a variety of genetic abnormalities lead to the development of this disorder. Dense granule deficiencies can be subdivided into deficiency states associated with albinism and those in otherwise normal individuals (nonalbinos).

In the platelets of nonalbinos, there is evidence for the presence of dense granule membranes in normal to near-normal numbers, which suggests that the disorder arises from an inability to package the dense granule contents.[43,44] Serotonin accumulates in normal dense granules by an active uptake mechanism in which plasma serotonin is transported by a specific carrier-mediated system across the plasma membrane into the cytoplasm, and a second carrier-mediated system in the dense granule membrane transports serotonin from the cytoplasm to the interior of the dense granules.[45] These transport mechanisms are used in the serotonin release assay employed to detect heparin-dependent antiplatelet antibodies (Chapter 40). In addition to serotonin transport mechanisms, a nucleotide transporter MRP4 (*ABCC4*) that is highly expressed in platelets and dense granules has been identified. It would be expected that mutations in the gene for this transporter could affect nucleotide accumulation in dense granules.[46]

As an isolated abnormality, dense granule deficiency does not typically result in a serious hemorrhagic problem. Bleeding is usually mild and most often is limited to easy bruisability.

Dense granule deficiency affects the results of platelet aggregation tests. Dense granules are intracellular storage sites for ADP, adenosine triphosphate, calcium, pyrophosphate, and serotonin. The contents of these granules are extruded when platelet secretion is induced, and secreted ADP plays a major

---

BOX 41-3 Platelet Storage Pool Diseases

Dense granule deficiencies
Hermansky-Pudlak syndrome
Chédiak-Higashi syndrome
Wiskott-Aldrich syndrome
Thrombocytopenia–absent radius (TAR) syndrome

α-Granule deficiencies
Gray platelet syndrome

role in the propagation of platelet activation, recruitment, and aggregation and growth of the hemostatic plug.

In patients with dense granule deficiency, addition of arachidonic acid to platelet-rich plasma fails to induce an aggregation response (Chapter 42). Epinephrine and low-dose ADP induce a primary wave of aggregation, but a secondary wave is missing. Responses to low concentrations of collagen are decreased to absent, but a high concentration of collagen may induce a near-normal aggregation response.[42,45] This aggregation pattern is caused by the lack of ADP secretion and is almost identical to the pattern observed in patients taking aspirin.

Hermansky-Pudlak Syndrome. In addition to occurring as an isolated problem, dense granule deficiency is found in association with several disorders. *Hermansky-Pudlak syndrome* is an autosomal recessive disorder characterized by tyrosinase-positive oculocutaneous albinism, defective lysosomal function in a variety of cell types, ceroid-like deposition in the cells of the reticuloendothelial system, and a profound platelet dense granule deficiency.[47] Several of the mutations responsible for Hermansky-Pudlak syndrome have been mapped to chromosome 19. Mutations in at least seven genes individually can give rise to Hermansky-Pudlak syndrome. These genes encode for proteins that are involved in intracellular vesicular trafficking and are active in the biogenesis of organelles.[48] Whereas the bleeding associated with most dense granule deficiencies is rarely severe, Hermansky-Pudlak syndrome seems to be an exception. Most bleeding episodes in Hermansky-Pudlak syndrome are not severe; however, lethal hemorrhage has been reported, and in one series hemorrhage accounted for 16% of deaths in patients with Hermansky-Pudlak syndrome. A unique morphologic abnormality has been described in the platelets of four families with Hermansky-Pudlak syndrome. This abnormality consists of marked dilation and tortuosity of the surface-connecting tubular system (the so-called Swiss cheese platelet).[2,10,20,49]

Chédiak-Higashi Syndrome. This is a rare autosomal recessive disorder characterized by partial oculocutaneous albinism, frequent pyogenic bacterial infections, giant lysosomal granules in cells of hematologic (Figure 29-4) and nonhematologic origin, platelet dense granule deficiency, and hemorrhage.

The *Chédiak-Higashi syndrome* protein gene is located on chromosome 13, and a series of nonsense and frameshift mutations all result in a truncated Chédiak-Higashi syndrome protein that gives rise to a disorder of generalized cellular dysfunction involving fusion of cytoplasmic granules.

The disorder progresses to an accelerated phase in 85% of patients with Chédiak-Higashi syndrome and is marked by lymphocytic proliferation in the liver, spleen, and marrow and macrophage accumulation in tissues. During this stage, the pancytopenia worsens, which leads to hemorrhage and ever-increasing susceptibility to infection; the result is death at an early age. Initially, bleeding is increased because of dense granule deficiency and consequent defective platelet function. During the accelerated phase, however, the thrombocytopenia also contributes to a prolonged bleeding tendency. Bleeding episodes vary from mild to moderate but worsen as the platelet count decreases.[10,20]

Wiskott-Aldrich Syndrome. This is a rare X-linked disease caused by mutations in the gene that encodes for a 502-amino acid protein—the *Wiskott-Aldrich syndrome* protein (WASp)—that is found exclusively in hematopoietic cells, including lymphocytes. WASp plays a crucial role in actin cytoskeleton remodeling. T cell function is defective due to abnormal cytoskeletal reorganization, leading to impaired migration, adhesion, and insufficient interaction with other cells. There is a wide range of disease severity associated with Wiskott-Aldrich syndrome (WAS) gene mutations that range from the classic form of WAS with autoimmunity and/or malignancy to a milder form with isolated microthrombocytopenia (X-linked thrombocytopenia; XLT) (Chapter 40) to X-linked neutropenia (XLN). Approximately 50% of patients with WAS gene mutations have the WAS phenotype, and the other half have the XLT phenotype. WAS gene mutations causing XLN are very rare.[50] Homozygous mutations of the WIPF1 gene on chromosome 2 that encodes WASp-interacting protein (WIP)—a cytoplasmic protein required to stabilize WASp—can also cause a WAS phenotype.[51]

The classic form of WAS is characterized by susceptibility to infections associated with immune dysfunction with recurrent bacterial, viral, and fungal infections, microthrombocytopenia, and severe eczema. Thrombocytopenia is present at birth, but the full expression of WAS develops over the first 2 years of life. Individuals with this disorder lack the ability to make antipolysaccharide antibodies, which results in a propensity for pneumococcal sepsis. Patients with classic WAS tend to develop autoimmune disorders, lymphoma, or other malignancies, often leading to early death. Bleeding episodes are typically moderate to severe. In WAS, a combination of ineffective thrombocytopoiesis and increased platelet sequestration and destruction accounts for the thrombocytopenia. As with all X-linked recessive disorders, it is found primarily in males.[9,10,20,33,52]

Wiskott-Aldrich platelets are also structurally abnormal. The number of dense granules is decreased, and the platelets are small, a feature of diagnostic importance. Other than in WAS, such small platelets are seen only in TORCH (*T*oxoplasma, *o*ther agents, *r*ubella virus, *c*ytomegalovirus, *h*erpesvirus) infections. Diminished levels of stored adenine nucleotides are reflected in the lack of dense granules observed on transmission electron micrographs. The platelet aggregation pattern in WAS is typical of a storage pool deficiency. The platelets show a decreased aggregation response to ADP, collagen, and epinephrine and lack a secondary wave of aggregation in response to these agonists (Chapter 42). The response to thrombin is normal, however.[10,20] The most effective treatment for the thrombocytopenia seems to be splenectomy, which would be consistent with peripheral destruction of platelets. Platelet transfusions may be needed to treat hemorrhagic episodes. Bone marrow transplantation also has been attempted with some success.[20,53]

Thrombocytopenia with absent radii syndrome. *TAR* (Chapter 40) is a rare autosomal recessive disorder characterized by the congenital absence of the radial bones (the most pronounced skeletal abnormality), numerous cardiac and other skeletal abnormalities, and thrombocytopenia (90% of cases). It is mentioned here because the platelets have structural defects in dense granules with corresponding abnormal aggregation responses. Marrow megakaryocytes may be decreased in number, immature, or normal.[10,54]

α-Granule Deficiency: Gray Platelet Syndrome.

The α-granules are the storage site for proteins (Chapter 13) produced by the megakaryocyte (e.g., platelet-derived growth factor, thrombospondin, and platelet factor 4) or present in plasma and taken up by platelets and transported to α-granules for storage (e.g., albumin, immunoglobulin G [IgG], and fibrinogen). There are 50 to 80 α-granules per platelet, which are primarily responsible for the granular appearance of platelets on stained blood films.

Gray platelet syndrome, a rare disorder first described in 1971, is characterized by the specific absence of morphologically recognizable α-granules in platelets. The disorder is inherited in an autosomal recessive fashion. Clinically, gray platelet syndrome is characterized by lifelong mild bleeding tendencies, moderate thrombocytopenia, fibrosis of the marrow, and large platelets whose gray appearance on a Wright-stained blood film is the source of the name of this disorder.[2,8,10,55] More recently, a mutation in region 3p21 involving the gene NBEAL2 has been identified. This gene is crucial in the development of α-granules.[56,57]

In electron photomicrographs of platelets and megakaryocytes, the platelets appear to have virtually no α-granules, although they do contain vacuoles and small α-granule precursors that stain positive for VWF and fibrinogen. Other types of granules are present in normal numbers. The membranes of the vacuoles and the α-granule precursors have P-selectin (CD62) and GP IIb/IIIa, and these proteins can be translocated to the cell membrane on stimulation with thrombin. This indicates that these structures are α-granules that cannot store the typical α-granule proteins. This may provide an explanation for the observation that, in gray platelet syndrome, the plasma levels of platelet factor 4 and β-thromboglobulin are increased because while the proteins normally contained in α-granules are produced, storage in those granules is not possible. As a result, they are released into the circulation. Most patients develop early-onset myelofibrosis, which can be attributed to the inability of megakaryocytes to store newly synthesized platelet-derived growth factors.[44]

Treatment of severe bleeding episodes may require platelet transfusions. Few other treatments are available for these patients. Cryoprecipitate has been used to control bleeding. Desmopressin acetate was found to shorten the bleeding time and has been used as successful prophylaxis in a dental extraction procedure. Some authors believe that desmopressin acetate should be the initial therapy of choice.[2,8,44,58,59]

Other Storage Pool Diseases.

A rare disorder in which both α-granules and dense granules are deficient is known as α-dense storage pool deficiency. It seems to be inherited as an autosomal dominant characteristic. In these patients, other membrane abnormalities also have been described.[33]

Quebec platelet disorder is an autosomal dominant bleeding disorder that results from a deficiency of multimerin (a multimeric protein that is stored complexed with factor V in α-granules) and shows protease-related degradation of many α-granule proteins, even though α-granule structure is maintained. Thrombocytopenia may be present, although it is not a consistent feature.[33]

Thromboxane Pathway Disorders: Aspirin-Like Effects

Platelet secretion requires the activation of several biochemical pathways. One such pathway is the one leading to thromboxane formation. A series of phospholipases catalyze the release of arachidonic acid and several other compounds from membrane phospholipids. Arachidonic acid is converted to intermediate prostaglandins by cyclooxygenase and to thromboxane A_2 by thromboxane synthase (Figure 13-20). Thromboxane A_2 and other substances generated during platelet activation cause mobilization of ionic calcium from internal stores into the cytoplasm, occupancy of several activation receptors, and initiation of a cascade of events resulting in secretion and aggregation of platelets (Figure 13-21).[60]

Several acquired or congenital disorders of platelet secretion can be traced to structural and functional modifications of arachidonic acid pathway enzymes. Inhibition of cyclooxygenase occurs on ingestion of drugs such as aspirin and ibuprofen. As a result, the amount of thromboxane A_2 produced from arachidonic acid depends on the degree of inhibition. Thromboxane A_2 is required for storage granule secretion and maximal platelet aggregation in response to epinephrine, ADP, and low concentrations of collagen.[6,10,20,61]

Hereditary absence or abnormalities of the components of the thromboxane pathway are usually termed aspirin-like defects because the clinical and laboratory manifestations resemble those that follow aspirin ingestion. Platelet aggregation responses are similar to those in dense granule storage pool disorders (see earlier). Unlike in storage pool disorders, however, ultrastructure and granular contents are normal. Deficiencies of the enzymes cyclooxygenase and thromboxane synthase are well documented, and dysfunction or deficiency of thromboxane receptors is known.[44]

Inherited Disorders of Other Receptors and Signaling Pathways

Collagen Receptors

The $\alpha_2\beta_1$ (GP Ia/IIa) integrin is one of the collagen receptors in the platelet membrane. A deficiency of this receptor has been reported in a patient who lacked an aggregation response to collagen, whose platelets did not adhere to collagen, and who had a lifelong mild bleeding disorder.[62] A deficiency in another collagen receptor, GP VI, also has been reported in patients with mild bleeding. The platelets of these patients failed to aggregate in response to collagen, and adhesion to collagen also was impaired.[63] A family with gray platelet syndrome and defective collagen adhesion has been described.

Affected members of the family have a severe deficiency of GP VI.[64]

ADP Receptors

Platelets seem to contain at least three receptors for ADP. $P2X_1$ is linked to an ion channel that facilitates calcium ion influx. $P2Y_1$ and $P2Y_{12}$ ($P2T_{AC}$) are members of the seven-transmembrane domain (STD) family of G protein–linked receptors (Chapter 13). $P2Y_1$ is thought to mediate calcium mobilization and shape change in response to ADP. Pathology of the $P2Y_1$ receptor has not yet been reported. $P2Y_{12}$ is thought to be responsible for macroscopic platelet aggregation and is coupled to adenylate cyclase through a G-inhibitory (G_i) protein complex.[65] Some patients have been reported to have decreased platelet aggregation in response to ADP but normal platelet shape change and calcium mobilization. These patients have an inherited deficiency of the $P2Y_{12}$ receptor.[66-68] Bleeding problems seem to be relatively mild in these patients, but the only treatment for severe bleeding is platelet transfusion.

Epinephrine Receptors

Congenital defects of the α_2-adrenergic (epinephrine) receptor associated with decreased platelet activation and aggregation in response to epinephrine are known. The receptors that mediate aggregation in response to epinephrine, ADP, and collagen are STD receptors, as are the protease-activated receptors (PARs) for thrombin. So far, defects in the PAR receptors have not been described.[33]

Calcium Mobilization Defects

A group of intracellular defects that affect platelet function includes defects in which all elements of the thromboxane pathway are normal, but insufficient calcium is released from the dense tubular system, and the cytoplasmic concentration of ionic calcium in the cytoplasm never reaches levels high enough to support secretion. This group of disorders is often referred to as *calcium mobilization defects*. These represent a heterogeneous group of disorders in which the defects reside in the various intracellular signaling pathways, including defects in G protein subunits and phospholipase C isoenzymes.[20,69,70]

Scott Syndrome

Scott syndrome is a rare autosomal recessive disorder of calcium-induced membrane phospholipid scrambling (necessary for coagulation factor assembly) and thrombin generation on platelets. Platelets secrete and aggregate normally but do not transport phosphatidylserine and phosphatidylethanolamine from the inner leaflet to the outer leaflet of the plasma membrane. This phospholipid "flip" normally occurs during platelet activation and is essential for the binding of vitamin K–dependent clotting factors. In the membrane of resting platelets, phosphatidylserine and phosphatidylethanolamine are restricted to the inner leaflet of the plasma membrane, and phosphatidylcholine is expressed on the outer leaflet. This asymmetry is maintained by the enzyme aminophospholipid translocase.[71] When platelets are activated, the asymmetry is lost, and phosphatidylserine and phosphatidylethanolamine flip to the outer leaflet and facilitate the assembly of clotting factor complexes. The phospholipid flip is mediated by a calcium-dependent enzyme, scramblase.[72] In Scott syndrome, platelet plug formation (including adhesion, aggregation, and secretion) occurs normally, but clotting factor complexes do not assemble on the activated platelet surface, and thrombin generation is absent or much reduced. Because lack of thrombin generation leads to inadequate fibrin, the platelet plug is not stabilized, and a bleeding diathesis results.[73,74]

Stormorken Syndrome

Lastly, *Stormorken syndrome* is a condition in which platelets are always in an "activated" state and express phosphatidylserine on the outer leaflet of the membrane without prior activation. It has been postulated that patients with this syndrome have a defective aminophospholipid translocase.[75]

Acquired Defects of Platelet Function

Therapeutic drugs have been developed with the target to inhibit platelet function. Other drugs and certain agents have been identified that also affect platelet function. The agents that will be discussed are summarized in Table 41-1.

Drug-Induced Defects

Drugs That Inhibit the Prostaglandin Pathway. Unlike inherited disorders of platelet function, which are rare, acquired disorders of platelet function are commonly encountered. The most frequent cause of acquired platelet dysfunction is drug ingestion, with aspirin and other drugs that inhibit the platelet prostaglandin synthesis pathways being the most common culprits.

TABLE 41-1 Antiplatelet Agents

Drug	Mechanism of Action
Therapeutic Antiplatelet Agents	
Aspirin	Irreversible inhibition of COX1
Naproxen	Reversible inhibition of COX1
Sulfinpyrazone	Reversible inhibition of COX1
Ibuprofen (and related)	Reversible inhibition of COX1
Clopidogrel	Irreversible inhibition of $P2Y_{12}$ receptors
Prasugrel receptors	Irreversible inhibition of $P2Y_{12}$ receptors
Ticagrelor receptors	Reversible inhibition of $P2Y_{12}$ receptors
Abciximab	Inhibition of GP IIb/IIIa (α_{IIb}/β_3)
Eptifibatide	Inhibition of GP IIb/IIIa (α_{IIb}/β_3)
Tirofiban	Inhibition of GP IIb/IIIa (α_{IIb}/β_3)
Dipyridamole	Inhibition of PDE (and cAMP breakdown)
Aggrenox	Inhibition of COX1 and PDE

Drugs with Antiplatelet Effects

Alcohol	Inhibition of thromboxane synthesis (?)
Nitrofurantoin	Unknown
Dextrans	Interference with membrane function
Hydroxyethyl (HETA) starch	Interference with membrane function

A single 200-mg dose of *acetylsalicylic acid* (*aspirin*) can irreversibly acetylate 90% of the platelet cyclooxygenase (Figure 13-20). In platelets the acetylated cyclooxygenase (cyclooxygenase-1, or COX-1) enzyme is completely inactive. Platelets lack a nucleus and cannot synthesize new enzymes. The inhibitory effect is permanent for the circulatory life span of the platelet (7 to 10 days).

Endothelial cells synthesize new cyclooxygenase, and endothelial cell cyclooxygenase seems to be less sensitive to aspirin than the platelet enzyme, at least at low dosages. This has led to the view that low dosages of aspirin may be better than higher dosages for cardiovascular protection, because platelet thromboxane production is inhibited, whereas endothelial cells recover prostacyclin production with its accompanying antiplatelet effects. Others argue that inhibition of platelet function is the more important effect and that higher dosages of aspirin are better for this purpose. For these reasons, there are wide-ranging opinions as to the optimal dosage of aspirin.

What is lost in these arguments is that endothelial cells also produce another potent platelet inhibitor, nitric oxide (NO), and its production is not affected by aspirin. Although aspirin may inhibit a proaggregatory mechanism (thromboxane production) and an antiaggregatory mechanism (prostacyclin production) in endothelial cells, the NO platelet inhibitory mechanism is not affected.

It may be necessary to define a test system to determine the optimal dosage of aspirin for cardiovascular protection on an individual basis because some patients have, or develop, *aspirin resistance*, and a dosage that previously was sufficient to inhibit platelet function effectively may no longer be able to produce that effect. In addition, unlike the practice with almost all other therapeutic agents, a single dose of aspirin is usually prescribed in a "one dose fits all" fashion (e.g., 325 mg) without regard to the patient's weight, age, health status, or other measurable parameters. This practice is based on the assumption that the biologic effect will be the same in all patients. Evidence is emerging, however, that there are considerable interindividual differences in the response to a single dose of aspirin.[3,20,76-78] One study has shown that patients who do not respond well to aspirin have worse cardiovascular outcomes than patients who respond well.[79] The VerifyNow (Accumetrics, San Diego, CA) is one system that provides measurement of a patient's response to antiplatelet medication (Chapters 42 and 44). Individual tests for aspirin, P2Y$_{12}$ receptor inhibitors (clopidogrel, prasugrel, ticagrelor), or GP IIb/IIIa receptor inhibitors (abciximab, eptifibatide, tirofiban) are available on the VerifyNow.

Individuals known to have a defect in their hemostatic mechanism, such as a storage pool deficiency, thrombocytopenia, a vascular disorder, or VWD, may experience a marked increase in bleeding tendency after aspirin ingestion, and such individuals should be advised to avoid the use of aspirin and related agents.[20]

The list of drugs affecting the prostaglandin pathway that converts arachidonic acid to thromboxane is long and beyond the scope of this chapter. Many of these drugs inhibit cyclooxygenase, but, unlike with aspirin and closely related compounds, the inhibition is reversible. These drugs are said to be *competitive inhibitors of cyclooxygenase*, and as the blood concentration of the drug decreases, platelet function is recovered. This group of drugs includes *ibuprofen and related compounds*, such as ketoprofen and fenoprofen, naproxen, and sulfinpyrazone. In contrast to aspirin, most of these agents have little effect on the platelet function tests (Chapters 42 and 44). Except for their potential to irritate the gastric mucosa, these drugs have not been reported to cause clinically important bleeding.[6,11,20,80] Interestingly, ibuprofen appears to have a prothrombotic effect when ingested within 2 hours of aspirin because it blocks the acetylation site for aspirin on COX-1. Patients taking aspirin should be cautioned to avoid ibuprofen and related drugs near the time of aspirin ingestion.

The association of *chronic alcohol consumption* with thrombocytopenia is well known. Chronic, periodic, and even acute alcohol consumption may result in a transient decrease in platelet function, however, and the inhibitory effect seems to be more pronounced when alcohol is consumed in excess. Most patients who are scheduled to undergo a medical procedure in which there may be hemostatic challenge are advised to abstain from alcohol consumption for about 3 days before the procedure. The impaired platelet function seems to be related at least in part to inhibition of thromboxane synthesis. A reduced platelet count and impaired platelet function may contribute to the increased incidence of gastrointestinal hemorrhage associated with chronic excessive alcohol intake.[6,20,81,82]

Drugs That Inhibit Membrane Function.   Many drugs interact with the platelet membrane and cause a clinically significant platelet function defect that may lead to hemorrhage. Some of these drugs are useful antiplatelet agents, whereas for many other drugs, their effects on the platelet membrane are an adverse side effect.[60]

P2Y$_{12}$ (ADP) Receptor Inhibitors.   The *thienopyridine derivatives* clopidogrel, prasugrel, their predecessor ticlopidine, and the nucleoside *ticagrelor* are antiplatelet agents that bind to the P2Y$_{12}$ platelet receptor thus inhibiting platelet function. These drugs are for treatment of patients with arterial occlusive disease for prevention of myocardial infarction, for patients with cerebrovascular disease for reduction of the risk of thrombotic stroke, for stroke and myocardial infarction prophylaxis, and for patients who are intolerant of aspirin.

In contrast to the effects of aspirin, the effects of these agents do not reach a steady state for 3 to 5 days, although a steady state can be reached sooner with a loading dose. As prophylactic agents, they have been shown to be as efficacious as aspirin. P2Y$_{12}$ inhibitors and aspirin are often used in combination to prevent arterial thrombosis, primarily based on the synergistic action of these two drugs, which inhibit platelet function by different mechanisms.

The mechanism of action for P2Y$_{12}$ inhibitors is binding to the platelet membrane STD receptors for ADP and the prevention of ADP binding to those receptors.[66] As with aspirin inhibition of cyclooxygenase, the effect of the irreversible thienopyridines on platelet recovery of function following drug cessation is 50% of normal at 3 days, and complete at 7 to 10 days.[83]

The major effect of the binding of these drugs to $P2Y_{12}$ receptors appears to be inhibition of stimulus-response coupling between those receptors and fibrinogen binding to GP IIb/IIIa. As a consequence, platelet activation and aggregation induced by ADP are markedly inhibited, and responses to other aggregating agents, such as collagen, are reduced.

Clopidogrel (Plavix), a second-generation thienopyridine derivative, is an effective antiplatelet agent for a variety of clinical applications, though its clinical effectiveness varies from patient to patient based on metabolism to the active drug. Clopidogrel is a pro-drug and requires conversion to the active drug by the P450 enzyme systems of the liver. For clopidogrel, the isoform of P450 involved in clopidogrel metabolism is 2C19 (a.k.a. *CYP2C19*). There are numerous mutations in *CYP2C19* that result in decreased activity of the enzyme and therefore inhibit the conversion of clopidogrel to the active drug. *CYP2C19*1/*1* (wild type) represents two normal functioning alleles and normal metabolism of clopidogrel to the active drug. Hypofunctional alleles are *CYP2C19*2* to *10*, while *CYP2C19*17* is a hyperfunctional allele. Patients with one of the mutations resulting in decreased activity (e.g., *CYP2C19*1/*2*) are considered intermediate metabolizers, and the usual dose of clopidogrel does not achieve the degree of platelet inhibition desired. These individuals remain at increased risk for thromboembolic events. Increasing the dose of clopidogrel may increase the degree of platelet inhibition, but it does not decrease the thromboembolic risk. Those who have two hypofunctional alleles (*CYP2C19*2/*2, *2/*3*, or any combination of two hypofunctional alleles) are poor metabolizers and do not derive significant benefit from clopidogrel therapy. Approximately 25% of individuals have one or two hypofuctional alleles of *CYP2C19* and are considered to be *clopidogrel resistant*. In contrast, those with a *17* allele are rapid metabolizers and convert clopidogrel to the active drug at a faster rate. This results in increased blood levels of the active drug following a dose of clopidogrel and an increased risk of bleeding. Those with one normal allele and one *17* allele (*1/*17*) are considered to be rapid metabolizers and those who are *17/*17* are ultra-rapid metabolizers. Finally, individuals with one hypofunctional and one hyperfunctional allele (e.g., *2/*17*) have normal to intermediate clopidogrel metabolism. There are a variety of molecular methods available to test for the most common alleles of *CYP2C19*. Although the FDA has recommended pharmacogenetic testing for these alleles, it is not a common practice.

Clopidogrel has more effect on the platelet function tests than aspirin, although there is little difference in the risk of clinical bleeding.[84] Clopidogrel can occasionally produce major side effects in some patients, including long-lasting neutropenia, aplastic anemia, thrombocytopenia, gastrointestinal distress, and diarrhea.

Prasugrel (Effient) is a third-generation thienopyridine derivative. It has the same mechanism of action as clopidogrel. It is also a pro-drug, but its metabolism to the active form does not require *CYP2C19*. Instead, it is metabolized to the active drug by several enzymes of the cytochrome P450 system, including *CYP3A4* and *CYP2B6*. Because it is activated by several enzymes, mutations that result in decreased function of one or more of these enzyme have less impact, and the response is much more uniform than clopidogrel. Pharmacogenetic testing for mutations affecting prasugrel activation is not recommended.

Ticagrelor (Brilinta) is a nuceloside and the newest of the $P2Y_{12}$ inhibitors. While its antiplatelet effect is similar, it has two important differences from prasugrel and clopidogrel. First, it is not a pro-drug and therefore does not require bioactivation. Because it is rapidly absorbed, its antiplatelet effect is predictable and achieved in a short period of time. In addition, ticagrelor binds to a slightly different site on the $P2Y_{12}$ (ADP) receptor than clopidogrel or prasugrel. This difference results in reversible binding. Therefore, unlike clopidogrel and prasugrel whose effects are irreversible, platelet function returns quite rapidly with cessation of ticagrelor. However, this short half-life (7 to 9 hours) requires twice-daily dosing and may be a compliance issue for some patients.

GP IIb/IIIa (α_{IIb}/β_3) receptor inhibitors. Another target for antiplatelet agents to reduce cardiovascular thrombotic risk is the platelet membrane GP IIb/IIIa (α_{IIb}/β_3) receptor. Interference with the ability of this receptor to bind fibrinogen inhibits platelet aggregation stimulated in response to all of the usual platelet aggregating agents. Results of platelet function studies on platelets from patients receiving therapeutic doses of these drugs essentially mimic those of a mild form of Glanzmann thrombasthenia.

Two different types of agents are included in this group. The first such agent approved for clinical use in the United States was the Fab fragment of the mouse/human chimeric monoclonal antibody 7E3 (c7E3 Fab; *abciximab* [ReoPro]), which binds to GP IIb/IIIa, prevents the binding of fibrinogen, and prevents platelet aggregation. Numerous studies have shown the efficacy of this drug as an antiplatelet and antithrombotic agent.

The second type of agent in this group targets a GP IIb/IIIa recognition site for an arginine–glycine–aspartic acid (RGD) sequence found in fibrinogen and several adhesive proteins. These agents bind to the RGD recognition site, prevent the binding of fibrinogen, and consequently prevent platelet aggregation. These compounds are relatively easily synthesized. *Tirofiban* (Aggrastat) is a nonpeptide RGD mimetic, and *eptifibatide* (Integrilin) is a cyclic heptapeptide that is also an RGD mimetic. When the receptor site is occupied by the drug, GP IIb/IIIa is no longer able to bind fibrinogen or other adhesive proteins and is no longer functional as the aggregation receptor.

The goal of therapy with these drugs is to induce a controlled thrombasthenia-like state. At present, these agents are primarily used in patients undergoing percutaneous coronary intervention and are administered concurrently with heparin and other antiplatelet agents. The use of these agents is limited by the need to administer them by constant intravenous infusion and by their short half-lives. There have been attempts to make an orally active agent of this type, but none has been approved for use.[85-87]

Other Therapeutic Drugs That Inhibit Platelet Function.
Dipyridamole is an inhibitor of platelet phosphodiesterase, the

enzyme responsible for converting cyclic adenosine monophosphate (cAMP) to AMP. Elevation of cytoplasmic cAMP is inhibitory to platelet function, and inhibition of phosphodiesterase allows the accumulation of cAMP in the cytoplasm (Figure 13-21). Dipyridamole alone does not inhibit platelet aggregation in response to the usual platelet agonists, but it promotes inhibition of agents that stimulate cAMP formation, such as prostacyclin, stable analogues of prostacyclin, and NO. At one time, dipyridamole, alone or in combination with aspirin, was widely used. By the 1990s, interest in dipyridamole had waned. There has been a resurgence of interest in dipyridamole, however, as a combination agent compounded with aspirin (*Aggrenox*).

Miscellaneous Agents That Inhibit Platelet Function.
Well known for their ability to interfere with platelet function are *antibiotics*. Most of the drugs with this effect contain the β-lactam ring and are either a penicillin or a cephalosporin (Figure 41-4). These drugs can inhibit platelet function tests, but this effect is seen only in patients receiving large parenteral doses and is thus only a problem for hospitalized patients. One postulated mechanism for the antiplatelet effect of these drugs is that they associate with the membrane via a lipophilic reaction and block receptor-agonist interactions or stimulus-response coupling between receptors and fibrinogen binding to GP IIb/IIIa. They also may inhibit calcium influx in response to thrombin stimulation, reducing the ability of thrombin to activate platelets. Although these drugs may prolong the bleeding time test and in vitro aggregation responses to certain agonists, their association with a hemostatic defect severe enough to cause clinical hemorrhage is uncertain and is not predicted by the bleeding time test results.[3,11,61,88]

Nitrofurantoin is an antibiotic that is not related to the β-lactam drugs but may inhibit platelet aggregation when high concentrations are present in the blood. This drug is not known to cause clinical bleeding, however.[88]

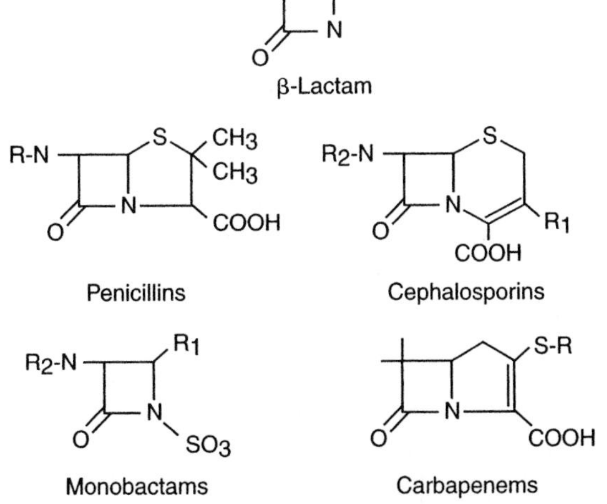

The *dextrans*, another class of commonly used drugs, can inhibit platelet aggregation, and impair platelet procoagulant activity when given as an intravenous infusion. These drugs have no effect on platelet function, however, when added directly to platelet-rich plasma. Dextrans are partially hydrolyzed, branched-chain polysaccharides of glucose. The two most commonly used are dextran 70 (molecular mass of 70,000 to 75,000 Daltons) and dextran 40 (molecular mass of 40,000 Daltons), also known as low-molecular-weight dextran. Both drugs are effective plasma expanders and are commonly used for this purpose. Because of their effects on platelets, they have been extensively used as antithrombotic agents. There does not seem to be any increased risk of hemorrhage associated with the use of these agents, but their efficacy in preventing postoperative pulmonary embolism is equal to that of low-dose subcutaneous heparin.[6,52,81,88]

Hydroxyethyl starch, or hetastarch, is a synthetic glucose polymer with a mean molecular mass of 450,000 Daltons that also is used as a plasma expander. It has effects similar to those of the dextrans. The mechanism of action of these drugs has not been clearly elucidated but is presumed to involve interaction with the platelet membrane.[6,52,81]

Several other agents of diverse chemical structure and function are known to inhibit platelet function. The mechanisms by which they induce platelet dysfunction are largely unknown. Nitroglycerin, nitroprusside, propranolol, and isosorbide dinitrate are drugs used to regulate cardiovascular function that seem to be able to cause a decrease in platelet secretion and aggregation. Patients taking phenothiazine or tricyclic antidepressants may have decreased secretion and aggregation responses, but these effects are not associated with an increased risk for hemorrhage. Local and general anesthetics may impair in vitro aggregation responses. The same is true of antihistamines. Finally, some radiographic contrast agents are known to inhibit platelet function.[88]

Disorders That Affect Platelet Function
Myeloproliferative Neoplasms.
Chronic myeloproliferative neoplasms (MPNs) include *polycythemia vera, chronic myelogenous leukemia, essential thrombocythemia,* and *myelofibrosis with myeloid metaplasia* (Chapter 33). Platelet dysfunction is a common finding in patients with these disorders. Hemorrhagic complications occur in about one third, thrombosis occurs in another third, and, although it is uncommon, both develop in some patients. These complications are serious causes of morbidity and mortality.

Although the occurrence of hemorrhage or thrombosis in MPN patients is largely unpredictable, certain patterns have emerged. Hemorrhage and thrombosis are less common in chronic myelogenous leukemia than in the other MPNs. Bleeding seems to be more common in myelofibrosis with myeloid metaplasia, but thrombosis is more common in the other MPNs.

Abnormal platelet function has been postulated as a contributing cause. This hypothesis is supported by the observation that bleeding is usually mucocutaneous in nature, and thrombosis may be arterial or venous.

Figure 41-4 Chemical structure of major classes of β-lactam antibiotics. *R*, Nonspecified side chain. (From Mahon CR, Lehman DE, Manuselis G: *Textbook of diagnostic microbiology*, ed 4, St. Louis, 2011, Saunders.)

In patients with these disorders, thrombosis may occur in unusual sites, including the mesenteric, hepatic, and portal circulations. Patients with essential thrombocythemia may develop digital artery thrombosis and ischemia of the fingers and toes, occlusions of the microvasculature of the heart, and cerebrovascular occlusions that result in neurologic symptoms.[88]

In MPNs, a variety of platelet function defects have been described, but their clinical importance is uncertain. Platelets have been reported to have abnormal shapes, decreased procoagulant activity, and a decreased number of secretory granules. In essential thrombocythemia, platelet survival may be shortened. The bleeding time is prolonged in only a few patients, and hemorrhage can occur in patients with a normal bleeding time. The risk of thrombosis or hemorrhage correlates poorly with the elevation of the platelet count.

The most common abnormalities are decreased aggregation and secretion in response to epinephrine, ADP, and collagen.[89] Possible causes of the platelet dysfunction include loss of platelet surface membrane α-adrenergic (epinephrine) receptors, impaired release of arachidonic acid from membrane phospholipids in response to stimulation by agonists, impaired oxidation of arachidonic acid by the cyclooxygenase and lipoxygenase pathways, a decrease in the contents of dense granules and α-granules, and loss of a variety of platelet membrane receptors for adhesion and activation. There seems to be no correlation between a given MPN and the type of platelet dysfunction observed, with the exception that most patients with essential thrombocythemia lack an in vitro platelet aggregation response to epinephrine. This observation may be helpful in the differential diagnosis.[6,11,88,90]

Multiple Myeloma and Waldenström Macroglobulinemia.

Platelet dysfunction is observed in approximately one third of patients with *IgA myeloma* or *Waldenström macroglobulinemia*, a much smaller percentage of patients with *IgG multiple myeloma*, and only occasionally in patients with *monoclonal gammopathy* of undetermined significance.

Platelet dysfunction results from coating of the platelet membranes by paraprotein and does not depend on the type of paraprotein present. In addition to interacting with platelets, the paraprotein may interfere with fibrin polymerization and the function of other coagulation proteins.

Almost all patients with malignant paraprotein disorders have clinically significant bleeding, but thrombocytopenia is still the most likely cause of bleeding in these patients. Other causes of bleeding include hyperviscosity syndrome, complications of amyloidosis (e.g., acquired factor X deficiency), and, in rare instances, presence of a circulating heparin-like anticoagulant or fibrinolysis.[9,81,88]

Cardiopulmonary Bypass Surgery.

The use of the *cardiopulmonary bypass machine* (CPB; heart-lung machine) during cardiac surgery induces thrombocytopenia and a severe platelet function defect that assumes major importance in bleeding after surgery. The function defect most likely results from platelet activation and fragmentation in the extracorporeal circuit.

Causes of platelet activation include adherence and aggregation of platelets to fibrinogen (adsorbed onto the surfaces of the bypass circuit material), mechanical trauma and shear stresses, use of blood conservation devices and bypass pump-priming solutions during surgery, hypothermia, complement activation, and exposure of platelets to the blood-air interface in bubble oxygenators.

Some degree of platelet degranulation typically is found after cardiac surgery using the cardiopulmonary bypass machine, which indicates that platelet activation and secretion have occurred during the operation. Platelet membrane fragments, or "microparticles," are found consistently in the blood of these surgical patients, providing additional evidence of the severe mechanical stress encountered by platelets during these procedures.

The severity of the platelet function defect closely correlates with the length of time on the bypass machine. After an uncomplicated surgical procedure, normal platelet function returns in about 1 hour, although the platelet count does not return to normal for several days. Thrombocytopenia is caused by hemodilution, accumulation of platelets on the surfaces of the bypass materials, sequestration or removal of damaged platelets by the liver and reticuloendothelial system, and consumption associated with normal hemostatic processes after surgery.[81,88]

Liver Disease.

Moderate to severe *liver disease* is reported to be associated with a variety of hemostatic abnormalities, including reduction in clotting proteins, reduction of proteins in the natural anticoagulant pathways, dysfibrinogenemia, and excessive fibrinolysis (Chapter 38). Mild to moderate thrombocytopenia is seen in approximately one third of patients with chronic liver disease in association with hypersplenism or as a result of alcohol toxicity.[8,88]

Abnormal platelet function test results seen in patients with chronic liver disease include reduced platelet adhesion, abnormal platelet aggregation (in response to ADP, epinephrine, and thrombin), abnormal platelet factor 3 (phospholipids) availability, and reduced procoagulant activity. An acquired storage pool deficiency also has been suggested. The abnormal platelet function in these patients may respond to infusion of desmopressin acetate. It is unclear, however, whether desmopressin acetate provides a benefit in preventing bleeding in these patients or is simply correcting an abnormal laboratory test result.

In *chronic alcoholic cirrhosis*, the thrombocytopenia and platelet abnormalities may result from the direct toxic effects of alcohol on bone marrow megakaryocytes. The severe bleeding diathesis associated with end-stage liver disease has many causes, such as markedly decreased or negligible coagulation factor production, excessive fibrinolysis, dysfibrinogenemia, thrombocytopenia, and (occasionally) disseminated intravascular coagulation. Upper gastrointestinal tract bleeding is a relatively common feature of cirrhosis, particularly alcoholic cirrhosis, and recombinant factor VIIa (rVIIa, NovoSeven, Novo Nordisk Inc, Princeton, NJ) has been shown to be effective treatment in some patients.[91]

Uremia. This is commonly accompanied by bleeding caused by platelet dysfunction. In *uremia*, guanidinosuccinic acid (GSA) is present in the circulation in higher than normal levels as a result of inhibition of the urea cycle. GSA is dialyzable, and dialysis (peritoneal dialysis or hemodialysis) is usually effective in correcting the prolonged bleeding time test and the abnormal platelet function characteristic of uremia. NO diffuses into platelets; activates soluble guanylate cyclase; and inhibits platelet adhesion, activation, and aggregation.[92] Because GSA is an NO donor, NO is present in the circulation at higher than normal levels in uremia. Abnormal platelet function is far more common than clinically significant bleeding in uremic patients.[2,60,62]

Platelet aggregation pattern abnormalities are not uniform, and any combination of defects may be seen. There is evidence of a deficient release reaction, such as lack of primary ADP-induced aggregation, and subnormal platelet procoagulant activity. The bleeding time test is characteristically prolonged in uremia and seems to correlate with the severity of renal failure in these patients. There does not seem to be any significant correlation, however, between the bleeding time test and the risk of clinically significant bleeding. Anemia is an independent cause of prolonged bleeding time, and the severity of anemia in uremic patients correlates with the severity of renal failure. Many uremic patients are treated with recombinant erythropoietin to increase their hematocrit. Maintenance of the hematocrit at greater than 30% also may help to normalize the bleeding times.[2,81,84]

Bleeding is uncommon in uremic patients and is seen more often with concurrent use of drugs that interfere with platelet function or in association with heparin use in hemodialysis. Platelet concentrates often are used to treat severe hemorrhagic episodes in patients with uremia but usually do not correct the bleeding. Other therapies that are sometimes effective include cryoprecipitate, desmopressin acetate, and conjugated estrogen.[2,81,84]

Hereditary Afibrinogenemia. Hereditary afibrinogenemia has been documented in more than 150 families. Although it is not truly a platelet function disorder, platelets do not exhibit normal function in the absence or near-absence of fibrinogen. In most patients, the bleeding time is prolonged, and because fibrinogen is essential for normal platelet aggregation, platelet aggregation test results are abnormal. Abnormal results on platelet retention and adhesion studies involving the use of glass beads also have been documented. In addition, results of all clot-based tests (including partial thromboplastin time, prothrombin time, reptilase time, thrombin time, and whole-blood clotting time) are abnormal. Addition of fibrinogen to samples or infusion of fibrinogen into the patient results in correction of the abnormal test results.[2,93]

A high incidence of hemorrhagic manifestations is found in patients with afibrinogenemia (or severe hypofibrinogenemia). Bleeding is the cause of death in about one third of such patients. Cryoprecipitate or fibrinogen concentrates can be used to treat bleeding episodes. Some patients develop antibodies to fibrinogen, and this treatment then becomes ineffective.[93]

Hyperaggregable Platelets

Patients with a variety of disorders associated with thrombosis or increased risk for thrombosis, including hyperlipidemia, diabetes mellitus, peripheral arterial occlusive disease, acute arterial occlusion, myocardial infarction, and stroke, have been reported to have increased platelet reactivity. Platelets from these patients tend to aggregate at lower concentrations of aggregating agents than do platelets from individuals without these conditions.

Sticky platelet syndrome is an inherited disorder with autosomal dominant characteristics and is associated with venous and arterial thromboembolic events. The disorder is characterized by hyperaggregable platelets in response to ADP, epinephrine, or both. In these patients, venous and/or arterial thrombotic events are often associated with emotional stress. Prophylactic treatment of these patients with low-dose aspirin reverses clinical symptoms and normalizes hyperaggregable responses to aggregating agents in the laboratory.

Spontaneous aggregation (aggregation in response to in vitro stirring only) is also an indicator of abnormally increased platelet reactivity and often accompanies increased sensitivity to platelet agonists. The presence of spontaneous aggregation by itself is considered to be consistent with the presence of a hyperaggregable state. Because participation of platelets is necessary for the development of arterial thrombosis, the presence of hyperaggregable platelets is often an indication that an antiplatelet agent should be used as part of a therapeutic or prophylactic regimen for arterial thrombosis.[81,94,95]

Acquired platelet function defects are seen occasionally in patients with autoimmune disorders, including systemic lupus erythematosus, rheumatoid arthritis, scleroderma, and the immune thrombocytopenias, such as immune thrombocytopenic purpura.[88]

Purified fibrin degradation products can induce platelet dysfunction in vitro. The pathophysiologic relevance of this observation is uncertain because the concentrations of fibrin degradation products required are unlikely to be reached in vivo. Patients with disseminated intravascular coagulation may have reduced platelet function, however, as a result of in vivo stimulation by thrombin and other agonists resulting in in vivo release of granule contents. This has been called *acquired storage pool disease*; the term *exhausted platelets* may be more appropriate.[96]

VASCULAR DISORDERS

The pathophysiology of disorders of vessels and their supporting tissues is obscure. Laboratory studies of platelets and blood coagulation usually yield normal results. The diagnosis is often based on medical history and is made by ruling out other sources of bleeding disorders. The usual clinical sign is the tendency to bruise easily or to bleed spontaneously, especially from mucosal surfaces. Vascular disorders are summarized in Box 41-4.

Hereditary Vascular Disorders
Hereditary Hemorrhagic Telangiectasia (Rendu-Osler-Weber Syndrome)

The mode of inheritance of *hereditary hemorrhagic telangiectasia* is autosomal dominant. The vascular defect of this disorder is characterized by thin-walled blood vessels with a discontinuous endothelium, inadequate smooth muscle, and inadequate or missing elastin in the surrounding stroma. Telangiectasias (dilated superficial blood vessels that create small, focal red lesions) occur throughout the body but are most obvious on the face, lips, tongue, conjunctiva, nasal mucosa, fingers, toes, and trunk and under the tongue. The lesions blanch when pressure is applied. The disorder usually becomes manifest by puberty and progresses throughout life. Telangiectasias are fragile and prone to rupture. Epistaxis is an almost universal finding, and symptoms almost always worsen with age. The age at which nosebleeds begin is a good gauge of the severity of the disorder. Although the oral cavity, gastrointestinal tract, and urogenital tract are common sites of bleeding, bleeding can occur in virtually every organ.[97]

The diagnosis of hereditary hemorrhagic telangiectasia is based on the characteristic skin or mucous membrane lesions, a history of repeated hemorrhage, and a family history of a similar disorder.

Patients with hereditary hemorrhagic telangiectasia do well despite the lack of specific therapy and the seriousness of their hemorrhagic manifestations.[2,10,97] There are several other disorders and conditions in which telangiectasias are present, including cherry-red hemangiomas (common in older men and women), ataxia-telangiectasia (Louis-Bar syndrome), and chronic actinic telangiectasia; they also are seen in association with chronic liver disease and pregnancy.[97]

Hemangioma-Thrombocytopenia Syndrome (Kasabach-Merritt Syndrome)

Kasabach and Merritt originally described the association of a giant cavernous hemangioma (vascular tumor), thrombocytopenia,

and a bleeding diathesis. The hemangiomas are visceral or subcutaneous, but rarely both. External hemangiomas may become engorged with blood and resemble hematomas. Other well-recognized features of *Kasabach-Merritt syndrome* include acute or chronic disseminated intravascular coagulation (Chapters 38 and 39) and microangiopathic hemolytic anemia. A hereditary basis for this syndrome has not been established, but the condition is present at birth. Several treatment modalities are available for the angiomas and the associated coagulopathy and range from corticosteroid therapy to surgery.[10,98]

Ehlers-Danlos Syndrome and Other Genetic Disorders

Ehlers-Danlos syndrome may be transmitted as an autosomal dominant, recessive, or X-linked trait. It is manifested by hyperextensible skin, hypermobile joints, joint laxity, fragile tissues, and a bleeding tendency, primarily subcutaneous hematoma formation. Eleven distinct varieties of the disorder are recognized. The severity of bleeding ranges from easy bruisability to arterial rupture. The disorder generally can be ascribed to defects in collagen production, structure, or cross-linking, with resulting inadequacy of the connective tissues. Platelet abnormalities have been reported in some patients.[10]

Other inherited vascular disorders include pseudoxanthoma elasticum and homocystinuria (autosomal recessive disorders), and Marfan syndrome and osteogenesis imperfecta (autosomal dominant disorders). In addition to vascular defects, Marfan syndrome is characterized by skeletal and ocular defects.[10]

Acquired Vascular Disorders
Allergic Purpura (Henoch-Schönlein Purpura)

The term *allergic purpura* or *anaphylactoid purpura* generally is applied to a group of nonthrombocytopenic purpuras characterized by apparently allergic manifestations, including skin rash and edema. Allergic purpura has been associated with certain foods and drugs, cold, insect bites, and vaccinations. The term *Henoch-Schönlein purpura* is applied when the condition is accompanied by transient arthralgia, nephritis, abdominal pain, and purpuric skin lesions, which are frequently confused with the hemorrhagic rash of immune thrombocytopenic purpura.[2,10,52]

General evidence implicates autoimmune vascular injury, but the pathophysiology of the disorder is unclear. Preliminary evidence indicates that the vasculitis is mediated by immune complexes containing IgA antibodies. It has been suggested that allergic purpura may represent autoimmunity to components of vessel walls.[2,10]

Henoch-Schönlein purpura is primarily a disease of children, occurring most commonly in children 3 to 7 years of age. It is relatively uncommon among individuals younger than age 2 and older than age 20. Twice as many boys as girls are affected. The onset of the disease is sudden, often following an upper respiratory tract infection. The infectious organism may damage the endothelial lining of blood vessels, which results in vasculitis. Attempts have been made to implicate a specific infectious agent, particularly β-hemolytic streptococcus.[2,10]

Malaise, headache, fever, and rash may be the presenting symptoms. The delay in the appearance of the skin rash often poses a difficult problem in differential diagnosis. The skin lesions are urticarial and gradually become pinkish, then red, and finally hemorrhagic. The appearance of the lesions may be very rapid and accompanied by itching. The lesions have been described as "palpable purpura," in contrast to the perfectly flat lesions of thrombocytopenia and most other forms of vascular purpura. These lesions are most commonly found on the feet, elbows, knees, buttocks, and chest. Ultimately, a brownish-red eruption is seen. Petechiae also may be present.[2,10]

As the disease progresses, abdominal pain, polyarthralgia, headaches, and renal disease may develop. Renal lesions are present in 60% of patients during the second to third week of the disorder. Proteinuria and hematuria are commonly present.[2,8,10]

The platelet count is normal. Tests of hemostasis, including the bleeding time, and tests of blood coagulation, usually yield normal results in patients with allergic purpura. Anemia generally is not present unless the hemorrhagic manifestations have been severe. The white blood cell count and the erythrocyte sedimentation rate are usually elevated. The disease must be distinguished from other forms of nonthrombocytopenic purpura. Numerous infectious diseases that may be associated with purpura also must be considered in the differential diagnosis. Drugs or chemicals sometimes may be implicated.[2,10]

In the pediatric age group, the average duration of the initial episode is about 4 weeks. Relapses are frequent, usually after a period of apparent well-being. Except for patients in whom chronic renal disease develops, the prognosis is usually good. Occasionally, death from renal failure has occurred. Management is directed primarily at symptomatic relief, because there currently is no effective treatment. Corticosteroids sometimes have been helpful in alleviating symptoms. Most patients recover without treatment.[2,10]

Paraproteinemia and Amyloidosis

Platelet function can be inhibited by *myeloma proteins*. Abnormalities in platelet aggregation, secretion, and procoagulant activity (Chapter 42) correlate with the concentration of the plasma paraprotein and are likely due to coating of the platelet membrane with the paraprotein. Under these conditions, platelet adhesion and activation receptor functions are inhibited, and the paraprotein coating also inhibits assembly of clotting factors on the platelet surface. High concentrations of paraprotein can cause severe hemorrhagic manifestations as a result of a combination of hyperviscosity and platelet dysfunction. About one third of patients with *IgA myeloma* and *Waldenström macroglobulinemia* and approximately 5% of patients with *IgG myeloma* (usually IgG3) exhibit platelet function abnormalities. Finally, the paraprotein may contribute further to bleeding by inhibiting fibrin polymerization. In these patients, there is poor correlation between abnormal results on laboratory tests (e.g., prothrombin time, activated partial thromboplastin time, thrombin time, bleeding time) and evidence of clinical bleeding. Treatment for the bleeding complications of these disorders is primarily reduction in the level of the paraprotein. This can be accomplished quickly, albeit transiently, by plasmapheresis. Longer-term treatment is usually chemotherapy for the underlying plasma cell malignancy.[88,99]

Amyloid is a fibrous protein consisting of rigid, linear, non-branching, aggregated fibrils approximately 7.5 to 10 nm wide and of indefinite length. Amyloid is deposited extracellularly and may lead to damage of normal tissues. Various proteins can serve as subunits of the fibril, including monoclonal light chains (λ more frequently than κ). Amyloidosis, the deposition of abnormal quantities of amyloid in tissues, may be primary or secondary and localized or systemic. A discussion of the clinical spectrum of amyloidosis is beyond the scope of this chapter. Purpura, hemorrhage, and thrombosis may be a part of the clinical presentation of patients with amyloidosis, however. Thrombosis and hemorrhage have been ascribed to amyloid deposition in the vascular wall and surrounding tissues. Platelet function has been shown to be abnormal in a few cases, and in rare cases patients may have thrombocytopenia. Current treatments for amyloidosis are not effective.[100]

Senile Purpura

Senile purpura occurs more commonly in elderly men than in women and is due to a lack of collagen support for small blood vessels and loss of subcutaneous fat and elastic fibers. The incidence increases with advancing age. The dark blotches are flattened, are about 1 to 10 mm in diameter, do not blanch with pressure, and resolve slowly, often leaving a brown stain in the skin (age spots). The lesions are limited mostly to the extensor surfaces of the forearms and backs of the hands and occasionally occur on the face and neck. With the exception of increased capillary fragility, results of laboratory tests are normal, and no other bleeding manifestations are present.[2,10]

Drug-Induced Vascular Purpuras

Purpura associated with *drug-induced vasculitis* occurs in the presence of functionally adequate platelets. A variety of drugs are known to cause *vascular purpura*, including aspirin, warfarin, barbiturates, diuretics, digoxin, methyldopa, and several antibiotics. Sulfonamides and iodides have been implicated most frequently. The lesions vary from a few petechiae to massive, generalized petechial eruptions. Mechanisms include development of antibodies to vessel wall components, development of immune complexes, and changes in vessel wall permeability. As soon as the disorder is recognized, the offending drug should be discontinued. No other treatment is necessary.[10]

Miscellaneous Causes of Vascular Purpura

Insufficient dietary intake of vitamin C (ascorbic acid) results in *scurvy* and decreased synthesis of collagen, with weakening of capillary walls and the appearance of purpuric lesions.[10] A diagnosis of *purpura simplex* (simple vascular purpura) or *vascular fragility* is made when a cause for purpura cannot be found. The ecchymoses are superficial, bleeding is usually mild, and laboratory test results are most often normal.[10] Cutaneous bleeding and bruising through intact skin has been observed in patients in whom no vascular or platelet dysfunction can be detected. Most such cases involve women with emotional problems, and the bruising is often accompanied by nausea, vomiting, or fever. Evidence for a psychosomatic origin is equivocal. Laboratory test results are invariably normal.[10]

SUMMARY

- Inherited qualitative platelet disorders can cause bleeding disorders ranging from mild to severe.
- Bernard-Soulier syndrome is caused by the lack of expression of GP Ib/IX/V complexes on the platelet surface. This receptor complex is responsible for platelet adhesion and its absence results in a severe bleeding disorder.
- Glanzmann thrombasthenia is caused by the lack of expression of GP IIb/IIIa complexes on the platelet surface. This complex is known as the *platelet aggregation receptor,* and its absence is associated with a severe bleeding disorder.
- Storage pool disorders result from the absence of intraplatelet α-granules, dense granules, or both. Platelet dysfunction associated with these disorders is generally mild; bleeding symptoms also are usually mild.
- Aspirin-like effects result from defects in elements of the arachidonic acid metabolic pathway. Platelet dysfunction mimics that seen after aspirin ingestion.
- Deficiencies of several of the receptors for platelet-activating substances have been documented, and bleeding symptoms of varying severity are associated with these deficiencies.

- Drugs are the most common cause of acquired platelet dysfunction, and aspirin is the most frequent culprit. Several new classes of antiplatelet agents with effects different from aspirin are now available and gaining in popularity.
- A variety of pathologic conditions can result in platelet dysfunction and range from hematologic malignancies to kidney disease and liver disease.
- Vascular disorders that result in bleeding are uncommon. There are a few well-recognized inherited disorders, however, such as Ehlers-Danlos syndrome and hereditary hemorrhagic telangiectasia that can result in substantial blood loss.
- Vascular disorders can be acquired, and these are much more common than inherited disorders. Causes range from the effects of aging to drug effects to allergic reaction.

Now that you have completed this chapter, go back and read again the case study at the beginning and respond to the questions presented.

REVIEW QUESTIONS

Answers can be found in the Appendix.

1. The clinical presentation of platelet-related bleeding may include all of the following *except:*
   a. Bruising
   b. Nosebleeds
   c. Gastrointestinal bleeding
   d. Bleeding into the joints (hemarthroses)

2. A defect in GP IIb/IIIa causes:
   a. Glanzmann thrombasthenia
   b. Bernard-Soulier syndrome
   c. Gray platelet syndrome
   d. Storage pool disease

3. Aspirin ingestion blocks the synthesis of:
   a. Thromboxane A_2
   b. Ionized calcium
   c. Collagen
   d. ADP

4. Patients with Bernard-Soulier syndrome have which of the following laboratory test findings?
   a. Abnormal platelet response to arachidonic acid
   b. Abnormal platelet response to ristocetin
   c. Abnormal platelet response to collagen
   d. Thrombocytosis

5. Which of the following is the most common of the hereditary platelet function defects?
   a. Glanzmann thrombasthenia
   b. Bernard-Soulier syndrome
   c. Storage pool defects
   d. Multiple myeloma

6. A mechanism of antiplatelet drugs targeting GP IIb/IIIa function is:
   a. Interference with platelet adhesion to the subendothelium by blocking of the collagen binding site
   b. Inhibition of transcription of the GP IIb/IIIa gene
   c. Direct binding to GP IIb/IIIa
   d. Interference with platelet secretion

7. The impaired platelet function in myeloproliferative neoplasms results from:
   a. Abnormally shaped platelets
   b. Extended platelet life span
   c. Increased procoagulant activity
   d. Decreased numbers of α- and dense granules

8. Which is a *congenital* qualitative platelet disorder?
   a. Senile purpura
   b. Ehlers-Danlos syndrome
   c. Henoch-Schönlein purpura
   d. Waldenström macroglobulinemia

9. In uremia, platelet function is impaired by higher than normal levels of:
   a. Urea
   b. Uric acid
   c. Creatinine
   d. NO

10. The platelet defect associated with increased paraproteins is:
    a. Impaired membrane activation owing to protein coating
    b. Hypercoagulability owing to antibody binding and membrane activation
    c. Impaired aggregation because the hyperviscous plasma prevents platelet-endothelium interaction
    d. Hypercoagulability because the increased proteins bring platelets closer together, which leads to inappropriate aggregation

REFERENCES

1. Triplett, D. A. (1978). How to evaluate platelet function. *Lab Med Pract Phys*, July-Aug, 37–43.
2. Thorup, O. A. (1987). *Leavell and Thorup's Fundamentals of Clinical Hematology*. (5th ed.). Philadelphia: Saunders.
3. Thompson, A. R., & Harker, L. A. (1983). *Manual of Hemostasis and Thrombosis*. (3rd ed.). Philadelphia: FA Davis.
4. Colvin, B. T. (1985). Thrombocytopenia, *Clin Haematol, 14*, 661–681.
5. Nurden, P., & Nurder, A. T. (2008). Congenital disorders associated with platelet dysfunctions. *Thromb Haemost, 99*, 253–263.
6. George, J. N., & Shattil, S. J. (1991). The clinical importance of acquired abnormalities of platelet function. *N Engl J Med, 324*, 27–39.
7. Caen, J. P. (1989). Glanzmann's thrombasthenia. *Baillieres Clin Haematol, 2*, 609–623.
8. Coller, B. S., Mitchell, W. B., & French, D. L. (2006). Hereditary qualitative platelet disorders. In Lichtman, M. A., Beutler, E., Kipps, T. J., et al., (Eds.), *Williams Hematology*. (7th ed., pp. 1795–1832). New York: McGraw-Hill.
9. Triplett, D. A., (Ed.). (1978). *Platelet Function: Laboratory Evaluation and Clinical Application*. Chicago: American Society of Clinical Pathologists.
10. Powers, L. W. (1989). *Diagnostic Hematology: Clinical and Technical Principles*. St Louis: Mosby.
11. Rapaport, S. I. (1987). *Introduction to Hematology*. (2nd ed.). Philadelphia: JB Lippincott.
12. Meyer, M., Kirchmaier, C. M., Schirmer, A., et al. (1991). Acquired disorder of platelet function associated with autoantibodies against membrane glycoprotein IIb-IIIa complex: 1. Glycoprotein analysis. *Thromb Haemost, 65*, 491–496.
13. Tarantino, M. D., Corrigan, J. J., Jr, Glasser, L., et al. (1991). A variant form of thrombasthenia. *Am J Dis Child, 145*, 1053–1057.
14. Friedlander, M., Brooks, P. C., Shaffer, R. W., et al. (1995). Definition of two angiogenic pathways by distinct a_v integrins. *Science, 270*, 1500–1502.
15. Nurden, A. T., & George, J. N. (2006). Inherited disorders of the platelet membrane: Glanzmann thrombasthenia, Bernard-Soulier syndrome and other disorders. In Colman, R. W., Marder, V. J., Clowes, A. W., et al., (Eds.), *Hemostasis and Thrombosis: basic Principles and Clinical Practice*. (5th ed., pp. 987–1010). Philadelphia: Lippincott Williams & Wilkins.
16. Nurden, A. T. (2005). Qualitative disorders of platelets and megakaryocytes. *J Thromb Haemost, 3*, 1773–1782.
17. Nurden, A. T., Fiore, M., Nurden, P., et al. (2011). Glanzmann thrombasthenia: a review of *ITGA2B* and *ITGB3* defects with emphasis on variants, phenotypic variability, and mouse models. *Blood, 118*(23), 5996–6005.
18. Coller, B. S., Cheresh, D. A., Asch, E., et al. (1991). Platelet vitronectin receptor expression differentiates Iraqi-Jewish from Arab patients with Glanzmann thrombasthenia in Israel. *Blood, 77*, 75–83.
19. French, D. L. (1998). The molecular genetics of Glanzmann's thrombasthenia. *Platelets, 9*, 5–20.
20. Corriveau, D. M., & Fritsma, G. A. (1988). *Hemostasis and Thrombosis in the Clinical Laboratory*. Philadelphia: JB Lippincott.
21. Rosa, J. P., Artçanuthurry, V., Grelac, F., et al. (1997). Reassessment of protein tyrosine phosphorylation in thrombasthenic platelets: evidence that phosphorylation of cortactin and a 64 kD protein is dependent on thrombin activation and integrin αIIbβ3. *Thromb Haemost, 89*, 4385–4392.
22. Byzova, T. V., & Plow, E. F. (1997). Networking in the hemostatic system: integrin αIIbβ3 binds prothrombin and influences its activation. *J Biol Chem, 272*, 27183–27188.
23. Gemmell, C. H., Sefton, M. V., & Yeo, E. L. (1993). Platelet-derived microparticle formation involves glycoprotein IIb-IIIa: inhibition by RGDs and a Glanzmann's thrombasthenia defect. *J Biol Chem, 268*, 14586–14589.
24. Reverter, J. C., Beguin, S., Kessels, H., et al. (1996). Inhibition of platelet-mediated tissue factor-induced thrombin generation by the mouse/human chimeric 7E3 antibody: potential implications for the effect of c7E3 Fab treatment on acute thrombosis and "clinical restenosis." *J Clin Invest, 98*, 863–874.
25. Caen, J. P. (1972). Glanzmann's thrombasthenia. *Clin Hematol, 1*, 383–392.
26. George, J. N., Caen, J. P., & Nurden, A. T. (1990). Glanzmann's thrombasthenia: the spectrum of clinical disease. *Blood, 75*, 1383–1395.
27. Jennings, L. K., Wang, W. C., Jackson, C. W., et al. (1991). Hemostasis in Glanzmann's thrombasthenia (GT): GT platelets interfere with the aggregation of normal platelets. *Am J Pediatr Hematol Oncol, 13*, 84–90.
28. Poon, M. C., d'Oiron, R., Von Depka, M., et al. (2004). International Data Collection on Recombinant Factor VIIa and Congenital Platelet Disorders Study Group: Prophylactic and therapeutic recombinant factor VIIa administration to patients with Glanzmann's thrombasthenia: results of an international survey. *J Thromb Haemost, 2*, 1096–1103.
29. Lisman, T., Adelmaier, J., Heijnen, H. F. G., et al. (2004). Recombinant factor VIIa restores aggregation of αIIb/β3-deficient platelets via tissue factor-independent fibrin generation. *Blood, 103*, 1720–1727.
30. Geddis, A. E., & Kaushansky, K. (2004). Inherited thrombocytopenias: toward a better molecular understanding of disorders of platelet production. *Curr Opin Pediatr, 16*, 15–24.
31. Nurden, P., & Nurden, A. (1996). Giant platelets, megakaryocytes and the expression of glycoprotein Ib-IX complexes. *C R Acad Sci III, 319*, 717–726.
32. Clementson, K. J. (1997). Platelet GP Ib-V-IX complex. *Thromb Haemost, 78*, 266–270.
33. Nurden, A. T. (1998). Inherited abnormalities of platelets. *Thromb Haemost, 82*, 468–480.
34. Lopez, J. A., Andrews, R. K., Afshar-Kharghan, V., et al. (1998). Bernard-Soulier syndrome. *Blood, 91*, 4397–4418.
35. Savoia, A., Pastore, A., De Rocco, D., et al. (2011). Clinical and genetic aspects of Bernard-Soulier syndrome: searching for genotype/phenotype correlations. *Haematologica, 96*(3), 417–423.

36. Sumitha, E., Jayandharan, G. R., David, S., et al. (2011). Molecular basis of Bernard-Soulier syndrome in 27 patients from India. *J Thromb Haemost, 9*(8), 1590.

37. Takahashi, H., Murata, M., Moriki, T., et al. (1995). Substitution of Val for Met at residue 239 of platelet glycoprotein Ib alpha in Japanese patients with platelet-type von Willebrand disease. *Blood, 85*, 727–733.

38. Matsubara, Y., Murata, M., Sugita, K., et al. (2003). Identification of a novel point mutation in platelet glycoprotein Ibα, Gly to Ser at residue 233, in a Japanese family with platelet-type von Willebrand disease. *J Thromb Haemost, 1*, 2198–2205.

39. Othman, M., Elbatarny, H. S., Notley, C., et al. (2004). Identification and functional characterization of a novel 27 bp deletion in the macroglycopeptide-coding region of the GPIbα gene resulting in platelet-type von Willebrand disease. *Blood, 104*(abstract 1023).

40. Mhawech, P., & Saleem, A. (2000). Inherited giant platelet disorders: classification and literature review. *AJCP, 113*, 176–190.

41. Pati, H., & Saraya, A. K. (1986). Platelet storage pool disease. *Indian J Med Res, 84*, 617–620.

42. Rao, A. K. (2006). Hereditary disorders of platelet secretion and signal transduction. In Colman, R. W., Marder, V. J., Clowes, A. W., et al., (Eds.), *Hemostasis and Thrombosis: Basic Principles and Clinical Practice.* (5th ed., pp. 961–974). Philadelphia: Lippincott Williams & Wilkins.

43. Weiss, H. J., Lages, B., Vicic, W., et al. (1993). Heterogeneous abnormalities of platelet dense granule ultrastructure in 20 patients with congenital storage pool deficiency. *Br J Haematol, 83*, 282–295.

44. Bennett, J. S. (2005). Hereditary disorders of platelet function. In Hoffman, R., Benz, E. J., Jr., Shattil, S. J., et al., (Eds.), *Hematology: Basic Principles and Practice.* (4th ed., pp. 2327–2345). Philadelphia: Churchill Livingstone.

45. Abrams, C. S., & Brass, L. F. (2006). Platelet signal transduction. In Colman, R. W., Marder, V. J., Clowes, A. W., et al., (Eds.), *Hemostasis and Thrombosis: Basic Principles and Clinical Practice.* (5th ed., pp. 617–630). Philadelphia: Lippincott Williams & Wilkins.

46. Jedlitschky, G., Tirwschmann, K., Lubenow, L. E., et al. (2004). The nucleotide transporter MRP4 (*ABCC4*) is highly expressed in human platelets and present in dense granules, indicating a role in mediator storage. *Blood, 104*, 3603–3610.

47. Spritz, R. A. (1998). Molecular genetics of the Hermansky-Pudlak and Chédiak-Higashi syndromes. *Platelets, 9*, 21–29.

48. Dell'Angellica, E. C., Aguilar, R. C., Wolins, N., et al. (2000). Molecular characterization of the protein encoded by the Hermansky-Pudlak syndrome type 1 gene. *J Biol Chem, 275*, 1300–1306.

49. White, J. G. (1987). Inherited abnormalities of the platelet membrane and secretory granules. *Hum Pathol, 18*, 123–139.

50. Villa, A., Notarangelo, L., Macchi, P., et al. (1995). X-linked thrombocytopenia and Wiskott-Aldrich syndrome are allelic diseases with mutations in the *WASP* gene. *Nat Genet, 9*(4), 414.

51. Lanzi, G., Moratto, D., Vairo, D., et al. (2012, Jan). A novel primary human immunodeficiency due to deficiency in the WASP-interacting protein WIP. *J Exp Med, 209*(1), 29–34.

52. Quick, A. J. (1966). *Hemorrhagic Diseases and Thrombosis.* (2nd ed.). Philadelphia: Lea & Febiger.

53. Cleary, A. M., Insel, R. A., & Lewis, D. B. (2005). Disorders of lymphocyte function. In Hoffman, R., Benz, E. J., Jr., Shattil, S. J., et al., (Eds.), *Hematology: Basic Principles and Practice.* (4th ed., pp. 831–855). Philadelphia: Churchill Livingstone.

54. de Alarcon, P. A., Graeve, J. A., Levine, R. F., et al. (1991). Thrombocytopenia and absent radii syndrome: defective megakaryocytopoiesis-thrombocytopoiesis. *Am J Pediatr Hematol Oncol, 13*, 77–83.

55. Raccuglia, G. (1971). Gray platelet syndrome: a variety of qualitative platelet disorder. *Am J Med, 51*, 818–828.

56. Gunay-Aygun, M., Zivony-Elboum, Y., Gumruk, F., et al. (2010). Gray platelet syndrome: natural history of a large patient cohort and locus assignment to chromosome 3p. *Blood, 116*(23), 4990.

57. Gunay-Aygun, M., Falik-Zaccai, T. C., Vilboux, T., et al. (2011). *NBEAL2* is mutated in gray platelet syndrome and is required for biogenesis of platelet α granules. *Nat Genet, 43*(8), 732.

58. Berrebi, A., Klepfish, A., Varon, D., et al. (1988). Gray platelet syndrome in the elderly. *Am J Hematol, 28*, 270–272.

59. Pfueller, S. L., Howard, M. A., White, J. G., et al. (1987). Shortening of the bleeding time by 1-deamino-8-arginine vasopressin (DDAVP) in the absence of platelet von Willebrand factor in gray platelet syndrome. *Thromb Haemost, 58*, 1060–1063.

60. Brace, L. D., Venton, D. L., Le Breton, G. C. (1985). Thromboxane A$_2$/prostaglandin H$_2$ mobilizes calcium in human blood platelets. *Am J Physiol, 249*, H1–H7.

61. Moake, J. L., & Funicella, T. (1983). Common bleeding problems. *Clin Symp, 35*, 1–32.

62. Nieuwenhuis, H. K., Sakariassen, K. S., Houdijk, W. P. M., et al. (1986). Deficiency of platelet membrane glycoprotein Ia associated with a decreased platelet adhesion to subendothelium: a defect in platelet spreading. *Blood, 68*, 692–695.

63. Moroi, M., Jung, S. M., Okuma, M., et al. (1989). A patient with platelets deficient in glycoprotein VI that lack both collagen-induced aggregation and adhesion. *J Clin Invest, 84*, 1440–1445.

64. Nurden, P., Jandrot-Perrus, M., Combrie, R., et al. (2004). Severe deficiency of glycoprotein VI in a patient with gray platelet syndrome. *Blood, 104*, 107–114.

65. Cattaneo, M. (2003). Inherited platelet-based bleeding disorders. *J Thromb Haemost, 1*, 1628–1636.

66. Daniel, J. L., Dangelmaier, C., Jin, J., et al. (1998). Molecular basis for ADP-induced platelet activation: I. Evidence for three distinct ADP receptors on human platelets. *J Biol Chem, 273*, 2024–2029.

67. Nurden, P., Savi, P., Heilmann, E., et al. (1995). An inherited bleeding disorder linked to a defective interaction between ADP and its receptor on platelets. *J Clin Invest, 95*, 1612–1622.

68. Cattaneo, M., Zighetti, M. L., Lombardi, R., et al. (2003). Molecular basis of defective signal transduction in the platelet P2Y12 receptor of a patient with congenital bleeding. *Proc Natl Acad Sci U S A, 100*, 1978–1983.

69. Rao, A. K. (1998). Congenital disorders of platelet function: disorders of signal transduction and secretion. *Am J Med Sci, 316*, 69–76.

70. Rao, A. K. (2003). Inherited defects in platelet signaling mechanisms. *J Thromb Haemost, 1*, 671–681.

71. Zhou, Q., Sims, P. J., & Wiedmer, T. (1998). Expression of proteins controlling transbilayer movement of plasma membrane phospholipids in B lymphocytes from a patient with Scott syndrome. *Blood, 92*, 1707–1712.

72. Zhou, Q., Zhao, J., Stout, J. G., et al. (1997). Molecular cloning of human plasma membrane phospholipid scramblase: a protein mediating transbilayer movement of plasma membrane phospholipids. *J Biol Chem, 272*, 18240–18244.

73. Zwaal, R. F., Comfurius, P., & Bevers, E. M. (2004). Scott syndrome, a bleeding disorder caused by a defective scrambling of membrane phospholipids. *Biochim Biophys Acta, 1636*, 119–128.

74. Sims, P., & Wiedmer, T. (2001). Unraveling the mysteries of phospholipid scrambling. *Thromb Haemost, 86*, 266–275.

75. Stormorken, H., Holmsen, H., Sund, R., et al. (1995). Studies on the haemostatic defect in a complicated syndrome: an inverse Scott syndrome platelet membrane abnormality? *Thromb Haemost, 74*, 1244–1251.

76. Helgason, C. M., Bolin, K. M., Hoff, J. A., et al. (1994). Development of aspirin resistance in persons with previous ischemic stroke. *Stroke, 25*, 2331–2336.

77. Helgason, C. M., Tortorice, K. L., Winkler, S. R., et al. (1993). Aspirin response and failure in cerebral infarction. *Stroke, 24,* 345–350.

78. Beardsley, D. S. (1991). Hemostasis in the perinatal period: approach to the diagnosis of coagulation disorders. *Semin Perinatol, 15*(Suppl. 2), 25–34.

79. Eikelboom, J. W., Hirsh, J., Weitz, J., et al. (2002). Aspirin-resistant thromboxane biosynthesis and the risk of myocardial infarction, stroke, or cardiovascular death in patients at high risk for cardiovascular events. *Circulation, 105,* 1650–1655.

80. Green, D. (1988). Diagnosis and management of bleeding disorders. *Compr Ther, 14,* 31–36.

81. Bick, R. L., & Scates, S. M. (1992). Qualitative platelet defects. *Lab Med, 23,* 95–103.

82. Haut, M. J., & Cowan, D. H. (1974). The effect of ethanol on hemostatic properties of human blood platelets. *Am J Med, 56,* 22–33.

83. Schleinitz, M. D., & Heidenreich, P. A. (2005). A cost-effectiveness analysis of combination antiplatelet therapy of high-risk acute coronary syndromes: clopidogrel plus aspirin versus aspirin alone. *Ann Intern Med, 142,* 251–259.

84. Wilhite, D. B., Comerota, A. J., Schmieder, F. A., et al. (2003). Managing PAD with multiple platelet inhibitors: the effect of combination therapy on bleeding time. *J Vasc Surg, 38,* 710–713.

85. Coller, B. S. (1997). GPIIb/IIIa antagonists: pathophysiologic and therapeutic insights from studies of c7E3 Fab. *Thromb Haemost, 78,* 730–735.

86. Tcheng, J. E. (1997). Platelet glycoprotein IIb/IIIa integrin blockade: recent clinical trials in interventional cardiology. *Thromb Haemost, 78,* 205–209.

87. Van de Werf, F. (1997). Clinical trials with glycoprotein IIb/IIIa receptor antagonists in acute coronary syndromes. *Thromb Haemost, 78,* 210–213.

88. Lopez, J., & Thiagarajan, P. (2005). Acquired disorders of platelet function. In Hoffman, R., Benz, E. J., Jr., & Shattil, S. J., (Eds.), *Hematology: Basic Principles and Practice,* (4th ed., pp. 2347–2367). Philadelphia: Churchill Livingstone.

89. Landolfi, R., Marchioli, R., & Patrono, C. (1997). Mechanisms of bleeding and thrombosis in myeloproliferative disorders. *Thromb Haemost, 78,* 617–621.

90. Swart, S. S., Pearson, D., Wood, J. K., et al. (1984). Functional significance of the platelet alpha$_2$-adrenoreceptor: studies in patients with myeloproliferative disorders. *Thromb Res, 33,* 531–541.

91. Bosch, J., Thabut, D., Bendtsen, F., et al. (2004). Recombinant factor VIIa for upper gastrointestinal bleeding in patients with cirrhosis: a randomized, double-blind trial. *Gastroenterology, 127,* 1123–1130.

92. Boccardo, P., Remuzzi, G., & Galbusera, M. (2004). Platelet dysfunction in renal failure. *Semin Thromb Hemost, 30,* 579–589.

93. Martinez, J., & Ferber, A. (2005). Disorders of fibrinogen. In Hoffman, R., Benz, E. J., Jr., Shattil, S. J., et al., (Eds.), *Hematology: Basic Principles and Practice.* (4th ed., pp. 2097–2109). Philadelphia: Churchill Livingstone.

94. Eldrup-Jorgensen, J., Flanigan, D. P., Brace, L. D., et al. (1989). Hypercoagulable states and lower limb ischemia in young adults. *J Vasc Surg, 9,* 334–341.

95. Helgason, C. M., Hoff, J. A., Kondos, G. T., et al. (1993). Platelet aggregation in patients with atrial fibrillation taking aspirin or warfarin. *Stroke, 24,* 1458–1461.

96. Pareti, F. I., Capitanio, A., Mannucci, L., et al. (1980). Acquired dysfunction due to circulation of "exhausted" platelets. *Am J Med, 69,* 235–240.

97. Coller, B. S., & Schneiderman, P. I. (2005). Clinical evaluation of hemorrhagic disorders: the bleeding history and differential diagnosis of purpura. In Hoffman, R., Benz, E. J., Jr., Shattil, S. J., et al., (Eds.), *Hematology: Basic Principles and Practice.* (4th ed., pp. 1824–1840). Philadelphia: Churchill Livingstone.

98. Maceyko, R. F., & Camisa, C. (1991). Kasabach-Merritt syndrome. *Pediatr Dermatol, 8,* 133–136.

99. Brace, L. D. (1981). The multiple myelomas: a review of selected aspects. *Allied Health Behav Sci, 3,* 47–61.

100. Gertz, M. A., Lacy, M. Q., & Dispenzieri, A. (2005). Amyloidosis. In Hoffman, R., Benz, E. J., Jr., Shattil, S. J., et al., (Eds.), *Hematology: Basic Principles and Practice.* (4th ed., pp. 1537–1560). Philadelphia: Churchill Livingstone.

42

Laboratory Evaluation of Hemostasis

George A. Fritsma

OBJECTIVES

After completion of this chapter, the reader will be able to:

1. Properly collect and transport hemostasis blood specimens.
2. Reject hemostasis blood specimens due to clots, short draws, or hemolysis.
3. Prepare hemostasis blood specimens for analysis.
4. Describe the principles of platelet aggregometry.
5. Apply appropriate platelet function tests in a variety of conditions and interpret their results.
6. Diagnose von Willebrand disease and monitor its treatment.
7. Analyze plasma markers of platelet activation platelet factor 4 and β-thromboglobulin.
8. Describe the principle of, appropriately select, and correctly interpret the results of clot-based coagulation screening tests, including activated clotting time, prothrombin time, partial thromboplastin time, and the thrombin clotting time.
9. Interpret clot-based screening test results collectively to reach presumptive diagnoses, and then recommend and perform confirmatory tests.
10. Perform partial thromboplastin time mixing studies to detect factor deficiencies, lupus anticoagulants, and specific factor inhibitors.
11. Describe the principle of, appropriately select, and correctly interpret coagulation factor assays.
12. Describe the principle of and correctly interpret Bethesda titers for coagulation factor inhibitors.
13. Describe the principle of, appropriately select, and correctly interpret tests of fibrinolysis, including assays for D-dimer, plasminogen, plasminogen activators, and plasminogen activator inhibitors.
14. Interpret global coagulation assay tracings: Thromboelastograph and ROTEM.

CASE STUDY

After studying the material in this chapter, the reader should be able to respond to the following case study:

A 54-year-old woman experienced a pulmonary embolism on September 26 and began oral anticoagulant therapy. Monthly PT values were collected to monitor therapy. From October through January, her INR was stable at 2.4, but on February 1, her INR was 1.3. The reduced INR was reported to her physician.

On questioning, the patient reported that there had been no change in her warfarin (Coumadin) dosage or in her diet. She recalled, however, that the phlebotomist had used a tube with a red-and-black stopper. She had thought this to be out of the ordinary and had remarked about it to the phlebotomist, who made no response. The medical laboratory practitioner who had performed the PT assay reexamined the blood specimen and saw that it was in a blue-topped tube.

1. What did the phlebotomist do?
2. What was the consequence of this action?
3. What else could cause an unexpectedly short PT?

HEMOSTASIS SPECIMEN COLLECTION

Most hemostasis laboratory procedures are performed on venous whole blood collected by venipuncture and mixed 9:1 with a 3.2% solution of sodium citrate anticoagulant. The specimen is maintained as well-mixed whole blood for platelet function testing or centrifuged to provide platelet-poor plasma (PPP) for other procedures. Phlebotomists, patient care technicians, nurses, medical laboratory practitioners, and other health personnel who collect blood specimens must adhere closely to published protocols for specimen collection and management. The nursing or laboratory supervisor is responsible for the current validity of specimen collection and handling protocols and ensures that personnel employ approved techniques.[1]

Patient Management During Hemostasis Specimen Collection

Patients need not fast, but they should avoid vigorous activities and should rest quietly for 30 minutes prior to collection for hemostasis testing. Little additional preparation is necessary; however, there are numerous drugs that affect the outcomes of coagulation tests. For example, aspirin suppresses most platelet function, and Coumadin (warfarin) reduces the activities of factor II (prothrombin), factor VII, factor IX, factor X, protein C, protein S, and protein Z and prolongs the prothrombin time (PT) test. The phlebotomist should attempt to record all drugs the patient is currently taking, and patients should be instructed by their physicians to discontinue drugs that may interfere with coagulation test results before testing.

Phlebotomists may manage patients using standard protocols for identification, cleansing, tourniquet use, and venipuncture (Chapter 3). If there is a reason to anticipate excessive bleeding—for instance, if the patient has multiple bruises or mentions a tendency to bleed—the phlebotomist should extend the time for observing the venipuncture site from 1 to 5 minutes and should apply a pressure bandage before dismissing the patient.

Hemostasis Specimen Collection Tubes

Most hemostasis specimens are collected in *plastic blue-stopper* (blue-top, blue-closure) *sterile evacuated blood collection tubes* containing a measured volume of 0.105 to 0.109 M (3.2%) buffered sodium citrate anticoagulant.[2] Tubes of uncoated soda-lime glass are unsuitable because their negative surface charge activates platelets and plasma procoagulants. *Siliconized* (plastic-coated) glass tubes are available, but their use is waning because of concern for potential breakage, with consequent risk of exposure to bloodborne pathogens.[3]

Hemostasis Specimen Collection Protocol

Laboratory directors typically prefer evacuated blood collection tube systems for hemostasis blood collections; however, many directors may require syringe collection and initial "discard tubes" in special circumstances. Table 42-1 provides a list of collection errors.

- If the hemostasis specimen is part of a *series of tubes* to be filled from a single venipuncture site, it must be collected *first* or immediately after a *nonadditive tube*. The hemostasis tube may not immediately follow a tube that contains heparin (green stopper), ethylenediamine tetraacetic acid (EDTA,

TABLE 42-1 Hemostasis Specimen Collection Errors That Require Collection of a New Specimen

Error	Comments
Short draw	Whole-blood volume less than 90% of required volume or less than manufacturer specified minimum.
Clot in specimen	Each specimen must be visually inspected prior to centrifugation; the presence of even a small clot requires that the specimen be recollected.
Visible hemolysis	Hemolysis, pink or red plasma indicates in vitro activation of platelets and coagulation. Results are unreliable.
Lipemia or icterus	Optical instruments may not measure clots in cloudy or highly colored specimens, especially chromogenic substrate methods. The practitioner must employ a mechanical instrument.
Prolonged tourniquet application	Stasis elevates the concentration of von Willebrand factor and factor VIII; falsely decreases fibrinolytic parameters; and falsely shortens clot-based test results.
Specimen storage at 1° C to 6° C	Storage at refrigerator temperatures causes precipitation of large von Willebrand factor multimers, activation of coagulation factor VII, and destroys platelet integrity.
Specimen storage at more than 25° C	Storage at above standard room temperature causes coagulation factors V and VIII to deteriorate.

lavender stopper), sodium fluoride (gray stopper), or clot-promoting *silica* particles as contained in plastic red-topped or serum separator (gel) tubes. These additives may become transferred to the hemostasis specimen on the stopper needle and invalidate all hemostasis test results. Nonadditive tubes include red-topped glass tubes and clear-topped or red-and-gray marble-topped tubes. If nonadditive tubes are unavailable, the phlebotomist may use and discard a preliminary blue-topped tube.[4] Some hemostasis laboratory directors specify that a nonadditive tube be collected and discarded prior to the hemostasis specimen when the specimen is intended for platelet function studies or specialized coagulation assays. Their purpose is to ensure the absence of tissue contaminants in the specimen.

- The ratio of whole blood to anticoagulant must be 9 parts blood to 1 part anticoagulant. Evacuated tubes are designed so that the negative internal pressure draws the correct volume of blood from the vein. Collection tube manufacturers indicate the allowable range of collection volume error in package inserts and provide a minimum volume line on each tube. In most cases, the volume of blood collected must be within 90% of the calibrated volume. A *short draw*—that is, a specimen with a smaller volume than the minimum specified by the manufacturer—generates erroneously prolonged clot-based coagulation test results because the excess anticoagulant relative to blood volume neutralizes test reagent calcium.[5] Short-draw specimens are consistently discarded, and a fresh specimen is collected from the patient. Most plastic blue-topped tubes collect 2.7 mL of whole blood; the smaller the collection tube, the narrower the tolerance for short draws.

- When specimens are collected using *winged-needle butterfly sets,* the phlebotomist must compensate for the internal volume of the tubing, which is usually 12 inches long and contains approximately 0.5 mL of air. The phlebotomist must first collect and discard a nonadditive tube or an identical blue-topped tube. This step ensures that the needle set tubing is filled with fresh patient blood before the hemostasis specimen is collected.[6]

- *Clotted specimens* are useless for hemostasis testing, even if the clot is small. A few seconds after collection, the phlebotomist must gently invert the specimen at least *five times* to mix the blood with the anticoagulant and prevent clot formation. If possible, the medical laboratory practitioner must visually examine for clots just before centrifugation and testing. Many coagulometers are equipped to detect the presence of clots. Clotted specimens are discarded, and a new specimen is collected from the patient.

- Excessive specimen agitation causes hemolysis (RBC rupture), procoagulant activation, and platelet activation. The phlebotomist must *never shake the tube.* The test results from visibly hemolyzed specimens are unreliable, and the specimen must be recollected.[7]

- Excess needle manipulation may promote the release of procoagulant substances from the skin and connective tissue, which contaminate the specimen and cause clotting

factor activation. Consequently, test results from specimens collected during a *traumatic* venipuncture may be falsely shortened and unreliable.[8]

- During blood collection, the phlebotomist must remove the tourniquet within 1 minute of its application to avoid blood *stasis.*[9] Stasis is a condition in which venous flow is slowed. Stasis results in the local accumulation of coagulation factor VIII and von Willebrand factor (VWF), which may result in false shortening of clot-based coagulation test results.

Specimen Collection Using Syringes and Winged-Needle Sets

Managers of many hemostasis specialty laboratories insist that specimens from patients with difficult venous access and patients whose veins are small, fragile, or scarred by repeated venipunctures be collected by syringe. Additionally, in an effort to reduce the activation of platelets and coagulation, specimens for specialized tests such as platelet aggregometry are collected by syringe. Many hemostasis laboratories employ medical laboratory practitioners and phlebotomists who are specially trained in specimen collection to ensure the integrity of the specimen. The use of syringes presents additional needle-stick risk to the phlebotomist, so careful training and handling are essential.[10]

The phlebotomist selects sterile syringes of 20 mL capacity or less with nonthreaded Luer-slip hubs. The phlebotomist assembles syringes, a winged needle set (Figure 42-1), a tubing clamp, and standard venipuncture materials. The phlebotomist then uses the following protocol:

1. Use standard patient identification and standard blood specimen management precautions (Chapter 3).
2. Most syringes are delivered with the plunger withdrawn about 1 mm from the end of the barrel. Move the plunger outward and inward within the barrel. Expel all air from the barrel and affix the needle set to the Luer-slip hub.
3. Cleanse the venipuncture site, affix the tourniquet, and insert the winged needle. Immobilize the needle set by loosely taping the tube to the arm about 2 inches from the needle.
4. Fill the syringe using a gentle, even pressure.
5. Place the syringe on a clean surface and clamp the tubing with a hemostat near the needle hub.
6. Remove the first syringe and discard to avoid tissue contamination of the hemostasis specimen. The phlebotomist may use this specimen for chemistry or other tests. Attach a second syringe for collection of the hemostasis specimen; release the clamp and fill the second syringe. Repeat if needed.
7. Replace the clamp, remove the needle set, and immediately activate the needle cover.

After seeing to the patient's welfare, the phlebotomist cautiously transfers the blood specimen to sealed evacuated tubes by affixing a safety transfer device. The specimen is allowed to flow gently down the side of the tube. The specimen is not pushed forcibly into the tube, because agitation causes hemolysis and platelet activation. The phlebotomist must transfer the specimen within a few seconds of the time the syringe is filled, and the tube

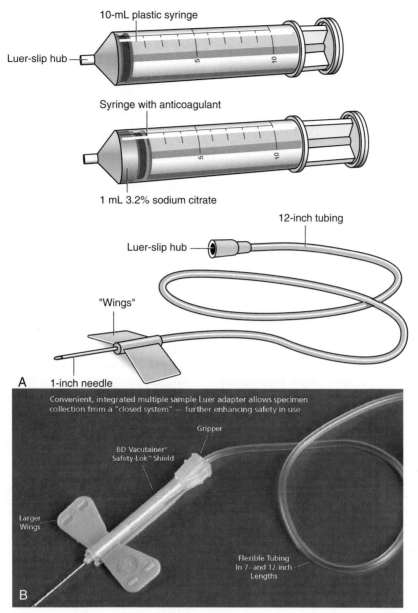

Figure 42-1 **A,** Winged needle set and syringe for collecting special hemostasis specimens. The phlebotomist may use the option of drawing the desired volume of anticoagulant into the syringe prior to blood collection. **B,** Winged needle illustrating needle-covering safety interlock.

must be gently inverted at least five times. The specimen volume must be correct for the proper ratio of blood to sodium citrate.

Selection of Needles for Hemostasis Specimens

Whether evacuated collection tubes or syringes are used, the bore of the needle should be sufficient to prevent hemolysis and activation of platelets and plasma procoagulants. If the overall specimen is 25 mL or less, a 20- or 21-gauge thin-walled needle is used (Table 42-2). For a larger specimen, a 19-gauge needle is required. A 23-gauge needle is acceptable for pediatric patients or patients whose veins are small, but the negative collection pressure must be reduced. All needles provide safety

closures that either cover or blunt the needle immediately after completion of the venipuncture.

Specimen Collection from Vascular Access Devices

Blood specimens may be drawn from heparin or saline locks, ports in intravenous lines, peripherally inserted central catheters (PICC tubes), central venous catheters, or dialysis catheters. Vascular access device management requires strict adherence to protocol to ensure sterility, prevent emboli, and prevent damage to the device. Personnel must be trained and must recognize the signs of complications and take appropriate action. Institutional protocol may limit vascular

TABLE 42-2 Selection of Needles for Hemostasis Specimens

Application	Preferred Needle Gauge and Length
Adult with good veins, specimen ≤25 mL	20 or 21 gauge, thin-walled, 1.0 or 1.25 inches long
Adult with good veins, specimen ≥25 mL	19 gauge, 1.0 or 1.25 inches long
Child or adult with small, friable, or hardened veins	23 gauge, winged-needle set; apply minimal negative pressure
Transfer of blood from syringe to tube	19 gauge, slowly inject through tube closure
Syringe with winged-needle set	20, 21, or 23 gauge, thin-walled; use only for small, friable, or hardened veins or specialized coagulation testing

access device blood collection to physicians and nurses. Before blood is collected for hemostasis testing, the line must be flushed with 5 mL of saline, and the first 5 mL of blood, or six times the volume of the tube, must be collected and discarded. The phlebotomist *must not flush with heparin.* Blood is collected into a syringe and transferred to an evacuated tube as described in the prior section on hemostasis specimen collection with syringes and winged needle sets.[11]

Specimen Collection Using Capillary Puncture

Several near-patient testing (point-of-care) coagulometers (Chapter 44) generate PT results from a specimen consisting of 10 to 50 μL of whole blood. These instruments are designed to test either anticoagulated venous whole blood or capillary (finger-stick) blood and represent a significant convenience to patients and to anticoagulation clinics.[12] Many are designed for patient self-testing and pediatric or neonatal testing, and laboratory practitioners are often charged with training patients in proper capillary puncture technique.[13]

Capillary specimen punctures are made using sterile spring-loaded lancets designed to make a cut of standard depth and width, while avoiding injury (Chapter 3). The phlebotomist or patient selects and cleanses the middle or fourth (ring) finger and activates the device so that it produces a puncture that is just off-center of the fingertip and perpendicular to the fingerprint lines. After wiping away the first drop of blood, which is likely to be contaminated by tissue fluid, the phlebotomist places the collection device directly adjacent to the free-flowing blood and allows the device to fill. The phlebotomist wipes excess blood from the outside of the device and introduces it to the coagulometer to complete the assay. The phlebotomist then presses a gauze pad to the wound and instructs the patient to maintain pressure until bleeding ceases. The phlebotomist then provides a spot bandage to cover the wound.

The key to accurate PT measurement is a free-flowing puncture. Often it is necessary for the phlebotomist to warm the patient's hand to increase blood flow to the fingertips. Blood collection device distributors provide dry, disposable warming devices for this purpose. The phlebotomist avoids squeezing ("milking") the finger, because this renders the blood specimen inaccurate by raising the concentration of tissue fluid relative to blood cells.[14]

Anticoagulants Used for Hemostasis Specimens

Sodium Citrate (Primary Hemostasis Anticoagulant)

The anticoagulant used for hemostasis testing is buffered 3.2% (0.105 to 0.109 M) sodium citrate, $Na_3C_6H_5O_7 \cdot 2H_2O$, molecular weight 294.1 Daltons. Sodium citrate binds calcium ions to prevent coagulation, and the buffer stabilizes specimen pH as long as the tube stopper remains in place.[15]

The anticoagulant solution is mixed with blood to produce a 9:1 ratio: 9 parts whole blood to 1 part anticoagulant. In most cases, 0.3 mL of anticoagulant is mixed with 2.7 mL of whole blood, which are the volumes in the most commonly used evacuated plastic collection tubes, but any volumes are valid, provided that the 9:1 ratio is maintained. The ratio yields a final citrate concentration of 10.5 to 10.9 mM of anticoagulant in whole blood.[16] Some laboratory practitioners prepare specimen tubes locally for special hemostasis testing.

Adjustment of Sodium Citrate Volume for Elevated Hematocrits

The 9:1 blood-to-anticoagulant ratio is effective, provided the patient's hematocrit is 55% or less. In polycythemia, the decrease in plasma volume relative to whole blood unacceptably raises the anticoagulant-to-plasma ratio, which causes falsely prolonged results for clot-based coagulation tests. The phlebotomist must provide tubes with relatively reduced anticoagulant volumes for collection of blood from a patient whose hematocrit is known to be 55% or higher. The amount of anticoagulant needed may be computed for a 5 mL total specimen volume by using the graph in Figure 42-2 or the following formula, which is valid for any total volume:

$$C = (1.85 \times 10^{-3})(100 - H)V$$

where C is the volume of sodium citrate in milliliters, V is volume of whole blood-sodium citrate solution in milliliters, and H is the hematocrit in percent.

For example, to collect 3 mL of blood and anticoagulant mixture from a patient who has a hematocrit of 65%, calculate the volume of sodium citrate as follows:

$$C = (1.85 \times 10^{-3})(100 - 65\%) \times 3.0 \text{ mL}$$
$$C = (1.85 \times 10^{-3})(35\%) \times 3.0 \text{ mL}$$
$$C = 0.19 \text{ mL of } 3.2\% \text{ sodium citrate}$$

Remove the stopper from the blue closure collection tube, pipette and discard 0.11 mL from the 0.3 mL of anticoagulant, leaving 0.19 mL. Collect blood in a syringe and transfer

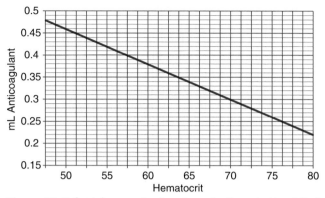

Figure 42-2 Graph for computing the volume of anticoagulant in a 5.0 mL specimen when the patient's hematocrit is 55% or greater. (From Ingram GIC, Brozovic M, Slater NGP: *Bleeding disorders, investigations, and management*, ed 2, Oxford, 1982, Blackwell, pp. 244-245.)

2.81 (2.8) mL of blood to the tube, replace the stopper, and immediately mix by gently inverting four times. Alternatively, the laboratory practitioner can prepare for collection of 10 mL of blood and anticoagulant solution in a 12 mL centrifuge tube as follows:

$$C = (1.85 \times 10^{-3})(35\%) \times 10.0 \text{ mL}$$
$$C = 0.64 \text{ mL of 3.2\% sodium citrate}$$

In this instance, 0.64 mL of sodium citrate is pipetted into the tube, and 9.36 (9.4) mL of whole blood is transferred from the collection syringe. There is no evidence suggesting a need for increasing the volume of anticoagulant for specimens from patients with anemia, even when the hematocrit is less than 20%.

Other Anticoagulants Used for Hemostasis Specimens

EDTA-anticoagulated specimens are not used for coagulation testing because calcium ion chelation by EDTA is irreversible, interfering with coagulation assays.[17] Calcium ion chelation with citrate, on the other hand, is reversed with the addition of calcium. EDTA is the anticoagulant used in collecting specimens for complete blood counts, including platelet counts.

EDTA may be required for specimens used for *molecular* diagnostic testing, such as testing for *factor V Leiden mutation* or the *prothrombin G20210A mutation*. Likewise, acid citrate dextrose (ACD, yellow stopper) and dipotassium EDTA (K_2EDTA) with gel (white stopper) tubes may be used for molecular diagnosis, as specified by institutional protocol. Heparinized specimens have never been validated for use in plasma coagulation testing but may be necessary in cases of platelet satellitosis (satellitism) as a substitute for specimens collected in EDTA or sodium citrate. *Citrate theophylline adenosine dipyridamole* (CTAD, blue stopper) tubes are used to halt in vitro platelet or coagulation activation for specialty assays such as those for the platelet activation markers *platelet factor 4* (PF4) and platelet surface membrane *P-selectin* (measured by flow cytometry) or the coagulation activation markers *prothrombin fragment 1+2* and *thrombin-antithrombin complex.*

HEMOSTASIS SPECIMEN MANAGEMENT

Hemostasis Specimen Storage Temperature

Sodium citrate-anticoagulated whole blood specimens are placed in a rack and allowed to stand in a vertical position with the stopper intact and uppermost. The pH remains constant as long as the specimen is sealed. Specimens are maintained at 18° C to 24° C (ambient temperature), never at refrigerator temperatures (Table 42-3). Storage at 1° C to 6° C activates factor VII, destroys platelet activity through uncontrolled activation, and causes the cryoprecipitation of large VWF multimers.[18,19] Also, specimens should never be stored at temperatures greater than 24° C because heat causes deterioration of coagulation factors V and VIII.

Hemostasis Specimen Storage Time

Specimens collected for PT testing may be held at 18° C to 24° C and tested within 24 hours of the time of collection. Specimens collected for partial thromboplastin time (PTT) testing also may be held at 18° C to 24° C, but they must be tested within 4 hours of the time of collection, provided that the specimen does not contain unfractionated heparin anticoagulant. If a patient is getting unfractionated heparin therapy, specimens for PTT testing must be centrifuged within 1 hour of the time of collection, and the plasma, which should be PPP, must be tested within 4 hours of the time of collection.[20]

TABLE 42-3 Hemostasis Specimen Storage Times and Temperatures

Application	Temperature	Time
PT with no unfractionated heparin present in specimen	18–24° C	24 hours
PTT with no unfractionated heparin present in specimen	18–24° C	4 hours
PTT for monitoring unfractionated heparin therapy	18–24° C	Separate within 1 hour, test within 4 hours
PT when unfractionated heparin is present in specimen	18–24° C	Separate within 1 hour, test within 4 hours
Factor assays	18–24° C	4 hours
Optical platelet aggregometry using platelet-rich plasma	18–24° C	Wait 30 min after centrifugation, test within 4 hours of collection
Whole-blood aggregometry	18–24° C	Test within 3 hours of collection
Storage in household freezer	−20° C	2 weeks
Storage for 6 months	−70° C	6 months

PT, Prothrombin time; *PTT,* partial thromboplastin time.

Preparation of Hemostasis Specimens for Assay

Whole-Blood Specimens Used for Platelet Aggregometry

Blood for whole-blood platelet aggregometry or lumiaggregometry must be collected with 3.2% sodium citrate and held at 18° C to 24° C until testing. Chilling destroys platelet activity. Aggregometry should be started immediately and must be completed within 4 hours of specimen collection. The practitioner mixes the specimen by gentle inversion, checks for clots just before testing, and rejects specimens with clots. Most specimens for whole-blood aggregometry are mixed 1:1 with normal saline before testing, although if the platelet count is less than 100,000/μL the specimen is tested undiluted.[21]

Platelet-Rich Plasma Specimens Used for Platelet Aggregometry

Light-transmittance (optical) platelet aggregometers are designed to test platelet-rich plasma (PRP), plasma with a platelet count of 200,000 to 300,000/μL. Sodium citrate–anticoagulated blood is first checked visually for clots and then centrifuged at 50 *xg* for 30 minutes with the stopper in place to maintain the pH. The supernatant PRP is transferred by a plastic pipette to a clean plastic tube, and the tube is sealed and stored at 18° C to 24° C (ambient temperature) until the test is begun. PRP-based light-transmittance aggregometry is initiated no less than 30 minutes after the specimen is centrifuged and completed within 4 hours of the time of collection. To produce sufficient PRP, the original specimen must measure 9 to 12 mL of whole blood. Light-transmittance aggregometry is unreliable when the patient's whole-blood platelet count is less than 100,000/μL.

Platelet-Poor Plasma Required for Clot-Based Testing

Clot-based plasma coagulation tests require PPP-plasma with a platelet count of less than 10,000/μL.[22] Sodium citrate-anticoagulated whole blood is centrifuged at 1500 *xg* for 15 minutes in a *swinging bucket* centrifuge to produce supernatant PPP. Alternatively, the *angle-head* StatSpin Express 2 (Iris Sample Processing, Inc., Westwood, MA) generates 4400 *xg* and can produce PPP within 3 minutes. Both make it possible for automated coagulometers to sample from the supernatant plasma of the primary blood collection tube. The advantage of the slower swinging bucket centrifuge head is that it produces a straight, level plasma-blood cell interface, whereas angle-head centrifuge heads cause platelets to adhere to the side of the tube. If the "angle-spun" tube is allowed to stand, the adherent platelets drift back into the plasma and release granule contents. Each hemostasis laboratory manager establishes the correct centrifugation speed and times for the local laboratory. Centrifugation must yield PPP from specimens with high initial platelet counts.

In the special hemostasis laboratory the manager may choose a *double-spin* approach. The primary tube is centrifuged using a swinging bucket centrifuge, and the plasma is transferred to a secondary plastic tube, which is labeled and centrifuged again. The double-spin approach may be used to produce PPP with a plasma platelet count of less than 5000/μL, which some laboratory directors prefer for lupus anticoagulant (LA) testing and for preparation of frozen plasma.

The presence of greater than 10,000 platelets/μL in plasma affects clot-based test results. Platelets are likely to become activated in vitro and release the membrane phospholipid *phosphatidylserine*, which triggers plasma coagulation and neutralizes LA if present, interfering with LA testing. Platelets also secrete fibrinogen, factors V and VIII, and VWF (Chapter 13). These may desensitize PT and PTT assays and interfere with clot-based coagulation assays. In addition, platelets release platelet factor 4 (PF4), a protein that binds and neutralizes therapeutic heparin in vitro, falsely shortening the PTT and interfering with heparin management.

The hemostasis laboratory manager arranges to perform plasma platelet counts on coagulation plasmas at regular intervals to ensure that they are consistently platelet poor. Many managers select 10 to 12 specimens from each centrifuge every 6 months, perform plasma platelet counts, and document that their samples remain appropriately platelet poor, even if the initial platelet count is elevated.

Laboratory practitioners inspect hemostasis plasmas for hemolysis (red), lipemia (cloudy, milky), and icterus (golden yellow from bilirubin). Visible hemolysis implies platelet or coagulation pathway activation. Visibly hemolyzed specimens are rejected, and new specimens must be obtained. Lipemia and icterus may affect the end-point results of optical coagulation instruments. The hemostasis laboratory manager may choose to maintain a separate mechanical end-point coagulometer to substitute for the optical instrument if the specimen is too cloudy for optical determinations. Conversely, some optical instruments detect and compensate for lipemia and icterus via spectrophotometric analysis.[23]

Specimen Storage

Specimens for PT assay only may be held uncentrifuged at 18° C to 24° C for up to 24 hours, provided the tubes remain closed. Likewise, specimens for PTT measurement may be held uncentrifuged for up to 4 hours. However, specimens from patients receiving unfractionated heparin collected for PTT heparin monitoring must be centrifuged, and the supernatant PPP must be sampled or transferred within 1 hour to avoid false shortening of the PTT as platelet granule PF4 neutralizes the heparin.

If the hemostasis test cannot be completed within the prescribed interval, the laboratory practitioner must immediately centrifuge the specimen. The supernatant PPP must be transferred by plastic pipette to a plastic freezer tube (nonsiliconized glass materials are never used with plasma handling as it activates the coagulation cascade), sealed, and frozen and may be stored at –20° C for up to 2 weeks or at –70° C for up to 6 months. At the time the test is performed, the specimen must be thawed rapidly at 37° C, mixed well, and tested within 1 hour of the time it is removed from the freezer. If it cannot be tested immediately, the specimen may be stored at 1° C to 6° C for 2 hours after thawing. To avoid cryoprecipitation of VWF, specimens may not be frozen and thawed more than once.

PLATELET FUNCTION TESTS

Platelet function tests are designed to detect qualitative (functional) platelet abnormalities in patients who are experiencing the symptoms of mucocutaneous bleeding (Chapter 41). A platelet count is performed, and the blood film is reviewed before platelet function tests are begun, because thrombocytopenia is a common cause of hemorrhage (Chapter 40).[24] Qualitative platelet abnormalities are suspected only when bleeding symptoms are present and the platelet count exceeds 50,000/μL.

Although hereditary platelet function disorders are rare, acquired defects are common.[25] Acquired platelet defects are associated with liver disease, renal disease, myeloproliferative neoplasms, myelodysplastic syndromes, myeloma, uremia, autoimmune disorders, anemias, and drug therapy. Platelet morphology is often a clue; for instance, in Bernard-Soulier syndrome, the blood film reveals mild thrombocytopenia and large gray platelets (Figure 41-3). Similarly, the presence of large platelets on the blood film associated with elevated mean platelet volume often indicates rapid platelet turnover, such as what occurs in *immune thrombocytopenic purpura* or *thrombotic thrombocytopenic purpura*. Giant or dysplastic platelets are seen in myeloproliferative neoplasms, acute leukemia, and myelodysplastic syndromes.

Bleeding Time Test for Platelet Function

The *bleeding time* test was the original test of platelet function, although it is now largely replaced by near-patient analysis of platelet function using the PFA-100 (Siemens Healthcare Diagnostics, Inc., Deerfield, IL), the Multiplate (DiaPharma, West Chester, OH), or platelet aggregometry.[26] To perform the test, the phlebotomist uses a lancet to make a small, controlled puncture wound and records the duration of bleeding, comparing the results with the universally accepted reference interval of 2 to 9 minutes. The bleeding time test was first described by Duke[27] in 1912 and modified by Ivy[28] in 1941. In 1978 some standardization was attempted. A blood pressure cuff was inflated to 40 mm Hg, a calibrated spring-loaded lancet (Surgicutt Bleeding Time Device; International Technidyne Corp., Edison, NJ) was triggered on the volar surface of the forearm a few inches distal to the antecubital crease, and the resulting wound was blotted every 30 seconds with filter paper until bleeding stopped.[29,30]

A prolonged bleeding time could theoretically signal a functional platelet disorder such as von Willebrand disease (VWD) or a vascular disorder such as scurvy or vasculitis, and was a characteristic result of therapy with aspirin and other nonsteroidal anti-inflammatory drugs (NSAIDs). Measurement of the bleeding time was often requested by surgeons at admission in an attempt to predict surgical bleeding, but a series of studies in the 1990s revealed that the test has inadequate predictive value. The bleeding time is affected by the nonplatelet variables of intracapillary pressure, skin thickness at the puncture site, and size and depth of the wound, all of which interfere with accurate interpretation of the test results. Owing to its poor predictive value for bleeding and its tendency to scar the forearm, use of the bleeding time assay has been discontinued at most institutions.

Platelet Aggregometry and Lumiaggregometry

Functional platelets *adhere* to subendothelial collagen, *aggregate* with one another, and *secrete* the contents of their α-granules and dense granules (Chapter 13). Normal adhesion requires intact platelet membranes and functional plasma VWF. Normal aggregation requires that platelet membranes and platelet activation pathways are intact, that the plasma fibrinogen concentration is normal, and that normal secretions are released from platelet granules. Platelet adhesion, aggregation, and secretion are assessed using in vitro platelet aggregometry.

An aggregometer is an instrument designed to measure platelet aggregation in a suspension of citrated whole blood or PRP. Specimens are collected and managed in compliance with standard laboratory protocol as described in the section entitled Preparation of Hemostasis Specimens for Assay, and maintained at ambient temperature (18° C to 24° C) until testing begins. Specimens for PRP-based light-transmittance aggregometry must stand undisturbed for 30 minutes after centrifugation while the platelets regain their responsiveness. Specimens for impedance whole blood aggregometry are diluted 1:1 with normal saline and tested immediately. Specimens must be tested within 4 hours of collection to avoid spontaneous in vitro platelet activation and loss of normal activity. Platelet aggregometry is a high-complexity laboratory test requiring a skilled, experienced operator.

Platelet Aggregometry Using Platelet-Rich Plasma

PRP aggregometry is performed using a specialized photometer called a *light-transmittance aggregometer* (PAP-8E Platelet Aggregation Profiler; Bio/Data Corp., Horsham, PA).[31] After calibrating the instrument in accordance with manufacturer instructions, the operator pipettes the PRP to instrument-compatible cuvettes, usually 500 μL; drops in one clean plasticized stir bar per sample; places the cuvettes in incubation wells; and allows the samples to warm to 37° C for 5 minutes. The operator then transfers the first cuvette, containing specimen and stir bar, to the instrument's reaction well and starts the stirring device and the recording computer. The stirring device turns the stir bar at 800 to 1200 rpm, a gentle speed that keeps the platelets in suspension. The instrument directs focused light through the sample cuvette to a photodetector (Figure 42-3). As the PRP is stirred, the recorder tracing first stabilizes to generate a baseline, near 0% light transmittance. After a few seconds, the operator pipettes an agonist (aggregating agent) directly into the sample to trigger aggregation. In a normal specimen, after the agonist is added, the shape of the suspended platelets changes from discoid to spherical, and the intensity of light transmittance initially (and briefly) decreases, then increases in proportion to the degree of shape change. Percent light transmittance is monitored continuously and recorded (Figure 42-4). As platelet aggregates form, more light passes through the PRP, and the tracing begins to move toward 100% light transmittance. Platelet function deficiencies are reflected in diminished or absent aggregation; many laboratory directors choose 40% aggregation as the lower limit of normal.

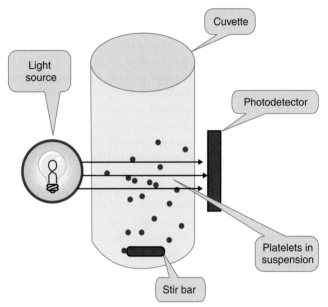

Figure 42-3 Analysis of platelet-rich plasma in an optical aggregometer. Desired platelet count is approximately 200,000/µL. Platelets are maintained in suspension by a magnetic stir bar turning at 800 to 1200 rpm. (Courtesy Kathy Jacobs, Chrono-log Corp., Havertown, PA.)

Whole-Blood Platelet Aggregometry

In whole-blood platelet aggregometry, platelet aggregation is measured by electrical impedance using a 1:1 saline–whole blood suspension (Model 700 Whole Blood/Optical Lumi-Aggregometer; Chrono-log Corp., Havertown, PA).[32] The operator pipettes aliquots of properly mixed whole blood to cuvettes and adds equal volumes of physiologic saline. Suspension volume may be 300 to 500 µL. The operator drops in one stir bar per cuvette and places the cuvettes in 37° C incubation wells for 5 minutes. The operator transfers the first cuvette to a reaction well, pipettes an agonist directly into the specimen, and suspends a pair of low-voltage cartridge-mounted disposable direct current (DC) electrodes in the mixture. As aggregation occurs, platelets adhere to the electrodes and one another, impeding the DC current (Figure 42-5). The rise in impedance, which is directly proportional to platelet aggregation, is amplified and recorded by instrument circuitry. A whole-blood aggregometry tracing closely resembles a PRP-based light-transmittance aggregometry tracing, as shown in Figure 42-4.

Platelet Lumiaggregometry

The Chrono-log Whole Blood/Optical Lumi-Aggregometer may also be used for simultaneous measurement of platelet aggregation

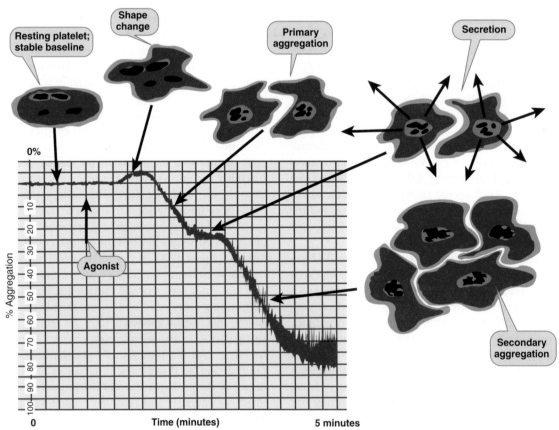

Figure 42-4 Optical aggregometry tracing showing five phases of platelet aggregation: baseline at 0% aggregation, shape change after the addition of the agonist, primary aggregation, release of adenosine diphosphate and adenosine triphosphate, and second-wave aggregation that forms large clumps. The % aggregation is measured by amount of light transmittance through the test sample. (Courtesy Kathy Jacobs, Chrono-log Corp., Havertown, PA.)

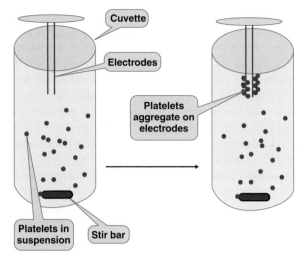

Figure 42-5 In whole-blood platelet aggregometry, aggregating platelets form a layer on the electrodes and the platelet layer impedes current. Resistance (in ohms) is proportional to aggregation, and a tracing is provided that resembles the tracing obtained using optical aggregometry. (Courtesy Kathy Jacobs, Chrono-log Corp., Havertown, PA.)

TABLE 42-4 Typical Normal Ranges in Platelet Lumiaggregometry

Agonist	Final Concentration	Aggregation Recorded as Impedance	ATP Secretion
Thrombin	1 unit/mL	Not recorded, as thrombin often causes clotting	1.0–2.0 nM
TRAP	10, 50, 100 µM	15–27 Ω	1.0–2.0 nM
Collagen	1 µg/mL	15–27 Ω	0.5–1.7 nM
	5 µg/mL	15–31 Ω	0.9–1.7 nM
ADP	5 µM	1–17 Ω	0.0–0.7 nM
	10 µM	6–24 Ω	0.4–1.7 nM
Arachidonic acid	500 µM	5–17 Ω	0.6–1.4 nM
Ristocetin	1 mg/mL	>10 Ω	Not recorded

TRAP, Thrombin receptor-activating peptide; *ATP*, adenosine triphosphate; *ADP*, adenosine diphosphate.

and the secretion of adenosine triphosphate (ATP) from activated platelet dense granules.[33] The procedure for *lumiaggregometry* differs little from that for conventional aggregometry and simplifies the diagnosis of platelet dysfunction.[34] As ATP is released, it oxidizes a firefly-derived luciferin-luciferase reagent (Chrono-lume; Chrono-log Corp.) to generate cold chemiluminescence proportional to the ATP concentration. A photodetector amplifies the luminescence, which is recorded as a second tracing on the aggregation report.[35]

Lumiaggregometry may be performed using whole blood or PRP.[36] To perform lumiaggregometry, the operator adds an ATP standard to the first sample, then adds luciferin-luciferase and tests for full luminescence. The operator then adds luciferin-luciferase and an agonist to the second sample; the instrument monitors for aggregation and secretion simultaneously. *Thrombin* is typically the first agonist used because thrombin induces full secretion. The luminescence induced by thrombin is measured, recorded, and used for comparison with the luminescence produced by the additional agonists. Normal secretion induced by agonists other than thrombin produces luminescence at a level of about 50% of that resulting from thrombin (Table 42-4). Figure 42-6 depicts simultaneous aggregation and secretion responses to thrombin; Figure 42-7 is a scanning electron micrograph of resting and activated platelets.

Platelet Agonists (Activating Agents) Used in Aggregometry

The optical PRP-based aggregation method is employed most frequently in clinical practice, and the agonists used are thrombin or synthetic *thrombin receptor-activating peptide* (TRAP), adenosine diphosphate (ADP), epinephrine, collagen, arachidonic acid, and ristocetin. Table 42-5 lists representative concentrations and platelet activation pathways tested by each agonist. Small volumes (2 to 5 µL) of concentrated agonist are

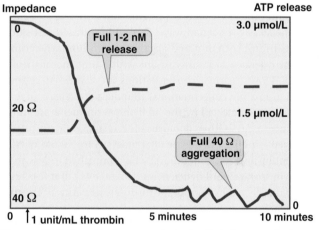

Figure 42-6 Normal lumiaggregometry tracing illustrating monophasic aggregation curve with superimposed release (secretion) reaction curve. Aggregation is measured in ohms (Ω) using the left *y*-axis scale; release is measured in µM of adenosine triphosphate (ATP) based on luminescence using the right *y*-axis scale. Curve illustrates full aggregation and secretion response to 1 unit/mL of thrombin. (Courtesy Margaret Fritsma, University of Alabama at Birmingham.)

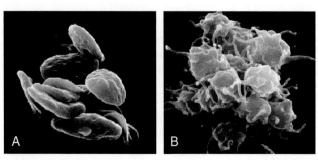

Figure 42-7 Scanning electron micrograph of resting **(A)** and activated **(B)** platelets.

TABLE 42-5 Platelet Aggregometry Agonists, Reaction Concentrations, and Platelet Receptors

Agonist	Typical Final Concentration	Platelet Membrane Receptors
Thrombin	1 unit/mL	PAR1 and PAR4; GP Ibα and GP V
ADP	1–10 μM	P2Y$_1$, P2Y$_{12}$
Epinephrine	2–10 μg/mL	α$_2$-adrenergic receptor
Collagen	5 μg/mL	GP Ia/IIa, GP VI
Arachidonic acid	500 μM	TPα, TPβ
Ristocetin	1 mg/mL	GP Ib/IX/V in association with von Willebrand factor

GP, Glycoprotein; PAR, protease-activatable receptor; P2Y, platelet membrane ADP-receptor; TP, thromboxane receptor.

used so that they have little dilutional effect in the reaction system.[37]

Thrombin (or *TRAP*) cleaves two platelet membrane protease-activatable receptors (PARs), PAR-1 and PAR-2, both members of the seven-transmembrane repeat receptor family (Chapter 13). Thrombin or TRAP also cleaves glycoprotein (GP) 1bα and GP V. Internal platelet activation is effected by membrane-associated G proteins and both the *eicosanoid* and the *diacylglycerol* pathways. Thrombin-induced activation results in full secretion and aggregation. In lumiaggregometry, the operator ordinarily begins with 1 unit/mL of thrombin or TRAP (agonist concentrations are expressed as final reaction mixture concentrations) to induce the release of 1 to 2 nM of ATP, detected by the firefly luciferin-luciferase luminescence assay. Other agonists—for instance, 5 μg/mL of collagen—induce the release of at most 0.5 to 1.0 nM of ATP. Thrombin-induced secretion may be diminished to less than 1 nM in storage pool deficiencies (Chapter 41), but it is relatively unaffected by membrane disorders or pathway enzyme deficiencies.

Reagent thrombin is stored dry at –20° C and is reconstituted with physiologic saline immediately before use. Leftover reconstituted thrombin may be divided into aliquots, frozen, and thawed for later use. Thrombin has the disadvantage that it often triggers coagulation (fibrin formation) simultaneously with aggregation. The use of TRAP avoids this pitfall.

ADP binds platelet membrane receptors P2Y$_1$ and P2Y$_{12}$, also members of the seven-transmembrane repeat receptor family. ADP-induced platelet activation relies on the physiologic response of membrane-associated G protein and the eicosanoid synthesis pathway. The end product of eicosanoid synthesis, thromboxane A$_2$, raises cytosolic free calcium, which mediates platelet activation and induces secretion of ADP stored in dense granules. The secreted ADP activates neighboring platelets.

ADP is the most commonly used agonist, particularly in aggregometry systems that measure only aggregation and not luminescence. The operator adjusts the ADP concentration to between 1 and 10 μM to induce "biphasic" aggregation (Figure 42-4). At ADP concentrations near 1 μM, platelets achieve only *primary aggregation,* followed by disaggregation. The graph line deflects from the baseline for 1 to 2 minutes and then returns to baseline.

Primary aggregation involves shape change with formation of microaggregates, both reversible. *Secondary aggregation* is the formation of full platelet aggregates after release of platelet dense-granule ADP. At agonist ADP concentrations near 10 μM, there is simultaneous irreversible shape change, secretion, and formation of aggregates, resulting in a monophasic curve and full deflection of the tracing. ADP concentrations between 1 and 10 μM induce a biphasic curve: primary aggregation followed by a brief flattening of the curve called the *lag phase* and then secondary aggregation.

Operators expend considerable effort to discover the ADP concentration that generates a biphasic curve with a visible lag phase because the appropriate concentration varies among patients. This enables operators to use aggregometry alone to distinguish between membrane-associated platelet defects and storage pool or release defects.

Lumiaggregometry provides a clearer and more reproducible measure of platelet secretion, rendering the quest for the biphasic curve unnecessary. Secretion in response to ADP at 5 μM is diminished in platelet membrane disorders; eicosanoid synthesis pathway enzyme deficiencies; or aspirin, NSAID, or clopidogrel therapy. Secretion is absent in storage pool deficiency when thrombin or TRAP is used as the agonist.

Reagent ADP is stored at –20° C, reconstituted with physiologic saline, and used immediately after reconstitution. Leftover reconstituted ADP may be aliquotted and frozen for later use.

Epinephrine binds platelet α-adrenergic receptors, identical to muscle receptors, and activates the platelets through the same metabolic pathways as reagent ADP. The results of epinephrine-induced aggregation match those of ADP, except that epinephrine cannot induce aggregation in storage pool disorder or eicosanoid synthesis pathway defects no matter how high its concentration. Epinephrine does not work in whole-blood aggregometry.

Epinephrine is stored at 1° C to 6° C and reconstituted with distilled water immediately before it is used. Leftover reconstituted epinephrine may be aliquotted and frozen for later use.

Collagen binds GP Ia/IIa and GP VI, but it induces no primary aggregation. After a lag of 30 to 60 seconds, aggregation begins, and a monophasic curve develops. Aggregation induced by collagen at 5 μg/mL requires intact membrane receptors, functional membrane G proteins, and normal eicosanoid pathway function. Loss of collagen-induced aggregation may indicate a membrane abnormality, storage pool disorder, release defect, or the presence of aspirin.

Most laboratory managers purchase lyophilized fibrillar collagen preparations such as Chrono-Par Collagen (Chrono-log Corp.). Collagen is stored at 1° C to 6° C and used without further dilution. Collagen may not be frozen.

Arachidonic acid assesses the viability of the eicosanoid synthesis pathway. Free arachidonic acid agonist at 500 μM is added to induce a monophasic aggregometry curve with virtually no lag phase. Aggregation is independent of membrane integrity. Deficiencies in eicosanoid pathway enzymes, including deficient or aspirin-suppressed cyclooxygenase, result in reduced aggregation and secretion.

Arachidonic acid is readily oxidized and must be stored at –20° C in the dark. The operator dilutes arachidonic acid with a solution of bovine albumin for immediate use. Aliquots of bovine albumin–dissolved arachidonic acid may be frozen for later use.

Platelet Aggregometry Tests in von Willebrand Disease

Ristocetin-Induced Platelet Aggregation. Although this test is usually called the *ristocetin-induced platelet aggregation (RIPA) test*, ristocetin actually induces an *agglutination* reaction that involves little platelet shape change and little secretion. A normal RIPA result may imply that normal concentrations of functional VWF are present and that the platelets possess a functional VWF receptor, GP Ib/IX/V (Chapter 13).[38]

Using light transmittance aggregometry, ristocetin at 1 mg/mL final concentration induces a monophasic aggregation tracing from a normal specimen. Specimens from patients with VWD, except for subtype 2B VWD, produce a reduced or absent reaction, although all other agonists generate normal tracings (Table 38-4). Exogenous VWF from normal plasma restores a normal RIPA reaction, confirming the diagnosis (Chapter 38). In patients with Bernard-Soulier syndrome, a congenital abnormality of the GP Ib or IX portion of the GP Ib/IX/V receptor results in a diminished RIPA reaction that is not corrected by the addition of VWF (Chapter 41).

In VWD subtype 2B, a VWF gain-of-function mutation, aggregation occurs even when reduced ristocetin concentrations (down to 0.1 mg/mL final concentration) are added. This response illustrates the increased affinity of large VWF multimers for platelet receptors. The low-dose or low-concentration RIPA, sometimes called the *ristocetin response curve*, is used to diagnose type 2B VWD.

The RIPA test is qualitative and is diagnostic in only about 70% of cases. Most laboratory managers have dropped RIPA from their test menus because of its poor predictive value. There is considerable variation in laboratory results from one patient to another in the same kindred and from time-to-time in a single patient. Consequently, the laboratory director must include the *ristocetin cofactor test*, the *VWF antigen immunoassay*, and the *coagulation factor VIII activity assay* in the VWD profile. Many laboratories also offer the *VWF activity immunoassay* and the *VWF collagen-binding assay*. Ultimate confirmation and characterization of VWD is based on gel immunoelectrophoresis to characterize VWF monomers (Chapter 38).[39]

Ristocetin Cofactor Assay for von Willebrand Factor Activity. One essential refinement of ristocetin aggregometry is the substitution of formalin-fixed or lyophilized normal "reagent" platelets for the patient's platelets.[40] When reagent platelets are used, the test is called the *ristocetin cofactor* or *VWF activity assay*. The medical laboratory practitioner prepares the patient's PPP; mixes it with reagent platelets; adds ristocetin; and performs optical, not impedance, aggregometry. The ristocetin cofactor assay yields a proportional relationship between VWF activity and the aggregometry response of the reagent platelets. Comparison of the aggregation results for patients' PPP with those for standard dilutions of normal "reagent" PPP permits a quantitative expression of the VWF activity level. The

ristocetin cofactor test also is available as an automated assay on the BCT coagulometer and the BCS coagulometer (Siemens Healthcare Diagnostics, Deerfield, IL), which use latex particles in place of preserved platelets.

VWF Activity Immunoassay and VWF Activity Collagen Binding Assay. Although the ristocetin cofactor assay has been used for many years to measure VWF activity, it offers consistently poor precision, as illustrated by external quality assurance survey results.[41] Two additional assays, the VWF Activity Immunoassay (for instance, the REAADS von Willebrand Factor Activity enzyme immunoassay, DiaPharma, West Chester, OH) and the VWF Collagen Binding Assay (Technozym vWF:CBA ELISA Collagen Type I, DiaPharma, West Chester, OH) are available. The former employs a monoclonal antibody specific for an active VWF epitope, and the latter mimics VWF's in vivo collagen adhesion property. Both reflect VWF activity rather than concentration and offer improved precision when compared to the ristocetin cofactor assay.

Summary of Lumiaggregometry Agonist Responses in Various Circumstances

Thrombin produces maximum ATP release through at least two membrane-binding sites. Laboratory practitioners use collagen, ADP, and epinephrine to test for abnormalities of their respective membrane binding sites and the eicosanoid synthesis pathway. Arachidonic acid is the agonist that practitioners use to check for eicosanoid synthesis deficiencies. Ristocetin is used to check for abnormalities of plasma VWF in VWD. The following conditions may be detected through platelet lumiaggregometry.

Therapy with Aspirin, Other Nonsteroidal Anti-Inflammatory Drugs, and Clopidogrel. NSAIDs such as aspirin, ibuprofen, indomethacin, and sulfinpyrazone permanently inactivate or temporarily inhibit cyclooxygenase. The thienopyridine antiplatelet drugs *clopidogrel* and *prasugrel* irreversibly occupy the ADP receptor $P2Y_{12}$ whereas the *nucleoside ticagrelor* is reversibly bound (Chapter 41). The NSAIDs limit or eliminate the aggregation and secretion responses to arachidonic acid and collagen. The $P2Y_{12}$ inhibitors suppress aggregation and secretion responses to ADP.[42] Platelet aggregometry is employed to monitor response to these antiplatelet drugs (Chapter 41).[43] The VerifyNow system (Accumetrics, San Diego, CA) with specific assays for monitoring the effect of aspirin, the $P2Y_{12}$ inhibitors, and the GP IIb/IIIa inhibitor antiplatelet drugs is gaining favor in point-of-care settings (Chapter 44). The physician or medical laboratory practitioner must instruct the patient to discontinue all antiplatelet drugs at least 1 week before blood is collected for aggregometry unless aggregometry is ordered to monitor the effects of these drugs.

Platelet Release (Secretion) Defects: Eicosanoid Pathway Enzyme Deficiencies. Congenital or acquired deficiencies of cyclooxygenase, thromboxane synthase, protein kinase C, or any enzyme in the eicosanoid activation pathway limit or prevent secretion. Thrombin may induce normal responses, but secretion and aggregation are diminished in response to ADP, collagen, and arachidonic acid. Because the aggregation responses resemble the responses seen during the use of NSAIDs, release defects are often called *aspirin-like disorders.*

Storage Pool Deficiency.
Storage Pool Deficiency. In a congenital or acquired storage pool defect, dense granules are empty or missing. ATP release in response to thrombin is reduced, as it is in response to ADP, arachidonic acid, and collagen (Table 42-6).

Platelet Membrane Defects: Thrombasthenia. Glanzmann thrombasthenia, a membrane defect characterized by dysfunction or loss of the GP IIb/IIIa receptor site, may be diagnosed by its characteristically diminished secretion and aggregation responses to all agonists except thrombin or its modest response to arachidonic acid.

Acquired Platelet Disorders. Platelets may become either dysfunctional or hyperactive in acquired hematologic and systemic disorders such as acute leukemia, aplastic anemia, myeloproliferative neoplasms, myelodysplastic syndromes, myeloma, uremia, liver disease, and chronic alcohol abuse. The physician looks for these disorders in any case where aggregation is abnormal and no other explanation is available. Platelet aggregometry results may predict the risk of bleeding or thrombosis in the patient with acquired platelet function disorders.[44]

Testing for Heparin-Induced Thrombocytopenia

A description of the clinical manifestations and mechanism of heparin-induced thrombocytopenia (HIT) is provided in Chapter 39, and a summary of laboratory tests for HIT is provided in Chapter 40. Aggregation tests for HIT include light-transmittance aggregometry, washed platelet light-transmittance aggregometry, washed platelet lumiaggregometry, and whole-blood lumiaggregometry.[45-47] The washed platelet carbon-14 (^{14}C) serotonin release assay (SRA) is based on platelet activation and secretion. All these tests employ unfractionated heparin as their agonist. The ^{14}C-SRA is available from specialized reference laboratories and is regarded as the reference confirmatory method. Few local institutions

TABLE 42-6 Expected Platelet Lumiaggregometry Results in Storage Pool Disorder for a Variety of Agonists

Agonist	Final Concentration	Aggregation Recorded as Impedance	ATP Secretion
Thrombin	1 unit/mL	Not recorded*	<0.1 nM
TRAP	10, 50, 100 μM	20 Ω	<0.1 nM
Collagen	5 μg/mL	20 Ω	<0.1 nM
Arachidonic acid	500 μM	12 Ω	<0.1 nM

*Thrombin aggregation is not recorded as thrombin typically causes clotting, which interferes with the aggregation response. TRAP avoids the clotting response.
ATP, Adenosine triphosphate.

provide the ^{14}C-SRA, because a radionuclide license is required. Except for the ^{14}C-SRA, aggregometry and lumiaggregometry tests for HIT have proven to be insensitive and have been largely discontinued.

QUANTITATIVE MEASUREMENT OF PLATELET MARKERS

Immunoassay for the Anti–Platelet Factor 4 (Heparin-Induced Thrombocytopenia) Antibody

Amiral and colleagues developed a HIT screening immunoassay based on their discovery that PF4 is the target for the heparin-dependent antiplatelet antibody that causes HIT (Chapter 40).[48] One adaptation of this principle is the PF4 Enhanced Solid Phase ELISA (Hologic Gen-Probe Inc., San Diego, CA). Patient plasma is incubated in microtiter plate wells that are coated with a solid-phase complex of purified PF4 and polysulfonate, a plastic molecule integral to plate construction that resembles heparin. Heparin-dependent anti-PF4 antibodies bind the PF4-polysulfonate complex. Bound antibodies are detected using enzyme-conjugated anti–human immunoglobulin G (IgG), IgA, and IgM antibodies and a substrate chromophore. This test is more sensitive than the ^{14}C-SRA and detects antibodies early in the development of HIT, but it may detect antibodies that are unaccompanied by clinical symptoms, known as *biologic false positives.*[49] A second kit that uses only enzyme-conjugated anti-human IgG is more specific. Other immunoassay kits employ PF4-heparin in place of PF4-polysulfonate and have similar sensitivity and specificity characteristics.

Assays for Platelet Activation Markers

Elevated plasma levels of the platelet-specific proteins β-thromboglobulin and PF4 may accompany thrombotic stroke or coronary thrombosis.[50] The implication that in vivo platelet activation contributes to the condition or that the measurement of these proteins is of diagnostic or prognostic significance is under investigation.[51] Diagnostica Stago, Inc. (Parsippany, NJ) produces enzyme immunoassay kits for PF4 and β-thromboglobulin (β-TG) under the brand names Asserachrom PF4 and Asserachrom β-TG. Special collection techniques are necessary because PF4 and β-TG test results may be invalidated by platelet activation during and even subsequent to specimen collection.[52] CTAD tubes (refer to the section on Hemostasis Specimen Collection above) are required for specimen collection for PF4 and β-TG assays. Plasma must undergo extraction before PF4 and β-TG assays are performed because several eicosanoids cross-react with kit antibodies and falsely raise the results.

Thromboxane A2, the active product of the eicosanoid pathway, has a half-life of 30 seconds, diffuses from the platelet, and spontaneously reduces to thromboxane B2, a stable, measurable plasma metabolite (Chapter 13). Efforts to produce a clinical assay for plasma thromboxane B2 have been unsuccessful because specimens must be collected in CTAD tubes to prevent in vitro platelet activation and must undergo an extraction step before the assay is performed. Thromboxane B2 is acted on by liver enzymes to produce an array of soluble urine metabolites, including 11-dehydrothromboxane B2, which is stable and measurable.[53] Immunoassays of urine 11-dehydrothromboxane B2 are employed to characterize in vivo platelet activation.[54] These assays require no special specimen management and can be performed on random urine specimens. The urinary 11-dehydrothromboxane B2 assay also may be used to monitor aspirin therapy and to identify cases of therapy failure or aspirin resistance.[55]

CLOT-BASED PLASMA PROCOAGULANT SCREENS

The Lee-White whole-blood coagulation time test, described in 1913, was the first laboratory procedure designed to assess coagulation.[56] The Lee-White test is no longer used, but it was the first in vitro clot procedure that employed the principle that the time interval from the initiation of clotting to visible clot formation reflects the condition of the coagulation mechanism. A prolonged clotting time indicates a coagulopathy (coagulation deficiency). A 1953 modification, the *activated clotting time* (ACT) test, utilizes a particulate clot activator in the test tube, which speeds the clotting process. The ACT is still widely used as a point-of-care assay to monitor heparin therapy in high-dosage applications such as percutaneous intervention (cardiac catheterization) and coronary artery bypass graft surgery (Chapter 43).

The standard clot-based coagulation screening tests—PT, PTT, fibrinogen assay, and thrombin clotting time (TCT)—use the clotting time principle of the Lee-White test. Many specialized tests, such as coagulation factor assays, tests of fibrinolysis, inhibitor assays, reptilase time, Russell viper venom time, and dilute Russell viper venom time, are also based on the relationship between time to clot formation and coagulation function.

Prothrombin Time
Prothrombin Time Principle

PT reagents, often called *thromboplastin* or *tissue thromboplastin,* are prepared from recombinant or affinity-purified *tissue factor* suspended in phospholipids mixed with a buffered 0.025 M solution of calcium chloride.[57] A few less responsive thromboplastins are organic extracts of emulsified rabbit brain or lung suspended in calcium chloride. When mixed with citrated PPP, the PT reagent triggers fibrin polymerization by activating plasma factor VII (Figure 42-8). Calcium and phospholipids participate in the formation of the tissue factor–factor VIIa complex, the factor VIIIa–factor IXa complex, and the factor Va–factor Xa complex. The clot is detectable visually or by optical or electromechanical sensors. Although the coagulation pathway implies that the PT would be prolonged in deficiencies of fibrinogen, prothrombin, and factors V, VII, VIII, IX, and X, the procedure is most sensitive to factor VII deficiencies, moderately sensitive to factor V and X deficiencies, sensitive to severe fibrinogen and prothrombin deficiencies, and insensitive to deficiencies of factors VIII and IX.[58,59] The PT is prolonged in multiple factor deficiencies that include deficiencies of factors VII and X and is used most often to monitor the effects of therapy with the oral anticoagulant Coumadin (Chapter 43).

Prothrombin Time Procedure

The tissue factor-phospholipid-calcium chloride reagent is warmed to 37° C. An aliquot of test PPP, 50 or 100 μL, is transferred to the reaction vessel, which also is maintained at 37° C. The PPP aliquot is incubated at 37° C for at least 3 and for no more than 10 minutes. Aliquots that are incubated longer than 10 minutes become prolonged as coagulation factors begin to deteriorate or are affected by evaporation and pH change. A premeasured volume of reagent, 100 or 200 μL, is directly and quickly added to the PPP aliquot, and a timer is started. As the

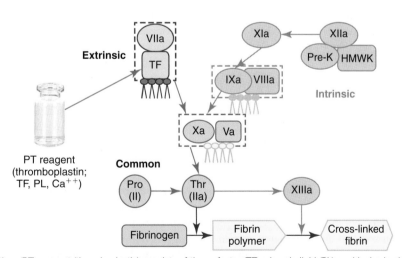

Figure 42-8 Prothrombin time (PT) reagent (thromboplastin) consists of tissue factor (TF), phospholipid (PL), and ionized calcium (Ca^{++}). The reagent activates the extrinsic and common pathways of the coagulation mechanism beginning with factor VII (see colored area in figure). The PT is prolonged by deficiencies of factors VII, X, and V; prothrombin; and fibrinogen when the fibrinogen level is less than 100 mg/dL. The PT is prolonged in Coumadin therapy because Coumadin suppresses production of factor VII, factor X, and prothrombin. Factor VII has a 6-hour half-life and has the earliest effect on the PT. The PT does not detect factor XIII deficiency. *HMWK,* High-molecular-weight kininogen (Fitzgerald factor); *Pre-K,* prekallikrein (Fletcher factor); *Pro,* prothrombin (II, zymogen); *Thr,* thrombin (activated factor II, or IIa; serine protease); *Va, VIIIa,* activated factors V and VIII (serine protease cofactors); *VIIa, IXa, Xa, XIa,* activated factors VII, IX, X, XI (serine proteases); *XIIa,* activated factor XII (serine protease, but not part of in vivo coagulation); *XIIIa,* activated factor XIII (transglutaminase).

clot forms, the timer stops, and the elapsed time is recorded. If the procedure is performed in duplicate, the duplicate values must be within 10% of their mean or the test is repeated for a third time. Most laboratory practitioners perform PTs using automated instruments that strictly control temperature, pipetting, and interval timing (Chapter 44). With automated instruments, duplicate testing is unnecessary.

Prothrombin Time Quality Control

The medical laboratory practitioner tests normal and prolonged control PPP specimens at the beginning of each 8-hour shift or with each change of reagent. Although lyophilized control PPPs are commercially available, the laboratory manager may choose to collect and pool PPP specimens from designated subjects to make "laboratory-developed" controls. In this case, the specimens must be collected and managed using the same tubes, anticoagulant, and protocol that are used for patient plasma specimen collection. The samples are pooled, tested, and aliquotted. Regardless of whether commercial or locally prepared controls are used, the control is tested alongside patient specimens using the same protocol as for patient PPP testing.

The normal control result should be within the reference interval, and the prolonged control result should be within the therapeutic range for Coumadin. If the control results fall within the stated limits provided in the laboratory protocol, the test results are considered valid. If the results fall outside the control limits, the reagents, control, and equipment are checked; the problem is corrected; and the control and patient specimens are retested. The operator records all the actions taken. Control results are recorded and analyzed at regular intervals to determine the long-term validity of results.

Reporting of Prothrombin Time Results and the International Normalized Ratio

The medical laboratory practitioner reports PT results to the nearest tenth of a second, along with the PT reference interval. If the PT assay is performed in duplicate, the results are averaged, and the average is reported.

For Coumadin monitoring, to compensate for the inherent variations among thromboplastin reagents, most laboratories report the *international normalized ratio* (INR) for patients with a stable anticoagulation response using the following formula:[60]

$$INR = \left(PT_{patient}/PT_{geometric\ mean\ of\ normal}\right)^{ISI}$$

where $PT_{patient}$ is the PT of the patient in seconds, $PT_{geometric\ mean\ of\ normal}$ is the PT of the geometric mean of the reference interval, and *ISI* is the *international sensitivity index*. Reagent producers generate the ISI for their thromboplastin by performing an orthogonal regression analysis comparing its PT results on a set of plasmas, with the results obtained using the international reference thromboplastin preparation (World Health Organization human brain thromboplastin). Most responsive thromboplastin reagents have ISIs near 1, the assigned ISI of the

WHO reagent. Automated coagulation instruments "request" the reagent ISI from the operator or incorporate it from the reagent label bar code and compute the INR for each specimen. INRs are meant to be computed only for samples from patients who have achieved a stable anticoagulation response with Coumadin. During the first week of Coumadin therapy, the physician should interpret PT results in seconds, comparing them with the reference interval. Chapter 43 provides a full discussion of Coumadin therapy monitoring.

Localized ISI calibration is replacing reagent manufacturer-generated ISIs as it produces a laboratory-specific ISI value that is likely to be more accurate than a distributor-provided ISI.[61] The laboratory practitioner performs PTs on a set of four to five calibrator plasmas—for instance, ISI Calibrate (Instrumentation Laboratory, Bedford, MA). The calibrators arrive with predetermined PT values. If calibrators are not available, the practitioner may use a series of 100 patient specimens. The practitioner prepares a linear graph with the preestablished calibrator PTs or the PT values of the 100 patient specimens using the lab's current PT reagent on the Y scale and local PTs using the new reagent on the X scale and computes the slope. The reference ISI provided by the manufacturer for the new PT reagent is multiplied by the slope value to produce the local ISI of the new PT reagent.

The same approach may be applied to lot-to-lot calibrations of PT reagents; however, in most lot-to-lot validations the operator need only assay a three-level validation plasma set—for instance, ISI Validate (Instrumentation Laboratory, Bedford, MA). If the lot values determined using the new reagent are within predetermined limits, the lot may be placed in everyday operation without a change; if not, it is necessary to recalibrate the ISI value of the new lot of the PT reagent.

Prothrombin Time Reference Interval

The PT reference interval, computed from PT values of healthy individuals, varies from site to site, depending on the patient population, type of thromboplastin used, type of instrument used, and pH and purity of the reagent diluent. Each center must establish its own range for each new lot of reagents, or at least once a year. This may be done by testing a sample of at least 30 specimens from healthy donors of both sexes spanning the adult age range over several days and computing the 95% confidence interval of the results. A typical PT reference interval is 12.6 to 14.6 seconds.

The Prothrombin Time as a Diagnostic Assay

The PT is performed diagnostically when any coagulopathy is suspected. Acquired multiple deficiencies such as disseminated intravascular coagulation (DIC), liver disease, and vitamin K deficiency all affect factor VII activity and are detected through prolonged PT results. The PT is particularly sensitive to liver disease, which causes factor VII levels to become rapidly diminished (Chapter 38).

Vitamin K deficiency is seen in severe malnutrition, during use of broad-spectrum antibiotics that destroy gut flora, with parenteral nutrition, and in malabsorption syndromes. Vitamin K levels are low in newborns, in which bacterial colonization of the gut has not begun. Hemorrhage is likely in vitamin K deficiency, and the PT is the best indicator. To distinguish between vitamin K deficiency and liver disease, the laboratory practitioner determines factor V and factor VII levels. Both factor V and factor VII are reduced in liver disease; only factor VII is reduced in vitamin K deficiency. Chapter 38 provides details regarding liver disease and vitamin K deficiency.

The PT is prolonged in congenital single-factor deficiencies of factor X, VII, or V; profound prothrombin deficiency; and fibrinogen deficiency when the fibrinogen level is 100 mg/dL or less. When the PT is prolonged but the PTT and thrombin clotting time (TCT) test results are normal, factor VII activity may be deficient. Any suspected single-factor deficiency is confirmed with a factor assay. The PT is not affected by factor VIII or IX deficiency, because the concentration of tissue factor in the reagent is high, and those factors are bypassed in thrombin generation.

Minimal Effectiveness of Prothrombin Time as a Screening Tool

Preoperative PT screening of asymptomatic surgical patients to predict intraoperative hemorrhage is not supported by prevalence studies, unless the patient is a member of a high-risk population.[62,63] No clinical data support the use of the PT as a general screening test for individuals at low risk of bleeding, and the PT is not useful for establishing baseline values in Coumadin therapy.[64] The therapeutic target range for Coumadin therapy is based on the INR, not the baseline PT result or PT control value.

Limitations of the Prothrombin Time

Specimen variations profoundly affect PT results (Table 42-7). The ratio of whole blood to anticoagulant is crucial, so collection tubes must be filled to within tube manufacturers' specifications

and not underfilled or overfilled. Anticoagulant volume must be adjusted when the hematocrit is greater than 55% to avoid false prolongation of the results. Specimens must be inverted five times immediately after collection to ensure good anticoagulation, but the mixing must be gentle. Practitioners must reject clotted and visibly hemolyzed specimens because they give unreliable results. Plasma lipemia or icterus may affect the results obtained with optical instrumentation.

Heparin may prolong the PT. If the patient is receiving therapeutic heparin, it should be noted on the order and commented on when the results are reported. The laboratory manager selects thromboplastin reagents that are maximally sensitive to oral anticoagulant therapy and insensitive to heparin. Many reagent manufacturers incorporate polybrene (5-dimethyl-1,5-diazaundecamethylene polymethobromide, hexadimethrine bromide, Sigma-Aldrich, St. Louis, MO) in their thromboplastin reagent to neutralize heparin. The medical laboratory practitioner may detect unexpected heparin by using the TCT test, which is described subsequently.

Lupus anticoagulants (LAs) prolong some thromboplastins. LAs are members of the antiphospholipid antibody family and may partially neutralize PT reagent phospholipids. Coumadin often is prescribed to prevent thrombosis in patients with LAs, but the PT may be an unreliable monitor of therapy in such cases. Patients who have an LA and are taking Coumadin should be monitored using an alternative system, such as the chromogenic factor X assay.[65,66]

Reagents must be reconstituted with the correct diluents and volumes following manufacturer instructions. Reagents must be stored and shipped according to manufacturer instructions and never used after the expiration date.

Partial Thromboplastin Time
Partial Thromboplastin Time Principle

The PTT (also called the *activated partial thromboplastin time,* or APTT) is performed to monitor the effects of unfractionated heparin therapy and to detect LA and specific anticoagulation factor antibodies such as anti-factor VIII antibody. The PTT is also prolonged in all congenital and acquired procoagulant deficiencies, except for deficiencies of factor VII or XIII.[67]

The PTT reagent contains phospholipid (previously called *partial thromboplastin*) and a negatively charged particulate activator such as silica, kaolin, ellagic acid, or celite in suspension. The phospholipid mixture, which was historically extracted from rabbit brain, is now produced synthetically. The activator provides a surface that mediates a conformational change in plasma factor XII that results in its activation (Figure 42-9). Factor XIIa forms a complex with two other plasma components: high-molecular-weight kininogen (*Fitzgerald factor*) and prekallikrein (*Fletcher factor*). These three plasma glycoproteins, termed the *contact activation factors,* initiate in vitro clot formation through the *intrinsic* pathway but are not part of in vivo coagulation. Factor XIIa, a serine protease, activates factor XI (XIa), which activates factor IX (IXa) (Chapter 37).

Factor IXa binds calcium, phospholipid, and factor VIIIa to form a complex. In the PTT reaction system, ionic calcium and

TABLE 42-7 Factors That Interfere with the Validity of Clot-based Test Results

Problem	Solution
Blood collection volume less than specified minimum	PT falsely prolonged; recollect specimen.
Hematocrit ≥55%	Adjust anticoagulant volume using formula and recollect specimen using new anticoagulant volume.
Clot in specimen	All results are affected unpredictably; recollect specimen.
Visible hemolysis	PT falsely shortened; recollect specimen.
Icterus or lipemia	Measure PT using a mechanical coagulometer.
Heparin therapy	Use reagent known to be insensitive to heparin or one that includes a heparin neutralizer such as polybrene.
Lupus anticoagulant	PT result is invalid; use chromogenic factor X assay instead of PT.
Incorrect calibration, incorrect dilution of reagents	Correct analytical error and repeat test.

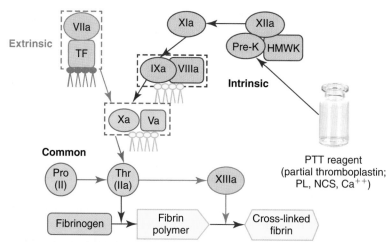

Figure 42-9 Partial thromboplastin time (PTT) reagent (partial thromboplastin) consists of phospholipid (PL), a negatively charged particulate activator (NCS), and ionized calcium. It activates the intrinsic and common pathways of the coagulation mechanism through the contact factors XII, prekallikrein (Pre-K; also called *Fletcher factor*), and high-molecular-weight kininogen (HMWK; also called *Fitzgerald factor*), none of which is significant in the in vivo coagulation mechanism (see colored area in figure). The PTT is prolonged by deficiencies in Pre-K; HMWK; factors XII, XI, IX, VIII, X, and prothrombin; and fibrinogen when the fibrinogen level is less than 100 mg/dL. The deficiencies for which the PTT reagent is specifically calibrated are factors VIII, IX, and XI. The PTT is prolonged in heparin therapy because heparin activates plasma antithrombin, which neutralizes all the plasma serine proteases, particularly thrombin (IIa) and activated factor X (Xa). The PTT is prolonged in the presence of lupus anticoagulant because the anticoagulant neutralizes essential reagent phospholipids. The PTT does not detect factor XIII deficiency. *TF,* Tissue factor; *Pro,* prothrombin (II, zymogen); *Thr,* thrombin (activated factor II, or IIa; serine protease); *Va, VIIIa,* activated factors V and VIII (serine protease cofactors); *VIIa, IXa, Xa, XIa,* activated factors VII, IX, X, XI (serine proteases); *XIIa,* activated factor XII (serine protease, but not part of in vivo coagulation); *XIIIa,* activated factor XIII (transglutaminase).

phospholipid are supplied in the reagent. The factor IXa–calcium–factor VIIIa–phospholipid complex catalyzes factor X (Xa). Factor Xa forms another complex with calcium, phospholipid, and factor Va, catalyzing the conversion of prothrombin to thrombin. Thrombin catalyzes the polymerization of fibrinogen and the formation of the fibrin clot, which is the endpoint of the PTT.

The factors whose deficiencies are associated with hemorrhage and are reflected in prolonged PTT results, taken in the order of reaction, are XI, IX, VIII, X, and V; prothrombin; and fibrinogen, when fibrinogen is 100 mg/dL or less. Most PTT reagents are designed so that the PTT is prolonged when the test PPP has less than approximately 0.3 units/mL (30% of normal) of VIII, IX, or XI.[68] The PTT also is prolonged in the presence of LA, an immunoglobulin with affinity for phospholipid-bound proteins, and is prolonged by anti-factor VIII antibody, antibodies to factor IX and other coagulation factors, and therapeutic heparin. Factor VII and factor XIII deficiencies have no effect on the PTT. Deficiencies of factor XII, prekallikrein, or high-molecular-weight kininogen prolong the PTT but do not cause bleeding.

Partial Thromboplastin Time Procedure

To initiate contact activation, 50 or 100 μL of warmed (37° C) reagent consisting of phospholipid and particulate activator is mixed with an equal volume of warmed PPP. The mixture is allowed to incubate for the exact manufacturer-specified time, usually 3 minutes. Next, 50 or 100 μL of warmed 0.025 M calcium chloride is forcibly added to the mixture, and a timer is started. When a fibrin clot forms, the timer stops, and the interval is recorded. Timing may be done with a stopwatch

or by an automatic electromechanical or photo-optical device. If the PTT is performed manually, the test should be done in duplicate, and the two results must match within 10%.

Partial Thromboplastin Time Quality Control

The medical laboratory practitioner tests normal and prolonged control plasma specimens at the beginning of each 8-hour shift or with each new batch of reagent. The laboratory director may require more frequent use of controls. Controls are tested using the protocol for patient plasma testing.

The normal control result should be within the reference interval, and the abnormal control result should be within the therapeutic range for unfractionated heparin (Chapter 43). If the control results fall within the stated limits in the laboratory protocol, the test results are considered valid. If the results fall outside the control limits, the reagents, control, and equipment are checked; the problem is corrected; and the control and patient specimens are retested. The operator records each control run and all the actions taken. Control results are recorded and analyzed at regular intervals to determine the long-term validity of results.

Reagents must be reconstituted with the correct diluents and volumes following manufacturer instructions. Reagents must be stored and shipped according to manufacturer instructions and never used after the expiration date.

Specimen errors that affect the PT similarly affect the PTT (Table 42-7).

Partial Thromboplastin Time Reference Interval

The PTT reference interval varies from site to site, depending on the patient population, type of reagent, type of instrument, and pH and purity of the diluent. One medical center laboratory has established 26 to 38 seconds as its reference interval. This range is typical, but each center must establish its own interval for each new lot of reagent, or at least once a year. This may be done by testing a sample of 30 or more specimens from healthy donors of both sexes spanning the adult age range over several days and computing the 95% confidence interval of the results.

Monitoring of Heparin Therapy with Partial Thromboplastin Time

Since the early 1970s, the PTT has been the standard method for monitoring unfractionated heparin therapy, which is used to treat patients with venous thrombosis, pulmonary embolism, myocardial infarction, and several other medical conditions.[69] The laboratory practitioner establishes a PTT therapeutic range and publishes it to all inpatient units. A typical therapeutic range is 60 to 100 seconds; however, the range varies widely and must be established locally.[70] The range must be reestablished with each change of PTT reagent, including each lot change, and upon instrument recalibration. Details on monitoring of heparin therapy and establishment of the PTT therapeutic range are provided in Chapter 43.

The Partial Thromboplastin Time as a Diagnostic Assay

The physician orders a PTT assay when a hemorrhagic disorder is suspected or when recurrent thrombosis or the presence of an autoimmune disorder points to the possibility of an LA.[71] The PTT result is prolonged when there is a deficiency of one or more of the following coagulation factors: prothrombin; factor V, VIII, IX, X, XI, or XII; or fibrinogen when the fibrinogen level is 100 mg/dL or less. The PTT also is prolonged in the presence of a specific inhibitor, such as anti-factor VIII or anti-factor IX; a non-specific inhibitor, such as LA; and interfering substances, such as fibrin degradation products (FDPs) or paraproteins, which are present in myeloma.

DIC prolongs PTT results because of consumption of procoagulants, but the PTT results alone are not definitive for the diagnosis of DIC. Vitamin K deficiency results in diminished levels of procoagulant factors II (prothrombin), VII, IX, and X, and the PTT is eventually prolonged. Because factor VII deficiency does not affect the PTT, however, and because it is the first coagulation factor to become deficient, the PTT is not as sensitive to vitamin K deficiency or Coumadin therapy as the PT. The PTT is not prolonged in deficiencies of factor VII or XIII. No clinical data support the use of the PTT as a general screening test for individuals at low risk of bleeding.[72]

Partial Thromboplastin Time Mixing Studies
Lupus Anticoagulants

LAs are IgG immunoglobulins directed against a number of phospholipid-protein complexes.[72] LAs prolong the phospholipid-dependent PTT reaction. Most laboratories employ a moderate-phospholipid or high-phospholipid PTT reagent in their primary PTT assay to monitor heparin therapy and detect coagulopathies. Laboratories use a second low-phospholipid

PTT reagent such as PTT-LA (Diagnostica Stago, Parsippany, NJ), which is more sensitive to LA, as their LA screen (Chapter 39). Because they have a variety of target antigens, LAs are called *nonspecific inhibitors*. Chronic presence of LAs confers a 30% risk of arterial or venous thrombosis; every acute care laboratory must provide a means for their detection. Together, chronic and transient LAs are found in 1% to 2% of randomly selected individuals.

Specific Factor Inhibitors

Specific factor inhibitors are IgG immunoglobulins directed against coagulation factors. Specific inhibitors arise in severe congenital factor deficiencies during factor concentrate treatment. Anti-factor VIII, the most common of the specific inhibitors, is detected in 10% to 20% of patients with severe hemophilia, and anti-factor IX is detected in 1% to 3% of factor IX-deficient patients. Autoantibodies to factor VIII occasionally may arise in individuals without hemophilia, usually in young women, where they are associated with a postpartum bleeding syndrome or in patients over 60 with autoimmune disorders. The presence of these types of antibodies is called *acquired hemophilia* (Chapter 38). Alloantibodies and autoantibodies to factor VIII are associated with severe anatomic hemorrhage.

Detection and Identification of Lupus Anticoagulants and Specific Inhibitors

LA testing is part of every thrombophilia profile (Chapter 39). An unexpectedly prolonged screening PTT may also trigger an LA investigation. PTT mixing studies are necessary for the initial detection of LAs.[73] Mixing studies also distinguish LAs from specific inhibitors and factor deficiencies and should be available in all coagulation laboratories.[74]

When the initial PTT is prolonged beyond the upper limit of the reference interval, the laboratory practitioner first determines if heparin is present by performing the TCT. A TCT result that exceeds the upper limit of the TCT reference interval is evidence for the presence of heparin. In fact, heparin often prolongs the TCT to 30 to 40 seconds. Heparin may be neutralized using polybrene or heparinase (Hepzyme; Siemens Healthcare Diagnostics, Tarrytown, NY), and the treated sample may be used for PTT mixing studies.

The heparin-free or heparin-neutralized patient plasma is then mixed 1:1 with *reagent platelet-poor normal plasma* (PNP; Figure 39-1). Several manufacturers make PNP—for example, frozen Cryo*check* Normal Reference Plasma (Precision BioLogic, Inc, Dartmouth, Nova Scotia). A new PTT is performed immediately on the 1:1 mixture. If the mixture PTT corrects to within 10% of the PNP PTT (or to within the reference interval) and the patient is experiencing bleeding, a coagulation factor deficiency (coagulopathy) is presumed.[75]

Some LAs are time dependent and temperature dependent. Most anti-factor VIII inhibitors are temperature-dependent IgG4-class antibodies. If the immediate PTT corrects, a new mixture is prepared and incubated 1 to 2 hours at 37° C. If the incubated mixture's PTT fails to correct to within 10% of the incubated PNP PTT, an inhibitor may be present. If the patient is bleeding, a specific inhibitor such as anti-factor VIII is suspected, and a factor VIII activity assay is performed. Although anti-factor IX and other inhibitors have been documented, anti-factor VIII is the most common. The Bethesda titer procedure, discussed later in this chapter, is used to confirm the presence of specific anti-coagulation factor antibodies.

If the PTT of the initial or incubated mixture fails to correct and the patient is not bleeding, the laboratory practitioner suspects LA and automatically orders an LA profile, as described in Chapter 39. LA profiles are available from tertiary care facilities and specialty reference laboratories.

Thrombin Clotting Time

Thrombin Clotting Time Reagent and Principle

Commercially prepared bovine thrombin reagent at 5 National Institutes of Health (NIH) units/mL cleaves fibrinopeptides A and B from plasma fibrinogen to form a detectable fibrin polymer (Figure 42-10).

Thrombin Clotting Time Procedure

Reagent thrombin is warmed to 37° C for a minimum of 3 and a maximum of 10 minutes. Thrombin deteriorates during incubation and must be used within 10 minutes of the time incubation is begun. An aliquot of PPP, usually 100 μL, is also incubated at 37° C for a minimum of 3 and a maximum of 10 minutes. The operator pipettes 200 μL of thrombin into the PPP aliquot, starts a timer, and records the interval to clot formation. TCT tests may be performed in duplicate and the results averaged.

Thrombin Clotting Time Quality Control

The medical laboratory practitioner tests a normal control sample and an abnormal control sample with each batch of TCT assays and records the results. The normal control results should fall within the laboratory's reference interval. The abnormal control results should be prolonged to the range reached by the TCT in moderate hypofibrinogenemia. If the results fall outside the laboratory protocol's control limits, the reagents, control, and equipment are checked; the problem is corrected; and the control is retested. The actions taken to correct out-of-limit tests are recorded. Control results are analyzed at regular intervals (weekly is typical) to determine the longitudinal validity of the procedure.

Specimen errors that affect the PT likewise affect the TCT (Table 42-7).

Reporting of Thrombin Clotting Time Results and Clinical Utility

A typical TCT reference interval is 15 to 20 seconds, although the reference interval should be established locally. The TCT is prolonged when the fibrinogen level is less than 100 mg/dL (hypofibrinogenemia) or in the presence of antithrombotic materials such as FDPs, paraproteins, or heparin. Afibrinogenemia (absence of fibrinogen) and dysfibrinogenemia (presence of fibrinogen that is biochemically abnormal and nonfunctional) also cause a prolonged TCT. Before a prolonged TCT may be considered as evidence of diminished or abnormal fibrinogen, the presence of antithrombotic substances, such as heparin, FDPs, or paraproteins, must be ruled out. The TCT is part of the PTT mixing study protocol and is used to determine whether heparin is present whenever the PTT is prolonged.[76]

The TCT may also assess the presence of the oral direct thrombin inhibitor dabigatran. The TCT provides binary (qualitative) evidence for dabigatran; if drug is present, the TCT is markedly prolonged. A normal TCT rules out dabigatran.

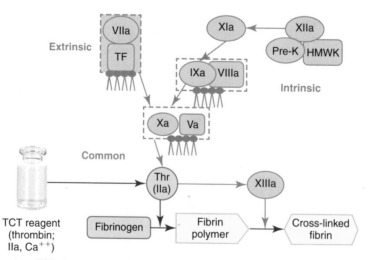

Figure 42-10 Thrombin clotting time (TCT, also reptilase time) coagulation pathway. The reagent activates the coagulation pathway at the level of thrombin and tests for the polymerization of fibrinogen (see colored area in figure). The TCT is prolonged by unfractionated heparin; direct thrombin inhibitors; fibrin degradation products; M-proteins; and dysfibrinogenemia, hypofibrinogenemia, and afibrinogenemia. The reptilase time is unaffected by heparin but is prolonged by dysfibrinogenemia, hypofibrinogenemia, and afibrinogenemia. Neither the TCT nor reptilase time detects factor XIII deficiency. *HMWK,* High-molecular-weight kininogen (Fitzgerald factor); *NCS,* negatively charged surface; *Pre-K,* prekallikrein (Fletcher factor); *PL,* phospholipid; *TF,* tissue factor; *Thr,* thrombin (activated factor II, or IIa; serine protease); *Va, VIIIa,* activated factors V and VIII (serine protease cofactors); *VIIa, IXa, Xa, XIa,* activated factors VII, IX, X, XI (serine proteases); *XIIa,* activated factor XII (serine protease, but not part of in vivo coagulation); *XIIIa,* activated factor XIII (transglutaminase).

A TCT modification, the plasma-diluted TCT, provides a quantitative measure of dabigatran when used with calibrators of specific drug concentrations.[77]

The fibrinogen assay described in a subsequent section is a simple modification of the TCT. In the fibrinogen assay, the concentration of reagent thrombin is 50 NIH units/mL, or about 10 times that used in the TCT, and the patient specimen is diluted 1:10. This dilution minimizes the effects of heparin or antithrombotic proteins. The reptilase time procedure described below is identical to the TCT procedure, except that the reptilase reagent is insensitive to the effects of heparin.

Reptilase Time
Reptilase Time Reagent and Principle
Reptilase is a thrombin-like enzyme isolated from the venom of *Bothrops atrox* that catalyzes the conversion of fibrinogen to fibrin (Pefakit Reptilase Time; Pentapharm, Inc., Basel, Switzerland). In contrast to thrombin, this enzyme cleaves only fibrinopeptide A from the fibrinogen molecule, whereas thrombin cleaves both fibrinopeptides A and B.[78] The specimen requirements, procedure, and quality assurance protocol for the reptilase time test are the same as those for the TCT. The reagent is reconstituted with distilled water and is stable for 1 month when stored at 1° C to 6° C. Reptilase time reagent is a poison that may be fatal if it directly enters the bloodstream.

Reptilase Time Clinical Utility
Reptilase is insensitive to heparin but is sensitive to dysfibrinogenemia, which profoundly prolongs the assay time. The reptilase time test is also useful for detecting hypofibrinogenemia or dysfibrinogenemia in patients receiving heparin therapy. The reptilase time is prolonged in the presence of FDPs and paraproteins.

Russell Viper Venom
Russell viper venom (RVV) from the *Daboia russelii* viper, which triggers coagulation at the level of factor X, was once used as an alternative to the prothrombin time. The assay was named the Stypven time, but is now obsolete. Russell viper venom is used in a dilute form to detect and confirm lupus anticoagulant, an assay called the dilute Russell viper venom time described in Chapter 39.

COAGULATION FACTOR ASSAYS

Fibrinogen Assay
Fibrinogen Assay Principle
The clot-based method of Clauss, a modification of the TCT, is the recommended procedure for estimating the functional fibrinogen level.[79,80] The operator adds reagent bovine thrombin to dilute PPP, catalyzing the conversion of fibrinogen to fibrin polymer. In the fibrinogen assay, the thrombin reagent concentration is 50 NIH units/mL. The PPP to be tested is diluted 1:10 with Owren buffer. There is an inverse relationship between the interval to clot formation and the concentration of functional fibrinogen. Because the thrombin reagent is

concentrated and the PPP is diluted, the relationship is linear when the fibrinogen concentration is 100 to 400 mg/dL. Diluting the PPP also minimizes the antithrombotic effects of heparin, FDPs, and paraproteins; heparin levels less than 0.6 units/mL and FDP levels less than 100 μg/dL do not affect the results of the fibrinogen assay provided the fibrinogen concentration is 150 mg/dL or greater.

The interval to clot formation is compared with the results for fibrinogen calibrators. A calibration curve is prepared in each laboratory and updated regularly.

Fibrinogen Assay Procedure
Fibrinogen Assay Thrombin Reagent. Most laboratory managers prefer commercially manufactured diagnostic lyophilized bovine thrombin reagent for fibrinogen assays. Pharmaceutical topical thrombin also may be used. The reagent is reconstituted according to manufacturer instructions and used immediately or aliquotted and frozen. If thrombin is to be frozen, it should be prepared in a stock solution of 1000 NIH units/mL and frozen at –70° C until it is ready for use. When thawed, the thrombin is diluted 1:2 with buffer, is stable for only a few hours, and cannot be refrozen.

Fibrinogen Assay Calibration Curve. The laboratory practitioner prepares a calibration curve every 6 months at a minimum and with each change of reagent lot numbers, with a shift in QC, and after major maintenance. The curve is prepared by reconstituting commercially available lyophilized fibrinogen calibration plasma. Using Owren buffer, five dilutions of the calibration plasma are prepared: 1:5, 1:10, 1:15, 1:20, and 1:40. An aliquot of each dilution, usually 200 μL, is transferred to each of three reaction tubes or cups, warmed to 37° C, and tested by adding 100 μL of working thrombin reagent at 50 NIH units/mL. Time from addition of thrombin to clot formation is recorded, results of duplicate tests are averaged, and the values in seconds are graphed against fibrinogen concentration (Figure 42-11). Because patient PPPs are diluted 1:10 before testing, the 1:10 calibration plasma dilution is assigned the same fibrinogen concentration value as that of the undiluted reconstituted calibration plasma.

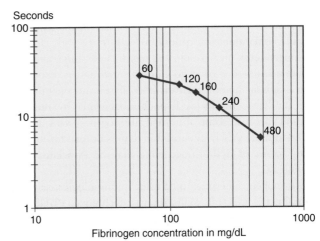

Figure 42-11 Fibrinogen calibrator curve plotted on log-log axes.

Fibrinogen Assay Test Protocol. The laboratory practitioner prepares a 1:10 dilution of each patient PPP and control with Owren buffer. Then 200 µL of each of the diluted PPPs is warmed to 37° C in each of two reaction tubes or cups for 3 minutes. After incubation, 100 µL of thrombin reagent is added, a timer is started, and the mixture is observed until a clot forms. The timer is stopped, values for duplicate runs are averaged, and the interval in seconds is compared with the graph. Results are reported in mg/dL of fibrinogen.

If the clotting time of the patient PPP dilution is short, indicating a fibrinogen level greater than 480 mg/dL, a 1:20 dilution is prepared and tested. The resulting fibrinogen concentration from the graph must be multiplied by 2 to compensate for the dilution. If the clotting time of the original 1:10 patient PPP dilution is prolonged, indicating less than 200 mg/dL of fibrinogen, a 1:5 dilution is prepared. The operator divides the resulting concentration reading from the graph by 2 to compensate for the greater concentration of the specimen.

Fibrinogen Assay Quality Control

All results for duplicate tests must agree within a coefficient of variation of less than 7%. The medical laboratory practitioner tests a normal control sample and an abnormal control sample with each batch of specimens for which fibrinogen levels are measured and records the results. The normal control results should be within the laboratory's reference interval. The abnormal control results should be less than 100 mg/dL. If either control result falls outside the control limits, the reagents, control, and equipment are checked; the problem is corrected; and the control is retested. The actions taken to correct out-of-limit tests are recorded. Control results are analyzed at regular intervals (weekly is typical) to determine the longitudinal validity of the procedure.

Specimen errors that affect the PTT likewise affect the fibrinogen assay and all factor assays (Table 42-7).

Fibrinogen Assay Results and Clinical Utility

One institution's reference interval for fibrinogen concentration is 220 to 498 mg/dL, although each local institution prepares its own interval. Hypofibrinogenemia, a fibrinogen level of less than 220 mg/dL, is associated with DIC and severe liver disease. Moderately severe liver disease, pregnancy, and a chronic inflammatory condition may cause an elevated fibrinogen level, greater than 498 mg/dL. Congenital afibrinogenemia leads to prolonged clotting times and is associated with a variable hemorrhagic disorder. Dysfibrinogenemia may give the same results as hypofibrinogenemia by this test method, because some abnormal fibrinogen species are hydrolyzed more slowly by thrombin than is normal fibrinogen. Some forms of dysfibrinogenemia may be associated with thrombosis.[81]

Fibrinogen values measured using immunologic assays and turbidimetric methods (Ellis-Stransky technique; PT-Fibrinogen HS Plus, Instrumentation Laboratory, Bedford, MA) are normal in dysfibrinogenemia. The fibrinogen concentration is estimated from reaction mixture turbidity and reported with each PT.

Fibrinogen Assay Limitations

Although antithrombotic effects are minimized by the dilution of PPP specimens, heparin levels greater than 0.6 units/mL and FDP levels greater than 100 µg/mL prolong the results and give falsely lowered fibrinogen results. The operator ensures that the thrombin reagent is pure and has not degenerated. Exposure to sunlight or oxidation results in rapid breakdown. The working dilution lasts only 1 hour at 1° C to 6° C and should remain cold until just before testing.

Single-Factor Assays Using the Partial Thromboplastin Time Test

Principle of Single-Factor Assays Based on Partial Thromboplastin Time

If the PTT is prolonged and the PT and TCT are normal, and there is no ready explanation for the prolonged PTT such as heparin therapy, LA, or a factor-specific inhibitor, the medical laboratory practitioner may suspect a congenital single-factor deficiency. Three factor deficiencies that give this reaction pattern and cause hemorrhage are factor VIII deficiency (hemophilia A), factor IX deficiency (hemophilia B), and factor XI deficiency, which causes a mild intermittent bleeding disorder called *Rosenthal syndrome* found primarily in Ashkenazi Jews.[82,83] These deficiencies are most often detected in childhood. The next step in diagnosis of a congenital single-factor deficiency is the performance of a one-stage single-factor assay based on the PTT system.

Although necessary for diagnosis, PTT-based single-factor assays are most often performed on specimens from patients with previously identified single-factor deficiencies. Their purpose is to monitor supportive therapy during bleeding episodes or invasive procedures. Because hemophilia A is the most common single-factor deficiency disorder, this discussion is confined to the factor VIII assay; however, the protocol may be generalized to the assays for factors IX and XI.

The medical laboratory practitioner uses the PTT system to estimate the concentration of functional factor VIII by incorporating commercially prepared factor VIII-depleted PPP in the test system (Cryo*check* Factor VIII Deficient Plasma; Precision BioLogic Inc, Dartmouth, Nova Scotia). Distributors collect plasma from normal donors and employ *immunodepletion*, relying on a monoclonal anti-factor VIII antibody bound to a separatory column, to prepare factor VIII-depleted plasma.[84]

In the PTT-based factor assay system, factor VIII-depleted PPP provides normal activity of all procoagulants except factor VIII. Tested alone, factor VIII-depleted PPP has a prolonged PTT, but when normal PPP is added, the PTT reverts to normal. In contrast, a prolonged result for a mixture of patient PPP and factor VIII-depleted PPP implies that the patient PPP is factor VIII deficient. The clotting time interval for the mixture of patient PPP and factor VIII-depleted PPP may be compared with a previously prepared reference curve to estimate the level of factor VIII activity in the patient PPP. The quantitative factor assay is typically performed on three or four dilutions of patient PPP—for instance, 1:10, 1:20, 1:40, and 1:80—and the results compared with mathematical manipulation. Multiple dilutions contribute to the accuracy of the results.

Factor VIII Assay Reference Curve

To prepare a reference curve for the factor VIII assay, the laboratory practitioner obtains a reference plasma such as CAP FVIIIc RM (College of American Pathologists, Northfield, IL) and prepares a series of dilutions with buffered saline.[85] Although laboratory protocols vary, most laboratory practitioners prepare a series of five dilutions, from 1:5 to 1:500. Each dilution is mixed with reagent factor VIII-depleted plasma and tested in duplicate using the PTT system. The duplicate results are averaged and plotted on log-log or log-linear graph paper (Figure 42-12). The 1:10 dilution is assigned the factor VIII assay activity value found on the package insert. When patient PPP is tested, the time interval obtained is entered on the vertical coordinate and converted to a percentage.[86]

Factor VIII Assay Procedure

The medical laboratory practitioner (or the automated coagulometer) prepares 1:10, 1:20, 1:40, and 1:80 dilutions of each patient PPP and control specimen and then mixes each dilution with equal volumes of factor VIII-depleted plasma and PTT reagent. In most cases, 100 μL of PTT reagent is mixed with 100 μL each of patient PPP dilution and factor VIII-depleted plasma mixture. All dilutions of each specimen or control are tested in duplicate. After incubation at 37° C for the manufacturer-specified time, typically 3 minutes, 100 μL of 0.025 M calcium chloride is added, and a timer is started. The interval is recorded in seconds, duplicates are averaged, the mean result is compared with the reference curve, and the percentage of factor VIII activity is reported. Factor activity results for the 1:20, 1:40, and 1:80 dilutions are multiplied by 2, 4, and 8, respectively, to compensate for the dilutions and should match the results of the 1:10 dilutions within 10%. If the results of the dilutions do not match within 10%, they are considered to be *nonparallel*. An LA may be present, and the assay cannot provide a reliable estimate of factor VIII activity.

Tests for factors IX and XI are performed using the same approach, except that the appropriate factor-depleted plasma is substituted for factor VIII-depleted plasma. Tests for the contact factors XII, prekallikrein, and high-molecular-weight kininogen are seldom requested because deficiencies are not associated with bleeding disorders. Acquired and congenital contact factor deficiencies are relatively common, however, and cause PTT prolongation. Factor XII, prekallikrein, and high-molecular-weight kininogen assays are available from hemostasis reference laboratories, and their use may be necessary to account for an unexplained prolonged PTT.

Expected Results and Clinical Utility of Single-Factor Assays

The reference interval for factor VIII activity is 50% to 186%. Spontaneous symptoms of hemophilia are evident at activity levels of 10% or less. The test is used most often to estimate the plasma level of factor VIII activity during therapy (Chapter 38). Chronically elevated factor VIII predicts an elevated risk of venous thrombotic disease (Chapter 39).

Single-Factor Assay Quality Control

All duplicate results must agree within 10%. The medical laboratory practitioner tests a normal and a deficient control specimen with each assay and records the results. The normal control results should fall within the reference interval. The deficient control results should be in the range of 10% factor VIII activity or below. If either control result falls outside the control limits, the reagents, control, and equipment are checked; the problem is corrected; and the control is retested. The practitioner records all actions taken to correct out-of-limit tests. Control results are analyzed at regular intervals (weekly is typical) to determine the longitudinal validity of the procedure.

Limitations of Single-Factor Assays

Interlaboratory coefficients of variation for the factor VIII assay reach 80%, which implies undesirable variation in the interpretation of therapeutic monitoring results from unrelated institutions. To reduce inherent variation, the medical laboratory practitioner uses assayed commercial plasma to prepare the reference curve and selects reference dilutions that correspond to only the linear portion of the curve. The laboratory must assay three or more dilutions of patient PPP to check for inhibitors. The practitioner also selects a matching reagent-instrument system with a demonstrated coefficient of variation of less than 5% and uses factor-depleted substrates with no trace of the depleted factor.[87] As with the PTT test, good specimen management is essential. Clotted, hemolyzed, icteric, or lipemic specimens are rejected because they give unreliable results. Reagents must be reconstituted with the correct diluents and volumes following manufacturer instructions. Reagents must be stored and shipped in accordance with manufacturer instructions and never used after the expiration date.

Bethesda Titer for Anti–Factor VIII Inhibitor

The Bethesda titer is used to confirm the presence of and quantify an anti-factor VIII inhibitor, which is typically an IgG4-class immunoglobulin.[88] In this method, 200 μL of patient PPP is incubated with 200 μL of reagent normal plasma for 2 hours at 37° C. A control specimen consisting of 200 μL of imidazole buffer at pH 7.4 mixed with 200 μL of reagent normal plasma is incubated simultaneously. During the incubation period,

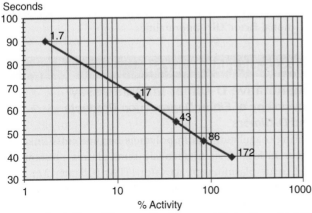

Seconds

Figure 42-12 Factor VIII assay calibrator curve plotted on linear-log axes.

anti-factor VIII from the patient PPP neutralizes a percentage of the reagent normal plasma factor VIII activity. The degree of factor VIII activity neutralized is proportional to the level of inhibitor activity. After incubation, residual factor VIII activity in the patient PPP–reagent normal plasma mixture is measured using the specific factor activity assay as described in the section on factor assays using the PTT system.

The titer of inhibitor is expressed as a percentage of the control. If the patient PPP-reagent normal plasma mixture retains 75% of the residual factor VIII activity of the control, no factor VIII inhibitor is present. If the residual factor VIII level is 25% that of the control, the patient PPP factor VIII inhibitor level is titered using several dilutions of the patient specimen in reagent normal PPP. One Bethesda unit of activity is the amount of antibody that leaves 50% residual factor VIII activity in the mixture.

Single-Factor Assays Using the Prothrombin Time Test

If the PTT and the PT are both prolonged, the TCT is normal, and there is no ready explanation for the prolonged test results, such as liver disease, vitamin K deficiency, DIC, or Coumadin therapy, the medical laboratory practitioner may suspect a congenital single-factor deficiency of the common pathway (Chapter 37). Three relatively rare factor deficiencies that give this reaction pattern and cause hemorrhage are prothrombin deficiency, factor V deficiency, and factor X deficiency. If the PT is prolonged and all other test results are normal, factor VII deficiency is suspected. The next step is the performance of a one-stage single-factor assay based on the PT test system, which is a relatively rare event. The principles and procedure described in the section on single-factor assay using the PTT system may be applied except that PT reagent replaces the PTT reagent in the test system, and the PT protocol is followed. Factor II (prothrombin)-depleted, factor V-depleted, factor VII-depleted, and factor X-depleted plasmas are available (Table 42-8).

Factor XIII Assay

Coagulation factor XIII is a transglutaminase that catalyzes covalent cross-links between the α and γ chains of fibrin polymer.[89] Cross-linking strengthens the fibrin clot and renders it

TABLE 42-8   Factor Assays Using the TCT, PT, and PTT Test Systems

Factor	System
Fibrinogen (I)	Clauss method: modified thrombin clotting time
Prothrombin (II)	Prothrombin time
Factor V	Prothrombin time
Factor VII	Prothrombin time
Factor VIII	Partial thromboplastin time
Factor IX	Partial thromboplastin time
Factor X	Prothrombin time
Factor XI	Partial thromboplastin time
Factor XIII	Chromogenic assay

PT, prothrombin time; *PTT,* partial thromboplastin time; *TCT,* thrombin clotting time.

resistant to proteases. This is the final event in coagulation, and it is essential for normal hemostasis and normal wound healing. Factor XIII from plasma, platelets, and tissue function identically. Neither the PT nor the PTT is prolonged by factor XIII deficiency.

Inherited factor XIII deficiency, an autosomal recessive disorder, affects both sexes in all races. The first report of the deficiency appeared in 1960, and the frequency is estimated at 1 in 2 million. Factor XIII levels also may be low in chronic DIC secondary to Crohn disease, leukemias, ulcerative colitis, sepsis, inflammatory bowel disease, surgery, and Henoch-Schönlein purpura. In these cases, the factor XIII level decreases to 50% of normal, not low enough to create symptoms, although occasionally acquired factor XIII deficiencies produce low enough levels to cause mild bleeding. Acquired factor XIII inhibitors have been described in patients treated with isoniazid, penicillin, valproate, and phenytoin.[90] These drugs may cause complete absence of factor XIII.

Factor XIII activity levels lower than 5% result in hemorrhage. In congenital factor XIII deficiency, bleeding is evident in infants, with seepage at the umbilical stump.[91] In adults, bleeding is slow but progressive, accompanied by poor wound healing and slowly resolving hematomas. Recurrent spontaneous abortion and posttraumatic hemorrhage are common. Acquired factor XIII inhibitors cause severe bleeding that does not respond to therapy.

When a patient comes for treatment of bleeding and poor wound healing and the PTT, PT, platelet count, and fibrinogen level are normal, the laboratory practitioner may recommend a factor XIII assay such as the Technochrom Factor XIII (DiaPharma Group, Inc., West Chester, OH).[92] In this representative assay, quantitation of factor XIII activity is based on the measurement of ammonia released during an in vitro transglutaminase reaction. Plasma factor XIII is first activated by reagent thrombin. The resultant factor XIIIa then cross-links the fibrin amine substrate glycine ethyl ester to the glutamine residue of a peptide substrate, releasing ammonia. The concentration of ammonia is monitored in a glutamate dehydrogenase–catalyzed reaction that depends on NADPH, the reduced form of nicotinamide adenine dinucleotide phosphate. NADPH consumption is measured by the decrease of absorbance at 340 nm. The absorbance is inversely proportional to factor XIII activity. Several manufacturers market immunoassays for factor XIII, which provide factor XIII concentration but do not identify functional factor XIII abnormalities.

TESTS OF FIBRINOLYSIS

Quantitative D-Dimer Immunoassay
Physiology of Fibrin Degradation Products and D-Dimers

During coagulation, fibrin polymers become cross-linked by factor XIIIa and simultaneously bind plasma plasminogen and tissue plasminogen activator (TPA) (Chapter 37). Over several hours, bound TPA activates nearby plasminogen to form plasmin. The bound plasmin cleaves fibrin and yields the FDPs D, E, X, and Y and D-dimer. The FDPs represent original fibrinogen domains, and D-dimers are covalently linked D domains reflecting the cross-linking effects of factor XIIIa. Assays for FDPs, including D-dimer, are convenient for detecting active fibrinolysis, which indirectly implies the occurrence of thrombosis. Normally, FDPs, including D-dimer, circulate at concentrations of less than 2 ng/mL. Fibrinolysis yields FDPs and D-dimer at concentrations greater than 200 ng/mL. Increased FDP and D-dimer concentrations are characteristic of acute and chronic DIC, systemic fibrinolysis, deep vein thrombosis, and pulmonary embolism.[93] FDPs, including D-dimer, also are detected in plasma after thrombolytic therapy.[94]

Principle of the Quantitative D-Dimer Assay

Plasma D-dimer immunoassays abound, and several diagnostics distributors offer automated quantitative immunoassays for plasma D-dimers that generate results within 30 minutes.[95] Microlatex particles in buffered saline are coated with monoclonal anti–D-dimer antibodies. The coated particles are agglutinated by patient plasma D-dimer; the resultant turbidity is measured using turbidometric or nephelometric technology. Sensitivity varies, depending on the avidity of the monoclonal anti–D-dimer and the detection method; however, most methods detect concentrations as low as 10 ng/mL.

Clinical Value of the Quantitative D-Dimer Assay

The quantitative D-dimer assay is essential for ruling out venous thromboembolic disease in patients with low pretest probability and is required for detecting and monitoring DIC (Chapter 39).[96] The D-dimer assay helps rule out acute myocardial infarction and ischemic stroke and may be used to monitor the efficacy of Coumadin therapy.[97] The various quantitative D-dimer assays have negative predictive values of 90% to 95% and may be used to rule out deep vein thrombosis and pulmonary thrombotic emboli in patients at low risk without resorting to compression ultrasonography, tomography, or venous imaging.[98,99] Because of the high sensitivity but low specificity (60% to 70%) of the quantitative D-dimer assay, laboratory practitioners do not use this assay to positively diagnose venous thromboembolic disease but only to rule it out. Because any chronic or acute inflammation is accompanied by elevated D-dimer concentrations, the assay cannot be used to "rule in" thromboembolic disease. The upper limit of the reference interval for the quantitative D-dimer assay varies with the methodology, ranging from 250 ng/mL to 500 ng/mL. In DIC, D-dimer levels may reach 10,000 to 20,000 ng/mL.

Qualitative D-Dimer Assay

The automated quantitative D-dimer assay has largely replaced manual D-dimer or FDP assays. The SimpliRED D-dimer assay (BBInternational, Inc., Dundee, United Kingdom) is a manual method that uses visible latex particles coated with monoclonal antibody. The SimpliRED D-dimer assay is suited to low-volume or near-patient (point-of-care) applications. The manufacturer reports the clinical sensitivity for pulmonary embolus to be 94% and the specificity to be 67%.[100]

Fibrin Degradation Product Immunoassay

Although the FDP assay has largely been replaced by the automated quantitative D-dimer assay or the manual semiquantitative D-dimer assay, FDPs may be detected using a semiquantitative visible agglutination immunoassay.[101] One such method is the 1972 Thrombo-Wellcotest (Remel, Inc., Lenexa, KS).[102] Polystyrene latex particles in buffered saline are coated with polyclonal antibodies specific for D and E fragments calibrated to detect FDPs at a concentration of 2 µg/mL or greater. The assay usually is performed on serum collected in special tubes that promote clotting and prevent in vitro fibrinolysis, although plasma-based assays are also available.

Plasminogen Chromogenic Substrate Assay

Excessive fibrinolytic activity occurs in a variety of conditions. Inflammation and trauma may be reflected in a radical increase in circulating plasmin that has the potential to cause hemorrhage. Bone trauma, fractures, and surgical dissection of bone, as in cardiac surgery, may raise fibrinolysis activity.[103] Fibrinolysis deficiencies occur when TPA or plasminogen levels become depleted or when excess secretion of PAI-1 depresses TPA activity. Plasminogen, the precursor of the trypsin-like proteolytic enzyme plasmin, is produced in the liver and circulates as a single-chain glycoprotein (Chapter 37). When bound to fibrin, plasminogen is converted to plasmin by the action of nearby TPA. Bound plasmin degrades fibrin, whereas a circulating inhibitor, α_2-antiplasmin, rapidly inactivates free plasmin.

Congenital plasminogen deficiencies are associated with thrombosis in some families.[104] Acquired plasminogen deficiencies are seen in DIC and acute promyelocytic leukemia.[105] Thrombolytic therapy is ineffective when plasminogen activity is low. Plasminogen is readily measured in PPP using a chromogenic substrate assay, available from several manufacturers.

Principle of the Plasminogen Chromogenic Substrate Assay

Chromogenic substrates employ synthetic oligopeptides whose amino acid sequences are designed to be specific for their chosen enzymes. Plasmin hydrolyzes a bond in the oligopeptide sequence valine-leucine-lysine (Val-Leu-Lys). A fluorophore or a chromophore such as para-nitroaniline (pNA) is covalently bound to the carboxyl terminus of the oligopeptide and may be released on digestion. S-2251, composed of H-D-Val-Leu-Lys-pNA, is a chromogenic substrate for plasmin. On plasmin digestion, the pNA is released and transforms from a colorless liquid to yellow (Figure 42-13).

Streptokinase is an exogenous plasminogen activator derived from cultures of β-hemolytic streptococci. Streptokinase is added to patient PPP, where it binds and activates plasminogen. The resulting streptokinase-plasmin complex reacts with a chromogenic substrate such as S-2251 to release a color whose intensity is proportional to the plasminogen concentration. Several analogous chromogenic and fluorogenic substrates are suitable for plasminogen measurement. Control plasma is tested with the patient plasma, and the results are recorded.

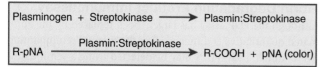

Figure 42-13 Assay of plasma plasminogen using the chromogenic substrate method. Reagent streptokinase activates plasminogen to form plasmin. *R-pNA* designates a chromogenic substrate, where *R* indicates one of several choices of peptide sequence and *pNA* (para-nitroaniline) is the chromophore. In the case of plasminogen, the *R* represents the peptide sequence valine-leucine-lysine (Val-Leu-Lys). Plasmin recognizes the Val-Leu-Lys amide sequence as its enzymatic cleavage site, releasing the pNA, which generates a yellow color.

Results and Clinical Utility of the Plasminogen Chromogenic Substrate Assay

The plasminogen reference interval is 5 to 13.5 mg/dL. Plasminogen levels are decreased in thrombolytic therapy, DIC, hepatitis, and cancer. Hereditary deficiencies have also been recorded.[101] Decreased plasminogen is associated with thrombosis. Plasminogen rises in inflammation and during pregnancy, and high levels may be associated with hemorrhage. Plasminogen levels may also be elevated in systemic fibrinolysis. Plasminogen assays are seldom offered in acute care facilities but are readily available at specialty reference laboratories.

Tissue Plasminogen Activator Assay
Physiology of Tissue Plasminogen Activator

The two physiologic human plasminogen activators are TPA and urokinase.[106,107] TPA is synthesized in vascular endothelial cells and released into the circulation, where its half-life is approximately 3 minutes and its plasma concentration averages 5 ng/mL. Urokinase is produced in the kidney and vascular endothelial cells and has a half-life of approximately 7 minutes and a concentration of 2 to 4 ng/mL. Both activators are serine proteases that form ternary complexes with bound plasminogen at the surface of fibrin, activating the plasminogen and initiating thrombus degradation. The endothelial secretion *plasminogen activator inhibitor-1* (PAI-1) covalently inactivates both.

Clinical Significance of Tissue Plasminogen Activator

The reference interval upper limit for TPA *activity* is 1.1 units/mL, and the upper limit for TPA *antigen* is 14 ng/mL. TPA is the primary mediator of fibrinolysis and is the model for synthetic TPA (Activase; Genentech, Inc., South San Francisco, CA). Decreased TPA levels may indicate increased risk of myocardial infarction, stroke, or deep vein thrombosis, although more data are needed to verify a relationship.[108] Impaired fibrinolysis in the form of TPA deficiency or PAI-1 excess also is associated with deep vein thrombosis and myocardial infarction.[109]

Specimen Collection for the Tissue Plasminogen Activator Assay

TPA activity exhibits diurnal variation and rises upon exercise. Further, TPA is unstable in vitro because it rapidly binds PAI-1 after collection. For specimen collection, patients should be at rest, tourniquet application should be minimal, the phlebotomist should record the collection time, and immediate acidification of the specimen in acetate buffer is necessary.[110] Acidification may be accomplished using the Stabilyte acidified citrate tube (Diagnostica Stago, Inc., Parsippany, NJ). Supernatant PPP may be frozen at –70° C until the assay is performed.

Principle of the Tissue Plasminogen Activator Assay

Plasma concentration of TPA antigen may be estimated by enzyme immunoassay. To measure TPA activity, a specified concentration of reagent plasminogen is added to the patient plasma (Chromolyse TPA Activity; Diagnostica Stago, Inc, Parsippany, NJ). Plasma TPA activates the plasminogen, and the resultant plasmin activity is measured using a chromogenic substrate. The resulting color intensity is proportional to TPA activity (Figure 42-14). The system may incorporate soluble fibrin to increase TPA activity.

Plasminogen Activator Inhibitor-1 Assay

PAI-1 is produced by vascular endothelial cells and hepatocytes and circulates in plasma bound to vitronectin at an average concentration of 10 μg/L with diurnal variations.[111] An inactive form of PAI-1 circulates in high concentrations in platelets.[112] PAI-1 inactivates free TPA by covalent binding. Elevated PAI-1 is associated with venous thrombosis and may be a cardiovascular risk factor (Chapter 39). A few cases of PAI-1 deficiency have been reported; however, hemorrhage apparently occurs only in the complete absence of PAI-1.

Blood is collected from patients at rest into an acidified citrate tube (Stabilyte) and centrifuged immediately to make PPP; this avoids in vitro release of platelet PAI-1. Several immunometric and chromogenic substrate methods are available for estimation of PAI-1 antigen and PAI-1 activity, respectively. One enzyme immunoassay for functional PAI-1 uses urokinase to bind PAI-1. The urokinase–PAI-1 complex is immobilized with solid-phase monoclonal anti–PAI-1 and is measured using monoclonal anti-urokinase immunoglobulin as the detecting antibody.[113,114]

Most chromogenic substrate kits for PAI-1 use an indirect measurement approach (Spectrolyse PAI-1; Diagnostica Stago, Inc, Parsippany, NJ). Patient PPP is mixed with a measured amount of reagent TPA. Residual TPA is assayed in the

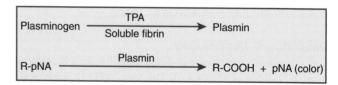

Figure 42-14 To assay tissue plasminogen activator (TPA), plasma that contains TPA is added to plasminogen to produce plasmin. Plasmin activity is measured using the same chromogenic substrate system as in the plasminogen assay illustrated in Figure 42-13. The intensity of color is proportional to TPA activity. *pNA*, Para-nitroaniline; *R*, variable peptide sequence.

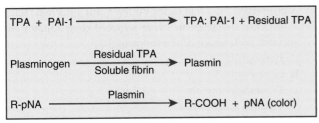

Figure 42-15 To assay plasminogen activator inhibitor 1 (PAI-1) activity, plasma containing PAI-1 is added to reagent tissue plasminogen activator (TPA) of known concentration. The residual TPA is assayed, as shown in Figure 42-14. The intensity of color is inversely proportional to PAI-1 level. *pNA*, Para-nitroaniline; *R*, variable peptide sequence.

plasminogen system as shown in Figure 42-15. The resulting color intensity is inversely proportional to plasma PAI-1 activity.

Confirmation of total PAI-1 deficiency may be accomplished using the *serum* PAI-1 assay. In serum, platelet PAI-1 is expressed in excess. In true PAI-1 absence, no PAI-1 is detectable in serum.

GLOBAL COAGULATION ASSAYS

The TEG Thromboelastograph Hemostasis Analyzer (Haemoscope Corporation, Niles, IL, a division of Haemonetics Corporation) and the ROTEM (Tem, Inc, Durham, NC) are global whole-blood analyzers that measure clotting time and dynamics, clot strength, antithrombotic effects, platelet effects on clot dynamics and strength, and fibrinolysis.[115] Both are used as a manual coagulometers, mainly in liver and cardiac surgeries and are described in detail in Chapter 44.

SUMMARY

- Proper hemostasis specimen collection, transport, storage, and centrifugation ensure a valid test result.
- Specimens that are short draws, clotted, or hemolyzed are rejected.
- Platelet aggregometry helps determine the cause of nonthrombocytopenic mucocutaneous bleeding.
- VWD is diagnosed and monitored through the judicious selection and performance of platelet-based laboratory tests.
- The plasma markers PF4 and β-thromboglobulin are research applications used to assess platelet activation.
- Clot-based coagulation screening tests include the ACT, PT, PTT, and TCT.
- Mixing studies are used to detect factor deficiencies, LAs, and specific factor inhibitors.

- Coagulation factor assays are used to detect and measure coagulation factor deficiencies.
- Bethesda titers are used to detect and measure coagulation factor inhibitors.
- Tests of fibrinolysis include assays for FDPs, D-dimer, plasminogen, TPA, and PAI-1.
- Thromboelastography and thromboelastometry are widely used global hemostasis assay methods.

Now that you have completed this chapter, go back and read again the case study at the beginning and respond to the questions presented.

REVIEW QUESTIONS

Answers can be found in the Appendix.

1. What happens if a coagulation specimen collection tube is underfilled?
   a. The specimen clots and is useless
   b. The specimen is hemolyzed and is useless
   c. Clot-based test results are falsely prolonged
   d. Chromogenic test results are falsely decreased

2. If you collect blood into a series of tubes, when in the sequence should the hemostasis (blue stopper) tube be filled?
   a. After a lavender-topped or green-topped tube
   b. First, or after a nonadditive tube
   c. After a serum separator tube
   d. Last

3. What is the effect of hemolysis on a hemostasis specimen?
   a. In vitro platelet and coagulation activation occur
   b. The specimen is icteric or lipemic
   c. Hemolysis has no effect
   d. The specimen is clotted

4. Most coagulation testing must be performed on PPP, which is plasma with a platelet count less than:
   a. 1000/μL
   b. 10,000/μL
   c. 100,000/μL
   d. 1,000,000/μL

5. You wish to obtain a 5-mL specimen of whole-blood/anticoagulant mixture. The patient's hematocrit is 65%. What volume of anticoagulant should you use?
   a. 0.32 mL
   b. 0.5 mL
   c. 0.64 mL
   d. 0.68 mL

6. You perform whole-blood lumiaggregometry on a specimen from a patient who complains of easy bruising. Aggregation and secretion are diminished when the agonists, thrombin, ADP, arachidonic acid, and collagen are used. What is the most likely platelet abnormality?
   a. Storage pool disorder
   b. Aspirin-like syndrome
   c. ADP receptor anomaly
   d. Glanzmann thrombasthenia

7. What is the reference assay for HIT?
   a. Enzyme immunoassay
   b. Serotonin release assay
   c. Platelet lumiaggregometry
   d. Washed platelet aggregation

8. What agonist is used in platelet aggregometry to detect VWD?
   a. Arachidonic acid
   b. Ristocetin
   c. Collagen
   d. ADP

9. Deficiency of which single factor is likely when the PT result is prolonged and the PTT result is normal?
   a. Factor V
   b. Factor VII
   c. Factor VIII
   d. Prothrombin

10. A prolonged PT, a low factor VII level, but a normal factor V level are characteristic of an acquired coagulopathy associated with which of the following?
    a. Hemophilia
    b. Liver disease
    c. Thrombocytopenia
    d. Vitamin K deficiency

11. The patient has deep vein thrombosis. The PTT is prolonged and is not corrected in an immediate mix of patient plasma with an equal part of normal plasma. What is the presumed condition?
    a. Factor VIII inhibitor
    b. Lupus anticoagulant
    c. Factor VIII deficiency
    d. Factor V Leiden mutation

12. What condition causes the most pronounced elevation in the result of the quantitative D-dimer assay?
    a. Deep vein thrombosis
    b. Fibrinogen deficiency
    c. Paraproteinemia
    d. DIC

13. What is the name given to the type of assay that uses a synthetic polypeptide substrate that releases a chromophore on digestion by its serine protease?
    a. Clot-based assay
    b. Molecular diagnostic assay
    c. Fluorescence immunoassay
    d. Chromogenic substrate assay

14. What component of the fibrinolytic process binds and neutralizes free plasmin?
    a. PAI-1
    b. TPA
    c. α_2-Antiplasmin
    d. Urokinase

REFERENCES

1. Clinical and Laboratory Standards Institute. (2008). *Collection, Transport, and Processing of Blood Specimens for Testing Plasma-Based Coagulation Assays: Approved Guideline.* (5th ed.). CLSI Document H21-A5, Wayne, PA: Clinical and Laboratory Standards Institute.
2. Clinical and Laboratory Standards Institute. (2007). *Procedures for the Collection of Diagnostic Blood Specimens by Venipuncture: Approved Standard.* (6th ed.). CLSI Document GP41-A6, Wayne, PA: Clinical and Laboratory Standards Institute.
3. Clinical and Laboratory Standards Institute. (2010). *Tubes and Additives for Venous Blood Specimen Collection: Approved Standard.* (6th ed.). CLSI Document GP39-A6, Wayne, PA: Clinical and Laboratory Standards Institute.
4. McGlasson, D. L., More, L., Best, H. A., Norris, W. L., Doe, R. H., & Ray, H. (1999). Drawing specimens for coagulation testing: is a second tube necessary? *Clin Lab Sci, 12,* 137–139.
5. Adcock, D. M., Kressin, D. C., & Marlar, R. A. (1998). Minimum specimen volume requirements for routine coagulation testing. *Am J Clin Pathol, 109,* 595–599.
6. Ernst, D. J. (2008). *Blood Specimen Collection FAQs.* Ramsey, IN: Center for Phlebotomy Education.
7. Marcus, N. (2010). Coagulation testing in the context of the automated hospital lab and optimizing for the effects of common interferences. *Clin Chem, 56*(Suppl.), A172 (abstract).
8. Marques, M., & Fritsma, G. A. (2009). *Quick Guide to Coagulation Testing.* (2nd ed.). Washington, DC: AACC Press.
9. Bennett, A., & Fritsma, G. A. (2010). *Quick Guide to Venipuncture.* Washington, DC: AACC Press.
10. McCall, R., & Tankersley, C. (2007). *Phlebotomy Essentials.* (4th ed.). Philadelphia: Lippincott Williams & Wilkins.
11. Ernst, C., & Ernst, D. J. (2001). *Phlebotomy for Nurses and Nursing Personnel.* Ramsey, IN: Center for Phlebotomy Education.
12. Sunderji, R., Gin, K., Shalansky, K., et al. (2005). Clinical impact of point-of-care vs. laboratory measurement of anticoagulation. *Am J Clin Pathol, 123,* 184–188.
13. McGlasson, D. L., Paul, J., & Shaffer, K. M. (1993). Whole blood coagulation testing in neonates. *Clin Lab Sci, 6,* 76–77.

14. Clinical and Laboratory Standards Institute. (2008). *Procedures and Devices for the Collection of Diagnostic Capillary Blood Specimens; Approved Standard.* (6th ed.). CLSI Document GP64-A6, Wayne, PA: Clinical and Laboratory Standards Institute.

15. Adcock, D. M., Kressin, D. C., & Marlar, R. A. (1998). Minimum specimen volume requirements for routine coagulation testing: dependence on citrate concentration. *Am J Clin Pathol,* 109595–109599.

16. van den Besselaar, A. M., Meeuwisse-Braun, J., Schaefer-van Mansfeld, H., et al. (1997). Influence of plasma volumetric errors on the prothrombin time ratio and international sensitivity index. *Blood Coagul Fibrinolysis, 8,* 431–435.

17. Horsti, J. (2001). Use of EDTA samples for prothrombin time measurement in patients receiving oral anticoagulants. *Haematologica, 86,* 851–855.

18. National Heart, Lung, and Blood Institute. (2007). *The Diagnosis, Evaluation, and Management of Von Willebrand Disease.* NIH Publication No. 08-5832, Bethesda, MD: US Department of Health and Human Services, National Institutes of Health.

19. Ens, G. E., & Newlin, F. (1995). Spurious protein S deficiency as a result of elevated factor VII levels. *Clin Hemost Rev, 9,* 18.

20. Adcock, D., Kressin, D., & Marlar, R. A. (1998). The effect of time and temperature variables on routine coagulation tests. *Blood Coagul Fibrinolysis, 9,* 463–470.

21. Dyszkiewicz-Korpanty, A. M., Frenkel, E. P., Ravindra Sarode, R. (2005). Approach to the assessment of platelet function: comparison between optical-based platelet-rich plasma and impedance-based whole blood platelet aggregation methods. *Clin Appl Thromb Hemost, 11,* 25–35.

22. Pierangeli, S. S., & Harris, E. N. (2005). Clinical laboratory testing for the antiphospholipid syndrome. *Clin Chim Acta, 357,* 17–33.

23. Lippi, G., Plebani, M., & Favaloro, E. J. (2013). Interference in coagulation testing: focus on spurious hemolysis, icterus, and lipemia. *Semin Thromb Hemost, 39,* 258–266.

24. Matthews, D. C. (2013). Inherited disorders of platelet function. *Pediatr Clin North Am, 60,* 1475–1478.

25. Dlott, J. S. (2001). Acquired platelet function disorders. In Goodnight, S. H., & Hathaway, W. E., (Eds.), *Disorders of Hemostasis and Thrombosis.* (2nd ed.). New York: McGraw-Hill.

26. Lind, S. E. (1991). The bleeding time does not predict surgical bleeding. *Blood, 77,* 2547–2552.

27. Duke, W. W. (1912). The pathogenesis of purpura haemorrhagica with especial reference to the part played by the blood platelets. *Arch Intern Med, 10,* 445.

28. Ivy, A. C., Nelson, D., & Bucher, G. (1941). The standardization of certain factors in the cutaneous "venostasis" bleeding time technique. *J Lab Clin Med, 26,* 1812.

29. Kumar, R., Ansell, J. E., Canoso, R. T., et al. (1978). Clinical trial of a new bleeding device. *Am J Clin Pathol, 70,* 642–645.

30. Mielke, C. H., Jr., Kaneshiro, M. M., Maher, I. A., et al. (1969). The standardized normal Ivy bleeding time and its prolongation by aspirin. *Blood, 34,* 204–215.

31. Cattaneo, M. (2009). Light transmission aggregometry and ATP release for the diagnostic assessment of platelet function. *Semin Thromb Hemost, 35,* 158–167.

32. McGlasson, D. L., & Fritsma, G. A. (2009). Whole blood platelet aggregometry and platelet function testing. *Semin Thromb Hemost, 35,* 168–180.

33. Rand, M. L., Leung, R., & Packham, M. A. (2003). Platelet function assays. *Transfus Apher Sci, 28,* 307–317.

34. Goldenberg, S. J., Veriabo, N. J., & Soslau, G. (2001). A micromethod to measure platelet aggregation and ATP release by impedance. *Thromb Res, 103,* 57–61.

35. Dyszkiewicz-Korpanty, A. M., Frenkel, E. P., & Sarode, R. (2005). Approach to the assessment of platelet function: comparison between optical-based platelet-rich plasma and impedance-based whole blood platelet aggregation methods. *Clin Appl Thromb Hemost, 11,* 25–35.

36. White, M. M., Foust, J. T., Mauer, A. M., et al. (1992). Assessment of lumiaggregometry for research and clinical laboratories. *Thromb Haemost, 67,* 572–577.

37. Ren, Q., Ye, S., & Whiteheart, S. W. (2008). The platelet release reaction: just when you thought platelet secretion was simple. *Curr Opin Hematol, 15,* 537–541.

38. Michiels, J. J., Gadisseur, A., Budde, U., et al. (2005). Characterization, classification, and treatment of von Willebrand disease: a critical appraisal of the literature and personal experiences. *Semin Thromb Hemost, 31,* 577–601.

39. Budde, U., Drewke, E., Mainusch, K., et al. (2002). Laboratory diagnosis of congenital von Willebrand disease. *Semin Thromb Hemost, 28,* 173–190.

40. Redaelli, R., Corno, A. R., Borroni, L., et al. (2005). von Willebrand factor ristocetin cofactor (VWF:RCo) assay: implementation on an automated coagulometer (ACL). *J Thromb Haemost, 3,* 2684–2688.

41. Hayes, T. E., Brandt, J. T., Chandler, W. L., et al. (2006). External peer review quality assurance testing in von Willebrand disease: the recent experience of the United States College of American Pathologists proficiency testing program. *Semin Thromb Hemost, 32,* 499–504.

42. Sharma, R. K., Reddy, H. K., Singh, V. N., et al. (2009). Aspirin and clopidogrel hyporesponsiveness and nonresponsiveness in patients with coronary artery stenting. *Vasc Health Risk Manag, 5,* 965–972.

43. Raichand, S., Moore, D., Riley, R. D., et al. (2013). Protocol for a systematic review of the diagnostic and prognostic utility of tests currently available for the detection of aspirin resistance in patients with established cardiovascular or cerebrovascular disease. *Syst Rev, 26,* 2–16. doi: 10.1186/2046-4053-2-16.

44. Manoharan, A., Brighton, T., Gemmell, R., et al. (2002). Platelet dysfunction in myelodysplastic syndromes: a clinicopathological study. *Int J Hematol, 76,* 272–278.

45. Brace, L. D. (1992). Testing for heparin-induced thrombocytopenia by platelet aggregometry. *Clin Lab Sci, 5,* 80–81.

46. Warkentin, T. (2013). Heparin-induced thrombocytopenia. In Kitchens, C. S., Kessler, C. M., & Konkle, B. A. *Consultative Hemostasis and Thrombosis.* (3rd ed., pp. 442–476). Elsevier, St. Louis.

47. Warkentin, T. E., Pai, M., Sheppard, J. I., et al. (2011). Fondaparinux treatment of acute heparin-induced thrombocytopenia confirmed by the serotonin-release assay: a 30-month, 16-patient case series. *J Thromb Hemostas, 9,* 2389–2396.

48. McFarland, J., Lochowicz, A., Aster, R., Chappell, B., & Curtis, B. (2012). Improving the specificity of the PF4 ELISA in diagnosing heparin-induced thrombocytopenia. *Am J Hematol, 87,* 776–781.

49. Hassell, K. (2008). Heparin-induced thrombocytopenia: diagnosis and management. *Thromb Res, 123*(Suppl. 1), S16–S21.

50. Ferroni, P., Riondino, S., Vazzana, N., et al. (2012). Biomarkers of platelet activation in acute coronary syndromes. *Thromb Haemost, 108,* 1109–1123.

51. Darling, C. E., Michelson, A. D., Volturo, G. A., et al. (2009). Platelet reactivity and the identification of acute coronary syndromes in the emergency department. *J Thromb Thrombolysis, 28,* 31–37.

52. Rand, M. L., Leung, R., & Packham, M. A. (2003). Platelet function assays. *Transfus Apher Sci, 28,* 307–317.

53. Fritsma, G. A., Ens, G. E., Alvord, M. A., et al. (2001). Monitoring the antiplatelet action of aspirin. *JAAPA, 14,* 57–62.

54. Eikelboom, J. W., & Hankey, G. J. (2004). Failure of aspirin to prevent atherothrombosis: potential mechanisms and implications for clinical practice. *Am J Cardiovasc Drugs, 4,* 57–67.

55. Eikelboom, J. W., Hankey, G. J., Thom, J., et al. (2008). Incomplete inhibition of thromboxane biosynthesis by acetylsalicylic acid: determinants and effect on cardiovascular risk. *Circulation, 118,* 1705–1712.

56. Lee, R. I., & White, P. D. (1913). A clinical study of the coagulation time of blood. *Am J Med Sci, 243,* 279–285.

57. Clinical and Laboratory Standards Institute. (2008). *One-Stage Prothrombin Time (PT) Test and Activated Partial Thromboplastin*

Time (APTT) Test; Approved Guideline. (2nd ed.). CLSI Document H47-A2, Wayne, PA: CLSI.

58. Mannucci, P. M., & Tripodi, A. (2012). Hemostatic defects in liver and renal dysfunction. *Am Soc Hematol Educ Program, 2012*, 168–173.

59. Biggs, R., & MacFarlane, R. G. (1951). Reaction of haemophilic plasma to thromboplastin. *J Clin Pathol, 4*, 445–459.

60. Poller, L. (1986). Laboratory control of anticoagulant therapy. *Semin Thromb Hemost, 12*, 13–19.

61. Ibrahim, S. A., Jespersen, J., Pattison, A., & Poller, L. (2011). European Concerted Action on Anticoagulation. Evaluation of European Concerted Action on Anticoagulation lyophilized plasmas for INR derivation using the PT/INR line. *Am J Clin Pathol, 135*, 732–740.

62. Eisenberg, J. M., Clarke, J. R., & Sussman, S. A. (1982). Prothrombin and partial thromboplastin times as preoperative screening tests. *Arch Surg, 117*, 48–51.

63. Gravlee, G. P., Arora, S., Lavender, S. W., et al. (1994). Predictive value of blood clotting tests in cardiac surgical patients. *Ann Thorac Surg, 58*, 216–221.

64. McKinly, L., & Wrenn, K. (1993). Are baseline prothrombin time/partial thromboplastin time values necessary before instituting anticoagulation? *Ann Emerg Med, 22*, 697–702.

65. Rosborough, T. K., Jacobsen, J. M., & Shepherd, M. F. (2009). Relationship between chromogenic factor X and international normalized ratio differs during early warfarin initiation compared with chronic warfarin administration. *Blood Coagul Fibrinolysis, 20*, 433–435.

66. McGlasson, D. L., Romick, B. G., & Rubal, B. J. (2008). Comparison of a chromogenic factor X assay with international normalized ratio for monitoring oral anticoagulation therapy. *Blood Coagul Fibrinolysis, 19*, 513–517.

67. Lusher, J. M. (1996). Screening and diagnosis of coagulation disorders. *Am J Obstet Gynecol, 175*, 778–783.

68. Lawrie, A. S., Kitchen, S., Efthymiou, M., Mackie, I. J., & Machin, S. J. (2013). Determination of APTT factor sensitivity—the misguiding guideline. *Int J Lab Hematol, 35*, 652–657.

69. Triplett, D. A., Harms, C. S., & Koepke, J. A. (1978). The effect of heparin on the partial thromboplastin time. *Am J Clin Pathol, 70*(Suppl.), 556–559.

70. Brill-Edwards, P., Ginsberg, J. S., Johnston, M., et al. (1993). Establishing a therapeutic range for heparin therapy. *Ann Intern Med, 119*, 104–109.

71. Hayward, C. P., Moffat, K. A., & Liu, Y. (2012). Laboratory investigations for bleeding disorders. *Semin Thromb Hemost, 38*, 742–752.

72. McKinly, L., & Wrenn, K. (1993). Are baseline prothrombin time/partial thromboplastin time values necessary before instituting anticoagulation? *Ann Emerg Med, 22*, 697–702.

73. McNeil, H. P., Simpson, R. J., Chesterman, C. N., et al. (1990). Antiphospholipid antibodies are directed against a complex antigen that includes a lipid-binding inhibitor of coagulation: β-2-glycoprotein I. *Proc Natl Acad Sci USA, 87*, 4120–4124.

74. Ledford-Kraemer, M. R. (2008). Laboratory testing for lupus anticoagulants: pre-examination variables, mixing studies, and diagnostic criteria. *Semin Thromb Hemost, 34*, 380–388.

75. Pengo, V., Tripodi, A., & Reber, G. (2009). Update of the guidelines for lupus anticoagulant detection. Subcommittee on Lupus Anticoagulant/Antiphospholipid Antibody of the Scientific and Standardisation Committee of the International Society on Thrombosis and Haemostasis. *J Thromb Haemost, 7*, 1737–1740.

76. Eika, C., Godal, H. C., & Kierulf, P. (1972). Detection of small amounts of heparin by the thrombin clotting-time. *Lancet, 300*, 376–377.

77. Winkler, A. M., & Tormey, C. A. (2013). Education Committee of the Academy of Clinical Laboratory Physicians and Scientists. Pathology consultation on monitoring direct thrombin inhibitors and overcoming their effects in bleeding patients. *Am J Clin Pathol, 140*, 610–62.

78. Meh, D. A., Siebenlist, K. R., Bergtrom, G., et al. (1995). Sequence of release of fibrinopeptide A from fibrinogen molecules by thrombin or Atroxin. *J Lab Clin Med, 125*, 384–391.

79. Clinical and Laboratory Standards Institute. (2001). *Procedure for the Determination of Fibrinogen in Plasma: Approved Guideline.* (2nd ed.). CLSI Document H30-A2, Wayne, PA: Clinical and Laboratory Standards Institute.

80. Poller, L., Thomson, J. M., & Yee, K. F. (1980). Fibrinogen determination in a series of proficiency studies. *Clin Lab Haematol, 2*, 43–51.

81. Comp, P. C. (1990). Overview of the hypercoagulable states. *Semin Thromb Hemost, 16*, 158–161.

82. Seligsohn, U. (1978). High gene frequency of factor XI (PTA) deficiency in Ashkenazi Jews. *Blood, 51*, 1223–1228.

83. James, P., Salomon, O., Mikovic, D., & Peyvandi, F. (2014). Rare bleeding disorders—bleeding assessment tools, laboratory aspects and phenotype and therapy of FXI deficiency. *Haemophilia, 20*(Suppl. 4), 71–75.

84. Takeyama, M., Nogami, K., Okuda, M., et al. (2008). Selective factor VIII and V inactivation by iminodiacetate ion exchange resin through metal ion adsorption. *Br J Haematol, 142*, 962–970.

85. Arkin, C. F., Bovill, E. G., Brandt, J. T., et al. (1992). Factors affecting the performance of factor VIII coagulant activity assays: results of proficiency surveys of the College of American Pathologists. *Arch Pathol Lab Med, 116*, 908–915.

86. Bowyer, A. E., Van Veen, J. J., Goodeve, A. C., Kitchen, S., & Makris, M. (2013). Specific and global coagulation assays in the diagnosis of discrepant mild hemophilia A. *Haematologica, 98*, 1980–1987.

87. Hirst, C. F., Hewitt, J., & Poller, L. (1992). Trace levels of factor VIII in substrate plasma. *Br J Haematol, 81*, 305–306.

88. Kershaw, G., Jayakodi, D., & Dunkley, S. (2009). Laboratory identification of factor inhibitors: the perspective of a large tertiary hemophilia center. *Semin Thromb Hemost, 35*, 760–768.

89. Duval, C., Philippou, H., & Ariens, R. A. S. (2013). Factor XIII. In Marder, V. J., Aird, W. C., Bennett, J. S., Schulman, S., & White G. C., II, (Eds.), *Hemostasis and Thrombosis: Basic Principles and Clinical Practice.* (6th ed., pp. 272–285). Philadelphia: Lippincott Williams & Wilkins.

90. Krumdieck, R., Shaw, D. R., Huang, S. T., et al. (1991). Hemorrhagic disorder due to an isoniazid-associated acquired factor XIII inhibitor in a patient with Waldenström's macroglobulinemia. *Am J Med, 90*, 639–645.

91. Karimi, M., Bereczky, Z., Cohan, N., et al. (2009). Factor XIII deficiency. *Semin Thromb Hemost, 35*, 426–438.

92. Schroeder, V., & Kohler, H. P. (2013). Factor XIII deficiency: an update. *Semin Thromb Hemost, 39*, 632–641.

93. Southern, D. K. (1992). Serum FDP and plasma D-dimer testing: what are they measuring? *Clin Lab Sci, 5*, 332–333.

94. Lawler, C. M., Bovill, E. G., Stump, D. C., et al. (1990). Fibrin fragment D-dimer and fibrinogen B beta peptides in plasma as markers of clot lysis during thrombolytic therapy in acute myocardial infarction. *Blood, 76*, 1341–1348.

95. Waser, G., Kathriner, S., Wuillemin, W. A. (2005). Performance of the automated and rapid STA Liatest D-dimer on the STA-R analyzer. *Thromb Res, 116*, 165–170.

96. Reber, G., Bounameaux, H., Perrier, A., et al. (2002). Evaluation of advanced D-dimer assay for the exclusion of venous thromboembolism. *Thromb Res, 107*, 197–200.

97. Sadanaga, T., Sadanaga, M., & Ogawa, S. (2010). Evidence that D-dimer levels predict subsequent thromboembolic and cardiovascular events in patients with atrial fibrillation during oral anticoagulant therapy. *J Am Coll Cardiol, 55*, 2225–2231.

98. Khoury, J. D., Adcock, D. M., Chan, F., et al. (2010). Increases in quantitative D-dimer levels correlate with progressive disease better than circulating tumor cell counts in patients with refractory prostate cancer. *Am J Clin Pathol, 134*, 964–969.

99. Stein, P. D., Hull, R. D., Patel, K. C., et al. (2004). D-dimer for the exclusion of acute venous thrombosis and pulmonary embolism: a systematic review. *Ann Intern Med, 140*, 589–602.

100. Kline, J. A., Israel, E. G., & Michelson, E. A. (2001). Diagnostic accuracy of a bedside D-dimer assay and alveolar dead-space measurement for rapid exclusion of pulmonary embolism: a multicenter study. *JAMA, 285*, 761–768.

101. Drewinko, B., Surgeon, J., Cobb, P., et al. (1985). Comparative sensitivity of different methods to detect and quantify circulating fibrinogen/fibrin split products. *Am J Clin Pathol, 84*, 58–66.

102. Garvey, M. B., & Black, J. M. (1972). The detection of fibrinogen-fibrin degradation products by means of a new antibody-coated latex particle. *J Clin Pathol, 25*, 680–682.

103. Schuster, V., Hügle, B., & Tefs, K. (2007). Plasminogen deficiency. *J Thromb Haemost, 5*, 2315–2322.

104. Mehta, R., & Shapiro, A. D. (2008). Plasminogen deficiency. *Haemophilia, 14*, 1261–1268.

105. Mutch, N. J., & Booth, N. A. (2013). Plasminogen activation and regulation of fibrinolysis. In Marder, V. J., Aird, W. C., Bennett, J. S., Schulman, S., White G. C., II, (Eds.), *Hemostasis and Thrombosis: Basic Principles and Clinical Practice.* (6th ed., pp. 314–333). Philadelphia: Lippincott Williams & Wilkins.

106. Gebbink, M. F. (2011). Tissue-type plasminogen activator-mediated plasminogen activation and contact activation, implications in and beyond haemostasis. *J Thromb Haemost, 9*(Suppl. 1), 174–181.

107. Patrassi, G. M., Sartori, M. T., Casonato, A., et al. (1992). Urokinase-type plasminogen activator release after DDAVP in von Willebrand disease: different behaviour of plasminogen activators according to the synthesis of von Willebrand factor. *Thromb Res, 66*, 517–526.

108. Vemulapalli, S., & Becker, R. C. (2013). Aspects of cardiovascular medicine. In Kitchens, C. A., Kessler, C. M., & Konkle, B. A., (Eds.), *Consultative Hemostasis and Thrombosis.* (3rd ed., pp. 342–394). Philadelphia: Elsevier.

109. Nicholl, S. M., Roztocil, E., & Davies, M. G. (2006). Plasminogen activator system and vascular disease. *Curr Vasc Pharmacol, 4*, 101–116.

110. Chandler, W. L., Schmer, G., & Stratton, J. R. (1989). Optimum conditions for the stabilization and measurement of tissue plasminogen activator activity in human plasma. *J Lab Clin Med, 113*, 362–371.

111. Oishi, K. (2009). Plasminogen activator inhibitor-1 and the circadian clock in metabolic disorders. *Clin Exp Hypertens, 31*, 208–219.

112. Levi, M., de Jonge, E., van der Poll, T. (2004). New treatment strategies for disseminated intravascular coagulation based on current understanding of the pathophysiology. *Ann Med, 36*, 41–49.

113. Macy, E. M., Meilahn, E. N., Declerck, P. J., et al. (1993). Sample preparation for plasma measurement of plasminogen activator inhibitor-1 antigen in large population studies. *Arch Pathol Lab Med, 117*, 67–70.

114. Philips, M., Juul, A., Selmer, J., et al. (1992). A specific immunologic assay for functional plasminogen activator inhibitor 1 in plasma standardized measurements of the inhibitor and related parameters in patients with venous thromboembolic disease. *Thromb Haemost, 68*, 486–494.

115. Whiting, D., & DiNardo, J. A. (2014). TEG and ROTEM: technology and clinical applications. *Am J Hematol, 89*, 228–232.

43

Antithrombotic Therapies and Their Laboratory Assessment

George A. Fritsma

OBJECTIVES

After completion of this chapter, the reader will be able to:

1. Describe the purpose of antithrombotic drug administration and distinguish between anticoagulants and antiplatelet therapy.
2. Describe the indications for, dosage of, and management of Coumadin therapy, including how to detect and manage Coumadin overdose.
3. Monitor Coumadin therapy using the prothrombin time and international normalized ratio, and compare these tests with the chromogenic factor X assay.
4. Perform and interpret prothrombin times with international normalized ratios using point-of-care instruments.
5. Describe the indications for, dosage of, and laboratory monitoring of unfractionated heparin therapy, including how to establish the unfractionated heparin partial thromboplastin time therapeutic range.
6. Perform and interpret the results of the partial thromboplastin time and activated clotting time assays for monitoring unfractionated heparin therapy, and compare these tests with the chromogenic anti-factor Xa heparin assay.
7. Describe the indications, dosage, and laboratory measurement of low-molecular-weight heparin therapy and fondaparinux therapy.
8. Perform and interpret the results of the chromogenic anti-factor Xa assay for measuring unfractionated heparin, low-molecular-weight heparin, fondaparinux, rivaroxaban, apixaban, and edoxaban therapy.
9. Measure direct thrombin inhibitor therapy, including dabigatran, using the partial thromboplastin time, ecarin clotting time, ecarin chromogenic assay, and plasma-diluted thrombin time.
10. Describe the indications for intravenous platelet glycoprotein IIb/IIIa inhibitors abciximab, eptifibatide, and tirofiban and describe how their effects are measured.
11. Describe the indications for oral platelet inhibitors aspirin, clopidogrel, prasugrel, and ticagrelor, and describe how their effects are measured.

CASE STUDY

After studying the material in this chapter, the reader should be able to respond to the following case study:

A 71-year-old woman with atrial fibrillation has been taking 5 mg of Coumadin (warfarin sodium) per day for 8 years. Her monthly prothrombin time and international normalized ratio (PT/INR) has been maintained consistently within the standard therapeutic range, 2 to 3. Last Monday, however, her INR was 6.5. For several days earlier she had noticed that her gums bled after she brushed her teeth.

1. What could cause this change in the PT/INR result?
2. What should be done about her PT/INR and symptoms?
3. What alternative test may be used to monitor Coumadin therapy?

Thrombosis, described in detail in the introduction to Chapter 39, is the pathological formation of blood clots in veins or arteries that obstruct flow and cause tissue ischemia and necrosis. Antithrombotic drugs have been employed to treat and prevent thrombosis since heparin was first developed in 1916 and then was FDA-cleared in 1936.[1] Antithrombotics include *anticoagulants*, which suppress coagulation and reduce thrombin formation, and *antiplatelet drugs*, which suppress platelet activation. Fibrinolytics are also employed to disperse or reduce existing clots clogging veins and arteries. Table 43-1 provides a list of current antithrombotics with their indications.

Venous thromboembolic disease (VTE, venous thromboembolism; Chapter 39) includes superficial and *deep vein thrombosis* (DVT) and *pulmonary embolism* (PE). VTE is treated using intravenous standard unfractionated heparin (UFH), subcutaneous low-molecular-weight heparin (LMWH, enoxaparin, tinzaparin), subcutaneous synthetic pentasaccharide (fondaparinux), or the oral direct factor Xa inhibitor, rivaroxaban. VTE is also treated using the oral vitamin K antagonist Coumadin (warfarin sodium). These anticoagulants are also used to prevent VTE subsequent to total hip and total knee replacement surgery, orthopedic repair surgery, and in several medical conditions.

The *direct thrombin inhibitors* (DTIs) *argatroban* and *bivalirudin* are intravenous anticoagulants that are substituted for UFH in patients who have developed *heparin-induced thrombocytopenia with thrombosis* (HIT), a devastating arterial and venous thrombotic side effect of UFH therapy (Chapters 39 and 40). Dabigatran is an oral DTI cleared in 2010 to prevent ischemic stroke, a common side effect for patients who suffer nonvalvular atrial fibrillation. The direct anti-factor Xa anticoagulants rivaroxaban and apixaban are also available to prevent ischemic stroke in atrial fibrillation.

Arterial thrombosis includes *acute myocardial infarction* (AMI), ischemic *cerebrovascular accident* (CVA, stroke), *transient ischemic attack* (TIA), and *peripheral arterial occlusion* (PAO or peripheral artery disease, PAD) and is managed with UFH, LMWH, fondaparinux, Coumadin, the intravenous DTIs, and the antiplatelet drugs aspirin, clopidogrel, prasugrel, and ticagrelor. Aspirin is taken prophylactically by many healthy people at less than 100 mg/day and is particularly effective in reducing mortality when taken within minutes of the acute onset of stroke or cardiac symptoms.[2] The intravenous platelet *glycoprotein IIb/IIIa inhibitor* (GPI) drugs eptifibatide, abciximab, and tirofiban are used to prevent thrombosis during cardiac catheterization procedures.

Thrombolytic therapy may be used to resolve DVT, PE, PAO, AMI, and stroke, particularly when used 3 to 4 hours after the onset of symptoms. Thrombolytic therapy employs recombinant forms of *tissue plasminogen activator* (reteplase, alteplase, and tenecteplase). Thrombolytic therapy raises the risk of hemorrhage, particularly intracranial hemorrhage. Because thrombolytic therapy is not measured by laboratory tests (although fibrinogen levels can be checked), it is not further discussed in this chapter.

Many lives have been saved through the judicious use of antithrombotic therapy, and countless more healthy individuals have been spared thrombotic disease through long-term antithrombotic prophylaxis in moderate-risk circumstances and conditions. However, antithrombotics are dangerous because their effective dosage ranges are narrow.[3] Overdose is critical and leads to emergency department visits for uncontrolled bleeding; inadequate dosages lead to secondary (repeat), often fatal, thrombotic events. Dosages and half-lives differ among the antithrombotics because of variations in formulation and metabolism.[4,5]

Because of these risks, laboratory monitoring or measurement of anticoagulant therapy is essential. Coagulation laboratory scientists and technicians perform countless prothrombin time (PT) assays, partial thromboplastin time (PTT, synonymous with activated partial thromboplastin time, APTT) assays, and chromogenic anti-factor Xa heparin assays to measure or monitor anticoagulant therapy; meanwhile, physicians and nurses regularly modify Coumadin and UFH dosages in response to laboratory outcomes. Although anticoagulant therapy measurement or monitoring may seem routine, vigilance is essential to provide consistently valid results in a dangerous therapeutic world.[6]

The antiplatelet drugs aspirin, clopidogrel, prasugrel, and ticagrelor, as well as LMWH, fondaparinux, and the direct oral anticoagulants (dabigatran, rivaroxaban, apixaban, and edoxaban), have fixed dose-response characteristics and do not require regular monitoring or laboratory-directed dose adjustment. However, though routine monitoring and dose adjustment may be unnecessary, these drugs require measurement in the conditions listed in Box 43-1.

COUMADIN THERAPY AND THE PROTHROMBIN TIME

Coumadin Is a Vitamin K Antagonist

As detailed in Chapter 37, the coagulation factors II (prothrombin), VII, IX, and X depend on vitamin K for normal production, as do coagulation control proteins C, S, and Z. Vitamin K is responsible for the

Table 43-1 Current Antithrombotics, Mode of Action, Measurement, Reversal

Antithrombotic	Indication	Mode of Action	Half-Life	Measurement	Reversal	FDA Cleared
Coumadin	Prevent post-VTE rethrombosis, ischemic stroke	Oral VK antagonist	5 d	Monitor: PT/INR; CFX	Vitamin K, PCC, rFVIIa	1954
UFH	Prevent post-VTE and ACS rethrombosis; intraoperative anticoagulation	IV AT activation, anti-IIa & anti-Xa	1–2 h	Monitor: PTT, anti-Xa, ACT	PS	1936
LMWH	Prevent thrombosis after surgery, in medical conditions or in ACS; DVT/PE treatment	SC AT activation, anti-Xa	3–5 h	Anti-Xa	PS (partial)	1993
Fondaparinux			12–17 h	Anti-Xa	None	2001
Rivaroxaban	Prevent ischemic stroke, prevent thrombosis after orthopedic surgery, prevent post-VTE rethrombosis	Oral direct anti-Xa	12–15 h	PT?, anti-Xa	4-factor PCC, FEIBA, rFVIIa	2011
Apixaban	Prevent ischemic stroke		12–15 h			2012
Edoxaban			12 h		Clinical trials in progress	
Argatroban	Anticoagulation in HIT	IV DTI	50 min	PTT	Discontinue	1997
Bivalirudin		IV DTI	25 min		Discontinue	2000
Dabigatran	Prevent ischemic stroke	Oral DTI	17 h	PTT, ECT, ECA, DTT	None	2010
Aspirin	Prevent acute coronary syndrome recurrence	Oral antiplatelet COX inhibitor		VerifyNow Aspirin, AspirinWorks, platelet aggregation	Discontinue	1900
Clopidogrel		Oral, binds platelet P2Y$_{12}$		VerifyNow P2Y	Discontinue	2000
Prasugrel		Oral, binds platelet P2Y$_{12}$		VerifyNow P2Y	Discontinue	2009
Ticagrelor		Oral, binds platelet P2Y$_{12}$		VerifyNow P2Y	Discontinue	2011
Eptifibatide	Maintain vascular patency during PCI and medical therapy for acute coronary syndrome	IV, binds platelet GP IIb/IIIa	2.5 h	VerifyNow GPI	Discontinue	1998
Abciximab		GP IIb/IIIa	12–24 h	VerifyNow GPI	Discontinue	1993
Tirofiban			2.5 h			1998

ACS, acute coronary syndrome; *ACT,* activated clotting time; *AT,* antithrombin; *CFX,* chromogenic factor X activity; *COX,* cyclooxygenase; *DTI,* direct thrombin inhibitor; *DTT,* plasma-diluted thrombin time; *ECA,* ecarin chromogenic assay; *ECT,* ecarin clotting time; *FEIBA,* factor VIII inhibitor bypassing activity; *GPI,* glycoprotein inhibitor; *INR,* international normalized ratio; *IV,* intravenous; *PCC,* prothrombin complex concentrate; *PT,* prothrombin time; *PTT,* partial thromboplastin time; *PS,* protamine sulfate; *rFVIIa,* recombinant activated factor VII; *SC,* subcutaneous; *VK,* Vitamin K.

γ-carboxylation of a linear series of 12 to 18 glutamic acids near each molecule's N-terminus (amino terminus), a posttranslational modification that enables these coagulation factors and coagulation control proteins to bind ionic calcium (Ca^{2+}) and cell membrane phospholipids, especially phosphatidylserine (Figure 37-9). Vitamin K is concentrated in green tea, avocados, and green leafy vegetables and is produced by gut flora; its absence results in the production of nonfunctional *des-γ carboxyl* forms of factors II, VII, IX, and X and proteins C, S, and Z.

Coumadin (4-hydroxycoumarin, warfarin sodium) is a member of the coumarin drug family and is the formulation of coumarin most often used in North America.[7] Another coumarin is dicoumarol (3,3′-methylenebis-[4-hydroxycoumarin]), the original anticoagulant extracted from moldy sweet clover, described in 1940, and used for many years as a rodenticide.[8] Coumadin is a vitamin K antagonist that suppresses γ-carboxylation of glutamic acid by slowing the activity of the enzyme *vitamin K epoxide reductase* (Figure 37-9). During Coumadin therapy, the activities of factors II, VII, IX, and X and proteins C, S, and Z become reduced as the nonfunctional des-carboxyl proteins are produced in their place. These are sometimes called *proteins induced by vitamin K antagonists* (PIVKAs); they bind few calcium ions, do not assemble on phospholipid surfaces with their substrates, and therefore do not participate in coagulation. Despite several developmental efforts, until 2009, Coumadin was the only oral anticoagulant in the United States, so Coumadin therapy has often been called *oral anticoagulant therapy (OAT).* The new direct-acting oral anticoagulants rivaroxaban, apixaban, edoxaban, and dabigatran have broadened the meaning of "OAT."

Coumadin Prophylaxis and Therapy

Physicians prescribe Coumadin prophylactically to prevent TIAs and strokes in patients with nonvalvular atrial fibrillation

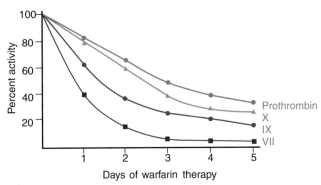

Figure 43-1 Factor VII activity decreases to 50% of normal 6 hours after Coumadin therapy is begun, prolonging the factor VIIa–sensitive prothrombin time to near the therapeutic INR of 2 to 3. The half-lives of factors II (prothrombin), IX, and X are longer than that of VII; factor II activity requires at least 3 days to decline by 50%. The patient gains full anticoagulation effects approximately 5 days after the start of Coumadin therapy.

TABLE 43-2 Plasma Half-Life, Normal Plasma Level, and Minimum Effective Hemostatic Level as a Percentage of Normal Level for the Coagulation Factors

Factor	Half-Life	Plasma Level	Hemostatic Level
Fibrinogen	4 days	280 mg/dL	50 mg/dL
Prothrombin	60 hr	1300 µg/mL	20%
V	16 hr	680 µg/mL	25%
VII	6 hr	120 µg/mL	20%
VIII	12 hr	0.24 µg/mL	30%
IX	24 hr	5 µg/mL	30%
X	30 hr	1 mg/dL	25%
XI	2–3 days	6 µg/mL	25%
XIII	7–10 days	290 µg/mL	2%–3%
Von Willebrand factor	30 hr	6 µg/mL	50%

and to prevent VTE after trauma, orthopedic surgery, and general surgery, and in a number of chronic medical conditions. They also prescribe Coumadin therapeutically to prevent DVT or PE recurrence. Coumadin is also used therapeutically after AMI if the event is complicated by congestive heart failure or coronary insufficiency and to control clotting in patients with mechanical heart valves. Coumadin is among the 20 most commonly prescribed drugs in North America.

Whether prescribed prophylactically or therapeutically, the standard Coumadin regimen begins with a 5-mg daily oral dose. The starting dosage for people over 70 and people who are debilitated, malnourished, or have congestive heart failure is 2 mg/day. For people simultaneously taking drugs that are known to raise Coumadin sensitivity, the starting dosage is 2 mg/day, and 2 mg/day is also the dosage used for those with inherited Coumadin sensitivity. There is no loading dose, and subsequent dosing is based on patient response as measured by the PT (next section). The activity of each of the vitamin K–dependent coagulation factors begins to decline immediately but at different rates (Figure 43-1), and it takes about 5 days for all the factors to reach therapeutic levels. Table 43-2 lists the plasma half-life, plasma concentration, and minimum effective plasma percentage of normal factor activity for the coagulation factors.

Control protein activities also become reduced, especially the activity of protein C, which has a 6-hour half-life, so for the first 2 or 3 days of Coumadin therapy the patient actually incurs the risk of thrombosis. For this reason, Coumadin therapy is "covered" by UFH, LMWH, or fondaparinux therapy for at least 5 days. Failure to provide anticoagulant therapy during this period may result in *warfarin skin necrosis*, a severe thrombotic reaction requiring débridement of dead tissue.[9]

Monitoring Coumadin Therapy Using the Prothrombin Time Assay

The PT effectively monitors Coumadin therapy because it is sensitive to reductions of factors II, VII, and X (Figure 43-2) (Chapter 42). The PT reagent consists of tissue factor, phospholipid, and ionic calcium, so it triggers the coagulation pathway at the level of factor VII. Owing to the 6-hour half-life of factor VII, the PT begins to prolong within 6 to 8 hours; however, anticoagulation becomes therapeutic only when the activities of factors II and X decrease to less than 50% of normal, which takes approximately 5 days.

The first PT is collected and performed 24 hours after therapy is initiated; subsequent PTs are performed daily until at least two consecutive results are within the target therapeutic range. Monitoring continues every 4 to 12 weeks until the completion of therapy, which often lasts for 6 months following a thrombotic event.[10] Coumadin therapy for stroke prevention in atrial fibrillation is indefinite, possibly lifelong. Because the therapeutic range is narrow, close monitoring is essential for successful Coumadin therapy. Under-anticoagulation signals

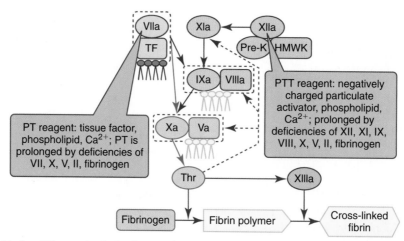

Figure 43-2 The prothrombin time (PT) reagent activates the extrinsic coagulation pathway beginning with factor VII. The PT is prolonged by deficiencies of factors VII, X, V, II (prothrombin), and fibrinogen when the fibrinogen concentration is less than 100 mg/dL. The PT is prolonged in Coumadin therapy because it responds to the reduced VII, X, and prothrombin activity. The partial thromboplastin time (PTT) reagent activates the intrinsic coagulation pathway through factor XII, in association with prekallikrein (pre-K) and high-molecular-weight kininogen (HMWK). The PTT is prolonged by deficiencies of pre-K; HMWK; factors XII, XI, IX, VIII, and X; prothrombin; and fibrinogen when the fibrinogen concentration is less than 100 mg/dL. The PTT is prolonged in unfractionated heparin (UFH) therapy because UFH activates the plasma control protein antithrombin, which neutralizes the serine proteases XIIa, XIa, Xa, IXa, and IIa (thrombin [Thr]). The PTT is also prolonged by lupus anticoagulant. *TF,* Tissue factor.

the danger of thrombosis or secondary thrombosis (rethrombosis); overdose carries the danger of hemorrhage.

Reporting Prothrombin Time Results and the International Normalized Ratio

The medical laboratory technician or scientist reports PT results to the nearest tenth of a second and provides the PT reference interval in seconds for comparison. In view of the inherent variations among thromboplastin reagents and to accomplish interlaboratory normalization, all laboratories report the international normalized ratio (INR) for patients who have reached a stable response to Coumadin therapy. Laboratory practitioners use the following formula:[11]

$$INR = (PT_{patient}/PT_{normal})ISI$$

where $PT_{patient}$ is the PT of the patient in seconds, PT_{normal} is the *geometric mean* of the PT reference interval in seconds, and *ISI* is the international sensitivity index applied as an exponent.

Thromboplastin producers generate the ISI by performing an orthogonal regression analysis comparing the results of their PT reagents for 50 or more Coumadin plasma specimens and 10 or more normal specimens with the results of the *international reference thromboplastin* (World Health Organization human brain thromboplastin) on the same plasmas.[12] Most manufacturers provide ISIs for a variety of coagulation instruments, because each coagulometer may respond differently to their thromboplastins; for instance, some coagulometers rely on photometric plasma changes, whereas others use an electromechanical system (Chapter 44). Most thromboplastin reagents have ISIs near 1.0, matching the ISI of the World Health Organization's international reference thromboplastin. Automated coagulometers "request" the reagent ISI from the operator or obtain it electronically from a reagent vial label bar code, and compute the

INR for each assay result. Although INRs are meant to be computed only for patients in whom the response to Coumadin has stabilized, they typically are reported for all patients, even those who are not taking Coumadin. During the first 5 days of Coumadin therapy, the astute physician and medical laboratory practitioner ignore the INR as unreliable and interpret the PT results in seconds, comparing it with the reference interval.

Coumadin International Normalized Ratio Therapeutic Range

The physician adjusts the Coumadin dosage to achieve the desired INR of 2 to 3, or 2.5 to 3.5 if the patient has a mechanical heart valve. INRs greater than 4 are associated with increased risk of hemorrhage and require immediate communication with the clinician who is managing the patient's case.[13] Dosage adjustments are made conservatively because the INR requires 4 to 7 days to stabilize, but an elevated INR accompanied by the symptoms of anatomic bleeding is a medical emergency.

Monitoring Coumadin Therapy Using the Chromogenic Factor X Assay

The chromogenic coagulation factor X assay (not to be confused with the chromogenic anti-factor Xa heparin assay) may be used as an alternative to the PT/INR system, eliminating the necessity for normalization.[14] The therapeutic range is determined locally by comparison to the INR and typically is close to 20% to 40% of normal factor X activity.[15] The chromogenic factor X assay is useful when the PT is compromised by lupus anticoagulant, a factor inhibitor, or a coagulation factor deficiency.[16]

Effect of Diet and Drugs on Coumadin Therapy

Dietary vitamin K decreases Coumadin's effectiveness and reduces the INR. Green vegetables are an important source of vitamin K, but vitamin K also is concentrated in green tea, cauliflower, liver, avocados, parenteral nutrition formulations, multivitamins, red wine, over-the-counter nutrition drinks, and over-the-counter dietary supplements. A patient who is taking Coumadin is counseled to maintain a regular balanced diet, avoid supplements, and to follow up dietary changes or dietary supplement changes with additional PT assays and dosage adjustments, if indicated.

Coumadin is metabolized in the mitochondrial cytochrome P-450 (CYP 2C9) pathway of hepatocytes—the "disposal system" for at least 80 drugs. Theoretically, use of any drug metabolized through the CYP 2C9 pathway may unpredictably suppress or enhance the effects of Coumadin. Amiodarone, metronidazole, and cimetidine typically double or triple the INR. Any change in drug therapy, like a change in diet, must be followed up with additional PT assays and dosage adjustments.

Coumadin is contraindicated during pregnancy because it causes birth defects. When anticoagulation is desired during pregnancy—for instance, in women who possess a thrombosis risk factor—LMWH or fondaparinux is prescribed. There are no current recommendations for the direct oral anticoagulants during pregnancy.

Effect of Polymorphisms on Coumadin Therapy

Two genetic polymorphisms generate variations in enzymes of the cytochrome P-450 pathway. These are *CYP2C9*2* and *CYP2C9*3*, which reduce enzyme pathway activity and slow the metabolic breakdown of Coumadin. Likewise, there is a polymorphism that affects the key enzyme of vitamin K metabolism, *vitamin K epoxide reductase*. This polymorphism, named *VKORC1*, slows vitamin K reduction, which makes the patient more sensitive to Coumadin.[17] In patients possessing one, two, or all three of these polymorphisms, Coumadin therapy should begin at 2 mg/day and should be adjusted and monitored daily until the INR remains consistently in the therapeutic range. The standard 5 mg/day regimen risks hemorrhage in patients who possess these polymorphisms. In 2007, the FDA required that drug manufacturers add a statement on all vials of Coumadin recommending that physicians screen patients for these common dosage-affecting polymorphisms. Although the FDA recommendation does not carry the weight of a black box warning issued by the FDA for drug use, numerous molecular diagnostics manufacturers have developed short turnaround assays for these three polymorphisms. Screening for these polymorphisms is the first and most public example of pharmacogenomic laboratory testing, although not universally endorsed.[18]

Conversely, *Coumadin receptor insufficiency* may render the patient resistant to Coumadin therapy. Some patients require dosages of 20 mg/day or higher to achieve a therapeutic INR. The search is on for polymorphisms of the vitamin K reductase pathway responsible for "Coumadin resistance."[19]

Effect of Direct Thrombin Inhibitors on the Prothrombin Time

The intravenously administered DTIs argatroban and bivalirudin, which are used in place of heparin as a life-saving measure

TABLE 43-3 Recommendations for the Reversal of Coumadin Overdose Based on International Normalized Ratio (INR) and Bleeding

Bleeding	INR	Intervention
No significant bleeding	3–5	Reduce dosage or omit one dose, monitor INR frequently
	5–9	Omit Coumadin, monitor INR frequently, consider oral vitamin K (≤5 mg) if high risk for bleeding (surgery)
	>9	Stop Coumadin, give 5–10 mg oral vitamin K, monitor INR frequently
Serious bleeding	Any INR	Stop Coumadin; give 10 mg vitamin K by intravenous push, may repeat every 12 hr; give thawed fresh-frozen plasma, prothrombin complex concentrate, or recombinant factor VIIa
Life-threatening bleeding	Any INR	Same as for serious bleeding, except stronger indication for recombinant factor VIIa

for patients with HIT, and the anti-factor Xa direct oral anticoagulants rivaroxaban and apixaban, may prolong the PT (depending on the PT reagent). In switching to Coumadin therapy, the combination of a DTI or direct oral anticoagulant and Coumadin can nearly double the PT for the duration of action of the DTI or direct oral anticoagulant, which may extend 3 or 4 days.[20] The chromogenic factor X assay is an effective means for monitoring Coumadin dosage during the crossover period.

Reversing Bleeding Caused by a Coumadin Overdose

Table 43-3 provides recommendations for the reversal of a Coumadin overdose based on INR and clinical evidence of bleeding. Reversal requires oral or intravenous vitamin K and, if bleeding is severe, a means for substituting active coagulation factors such as fresh-frozen plasma, recombinant activated factor VII (NovoSeven, Novo Nordisk, Princeton, NJ), activated three-factor prothrombin complex concentrate (FEIBA FH, Baxter Healthcare Corporation, Westlake Village, CA), three-factor prothrombin complex concentrate ("non-activated" Profilnine SD; Grifols Biologicals, Inc., Los Angeles, CA), or four-factor prothrombin complex concentrate (4F-PCC, Kcentra; CSL Behring, King of Prussia, PA).[21]

UNFRACTIONATED HEPARIN THERAPY AND THE PARTIAL THROMBOPLASTIN TIME

Heparin Is a Catalyst That Activates Antithrombin to Neutralize Serine Proteases

Standard UFH is a biological substance, first described in 1916. It is a mixture of sulfated glycosaminoglycans (polysaccharides) extracted from porcine mucosa. The molecular weight of UFH ranges from 3000 to 30,000 Daltons (average molecular weight 15,000 Daltons). Approximately one third of its molecules support somewhere on their length a high-affinity pentasaccharide that binds plasma antithrombin. The anticoagulant action of UFH is indirect and catalytic, relying on antithrombin. The pentasaccharide-bound antithrombin undergoes a steric change (allostery), exposing an anticoagulant site that covalently binds and inactivates the coagulation pathway serine proteases, factors IIa (thrombin), IXa, Xa, XIa, and XIIa (Chapter 37). Laboratory practitioners call activated antithrombin a *serine protease inhibitor* (SERPIN), and the protease-binding reaction yields, among other products, the measurable inactive plasma complex thrombin-antithrombin (TAT).

Heparin supports the thrombin-antithrombin reaction through a "bridging" mechanism (Figure 43-3). If the heparin molecule exceeds 17 linear saccharide units, thrombin assembles on the heparin molecule near the activated antithrombin. Bridging drives the thrombin-antithrombin reaction at a rate four times that of the factor Xa-antithrombin reaction, because factor Xa becomes inactivated only through antithrombin's steric modification, and its covalent binding is not enhanced by bridging.

UFH preparations vary in average molecular weight, molecule length, and efficacy. Individual patient heparin dose-responses diverge markedly, because numerous plasma and cellular proteins bind UFH at varying rates. Consequently, laboratory monitoring is essential.[22]

Unfractionated Heparin Therapy

Physicians administer UFH intravenously to treat VTE, to provide initial treatment of AMI, to prevent reocclusion after stent placement, and to maintain vascular patency during cardiac surgery using cardiopulmonary bypass (CPB) with extracorporeal circulation. Different dosing regimens are used in various settings. For VTE treatment, therapy begins with a bolus of 5000 to 10,000 units, followed by continuous infusion at approximately 1300 units/hour, adjusted to patient weight. UFH therapy is discontinued when the acute clinical state has resolved or after the procedure or surgery. If necessary the patient will be switched to a non-intravenous anticoagulant to prevent future thrombotic events. To avoid HIT (Chapters 39 and 40), LMWH or other anticoagulants are used in place of UFH where possible.

Monitoring Unfractionated Heparin Therapy Using the Partial Thromboplastin Time

Because of its inherent pharmacologic variations and narrow therapeutic range, UFH therapy is diligently monitored using the PTT (Figure 43-2). Blood is collected and assayed before therapy is begun to ensure that the baseline PTT is normal.[23] A prolonged baseline PTT may indicate the presence of a lupus anticoagulant, factor inhibitor, or a factor deficiency and confuses the therapeutic interpretation. In such cases, the laboratory practitioner switches to the chromogenic anti-factor Xa heparin assay throughout the duration of therapy (discussed later in the chapter).

A second specimen is collected at least 4 to 6 hours but not longer than 24 hours after the initial bolus and a PTT is measured on this specimen. The PTT becomes prolonged within minutes of UFH administration, which reflects the immediate anticoagulation effect of UFH. The result for this specimen should fall within the therapeutic range, which is established by the laboratory practitioner (next section) and reported with the result. The physician or nurse adjusts the infusion rate to ensure that the PTT result is within the target range. PTT measurement is subsequently repeated every 24 hours, and the dosage is continually readjusted until UFH anticoagulation is complete. The physician also monitors the platelet count daily. A 40% or greater reduction in the platelet count, even within the reference interval, is evidence for HIT (see the discussion of the "4Ts" HIT diagnosis system in Chapter 39). If HIT is suspected, UFH therapy is immediately discontinued and replaced with DTI therapy.

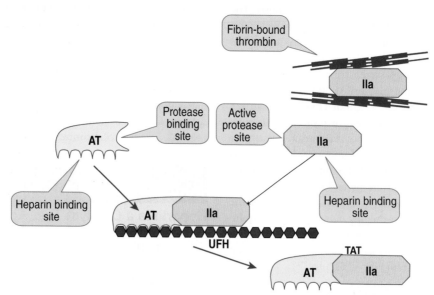

Figure 43-3 The heparin binding site of antithrombin (AT) binds a specific pentasaccharide, producing an allosteric change that activates AT. Factor IIa (thrombin) assembles on the heparin surface, provided the molecule is at least 17 saccharide units long. AT binds factor IIa, and the complex is released from unfractionated heparin (UFH) to form the soluble, measurable thrombin-antithrombin (TAT) complex. The UFH recycles. Fibrin-bound IIa does not enter the reaction.

Determining the Partial Thromboplastin Time Therapeutic Range for Unfractionated Heparin Therapy

The hemostasis laboratory is required to establish and communicate a PTT therapeutic range to monitor and manage UFH therapy. The medical laboratory technician or scientist collects 20 to 30 plasma specimens from patients being infused with UFH at all levels of anticoagulation, ensuring that fewer than 10% of the specimens are collected from the same patient, and measures PTT for all.[24] The specimens must be from patients who are not receiving simultaneous Coumadin therapy; that is, their PT results must be normal. Chromogenic anti-factor Xa heparin assays are performed on all specimens, plus at least 10 specimens from healthy normal subjects, and the paired results are displayed on a linear graph (Figure 43-4). The range in seconds of PTT results that corresponds to 0.3 to 0.7 chromogenic anti-factor Xa heparin units/mL is the therapeutic range.[25] This is known as the *ex vivo* or *Brill-Edwards method* for establishing the heparin therapeutic range of the PTT, and its use is required by laboratory certification and licensing agencies. Other approaches to determining the PTT therapeutic range for UFH therapy are discouraged. For instance, experts once recommended that the PTT therapeutic range be established as 1.5 to 2.5 times the mean of the reference interval. This approach, however, must be avoided as it consistently results in under-anticoagulation, which raises the risk of a secondary thrombotic event. In addition, the practice of developing a therapeutic range by "spiking" normal plasma with measured volumes of heparin is prohibited because the curve that is generated tends to flatten at higher concentrations.[26]

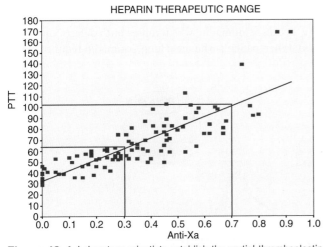

Figure 43-4 Laboratory scientists establish the partial thromboplastin time (PTT) therapeutic range for unfractionated heparin (UFH) by collecting specimens from 20 to 30 patients receiving UFH at representative dosages who have normal PTs and at least 10 individuals not receiving heparin. PTT and chromogenic anti-factor Xa heparin assays are performed on all specimens, and a linear graph of paired results is prepared with PTT on the vertical scale. The PTT range in seconds is correlated with the chromogenic anti-factor Xa therapeutic range of 0.3 to 0.7 units/mL or the prophylactic range of 0.1 to 0.4 units/mL.

Clinical Utility of Monitoring Unfractionated Heparin Therapy Using the Partial Thromboplastin Time

The medical laboratory practitioner reports the PTT results, the reference interval, and the UFH therapeutic range to the clinician (physician, nurse, or pharmacist) who is managing the patient's UFH dosage. Because reagent sensitivity varies among producers and among individual producers' reagent lots, the clinician must evaluate PTT results in relation to the institution's current published therapeutic range and reference interval.[27] No system analogous to the INR exists for normalizing PTT results, because reagents and patient responses are too variable.[28] While the PTT is used most often to measure the effects of UFH therapy, LMWH (next section) selectively catalyzes the neutralization of factor Xa more avidly than the neutralization of thrombin, thus its effects cannot be measured using the PTT. However, the chromogenic anti-factor Xa heparin assay may be used to assay UFH, LMWH, and fondaparinux.

Limitations of Monitoring Unfractionated Heparin Therapy Using the Partial Thromboplastin Time

Several conditions render the patient unresponsive to heparin therapy, a circumstance called *heparin resistance.*[29] Inflammation typically is accompanied by fibrinogen levels raised to greater than 500 mg/dL and coagulation factor VIII activities of greater than 190% above the mean of the reference interval. Both elevations render the PTT less sensitive to the effects of heparin. Further, in many patients, antithrombin activity becomes depleted as a result of prolonged therapy or an underlying deficiency secondary to chronic inflammation. In this instance, the PTT result remains below the therapeutic range, becoming only modestly prolonged despite ever-increasing heparin dosages. Inflammation may be reduced through administration of steroids and aspirin or nonsteroidal anti-inflammatory drugs, and antithrombin concentrate may be administered. In the interim, however, it is necessary to use an alternative assay such as the chromogenic anti-factor Xa heparin assay.

Platelets in anticoagulated whole-blood specimens release platelet factor 4, a heparin-neutralizing protein (Chapter 13). In specimens from patients receiving heparin therapy, the PTT begins to shorten as soon as 1 hour after collection because of in vitro platelet factor 4 release unless the specimen is centrifuged and the platelet-poor plasma is removed from the cells (Chapter 42).[30] Hypofibrinogenemia, factor deficiencies, and the presence of lupus anticoagulant, fibrin degradation products, or paraproteins prolong the PTT independent of heparin levels.[31]

Monitoring Unfractionated Heparin Therapy Using the Activated Clotting Time

The ACT is a 1966 modification of the time-honored but obsolete Lee-White whole blood clotting time test. The ACT is a popular point of care assay that is used in clinics, at the inpatient's bedside, in the cardiac catheterization laboratory, or in the surgical suite, and it is particularly useful at the high UFH dosages, 1 to 2 units/mL, used in percutaneous intervention (PCI, cardiac catheterization) and in cardiac surgery using extracorporeal circulation.[32]

ACT assay distributors such as International Technidyne Corporation, Edison, NJ, the makers of the Hemochron Response (Chapter 44), provide evacuated blood specimen collection tubes that contain 12 mg of diatomaceous earth, a particulate clot activator. The negative pressure within the tube is calibrated to collect 2 mL of blood. As soon as the specimen is collected, the tube is placed in the instrument cuvette well, where it is rotated and continuously monitored. When a clot forms, a magnet positioned within the sample is pulled away from a sensing device, which stops the timer. The time interval to clot formation is recorded automatically. The results of the ACT assay are comparable to those of the PTT assay for UFH monitoring, provided adequate quality control steps are taken. The median of the ACT reference interval is 98 seconds. Heparin is administered to yield results of 200 to 240 seconds in PCI or 400 to 450 seconds during cardiac surgery, levels at which the PTT is ineffective.

Reversal of Unfractionated Heparin Overdose Using Protamine Sulfate

At completion of cardiac surgery when the extracorporeal circuit is to be terminated, heparin anticoagulation needs to be quickly reversed. In other settings, a UFH overdose, or co-administration with aspirin, fibrinolytic therapy, or a GPI, may raise the risk of bleeding. Protamine sulfate, a cationic protein extracted from salmon sperm, neutralizes UFH at a ratio of 100 units of heparin per milligram of protamine sulfate. The health care provider administers protamine sulfate slowly by intravenous push. The effect of the protamine sulfate may be detected by the shortening of the PTT or ACT. Protamine sulfate also neutralizes LMWH, although the neutralization is incompletely reflected in the results of the chromogenic anti-factor Xa heparin assay described in the following paragraphs.

Protamine sulfate has also been implicated as causing a delayed form of HIT, consequently, platelet counts for patients who have received protamine sulfate are routinely monitored.[33,34]

LOW-MOLECULAR-WEIGHT HEPARIN THERAPY AND THE CHROMOGENIC ANTI–FACTOR Xa HEPARIN ASSAY

Low-Molecular-Weight Heparin Is Produced from Unfractionated Heparin

Uncertainty about UFH dose response and the ever-present threat of HIT led to the development of LMWH, which was cleared for anticoagulant prophylaxis in the United States and Canada in 1993.[35] LMWH is prepared from UFH using chemical (enoxaparin, Lovenox, Sanofi-Aventis, Bridgewater, NJ) or enzymatic fractionation (tinzaparin sodium, Innohep, LEO Pharmaceutical Products, Ballerup, Denmark).[36] Fractionation yields a product with a mean molecular weight of 4500 to 5000 Daltons, about one third the mass of UFH. LMWH possesses the same active pentasaccharide sequence as UFH; however, the overall shorter polysaccharide chains provide little space for thrombin bridging, so the thrombin neutralization response is reduced (Figure 43-5). The factor Xa neutralization response is unchanged, however, because this reaction does not rely on factor Xa binding to heparin's polysaccharide chain, so LMWH provides nearly the same anticoagulant efficacy as UFH, although predominantly through factor Xa inhibition.

LMWH is administered by subcutaneous injection once or twice a day using premeasured syringes at selected dosages—for instance, 30 mg subcutaneously every 12 hours or 40 mg subcutaneously once daily. Prophylactic applications provide coverage during or after general and orthopedic surgery and trauma, typically for 14 days from the time of the event. LMWH also is used to treat DVT, PE, and unstable angina. LMWH is indicated during pregnancy for women at risk of VTE, because Coumadin, which causes birth defects, cannot be used. When patients who are taking Coumadin require surgery

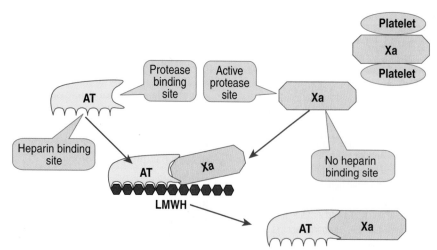

Figure 43-5 The antithrombin (AT) binding site binds a specific heparin pentasaccharide, producing an allosteric change that activates AT. The low-molecular-weight heparin (LMWH) molecule is too short to support a factor IIa-AT reaction; however, the activated AT binds factor Xa independently of the bridging phenomenon, producing a soluble AT-factor Xa complex. The LMWH recycles.

it is discontinued for up to a week before the procedure and replaced with LMWH.[37]

The advantages of LMWH are rapid bioavailability after subcutaneous injection, making intravenous administration unnecessary; a half-life of 3 to 5 hours compared with 60 to 90 minutes for UFH; and a fixed dose response that eliminates the need for laboratory monitoring, although laboratory measurement is still required in the conditions listed in Box 43-1. The risk of HIT is reduced by 90% in people who have never received heparin before; however, LMWH may cross-react with previously formed antibodies against heparin-platelet factor 4. Consequently, LMWH is contraindicated in patients who developed HIT after UFH therapy. The risk of LMWH-induced bleeding is less than that for UFH.

Measuring Low-Molecular-Weight Heparin Therapy

The kidneys alone clear LMWH, so it accumulates in renal insufficiency. Laboratory measurement of LMWH therapy is necessary when the creatinine clearance is less than 30 mL/min or the serum creatinine is greater than 4 mg/dL. During LMWH therapy, creatinine assays are performed periodically to document kidney function and avoid the risk of LMWH accumulation in plasma. LMWH therapy in children, adults under 50 kg, adults over 150 kg, and during pregnancy also requires measurement because of fluid compartment imbalances or unstable coagulation (Box 43-1).

The phlebotomist collects a blood specimen 4 hours after subcutaneous injection, and the plasma is tested using the chromogenic anti-factor Xa heparin assay. The PTT is insensitive to LMWH. The chromogenic anti-factor Xa heparin assay employs a reagent that provides a fixed concentration of factor Xa and substrate specific to factor Xa (Figure 43-6). Some distributors add fixed concentrations of antithrombin, and others none; the latter rely on the patient's plasma antithrombin and provide sensitivity to antithrombin depletion or deficiency. Heparin forms a complex with reagent factor Xa and antithrombin; a measured excess of factor Xa digests the substrate,

yielding a colored product whose intensity is inversely proportional to heparin concentration.

To prepare a standard curve, the laboratory practitioner obtains the characteristic UFH or LMWH calibrators from distributors, then computes and prepares dilutions that "bracket" the reference and the therapeutic range. If the chromogenic anti-factor Xa heparin assay is to be used to monitor UFH and LMWH, a single hybrid standard curve may be prepared.[38,39] A separate curve is necessary to monitor the pentasaccharide fondaparinux (next section). The prophylactic range for LMWH is 0.2 to 0.5 unit/mL, and the therapeutic range is 0.5 to 1.2 units/mL.[24]

The chromogenic anti-factor Xa heparin assay is the primary assay available to measure LMWH and fondaparinux. It may also be used in place of the PTT to assay UFH with little or no modification, and it substitutes for the PTT when clinical or laboratory conditions render PTT results unreliable. The chromogenic anti-factor Xa heparin assay is "tertiary" in the sense that it measures the heparin concentration and not heparin's anticoagulant effects; however, the assay is precise and, in contrast to the PTT, is affected by few interferences. The chromogenic anti-factor Xa heparin assay is also the reference method for establishing the PTT therapeutic range. Laboratory directors have begun to recognize the merits of the chromogenic anti-factor Xa heparin assay and substitute it for the PTT in monitoring all UFH therapy, as well as in measuring therapy levels of LMWH and fondaparinux.

MEASURING PENTASACCHARIDE THERAPY USING THE CHROMOGENIC ANTI–FACTOR Xa HEPARIN ASSAY

Fondaparinux sodium (Arixtra; GlaxoSmithKline, Research Triangle Park, NC) is a synthetic formulation of the active pentasaccharide sequence in UFH and LMWH (Figure 43-7). Fondaparinux raises antithrombin activity 400-fold.[40] It is equivalent in clinical efficacy to LMWH with a reduced major bleeding effect and has a reproducible dose response and a

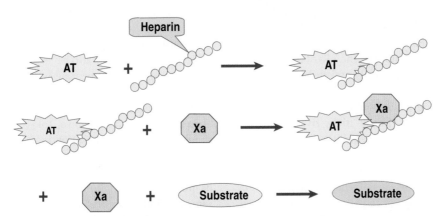

Figure 43-6 The chromogenic anti-factor Xa heparin assay. The reagent is a mixture of antithrombin (AT) and a measured excess of Xa. Most kits do not provide AT and rely solely on patient plasma AT. AT binds heparin, and this complex binds factor Xa. Excess free factor Xa digests its substrate to produce a colored end product. The color intensity of the product is inversely proportional to plasma heparin. This assay is used for unfractionated heparin, low-molecular-weight heparin, and pentasaccharide fondaparinux; a dedicated standard curve is required for fondaparinux.

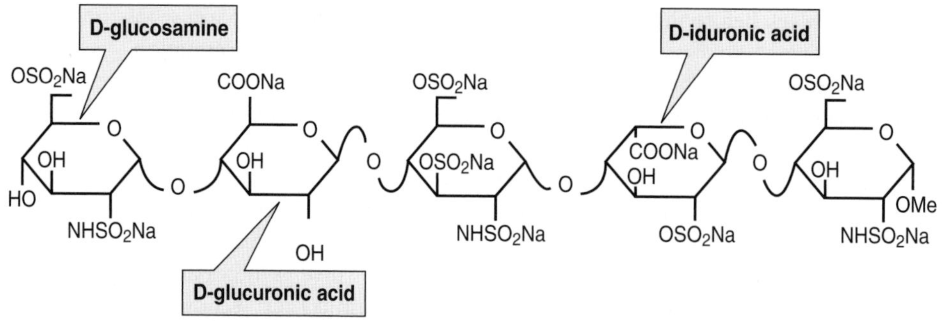

Figure 43-7 The specific saccharide sequence in unfractionated heparin and low-molecular-weight heparin (glucosamine, glucuronic acid, glucosamine, iduronic acid, glucosamine) is synthesized to make fondaparinux, which binds and activates the heparin-binding site of antithrombin. (From Turpie AGG: Pentasaccharides. *Semin Hematol* 39:159-171, 2002.)

desirable half-life of 17 to 21 hours. Because of the extended half-life, fondaparinux is administered in once-a-day subcutaneous injections of 2.5 to 7.5 mg.[41] Fondaparinux is FDA-cleared for prevention of VTE after orthopedic and abdominal surgery and for treatment of acute VTE events, but its use is contraindicated in patients with creatinine clearance values of less than 30 mL/min.[42]

The chromogenic anti-factor Xa heparin assay is used to measure fondaparinux therapy in children, adults below 50 kg or over 150 kg, patients receiving treatment for more than 7 to 8 days, and pregnant women.[43-45] Blood is collected 4 hours after injection, and the target range, derived from clinical studies, though not confirmed by outcome studies, is 0.2 to 0.4 mg/mL for a 2.5 mg dose and 0.5 to 1.5 mg/mL for a 7.5 mg dose. The operator prepares a calibration curve using fondaparinux—not UFH, LMWH, or a hybrid calibrator—because concentrations are expressed in mg/mL, not units per mL. The PTT is not sensitive to the effects of fondaparinux because, although fondaparinux reacts with antithrombin and factor Xa, it does not inhibit thrombin or factors IXa, XIa, or XIIa.

In the event of bleeding associated with fondaparinux overdose, protamine sulfate is ineffective. Recombinant activated factor VII (rFVIIa, NovoSeven; Novo Nordisk, Princeton, NJ) may partially reverse the effects of fondaparinux.[46]

MEASURING ORAL DIRECT FACTOR Xa INHIBITORS

Oral rivaroxaban (Xarelto; Bayer Healthcare AG, Leverkusen, Germany; Janssen Pharmaceuticals, Inc., Raritan, NJ) is an oxazolidinone derivative that directly and stoichiometrically inhibits factor Xa.[47,48] It inhibits free factor Xa, factor Xa that is bound by factor IXa, and clot-bound factor Xa.[45] As established by results of several clinical trials, rivaroxaban has efficacy and safety characteristics equivalent to LMWH or Coumadin.

Rivaroxaban was cleared in September 2008 by both Health Canada and the European Medicines Agency and in July 2011 by the U.S. FDA for VTE prophylaxis in patients who are undergoing total knee or total hip replacement surgery. The FDA also cleared rivaroxaban in November 2011 for prevention of ischemic stroke in patients with chronic nonvalvular atrial fibrillation at 20 mg/day and for prevention of secondary thrombosis

subsequent to DVT or PE at 15 mg twice a day in December 2012.[49,50] The European Medicines Agency cleared rivaroxaban at 2.5 mg/day for prevention of secondary thrombosis following acute myocardial infarction in March 2013, but that same month the FDA deferred clearance for the same indication having considered a dosage of 10 mg/day.[47,51] The distributor re-filed in August 2013. As of June 2014, rivaroxaban has not been approved for use in patients with MI.

Rivaroxaban slightly prolongs the PT, as reported in several clinical trials, but to a lesser extent than Coumadin. Attempts to correlate PT results with dosage have revealed variability among PT thromboplastin reagents, rendering the PT only partially valid as a means to measure rivaroxaban.[52-54] Rivaroxaban may also be assayed using a version of the chromogenic anti-factor Xa heparin assay. The assay must be calibrated using rivaroxaban in place of UFH, LMWH, or fondaparinux.[55] Using either PT or anti-factor Xa, laboratory practitioners are working to correlate laboratory results with clinical outcomes in an effort to provide a therapeutic range.[56]

Like rivaroxaban, oral apixaban (Eliquis; Pfizer, New York, NY; Bristol-Myers Squibb, New York, NY) is a small oxazolidinone-derived direct stoichiometric factor Xa-inhibiting anticoagulant. The results of clinical trials reveal that apixaban actually improves on the efficacy and safety of Coumadin. The FDA cleared apixaban in December 2012 for the prevention of ischemic stroke in atrial fibrillation. The dosage for this indication is 2.5 mg twice a day. Apixaban has a weaker effect on the PT than rivaroxaban and Coumadin but may be measured using the PT, provided the operator first determines the sensitivity of the reagent. The chromogenic anti-factor Xa may also be used to measure apixaban when controls and calibrators become available in the North American market.[57]

A third oral direct-acting anti-factor Xa anticoagulant, edoxaban (Lixiana; Daiichi-Sankyo, Tokyo, Japan), cleared in Japan in July 2011 for clot prevention in patients who have had total knee or hip replacement, is currently in phase III trials worldwide. Its characteristics mirror rivaroxaban and apixaban, and its plasma concentration may likely be measured using the same methods, but this has not yet been determined.[58]

The oral direct anti-factor Xa inhibitors rivaroxaban, apixaban, and edoxaban all possess half-lives of approximately 12 hours. Apixaban may have an advantage in that 70% of the active drug is cleared by the liver and only 30% by the kidney, so dosage is relatively unaffected by renal insufficiency. There is no current recommended reversal agent for hemorrhages caused by overdoses of these drugs; however, some clinicians report normalization of laboratory test results by the use of factor eight inhibitor bypassing agent (FEIBA; Baxter, Deerfield, IL), four-factor (II, VII, IX, and X) prothrombin complex concentrate (Kcentra; DSL Behring, King of Prussia, PA), or recombinant activated factor FVII (rFVIIa, NovoSeven; Novo Nordisk, Princeton, NJ). All oral direct factor Xa inhibitors are prescribed with no monitoring (contrary to Coumadin); however, the clinical conditions listed in Box 43-1 may dictate the need to measure drug levels at specific times. A drug-specific chromogenic anti-factor Xa assay, utilizing a sodium citrate plasma sample, will likely be the assay of choice in most laboratories. Although the anti-factor Xa assay has been used for several years to monitor UFH and measure LMWH and fondaparinux, it awaits FDA clearance and is currently classified as *research use only* when applied to measuring rivaroxaban, apixaban, and edoxaban.

DIRECT THROMBIN INHIBITORS

Argatroban

The intravenous use DTIs argatroban and bivalirudin reversibly bind and inactivate free and clot-bound thrombin (Figure 43-8). DTIs are substituted for UFH or LMWH when HIT is suspected or confirmed using the "4Ts" assessment system (Chapter 39). Without the use of an intravenous DTI, the risk of thrombosis is 50% for 30 days after heparin is discontinued. In HIT, Coumadin, UFH, and LMWH are contraindicated.

Argatroban (Novostan; GlaxoSmithKline, Research Triangle Park, NC) is a non-protein L-arginine derivative with a molecular weight of 527 Daltons. Argatroban was FDA-cleared in 1997 for thrombosis prophylaxis and treatment and for anticoagulation during cardiac catheterization for patients with HIT.[59,60]

For patients with HIT, the physician initiates the argatroban intravenous infusion at 2 µg/kg/min or in patients with hepatic disease at 0.5 µg/kg/min. During percutaneous cardiac intervention, a bolus of 350 µg/kg is given over 3 to 5 minutes, followed by an infusion at 25 µg/kg/min. Argatroban is cleared by the liver and excreted in stool. There is a 5% general bleeding risk and no direct reversal agent; however, the half-life is 50 minutes, and argatroban clears completely in 2 to 4 hours.

Bivalirudin, a Recombinant Analogue of Leech Saliva Hirudin

Bivalirudin (Angiomax; The Medicines Company, Parsippany, NJ) is a synthetic 20-amino acid (2180 Daltons molecular weight) peptide derivative of the active site of hirudin, an anticoagulant produced in trace amounts by the medicinal leech *Hirudo medicinalis*. Bivalirudin was cleared by the FDA in 2000 for use as an anticoagulant in patients with unstable angina at risk for HIT who are undergoing percutaneous coronary intervention.[61]

Bivalirudin is intended for use with concurrent aspirin therapy at a dosage of 325 mg/day and has been studied only in patients receiving aspirin.[62] Physicians provide an intravenous bolus dose of 0.75 mg/kg bivalirudin, followed by an infusion of 1.75 mg/kg/hr for the duration of the percutaneous cardiac intervention. After 4 hours, an additional intravenous infusion may be given at a rate of 0.2 mg/kg/hr for 20 hours.

The rate of major hemorrhage with bivalirudin is 4%. There is no reversal agent; however, in patients with normal renal function, the half-life is 25 minutes. The dosage is decreased in patients with reduced creatinine clearance or elevated serum creatinine.[63,64]

Dabigatran, an Oral Direct Thrombin Inhibitor

Oral dabigatran etexilate (Pradaxa; Boehringer Ingelheim, Ingelheim, Germany) is a prodrug that converts upon ingestion to active dabigatran, a reversible DTI that binds both free and clot-bound thrombin. Dabigatran's efficacy and safety appear to match those of LMWH and Coumadin, and it has no known interaction with food. It is cleared by the kidneys, has a half-life

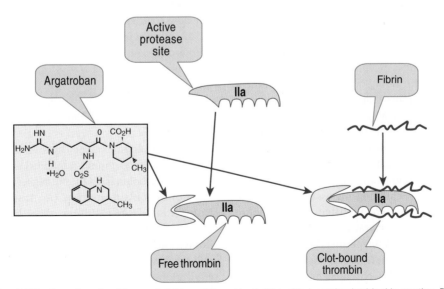

Figure 43-8 Argatroban inhibits the active site of free and clot-bound thrombin. Antithrombin is not involved in this reaction. Bivalirudin and dabigatran inhibit thrombin by interacting at the same site but with their own specific binding characteristics.

of 12 to 17 hours, and is not metabolized by liver cytochrome enzymes; however, it does affect the P-glycoprotein transport system, which can impact drug-drug interactions.[65] Dabigatran was cleared by the European Medicines Agency and Canada Health in the spring of 2008 for VTE prophylaxis following total knee or total hip replacement surgery at dosages of 220 mg/day, or 150 mg/day in the elderly or those with moderate renal impairment. In October 2010, the U.S. FDA cleared dabigatran for prevention of ischemic stroke in nonvalvular atrial fibrillation. In renal disease the half-life may be prolonged to as much as 60 hours, and in overdose-caused hemorrhage there is no known reversal agent.[66-70]

Measuring Direct Thrombin Inhibitor Therapy

Argatroban and bivalirudin prolong the thrombin time, PT, PTT, and ACT.[71] For nonsurgical therapy, distributors recommend assaying with the PTT using the target therapeutic range of 1.5 to 3 times the mean of the laboratory reference interval (but not more than 90 seconds). Blood is collected 2 hours after the initiation of intravenous therapy for argatroban and 4 hours after therapy initiation for bivalirudin, and the dosage is adjusted to achieve a PTT within the therapeutic range. The ACT may be employed during cardiac catheterization or cardiac surgery. During these procedures, the target ACT for bivalirudin therapy is 320 to 400 seconds (median normal value, 98 seconds).

In instances in which the baseline PTT is prolonged by lupus anticoagulant, factor inhibitors, or factor deficiencies, the ecarin clotting time (ECT) is a potential alternative for assaying argatroban and bivalirudin. Ecarin (Ecarinase; Pentapharm, Basel, Switzerland) is an enzyme extracted from *Echis carinatus* venom that converts prothrombin to intermediate *meizothrombin*, which converts fibrinogen to fibrin. Argatroban and bivalirudin bind meizothrombin and generate a linear, dose-dependent prolongation of the ECT. Aside from DTIs, the ECT is prolonged only by abnormally low prothrombin or fibrinogen activity.

The oral direct thrombin inhibitor dabigatran is prescribed without routine monitoring. The clinical situations listed in Box 43-1, however, may necessitate measuring dabigatran drug levels. Dabigatran prolongs the thrombin time, PTT, and ECT.[72] The standard thrombin time is exceptionally sensitive to dabigatran and is convenient for ruling out dabigatran, because a normal thrombin time indicates that no dabigatran is present. A prolonged thrombin time may indicate that dabigatran is present, but it does not indicate the plasma concentration. The PTT generates a "curvilinear" response to dabigatran and is unreliable at low levels; additionally, there is considerable variability in sensitivity to dabigatran among PTT reagents.[73]

The ECT and the ecarin chromogenic assay (ECA; Stago, Asnières sur Seine, France) provide a reliable, linear response to dabigatran, except at low concentrations.[74] Also, a modification of the thrombin time called the plasma-diluted thrombin time (Hemoclot Direct Thrombin Inhibitor Assay; Aniara Hyphen, West Chester, OH) and a chromogenic assay that is based on the thrombin time (Biophen DTI [chromogenic] Assay; Aniara Hyphen, West Chester, OH) are available.[75] ECT,

ECA, plasma-diluted thrombin time, and Biophen DTI, all of which require a sodium citrate plasma sample, await FDA clearance and are currently restricted to *research use only*.[76-78]

MEASURING ANTIPLATELET THERAPY USING PLATELET ACTIVITY ASSAYS

Intravenous Glycoprotein IIb/IIIa Inhibitors Are Used During Cardiac Catheterization

Glycoprotein IIb (α_{IIb}) and glycoprotein IIIa (β_3) are present on the membrane of resting platelets. Upon activation by any agonist, these molecules join to form glycoprotein IIb/IIIa ($\alpha_{IIb}\beta_3$) heterodimers, receptors that bind fibrinogen and von Willebrand factor through their arginine–glycine–aspartic acid (RGD) sequences. Fibrinogen binding to $\alpha_{IIb}\beta_3$ supports the key step of in vivo platelet aggregation (Chapter 13). The intravenous glycoprotein IIb/IIIa inhibitors (GPIs) abciximab, eptifibatide, and tirofiban fill $\alpha_{IIb}\beta_3$ receptor sites and block fibrinogen or von Willebrand factor binding, thereby preventing platelet aggregation[79] (Figure 43-9). Cardiologists use intravenous GPIs to maintain vascular patency during cardiac catheterization and intracoronary stent placement.[80]

Before GPI infusion, the PT, PTT, ACT, hemoglobin, hematocrit, and platelet count are determined to detect any hemostatic or hematologic abnormality.[81] During infusion, the PTT and ACT are maintained within the UFH therapeutic range as determined by the laboratory. Platelet counts are performed at 2 hours, 4 hours, and 24 hours following the initial bolus. If the platelet count drops by 25% or more, UFH and GPI are discontinued and the platelet count is monitored daily until it returns to within the reference interval. GPI efficacy may be measured using the Multiplate analyzer (DiaPharma, West Chester, OH; Roche Diagnostics Corporation, Indianapolis, IN) or VerifyNow IIb/IIIa assay (Accumetrics, San Diego, CA; International Technidyne Corporation, Edison, NJ).

Abciximab (ReoPro; Eli Lilly and Company, Indianapolis, IN) is the 47,615 Dalton Fab fragment of a mouse monoclonal antibody specific for $\alpha_{IIb}\beta_3$ that effectively fills the receptor site.[82] The dose is 0.25 mg/kg given by intravenous bolus administered 10 to 60 minutes before the start of cardiac catheterization, followed by continuous infusion of 0.125 μg/kg/min for up to 12 hours. Abciximab is always coadministered with UFH and aspirin.

Eptifibatide (Integrilin; Schering Corporation, Kenilworth, NJ) is an 832 Dalton heptapeptide GPI. It is coadministered with aspirin and UFH. An intravenous bolus of 180 μg/kg is given as soon as possible after initial diagnosis, and a continuous intravenous drip of 2 μg/kg/min is continued for up to 96 hours following the initial bolus, including throughout cardiac catheterization.

Tirofiban hydrochloride (Aggrastat; Baxter Healthcare Corporation, Deerfield, IL) is a 495 Dalton non-protein GPI that is coadministered with aspirin and UFH. It is administered intravenously at an initial rate of 0.4 μg/kg/min for 30 minutes and then continued at 0.1 μg/kg/min throughout cardiac catheterization and for 12 to 24 hours after catheterization. Tirofiban is excreted through the kidney, so the dosage is halved when the creatinine clearance is less than 30 mL/min.

Aspirin, Clopidogrel, Prasugrel, and Ticagrelor Reduce the Incidence of Arterial Thrombosis

The most commonly prescribed oral antiplatelet drugs are aspirin, clopidogrel (Plavix; Sanofi-Aventis, Bridgewater, NJ; Bristol-Myers Squibb, New York, NY), prasugrel (Effient; Eli Lilly and Company, Indianapolis, IN), and ticagrelor (Brilinta; AstraZeneca, Wilmington, DE). Aspirin irreversibly acetylates the platelet enzyme cyclooxygenase at the serine in position 529 (Figure 43-9). The serine-bound acetyl group sterically hinders the access of arachidonic acid to its reactive site within the cyclooxygenase molecule. This prevents production of platelet-activating thromboxane A_2 through the eicosanoid synthesis pathway (Chapter 13).[83] Acetylation is irreversible; the eicosanoid synthesis pathway is shut down for the remainder of the life of the platelet.

In contrast, clopidogrel, prasugrel, and ticagrelor are generally considered to be members of the thienopyridine drug family, though ticagrelor is actually a purine analogue. Thienopyridines occupy the platelet membrane adenosine diphosphate (ADP) receptor $P2Y_{12}$, suppressing the normal platelet aggregation and secretion response to the activating ligand (agonist) ADP. Clopidogrel and prasugrel are irreversible inhibitors, whereas ticagrelor is a reversible inhibitor.

Aspirin is often prescribed alone at 81 or 325 mg/day to prevent myocardial infarction and ischemic cerebrovascular disease in patients with stable or unstable angina,[84,85] AMI,[86] transient cerebral ischemia,[87] peripheral vascular disease,[88] or stroke.[89,90] In healthy people, aspirin prophylaxis annually prevents four thrombotic events per 1000 individuals treated, although it carries a risk of bleeding.[91-93]

Clopidogrel is prescribed at 75 mg/day together with aspirin at 81 or 325 mg/day. Clopidogrel is a prodrug, and patients appear to have varying responses to the fixed dose of clopidogrel, which raises the need for routine laboratory measuring using platelet function assays. Patients who possess a genetic variant of the CYP2C19 liver enzyme that activates clopidogrel may not get the full therapeutic effect. The variant polymorphism may be identified via molecular diagnostic techniques or phenotypically, as described in the next section.

Prasugrel was cleared by the FDA in July 2009.[94] It is administered as an oral prodrug that is converted in the liver via several cytochrome P-450 pathways to an active metabolite whose elimination half-life is about 7 hours. Treatment begins with a single 60-mg oral loading dose and continues at 10 mg daily, or 5 mg daily for patients who weigh less than 60 kg. Prasugrel is to be taken with aspirin at 81 mg or 325 mg daily and appears to require no laboratory measuring. However, up to 14% of patients may not achieve the full effect of prasugrel due to a genetic variant of the CYP2C19 liver enzyme needed to activate the drug. Drug interactions that increase or decrease the activity of prasugrel are important to identify. Prasugrel carries a higher risk of bleeding than clopidogrel and may be associated with an increased risk of solid tumors.

Ticagrelor was cleared in July 2011 to be coadministered with aspirin. Ticagrelor is a prodrug whose main active metabolite is formed rapidly via the CYP3A4 liver enzyme. It is provided in 90-mg tablets. Therapy is begun with two tablets totaling 180 mg, taken with one 325-mg aspirin tablet, followed by 90 mg of ticagrelor twice a day and one aspirin a day, not to exceed 100 mg. Ticagrelor reaches full effectiveness in 1.5 hours and maintains steady state for at least 8 hours. Drug interactions that increase or decrease the activity of ticagrelor are important to identify.

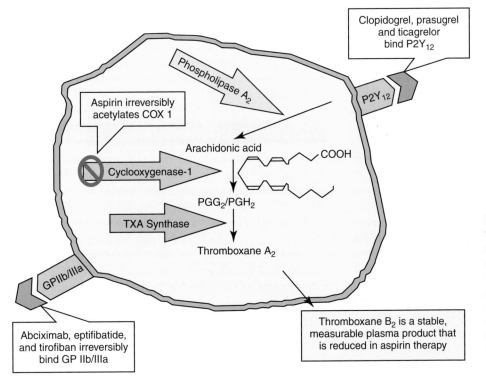

Figure 43-9 Antiplatelet drugs employ three mechanisms to inactivate platelets. Aspirin irreversibly acetylates and inactivates cyclooxygenase 1 (COX-1). Clopidogrel (irreversible), prasugrel (irreversible), and ticagrelor (reversible) bind the adenosine diphosphate (ADP) receptor, $P2Y_{12}$. Intravenous abciximab, eptifibatide, and tirofiban bind the fibrinogen binding site, glycoprotein (GP) IIb/IIIa. *PGG$_2$*, Prostaglandin G$_2$; *PGH2*, prostaglandin H$_2$; *TXA synthase*, thromboxane A$_2$ synthase.

Variable Aspirin and Clopidogrel Response and Laboratory Measuring of Antiplatelet Resistance

Several investigations confirm that 10% to 20% of people who are taking aspirin generate an inadequate response as measured in the laboratory by light transmittance platelet aggregometry or whole-blood impedance aggregometry using arachidonic acid as the agonist. Inadequate response to aspirin has been termed *aspirin resistance*.[95-98] Likewise, the response to clopidogrel as measured by aggregometry using ADP as the agonist varies markedly among patients, and the results of this assay may be used to adjust clopidogrel dosage.[99] Mechanisms that explain aspirin resistance and clopidogrel response variation are currently under study. Unlike treatment with aspirin and clopidogrel, prasugrel and ticagrelor therapy may show less interpatient variation. Aggregometry is the reference method for determining aspirin and clopidogrel responses, but several more rapid assays are available.

- VerifyNow: The Accumetrics VerifyNow (Accumetrics, San Diego, CA; International Technidyne Corporation, Edison, NJ) system is designed for point-of-care testing and uses light transmittance aggregometry to individually test for platelet aggregation responses to aspirin, clopidogrel, prasugrel, ticagrelor, and GPIs.[100] For each assay a cartridge is provided that contains the desired agonist and fibrinogen-coated beads. VerifyNow Aspirin uses arachidonic acid as its agonist. VerifyNow P2Y$_{12}$ uses ADP. VerifyNow IIb/IIIa uses thrombin receptor–activating polypeptide (TRAP), which activates platelets by binding to the thrombin receptor *protease-activated receptor 1* (PAR1; Chapter 13). The laboratory establishes reference interval limits and therapeutic target limits for each assay. Results that are outside the therapeutic target range indicate possible treatment failure and the need to revise dosage or change to a new antiplatelet drug. All three Accumetrics VerifyNow systems are FDA cleared.

- Multiplate: The Multiplate (DiaPharma, West Chester, OH; Roche Diagnostics Corporation, Indianapolis, IN) analyzer is automated for point-of-care testing and uses impedance aggregometry to simultaneously or individually test for platelet aggregation responses to aspirin, thienopyridines, and GPIs. The Multiplate requires 300 µL of whole blood. The aspirin resistance assay uses arachidonic acid as its agonist, the thienopyridine response assay uses ADP, and the GPI response uses TRAP. The instrument integrates three aggregometry parameters—*aggregation velocity, maximum aggregation,* and *area under the aggregation curve*—to produce measurement units. The local laboratory establishes reference interval limits and expected therapeutic target ranges. Results that are outside the therapeutic target range indicate possible treatment failure and the need to revise dosage or change to a new antiplatelet drug. The Multiplate is available in Europe and was cleared by the FDA for use in the United States in August 2012.

- Plateletworks: The Plateletworks assay from Helena Laboratories (Beaumont, TX) determines the percent platelet aggregation in whole blood. Whole blood is added to EDTA tubes coated with the agonists ADP or collagen, plus plain EDTA tubes. The practitioner performs platelet counts on the plain tube (baseline) and the agonist-treated EDTA tubes using an impedance-based electronic cell counter. The differences, expressed as percentages, indicate the degree of platelet aggregation triggered by each agonist. An expected effect of antiplatelet drug therapy would be a platelet aggregation response that is reduced 40% to 60% from a normal response.

- PFA-100 (Siemens Medical Solutions USA, Inc., Malvern, PA). The PFA-100 system uses two cartridges. The first provides an aperture impregnated with collagen and epinephrine, and the second provides an aperture impregnated with collagen and ADP. The operator pipettes 800 µL whole blood per cartridge and places the cartridge on the instrument.[101] The specimen passes through the aperture until activation by the agonist causes occlusion of the aperture, generating a parameter called *closure time*. The PFA-100 tests only for aspirin resistance. A closure time that is shorter than the anticipated therapeutic range for aspirin indicates resistance.

- AspirinWorks (Corgenix Medical Corporation, Broomfield, CO): The AspirinWorks immunoassay measures a urine metabolite of platelet eicosanoid synthesis and thromboxane A$_2$ activation (Chapter 13). Hepatocyte *11-hydroxythromboxane dehydrogenase* acts upon stable platelet-derived plasma thromboxane B$_2$, the end product of eicosanoid synthesis and the stable analogue of thromboxane A$_2$, to produce water-soluble 11-dehydrothromboxane B$_2$.[99] The urine concentration of 11-dehydrothromboxane B$_2$ is sufficient for measurement without extraction and, because platelets seem to be its primary source, proportionally reflects platelet activity within the previous 12 hours. Urine levels of 11-dehydrothromboxane B$_2$ frequently are elevated in atherosclerosis; after stroke, transient ischemic attack, or intracerebral hemorrhage; and in atrial fibrillation. Levels of 11-dehydrothromboxane B$_2$ typically are decreased in patients receiving aspirin therapy, even in those with atherosclerosis, myocardial infarction, and atrial fibrillation, but appear to remain normal in patients who have aspirin resistance.

FUTURE OF ANTITHROMBOTIC THERAPY

Antithrombotic therapy, unchanged for more than 50 years, is likely to see further changes between 2014 and 2020. Several oral anticoagulants currently under development or awaiting clearance are likely to replace Coumadin, the heparins, and fondaparinux. Likewise, a series of new and emerging antiplatelet drugs will augment the time-honored aspirin tablet. The work of the clinical laboratory will reflect these changes, moving from the PT and PTT to chromogenic anti-factor Xa, modifications of the thrombin time, the ecarin clotting time, chromogenic assays, and new molecular assays. Antiplatelet response measuring will grow in convenience and take advantage of flow cytometry, immunoassays, and molecular assays that are currently in development.

SUMMARY

- Coumadin was developed in 1940 by Link and was first used in 1952. It prevents VTE, but it has a narrow therapeutic range, and an overdose causes hemorrhage. Coumadin therapy is monitored by the PT assay and reported as an INR. PT measurement is available on portable point-of-care instrumentation. Anticoagulation clinics are available to facilitate Coumadin monitoring and provide patient education and support.

- UFH is administered intravenously to provide immediate control of coagulation. Its therapeutic effect is monitored using the PTT, which requires the laboratory practitioner to develop a therapeutic range in seconds keyed to the chromogenic anti-factor Xa heparin assay. PTT results are subject to several interferences. Heparin is also used during cardiac catheterization or cardiac surgery that requires extracorporeal circulation. In these acute settings it is monitored by the ACT for its point-of-care and sensitivity to high heparin dose capabilities.

- LMWH and fondaparinux substitute for UFH and are administered subcutaneously for both prophylaxis and therapy. Both provide near-complete bioavailability, predictable dose response, and longer half-lives than UFH. LMWH and fondaparinux therapy require laboratory measurement only in patients with renal insufficiency, pregnant women, obese patients, children, and underweight adults using the chromogenic anti-factor Xa heparin assay.

- Rivaroxaban, apixaban, and edoxaban are the first to come to market of several oral direct-acting anti-factor Xa anticoagulants that require little laboratory measurement. New measurement techniques include the chromogenic anti-factor Xa assays using rivaroxaban, apixaban, and edoxaban calibrators and controls.

- The intravenous DTIs argatroban and bivalirudin directly bind thrombin without involving antithrombin and are substituted for heparin in patients with HIT. Intravenous DTI therapy is monitored using the PTT or ECT, and all affect the PT results during switchover to Coumadin therapy. At higher doses, as used during interventional procedures, these drugs are monitored by the ACT.

- Dabigatran is an oral DTI that requires minimal laboratory measurement. Dabigatran may be measured using the PTT, ECT, ECA, and plasma-diluted thrombin time.

- The antiplatelet drugs aspirin, clopidogrel, prasugrel, and ticagrelor are used after arterial thrombotic events to prevent repeat AMI, stroke, and PAO. Patient responses to aspirin and clopidogrel therapy vary. Response variation is detected using platelet aggregometry, the Accumetrics Verify*Now* system, the Multiplate system, Helena's Plateletworks, the PFA-100 or the AspirinWorks assay; the latter two measure aspirin only.

- The intravenous antiplatelet drugs abciximab, eptifibatide, and tirofiban are used during cardiac catheterization to maintain vascular patency. Because they may cause thrombocytopenia, the platelet count is monitored carefully. Their efficacy may be monitored using the Accumetrics VerifyNow system, Helena's Plateletworks, or the Multiplate system.

Now that you have completed this chapter, go back and read again the case study at the beginning and respond to the questions presented.

REVIEW QUESTIONS

Answers can be found in the Appendix.

1. What is the PT/INR therapeutic range for Coumadin therapy when a patient has a mechanical heart valve?
   a. 1 to 2
   b. 2 to 3
   c. 2.5 to 3.5
   d. Coumadin is not indicated for patients with mechanical heart valves

2. Monitoring of a patient taking Coumadin showed that her anticoagulation results remained stable over a period of about 7 months. The frequency of her visits to the laboratory began to decrease, so the period between testing averaged 6 weeks. This new testing interval is:
   a. Acceptable for a patient with stable anticoagulation results after 6 months
   b. Unnecessary, because monitoring for patients taking oral anticoagulants can be discontinued entirely after 4 months of stable test results

   c. Too long even for a patient with previously stable test results; 4 weeks is the standard
   d. Acceptable as long as the patient performs self-monitoring daily using an approved home testing instrument and reports unacceptable results promptly to her physician

3. What is the greatest advantage of point-of-care PT testing?
   a. It permits self-dosing of Coumadin
   b. It is inexpensive
   c. It is convenient
   d. It is precise

4. You collect a citrated whole-blood specimen to monitor UFH therapy. What is the longest it may stand before the plasma must be separated from the cells?
   a. 1 hour
   b. 4 hours
   c. 24 hours
   d. Indefinitely

5. What test is used to monitor high-dose UFH therapy in the cardiac catheterization lab?
   a. PT
   b. PTT
   c. Bleeding time
   d. ACT

6. What test is used most often to monitor UFH therapy in the central laboratory?
   a. PT
   b. PTT
   c. ACT
   d. Chromogenic anti-factor Xa heparin assay

7. What test is used most often to monitor LMWH therapy in the central laboratory?
   a. PT
   b. PTT
   c. ACT
   d. Chromogenic anti-factor Xa heparin assay

8. What is an advantage of LMWH therapy over UFH therapy?
   a. It is cheaper
   b. It causes no bleeding
   c. It has a stable dose response
   d. There is no risk of HIT

9. In what situation is an intravenous DTI used?
   a. DVT
   b. HIT
   c. Any situation in which Coumadin could be used
   d. Uncomplicated AMI

10. What laboratory test may be used to monitor intravenous DTI therapy when PTT results are unreliable?
    a. PT
    b. ECT
    c. Reptilase clotting time
    d. Chromogenic anti-factor Xa heparin assay

11. What is the reference method for detecting aspirin or clopidogrel resistance?
    a. Platelet aggregometry
    b. AspirinWorks
    c. VerifyNow
    d. PFA-100

12. What is the name of the measurable platelet activation metabolite used in the AspirinWorks assay to monitor aspirin resistance?
    a. 11-dehydrothromboxane B_2
    b. Arachidonic acid
    c. Thromboxane A_2
    d. Cyclooxygenase

13. Which of the following is an intravenous antiplatelet drug used in the cardiac catheterization laboratory?
    a. Abciximab
    b. Ticagrelor
    c. Prasugrel
    d. Clopidogrel

14. Which of the following is a newly developed oral anticoagulant?
    a. Argatroban
    b. Lepirudin
    c. Bivalirudin
    d. Rivaroxaban

15. Which of the following is *not* a point-of-care instrument for the measurement of PT?
    a. CoaguChek XS PT
    b. Gem PCL Plus
    c. Cascade POC
    d. Multiplate

REFERENCES

1. Galanaud, J. P., Laroche, J. P., & Righini, M. (2013). The history and historical treatments of deep vein thrombosis. *J Thromb Haemost, 11,* 402–411.
2. Shannon, A. W., & Harrigan, R. A. (2001). General pharmacologic treatment of acute myocardial infarction. *Emerg Med Clin North Am, 19,* 417–431.
3. Whitlock, R. P., Sun, J. C., Fremes, S. E., Rubens, F. D., & Teoh, K. H. (2012). Antithrombotic and thrombolytic therapy for valvular disease: antithrombotic therapy and prevention of thrombosis, 9th ed. American College of Chest Physicians Evidence-Based Clinical Practice Guidelines. *Chest, 141* (Suppl. 2), e576–e600s.
4. Patriquin, C., & Crowther, M. (2013). Antithrombotic agents. In Kitchens, C. S., Kessler, C. M., Konkle, B. A., (Eds.), *Consultative Hemostasis and Thrombosis.* (3rd ed., pp. 477–495). Philadelphia: Saunders.
5. Marder, V. J. (2013). Thrombolytic therapy. In Kitchens, C. S., Kessler, C. M., & Konkle, B. A., (Eds.), *Consultative Hemostasis and Thrombosis.* (3rd ed., pp. 526–537). Philadelphia: Saunders.
6. Adverse events and deaths associated with laboratory errors at a hospital—Pennsylvania. (2001). *MMWR Morb Mortal Wkly Rep, 50,* 710–711.
7. Ageno, W., Gallus, A. S., Wittkowsky, A., et al. (2012). Oral anticoagulant therapy: antithrombotic therapy and prevention of thrombosis: American College of Chest Physicians Evidence-Based Clinical Practice Guidelines (9th edition). *Chest, 141,* e44S–e88S.
8. Duxbury, B. M., & Poller, L. (2001). The oral anticoagulant saga: past, present, and future. *Clin Appl Thromb Hemost, 7,* 269–275.
9. Nazarian, R. M., Van Cott, E. M., Zembowicz, A., et al. (2009). Warfarin-induced skin necrosis. *J Am Acad Dermatol, 61,* 325–332.

10. Witt, D. M. (2012). Approaches to optimal dosing of vitamin K antagonists. *Semin Thromb Hemost, 38,* 667–672.

11. Ng, V. L. (2009). Anticoagulation monitoring. *Clin Lab Med, 29,* 283–304.

12. Kitchen, S., & Preston, F. E. (1999). Standardization of prothrombin time for laboratory control of oral anticoagulant therapy. *Semin Thromb Hemost, 25,* 17–25.

13. Turpie, A. G. G. (2008). New oral anticoagulants in atrial fibrillation. *Eur Heart J, 29,* 155–165.

14. Rosborough, T. K., Jacobsen, J. M., & Shepherd, M. F. (2009). Relationship between chromogenic factor X and INR differs during early Coumadin initiation compared with chronic warfarin administration. *Blood Coagul Fibrinolysis, 20,* 433–435.

15. McGlasson, D. L., Romick, B. G., & Rubal, B. J. (2008). Comparison of a chromogenic factor X assay with INR for monitoring oral anticoagulation therapy. *Blood Coagul Fibrinolysis, 19,* 513–517.

16. Rosborough, T. K., & Shepherd, M. F. (2004). Unreliability of international normalized ratio for monitoring warfarin therapy in patients with lupus anticoagulant. *Pharmacotherapy, 24,* 838–842.

17. Caldwell, M. D., Awad, T., & Johnson, J. A. (2008). CYP4F2 genetic variant alters required warfarin dose. *Blood, 111,* 4106–4112.

18. Cavallari, L. H., & Limdi, N. A. (2009). Warfarin pharmacogenomics. *Curr Opin Mol Ther, 11,* 243–251.

19. Osinbowale, O., Al Malki, M., Schade, A., et al. (2009). An algorithm for managing warfarin resistance. *Cleve Clin J Med, 76,* 724–730.

20. Linkins, L. A., Dans, A. L., Moores, L. K., et al. (2012). Treatment and prevention of heparin-induced thrombocytopenia: antithrombotic therapy and prevention of thrombosis: American College of Chest Physicians Evidence-Based Clinical Practice Guidelines (9th ed.). *Chest, 141,* e495S–e530S.

21. Pabinger-Fasching, I. (2008). Warfarin-reversal: results of a phase III study with pasteurized, nanofiltrated prothrombin complex concentrate. *Thromb Res, 122*(Suppl. 2), S19–S22.

22. Garcia, D. A., Baglin, T. P., Weitz, J. I., & Samama, M. M. (2012). Parenteral anticoagulants: antithrombotic therapy and prevention of thrombosis: American College of Chest Physicians Evidence-Based Clinical Practice Guidelines (9th ed.). *Chest, 141,* e24S–e43S.

23. Olson, J. D., Arkin, C. F., Brandt, J. T., et al., (Eds.). (1998). College of American Pathologists Conference XXXI on laboratory monitoring of anticoagulant therapy: laboratory monitoring of unfractionated heparin therapy. *Arch Pathol Lab Med, 122,* 782–798.

24. Marlar, R. A., & Gausman, J. (2013). The optimum number and type of plasma samples necessary for an accurate activated partial thromboplastin time-based heparin therapeutic range. *Arch Pathol Lab Med, 137,* 77–82.

25. Brill-Edwards, P., Ginsberg, J. S., Johnston, M., et al. (1993). Establishing a therapeutic interval for heparin therapy. *Ann Intern Med, 119,* 104–109.

26. CLSI. (2008). *One-stage prothrombin time (PT) test and activated partial thromboplastin time (APTT) test; approved guideline.* (2nd ed.). CLSI Document H27-A2, Wayne, Penn: Clinical and Laboratory Standards Institute.

27. Eikelboom, J. W., & Hirsh, J. (2006). Monitoring unfractionated heparin with the aPTT: time for a fresh look. *Thromb Haemost, 96,* 547–552.

28. Tripodi, A., van den Besselaar, A. (2009). Laboratory monitoring of anticoagulation: where do we stand? *Semin Thromb Hemost, 35,* 34–41.

29. Bharadwaj, J., Jayaraman, C., & Shrivastava, R. (2003). Heparin resistance. *Lab Hematol, 9,* 125–131.

30. Adcock, D. M., Kressin, D. C., & Marlar, R. A. (1998). The effect of time and temperature variables on routine coagulation tests. *Blood Coagul Fibrinolysis, 9,* 463–470.

31. Estry, D. W., & Wright, L. (1988). Laboratory assessment of anticoagulant therapy. *Clin Lab Sci, 1,* 161–164.

32. Slight, R. D., Buell, R., Nzewi, O. C., et al. (2008). A comparison of activated coagulation time–based techniques for anticoagulation during cardiac surgery with cardiopulmonary bypass. *J Cardiothorac Vasc Anesth, 22,* 47–52.

33. Bakchoul, T., Zoliner, H., Amiral, J., et al. (2013). Anti-protamine-heparin antibodies: incidence, clinical relevance, and pathogenesis. *Blood, 121,* 2821–2827.

34. Warkentin, T. E., & Linkins, L. A. (2009). Immunoassays are not created equal. *J Thromb Haemost, 7,* 1256–1269.

35. Hull, R. D., Raskob, G. E., Pineo, G. F., et al. (1992). Subcutaneous low molecular weight heparin compared with continuous intravenous heparin in the treatment of proximal-vein thrombosis. *N Engl J Med, 326,* 975–982.

36. Cheer, S. M., Dunn, C. J., & Foster, R. (2004). Tinzaparin sodium: a review of its pharmacology and clinical use in the prophylaxis and treatment of thromboembolic disease. *Drugs, 64,* 1479–1502.

37. Douketis, J. D., Spyropoulos, A. C., Spencer, F. A., et al. (2012). Perioperative management of antithrombotic therapy: antithrombotic therapy and prevention of thrombosis: American College of Chest Physicians Evidence-Based Clinical Practice Guidelines (9th ed.). *Chest, 141,* e326S–e350S.

38. McGlasson, D. L., Kaczor, D. A., Krasuski, R. A., et al. (2005). Effects of pre-analytical variables on the anti–activated factor X chromogenic assay when monitoring unfractionated heparin and low molecular weight heparin anticoagulation. *Blood Coagul Fibrinolysis, 16,* 173–176.

39. McGlasson, D. L. (2005). Using a single calibration curve with the anti-Xa chromogenic assay for monitoring heparin anticoagulation. *Lab Med, 36,* 297–299.

40. Turpie, A. G. G. (2002). Pentasaccharides. *Semin Hematol, 39,* 158–171.

41. Heit, J. A. (2002). The potential role of fondaparinux as venous thromboembolism prophylaxis after total hip or knee replacement of hip fracture surgery. *Arch Intern Med, 162,* 1806–1808.

42. Samama, M. M., & Gerotziafas, G. T. (2010). Newer anticoagulants in 2009. *J Thromb Thrombolysis, 29,* 92–104.

43. Turpie, A. G. G., Bauer, K. A., Eriksson, B. I., & Lassen, M. R. (2002). Fondaparinux vs. enoxaparin for the prevention of venous thromboembolism in major orthopedic surgery: a meta-analysis of 4 randomized double-blind studies. *Arch Intern Med, 162,* 1833–1840.

44. Fuji, T., Fujita, S., Tachibana, S., et al. (2008). Randomized, double-blind, multi-dose efficacy, safety and biomarker study of the oral factor Xa inhibitor DU-176b compared with placebo for prevention of venous thromboembolism in patients after total knee arthroplasty. ASH Annual Meeting Abstracts. *Blood, 112,* 34.

45. Bauer, K. A., Homering, M., & Berkowitz, S. D. (2008). Effects of age, weight, gender and renal function in a pooled analysis of four phase III studies of rivaroxaban for prevention of venous thromboembolism after major orthopedic surgery. *Blood, 112,* Abstract 436.

46. Bijsterveld, N. R., Moons, A. H., Boekholdt, S. M., et al. (2002). Ability of recombinant factor VIIa to reverse the anticoagulant effect of the pentasaccharide fondaparinux in healthy volunteers. *Circulation, 106,* 2550–2554.

47. Laux, V., Perzborn, E., Kubitza, D., & Misselwitz, F. (2007). Preclinical and clinical characteristics of rivaroxaban: a novel, oral, direct factor Xa inhibitor. *Semin Thromb Hemost, 33,* 5115–5123.

48. US Dept of HHS Agency for Healthcare Research and Quality. (2008). Retrieved from http://www.ahrq.gov/qual/vtguide/vtguideapa.htm. Accessed 05.07.13.

49. Mayo Foundation for Medical Education and Research. (2014). http://www.mayoclinic.org/atrial-fibrillation/treatment.html. Accessed 05.07.13.

50. Go, A. S., Hylek, E. M., Phillips, K. A., et al. (2001). Prevalence of diagnosed atrial fibrillation in adults: national implications for rhythm management and stroke prevention: the AnTicoagulation and Risk Factors in Atrial Fibrillation (ATRIA) Study. *JAMA, 285,* 2370–2375.

51. FDA application and approval history for Xarelto (rivaroxaban) supplied by Janssen Pharmaceuticals, Inc. Retrived from http://www.drugs.com. Accessed 18.12.14.

52. Baglin, T., Hillarp, A., Tripodi, A., et al. (2013). Measuring oral direct inhibitors of thrombin and factor Xa: a recommendation from the Subcommittee on Control of Anticoagulation of the SSC of the ISTH. *J Thromb Haemost, 11,* 756–760.

53. Tripodi, A., Chantarangkul, V., Guinet, C., & Samama, M. M. (2011). The international normalized ratio calibrated for rivaroxaban has the potential to normalize prothrombin time results for rivaroxaban-treated patients: results of an in vitro study. *J Thromb Haemost, 9,* 226–228.

54. Tripodi, A. (2013). Which test to use to measure the anticoagulant effect of rivaroxaban: the prothrombin time test. *J Thromb Haemostas, 11,* 576–578.

55. Samama, M. M. (2013). Which test to use to measure the anticoagulant effect of rivaroxaban: the anti-factor Xa assay. *J Thromb Haemostas, 11,* 579–580.

56. Favaloro, E. J., & Lippi, G. (2012). The new oral anticoagulants and the future of haemostasis laboratory testing. *Biochemia Medica, 22,* 329–341.

57. Quinlan, D. J., & Eriksson, B. I. (2013). Novel oral anticoagulants for thromboprophylaxis after orthopaedic surgery. *Best Pract Res Clin Haematol, 26,* 171–182.

58. Shirasaki, Y., Morishima, Y., & Shibano, T. (2013, Aug 6). Comparison of the effect of edoxaban, a direct factor Xa inhibitor, with a direct thrombin inhibitor, melagatran, and heparin on intracerebral hemorrhage induced by collagenase in rats. *Thromb Res,* doi:pii:S0049-3848(13)00293-4. 10.1016/j.thromres.2013.07.015.

59. Yeh, R. W., & Jang, I. K. (2006). Argatroban: update. *Am Heart J, 151,* 1131–1138.

60. Shantsila, E., Lip, G. Y., & Chong, B. H. (2009). Heparin-induced thrombocytopenia. A contemporary clinical approach to diagnosis and management. *Chest, 135,* 1651–1654.

61. Schulman, S., & Spencer, F. A. (2010). Antithrombotic drugs in coronary artery disease: risk benefit ratio and bleeding. *J Thromb Haemost, 8,* 641–650.

62. Curran, M. P. (2010). Bivalirudin: in patients with ST-segment elevation myocardial infarction. *Drugs, 70,* 909–918.

63. Kaplan, K. L., & Francis, C. W. (2002). Direct thrombin inhibitors. *Semin Hematol, 39,* 187–196.

64. Prechel, M., & Walenga, J. M. (2008). The laboratory diagnosis and clinical management of patients with heparin-induced thrombocytopenia: an update. *Semin Thromb Hemostas, 34,* 86–96.

65. Wittkowsky, A. K. (2010). New oral anticoagulants: a practical guide for clinicians. *J Thromb Thrombolysis, 29,* 182–191.

66. Heidbuchel, H., Verhamme, P., Alings, M., et al. (2013). European Heart Rhythm Association practical guide on the use of new oral anticoagulants in patients with nonvalvular atrial fibrillation. *Europace, 15,* 625–651.

67. Khadzhynov, D., Wagner, F., Formella, S., et al. (2013). Effective elimination of dabigatran by haemodialysis; A phase I single-centre study in patients with end-stage renal disease. *Thromb Haemost, 109,* 596–60.

68. Laulicht, B., Bakhru, S., Jiang, X., et al. (2013). Antidote for new oral anticoagulants: mechanism of action and binding specificity of PER977. *J Thromb Haemostas, 11*(Suppl. 2), ISTH Abstract AS 47.1.

69. Crowther, M., Kitt, M., Lorenz, T., et al. (2013). A phase 2 randomized, double-blind, placebo controlled trial of PRT064445, a novel, universal antidote for direct and indirect factor Xa inhibitors. *J Thromb Haemostas, 11*(Suppl. 2), Abstr OC 20.1.

70. Levi, M., Moore, T., Castillejos, C. F., et al. (2013). Effects of 3-factor and 4-factor prothrombin complex concentrates on the pharmacodynamics of rivaroxaban. *J Thromb Haemostas, 11*(Suppl. 2), Abstr OC 36.5.

71. Chia, S., Van Cott, E. M., Raffel, O. C., et al. (2009). Comparison of activated clotting times obtained using Hemochron and Medtronic analyzers in patients receiving anti-thrombin therapy during cardiac catheterization. *Thromb Haemost, 101,* 535–540.

72. Van Ryn, J., Stangier, J., Haertter, S., et al. (2010). Dabigatran etexilate—a novel, reversible, oral direct thrombin inhibitor: interpretation of coagulation assays and reversal of anticoagulant activity. *Thromb Haemostas, 103,* 1116–1127.

73. Harenberg, J., Giese, C., Marx, S., Math, M., & Kramer, R. (2012). Determination of dabigatran in human plasma samples. *Semin Thromb Hemost, 38,* 16–22.

74. Antovic, J. P., Skeppholm, M., Eintrei, J., et al. (2013). How to monitor dabigatran when needed: comparison of coagulation laboratory methods and dabigatran concentrations in plasma. *J Thromb Haemostas, 11*(Suppl. 2), Abstr AS 02-3.

75. Avecilla, S. T., Ferrell, C., Chandler, W. L., & Reyes, M. (2012). Plasma-diluted thrombin time to measure dabigatran concentrations during dabigatran etexilate therapy. *Am J Clin Pathol, 137,* 572–574.

76. Love, J. E., Ferrell, C., & Chandler, W. (2007). Monitoring direct thrombin inhibitors with a plasma diluted thrombin time. *Thromb Haemost, 98,* 234–242.

77. Chandler, W. (2013). Assays for antithrombotic drugs. *J Thromb Haemostas, 11*(Suppl. 2), ISTH Abstract AS 02.

78. Baglin, T., Hillarp, A., Tripodi, A., et al. (2013). Measuring oral direct inhibitors of thrombin and factor Xa: a recommendation from the Subcommittee on Control of Anticoagulation of the Scientific and Standardization Committee of the International Society on Thrombosis and Haemostasis. *J Thromb Haemost, 11,* 756–760.

79. Lincoff, A. M., Tcheng, J. E., Califf, R. M., et al. (1999). For the EPILOG Investigators. Sustained suppression of ischemic complications of coronary intervention by platelet GP IIb/IIIa blockade with abciximab. *Circulation, 99,* 1951–1958.

80. Muhlestein, J. B. (2010). Effect of antiplatelet therapy on inflammatory markers in atherothrombotic patients. *Thromb Haemost, 103,* 71–82.

81. CAPTURE Investigators. (1997). Randomised placebo-controlled trial of abciximab before, during and after coronary intervention in refractory unstable angina: the CAPTURE study. *Lancet, 349,* 1429–1435.

82. van't Hof, A. W., & Valgimigli, M. (2009). Defining the role of platelet glycoprotein receptor inhibitors in STEMI: focus on tirofiban. *Drugs, 69,* 85–100.

83. Gilroy, D. W. (2010). Eicosanoids and the endogenous control of acute inflammatory resolution. *Int J Biochem Cell Biol, 42,* 524–528.

84. Juul-Moller, S., Edvardsson, N., Jahnmatz, B., et al. (1992). Double-blind trial of aspirin in primary prevention of myocardial infarction in patients with stable chronic angina pectoris. *Lancet, 340,* 1421–1425.

85. The RISC Group. (1990). Risk of myocardial infarction and death during treatment with low dose aspirin and intravenous heparin in men with unstable coronary artery disease. *Lancet, 336,* 827–830.

86. ISIS-2 Collaborative Group. (1988). Randomised trial of intravenous streptokinase, oral aspirin, both or neither among 17,187 cases of suspected acute myocardial infarction: ISIS-2. *Lancet, 2,* 349–360.

87. The Dutch TIA Study Group. (1991). A comparison of two doses of aspirin (30 mg vs. 283 mg a day) in patients after a transient ischemic attack or minor ischemic stroke. *N Engl J Med, 325,* 1261–1262.

88. Hirsh, J., Dalen, J. E., Fuster, V., et al. (1995). Aspirin and other platelet-active drugs: the relationship among dose, effectiveness, and side effects. *Chest, 108*, 247S–257S.

89. International Stroke Trial Collaborative Group. (1997). The International Stroke Trial (IST): a randomised trial of aspirin, subcutaneous heparin, both, or neither among 19,435 patients with acute ischemic stroke. *Lancet, 349*, 1569–1581.

90. CAST (Chinese Acute Stroke Trial) Collaborative Group. (1997). CAST: randomised placebo-controlled trial of early aspirin use in 20,000 patients with acute ischemic stroke. *Lancet, 349*, 1641–1649.

91. Antiplatelet Trialists' Collaboration. (1994). Collaborative overview of randomized trials of antiplatelet therapy: I. prevention of death, myocardial infarction, and stroke by prolonged antiplatelet therapy in various categories of patients. *Br Med J, 308*, 81–106.

92. Hennekens, C. H., Peto, R., Hutchison, G. B., et al. (1988). An overview of the British and American aspirin studies. *N Engl J Med, 318*, 923–924.

93. Manson, J. E., Stampfer, M. J., Colditz, G. A., et al. (1991). A prospective study of aspirin use and primary prevention of cardiovascular disease in women. *JAMA, 266*, 521–527.

94. Freeman, M. K. (2010). Thienopyridine antiplatelet agents: focus on prasugrel. *Consult Pharm, 25*, 241–257.

95. Eikelboom, J. W., Hirsh, J., Weitz, J. I., et al. (2002). Aspirin-resistant thromboxane biosynthesis and the risk of myocardial infarction, stroke, or cardiovascular death in patients at high risk for cardiovascular events. *Circulation, 105*, 1650–1655.

96. Gum, P. A., Kottke-Marchant, K., Welsh, P. A., et al. (2003). A prospective, blinded determination of the natural history of aspirin resistance among stable patients with cardiovascular disease. *J Am Coll Cardiol, 41*, 961–965.

97. Chen, W. H. (2006). Antiplatelet resistance with aspirin and clopidogrel: is it real and does it matter? *Curr Cardiol Rep, 8*, 301–306.

98. Knoepp, S. M., & Laposata, M. (2005). Aspirin resistance: moving forward with multiple definitions, different assays, and a clinical imperative. *Am J Clin Pathol, 123*, S125–S132.

99. van Werkum, J. W., Harmsze, A. M., Elsenberg, E. H., et al. (2008). The use of the VerifyNow system to monitor antiplatelet therapy: a review of the current evidence. *Platelets, 19*, 479–488.

100. Mueller, T., Dieplinger, B., Poelz, W., et al. (2009). Utility of the PFA-100 instrument and the novel Multiplate analyzer for the assessment of aspirin and clopidogrel effects on platelet function in patients with cardiovascular disease. *Clin Appl Thromb Hemost, 15*, 652–659.

101. McGlasson, D. L., Chen, M., & Fritsma, G. A. (2005). Urinary 11-dehydrothromboxane B$_2$ levels in healthy individuals following a single dose response to two concentrations of aspirin. *J Clin Ligand Assay, 28*, 147–150.

44

Hemostasis and Coagulation Instrumentation

*Debra A. Hoppensteadt and JoAnn Molnar**

OBJECTIVES

After completion of this chapter, the reader will be able to:

1. Describe testing methodologies previously considered as specialized that are now routinely available on coagulation analyzers.
2. Identify testing applications for various coagulation analyzers.
3. Explain the methods of clot detection used by each type of coagulation analyzer presented.
4. List common instrument flags that alert operators to specimen and instrument problems.
5. Describe the advantages and disadvantages of each method of clot detection.
6. Distinguish the characteristics of manual, semiautomated, and automated coagulation analyzers.
7. Identify key performance characteristics that should be evaluated when selecting the most appropriate coagulation analyzer for an individual laboratory setting.
8. Explain the purpose of incorporating platelet function testing analyzers into the routine coagulation laboratory.
9. Identify the role of platelet aggregation in the coagulation laboratory.
10. Describe the methods available for molecular testing in the clinical lab and the analytes that can be measured using these techniques.
11. Develop a model plan of action for objective evaluation of coagulation analyzers for purchase.
12. Explain the main purpose of point-of-care coagulation testing.

CASE STUDY

After studying the material in this chapter, the reader should be able to respond to the following case study:

A 35-year-old white man was admitted to the hospital with abdominal pain and tenderness, malaise, and a low-grade fever. A tentative diagnosis of cholecystitis was made, with possible surgical intervention considered. Pertinent medical history included tonsillectomy at age 6 and appendectomy at age 18 with no abnormal bleeding symptoms noted. The patient reported that he was taking no medications at this time. In anticipation of surgery, routine coagulation studies were ordered. When the specimen arrived in the laboratory, it was centrifuged, and it was noted that the plasma had a whitish, milky appearance. The specimen was processed by an automated analyzer using photo-optical end-point detection methodology, and the following results were obtained:

Test	Results	Reference Interval	Flags
Prothrombin time	16.7 sec	10.9–13.0 sec	Lipemia
Partial thromboplastin time	>150 sec	30.6–35.0 sec	Lipemia
Fibrinogen	245 mg/dL	190–410 mg/dL	Lipemia

Because the laboratory's policy is to retest after all abnormal coagulation results, the prothrombin time and partial thromboplastin time assays were repeated, and similar values were obtained.

1. Should the operator report the test results as shown?
2. What action should the operator take to address the lipemia flagging of this specimen?
3. Would you expect this patient to be at risk for bleeding based on these test results?

*The authors acknowledge the substantial contributions of David L. McGlasson, MS, MLS(ASCP), to Chapter 47 of the fourth edition of this textbook, many of which continue in this edition.

The coagulation laboratory is an ever-changing environment populated by automated analyzers that offer advances in both volume and variety of tests.[1] Hardware and software innovations provide for random access testing with multitest profiles. In the past, the routine coagulation test menu consisted of prothrombin time (PT) with the international normalized ratio (INR), partial thromboplastin time (PTT; also referred to as the activated partial thromboplastin time [APTT]), fibrinogen, thrombin time, and D-dimer assays. More specialized testing was performed in tertiary care institutions or reference laboratories employing medical laboratory scientists with specialized training. With the introduction of new instrumentation and test methodologies, coagulation testing capabilities have expanded significantly, so many formerly "specialized" tests can be performed easily by general medical laboratory staff. New instrumentation has made coagulation testing more standardized, consistent, and cost effective. Automation has not advanced, however, to the point of making coagulation testing foolproof or an exact science. Operators must develop expertise in correlating critical test results with the patient's diagnosis and when monitoring antithrombotic therapy. Good method validation of procedures, cognitive ability, and theoretical understanding of the hemostatic mechanisms are still required to ensure the accuracy and validity of test results so that the physician can make an informed decision about patient care.

HISTORICAL PERSPECTIVE

Visual clot-based testing began in the eighteenth century. The first observation of blood clotting was from blood taken from the vein of a dog that was completely "jellied" in about 7 minutes. In 1780, Hewson measured that human blood clotted in 7 minutes using a basin to collect the blood. With the discovery of the microscope, scientists were able to observe visible clot formation and turbidity.

Many advances took place from 1822 to 1921. These included temperature control during clot formation, passing objects such as a fine needle through the blood to detect resistance, and using different sizes and shapes of glass tubes to view clot formation. In the early 1900s, researchers monitored the length of time it took whole blood to clot in a glass tube while it was being tilted, a precursor to the Lee-White clotting time (1913). These early clotting time tests depended on observing the clot directly (visually) or microscopically.

In 1910, the first clot detection instrument, the "Koaguloviskosimeter," was developed by Kottman. This apparatus measured the change in viscosity of blood as it clotted. This process generated a voltage change that was recorded by a direct readout system. Voltage changes were plotted against time to measure clot formation.

Except for point-of-care testing and whole-blood platelet aggregometry, citrated plasma (usually platelet-poor plasma, plasma with a platelet count of less than 10,000/μL) has now replaced whole blood in coagulation instruments. However, the principle of interval to clot formation lives on.[1,2]

Plasma coagulation testing began in 1920 when Gram added calcium chloride to anticoagulated plasma at 37° C. He measured the increasing viscosity of the blood during fibrin monomer polymerization, a principle used today in thromboelastography (TEG) and sonar clot detection, laying the groundwork for the PT and PTT (Chapter 42).[3]

In these early days and for many years hence, coagulation testing was typically performed by adding plasma and reagents to a glass tube held in a 37° C water bath. Clot formation was determined by visual inspection of the plasma as the tube was tilted, and a stopwatch was used to determine the time to clot formation. This is referred to as the "tilt-tube technique."

Nephelometers, developed in 1920, were the first instruments for coagulation testing. These devices measure 90-degree light dispersion of a colloidal suspension. As plasma clots, a change in light scatter can be measured over time—a principle still in use today. Subsequent twentieth-century developments in clot detectors include manual loops, an electromechanical end-point using a movable electrode (BBL Fibrometer) or a rolling steel ball (Diagnostica Stago ST-4), and photo-optical clot detection (Coag-A-Mate, originally manufactured by General Diagnostics).

The 1950s saw the development of the BBL Fibrometer, an instrument that can still be found in coagulation laboratories, although it is no longer being manufactured. This instrument employed an electromechanical clot detection methodology that allowed laboratories to transition from the manual tilt tube or wire loop method to a more accurate semiautomated testing process.

Current coagulation instruments apply many of the clot detection principles of these early analytical systems. They either "observe" the clot formation (optical, nephelometric devices) or they detect the clot by "feel" (mechanical, viscosity-based devices). Although the detection principles remain the same, current instrumentation has been enhanced to eliminate variations in pipetting and end-point detection. They also allow multiple analyses to be performed simultaneously on a single specimen.[4]

The introduction of new coagulation methodologies as will be described below has further improved testing capabilities in the coagulation laboratory. Refinement of these methodologies has allowed the use of synthetic substrates and measurements of single proenzymes, enzymes, and monoclonal antibodies, which increases the ability to recognize the causes of disorders of hemostasis and thrombosis.[5]

ASSAY END-POINT DETECTION PRINCIPLES

The available coagulometers are automated or semiautomated. Semiautomated coagulometers require the operator to deliver test plasma and reagents manually to the reaction cuvette and limit testing to one or two specimens at a time. These are relatively inexpensive instruments, but their use requires considerable operator expertise.

Fully automated analyzers provide pipetting systems that automatically transfer reagents and test plasma to reaction vessels and measure the end-point without operator intervention (Table 44-1). Multiple specimens can be tested simultaneously.

TABLE 44-1 Levels of Coagulation Automation

Level	Description	Examples
Manual	All reagents and specimens are transferred manually by the operator. Temperature is maintained by a water bath or heat block; external measurement by operator may be required. End-point is determined visually by the operator. Timer is initiated and stopped by the operator.	Tilt tube Wire loop
Semiautomated	All reagents and specimens are transferred manually by the operator. Instrument usually contains a device for maintaining constant 37° C temperature. Analyzer may internally monitor temperature. Instrument has mechanism to initiate timing device automatically on addition of final reagent and mechanism for detecting clot formation and stopping the timer.	Fibrometer STart 4 Cascade M and M-4 BFT-II KC1 and KC4
Automated	All reagents are automatically pipetted by the instrument. Specimens may or may not be automatically pipetted. Analyzer contains monitoring devices and internal mechanism to maintain and monitor constant 37° C temperature throughout testing sequence. Timers are initiated and clot formation is detected automatically.	ACL TOP STA-R Evolution STA Compact and Compact CT Sysmex CA-530, CA-560, CA-620, CA-660, CA-1500, CA-7000 BCS XP CoaLAB

Automated coagulometers are expensive, and laboratory staff require specialized training to operate and maintain them. Regardless of technology, all semiautomated and automated analyzers offer better coagulation testing accuracy and precision than the manual methods.

Instrument methodologies used for coagulation testing are classified into five groups based on the end-point detection principle:

1. Mechanical
2. Photo-optical (turbidometric)
3. Nephelometric
4. Chromogenic (amidolytic)
5. Immunologic

Historically, clot detecting instruments were limited to a single type of end-point detection system such as the mechanical or photo-optical detection. Photo-optical detection in instruments that read at a fixed wavelength between 500 nm and 600 nm has become the most commonly used system in today's clinical instruments. With the advancements in coagulation testing, a second type of instrument was designed to read at 405 nm to perform the chromogenic (colorimetric) assays. With advancements in technology, changes made it possible to automate advanced procedures. However, laboratories were required to purchase multiple analyzers if they wanted to offer the wider range of clot-based and chromogenic testing methods. Since 1990, instrument manufacturers have successfully incorporated multiple detection methods into single analyzers, which allows a laboratory to purchase and train on only one instrument while still providing specialized testing capabilities.[4] Immunologics have recently been incorporated into coagulation laboratories for specific analyte measurements.

Mechanical End-Point Detection

Electromechanical clot detection systems measure a change in conductivity between two metal electrodes in plasma. The BBL Fibrometer was the first semiautomated instrument to be used routinely in the coagulation laboratory. The probe of this instrument has one stationary and one moving electrode. During clotting, the moving electrode enters and leaves the plasma at regular intervals. The current between the electrodes is broken as the moving electrode leaves the plasma. When a clot forms, the fibrin strand conducts current between the electrodes even when the moving electrode exits the solution. The current completes a circuit and stops the timer.[6]

Another mechanical clot detection method employs a magnetic sensor that monitors the movement of a steel ball within the test plasma. Two principles are used for the mechanical clot detection in the routinely used coagulation instruments. In one system, an electromagnetic field detects the oscillation of a steel ball within the plasma-reagent solution.[3] As fibrin strands form, the viscosity starts to increase, slowing the movement (Figure 44-1). When the oscillation decreases to a predefined rate, the timer stops, indicating the clotting time of the plasma. This methodology is found on all Diagnostica Stago analyzers.

In the second system, a steel ball is positioned in an inclined well. The position of the ball is detected by a magnetic sensor. As the well rotates, the ball remains positioned on the incline. When fibrin forms, the ball is swept out of position. As it moves away from the sensor, there is a break in the circuit, which stops the timer. This technology can be found on AMAX and Destiny instruments distributed by Tcoag US, a division of Diagnostica Stago, as well as on the original Hemochron ACT instruments.

Mechanical methods are not affected by icteric or lipemic plasma. Mechanical methods also provide a sensitive end-point able to detect weak clots such as those formed in plasmas with low fibrinogen or a factor XIII deficiency where clots are not stabilized.

Photo-Optical End-Point Detection

Photo-optical (turbidometric) coagulometers detect a change in plasma optical density (OD, light transmittance) during

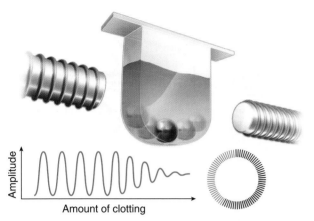

Figure 44-1 Viscosimetric (electromechanical) clot detection in a Diagnostica Stago analyzer. A steel ball oscillates in an arc from one side of the cuvette to the other. Movement is monitored continuously within a magnetic field. As the sample clots, viscosity rises and movement of the steel ball is impeded. Variation in amplitude stops the timer, and the interval is the clotting time.

clotting. Light of a specified wavelength passes through plasma, and its intensity (OD) is recorded by a photodetector. The OD depends on the color and clarity of the sample and is established as the baseline. Formation of fibrin strands causes light to scatter, allowing less light to fall on the photodetector, thus generating an increase in OD. When the OD rises to a predetermined variance from baseline, the timer stops indicating clot formation. Because the baseline OD is subtracted from the final OD, effects of lipemia and icterus are minimized. Many optical systems employ multiple wavelengths that discriminate and filter out the effects of icterus and lipemia. Most of the automated and semiautomated coagulation instruments developed since 1970 use photo-optical clot detection (Figure 44-2).

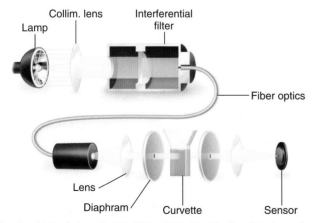

Figure 44-2 Photo-optical (turbidometric) clot detection. Polychromatic light is focused by a collimator and filtered to transmit a selected wavelength. Monochromatic light is transmitted by fiber optics and focused on the reaction cuvette. As fibrin forms, opacity increases and the intensity of light reaching the sensor decreases. *Collim.,* Collimator.

Nephelometric End-Point Detection

Nephelometry is a modification of photo-optical end-point detection in which 90-degree or forward-angle light scatter, rather than OD, is measured. A light-emitting diode produces incident light at approximately 600 nm, and a photodetector detects variations in light scatter at 90 degrees (side scatter) and 180 degrees (forward-angle scatter). As fibrin polymers form, side scatter and forward-angle scatter rise (Figure 44-3).[4,7,8] The timer stops when scatter reaches a predetermined intensity, and the interval is recorded.

Nephelometry can be adapted to dynamic clot measurement. Continuous readings are taken throughout clotting, measuring the entire clotting sequence to completion and producing a clot curve or "signature."

Nephelometry was first applied to immunoassays. As antigen-antibody complexes (immune complexes) precipitate, the resulting turbidity scatters incident light.[9] In reactions in which the immune complexes are known to be too small for detection, the antibodies are first attached to microlatex particles. In coagulation, coagulation factor immunoassays employ specific factor antibodies bound to latex particles. Nephelometry provides a quantitative, but not functional, assay of coagulation factors. Nephelometry is often employed in complex automated coagulometers because it allows for both clot-based assays and immunoassays. Nephelometry-style analyzers can be used to produce high-volume multiple-assay coagulation profiles.

Chromogenic End-Point Detection

Chromogenic (synthetic substrate, amidolytic) methodology employs a synthetic oligopeptide substrate conjugated to a chromophore, usually para-nitroaniline (pNA) (Chapter 42). Chromogenic analysis is a means for measuring specific coagulation factor activity because it exploits the factor's enzymatic (protease) properties. The oligopeptide is a series of amino acids whose sequence matches the natural substrate of the protease being measured.[10-13] Protease cleaves the chromogenic substrate at the site binding the oligopeptide to the pNA, freeing the pNA. Free pNA is yellow; the OD of the solution is proportional to protease activity and is measured by a photodetector at 405 nm (Figure 44-4).

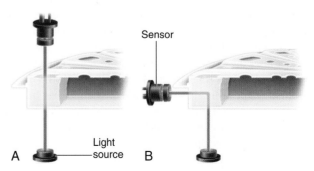

Figure 44-3 Nephelometric clot detection. **A,** Light from below passes through the sample in a cuvette to the detector above. **B,** As fibrin polymerizes, light is deflected and is detected at an angle from the original path.

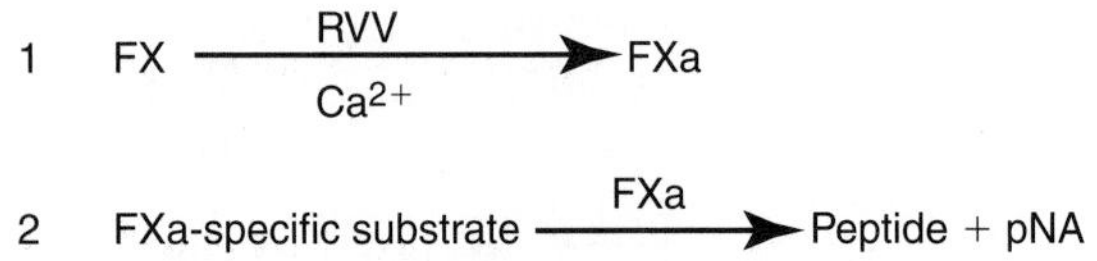

1 FX $\xrightarrow[Ca^{2+}]{RVV}$ FXa

2 FXa-specific substrate $\xrightarrow{FXa}$ Peptide + pNA

Figure 44-4 Method used in the DiaPharma chromogenic factor X assay as an example of a direct chromogenic assay. The method involves two stages. In stage 1, the activator Russell viper venom (RVV) activates factor X (FX) in the presence of calcium to factor Xa (FXa). In stage 2, the generated FXa hydrolyzes the chromogenic substrate S-2765, liberating the chromophore group para-nitroaniline (pNA). Free pNA is yellow in color. The color is then read photometrically at 405 nm. The amount of FXa generated, and thus the intensity of the color, is proportional to the FX activity in the sample over the assay range.

Assays based on a chromogenic end-point (rather than a clot-based assay) are useful to evaluate specimens from patients who have circulating inhibitors or who are on anticoagulant treatment because the inhibitors do not interfere in the chromogenic assay. For clot-based assays, the entire coagulation cascade is part of the test system. For chromogenic assays, the test is isolated to the specific chemical reaction in question.

The activity of coagulation factors and many other enzymes are measured by the chromogenic method directly or indirectly:

- *Direct chromogenic measurement:* OD is proportional to the activity of the substance being measured—for instance, protein C activity measured by a synthetic chromogenic substrate specific for protein C.
- *Indirect chromogenic measurement:* The protein or analyte being measured inhibits a target enzyme. It is the target enzyme that has activity directed toward the synthetic chromogenic substrate. The change in OD is inversely proportional to the concentration or activity of the substance being measured—for example, heparin in the anti-factor Xa assay.

Immunologic Light Absorbance End-Point Detection

Immunologic assays are the newest assays available in coagulation laboratories and are based on antigen-antibody reactions similar to those used in nephelometry as described previously. Latex microparticles are coated with antibodies directed against the selected analyte (antigen). Monochromatic light passes through the suspension of latex microparticles. When the wavelength is greater than the diameter of the particles, only a small amount of light is absorbed.[14] When the coated latex microparticles come into contact with their antigen, however, the antigen attaches to the antibody and forms "bridges," which causes the particles to agglutinate. As the diameter of the agglutinates increases relative to the wavelength of the monochromatic light beam, light is absorbed. The increase in light absorbance is proportional to the size of the agglutinates, which in turn is proportional to the antigen level.

Immunoassay technology became available on coagulometers in the 1990s and is used to measure a growing number of coagulation factors and proteins, such as D-dimer. These assays, which used to take hours or days to perform using traditional antigen-antibody detection methodologies such as enzyme-linked immunosorbent assay or electrophoresis, now can be done in minutes on an automated analyzer.

ADVANCES IN COAGULATION TECHNOLOGY

Significant advances have been made in the capability and flexibility of coagulation instrumentation. Instruments previously required manual pipetting, recording, and calculating the results, which necessitated significant operator expertise, intervention, and time. Current technology allows a "walkaway" environment in which, after specimens and reagents are loaded and the testing sequence is initiated, the operator can move on to perform other tasks.

Clot detection methods have remained consistent, but with the advent of chromogenic- and immunologic-based assays other instrumentation needed to be incorporated into the coagulation laboratory. Multiple methodologies became incorporated into single analyzers to expand their test menu options. From instruments that performed only clot-based assays, clinical laboratory instruments were developed that could perform both clot-based and chromogenic-based assays on one platform.[12,15-17] The next step was the development of a single instrument that could perform clotting and chromogenic and immunologic assays. Additional advances have included improved specimen and reagent storage and processing, increased throughput, and enhanced data management and result traceability.

Improved Accuracy and Precision

In the days of visual methods, coagulation assays were performed in duplicate to reduce the coefficient of variation, which generally exceeded 20%. Semiautomated instruments have improved upon precision, but the requirement for manual pipetting of plasma and reagents continues to necessitate duplicate testing. With the advent of fully automated instruments, precision has improved to the extent that single testing can be performed with confidence, halving material and reagent costs. Coefficients of variation of less than 5%, and even less than 1% for some tests, have been achieved. Initial accuracy and precision are established by in-lab method validation for all instrument and reagent combinations.

Random Access Testing

Automated coagulometers now provide random access testing. Through simple programming, a variety of tests can be run in any order on single or multiple specimens within a testing sequence. Previous automated analyzers were capable of running only one or two assays at a time, so batching was necessary. The disadvantage was that specimens with multiple orders had to be handled multiple times. For current automated analyzers, the ability to run multiple tests is limited only by the number of reagents that can be stored in the analyzer and the instrument's ability to interweave tests requiring different end-point detection methodologies simultaneously, such as clot-based, chromogenic, and immunologic methods. Random access promotes profiling.

Improved Reagent Handling

Reduced Reagent and Specimen Volumes. Automated and semiautomated coagulometers now have the capability to perform tests on smaller sample volumes. Traditionally, PT assays required 0.1 mL of patient plasma and 0.2 mL of thromboplastin/calcium chloride reagent. PTT was measured using 0.1 mL of plasma, 0.1 mL of activated partial thromboplastin, and 0.1 mL of calcium chloride. Current analyzers can perform the same tests using one half or even one quarter the traditional volumes of reagents and patient specimens. This promotes the use of smaller specimen volumes, especially from pediatric patients or those from whom specimens are difficult to draw, and further reduces reagent costs.

Open Reagent Systems

A variety of reagents from numerous distributors are available for coagulation testing, and laboratory directors want the flexibility of selecting the reagents that best suit their needs without being restricted in their choices by the analyzers being used. Recognizing that the ability to select reagents independently of the test system is a high priority, instrument manufacturers have responded by developing systems that provide optimal performance with alternative manufacturer's reagents, provided that the reagents are compatible with the instrument's methodology.

Reagent Tracking

Many automated instruments keep records of reagent lot numbers and expiration dates, which makes it easier for the laboratory to maintain reagent integrity and comply with regulatory requirements. Additional features often include on-board monitoring of reagent volumes with flagging systems to alert the operator when an insufficient volume of reagent is present in relation to the number of specimens programmed to be run. Reagent bar coding supports record keeping because it tracks reagent properties and enables the operator to load coagulometers without stopping specimen analyses.

Improved Specimen Management
Primary Tube Sampling

Many coagulometers encourage the operator to place the primary collection tube on the instrument after centrifugation, which eliminates the need to separate the plasma into a secondary tube. In addition, instruments often accommodate multiple tube sizes. Significant time savings occur as a result of elimination of the extra specimen preparation step, and errors resulting from mislabeling of the aliquot tube are reduced.

Closed-Tube Sampling

Closed-tube sampling has improved the safety and efficiency of coagulation testing. After centrifugation, the tube is placed on the analyzer without removing the blue stopper. The cap is pierced by a needle that aspirates plasma without disturbing the red blood cell layer. Not only does closed-tube sampling save staff time, it also reduces the risk of specimen exposure through aerosols or spillage. Closure also promotes plasma pH stabilization. When closed-tube sampling is used, specimens are visually checked for clots after centrifugation by looking for the presence of fibrin strands. For example, if the assay result is a short clotting time (or the corresponding coagulation tracing available on some instruments) is abnormal then the sample will be rimmed with wooden sticks to determine if a clot is present.

Flagging for Specimen Interferences

Some analyzers monitor the quality of the test specimen for interfering substances or unusual testing characteristics, such as hemolysis, lipemia, bilirubinemia (icterus), abnormal clotting patterns, or results that fall outside the linear range of the reference curve (values above the top point or below the bottom point of the calibration line). Flags warn the operator of potential errors so that problems can be resolved in a timely manner (see later).

Automatic Dilutions

Many instruments perform multiple dilutions on patient specimens, calibrators, or controls, eliminating the need for the operator to perform this task manually and reducing the potential for dilution errors. These conditions can be automatically programmed into the individual test setups on the analyzers being used.

Expanded Computer Capabilities

The computer circuitry of analyzers now incorporates internal data storage and retrieval systems. Hundreds of results can be stored, retrieved, and compiled into cumulative reports. Multiple calibration curves can be stored and accessed. Quality control files can be stored, which eliminates the time-consuming task of manually logging and graphing quality control values. Westgard rules can be applied, and failures are automatically flagged. Some analyzers feature automatic repeat testing when failures occur on the initial run. The quality control files can be reviewed or printed on a regular basis to meet regulatory requirements.

The programming flexibility of modern analyzers has enhanced the laboratory's opportunities to provide expanded test menus. Most advanced analyzers are preprogrammed with several routine test protocols ready for use. Specimen and reagent volumes, incubation times, and other testing parameters do not need to be predetermined by the operator but can be changed easily when necessary. Additional tests can be programmed into the analyzer by the user whenever needed, which allows for enhanced flexibility of the analyzer and reduces the need for laboratories to have multiple instruments.

Instrument interfacing to laboratory information systems and specimen bar coding capabilities have become a priority as facilities of all sizes endeavor to reduce dependence on manual record keeping. Bidirectional interfaces improve efficiency through the ability of the instrument to send specimen bar code information to the laboratory information systems and receive a response listing the tests that have been ordered. This eliminates the need for the operator to program each specimen and test.

Other Automated Features

A few additional features offered by current coagulation analyzers should be mentioned:

Improved flagging capabilities alert the operator when preset criteria have been exceeded (Box 44-1). Flags may indicate instrument malfunction such as cuvette jams, low reagent volume, and temperature errors, or a problem with the results such as values that exceed critical limits, inability to detect an accurate end-point, or values outside of the linear range.

Reflex testing is the automatic ordering of tests based on preset parameters or the results of prior tests. Instruments may make additional dilutions if the initial result is outside of the linearity limits, or supplementary tests can be run automatically if clinically indicated by the initial test result. The first result does not need to wait for review by the operator before follow-up action is taken.

Graphing of clot formation is provided on analyzers such as the ACL TOP (Instrumentation Laboratory). The graph is generated by an algorithm, a formula used to convert raw optical measurements into a clotting time. Besides determining the clotting time, it also smooths the raw data into a visible curve and uses the curve to check for clot integrity. Multiple checks are performed to ensure an accurate and reproducible result. Should the data not meet all of the acceptable criteria, an error flag is generated. The clot curve is examined to troubleshoot potential technical aberrations. The clot formation graph may also be used as a "signature" that correlates with the disease state. Figure 44-5 shows an example of a typical clot curve.

Specimen Quality Set Points

Specimen quality flags, such as the following, can be included on some coagulation instrumentation:

- *Clotted:* will cause falsely shortened clotting times because of premature activation of coagulation factors and platelets that generate FVIIa and thrombin.
- *Lipemia:* may cause falsely prolonged clotting times on OD instruments because of interference with light transmittance.
- *Hemolysis:* may cause falsely shortened clotting times because of premature activation of coagulation factors and platelets that generate FVIIa and thrombin.[18]

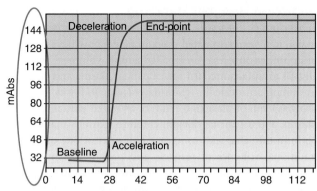

Figure 44-5 Clot signature produced by the ACL TOP analyzer (Instrumentation Laboratory). The clot curve consists of baseline, acceleration phase, deceleration phase, and end-point. The baseline is recorded before clotting occurs. Acceleration reflects clotting and is normally steep because clotting is rapid. The deceleration phase represents the decreasing rate of clot formation as all available fibrinogen converts to fibrin. The end-point is flat and stable, reflecting consumption of all fibrinogen. A key component in evaluating the clot curve is the y-axis, absorbance, which provides the clot interval when it reaches a defined minimum. Absorbance adjusts to compensate for baseline fibrinogen and interferences such as lipemia or icterus. (Image courtesy of Beckman-Coulter, Brea, CA.)

- *Icterus (bilirubinemia):* indicates liver dysfunction that may lead to prolonged clotting times because of inadequate clotting factor production; also may interfere with OD instruments.
- *Abnormal clot formation:* may lead to falsely elevated clotting times because of instrument inability to detect an end-point.
- *No end-point detected:* indicates that the instrument was unable to detect clot formation; the specimen may need to be tested using an alternate methodology.

Instrument Malfunction Flags

Instrument malfunction flags, such as the following, can be included on some instrumentation:
- Temperature error
- Photo-optics error
- Mechanical movement error
- Probe not aspirating
- No end-point detected
- Specimen track error
- Cuvette jams

ADVANTAGES AND DISADVANTAGES OF DETECTION METHODS

Photo-optical end-point detection may be confounded by icterus or lipemia, which erroneously prolongs the clotting time because the change in OD is masked by the color or turbidity of the specimen. Some coagulation instruments may be unable to employ synthetic reagents because they are more translucent than reagents used to optimize the end-point detectors.[19]

All coagulation tests that use clot-based end-points need special considerations when interpreting results. There are many preanalytical variables that affect coagulation function, and the integrity of the entire coagulation cascade is relevant to

---

BOX 44-1 Warning Flags Available on Coagulometers

Instrument Malfunction Flags
Temperature error
Photo-optics error
Mechanical movement error
Probe not aspirating

Sample Quality Flags
Lipemia
Hemolysis
Icterus
Abnormal clot formation
No end-point detected

the final test result. Thus these assays are not highly specific. This would not be a function of chromogenic or immunologic end-point assays that do not rely on the cascade but rather are single analyte specific. Table 44-2 summarizes the advantages and disadvantages of each detection methodology.

POINT-OF-CARE TESTING

Point-of-care coagulation testing has been used since 1966 in the setting of cardiac surgery using the whole-blood activated clotting time (ACT) for heparin monitoring in the operating room (Chapter 43). Today point-of-care testing has expanded beyond the ACT. Most point-of-care instruments are hand-held and permit near-patient testing, bedside testing, self-testing, and testing of infants. The instantaneous turnaround time of results, small sample volume, and portability of the instruments are conveniences appreciated by physicians and patients.

Anticoagulation clinics can be high-volume users of point-of-care testing. Patients on oral anticoagulant therapy with vitamin K antagonists need to be monitored monthly (Chapter 43). Anticoagulation clinics provide this service in the outpatient setting using the prothrombin time/international normalized ratio (PT/INR) test on a point-of-care instrument. Quick test resulting allows for dose adjustments at the same clinic visit, eliminates patient waiting time, and allows time for patient education.

Other point-of-care coagulation tests include the PTT and thrombin clotting time with other assays such as fibrinogen likely available in the future.

Table 44-3 summarizes the variety of FDA-cleared point-of-care instruments and assays available.[20] Various end-point detection techniques are employed. Each instrument uses individual patented technology. The newer versions of these point-of-care instruments include touch screen, wireless transmission of results in real-time, and micro-blood volumes.

Point-of-care coagulation analyzers employ capillary (fingerstick) or anticoagulated whole blood (venipuncture). Typically a 10- to 50-μL sample is transferred to a test cartridge and the cartridge is inserted into the test module. Other instruments

TABLE 44-2 Advantages and Disadvantages of Detection Systems

End-Point Detection Method	Advantages	Disadvantages
Mechanical	No interference from specimen lipemia or bilirubinemia (icterus) Ability to use specimen and reagent volumes as small as 25 μL in some instruments Able to detect weak clots	Reliance on the integrity of the entire coagulation cascade Inability to observe graph of clot formation
Photo-optical	Good precision Increased test menu flexibility and specimen quality information when multiple wavelengths are used Ability to observe graph of clot formation with some instrumentation	Interference from lipemia, hemolysis, bilirubinemia, and increased plasma proteins; this issue has been addressed by some manufacturers with readings from multiple wavelengths May not detect short clotting times owing to long lag phase May not detect small friable clots that are translucent
Chromogenic	Ability to measure proteins that do not clot More specific than clot-based assays Expanded menu options to replace clottable assays affected by preanalytical variables such as heparin, thrombin inhibitors (e.g., argatroban, dabigatran) or FXa inhibitors (e.g., rivaroxaban) Most automated systems now have cost-effective chromogenic capabilities	Limited by wavelength capabilities of some instruments May need large test volume to be cost effective
Immunologic	Ability to automate tests previously available only with manual, time-consuming methods, such as enzyme-linked immunosorbent assays Expanded test menu capabilities	Limited number of automated tests available Higher cost of instruments and reagents May need to have additional instruments available to run routine tests in laboratories without automated coagulation analyzers that have random access capability
Nephelometric	Ability to measure antigen-antibody reactions for proteins present in small concentrations	Limited number of tests available Higher cost of reagents Need for special staff training

TABLE 44-3 A Comparison of Point-of-Care Instruments for Coagulation Testing

Manufacturer/Instrument	Year	Testing	Specimen	Clot Detection	Includes QC
Abbott/iSTAT	2000	PT/INR, PTT, ACT	Whole Blood	Electrogenic	Yes
Alere/INRatio/INRatio2	2003/2008	PT/INR	Fingerstick	Electrochemical, impedance	Yes
Helena/Cascade POC	2000	PT/INR, PTT, ACT, low molecular weight heparin	Whole Blood/Fingerstick	Photo-mechanical	Yes
Helena/Actalyke Mini II	2004	ACT	Whole Blood	2-point electromechanical	Yes
Helena/Actalyke XL	2002	ACT	Whole Blood	2-point electromechanical	Yes
Instrumentation Lab/Gem PCL Plus	2003	PT/INR, PTT, ACT	Whole Blood/Fingerstick	Mechanical end-point monitored optically	Yes
ITC/ProTime Micro Coagulation System	1995/2003/2006	PT/INR	Fingerstick	Mechanical clot	Yes
ITC/Hemochron Signature Elite	2005	PT/INR, PTT, ACT	Whole Blood/Fingerstick	Mechanical clot	Yes
ITC/Hemochron Signature +	2002	PT/INR, PTT, ACT	Whole Blood/Fingerstick	Mechanical clot	Yes
ITC/Hemochron Response	2000	PT/INR, PTT, ACT, TT	Whole Blood/Fingerstick	Mechanical clot	Yes
Medtronics/HMS Plus	1999	ACT, protamine titration	Whole Blood	Mechanical clot	Yes
Medtronics/ACT Plus	2003	ACT	Whole Blood	Mechanical clot	Yes
Roche/CoaguCheck XS PT Test System	2007	PT/INR	Whole Blood/Fingerstick	Amperometric	No
Roche/CoaguCheck XS Plus PT Test System	2007	PT/INR	Whole Blood/Fingerstick	Amperometric	Yes
Roche/CoaguCheck XS Pro PT Test System	2010	PT/INR	Whole Blood/Fingerstick	Amperometric	Yes
CoaguSense PT/INR Monitoring System	2010	PT/INR	Fingerstick	Mechanical	Yes

require nonanticoagulated whole blood, so higher volumes of blood are needed.

Before point-of-care instruments are placed in service, laboratory scientists validate the units against a reference method in a central lab using the plasma-based assays (Chapter 5). Because point-of-care assays and the plasma-based central laboratory assays can show a weak correlation, care must be taken to understand the differences between point-of-care and central lab results and to ensure that clinical decisions are consistent. In the case of the anticoagulation clinic, an INR that exceeds 4.0 or any unexpected INR change is confirmed with a venipuncture blood specimen tested by the plasma-based assay in the central lab.

WHOLE-BLOOD CLOTTING ASSAYS

The *TEG Thromboelastograph Hemostasis Analyzer System* (Haemoscope, Niles, IL, a division of Haemonetics) is an operator-dependent system that provides global hemostasis assessment. The TEG assesses both bleeding and thrombosis risk in patients. TEG analysis is useful in patients with hepatic disease, having liver transplant surgery, undergoing cardiac surgery, obstetrics patients, and trauma patients. Computerization of TEG facilitates its usefulness in intraoperative hemostasis management, where it helps to predict the need for and to monitor clotting factor administration, platelet transfusion, fibrinolytic therapy, and antiplatelet therapy with medications such as aspirin or clopidogrel.

Citrated whole blood is pipetted into a cylindrical cup that oscillates by 4.75°. A stationary pin with a diameter 1 mm smaller than the cup's is suspended by a torsion wire in the cup. Kaolin (or another activator) is added to trigger clotting. As the blood clots, fibrin links the pin to the cup, and viscoelasticity changes are transmitted to the pin. The resulting pin torque generates an electrical signal from the torsion wire that is plotted as a function of time to produce a TEG tracing (Figure 44-6). The tracing is analyzed to determine the speed, strength, and stability of clot formation and the downstream effect of fibrinolysis. Viscoelasticity depends on procoagulant activity, cellular components (red blood cells, white blood cells, and platelets), and fibrinolysis and the interactions between these components. The trace furnishes real-time information about the evolving clot from platelet activation to initial fibrin formation, fibrin cross-linkage, and fibrinolysis.[21] This is the only available whole blood assay that provides a comprehensive, global evaluation of functional hemostasis.

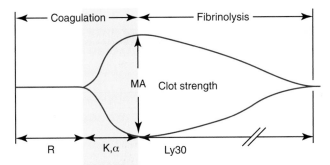

Figure 44-6 Thromboelastograph (TEG) tracing from the TEG 5000 Hemostasis Analyzer System. The TEG® analyzer produces results that document the interaction of platelets with proteins (enzymes, inhibitors, cofactors) of the coagulation pathway and the fibrinolytic system as a whole blood clot forms and eventually breaks down. The R value reflects the initial generation of thrombin and fibrin formation. The K value and angle reflect the rate of initial clot formation mediated by thrombin-activated platelets, fibrin generation, fibrin polymerization, and the developing strength and stabilization of the clot due to platelet function, fibrinogen level, and FXIII. The MA value is an indicator of fibrin-platelet interaction, and overall clot firmness and stability. LY is a kinetic measure of time to and extent of clot lysis. (This image is used with permission of the Haemoscope Corporation, a division of Haemonetics, Niles, IL.)

A newer version is the *ROTEM* (Tem Innovations GmbH, Munich, Germany). The enhancement of the *ROTEM* is that it is not sensitive to vibrations. In the *ROTEM*, a whole-blood sample is placed in a cuvette, and a suspended pin is immersed into the blood. One of various activators is added to trigger clotting. The pin rotates (the cup is stationary), and upon clot formation, the increased tension from fibrin binding the cup to the pin is detected by sensors. *ROTEM* parameters are the same as those described above for TEG.[22] *ROTEM* reagents are available to assess factor and fibrinogen deficiency, platelet function, fibrinolysis, and anticoagulant influence on hemostasis.

PLATELET FUNCTION TESTING

The demand for rapid, cost-effective methods for the evaluation of platelet function has increased due to the need to monitor the efficacy of antiplatelet therapy such as aspirin, clopidogrel, and glycoprotein IIb/IIIa inhibitors used in cardiovascular patients. In addition, preoperative evaluation of platelet function is important in hemostatic management, particularly if the patient has a history of bleeding or if the patient is on antiplatelet medication.[23] Platelet function testing has been a challenge for the clinical laboratory because of the lack of reliable, accurate, and easy-to-perform methods. In addition, specimen procurement for platelet function testing plays an important role in the reliability and accuracy of the test. Platelet function historically has been assessed by the bleeding time test and platelet aggregation assays (Chapter 42). The bleeding time is technically demanding and is highly dependent on the technician performing the test. In addition, it fails

to correlate with intraoperative bleeding risk[24-27] and thus has been discontinued in most institutions. New platelet aggregometers and several new devices are making it easier to assess platelet function.

Platelet Aggregometers

Classical platelet aggregometry using the light transmission principle was developed in the 1960s by Born. This test system measures the increase in light transmission that occurs in direct proportion to platelet aggregation (Figures 42-3 and 42-4) induced by various agonists (e.g., collagen, adenosine diphosphate [ADP], epinephrine) that stimulate different platelet receptors. The test sample is patient platelet-rich plasma (PRP) produced by differential centrifugation of a whole-blood specimen to isolate platelets in plasma with platelet-poor plasma (PPP) as a control. Since its inception, platelet aggregation has been the primary assay to determine alterations in platelet function.

Several newer devices to detect platelet aggregation based on whole-blood impedance, luminescence, and light scatter have since been developed. Table 44-4 compares the newest FDA-cleared platelet aggregometers.

The *Multiplate Analyzer*, also called the *Whole-Blood Multiple Electrode Platelet Aggregometer* (MEA; Dynabyte, Munich, Germany, distributed by DiaPharma Group, West Chester, OH), monitors platelet function by impedance.[28] The multiplate has 5 channels with duplicate electrodes per channel. Small whole blood sample volumes are required (300 μL). The multiplate analysis is based on the principle that upon activation, platelets become sticky and adhere to metal sensor wires (electrodes) (Figure 42-5). The change in electrical resistance between the electrodes is detected and recorded. Three parameters are calculated from each sample: aggregation, area under the curve, and velocity.[28] Tests for the therapeutic efficacy of aspirin, clopidogrel, and glycoprotein IIb/IIIa antagonists using arachidonic acid, ADP, and TRAP, respectively, are pending FDA approval. Other applications for platelet function testing are available on this device.

The *AggRAM* (Helena Laboratories Corporation, Beaumont, TX) is a modular system for platelet aggregation and ristocetin cofactor testing that has advanced laser optics utilizing a laser diode measuring at a wavelength of 650 nm to enhance precision of the measured aggregation tracing.[29] The *AggRAM* has four channels capable of micro-volume testing, customized result reporting, and internal quality control programs.

The *PAP-8E* from BioData Corporation (Horsham, PA) is an eight-channel platelet aggregometer with a touch screen and on-screen procedure templates (Figure 44-7). It has a programmable pipette and an optional bar code scanner. The *PAP-8E* utilizes light transmission aggregometry and requires a low sample volume (225 μL). BioData also has a Platelet Function Centrifuge that has been validated for platelet function testing (Figure 44-8).[30] PRP is prepared in 30 seconds, and PPP can be prepared in 120 seconds. Platelet-free plasma (PFP) is prepared in 180 seconds.

Chrono-Log Corporation (Havertown, PA) has a *Whole Blood–Optical Lumi–Aggregation System*. The Model 700 aggregometer

TABLE 44-4 A Comparison of Platelet Aggregometers

Parameter	Bio/Data Corp.	ChronoLog Corp.	Helena Laboratories
Instrument name (first year sold)	Platelet Aggregation Profiler, Model PAP-8E (2005)	Whole Blood–Optical Lumi–Aggregation System, Model 700-2/700-4 (2006)	AggRAM (2005)
Operational type	Batch, random access	Batch, random access	Batch, random access
Reagent type	Open reagent system, assay kits, reagents, controls, diluents, buffers	Open reagent system, assay kits, reference plasma, controls	Open reagent system
Operates on whole blood or spun plasma	Spun plasma, optional centrifugation with PDQ to obtain PRP in 3 minutes	Whole blood, spun plasma	Spun plasma
Plasma volume/test	225 μL	225 μL	225 μL
Model type	Benchtop	Benchtop	Benchtop
Number of channels	8	2–4	4–8
Time required for maintenance by lab staff	Weekly:15 minutes; monthly: 30 minutes	30 minutes when optical calibration required	Daily: 15 minutes; weekly: 15 minutes; monthly: 1 hour

provides platelet aggregation in whole blood or PRP, while simultaneously measuring secretion (Figure 42-6). This aggregometer uses electrical impedance in whole blood and optical density for measuring luminescence. It can be configured as either a two- or four-channel aggregometer.[31] Either disposable or reusable electrodes can be used for impedance measurements. In addition, Chrono-Log has several other optical and impedance-based instruments. The advantage of whole-blood aggregometry is that it is a more physiological test due to the ability to measure platelet aggregation in the presence of erythrocytes and leukocytes.

Platelet Function Analyzers

The *PFA-100 Platelet Function Analyzer* (Siemens, Deerfield, IL) is a rapid, automated instrument that is sensitive to quantitative and qualitative platelet abnormalities. Test cartridges contain membranes coated with collagen/epinephrine or collagen/ADP to stimulate platelet aggregation. Whole blood is aspirated under controlled flow conditions through a microscopic aperture

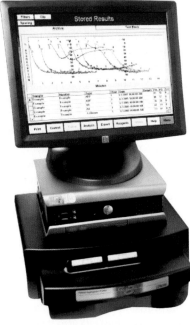

Figure 44-7 PAP-8E from BioData Corporation. An eight-channel aggregometer with a touch screen and a programmable pipet. This instrument requires a sample volume of 225 μL per test and allows for the analysis of routine platelet aggregation testing, measurement of ristocetin cofactor activity, the monitoring of patients with platelet function abnormalities, and the management of antiplatelet therapy. (Photo courtesy of BioData Corp, Horsham, PA.)

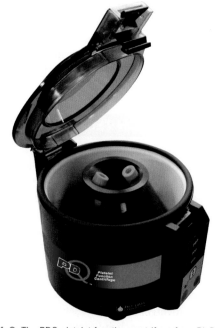

Figure 44-8 The PDQ platelet function centrifuge from BioData Corporation is an optional unit to the PAP-8E. The centrifuge is validated for platelet function testing. The PDQ provides platelet-rich plasma, platelet-poor plasma and platelet-free plasma within 5 minutes. (Photo courtesy of BioData Corp, Horsham, PA.)

in the membrane. The time required for a platelet plug to occlude the aperture is an indication of platelet function.[32,33] The PFA-100 system is successful at detecting von Willebrand disease and the efficacy of aspirin therapy.[33,34]

The Accumetrics *VerifyNow System* (San Diego, CA) is an optical detection system that measures platelet-induced aggregation by microbead agglutination. The system employs a disposable cartridge that contains lyophilized fibrinogen-coated beads and a platelet agonist specific for the test. Whole blood is dispensed from the blood collection tube into the assay device, with no blood handling required by the operator. The instrument provides an aspirin assay using arachidonic acid as the test reagent, a glycoprotein IIb/IIIa inhibitor (abciximab, tirofiban, eptifibatide) assay using thrombin receptor activation peptide (TRAP) as the test reagent, and a P2Y$_{12}$ inhibitor (clopidogrel, prasugrel, ticagrelor) assay using ADP as the test reagent.[35-38]

The Plateletworks platelet function assay is available from Helena Laboratories (Beaumont, TX). This assay kit can be run on any standard impedance cell counter found in the hematology laboratory. Aggregation results are based on a platelet count before (high count) and after (lower count) platelet activation using one of the agonist-filled tubes provided in the kit. Testing requires 1 mL of whole blood for baseline count and 1 mL for each additional agonist-containing reagent tube. Results can be obtained in 2 minutes. The *Plateletworks* platelet function kit can be used for presurgical screening and to monitor antiplatelet therapy.[39]

MOLECULAR COAGULATION TESTING

Molecular testing in the coagulation laboratory is available for patients with thrombophilia (Chapter 39). Molecular testing has become readily available for gene mutations of factor V (FV Leiden) and prothrombin (prothrombin G20210A). Testing for methylene-tetrahydrofolate reductase (MTHFR) is also commonly performed for patients with thrombophilia. However, the clinical utility of MTHFR testing is not clear, and the American College of Medical Genetics and Genomics (ACMG) has recommended that MTHFR testing should not be routinely performed for the workup of patients with thrombophilia.[40]

There are several methods available for the clinical laboratory. Cost and labor usually are considered when evaluating which test system to use in the clinical laboratory. The most common methods used are polymerase chain reaction (PCR)-based assays. PCR is accurate for the detection of both point mutations and single-nucleotide polymorphisms. FV Leiden and prothrombin G20210A, and the MTHFR mutations have been shown to be detectable using this method (Table 44-5). A common method to analyze PCR products is restriction fragment-length polymorphism (RFLP) analysis. However, RFLP analysis is not a high-throughput method and is not suitable for high volume laboratories. Other methods that are PCR-based and some non-PCR-based methods, which no longer require restriction digestion, are also used.[41-43] A popular non-PCR based method is the Invader assay which uses allele-specific hybridization in a high-throughput format.

TABLE 44-5 Molecular Techniques for the Evaluation of Hypercoagulable States

Assay	Accuracy	Throughput	Current Clinical Applications
PCR/RFLP	Good	Limited	Factor V Leiden, prothrombin G20210A, MTHFR
PCR/ARMS	Excellent	Intermediate	Factor V Leiden, prothrombin G20210A, MTHFR
Light cycler	Excellent	Intermediate	Factor V Leiden, prothrombin G20210A, MTHFR
Array technology	Excellent	Very high	Factor V Leiden, prothrombin G20210A, MTHFR
Invader assays	Excellent	Limited	Factor V Leiden, prothrombin G20210A, MTHFR
Ligand-based technologies	Excellent	Very high	Factor V Leiden, prothrombin G20210A, MTHFR

MTHFR, Methylene-tetrahydrofolate reductase.

In order to obtain rapid and reliable results, sequence-specific primers, allele-specific oligonucleotides, hybridization, rapid-cycle PCR using LightCycler instrumentation, and nanochips have become available for molecular testing. The major advantages of molecular testing are the increase in sensitivity and specificity and lack of interference by anticoagulants or inhibitors.[41,42]

Molecular diagnostics in hemophilia and von Willebrand disease are currently limited; however, this is an area that is under development. There is a strong potential for utilization of these assays for the diagnosis and classification of the subgroups of von Willebrand disease. Molecular diagnostics also may have a role in the diagnosis of hemophilia and the mutations involved in both factor VIII and factor IX genes.[42] Testing for these disorders will become more accessible with the rapid decrease in cost of sequencing and availability of high-throughput next generation sequencing technologies.

The role of molecular diagnostics in thrombophilia workups will continue to grow due to the identification of new genetic mutations and polymorphisms in coagulation disorders. The challenge is for the laboratory to determine which tests to offer and their relevance to patient care.

SELECTION OF COAGULATION INSTRUMENTATION

In today's laboratory, more than ever before, cost effectiveness, testing capabilities, and standardization are top priorities. As an increasing number of tests become available, laboratories must determine what tests to incorporate to provide guidance to physicians in diagnosis and treatment. Identification of testing needs based on patient population should be the first step in the process. The decisions regarding which tests are the most appropriate for the clinical situations encountered by each laboratory should be made in conjunction with the medical staff. When that input has been obtained, the laboratory can determine the availability and cost of instruments that would meet those requirements.

An instrument should be matched to the anticipated workload. It may not be necessary to purchase a highly sophisticated analyzer capable of performing a large menu of tests if the setting is a small hospital laboratory ordering very few of the more "esoteric" test options available on the instrument under consideration. A batch analyzer with high throughput may be more appropriate for this situation. The option to send out esoteric tests and/or low-volume tests to a reference lab is always available.

Instrument selection criteria may include, but are not limited to, the following:

- Instrument cost
- Consumables cost
- Service response time
- Reliability and downtime
- Maintenance requirements and time
- Operator ease of use
- Breadth of testing menu
- Ability to add new testing protocols
- Reagent lot to lot variation

- Throughput for high-volume testing
- Laboratory information systems (LIS) interface capabilities
- Footprint (the space the instrument occupies; benchtop or floor model)
- Special requirements (water, power, waste drain)
- Flexibility in using other manufacturers' reagents
- Availability of a training program and continued training support

When the choices have been narrowed based on the most desirable criteria, consideration should be given to additional features. Because no instrument has all the desired features, prioritizing helps the laboratory focus on the capabilities that would be the most advantageous for them. Box 44-2 summarizes several of these specialized features.

CURRENTLY AVAILABLE INSTRUMENTS

A variety of coagulometers address the increasing demand for test volume, random access testing, and test variety. All analyzers perform routine testing quickly and efficiently. The challenge lies in determining which instruments should be considered for a particular laboratory setting and in developing an organized approach for their evaluation. Table 44-6 lists several of the coagulation analyzers currently available, the type of end-point detection offered, and selected specialized features highlighted by the manufacturers in their product information.[44,45]

BOX 44-2 Specialized Coagulometer Features

Random access: A variety of tests can be performed on a single specimen or multiple specimens in any order as determined by the operator.

Primary tube sampling: Plasma is directly aspirated from an open or capped centrifuged primary collection tube on the analyzer.

Cap piercing: Analyzer aspirates plasma from the closed centrifuged primary collection tube.

Bar coding: Reagents and specimens are identified with a bar code; eliminates manual information entry.

Bidirectional laboratory information system (LIS) interface: Analyzer queries the host computer (LIS) to determine which tests have been ordered. Results are returned to the LIS after verification.

Specimen and instrument flagging: Automated alerts indicate problems with specimen integrity or instrument malfunction.

Liquid level sensing: Operator is alerted when there is inadequate specimen or reagent volume. An alert is also given when the instrument fails to aspirate the required sample volume. Volume is verified each time a specimen or reagent is aspirated.

On-board quality control: Instrument stores and organizes quality control data; may include application of Westgard rules for flagging out-of-range results; instrument may transmit quality control data to the LIS.

Stat capabilities: Operator can interrupt a testing sequence to place a stat specimen next in line for testing.

On-board refrigeration of specimens and reagents: Refrigeration maintains the integrity of specimens and reagents throughout testing and allows reagents to be kept in the analyzer for extended periods, which reduces setup time for less frequently performed tests.

On-board specimen storage capacity: Indicates the number of specimens that can be loaded at a time.

Reflex testing: Instrument can be programmed to perform repeat or additional testing under operator-defined circumstances.

Patient data storage: Test results can be stored for future retrieval; clot formation graphs may be included.

Throughput: Number of tests that can be processed within a specified interval, usually the number of tests per hour; depends on test mix and methodologies.

Total testing (dwell) time: Length of time from specimen placement in the analyzer until testing is completed; depends on the type and complexity of the procedure.

Graph of clot formation: Operator can visualize how the clot is formed over time.

TABLE 44-6 Comparison of the Available Coagulation Analyzers

Instrument Name/ Manufacturer	Sample Handling System	FDA-Cleared Clot-Based Tests	FDA-Cleared Chromogenic Tests	FDA-Cleared Immunologic Tests	Methodologies Supported	Number of Different Assays Onboard Simultaneously	Standard Specimen Volume PT/ PTT	Detection of Hemolysis/ Turbidity	Onboard Patient Dilutions
American Labor Lab A.C.M.	Cuvette, semi automated	PT, PTT, fibrinogen, any clot-based assay	None	None	Clot detection, optical	2	Manual pipetting	No/no	No
Diagnostica Stago STA Satellite	Carousel—primary tube	PT, PTT, fibrinogen	Heparin (UFH, LMWH), AT	D-dimer	Clot detection, mechanical; chromogenic; immunologic	80	5 μL	No/no (mechanical method)	Yes
Diagnostica Stago STA-R Evolution	Rack with continuous access	PT, PTT, TT, fibrinogen, reptilase, factors, protein C, protein S, lupus anticoagulant, DRVVT screen and confirm	Heparin (UFH, LMWH), protein C, AT, plasminogen, antiplasmin	D-dimer, VWF, total and free protein S, AT antigen	Clot detection, mechanical; chromogenic; immunologic	200	5 μL	No/no (mechanical method)	Yes
Diagnostica Stago STA Compact, CT	Continuous specimen access—primary tube	PT, PTT, TT, fibrinogen, reptilase, factors, protein C, protein S, lupus anticoagulant, DRVVT	None	None	Clot detection, mechanical	80	5 μL	No/no (mechanical method)	Yes
Diagnostica Stago Start4 Hemostasis	Manual	PT, PTT, TT, fibrinogen, reptilase, factors, protein C, protein S, lupus anticoagulant	None	None	Clot detection	1	25 μL	No/no (mechanical method)	No
Diagnostica Stago STA Compact	Continuous specimen access—primary tube	PT, PTT, TT, fibrinogen, reptilase, factors, protein C, protein S, lupus anticoagulant, DRVVT screen and confirm	Heparin (UFH and LMWH), protein C, AT, plasminogen, antiplasmin	D-dimer, VWF, total and free protein S, AT antigen	Clot detection; chromogenic; immunologic	80	50 μL/5 μL	No/no (mechanical method)	Yes
Diagnostica Stago STA Compact Plus	Continuous specimen access—primary tube	PT, PTT, TT, fibrinogen, reptilase, factors, protein C, protein S, lupus anticoagulant, DRVVT screen and confirm	Heparin (UFH and LMWH), protein C, AT, plasminogen, antiplasmin	D-dimer, VWF, total and free protein S, AT antigen	Clot detection, mechanical; chromogenic; immunologic	80	50 μL/5 μL	No/no (mechanical method)	Yes

Continued

TABLE 44-6 Comparison of the Available Coagulation Analyzers—cont'd

Instrument Name/ Manufacturer	Sample Handling System	FDA-Cleared Clot-Based Tests	FDA-Cleared Chromogenic Tests	FDA-Cleared Immunologic Tests	Methodologies Supported	Number of Different Assays Onboard Simultaneously	Standard Specimen Volume PT/ PTT	Detection of Hemolysis/ Turbidity	Onboard Patient Dilutions
Diagnostica Stago Destiny Plus	Continuous rack loading	Open system: all clottable assays; PT, PTT, fibrinogen, TT, factors, venom time, protein C, protein S, aPCR, lupus screen and confirm	Open system: all chromogenic assays (protein C, AT FIIa and FXa based, heparin anti-FXa, plasminogen)	Open system: all latex immuno-assays (D-dimer)	Clot detection, mechanical and optical (turbidometric); chromogenic; immunologic	10	25 μL/ 10 μL	Not necessary	Yes
Diagnostica Stago Destiny Max	Continuous rack loading	Open system: all clottable assays; PT, PTT, fibrinogen, TT, factors, venom time, protein C, protein S, aPCR, lupus screen and confirm	Open system: all chromogenic assays (protein C, AT FIIa and FXa based, heparin anti-FXa, plasminogen)	Open system: all latex immuno-assays (D-dimer)	Clot detection, mechanical and optical; chromogenic; immunologic	Unlimited	25 μL/ 10 μL	Not necessary	Yes
Helena Laboratories Cascade M-4	Manual	PT, PTT, fibrinogen, TT, factors II, V, VII to XII	None	None	Clot detection, optical, turbidometric	4	100 μL	No/no	No
Helena Laboratories Cascade M	Manual	PT, PTT, fibrinogen, TT, factors II, V, VII to XII	None	None	Clot detection, optical, turbidometric	1	100 μL	No/no	No
Instrumentation Laboratory ACL 300	Continuous rack loading	PT, PTT, fibrinogen, TT, factors, FVIII (with VWF)		D-dimer HS		500		No/no	Yes
Instrumentation Laboratory ACL 500	Continuous rack loading	PT, PTT, fibrinogen, TT, factors, lupus (SCT and DRVVT), protein C, protein S, aPCR-V, FVIII (with VWF)	Heparin anti-FXa, protein C, AT, plasminogen, antiplasmin	D-dimer, D-dimer HS, VWF (activity and antigen), free protein S, FXIII antigen, homocysteine	Clot detection, LED optical; chromogenic; immunologic (turbidometric)	500	PT and PTT: 50 μL; FVIII: 25 μL	No/no	Yes
Instrumentation Laboratory ACL 700	Continuous rack loading	PT, PTT, fibrinogen, TT, factors, lupus (SCT and DRVVT), aPCR-V, protein C, protein S, FVIII (with VWF)	Heparin anti-FXa, protein C, AT, plasminogen, antiplasmin	D-dimer, D-dimer HS, VWF (activity and antigen), free protein S, FXIII antigen, homocysteine	Clot detection, LED optical; chromogenic; immunologic	500	PT and PTT: 50 μL; FVIII: 25 μL	No/no	Yes

TABLE 44-6 Comparison of the Available Coagulation Analyzers—cont'd

Instrument Name/Manufacturer	Sample Handling System	FDA-Cleared Clot-Based Tests	FDA-Cleared Chromogenic Tests	FDA-Cleared Immunologic Tests	Methodologies Supported	Number of Different Assays Onboard Simultaneously	Standard Specimen Volume PT/PTT	Detection of Hemolysis/Turbidity	Onboard Patient Dilutions
Instrumentation Laboratory ACL Elite Series	Tray-primary tubes	PT, PTT, fibrinogen, TT, factors, protein C, protein S, lupus (SCT and DRVVT), aPCR-V	Heparin anti-FXa, protein C, AT, plasminogen, antiplasmin, FVIII	D-dimer, VWF (activity and antigen), free protein S, FXIII antigen, homocysteine	Clot detection, LED optical (nephelometric); chromogenic; immunologic	22	PT and PTT: 60 µL; FVIII: 18 µL	No/no	Yes
Siemens BFT II	Manual	PT, PTT, fibrinogen	None	None	Turbodensitometric	1	50 µL	No/no	No
Siemens CA-1500	10-Tube position sample rack × 5	PT, PTT, fibrinogen, TT, reptilase time, DRVVT factors, DRVVT screen and confirm, FV Leiden, protein C clot, protein S activity	Innovance AT, Berichrom AT, plasminogen, FVIII chromogenic; anti-plasmin, protein C chromogenic, heparin	Innovance D-dimer	Clot detection, optical, turbidometric; chromogenic; immunologic	15	50 µL/5 µL	No/yes	Yes
Siemens CA-7000	Rack	PT, PTT, fibrinogen, TT, reptilase time, factors, DRVVT screen and confirm, FV Leiden, protein C clot, protein S activity	Innovance AT, Berichrom AT, plasminogen, FVIII chromogenic; anti-plasmin, protein C chromogenic, heparin	Innovance D-dimer	Clot detection, optical, turbidometric; chromogenic; immunologic	20	50 µL/5 µL	No/yes	Yes
Siemens BCS XP	10-Tube position sample rack	PT, PTT, fibrinogen, TT, reptilase time, factors, DRVVT screen and confirm, FV Leiden, protein C clot, protein S activity	Innovance AT, Berichrom AT, plasminogen, FVIII chromogenic; anti-plasmin, protein C chromogenic, heparin	Innovance D-dimer	Clot detection, optical (xenon flasher lamp); chromogenic; immunologic	>100	50 µL/20 µL min. 100 µL (includes dead volume/50 µL	Yes/no	Yes
Siemens CA-600	10-Tube position sample rack	PT, PTT, fibrinogen, TT, reptilase time, protein C clot, factor assays	Innovance AT, Berichrom AT, protein C chromogenic, heparin	Innovance D-dimer	Clot detection, optical; turbidometric; chromogenic; immunologic	5	50 µL/5 µL	No/yes	Yes
LABiTech GmbH CoaData 2004	Semiautomated manual pipette-auto start	PT, PTT	None	None	Clot detection, optical; turbodensitometric	1	50 µL	No/no	No

aPCR, Activated protein C resistance; AT, antithrombin; DRVVT, dilute Russell viper venom test; F, factor; LMWH, low molecular weight heparin; HS, high sensitivity; PT, prothrombin time; PTT, partial thromboplastin time; SCT, silica clotting test; TT, thrombin clotting time; UFH, unfractionated heparin; VWF, von Willebrand factor.

SUMMARY

- Advanced technology used in semiautomated and automated analyzers has greatly improved coagulation testing accuracy and precision.
- End-point detection methodologies employed by modern coagulation analyzers include mechanical, photo-optical, nephelometric, chromogenic, and immunologic methods.
- Advances in end-point detection methodologies have greatly expanded the testing capabilities available in the routine coagulation laboratory.
- Markedly improved instrument precision and reduced reagent volume requirements have led to substantial cost savings in coagulation testing.
- Instrument manufacturers have incorporated many features that have enhanced efficiency, safety, and diagnostic capabilities in hemostasis testing.
- Coagulation analyzer flagging alert functions warn the operator when sample or instrument conditions exist that might lead to invalid test results so that appropriate actions can be taken to ensure test accuracy.

- Each method of end-point detection has advantages and disadvantages that must be recognized and understood to ensure the validity of test results.
- Several methods to evaluate platelet function are available for both general platelet function testing and antiplatelet drug monitoring.
- The role of molecular diagnostics will continue to grow to identify new mutations and polymorphisms associated with bleeding and clotting disorders.
- Coagulation testing has been incorporated into the arena of point-of-care testing primarily to enhance the patient's and physician's ability to monitor oral anticoagulant therapy.
- A systematic approach to the evaluation and selection of a new coagulation analyzer should be developed and followed to determine the best instrument for a specific laboratory setting.

Now that you have completed this chapter, go back and read again the case study at the beginning and respond to the questions presented.

REVIEW QUESTIONS

Answers can be found in the Appendix.

1. The photo-optical method of end-point detection can be described as:
   a. Measurement of a color-producing chromophore at a wavelength of 405 nm
   b. Measurement of the change in OD of a test solution as a result of fibrin formation
   c. Application of an electromagnetic field to the test cuvette to detect the decreased motion of an iron ball within the cuvette
   d. Measurement of the turbidity of a test solution resulting from the formation of antigen-antibody complexes using latex particles

2. Modern coagulation analyzers have greatly enhanced the ability to perform coagulation testing as a result of which of the following?
   a. Maintenance of a level of accuracy and precision similar to that of manual methods
   b. Increase in reagent volume capabilities to improve sensitivity
   c. Automatic adjustment of results for interfering substances
   d. Improved flagging capabilities to identify problems in sample quality or instrument function

3. Which of the following is considered to be an advantage of the mechanical end-point detection methodology?
   a. It is not affected by lipemia in the test sample
   b. It has the ability to provide a graph of clot formation
   c. It can incorporate multiple wavelengths into a single testing sequence
   d. It can measure proteins that do not have fibrin formation as the end-point

4. Which of the following methods use the principle of changes in light scatter or transmission to detect the end-point of the reaction?
   a. Immunologic, mechanical, photo-optical
   b. Photo-optical, nephelometric, mechanical
   c. Photo-optical, nephelometric, immunologic
   d. Chromogenic, immunologic, mechanical

5. Which of the following is a feature of semiautomated coagulation testing analyzers?
   a. The temperature is maintained externally by a heat block or water bath
   b. Reagents and samples usually are added manually by the operator
   c. Timers are automatically started as soon as the analyzer adds reagents to the test cuvette
   d. The end-point must be detected by the operator

6. When a sample has been flagged as being icteric by an automated coagulation analyzer, which method would be most susceptible to erroneous results because of the interfering substance?
   a. Mechanical clot detection
   b. Immunologic antigen-antibody reaction detection
   c. Photo-optical clot detection
   d. Chromogenic end-point detection

7. Platelet function testing has been incorporated into the routine coagulation laboratory in recent years as a result of:
   a. Increased use of drugs that stimulate platelet production in patients receiving chemotherapy
   b. The convenience of being able to do the testing on the same instrument that performs the coagulation testing
   c. Increased therapeutic use of aspirin in the treatment of heart disease
   d. Increased outpatient/outreach testing that prevents the laboratory from having access to patients to do bleeding time tests

8. All of the following are performance characteristics to consider in the selection of a coagulation analyzer *except:*
   a. Location of the manufacturer's home office
   b. Instrument footprint
   c. Ease of use for the operator
   d. Variety of tests the instrument can perform

9. The PFA-100 measures platelet function by:
   a. Detecting the change in blood flow pressure along a small tube when a clot impairs blood flow
   b. Detecting the aggregation of latex beads coated with platelet activators
   c. Graphing the transmittance of light through platelet-rich plasma over time after addition of platelet activators
   d. Detecting the time it takes for a clot to form as blood flows through a small aperture in a tube coated with platelet activators

10. Point-of-care coagulation testing is used mainly:
    a. To monitor patients receiving oral anticoagulant therapy
    b. To monitor patients taking platelet inhibitors such as aspirin
    c. To provide a baseline for all subsequent patient test result comparisons when the patient starts any kind of anticoagulant therapy
    d. To monitor obstetric patients at risk of fetal loss

REFERENCES

1. McGlinchey, K. (2009). Sophistication in coagulation platforms. *Adv Med Lab Prof, 20,* 20-21.
2. Owen, C. A. (2002). History of blood coagulation. *JAMA, 87,* 1051-1052.
3. Bender, G. T. (1998). *Principles of Chemical Instrumentation: STA-R Operator's Manual* (pp.119-124). Parsippany, NJ: Diagnostica Stago.
4. Johns, C. S. (2007). Coagulation instrumentation. In Rodak, B. G., Fritsma, G. A., & Doig, K., (Eds.), *Hematology: clinical principles and applications.* (3rd ed., pp. 714–728). St Louis, Saunders.
5. Gram, J., & Jespersen, J. (1999). Introduction to laboratory assays in haemostasis and thrombosis. In Jepersen, J., Bertina, R. M., & Haverkate, F., (Eds.), *Laboratory Techniques in Thrombosis—a manual.* (2nd ed., pp. 1–7). Boston: Kluwer Academic Publishers.
6. *BBL FibroSystem Manual.* (1992). Sparks, MD: BD Diagnostics Systems.
7. Thomas, L. C., & Sochynsky, C. L. (1999). Multiple measuring modes of coagulation instruments. *Clin Hemost Rev, 13,* 8.
8. *Behring Nephelometer 100 Operator's manual.* (1995). Deerfield, IL: Dade Behring, Inc.
9. Schueter, A., & Olson, J. D. (2002). Coagulation instrumentation: the hospital laboratory to the home. *Adv Lab Methods Haematol,* 316–336.
10. *DiaPharma factor X kit.* (2005). West Chester, Ohio: DiaPharma Group (package insert).
11. Abildgaard, U., Lie, M., & Odegard, O. R. (1976). A simple amidolytic method for the determination of functionally active antithrombin III. *Scand J Clin Lab Invest. 36,* 109-115.
12. Walenga, J., Fareed, J., & Bermes, E. W. Jr. (1983). Automated instrumentation and the laboratory diagnosis of bleeding and thrombotic disorders. *Semin Thromb Hemost, 9,* 172-193.
13. Fareed, J., Messmore, H. L., Walenga, J. M., & Bermes, E. W. Jr. (1983). Diagnostic efficacy of newer synthetic-substrates methods for assessing coagulation variables: a critical overview. *Clin Chem, 29,* 225-236.
14. STA Liatest D-Di. Parsippany, NJ, 2005, Diagnostica Stago (package insert).
15. Fareed, J., Bermes, E. W. Jr, & Walenga, J. (1984). Automation in coagulation testing. *J Clin Lab Auto, 4,* 415-425.
16. Fareed, J., & Walenga, J. (1983). Current trends in hemostatic testing. *Semin Thromb Hemost, 9,* 379-391.
17. Fareed, J., Bick, R. L., Squillaci, G., Walenga, J. M., & Bermes, E. W. Jr. (1983). Molecular markers of hemostatic disorders: implications in the diagnosis and therapeutic management of thrombotic and bleeding disorders. *Clin Chem, 29,* 1641-1658.
18. Laga, A. C., Cheves, T. A., & Sweeney, J. D. (2006). The effect of specimen hemolysis on coagulation test results. *Am J Clin Pathol, 126,* 748-756.
19. Allen, R., & Sheridan, B. (1999, Jan). Service above all. *CAP Today* (pp. 39-60).
20. Dabkowski, B. (2012, May). Coagulation analyzers—point of care, self monitoring. *CAP Today* (pp. 20-30).
21. Hobson, A. R., Agarwala, R. A., Swallow, K. D., et al. (2006). Thromboelastography: Current clinical applications and its potential role in interventional cardiology. *Platelets, 17,* 509-518.
22. ROTEM *delta* Manual. (2011). Tem Innovations GmbH.
23. Harrison, P., & Mumford, A. (2009). Screening tests of platelet function: update on their appropriate uses for diagnostic testing. *Semin Thromb Hemost, 35,* 150–157.
24. Rodgers, R. P. C., & Levin, J. (1990). A critical reappraisal of the bleeding time. *Semin Thromb Hemost, 16,* 1–20.
25. Lind, D. E. (1991). The bleeding time does not predict surgical bleeding. *Blood, 77,* 2547–2552.

26. Gerwitz, A. S., Miller, M. L., & Keys, T. F. (1996). The clinical usefulness of the preoperative bleeding time. *Arch Pathol Lab Med, 120,* 353–356.

27. Peterson, P., Hayes, T. C., Arkin, C. F., et al. (1998). The preoperative bleeding time test lacks clinical benefit: College of American Pathologists' and American Society of Clinical Pathologists' position article. *Arch Surg, 133,* 134–139.

28. *Multiplate 5.0 analyzer product information.* (2013). West Chester, OH: DiaPharma Corporation.

29. *AggRAM product information.* (2005). Beaumont, TX: Helena Laboratories.

30. *PAP-8E product information.* (2005). Horsham, PA: BioData Corporation.

31. *Model 700 aggregometer product information.* (2006). Havertown, PA; Chrono-Log Corporation.

32. Kundu, S. K., Heilmann, E. F., Sio, R., et al. (1996). Characterization of an in vitro platelet function analyzer, PFA-100. *Clin Appl Thromb Hemost, 2,* 241–249.

33. Franchini, M. (2005). The platelet function analyzer (PFA-100): an update on its clinical use. *Clin Lab, 51,* 367–372.

34. Favaloro, E. J. (2008). Clinical utility of the PFA-100. *Semin Thromb Hemost, 34,* 709–733.

35. McKee, S. A., Sane, D. C., & Deliargyris, E. N. (2002). Aspirin resistance in cardiovascular disease: A review of prevalence, mechanisms, and clinical significance. *Thromb Haemost, 88,* 711–715.

36. Lordkipanidze, M., Pharand, C., Schampaert, E., et al. (2007). A comparison of six major platelet function tests to determine the prevalence of aspirin resistance in patients with stable coronary artery disease. *Eur Heart J, 28,* 1702–1708.

37. Dyskiewicz-Korpanty, D. M., Kim, A., Durner, J. D., et al. (2007). Comparison of a rapid platelet function assay—VerifyNow Aspirin—for the detection of aspirin resistance. *Thromb Res, 120,* 485–488.

38. McGlasson, D. L., & Fritsma, G. A. (2008). Comparison of four laboratory methods to assess aspirin sensitivity. *Blood Coagul Fibrinolysis, 19,* 120–123.

39. Hussein, H. M., Emiru, T., Georgiadis, A. L., & Qureshi, A. I. (2013). Assessment of platelet inhibition by point-of-care testing in neuroendovascular procedures. *Am J Neuroradiol, 34,* 700–706.

40. Hickey, S. E., Curry, C. J., & Toriello, H. V. (2013). ACMG Practice Guideline: lack of evidence for MTHFR polymorphism testing. *Genet Med, 15,* 153-156.

41. Nagy, P. L., Schrijver, I., & Zehnder, J. L. (2004). Molecular diagnosis of hypercoagulable states. *Lab Med, 35,* 214-221.

42. Ballestros, E. (2006). Molecular diagnostics in coagulation. In Coleman, W. B., & Tsongalis, J., (Eds.), *Molecular Diagnostics: For the Clinical Laboratorian.* (2nd ed., pp. 311–320). New York: Humana Press.

43. Perrotta, P. L., & Svensson, A. M. (2009). Molecular diagnostics in hemostatic disorders. *Clin Lab Med, 29,* 367-90.

44. Dabkowski, B. (2013, Jan). Coagulation analyzers. CAP Today (pp. 14–24).

45. Dabkowski, B. (2009, Jan). Coagulation analyzers offering speed, full menus and more. *CAP Today* (pp. 19–29).

Pediatric and Geriatric Hematology and Hemostasis

45

Linda H. Goossen

OUTLINE

OBJECTIVES

After completion of this chapter, the reader will be able to:

1. Describe the major differences in reference intervals for the complete blood count, reticulocyte count, and nucleated red blood cells (NRBCs) in preterm newborns, full-term newborns, infants, children, adults, and elderly adults.
2. Explain the cause of physiologic anemia of infancy and the time frame in which it is expected.
3. Describe normal RBC morphology in neonates.
4. Compare the RBC survival in preterm and full-term infants with that in adults.
5. Recognize and list factors affecting sample collection that can have an impact on the interpretation of hematology values in newborns.
6. Compare and contrast the morphology of lymphocytes in children and in adults, and indicate reasons for differences.
7. Describe the general association between age and hemoglobin levels in the elderly.
8. Explain the clinical significance of anemia in the elderly.
9. Name the two most common anemias seen in the elderly and their common causes in this age group.
10. List other anemias affecting elderly individuals.
11. Compare the frequency of acute lymphoblastic leukemias and chronic lymphocytic leukemias in children and the elderly.
12. Compare the hemostatic systems of newborns, children, adults, and the elderly, including the risk of bleeding and thrombosis.
13. Name hematologic malignancies that are more common in the elderly than in other age groups.

CASE STUDY

After studying this chapter, the reader should be able to respond to the following case study:

A full-term newborn infant in no apparent distress had a complete blood count (CBC) performed as part of a panel of testing for infants born to mothers who received no prenatal care. Results were as follows:

	Patient Results	Reference Intervals
WBCs (×10⁹/L)	18.0	9.0–37.0
RBCs (×10¹²/L)	5.28	4.10–6.10
HGB (g/dL)	18.5	16.5–21.5
HCT (%)	55.5	48–68
MCV (fL)	105.1	95–125

WBC differential: 50% neutrophils and 50% lymphocytes
RBC morphology: Macrocytic with slight to moderate polychromasia. There were 7 NRBCs/100 WBCs.

1. Are the results for hemoglobin and hematocrit within the reference intervals expected for a newborn?
2. What is the significance of the elevated MCV, NRBCs, and polychromasia?
3. Comment on the WBC and differential count.

Hematologic values are fairly stable throughout adult life, but significant differences exist in the pediatric and, to some extent, in the geriatric populations. This chapter focuses on the more significant differences.

PEDIATRIC HEMATOLOGY AND HEMOSTASIS

Children are not merely "small adults." The newborn infant, older child, and adult exhibit profound hematologic differences from one another. Because children mature at different rates, it is inappropriate to use adult reference intervals for the assessment of pediatric blood values. Historically, pediatric reference intervals were inferentially established from adult data because of the limitations in attaining analyzable data. Pediatric procedures required large blood draws and tedious methodologies and lacked standardization. The implementation of child-friendly phlebotomy techniques and micropediatric procedures has revolutionized laboratory testing. Pediatric hematology has emerged as a specialized science with age-specific reference intervals that correlate with the hematopoietic, immunologic, and chemical changes in a developing child.

Dramatic changes occur in the blood and bone marrow of the newborn infant during the first hours and days after birth, and there are rapid fluctuations in the quantities of all hematologic elements. Significant hematologic differences are seen between term and preterm infants and among newborns, infants, young children, and older children. This chapter reviews neonatal hematopoiesis, which is discussed in detail in Chapter 7, as a prerequisite to understanding the changes in pediatric hematologic reference intervals, morphologic features, and age-specific physiology.

Prenatal Hematopoiesis

Hematopoiesis, the formation and development of blood cells from hematopoietic stem cells, begins in the first weeks of embryonic development and proceeds systematically through three phases of development: mesoblastic (yolk sac), hepatic (liver), and myeloid (bone marrow). The first cells produced in the developing embryo are primitive erythroblasts formed in the yolk sac. These cells appear megaloblastic and circulate as large nucleated cells, synthesizing embryonic hemoglobins. A second wave of yolk-sac derived erythroid progenitor cells, termed *burst forming units–erythroid* (BFU-E), appear around four weeks and are thought to seed the fetal liver.[1-6]

By the second month of gestation, hematopoiesis ceases in the yolk sac, and the liver becomes the center for hematopoiesis, reaching its peak activity during the third and fourth gestational months. Leukocytes of each cell type systematically make their appearance. In week 9 of gestation, lymphocytes can be detected in the region of the thymus. They are subsequently found in the spleen and lymph nodes. During the fourth and fifth gestational months, the bone marrow emerges as a major site of blood cell production, and it becomes the primary site by birth (Chapter 7).[1-6]

Hematopoiesis of the Newborn

Hematopoietically active bone marrow is referred to as *red marrow,* as opposed to inactive *yellow* (fatty) *marrow.* At the time of birth, the bone marrow is fully active and almost completely cellular, with all hematopoietic cell lineages undergoing cellular differentiation and amplification. In addition to the mature cells in fetal blood, there are significant numbers of circulating progenitor cells in cord blood.[7,8]

In a full-term infant, hepatic hematopoiesis has ceased except in widely scattered small foci that become inactive soon after birth.[1-6] Postembryonic extramedullary hematopoiesis is abnormal in a full-term infant. In a premature infant, foci of hematopoiesis are frequently seen in the liver and occasionally observed in the spleen, lymph nodes, or thymus.[1-10]

Pediatric Developmental Stages

Pediatric hematologic values change markedly in the first weeks and months of life, and many variables influence the interpretation of what might be considered healthy at the time of birth. Thus it is important to provide age-appropriate pediatric hematology reference intervals that extend from neonatal life through adolescence. The pediatric population can be categorized with reference to three different developmental stages: the neonatal period, which represents the first 4 weeks of life; infancy, which incorporates the first year of life; and childhood, which spans age 1 to puberty (age 8 to 12 years).

Preterm, low-birth-weight infants are more apt to develop health problems than are other newborns. Since the 1970s, the rising quality of medical care in neonatal intensive care units in the United States and other industrialized countries has improved markedly the survival of smaller infants born at younger gestational ages with less mature hematopoietic systems.

Gestational Age and Birth Weight

Hematologic values obtained from full-term infants generally do not apply to preterm infants, and laboratory values for low-birth-weight preterm infants differ from values for extremely low-birth-weight infants. A full-term infant is defined as an infant who has completed 37 to 42 weeks of gestation. Infants born before 37 weeks' gestation are referred to as *premature* or *preterm,* whereas infants delivered after 42 weeks are considered *postterm.*[11,12] Infants can be subcategorized further by birth weight as (1) appropriate size for gestational age; (2) small for gestational age, including low-birth-weight infants (2500 g or less); (3) very low-birth-weight infants (1500 g or less); (4) extremely low-birth-weight micropreemies (1000 g or less); and (5) large for gestational age (more than 4000 g).[11,12]

Red Blood Cell Values at Birth

Neonatal hematologic values are affected by the gestational age of the infant, birth weight, the age in hours after delivery, the presence of illness, and the level of support required. Other important variables to be considered when evaluating laboratory data include site of sampling and technique (capillary versus venous puncture, warm or unwarmed extremity), timing of sampling, and conditions such as the course of labor and the treatment of the umbilical vessels, and maternal drug use.[1,2,13] The presence of fetal hemoglobin (Hb F), bilirubin, and lipids in newborns can also interfere with hematology laboratory testing.[14-17] As with all laboratory testing, each laboratory should establish reference intervals based on its instrumentation, methods, and patient population (Chapter 5).

Red Blood Cell Count

Refer to the inside front cover of this book for red blood cell (RBC) reference intervals. The RBC count increases during the first 24 hours of life, remains at this plateau for about 2 weeks, and then slowly declines. This "polycythemia" of the newborn[18] may be explained by in utero hypoxia, which becomes more pronounced as the fetus grows. Hypoxia, the trigger for increased secretion of erythropoietin, stimulates erythropoiesis.[19] At birth, the physiologic environment changes, and the fetus makes the transition from its placenta-dependent oxygenation to the increased tissue oxygenation by the lungs. This increased oxygen tension suppresses erythropoietin production, which is followed by a decrease in RBC and hemoglobin production. Studies show that erythropoietin levels before birth are equal to or greater than adult levels with a gradual drop to near zero a few weeks after birth.[20-24] This decline corresponds to the physiologic anemia seen at 5 to 8 weeks of life, with the RBCs reaching their lowest count at 7 weeks of age and hemoglobin reaching its lowest concentration at 9 weeks of age.[19]

Erythrocyte Morphology of the Neonate. Early normoblasts are megaloblastic, hypochromic, and irregularly shaped. During hepatic hematopoiesis, normoblasts are smaller than the megaloblasts of the yolk sac but are still macrocytic. Erythrocytes remain macrocytic from the first 11 weeks of gestation until day 5 of postnatal life (Figure 45-1).[1,2,13,20,21,24,25]

The macrocytic RBC morphology gradually changes to the characteristic normocytic, normochromic morphology. Orthochromic normoblasts frequently are observed in the full-term infant on the first day of life but disappear within postnatal days 3 to 5. These nucleated RBCs (NRBCs) may persist longer than a week in immature infants. The average number of NRBCs ranges from 3 to 10 per 100 white blood cells (WBCs) in a healthy full-term infant to 25 NRBCs per 100 WBCs in a premature infant. The presence of NRBCs for more than 5 days suggests hemolysis, hypoxic stress, or acute infection.[1,2,6,13,20-24]

The erythrocytes of newborns show additional morphologic differences. The number of biconcave discs relative to stomatocytes is reduced in neonates (43% discs, 40% stomatocytes) compared with adults (78% discs, 18% stomatocytes).[26] In addition, increased numbers of pitted cells, burr cells, spherocytes, and other abnormally shaped erythrocytes are seen in neonates. The number of these "dysmorphic" cells is even higher in premature infants. Zipursky and colleagues found 40% discs, 30% stomatocytes, and 27% additional poikilocytes in premature infants.[1,26]

Reticulocyte Count

An apparent reticulocytosis exists during gestation, decreasing from 90% reticulocytes at 12 weeks' gestation to 15% at 6 months' gestation and ultimately to 4% to 6% at birth. Reticulocytosis persists for about 3 days after birth and then declines abruptly to 0.8% reticulocytes on postnatal days 4 to 7. At 2 months, the number of reticulocytes increases slightly, followed by a slight decline from 3 months to 2 years, when adult levels of 0.5% to 2.5% are attained.[1,2,6,13,20-24] The reticulocyte count of premature infants is typically higher than that of term infants; however, the count can vary dramatically, depending on the extent of illness in the newborn. Significant polychromasia seen on a Wright-stained blood film is indicative of postnatal reticulocytosis (Figure 45-2).

Hemoglobin

Full-Term Infants. Hemoglobin synthesis results from an orderly evolution of a series of embryonic, fetal, and adult hemoglobins. At birth Hb F constitutes 60% to 90% of the total hemoglobin.[27] Hb F declines from 90% to 95% at 30 weeks' gestation to approximately 7% at 12 weeks after birth and stabilizes at 3.2 ± 2.1% at 16 to 20 weeks after birth.[28] The switch

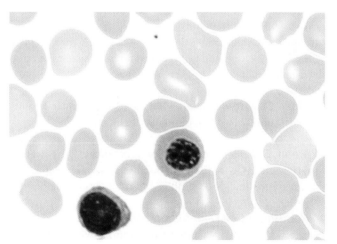

Figure 45-1 Peripheral blood from a healthy newborn demonstrating a normal lymphocyte, macrocytes, polychromasia, and one nucleated red blood cell (×1000).

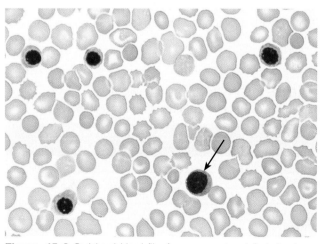

Figure 45-2 Peripheral blood film from a premature infant showing a normal lymphocyte (arrow), four nucleated red blood cells, and increased polychromasia (×500).

from Hb F to Hb A is genetically controlled and determined by gestational age; it does not appear to be influenced by the age at which birth occurs.[24,29] Chapter 10 provides an in-depth discussion of the ontogeny, structure, and types of hemoglobin.

The concentration of hemoglobin fluctuates dramatically in the weeks and months after birth as a result of physiologic changes, and various factors must be considered when analyzing pediatric hematologic values. The site of sampling, gestational age, and time interval between delivery and clamping of the umbilical cord can influence the hemoglobin level in newborn infants.[1,2,6,9-11] In addition, there are significant differences between capillary and venous blood hemoglobin levels. Capillary samples in newborns generally have a higher hemoglobin concentration than venous samples, which can be attributed to circulatory factors.[14,20-22,24,25] Racial differences must also be considered when evaluating hemoglobin levels in children. Black children have hemoglobin levels averaging 0.5 g/dL lower than those in white children.[30]

The reference interval for hemoglobin for a full-term infant at birth is 16.5 to 21.5 g/dL; levels less than 14 g/dL are considered abnormal.[2,20,21] The average hemoglobin value for a preterm infant who is small for gestational age is 17.1 g/dL, lower than that for a full-term infant; hemoglobin values less than 13.7 g/dL are considered abnormal in preterm infants.[20,21]

Physiologic Anemia of the Neonate.   The hemoglobin concentration of term infants decreases during the first 5 to 8 weeks of life, a condition known as *physiologic anemia of infancy*. Infants born prematurely also experience a decrease in hemoglobin concentration, which is termed *physiologic anemia of prematurity*.[2,32-34] Along with a decrease in hemoglobin, there is a reduction in the number of RBCs, a decrease in the reticulocyte percentages (Table 45-1), and undetectable levels of erythropoietin associated with the transition from the placenta to the lungs as a source of oxygen. When the hemoglobin concentration decreases to approximately 11 g/dL, erythropoietic activity increases until it reaches its adult levels by 14 years of age.[18,35-40] Also contributing to the physiologic anemia is the shortened life span of the fetal RBC. Studies of chromium-labeled newborn RBCs estimate a survival time of 60 to 70 days, with correction for the elution rate of chromium from

newborn cells.[1] The life span of RBCs in premature infants is about 35 to 50 days.[1] The more immature the infant, the greater the degree of reduction.[1,21,24] The reasons for the shortened life span of the erythrocytes are unclear. This physiologic anemia is not known to be associated with any abnormalities in the infant.

The hemoglobin levels of premature infants are typically 1 g/dL or more below the values of full-term infants. Thereafter, a gradual recovery occurs, which results in values approximating those of healthy full-term infants by about 1 year of age.[15,18,23,35,36,40] Very low-birth-weight infants (less than 1500 g) show a progressive decline in hemoglobin, RBC count, mean cell volume (MCV), mean cell hemoglobin (MCH), and mean cell hemoglobin concentration (MCHC) and have a slower recovery than other preterm and term infants.

Hematocrit

The average capillary hematocrit (HCT) at birth for healthy full-term infants is 61% (reference interval, 48% to 68%).[1,2,24] Frequently, newborns with increased hematocrits, especially values greater than 65%, experience hyperviscosity of the blood. This can cause problems in producing a high-quality peripheral blood film.

The hematocrit usually increases approximately 5% during the first 48 postnatal hours; this is followed by a slow linear decline to 46% to 62% at 2 weeks and 32% to 40% between the second and fourth months.[1,2,25] Adult values of 47% for males and 42% for females are achieved during adolescence. Very low-birth-weight preterm infants are frequently anemic at birth (Table 45-1). Many require transfusions or erythropoietin injections or both.

Red Blood Cell Indices

The RBC indices and RBC distribution width (RDW) provide one means for assessing the type of anemia (Chapter 19).

Mean Cell Volume.   The erythrocytes of newborn infants are markedly macrocytic at birth. The average MCV for full-term infants is 119 ± 9.4 fL; however, a sharp decrease occurs during the first 24 hours of life.[1,2] The MCV continues to decrease to 90 ± 12 fL in 3 to 4 months.[2,18,37] The more premature the infant, the higher the MCV. A newborn with an MCV of less than 94 fL should be evaluated for α-thalassemia or iron deficiency.[1,41]

Mean Cell Hemoglobin.   MCH is 30 to 42 pg in healthy neonates and 27 to 41 pg in premature infants.[18,37]

Mean Cell Hemoglobin Concentration.   The average MCHC is the same for full-term infants, premature infants, and adults: approximately 33 g/dL.

Red Blood Cell Distribution Width.   The red blood cell distribution width is elevated in newborns, with a reference interval of 14.2% to 17.8% the first 30 days of life. After that it gradually decreases and reaches the adult reference interval by 6 months of age.[25]

TABLE 45-1 Hematologic Values for Very Low-Birth-Weight Infants During the First 6 Weeks of Life

Hematologic Value	AGE OF INFANT (DAYS)			
	3	12–14	24–26	40–42
Hemoglobin (g/dL)	15.6	14.4	12.4	10.6
Hematocrit (%)	47	44	39	33
Red blood cells (×10^{12}/L)	4.2	4.1	3.8	3.4
Reticulocytes (%)	7.1	1.7	1.5	1.8
Platelets (×10^9/L)	203.5	318	338	357
White blood cells (×10^9/L)	9.5	12.3	10.4	9.1

Modified from Obladen M, Diepold K, Maier RF, et al: Venous and arterial hematologic profiles of very low birth weight infants, *Pediatrics* 106:707-711, 2000.

TABLE 45-2 Leukocyte Count Reference Intervals by Age*

Age	NEUTROPHILS† Mean	NEUTROPHILS† Range	NEUTROPHILS† %	LYMPHOCYTES Mean	LYMPHOCYTES Range	LYMPHOCYTES %	EOSINOPHILS Mean	EOSINOPHILS %	MONOCYTES Mean	MONOCYTES %	TOTAL WBC COUNT Mean	TOTAL WBC COUNT Range
Birth	4.0	2.0–6.0	—	4.2	2.0–7.3	—	0.1	—	0.6	—	—‡	—
12 hr	11.0	7.8–14.5	—	4.2	2.0–7.3	—	0.1	—	0.6	—	—	—
24 hr	9.0	7.0–12.0	—	4.2	2.0–7.3	—	0.1	—	0.6	—	—	—
1–4 wk	3.6	1.8–5.4	—	5.6	2.9–9.1	—	0.2	—	0.7	—	—	—
6 mo	3.8	1.0–8.5	32	7.3	4.0–13.5	61	0.3	3	0.6	5	11.9	6.0–17.5
1 yr	3.5	1.5–8.5	31	7.0	4.0–10.5	61	0.3	3	0.6	5	11.4	6.0–17.5
2 yr	3.5	1.5–8.5	33	6.3	3.0–9.5	59	0.3	3	0.5	5	10.6	6.0–17.0
4 yr	3.8	1.5–8.5	42	4.5	2.0–8.0	50	0.3	3	0.5	5	9.1	5.5–15.5
6 yr	4.3	1.5–8.0	51	3.5	1.5–7.0	42	0.2	3	0.4	5	8.5	5.0–14.5
8 yr	4.4	1.5–8.0	53	3.3	1.5–6.8	39	0.2	2	0.4	4	8.3	4.5–13.5
10 yr	4.4	1.8–8.0	54	3.1	1.5–6.5	38	0.2	2	0.4	4	8.1	4.5–13.5
16 yr	4.4	1.8–8.0	57	2.8	1.2–5.2	35	0.2	3	0.4	5	7.8	4.5–13.0

Data from Cairo MS, Bracho F: White blood cells. In Rudolph CD, Rudolph AM, Hostetter MK, et al, editors: *Rudolph's pediatrics*, ed 21, New York, 2003, McGraw-Hill, p 1548.
*Numbers of leukocytes are $\times 10^9$/L (or thousands per microliter), ranges are estimates of 95% confidence limits, and percentages refer to differential counts.
†Neutrophils include band cells at all ages and a small number of metamyelocytes and myelocytes in the first few days of life. WBC, white blood cell.
‡Dashes indicate insufficient data for a reliable estimate.

Anemia in Infants and Children

Nutritional deficiencies in infants and children can result in iron deficiency anemia and, rarely, in megaloblastic anemia (Chapters 20 and 21), particularly in low-birth-weight and premature infants. These anemias are associated with abnormal psychomotor development; however, they can easily be treated with dietary fortification.[42-46]

Iron Deficiency Anemia.

Iron deficiency anemia is the most common pediatric hematologic disorder and the most frequent cause of anemia in childhood.[47] The occurrence of iron deficiency anemia in infants has decreased in the United States due to iron fortification of infant formula and increased rates of breastfeeding.[48] However, the prevalence is still 2% in toddlers 1 to 2 years of age and 3% in children 3 to 5 years of age[49] and is related to early introduction and excessive intake of whole cow's milk.[42,50] Chapter 20 provides an in-depth discussion of iron deficiency anemia.

Ancillary Tests for Anemia in Infants and Children.

The differential diagnosis of anemia in infants and children relies on a variety of ancillary tests. The reference intervals for a number of these tests differ from those for adults. Haptoglobin levels are so low as to be undetectable in neonates, which makes it unreliable as a marker of infant hemolysis.[51] Transferrin levels are also lower in neonates, increasing rapidly after birth and reaching adult levels at 6 months.[51] Both serum ferritin and serum iron are high at birth, rise during the first month, drop to their lowest level between 6 months and 4 years of age, and remain low throughout childhood.[52-54] Consideration of these differences is important when interpreting hematology laboratory results for infants and children.

White Blood Cell Values in the Newborn

Fluctuations in the number of WBCs are common at all ages but are greatest in infants (Table 45-2). Leukocytosis is typical at birth for full-term and preterm infants, with a wide reference interval.[18] There is an excess of segmented neutrophils and bands, and an occasional metamyelocyte, with no evidence of disease. The absolute neutrophil count rises within the first 8 to 12 hours following birth and then declines by 12 hours to a constant level.[2,18,55,56]

Neutrophilic Leukocytes

Refer to Table 45-2 and the inside front cover for the leukocyte reference intervals for healthy full-term infants. Term and premature infants show a greater absolute neutrophil count than that found in older children, who characteristically maintain a predominance of lymphocytes. Band forms are also higher for the first 3 to 4 days after birth (Table 45-3).

TABLE 45-3 Neutrophil and Band Counts for Newborns During the First 2 Days of Life*

Age	Absolute Neutrophil Count ($\times 10^9$/L)	Absolute Band Count ($\times 10^9$/L)
Birth	3.5–6.0	1.3
12 hr	8.0–15.0	1.3
24 hr	7.0–13.0	1.3
36 hr	5.0–9.0	0.7
48 hr	3.5–5.2	0.7

Modified from Luchtman-Jones L, Wilson DB: The blood and hematopoietic system. In Martin RJ, Fanaroff AA, Walsh MC, editors: *Fanaroff and Martin's neonatal-perinatal medicine*, ed 9, Philadelphia, 2011, Elsevier Mosby, p 1325.
*Reference intervals were obtained from the assessment of 3100 separate white blood cell counts obtained from 965 infants; 513 counts were from infants considered to be completely healthy at the time the count was obtained and for the preceding and subsequent 48 hours. There was no difference in the reference intervals when values were stratified by infant birth weight or gestational age.

Newborn females have absolute neutrophil counts averaging 2000 cells/μL higher than those of males; neonates whose mothers have undergone labor have higher counts than neonates delivered by cesarean section with no preceding maternal labor.[55,56] There is some evidence that absolute neutrophil counts are lower in healthy black children than in white children.[57,58]

Premature Infants. At birth, preterm infants exhibit a left shift, with promyelocytes and myelocytes frequently observed. The trend to lymphocyte predominance occurs later than in full-term infants. The neutrophil counts in premature infants are similar to or slightly lower than the neutrophil counts in full-term infants during the first 5 days of life; however, the count gradually declines to 2.5×10^9/L (1.1 to 6.0 × 10^9/L) at 4 weeks.[59] There is no significant difference in the absolute neutrophil count of infants by birth weight or gestational age; however, very low-birth-weight infants have a significantly lower limit (1.0×10^9/L) compared with larger infants.[59-61]

Neutropenia. Neutropenia is defined as a reduction in the number of circulating neutrophils to less than 1.5×10^9/L. Neutropenia accompanied by bands and metamyelocytes is often associated with infection, particularly in preterm neonates. Neutropenia represents a decrease in neutrophil production or an increase in consumption.[62]

Neutrophilia. Neutrophilia refers to an increase in the absolute number of neutrophils to greater than 8.0×10^9/L. Morphologic changes associated with infection include Döhle bodies, vacuoles, and toxic granulation.[63]

Eosinophils and Basophils

The percentages of eosinophils and basophils remain consistent throughout infancy and childhood. Refer to the inside front cover of this book for reference intervals.

Lymphocytes

Lymphocytes constitute about 30% of the leukocytes at birth and increase to 60% at 4 to 6 months. They decrease to 50% by 4 years, to 40% by 6 years, and to 30% by 8 years.[13,20] Benign immature B cells (hematogones), although predominantly found in the bone marrow, can sometimes be seen in the peripheral blood of newborns. These lymphocytes are primarily mid-stage B cells[64,65] and are frequently referred to as "baby" or "kiddie" lymphocytes. They vary in diameter from 10 to 20 μm, have scant cytoplasm and condensed but homogeneous nuclear chromatin, and may have small, indistinct nucleoli (Figures 45-3 and 45-4.[66-68] Although these lymphocytes may be similar in appearance to the malignant cells seen in childhood acute lymphoblastic leukemia (ALL), these benign cells lack the asynchronous or aberrant antigen expression seen in ALL and thus can be differentiated from the lymphocytes of infant ALL by immunophenotyping (Chapter 32).[69,70]

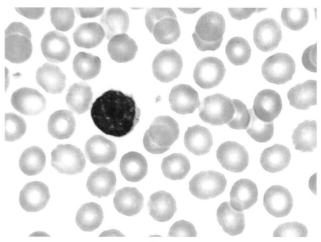

Figure 45-3 Peripheral blood film from a healthy newborn showing a benign lymphocyte (×1000).

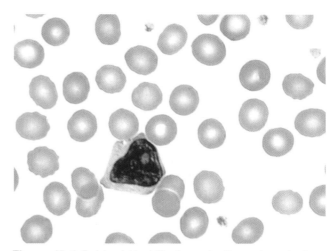

Figure 45-4 Peripheral blood film from a healthy newborn showing a benign lymphocyte with visible nucleoli (×1000).

Monocytes

The mean monocyte count of neonates is higher than adult values. At birth the average proportion of monocytes is 6%. During infancy and childhood, an average of 5% is maintained, except in the second and third weeks, when the proportion increases to around 9%. The count reaches adult levels at 3 to 5 months.[25]

Neonatal Hematologic Response to Infection. The immune response of newborns is considered "immature," with decreased responsiveness to agonists. This distinct immune response is postulated to be related to the demands of the fetal environment and the need to avoid response to maternal antigens.[71] Sepsis in neonates is a common cause of morbidity, particularly in premature and low-birth-weight infants.[72-76] Defective B cell response against polysaccharide agents, as well as abnormal cytokine release by neutrophils and monocytes, has been implicated.[77-80] Because of the transient neutrophilia that occurs during the first 24 hours after birth, followed by a rapid decline, the neutrophil count is not a satisfactory index of infection in the newborn.[81] Newborns with bacterial infections frequently have neutrophil counts within or below the reference interval with a shift to the left. Thus many practitioners depend on the band count and its derived immature-to-total neutrophil ratio as an indicator of sepsis in neonates,[82] although CD64 index, C-reactive protein, and procalcitonin levels have been suggested as more sensitive markers of sepsis in infants and children.[82,83]

Platelet Values in the Newborn

The platelet count usually ranges from 150 to 400 $\times 10^9$/L for full-term and preterm infants, comparable to adult values (Table 45-4).[84,85] Thrombocytopenia of fewer than 100 $\times 10^9$ platelets/L may be seen in high-risk infants with sepsis or respiratory distress and neonates with trisomy syndromes, and investigation should be undertaken for underlying pathology.[86,87] Platelets of a newborn infant show great variation in size and shape. Neonatal thrombocytopenia is discussed in Chapter 40.

Neonatal Hemostasis

The physiology of the hemostatic system in infants and children is different from that in adults (Chapter 37). The vitamin K–dependent coagulation factors (factors II, VII, IX, and X) are at about 30% of adult values at birth; they reach adult values after 2 to 6 months, although the mean values remain lower in children than in adults. Levels of factor XI, factor XII, prekallikrein, and high-molecular-weight kininogen are between 35% and 55% of adult values at birth, reaching adult values after 4 to 6 months. In contrast, the levels of fibrinogen, factor VIII, and von Willebrand factor are similar to adult values throughout childhood.[88,89] Factor V decreases during childhood, with lower levels during the teen years as compared with adults. The physiologic anticoagulants and inhibitors of coagulation (protein C, protein S, and antithrombin) and a disintegrin and metalloproteinase with a thrombospondin type 1 motif, member 13 (ADAMTS-13) that cleaves ultra-long von Willebrand factor multimers are reduced to about 30% to 40% at birth. Antithrombin reaches adult values by 3 months, whereas protein C does not reach adult levels until after 6 months.[88] In the fibrinolytic system, levels of plasminogen and α_2-antiplasmin are similar to adult levels at birth, whereas levels of tissue plasminogen activator are low and levels of plasminogen activator inhibitor 1 (PAI-1) are increased (Table 45-5).[89] The hemostatic components are not only changing in concentration over the first few weeks to months of life, but their values are also dependent on the gestational age of the child, and premature infants have different values at birth than term infants (Table 45-6).

Bleeding and Thrombosis

The reference intervals for the prothrombin time and partial thromboplastin time for neonates extend higher than those for adults; however, these values reach adult reference intervals by 6 months (Table 45-5). The risk of bleeding is not increased in a healthy newborn despite the decreased levels of the vitamin K–dependent coagulation factors, which is primarily related to the reduced levels of the physiologic anticoagulants protein C and protein S.[90]

The risk of thrombosis is considerably less in neonates and children than in adults. However, two age-related peaks in frequency occur, the first in the neonatal period and the second in postpuberty adolescence.[91] Central venous catheters, cancer, and chemotherapy are the most common risk factors in both of these groups.[92-95] Hemorrhagic and thrombotic disorders are discussed in Chapters 38 and 39, respectively.

GERIATRIC HEMATOLOGY AND HEMOSTASIS

In 2010, there were 40 million people in the United States aged 65 and over, accounting for 13% of the population. The older population in 2030 is projected to be twice as large as in 2000, growing from 35 million to 75 million and representing 20% of the total U.S. population.[96] The life expectancy and quality of life of the elderly have improved dramatically in recent decades. Americans are living longer than ever before. Life expectancies at both age 65 and age 85 have increased. Under current conditions, people who survive to age 65 can expect to live an average of 19.2 more years—almost 5 years longer than people aged 65 in 1960. In 2009, the life expectancy of people who survived to age 85 was 7 years for women and 5.9 years for men.[96]

Disease and disabilities are not a function of age, although age is a risk factor for many diseases. However, with the increase in the aging population, the incidence of age-related health conditions also is likely to increase. Thus the care of the elderly has become a growing concern as the life expectancy of the population continues to increase.

The elderly can be roughly divided into three age categories: the "young-old," aged 65 to 74; the "old-old," aged 74 to 84; and the "very old," aged 85 and older.[97] The 85 and older age group is the fastest-growing segment of the elderly population.

Geriatric medicine is a rapidly growing branch of medicine. The use of inappropriate reference intervals may lead to unnecessary testing and investigations or, more importantly, result in failure to detect a critical underlying disease. The growing concern about the interpretation of hematologic data in reference to age is due partly to the tremendous heterogeneity in the aging process and partly to the difficulty in separating the effects of age from the effects of occult diseases that accompany aging.[98]

TABLE 45-4 Platelet Count Reference Intervals for Full-Term and Preterm Infants

Age	Platelet Count ($\times 10^9$/L; mean $\pm$ 1 SD)
Preterm infants, 27–31 wk	275 $\pm$ 60
Preterm infants, 32–36 wk	290 $\pm$ 70
Term infants	310 $\pm$ 68
Healthy child/adult	300 $\pm$ 50

Adapted from Oski FA, Naiman JL: Normal blood values in the newborn period. In *Hematologic problems in the newborn*, Philadelphia, 1982, WB Saunders. *SD*, Standard deviation.

TABLE 45-5 Reference Intervals for Coagulation Tests in the Healthy Full-Term Infant During the First 6 Months of Life

	Day 1	Day 5	Day 30	Day 90	Day 180	Adult
Screening Tests						
PT (Sec)	10.1–15.9	10.0–15.3	10.0–14.3	10.0–14.2	10.7–13.9	10.8–13.9
PT (INR)	0.53–1.62	0.53–1.48	0.53–1.26	0.53–1.26	0.61–1.17	0.64–1.17
PTT (Sec)	31.3–54.3	25.4–59.8	32.0–55.2	29.0–50.1	28.1–42.9	26.6–40.3
TCT (Sec)	19.0–28.3	18.0–29.2	19.4–29.2	20.5–29.7	19.8–31.2	19.7–30.3
Factor Assays						
Fibrinogen (mg/dL)	167–399	162–462	162–378	150–379	150–387	156–400
II (%)	26–70	33–93	34–102	45–105	60–116	70–146
V (%)	34–108	45–145	62–134	48–132	55–127	62–150
VII (%)	28–104	35–143	42–138	39–143	47–127	67–143
VIII (%)	50–178	50–154	50–157	50–125	50–109	50–149
VWF (%)	50–287	50–254	50–246	50–206	50–197	50–158
IX (%)	15–91	15–91	21–81	21–113	36–136	55–163
X (%)	12–68	19–79	31–87	35–107	38–118	70–152
XI (%)	10–66	23–87	27–79	41–97	49–134	67–127
XII (%)	13–93	11–83	17–81	25–109	39–115	52–164
PK (Fletcher, %)	18–69	20–76	23–91	41–105	56–116	62–162
HMWK (Fitzgerald, %)	6–102	16–132	33–121	30–146	36–128	50–136
XIIIa (%)	27–131	44–144	39–147	36–172	46–162	55–155
XIIIb (%)	30–122	32–180	39–173	48–184	20–170	57–137
Control Proteins						
Antithrombin (%)	39–87	41–93	48–108	73–121	84–124	79–131
α_2-Macroglobulin (%)	95–183	98–198	106–194	126–226	149–233	52–120
C_1 Inhibitor (%)	36–108	60–120	47–131	71–159	89–193	71–131
α_1-Antitrypsin (%)	49–137	49–129	36–88	42–102	47–107	55–131
Heparin Cofactor II (%)	10–93	0–96	10–87	10–146	50–190	66–126
Protein C (%)	17–53	20–64	21–65	28–80	37–81	64–128
Protein S (%)	12–60	22–78	33–93	54–118	55–119	60–124
Fibrinolytic Proteins						
Plasminogen (%)	125–265	141–293	126–270	174–322	221–381	248–424
Tissue Plasminogen Activator (ng/mL)	5.0–18.9	4.0–10.0	1.0–6.0	1.0–5.0	1.0–6.0	1.4–8.4
α_2-Antiplasmin (%)	55–115	70–130	76–124	76–140	83–139	68–136
Plasminogen Activator Inhibitor 1 (%)	20–151	0–81	0–88	10–153	60–130	0–110

From Andrew M, Paes B, Johnston M: Development of the hemostatic system in the neonate and young infant, *Am J Pediatr Hematol Oncol* 12(1):95-104, 1990.
HMWK, High-molecular-weight kininogen; *INR,* international normalized ratio; *PK,* prekallikrein; *PT,* prothrombin time; *PTT,* partial thromboplastin time; *TCT,* thrombin clotting time; *VWF,* von Willebrand factor.

This section focuses on hematologic changes in the elderly and discusses hematologic reference intervals for various geriatric age groups as well as hematopathologic conditions seen in the geriatric population.

Aging and Hematopoiesis

The aging process is associated with the functional decline of several organ systems, such as cardiovascular, renal, musculoskeletal, pulmonary, and bone marrow reserve. Certain cells lose their ability to divide (e.g., nervous tissue, muscles), whereas others, such as bone marrow and the gastrointestinal mucosa, remain mitotic. Marrow cellularity begins at 80% to 100% in infancy and decreases to about 50% after 30 years, followed by

a decline to 30% after age 65.[99-101] These changes may be due to a reduction in the volume of cancellous (trabecular or spongy) bone, along with an increase in fat, rather than to a decrease in hematopoietic tissue.[101] Telomere shortening, which determines the number of divisions a cell undergoes, has not been definitively correlated to age-related hematopoietic stem cell exhaustion in humans[102]; however, it is speculated to be associated with hematopoietic stem cell differentiation.[103]

Assessment of Hematologic Parameters in Healthy Elderly Adults

In 1930, Wintrobe published hematologic reference intervals that are still in use today. These were derived from healthy

TABLE 45-6　Reference Intervals for Coagulation Tests in the Healthy Premature Infant of 30 to 36 Weeks' Gestation During the First 6 Months of Life

	Day 1	Day 5	Day 30	Day 90	Day 180	Adult
Screening Tests						
PT (Sec)	10.6–16.2	10.0–15.3	10.0–13.6	10.0–14.6	10.0–15.0	10.8–13.9
PT (INR)	0.61–1.70	0.53–1.48	0.53–1.11	0.53–1.32	0.50–1.48	0.64–1.17
PTT (Sec)	27.5–79.4	26.9–74.1	26.9–62.5	28.3–50.7	27.2–53.3	26.6–40.3
TCT (Sec)	19.2–30.4	18.8–29.4	18.8–29.9	19.4–30.8	18.9–31.5	19.7–30.3
Factor Assays						
Fibrinogen (mg/dL)	150–373	160–418	150–414	150–352	150–360	156–400
II (%)	20–77	29–85	36–95	30–106	51–123	70–146
V (%)	41–144	46–154	48–156	59–139	58–146	62–150
VII (%)	21–113	30–138	21–145	31–143	47–151	67–143
VIII (%)	50–213	53–205	50–199	58–188	50–187	50–149
VWF (%)	78–210	72–219	66–216	75–184	54–158	50–158
IX (%)	19–65	14–74	13–80	25–93	50–120	55–163
X (%)	11–71	19–83	20–92	35–99	35–119	70–152
XI (%)	8–52	13–69	15–71	25–93	46–110	67–127
XII (%)	10–66	9–69	11–75	15–107	22–142	52–164
PK (Fletcher, %)	9–57	25–75	31–87	37–121	40–116	62–162
HMWK (Fitzgerald, %)	9–89	24–100	16–112	32–124	41–125	50–136
XIIIa (%)	32–108	57–145	39–147	71–155	65–161	55–155
XIIIb (%)	35–127	68–158	57–157	75–167	67–163	57–137

From Andrew M, Paes B, Milner R, et al: Development of the human coagulation system in the healthy premature infant, *Blood* 72(5):1651-1657, 1988.
HMWK, High-molecular-weight kininogen; *INR,* international normalized ratio; *PK,* prekallikrein; *PT,* prothrombin time; *PTT,* partial thromboplastin time; *TCT,* thrombin clotting time; *VWF,* von Willebrand factor.

young adults, mostly medical students and nurses. What constitutes "normal" for elderly patients is a matter of considerable debate. There is controversy concerning the assignment of geriatric age-specific reference intervals, especially because aging is often accompanied by physiologic changes, and the prevalence of disease increases markedly. The baseline values for the elderly are the same reference intervals used for healthy adults. Proper interpretation of hematologic data, however, requires a complete understanding of the association between disease and older age. The next section highlights hematologic reference intervals for healthy elderly individuals with and without evidence of underlying disease.

Red Blood Cells

Most RBC parameters (e.g., RBC count, indices, and RDW) for healthy elderly do not show significant deviations from those for younger adults. There is a gradual decline in hemoglobin starting at middle age, with the mean level decreasing by about 1 g/dL during the sixth through eighth decades.[104] Men older than 60 years have average hemoglobin levels of 12.4 to 15.3 g/dL, whereas men aged 96 to 106 years have a mean hemoglobin level of 12.4 g/dL.[105,106] The hemoglobin levels in women may increase slightly with age or remain unchanged. Elderly women have hemoglobin concentrations ranging from 11.7 to 13.8 g/dL. Males characteristically have higher hemoglobin levels than females, owing to the stimulating effect of androgens on erythropoiesis; however, the difference narrows as androgen levels decrease in elderly men and estrogen levels

decrease in older women.[107] Characteristically, the lowest hemoglobin levels are found in the oldest patients (Table 45-7).

Leukocytes

In the absence of any underlying pathologic condition, there are no statistically significant differences between the total leukocyte count and WBC differential for the young-old and old-old and those for middle-aged adults.[106] Some investigators, however, have reported a lower leukocyte count—3.1 to 8.5 × 10⁹/L—in individuals older than age 65, owing primarily to a decrease in the lymphocyte count. Others have reported a decrease in the lymphocyte and the neutrophil counts in women, but not in men, older than age 50.[107]

Immune Response in the Elderly.　Infectious diseases are an important cause of morbidity and mortality in the elderly. Aged adults are more susceptible to infection, take longer to recover from infection, and are often less responsive to vaccination.[108] The adverse changes that occur in the function of the immune system with age are called *immunosenescence.*[109] Although all components of immunity are affected, T cells appear to be the most susceptible.[110] The thymus disappears by early middle age, and adults must then depend on their T-lymphocyte pool in the secondary tissues to mediate T cell–dependent immune responses.[111,112] The number of naive T cells decreases in the elderly, which increases the dependence on memory T cells. T cells of the elderly have impaired responsiveness to mitogens and antigens as a result of decreased

TABLE 45-7 Hematologic Values in Ambulatory Healthy Adults*

	84–98 yr	30–50 yr
Red Blood Cells (×10^{12}/L)		
Males	4.8 ± 0.4	5.1 ± 0.2
Females	4.5 ± 0.3	4.6 ± 0.3
Hemoglobin (g/dL)		
Males	14.8 ± 1.1	15.6 ± 0.7
Females	13.6 ± 1.0	14.0 ± 0.8
Hematocrit (%)		
Males	43.8 ± 3.3	45.3 ± 2.2
Females	40.7 ± 2.9	41.6 ± 2.3
Mean Cell Volume (fL)		
Males	91.3 ± 5.4	87.8 ± 2.8
Females	90.5 ± 4.1	90.5 ± 5.0
Mean Cell Hemoglobin (pg)		
Males	31.0 ± 2.0	30.1 ± 1.6
Females	30.2 ± 1.2	30.3 ± 2.1
Mean Cell Hemoglobin Concentration (g/dL)		
Males	33.7 ± 1.5	34.2 ± 1.5
Females	33.4 ± 1.2	33.5 ± 1.5
White Blood Cells (×10^9/L)		
	7.6 ± 0.5	8.8 ± 0.4
Platelets (×10^9/L)		
	277 ± 21	361 ± 38
Neutrophils (×10^9/L)		
	4.5 ± 0.3	5.9 ± 0.3
Lymphocytes (×10^9/L)		
	1.9 ± 0.3	1.9 ± 0.8

Adapted from Zauber NP, Zauber AG: Hematologic data of healthy very old people, *JAMA* 357:2181-2184, 1987; and Chatta GS, Lipschitz DA: Aging of the hematopoietic system. In Hazzard WR, Blass JP, Halter JB, et al: *Principles of geriatric medicine and gerontology*, ed 5, New York, 2003, McGraw-Hill, p 767.
*Mean values ± 1 standard deviation.

expression of costimulator CD28. There is also an alteration of T cell signaling with aging.[113-115] B-lymphocyte function depends on T cell interaction. Thus the decreased ability to generate antibody responses, especially to primary antigens, may be the result of T cell changes rather than intrinsic defects in B lymphocytes.[111,112,116,117]

Many neutrophil functions are decreased in the elderly, including chemotaxis, phagocytosis of microorganisms, and generation of superoxide. Studies indicate that these defects may be associated with changes to the cell membrane and/or to receptor signaling.[108]

Monocytes and Macrophages

The aging process does not significantly affect the number of monocytes. Information on the effects of aging on monocyte and macrophage function is limited and often conflicting.[108] Recent studies provide evidence for defects in the toll-like receptor (TLR) function in monocytes and macrophages in older individuals.[108] The TLRs play a crucial role in the immune response.[118]

Platelets

The platelet count does not significantly change with age. There have been reports of increased levels of β-thromboglobulin and platelet factor 4 in the α-granules and increased platelet phospholipid content.[119,120] Thrombocytopenia may be drug induced or secondary to marrow infiltration of metastatic cancer, lymphoma, or leukemia (Chapter 40). Thrombocytosis can be categorized into primary and secondary (Chapter 40). Essential thrombocythemia is a myeloproliferative neoplasm characterized by sustained proliferation of megakaryocytes, resulting in platelet counts of 450 × 10^9/L or greater (Chapter 33).[121] Primary thrombocytosis can also be seen in chronic myelogenous leukemia. Secondary thrombocytosis, or reactive thrombocytosis, is associated with infections, rheumatoid arthritis, chronic inflammatory bowel disease, iron deficiency anemia, sickle cell anemia, and splenectomy.[122-124]

Anemia and the Elderly

Anemia is common in the elderly and its prevalence increases with age; however, anemia should not be viewed as an inevitable consequence of aging.[125,126] Although anemia in the elderly is typically mild, it has been associated with substantial morbidity and mortality.[127,128] WHO defines anemia as hemoglobin less than 13 g/dL in males and less than 12 g/dL in females. Using the WHO definition of anemia, the Third National Health and Nutrition Examination Survey (NHANES III), a national study that samples clinical specimens, found the prevalence of anemia in the United States in individuals over the age of 65 to be 11% in men and 10.2% in women. This proportion doubles in those aged 85 and above.[126] However, studies of the prevalence of anemia in the elderly show great variability in the definitions of anemia used, as well as differences in sample sizes, patient populations studied, countries in which the study was conducted, and study design. Thus estimates of the prevalence of anemia vary from 2.9% to 61% in elderly men and from 3.3% to 41% in elderly women.[129]

The factors contributing to anemia include a decrease in bone marrow function, a decline in physical activity, nutritional deficiencies, cardiovascular disease, and chronic inflammatory disorders. Unexplained anemia, anemia due to hematologic malignancies, iron deficiency anemia, anemia related to therapy for nonhematologic malignancies, and anemia of chronic inflammation are the most common causes of anemia in the elderly.[130]

Ineffective erythropoiesis and hypoproliferation are also seen in the elderly. Ineffective erythropoiesis is associated with vitamin B$_{12}$ or folate deficiency, myelodysplastic syndrome, sideroblastic anemia, and thalassemia. Hypoproliferative anemia often occurs secondary to iron deficiency, vitamin B$_{12}$ or folate deficiency, renal failure, hypothyroidism, chronic inflammation, or endocrine disease.[130,131] To a lesser extent, the elderly are prone to anemias such as aplastic anemia, hemolytic anemia, myelophthisic anemia, and anemia due to protein-calorie malnutrition.

The initial laboratory evaluation of anemia should include a complete blood count (CBC), a reticulocyte count, peripheral blood film review, and chemistry panel, along with other diagnostic tools, including iron studies (with ferritin), vitamin B_{12}, and folate levels. Table 45-8 indicates the types of anemia suggested by MCV and RDW results. In addition, assessment for signs of gastrointestinal blood loss, hemolysis, nutritional deficiencies, malignancy, chronic infection, renal or hepatic disease, or other chronic disease can provide important information for the evaluation of anemia in the elderly.

Anemia of Chronic Inflammation

Anemia of chronic inflammation, also known as *anemia of chronic disease*, frequently occurs with inflammatory disorders (e.g., rheumatoid arthritis, renal failure, liver disease), chronic infections, bedsores, collagen vascular disease, protein malnutrition, endocrine disorders, vitamin C deficiency, and neoplastic disorders.[131-139] This hypoproliferative anemia is the most common form of anemia in the hospitalized geriatric population.[140] The severity of the anemia generally correlates with the severity of the underlying disease.[141] Hepcidin-induced inhibition of iron absorption in the intestines and iron mobilization from macrophages and hepatocytes, and impaired erythropoietin-dependent erythropoiesis triggered by inflammatory cytokines is involved in the pathogenesis of anemia of chronic inflammation (Chapter 20).[142,143]

Iron Deficiency Anemia

Iron deficiency anemia is common in the elderly. Iron deficiency affects not only erythrocytes but also the metabolic pathways of iron-dependent tissue enzymes.[136] Hemoglobin synthesis is reduced, and even a minimal decrease can cause

profound functional disabilities in an elderly patient. The serum iron level decreases progressively with each decade of life, particularly in females. Nevertheless, healthy elderly adults usually have serum iron levels within the adult reference interval.

Iron deficiency anemia in the elderly is rarely due to dietary deficiency in industrialized nations because of the prevalence of iron fortification of grains, as well as a diet that includes meats containing heme iron. Iron deficiency in the elderly most frequently results from conditions leading to chronic gastrointestinal blood loss, including long-term use of nonsteroidal anti-inflammatory medications, gastritis, peptic ulcer disease, gastroesophageal reflux disease with esophagitis, colon cancer, and angiodysplasia.[144-146] It also may be due to poor diet in an elderly individual who has lost the taste or desire for food or is unable to prepare nutritious meals. Chapter 20 discusses iron disorders in detail.

Ineffective Erythropoiesis

Ineffective erythropoiesis has been attributed not only to maturation disorders such as vitamin B_{12} and folic acid deficiency but also to sideroblastic anemia, thalassemia, and myelodysplastic syndrome. Sideroblastic anemias are characterized by impaired heme synthesis, and abnormal globin synthesis occurs in the thalassemias (Chapters 20 and 28). Megaloblastic anemia results from defective synthesis of deoxyribonucleic acid (DNA) (Chapter 21) with compromised cell division but normal cytoplasmic development (i.e., asynchrony).[147-149] These megaloblastic cells are more prone to destruction in the bone marrow, which results in ineffective erythropoiesis. Two causes of megaloblastic anemia are vitamin B_{12} deficiency and folate deficiency. Myelodysplastic syndrome results in ineffective hematopoiesis due to mutations in hematopoietic stem cells and progenitor cells. It is more common in the elderly and is discussed below.

Vitamin B_{12} Deficiency. Vitamin B_{12} (cobalamin) deficiency causes a megaloblastic disorder in 5% to 10% of the elderly.[131] It may be difficult to detect because anemia is present in only about 60% of patients.[150] Neurologic complications are found in 75% to 90% of individuals with clinically apparent vitamin B_{12} deficiency.[151,152] In the absence of anemia, neurologic symptoms may be the only indication. Even when anemia is present, it does not always manifest with the classic macrocytic and megaloblastic picture but may be normocytic.

Vitamin B_{12} deficiency in the elderly has been attributed to inadequate intestinal absorption of food-bound vitamin B_{12} rather than pernicious anemia or inadequate intake.[143,153] Many elderly individuals have atrophic gastritis resulting in decreased gastric production of acid. In this condition there is low vitamin B_{12} absorption because protein-bound vitamin B_{12} is not dissociated from food proteins and therefore cannot bind to intrinsic factor for absorption. In addition, the loss of gastric acid can result in bacterial overgrowth, particularly with *Helicobacter pylori*, which also interferes with vitamin B_{12} absorption.[154,155] Inadequate vitamin B_{12} absorption in the

TABLE 45-8 Classification of Geriatric Anemia Based on Typical Mean Cell Volume (MCV) and Red Cell Distribution Width (RDW)

MCV	RDW	Anemia
Normal	Normal	Anemia of chronic inflammation (some)
		Hemorrhagic anemia
		Leukemia-associated anemia
	High	Early iron deficiency anemia
		Mixed deficiency anemia (e.g., vitamin B_{12} and iron)
		Sideroblastic anemia
Low	Normal	Anemia of chronic inflammation (some)
	High	Iron deficiency anemia
High	Normal	Anemia associated with myelodysplastic syndrome
	High	Vitamin B_{12} deficiency anemia
		Folate deficiency anemia
		Hemolytic anemia

Note that this classification is not absolute because there can be an overlap of RDW values among some of the conditions in each MCV category.

elderly has also been reported in other infrequent conditions such as small bowel disorder, gastric resection, pancreatic insufficiency, resection of the terminal ileum, blind loop syndrome, and tropical sprue.[156] Pernicious anemia develops slowly and insidiously in patients when autoimmune antibodies to intrinsic factor or to parietal cells destroy their parietal cells so that they are left without intrinsic factor.[157] Given the high risk of vitamin B_{12} deficiency in the aged and the risks of the condition, some authors have proposed that all elderly adults be screened periodically for vitamin B_{12} deficiency.[158,159] Chapter 21 discusses megaloblastic anemias.

Folate Deficiency.

A second megaloblastic anemia that may be seen in the elderly results from folate deficiency. In contrast to vitamin B_{12} deficiency, folic acid deficiency usually develops from inadequate dietary intake because the body stores little folate.[160] However, the incidence of low serum and RBC folate levels has declined in all age groups, including the elderly, since countries began to fortify their grains with folic acid in the 1990s.[161] Alcoholic elderly patients are particularly prone to folic acid deficiency because alcohol interferes with folate absorption, enterohepatic recycling, metabolism, breakdown, and excretion (Chapter 21).[162,163]

Hemolytic Anemia

Hemolytic anemias are characterized by a shortened RBC survival time. The three major types of hemolytic anemias are those caused by immunologic mechanisms; those due to intrinsic defects, such as an RBC membrane defect, abnormal hemoglobins, or RBC enzyme defects; and those resulting from extrinsic factors, such as mechanical or lytic processes.[132,164] The elderly are at risk for drug-induced hemolytic anemia because they may take multiple medications. Drug-induced hemolytic anemia has been associated with high doses of antibiotics (penicillin, chloramphenicol, cephalosporins), several nonsteroidal anti-inflammatory drugs, quinidine, phenacetin, and others. Hemolytic anemias in the elderly also can result from collagen vascular diseases, infections, and chronic lymphocytic leukemia. The hemolytic anemias are discussed in Chapters 23 to 28.

Hematologic Neoplasia in Older Individuals

Although hematologic malignancies may occur at any age, certain disorders are common in those older than 50 years. A brief overview of these disorders is included in this chapter, with references to more detailed discussions.

Chronic Myeloid Neoplasms

The 2008 WHO classification of adult chronic myeloid neoplasms includes four broad categories: myelodysplastic syndrome; myeloproliferative neoplasms; myelodysplastic/myeloproliferative neoplasms; and myeloid and lymphoid neoplasms associated with eosinophilia and abnormalities of platelet-derived growth factor receptor α, platelet-derived growth factor receptor β, or fibroblast growth factor receptor 1. The chronic myeloid neoplasms show increased incidence in the elderly.

Myelodysplastic Syndrome.

Myelodysplastic syndrome represents a heterogeneous group of clonal bone marrow disorders that may affect multiple cell lineages. Myelodysplastic syndrome is the most common hematologic malignancy in the elderly.[130,165] The incidence of myelodysplastic syndrome increases from 6.6 cases per 100,000 for individuals aged 60 to 64 to 20.9 per 100,000 for those aged 70 to 74, and is 51.2 per 100,000 for those age 85 and older.[166] Typical features include progressive cytopenias, dyspoiesis in one or more cell lines, and an increase in blasts in the peripheral blood and bone marrow. Chapter 34 provides a complete discussion of myelodysplastic syndrome.

Myeloproliferative Neoplasms.

Myeloproliferative neoplasms are monoclonal proliferations of hematopoietic stem cells with overaccumulation of RBCs, WBCs, or platelets in various combinations. Myeloproliferative disorders include chronic myelogenous leukemia, polycythemia vera, essential thrombocythemia, primary myelofibrosis, chronic eosinophilic leukemia not otherwise classified, mastocytosis, chronic neutrophilic leukemia, and unclassifiable myeloproliferative neoplasms. The incidence of myeloproliferative neoplasms increases from 6.1 per 100,000 for individuals aged 60 to 64, to 11.5 per 100,000 for those aged 70 to 74, and to 15.8 per 100,000 for those 85 years of age and older.[166] Chapter 33 discusses the myeloproliferative neoplasms.

Leukemia

Leukemia is a neoplastic disease characterized by a malignant proliferation of hematopoietic stem cells in the bone marrow, peripheral blood, and often other organs. Leukemia is broadly classified on the basis of the cell type involved (lymphoid or myeloid) and the stage of maturity of the leukemic cells (acute or chronic). Although the overall incidence of leukemia has decreased in the past 5 decades, there has been a disproportionately greater incidence of leukemia in the elderly (Table 45-9). The peaks in leukemia incidence seem to occur in the very young (age 1 to 4 years) and the very old (age 70 or older,

TABLE 45-9 SEER Incidence of Leukemia in the Elderly in the United States per 100,000 (2000–2010)*

Age at Diagnosis	All Leukemias	ALL	CLL	AML	CML	AMoL
65–69 yr	36.8	1.3	16.7	10.4	4.4	0.7
70–74 yr	49.4	1.4	21.9	14.9	5.7	0.9
75–79 yr	65.7	1.5	28.5	19.7	7.9	1.2
80–84 yr	77.8	1.6	32.4	23.2	9.7	1.4
≥85 yr	88.5	1.8	37.5	22.7	10.1	1.5

Adapted from Howlader N, Noone AM, Krapcho M, et al, editors: SEER cancer statistics review, 1975-2010, Bethesda, Md, 2010, National Cancer Institute. Based on November 2012 SEER data submission, posted to the SEER website in 2013. Available at: http://seer.cancer.gov/csr/1975_2010/. Accessed July 10, 2013.
ALL, Acute lymphoblastic leukemia; *AML*, acute myeloid leukemia; *AMoL*, acute monocytic leukemia; *CLL*, chronic lymphocytic leukemia; *CML*, chronic myelogenous leukemia.
*Surveillance, Epidemiology, and End Results (SEER) Incidence Source: SEER 18 areas.

especially men). Acute myelogenous leukemia (Chapter 35) and chronic lymphocytic leukemia (Chapter 36) show the most dramatic age-related increase in incidence.[166]

Geriatric Hemostasis

Age-related changes occur in the vascular and hemostatic systems, including alterations in platelets, coagulation, and fibrinolytic factors. These changes are thought to contribute to the increased incidence of thrombosis in the elderly. The rate of venous thromboembolism, for example, increases from 1 per 10,000 in the young (25 to 30 years of age) to 8 per 1000 in the elderly (85 years and older).[167] Approximately 60% of venous thrombosis events occur in those aged 70 years and older (Chapter 39).[168]

Fibrinogen, factor V, factor VII, factor VIII, factor IX, factor XIII, high-molecular-weight kininogen, and prekallikrein increase in healthy individuals as they age.[169] Fibrinogen, which has been implicated as a primary risk factor for thrombotic disorders, increases approximately 10 mg/dL per decade in the elderly (65 to 79 years),[170] from 280 mg/dL to over 300 mg/dL.

Elevated levels of factor VIII also have been associated with increased risk of venous thrombosis.[171] Studies of the association between factor VII and venous thrombosis have yielded conflicting findings.[169]

PAI-1, the major inhibitor of fibrinolysis, increases with aging. PAI-1 has been shown to promote age-dependent thrombosis in animal models and could play an important role in causing hypercoagulability in the elderly.[172-174]

Platelets increase in activity with age, as evidenced by a decrease in bleeding time as males age from 11 to 70 years[175] and an increase in markers of platelet activation, platelet β-thromboglobulin, and platelet factor 4.[176] Increased platelet activity with aging is also associated with increased platelet phospholipids, which suggests an age-related increase in platelet transmembrane signaling.[177]

Many conventional risk factors associated with venous thrombosis are likely to also increase the risk of thrombosis in the elderly. These factors include immobility, malignant disease, comorbidities, and prescription drugs that influence coagulation or platelet function.[143,167]

SUMMARY

- The newborn infant, preadolescent child, and elderly adult exhibit profound hematologic differences from one another.
- Newborn hematologic parameters continue to change and evolve over the first few days, weeks, and months of life. Laboratory results must be assessed in light of gestational age, birth weight, and developmental differences between newborns and older infants.
- The erythrocytes of newborn infants are markedly macrocytic at birth. A condition known as *physiologic anemia of infancy* occurs after the first few weeks of life. Infants born prematurely also experience a decrease in hemoglobin concentration, which is termed *physiologic anemia of prematurity.*
- Iron deficiency is the most frequent cause of anemia in children.
- Fluctuations in the number of WBCs are common at all ages but are greatest in infants. Leukocytosis is typical at birth for healthy full-term and preterm infants, with a mean of 22×10^9 cells/L (range, 9 to 30×10^9 cells/L) at 12 hours of life. There is an increase in segmented neutrophils, bands, and occasional metamyelocytes with no evidence of disease.
- Sepsis in neonates is a common cause of morbidity, particularly in premature and low-birth-weight infants. Defective B cell response against polysaccharide agents, as well as abnormal cytokine release by neutrophils and monocytes, have been implicated.

- Although hemostatic values are different in infants and children from those in adults, this population is not at increased risk of bleeding or thrombosis.
- There is a gradual decline in hemoglobin starting at middle age, and the mean level decreases by about 1 g/dL during the sixth through eighth decades.
- Although anemia is common in elderly patients, it is not a normal occurrence in the aging process. The cause of anemia may be multifactorial in elderly patients.
- Iron deficiency anemia, anemia of chronic inflammation, and megaloblastic anemia related to vitamin B_{12} deficiency are the most common anemias seen in the elderly.
- *Immunosenescence* refers to the adverse changes in the immune system associated with aging.
- The elderly experience an increased frequency of many neoplastic and malignant disorders, such as acute and chronic leukemia, myelodysplastic syndromes, and myeloproliferative neoplasms.
- The elderly are at an increased risk of thrombosis associated with age-related changes in the vascular and hemostatic systems.

Now that you have completed this chapter, go back and read again the case study at the beginning and respond to the questions presented.

REVIEW QUESTIONS

Answers can be found in the Appendix.

1. The CBC results for children (aged 3 to 12 years) differ from those of adults chiefly in what respect?
   a. NRBCs are present.
   b. Notable polychromasia is seen, indicating increased reticulocytosis.
   c. Platelet count is lower.
   d. The percentage of lymphocytes is higher.

2. Physiologic anemia of infancy results from:
   a. Iron deficiency caused by a milk-only diet during the early neonatal period
   b. Increased oxygenation of blood and decreased erythropoietin
   c. Replacement of active marrow with fat soon after birth
   d. Hb F and its diminished oxygen delivery to tissues

3. The CBC report on a 3-day-old neonate who was born 6 weeks prematurely shows a decrease in hemoglobin compared with the value obtained 2 days earlier. Which of the following should be considered as an explanation for this result when no apparent source of hemolysis or bleeding is evident?
   a. The sample was collected from a vein at the time that an intravenous line was inserted.
   b. The sample was collected by heel puncture rather than finger puncture because of the infant's small size.
   c. The umbilical cord was clamped quickly to begin appropriate treatment for a preterm infant.
   d. The infant has become dehydrated.

4. Morphologically, the hematogones in newborns are:
   a. Similar to those seen in megaloblastic anemia
   b. Easily confused with leukemic blasts
   c. Monocytoid in appearance
   d. Similar to adult lymphocytes

5. The most frequent cause of anemia in childhood is:
   a. Vitamin B_{12} deficiency
   b. Drug-related hemolysis
   c. Iron deficiency
   d. Folate deficiency

6. As age increases, the hemoglobin level of elderly adults:
   a. Remains unchanged from that of middle-aged adults
   b. Increases due to diminished respiration and poor tissue oxygenation
   c. Decreases for reasons that are unclear
   d. Becomes comparable to that of newborns

7. Which of the following are the most common anemias in the elderly population?
   a. Megaloblastic anemia and iron deficiency anemia
   b. Sideroblastic anemia and megaloblastic anemia
   c. Myelophthisic anemia and anemia of chronic inflammation
   d. Iron deficiency anemia and anemia of chronic inflammation

8. When iron deficiency is recognized in an elderly individual, the cause is usually:
   a. An iron-deficient diet
   b. Gastrointestinal bleeding
   c. Diminished absorption
   d. Impaired incorporation of iron into heme as a result of telomere loss

9. Which of the following conditions is least likely in an elderly individual?
   a. Acute lymphoblastic leukemia
   b. Multiple myeloma
   c. Myelodysplasia
   d. Chronic lymphocytic leukemia

10. The multiple medications used by the elderly makes this population more prone to:
    a. Anemia of chronic inflammation
    b. Megaloblastic anemia
    c. Hemolytic anemia
    d. Iron deficiency anemia

REFERENCES

1. Brugnara, C., & Platt, O. S. (2009). The neonatal erythrocyte and its disorders. In Orkin, S. H., Nathan, D. G., Ginsburg, D., et al., (Eds.), *Nathan and Oski's Hematology of Infancy and Childhood.* (7th ed., pp. 21–66). Philadelphia: Saunders.
2. Palis, J., & Segal, G. B. (2010). Hematology of the fetus and newborn. In Kaushansky, K., Lichtman, M. A., Beutler, E., et al., (Eds.), *Williams Hematology.* (8th ed., pp. 87–104). New York: McGraw-Hill.
3. Hann, I. M., Bodger, M. P., & Hoffbrand, A. V. (1983). Development of pluripotent hematopoietic progenitor cells in the human fetus. *Blood, 62,* 118–123.
4. Forestier, F., Daffos, F., Catherine, N., et al. (1991). Developmental hematopoiesis in normal human fetal blood. *Blood, 77,* 2360–2363.
5. Christensen, R. D., & Ohls, R. K. (2011). Development of the hematopoietic system. In Kliegman, R., Stanton, B. F., Geme J. W., III, et al., (Eds.), *Nelson Textbook of Pediatrics.* (19th ed., pp. 1648–1651). Philadelphia: Elsevier Saunders.
6. Christensen, R. D. (1989). Hematopoiesis in the fetus and neonate. *Pediatr Res, 26,* 531–535.
7. Linch, D. C., Knott, L. J., Rodeck, C. H., et al. (1982). Studies of circulating hematopoietic progenitor cells in human fetal blood. *Blood, 59,* 976–979.

8. Christensen, R. D. (1987). Circulating pluripotent hematopoietic progenitor cells in neonates. *J Pediatr, 110*, 622–625.

9. Yoder, M. C. (2002). Embryonic hematopoiesis. In Christensen, R. D., (Ed.), *Hematologic Problems of the Neonate* (pp. 3–20). Philadelphia: Saunders.

10. Tavassoli, M. (1991). Embryonic and fetal hemopoiesis: an overview. *Blood Cells, 1*, 269–281.

11. Waldemar, A. C. (2011). The high risk infant. In Kliegman, R., Stanton, B. F., Geme J. W., III, et al., (Eds.), *Nelson Textbook of Pediatrics*. (19th ed., pp. 552–565). Philadelphia: Elsevier Saunders.

12. Peterec, S. M., & Warshaw, J. B. (2006). The premature newborn. In McMillan, J. A., (Ed.), *Oski's Pediatrics*. (4th ed., pp. 220–235). Philadelphia: Lippincott Williams & Wilkins.

13. Oski, F. A., & Naiman, J. L. (1982). Normal blood values in the newborn period. In Oski, F. A., & Naiman, J. L., (Eds.). *Hematologic Problems in the Newborn*. (3rd ed., pp. 1–31). Philadelphia: WB Saunders.

14. Maheshwari, A., & Carlo, W. A. (2011). Anemia in the newborn infant. In Kliegman, R., Stanton, B. F., Geme, J. W., III, et al., (Eds.), *Nelson Textbook of Pediatrics*. (19th ed., pp. 612–621). Philadelphia: Elsevier Saunders.

15. Speakman, E. D., Boyd, J. C., & Bruns, D. E. (1995). Measurement of methemoglobin in neonatal samples containing fetal hemoglobin. *Clin Chem, 41*, 458–461.

16. Puukka, R., & Puukka, M. (1994). Effect of hemoglobin F on measurements of hemoglobin A_{1c} with physicians' office analyzers. *Clin Chem, 40*, 342–343.

17. Sandberg, S., Sonstabo, K., & Christensen, G. (1989). Influence of lipid and leukocytes on the haemoglobin determination by Coulter Counter S Plus III, Technicon H 6000, Technicon H1, LK 540, Reflotron and Hemocap. *Scand J Clin Lab Invest, 49*, 145–148.

18. Geaghan, S. M. (1999). Hematologic values and appearances in the healthy fetus, neonate, and child. *Clin Lab Med, 19*, 1–37.

19. Matoth, Y., Zaizov, R., & Varsano, I. (1971). Postnatal changes in some red cell parameters. *Acta Paediatr Scand, 60*, 317–323.

20. Christensen, R. D., & Ohls, R. K. (2012). Anemia in the neonatal period. In Buonocore, G., Bracci, R., & Weingling, M., (Eds.), *Neonatology a Practical Approach to Neonatal Diseases* (pp. 784–798). Milan: Springer.

21. Zaizov, R., & Matoth, Y. (1976). Red cell values on the first postnatal day during the last 16 weeks of gestation. *Am J Hematol, 1*, 275–278.

22. Thomas, R. M., Canning, C. E., Cotes, P. M., et al. (1983). Erythropoietin and cord blood hemoglobin in the regulation of human fetal erythropoiesis. *Br J Obstet Gynaecol, 90*, 795–800.

23. Pahal, G. S., Jauniaux, E., Kinnon, C., et al. (2000). Normal development of human fetal hematopoiesis between eight and seventeen weeks' gestation. *Am J Obstet Gynecol, 183*, 1029–1034.

24. Luchtman-Jones, L., & Wilson, D. B. (2011). The blood and hematopoietic system. In Martin, R. J., Fanaroff, A. A., & Walsh, M. C., (Eds.), *Neonatal-Perinatal Medicine*. (9th ed., pp. 1303–1360). St Louis: Saunders Elsevier.

25. Soldin, S., Wong, E. C., Brugnara, C., et al., (Eds.). (2011). *Pediatric Reference Intervals*. (7th ed.). Washington, DC: AACC Press.

26. Zipursky, M. D., Brown, E., Palko, J., et al. (1983). The erythrocyte differential count in newborn infants. *Am J Pediatr Hematol Oncol, 3*, 45–51.

27. Cook, C. D., Brodie, H. R., & Allen, D. W. (1957). Measurement of fetal hemoglobin in premature infants: correlation with gestational age and intrauterine hypoxia. *Pediatrics, 20*, 272–278.

28. Bard, H. (1975). The postnatal decline of hemoglobin F in normal full-term infants. *J Clin Invest, 55*, 395–398.

29. Bard, H. (1973). Postnatal fetal and adult hemoglobin synthesis in early preterm newborn infants. *J Clin Invest, 52*, 1789–1795.

30. Dallman, P. R., George, D. B., Allen, C. M., et al. (1978). Hemoglobin concentration in white, black, and oriental children: is there a need for separate criteria in screening for anemia? *Am J Clin Nutr, 31*, 377–380.

31. Alur, P., Satish, S., Super, D. M., et al. (2000). Impact of race and gestational age on red blood cell indices in very low birth weight infants. *Pediatrics, 106*, 306–310.

32. Doyle, J. J. (1997). The role of erythropoietin in the anemia of prematurity. *Semin Perinatol, 21*, 20–27.

33. Strauss, R. G. (1997). Recombinant erythropoietin for the anemia of prematurity: still a promise, not a panacea. *J Pediatr, 131*, 653–655.

34. Garby, L., Sjölin, S., & Vuille, J. (1963). Studies of erythrokinetics in infancy. III. Disappearance from plasma and red cell uptake of radioactive iron injected intravenously. *Acta Paediatr, 52*, 537–553.

35. O'Brien, R. T., & Pearson, H. A. (1971). Physiologic anemia of the newborn infant. *J Pediatr, 79*, 132–138.

36. McIntosh, N., Kempson, C., & Tyler, R. M. (1988). Blood counts in extremely low birth weight infants. *Arch Dis Child, 63*, 74–76.

37. Cavaliere, T. A. (2004). Red blood cell indices: implications for practice. *Newborn Infant Nurs Rev, 4*, 231–239.

38. Obladen, M., Diepold, K., & Maier, R. F. (2000). Venous and arterial hematologic profiles of very low birth weight infants. *Pediatrics, 106*, 707–711.

39. Halvorsen, S., & Finne, P. H. (1968). Erythropoietin reduction in the human fetus and newborn. *Ann N Y Acad Sci, 149*, 576–577.

40. Mann, D. L., Sites, M. L., & Donati, R. M. (1965). Erythropoietic stimulating activity during the first ninety days of life. *Proc Soc Exp Biol Med, 118*, 212–214.

41. Means, R. T., & Glader, B. (2009). Anemia: general considerations. In Greer, J. P., Foerster, J., Rodgers, G. M., et al., (Eds.), *Wintrobe's Clinical Hematology*. (12th ed., pp. 779–809). Philadelphia: Wolters Kluwer Health/Lippincott Williams & Wilkins.

42. Nickerson, H. J., Silberman, T., Park, R. W., et al. (2000). Treatment of iron deficiency anemia and associated protein-losing enteropathy in children. *J Pediatr Hematol Oncol, 22*, 50–54.

43. Dagnelie, P. C., Van Staveren, W. A., & Hautvast, J. G. (1991). Stunting and nutrient deficiencies in children on alternative diets. *Acta Paediatr Scand, 374*, 111–118.

44. Schneede, J., Dagnelie, P. C., Van Staveren, W. A., et al. (1994). Methylmalonic acid and homocysteine in plasma as indicators of functional cobalamin deficiency in infants on macrobiotic diets. *Pediatr Res, 36*, 194–201.

45. Walter, T., DeAndraca, I., Chadud, P., et al. (1989). Iron deficiency anemia: adverse effects on infant psychomotor development. *Pediatrics, 84*, 7–17.

46. Bridges, K. R., & Pearson, H. A. (2008). *Anemias and other red cell disorders* (pp. 99–100). New York: McGraw-Hill.

47. Will, A. M. (2006). Disorders of iron metabolism: iron deficiency, iron overload and the sideroblastic anemias. In Arceci, R. J., Hann, I. M., & Smith, O. P., (Eds.), *Pediatric Hematology*. (3rd ed., pp. 79–104). Malden, Mass: Blackwell.

48. Andrews, N. C., Ulrich, C. K., & Fleming, M. D. (2009). Disorders of iron metabolism and sideroblastic anemia. In Orkin, S. H., Nathan, D. G., Ginsburg, D., et al., (Eds.), *Nathan and Oski's Hematology of Infancy and Childhood*. (7th ed., pp. 521–570). Philadelphia: Saunders.

49. Looker, A. (2002). Iron deficiency—United States, 1999-2000. *MMWR Morb Mortal Wkly Rep, 51*, 897–899.

50. Gartner, L. M., Morton, J., Lawrence, R. A., et al; American Academy of Pediatrics Section on Breastfeeding. (2005). Breastfeeding and the use of human milk. *Pediatrics, 115*, 496–506.

51. Kanakoudi, F., Drossou, V., Tzimouli, V., et al. (1995). Serum concentrations of 10 acute-phase proteins in healthy term

and preterm infants from birth to age 6 months. *Clin Chem*, *41*, 605–608.

52. Minder, N., & Cohn, J. (1984). Serum iron, serum transferrin and transferrin saturation in healthy children without iron deficiency. *Eur J Pediatr*, *143*, 96–98.

53. Saarinen, U. M., & Siimes, M. A. (1978). Serum ferritin in assessment of iron nutrition in healthy infants. *Acta Paediatr Scand*, *67*, 745–751.

54. Siimes, M. A., Addiego, J. E., & Dall, P. R. (1974). Ferritin in serum: diagnosis of iron deficiency and iron overload in infants and children. *Blood*, *43*, 581–590.

55. Schmutz, N., Henry, E., Jopling, J., et al. (2008). Expected ranges for blood neutrophil concentrations of neonates: the Manroe and Mouzinho charts revisited. *J Perinatol*, *28*, 275–281.

56. Christensen, R. D., Henry, E., Jopling, J., et al. (2009). The CBC: reference ranges for neonates. *Semin Perinatol*, *33*, 3–11.

57. Caramihai, E., Karayalein, G., Aballi, A. J., et al. (1975). Leukocyte count differences in healthy white and black children 1 to 5 years of age. *J Pediatr*, *86*, 252–254.

58. Castro, O. L., Haddy, T. B., & Rana, S. R. (1987). Age- and sex-related blood cell values in healthy black Americans. *Public Health Reports*, *102*, 232–237.

59. Monroe, B. L., Weinberg, A. G., & Rosenfeld, C. R. (1976). The neonatal blood count in health and disease: I. reference values for neutrophilic cells. *J Pediatr*, *95*, 89–98.

60. Mouzinho, A., Rosenfeld, C. R., Sanchez, P. J., et al. (1994). Revised reference ranges for circulating neutrophils in very-low-birth-weight neonates. *Pediatrics*, *94*, 76–82.

61. Alexander, G. R., Kogan, M., Bader, G., et al. (2003). US birth weight/gestational age–specific neonatal mortality: 1995-1997 rates for whites, Hispanics and blacks. *Pediatrics*, *111*, e61–e66.

62. Dinauer, M. C., & Newburger, P. E. (2009). The phagocyte system and disorders of granulopoiesis and granulocyte function. In Orkin, S. H., Nathan, D. G., Ginsburg, D., et al., (Eds.), *Nathan and Oski's Hematology of Infancy and Childhood.* (7th ed., pp. 1109–1217). Philadelphia: Saunders.

63. Ezekowitz, R. A. B. (2009). Hematologic manifestations of systemic diseases. In Orkin, S. H., Nathan, D. G., Ginsburg, D., et al., (Eds.), *Nathan and Oski's Hematology of Infancy and Childhood.* (7th ed., pp. 1680–1739). Philadelphia: Saunders.

64. Wright, B., McKenna, R. W., Asplund, S. L., et al. (2002). Maturing B-cell precursors in bone marrow: a detailed subset analysis of 141 cases by 4-color flow cytometry. *Mod Pathol*, *15*, 270A.

65. Rimsza, L. M., Douglas, V. K., Tighe, P., et al. (2004). Benign B-cell precursors (hematogones) are the predominant lymphoid population in the bone marrow of preterm infants. *Biol Neonate*, *86*, 247–253.

66. Vogel, P., & Erf, L. A. (1937). Hematological observations on bone marrow obtained by sternal punctures. *Am J Clin Pathol*, *7*, 436–447.

67. Muehleck, S. D., McKenna, R. W., Gale, P. F., et al. (1983). Terminal deoxynucleotidyl transferase (TdT)–positive cells in bone marrow in the absence of hematologic malignancy. *Am J Clin Pathol*, *79*, 277–284.

68. Brunning, R. D., McKenna, R. W. (1994). *Tumors of the bone marrow*. Washington DC: Armed Forces Institute of Pathology.

69. McKenna, R. W., Washington, L. T., Aquino, D. B., et al. (2001). Immunophenotypic analysis of hematogones (B-lymphocyte precursors) in 662 consecutive bone marrow specimens by 4-color flow cytometry. *Blood*, *98*, 2498–2507.

70. Intermesoli, T., Mangili, G., Salvi, A., et al. (2007). Abnormally expanded pro-B hematogones associated with congenital cytomegalovirus infection. *Am J Hematol*, *82*, 934–936.

71. Cuenca, A. G., Wynn, J. J., Moldawer, I. L., et al. (2013). Role of innate immunity in neonatal infection. *Am J Perinat*, *30*, 105–112.

72. Chirico, G., Ciardelli, L., & Gasparoni, A. (1997). Clinical and experimental aspects on the use of granulocyte colony stimulating factor (G-CSF) in the neonate. In Bellanti, J. A., Bracci, R., Prindull, G., et al., (Eds.), *Neonatal Hematology and Immunology III* (pp. 33–38). Amsterdam: Elsevier Science.

73. Weimann, E., Rutkowski, S., & Reisbach, G. (1998). G-CSF, GM-CSF and IL-6 levels in cord blood: diminished increase of G-CSF and IL-6 in preterms with perinatal infection compared to term neonates. *J Perinat Med*, *26*, 211–218.

74. Squire, E., Favara, B., & Todd, J. (1979). Diagnosis of neonatal bacterial infection: hematologic and pathologic findings in fatal and nonfatal cases. *Pediatrics*, *64*, 60–64.

75. Garra, G., Cunningham, S. J., & Crain, E. F. (2005). Reappraisal of criteria used to predict serious bacterial illness in febrile infants less than 8 weeks of age. *Acad Emerg Med*, *12*, 921–925.

76. Jaskiewicz, J. A., McCarthy, C. A., Richardson, A. C., et al. (1994). Febrile infants at low risk for serious bacterial infection—an appraisal of the Rochester criteria and implications for management. Febrile Infant Collaborative Study Group. *Pediatrics*, *94*, 390–396.

77. Timens, W., Rozeboom, T., & Poppema, S. (1987). Fetal and neonatal development of human spleen: an immunohistological study. *Immunology*, *60*, 603–609.

78. Davidson, D., Miskolci, V., Clark, D. C., et al. (2007). Interleukin-10 production after pro-inflammatory stimulation of neutrophils and monocytic cells of the newborn. *Neonatology*, *92*, 127–133.

79. Rondini, G., & Chirico, G. (1999). Hematopoietic growth factor levels in term and preterm infants. *Curr Opin Hematol*, *6*, 192–197.

80. Kotiranta-Ainamo, A., Rautonen, J., & Rautonen, N. (2004). Imbalanced cytokine secretion in newborns. *Biol Neonate*, *85*, 55–60.

81. Akenzua, G. I., Hui, Y. T., Milner, R., et al. (1974). Neutrophil and band counts in the diagnosis of neonatal infection. *Pediatrics*, *54*, 38–42.

82. Bhandari, V., Wang, C., Rinder, C., et al. (2008). Hematologic profile of sepsis in neonates: neutrophil CD64 as a diagnostic marker. *Pediatrics*, *121*, 129–134.

83. Rey, C., Los Arcos, M., Concha, A., et al. (2007). Procalcitonin and C-reactive protein as markers of systemic inflammatory response syndrome severity in critically ill children. *Intensive Care Med*, *33*, 477–484.

84. Fogel, B. J., Arais, D., & Kung, F. (1968). Platelet counts in healthy premature infants. *J Pediatr*, *73*, 108–110.

85. Sell, E. J., & Corrigan, J. J. (1973). Platelet counts, fibrinogen concentrations and factor V and factor VIII levels in healthy infants according to gestational age. *J Pediatr*, *82*, 1028–1032.

86. Mehta, P., Vasa, R., Neumann, L., et al. (1980). Thrombocytopenia in the high-risk infant. *J Pediatr*, *97*, 791–794.

87. Meberg, A., Halvorsen, S., & Orstavik, I. (1977). Transitory thrombocytopenia in small-for-dates infants, possibly related to maternal smoking. *Lancet*, *2*, 303–304.

88. Andrew, M., Paes, B., Milner, R., et al. (1987). Development of the human coagulation system in the full-term infant. *Blood*, *70*, 165–172.

89. Andrew, M., Vegh, P., Johnston, M., et al. (1992). Maturation of the hemostatic system during childhood. *Blood*, *80*, 1998–2005.

90. Manno, C. S. (2005). Management of bleeding disorders in children. *Hematology Am Soc Hematol Educ Program*, 416–422.

91. Pabinger, I., & Schneider, B. (1996). Thrombotic risk in hereditary antithrombin III, protein C, or protein S deficiency. A cooperative, retrospective study. Gesellschaft für Thrombose- und

Hamostaseforschung (GTH) Study Group on Natural Inhibitors. *Arterioscler Thromb Vasc Biol, 12*, 742–748.

92. Worly, F. M., Fortenberry, J. D., Hansen, I., et al. (2004). Deep venous thrombosis in children with diabetic ketoacidosis and femoral central venous catheters. *Pediatrics, 113*, 57–60.

93. Gutierrez, J. A., Bagatell, R., Samson, M. P., et al. (2003). Femoral central venous catheter–associated deep venous thrombosis in children with diabetic ketoacidosis. *Crit Care Med, 31*, 80–83.

94. Ruud, E., Holmstrom, H., Natvig, S., et al. (2002). Prevalence of thrombophilia and central venous catheter–associated neck vein thrombosis in 41 children with cancer: a prospective study. *Med Pediatr Oncol, 38*, 405–410.

95. Parasuraman, S., & Goldhaber, S. Z. (2006). Venous thromboembolism in children. *Circulation, 113*, e12–e16.

96. Federal Interagency Forum on Aging Related Statistics. (2012). *Older Americans 2012: key indicators of well-being*. Retrieved from http://www.AgingStats.gov. Accessed 28.06.13.

97. Zauber, N. P., & Zauber, A. G. (1987). Hematologic data of healthy old people. *JAMA, 257*, 2181–2184.

98. Chatta, G. S., & Dale, D. C. (1996). Aging and haemopoiesis: implications for treatment with haemopoietic growth factors. *Drugs Aging, 9*, 37–47.

99. Lansdorp, P. M. (1997). Self-renewal of stem cells. *Biol Blood Marrow Transplant, 3*, 171–178.

100. Hartstock, R. J., Smith, E. B., & Petty, C. S. (1965). Normal variation with aging of the amount of hematopoietic tissue in bone marrow from the anterior iliac crest. *Am J Clin Pathol, 43*, 326–331.

101. Ricci, C., Cova, M., Kang, Y., et al. (1990). Normal age-related pattern of cellular and fatty bone marrow distribution in the axial skeleton: MR imaging study. *Radiology, 177*, 83–88.

102. Frenck, R. W., Jr., Blackburn, E. H., & Shannon, K. M. (1998). The rate of telomere sequence loss in human leukocyte varies with age. *Proc Natl Acad Sci U S A, 95*, 5607–5610.

103. Sahin, E., & DePinho, R. A. (2010). Linking functional decline of telomeres, mitochondria and stem cells during ageing. *Nature, 464*, 520–528.

104. Nilsson-Ehle, H., Jagenburg, R., Landahl, S., et al. (2000). Blood haemoglobin values in the elderly: implications for reference intervals from age 70 to 88. *Eur J Haematol, 65*, 296–305.

105. Myers, A. M., Saunders, C. R., & Chalmers, D. G. (1968). The haemoglobin level of fit elderly people. *Lancet, 2*, 261–263.

106. Salive, M. E., Cornoni-Huntley, J., Guralnik, J. M., et al. (1992). Anemia and hemoglobin level in older persons: relationship with age, gender and health status. *J Am Geriatr Soc, 40*, 489–496.

107. Allan, R. N., & Alexander, M. K. (1965). A sex difference in the leukocyte count. *J Clin Pathol, 21*, 691–694.

108. Panda, A., Arjona, A., Sapey, E., et al. (2009). Human innate immunosenescence: causes and consequences for immunity in old age. *Trends Immunol, 30*, 325–333.

109. Fulop, T., Pawalec, G., Castle, S., & Loeb, M. (2009). Immunosenescence and vaccination in nursing home residents. *Clin Infect Dis, 48*, 443–448.

110. Fulop, T., Larbi, A., Wikby, A., et al. (2005). Dysregulation of T cell function in the elderly: scientific basis and clinical implications. *Drugs Aging, 22*, 589–603.

111. Mangolas, S. C., & Jilka, R. L. (1995). Bone marrow, cytokines and bone remodeling. *N Engl J Med, 332*, 302–311.

112. Globerson, A. (1995). T lymphocytes and aging. *Int Arch Allergy Immunol, 107*, 491–497.

113. Nel, A. E., & Slaughter, N. (2002). T-cell activation through the antigen receptor, part 2: role of signaling cascades in T-cell differentiation, anergy, immune senescence, and development of immunotherapy. *J Allergy Clin Immunol, 109*, 901–915.

114. Larbi, A., Douziech, N., Dupuis, G., et al. (2004). Age-associated alterations in the recruitment of signal transduction proteins to lipid rafts in human T lymphocytes. *J Leukoc Biol, 75*, 373–381.

115. Larbi, A., Dupuis, G., Khalil, A., et al. (2006). Differential role of lipid rafts in the functions of CD4+ and CD8+ human T lymphocytes with aging. *Cell Signal, 18*, 1017–1030.

116. Song, L., Kim, Y. H., Chopra, R. K., et al. (1993). Age related effects in T cell activation and proliferation. *Exp Gerontol, 28*, 313–321.

117. Wick, G., & Grubeck-Lobenstein, B. (1997). The aging immune system: primary and secondary alterations of immune reactivity in the elderly. *Exp Gerontol, 32*, 401–413.

118. Kawai, T., Akira, S. (2007). TLR signaling. *Semin Immunol, 19*, 24–32.

119. Sansoni, P., Cossarizza, A., Brianti, V., et al. (1993). Lymphocyte subsets and natural killer cell activity in healthy old people and centenarians. *Blood, 82*, 2767–2773.

120. Grubeck-Lobenstein, B. (1997). Changes in the aging immune system. *Biologicals, 25*, 205–208.

121. Tefferi, A., Thiele, J., Orazi, A., et al. (2007). Proposals and rationale for revision of the World Health Organization diagnostic criteria for polycythemia vera, essential thrombocythemia, and primary myelofibrosis: recommendation from an ad hoc international expert panel. *Blood, 110*, 1092–1097.

122. Zahavi, J., Jones, N. A., Leyton, J., et al. (1980). Enhanced in vivo platelet "release reaction" in old healthy individuals. *Thromb Res, 17*, 329–336.

123. Chong, B. H. (1995). Heparin-induced thrombocytopenia. *Br J Haematol, 89*, 431–439.

124. Cortelazzo, S., Finazzi, G., Ruggeri, M., et al. (1995). Hydroxyurea for patients with essential thrombocythemia and a high risk for thrombosis. *N Engl J Med, 332*, 1132–1136.

125. Balducci, L. (2003). Anemia, cancer, and aging. *Cancer Control, 10*, 478–486.

126. Guralnik, J., Eisenstaedt, R., Ferrucci, L., et al. (2004). Prevalence of anemia in persons 65 years and older in the United States: evidence for a high rate of unexplained anemia. *Blood, 104*, 2263–2268.

127. Izaka, G. J., Westendorp, R. G., & Knook, D. L. (1999). The definition of anemia in older persons. *JAMA, 281*, 1714–1717.

128. Lipschitz, D. (2003). Medical and functional consequences of anemia in the elderly. *J Am Geriatr Soc, 51*(Suppl), 10–13.

129. Beghé, C., Wilson, A., & Ershler, W. B. (2004). Prevalence and outcomes of anemia in geriatrics: a systematic review of the literature. *Am J Med, 116*, 3S–10S.

130. Price, E. A., Mehra, R., Holmes, T. H., et al. (2011). Anemia in older persons: etiology and evaluation. *Blood Cell Mol Dis, 46*, 159–165.

131. Howe, R. B. (1983). Anemia in the elderly. *Postgrad Med, 73*, 153–160.

132. Timiras, M. L., & Brownstein, H. (1987). Prevalence of anemia and correlation of hemoglobin with age in a geriatric screening clinic population. *J Am Geriatr Soc, 35*, 639–643.

133. Ania, B. J., Suman, V. J., Fairbanks, V. F., et al. (1994). Prevalence of anemia in medical practice: community versus referral patients. *Mayo Clin Proc, 69*, 730–735.

134. Smith, D. (2002). Management and treatment of anemia in the elderly. *Clin Geriatr, 10*, 8.

135. Daly, M. P. (1989). Anemia in the elderly. *Am Fam Physician, 39*, 129–136.

136. Walsh, J. R. (1997). Hematologic problems. In Cassel, C. K., Cohen, H. J., Larson, E. B., et al., (Eds.), *Geriatric Medicine*. (3rd ed., pp. 627–636). New York: Springer Verlag.

137. Lipschitz, D. A. (1990). The anemia of chronic disease. *J Am Geriatr Soc, 38*, 1258–1264.

138. Gardner, L. B., & Benz, E. J. (2009). Anemia of chronic diseases. In Hoffman, R., Furie, B., Benz, E. J., Jr., et al., (Eds.),

Hematology Basic Principles and Practices. (5th ed.). Philadelphia: Saunders.

139. Cash, J., Sears, D. A. (1989). The anemia of chronic disease: spectrum of associated disease in a series of unselected hospitalized patients. *Am J Med, 87,* 638–644.

140. Joosten, E. (2004). Strategies for the laboratory diagnosis of some common causes of anaemia in elderly patients. *Gerontology, 50,* 49–56.

141. Ania, B. J., Suman, V. J., Fairbanks, V. F., et al. (1994). Prevalence of anemia in medical practice: community versus referral patients. *Mayo Clin Proc, 69,* 730–735.

142. Means, R. T. (2000). The anaemia of infection. *Baillieres Clin Haematol, 13,* 151–162.

143. Kanapuru, B., & Ershler, W. B. (2010). Blood disorders in the elderly. On Fillit, H. M., Rockwood, K., & Woodhouse, K., (Eds.), *Brocklehurst's Textbook of Geriatric Medicine and Gerontology.* (7th ed., pp. 775–790). Philadelphia: Saunders Elsevier.

144. Smith, D. I. (2000). Anemia in the elderly. *Am Fam Physician, 62,* 1565–1572.

145. Chiari, M. M., Bagnoli, R., DeLuca, P., et al. (1995). Influence of acute inflammation on iron and nutritional status indexes in older inpatients. *J Am Geriatr Soc, 43,* 767–771.

146. Daly, M. P. (1989). Anemia in the elderly. *Am Fam Physician, 39,* 129–136.

147. Pennypacker, L. C., Allen, R. H., Kelly, J. P., et al. (1992). High prevalence of cobalamin deficiency in elderly outpatients. *J Am Geriatr Soc, 40,* 1197–1204.

148. Stabler, S. P. (1998). Vitamin B$_{12}$ deficiency in older people: improving diagnosis and preventing disability. *J Am Geriatr Soc, 46,* 1317–1319.

149. Nexo, E., Hansen, M., Rasmussen, K., et al. (1994). How to diagnosis cobalamin deficiency. *Scand J Clin Lab Invest Suppl, 219,* 61–76.

150. Powell, D. E., & Thomas, J. H. (1969). The iron binding capacity of serum in elderly hospital patients. *Gerontol Clin (Basel), 11,* 36–47.

151. Healton, E. B., Savage, D. G., Brust, J. C., et al. (1991). Neurologic aspects of cobalamin deficiency. *Medicine, 70,* 229–244.

152. Savage, D. G., & Lindenbaum, J. (1995). Neurological complications of acquired cobalamin deficiency: clinical aspects. *Baillieres Clin Haematol, 8,* 657–678.

153. Matthews, J. H. (1999). Cobalamin and folate deficiency in the elderly. *Baillieres Clin Haematol, 54,* 245–253.

154. Doscherholmen, A., & Swaim, W. R. (1973). Impaired assimilation of egg ^{57}Co vitamin B$_{12}$ in patients with hypochlorhydria and achlorhydria and after gastric resection. *Gastroenterology, 64,* 913–919.

155. Suter, P. M., Golner, B. B., Goldin, B. R., et al. (1991). Reversal of protein-bound vitamin B$_{12}$ malabsorption with antibiotics in atrophic gastritis. *Gastroenterology, 101,* 1039–1045.

156. Baik, H. W., & Russell, R. M. (1999). Vitamin B$_{12}$ deficiency in the elderly. *Annu Rev Nutr, 19,* 357–377.

157. Carmel, R. (1996). Prevalence of undiagnosed pernicious anemia in the elderly. *Arch Intern Med, 156,* 1097–1100.

158. Norman, E. J., & Morrison, J. A. (1993). Screening elderly populations for cobalamin (vitamin B$_{12}$) deficiency using the urinary methymalonic acid assay by gas chromatography mass spectrometry. *Am J Med, 94,* 489–494.

159. Loikas, S., Koskinen, P., Irjala, K., et al. (2007). Vitamin B$_{12}$ deficiency in the aged: a population-based study. *Age Ageing, 36,* 177–183.

160. Karnaze, D. S., & Carmel, R. (1987). Low serum cobalamin levels in primary degenerative dementia. *Arch Intern Med, 17,* 429–431.

161. Pfeiffer, C. M., Johnson, C. L., Jain, R. B., et al. (2007). Trends in blood folate and vitamin B-12 concentrations in the United States, 1988-2004. *Am J Clin Nutr, 86,* 718–727.

162. Andrews, N. C., & Schmidt, P. J. (2007). Iron homeostasis. *Annu Rev Physiol, 69,* 69–85.

163. Lindenbaum, J. (1980). Folate and vitamin B$_{12}$ deficiencies in alcoholism. *Semin Hematol, 17,* 119–128.

164. Petz, L. D. (1980). Drug-induced immune haemolytic anaemia. *Clin Haematol, 9,* 455–482.

165. Saba, H. A. (2001). Myelodysplastic syndromes in the elderly. *Cancer Control, 8*(1), 79–102. Retrieved from http://www .moffitt.org/research—clinical-trials/cancer-control-journal/ oncologic-support-and-care. Accessed 10.07.13.

166. Howlander, N., Noone, A. M., Krapcho, M., et al., (Eds.). (2010). *SEER Cancer Statistics Review, 1975-2010.* Bethesda, Md: National Cancer Institute. Based on November 2012 SEER data submission, posted to the SEER website 2013. Retrieved from http://seer.cancer.gov/csr/1975_2010/. Accessed 10.07.13.

167. Engbers, M. J., Van Hylckama Vlieg, A., Rosendall, F. R. (2010). Venous thrombosis in the elderly: incidence, risk factors and risk groups. *J Thromb Haemost, 8,* 2105–2112.

168. Naess, I. A., Christiansen, S. C., Romendstad, P., et al. (2007). Incidence and mortality of venous thrombosis: a population-based study. *J Thromb Haemost, 5,* 692–699.

169. Franchini, M. (2006). Hemostasis and aging. *Crit Rev Oncol Hematol, 60,* 144–151.

170. Kannel, W. B., Wolf, P. A., Castelli, W. P., et al. (1987). Fibrinogen and risk of cardiovascular disease. The Framingham Study. *JAMA, 258,* 1183–1186.

171. Koster, T., Blann, A. D., Briët, E., et al. (1995). Role of clotting factor VIII in effect of von Willebrand factor on occurrence of deep-vein thrombosis. *Lancet, 345,* 152–155.

172. Cushman, M., Lemaitre, R. N., Kuller, L. H., et al. (1999). Fibrinolytic activation markers predict myocardial infarction in the elderly. The Cardiovascular Health Study. *Arterioscler Thromb Vasc Biol, 19,* 493–498.

173. Yamamoto, K., Takeshita, K., Shimokawa, T., et al. (2002). Plasminogen activator inhibitor-1 is a major stress-regulated gene: implications for stress-induced thrombosis in aged individuals. *Proc Natl Acad Sci U S A, 99,* 890–895.

174. Yamamoto, K., Takeshita, K., Kojima, T., et al. (2005). Aging and plasminogen activator inhibitor-1 (PAI-1) regulation: implication in the pathogenesis of thrombotic disorders in the elderly. *Cardiovasc Res, 66,* 276–285.

175. Jørgensen, K. A., Dyerberg, J., Olesen, A. S., et al. (1980). Acetylsalicylic acid, bleeding time and age. *Thromb Res, 19,* 799–805.

176. Zahavi, J., Jones, N. A., Leyton, J., et al. (1980). Enhanced in vivo platelet "release reaction" in old healthy individuals. *Thromb Res, 17,* 329–336.

177. Bastyr, E. J., 3rd., Kadrofske, M. M., & Vinik, A. I. (1990). Platelet activity and phosphoinositide turnover increase with advancing age. *Am J Med, 88,* 601–606.

Answers

CHAPTER 2

Case Study

1. This item describes two deficiencies. First, the hematology laboratory scientist should have washed his/her hands after removing the gloves and before leaving the laboratory. Second, the hematology laboratory scientist should have removed his/her laboratory coat before going to the meeting.
2. This item describes a deficiency. Storage of food in a specimen refrigerator is prohibited.
3. This may or may not be a deficiency. The laboratory employees may have had on a personal laboratory coat. A second laboratory coat could have been obtained by the employees to wear in public areas. Some laboratories require different colored lab coats for public areas.
4. No deficiency is indicated. Fire extinguishers should be placed every 75 feet.
5. This item describes a deficiency. Fire extinguishers should be inspected monthly and maintained annually.
6. This item represents a deficiency. All chemicals should be labeled.
7. This item represents a deficiency. The 1:10 bleach solution should be made fresh daily.
8. No deficiency is indicated. Gloves should be worn by all personnel handling specimens.
9. No deficiency is indicated. Safety data sheets can be received by fax.
10. This item describes a deficiency. Chemicals should not be stored alphabetically, but according to storage requirements specified in the safety data sheets.

Review Questions

1. d; 2. b; 3. c; 4. c; 5. a; 6. b; 7. c; 8. b; 9. b; 10. b; 11. d

CHAPTER 3

Case Studies

Case 1

The proper procedure is to ask the patient to state his/her full name and then confirm by asking his/her birth date and/or address. The phlebotomist should not prelabel tubes; tubes should be labeled after the blood is drawn and before leaving the patient.

Case 2

Test results that can be affected by this selection of tubes and order of draw include the prothrombin time (PT), potassium, and type and screen.

- The light blue stopper tube for the PT should not have been collected after the serum separator tube (which contains an inert gel and clot activator). The clot activator could contaminate the blue stopper tube, activate coagulation factors, and cause an error in the PT results.

- The green stopper tube for potassium should not have been collected after a lavender stopper tube (which contains EDTA, usually as a potassium salt). The potassium-EDTA could be carried over into the green stopper tube and falsely elevate the potassium level. The potassium could, however, be assayed in the serum separator tube.
- The type and screen cannot be done on blood from the serum separator tube because the gel interferes with blood bank procedures; the lavender stopper tube, however, could be used for the type and screen. Box 3-2 contains the correct order of draw for evacuated tubes.

Review Questions

1. a; 2. b; 3. b; 4. c; 5. b; 6. b; 7. b; 8. d; 9. b; 10. c; 11. c; 12. a

CHAPTER 4

Case Study

The following things should be checked:

Is the slide right side up? This is the most common cause of inability to focus a slide under oil when it has been focused under $10\times$ and $40\times$ objectives.

If the slide is right side up, continue by checking the following:

- Is there sufficient oil on the slide? If not, clean off all the residual oil first and then apply another drop of oil.
- Is the objective screwed in tightly? If not, tighten the objective.
- If the slide has a coverslip, is there more than one coverslip on the slide? If so, gently remove the top coverslip.
- Has oil seeped into the seal on the oil objective? Examine by removing the objective and use an inverted eyepiece as a magnifier to check the seal. If the seal is broken, the objective must be replaced.

Review Questions

1. b; 2. c; 3. a; 4. b; 5. c; 6. c; 7. d; 8. a; 9. c; 10. d; 11. b

CHAPTER 5

Case Study

1. This is a systematic error because the magnitude of error remains constant at three ranges of test results.
2. It is not acceptable to continue using the instrument or to simply subtract the systematic error from test sample results. All the samples in a two out-of-control test run must be re-assayed after the error is corrected.
3. Determine from the quality control charts at what moment the error occurred. Investigate potential changes in instrument settings, calibration, reagent changes, or instrument malfunction that may have occurred at the time the error was recorded.

Review Questions

1. d; 2. c; 3. b; 4. b; 5. b; 6. a; 7. d; 8. d; 9. c; 10. c; 11. c; 12. a; 13. b; 14. c; 15. a; 16. b

---

CHAPTER 6

Review Questions

1. b; 2. b; 3. a; 4. b; 5. c; 6. a; 7. d; 8. d; 9. c; 10. b; 11. a; 12. d; 13. b; 14. a

---

CHAPTER 7

Review Questions

1. a; 2. d; 3. c; 4. a; 5. b; 6. c; 7. c; 8. b; 9. a; 10. d; 11. a; 12. b

---

CHAPTER 8

Case Study

1. When the blood is not well oxygenated, the bone marrow responds by producing more red blood cells to carry more oxygen.
2. The hormone that stimulates RBC production is erythropoietin (EPO). The peritubular cells of the kidney detect hypoxia. A hypoxia-sensitive transcription factor is produced that moves to the peritubular cell nucleus and upregulates transcription of the EPO gene. EPO acts by preventing apoptosis of the erythroid colony-forming unit. In RBC precursors, it also shortens the cell cycle time between mitoses and reduces the number of mitotic divisions; and it promotes early release of reticulocytes from the bone marrow.
3. Once the patient was receiving oxygen therapy, hypoxia diminished and EPO production also declined. Thus, production of new RBCs slowed. At the same time, RBCs reaching 120 days of age were removed from the circulation. Thus the total number of circulating RBCs decreased.

Review Questions

1. c; 2. a; 3. d; 4. b; 5. b; 6. d; 7. a; 8. d; 9. a; 10. c; 11. b; 12. b

---

CHAPTER 9

Case Study

1. A reducing agent is able to donate an electron to an oxidized compound so that the oxidized compound has one fewer unpaired proton. The compound receiving the electron becomes reduced and the donating compound becomes oxidized.
2. When heme iron is oxidized, the molecule cannot carry oxygen and patients become cyanotic. Because vitamin C eliminated the cyanosis, it must be able to reduce methemoglobin and restore the oxygen-carrying capacity of the blood.
3. Because this condition affected brothers, a hereditary condition was suggested in which hemoglobin became oxidized more than is usual. (The condition affecting these brothers was later identified as a hereditary deficiency of methemoglobin reductase.)

Review Questions

1. a; 2. c; 3. b; 4. d; 5. b; 6. b; 7. a; 8. c; 9. a; 10. a; 11. a; 12. a

---

CHAPTER 10

Case Study

1. The mother's and infant's hemoglobin results were within the reference intervals. (Reference intervals: adult women, 12.0 to 15.0 g/dL; newborns, 16.5 to 21.5 g/dL.)

2. The major hemoglobin at birth is Hb F. It has a high oxygen affinity because it weakly binds 2,3-BPG resulting in decreased delivery of oxygen to the tissues. The hypoxia triggers an increase in secretion of erythropoietin by the fetal kidney, which results in an increase in the production and release of red blood cells from the fetal bone marrow. The resultant increase in red blood cell count, hemoglobin concentration, and hematocrit compensates for the high Hb F oxygen affinity and reduced oxygen transfer to tissues. The Hb F concentration gradually decreases to adult physiologic levels by 1 to 2 years of age as most of the Hb F is replaced by Hb A.
3. The hemoglobin assay measures concentration; high performance liquid chromatography (and hemoglobin electrophoresis) identifies and quantifies hemoglobin types.
4. These are the expected results for hemoglobin fractions for a healthy mother and infant. In the second and third trimesters of fetal life, the α- and γ-globin genes are activated producing α and γ globin chains that combine to form Hb F. In late fetal life, γ-β switching begins in which transcription of the β-globin gene begins to be activated and the γ-globin gene begins to be repressed. With the activation of the β-globin gene, the β chains combine with the α chains to form Hb A. The Hb F level decreases from 60% to 90% at birth to 1% to 2% by 1 to 2 years of age, while the Hb A increases from 10% to 40% at birth to greater than 95% at 1 to 2 years of age and throughout life. The synthesis of Hb A_2 begins shortly before birth and remains at less than 3.5% throughout life.

Review Questions

1. d; 2. a; 3. a; 4. a; 5. a; 6. d; 7. c; 8. b; 9. d; 10. b; 11. c

---

CHAPTER 11

Case Study

1. Iron loss via blood donations and normal physiologic loss was not compensated by diet or supplementation.
2. Adaptation to the low iron levels. Iron stores of ferritin were mobilized first. But when storage iron declined, hepcidin levels declined, and as a result, duodenal iron absorption increased.
3. Ferritin
4. Transferrin saturation reflects the proportion of transferrin binding sites for iron that are actually filled with iron during transit in the plasma. Transferrin level is an indirect indicator of the iron storage compartment while serum iron is the transport compartment, so transferrin saturation effectively reflects both compartments.

Review Questions

1. c; 2. b; 3. c; 4. c; 5. c; 6. b; 7. d; 8. b; 9. d; 10. c; 11. b; 12. d

---

CHAPTER 12

Case Study

1. The patient had an asthmatic attack. Eosinophils play an important role in the initiation and maintenance of symptoms. Eosinophils release basic proteins, lipid mediators, and reactive oxygen species that cause inflammation and damage to the mucosal cells lining the airway.
2. Eosinophils are typically elevated in the peripheral blood and also in the sputum of asthmatic patients. The number of eosinophils in the blood correlates with the severity of the case.
3. IL-5 plays an important role in the differentiation and proliferation of eosinophils. Monoclonal antibodies to IL-5 block eosinophil development. Since eosinophils are reduced, the symptoms of asthma are controlled.

Review Questions

1. b; 2. d; 3. a; 4. c; 5. b; 6. c; 7. c; 8. a; 9. b; 10. d

CHAPTER 13

Case Study

1. Bleeding characterized by petechiae, purpura, and ecchymoses is known as *mucocutaneous bleeding,* also called *systemic bleeding.* By contrast, *anatomic bleeding* is bleeding into soft tissue, muscles, joints, or body cavities.
2. *Thrombocytopenia,* or low platelet count, is a common cause of mucocutaneous bleeding. Another is diseases that weaken vascular collagen such as scurvy.
3. No, the bone marrow megakaryocyte estimate is high, indicating an increase in platelet production.
4. *Thrombopoietin* and *interleukin-11* have the greatest effect on recruitment and proliferation of megakaryocytes and their progenitors. Also involved in early progenitor recruitment are interleukin-3 and interleukin-6. Other cytokines and hormones that participate synergistically with thrombopoietin and the interleukins are KIT ligand, also called *stem cell factor* or *mast cell growth factor;* granulocyte-macrophage colony-stimulating factor; granulocyte colony-stimulating factor; and erythropoietin.

Review Questions

1. d; 2. d; 3. c; 4. b; 5. d; 6. d; 7. a; 8. a; 9. c; 10. d

CHAPTER 14

Case Studies

Case 1

1. HGB × 3 = HCT ± 3
   15 × 3 = 45 ± 3 (42−48)
2. Hemoglobin can be falsely elevated by lipemia, increased WBC count, or presence of Hb S or Hb C. Hematocrit can be falsely decreased by a short draw in an EDTA-anticoagulated tube causing RBC shrinkage, or contamination of the specimen with intravenous fluids. In the microhematocrit method, false decreases can be caused by improper sealing of the capillary tube, errors in reading the microhematocrit reader, excessive centrifugation, and improper mixing of the specimen.
3. For lipemia, replace lipemic plasma with an equal amount of saline and retest; or use a plasma blank. For increased WBC count, centrifuge the hemoglobin/reagent solution and read the % T of the supernatant (manual procedure). For specimens with Hb S or Hb C, make a 1 : 2 dilution of blood with distilled water and multiply the result by 2. For the microhematocrit, check if the specimen tube was filled to the proper level, and ensure the procedure is performed correctly.

Case 2

1. MCV = 59 fL; MCH = 18.1 pg; MCHC = 30.7 g/dL.
2. Microcytic, hypochromic red blood cells
3. Examine the patient's peripheral blood film

Case 3

1. The sodium concentration could affect the hematocrit. The sample electrolyte concentration is used to correct the measured conductivity prior to reporting hematocrit results. Factors that affect sodium concentration will therefore also affect the hematocrit.
2. A high sodium concentration would falsely decrease the hematocrit.
3. Factors that decrease the hematocrit by this method are low total protein, settling of red blood cells in the collection device, presence of cold agglutinins, and specimen contamination by intravenous solutions.

Review Questions

1. b; 2. c; 3. c; 4. d; 5. d; 6. b; 7. c; 8. c; 9. a; 10. d

CHAPTER 15

Review Questions

1. d; 2. a; 3. d; 4. c; 5. c; 6. Impedance - c; RF - b; optical scatter - a; 7. b; 8. b; 9. c; 10. Abbott CELL-DYN Sapphire - b; Siemens ADVIA 2120i - c; Sysmex XN-1000 - d; Beckman Coulter UniCel DxH 800 - a.

CHAPTER 16

Case Study

1. The patient's hemoglobin shows neither anemia or polycythemia; hence it is normal. Red blood cells are normocytic and normochromic with no anisocytosis. The blood picture shows leukocytosis and thrombocytopenia. The mean platelet volume is slightly low, which suggests small average platelet volume. There is no white blood cell (WBC) differential.
2. The platelet count and WBC count should be questioned because of platelet clumping. EDTA-induced pseudothrombocytopenia and pseudoleukocytosis most likely occurred.
3. The specimen should be redrawn in sodium citrate and processed through the automated analyzer. The new WBC and platelet counts should then be adjusted for the sodium citrate dilution by multiplying the results by the dilution factor 10/9 or 1.1. The following are the new results:
   a. WBCs for specimen drawn in sodium citrate: $(8.4 \times 10^9/L) \times 1.1 = 9.2 \times 10^9/L$ (the corrected WBC count)
   b. Platelets for specimen drawn in sodium citrate: $(231 \times 10^9/L) \times 1.1 = 254 \times 10^9/L$ (the corrected platelet count)

Review Questions

1. d; 2. c; 3. a; 4. c; 5. b; 6. c; 7. a; 8. b; 9. b; 10. a

CHAPTER 17

Case Study

1. Bone marrow cellularity, estimated from the core biopsy specimen, or the aspirate if a biopsy specimen is unavailable, provides information on blood cell production.
2. The ratio is 9:1, which indicates myeloid hyperplasia.
3. When a bone marrow aspirate or core biopsy specimen is reviewed, the normal megakaryocyte distribution is 2 to 10 per low-power field. Counts outside these limits are characterized as decreased or increased megakaryocytes. Megakaryocyte morphology is also reviewed for diameter, granularity, and nuclear lobularity.

Review Questions

1. c; 2. b; 3. c; 4. a; 5. d; 6. c; 7. d; 8. b; 9. b; 10. b; 11. b

CHAPTER 18

Case Study

1. Tube 3 or the least bloody tube.
2. A 1:53 dilution with saline is necessary for a satisfactory cytocentrifuge slide.
3. Bacteria.
4. The most likely diagnosis is bacterial meningitis.

Review Questions

1. b; 2. a; 3. c; 4. b; 5. a; 6. b; 7. c; 8. d; 9. c; 10. a

CHAPTER 19

Case Study

1. Anemia is not a disease or diagnosis in itself but is the symptom of an underlying disorder. A complete history and physical examination are necessary to help identify the cause(s) of the anemia. If the underlying cause is not determined and corrected, the patient will continue to be anemic. Questions regarding lifestyle, medications, and bleeding history are only some of the questions that should be asked.

2. The reticulocyte count differentiates anemias into those involving impaired production (decreased reticulocyte count) and increased destruction (increased reticulocyte count). Anemia can also be classified on the basis of mean cell volume into normocytic, microcytic, or macrocytic. With that knowledge, appropriate laboratory testing can be ordered to determine the cause.

3. The peripheral blood film yields valuable information about the volume and hemoglobin content of the erythrocytes as well as any abnormal shapes, which may be correlated with specific causes. Some anemias are also associated with white blood cell and/or platelet abnormalities, which may be noted on the blood film.

Review Questions

1. c; 2. b; 3. d; 4. c; 5. c; 6. b; 7. c; 8. d; 9. b; 10. c; 11. d

CHAPTER 20

Case Study

1. The patient's results demonstrate a severe hypochromic, microcytic anemia with anisocytosis. There is no evidence of a bone marrow response as there is no polychromasia mentioned in the morphology which does note unspecified poikilocytosis, anisocytosis, hypochromia, and microcytosis, all consistent with the numerical values. The white blood cells are unremarkable in number, distribution, and morphology as are the platelets.

2. Hypochromic, microcytic anemias to be considered include iron deficiency anemia, thalassemia, hemoglobin E disease, sideroblastic anemias, and possibly, anemia of chronic inflammation.

3. Thalassemia and hemoglobin E disease can be eliminated because they are not conditions that would be acquired late in life.

4. Anemia of chronic inflammation could be eliminated in this case because the woman is otherwise healthy. Although iron deficiency anemia is not as common in women after menopause, it is probably the most likely of the remaining possibilities for an anemia that is this severe.

5. Iron studies, including ferritin, would be useful in clarifying the patient's diagnosis. Assuming that she is iron deficient, the ferritin, total serum iron, and percent saturation should all be decreased, whereas total iron-binding capacity (TIBC) would be expected to be increased. Upon hospitalization, the patient was immediately placed on oxygen while laboratory tests were ordered. With the confirmation by the hospital laboratory of a dangerously low hemoglobin, transfusions were ordered, and the patient received 3 units of packed cells over the first 2 days of hospitalization. The transfusions were administered very slowly so as not to stress her cardiovascular system with added volume. Noting the hypochromic, microcytic blood picture, the physician ordered iron studies on blood specimens drawn before the transfusions. The results

were as follows: serum iron decreased, TIBC increased, percent saturation decreased, and ferritin decreased. The possibility of gastrointestinal bleeding as a cause for iron deficiency was investigated. Results of tests for occult blood in the stool were negative. The hospital dietitian assessed the patient's usual diet of tea, toast, canned soup, and crackers and determined that it was quite inadequate not only in iron, but also in other important nutrients. The physician concluded that the patient's dietary iron deficiency had developed slowly, which had allowed her to adapt to the exceedingly low hemoglobin level. Furthermore, her low level of activity meant that she rarely experienced the effects of the anemia. She was started on a course of oral iron supplementation and arrangements were made for her to receive one balanced meal daily from the Meals on Wheels program sponsored through a community service organization for senior citizens. She was quite responsible about taking her iron supplements, and her hemoglobin was within the reference interval within 3 months.

Review Questions

1. b; 2. a; 3. d; 4. a; 5. c; 6. a; 7. d; 8. c; 9. b; 10. d; 11. b; 12. d

CHAPTER 21

Case Study

1. The complete blood count findings for this patient (notably macrocytic, normochromic anemia; pancytopenia; hypersegmentation of neutrophils; and oval macrocytes) were consistent with the physician's suspicion of megaloblastic anemia as suggested by the clinical findings.

2. Although the relative reticulocyte count was within the reference interval of 0.5% to 2.5%, and the calculated absolute reticulocyte count (approximately $40 \times 10^9/L$) was within the reference interval of 20 to $115 \times 10^9/L$, the calculated reticulocyte production index was 0.5, which was clearly inadequate to compensate for a substantial anemia (Chapter 14).

3. The patient's vitamin assays point to a deficiency of vitamin B_{12}, substantiated by an increase in serum methylmalonic acid.

4. Based on these results, a test for intrinsic factor blocking antibodies would be appropriate. However, the physician also inquired further about the patient's dietary habits and learned that he enjoyed dishes of raw fish obtained from the surrounding lakes. Therefore, the physician ordered a stool analysis for ova and parasites. The study indicated the presence in the stool of both eggs and proglottids of the fish tapeworm *Diphyllobothrium latum*. The patient was treated with a suitable purgative, and the scolex of the tapeworm was discovered in a stool sample after a single treatment. The patient was counseled on the proper preparation of fresh fish to avoid reinfection. He received injections of cyanocobalamin to replenish his vitamin B_{12} stores. His hemoglobin returned to normal over the next month, and his neurologic symptoms subsided.

Review Questions

1. d; 2. c; 3. c; 4. b; 5. a; 6. b; 7. c; 8. d; 9. a; 10. c

CHAPTER 22

Case Study

1. The term used to describe a decrease in all cell lines is *pancytopenia*.

2. Acquired aplastic anemia should be considered due to the pancytopenia, reticulocytopenia, bone marrow hypocellularity, normal vitamin B_{12} and folate levels, absence of blasts and abnormal cells

in the bone marrow and peripheral blood, normal myelopoiesis and megakaryopoiesis, and history of autoimmune hepatitis.

3. An increase in blasts or reticulin in the bone marrow suggests a diagnosis of myelodysplasia or leukemia.

4. The extent of the patient's bone marrow hypocellularity, her hemoglobin concentration, and neutrophil and platelet counts place her disorder in the severe aplastic anemia category.

5. Because of her age and the severity of her aplastic anemia, hematopoietic stem cell transplant is the treatment of choice if she has an HLA-identical sibling. If an HLA-identical sibling is not available, an HLA-matched unrelated donor or immunosuppressive therapy (anthymocyte globulin and cyclosporine) may be considered. Blood product replacement should be given judiciously to avoid alloimmunization. In general, red blood cells would be transfused if the patient had symptoms of anemia, whereas platelet transfusions would be given if her platelet count fell below $10 \times 10^9/L$.

Review Questions

1. c; 2. d; 3. b; 4. d; 5. b; 6. d; 7. c; 8. d; 9. c; 10. d; 11. a

CHAPTER 23

Case Study

1. Intravascular hemolysis is suspected in the patient because the color of the urine suggests oxidized hemoglobin.

2. Tests for serum haptoglobin, serum unconjugated (indirect) bilirubin, serum lactate dehydrogenase, plasma hemoglobin, and urine hemoglobin and examination of a peripheral blood film can differentiate the mechanism of hemolysis as fragmentation or macrophage-mediated.

3. Due to the likelihood that the patient had hemoglobinuria, fragmentation hemolysis was suspected. Therefore, the serum haptoglobin would be markedly decreased, while the serum lactate dehydrogenase and plasma hemoglobin levels would be increased, if measured. Routine urinalysis should yield positive results for blood on the test strip with no intact red blood cells in the urine sediment. The serum indirect bilirubin does not increase immediately after an episode of intravascular hemolysis, but should begin to increase within several days. The peripheral blood film may demonstrate schistocytes immediately, but reticulocytosis several days later.

Review Questions

1. a; 2. b; 3. d; 4. b; 5. c; 6. a; 7. d; 8. b; 9. c; 10. c

CHAPTER 24

Case Study

1. On the basis of the patient's jaundice and splenomegaly, history of gallstones, family history of anemia, low hemoglobin, increased mean cell hemoglobin concentration and red cell distribution width, and spherocytes and polychromasia on the peripheral blood film, hereditary spherocytosis (HS) is suspected.

2. Additional laboratory tests to confirm HS should demonstrate increased hemolysis (increased serum indirect bilirubin level and lactate dehydrogenase activity, decreased serum haptoglobin level), increased erythropoiesis to compensate for the premature hemolysis (increased reticulocyte count), and the nonimmune nature of the hemolysis (negative result on the direct antiglobulin test). Testing family members to establish a mode of inheritance is desirable. The osmotic fragility test is expected to show increased fragility and the eosin-5'-maleimide (EMA) binding test is expected to show low mean fluorescence intensity of the red blood cells when measured in a flow cytometer. However, special tests are not required for diagnosis of HS in a patient with a familial inheritance pattern and the typical clinical and laboratory findings.

3. HS is an inherited intrinsic hemolytic anemia caused by a mutation that disrupts the vertical protein interactions in the red blood cell (RBC) membrane. Various mutations in five known genes can result in the HS phenotype. The defective membrane protein causes the RBCs to lose unsupported lipid membrane over time due to a local disconnection between transmembrane proteins and the cytoskeleton. The loss of membrane with minimal loss of cell volume results in a decreased surface area-to-volume ratio and the formation of spherocytes. Spherocytes do not have the deformability of normal biconcave discoid RBCs. As the cells repeatedly go through the spleen, they lose more membrane due to splenic conditioning and eventually become trapped in the spleen and removed by the splenic macrophages. The RBC membrane also has abnormal permeability to cations, particularly sodium and potassium, likely due to the disruption of the cytoskeleton by the mutated protein.

Review Questions

1. b; 2. a; 3. a; 4. b; 5. a; 6. d; 7. a; 8. b; 9. b; 10. a; 11. d

CHAPTER 25

Case Study

1. Many malarial ring forms, with multiple ring forms in individual red blood cells (RBCs), are present in the thin peripheral blood film. Many ring forms and a crescent-shaped gametocyte are also present in the thick peripheral blood film.

2. The high parasitemia, the presence of multiple ring forms in individual RBCs, the crescent-shaped gametocyte on the thick film, and the absence of other parasite stages in the thin and thick peripheral blood films suggest a diagnosis of malaria due to *Plasmodium falciparum*.

3. The patient had typical symptoms of malaria after a recent 3-week trip to Ghana in West Africa. Malaria is endemic in Ghana, and according to the Centers for Disease Control and Prevention,[52] most of the malaria cases in Ghana are due to *P. falciparum*.

4. The only forms of *P. falciparum* that are seen on a peripheral blood film are ring forms and gametocytes, and the latter are characteristically crescent-shaped.

5. Anemia in malaria is due to direct lysis of infected RBCs during schizogony; immune destruction of infected and noninfected RBCs by macrophages in the spleen; and inhibition of erythropoiesis and ineffective erythropoiesis.

Review Questions

1. c; 2. a; 3. b; 4. b; 5. c; 6. b; 7. c; 8. c; 9. c; 10. d; 11. c

CHAPTER 26

Case Study

1. The WBC can be elevated due to an underlying infection or the autoimmune response itself (inflammation). The MCV is elevated due to the reticulocytosis; the RDW is slightly elevated due to the anisocytosis and occasional schistocytes. The reticulocyte count is increased due to a surge in RBC production in the bone marrow in response to the anemia.

2. In this immune process, spherocytes develop from IgG-sensitized RBCs that have had the immune complex (and a part of the cell membrane) removed by macrophages. The membranes seal and the cells become spherocytic. The red pulp of the spleen eventually entraps the spherocytes, which are less deformable, and macrophages engulf and digest them, thus shortening their life span.

3. The direct antiglobulin test detected an IgG autoantibody which attached to the patient's RBCs in vivo, which is a hallmark of WAIHA. The IgG autoantibody was also detected in the serum with the antibody screen using the indirect antiglobulin test. The patient's RBCs, sensitized with IgG autoantibody, were prematurely ingested and destroyed by macrophages (extravascular hemolysis); within the macrophages hemoglobin is degraded to polypeptide chains, iron, and the protoporphyrin ring. The protoporphyrin is converted to unconjugated bilirubin and is transported to the liver where it is conjugated with glucuronic acid to form conjugated bilirubin. When there is excessive hemolysis, the liver cannot process all the excess unconjugated bilirubin that is being formed, so it accumulates in the serum. The excess conjugated bilirubin formed in the liver is excreted through the bile duct to the intestines where it is converted to urobilinogen. Because of the increased urobilinogen produced in the intestines, an increased amount is reabsorbed into the blood, and an increased amount is excreted in the urine. There is also an increase in intravascular hemolysis which liberates lactate dehydrogenase and elevates the level in serum. Free hemoglobin is also liberated and is bound by haptoglobin. The hemoglobin-haptoglobin complex is taken up and degraded by macrophages, resulting in a decrease in serum haptoglobin. When the serum haptoglobin is depleted, the excess hemoglobin accumulates in the plasma. Some is salvaged by hemopexin, but the excess is filtered by the kidney. Some hemoglobin is absorbed by the proximal tubular cells; the iron is removed and converted to hemosiderin. When the tubular cells slough off into the urine, the hemosiderin can be detected. The excess hemoglobin that is not absorbed by the tubular cells flows into the urine resulting in hemoglobinuria.

4. Prednisone is a glucocorticosteroid with immunosuppressive properties, such as reducing WBC response to inflammation and production of inflammatory cytokines. When a patient with an autoimmune disorder is given prednisone, most of these inflammatory mechanisms are switched off or slowed down, which in turn reduces the body's autoimmune response. The patient probably had an acute form of WAIHA because the symptoms and severe anemia developed suddenly and there was no evidence of an underlying condition.

Review Questions

1. b; 2. a; 3. a; 4. d; 5. d; 6. d; 7. a; 8. c; 9. c; 10. c; 11. c

CHAPTER 27

Case Study

1. The confirmatory test that should be performed is citrate agar electrophoresis at a pH between 6.0 and 6.2. In the citrate agar test, Hb C is separated from Hb A$_2$, Hb O, and Hb E, and Hb S is separated from Hb D and Hb G (see Figure 27-7).

2. The characteristic morphologic feature on the peripheral blood film is a Hb SC crystal. They appear as fingerlike or quartzlike crystals of dense hemoglobin protruding from the RBC membrane.

3. On the basis of the electrophoretic pattern and RBC morphology, Hb SC disease is likely.

4. With parents of the genotypes SC and AS, 25% of the offspring would have each of the following genotypes: AS, SS, AC, and SC.

Review Questions

1. d; 2. b; 3. c; 4. b; 5. d; 6. b; 7. a; 8. b; 9. c; 10. a; 11. b; 12. d; 13. d; 14. b; 15. c; 16. d

CHAPTER 28

Case Study

1. The family history revealed a Mediterranean ethnic background; both α- and β-thalassemia are common in the Mediterranean population. The student's mother had always been anemic, and her gallbladder "attacks" were probably caused by pigmented gallstones (calcium bilirubinate), which resulted from the mild hemolytic anemia of heterozygous β-thalassemia. A cousin on the mother's side had children with thalassemia major. Because of the family history, it is quite likely that the student has β-thalassemia minor. Note that his mother was periodically given iron therapy. It is a common mistake to treat a thalassemic individual for iron deficiency anemia, especially in areas in which thalassemia is not common in the general population, because both iron deficiency anemia and thalassemia are microcytic, hypochromic anemias.

2. The student had a mild hypochromic (decreased mean cell hemoglobin concentration) and microcytic (decreased mean cell volume) anemia with target cells and basophilic stippling on his peripheral blood film. He had an elevated level of hemoglobin A$_2$, which is a marker for β-thalassemia minor. His serum ferritin level was within the reference interval, which ruled out a diagnosis of iron deficiency anemia.

3. A microcytic, hypochromic anemia could be due to α- or β-thalassemia, Hb E disease or trait, iron deficiency anemia, or, more rarely, sideroblastic anemia (including lead poisoning) or anemia of chronic inflammation (see Figure 19-2). Iron deficiency anemia is the most common of these. Iron studies can differentiate these conditions. An incorrect presumption that a patient has iron deficiency may lead to inappropriate iron therapy or to unnecessary diagnostic procedures.

4. The potential mother should be screened for β-thalassemia trait, and if she is heterozygous for a β-thalassemia gene mutation, the couple should be advised that there is a 25% chance of having a baby with β-thalassemia major (homozygous or compound heterozygous for a β-thalassemia mutation). In addition, there is a 25% chance of having a baby who is homozygous for normal β-globin genes, and a 50% chance of having a baby heterozygous for a β-thalassemia mutation (β-thalassemia trait). Molecular genetic testing of the *HBB* gene is performed for carrier detection in couples seeking preconception counseling.

Review Questions

1. b; 2. c; 3. a; 4. d; 5. a; 6. c; 7. a; 8. c; 9. d; 10. a; 11. d; 12. b; 13. c; 14. d; 15. c

CHAPTER 29

Case Studies
Case 1

1. Chronic granulomatous disease.

2. Patient neutrophils are unable to form reactive oxygen species such as hydrogen peroxide.

3. Aggressive treatment of infections and use of antifungal agents have greatly increased survival rates so that the majority of patients survive into adulthood.
4. The majority of cases are X-linked.

Case 2
1. Because of the reactive monocytosis, the blood film should be examined for possible circulating macrophages.
2. On the edges of the blood film, because macrophages are very large cells.
3. Circulating macrophages indicate sepsis.
4. A buffy coat preparation, which concentrates nucleated cells.

Review Questions
1. a; 2. d; 3. c; 4. b; 5. d; 6. c; 7. d; 8. c; 9. b; 10. c

CHAPTER 30

Case Study
1. G banding utilizes Giemsa staining to differentiate chromosomes into bands for identification of specific chromosomes. The chromosomes must be pretreated with the proteolytic enzyme trypsin.
2. The mutation is an example of a structural rearrangement between chromosomes 9 and 22, called the *Philadelphia chromosome*. The Philadelphia chromosome represents a balanced translocation between the long arms of chromosomes 9 and 22. At the molecular level, the gene for *ABL1*, an oncogene, joins a gene on chromosome 22 named *BCR*. The result of the fusion of these two genes is a new fusion protein.
3. Fluorescence in situ hybridization (FISH) is a molecular technique that uses DNA or RNA probes labeled directly with a fluorescent nucleotide or with a hapten (e.g., dinitrophenyl, digoxigenin, or biotin). Both the probe and either metaphase or interphase cells are made single-stranded (denatured) and then hybridized together. Cells hybridized with a direct-label probe are viewed with a fluorescence microscope. If the probe was labeled with a hapten, antibodies to the hapten, carrying a fluorescent tag, are applied to the cells. Once the antibodies bind to the RNA or DNA probe, the cells can be viewed using a fluorescence microscope. FISH complements standard chromosome analysis by confirming the G-band analysis and by improving resolution, which allows for analysis at the molecular level.

Review Questions
1. c; 2. d; 3. a; 4. d; 5. a; 6. c; 7. d; 8. c; 9. c; 10. b

CHAPTER 31

Case Study
1. DNA isolation for the detection of inherited mutations requires whole blood collected in a lavender stopper tube containing EDTA to preserve white blood cells.
2. The correct controls are present and include a positive control (Lane B), a negative control (Lane D), and a "no-DNA" control (Lane E). The no-DNA control is essential when any polymerase chain reaction (PCR) test is performed in the clinical laboratory. This control will demonstrate whether cross-contamination occurred during the setup of the PCR procedure. The no-DNA control region of the gel should lack a banding pattern, as seen in Figure 31-1. If a banding pattern is present in the no-DNA control region or this control is missing, the test must be repeated before reporting patient results.

3. Bands in the patient's sample (Lane C) appear at 141, 104, and 82 bp.
4. The following band sizes are expected in factor V Leiden DNA analysis:
   - Normal: 104 and 82 bp (37 bp is sometimes barely visible, as well)
   - Heterozygous: 141, 104, and 82 bp (37 bp is sometimes barely visible, as well)
   - Homozygous: 141 and 82 bp
5. The three bands in the patient sample indicate that this patient is heterozygous for the factor V Leiden mutation.

Review Questions
1. d; 2. b; 3. d; 4. b; 5. b; 6. c; 7. a; 8. a; 9. b; 10. b

CHAPTER 32

Case Studies
Case 1
1. The lymphoid population is the most prominent. Forward scatter demonstrates small to medium-sized cells. These cells are characterized by low side scatter indicative of sparse agranular cytoplasm.
2. The majority of cells express CD19, CD10, and κ light chain. There is also a small population of T cells positive for CD5 and negative for CD19 antigen.
3. Prominent κ light chain expression indicates a monoclonal B-cell population that is characteristic of lymphoma.

Case 2
1. The low density of CD45 antigen coupled with relatively low side scatter is characteristic of a blast population. Such a prominent blast population can only be seen in acute leukemias.
2. The expression of immature markers (CD34 and HLA-DR) coupled with positivity for myeloid and megakaryoblastic antigens (CD33, CD41, and CD61) is seen in acute megakaryoblastic leukemias.

Review Questions
1. c; 2. b; 3. a; 4. d; 5. b; 6. a; 7. a; 8. a; 9. c; 10. a; 11. b

CHAPTER 33

Case Study
1. An elevated white blood cell (WBC) count with a left shift suggests a myeloproliferative neoplasm or a leukemoid reaction (reactive neutrophilia). However, in this patient the WBC count was extremely elevated, the left shift was rather deep (presence of promyelocytes and blasts), and basophilia was present, which suggests that a myeloproliferative neoplasm is likely present. Chronic myelogenous leukemia (CML) is the most likely cause of these laboratory findings.
2. The leukocyte alkaline phosphatase (LAP) score is low in CML due to inappropriate LAP synthesis in the secondary granules, whereas LAP is elevated in bacterial infections due to activation of enzyme synthesis.
3. The *BCR/ABL1* fusion gene must be identified to confirm the diagnosis of CML. *BCR/ABL1* can be demonstrated from a karyotype analysis showing the t(9;22) reciprocal translocation known as the *Philadelphia chromosome* (Chapter 30), by demonstration of the *BCR/ABL1* fusion gene using fluorescence in situ hybridization (Chapter 30), or by demonstration of the BCR/ABL1 fusion mRNA

by qualitative reverse transcriptase polymerase chain reaction (Chapter 31). Patients who have complete blood count and differential results that resemble those in CML but test negative for *BCR/ABL1* are considered to have atypical CML, and the disorder is classified as myelodysplastic syndrome/myeloproliferative neoplasm (Chapter 34).

4. Cytogenetic studies are likely to show the t(9;22) mutation.

5. The t(9;22) translocation produces the *BCR/ABL1* chimeric gene, which is observed in four primary molecular forms that produce three versions of the BCR/ABL chimeric protein: p190, p210, and p230.

6. First-line therapy for CML is the tyrosine kinase inhibitor imatinib mesylate (Gleevec). Allogeneic stem cell transplantation should be considered for all CML patients, because it is the only potentially curative treatment for CML. However, few CML patients qualify for allogeneic stem cell transplantation, because most do not meet the criteria for low risk: age younger than 40 years, disease in the chronic phase, transplantation within 1 year of diagnosis, and availability of an HLA-matched donor. For those patients who qualify for allogeneic stem cell transplantation, imatinib is used to induce remission prior to transplant, to treat minimum residual disease, and to provide rescue therapy if the transplant fails. Imatinib is continued as lifelong therapy until drug resistance is detected.

7. The majority of cases of imatinib resistance result from two primary causes: acquisition of additional *BCR/ABL1* mutations and expression of point mutations in the adenosine triphosphate (ATP) binding site. Additional *BCR/ABL1* mutations can occur through the usual translocation of the remaining unaffected chromosomes 9 and 22, which converts the hematopoietic stem cell from heterozygous to homozygous for the *BCR/ABL1* mutation. A double dose of *BCR/ABL1* can also be acquired from gene duplication during mitosis and accounts for 10% of secondary mutations. An additional *BCR/ABL1* mutation will double the tyrosine kinase activity, which makes the imatinib dosage inadequate. In these cases higher dosages of imatinib will restore remission in most patients. Over 60 mutations have been identified in the ATP binding site, and these account for the remaining 50% to 90% of secondary mutations. Mutations in the ATP binding site reduce the binding affinity of imatinib, producing some level of resistance.

Review Questions

1. b; 2. c; 3. d; 4. c; 5. c; 6. c; 7. b; 8. d; 9. a; 10. c

CHAPTER 34

Case Study

1. The differential diagnosis of patients with pancytopenia should include megaloblastic anemia (vitamin B_{12} or folate deficiency), aplastic anemia, liver disease, alcoholism, and myelodysplastic syndrome (MDS).

2. The probable diagnosis is MDS.

3. This patient's MDS should be classified as refractory anemia with ringed sideroblasts (RARS).

Review Questions

1. d; 2. a; 3. b; 4. b; 5. c; 6. c; 7. a; 8. d; 9. c; 10. c

CHAPTER 35

Case Study

1. Due to the presence of blasts on the peripheral blood film, the most likely diagnosis is acute leukemia. The thrombocytopenia and

anemia support that diagnosis. According to the WHO classification, ≥ 20% blasts in the bone marrow is required for diagnosis of acute leukemia; an exception to this criterion are those cases that have specific genetic abnormalities (delineated in the WHO classification) that are diagnostic, regardless of blast count. Acute lymphoblastic leukemia (ALL) is more common in children. Immunophenotyping by flow cytometry determines the lineage and maturation stage of the blasts. Testing for genetic abnormalities is required for diagnosis and prognosis.

2. This child has clinical and laboratory features indicative of a favorable prognosis: young age, a white blood cell count less than $20 \times 10^9/L$ (i.e., low tumor burden), and hyperdiploidy. The strongest predictor of patient outcome is the presence of certain genetic abnormalities; the immunophenotype also contributes to the prognosis.

3. Hyperdiploidy carries a favorable prognosis in B-cell ALL in children.

Review Questions

1. b; 2. b; 3. a; 4. d; 5. b; 6. d; 7. c; 8. c; 9. b; 10. b; 11. b; 12. b

CHAPTER 36

Case Study

1. Diffuse large B-cell lymphoma (DLBCL).

2. This lesion is expected to show exclusive (clonal) κ or λ light chain expression. Flow cytometry is particularly sensitive in detecting surface and cytoplasmic immunoglobulin light chains and is commonly used to confirm clonality of lymphoproliferative disorders. In addition, other pan–B-cell markers can be studied by flow cytometry (e.g., CD19, CD22, and FMC7 antigens) to demonstrate the B-cell origin of this lymphoma.

3. Most often DLBCL presents as a localized disease involving a group of lymph nodes. Bone marrow involvement is rare at presentation; however, it can occur later in the course of the disease.

Review Questions

1. d; 2. c; 3. d; 4. d; 5. b; 6. b; 7. b; 8. a; 9. c; 10. a

CHAPTER 37

Case Study

1. Given the family history, this may be an inherited condition, although pregnancy is an independent risk factor for thrombosis.

2. Thrombosis is probably caused by the deficiency of a coagulation inhibitor such as protein C, protein S, or antithrombin. It may be caused by a procoagulant gain-of-function mutation such as the factor V Leiden mutation or the prothrombin G20210A mutation.

Review Questions

1. b; 2. c; 3. b; 4. d; 5. b; 6. d; 7. b; 8. c; 9. a; 10. a

CHAPTER 38

Case Study

1. The combination of thrombocytopenia and prolonged prothrombin time (PT) and partial thromboplastin time (PTT) indicate probable liver disease. In the absence of a full medical history, the patient's hemarthroses and description of himself as a "bleeder" lead to the presumption of hemophilia, possibly hemophilia A. It is possible that he contracted hepatitis C from an untreated blood product. Treatment of factor concentrates for viral disease began in

1984. Prior to 1984 most hemophilia patients eventually developed hepatitis B or C from factor concentrates. Hepatitis A is also a possibility. Liver disease may be confirmed using bilirubin and liver enzyme assays.

In advanced liver disease, poor liver circulation causes pressure in the portal circulation. This enlarges the spleen (splenomegaly). The enlarged spleen sequesters and clears platelets more rapidly than normal, a condition called *hypersplenism,* which causes thrombocytopenia. In most cases, platelet function is reduced. This reduced platelet function can be demonstrated in the laboratory using platelet aggregometry and is the reason for the patient's epistaxis.

Vitamin K deficiency is also a possibility. To differentiate vitamin K deficiency from liver disease, a factor V and VII activity assay is performed. In vitamin K deficiency factor VII activity is reduced but factor V activity is normal. In liver disease, both are reduced.

2. In early liver disease the vitamin K–dependent factors II (prothrombin), VII, IX, and X are produced with diminished function. This can be corrected with a trial dose of oral or intravenous vitamin K. In people with true vitamin K deficiency secondary to an altered diet, the vitamin K therapy corrects bleeding and normalizes the PT and PTT, but in liver disease vitamin K may not have a lasting effect. This is because the liver cannot process the vitamin K normally.

In addition to vitamin K therapy, thawed frozen plasma (FP) transfusion at 1 to 2 units/day is effective in supplementing the liver's production of all the coagulation factors. Cryoprecipitate may also be used to raise the fibrinogen concentration, and platelet concentrate may be used if the platelet count drops to below 50,000/μL and there is continued evidence of mucocutaneous bleeding.

Administration of vitamin K, FP, cryoprecipitate, and platelets does not cure liver disease; these therapies only treat the bleeding symptoms. Additional treatment may include antibiotics, antivirals, and anti-inflammatory drugs.

Review Questions

1. c; 2. d; 3. b; 4. c; 5. b; 6. b; 7. d; 8. a; 9. a; 10. c; 11. c

CHAPTER 39

Case Study

1. The following tests for congenital and acquired risk factors are included in a thrombophilia profile. Results for the items with asterisks are valid only when the test is performed 10 to 14 days after termination of antithrombotic therapy or resolution of a thrombotic event.
   - Homocysteine
   - Lupus anticoagulant profile*
   - Prothrombin G20210A mutation
   - Activated protein C resistance*
   - Factor V Leiden mutation (confirmatory for activated protein C resistance)
   - Anticardiolipin antibodies by immunoassay
   - Protein C functional assay and follow-up immunoassay*
   - Protein S functional assay and follow-up immunoassay*
   - Antithrombin functional assay and follow-up immunoassay*
2. The most common acquired thrombotic risk factors are antiphospholipid antibodies and lupus anticoagulant, and these are most often implicated in a thrombotic event.
3. Patients with thrombotic risk factors may be instructed to avoid situations and practices that may trigger thrombosis, such as immobilization, smoking, and use of oral contraceptives or

hormone replacement therapy. They may be provided with prophylactic antithrombotic therapy at times when circumstances increasing thrombotic risk cannot be avoided, such as when undergoing orthopedic surgery.

Review Questions

1. b; 2. a; 3. d; 4. c; 5. a; 6. b; 7. a; 8. a; 9. c; 10. d; 11. d; 12. d; 13. d; 14. c

CHAPTER 40

Case Study

1. Yes, the heparin is significant.
2. Heparin-induced platelet aggregation assay, serotonin release assay, or enzyme-linked immunosorbent assay (ELISA) should be ordered.

   An ELISA was performed to look for the presence of heparin-induced antibodies. Results gave an optical density of 0.650, with a reference interval of less than 0.400 optical density. The patient was found to have clinically significant levels of heparin-induced antibodies.

   The patient underwent an above-knee amputation of her right leg. No heparin or low molecular weight heparin was used during or after the procedure. The grafting surgeries were successful, and the patient recovered.

Review Questions

1. b; 2. d; 3. b; 4. c; 5. b; 6. b; 7. b; 8. c; 9. d; 10. a

CHAPTER 41

Case Study

1. Storage pool disease, aspirin-like defects, and use of antiplatelet agents such as aspirin are possibilities.
2. Storage pool disease or aspirin-like defects seem most likely.
3. Based on the results of the quantitative test for adenosine triphosphate release, the likely cause is dense granule storage pool disease.

   These results were confirmed by the findings of electron microscopy of the patient's platelets, which revealed the absence of detectable dense granules. Because the patient's bleeding problems are due to an inherited abnormality that typically results in only mild bleeding problems, the patient was counseled to avoid antiplatelet agents, particularly aspirin, since they are known to exacerbate the bleeding problems encountered by patients with dense granule deficiency.

Review Questions

1. d; 2. a; 3. a; 4. b; 5. c; 6. c; 7. d; 8. b; 9. d; 10. a

CHAPTER 42

Case Study

1. The laboratory director questioned the phlebotomist about the problem. The phlebotomist admitted that he had erroneously collected blood in a red- and gray-stoppered "tiger-top" tube and, responding to the patient's remark, had immediately poured the blood into a blue-stoppered tube for analysis. He thought the specimen would be okay because it had not clotted yet.
2. The red and gray marbleized stopper designates a serum separator tube. The phlebotomist poured the blood into the blue-stoppered tube before it had begun to clot; however, the activator from the

tiger-top tube shortened the clotting time on the prothrombin time (PT) test, thus causing an erroneously short PT and low international normalized ratio (INR).

3. Unexpectedly short PTs during oral anticoagulant therapy are generally indicators of patient non-compliance to the drug regimen. The second most common circumstance that affects the PT is dietary changes, most often an increased intake of vitamin K–rich foods such as green leafy vegetables, liver, or avocado. In this instance the patient had been fully compliant, carefully following the prescribed dosage and timing, and her diet had not changed. These facts led the laboratory director to consider a specimen collection error.

Specimens collected in 3.2% sodium citrate may be stored for up to 24 hours at room temperature without a change in the PT. However, specimens stored at higher than 24° C deteriorate rapidly, which causes prolongation of the PT and increase in the INR. Prolonged storage at 2° to 4° C may activate factor VII, which slightly shortens the PT and slightly decreases the INR.

Many serum separator tubes contain particulate materials that hasten in vitro clotting. Core laboratory managers select these tubes to improve test result turnaround time when the required sample is serum. When blood is collected into a series of tubes that includes a blue-stoppered tube for hemostasis testing, the blue-stoppered tube should be filled first or should be filled after a tube without additives. It should not be filled immediately after filling a serum separator tube with clot activators, because the activators may carry over to the hemostasis specimen and affect test results.

In this case, an observant patient provided clues that led to identification of the pre-analytical error. The phlebotomist was carefully counseled about the effects of tube additives on hemostasis tests.

Review Questions

1. c; 2. b; 3. a; 4. b; 5. a; 6. a; 7. b; 8. b; 9. b; 10. d; 11. b; 12. d; 13. d; 14. c

CHAPTER 43

Case Study

1. The increase in anticoagulation could be caused by a change in diet, dietary supplements, or drugs. Any new drug that interferes with the cytochrome oxidase P-450 enzyme 2C9 pathway could reduce warfarin breakdown and excretion, and increase its effectiveness.
2. Determine what has caused the change in warfarin efficacy and eliminate it if possible, adjust the warfarin dosage, or give vitamin K orally or intravenously to stop bleeding if necessary.
3. The chromogenic factor X assay.

Review Questions

1. c; 2. c; 3. c; 4. a; 5. d; 6. b; 7. d; 8. c; 9. b; 10. b; 11. a; 12. a; 13. a; 14. d; 15. d

CHAPTER 44

Case Study

1. No. The description of the sample and the instrument flags indicating lipemia should alert the operator to a potentially invalid test result because lipemia is known to cause erroneous results on some photo-optical coagulation analyzers.
2. Two options are available to negate the effect of the lipemia and obtain valid test results:
   a. Remove the lipids from the plasma by high-speed centrifugation or ultracentrifugation.
   b. Perform testing using an endpoint detection method that is not susceptible to lipemia in the sample, such as mechanical clot detection.
3. Because the patient history includes previous surgical procedures without bleeding symptoms and there is no other indication of abnormal bleeding tendencies for this patient, it is probably safe to consider that the prolonged prothrombin time and activated partial thromboplastin time results are due to the lipemic nature of the sample. The patient would most likely not be at risk for bleeding during the surgery, and it would be anticipated that repeat testing using one of the options listed previously would yield test results within the reference interval.

Review Questions

1. b; 2. d; 3. a; 4. c; 5. b; 6. c; 7. c; 8. a; 9. d; 10. a

CHAPTER 45

Case Study

1. Yes, the newborn reference interval for hemoglobin is 16.5 to 21.5 g/dL and for the hematocrit is 48% to 68%.
2. These values are normal for newborns. Erythrocytes of a newborn are markedly macrocytic. There may be 2 to 24 nucleated red blood cells on the first postnatal day, but they are not present by day 5. The polychromasia reflects the reticulocytosis that persists for about 4 days.
3. These values are within the reference intervals for newborns. The white blood cell count of a newborn fluctuates a great deal with a reference interval of 9.0 to 37.0 × 10^9/L, and leukocytosis without evidence of infection is common. The differential may show an increase in neutrophils rather than the lymphocyte predominance seen after 2 weeks. In this case the neutrophils and lymphocytes were present in equal amounts, but no immature neutrophils were seen.

Review Questions

1. d; 2. b; 3. a; 4. b; 5. c; 6. c; 7. d; 8. b; 9. a; 10. c

Glossary

a-β-lipoproteinemia Autosomal recessive disorder of lipoprotein metabolism in which lipoproteins containing apolipoprotein B (chylomicrons, very-low-density lipoproteins, and low-density lipoproteins) are not synthesized. Characterized by the presence of peripheral blood film acanthocytes and low plasma cholesterol levels.

absolute neutrophil count (ANC) Total of neutrophils per liter of blood. The absolute neutrophil count is calculated by multiplying the total white blood cell count by the percentage of segmented neutrophils and bands or may be counted directly using an automated hematology analyzer.

absolute reticulocyte count (ARC) Reticulocytes per liter. The absolute reticulocyte count is calculated by multiplying the patient's visual reticulocyte count (reticulocyte percentage, VRET%) by the red blood cell count or may be measured directly using an automated hematology analyzer.

acanthocyte Red blood cell with spiny projections of varying lengths distributed irregularly over its surface, associated with lipid imbalance. Contrast with the echinocyte, which has regular projections of uniform length.

acanthocytosis Presence of acanthocytes in the blood. Associated with abetalipoproteinemia or abnormalities of lipid metabolism, such as abnormalities occurring in liver disease.

accuracy Extent to which an assay result matches its true value. Accuracy is computed by comparing assay results with the results from an established reference assay or a primary standard.

achlorhydria Pathologic absence of free hydrochloric acid from gastric secretions following stimulation.

acid elution slide test (Kleihauer-Betke stain) Test for detecting fetal red blood cells (RBCs) in the maternal circulation. Blood films are immersed in an acid buffer, which causes adult hemoglobin (Hb A) to be eluted from RBCs. The film is stained, and RBCs that have fetal hemoglobin (Hb F) take up the stain.

acquired immunodeficiency syndrome (AIDS) Late-stage immune system suppression characterized by depletion of CD4$^+$ T lymphocytes and depression of cellular immunity causing susceptibility to opportunistic infections and neoplasms. Caused by infection with human immunodeficiency virus (HIV), a retrovirus.

acrocentric Describes the appearance of a metaphase chromosome with the centromere near one end, which causes the q arm to be much longer than the p arm.

acrocyanosis (Raynaud phenomenon) Persistent symmetrical cyanosis (blotchy blue or red discoloration) in the skin of the digits, palm, wrists, and ankles, and less frequently the nose and ears, upon prolonged exposure to cold.

activated coagulation time (ACT) Whole-blood clotting time test often used in cardiac surgical suites. A particulate activator is added to blood, the mixture is rocked, and the interval to clotting is recorded. Employed to monitor high-dose unfractionated heparin therapy during cardiac catheterization or coronary artery bypass graft surgery.

activated partial thromboplastin time (APTT, partial thromboplastin time, PTT) Clot-based screening test for intrinsic coagulation that is prolonged in deficiencies of prekallikrein, high-molecular-weight kininogen, factors XII, XI, IX, VIII, X, V, and II (prothrombin), and fibrinogen. Calcium chloride, phospholipid, and negatively charged particulate activator are added to patient plasma. The interval from the addition of reagent to clot formation is recorded. The test is used to monitor unfractionated heparin therapy and to screen for intrinsic and common pathway deficiencies, specific factor inhibitors, and lupus anticoagulant.

activated protein C (APC) Coagulation pathway regulatory protein activated by the thrombin-thrombomodulin complex that, when bound and stabilized by protein S, hydrolyzes and inactivates factor Va and factor VIIIa.

activated protein C resistance (APCR) Inherited condition in which activated coagulation factor V (Va) resists activated protein C digestion, which results in an increased risk of venous thrombosis. In 90% of cases, activated protein C resistance is caused by the factor V Leiden mutation.

activated prothrombin complex concentrate Therapeutic plasma preparation that bypasses factor VIII activation, used to treat bleeding episodes in hemophilic patients who have developed factor VIII inhibitor. Contains activated factors II (prothrombin), VII, IX, and X. Also known as *prothrombin complex concentrate, factor eight inhibitor bypassing activity* (FEIBA; Baxter Healthcare Corporation, Deerfield, IL).

acute Describes diseases whose symptoms begin abruptly with marked intensity and then subside after a relatively short period.

acute leukemia Malignant, unregulated proliferation of hematopoietic progenitors of the myeloid or lymphoid cell lines. Characterized by abrupt onset of symptoms and, if left untreated, death within months of the time of diagnosis.

acute myocardial infarction (AMI) Occlusion of a coronary artery by a clot, causing ischemia and necrosis (tissue death) of surrounding heart muscle. Commonly called a *heart attack*.

acute phase reactant Serum protein produced by the liver whose level rises during inflammation. Examples include C-reactive protein, ferritin, and fibrinogen.

adenopathy Enlargement of one or more lymph nodes.

adenosine diphosphate (ADP) Purine nucleotide that activates platelets by binding platelet receptor P2Y$_1$ and P2Y$_{12}$. Produced by hydrolysis of adenosine triphosphate.

adenosine triphosphate (ATP) Purine nucleotide that stores energy in the form of high-energy phosphate bonds, releasing energy upon hydrolysis to drive metabolic reactions.

adhesion Property of binding or remaining in proximity; for example, attachment of platelets to surfaces such as subendothelial collagen.

adipocyte Fat cell; adipocytes make up adipose tissue and the yellow portion of the bone marrow.

afibrinogenemia Complete absence of plasma fibrinogen.

agammaglobulinemia Immunodeficiency characterized by an absence or extremely reduced level of plasma gamma globulin and reduced levels of immunoglobulins. Associated with increased risk of infection.

agglutination Cross-linking of antigen-bearing cells or particles by a specific antibody to form visible clumps.

aggregation Cluster or clump of similar cell types or particles; for example, attachment of platelets to other platelets, red blood cell clumping.

agnogenic Of idiopathic or unknown origin.

agranulocytosis Any condition involving decreased numbers of granulocytes (segmented neutrophils or band neutrophils).

albinism Hereditary condition characterized by partial or total lack of melanin pigment in the body; skin, hair, and eyes may be affected. Individuals with total albinism have pale skin that does not tan, white hair, and pink eyes. Albinism is often associated with platelet storage pool deficiency.

Alder-Reilly anomaly Autosomal dominant polysaccharide metabolism disorder in which white blood cells (WBCs) of the myelocytic series, and sometimes all WBCs, contain coarse azurophilic mucopolysaccharide granules.

allele One of two or more alternative forms of a gene that occupy corresponding loci on homologous chromosomes. Each allele encodes a certain inherited characteristic. An individual normally has two alleles for each gene, one contributed by the mother and one by the father. If both alleles are the same, the individual is homozygous, but if the alleles are different, the individual is heterozygous. In heterozygous individuals, one of the alleles may be dominant and the other recessive.

alloantibody (isoantibody) Antibody that is produced in response to the presence of foreign antigens; for instance, an antibody to a therapeutic coagulation factor that may render factor therapy ineffective.

alloimmune Producing antibodies to antigens derived from a genetically dissimilar individual of the same species.

alloimmune hemolytic anemia Anemia caused by antibodies stimulated by exposure to foreign red blood cell (RBC) antigens. Antibodies coat and shorten the life span of circulating RBCs. This is the basis for hemolytic disease of the newborn.

α-granules Platelet granules that store and release a variety of hemostasis proteins. There are 50 to 80 α-granules per platelet. In transmission electron microscopy, α-granules appear light gray, in contrast to δ-granules (dense bodies), which appear black.

α-thalassemia Moderate to severe inherited anemia caused by a decreased or absent production of the α-globin chains of hemoglobin.

amyloidosis Disease in which a waxy, starchlike glycoprotein (amyloid) accumulates in tissues and organs, impairing their function.

analogue drugs Drugs that are chemically similar to one another but, because of minor structural differences, may have different physiologic actions.

anaplastic Characterized by loss of differentiation and growth without structure or form. Anaplasia is a characteristic of cancer.

anatomic bleeding disorder Chronic episodic bleeding into soft tissue, joints, and body cavities. Indicates a secondary coagulopathy such as hemophilia or an acquired coagulation factor deficiency.

anemia Diminished delivery of oxygen to tissues, as evidenced by pallor, malaise, and dyspnea. May be caused by blood loss, decreased red blood cell (RBC) production, increased RBC destruction (shortened life span).

aneuploid Having a chromosome number that is not an exact multiple of the normal diploid number (46 in humans) so that there are fewer or more chromosomes than normal.

anisocytosis Abnormal red blood cell (RBC) morphology characterized by considerable variation in RBC volume or RBC diameter on a blood film.

annular diaphragm Device used in phase microscopy that, together with a phase-shifting element, produces contrast between an unstained cell and its dark background.

anoxia Inadequate tissue oxygenation caused by poor lung perfusion or a diminished blood supply.

antagonist Drug that nullifies the action of another drug or that reduces a normal cellular response. Aspirin is a platelet antagonist because it reduces platelet activation.

antecubital fossa Concavity opposite the elbow.

antibody (Ab) Specialized protein (immunoglobulin) that is produced by B lymphocytes and plasma cells when the immune system is exposed to foreign antigens from bacteria, viruses, or other biologic materials. An antibody molecule has a specific amino acid sequence in its variable region that matches it to the antigen that originally stimulated its production.

anticardiolipin antibody (ACL, ACA) Member of the antiphospholipid antibody family that includes anti–β2-glycoprotein 1 and lupus anticoagulant. An ACL antibody is an autoantibody detected in a solid-phase immunoassay system using cardiolipin as the target antigen. The chronic presence of ACL antibodies is associated with venous and arterial thrombotic disease.

anticoagulant Therapeutic agent that delays blood coagulation, such as heparin or warfarin, used to prevent thrombotic events in patients who are at risk. Additive to blood specimen collection tubes that prevents in vitro blood clotting such as sodium citrate.

antigen Molecule that the immune system recognizes as foreign and that subsequently evokes an immune response.

antihemophilic factor (AHF) Therapeutic concentration of coagulation factor VIII produced through chemical fractionation, immunoaffinity column, or recombinant synthesis. Antihemophilic factor is prescribed in the treatment of hemophilia A, a hereditary deficiency of factor VIII.

antineoplastic Chemotherapeutic agent that controls or kills cancer cells.

antiphospholipid antibody (APL, APA) Member of the antibody family that includes anticardiolipin, anti–β2-glycoprotein I, and lupus anticoagulant. APL antibodies bind phospholipid-binding proteins, such as β2-glycoprotein. The presence of an APL antibody is associated with venous and arterial thrombotic disease.

antiphospholipid syndrome (APS) Group of thrombotic disorders related to the chronic presence of an antiphospholipid antibody, such as anticardiolipin, anti–β2-glycoprotein I, or lupus anticoagulant. Manifestations include migraine, transient ischemic attacks, strokes, acute myocardial infarction, peripheral artery disease, venous thromboembolic disease, and spontaneous abortion.

antithrombin (AT, antithrombin III, AT III) Plasma serine protease inhibitor produced in the liver and activated by therapeutic heparin or vascular heparan sulfate. When activated, antithrombin controls the coagulation pathway, because it neutralizes all the serine proteases except factor VIIa, most importantly factors IIa (thrombin) and Xa.

aperture Optical device in a microscope substage light path that controls the diameter of the light column that reaches the specimen. The aperture may be adjusted to improve specimen clarity.

aplasia Failure of the normal process of cell generation and development. Bone marrow aplasia is the loss of all bone marrow cellular elements.

aplastic anemia Deficiency of all of the formed elements of blood, representing a failure of the blood cell–generating capacity of bone marrow.

apoferritin Protein component of the ferritin molecule consisting of 24 identical spherical subunits that surround iron in the ferric valence form.

apoptosis Natural cell death characterized by nuclear condensation and loss of cytoplasmic integrity. Apoptosis is a mechanism that prevents proliferation of dysplastic or mutated cells.

aspirin (acetylsalicylic acid, ASA) Acetylsalicylic acid in tablet form; irreversibly acetylates platelet cyclooxygenase and reduces platelet activation. Aspirin is used for its antithrombotic properties.

asynchrony Disturbance of coordination that causes processes to occur at abnormal times. In hematopoietic cell development, a difference in rate between cytoplasmic and nuclear maturation.

atrial fibrillation (AFIB) Uncontrolled and ineffective atrial heartbeat that affects at least 2 million U.S. citizens. Atrial fibrillation raises the risk for stroke. The risk is controlled using long-term anticoagulation therapy, such as warfarin.

atypical lymphocytes (transformed, reactive, or variant lymphocytes) Lymphocytes whose altered morphology includes stormy blue cytoplasm and lobular or irregular nuclei. Variant lymphocytes indicate stimulation by a virus, particularly Epstein-Barr virus, which causes infectious mononucleosis.

Auer rod Abnormal needle-shaped or round pink to purple inclusion in the cytoplasm of myeloblasts and promyelocytes; composed of condensed primary granules. Indicates acute myeloid leukemia.

autoantibody Antibody produced by an individual that recognizes and binds an antigen on the individual's own tissues.

autoimmune Describes an immune response in which an antibody forms to one's own tissues; for instance, antinuclear antibody in lupus erythematosus.

autoimmune hemolytic anemia Anemia characterized by premature red blood cell (RBC) destruction. Autoantibodies to RBC surface antigens bind the membrane, causing rapid splenic clearance and hemolysis.

autologous Related to self or belonging to the same organism; for example, used to describe blood that is donated by patients before surgery for the purpose of transfusion to themselves during or after surgery.

autosomal dominant inheritance Pattern of inheritance in which the transmission of a dominant allele on an autosome causes a trait to be expressed in heterozygotes.

autosomal inheritance Inheritance of traits located on non–sex-related chromosomes.

autosomal recessive inheritance Pattern of inheritance resulting from the transmission of a recessive allele that is not expressed in heterozygotes.

autosome Any of the 22 pairs of chromosomes in humans other than the sex chromosomes X and Y.

autosplenectomy Disappearance of the spleen through progressive fibrosis and shrinkage secondary to a hemolytic anemia such as sickle cell anemia.

azurophilic Having cellular structures that stain blue with Giemsa stain and red-purple with Wright stain.

azurophilic granules Primary cytoplasmic granules in myelocytic cells that, when stained with Wright stain, appear reddish purple. Azurophilic granules of different composition may also appear in a minority of lymphocytes.

B cell Any of a family of lymphocytes that produce antibodies. The end product of B-cell maturation is the plasma cell.

Babesia Protozoal parasite transmitted by ticks that infects human red blood cells and causes babesiosis, a malaria-like illness. The parasite is an intracellular ringlike structure 2 to 3 µm in diameter.

band neutrophil (band) Immediate precursor of the mature segmented neutrophil. Band neutrophils have a nonsegmented, usually curved, nucleus and are present in the bone marrow and peripheral blood.

bartonellosis Acute febrile infection caused by the bacterium *Bartonella bacilliformis*, which is transmitted by the bite of a sandfly. The first stage of the disease is associated with severe hemolytic anemia.

base pair Pair of nucleotides in the complementary strands of a DNA molecule that interact through hydrogen bonding across the axis of the DNA helix. One of the nucleotides in each pair is a purine (either adenine or guanine), and the other is a pyrimidine (either thymine or cytosine). Adenine always pairs with thymine, and guanine always pairs with cytosine.

basophil (baso) Granulocytic white blood cell characterized by cytoplasmic granules that stain bluish black when exposed to a basic dye. Cytoplasmic granules of basophils are of variable size and may obscure the nucleus.

basophilia Abnormal increase of basophils in the blood.

basophilic normoblast (prorubricyte) Second identifiable stage in bone marrow erythrocytic maturation; it is derived from the pronormoblast (rubriblast). Typically 10 to 15 µm in diameter, the basophilic normoblast (prorubricyte) has cytoplasm that stains dark blue with Wright stain.

basophilic stippling Barely visible dark blue to purple granules evenly distributed within a red blood cell stained with Wright stain. Composed of precipitated ribosomal protein and RNA.

Bence Jones protein Protein found almost exclusively in the urine of patients with multiple myeloma, consisting of the light chain of the abnormal immunoglobulins produced.

benign Noncancerous or nonmalignant.

Bernard-Soulier syndrome (BSS) Mild to moderate mucocutaneous bleeding disorder caused by one of a series of mutations to platelet glycoprotein Ib (GP Ib) or GP IX, part of the GP Ib/IX/V von Willebrand factor receptor complex. The disorder is a defect of platelet adhesion.

β_2-glycoprotein I (β_2-GPI) Plasma globulin that is a target of the antiphospholipid antibody anti–β_2-glycoprotein I.

β-thalassemia Inherited anemia caused by diminished synthesis of the β-globin chains of hemoglobin.

β-thromboglobulin (β-TG) Heparin-neutralizing protein that is stored and secreted by platelet α-granules.

bilirubin Gold-red-brown pigment, the main component of bile and a major metabolic product of the heme portion of hemoglobin, released from senescent red blood cells. Elevated bilirubin imparts a gold color to plasma and urine and may indicate hemolytic anemia, liver disease, or bile duct occlusion.

bilirubinemia (icterus, hyperbilirubinemia) Excess bilirubin in plasma. It imparts a gold color to plasma and may indicate hemolytic anemia, liver disease, or bile duct occlusion.

2,3-bisphosphoglycerate (2,3-BPG, 2,3-diphosphoglycerate, 2,3-DPG) Product of red blood cell glycolysis that is generated in the Rapoport-Luebering shunt. 2,3-BPG is one of the main regulators of oxygen uptake and delivery by hemoglobin. 2,3-BPG decreases hemoglobin's affinity for oxygen, which enables it to more readily release oxygen to the target tissues.

blast Earliest, least differentiated stage of hematopoietic maturation that can be identified by its morphology in a Wright-stained bone marrow smear; for example, myeloblast, pronormoblast (rubriblast), lymphoblast.

bleeding time (BT) Time interval required for blood to stop flowing from a puncture wound 2 mm long and 1 mm deep on the volar surface of the forearm. Largely of historical interest, the bleeding time test was performed to evaluate vascular and platelet function.

Bohr effect Effect of carbon dioxide and hydrogen ions on the affinity of hemoglobin for oxygen. Increasing carbon dioxide and hydrogen ion concentrations (lower pH) decrease oxygen saturation; decreasing concentrations increase oxygen saturation.

bone marrow Gelatinous red and yellow tissue filling the medullary cavities of bones. Red marrow is found in most bones of infants and children and in the ends of long bones and the cavities of flat bones in adults. Diagnostic marrow specimens are collected from the anterior or posterior iliac crest or sternum in adults. Fatty yellow marrow is found in the medullary cavity of most adult long bones.

bone marrow aspirate specimen A 1- to 1.5-mL aliquot of gelatinous red marrow obtained by passing a needle into the marrow cavity and applying negative pressure. The aspirate specimen is spread as a smear on a microscope slide, stained, and examined for hematologic or systemic disease. The aspirate specimen provides for analysis of individual cell morphology.

bone marrow biopsy specimen A 1- to 2-cm cylinder of gelatinous red marrow obtained by passing a biopsy cannula into the marrow cavity, rotating, and withdrawing. The cylinder is fixed in formalin, sectioned, stained, and examined for hematologic or systemic disease. The biopsy specimen provides for analysis of bone marrow architecture.

buffy coat Gray-white layer of white blood cells (WBCs) and platelets that accumulates at the red blood cell–plasma interface when a tube of anticoagulated blood is allowed to stand or is centrifuged. The buffy coat may be used to harvest WBCs for microscopic analysis when the WBC count is low, and an enlarged buffy coat may indicate leukemia.

Burkitt lymphoma Lymphatic solid tissue tumor composed of mature B lymphocytes with a characteristic morphology, called *Burkitt cells*. Burkitt cells appear in lymph node biopsies, bone marrow, and occasionally in peripheral blood and have dark blue cytoplasm with multiple vacuoles creating a "starry sky" pattern.

burst-forming unit (BFU) Early hematopoietic progenitor cell stages of the erythroid and megakaryocytic cell lines characterized by their tissue culture growth pattern in which large colonies are produced. Contrast with the more differentiated colony-forming units, which produce smaller colonies.

C banding In cytogenetic analysis, a specialized Giemsa stain technique employing first an acid and then a basic buffer, which highlights the centromeres of chromosomes. The stained centromere is the C band, which helps to identify the chromosome.

Cabot rings Threadlike structures that appear as purple-blue loops or rings in Wright-stained red blood cell cytoplasm. They are remnants of mitotic spindle fibers that indicate hematologic disease such as megaloblastic or refractory anemia.

calibrator (secondary standard) Preserved material in which the analyte concentration has been assigned by reference to a primary standard or by controlled reference assays in expert laboratories. Calibrators are used for assays in which there are no primary standards, such as blood cell counts or coagulation assays.

carboxyhemoglobin Hemoglobin that has bound carbon monoxide, which prevents normal oxygen exchange. Carboxyhemoglobin imparts a cherry-red color to venous blood, and its reduced oxygen capacity is the basis for carbon monoxide poisoning.

carcinoma Malignant neoplasm of epithelial cell origin that invades surrounding tissue and may metastasize to distant regions of the body.

cell membrane Cell surface composed of two layers of phospholipids intermixed with cholesterol and a variety of specialized glycoproteins that support cell structure, signaling, and ion transport.

cellular immunity (cell-mediated immunity, CMI) Immune response initiated and mediated by T-lymphocyte secretions called *cytokines*, natural killer cells, and macrophages; the mechanism of acquired immunity characterized by the dominant role of the T lymphocytes. Cellular immunity is the basis for graft rejection, delayed hypersensitivity, and responses to viral infections and tumors.

centriole Cylindrical organelle composed of microtubules. Two centrioles typically orient perpendicular to each other forming the centrosome, located near the nucleus. During mitosis they replicate and move to opposite ends of the cell where they bind to spindle fibers that attach to the centromeres of chromosomes and effect their movement during metaphase.

centromere Constricted portion of a chromosome that attaches to a spindle fiber to effect movement during metaphase. Centromeres are categorized by their location as acrocentric (near one end), metacentric (near the center), or submetacentric (off center).

cerebrospinal fluid (CSF) Fluid that flows through and protects the four ventricles of the brain, the subarachnoid spaces, and the spinal canal. CSF is derived from plasma and is the site of bacterial and viral infections called *meningitis* or *encephalitis*. CSF is sampled by lumbar puncture.

cerebrovascular accident (CVA) Stroke; occlusion of an artery of the brain or brain hemorrhage resulting in necrosis of brain tissue and loss of function.

Charcot-Leyden crystals Crystalline structures that are shaped like narrow double pyramids and are found in the sputum of asthma patients and the feces of dysentery patients. Formed from the granules of disintegrating eosinophils.

Chédiak-Higashi anomaly Autosomal recessive disorder characterized by partial albinism, photophobia, susceptibility to infection, and the presence of giant blue granules in the cytoplasm of Wright-stained white blood cells and platelets.

chelation Chemical formation of a ring-shaped molecular complex in which a metal ion is covalently bound. Chelating agents such as ethylenediaminetetraacetic acid (EDTA) or sodium citrate trap calcium ions and are used as blood specimen anticoagulants. Chelators are also used to treat lead poisoning or iron overload.

chemotaxis Cellular movement toward or away from a chemical stimulus. Characteristic of neutrophils and monocytes, whose phagocytic activity is influenced by chemical factors released by invading microorganisms.

chemotherapy Treatment of neoplastic disease (cancer) by chemical agents.

chromogen Chemical that absorbs light and produces color. Chromogens are used in laboratory analysis by spectrophotometry.

chromophore The portion of a molecule that absorbs incident light and emits colored light, usually as a result of the presence of 10 or more double bands or aromatic rings. Chromophores are the colored portions of chromogens and are synthesized in molecules to provide measurable color in laboratory assays.

chromosome Threadlike nuclear structure composed of condensed DNA that transmits genetic information. In humans there are 46 chromosomes, including 22 homologous pairs of autosomes and 1 pair of sex chromosomes, X and Y.

chronic Persisting over a long period of time, often for the remainder of a person's life.

chronic leukemia Malignant, unregulated proliferation of myelocytic or lymphocytic cells that appear at several stages of differentiation in peripheral blood. Characterized by slow onset and progression of symptoms.

Clinical and Laboratory Standards Institute (CLSI) Global nonprofit agency that uses consensus to develop and publish healthcare guidelines and standards.

Clinical Laboratory Improvement Amendments (CLIA) of 1988 Law establishing the Clinical Laboratory Improvement Amendments Committee (CLIAC), which sets and enforces standards for quality testing in the clinical laboratory.

clone Group of genetically identical cells derived from a single common cell through mitosis.

Clostridium perfringens Anaerobic gram-positive bacteria that cause gangrene in humans. Symptoms of gangrene include intravascular hemolysis and thrombosis.

cluster of differentiation (CD) Cell surface membrane receptors or markers used to characterize cells by their functions. CD profiles are used in flow cytometry to identify cell types. CDs are used in hematology to identify cell clones associated with lymphoid and myelogenous leukemias and lymphomas.

coagulation Series of enzymatic reactions beginning with activation of factor VII by tissue factor (extrinsic/in vivo) or factor XII by a negatively charged surface (intrinsic/in vitro) and proceeding through the common pathway to the formation of an insoluble fibrin clot.

coagulation cascade Series of enzymatic reactions beginning with activation of factor VII by tissue factor (extrinsic/in vivo) or factor XII by a negatively charged surface (intrinsic/in vitro) and proceeding through the common pathway to the formation of an insoluble fibrin clot.

coagulation factors Plasma proteins, also called *procoagulants*, that circulate as inactive forms. When activated in the process of coagulation, procoagulants participate in the coagulation cascade to form a fibrin clot.

codocyte (target cell) Poorly hemoglobinized red blood cell (RBC) that appears in hemoglobinopathies, thalassemia, and liver disease. In a Wright-stained peripheral blood film, hemoglobin concentrates in the center of the RBC and around the periphery, causing the cell to resemble a "bull's-eye."

coefficient of variation (CV, percent CV, CV%) Statistical measure of the deviation of a variable from its mean divided by the mean, usually expressed as a percentage.

colchicine Alkaloid that blocks microtubule formation and prevents cell division. Used in cytogenetic studies to arrest mitosis in metaphase so that chromosomes may be karyotyped. Colchicine is also a component of a drug used to treat gout. Colcemid is the trademark for a colchicine derivative used in preparing chromosomes for karyotyping.

cold agglutinin IgM autoantibody specific for red blood cell surface membrane antigens usually of the Ii system that typically reacts at temperatures below 30° C.

cold agglutinin disease Acquired autoimmune hemolytic anemia resulting from red blood cell (RBC) agglutination by IgM autoantibodies that react with RBCs at temperatures above 30° C.

Patients with cold agglutinin disease experience *Raynaud phenomenon*, characterized by pallor, cyanosis, and pain in the fingers, palms, wrists, and ankles after exposure to cold.

colony-forming unit (CFU) Hematopoietic progenitor cells that are derived from the pluripotential hematopoietic stem cell and give rise to the different cell lineages of the bone marrow. Named because of their ability to form colonies in tissue culture.

colony-forming unit–granulocyte, erythrocyte, monocyte, and megakaryocyte (CFU-GEMM) Hematopoietic progenitor cell capable of differentiating into the granulocytic (myelocytic), erythrocytic (normoblastic), monocytic, or megakaryocytic cell lines.

colony-stimulating factor (CSF) Cytokine that promotes the division and differentiation of hematopoietic cells.

common coagulation pathway The steps in the coagulation cascade from the activation of factor X through the conversion of fibrinogen to fibrin. The common pathway begins at the junction of the intrinsic and extrinsic pathways and involves factors X, V, and II (prothrombin) and fibrinogen, in order of reaction.

complement (C) System of at least 20 serum enzymes. The complement system responds to antigen-antibody reaction to stimulate white blood cell chemotaxis, generate inflammation, and cause red blood cell lysis.

condenser Substage microscope device that focuses light on the slide-mounted specimen to promote visual clarity.

confidence interval (CI) Range of values expected to contain the measured value (parameter) with a predetermined degree of statistical confidence. For instance, the 95% confidence interval is expected to include 95% of all values of a parameter measured in a normal population, which corresponds closely to ±2 standard deviations.

congenital Describes a condition that exists at, and presumably before, birth. Often refers to a hereditary condition.

Coombs test (direct antiglobulin test, DAT) Screening procedure in which antihuman globulin is used to detect antibodies and complement bound to red blood cells in vivo.

coronary artery bypass grafting (CABG) Cardiac surgery usually requiring cardiopulmonary bypass and extracorporeal circulation in which occluded sections of coronary arteries are replaced with grafts taken from nearby arteries, for example, the internal mammary artery.

corrected reticulocyte count Calculation performed to correct the visual reticulocyte count for specimens with a hematocrit below 45% to the equivalent reticulocyte count at a hematocrit of 45%. In anemia, the visual reticulocyte percentage is misleadingly elevated because whole blood contains fewer red blood cells relative to reticulocytes.

Coumadin (warfarin) Vitamin K antagonist used as an anticoagulant to prevent thrombosis in people with atrial fibrillation, venous thromboembolism, or cardiac insufficiency. Also used prophylactically after orthopedic surgery. Warfarin suppresses vitamin K and reduces the activity of the vitamin K–dependent coagulation factors II (prothrombin), VII, IX, and X.

cryoglobulin Any of numerous serum globulins, typically immunoglobulins, that precipitate at around 4° C and become resuspended at 37° C.

cryoprecipitate (CRYO) Therapeutic agent rich in fibrinogen, factor VIII, and factor XIII, used to treat bleeding disorders in fibrinogen deficiency, factor XIII deficiency, and hemorrhagic trauma. Cryoprecipitate is collected from human plasma that has been frozen and slowly thawed.

cyanosis Bluish discoloration of the skin, sclera, and mucous membranes caused by poor tissue oxygenation. Usually a sign of anemia.

cytochemical analysis Use of specialized stains to detect cellular enzymes and other chemicals in peripheral blood films and bone marrow aspirate smears. Used to differentiate hematologic diseases, especially leukemias.

cytogenetics Branch of genetics devoted to the laboratory study of visible chromosome abnormalities, such as deletions, translocations, and aneuploidy.

cytokine Cellular product that influences the function or activity of other cells. Cytokines include colony-stimulating factors, interferons, interleukins, and lymphokines.

cytomegalovirus (CMV) Group of DNA viruses of the family Herpesviridae. CMV infection is asymptomatic in adults but can be transmitted to a fetus in utero to cause a potentially fatal infection or reduced intelligence. CMV can be transmitted by blood transfusions and is detected using molecular diagnostic techniques.

cytopenia Reduced cell count in one or more of any blood cell line—red blood cells, white blood cells, or platelets.

cytosol Fluid portion of the cytoplasm, less granules and organelles, as separated by ultracentrifugation.

cytotoxic Describes a compound or agent that destroys or damages cells.

dacryocyte (teardrop cell) Red blood cell with a single pointed extension, resembling a teardrop. Dacryocytes are often seen in the myeloproliferative neoplasm termed *myelofibrosis with myeloid metaplasia.*

D-dimer (D:D, D-D) One of the fibrin degradation products. D-dimer is composed of two fibrin D fragments covalently joined by the enzymatic action of factor XIII. The D-dimer assay is used to rule out venous thromboembolic disease and disseminated intravascular coagulation, and may be used to monitor the efficacy and length of warfarin therapy.

deep vein thrombosis (DVT, deep venous thrombosis) Pathologic formation of a clot in a deep leg vein such as the femoral vein. A manifestation of venous thromboembolic disease that is associated with a number of acquired or congenital thrombotic risk factors, deep vein thrombosis raises the risk of a pulmonary embolus.

11-dehydrothromboxane B$_2$ (11-DHT) Measurable urine product of the platelet cyclooxygenase (eicosanoid) activation pathway. Employed clinically to measure in vivo platelet activation and aspirin resistance.

delayed hemolytic transfusion reaction Hemolysis that occurs days or weeks after a blood transfusion, caused by an anamnestic response to the transfused red blood cells in a patient alloimmunized from a previous pregnancy or transfusion.

δ check Quality control process in which a current analyte result is compared with the result for the same analyte from the previous specimen from the same patient.

dense granule (dense body, δ-body, δ-granule) Platelet organelle that contains and secretes the small molecules adenosine diphosphate, adenosine triphosphate, serotonin, calcium (Ca^{2+}), and magnesium (Mg^{2+}). There are two to seven dense granules per platelet, and they are named by their opaque appearance in transmission electron microscopy.

deoxyhemoglobin Hemoglobin that is not combined with oxygen, formed when oxyhemoglobin releases its oxygen to the tissues.

deoxyribonucleic acid (DNA) Double-stranded, helical nucleic acid that carries genetic information. DNA is composed of nucleotide sequences with four repeating bases: adenine, cytosine, guanine, and thymine. During mitosis, DNA condenses to form chromosomes.

des-γ-carboxy coagulation factors and coagulation control proteins Coagulation cascade procoagulants II, VII, IX, and X; and control proteins C, S, and Z that require vitamin K–catalyzed γ-carboxylation of glutamic acid. During anticoagulant therapy with warfarin (Coumadin), which suppresses vitamin K, these des-γ-carboxylated proteins cannot participate in coagulation.

desquamation Shedding of epithelial elements, chiefly of the skin, in scales or sheets.

Diamond-Blackfan anemia (DBA, congenital pure red cell aplasia) Rare congenital anemia due to mutations in DNA repair genes, and evident in the first 3 months of life. Anemia is severe and erythropoietin resistant; the reticulocyte count does not rise. Platelet and white blood cell counts are normal.

diapedesis Outward passage of white blood cells through intact vessel walls.

differential white blood cell count Review and tabulation of 100 to 200 white blood cells (WBCs) in a stained blood film. The different types of WBCs are counted and reported as absolute counts or percentages of total WBCs. In automated hematology analyzers, the differential WBC count is accomplished by counting thousands of WBCs using various technologies.

dilute Russell viper venom time (DRVVT) Coagulation test performed like a prothrombin time assay. Russell viper venom activates the common coagulation pathway at the level of factor X. In the DRVVT assay, the reagent is diluted 1:500. DRVVT is prolonged by lupus anticoagulant, and the test is used routinely in screening for this antibody.

diploid Having two sets of chromosomes, as normally found in nuclei of somatic cells. In humans, the normal diploid number is 46.

direct antiglobulin test (DAT, Coombs test) Screening procedure in which antihuman globulin is used to detect antibodies and complement bound to red blood cells in vivo.

direct thrombin inhibitors (DTIs) Class of intravenous therapeutic anticoagulants including argatroban, dabigatran, and bivalirudin that suppress coagulation by directly neutralizing thrombin. DTIs are used in place of heparin when heparin-induced thrombocytopenia with thrombosis is suspected. DTI therapy may be monitored using the partial thromboplastin time.

disseminated intravascular coagulation (DIC) Uncontrolled activation of thrombin and consumption of coagulation factors, platelets, and fibrinolytic proteins secondary to many initiating events, including infection, inflammation, shock, and trauma. Most commonly evidenced by diffuse mucocutaneous bleeding.

Döhle bodies In Wright-stained peripheral blood films, gray to light blue round or oval inclusions composed of ribosomal RNA found singly or in multiples near the inner membrane surface of granulocyte cytoplasm.

dominant Denoting an inherited allele whose trait is expressed whenever the gene is present, even in heterozygotes.

Donath-Landsteiner (D-L) autoantibody IgG autoantibody with anti-P specificity that binds red blood cells at temperatures below 20° C and causes hemolysis at 37° C. Donath-Landsteiner antibody causes hemolysis in patients with paroxysmal cold hemoglobinuria.

Down syndrome Congenital group of physical, mental, and functional abnormalities including distinctive facial features, congenital heart disease, muscular hypotonia, and mental retardation, all associated with trisomy 21. Approximately 10% of infants with Down syndrome are born with or develop transient myeloproliferative disease (TMD), which resembles chronic myelogenous leukemia but resolves spontaneously. Within a few weeks of TMD resolution, the child has a 10% to 30% chance of developing acute myeloid or acute lymphoblastic leukemia.

drepanocyte (sickle cell) Abnormal crescent-shaped red blood cell containing hemoglobin S, characteristic of sickle cell anemia.

drug-induced hemolytic anemia Hemolytic anemia caused directly by a drug or secondary to an antibody-mediated response stimulated by the drug.

dry tap Term used when an inadequate sample of bone marrow fluid is obtained during bone marrow aspiration. Dry taps occur when the marrow is packed, as in chronic myelogenous leukemia, or when it is fibrotic, as in myelofibrosis with myeloid metaplasia.

duodenum Proximal portion of the small intestine adjacent to the stomach.

dyscrasia Disorder of a hematologic cell line or lines.

dyserythropoiesis Deranged erythropoiesis producing cells with abnormal morphology; usually applied to congenital dyserythropoietic anemia and myelodysplastic syndrome.

dysfibrinogenemia Presence in the plasma of structurally abnormal fibrinogen; often a result of liver disease, occasionally congenital.

dysmegakaryopoiesis Defective megakaryocytic production and maturation characterized by cells with abnormal morphology and increased or decreased megakaryocyte counts.

dysmyelopoiesis Defective myelocytic production and maturation characterized by cells with abnormal morphology; often applied to myelodysplastic syndromes.

dysplasia Abnormal growth pattern; for example, enlarged skull in chronic anemia. Abnormal cervical epithelial cell histopathologic features.

dyspnea Difficult or painful breathing.

ecchymosis Hemorrhagic spot, 1 cm or larger in diameter, in the skin or mucous membranes, typically forming an irregular blue or purplish patch. Also known as a *bruise*.

echinocyte (burr cell, crenated red blood cell) Red blood cell (RBC) with short, equally spaced, spiny projections. Burr cells are found in uremia and pyruvate kinase deficiency, and observed in all fields of a peripheral blood film. Crenated RBCs are formed by cellular dehydration (drying artifact), and not observed in all fields.

eclampsia Potentially life-threatening disorder during pregnancy characterized by hypertension, generalized edema, proteinuria, and convulsions.

edema Accumulation of excess serous fluid in a fluid compartment or tissue.

effusion Seepage and accumulation of plasma-derived fluid into a body cavity from blood vessels as a result of blood vessel damage or hydrostatic pressure.

electronic impedance Opposition to the flow of electrical current. The impedance principle of cell counting is based on the detection and measurement of changes in electrical resistance produced by cells as they transverse a small aperture in a conducting solution.

electrophoresis Separation and identification of proteins, nucleic acids, and hemoglobin types based on their relative rates of migration through agarose or polyacrylamide gel in an applied electrical field. Depending on the component, the rate of migration may be based on molecular mass and/or net charge.

elliptocytes (ovalocytes) Oval red blood cells seen in the peripheral blood in the membrane disorder hereditary elliptocytosis. May be found in low numbers in healthy states and in other anemias such as iron deficiency and thalassemia.

elliptocytosis (ovalocytosis) Hereditary hematologic disorder characterized by the presence of elliptocytes; often asymptomatic but may be associated with slight anemia.

Embden-Meyerhof pathway (EMP, glycolysis) A series of enzymatically catalyzed reactions by which glucose and other sugars are metabolized to yield lactic acid (anaerobic glycolysis) or pyruvic acid (aerobic glycolysis). Metabolism releases energy in the form of adenosine triphosphate.

embolism Pathologic event in which an embolus (foreign object) travels through the bloodstream, becomes lodged in an artery, and obstructs blood flow. The embolus is often a blood clot, but it may be a fat globule, air bubble, piece of tissue, or clump of bacteria. Emboli occlude an artery and cause tissue ischemia, necrosis, and loss of function. A pulmonary embolism is an embolus in a lung artery and is often fatal.

endoplasmic reticulum (ER) Extensive network of membrane-enclosed tubules in the cytoplasm of cells. Rough endoplasmic reticulum is rich in ribosomes that synthesize proteins and provides a pathway for transport of membrane-bound protein through the cytoplasm.

endothelial cells Cell layer that lines the inner surface of all blood vessels. Intact endothelial cells prevent thrombosis because they present a smooth, nonactivating surface and secrete antiplatelet and anticoagulant substances. Injured endothelial cells promote clotting through expression of tissue factor and secretion of coagulation-promoting factors, such as von Willebrand factor.

enterocytes Epithelial cells that form the inner lining of the intestine. Enterocytes absorb nutrients from the intestinal lumen and transport them to the portal circulation.

eosinophil Granulocyte with large uniform cytoplasmic granules that stain orange to pink with Wright stain. Granules usually do not obscure the segmented nucleus.

eosinophilia Increase in the blood eosinophil count that is associated with allergies, parasitic infections, or hematologic disorders.

epiphyses Ends of long bones that normally contain hematopoietic tissue.

epistaxis Hemorrhage from the nose; a nosebleed that requires intervention.

Epstein-Barr virus (EBV) Herpesvirus that causes infectious mononucleosis and leads to the appearance of variant lymphocytes.

erythroblastosis fetalis (hemolytic disease of the fetus and newborn, HDFN) Alloimmune anemia caused by maternal immunoglobulin G antibody that crosses the placenta and binds fetal red blood cell antigens inherited from the father; for instance, maternal anti-A with fetal A antigen. The disorder is characterized by hemolytic anemia, hyperbilirubinemia, and extramedullary erythropoiesis.

erythrocyte (red blood cell, RBC) Nonnucleated biconcave disk-shaped peripheral blood cell containing hemoglobin. Its primary function is oxygen transport and delivery to tissues.

erythrocyte sedimentation rate (ESR) Distance that red blood cells fall in a column of anticoagulated blood in a specified time period. Elevated sedimentation rates are not specific for any disorder but indicate the presence of inflammation.

erythrocytosis Increase in the red blood cell count in peripheral blood.

erythroleukemia (Di Guglielmo disease, M6) Acute malignancy characterized by a proliferation of erythroid and myeloid precursors in bone marrow, with erythroblasts with bizarre lobulated nuclei and abnormal myeloblasts in peripheral blood.

erythron Total mass of red blood cells circulating in the peripheral blood and their bone marrow precursors.

erythropoiesis Bone marrow process of red blood cell production.

erythropoietin (EPO) Glycoprotein hormone synthesized primarily in the kidneys and released into the bloodstream in response to hypoxia. The hormone acts to stimulate and regulate the bone marrow production of red blood cells.

essential thrombocythemia Myeloproliferative neoplasm characterized by marked thrombocytosis and dysfunctional platelets. Patients may experience bleeding or thrombosis.

etiology Causes or origin of a disease, for instance, genetic factors, infection, toxins, or trauma. Contrast with *pathogenesis*, which is the physiologic and biochemical mechanisms by which a disease progresses.

euchromatin Portion of DNA that is active in gene expression and stains lightly with Wright stain.

euglobulin In the euglobulin lysis assay, the fraction of treated plasma that contains fibrinogen, plasmin, plasminogen, and plasminogen activators, but lacks fibrinolytic inhibitors.

exogenous Originating from outside the body or produced by external causes; used, for example, to describe a disease caused by a bacterial or viral agent foreign to the body.

exon Portion of a DNA molecule that becomes translated to form a protein product. Exons and introns are transcribed from DNA to heteronuclear RNA, where the introns are excised to form messenger RNA.

extramedullary hematopoiesis (myeloid metaplasia) Production of blood cells outside the bone marrow, such as in the spleen, liver, or lymph nodes. Extramedullary hematopoiesis usually occurs in response to bone marrow fibrosis and loss of bone marrow hematopoiesis.

extranodal Located outside a lymph node.

extravascular hemolysis Destruction of red blood cells outside of a blood vessel, typically by splenic macrophage phagocytosis. Also called *macrophage-mediated* hemolysis.

extrinsic coagulation pathway Primary in vivo coagulation pathway. Exposure of tissue factor activates factor VII. Factor VIIa activates factors IX and X, which triggers the common pathway of coagulation and formation of fibrin.

exudate Fluid that has effused into a body cavity in association with bacterial or viral infections, malignancy, pulmonary embolism, or systemic lupus erythematosus. An exudate is typically cloudy, because it contains cells and concentrated protein.

factor assay Clot-based or chromogenic assay for specific coagulation factor activity.

factor V Leiden mutation Substitution of arginine with glutamine at position 506 in the factor V protein. The resultant factor V resists digestion by activated protein C. The factor V Leiden mutation results in increased thrombin production and is a thrombosis risk factor.

Fanconi anemia Autosomal recessive or X-linked aplastic anemia manifesting in childhood or early adult life. Characterized by mental retardation, absence of the thumb and radius, small stature, hypogonadism, and patchy brown discoloration of the skin.

favism Acute hemolytic anemia caused by ingestion of fava beans or inhalation of the pollen of the plant. Usually occurs in individuals with an inherited deficiency of glucose-6-phosphate dehydrogenase in red blood cells.

ferritin Iron-apoferritin complex, a major form in which iron is stored in the liver.

ferrokinetics Study of iron metabolism, including the movement of iron among the storage, transport, and functional iron compartments.

fibrin Fibrillar protein produced by the action of thrombin on fibrinogen in the clotting process. Fibrin is responsible for the semisolid character of a blood clot.

fibrin degradation products (FDPs, fibrin split products, FSPs) Fibrin fragments X, Y, D, and E and D-dimer produced by the action of fibrin-bound plasmin during fibrinolysis.

fibrinogen Plasma glycoprotein that is converted to fibrin by thrombin digestion.

fibrinolysis Continual process of digestion of fibrin by bound plasmin that has been activated by bound plasminogen activator. Fibrinolysis is the normal mechanism for the removal of fibrin clots. Fibrin is digested into fragments X, Y, D, and E and D-dimer.

fibroblast Connective tissue cell that differentiates into numerous cells, which comprise the fibrous tissue of the body, for instance, tissue in the walls of arteries.

Fitzgerald factor (high-molecular-weight kininogen, HMWK) Member of the kinin inflammatory system that is digested and activated by kallikrein to form bradykinin. Fitzgerald factor is one of the in vitro contact activators of the coagulation system, which also include prekallikrein and factor XII.

Fletcher factor (prekallikrein, PK, pre-K) Member of the kinin inflammatory system that forms active kallikrein upon digestion by kininogen. Fletcher factor helps to trigger in vitro coagulation contact activation. Fletcher factor deficiency prolongs the partial thromboplastin time but has no clinical consequence.

flow cytometer Instrument in which cells suspended in fluid flow one at a time through a focused beam of light. The light is scattered in patterns characteristic of the cells and their components. A sensor detecting the scattered or emitted light measures the size and molecular characteristics of individual cells.

fluorescence in situ hybridization (FISH) Laboratory technique in which fluorescence-labeled nucleic acid probes hybridize to selected DNA or RNA sequences in fixed tissue. FISH allows for the visual microscopic detection of specific polymorphisms or mutations such as *BCR/ABL* in cell or tissue specimens.

fluorophore Portion of a molecule that absorbs incident light and emits fluorescent light. Fluorophores are synthesized in molecules to provide measurable fluorescence in laboratory assays.

free erythrocyte protoporphyrin (FEP) Porphyrin precursor of heme that is present in low concentrations in normal red blood cells (RBCs). Elevated RBC concentrations indicate iron deficiency or impaired iron insertion.

French-American-British (FAB) classification International classification system for acute leukemias, myeloproliferative neoplasms, and myelodysplastic syndromes developed in the 1970s and 1980s. Still in use, although it is being displaced by the World Health Organization classification.

fresh frozen plasma (FFP) Plasma that is separated by centrifugation from whole-blood donations and frozen within 8 hours of collection. FFP contains all of the plasma procoagulants and control proteins, including the labile factors V and VIII. FFP is used for replacement therapy in acquired multiple-factor deficiencies, or in single-factor deficiencies when factor concentrates are not available.

G banding (GTG banding) In cytogenetic analysis, a procedure in which metaphase chromosomes are treated with trypsin and then stained with Giemsa dye. The areas rich in adenine-thymine, called G+, stain intensely, whereas the areas rich in guanine-cytosine (G–) stain more lightly. The G+ bands correspond with Q bands in Q banding. Banding patterns are used for the identification of chromosomes.

gammopathy Plasma protein imbalance caused by markedly increased concentrations of gamma globulin. A monoclonal protein produced by myeloma tumor cells causes most gammopathies.

Gaucher disease Rare autosomal recessive disorder of fat metabolism caused by glucocerebrosidase deficiency and characterized by histiocytic hyperplasia in the liver, spleen, lymph nodes, and bone marrow. The characteristic Gaucher cells, which are lipid-filled macrophages whose cytoplasm resembles crumpled tissue paper, are found on the Wright-stained bone marrow aspirate smear.

Gaussian distribution Frequency distribution that approximates the distribution of many random variables and is portrayed graphically as a symmetric bell-shaped curve. The peak represents the mean of the distribution and the width of the curve represents the dispersion or variability, which is generally expressed in terms of standard deviation from the mean. Also called a *normal distribution.*

gene Segment of a DNA molecule that contains all the information required for synthesis of a protein, including both coding (exon) and noncoding (intron) sequences. Each gene occupies a specific position (locus) on a particular chromosome.

gene rearrangement Reorganization of the DNA sequences of a gene. Rearrangement of B-cell and T-cell genes produces an infinite variety of variable-region receptor and immunoglobulin sequences. *Clonal* gene rearrangements occur in lymphoma and lymphocytic leukemia and are detected by flow cytometry to identify these diseases.

gestational age Age of the fetus, usually expressed as the time elapsed from the first day of the mother's last menstrual period.

Glanzmann thrombasthenia (GT) Severe mucocutaneous bleeding disorder caused by one of a series of mutations in platelet glycoprotein (GP) IIb or IIIa. Normal GP IIb/IIIa recognizes and binds the arginine-glycine-aspartate peptide sequence receptor complex found in fibrinogen and von Willebrand factor. Glanzmann thrombasthenia causes a defect of fibrinogen-dependent platelet aggregation.

globin Protein constituent of hemoglobin. Two identical pairs of globin chains bind four heme molecules to form hemoglobin.

globulins Class of proteins that are insoluble in water or highly concentrated salt solutions but are soluble in moderately concentrated salt solutions. All plasma proteins are globulins except albumin and prealbumin.

glossitis Inflammation of the tongue that causes it to be red and smooth.

glucose-6-phosphate dehydrogenase (G6PD) First enzyme of the glucose monophosphate shunt from the Embden-Meyerhoff pathway. G6PD catalyzes the oxidation of glucose-6-phosphate to a lactone, converting the oxidized form of nicotinamide adenine dinucleotide phosphate (NADP) to the reduced form (NADPH).

glucose-6-phosphate dehydrogenase deficiency X-linked recessive deficiency of glucose-6-phosphate dehydrogenase characterized by episodes of acute intravascular hemolysis under conditions of oxidative stress, including exposure to oxidative drugs such as quinine.

glycocalyx Glycoprotein and polysaccharide covering that surrounds many cells. The platelet glycocalyx is thicker than that of other cells and provides a procoagulant environment.

glycolysis (Embden-Meyerhof pathway, EMP) A series of enzymatically catalyzed reactions by which glucose and other sugars are metabolized to yield lactic acid (anaerobic glycolysis) or pyruvic

acid (aerobic glycolysis). Metabolism releases energy in the form of adenosine triphosphate.

glycophorin Transmembrane red blood cell protein that carries several blood group antigens.

glycoprotein Conjugated protein containing one or more covalently linked carbohydrate residues.

glycoprotein IIb/IIIa (GP IIb/IIIa) Pair of glycoproteins that function as a receptor for the arginine-glycine-aspartate sequence in fibrinogen and von Willebrand factor. The combination of fibrinogen and glycoprotein IIb/IIIa is essential to platelet aggregation.

Golgi apparatus Rigid organelle comprised of numerous flattened sacs and associated vesicles. It is the location of the posttranslational modification and storage of glycoproteins, lipoproteins, membrane-bound proteins, and lysosomal enzymes.

gout Painful inflammation caused by excessive plasma uric acid, which becomes deposited as monosodium urate monohydrate in joint capsules and adjacent tendons.

graft-versus-host disease (GVHD) Condition including tissue rejection that occurs when immunologically competent cells or their precursors are transplanted into an immunocompromised host who is not histocompatible with the donor. The donor cells engraft and mount an immune response against the host.

granulocytes Class of white blood cells in peripheral blood characterized by cytoplasmic granules; includes basophils, eosinophils, and neutrophils.

granuloma Nodular, delimited aggregation of inflammatory cells, macrophages, and macrophage-derived multinucleate giant cells surrounded by a rim of lymphocytes and fibroblasts. Granulomas are major sites of cell-mediated immune response to particulate antigens, and they may occur in many organs in chronic granulomatous disease.

GTG banding (G banding) In cytogenetic analysis, a procedure in which metaphase chromosomes are treated with trypsin and then stained with Giemsa dye. The areas rich in adenine-thymine, called G+, stain intensely, whereas the areas rich in guanine-cytosine (G–) stain more lightly. The G+ bands correspond with Q bands in Q banding. Banding patterns are used for the identification of chromosomes.

guaiac test Test performed on stool emulsions to detect hemoglobin as evidence of gastrointestinal bleeding. Small amounts of blood may be invisible; therefore it is known as a test for occult (hidden) blood. The peroxidase activity of hemoglobin in blood reacts with guaiac to yield a blue color.

hairy cells Malignant B lymphocytes seen in the peripheral blood and bone marrow characterized by delicate gray cytoplasm with projections resembling hairs. These cells are seen in hairy cell leukemia.

haploid Referring to the number of chromosomes found in sperm or ova, which is only one of each pair of chromosomes found in somatic (diploid) cells. In humans, the haploid number is 23.

haptoglobin Plasma protein that irreversibly binds free hemoglobin, forming a complex that is removed by macrophages while conserving iron. Haptoglobin is decreased due to consumption in intravascular hemolysis.

Heinz bodies Round blue to purple inclusions attached to inner red blood cell membranes visible when stained with new methylene blue dye. Heinz bodies may be found in multiples and are composed of precipitated hemoglobin in unstable hemoglobin disorders and glucose-6-phosphate dehydrogenase deficiency.

helmet cell Helmet-shaped schistocyte that may appear in microangiopathic hemolytic anemia (fragmented red blood cell).

hemarthroses Chronic joint bleeds that cause inflammation and immobilization; a symptom of severe hemophilia.

hematemesis Vomiting of bright red blood.

hematocrit (HCT, packed cell volume, PCV) Proportion of whole blood that consists of red blood cells, expressed as a percentage of the total blood volume.

hematoidin Golden yellow, brown, or red crystals that are chemically similar to bilirubin. Hematoidin crystal in a tissue preparation indicates a hemorrhage site.

hematology Clinical study of blood cells and blood-forming tissues.

hematoma Localized collection of extravasated blood (blood that has escaped from vessel into tissue), usually clotted, in an organ space or tissue, giving the appearance of a bruise.

hematopathology Study of the diseases of blood cells and hematopoietic tissue.

hematopoiesis Formation and development of blood cells. Hematopoiesis occurs mostly in the bone marrow and peripheral lymphatic tissues.

hematopoietic microenvironment Matrix of bone marrow stromal cells and tissue that supports hematopoiesis both structurally and through the production of cytokines and colony-stimulating factors.

hematopoietic progenitor cell (HPC) Actively dividing cell that is committed to a single blood cell lineage and is not capable of self-renewal. Therapeutic hematopoietic progenitor cell products intended for transplantation provide both hematopoietic stem cells and progenitor cells.

hematopoietic stem cell (HSC) Actively dividing cell that is capable of self-renewal and of differentiation into any blood cell lineage.

hematuria Abnormal presence of intact red blood cells in the urine; indicative of kidney or urinary tract disease.

heme Pigmented iron-containing nonprotein part of the hemoglobin molecule. There are four heme groups in a hemoglobin molecule, each containing one ferrous ion in the center. Oxygen binds the ferrous ion and is transported from an area of high to low oxygen concentration.

hemochromatosis Disease of iron metabolism that is characterized by excess deposition of iron in the tissues. The disease may be inherited or may develop as a complication of a hemolytic anemia, such as β-thalassemia major.

hemoconcentration Elevation of the red blood cell, white blood cell, and platelet counts resulting from a decrease in plasma volume, for example, in dehydration.

hemocytometer (hemacytometer, counting chamber) Device used to perform visual blood and body fluid cell counts, consisting of a microscopic slide with a depression whose polished glass base is marked with grids and into which a measured volume of a sample of diluted blood is placed and covered with a cover glass. The number of cells in the squares is counted under a microscope and used as a representative sample for calculating the unit volume.

hemodialysis Extracorporeal circulation process that substitutes for the kidneys and removes wastes from the blood. Hemodialysis is used to treat patients with renal failure. The patient's blood is shunted from the body through a dialysis machine for diffusion and ultrafiltration and is then returned to the patient's circulation.

hemoglobin (Hb, HGB) Tetramer composed of two identical globin chains, each of which binds a heme molecule. Hemoglobin is the primary constituent of red blood cell cytoplasm and transports molecular oxygen from the lungs to the tissues.

hemoglobin C crystal Reddish hexagonal cytoplasmic red blood cell crystal described as a "gold bar," or "Washington monument." Typical of homozygous hemoglobin C disease, crystals form as deoxyhemoglobin C polymerizes.

hemoglobin electrophoresis Separation and identification of normal and abnormal hemoglobin types based on their relative rates of migration through agarose or polyacrylamide gel in an applied electric field. The rate of migration depends mainly on net charge. Examples of hemoglobin types include Hb A, Hb C, Hb F, and Hb S.

hemoglobin SC crystal Irregular reddish cytoplasmic red blood cell crystal described as a "glove" or "pistol." Typical of compound heterozygous hemoglobin SC disease, the crystals form as deoxyhemoglobin S and C polymerize.

hemoglobinemia Presence of free hemoglobin in the blood plasma; indicative of intravascular hemolysis.

hemoglobinopathy Condition characterized by structural variations in globin genes that result in the formation of abnormal globin chains. Examples are sickle cell anemia and hemoglobin C disease.

hemoglobinuria Visible reddish free hemoglobin in the urine; indicative of intravascular hemolysis.

hemolysis Disruption of red blood cell membrane integrity that destroys the cell and releases hemoglobin.

hemolytic anemia Anemia characterized by a shortened red blood cell (RBC) life span and inability of the bone marrow to adequately compensate by increasing RBC synthesis. Hemolytic anemia may be caused by extrinsic or intrinsic disorders.

hemolytic disease of the fetus and newborn (HDFN, erythroblastosis fetalis) Alloimmune anemia caused by maternal IgG antibody that crosses the placenta and binds fetal red blood cell antigens inherited from the father: for instance, maternal anti-A with fetal A antigen. HDFN is characterized by hemolytic anemia, hyperbilirubinemia, and extramedullary erythropoiesis.

hemolytic uremic syndrome (HUS) Severe microangiopathic hemolytic anemia that often follows infection of the gastrointestinal tract by *Escherichia coli* serotype O157:H7, which produces an exotoxin. It is characterized by renal failure, thrombocytopenia, the appearance of schistocytes on the peripheral blood film, and severe mucocutaneous hemorrhage.

hemopexin Plasma glycoprotein produced in the liver. Hemopexin binds free plasma heme in the absence of haptoglobin.

hemophilia Group of hereditary anatomic bleeding disorders caused by a deficiency of a single coagulation factor. The two most common forms are hemophilia A and hemophilia B, deficiencies of factors VIII and IX, respectively.

hemophilia A (classic hemophilia) Sex-linked recessive anatomic bleeding disorder caused by a deficiency of coagulation factor VIII.

hemophilia B (Christmas disease) Sex-linked recessive anatomic bleeding disorder caused by a deficiency of coagulation factor IX.

hemophilia C (Rosenthal syndrome) Autosomal anatomic bleeding disorder caused by a deficiency of coagulation factor XI.

hemorrhage Acute severe blood loss requiring intervention and transfusions.

hemorrhagic disease of the newborn Neonatal anatomic bleeding caused by vitamin K deficiency.

hemosiderin Intracellular storage form of iron found predominantly in liver, spleen, and bone marrow cells. Hemosiderin is a breakdown product of ferritin that appears in iron overload and hemochromatosis. Hemosiderin may be detected microscopically using the Prussian blue iron stain.

hemosiderinuria Presence in the urine of hemosiderin, which can be visualized using Prussian blue iron stain; most often an indicator of chronic intravascular hemolysis.

hemosiderosis Increased tissue iron stores without associated tissue damage; may progress to hemochromatosis.

hemostasis Process by which a series of platelet, endothelial cell, and plasma enzyme systems prevent blood loss through clot formation and maintain blood vessel patency.

heparin Naturally occurring mucopolysaccharide anticoagulant classified as a glycosaminoglycan. Heparin is produced by basophils and mast cells. Heparin extracted from porcine mucosa is used as a therapeutic anticoagulant.

heparin-induced thrombocytopenia with thrombosis (HIT) Morbid, often fatal effect of unfractionated heparin therapy. Up to 5% of patients receiving unfractionated heparin therapy for more than 5 days develop an antibody to the heparin-platelet factor 4 complex. The antibody and target antigen complex bind platelet Fc receptors and activate platelets, which causes a decrease in platelet count by greater than 30% and venous and arterial thrombosis.

hepatitis Inflammation of the liver that damages hepatocytes and releases bilirubin into the plasma.

hepatitis B virus (HBV) Causative agent of hepatitis B. The virus is transmitted by contaminated blood or blood products, by sexual contact with an infected person, or by the use of contaminated needles and instruments. Severe infection may cause prolonged illness, destruction of liver cells, cirrhosis, increased risk of liver cancer, or death.

hepatocyte Parenchymal liver cell.

hepatomegaly Abnormal enlargement of the liver; usually a sign of disease.

hepatosplenomegaly Abnormal enlargement of the spleen and liver.

hereditary elliptocytosis (ovalocytosis) Hereditary spectrin defect characterized by the presence of elliptocytes in the peripheral blood; often asymptomatic but may be associated with slight anemia.

hereditary pyropoikilocytosis Rare hereditary defect of spectrin that causes severe hemolytic anemia beginning in childhood and extreme poikilocytosis with red blood cell morphology resembling that seen in burn patients.

hereditary spherocytosis Hereditary defect in a cytoskeletal or transmembrane protein that results in loss of red blood cell membrane and causes hemolytic anemia characterized by numerous spherocytes on the peripheral blood film.

hereditary stomatocytosis Hereditary defect of the red blood cell membrane resulting in a complex group of diseases in which the hemolysis is mild to severe and stomatocytes are seen on the peripheral blood film.

hereditary xerocytosis Hereditary defect of the red blood cell membrane that results in hemolytic anemia with dehydrated red blood cells and the presence of stomatocytes, target cells, and macrocytes on the peripheral blood film.

heterochromatin Portion of DNA that is inactive during transcription to messenger RNA and stains deeply with Wright stain.

heterophile antibody Antibody that reacts with an antigen from a species other than that of the antigen that stimulated its production. For example, patients with infectious mononucleosis caused by the Epstein-Barr virus produce an antibody to the virus but also produce heterophile antibodies that react with sheep or horse red blood cells.

heterozygous Having two different alleles at corresponding loci on homologous chromosomes. An individual who is heterozygous for a trait has inherited an allele for that trait from one parent and an alternative allele from the other parent. A person who is heterozygous for a genetic disease will manifest the disorder if it is caused by a dominant allele but will remain asymptomatic if the disease is caused by a recessive allele.

high-molecular-weight kininogen (HMWK, Fitzgerald factor) Member of the kinin inflammatory system that is digested and activated by kallikrein to form bradykinin. HMWK is one of the in vitro contact activators of the coagulation system, which also include prekallikrein and factor XII.

histiocyte (macrophage) Mononuclear phagocyte found in all tissues; part of the immune system.

histochemical analysis Use of specialized stains to detect enzymes and other chemicals in tissues.

histocompatibility Quality or state of immunologic similarity that allows cells or tissues from one individual to be successfully transplanted into another individual. The degree of compatibility is controlled by white blood cell (WBC) surface markers of the human leukocyte antigen (HLA) system of the major histocompatibility complex. Grafts from donors of the immediate family are more compatible than those from unrelated donors.

histogram Graph of a frequency distribution. In hematology, a histogram is customarily a line graph generated by an automated analyzer that depicts the frequencies of platelet, white blood cell, or red blood cell volumes in a cell population.

histology Science concerned with the microscopic identification of cells and tissues used to identify cellular and tissue disease.

histone Nuclear protein that complexes with DNA to form chromatin. Histones provide for DNA folding and condensation and help regulate replication and transcription.

Hodgkin lymphoma Solid tumor characterized by painless, progressive hypertrophy of lymphoid tissue, first evident in cervical lymph nodes. Characterized by Reed-Sternberg cells and reactive white blood cells in lymphoid tissue and splenomegaly.

homocysteine Naturally occurring sulfur-containing amino acid formed in the metabolism of dietary methionine. Homocysteine concentration in plasma depends upon adequate intake of protein, vitamin B_6, vitamin B_{12}, and folate.

homocysteinemia Elevated plasma homocysteine, an independent risk factor for arterial thrombosis, typically caused by vitamin B_6, vitamin B_{12}, or folate deficiency.

homocysteinuria Increase or accumulation of homocysteine in urine; indicates an inherited error in an enzyme of the methionine-homocysteine metabolic pathway.

homozygous Having two identical alleles at corresponding loci on homologous chromosomes. An individual who is homozygous for a trait has inherited one identical allele for that trait from each parent. A person who is homozygous for a genetic disease caused by a pair of recessive alleles manifests the disorder.

Howell-Jolly (H-J) bodies Round blue to purple inclusions in red blood cells (RBCs), usually one per RBC, visible on Wright-stained peripheral blood films. Howell-Jolly bodies are composed of DNA and may indicate severe anemia or splenectomy.

human leukocyte antigens (HLA, major histocompatibility complex, MHC) Cell membrane glycoprotein system that forms the basis for antigen presentation in cellular and humoral immunity and enables the immune system to distinguish between self and nonself. HLA class I molecules (HLA-A, -B, -C) are found on most nucleated cells and on platelets. Class II antigens (HLA-DP, -DQ, -DR) are expressed on B lymphocytes, monocytes, macrophages, and dendritic cells.

humoral immunity Immune response mediated by B lymphocytes, which produce circulating antibodies (immunoglobulins) in reaction to infectious organisms and other foreign antigens.

hybridization In molecular biology, formation of a partially or wholly complementary nucleic acid duplex by association of single strands; used to detect and isolate specific nucleic acid sequences.

hydrops fetalis Gross edema of the entire body of a fetus or newborn infant, associated with severe anemia and occurring in hemolytic disease of the fetus and newborn.

hyperbilirubinemia (icterus, bilirubinemia) Excess bilirubin in the plasma, which imparts a gold color to the plasma; may indicate hemolytic anemia, liver disease, or bile duct occlusion.

hypercellular bone marrow Bone marrow showing an abnormal increase in the concentration of nucleated hematopoietic cells; potentially associated with leukemia or hemolytic anemia.

hypercoagulability (thrombophilia) Abnormally increased tendency to develop pathologic thromboses (clots) caused by a number of acquired and congenital factors.

hyperplasia Abnormally increased number of cells per unit volume of tissue caused by increased cellular division or abnormal retention. In bone marrow, hyperplasia is evident in hypercellularity. Such hyperplasia may cause enlarged joints or an enlarged forehead, called *frontal bossing*.

hypersegmented neutrophil Neutrophil with six or more nuclear lobes or segments; often associated with megaloblastic anemia.

hypersplenism Increased hemolytic activity of the spleen caused by splenomegaly, resulting in deficiency of peripheral blood cells and compensatory hypercellularity of the bone marrow.

hypertension Persistently elevated blood pressure.

hyperuricemia Excess of plasma uric acid or urates; sometimes associated with gout.

hypocellular bone marrow Abnormal decrease in the number of nucleated hematopoietic cells present in the bone marrow; may be associated with aplastic anemia or fibrosis.

hypochromia Abnormal decrease in the hemoglobin content of red blood cells so that they appear pale with a larger central pallor when stained with Wright stain. These cells are called *hypochromic*.

hypodiploid Having fewer than the normal number of somatic cell chromosomes; for example, fewer than 46 chromosomes in humans.

hypoplasia Underdevelopment of an organ or tissue, usually resulting from a fewer-than-normal number of cells. A hypoplastic bone marrow is one in which the distribution of nucleated hematopoietic cells is reduced, as in aplastic anemia or fibrosis.

hypoxia Diminished availability of oxygen to body tissues, usually secondary to decreased lung capacity or decreased oxygen-carrying capacity of the blood.

icterus (bilirubinemia, hyperbilirubinemia) Excess bilirubin in plasma, which imparts a gold color to the plasma; may indicate hemolytic anemia, liver disease, or bile duct occlusion.

idiopathic Without a known cause.

immediate transfusion reaction Hemolysis that begins within minutes or hours of a blood transfusion and is most commonly caused by an incompatibility of the ABO system.

immersion oil Optically clear oil placed in the space between a microscopic specimen and the microscope objective lens. Oil raises the refractive index, improving resolution.

immune hemolytic anemia Anemia resulting from shortened red blood cell (RBC) life span caused by antibodies to RBC membrane antigens or complement. The immunoglobulin- or complement-coated RBCs are cleared by splenic macrophages. Anemia results when the bone marrow fails to compensate for RBC consumption.

immune thrombocytopenic purpura (ITP, idiopathic thrombocytopenic purpura, autoimmune thrombocytopenic purpura, AITP) Mucocutaneous bleeding secondary to thrombocytopenia caused by a platelet-specific autoantibody that shortens platelet life span. Acute ITP occurs more often in children, while chronic ITP occurs more often in middle-aged adults, more commonly in women than in men.

immunoblast Large mitotically active T or B lymphocyte formed as a result of antigenic stimulation.

immunocompromised Unable to mount an adequate immune response due to disease or treatment with an immunosuppressive agent. An immunocompromised patient is susceptible to bacterial and viral infections.

immunocytochemical assays Laboratory tests in which antibodies labeled with chromophores or fluorophores hybridize specific cellular proteins or nucleic acids to produce a measurable color or fluorescent reaction.

immunoglobulin (antibody) Protein of the γ-globulin fraction produced by B lymphocytes and plasma cells that recognizes and binds a specific antigen. Immunoglobulins are the basis of humoral immunity.

immunophenotyping Classification of white blood cells and platelets by their membrane antigens. Synthetic antibodies, often monoclonal antibodies produced by hybridoma technology, are used to identify the antigens in flow cytometry.

immunosuppression Abnormal state of the immune system characterized by its inability to respond to antigenic stimuli. Immunosuppressive drugs are used to reduce immune responses, particularly in tissue transplant therapy.

infectious mononucleosis Acute infection caused by the Epstein-Barr virus, a herpesvirus. Characterized by fever, sore throat, lymphadenopathy, variant lymphocytes, splenomegaly, hepatomegaly, abnormal liver function, and bruising. Laboratory tests used to identify the disease include blood film review for variant lymphocytes, serologic mononucleosis testing, and molecular identification of Epstein-Barr virus.

integrin Any of a family of cell-adhesion receptors that mediate interactions between cells and between cells and the extracellular matrix.

interferon Natural glycoprotein produced by lymphocytes exposed to a virus or another foreign particle of nucleic acid. Interferon induces the production of translation inhibitory protein (TIP) in noninfected cells. TIP blocks the translation of viral RNA and thus gives other cells protection against the original as well as other viruses.

interleukin (IL) Any of a group of compounds that are synthesized by lymphocytes, macrophages, and matrix cells in the marrow and interact with cells to initiate, stimulate, or influence the maturation of blood cells.

international normalized ratio (INR) Index computed to normalize prothrombin time (PT) results worldwide. The activity of a PT reagent (thromboplastin) is characterized by manufacturers using the international sensitivity index (ISI), which compares the reagent to the international reference thromboplastin preparation provided by the World Health Organization. Local PTs are adjusted using the following formula: $INR = (PT_{patient}/PT_{normal})^{ISI}$, where $PT_{patient}$ is the individual patient's PT and PT_{normal} is the geometric mean of the PT reference interval.

international reference preparation (IRP) Human brain–derived thromboplastin maintained by the World Health Organization. Thromboplastin manufacturers worldwide compare their reagents' sensitivity with that of this reference preparation using orthogonal regression to generate an international sensitivity index (ISI) for their products.

international sensitivity index (ISI) Index comparing the sensitivity of a given thromboplastin preparation with the sensitivity of the international reference preparation as determined using orthogonal regression. The international sensitivity index is used as an exponent in the equation for calculating the international normalized ratio.

intracranial hemorrhage (ICH, hemorrhagic stroke) Bleeding into the brain causing tissue death. Fifteen percent of strokes are caused by intracranial hemorrhage; the remainder are caused by vascular occlusion (ischemia).

intramedullary hematopoiesis Formation and development of blood cells within the marrow cavity of a bone.

intramuscular (IM) Injected into muscle tissue.

intravascular hemolysis Red blood cell destruction that occurs within the blood vessels at a rate exceeding splenic macrophage clearance capacity, releasing hemoglobin into the plasma. Seen in acute hemolytic episodes such as those associated with transfusion reaction, glucose-6-phosphate dehydrogenase deficiency, and sickle cell anemia crisis.

intrinsic coagulation pathway Sequence of serine protease reactions leading to fibrin formation, beginning with the in vitro contact activation of factor XII, followed by the sequential activation of factors XI and IX, and resulting in the activation of factor X, which initiates the common pathway of coagulation.

intrinsic factor (IF) Glycoprotein secreted by parietal cells of the gastric mucosa that is essential for the intestinal absorption of vitamin B_{12}. A deficiency of, or antibody to, intrinsic factor results in B_{12} deficiency.

intron Nontranslated sequence in a gene. Introns are transcribed to heteronuclear RNA and are excised during the subsequent formation of messenger RNA.

inversion Structural chromosome alteration caused by breaks at two locations, reversal of direction of the detached sequence, and reattachment. Inversions have little effect on somatic DNA but cause loss of DNA information in offspring.

iron deficiency anemia Microcytic, hypochromic anemia caused by inadequate supplies of the iron needed to synthesize hemoglobin and characterized by pallor, fatigue, and weakness. Often caused by low dietary iron intake or chronic blood loss.

isoantibody (alloantibody) Antibody that is produced in response to the presence of foreign antigens; for instance, an antibody to a therapeutic coagulation factor that may render factor therapy ineffective.

jaundice Orange-yellow discoloration of the skin, mucous membranes, and sclera. Caused by elevated plasma bilirubin, which signals hepatitis, hemolytic anemia, or common bile duct obstruction.

karyorrhexis Nuclear necrosis in which the nucleus ruptures and chromatin disintegrates into formless granules.

karyotype Number, form, size, and arrangement of the chromosomes within the nucleus. In cytogenetic laboratory assays mitosis is halted in metaphase and the chromosomes are recorded in a photomicrograph to generate the karyotype.

kinin Any of a group of polypeptides that trigger inflammatory activity such as contraction of smooth muscle, vascular permeability, and vasodilation. Examples of kinins are bradykinin and kallidin.

kininogen Either of two plasma α_2-globulins that are kinin precursors, called *high-molecular-weight kininogen* and *low-molecular-weight kininogen*.

Kleihauer-Betke stain (acid elution slide test) Test for detecting fetal red blood cells (RBCs) in the maternal circulation. Blood films are immersed in an acid buffer, which causes adult hemoglobin (Hb A) to be eluted from RBCs. The film is stained, and RBCs that have fetal hemoglobin (Hb F) take up the stain.

Köhler illumination Light microscope illumination system that consists of a substage light source, field diaphragm, condenser, and aperture diaphragm. These are adjusted in sequence to optimize specimen illumination, resolution, contrast, and depth of field.

koilonychia Dystrophy of the fingernails in which they become thin, ridged, and concave. Associated with iron deficiency anemia.

Kupffer cells Fixed, highly phagocytic macrophages that line the liver sinusoids. Kupffer cells function like splenic macrophages (littoral cells) to clear senescent red blood cells, immune complexes, and foreign materials.

lactate dehydrogenase (LD) Enzyme that catalyzes the reversible conversion of lactate to pyruvate. It is widespread in tissues and is particularly abundant in the kidneys, skeletal muscle, liver, red blood cells, and myocardium. The lactate dehydrogenase assay may be used to detect and monitor cell necrosis in these organs, for instance, acute myocardial infarction or as an indicator of intravascular hemolysis.

Langerhans cell Immature dendritic macrophage (histiocyte) with an irregular nucleus and distinctive racquet-shaped cytoplasmic granules called *Birbeck bodies* normally found in the epidermis, oral and vaginal mucosa, and lungs. Langerhans cells have been identified as the cells of origin for a nonproliferating epidermal neoplasm known as *Langerhans cell histiocytosis.*

leptocyte Abnormal mature red blood cell that is thin and flat with hemoglobin at the periphery and increased central pallor.

leukemia Group of malignant neoplasms of hematopoietic tissues characterized by diffuse replacement of bone marrow or lymph nodes with abnormal proliferating white blood cells and the presence of leukemic cells in the peripheral blood. Leukemia may be chronic or acute and myeloid or lymphoid.

leukemoid reaction (LR) Clinical syndrome resembling leukemia in which the white blood cell count is elevated to greater than $50,000/\mu L$ in response to an allergen, inflammatory disease, infection, poison, hemorrhage, burn, or severe physical stress. Leukemoid reaction usually involves granulocytes and is distinguished from chronic myelogenous leukemia by the use of the leukocyte alkaline phosphatase staining of neutrophils.

leukocyte One of the formed elements of the blood. The five families of WBCs are lymphocytes, monocytes, neutrophils, basophils, and eosinophils. WBCs function as phagocytes of bacteria, fungi, and viruses; detoxifiers of toxic proteins that may be produced by allergic reactions and cellular injury; and immune system cells.

leukocytosis Abnormally elevated white blood cell count in peripheral blood.

leukoerythroblastic Characterized by the presence of immature red blood cells and granulocytes in the peripheral blood and bone marrow.

leukopenia Abnormal decrease in the white blood cell count in peripheral blood.

leukopoiesis Process by which white blood cells form and develop in the bone marrow and lymph nodes.

Levey-Jennings chart Quality control chart used to plot periodic test results for control specimens. The chart indicates the mean and the 1, 2, and 3 standard deviation intervals on both sides of the mean. Deviation from this standard distribution indicates the occurrence of a systematic analytical error.

ligand Molecule, ion, or group bound to the central atom of a chemical compound; for example, the oxygen molecule in hemoglobin, which is bound to the central iron atom. Also, a molecule that binds to another molecule; used especially to refer to a small molecule that specifically binds to a larger molecule.

littoral cells Fixed, highly phagocytic macrophages that line the sinusoid of the spleen. Littoral cells clear senescent red blood cells, immune complexes, and foreign materials.

low-molecular-weight heparin (LMWH) Heparin with an average molecular weight of 5000 to 8000 Daltons produced by enzymatic or chemical digestion of unfractionated heparin. LMWH is used for prophylaxis, and treatment monitoring is required only in conditions of fluid imbalance, such as obesity, renal disease, and pregnancy. LMWH therapy is monitored using the chromogenic anti–factor Xa heparin assay.

lupus anticoagulant (LA, LAC) Autoantibody to phospholipid-binding proteins such as β_2-glycoprotein I, annexin, and prothrombin. May be present as a primary condition or secondary to a collagen disorder such as systemic lupus erythematosus, Sjögren syndrome, or rheumatoid arthritis. Chronic lupus anticoagulant is associated with venous and arterial thrombosis and spontaneous abortion.

lymphadenopathy Any disorder characterized by a localized or generalized enlargement of the lymph nodes or lymph vessels.

lymphoblast Immature cell found in the bone marrow and lymph nodes, but not normally in the peripheral blood; the most primitive, morphologically recognizable precursor in the lymphocytic series, which develops into the prolymphocyte.

lymphocytes Mononuclear, nonphagocytic white blood cells found in the blood, lymph, and lymphoid tissues. Lymphocytes are categorized as B and T lymphocytes and natural killer cells. They are responsible for humoral and cellular immunity and tumor surveillance.

lymphocytopenia (lymphopenia) Abnormally reduced lymphocyte count in peripheral blood.

lymphocytosis Abnormally increased lymphocyte count in peripheral blood.

lymphoid Resembling or pertaining to lymph or tissue and cells of the lymphoid system.

lymphokines Biologic response mediators released by both B and T lymphocytes.

lymphoma Solid tumor neoplasm of lymphoid tissue categorized as Hodgkin or non-Hodgkin lymphoma and defined by lymphocyte morphology and the histologic features of the lymph nodes.

lymphopoiesis Formation and production of lymphocytes, predominantly in the lymph nodes.

lymphoproliferative Pertaining to the proliferation of lymphoid cells resulting in abnormally increased lymphocyte counts in peripheral blood, indicating a reactive or neoplastic condition.

lysosomes Membrane-bound sacs of varying size distributed randomly in the cytoplasm of granulocytes and platelets. Lysosomes contain hydrolytic enzymes that kill ingested bacteria and digest bacteria and other foreign materials.

macrocyte Red blood cell with an abnormally large diameter seen on a peripheral blood film and an elevated mean cell volume. Associated with folate and vitamin B_{12} deficiency, bone marrow failure, myelodysplastic syndrome, and chronic liver disease.

macroglobulin High-molecular-weight plasma globulin, such as α_2-macroglobulin or an immunoglobulin of the M isotype. Abnormal monoclonal IgM proteins seen in Waldenström macroglobulinemia.

macrophage (histiocyte) Mononuclear phagocyte found in all tissues; part of the immune system.

major histocompatibility complex (MHC, human leukocyte antigen, HLA) Cell membrane glycoprotein system that forms the basis for antigen presentation in cellular and humoral immunity and enables the immune system to distinguish between self and nonself. MHC class I molecules (HLA-A, -B, -C) are found on most nucleated cells and on platelets. Class II antigens (HLA-DP, -DQ, -DR) are expressed on B lymphocytes, monocytes, macrophages, and dendritic cells.

malaise Vague feeling of discomfort and fatigue, often associated with cancer or anemia.

malaria Infectious disease caused by one or more of five species of the protozoan genus *Plasmodium*. Malaria is transmitted from human to human by a bite from an infected *Anopheles* mosquito.

malignant Describes a cancerous disease that threatens life through its ability to metastasize.

marker chromosome In cytogenetic analysis, a chromosome of abnormal size or shape that is an early indicator of neoplastic disease, for instance, the Philadelphia chromosome in chronic myelogenous leukemia.

mast cell Connective tissue cell that has large basophilic granules containing heparin, serotonin, bradykinin, and histamine. These substances are released from the mast cell in response to immunoglobulin E stimulation.

May-Hegglin anomaly Rare autosomal dominant disorder characterized by thrombocytopenia and granulocytes that contain cytoplasmic inclusions similar to Döhle bodies.

mean Value that is derived by dividing the total of a set of values by the number of items in the set; the arithmetic average.

mean cell hemoglobin (MCH) Average red blood cell (RBC) hemoglobin mass in picograms computed from the RBC count and hemoglobin level.

mean cell hemoglobin concentration (MCHC) Average relative hemoglobin concentration per red blood cell (RBC), expressed in g/dL, computed from the hemoglobin and hematocrit. Relates to Wright-stained RBC color intensity.

mean cell volume (MCV) Average red blood cell (RBC) volume in femtoliters computed from the RBC count and hematocrit or directly measured by an automated hematology analyzer. Relates to Wright-stained RBC diameter.

megakaryoblast Least differentiated visually identifiable megakaryocyte precursor in a Wright-stained bone marrow aspirate smear. The megakaryoblast cannot be distinguished visually from the myeloblast but is identified using special immunochemical markers.

megakaryocyte Largest cell in the bone marrow, measuring 30 to 50 μm and having a multilobed nucleus. Its cytoplasm is composed of platelets, which are released to the blood through the extension of proplatelet processes. Megakaryocytes are identified and enumerated microscopically at low (10×) power on a bone marrow aspirate smear.

megakaryopoiesis (megakaryocytopoiesis) Production and development of megakaryocytes, the precursors to platelets, in the bone marrow.

megaloblast Abnormally large, nucleated, immature precursor of the erythrocytic series; an abnormal counterpart to the pronormoblast. Not only does it have a larger diameter, but the nucleus appears more immature than the cytoplasm. Megaloblasts give rise to macrocytic red blood cells and are associated with megaloblastic anemia, usually caused by folate or vitamin B$_{12}$ deficiency.

menorrhagia Abnormally heavy or prolonged menstrual periods.

metacentric Describes a mitotic chromosome having the centromere at the center, with one arm equal in length to the other.

metamyelocyte Stage in the development of the granulocyte series, located between the myelocyte stage and the band stage. Characterized by mature, granulated cytoplasm and a bean-shaped nucleus.

metaphase Second phase of mitosis in which the chromosomes are aligned at the equatorial plate. Chromosomes at metaphase are maximally contracted and are most easily identified in cytogenetic analysis.

metaplasia Conversion of normal tissue cells into another, less differentiated cell type in response to chronic stress or injury. For instance, *myeloid metaplasia* describes hematopoiesis in the spleen or liver.

metarubricyte (orthochromic normoblast) Fourth stage of bone marrow erythropoiesis and the last in which the cell retains a nucleus. The nucleus is fully condensed with no parachromatin, and the cytoplasm is 85% hemoglobinized and bluish-pink. When an orthochromic normoblast appears in the peripheral blood, it is called a *nucleated red blood cell.*

metastasis Extension or spread of tumor cells to distant parts of the body, usually through the lymphatics or blood vessels.

methemoglobin Abnormal form of hemoglobin in which the ferrous ion has become oxidized to the ferric state. Methemoglobin cannot carry oxygen.

microangiopathic hemolytic anemia (MAHA) Condition in which narrowing or obstruction of small blood vessels by fibrin or platelet aggregates results in distortion and fragmentation of red blood cells, hemolysis, and anemia. This causes the appearance of schistocytes on a Wright-stained blood film.

microcyte Small red blood cell (RBC) with reduced mean cell volume and reduced diameter on Wright-stained peripheral blood film. Microcytes are often associated with iron deficiency anemia and thalassemia.

microfilament Intracellular protein that supports the cytoskeleton and assists with cell motility.

microtubules Tubulin protein channels that maintain cellular shape, contribute to motility, and make up mitotic spindle fibers and centrioles.

mitochondria Round or oval structures distributed randomly in the cytoplasm of a cell. Mitochondria provide the cell's aerobic energy system by producing adenosine triphosphate.

mitosis Ordinary process of somatic cell division resulting in the production of two daughter cells that have identical diploid complements of chromosomes.

monoblast Most undifferentiated morphologically identifiable precursor of the bone marrow monocytic series; develops into the promonocyte.

monoclonal Pertaining to or designating a group of identical cells or organisms derived from a single cell or organism. Also used to describe products from a clone of cells, such as monoclonal antibodies.

monocyte Mononuclear phagocytic white blood cell having a round to horseshoe-shaped nucleus with abundant gray-blue cytoplasm filled with fine reddish granules. Circulating precursor to the macrophage, the primary phagocytic cell of most tissues.

monocytopenia Abnormally low monocyte count in peripheral blood.

monocytosis Abnormally elevated monocyte count in peripheral blood; may indicate infection or a neoplasm.

mononuclear Having only one nucleus. Used to describe cells such as monocytes or lymphocytes as distinct from neutrophils, which have nuclei that appear to be multiple and hence are called *segmented* or *polymorphonuclear.*

Mott cell Plasma cell containing colorless cytoplasmic inclusions of immunoglobulin called *Russell bodies* that appear similar to vacuoles.

multiple myeloma (now called **plasma cell myeloma**) Malignant neoplasm in which plasma cells proliferate in the bone marrow, destroying bone and resulting in pain, fractures, and excess production of a monoclonal plasma immunoglobulin.

mutation Permanent transmissible change in the DNA sequence of a single gene; includes substitution, loss, or gain of one or more nucleotides. Mutations cause the production of abnormal proteins or the loss of a protein.

myelo- Prefix relating to the bone marrow or spinal cord and used to identify granulocytic precursors of neutrophils.

myeloblast Least differentiated morphologically identifiable bone marrow precursor of the granulocytic series; develops into the promyelocyte. The appearance of myeloblasts in peripheral blood signals acute leukemia.

myelocyte Third stage of bone marrow granulocytic series differentiation, intermediate in development between a promyelocyte and a metamyelocyte. In this stage, differentiation of cytoplasmic granules has begun, so myelocytes may be basophilic, eosinophilic, or neutrophilic.

myelodysplastic syndromes (MDSs) Group of acquired clonal hematologic disorders characterized by progressive peripheral blood cytopenias that reflect defects in erythroid, myeloid, or megakaryocytic maturation.

myelofibrosis Replacement of bone marrow with fibrous connective tissue.

myeloid General term used to denote granulocytic cells and their precursors, including basophils, eosinophils, and neutrophils. Lymphoid and erythroid cell lines are excluded, and most morphologists also exclude the monocytic and megakaryocytic cell lines.

myeloid-to-erythroid (M:E) ratio Proportion of myeloid cells to nucleated erythroid precursors in bone marrow aspirate. The myeloid-to-erythroid ratio is used to evaluate hematologic cell production. Excluded from the myeloid cell count are monocytic and lymphoid precursors and plasma cells.

myelokathexis Inherited severe neutropenia and lymphopenia characterized by hypersegmented neutrophils and myeloid hyperplasia. Part of WHIM syndrome (*w*arts, *h*ypogammaglobulinemia, *i*nfections, and *m*yelokathexis).

myeloperoxidase (MPO) Enzyme that occurs in primary granules of promyelocytes, myelocytes, and neutrophils and exhibits bactericidal, fungicidal, and virucidal properties. Cytochemical stains that detect myeloperoxidase are used to identify myeloid precursors in acute leukemia.

myeloproliferative neoplasms (MPN, myeloproliferative disorders, MPD) Group of neoplasms characterized by proliferation of myeloid tissue and elevations in one or more myeloid cell types in the peripheral blood. Myeloproliferative neoplasms include myelofibrosis with myeloid metaplasia, essential thrombocythemia, polycythemia vera, and chronic myelogenous leukemia.

myoglobin Monomeric heme-containing protein in muscle. Combines with oxygen released by red blood cells, stores it, and transports it to the mitochondria of muscle cells, where it generates energy.

necrosis Localized tissue death that occurs in groups of cells in response to disease or injury.

neonatal Pertaining to the first 28 days after birth.

neoplasm Any abnormal growth of new tissue; can be malignant or benign. The term is usually applied to cancerous cells.

neuropathy Any disorder affecting the nervous system.

neutropenia Abnormally reduced neutrophil count in peripheral blood. Often associated with chemotherapy, it exposes the patient to the risk of infection.

neutrophil Mature segmented (polymorphonuclear) white blood cell with fine pink-staining cytoplasmic granules in a Wright-stained peripheral blood film. Neutrophils ingest bacteria and cellular debris.

neutrophilia Abnormally elevated neutrophil count in peripheral blood; often indicates bacterial infection and may be associated with chronic myelogenous leukemia.

nondisjunction Faulty distribution of chromosomal elements during mitosis or meiosis.

non-Hodgkin lymphoma (NHL) Solid tumors of lymphoid tissue classified by histologic features and lymphocytic morphology. Should be distinguished from Hodgkin lymphoma, which is caused by proliferation of Reed-Sternberg cells and accumulation of reactive peripheral blood cells.

nonsteroidal antiinflammatory drugs (NSAIDs) Antiinflammatory, analgesic, and antiplatelet drugs, other than steroids. NSAIDs include aspirin, which acetylates cyclooxygenase and reduces platelet activation, as well as naproxen, acetaminophen, and ibuprofen.

normochromic Describes a Wright-stained red blood cell with normal color and normal hemoglobin content with a mean cell hemoglobin concentration within the reference interval.

normocyte Normal, mature red blood cell with a mean cell volume within the reference interval.

nucleated red blood cell (NRBC) Red blood cell (RBC) in peripheral blood that possesses a nucleus; often an orthochromic normoblast (metarubricyte). Nucleated RBCs falsely raise manual white blood cell (WBC) counts, which requires a manual WBC count correction.

nucleolus Round or irregular pocket of messenger and ribosomal RNA in the nucleus. Nucleoli are observed by morphologists and are used to distinguish cell differentiation stages.

nucleoside Glycoside of purine and pyrimidine bases. In RNA and DNA, the glycosides are the pentoses ribose and deoxyribose.

nucleotide Phosphoric ester of a nucleoside. Allows for the formation of phosphodiesterase bridges between nucleotides to form RNA and DNA.

nucleus Cellular organelle containing DNA and RNA. Stores genetic information and controls cell functions.

nucleus-to-cytoplasm (N:C) ratio Estimated volume of a Wright-stained nucleus in comparison to the volume of the cytoplasm. The nucleus-to-cytoplasm ratio is used to differentiate cell developmental stages.

numerical aperture (NA) Number stamped on the barrel of a microscope lens designating the quality of the microscope objective. The higher the number, the greater the lens's resolution.

objective Microscope lens closest to the specimen. Most clinical grade microscopes provide 10× dry, 50× oil immersion, and 100× oil immersion objectives.

ocular Microscope lens, usually 10×, nearest the eye.

oncogene Gene capable, under certain conditions, of causing the initial and continuing conversion of normal cells into cancer cells. A mutated proto-oncogene.

opsonization Process by which an antibody or complement attaches itself to foreign material (bacteria), triggering or enhancing phagocytosis by white blood cells.

optical scatter Scattering of light caused by the interaction of absorption, diffraction, refraction, and reflection. Hematology analyzers that use both laser and nonlaser light apply the principle of light scatter to perform cell counting and identification. The angle of light scatter correlates with various cell features such as volume, density, and cellular complexity.

orthochromic normoblast (metarubricyte) Fourth stage of bone marrow erythropoiesis and the last in which the cell retains a nucleus. The nucleus is fully condensed with no parachromatin; the cytoplasm is 85% hemoglobinized and bluish-pink. When an orthochromic normoblast appears in the peripheral blood, it is called a *nucleated red blood cell.*

osmotic fragility test Assay in which whole blood is pipetted to each of a series of saline solutions of graduated concentration. The series begins with water and increases in concentration to normal (0.85%) saline. The osmotic fragility test is used to detect spherocytosis, because spherocytes rupture in saline concentrations near the normal level. It may also detect target cells, which, owing to their reduced hemoglobin content, are able to withstand osmotic stress and rupture only at very dilute saline concentrations.

osteoblast Bone-forming cell.

osteoclast Large multinuclear cell associated with the absorption and removal of bone. May be confused with a megakaryocyte.

oval macrocyte Oval red blood cell with an increased diameter seen in peripheral blood. Characteristic of megaloblastic anemia.

ovalocyte (elliptocyte) Oval red blood cell seen in peripheral blood in the membrane disorder hereditary elliptocytosis. May be found in low numbers in healthy states and in other anemias such as iron deficiency and thalassemia major.

oxygen affinity Ability of hemoglobin to bind oxygen molecules.

oxygen dissociation curve Graphic expression of the affinity between oxygen and hemoglobin or the concentration of oxygen bound at equilibrium to the hemoglobin in blood as a function of oxygen pressure.

oxyhemoglobin Hemoglobin that contains bound oxygen.

P arm Smaller (petite) arm of a chromosome.

packed cell volume (PCV, hematocrit, HCT) Proportion of whole blood that consists of red blood cells, expressed as a percentage of the total blood volume.

pallor Unnatural paleness or absence of color from the skin.

pancytopenia Marked reduction in the count of red blood cells, white blood cells, and platelets in peripheral blood.

Pappenheimer bodies (siderotic granules) Red blood cell inclusions composed of ferric iron. On Prussian blue iron stain preparations, they appear as multiple dark blue irregular granules. On Wright stain preparations they appear as pale blue clusters.

parachromatin Pale-staining portion of the nucleus, roughly equivalent to euchromatin.

parenteral Pertaining to administration of drugs or other compounds by means other than oral administration; includes intramuscular and intravenous administration.

paroxysmal cold hemoglobinuria (PCH) Rare acquired autoimmune hemolytic anemia in which the Donath-Landsteiner autoantibody binds red blood cells during exposure to cold, producing acute hemolysis and hematuria upon warming.

paroxysmal nocturnal hemoglobinuria (PNH) Acquired hemolytic anemia due to a stem cell clonal mutation that causes the cell to lack glycosylphosphatidylinositol-anchored proteins, including CD55 and CD59, two proteins that normally protect the red blood cell (RBC) from complement activation and hemolysis. RBCs therefore have an increased susceptibility to complement, which results in intravascular hemolysis and hemoglobinuria that occur in irregular episodes.

partial thromboplastin time (PTT, activated partial thromboplastin time, APTT) Clot-based screening test for intrinsic coagulation, which is prolonged in deficiencies of prekallikrein, high-molecular-weight kininogen, and factors XII, XI, IX, VIII, X, V, II, and fibrinogen. Calcium chloride, phospholipid, and activator are added to patient plasma. The interval from the addition of reagent to clot formation is recorded. The test is used to monitor unfractionated heparin therapy, to screen for intrinsic pathway deficiencies, and to screen for lupus anticoagulant.

pathogenesis Chemical and biologic events in cells and tissue by which disease occurs and progresses.

pathognomonic Specifically characteristic of a given disease; indicating a sign or symptom from which a diagnosis can be made.

Pelger-Huët anomaly Autosomal dominant asymptomatic anomaly of neutrophil nuclei, which fail to segment and appear dumbbell shaped or peanut shaped ("pince-nez" nuclei). Pelgeroid nuclei are more common and resemble the nuclei of Pelger-Huët anomaly, but may indicate myelodysplasia or may appear during chemotherapy.

percutaneous coronary intervention (PCI) Any catheter-based technique for the management of coronary artery occlusion, such as angiography, angioplasty, stent placement within a coronary artery, or cardiac catheterization.

peripheral artery occlusion (PAO) Blockage of a noncardiovascular, noncerebral artery—for example, a carotid or brachial artery—by thrombus formation.

pernicious anemia Progressive autoimmune disorder that results in megaloblastic macrocytic anemia due to a lack of, or antibodies to, parietal cells or intrinsic factor essential for the absorption of vitamin B_{12}.

personal protective equipment (PPE) Clothing that is used to prevent blood or other potentially infectious biologic substances from contacting clothing, eyes, mouth, or mucous membranes. Includes, for example, gloves, fluid-impermeable laboratory coats, and eye protection.

petechiae Pinpoint purple or red spots on the skin or mucous membranes, approximately 1 mm in diameter, indicating small bleeds within the dermal or submucosal layers. May indicate a systemic bleeding disorder.

phagocyte Cell that is able to surround, engulf, and digest microorganisms and cellular debris. Macrophages and neutrophils are phagocytes.

phagocytosis Ingestion of large particles or live microorganisms into a cell.

phagosome Membrane-bound cytoplasmic vesicle in a phagocyte containing the phagocytosed material.

Philadelphia chromosome Reciprocal translocation of the long arm of chromosome 22 to chromosome 9; definitive for the diagnosis of chronic myelogenous leukemia. The mutation results in the fusion of the *BCR* and *ABL* genes and abnormal tyrosine kinase production.

phlebotomy Use of a needle to puncture a vein and collect blood.

phytohemagglutinin (PHA) Lectin extracted from the red kidney bean that causes red blood cell agglutination by binding to *N*-acetyl-β-glucosamine. Also a mitogen that induces T-lymphocyte proliferation in culture.

pinocytosis Cellular ingestion of small particles or liquids.

pitting Removal by the spleen of material from within red blood cells (RBCs) without damage to the RBCs; for example, removal of nuclei or Howell-Jolly bodies.

plasma Fluid portion of the blood in which the formed elements (white blood cells, red blood cells, and platelets) are suspended.

plasma cell Fully differentiated B lymphocyte found in the bone marrow and lymphoid tissue, and occasionally in peripheral blood. It contains an eccentric nucleus with deeply staining chromatin and abundant dark blue cytoplasm. The Golgi apparatus produces a perinuclear halo due to its high lipid content. Plasma cells secrete antibody in the humoral immune response.

plasma frozen within 24 hours (FP24) Plasma that is separated from whole-blood donations and frozen within 24 hours of collection. FP24 contains all of the plasma procoagulants and control proteins, including adequate levels of the labile factors V and VIII. FP24 is used for replacement therapy in acquired multiple-factor deficiencies or in single-factor deficiencies when factor concentrates are not available.

plasmin Active form of plasminogen. Plasmin binds fibrin and, when activated by tissue plasminogen activator, digests fibrin to form fibrin degradation products in the fibrinolytic process.

plasminogen Inactive (zymogen) plasma precursor of plasmin.

plasminogen activator Substance that cleaves plasminogen and converts it into plasmin; includes urokinase, which is secreted by renal endothelial cells, and tissue plasminogen activator, which is secreted by all endothelia. Synthetic plasminogen activators are used therapeutically to clear coronary artery clots after acute myocardial infarction.

plasminogen activator inhibitor 1 (PAI-1) Endothelial cell inhibitor of tissue plasminogen activator; controls fibrinolysis.

platelet (thrombocyte) Smallest of the formed elements in blood; disk-shaped, 2 to 4 μm in diameter, nonnucleated cell formed in the bone marrow from the cytoplasm of megakaryocytes. Platelets trigger and control blood coagulation.

platelet adhesion Platelet attachment to subendothelial collagen, part of a sequential mechanism leading to the initiation and formation of a thrombus or hemostatic plug. Platelet adhesion requires von Willebrand factor and platelet receptor glycoprotein Ib/IX/V.

platelet aggregation Platelet-to-platelet binding, part of a sequential mechanism leading to the initiation and formation of a thrombus or hemostatic plug. Requires fibrinogen and platelet membrane receptor glycoprotein IIb/IIIa.

platelet factor 4 (PF4) Protein released from platelet α-granules that binds and inhibits heparin. The heparin-PF4 complex is implicated in heparin-induced thrombocytopenia with thrombosis.

platelet-poor plasma (PPP) Plasma centrifuged to achieve a platelet count of less than 10,000/μL. PPP is required for all coagulation testing, and only PPP may be frozen.

platelet-rich plasma (PRP) Plasma centrifuged at 50 x*g* to achieve a platelet count of 200,000/μL to 300,000/μL. Platelet-rich plasma is used for light-transmission platelet aggregometry.

platelet satellitosis (satellitism) Antibody-mediated in vitro adhesion of platelets to segmented neutrophils. Occurs primarily in specimens anticoagulated with ethylenediaminetetraacetic acid (EDTA) and causes pseudothrombocytopenia.

pleomorphic Occurring in various distinct forms; having the ability to exist in various forms and to change from one form to another.

pluripotential stem cell Stem cell that has the potential to differentiate into one of several types of hematopoietic progenitor cells, including lymphocytic, monocytic, granulocytic, megakaryocytic, and erythrocytic lineages and nonhematopoietic cells.

pneumatic tube system System of tubes for transporting blood specimens or other small materials in hospitals by forced air.

poikilocytosis Presence in the peripheral blood of red blood cells with varying or bizarre shapes.

point-of-care (POC) testing Rapid-turnaround clinical tests performed outside of the clinical laboratory at or near the patient; usually performed by nonlaboratory personnel but managed for quality by laboratory personnel.

polychromatic (polychromatophilic) Having a staining quality in which both acid and basic stains are incorporated. Usually used to denote a mixture of pink and blue in the cytoplasm of Wright-stained cells.

polychromatic normoblast (polychromatophilic normoblast, rubricyte) Precursor in the erythrocytic maturation series, intermediate between the basophilic normoblast (prorubricyte) and the orthochromic normoblast (metarubricyte). In this stage, differentiation is based on the decreasing cell diameter and the gray-blue cytoplasm as hemoglobin first becomes visible.

polychromatic or polychromatophilic red blood cell (reticulocyte) Immature but anucleate red blood cell (RBC) with bluish-pink cytoplasm on a Wright-stained blood film. When new methylene blue dye is used, the cytoplasm of these cells has a meshlike pattern of dark blue threads and particles, vestiges of the endoplasmic reticulum. Reticulocytosis or polychromatophilia indicates bone marrow regeneration activity in hemolytic anemia or acute blood loss.

polychromatophilia (reticulocytosis) Elevated reticulocyte count on a peripheral blood film stained with new methylene blue dye or increase in the number of polychromatophilic red blood cells on a Wright-stained blood film. Reticulocytosis or polychromatophilia indicates bone marrow regeneration activity in hemolytic anemia or acute blood loss.

polyclonal Describes a group of cells or organisms derived from several cells. Each cell is identical to its parent cells (i.e., a clone), but since all cells of the group did not derive from the same cell, the group of cells is mixed. A polyclonal antibody is developed within a laboratory animal and not a hybridoma.

polycythemia (erythrocytosis) Elevated red blood cell count, hemoglobin, and hematocrit in peripheral blood, usually in response to chronic hypoxia.

polycythemia vera (PV) Myeloproliferative neoplasm in which a somatic mutation leads to a marked increase in the red blood cell (RBC) count, hematocrit, hemoglobin, white blood cell count, platelet count, and red blood cell mass. RBC precursors are hypersensitive to erythropoietin.

polymerase chain reaction (PCR) Laboratory process in which a strand of DNA is replicated in a thermocycler to produce millions of copies within a few hours.

polymorphonuclear neutrophil (PMN, segmented neutrophil, seg) White blood cell whose nucleus is condensed into two to five segments or lobes connected by filaments. Distinguished from mononuclear cells such as monocytes and lymphocytes.

polyploid Having more than the characteristic diploid set of chromosomes; for example, triploid ($3\times$) or tetraploid ($4\times$).

porphyria Hereditary anemia caused by impaired heme synthesis with the accumulation of porphyrin and its precursors. Acquired porphyria may be seen in acute lead poisoning.

porphyrin Product of the metabolism of a group of iron- or magnesium-free pyrrole derivatives such as protoporphyrin and protoporphyrinogen that incorporates ferrous iron to form heme.

posttransfusion purpura Antibody-induced thrombocytopenia in patients who have received multiple transfusions of red blood cells or platelet concentrate. Antibodies to donor platelets cross-react with patient platelets to cause potentially life-threatening thrombocytopenia.

postmenstrual age Time elapsed between the first day of the mother's last menstrual period and birth (gestational age) plus the time elapsed after birth (chronologic age). For example, a preterm infant born at a gestational age of 32 weeks who is currently 10 weeks old (chronologic age) would have a postmenstrual age of 42 weeks.

precision Degree to which the results of replicate analyses of a sample parallel each other, often expressed as coefficient of variation or percent coefficient of variation.

precursor Differentiating (immature) hematopoietic cell stage that is morphologically identifiable as belonging to a given cell line; for example, pronormoblasts (rubriblasts) are precursors of basophilic normoblasts (prorubricytes) in erythropoiesis. *Precursor* may also refer to the inactive zymogen forms of coagulation factors; for example, prothrombin is a precursor of thrombin.

preeclampsia Pathologic condition of late pregnancy characterized by edema, proteinuria, and hypertension; may lead to eclampsia, which presents with seizures and is often fatal.

prekallikrein (PK, pre-K, Fletcher factor) Member of the kinin inflammatory system that forms active kallikrein upon digestion by kininogen. Pre-K helps to trigger in vitro coagulation contact activation. Pre-K deficiency prolongs the partial thromboplastin time but has no clinical consequence.

primary hemostasis First phase of hemostasis in which the blood vessels contract to seal the wound and platelets and von Willebrand factor fill the open space by forming a platelet plug.

primary standard Reference material that is of fixed and known composition and is capable of being prepared in essentially pure form.

primer Short piece of synthetic DNA complementary to a target DNA sequence. The primer acts as a point from which replication can proceed, as in a polymerase chain reaction.

procoagulant Coagulation (clotting) factor. During the coagulation process, inactive procoagulants become activated to form serine proteases or cofactors and function together to produce a localized thrombus.

progenitor Undifferentiated (immature) hematopoietic cell that is committed to a cell line but cannot be identified morphologically.

prolymphocyte Developmental form in the lymphocytic series that is intermediate between the lymphoblast and the lymphocyte.

promegakaryocyte Morphologically identifiable bone marrow cell stage that is intermediate between the megakaryoblast and the megakaryocyte.

promonocyte Precursor in the monocytic series; the cell stage intermediate in development between the monoblast and the monocyte.

promyelocyte Precursor in the granulocytic (myelocytic) series that is intermediate in development between a myeloblast and a myelocyte; contains primary granules.

pronormoblast (rubriblast) Undifferentiated (immature) hematopoietic cell that is the most primitive morphologically identifiable precursor in the erythrocytic series; differentiates into the basophilic normoblast (prorubricyte).

prorubricyte (basophilic normoblast) Second identifiable stage in bone marrow erythrocytic maturation; it is derived from the pronormoblast (rubriblast). Typically 10 to 15 μm in diameter, the prorubricyte has cytoplasm that stains dark blue with Wright stain.

prostaglandin (PG) Any of a family of unsaturated 20-carbon fatty acids that are cleaved from cell membrane phospholipids and serve as intracellular activators and inhibitors. The prostaglandins include thromboxane A_2, a platelet activator, and prostacyclin, a platelet inhibitor produced by endothelial cells.

protein C (PC) Vitamin K–dependent coagulation control protein. A plasma serine protease activated by thrombin-thrombomodulin and stabilized by its cofactor, protein S, protein C inhibits coagulation by inactivating factors Va and VIIIa.

protein S (PS) Vitamin K–dependent coagulation control protein. Serves as a stabilizing cofactor for protein C, enabling activated protein C, a serine protease, to inactivate factors Va and VIIIa.

proteins in vitamin K antagonism (PIVKA) Name given to the forms of factors II, VII, IX, and X and proteins C, S, and Z that, under conditions of vitamin K absence or antagonism, lack a second glutamic acid carboxyl group as required for binding to Ca^{2+} and phospholipid. Also called *des-γ-carboxyl coagulation factors*. The des-γ-carboxyl forms of these factors cannot participate in coagulation reactions. Vitamin K antagonism is the basis for oral anticoagulant therapy with warfarin (Coumadin).

proteolytic Pertaining to any substance that digests protein by hydrolyzing primary peptide bonds.

prothrombin (coagulation factor II) Plasma precursor of the coagulation factor thrombin. It is converted to thrombin by activated factor X complexed to factor V.

prothrombin time (protime, PT) Test to measure the activity of coagulation factors I (fibrinogen), II (prothrombin), V, VII, and X, which participate in the extrinsic and common pathways of coagulation. Thromboplastin and calcium are added to plasma and the clotting time is recorded. Widely used to monitor warfarin therapy.

proto-oncogene Normal gene controlling the cell cycle and other essential cell functions that, upon activation, may become an oncogene.

pseudo–Pelger-Huët cell (Pelgeroid cell) Hyposegmented, hypogranular neutrophils that resemble Pelger-Huët cells. Helpful in the diagnosis of leukemia, myeloproliferative neoplasms, and myelodysplastic syndromes.

pseudoleukocytosis Falsely increased white blood cell (WBC) count indicating mobilization of the marginal WBC pool caused by strenuous physical activity, cold, or fever. Also a falsely elevated WBC count due to interferences such as platelet clumping or lysis-resistant red blood cells.

pseudothrombocytopenia Falsely decreased platelet count often caused by platelet satellitosis.

pulmonary embolism (PE) Pathologic movement of a proximal fragment of clot from a deep vein thrombosis through the right side of the heart to the pulmonary circulation, where it lodges in an artery and causes infarction of the lung. Approximately one third of pulmonary emboli are fatal within 1 hour.

purpura Purple skin discoloration, typically rounded with a diameter greater than 3 mm, seen in mucocutaneous bleeding. Usually seen in thrombocytopenia, platelet disorders, von Willebrand disease, or vascular disorders such as scurvy.

pyknosis Degeneration of a cell in which the nucleus shrinks in size and the chromatin condenses to a solid, structureless mass or masses. Part of the process of apoptosis, or indicative of the effects of chemotherapy.

pyropoikilocytosis (hereditary pyropoikilocytosis) Rare hereditary defect of spectrin that causes severe hemolytic anemia beginning in childhood with extreme poikilocytosis in which the red blood cell morphology resembles that seen in burn patients.

pyruvate kinase (PK) Enzyme that converts phosphoenolpyruvate to pyruvate generating two molecules of ATP; essential for aerobic and anaerobic glycolysis.

pyruvate kinase deficiency Autosomal recessive disorder resulting in a deficiency of pyruvate kinase, the enzyme that converts phosphoenolpyruvate to pyruvate; causes hemolytic anemia by reducing red blood cell life span. It is the most common enzyme deficiency of the Embden-Meyerhof pathway.

Q arm Long arm of a chromosome.

Q banding (quinacrine banding) In cytogenetic analysis, a procedure in which metaphase chromosomes are stained with fluorescent quinacrine dye. The areas rich in adenine-thymine, called $Q+$, fluoresce intensely, whereas the areas rich in guanine-cytosine ($Q-$) fluoresce more lightly. The $Q+$ bands correspond with G bands in Giemsa stain–based G banding. Banding patterns are used to identify chromosomes.

qualitative analysis Study of a sample to determine the presence, but not the concentration, of specific chemicals.

quality control Term used to refer to the control and monitoring of the testing process to ensure that the results are valid and reproducible.

quantitative analysis Determination of the concentration of an analyte.

radiotherapy Treatment of neoplastic disease using x-rays or gamma rays to deter the proliferation of malignant cells by disrupting mitosis or impairing DNA synthesis.

Raynaud phenomenon (acrocyanosis) Persistent symmetrical cyanosis (blotchy blue or red discoloration) of the skin of the digits, palm, wrists, and ankles upon prolonged exposure to cold.

reactive lymphocytes (atypical, transformed, or variant lymphocytes) Lymphocytes whose altered morphology includes stormy blue cytoplasm and lobular or irregular nuclei. Variant lymphocytes indicate stimulation by a virus, particularly Epstein-Barr virus, which causes infectious mononucleosis.

recessive Denoting an allele whose product or effect is masked by a dominant allele at the corresponding locus. When an individual has two recessive genes, he or she is homozygous recessive, and the trait is expressed.

red blood cell (RBC) indices Numerical representations of average RBC volume (mean cell volume), hemoglobin mass (mean cell hemoglobin), and relative hemoglobin concentration (mean cell hemoglobin concentration). Indices are computed from the RBC count, hemoglobin, and hematocrit values. The mean cell volume is directly measured by some hematology analyzers.

red cell distribution width (RDW) Coefficient of variation of red blood cell volume. An increased red cell distribution width indicates anisocytosis.

red marrow Hematopoietic bone marrow, in contrast to yellow, fatty bone marrow.

Reed-Sternberg cell Giant, typically binucleate cell whose halves are mirror images. The nuclei are enclosed in abundant cytoplasm and contain prominent nucleoli. The presence of Reed-Sternberg cells is the definitive histologic characteristic of Hodgkin disease.

reference interval (RI) Range of test results for a given analyte that is seen in a healthy population of individuals, typically computed as the mean plus or minus two times the standard deviation. Each laboratory must define the reference interval for the instrument that is being used and for the population that is being served.

refractive index Speed at which light travels in air, divided by the speed at which light travels through another medium, such as immersion oil. The refractive index of oil is similar to the refractive index of glass.

reliability Extent to which a method is able to maintain both accuracy and precision over a defined period of time.

remission Partial or complete disappearance of the clinical and laboratory characteristics of a chronic or malignant disease.

replication DNA duplication or synthesis prior to mitosis; may also be used to refer to mitosis.

reptilase Thrombin-like enzyme isolated from the venom of *Bothrops atrox* that catalyzes the conversion of fibrinogen to fibrin in a manner similar to thrombin.

resheathing device Device that allows safe one-handed recapping of a blood collection needle to prevent needle stick injury.

resolution In microscopy, the smallest distance between which two adjacent objects can be distinguished. A measure of image and lens quality that relates to the smallest feature that can be seen with a set of lenses.

restriction endonuclease Enzyme that cleaves DNA at a specific nucleotide site.

reticulocyte (polychromatic or polychromatophilic red blood cell) Immature but anucleate red blood cell (RBC) that shows a meshlike pattern of dark blue threads and particles, vestiges of the endoplasmic reticulum, when stained with new methylene blue vital dye. In a Wright-stained blood film, no filaments are seen but the cytoplasm stains bluish-pink and the cell is called a *polychromatic* or *polychromatophilic RBC*. Reticulocytosis or polychromatophilia indicates bone marrow regeneration activity in hemolytic anemia or acute blood loss.

reticulocyte production index (RPI) Index calculated to correct for the presence of shift reticulocytes that otherwise may falsely elevate the visual reticulocyte count.

reticulocytosis (polychromatophilia) Elevated reticulocyte count on a peripheral blood film stained with new methylene blue dye or increase in the number of polychromatophilic red blood cells on a Wright-stained blood film. Reticulocytosis or polychromatophilia indicates bone marrow regeneration activity in hemolytic anemia or acute blood loss.

reticuloendothelial system (RES) System of fixed and motile phagocytic macrophages and their precursor monocytes engaged in primary efferent immunity. Macrophages are found in every organ and tissue.

retrovirus Any of a family of RNA viruses containing the enzyme reverse transcriptase.

reverse transcription polymerase chain reaction (RT-PCR) Polymerase chain reaction amplification process that produces complementary DNA from the messenger RNA present in an RNA sample extracted from patient cells.

Rh immune globulin (RhIg) Solution containing antibodies specific for the Rh(D) antigen given intramuscularly to an Rh(D)-negative mother with an Rh(D)-positive fetus or infant to prevent sensitization of the mother to the infant's D antigen. It is given antepartum at 28 weeks' gestation and again within 72 hours of delivery.

Rh-null disease Hemolytic anemia in persons who lack all Rh antigens (Rh null); marked by spherocytosis, stomatocytosis, and increased osmotic fragility.

ribonucleic acid (RNA) Single strand of polynucleotides connected by ribose molecules. RNA base sequences are transcribed from DNA and are the basis for translation to proteins. Major types of RNA include messenger RNA, ribosomal RNA, and transfer RNA.

ribosomes Granules embedded in the membranes of endoplasmic reticulum that are composed of protein and RNA. Ribosomes are the sites for primary protein translation from messenger and transfer RNA.

ring sideroblast Nucleated red blood cell precursor with at least five iron granules that circle at least one third of the nucleus. These cells, visible with Prussian blue stain, are the pathognomonic finding in refractory anemia with ring sideroblasts.

ristocetin Antibiotic no longer in clinical use that facilitates the in vitro interaction of von Willebrand factor with platelet membrane glycoprotein Ib/IX/V. Used as an agonist in platelet aggregation to test for von Willebrand disease.

Romanowsky stain Prototype of the many eosin–methylene blue stains for blood cells and malarial parasites, including Wright and Giemsa stain.

rouleaux Aggregation of stacked red blood cells caused by elevated plasma proteins and abnormal monoclonal proteins.

rubriblast (pronormoblast) Undifferentiated (immature) hematopoietic cell that is the most primitive morphologically identifiable precursor in the erythrocytic series; differentiates into the basophilic normoblast (prorubricyte).

rubricyte (polychromatic or polychromatophilic normoblast) Precursor in the erythrocytic maturation series that is intermediate between the basophilic normoblast (prorubricyte) and the orthochromic normoblast (metarubricyte). In this stage, differentiation is based on the decreasing cell diameter and the gray-blue cytoplasm as hemoglobin first becomes visible.

Russell bodies Plasma cell cytoplasmic inclusions that appear similar to vacuoles containing aggregates of immunoglobulins. Plasma cells with Russell bodies are called *Mott cells.*

Russell viper venom time Rarely used coagulation assay similar to the prothrombin time. Russell viper venom activates the coagulation factor common pathway at the level of factor X. The dilute Russell viper venom time assay is used routinely in lupus anticoagulant screening.

scatterplot Plot on rectangular coordinates of paired observations of two random variables, with each observation plotted as one point on the graph; the scatter or clustering of points provides an indication of the relationship between the two variables. In hematology a typical scatterplot graphs cell volume against cytoplasmic complexity.

schistocyte (schizocyte) Fragmented red blood cell characteristic of microangiopathic hemolytic anemia, severe burns, disseminated intravascular coagulation, and prosthetic mechanical trauma.

scurvy Deficiency of vitamin C (ascorbic acid) causing connective tissue breakdown. Marked by weakness, anemia, spongy gums, and a tendency to mucocutaneous bleeding.

secondary hemostasis Second phase of hemostasis involving the activation of plasma coagulation proteins to produce a fibrin clot.

secondary standard (calibrator) Calibration material for which the analyte concentration has been ascertained by reference to a primary standard or by controlled reference assays.

segmented neutrophil (seg, polymorphonuclear neutrophil, PMN) White blood cell whose nucleus is condensed into two to five segments connected by filaments. Distinguished from mononuclear cells such as monocytes and lymphocytes.

selectin Any of a family of cell adhesion molecules that mediate the binding of white blood cells and platelets to the vascular endothelium.

senescent Aging or growing old. A senescent red blood cell loses its deformability and is cleared by the spleen.

sensitivity In laboratory testing, the conditional probability that a person with a given disease will be correctly identified as having it by a clinical test (i.e., diagnostic sensitivity). Also, the lowest level of a substance that can be detected by a laboratory test procedure (i.e., analytical sensitivity).

sepsis (septicemia) Proliferation of pathologic organisms in the blood.

sequestration Transfer of blood cells from the circulation into a limited vascular area, such as the spleen. Platelets may be sequestered, which results in a decrease in their circulating numbers.

serine protease Any of a group of proteolytic enzymes of the trypsin family that include activated procoagulants (thrombin and factors VIIa, IXa, Xa, XIa, and XIIa) and activated inhibitors (antithrombin, activated protein C). Serine proteases are synthesized as inactive zymogens; activation occurs when the zymogen is cleaved at one or more specific sites by the action of another protease during the coagulation process.

serine protease inhibitor (serpin) Plasma proteins, for instance, antithrombin and heparin cofactor II, which control the coagulation cascade by inhibiting the serine proteases, particularly factors IIa and Xa.

serotonin Potent vasoconstrictor released from the dense granules of activated platelets.

Sézary cell Mononuclear cell with a cerebriform nucleus (resembling the surface of the cerebrum) and a narrow rim of cytoplasm. It is a characteristic finding in cutaneous T-cell lymphomas.

Sézary syndrome Cutaneous T-cell lymphoma characterized by exfoliative erythroderma, peripheral lymphadenopathy, and the presence of Sézary cells in the skin, lymph nodes, and peripheral blood.

shift reticulocyte Gray-blue red blood cell with increased diameter. The shift reticulocyte is a reticulocyte that has been released from the bone marrow prematurely to compensate for hemolytic anemia or acute blood loss. Shift reticulocytes require more than 1 day in the peripheral blood to lose residual RNA and gain a mature-looking reddish cytoplasm.

sickle cell (drepanocyte) Abnormal crescent-shaped red blood cell containing hemoglobin S, characteristic of sickle cell anemia.

sickle cell anemia (sickle cell disease) Severe chronic hemoglobinopathy in people who are homozygous for hemoglobin S. The abnormal hemoglobin results in distortion of red blood cells (sickle cells) and leads to crises characterized by joint pain, anemia, thrombosis, fever, and splenomegaly.

sickle cell crisis Any of several acute conditions occurring as part of sickle cell disease, such as aplastic crisis, which is temporary bone marrow aplasia; hemolytic crisis, which is acute red blood cell destruction; and vasoocclusive crisis, which is severe pain due to blockage of the blood vessels.

sickle cell trait Asymptomatic heterozygous condition characterized by the presence of both hemoglobin S and hemoglobin A.

sideroblast Bone marrow erythrocytic precursor that shows excessive iron granules (siderotic granules) with Prussian blue staining.

siderocyte Nonnucleated red blood cell in which particles of iron (siderotic granules) are visible with Prussian blue staining.

siderotic granules (Pappenheimer bodies) Red blood cell inclusions composed of ferric iron. With Prussian blue iron staining, they appear as multiple dark blue irregular granules. With Wright staining they appear as pale blue clusters.

Southern blotting Technique in which DNA fragments separated by gel electrophoresis are transferred to a nitrocellulose filter on which specific fragments can then be detected by their hybridization to probes.

specificity In laboratory testing, the conditional probability that a person who does not have a specific disease will be correctly identified as not having it by a clinical test (i.e., diagnostic specificity). Also used to describe the attribute of antibodies that are able to bind only with the antigen that stimulated their production.

spectrin Major cytoskeletal protein forming a lattice at the cytoplasmic surface of the cell membrane, providing lateral support to the membrane and thus maintaining its shape. Abnormalities in red blood cell spectrin account for hereditary spherocytosis, ovalocytosis, and pyropoikilocytosis.

spherocyte Abnormal spherical red blood cell with a decreased surface area-to-volume ratio. In Wright-stained peripheral blood films, spherocytes are dense, lack central pallor, and have a reduced diameter. Spherocytes appear most frequently in warm autoimmune hemolytic anemia and hereditary spherocytosis.

spleen Large organ in the upper left quadrant of the abdomen, just under the stomach. The spleen has the body's largest collection of macrophages, which are responsible for phagocytosis and elimination of senescent red blood cells. The spleen also houses many lymphoid cells.

splenectomy Excision of the spleen.

splenomegaly Enlargement of the spleen.

standard deviation Mathematic expression of the dispersion of a set of values or scores about the mean.

standard precautions (universal precautions) Practices to control blood-borne disease in which all human blood and body fluids are treated as if infectious. Infection is prevented by a series of protective methods including the use of sterile gloves, fluid-impermeable clothing, and eye protection.

steatorrhea Fat in the stool, usually due to malabsorption. Stool is green or colorless and foul smelling.

stem cell Undifferentiated mononuclear cell whose daughter cells may give rise to a variety of cell types and which is capable of renewing itself and thus maintaining a pool of cells that can differentiate into multiple other cell types.

stomatocyte Abnormal cup-shaped mature red blood cell that has a slitlike area of central pallor.

storage pool deficiency Inadequacy of platelet dense granules or dense granule contents that causes mucocutaneous bleeding. Usually hereditary and related to conditions with oculocutaneous albinism, such as Hermansky-Pudlak syndrome, Chédiak-Higashi syndrome, and Wiskott-Aldrich syndrome. Acquired storage pool disorder is sometimes associated with myelodysplastic syndrome.

stroma Supporting tissue or matrix of an organ.

subcutaneous (SC) Injected within the subdermal or dermal layer.

sulfhemoglobin Hemoglobin with a sulfur atom on one of its porphyrin rings, which makes it ineffective for transporting oxygen. Results from ingestion or exposure to drugs or chemicals containing sulfur.

supernatant Clear upper liquid part of a suspension after it has been centrifuged.

suppuration Formation or discharge of pus.

supravital stain (vital stain) Stain that colors living tissues or cells.

surface-connected canalicular system (SCCS, open canalicular system, OCS) System of channels that is distributed throughout platelets and extends the plasma membrane inward. The SCCS binds numerous coagulation factors and provides a route for secretion of the protein contents of α-granules.

syncope Brief lapse in consciousness; fainting.

systemic bleeding disorder Chronic episodic bleeding that is evidenced by bilateral petechiae and purpura, epistaxis, hematemesis, and menorrhagia. Indicates a primary coagulopathy such as thrombocytopenia, von Willebrand disease, or a qualitative platelet disorder.

systemic lupus erythematosus (SLE) Chronic autoimmune inflammatory disease manifested by severe vasculitis, renal involvement, and lesions of the skin and nervous system.

T cell (T lymphocyte) Lymphocyte that participates in cellular immunity, including cell-to-cell communication. The major T-cell categories are helper cells and suppressor-cytotoxic cells.

target cell (codocyte) Poorly hemoglobinized red blood cell (RBC) that is present in hemoglobinopathies, thalassemia, and liver disease. In a Wright-stained peripheral blood film, hemoglobin concentrates in the center of the RBC and around the periphery to resemble a "bull's-eye."

teardrop cell (dacryocyte) Red blood cell with a single pointed extension, resembling a teardrop. Dacryocytes are often seen in the myeloproliferative neoplasm called *myelofibrosis with myeloid metaplasia.*

telangiectasia Permanent dilation of capillaries, arterioles, and venules that creates focal red lesions, usually in the skin or mucous membranes.

telomere Repeating DNA sequences at a chromosome terminus.

tetraploid Possessing a double diploid chromosome complement, or four of each chromosome (4N).

thalassemia Production and hemolytic anemia characterized by microcytic, hypochromic red blood cells caused by deficient synthesis of α- or β-globin chains.

thrombin Primary serine protease of coagulation. Factors Xa and Va combine to cleave prothrombin to produce thrombin. Thrombin cleaves fibrinopeptides A and B from fibrinogen to initiate fibrin polymerization. Thrombin potentiates coagulation by activating platelets and factors XI, VIII, V, and XIII and also activates the coagulation control protein, protein C.

thrombin clotting time (TCT, thrombin time, TT) Coagulation test that measures the interval to clot formation after the addition of thrombin to plasma. Often used to test for the presence of heparin.

thrombocyte Platelet.

thrombocythemia Abnormally high platelet count with dysfunctional platelets; seen in the myeloproliferative neoplasm known as *essential thrombocythemia.*

thrombocytopenia Platelet count below the lower limit of the reference interval, usually 150,000/μL.

thrombocytosis Platelet count above the upper limit of the reference interval, usually 450,000/μL.

thrombophilia (hypercoagulability) Abnormally increased tendency to clotting caused by a number of acquired or congenital factors.

thrombopoietin Hormone produced by renal tissue that recruits stem cells to the megakaryocyte cell maturation line and stimulates megakaryocyte mitosis and maturation in response to thrombocytopenia.

thrombosis Formation, development, or presence of a clot in a blood vessel (i.e., a thrombus).

thrombospondin Adhesive glycoprotein secreted by endothelial cells and platelet α-granules.

thrombotic thrombocytopenic purpura (TTP) Congenital or acquired deficiency of ADAMTS-13, an endothelial cell von Willebrand factor–cleaving protease. Ultra-large von Willebrand factor multimers activate platelets to form white clots in the microvasculature, causing severe thrombocytopenia with mucocutaneous bleeding, microangiopathic hemolytic anemia, and neuropathy.

thromboxane A$_2$ Metabolically active product of the eicosanoid synthesis (cyclooxygenase, prostaglandin) pathway in platelets; binds platelet membrane receptor and activates platelets.

thromboxane B$_2$ Metabolically inactive measurable plasma product of the eicosanoid synthesis (cyclooxygenase, prostaglandin) pathway.

thrombus In vivo blood clot causing vascular occlusion and tissue ischemia.

tissue factor (TF) Constitutive membrane protein of the subendothelium. Exposure to tissue factor activates factor VII and the tissue factor (extrinsic) coagulation pathway. Tissue factor is expressed on monocytes and endothelial cells in chronic inflammation.

tissue plasminogen activator (TPA) Serine protease that is secreted by endothelial cells and binds fibrin. It activates nearby plasminogen molecules to trigger fibrinolysis, with the formation of fibrin degradation products.

toxic granulation Presence of abnormally large, dark-staining, or dominant primary granules in neutrophils associated with bacterial infections.

transcription Process by which messenger RNA is produced from a DNA template.

transferrin Plasma iron-transport protein that moves iron from sites of absorption and storage to hematopoietic tissue for incorporation into developing normoblasts.

transformed lymphocytes (atypical, variant, or reactive lymphocytes) Lymphocytes whose altered morphology includes stormy blue cytoplasm and lobular or irregular nuclei. Variant lymphocytes indicate stimulation by a virus, particularly Epstein-Barr virus, which causes infectious mononucleosis.

translation Process by which the genetic information carried by nucleotides in messenger RNA directs the sequence of amino acids in the synthesis of a specific polypeptide.

translocation Rearrangement of DNA within a chromosome or transfer of a segment of one chromosome to a nonhomologous one.

triploid Possessing a single addition chromosome complement, resulting in three of each chromosome (3N).

trisomy Presence of an extra chromosome in addition to a homologous pair; for example, trisomy 21 in Down syndrome.

tungsten-halogen light bulb Bulb used in brightfield microscopy consisting of a tungsten filament enclosed in a small quartz bulb filled with halogen gas. Tungsten creates a very bright yellow light.

unfractionated heparin (UFH, standard heparin) Heparin extracted from porcine mucosa and purified to yield molecular weights ranging from 7000 to 15,000 Daltons. Used routinely in cardiac surgery. Unfractionated heparin therapy requires monitoring with the partial thromboplastin time or activated clotting time assay.

universal precautions (now called **standard precautions**) Practices to control blood-borne disease in which all human blood and body fluids are treated as if infectious. Infection is prevented by a series of protective methods including the use of sterile gloves, fluid-impermeable clothing, and eye protection.

urobilinogen Colorless water-soluble compound formed in the intestine through the breakdown of bilirubin by bacteria; low levels appear in the urine in healthy states.

urokinase Enzyme produced by the kidney endothelial cells that acts as a plasminogen activator.

vacuole Any clear space or cavity formed in the cytoplasm of a cell.

vacuolization Formation of vacuoles.

vasoconstriction Reduction in blood vessel diameter due to smooth muscle constriction.

venipuncture Use of a needle to puncture a vein and collect blood.

vertigo Sensation of rotation or movement of oneself or one's surroundings; dizziness.

viscosity Resistance of a liquid to flow.

vital stain (supravital stain) Stain that colors living tissues or cells.

vitamin B$_{12}$ (cyanocobalamin) Complex vitamin involved in the metabolism of protein, fats, and carbohydrate; normal blood formation; and nerve function.

vitamin K Natural phylloquinone occurring in green leafy vegetables and liver and produced by commensal intestinal organisms. Vitamin K catalyzes the γ-carboxylation of glutamic acid in a number of calcium-binding proteins, including the vitamin K–dependent coagulation proteins factors II (prothrombin), VII, IX, and X and control proteins C, S, and Z.

vitamin K antagonist (VKA) Substance that inhibits the action of vitamin K; for example, warfarin (Coumadin), which is used in oral anticoagulant therapy.

von Willebrand disease Congenital autosomal dominant variable mucocutaneous bleeding disorder characterized by a deficiency of von Willebrand factor activity and antigen, and subsequent impairment of platelet adhesion.

waived testing Test classification defined by the Clinical Laboratory Improvement Amendments that includes tests that are simple and accurate and can be performed by noncertified personnel.

Waldenström macroglobulinemia Form of monoclonal gammopathy in which IgM is overproduced by the clone of a plasma cell. Increased viscosity of the blood may result in circulatory impairment, and normal immunoglobulin synthesis is decreased, which increases susceptibility to infections.

warfarin (Coumadin) Vitamin K antagonist used as an anticoagulant to prevent thrombosis in people with atrial fibrillation, venous thromboembolism, or cardiac insufficiency. Also used prophylactically after orthopedic surgery. Warfarin suppresses vitamin K and reduces the activity of the vitamin K–dependent coagulation factors II (prothrombin), VII, IX, and X.

warm antibody IgG antibody that reacts optimally at a temperature of 37° C.

warm autoimmune hemolytic anemia Most common autoimmune hemolytic anemia, which results from the reaction of IgG autoantibodies with red blood cells at an optimal temperature of 37° C.

Wiskott-Aldrich syndrome Immunodeficiency disorder characterized by oculocutaneous albinism, thrombocytopenia, inadequate T- and B-cell function, and an increased susceptibility to viral, bacterial, and fungal infections.

xanthochromic Having a yellowish color. Used to describe cerebrospinal fluid, in which xanthochromia indicates the presence of bilirubin and thus serves as evidence of a prior episode of bleeding into the brain.

X-linked Pertaining to genes or to the characteristics or conditions they transmit that are carried on the X chromosome.

X-linked recessive inheritance Pattern of inheritance in which a recessive allele is carried on the X chromosome; results in the carrier state in females and development of disease characteristics in males, since they do not have a normal X chromosome to compensate.

zymogen Inactive precursor that is converted to an active form by an enzyme. Zymogens are inactive coagulation factors, such as prothrombin.

Index

Note: Page numbers followed by f, t, and b indicate figures, tables, and boxes, respectively.

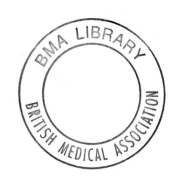